The Interface of Neurology & Internal Medicine

The Interface of Neurology & Internal Medicine

Editor-in-Chief

José Biller, MD, FACP, FAAN, FAHA

Professor
Departments of Neurology and Neurological Surgery
Chairman, Department of Neurology
Loyola University Chicago
Stritch School of Medicine
Maywood, Illinois

Wolters Kluwer Health | Lippincott Williams & Wilkins

Philadelphia • Baltimore • New York • London
Buenos Aires • Hong Kong • Sydney • Tokyo

Acquisitions Editor: Frances DeStefano
Managing Editor: Leanne McMillan
Marketing Manager: Kimberly Schonberger
Project Manager: Nicole Walz
Senior Manufacturing Manager: Ben Rivera
Design Coordinator: Stephen Druding
Cover Designer: Joseph DePinho
Production Services: Aptara, Inc.

530 Walnut Street
Philadelphia, PA 19106

Printed in the United States of America

Library of Congress Cataloging-in-Publication Data

The interface of neurology & internal medicine / editor-in-chief, José Biller.
p. ; cm.
Includes bibliographical references.
ISBN-13: 978-0-7817-7906-7
1. Nervous system—Diseases. 2. Neurologic manifestations of general diseases. 3. Internal medicine. I. Biller, José. II. Title: Interface of neurology and internal medicine.
[DNLM: 1. Neurologic Manifestations. 2. Internal Medicine. WL 340 I602 2007]
RC346. I53 2007
616.8—dc22

2007022710

Care has been taken to confirm the accuracy of the information presented and to describe generally accepted practices. However, the authors, editors, and publisher are not responsible for errors or omissions or for any consequences from application of the information in this book and make no warranty, expressed or implied, with respect to the currency, completeness, or accuracy of the contents of the publication. Application of this information in a particular situation remains the professional responsibility of the practitioner; the clinical treatments described and recommended may not be considered absolute and universal recommendations.

The authors, editors, and publisher have exerted every effort to ensure that drug selection and dosage set forth in this text are in accordance with current recommendations and practice at the time of publication. However, in view of ongoing research, changes in government regulations, and the constant flow of information relating to drug therapy and drug reactions, the reader is urged to check the package insert for each drug for any change in indications and dosage and for added warnings and precautions. This is particularly important when the recommended agent is a new or infrequently employed drug.

Some drugs and medical devices presented in this publication have Food and Drug Administration (FDA) clearance for limited use in restricted research settings. It is the responsibility of health care providers to ascertain the FDA status of each drug or device planned for use in their clinical practice.

The publishers have made every effort to trace copyright holders for borrowed material. If they have inadvertently overlooked any, they will be pleased to make the necessary arrangements at the first opportunity.

To purchase additional copies of this book, call our customer service department at (800) 638-3030 or fax orders to 1-301-223-2400. Lippincott Williams & Wilkins customer service representatives are available from 8:30 am to 6:00 pm, EST, Monday through Friday, for telephone access. Visit Lippincott Williams & Wilkins on the Internet: http://www.lww.com.

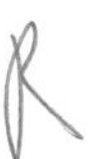

10 9 8 7 6 5 4 3 2 1

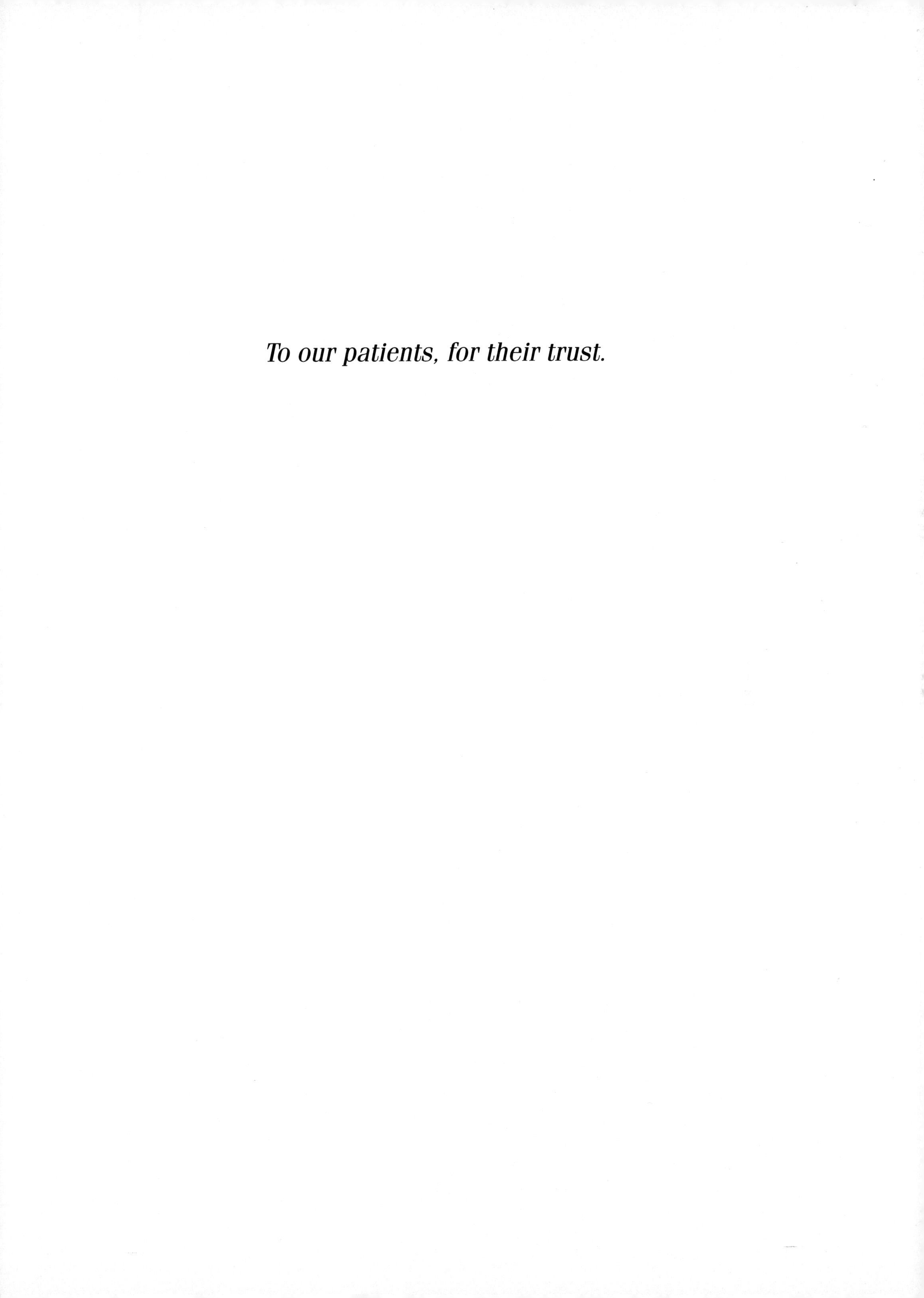

To our patients, for their trust.

CONTRIBUTORS

EDITOR-IN-CHIEF

José Biller, MD, FACP, FAAN, FAHA
Professor
Departments of Neurology and Neurological Surgery
Chairman, Department of Neurology
Loyola University Chicago
Stritch School of Medicine
Maywood, Illinois

SECTION EDITORS

PART I: Cardiovascular Diseases

José Biller, MD, FACP, FAAN, FAHA

David J. Wilber, MD
George M. Eisenberg Professor of Cardiovascular Science
Department of Medicine
Director, Cardiology and Cardiovascular Institute
Loyola University Chicago
Stritch School of Medicine
Maywood, Illinois

PART II: Pulmonary Diseases

Richard G. Wunderink, MD
Professor of Medicine
Pulmonary and Critical Care Division
Northwestern University, Feinberg School of Medicine
Chicago, Illinois

Richard A. Bernstein, MD, PhD
Associate Professor
Department of Neurology
Northwestern University
Attending Neurologist
Northwestern Memorial Hospital
Chicago, Illinois

PART III: Renal Diseases

Vinod K. Bansal, MD, FACP, FASN
Professor of Medicine
Division of Nephrology
Department of Medicine
Loyola University Chicago
Stritch School of Medicine
Maywood, Illinois

José Biller, MD, FACP, FAAN, FAHA

PART IV: Gastrointestinal Diseases

Ronald F. Pfeiffer, MD
Professor and Vice Chairman
Department of Neurology
University of Tennessee Health Science Center
Memphis, Tennessee

PART V: Liver Diseases/Biliary System

Benjamin H. Eidelman, MD, PhD
Professor of Neurology
Mayo Clinic College of Medicine
Department of Neurology
Mayo Clinic
Jacksonville, Florida

David J. Kramer, MD
Professor, Department of Medicine
Mayo Clinic College of Medicine
Director, Transplant Critical Care
Department of Transplantation
Mayo Clinic
Jacksonville, Florida

PART VI: Hematological Diseases

Gregory Gruener, MD, MBA
Professor, Associate Dean of Educational Affairs
Associate Chairman
Department of Neurology
Loyola University Chicago
Stritch School of Medicine
Maywood, Illinois

Harry L. Messmore, MD
Professor of Medicine, Emeritus
Department of Medicine
Loyola University Chicago
Stritch School of Medicine
Maywood, Illinois
Professor of Medicine, Emeritus
Department of Medicine
Edward J. Hines, Jr. VA Hospital
Hines, Illinois

PART VII: Oncologic Diseases

José Biller, MD, FACP, FAAN, FAHA

PART VIII: Metabolic Diseases

Roger E. Kelley, MD
Professor and Chairman
Department of Neurology
LSU Health Sciences Center-Shreveport
Chief of Neurology Service
Department of Neurology
LSU Health Sciences Center-Shreveport Hospital
Shreveport, Louisiana

PART IX: Nutritional Disorders

Rima M. Dafer, MD, MPH
Associate Professor
Department of Neurology
Loyola University Chicago
Stritch School of Medicine
Maywood, Illinois

PART X: Endocrine Diseases

Jorge C. Kattah, MD
Professor and Head
Department of Neurology
University of Illinois College of Medicine
Head of Neurology
Department of Neuroscience
Illinois Neurologic Institute, OSF Saint Francis Medical Center
Peoria, Illinois

PART XI: Musculoskeletal and Connective Tissue Disorders

Elaine M. Adams, MD
Professor of Medicine
Department of Medicine
Loyola University Chicago
Stritch School of Medicine
Maywood, Illinois

José Biller, MD, FACP, FAAN, FAHA

PART XII: Infectious Diseases

James J. Corbett, MD
McCarty Professor and Chairman for Neurology
Professor of Ophthalmology
Department of Neurology
University of Mississippi Medical Center
Jackson, Mississippi

Stanley W. Chapman, MD
Professor of Medicine
Department of Medicine
University of Mississippi Medical Center
Director, Division of Infectious Diseases
Department of Medicine
University of Mississippi Medical Center
Jackson, Mississippi

PART XIII: Substance Abuse

Michael A. Sloan, MD, MS
Professor of Neurology and Neurosurgery
Director, TGH/USF Stroke Program
Department of Neurology
University of South Florida
Tampa, Florida

Michael C. Beuhler, MD
Clinical Instructor, Department of Emergency Medicine
University of North Carolina at Chapel Hill
Chapel Hill, North Carolina
Medical Director
Carolinas Poison Center
Carolinas Medical Center
Charlotte, North Carolina

PART XIV: Environmental Disorders

Christopher Commichau, MD
Associate Professor
Department of Neurology and Neurosurgery
University of Vermont
Director, Neurocritical Care and Stroke
Department of Neurology
Fletcher Allen Health Care
Burlington, Vermont

PART XV: Dermatological Diseases

Robert M. Pascuzzi, MD
Professor and Chairman
Department of Neurology
Indiana University School of Medicine
Section Chief
Department of Neurology
Clarian Health Partners
Indianapolis, Indiana

Jeffrey B. Travers, MD, PhD
Kamped-Norins Professor and Chair
Department of Dermatology
Indiana University School of Medicine
Indianapolis, Indiana

PART XVI: Critical Care

Michael J. Schneck, MD
Associate Professor
Departments of Neurology and Neurological Surgery
Loyola University Chicago
Stritch School of Medicine
Maywood, Illinois

W. Scott Jellish, MD, PhD
Professor and Chairman
Department of Anesthesiology
Loyola University Chicago
Stritch School of Medicine
Maywood, Illinois

Richard L. Gamelli, MD, FACS
The Robert J. Freeark Professor and Chairman
Department of Surgery
Loyola University Chicago
Stritch School of Medicine
Maywood, Illinois

PART XVII: Ophthalmology

Michael P. Merchut, MD, FACP, FAAN
Professor
Department of Neurology
Loyola University Chicago
Stritch School of Medicine
Maywood, Illinois

Charles S. Bouchard, MD
Professor and Chairman
Department of Ophthalmology
Loyola University Chicago
Stritch School of Medicine
Maywood, Illinois

PART XVIII: Ear, Nose and Throat

James A. Stankiewicz, MD
Professor and Chairman
Department of Otolaryngology–Head and Neck Surgery
Loyola University Chicago
Stritch School of Medicine
Maywood, Illinois

PART XIX: Obstetrics and Gynecology

John G. Gianopoulos, MD
The Mary Isabelle Caestecker Professor and Chair
Department of Obstetrics and Gynecology
Loyola University Chicago
Stritch School of Medicine
Maywood, Illinois

Jorge J. Asconapé, MD
Professor
Department of Neurology
Loyola University Chicago
Stritch School of Medicine
Maywood, Illinois

PART XX: Pediatrics

John B. Bodensteiner, MD
Pilcher Chair of Pediatric Neurology
Department of Pediatrics
Children's Health Center and Barrow Neurologic Institute
Phoenix, Arizona
Professor of Clinical Pediatrics and Neurology
University of Arizona College of Medicine
Tucson, Arizona

PART XXI: Agents of Terror

Thomas P. Bleck, MD, FCCM
Vice-Chairman for Academic Programs
Department of Neurology
Professor of Neurology, Neurological Surgery and Medicine
Northwestern University Feinberg School of Medicine
Chicago, Illinois
Ruggles Chairman
Department of Neurology
Evanston Northwestern Healthcare
Evanston, Illinois

James A. Geiling, MD
Associate Professor
Department of Medicine
Dartmouth Medical School
Hanover, New Hampshire
Chief, Medical Service
VA Medical Center
White River Junction, Vermont

PART XXII: Psychiatry

Stephen C. Scheiber, MD
Clinical Professor
Department of Psychiatry and Behavioral Medicine
Medical College of Wisconsin
Milwaukee, Wisconsin
Attending Psychiatrist
Department of Psychiatry
Northwestern Evanston Health Care, Evanston Hospital
Branston, Illinois

PART XXIII: Miscellaneous

José Biller, MD, FACP, FAAN, FAHA

CONTRIBUTING AUTHORS

Carla Aamodt, MD
Assistant Professor
General and Geriatric Medicine
Kansas University Medical Center
Kansas City, Kansas

Robert M. Abrams, MD
Fellow, Maternal Fetal Medicine
Department of Obstetrics and Gynecology
Loyola University Chicago
Stritch School of Medicine
Maywood, Illinois

Elaine M. Adams, MD

Amjad Ahmad, MD
Assistant Professor
Department of Ophthalmology
Loyola University Chicago
Stritch School of Medicine
Maywood, Illinois
Edward J. Hines, Jr. VA Hospital
Hines, Illinois

Senda Ajroud-Driss, MD
Instructor
Department of Neurology
Feinberg School of Medicine, Northwestern University
Instructor
Department of Neurology
Northwestern Memorial Hospital
Chicago, Illinois

D. Adam Algren, MD
Clinical Instructor
Department of Emergency Medicine
Emory University School of Medicine
Medical Toxicology Fellow
Georgia Poison Center
Atlanta, Georgia

Latisha K. Ali, MD
Clinical Instructor
Department of Neurology
UCLA Stroke Center
University of California, Los Angeles
Los Angeles, California

Leslie Allen, DO
Pediatrics Resident
Department of Pediatrics
Joan C. Edwards School of Medicine at Marshall University
Huntington, West Virginia

David C. Anderson, MD
Professor and Head
Department of Neurology Residency Coordinator
University of Minnesota Medical School
Attending Physician
Department of Neurology
University of Minnesota Medical Center
Minneapolis, Minnesota

Elizabeth G. Araujo, MD
Assistant Professor
Department of Medicine
Loyola University Chicago
Stritch School of Medicine
Maywood, Illinois
Attending Rheumatologist
Department of Medicine
Edward J. Hines, Jr. VA Hospital
Hines, Illinois

Jorge J. Asconapé, MD

Fred K. Askari, MD, PhD
Associate Professor
Department of Internal Medicine
University of Michigan
Ann Arbor, Michigan
Director, Wilson Disease Program
Department of Internal Medicine, Division of Gastroenterology
University of Michigan Health System
Ann Arbor, Michigan

Hrayr P. Attarian, MD
Associate Professor
Neurology and Internal Medicine
University of Vermont
Director of Vermont Regional Sleep Center
Department of Neurology
Fletcher Allen Health Care
Burlington, Vermont

Taruna K. Aurora, MD
Assistant Professor
Departments of Emergency and Internal Medicine
Virginia Commonwealth University
Director, Clinical Decision Unit
Departments of Emergency and Internal Medicine
VCU Medical Center
Richmond, Virginia

Kurt Baker-Watson, MD
Assistant Professor
Department of Anesthesiology
Loyola University Chicago
Stritch School of Medicine
Maywood, Illinois

James F. Bale, Jr., MD
Professor and Associate Chair
Department of Pediatrics
University of Utah School of Medicine
Attending Physician
Department of Pediatrics
Primary Children's Medical Center
Salt Lake City, Utah

Vinod K. Bansal, MD, FACP, FASN

Richard J. Barohn, MD
Professor and Chair
Department of Neurology
University of Kansas Medical Center
Kansas City, Kansas

Sarice L. Bassin, MD
Assistant Professor
Department of Neurology
Northwestern University Feinberg School of Medicine
Staff
Department of Neurology and Critical Care
Northwestern Memorial Hospital
Chicago, Illinois

Robert P. Baughman, MD
Professor of Medicine
Department of Internal Medicine
University of Cincinnati
University of Cincinnati Medical Center
Cincinnati, Ohio

William E. Bell, MD
Professor Emeritus
Department of Pediatrics
University of Iowa College of Medicine
Iowa City, Iowa
Adjunct Clinical Professor
Department of Pediatrics
University of North Carolina School of Medicine
Chapel Hill, North Carolina

Jaime Belmares-Avalos, MD
Assistant Professor
Department of Medicine
Division of Infectious Diseases
Loyola University Chicago
Stritch School of Medicine
Maywood, Illinois

Eduardo E. Benarroch, MD, DSci
Professor
Department of Neurology
Mayo Clinic College of Medicine
Consultant
Department of Neurology
Mayo Clinic
Rochester, Minnesota

Oscar Benavente, MD, FRCPC
Associate Professor
Medicine/Neurology
University of Texas at San Antonio
Associate Professor
Medicine/Neurology
University of Texas Health Science Center at San Antonio
San Antonio, Texas

Sheldon Benjamin, MD
Professor of Psychiatry and Neurology
Department of Psychiatry
University of Massachusetts Medical School
Director of Neuropsychiatry
Director of Psychiatric Education & Training
Department of Psychiatry
UMass Memorial Healthcare
Worcester, Massachusetts

Joseph R. Berger, MD
Professor and Chairman
Department of Neurology
University of Kentucky
Lexington, Kentucky

Richard A. Bernstein, MD, PhD

Tulio E. Bertorini, MD
Professor
Departments of Neurology and Pathology
University of Tennessee Center for the Health Sciences
Chief, Department of Neurology
Methodist University Hospital
Wesley Neurology Clinic
Memphis, Tennessee

Richard E. Besinger, MD
Professor
Division Director
Department of Maternal-Fetal Medicine
Loyola University Chicago
Stritch School of Medicine
Maywood, Illinois

Michael C. Beuhler, MD

Nirmala Bhoopalam, MD
Professor
Department of Medicine
Loyola University Chicago
Stritch School of Medicine
Maywood, Illinois
Section Chief Hematology/Oncology
Department of Medicine
Edward J. Hines, Jr. VA Hospital
Hines, Illinois

José Biller, MD, FACP, FAAN, FAAA

Gretchen L. Birbeck, MD, MPH, DTMH
Director
International Neurologic and Psychiatric Epidemiology Program
Michigan State University
East Lansing, Michigan
Director
Epidemiology Program/Research Program
Chikankata Health Services
Mazabuka, Zambia

Andres T. Blei, MD
Professor of Medicine and Surgery
Division of Hepatology
Department of Medicine
Northwestern University Feinberg School of Medicine
Chicago, Illinois

Gregory M. Blume, MD
Clinical Assistant Professor
Department of Neurology
University of Illinois College of Medicine at Peoria
Staff Neurologist
Department of Neurology
OSF St. Francis Medical Center
Peoria, Illinois

John B. Bodensteiner, MD

David C. Bonovich, MD
Associate Professor of Neurology
Department of Neurology
University of California at San Francisco
Physician for Neurological Critical Care
Department of Neurology
Moffitt-Long Hospital, San Francisco General Hospital
San Francisco, California

Daniel J. Bonthius, MD, PhD
Associate Professor
Departments of Pediatrics and Neurology
University of Iowa
Iowa City, Iowa

James T. Boyd, MD
Assistant Professor
Department of Neurology
University of Vermont College of Medicine
Staff Neurologist
Department of Neurology
Fletcher Allen Health Care
Burlington, Vermont

Chris Braden, MD
Fellow
Department of Hematology and Oncology
Loyola University Chicago
Stritch School of Medicine
Maywood, Illinois

Steven U. Brint, MD
Associate Professor
Attending Physician
Department of Neurology
University of Illinois at Chicago
Chicago, Illinois

William R. Broderick, MD
Fellow
Department of Hematology and Oncology
Loyola University Chicago
Stritch School of Medicine
Maywood, Illinois

Beth L. Brogan, MD
Assistant Professor
Department of Dermatology
Indiana University School of Medicine
Indianapolis, Indiana

Terrence M. Brogan, MD
Resident
Department of Dermatology
Indiana University School of Medicine
Indianapolis, Indiana

David R. Chabolla, MD
Assistant Professor
Department of Neurology
Mayo Clinic College of Medicine
Jacksonville, Florida

Gar Ming Chan, MD
Assistant Clinical Professor of Emergency Medicine
Department of Emergency Medicine
New York University School of Medicine
New York, New York
Attending Physician
Department of Emergency Medicine
North Shore University Hospital
Manhasset, New York

Stanley W. Chapman, MD

Samuel T. Chao, MD
Associate Staff
Department of Radiation Oncology
Cleveland Clinic
Cleveland, Ohio

Jasvinder P.S. Chawla, MD
Assistant Professor
Department of Neurology
Loyola University Chicago
Stritch School of Medicine
Maywood, Illinois

Kathryn A. Coffman, MD
Department of Pediatrics
General Pediatric Attending
St. Joseph's Hospital and Medical Center
Phoenix, Arizona

Christopher Commichau, MD

James J. Corbett, MD

Thomas C. Corbridge, MD, FCCP
Associate Professor of Medicine
Associate Professor of Physical Medicine and Rehabilitation
Northwestern University, Feinberg School of Medicine
Director, Medical Intensive Care Unit
Northwestern Memorial Hospital
Chicago, Illinois

Richard Cowan, MD
Associate Professor
Clinical Director
Department of Neurology
Erie County Medical Center
Buffalo, New York

Bruce Crookes, MD, FACS
Assistant Professor of Surgery
Department of Surgery
University of Vermont College of Medicine
Director of Trauma
Department of Surgery
Fletcher Allen Hospital
Burlington, Vermont

Isam Daboul, MD
Chief, Department of Gastroenterology
University of Toledo Medical School
Toledo, Ohio

Rima M. Dafer, MD, MPH

Felipe De Alba, MD
Associate Professor
Department of Ophthalmology
Loyola University Chicago
Stritch School of Medicine
Maywood, Illinois

John K. DiBaise, MD
Associate Professor of Medicine
Department of Internal Medicine, Division of Gastroenterology and Hepatology
Mayo Clinic
Scottsdale, Arizona

Abigail L. Donovan, MD
Clinical Instructor
Department of Psychiatry
Harvard Medical School
Child Psychiatry Fellow
Department of Child Psychiatry
Massachusetts General Hospital
Boston, Massachusetts

Edward J. Dropcho, MD
Professor
Department of Neurology
Indiana University Medical Center
Indianapolis, Indiana

Steven L. Dubovsky, MD
Professor and Chair
Department of Psychiatry
University at Buffalo
Buffalo, New York
Adjunct Professor of Psychiatry and Medicine
University of Colorado
Denver, Colorado

Volker F. Eckardt, MD
Professor of Medicine
Department of Internal Medicine
Johannes Gutenberg Universität
Mainz, Germany
Chief
Gastroenterology
Deutsche Klinik Für Diagnostik
Wiesbaden, Germany

Steven B. Edelstein, MD
Associate Professor
Vice-Chairman, Medical Education
Department of Anesthesiology
Loyola University Chicago
Stritch School of Medicine
Maywood, Illinois

Benjamin H. Eidelman, MD, PhD

Baltazar R. Espiritu, MD
Associate Professor
Department of Medicine
Loyola University Chicago
Stritch School of Medicine
Maywood, Illinois

Camilo E. Fadul, MD
Associate Professor of Medicine
Department of Medicine
Dartmouth Medical School
Hanover, New Hampshire
Director, Neuro-oncology Program
Department of Medicine
Dartmouth-Hitchcock Medical Center
Lebanon, New Hampshire

Kathy L. Ferguson, DO
Fellow in Medical Toxicology
Department of Emergency Medicine
North Shore University Hospital
Manhasset, New York

Steven V. Fischel, MD, PhD
Assistant Professor
Department of Psychiatry
Tufts University School of Medicine
Boston, Massachusetts
Medical Director, Psychiatry Consultation Service
Department of Psychiatry
Baystate Medical Center
Springfield, Massachusetts

James D. Fleck, MD
Clinical Assistant Professor
Department of Neurology
Indiana University School of Medicine
Indianapolis, Indiana

Jeffrey J. Fletcher, MD
Clinical Instructor
Department of Medicine
Michigan State University
Neuro-Internist
Deparment of Neurology
Bronson Methodist Hospital
Kalamazoo, Michigan

Kere Frey, DO
Associate Professor
Staff Anesthesiologist
Department of Anesthesiology
Loyola University Chicago
Stritch School of Medicine
Maywood, Illinois

Minerva A. Galang, MD
Fellow
Division of Infectious Disease
Department of Medicine
Loyola University Chicago
Stritch School of Medicine
Maywood, Illinois

Edward R. Garrity, Jr., MD, MBA
Professor and Vice Chair of Clinical Operations
Department of Medicine
The University of Chicago
Chicago, Illinois

Paula Gerber, MD
Clinical Neurology and Epilepsy Fellow
Department of Neurology
Barrow Neurological Institute and St. Joseph's Health Center
Phoenix, Arizona

John G. Gianopoulos, MD

Jonathan Glass, MD
Professor of Medicine
Carroll W. Feist Professor of Cancer Research
Director, Feist-Weiller Cancer Center
Chief, Hematology-Oncology
Feist-Weiller Cancer Center, LSU Health Sciences Center
Shreveport, Louisiana

Harold W. Goforth, MD
Assistant Professor
Department of Psychiatry and Behavioral Sciences
Duke University Medical Center
Co-Director, Consult-Liaison Psychiatry
Department of Psychiatry
Durham Veterans' Administration Medical Center
Durham, North Carolina

Mark Gorman, MD
Associate Professor
Department of Neurology
University of Vermont College of Medicine
Burlington, Vermont
Staff Neurologist
Department of Neurology
Fletcher Allen Health Care
Burlington, Vermont

Ankush Gosain, MD, PhD
Resident
Department of Surgery
Loyola University Medical Center
Maywood, Illinois

Deborah M. Green, MD
Associate Clinical Professor
Department of Medicine
University of Hawaii/John A. Burns School of Medicine
Associate Director, Stroke Center; Staff Neurointensivist, Neuroscience Institute
The Queen's Medical Center
Honolulu, Hawaii

John E. Greenlee, MD
Professor and Interim Chair
Department of Neurology
University of Utah Health Science Center
Neurologist
Neurology Service
George E. Wahlen Veterans Affairs Medical Center
Salt Lake City, Utah

Charles Grose, MD
Professor
Department of Pediatrics
University of Iowa
Director
Division of Infectious Disease
Children's Hospital of Iowa
University of Iowa
Iowa City, Iowa

Gregory Gruener, MD, MBA

Marios Hadjivassiliou, MBcHB, MRCP, MD, FRCP
Honorary Senior Lecturer
Department of Neurology
University of Sheffield
Consultant Neurologist
Department of Neurology
The Royal Hallamshire Hospital
Sheffield, United Kingdom

DeVon C. Hale, MD
University of Utah Hospital
Professor
Department of Medicine and Pathology
University of Utah School of Medicine
Salt Lake City, Utah

Nancy Hammond, MD
Assistant Professor
Department of Neurology
University of Kansas
Kansas City, Kansas

Galen V. Henderson, MD
Assistant Professor
Department of Neurology
Harvard Medical School
Director of Neurocritical Care
Department of Neurology
Brigham and Womens Hospital
Boston, Massachusetts

Harold Henderson, MD
Professor of Medicine
Division of Infectious Diseases
University of Mississippi Medical Center
Director
HIV/AIDS Program
University of Mississippi Medical Center
Jackson, Mississippi

Alain Heroux, MD
Associate Professor
Section of Cardiology
Department of Medicine
Loyola University Chicago
Stritch School of Medicine
Maywood, Illinois

Wendy L. Hobson-Rohrer, MD, MSPH
Assistant Professor of Pediatrics
Department of Pediatrics
University of Utah
Salt Lake City, Utah

Christopher P. Holstege, MD
Associate Professor
Department of Emergency Medicine & Pediatrics
University of Virginia
Director
Division of Medical Toxicology
University of Virginia Health System
Charlottesville, Virginia

William J. Holubek, MD
Medical Toxicology Fellow
New York City Poison Control Center
Medical Toxicology Fellow
Emergency Medicine
New York University Medical Center/Bellevue
New York, New York

Susan H. Hou, MD
Professor
Department of Medicine
Medical Director, Renal Transplant Program
Loyola University Chicago
Stritch School of Medicine
Maywood, Illinois

Lisa M. Hurst, MD
Consultant
Department of Internal Medicine
Mayo Clinic Arizona
Phoenix, Arizona

Dan V. Iosifescu, MD, MSc
Assistant Professor of Psychiatry
Harvard Medical School
Director of Neurophysiology Research
Depression Clinical and Research Program
Massachusetts General Hospital
Boston, Massachusetts

Shehla P. Islam, MD
Clinical Assistant Professor
Department of Medicine, Division of Infectious Diseases
University of Florida
Shands at University of Florida
Gainesville, Florida

Michael Jacewicz, MD
Professor
Department of Neurology
University of Tennessee Health Science Center
Assistant Chief
Department of Neurology
VA Medical Center
Memphis, Tennessee

Alfredo F. Jacome, MD
Member
Publications and Health Committees
Academia Nacional de Medicina
Attending Physician
Outpatient Clinic
Asociación Colombiana de Diabetes
Bogotá, Colombia

Daniel E. Jacome, MD
Adjunct Associate Professor
Department of Medicine, Division of Neurology
Dartmouth Medical School
Hanover, New Hampshire
Consulting Staff
Department of Medicine
Franklin Medical Center
Greenfield, Massachusetts

W. Scott Jellish, MD, PhD

Vivekanand Jha, MD, DM
Additional Professor of Nephrology
Postgraduate Institute of Medical Education and Research
Chandigarh, India

Charlotte T. Jones, MD, PhD
Assistant Professor
Department of Pediatrics
Joan C. Edwards School of Medicine at Marshall University
Huntington, West Virginia

Wolfgang H. Jost, MD, PhD
Chief
Neurology
Deutsche Klinik Für Diagnostik
Wiesbaden, Germany
Professor, Department of Neurology
University of Saarland
Homburg/Saar, Germany

Vern C. Juel, MD
Associate Professor of Medicine
Department of Medicine, Division of Neurology
Duke University Medical Center
Durham, North Carolina

Marielle A. Kabbouche, MD
Assistant Professor in Pediatrics and Child Neurology
Pediatrics and Neurology
University of Cincinnati
Cincinnati Children's Hospital Medical Center
Cincinnati, Ohio

Arun A. Kalra, MD
Director of Pediatric Neurology
Associate Professor of Neurology and Pediatrics
Department of Neurology
LSU Health Sciences Center
Shreveport, Louisiana

Bahri Karaçay, PhD
Adjunct Assistant Professor
Department of Pediatrics
University of Iowa College of Medicine
Iowa City, Iowa

John Kashani, DO
Assistant Medical Director, New Jersey Poison Control
Assistant Professor
Department of Preventive Medicine and Public Health, Internal Medicine and Pediatrics
University of Medicine and Dentistry
Newark, New Jersey

Jorge C. Kattah, MD

William C. Kattah, MD
Internal Medicine and Endocrinology
Fundacion Santa Fe
Bogota, Colombia

Roger E. Kelley, MD

Anuradha Khanna, MD
Associate Professor
Department of Ophthalmology
Loyola University Chicago
Stritch School of Medicine
Maywood, Illinois
Director
Department of Ophthalmology
Edward J. Hines Jr. VA Hospital
Hines, Illinois

April E. Kilgore, MD
Resident Physician
Department of Pediatrics
Marshall University
Cabell Huntington Hospital
Huntington, West Virginia

Mark A. Kirk, MD
Associate Professor
Department of Emergency Medicine
University of Virginia
Charlottesville, Virginia

Hannah Klein de Licona, BS
Neuroscience Program, College of Medicine
University of Iowa College of Medicine
Iowa City, Iowa

Bruce Kleinman, MD
Professor
Department of Anesthesiology
Loyola University Chicago
Stritch School of Medicine
Maywood, Illinois

Laurie E. Knepper, MD
Clinical Associate Professor
Department of Neurology
University of Massachusetts Medical School
Worcester, Massachusetts
Attending Physician
Department of Neurology
Berkshire Medical Center
Pittsfield, Massachusetts

Michael Y. Ko, MD
Assistant Professor
Department of Neurology
Loyola University Chicago
Stritch School of Medicine
Maywood, Illinois

Boyd M. Koffman, MD, PhD
Assistant Professor
Department of Neurology
University of Toledo Health Science Campus
Staff Neurologist
Department of Neurology
University Medical Center
Toledo, Ohio

Isabelle Korn-Lubetzki, MD
Chief, Department of Neurology
Shaare Zedek Medical Center
Jerusalem, Israel

Athena Kostidis, MD
Assistant Professor
Department of Neurology
Loyola University Chicago
Stritch School of Medicine
Maywood, Illinois

Andreas H. Kramer, MD, FRCPC
Clinical Assistant Professor
Department of Critical Care Medicine and Clinical Neurosciences
University of Calgary
Calgary, Alberta

David J. Kramer, MD

Dorota Krezoiek, MD
Senior Fellow
Division of Infectious Diseases
Department of Medicine
Loyola University Chicago
Stritch School of Medicine
Maywood, Illinois

Leah Kroeger, MD
Private Practice
Manassas Neurology Associates
Manassas, Virginia

Jeffrey S. Kutcher, MD
Assistant Professor
Department of Neurology
University of Michigan
Service Chief
Department of Neurology
University of Michigan Health System
Ann Arbor, Michigan

Kenneth M. LeDez, MB, ChB, FRCPC
Chair, Discipline of Anesthesia; Associate Professor, Faculty of Medicine
Director, Centre for Offshore & Remote Medicine (MEDICOR)
Memorial University of Newfoundland
Staff Anesthesiologist & Director, Hyperbaric Medicine
Department of Anesthesia
Health Sciences Centre
St. John's, Newfoundland

David C. Lee, MD
Assistant Professor
Department of Emergency Medicine
New York University School of Medicine
New York, New York
Director of Research
Department of Emergency Medicine
North Shore University Hospital
Manhasset, New York

Kenneth V. Leeper, Jr., MD
Associate Professor
Department of Medicine
Emory University
Director of the MICU
Department of Medicine
Emory Crawford Long Hospital
Atlanta, Georgia

A. Arturo Leis, MD
Clinical Professor of Neurology
University of Mississippi Medical Center
Electrodiagnostic Consultant
Methodist Rehabilitation Center
Jackson, Mississippi

John P. Leonetti, MD
Professor and Vice-Chairman
Department of Otolaryngology, Head and Neck Surgery
Loyola University Chicago
Stritch School of Medicine
Maywood, Illinois

Steven N. Levine, MD
Chief, Section of Endocrinology and Metabolism
Department of Internal Medicine
Louisiana State University Health Sciences Center
Shreveport, Louisiana

William Levy, MD
Department of Cardiology
Berkshire Medical Center
Pittsfield, Massachusetts

Fred Leya, MD
Professor
Section of Cardiology
Department of Medicine
Loyola University Chicago
Stritch School of Medicine
Maywood, Illinois

Robert Lichtenberg, MD, FACC
Director, Adult Congenital Heart Clinic at the Illinois Medical District
Department of Pediatrics
Rush Presbyterian St. Lukes and the University of Illinois
Clinical Cardiologist, Department of Medicine
MacNeal Hospital
Berwyn, Illinois

Guillermo Linares-Tapia, MD
Neurologist
Department of Neurology
Cleveland Clinic
Cleveland, Ohio

Peter K. Linden, MD
Professor Critical Care Medicine
Director Abdominal Organ Transplant ICU
University of Pittsburgh Medical Center
Department of Critical Care Medicine
Pittsburgh, Pennsylvania

Benjamin Liptzin, MD
Professor and Deputy Chair
Department of Psychiatry
Tufts University School of Medicine
Boston, Massachusetts
Chair
Department of Psychiatry
Baystate Medical Center
Springfield, Massachusetts

Jacob A. Lohr, MD
Lohr Distinguished Professor of Pediatrics and Associate Chair
Department of Pediatrics
University of North Carolina School of Medicine
Attending Pediatrician
Department of Pediatrics
North Carolina Children's Hospital
Chapel Hill, North Carolina

Betsy B. Love, MD
Adjunct Associate Professor
Department of Neurology
Loyola University Chicago
Stritch School of Medicine
Maywood, Illinois

Charles W. Love, MD
Dermatologist
West Des Moines, Iowa

Fred A. Luchette, MD, FACS, FCCM
Ambrose and Gladys Bowyer Professor of Surgery
Chief, Division of Trauma, Surgical Critical Care and Burns
Department of Surgery
Loyola University Chicago
Stritch School of Medicine
Maywood, Illinois

Anne Mai, MD
Epilepsy EEG Fellow
Department of Neurology
Mayo Clinic Arizona
Phoenix, Arizona

Dan Major, MD, PhD
Chief Resident in Neurology
University of Washington
Seattle, Washington

Christopher R. Marino, MD
Chief, Medical Service
VA Medical Center
Professor
Medicine (Gastroenterology) and Physiology
University of Tennessee Health Science Center
Memphis, Tennessee

Lawrence A. Mark, MD, PhD
Assistant Professor
Department of Dermatology
Indiana University School of Medicine
Faculty Dermatologist
Department of Dermatology
Indiana University Hospital
Indianapolis, Indiana

Sam J. Marzo, MD
Associate Professor
Department of Otolaryngology-Head and Neck Surgery
Loyola University Chicago
Stritch School of Medicine
Maywood, Illinois

Glenn E. Mathisen, MD
Professor of Clinical Medicine
Department of Medicine
UCLA School of Medicine
Los Angeles, California
Chief, Infectious Disease
Department of Medicine
UCLA, Olive View Medical Center
Sylmar, California

Joseph Mattana, MD
Associate Professor of Medicine
Department of Medicine
Albert Einstein College of Medicine
Bronx, New York
Associate Chairman
Department of Medicine
Long Island Jewish Medical Center
New Hyde Park, New York

Peter J. Mazzone, MD, FRCPC, FCCP, MPH
Staff, Director of Lung Cancer Program
Department of Pulmonary, Allergy, and Critical Care Medicine
Cleveland Clinic
Cleveland, Ohio

Edward Melian, MD
Assistant Professor
Department of Radiation Oncology
Loyola University Chicago
Stritch School of Medicine
Maywood, Illinois

Michael P. Merchut, MD, FACP, FAAN

James R. Merikangas, MD
Clinical Professor
Departments of Psychiatry and Behavioral Sciences
George Washington University School of Medicine
Washington, District of Columbia

James F. Meschia, MD
Professor
Department of Neurology
Mayo Clinic
Jacksonville, Florida

Harry L. Messmore, MD

Ana-Claire L. Meyer, MD
VA/Robert Wood Johnson Clinical Scholar
Department of Neurology
University of California, Los Angeles
Fellow
Department of Neurology
Veteran's Administration West Los Angeles
Los Angeles, California

Laura C. Michaelis, MD
Assistant Professor
Division of Hematology/Oncology
Department of Medicine
Loyola University Chicago
Stritch School of Medicine
Maywood, Illinois

Federico E. Micheli, MD, PhD
Professor of Neurology
Facultad de Medicina
University of Buenos Aires
Director
Parkinson's Disease and Movement Disorders Unit
Hospital de Clínicas "Jose de San Martin"
Buenos Aires, Argentina

Mihaela Mihailescu, MD
Fellow
Department of Medicine/Rheumatology
University of Illinois at Chicago
Chicago, Illinois

Lisa A. Millsap, PharmD, ACNP, CCRN, CNRN
Lecturer
Marcella Niehoff School of Nursing
Loyola University Chicago
Maywood, Illinois

Augusto A. Miravalle, MD
Chief Resident
Department of Neurology
Loyola University Chicago
Stritch School of Medicine
Maywood, Illinois

Brian W. Mitchell, MD
Clinical Adjunct Professor
Department of Neurology
Medical College of Georgia
Augusta, Georgia
Medical Doctor
Department of Neurology
Athens Regional Medical Center
Athens, Georgia

Yair Molad, MD
Senior Lecturer
Department of Internal Medicine
Sackler School of Medicine, Tel Aviv University
Tel Aviv, Israel
Director
Rheumatology Unit
Rabin Medical Center, Beilinson Campus
Petah Tikva, Israel

John C. Morgan, MD, PhD
Assistant Professor
Movement Disorders Program, Department of Neurology
Medical College of Georgia
Augusta, Georgia

Gökhan M. Mutlu, MD
Associate Professor of Medicine
Department of Medicine, Division of Pulmonary and Critical Care Medicine
Northwestern University, Feinberg School of Medicine
Attending Physician
Department of Medicine, Division of Pulmonary and Critical Care Medicine
Northwestern Memorial Hospital
Chicago, Illinois

Andrew M. Naidech, MD, MSPH
Assistant Professor
Department of Neurology and Critical Care (Anesthesiology)
Northwestern University, Feinberg School of Medicine
Co-Director, Neurosciences ICU
Department of Neurology and Critical Care (Anesthesiology)
Northwestern Memorial Hospital
Chicago, Illinois

Sucha Nand, MD
Professor
Division of Hematology and Oncology
Department of Medicine
Loyola University Chicago
Stritch School of Medicine
Maywood, Illinois

Barnett R. Nathan, MD
Associate Professor
Departments of Neurology and Internal Medicine
Division of Neurocritical Care
University of Virginia
University of Virginia Health Sciences Center
Charlottesville, Virginia

Alexander J. Nemeth, MD
Assistant Professor
Section of Neuroradiology
Department of Radiology, Neuroradiology Section
Loyola University Chicago
Stritch School of Medicine
Maywood, Illinois

J. Paul O'Keefe, MD
Professor and Associate Chairman
Department of Medicine
Loyola University Chicago
Stritch School of Medicine
Maywood, Illinois

Ellen C. Omi, MD
Assistant Professor
Department of Surgery
Loyola University Chicago
Stritch School of Medicine
Maywood, Illinois

Mauna B. Pandya, MD
Fellow
Division of Hematology/Oncology
Department of Medicine
Loyola University Chicago
Stritch School of Medicine
Maywood, Illinois

Robert M. Pascuzzi, MD

Vijaya K. Patil, MD
Assistant Professor
Department of Neurology
Loyola University Chicago
Stritch School of Medicine
Maywood, Illinois
Staff Physician
Department of Neurology
Edward J. Hines, Jr. VA Hospital
Hines, Illinois

Angel S. Perez, MD
Neurology Resident
Department of Neurology
University of Tennessee Center of the Health Sciences
Resident
Wesley Neurology Clinic
Memphis, Tennessee

Gretchen Peyton, RD, LDN
Clinical Dietitian
Food and Nutrition Services
Loyola University Health System
Maywood, Illinois

Ronald F. Pfeiffer, MD

Istvan Pirko, MD
Assistant Professor
Department of Neurology
University of Cincinnati
Cincinnati, Ohio

Noor A. Pirzada, MD
Professor and Program Director
Department of Neurology
University of Toledo
Professor
Department of Neurology
Medical University Hospital
Toledo, Ohio

Subhash Popli, MD, FACP
Professor
Department of Medicine
Loyola University Chicago
Stritch School of Medicine
Maywood, Illinois
Director, Dialysis Unit
Department of Medicine/Renal
Edward J. Hines, Jr. VA Hospital
Hines, Illinois

Vikram C. Prabhu, MD, FACS
Assistant Professor
Departments of Neurological Surgery and Radiation Oncology
Loyola University Chicago
Stritch School of Medicine
Maywood, Illinois

J. Javier Provencio, MD
Assistant Professor of Medicine
Neuroinflammation Research Center/Neurological Institute
Cleveland Clinic Lerner College of Medicine
Neurointensivist
Cerebrovascular Center
Cleveland Clinic
Cleveland, Ohio

Adam D. Quick, MD
Fellow, Neuromuscular Disease
Department of Neurology
Fletcher Allen Health Care
Burlington, Vermont

Colin C. Quinn, MD
Neurology
University of Virginia School of Medicine
Charlottesvilie, Virginia

Stephen Raffanti, MD, MPH
Associate Professor, Division of Infectious Diseases
Department of Medicine
Vanderbilt University
Chief Medical Officer
Comprehensive Care Center
Nashville, Tennessee

Murali S. Rao, MD, DFAPA, FAPM
Associate Professor and Vice-Chair
Department of Psychiatry and Behavioral Neurosciences
Loyola University Chicago
Stritch School of Medicine
Maywood, Illinois

Timothy B. Rapp, MD
Assistant Professor
Department of Orthopaedic Surgery
Loyola University Chicago
Stritch School of Medicine
Maywood, Illinois

Sowjanya Reganti, MD
Fellow
Division of Hematology/Oncology
Department of Medicine
Loyola University Chicago
Stritch School of Medicine
Maywood, Illinois

Rosario Maria S. Riel-Romero, MD
Associate Professor of Neurology and Pediatrics
Department of Neurology
Louisiana State University Health Sciences Center, School of Medicine in Shreveport
Shreveport, Louisiana

John A. Robinson, MD
Professor of Medicine and Microbiology
Department of Medicine
Loyola University Chicago
Stritch School of Medicine
Maywood, Illinois

Adriana Rodriguez Quiñónez, MD
Epilepsy Fellow
Department of Neurology
Loyola University Chicago
Stritch School of Medicine
Maywood, Illinois

Joshua L. Roffman, MD
Instructor in Psychiatry
Department of Psychiatry
Harvard Medical School
Assistant in Psychiatry
Department of Psychiatry
Massachusetts General Hospital
Boston, Massachusetts

Ethel S. Rose, MD
Assistant Professor
Department of Neurology
University of Mississippi Medical Center
Assistant Chief
Department of Neurology
Jackson VA Medical Center
Jackson, Mississippi

Mark A. Ross, MD
Associate Professor
Department of Neurology
Mayo Clinic College of Medicine
Rochester, MN
Consultant
Department of Neurology
Mayo Clinic Hospital
Phoenix, Arizona

Beth K. Rush, PhD
Assistant Professor
Department of Psychiatry & Psychology
Mayo Clinic College of Medicine
Jacksonville, Florida

David S. Sanders, MD, FRCP, FACG
Honorary Reader in Gastroenterology
Department of Gastroenterology
University of Sheffield
Consultant Gastroenterologist
Royal Hallamshire Hospital
Sheffield, United Kingdom

John M. Santaniello, MD, FACS
Assistant Professor
Department of Surgery
Loyola University Chicago
Stritch School of Medicine
Maywood, Illinois

Maria E. Santiago, MD
Clinical Assistant Professor
Department of Neurology
University of Mississippi
Staff Neurologist
Department of Neurology
GV Montgomery VAMC
Jackson, Mississippi

Jeffrey L. Saver, MD
Professor of Neurology
Department of Neurology
Geffen School of Medicine, UCLA
Director, Stroke Center
UCLA Medical Center
Los Angeles, California

Robert R. Schade, MD, FACP, AGAF, FACG
Professor of Medicine
Department of Medicine
Medical College of Georgia
Chief, Division of Gastroenterology/Hepatology
Department of Gastroenterology/Hepatology
Medical College of Georgia Medical Center
Augusta, Georgia

Jeremiah M. Scharf, MD, PhD
Instructor
Department of Neurology
Harvard Medical School
Assistant in Neurology
Department of Neurology
Massachusetts General Hospital
Boston, Massachusetts

Carol R. Schermer, MD, MPH
Associate Professor
Department of Surgery
Loyola University Chicago
Stritch School of Medicine
Maywood, Illinois

Michael J. Schneck, MD

Rita Schuman, MD
Chief Resident
Department of Otolaryngology
Loyola University Chicago
Stritch School of Medicine
Maywood, Illinois

Robert Schwaner, MD
Attending in Emergency Medicine
North Shore University Hospital
Manhasset, New York

Jeffrey Schwartz, MD
Associate Professor
Department of Cardiovascular Surgery
Loyola University Chicago
Stritch School of Medicine
Maywood, Illinois

William D. Schweickert, MD
Fellow
Department of Medicine, Section of Pulmonary and Critical Care
University of Chicago
Chicago, Illinois

Joseph M. Scianna, MD
Assistant Professor
Department of Otolaryngology–Head and Neck Surgery
Loyola University Chicago
Stritch School of Medicine
Maywood, Illinois

Martha P. Seagrave, BSN, PA-C
Director of Predoctoral Programs
Department of Family Medicine
University of Vermont College of Medicine
Primary Care Clinician
Center for Health and Wellbeing
University of Vermont
Burlington, Vermont

Candice K. Sech, MD
Fellow
Heart Failure/Heart Transplant
Section of Cardiology
Department of Medicine
Loyola University Chicago
Stritch School of Medicine
Maywood, Illinois

Kapil D. Sethi, MD, FRCP(UK)
Movement Disorder Program, Department of Neurology
Medical College of Georgia
Augusta, Georgia

Hubert A. Shaffer, Jr., MD, FACR
Professor Emeritus
Department of Radiology
University of Virginia School of Medicine
Attending Radiologist
Department of Radiology
University of Virginia Health System
Charlottesville, Virginia

Hitesh H. Shah, MD, FACP, FASN
Assistant Professor
Department of Medicine
Albert Einstein College of Medicine
Bronx, New York
Director, Nephrology Fellowship Program
Department of Medicine
Long Island Jewish Medical Center
New Hyde Park, New York

Fergus Shanahan, MD, BSc, FRCPI, FRCP(UK), FACP, FRCP(C)
Professor and Chairman
Department of Medicine
University College Cork
Cork, Ireland

Brian Silver, MD, FRCPC
Assistant Professor
Department of Neurology
Wayne State University School of Medicine
Senior Staff Neurologist
Department of Neurology
Henry Ford Health Systems
Detroit, Michigan

Andrew Silverman, PharmD
Clinical Assistant Professor
School of Pharmacy
University of Florida
Pharmacotherapy Specialist in Abdominal Transplantation
Department of Pharmacy
Tampa General Hospital
Tampa, Florida

Monica Simionescu, MD
Cerebrovascular Fellow
Department of Neurology
Loyola University Chicago
Stritch School of Medicine
Maywood, Illinois

Michael D. Sirdofsky, MD
Associate Professor
Department of Neurology
Georgetown University Hospital
Washington, District of Columbia

Michael A. Sloan, MD, MS

Scott E. Smith, MD, PhD, FACP
Assistant Professor
Division of Hematology/Oncology
Department of Medicine
Loyola University Chicago
Stritch School of Medicine
Maywood, Illinois

Amanda Snodgrass, MD
Resident, Physician
Department of Pediatrics
Marshall University
Cabell Huntington Hospital
Huntington, West Virginia

William H. Spear, MD
Cardiology Fellow
Cardiovascular Institute
Loyola University Medical Center
Maywood, Illinois

James A. Stankiewicz, MD

Theodore A. Stern, MD
Professor of Psychiatry
Harvard Medical School
Chief
Psychiatry Consultation Service
Massachusetts General Hospital
Boston, Massachusetts

Joseph F. Stilwill, MD
Department of Medicine, Section of Hematology
Loyola University Chicago
Stritch School of Medicine
Maywood, Illinois

Jonathan Y. Streifler, MD
Senior Lecturer
Department of Neurology
Tel Aviv University
Tel Aviv, Israel
Head, Neurology Unit
Department of Neurology
Rabin Medical Center, Hasharon Hospital
Petach Tikva, Israel

Howard S. Sudak, MD
Clinical Professor
Department of Psychiatry
University of Pennsylvania
Professional Staff
Department of Psychiatry
The Pennsylvania Hospital
Philadelphia, Pennsylvania

John H. Suh, MD
Chairman
Department of Radiation Oncology
Cleveland Clinic
Cleveland, Ohio

Pawan Suri, MD
Assistant Professor
Departments of Emergency Medicine and Internal Medicine
VCU Medical Center
Director, Clinical Decision Unit
Department of Emergency Medicine
Virginia Commonwealth University Health Systems
Richmond, Virginia

William I. Swedler, MD
Associate Professor
Department of Internal Medicine
University of Illinois at Chicago
Interim Chief
Section of Rheumatology
University of Illinois Hospital
Chicago, Illinois

Edwin Swiatlo, MD, PhD
Associate Professor
Department of Medicine
University of Mississippi Medical Center
Associate Chief of Staff
Department of Research
VA Medical Center
Jackson, Mississippi

Terrie E. Taylor, DO
Professor
Department of Internal Medicine
College of Osteopathic Medicine, Michigan State University
East Lansing, Michigan
Director
Blantyre Malaria Project
Queen Elizabeth Central Hospital
Blantyre, Malawi

Maamoon Tammaa, MD
Neurology Resident
Department of Neurology
University of Tennessee Center for the Health Sciences
Resident
Wesley Neurology Clinic
Memphis, Tennessee

Rodney Tehrani, MD
Assistant Professor
Department of Medicine
Loyola University Chicago
Stritch School of Medicine
Maywood, Illinois

Alexander W. Thompson, MD, MBA
Acting Instructor
Department of Psychiatry and Behavioral Sciences
University of Washington
Seattle, Washington

Silvina B. Tonarelli, MD
Stroke Fellow
Medicine/Neurology
University of Texas at San Antonio
Stroke Fellow
Department of Internal Medicine/Neurology
The University of Texas Health Science Center at San Antonio
San Antonio, Texas

Amytis Towfighi, MD
Neurovascular Fellow
UCLA Stroke Center
Department of Neurology
University of California, Los Angeles
Los Angeles, California

Glenn Treisman, MD
Associate Professor
Department of Psychiatry
Johns Hopkins University
Director, AIDS Psychiatry
Johns Hopkins Hospital
Baltimore, Maryland

Joel M. Trugman, MD
Associate Professor
Department of Neurology
University of Virginia School of Medicine
Attending Neurologist
Department of Neurology
University of Virginia Health System
Charlottesville, Virginia

Hugo E. Vargas, MD
Professor of Medicine
Division of Transplant Medicine
Mayo Clinic Arizona
Scottsdale, Arizona
Professor of Medicine
Division of Transplant Medicine
Mayo Clinic Hospital
Phoenix, Arizona

John D. Wagner, MD, MBA
Associate Professor of Clinical Medicine
Department of Medicine
Albert Einstein College of Medicine
Bronx, New York
Head, Section of Dialysis
Department of Medicine, Division of Kidney Diseases and Hypertension
Long Island Jewish Medical Center
New Hyde Park, New York

Mervat Wahba, MD
Assistant Professor
Department of Neurology
University of Tennessee Health Science Center
Assistant Professor of Neurology
Department of Neurology
Semmes Murphy Clinic at Methodist University Hospital
Memphis, Tennessee

Yunxia Wang, MD
Assistant Professor
Department of Neurology
Kansas University Medical Center
Kansas City, Kansas

Risa M. Webb, MD, DTMH
Associate Professor
Department of Internal Medicine
University of Mississippi Medical Center
Infectious Disease Consultant/Hospital Epidemiologist
Department of Medicine
Jackson Veterans Administration Medical Center
Jackson, Mississippi

Karin Weissenborn, MD
Associate Professor
Department of Neurology
Medical School of Hannover
Hannover, Germany

William H. Wehrmacher, MD, FACP, FACC
Clinical Professor of Medicine and Adjunct Professor of Physiology
Departments of Medicine and Physiology
Loyola University Chicago
Stritch School of Medicine
Maywood, Illinois

Michael H. Whiteley, MD
Assistant Professor
Department of Anesthesiology
Loyola University Chicago
Stritch School of Medicine
Maywood, Illinois

David J. Wilber, MD

Thomas N. Wise, MD
Professor of Psychiatry
Department of Psychiatry and Behavioral Sciences
Johns Hopkins University School of Medicine
Baltimore, Maryland
Chairman, Department of Psychiatry
Inova Fairfax Hospital
Falls Church, Virginia

Lisa F. Wolfe, MD
Assistant Professor
Department of Medicine
Northwestern University Feinberg School of Medicine
Chicago, Illinois

Richard Wolin, MD
Department of Psychiatry
Buffalo Medical Group
Williamsville, New York

Richard G. Wunderink, MD

Daniel S. Yip, MD
Assistant Professor of Medicine
Department of Internal Medicine
Mayo Clinic College of Medicine
Medical Director, Heart Failure and Transplantation
Department of Transplantation
Mayo Clinic Transplantation Center
Jacksonville, Florida

Phyllis C. Zee, MD, PhD
Professor
Department of Neurology
Northwestern University Feinberg School of Medicine
Director, Sleep Disorders Center
Northwestern Memorial Hospital
Chicago, Illinois

Chad Zender, MD
Resident
Department of Otolaryngology–Head and Neck Surgery
Loyola University Chicago
Stritch School of Medicine
Maywood, Illinois

Saša Zivković, MD
Assistant Professor
Department of Neurology
University of Pittsburgh
Staff Physician
Department of Neurology
UPMC Presbyterian and VA Pittsburgh HCS
Pittsburgh, Pennsylvania

Richard A. Zuckerman, MD, MPH
Assistant Professor
Department of Medicine
Dartmouth Medical School
Hanover, New Hampshire
Director of Transplant Infectious Diseases
Section of Infectious Disease and International Health
Dartmouth-Hitchcock Medical Center
Lebanon, New Hampshire

CONTENTS

Part IV GASTROINTESTINAL DISEASES

Part V LIVER DISEASES/BILIARY SYSTEM

Part VI HEMATOLOGICAL DISEASES

Part VII ONCOLOGIC DISEASES

Part VIII METABOLIC DISEASES

Part XVIII EAR, NOSE AND THROAT

Part XIX OBSTETRICS AND GYNECOLOGY

Part XX PEDIATRICS

Part XXI AGENTS OF TERROR

Part XXII PSYCHIATRY

Part XXIII MISCELLANEOUS

PREFACE

It is true that these are exciting times in medicine. And it is well known, of course, that all fields of medicine are interrelated, and that the boundaries between different subspecialties are often imprecise and difficult to delineate. Versatility, team work, and permanent dialogue, by comparison, encircle all fields of specialization and are vital to the practice of quality medicine—period. It also seems clear that neurology is closer to internal medicine than any other subspecialty. Internists are 'initial neurologists,' and the same is probably true of neurologists—neurologists are initially 'internists' who focus on the nervous system. Justifiably, neurologists are reverting back to their role as internists of the nervous system. Accordingly, they need a broader understanding of general medicine and illnesses that are directly responsible for a significant number—not to mention frequently unique presentations—of neurological disease. With the foregoing propositions in mind, neurologists can no longer afford to overlook these interdependent relationships. Now that we are able to *do* more for our patients and those who seek our advice, we must *know* more. It is no longer possible to practice neurology in isolation: Neurology should be practiced as part of an inclusive and wide-ranging system of medicine that acknowledges the continuum between internal medicine and neurology itself.

Meaningful advances have been made in neurology and related disciplines. The field is vast, complex, rapidly expanding, and intellectually challenging. Randomized clinical trials that enrich our understanding and the publication of expanding guidelines have resulted in significant therapeutic developments. This growth, combined with workplace changes, and the exponentially increasing complexity of patients with multiple comorbidities, signify that busy clinicians will have to make greater efforts to keep up-to-date with medical knowledge, so as to be able to offer well-informed judgments in many fields. In this era of frequently competing demands, no health professional can become too complacent, or too relaxed, as it will not take long to fall behind. An appreciation of these facts and other practical concerns sparked the idea to take on this project: To provide a multidisciplinary, comprehensive, learning resource on the interface between neurology and internal medicine, to be used in various disciplines.

With the busy practitioner in mind, we divided our book into 171 chapters organized by organ system, which are further divided by specific conditions. The book examines the neurological manifestations of a wide range of medical conditions, spanning all or most areas of medicine; the neurological effects of drugs, organ transplantation, and other treatments; and the medical comorbidities or complications—iatrogenic or otherwise—that neurologists, internists, and other specialists must diagnose and treat in busy inpatient and/or outpatient practices.

Most chapters are coauthored by a neurologist and nonneurologist specialist(s). Each chapter presents information in an accessible format and includes a case vignette and the authors' recommendations for the case. All chapters have been uniformly organized in a 12-part format: Objectives; Case Vignette; Definition; Epidemiology; Etiology and Pathogenesis; Pathology; Clinical Manifestations; Diagnostic Approach; Treatment; Clinical Recommendation(s) of the Vignette; Summary; and References. In order to further enhance the clinical usefulness and practical focus of our book, a companion website provides multiple-choice questions for each chapter and a fully searchable text with additional comments and selected references. Using this linked approach should facilitate the learning process of the reader.

The birth of this book, more than two years in the making, was made possible through the efforts and collaboration of many dedicated and talented colleagues. During the course of editing it, I have been reminded of the importance of team effort.

We hope to receive constructive comments from our readership, to improve the content and/or layout of the textbook for forthcoming editions. We, therefore, welcome any comments or feedback regarding this text.

José Biller, MD, FACP, FAAN, FAHA

ACKNOWLEDGMENTS

I would like to express my gratitude for the efforts of the highly dedicated and talented team at Lippincott Williams & Wilkins who edited this book and are responsible for the final production.

I especially thank Frances DeStefano, Acquisitions Editor; Leanne McMillan, Associate Managing Editor; Kimberly Schonberger, Marketing Manager; Nicole Walz, Project Manager; Steve Druding, Design Coordinator; and Max Leckrone, Project Manager at Aptara, Inc., for their encouragement, energy, and professionalism. Writing this book was an extraordinary marathon, but all of you made it fun and worthwhile.

I am also forever grateful to Linda Turner for her wonderful secretarial and administrative support.

I also wish to express my sincere appreciation to the authors who shared their expertise and experience with us.

I would be remiss not to thank all my patients, who are "true living books," for contributing to my continued education, and by teaching us all many life lessons.

Finally, I also want to thank those in my family for their extraordinary patience.

José Biller, M.D., FACP, FAAN, FAHA
Professor
Departments of Neurology and Neurological Surgery
Chairman, Department of Neurology
Loyola University Chicago
Stritch School of Medicine
Maywood, Illinois

FOREWORD

The sphere of clinical neurology remains the domain of the skilled clinician. Few organ systems are so replete with such subtle, difficult to characterize, frequently confusing and challenging to associate signs, symptoms and findings than the nervous system. This is certainly the case in the early, prodromal stages of many neurologic diseases, per se. But it is also true of the neurologic signs and symptoms associated with the broad spectrum of other diseases which are not principally neurologic in origin.

The literature of medicine is rich in examples of neurologic diseases the presenting signs and symptoms of which are non-neurologic and richer still when the opposite occurs, that is, a manifest clinical syndrome appears primarily neurologic but is not. And the diagnostic challenge of sorting through a confusing clinical presentation is as daunting when the symptoms and signs are anatomically based as when they are functional and behavioral. We have likely not seen the last laparotomy for suspected gastrointestinal disease in a patient with visceral symptoms caused by diabetic neuropathy. Nor have we likely seen the last patient with adrenal cortical hyper function whose psychiatric or behavioral presentation is presumed to be functional and non-organic. Interestingly, the diagnostic challenge has not been rendered materially more straight-forward by the panoply of imaging and other diagnostic procedures and tests other than to tell the less-than-fully suspecting clinician what the presenting symptom complex is not. In fact, the injudicious use of the ever expanding array of diagnostic investigative options commonly takes one down a misleading path to a dead end.

At the basis of effective clinical problem solving, of course, is the systematic knowledge base of the common and less common presenting signs, symptoms and findings of underlying diseases regardless of the system of origin. And in focusing on the interplay of primarily neurologic and primarily non-neurologic diseases Dr. Biller, his associate editors and co-authors have created an interesting and useful clinical review for the skilled and for the aspiring diagnostician. This book, "The Interface of Neurology & Internal Medicine," is impressively comprehensive in its scope and depth. Its chapters are system based and written by experts in their respective disciplines calling upon both their appreciation of historic and current medical information and vast personal experience. This work is a compendium of diseases with neurologic and non-neurologic presentations and signs of which every competent physician should be mindful and vigilant. While its scope is encyclopedic it is its unique perspective on the functional interplay of Neurology and Internal Medicine that makes this first edition an important and well-written reference work.

To the credit of Dr. Biller and his collaborators this book is a practical and significant contribution to the body of clinical literature of both related disciplines and to the physicians and clinical scientists who work at their interface.

Anthony L. Barbato, M.D.
Professor of Medicine, Emeritus
Loyola University Chicago
Stritch School of Medicine

The Interface of Neurology & Internal Medicine

PART I Cardiovascular Diseases

CHAPTER 1

Cardiac Manifestations of Neurological Disorders

Betsy B. Love • José Biller • David J. Wilber

OBJECTIVES

- To discuss cardiac manifestations of cerebrovascular diseases (stroke and subarachnoid hemorrhage)
- To discuss cardiac manifestations of other neurological disorders, including migraine, epilepsy, multiple sclerosis, Parkinson's disease, dementias, neuromuscular disorders, Guillain-Barré syndrome, and diabetic autonomic neuropathy
- To discuss cardiac complications related to drugs used to treat neurological disorders
- To discuss prevention, diagnosis, and treatment of cardiac complications of neurological disorders

CASE VIGNETTE

A 32-year-old woman with no history of cardiac symptoms presents with a sudden, severe headache, followed by lethargy and left-sided weakness. Examination shows drowsiness, nuchal rigidity, and a moderate left hemiparesis. A computed tomographic (CT) scan without contrast shows subarachnoid blood in the cisterna lamina terminalis, the anterior pericallosal cistern, and the interhemispheric fissure. An electrocardiogram (ECG) shows sinus rhythm with a prolonged QT interval and T-wave inversion. Cerebral angiography reveals a 3 × 2 cm anterior communicating artery aneurysm. What is the likely cause of the ECG changes in this patient?

DEFINITION

It is well recognized that the central nervous system (CNS) regulates the function of the normal heart. It is not surprising, therefore, that central and peripheral neurological disorders can induce cardiac complications. The nervous system plays a role in the regulation of heart rate, blood pressure, vasomotor tone, and cardiac output. Some have described a probable role of the CNS in myocardial metabolism and cardiac contractility (1). The central and peripheral nervous system regulation of heart rate, rhythm, and contractility involves a hierarchical system of control, beginning in the hypothalamus, projecting to the medulla, through the intermediolateral cell column of the spinal cord and through cranial and peripheral autonomic nerves to synapse on the cardiac conduction system and cardiac muscle (2). A thorough review of the neuroanatomy of cardiovascular regulation is beyond the scope of this chapter, and the reader is referred elsewhere for a complete examination of this interaction (3). Because of the intimate brain–heart connection, certain neurological disorders can be associated with cardiac complications. Also, drugs used to treat neurological disorders can be associated with cardiac manifestations.

EPIDEMIOLOGY

Some of the cardiac changes that occur with neurological disorders can be mild and clinically insignificant, whereas others can be devastating, can cause an increase in morbidity and mortality, and can alter the prognosis of the neurological disorder. Examples of the latter are arrhythmias and cardiac arrest in association with epilepsy and subarachnoid hemorrhage (SAH).

Cardiac manifestations frequently occur in stroke, SAH, and epilepsy. ECG abnormalities are frequently seen in SAH (50% to 100%), stroke (90%), and epilepsy (40%, excluding sinus tachycardia). The incidence of serious, potentially life-threatening arrhythmias is 10% with stroke, 5% to 10% in SAH, and 10% in epilepsy. Sudden death occurs in 10% of those with SAH and 1.7% with epilepsy. The challenge that arises for the clinician is to distinguish between relatively benign cardiac changes and life-threatening cardiac dysfunction requiring immediate intervention.

ETIOLOGY, PATHOGENESIS, AND PATHOPHYSIOLOGY

Cardiac abnormalities frequently occur in association with cerebrovascular disorders, including SAH, ischemic stroke, and intracranial hemorrhage.

Cardiac injury and dysfunction after SAH is a well-recognized phenomenon. Cardiac complications after SAH can be divided into ECG changes, arrhythmias, myocardial enzyme abnormalities, cardiac troponin abnormalities, left ventricular dysfunction, the syndrome of neurogenic stunned myocardium, and cardiac arrest.

Electrocardiographic changes have been described in 50% to 100% of patients in the acute phase after SAH (4). Common ECG changes include depression or elevation of ST segments, prolongation of the QT interval corrected for rate (QTc) and T-wave inversion. These ECG changes, however, are not always indicative of myocardial damage or of underlying cardiac disease (5). Most patients require further testing to clarify the significance of ECG changes. ECG changes usually resolve after clinical recovery from SAH (6).

Arrhythmias are another potential complication after SAH. Life-threatening cardiac arrhythmias including malignant ventricular arrhythmias, ventricular tachycardia, torsade de pointes, and ventricular fibrillation have been described in approximately 5% to 10% of patients with SAH (5,7).

Elevation of the creatine kinase-MB (CK-MB) isoenzyme has been noted in SAH, but such elevations do not always indicate myocardial damage. Elevation of cardiac troponin I (cTI), which is detected in approximately 20% of patients with aneurysmal SAH, is more sensitive and specific for cardiac injury (8). Patients with SAH with more severe neurological injury, as graded by the Hunt-Hess grade, have a higher incidence of cTI release (9). In fact, a Hunt-Hess grade of ≥3 is highly predictive of cTI release (8).

Left ventricular (LV) dysfunction detected by echocardiographic evidence of diminished LV wall motion is identified in approximately 10% of patients with SAH (5). For unclear reasons, LV wall motion abnormalities are more common in women with SAH (10).

Reversible neurogenic LV dysfunction, also referred to as *neurogenic stunned myocardium*, is a rare condition that can occur with acute intracranial disorders, including SAH, that is characterized by reversible, globally diminished myocardial wall motion without a primary defect in myocardial perfusion. In addition to signs of LV failure, these patients may have decreased arterial blood pressure, ischemic ECG changes resembling an acute myocardial infarction (MI), elevated CK, CK-MB, and cTI levels, decreased cardiac output, and segmental wall motion abnormalities. Patients may have prominent heart failure and pulmonary edema requiring temporary mechanical support. Despite significant symptoms, the condition is uniformly reversible. It can be confusing clinically whether a patient with SAH has reversible neurogenic LV dysfunction or whether an acute MI has occurred. Some have proposed the following criteria to differentiate reversible neurogenic LV dysfunction with SAH from acute MI: (*a*) no history of cardiac problems; (*b*) new onset of abnormal cardiac function (ejection fraction [EF] <40%); (*c*) cardiac wall motion abnormalities on ECG that do not correlate with the coronary vasculature distribution noted on ECG; and (*d*) cardiac troponin levels less than 2.8 ng/mL in patients with an ejection fraction less than 40%. The presence of these factors would indicate reversible LV dysfunction (11). Some have recommended noninvasive technetium-99 m pyrophosphate myocardial infarct imaging to help differentiate MI from LV dysfunction (12). In some instances, coronary angiography may be necessary to rule out coronary artery disease.

Spontaneous SAH is the most frequent neurological disorder leading to out-of-hospital cardiac arrest, accounting for 4% of all cases of cardiac arrest before reaching the hospital in one series (13). Characteristics that are common with these dramatic presentations are female gender, age under 40 years, lack of comorbidity, headache before cardiac arrest, asystole or pulseless electrical activity as the initial cardiac rhythm, and no recovery of brainstem reflexes (13). Also, preictal hypertension can be a significant risk factor for development of cardiac arrest after SAH (7). Possible mechanisms for fatal cardiac arrest after SAH include a sudden increase in intracranial pressure, mass effect from a hematoma, intraventricular hemorrhage with acute fourth ventricle expansion, pulmonary edema, and cardiac dysrhythmia (14). Although a high mortality rate is seen among those with cardiac arrest after SAH, resuscitation in patients with in-hospital cardiac arrest is likely to be successful and the outcome of survivors of cardiac arrest is not worse than that for other patients without cardiac arrest after aneurysmal SAH (7). Withdrawal of life support should not be based on cardiac arrest alone (7).

The causes of cardiac dysfunction and abnormalities in SAH have been studied extensively, but the precise mechanisms underlying these cardiac manifestations have not been definitively determined. Suggested causes that have been investigated include hypokalemia, corticosteroid release, coronary artery disease, abnormal vagal tone, and local catecholamine toxicity (7). Of these potential factors, the data suggest that local catecholamine toxicity is likely the major causative factor (7). The pathophysiology of this disorder is postulated to be caused by oxygen-derived free radicals or transient calcium overload (15).

Cardiac comorbidities are frequent after ischemic stroke and account for approximately 20% of deaths in this population (16). Cardiac manifestations that can occur after acute ischemic stroke include ECG abnormalities, arrhythmias, elevation of CK-MB and of cardiac selective troponin levels, LV dysfunction, and MI.

All types of EEG changes are frequently reported, perhaps in as many as 90% of patients after acute ischemic stroke (17). ECG changes that have been reported with acute ischemic stroke include morphologic changes (T-wave changes, ST-segment depression or elevation, abnormal U waves, and QTc prolongation), cardiac conduction defects (heart block and bundle branch blocks), and arrhythmias (atrial fibrillation and ectopic beats). The most common ECG changes are nonspecific ST-segment changes (50%) and ST-segment depression (29%) (17). The most common arrhythmias after stroke are premature atrial and ventricular beats and atrial fibrillation (18).

Creatine kinase is elevated after stroke in approximately 45% of patients, with 11% of these demonstrating an elevated CK-MB (19). At times, CK-MB elevations in patients with stroke have not been associated with any clinically evident acute coronary syndrome. Because CK-MB is not entirely cardiac specific, some have suggested that CK-MB elevations in some patients with stroke may not be cardiac in origin and that CK-MB may be falsely elevated after stroke (20). Because troponin has superior sensitivity and specificity compared with CK-MB in revealing minor cardiac injury, it is more helpful in determining whether an MI has actually occurred. Troponin T (TnT) levels have been reported to be elevated in 17% of patients after ischemic stroke. Elevated troponin levels in patients with acute ischemic stroke are associated with a significantly higher risk of in-hospital cardiac complications and death (21). Approximately 13% of patients may present with a concomitant stroke and MI (22).

Similar cardiac manifestations as those described with ischemic stroke and SAH have been described with intracranial hemorrhage (ICH). These include ECG changes (60% to 70%), cardiac arrhythmias (98%), and sudden cardiac death (8%) (3,23). Increased intracranial pressure in acute intracranial processes can produce cardiovascular manifestations caused by the Cushing response, characterized by apnea, hypertension, and bradycardia. Cerebral trauma can produce cardiac effects similar to ICH.

Carotid endarterectomy (CEA) can be associated with fluctuations in blood pressure, MI, and congestive heart failure. Instability of blood pressure, with either hypertension or hypotension, can occur with CEA. The mechanism of these changes is postulated to be secondary to disruption of the carotid sinus baroreceptors during carotid surgery (24). The main cardiovascular complications of CEA in the North American Symptomatic Carotid Endarterectomy Trial (NASCET) were MI in 1.2% and congestive heart failure in 1.2% of patients (25).

Migraine headaches have been associated with ECG changes (26). Prolongations of the PR and QTc intervals are the most common findings (26). It is postulated that ECG changes result from a disruption in the autonomic innervation of the heart and coronary arteries, resulting in an imbalance between the sympathetic and parasympathetic nervous systems (27,28,29).

Epileptic seizures can have cardiac effects. The most common cardiac abnormality reported with both generalized and nongeneralized epileptic seizures is ictal sinus tachycardia. Sinus tachycardia has been reported in 100% of generalized seizures and in 64% to 100% of temporal lobe seizures (30). Although the heart rate may at times exceed 190 beats per minute, little clinical hemodynamic compromise appears to occur (31). Generalized seizures result in a significantly greater increase in heart rate compared with nongeneralized seizures, both during the ictus and postictally (30). Ictal bradycardia is less frequent, occurring in less than 6% of patients (32,33,34). In one large series, ECG changes other than sinus tachycardia were noted in 37% of patients with seizures (30). Most of these were benign abnormalities. Potentially serious ECG changes, however, occurred in 10% of patients, and included prominent ST-segment depression and T-wave inversion. Other cardiac abnormalities that have been described include severe bradycardia, asystole, bundle branch blocks, and QT-interval abnormalities (30). Seizure-induced asystole is very rare (35). A preexisting cardiac disorder can increase the risk for ictal asystole. Approximately 40% of patients with refractory epilepsy have one or more abnormalities in rhythm or repolarization during or immediately after seizures (36,37).

Cardiac disturbances might be one of the contributing factors in sudden unexplained death (SUD) in patients with epilepsy (SUD). SUD accounts for approximately 17% of mortality in patients with epilepsy and for approximately 50% of mortality among those with refractory epilepsy (38,39). Postulated mechanisms whereby seizures could result in lethal arrhythmias include excessive autonomic stimulation of the heart, structural damage to the heart from repetitive autonomic stimulation, and increased circulating catecholamines (30,40). The pathogenesis of SUD in patients with epilepsy has been studied extensively with many hypotheses, but the exact mechanism is unknown. It has been postulated that repetitive autonomic stimulation from multiple seizures might damage the heart, resulting in myocardial fibrosis and myofibrillar degeneration. Excessive autonomic discharges at the time of seizures, combined with an abnormal cardiac substrate, may result in lethal ventricular tachyarrhythmias (41).

Multiple sclerosis (MS) can be associated with autonomic symptoms, including orthostatic hypotension. Cardiovascular autonomic neuropathy (CAN) has been demonstrated in this population by reduced heart rate variation and decreased blood pressure responses on tilt table testing (42). Some evidence indicates that midbrain lesions in MS are associated with cardiovascular dysfunction (42). Also reported are cases of subclinical LV dysfunction by standard echocardiography, Doppler tissue imaging, and radionuclide ventriculography and, infrequently, of LV failure and pulmonary edema (43,44,45).

Parkinson's disease is associated with impairment of the autonomic nervous system, which can lead to impaired cardiovascular regulation in these patients. The main manifestation is orthostatic hypotension. A high prevalence is seen of decreased sympathetic innervation of the heart. Suppressed heart rate variability, which is a predictor of cardiac arrhythmia, is seen (46). Prolonged QT interval on ECG has been reported in patients with Parkinson's disease and multiple system atrophy and may be reflective of degeneration of cardioselective sympathetic and parasympathetic neurons (47).

Dementia and cognitive impairment have been associated with neurocardiovascular instability (NCVI) (48). NCVI encompasses disorders that are neurally mediated, causing hypotension with or without bradycardia, which are secondary to abnormal neural control of the cardiovascular system (48). NCVI is prevalent in patients with dementia and cognitive impairment who have falls. In patients with Lewy body dementia and Alzheimer's dementia, the most common disorders leading to NCVI are orthostatic hypotension and carotid sinus syndrome (48).

Cardiac manifestations are frequently associated with neuromuscular disorders, such as the muscular dystrophies, and the mitochondrial disorders. Each disorder has specific cardiac involvement, which can vary from mild ECG changes to congestive heart failure, lethal arrhythmias, and cardiac arrest (49). Because of the specific nature of possible ECG changes, and echocardiographic findings in neuromuscular disorders, the reader is referred to a complete review of this topic (49). ECG changes and arrhythmias in those with neuromuscular diseases are discussed in Chapter 8.

Guillain-Barré syndrome (GBS; acute inflammatory polyneuropathy) is associated with autonomic dysfunction. Cardiac manifestations that have been reported include sinus tachycardia, systolic hypertension, postural hypotension, ST changes on ECG, and an abnormally small R-R interval variation (50). In approximately 20% of patients, serious and potentially fatal disturbances of autonomic function, including arrhythmias and lability of arterial blood pressure, can occur (51). Labile changes in blood pressure and pulse and a reduced R-R interval variation should increase the suggestion of the occurrence of life-threatening arrhythmias. A number of arrhythmias have been reported, including bradycardia, asystole, ventricular fibrillation, ventricular tachycardia, and atrial fibrillation (50). Severe bradycardia can be preceded by extreme lability of systolic blood pressure and may require a cardiac pacemaker. Tracheal tube manipulation and tracheal suction have been associated with bradycardia and asystole in patients with GBS (52).

Patients with diabetes mellitus complicated by diabetic polyneuropathy usually have some degree of autonomic involvement. CAN, which is a result of damage to vagal and sympathetic nerves, is clinically evidenced by persistent sinus tachycardia, no variation in heart rate during activities, exercise intolerance, and bradycardia. Supine hypertension and orthostatic hypotension may be present. CAN may result in sympathetic imbalance, QT interval prolongation, arrhythmias, and primary cardiac arrest in this population (53,54).

Certain drugs used to treat neurological disorders have been associated with adverse cardiac effects. Carbamazepine (CBZ) has rarely been associated with sinoatrial or AV conduction disorders (55). These cardiac effects can occur with serum levels of CBZ in the therapeutic range. It should not be administered to patients with preexisting atrioventricular (AV) heart block. In addition, CBZ should be used cautiously in patients with a history of heart disease, including coronary artery disease, organic heart disease, or congestive heart failure. A cardiac examination and an ECG should be done in patients with a history of heart disease and in elderly patients to exclude AV block before initiation of CBZ (56). If syncope or a change in seizure type occurs in patients treated with CBZ, an evaluation of cardiac conduction is recommended (56).

Carbamazepine has been reported rarely to induce de novo hypertension in patients without predisposing factors (57). Aggravation of preexisting hypertension when CBZ is added to an established antihypertensive regimen is rare, but is described more frequently than new onset hypertension in the literature (57). Arterial blood pressure should be monitored carefully in hypertensive patients who begin taking carbamazepine. In addition, if new onset hypertension occurs during treatment with CBZ, it should be investigated as a possible cause.

Carbamazepine toxicity or overdose can be associated with a number of cardiac disturbances, including tachycardia, hypotension or hypertension, conduction disturbance with widening of the QRS complex, and fatal cardiac arrhythmias. Clinically significant cardiac toxicity, however, occurs only rarely in patients with toxic CBZ concentrations (58). Abrupt withdrawal of CBZ can increase sympathetic activity in sleep, thereby possibly predisposing to cardiac arrhythmias (59).

Phenytoin and fosphenytoin when administered intravenously (IV) can be associated with cardiac arrhythmias and hypotension. Well-established guidelines regarding the maximal infusion rate for the IV administration of these drugs should be followed.

Pergolide, an ergot-derived dopamine receptor agonist that is used to treat Parkinson's disease and restless legs syndrome, has been associated with drug-induced, restrictive valvular heart disease and pulmonary hypertension (60). Case reports are found of bromocriptine and cabergoline causing cardiac valvular disease (61,62). Patients need to be informed of the possible risk of valvular heart disease with these drugs. It is recommended that all patients taking pergolide have a thorough cardiovascular examination. Close clinical and ECG follow-up is mandatory. Detection of a new murmur with ECG confirmation of restrictive valvular heart disease in these patients requires the initiation of prophylaxis for endocarditis (60). Discontinuation of pergolide and switching to a nonergot drug should be considered if valvular disease is detected and no other cause is identified.

Mitoxantrone is an immunosuppressant agent with potent anti-inflammatory effects that is indicated to treat patients with multiple sclerosis (MS) who have worsening relapsing-remitting or secondary progressive MS despite prior therapy with interferons or glatiramer acetate. Mitoxantrone has been associated with cardiotoxicity, including irreversible cardiomyopathy, decreased EF and congestive heart failure. Recommendations are to measure the LV EF by ECG or multiple gated radionuclide angiography (MUGA) before administration of the initial dose and before each subsequent dose of mitoxantrone, as well as whenever the patient develops signs or symptoms of heart failure (63,64).

Reversible inhibitors of acetylcholinesterase, used in the management of Alzheimer's disease, are associated with bradycardia and cardiac conduction abnormalities. Donepezil is a piperidine-based, reversible inhibitor of acetylcholinesterase that has been associated with sinus bradycardia, complete AV block, and ventricular tachyarrhythmias (65). Donepezil should not be used in patients with sick sinus syndrome or supraventricular cardiac conduction abnormalities or in those with unexplained syncopal episodes. Rivastigmine, an inhibitor of acetylcholinesterase and butyrylcholinesterase, and galantamine hydrobromide, a reversible, competitive acetylcholinesterase inhibitor can cause bradycardia and AV block. Similar restrictions to those with donepezil apply to the use of these agents.

Treatment with L-dopa and dopamine agonists (bromocriptine, pergolide, pramipexole, ropinirole, and apomorphine) in Parkinson's disease can cause or aggravate orthostatic hypotension. Cardiovascular effects can be seen with L-dopa because of the β-adrenergic effect on the heart, causing sinus tachycardia, atrial and ventricular extrasystoles, atrial flutter and fibrillation, and ventricular tachycardia (66). Selegiline, a selective inhibitor of monoamine oxidase type B, diminishes autonomic responses, especially sympathetic responses, which may increase the risk of orthostatic hypotension (67).

Triptans (5-HT1B/1D agonists) used in the acute treatment of migraine have been associated with a variety of cardiac manifestations. The incidence of serious cardiovascular events with triptans, however, appears to be extremely low when appropriate warnings and contraindications are followed. Triptans are not to be used in patients with documented ischemic or vasospastic coronary artery disease. Triptans should not be given to patients with risk factors for coronary artery disease unless they are cleared by a cardiovascular evaluation. Cardiovascular manifestations that have been reported include chest pain, ECG changes, arrhythmias, MI, and rarely, cardiac arrest. Chest pain occurs in 3% to 10% of patients in long-term open label studies of triptans (68). It should be noted, however, that chest symptoms occurring during the use of triptans are generally not serious and may not represent ischemia in patients without known coronary artery disease (68). An evaluation, including history, physical examination, and ECG, should be obtained, however, in patients who experience chest pain with the use of triptans. The ECG changes that have been noted include ST-T segment elevation without identifiable cardiac injury and ST-T segment elevation with MI (69,70). Myocardial infarction has been reported with triptans, but it is extremely rare (70,71). Because the coronary vasculature has 5HT1B receptors, triptans may cause coronary artery vasospasm through this mechanism. Rare cases of serious arrhythmias, including ventricular fibrillation and cardiac arrest have been reported with use of these agents (72,73). Triptans can also cause hypertension. The use of triptans is contraindicated in patients with uncontrolled hypertension (systolic blood pressure ≥140 mm Hg, diastolic blood pressure ≥90 mm Hg).

Ergot alkaloid derivatives, such as dihydroergotamine and ergotamine tartrate, can cause hypertension owing to their potent vasoconstrictor effects. These agents should not be used in those with uncontrolled hypertension. Ergots have been associated with angina pectoris, Mi, and sudden death related to coronary artery spasm (74,75). Finally, ergotamine and methysergide maleate, a synthetic ergot alkaloid with antiserotonergic properties, have been reported to cause fibrotic valvular heart disease, most commonly involving the aortic and mitral valves (76). The valve dysfunction is caused by endocardial thickening and fibrosis, which causes valvular and chordae retraction and results in valvular stenosis or regurgitation (76,77).

Tricyclic antidepressant (TCA) medications are used frequently in the treatment of migraine headache. This class of drugs is associated with hypotension and orthostatic hypotension, tachycardia, and flattening or inversion of T waves on ECG. Overdose of TCA can cause early, transient hypertension by blockade of norepinephrine reuptake, sinus tachycardia caused by anticholinergic effects, hypotension, and orthostasis, and ECG changes (78). ECG changes noted in TCA overdose are sinus tachycardia, prolongation of the PR interval, QTc interval and QRS complex, and an R wave in aVR more than 3 mm. Arrhythmias, including ventricular tachycardia and ventricular fibrillation, may be seen in severe overdoses.

Drugs, such as beta-blockers (i.e., propranolol) and calcium channel blockers (i.e., verapamil), used in the treatment of migraine headaches can cause hypotension. Propranolol can be associated with bradycardia, congestive heart failure, and AV block (79). Verapamil can cause AV block and activation of accessory cardiac conduction pathways in patients with atrial fibrillation (79).

Pimozide, a diphenylbutylpiperidine derivative with neuroleptic properties, is used to treat tics, such as those occurring with Tourette's syndrome. Pimozide has been associated with ECG changes, including prolongation of the QT interval, flattening, notching, and inversion of the T wave, and the appearance of U waves (79). Also reported are ventricular tachyarrhythmias and sudden, unexpected death (80). Pimozide is contraindicated in patients with a history of cardiac arrhythmias, and in patients taking other drugs that prolong the QT interval. Methylphenidate, a sympathomimetic agent used in the treatment of attention-deficit hyperactivity disorder (ADHD) is associated with hypertension, increased heart rate, MI, and arrhythmias (81).

CLINICAL MANIFESTATIONS

In order to identify possible cardiac complications of neurologic disorders, it is necessary to have a high index of suspicion regarding their presence. On examination, patients may demonstrate alterations in blood pressure, either hypotension or hypertension. Orthostatic changes in blood pressure and pulse may be present. The heart rate may reveal tachycardia, bradycardia, and/or a disturbance in the rhythm. Cardiac examination findings are variable, and depend upon the particular cardiac disorder. A new cardiac murmur may be present in patients with drug-induced fibrotic valvular disease. Pulmonary examination may reveal signs of pulmonary edema in those with cardiac failure.

DIAGNOSTIC APPROACH

In patients with stroke or subarachnoid hemorrhage, a routine 12-lead ECG should be the initial test to evaluate for cardiac dysfunction. Continuous ECG monitoring is useful to detect arrhythmias in the first days after acute neurologic injury. Cardiac specific troponin levels may be useful within the first few days after stroke. Echocardiography may be indicated to evaluate for segmental wall motion abnormalities. More detailed cardiac testing may be indicated on a case-by-case basis.

In the patient with epilepsy, ECG monitoring should be performed routinely when the patient is admitted for video-EEG monitoring to identify serious ictal cardiac abnormalities, particularly in patients with refractory epilepsy (82). Patients with ictal cardiac arrhythmias should have a cardiac evaluation to uncover any serious underlying cardiac disorders, which may elevate the patient's risk of a lethal arrhythmia during a seizure. The occurrence of syncope or a change in apparent seizure type in patients with epilepsy should warrant an ECG and a cardiac evaluation.

In the patient with Guillain-Barré syndrome, continuous ECG monitoring is recommended in patients who are becoming severely affected until they have discontinued ventilatory support and have had their tracheostomy removed or until they have begun to recover without the need of either intervention (50). ECG monitoring may need to be continued longer in those who required artificial ventilation due to the higher incidence of arrhythmias in this population.

TREATMENT

Early diagnosis and management of cardiac complications in patients with neurologic disorders is paramount. A cardiology consultation should be obtained early in the course of most of these disorders. Specific treatment for these patients is tailored to the potential underlying cardiac disturbance. In general, arrhythmias are managed in a similar manner as in patients without neurologic disorders (see Chapter 8). Close attention should be paid to fluid and electrolyte status to prevent the precipitation of arrhythmias. If the cardiac disorder could be related to drugs used to treat the neurologic disorder, the potential offending drug should be discontinued, if possible, until the situation is clarified.

In the presence of significant orthostatic hypotension, risks and benefits should be weighed regarding the continued use of an offending drug. Since tracheal tube manipulation and suction have been associated with asystole in GBS patients with autonomic dysfunction, hyperoxygenation is advised before tracheal toilet and tracheal suction should be as gentle as possible (50).

CLINICAL RECOMMENDATIONS OF THE VIGNETTE

The patient described in the vignette needs further testing to clarify the etiology of the ECG changes. ECG findings such as

ST segment depression or elevation, QT prolongation and T-wave inversion are very common in the acute phase after SAH and are not necessarily indicative of myocardial infarction or underlying cardiac disease. Further testing that may be helpful may include continuous ECG monitoring, troponin levels, echocardiography and noninvasive technetium-99m pyrophosphate myocardial infarct imaging.

SUMMARY

Due to the intimate association between the heart and the brain, cardiac manifestations are observed in a number of neurologic disorders. Knowledge of the cardiac abnormalities occurring with neurologic disorders and with the drugs used to treat neurologic disorders is helpful in the management and prevention of complications in these patients.

REFERENCES

1. Talman WT. Cardiovascular regulation and lesions of the central nervous system. *Ann Neurol.* 1985;18:1–13.
2. Valeriano J, Elson J. Electrocardiographic changes in central nervous system disease. *Neurol Clin.* 1993;11:257–272.
3. Talman WT, Kelkar P. Neural control of the heart: Central and peripheral. *Neurol Clin.* 1993;11:239–256.
4. Mayer SA, Lin J, Homma S, et al. Myocardial injury and left ventricular performance after subarachnoid hemorrhage. *Stroke.* 1999;30:780–786.
5. Homma S, Grahame-Clarke C. Myocardial damage in patients with subarachnoid hemorrhage [Editorial Comment]. *Stroke.* 2004;35:552–553.
6. Gascon P, Ley TJ, Toltzis RJ, et al. Spontaneous subarachnoid hemorrhage simulating acute transmural myocardial infarction. *Am Heart J.* 1983;105:511–513.
7. Toussaint LG, 3rd, Friedman JA, Wijdicks EF, et al. Survival of cardiac arrest after aneurysmal subarachnoid hemorrhage. *Neurosurgery.* 2005;57:25–31.
8. Tung P, Kopelnik A, Banki N, et al. Predictors of neurocardiologic injury after subarachnoid hemorrhage. *Stroke.* 2004;35:548–552.
9. Parekh N, Venkatesh B, Cross D, et al. Cardiac troponin I predicts myocardial dysfunction in aneurysmal subarachnoid hemorrhage. *J Am Coll Cardiol.* 2000;36:1328–1335.
10. Sato K, Masuda T, Izumi T. Subarachnoid hemorrhage and myocardial damage clinical and experimental studies. *Jpn Heart J.* 1999;40:683–701.
11. Bulsara KR, McGirt MJ, Liao L, et al. Use of the peak troponin value to differentiate myocardial infarction from reversible neurogenic LV dysfunction associated with aneurysmal subarachnoid hemorrhage. *J Neurosurg.* 2003;98:524–528.
12. Chang PC, Lee SH, Hung HF, et al. Transient ST elevation and left ventricular asynergy associated with normal coronary artery and Tc-99 PYPm myocardial infarct scan in subarachnoid hemorrhage. *Int J Cardiol.* 1998;63:189–192.
13. Kurkciyan I, Meron G, Sterz F, et al. Spontaneous subarachnoid hemorrhage as a cause of out-of-hospital cardiac arrest. *Resuscitation.* 2001;51:27–32.
14. Schievink WI, Wijdicks EFM, Parisi JE, et al. Sudden death from aneurysmal subarachnoid hemorrhage. *Neurology.* 1995;45:871–874.
15. Bolli R, Marban E. Molecular and cellular mechanisms of myocardial stunning. *Physiol Rev.* 1999;79:609–634.
16. Silver FL, Norris JW, Lewis AJ, et al. Early mortality following stroke: A prospective review. *Stroke.* 1984;15:492–496.
17. Dogan A, Tunc E, Ozturk M, et al. Electrocardiographic changes in patients with ischemic stroke and their prognostic importance. *Int J Clin Pract.* 2004;58:436–440.
18. Norris JW, Froggatt GM, Hachinski VC. Cardiac arrhythmias in acute stroke. *Stroke.* 1978;9:392–396.
19. Norris JW, Hachinski VC, Myers MG, et al. Serum cardiac enzymes in stroke. *Stroke.* 1979;10:548–553.
20. Ay H, Arsava EM, Saribas O. Creatine kinase-MB elevation after stroke is not cardiac in origin: comparison to troponin T levels. *Stroke.* 2002;33:286–289.
21. Angelantonio E Di, Fiorelli M, Toni D, et al. Prognostic significance of admission levels of troponin I in patients with acute ischaemic stroke. *J Neurol Neurosurg Psychiatry.* 2005; 76:76–81.
22. Rolak LA, Rokey R. The patient with concomitant stroke and myocardial infarction: Clinical features. In: *Coronary and Cerebral Vascular Disease: A Practical Guide to Management of Patients with Atherosclerotic Vascular Disease of the Heart and Brain.* New York, NY: Futura; 1990:117–137.
23. Stober T, Sen S, Anstatt T, et al. Correlation of cardiac arrhythmias with brainstem compression in patients with intracerebral hemorrhage. *Stroke.* 1988;19:688–692.
24. Sigaudo-Roussel D, Evans DH, Naylor AR, et al. Deterioration in carotid baroreflex during carotid endarterectomy. *J Vasc Surg.* 2002;36:793–798.
25. North American Symptomatic Carotid Endarterectomy Trial Collaborators. Beneficial effect of carotid endarterectomy in symptomatic patients with high-grade carotid stenosis. *N Engl J Med.* 1991;325:445–453.
26. Aygun D, Altintop L, Doganay Z, et al. Electrocardiographic changes during migraine attacks. *Headache.* 2003;43:861–866.
27. Lafitte C, Even C, Henry-Lebras F, et al. Migraine and angina pectoris by coronary artery spasm. *Headache.* 1996;36:332–334.
28. Shechter A, Stewart WF, Silberstein SD, et al. Migraine and autonomic nervous system function: A population-based, case-control study. *Neurology.* 2002;58:422–427.
29. Appel S, Kuritzky A, Zahavi I, et al. Evidence for instability of the autonomic nervous system in patients with migraine headache. *Headache.* 1992;32:10–17.
30. Opherk C, Coromilas J, Hirsch LJ. Heart rate and EKG changes in 102 seizures: Analysis of influencing factors. *Epilepsy Res.* 2002;52:117–127.
31. Leutmezer F, Schernthaner C, Lurger S, et al. Electrocardiographic changes at the onset of epileptic seizures. *Epilepsia.* 2003;44:348–354.
32. Marshall DW, Westmorland BF, Sharbrough FW. Ictal tachycardia during temporal lobe seizures. *Mayo Clin Proc.* 1983;58:443–446.
33. Keilson MJ, Hauser WA, Magrill J. Electrocardiographic changes during electrographic seizures. *Arch Neurol.* 1989;46:1169–1170.
34. Blumhardt LD, Smith PE, Owen L. Electrocardiographic accompaniments of temporal lobe epileptic seizures. *Lancet.* 1986;1:1051–1056.
35. Rocamora R, Kurthen M, Lickfett L, et al. Cardiac asystole in epilepsy: Clinical and neurophysiologic features. *Epilepsia.* 2003;44:179–185.
36. Nei M, Ho RT, Sperling MR. EKG abnormalities during partial seizures in refractory epilepsy. *Epilepsia.* 2000;41:542–548.
37. Tigaran S, Molgaard H, McClelland R, et al. Evidence of cardiac ischemia during seizures in drug refractory epilepsy patients. *Neurology.* 2003;60:492–495.
38. Nashef L, Fish DR, Sander JW, et al. Incidence of sudden unexpected death in an adult outpatient cohort with epilepsy at a tertiary referral centre. *J Neurol Neurosurg Psychiatry.* 1995;58:462–464.
39. Lip GYH, Brodie MJ. Sudden death in epilepsy: An avoidable outcome? *J R Soc Med.* 1992;85:609–611.
40. Simon RP, Aminoff MJ, Benowitz NL. Changes in plasma catecholamines after tonic-clonic seizures. *Neurology.* 1984;34:255–257.
41. Nei M, Ho RT, Abou-Khalil BW, et al. EEG and ECG in sudden unexplained death in epilepsy. *Epilepsia.* 2004;45:338–345.
42. Saari A, Tolonen U, Paakko E, et al. Cardiovascular autonomic dysfunction correlates with brain MRI lesion load in MS. *Clin Neurophysiol.* 2004;115:1473–1478.
43. Akgul F, McLek I, Duman T, et al. Subclinical left ventricular dysfunction in multiple sclerosis. *Acta Neurol Scand.* 2006;114:114–118.
44. Beer M, Sandstede J, Weilbach F, et al. Cardiac metabolism and function in patients with multiple sclerosis: A combined 31P-MR-spectroscopy and MRI study. *RoFo.* 2001;173: 399–404.
45. Uriel N, Kaluski E, Hendler A, et al. Cardiogenic shock in young female with multiple sclerosis. *Resuscitation.* 2006;70:153–157.
46. Pursiainen V, Haapaniemi TH, Korpelainen JT, et al. Circadian heart rate variability in Parkinson's disease. *J Neurol.* 2002;249:1535–1540.
47. Deguchi K, Saski I, Tsukaguchi M. Abnormalities of rate-corrected QT intervals in Parkinson's disease—A comparison with multiple system atrophy and progressive supranuclear palsy. *J Neurol Sci.* 2002;199:31–37.
48. Kenny RAM, Kalaria RAJ, Ballard C. Neurocardiovascular instability in cognitive impairment and dementia. *Ann NY Acad Sci.* 2002;977:183–195.
49. Bhakta D, Groh WJ. Cardiac function tests in neuromuscular diseases. *Neurol Clin.* 2004;22:591–617.
50. Winer JB, Hughes RAC. Identification of patients at risk of arrhythmia in the Guillain-Barré syndrome. *Q J Med.* 1988;68:735–739.
51. Ropper AH, Wijdicks EFM, Truax BT. *Guillain-Barré Syndrome.* Philadelphia: FA Davis; 1991.
52. Pfeiffer G, Schiller B, Kruse J, et al. Indicators of dysautonomia in severe Guillain-Barré syndrome. *J Neurol.* 1999;246:1015–1022.
53. Kahn JK, Sisson JC, Vinik AI. QT interval prolongation and sudden cardiac death in diabetic autonomic neuropathy. *J Clin Endocrinol Metab.* 1987;64:751–754.
54. Whitsel EA, Boyko EJ, Rautaharju PM, et al. Electrocardiographic QT interval prolongation and risk of primary cardiac arrest in diabetic patients. *Diabetes Care.* 2005;28:2045–2047.
55. Puletti M, Iani C, Curione M, et al. Carbamazepine and the heart. *Ann Neurol.* 1991;29:575–576.
56. Boesen F, Andersen EB, Jensen EK, et al. Cardiac conduction disturbances during carbamazepine therapy. *Acta Neurol Scand.* 1983;68:49–52.
57. Jette N, Veregin T, Guberman A. Carbamazepine-induced hypertension. *Neurology.* 2002;59:275–276.
58. Apfelbaum JD, Caravati EM, Kerns WP II, et al. Cardiovascular effects of carbamazepine toxicity. *Ann Emerg Med.* 1995;25:631–635.
59. Hennessy MJ, Tighe MG, Binnie CD, et al. Sudden withdrawal of carbamazepine increases cardiac sympathetic activity in sleep. *Neurology.* 2001;57:1650–1654.
60. Van Camp G, Flamez A, Cosyns B, et al. Treatment of Parkinson's disease with pergolide and relation to restrictive valvular heart disease. *Lancet.* 2004;363:1179–1183.
61. Horvath J, Fross RD, Kleiner-Fisman G, et al. Severe multivalvular heart disease: A new complication of the ergot derivative dopamine agonists. *Mov Disord.* 2004;19:656–662.
62. Serratrice J, Disdier P, Habib G, et al. Fibrotic valvular heart disease subsequent to bromocriptine treatment. *Cardiol Rev.* 2002;10:334–336.
63. Cohen BA, Mikol DD. Mitoxantrone treatment of multiple sclerosis: Safety considerations. *Neurology.* 2004;63:S28–S32.
64. Pratt RG, Boehm GA, Kortepeter CM, et al. Mitoxantrone treatment of multiple sclerosis: Safety considerations [Correspondence]. *Neurology.* 2005:65:1997.
65. Suleyman T, Tevfik P, Abdulkadir G, et al. Complete atrioventricular block and ventricular tachyarrhythmia associated with donepezil. *Emerg Med J.* 2006;23:641–642.

66. Mars H, Krall J. L-dopa and cardiac arrhythmias. *N Engl J Med.* 1971;285:1437.
67. Turkka J, Suominen K, Tolonen U, et al. Selegiline diminishes cardiovascular autonomic responses in Parkinson's disease. *Neurology.* 1997;48:662–667.
68. Dodick D, Lipton RB, Martin V, et al. Consensus statement: Cardiovascular safety profile of triptans (5-HT1B/1D agonists) in the acute treatment of migraine. *Headache.* 2004;44:414–425.
69. Willett F, Curzen N, Adams J, et al. Coronary vasospasm induced by subcutaneous sumatriptan. *BMJ.* 1992;304:1415.
70. Ottervanger JP, Paalman HJA, Boxma GL, et al. Transmural myocardial infarction with sumatriptan. *Lancet.* 1993;341:861–862.
71. O'Connor P, Gladstone P. Oral sumatriptan-associated transmural myocardial infarction. *Neurology.* 1995;45:2274–2276.
72. Laine K, Raasakka T, Mantynen J, et al. Fatal cardiac arrhythmia after oral sumatriptan. *Headache.* 1999;39:511.
73. Kelly KM. Cardiac arrest following use of sumatriptan. *Neurology.* 1995;45:1211–1213.
74. Yasue H, Takizawa A, Nagao M. Acute myocardial infarction induced by ergotamine tartrate: Possible role of arterial spasm. *Angiology.* 1981;32:414–418.
75. Benedict CR, Robertson D. Angina pectoris and sudden death in the absence of atherosclerosis following ergotamine therapy for migraine. *Am J Med.* 1979;67:177–178.
76. Soler-Soler J, Galve E. Worldwide perspective of valve disease. *Heart.* 2000;83:721–725.
77. Redfield MM, Nicholson WJ, Edwards WD, et al. Valve disease associated with ergot alkaloid use: Echocardiographic and pathologic correlations. *Ann Intern Med.* 1992;117:50–52.
78. Frommer DA, Kulig KW, Mark JA, et al. Tricyclic antidepressant overdose. A review. *JAMA.* 1987;257:521–526.
79. Medical Economics Staff. *Physicians' Desk Reference,* 60th ed. Montvale, NJ: 2006.
80. Yap YG, Camm AJ. Drug induced QT prolongation and torsades de pointes, *Heart.* 2003;89:1363–1372.
81. Nissen SE. ADHD drugs and cardiovascular risk. *N Engl J Med.* 2006;354:1445–1448.
82. Devinsky O. Effects of seizures on autonomic and cardiovascular function. *Epilepsy Currents.* 2004;4:43.

CHAPTER **2**

Neurologic Manifestations of Congenital Heart Disease

Robert Lichtenberg • David C. Anderson

OBJECTIVES

- To review congenital heart disease and classify the type of patients that will present to the internist and neurologist involved with adult patients
- To discuss the pre- and postnatal factors involved in the neurologic and developmental outcomes of patients with congenital heart disease
- To review the genetic syndromes affecting both heart and brain
- To describe the neurologic risk to the adult with congenital heart disease because of residual defects or sequelae of the interventions according to their lesion
- To review the current information on cryptogenic stroke, and the role of the patent foramen ovale

CASE VIGNETTE

A 32-year-old woman with known cyanotic congenital heart disease presented with a 3-week history of fever, chills, and rapidly evolving delirium, agitation, and focal motor deficits. She had recently been incarcerated for 7 days. The patient has a history of alcohol and polysubstance abuse, but denied intravenous use.

Her cardiac defect has been labeled as an unbalanced atrioventricular (AV) canal with a double outlet right ventricle with severe pulmonary stenosis. The anatomy was not felt to be amenable to total surgical correction, and her only surgery had been a palliative shunt from the aorta to the pulmonary artery to increase pulmonary blood flow at 14 years of age. Examination demonstrated a fever of 39.4°C, nuchal rigidity, finger clubbing, with systemic saturations of 84% and a 4/6 harsh systolic murmur over the precordium. Multiple suspicious lesions were seen on the fingers, palms, and plantar aspect of her feet (Fig. 2-1). No needle tracks were seen. Computed tomographic (CT) scan showed multiple ring-enhancing lesions, predominantly in the left hemisphere with surrounding edema. Magnetic resonance imaging (MRI) showed multiple enhancing lesions in the left front, parietal, and occipital lobes involving the subcortical white matter, as well as the corticomedullary junction. Ring-enhancing lesions were seen in the parietal white matter. The largest lesion in the left frontal parietal region measured 2.1 cm by 1.9 cm. There was marked surrounding vasogenic edema. The lesions were interpreted as possible septic emboli with abscess formation (Fig. 2-2).

Echocardiogram showed a mobile vegetation on the atrioventricular valve (Fig. 2-3). Four of four blood cultures were positive for *Streptococcus viridans.*

DEFINITION

Adults with congenital heart disease represent a rapidly expanding population. Before the 1960s, <5% of infants born with congenital heart disease (CHD) would survive until age 21 years. Now, this same population of patients with CHD has earlier diagnosis and receives treatment, either palliative and or corrective, resulting in >95% survival into adulthood. This remarkable progress has resulted in a new challenge to the internist and neurologist treating adult patients with CHD. A systemic approach to these patients is important, starting with an understanding of the specific defect and any prior procedures. The procedures, such as stated above, have been life saving, but are not without sequelae, and, in most cases, they leave residual defects. This group of patients has been referred to as having GUCH (Grown Up Congenital Heart). This chapter will acquaint internists and neurologists with this challenging group of adult patients. Although sounding like something out of a Dr. Seuss book, these GUCH patients are pioneers and need insightful, caring physicians involved in their care. The adult patient with CHD will often fall into one of four categories:

1. No prior surgery and none likely to be required. An example of this would be the patient with a small restrictive ventricular septal defect. This represents approximately 10% of the adult population.
2. Prior surgical procedure performed that resulted in total correction of the defect, and a return to normal circulation with separation of the systemic venous return (directed to the pulmonary vascular bed) and the pulmonary venous return (directed to the systemic circulation). This group comprises most adult patients that the internist and neurologist will encounter. As an example, transposition of the great vessels demonstrates the complex-

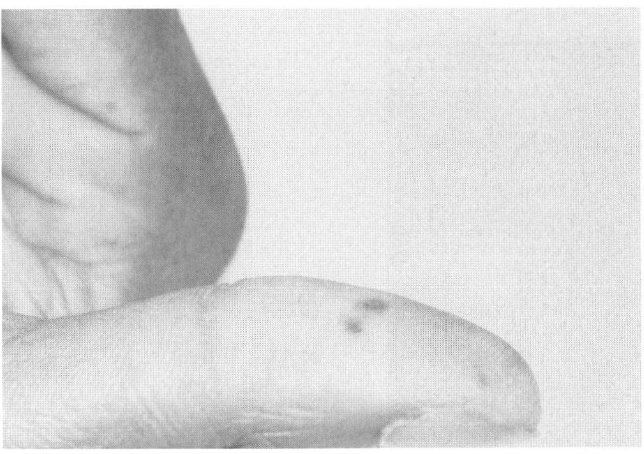

FIGURE 2-1. Peripheral manifestations of infective endocarditis Osler nodes.

ity of this population. Figure 2-4A represents the circulation at birth. As can be appreciated, the systemic circulation is separate from the pulmonary circulation with no mixing. This is not compatible with life and is uniformly fatal. The corrective procedure performed in the 1960s to 1980s, involved the redirection of blood at the atrial level, resulting in a physiologic, but not anatomic, correction. This procedure is known as the *atrial switch*; the two variations of it are called the *Mustard* and *Senning* procedures (Fig. 2-4B). Advancement in surgical techniques, with the ability to transfer the coronary arteries, has resulted in the development of the arterial switch (Fig. 2-4C). This results in both a physiologic and an anatomic correction. Both of these procedures are associated with consequences as a result of residual defects as well as sequelae of the procedure that present neurologic risk to the adult.

3. Prior palliative procedure. These procedures do not correct the underlying defect, but rather provide a partial correction to allow for survival. An example of this would be tetralogy of Fallot with a shunt placed from a systemic artery to the pulmonary artery to improve pulmonary blood flow (Fig. 2-5).
4. No surgery to date and none possible because of a missed opportunity to correct the defect before the development of severe complications. An example of this would be Eisenmenger syndrome and the development of severe fixed pulmonary hypertension because of an uncorrected left-to-right shunt, such as a ventricular septal defect or a patent ductus arteriosus.

EPIDEMIOLOGY

The incidence of CHD in the general population is 4 to 5 of 1,000 live births. If the bicuspid aortic valve, atrial septal aneurysm, and channelopathies such as prolonged QT syndrome, were included, the incidence would be as high as 50 of 1,000 live births (1). The neurologic manifestations of CHD involve many factors. Many genetic syndromes have both neurologic and cardiac defects, such as trisomy 21 or 22q11 microdeletions. Cerebral dysgenesis has been reported to be 10% to 29% in patients with CHD (2). The fetal cerebral circulation can be adversely affected by specific defects. The oxygenated blood returning to the right side of the heart through the ductus venosus is preferentially directed across the atrial

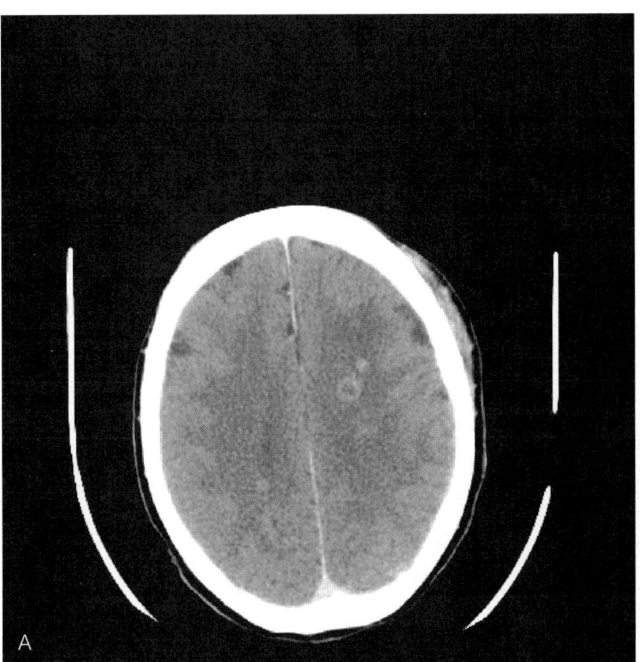

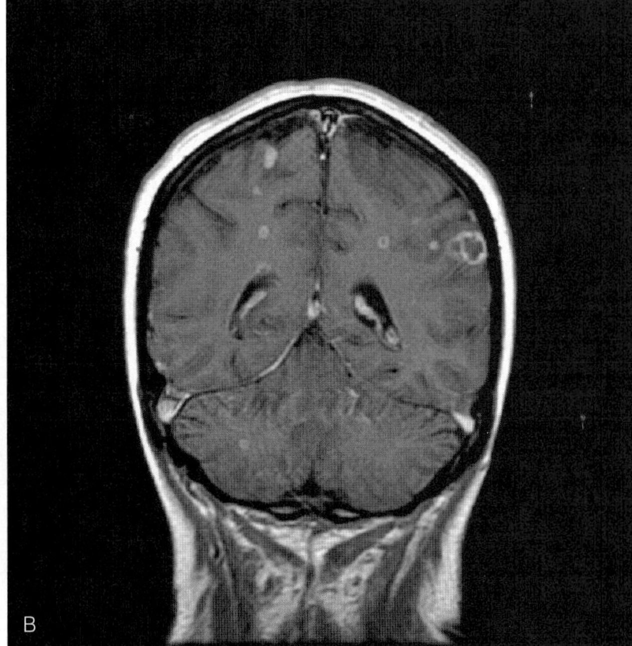

FIGURE 2-2. (**A**) Postcontrast axial computed tomography (CT) scan of the head at the level of the centrum semiovale shows multiple white matter ring-enhancing lesions measuring a few millimeters each. (**B**) Postcontrast coronal magnetic resonance image (MRI) of the head at the level of the choroid plexi of the lateral ventricles shows multiple ring-enhancing lesions in both hemispheres, most at the junction between gray and white matter, measuring between 3 and 10 mm; one lesion is present in the right cerebellar hemisphere.

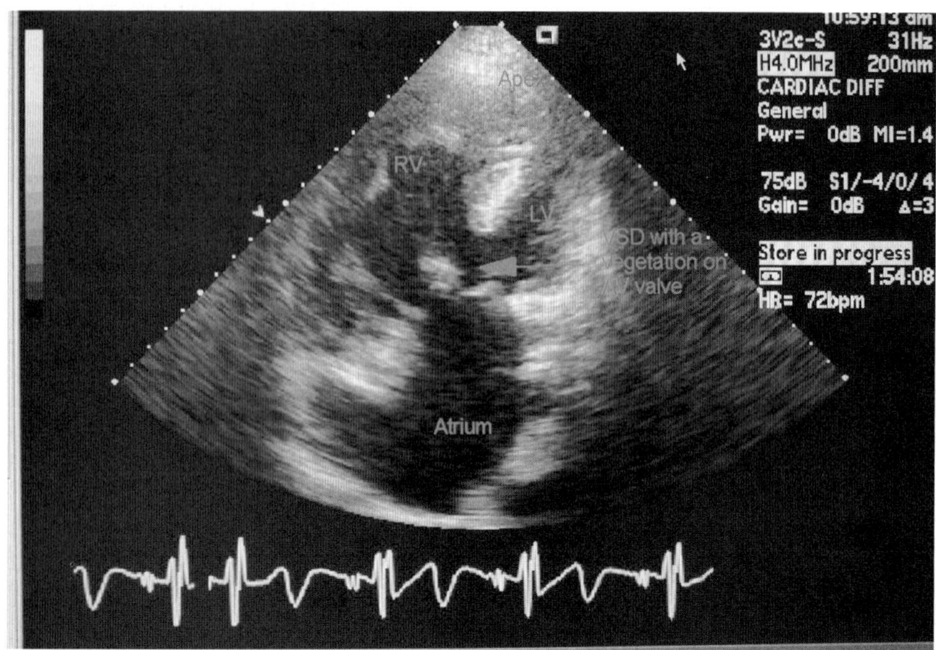

FIGURE 2-3. Echocardiogram with an apical view revealing a vegetation on the atrioventricular valve. LV, left ventricle; RV, right ventricle; VSD, ventricular septal defect, AV, atrioventricle.

septum to the left side of the heart, resulting in ascending aorta and cerebral delivery. Defects, such as premature closure of the fossa ovalis and hypoplastic left ventricle lesions, will result in decreased cerebral perfusion with oxygenated blood. Cerebral perfusion must occur retrograde from the descending aorta, which receives it blood supply from the ductus arteriosus and is desaturated as a result of mixing of desaturated and oxygenated blood. Many birth and postnatal factors have an impact on cerebral development. Chronic hypoxemia present in cyanotic congenital heart defects, despite compensatory erythrocytosis, has been associated with lower cognitive ability (3). It has also been shown that the earlier the correction of the cyanosis, the higher the cognitive ability (4,5). Operative intervention, however, is not without risk and includes embolic potential from palliative procedures (6), exposure to hypothermic, nonpulsatile cardiopulmonary bypass (7), and, commonly, severe hyperglycemia (8).

Congenital heart defects can be broadly classified at birth as cyanotic or acyanotic. For the physician treating adults, the original defect, repair, and residua and sequelae are important to understand. Table 2-1 outlines the most common congenital heart defects and their potential impact on the CNS.

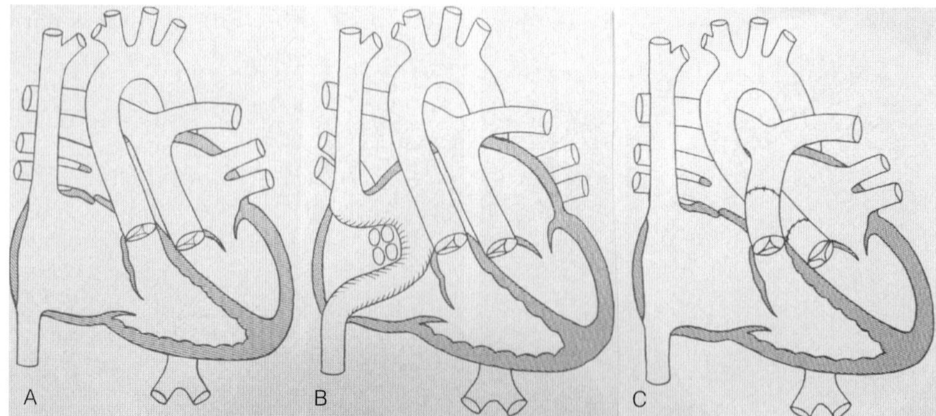

FIGURE 2-4. TGV–Atrial Switch–Arterial Switch: Transposition of Great Vessels. (**A**) At birth, the pulmonary and systemic circulations are in parallel, rather than series, not allowing for adequate mixing. The systemic circulation receives only unoxygenated blood that is recirculated without transit through the lungs for oxygenation. (**B**) The atrial switch (Mustard, Senning) procedure results in a physiologic, but not anatomic correction. The residual defect means that the right ventricle supports the systemic circulation. (**C**) The arterial switch (Jatene) procedure requires transecting the great vessels and mobilizing the coronary arteries for transfer. This results in an anatomic and physiologic correction, but with the sequela of circumferential suture and potential scar above both the pulmonary and aortic valves.

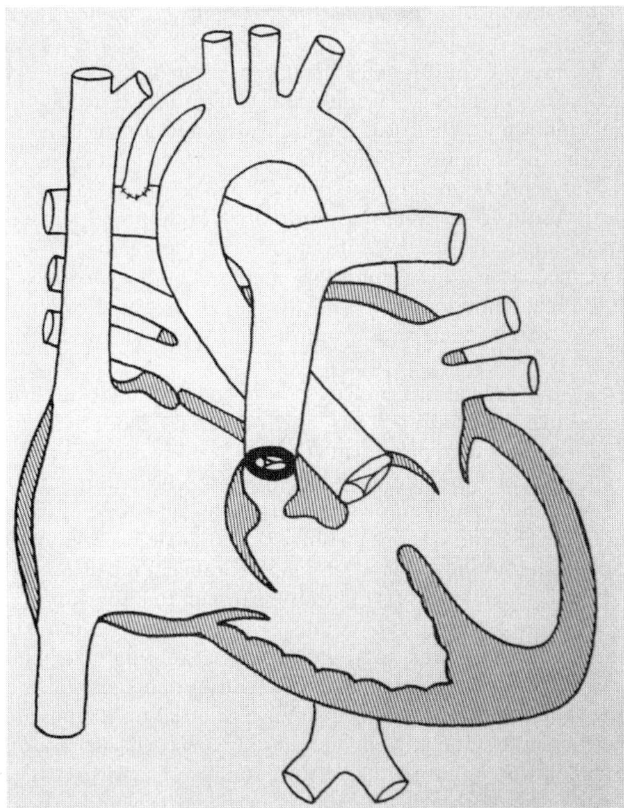

FIGURE 2-5. Tetralogy of Fallot: Palliative shunt. Blalock-Taussig procedure where the subclavian artery is ligated distally and the proximal segment is anastomosed to the pulmonary artery. The modified Blalock-Taussig shunt uses a graft placed between the subclavian artery and pulmonary artery and the distal vessel is left intact. (From *Congenital Heart Disease: A Diagrammatic Atlas,* Charles E. Mullens. John Wiley & Sons, with permission.)

ETIOLOGY AND PATHOGENESIS

SOURCES OF NEURODEVELOPMENTAL, COGNITIVE, AND NEUROLOGIC DEFICITS

Multiple factors potentially contribute to neurodevelopmental and cognitive deficits in children with CHD and GUCH. Congenital central nervous system (CNS) defects, either inherited or acquired in utero, can be associated with cardiac defects. Cardiovascular and metabolic instability from unpalliated CHD defects can also cause brain injuries before surgery can be performed. The palliative or corrective operative procedure itself or supporting management with hypothermic cardiac arrest or low flow bypass can be injurious to the brain. Postoperative medical issues and continuing vascular and hematologic derangements can cause harm. Finally, a childhood interrupted by illness, and health consciousness can limit opportunities for optimal growth.

The reported frequency of extracardiac congenital defects varies, reflecting varying sources of cases and means of study (9,10). Most cases of CHD (e.g., 90%) are not a part of a recognized malformation syndrome. Even so, 5% to 10% of these patients have a single major additional malformation, perhaps 1% to 2% involving the nervous system. A smaller percentage of patients with CHD (e.g., 10%) have a malformation syndrome (9). Many of the malformation syndromes include neurologic features and neurodevelopmental consequences. These may result from chromosomal or recognized single gene abnormalities, suspected gene defects, or in utero insults.

Neurodevelopmental and cardiac manifestations typically coexist in the chromosomal syndromes, including 13 (ventricular septal defect [VSD]), 18 (VSD), and 21 (AV canal defects) trisomies (11). Single gene syndromes with combined brain–heart defects include Noonan's (pulmonary stenosis), and Williams (supravalvular aortic stenosis). Embryopathies with neurodevelopmental consequences in which CHD may be a component include fetal alcohol syndrome (atrial septal defect [ASD], VSD) and rubella embryopathy (aortic and subaortic stenosis).

Children with severe CHD can acquire injuries that affect neurodevelopment because of marginal cerebral blood flow and oxygen delivery associated with unpalliated heart defects before operation. The lesions include periventricular leukomalacia and overt infarcts as detected by MRI (12,13) and cranial ultrasound (14) before surgical correction or palliation. Preoperative neurodevelopmental assessment has also detected deficits before surgery is undertaken in some of children with severe CHD (15).

Surgical advances have transformed the prospects for children with severe CHD. Survival is not only possible, but

TABLE 2-1. Most Common Congenital Heart Disorders and Potential Central Nervous System Impact

Defect	*Incidence and Associated Defects*	*Cyanotic* Pre	*Cyanotic* Post	*Arrythmias* Atrial	*Arrythmias* Vent	*Valvular Lesions*	*Endocarditis Risk*
Ventricular septal defect	30%	No	No	Low	Low	None	Low
Atrial septal defect	10%	No	No	Low	Low	Cleft mitral valve in the primum ASD	Low unless primum defect
Coarctation of aorta	7% Cerebral aneurysms	No	No	Low	Low	Aortic valve	Moderate with associated bicuspid aortic valve
Transposition of great vessels	4%	Yes	No	High	Low	Systemic AV valve insufficiency	Moderate to high
Atrial baffle							
Mustard arterial switch				Low	Low	Supravalvular aortic stenosis	
Tetralogy of Fallot	6%	Yes	No	Low	Mod	Pulmonary insufficiency	Moderate

ASD, atrial septal defect; AV, atrioventricular.

expected, for many defects that were uniformly fatal a half century ago. Attention has increasingly focused on improving the quality of life of the survivors. Hence, the refined goal is survival with neurodevelopmental and cognitive potential intact. Short and intermediate term follow-up of operated children show a high rate of neurodevelopmental, cognitive, and neurologic sequelae (10,12,13,16–37). Multiple operative, perioperative, and support issues have been examined in these outcome studies. Some suggestion is that use of cardiac arrest under deep hypothermia and duration of hypothermia, may be risk factors for neurodevelopmental deficits.

Several specific neurologic syndromes have been reported as complications of corrective surgery (38). Horner syndrome can be produced by interruption of preganglionic sympathetic fibers during aortic arch surgery (e.g., Blalock-Taussig shunts). Vocal cord paralysis is a rare complication of extensive aortic arch manipulation; for example, during patent ductus closure. Phrenic nerve palsy is usually, but not always, temporary after open heart surgery. Spinal cord injury is a rare but devastating complication of aortic arch surgery. The suspected mechanism is spinal cord ischemia caused by aortic cross-clamping. The subclavian steal syndrome has been reported following Blalock-Taussig shunt procedures for tetralogy of Fallot. This shunt is created by ligating the distal subclavian artery and anastomosing the proximal subclavian artery to the pulmonary artery. This procedure increases flow to the pulmonary circulation (Fig. 2-5). The distal subclavian artery may steal blood from the ipsilateral vertebral artery blood flow to supply the arm. Finally, a superior vena cava syndrome with intracranial venous hypertension can sometimes complicate the Mustard procedure performed to correct transpositions (Fig. 2-4B). The procedure creates a baffle that directs desaturated systemic blood to the left side of the heart and the pulmonary circuit. Obstructed venous return from the superior vena cava through the baffle occurs in up to 6% of patients. This was the procedure of choice throughout the 1960 to 1980 time span, thus, resulting in a large group of adults with CHD now reaching 30 to 50 years of age.

Common to almost all adults with CHD, whether uncorrected, palliated, or totally corrected, are ischemic and infectious processes. These will be covered next.

CLINICAL MANIFESTATIONS/SPECIAL SITUATIONS

STROKE

Focal brain ischemia is common in children who die because of CHD (39). "Silent" brain infarcts can contribute to neurodevelopmental and cognitive deficits. In children, most clinical strokes occur in those with cyanotic defects. It might be assumed that arterial distribution infarcts caused by paradoxical embolism would comprise the most common lesion and mechanism. They do not; instead, most common is venous thromboembolism (40,41). Reduced venous flow velocity, caused by erythrocytosis-related cellular hyperviscosity and decreased cerebral blood flow, and enhanced *clotting*, related to altered coagulation parameters, predispose to the formation of venous clots, as predicted by Virchow's triad. Parenthetically, it is prudent to recall that brain abscesses are notorious masqueraders for bland ischemic stroke among those patients with cyanotic CHD (42).

In cases of childhood clinical venous stroke, the clinical deficit often reflects parenchymal congestion and ischemic infarction caused by cortical vein involvement. Cortical venous infarcts are commonly complicated by seizures. Alternatively, the large intracranial venous sinuses may be the sites of occlusion resulting in a more gradually developing increased intracranial pressure. Manifestations include headache, somnolence, nausea, and vomiting. Sometimes, both a cortical vein and a major venous sinus are involved, leading to a combination of focal deficit and symptoms of increased intracranial pressure.

Several surgical procedures have been associated with arterial strokes in children. These include atrial balloon fenestration used as a temporary palliation before repairing transpositions (6) and the Fontan procedure for functional single ventricle (43). These procedures create a source of clot (damaged atrial septum, Fontan tunnel) and a clean pathway for embolism into the systemic circulation and cerebral arteries.

In the series by Oechslin et al. (44) from the Toronto Congenital Cardiac Centre for Adults, stroke accounted for >20% of the noncardiac cause of death. This relatively high incidence is in a population of patients at the end of a life-long journey into adulthood with a high incidence of atrial fibrillation and ventricular dysfunction. Yet perhaps unexpectedly, stroke is not particularly common in the functional and active GUCH. Again at first glance, adults with cyanotic CHD would seem to be prime candidates for stroke. They are cyanotic because of right-to-left shunting, and all patients with cyanosis, clinically detectable by measurement of saturations and clubbing, are at risk. They have erythrocytosis with associated hyperviscosity. Thus, it would seem that cerebral arterial paradoxical embolism and venous occlusions would abound. The actual rate of stroke caused by either venous or arterial thromboembolism, however, is relatively low (45). Patients with Eisenmenger syndrome should represent a high-risk group for paradoxical emboli, yet the annual risk of stroke is <1% (44–46).

In our adult congenital heart clinic there are 68 patients with Eisenmenger syndrome with >500 patient years of follow up. Only two strokes have occurred, however, with both of these occurring during hospitalization with testing involving intravenous access. Awareness of this potential risk and implementation of preventive measures are critical to navigating this patient population through hospitalization. A simple intravenous line or phlebotomy is a potential source of systemic embolization. This low incidence seems to be in conflict with the recently collected data in patients with cryptogenic stroke and patent foramen ovale where the annual incidence has been reported to be between 0.5% and 5% (47–51). These patients are at increased risk by the usual suspects: Atrial fibrillation, arterial hypertension, and, potentially, by iron deficiency anemia (41,46). Iron-deficient red blood cells have marked decreased deformability, thus resulting in increased viscosity despite their smaller size. Again, including all adults with cyanotic CHD, the stroke risk (1 of 100 patient-years) (46) is less than the stroke risk of even "low risk" atrial fibrillation (1% to 3%/year). This apparent protective mechanism may be related to the activated fibrinolytic system. Evidence suggests that this system is activated in patients with cyanotic CHD (52). Surgeons have known this for years, and often stated "TETS BLEED" in describing the operative field. Consequently, warfarin anticoagulation is not indicated, and actually is considered contraindicated for stroke prevention among adults with cyanotic CHD. As with warfarin, phlebotomy does not appear to be indicated on the grounds of ischemic stroke prevention, and it may also worsen the iron deficiency (52).

HYPERVISCOSITY

Patients with GUCH with Eisenmenger complex and other cyanotic defects have varying levels of erythrocytosis and associated increased cellular viscosity. Symptoms of hyperviscosity include dizziness, tinnitus, blurry vision, sluggish mentation, fatigue, headache, acral paresthesias, myalgias, nausea, and dyspnea (52).

Although phlebotomy does not have a role in stroke prevention among patients with cyanotic CHD, it has been used to counter symptoms of hyperviscosity. If phlebotomy is performed for this indication, the volume removed should be replenished with isotonic saline or colloid solutions to achieve maximal effect (52). Phlebotomy, however, can contribute to iron deficiency to which these patients seem predisposed. Of note, iron deficiency can contribute to hyperviscosity symptoms (53), although probably not to viscosity itself (54). Iron deficiency has also been identified as a risk factor for stroke in adults with cyanotic CHD (52). Consequently iron deficiency should be avoided. In patients who have already become iron deficient, oral iron therapy should be advanced slowly until a hematocrit response is just detected to avoid a rapid increase in hematocrit, which can precipitate hyperviscosity symptoms.

INFECTIVE ENDOCARDITIS

Congenital heart defects are at high risk for endocarditis. In fact, patients with complex cyanotic congenital heart defects, constructed systemic-to-pulmonary shunts, or those with congenital valvular defects, are in the highest risk group along with patients with prosthetic heart valves (55). The clinical diagnosis is made using the Duke criteria (55), which are outlined in Chapter 4. These criteria incorporate echocardiographic findings. It is important to recognize that many of the common sites involved with infective endocarditis are not visible on standard transthoracic and even transesophageal echocardiography. These include the systemic-to-pulmonary surgical shunts, as well as the extracardiac prosthetic heart valves. The clinician needs to be aware of this, and maintain a high index of suspicion when evaluating adults with CHD presenting with fever, especially in the setting of bacteremia.

Systemic embolization is a common occurrence, and the adult patient with CHD with right-to-left shunting is at an increased risk as a consequence of right-sided lesions having access to the systemic circulation. The CNS receives most of these emboli. Vegetation size, mobility, valve involved, infection with *Staphylococcus aureus* or fungal organisms are all predictors of a higher risk of embolization. Anticoagulation has never been demonstrated to be of benefit in these patients, and it is felt to result in a higher risk of hemorrhagic transformation in the first few weeks (55). Mycotic aneurysms arise as a result of septic embolization of vegetations to the nutrient vessels of the arterial system, the vasa vasorum. The resultant growth and spread of the infectious process results in a high-risk lesion associated with a 60% mortality (55). Patients may develop severe headache, altered sensorium, or focal neurologic deficits, which however, can also remain clinically silent before rupture.

ABSCESS

A brain abscess is usually thought to present subacutely, often with progressive focal neurologic deficits, symptoms of intracranial pressure, and fever. Acute onset of focal neurologic deficits in children and young adults with cyanotic CHD are almost as likely caused by a brain abscess or stroke (42). The suddenness of onset in cases of cyanotic CHD probably reflects the pathophysiology with initial embolism of infected material, local brain ischemia or anoxia conducive to growth of anaerobes, bacterial proliferation, and abscess formation (56). The hypoxemia caused by right-to-left shunting provides an ideal milieu for rapid growth of the lesion. Indeed, the hypoxia and ischemic tissues are critical factors for encouraging the growth of anaerobic streptococcus or other anaerobes, which are common organisms in cases of brain abscess. Early clinical suspicion and prompt diagnosis remain keys to successful medical management.

CEREBRAL ANEURYSMS

Coarctation of the aorta is amenable to surgical correction, but it is associated with a 28% mortality at a mean age of 38 years after repair (57). The association of coarctation with aortic valve disorders is well known, because up to 65% of patients have a bicuspid aortic valve. A strong association also exists with intracranial aneurysm, however (58–60). A recent report on a magnetic resonance angiographic study in 100 patients with coarctation of the aorta found that 10% had an intracranial aneurysm with a mean diameter of 3.5 mm with a range of 2 to 8 mm (59). This fivefold increased incidence compared with the general population suggests that screening for intracranial aneurysms should be done on all patients with coarctation of the aorta, even after surgical repair.

PARADOXICAL EMBOLISM AND THE PATENT FORAMEN OVALE

No doubt exists that the patent foramen ovale (PFO) can allow paradoxical emboli. This process has been caught in the act as evidenced by Figure 2-6. But data to suggest that all PFO should be closed as a primary or even secondary preventive measure are not definitively established. Clearly, the development of catheter-based closure devices has spearheaded this enthusiasm. Multiple reports demonstrate the enthusiasm and caution on this therapy (61–64). Ongoing trials, such as CLOSURE (randomized trial comparing transcatheter patent foramen ovale closure with the STARFlex septal occluder to best medical therapy) and RESPECT (randomized evaluation of recurrent stroke comparing PFO closure with established current standard of care treatment), it is hoped will provide data to address the defect found in up to 30% of everyone (65).

The adult with Eisenmenger syndrome caused by an atrial septal defect is not directly comparable to the patient with PFO for many reasons. Patients with Eisenmenger syndrome have compensatory erythrocytosis, splenomegaly with thrombocytopenia, and an activated thrombolytic system (52). The anatomy of the atrial septum can also play a pivotal role. The

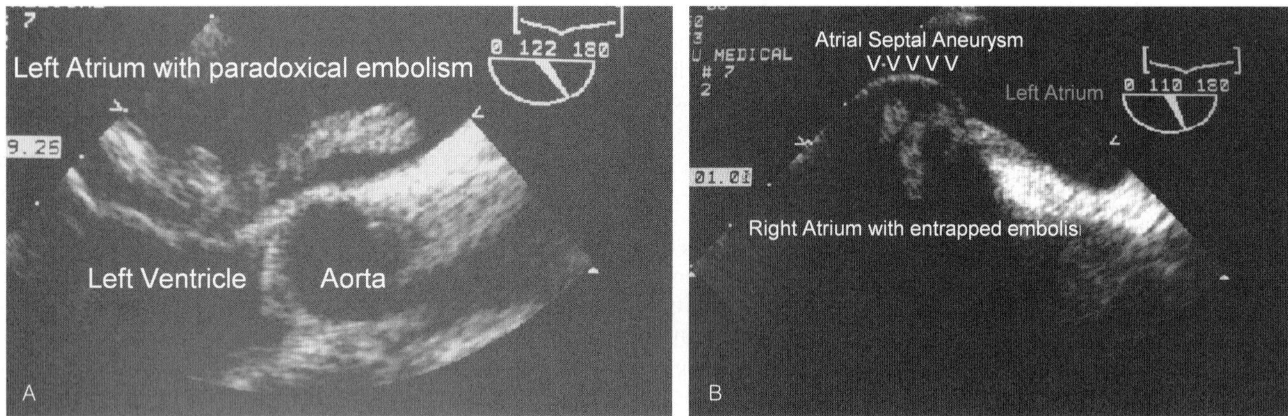

FIGURE 2-6. Large entrapped cast of a venous thrombus entrapped in a patent foramen ovale.

PFO often has a long tunnel, which creates a potential space for stasis and coagulation before entering the systemic circulation (Fig. 2-7). It may be this potential space that is critical in the apparent increased incidence of transient ischemic attacks and stroke in the PFO population.

DIAGNOSTIC APPROACH

The adult with CHD presenting with a neurologic disorder needs a thorough evaluation that starts with a detailed history, which must include as many of the details of the birth defect as well as the repairs, both palliative and corrective. Once the anatomy and circulation are properly understood, the residua and sequelae should be established. Table 2-1 should help with that task. A team approach is critical, and should involve the neurologist, cardiologist, internist, and surgical expertise that may involve cardiovascular and neurosurgical. Many of these patients will have implanted pacemakers and defibrillators, removing MR techniques from the diagnostic armamentarium. This places a heavier load on a precise history and detail-oriented physical examination. Awareness of the expected auscultation of the GUCH and attention for peripheral stigmata of infective endocarditis are essential.

CLINICAL RECOMMENDATIONS OF THE VIGNETTE

The patient had infective endocarditis with multiple septic emboli. She is cyanotic with prior palliative shunts and has high-risk lifestyle habits. Her incarceration allows for the establishment of an infectious process with resultant multiple emboli. The neurologic examination is consistent with a rapidly evolving process with both cerebral and meningeal signs. The echocardiogram reveals a high-risk lesion because of its mobility and size. Vegetations on the mitral valve >1 cm are at high risk for continued embolization. Medical therapy requires appropriate antibiotics and consultation with both neurosurgery and cardiovascular surgery. Anticoagulation is contraindicated in the early stages of active infective endocarditis.

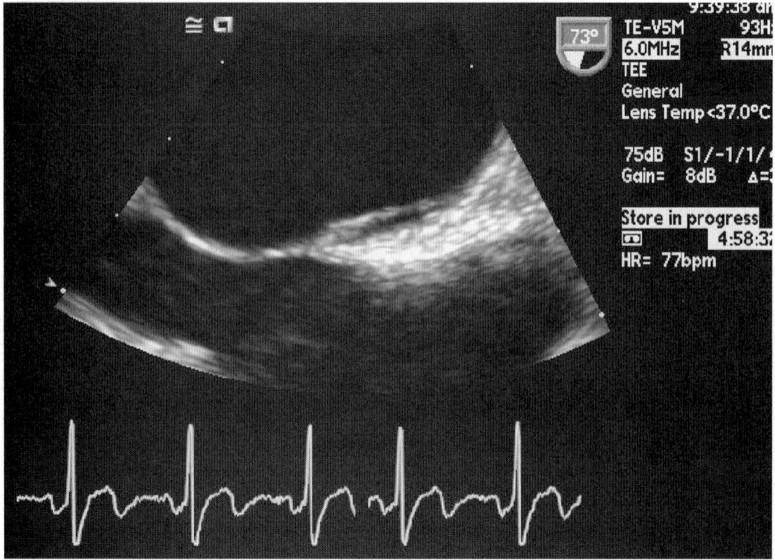

FIGURE 2-7. Long tunnel patent foramen ovale (PFO). The left atrium is on the **top** and the superior aspect is to the right on the image. The long tunnel is seen between the septum primum and septum secundum. This tunnel can result in stasis of flow for variable periods of time and subsequent release into the systemic circulation.

The patient had a stereotactic brain biopsy with surgical drainage of the largest lesion in the left frontal parietal region. Parenteral antibiotics are continued and a significant mitral and tricuspid valvular insufficiency did not develop. The patient completed a full course of antibiotics, with her only residual deficit being mild right leg paresis. Supportive efforts by the physician team, social work, and family are initiated.

SUMMARY

Patients with GUCH are warm, caring, and thankful for the medical developments to date and for ongoing insightful care. The adult with CHD represents an expanding population with unique anatomy and physiology. These adult patients, however, remain approachable with the standard tools available to the internist and neurologist with a few modifications. The history must be inclusive of the congenital defect from the prenatal perspective and inclusive of all procedures. This will be time intensive and likely take more than the usual allotted time for a new patient encounter or initial consultation. A 60- to 90-minute time span would be a suggested minimum. Examination must be detailed and best performed after an understanding of the anatomy and residual defects, as well as the sequelae of the corrective procedures. A team approach is essential and will serve these frontier patients well.

REFERENCES

1. Benson DW. The genetics of congenital heart disease: A point in the revolution. *Cardiol Clin.* 2002;20(5):385–394.
2. Jones, M. Anomalies of the brain and congenital heart disease: A study of 52 necropsy cases. *Pediatr Pathol.* 1991;11(5):721–736.
3. Aram DM, Ekelman BL, Ben-Schachar G. Intelligence and hypoxemia in children with congenital heart disease: Fact or artifact? *J Am Coll Cardiol.* 1985;6(4):889–893.
4. Finley KH, Buse ST, Popper RW. Intellectual functioning of children with tetralogy of Fallot: Influence of open heart surgery and earlier palliative operations. *J Pediatr.* 1984;85(40):318–323.
5. Newberger JW, Silber AR, Buckley LP, et al. Cognitive function and age of repair of transposition of the great arteries in children. *N Engl J Med.* 1984;310(23):1495–1499.
6. McQuillen PS, Hamrick SE, Perez MJ, et al. Balloon atrial septostomy is associated with preoperative stroke in neonates with transposition of the great arteries. *Circulation.* 2006;113(2):280–285.
7. Wypij D, Newburger JW, Pappaport LA, et al. The effect of duration of deep hypothermic circulatory arrest in infant heart surgery on late neurodevelopment: The Boston Circulatory Arrest Trial. *J Thorac Cardiovasc Surg.* 2003;126(11):1397–1403.
8. Lichtenberg RC, Goto M, Zeller WP. Lactic acid changes during and after hypothermic cardiopulmonary bypass in infants. *J Lab Clin Med.* 1993;121(6):697–705.
9. Kramer HH, Majewski F, Trampisch HJ, et al. Malformation patterns in children with congenital heart disease. *Am J Dis Child.* 1987;141(7):789–795.
10. Glauser TA, Rorke LB, Weinberg PM, et al. Acquired neuropathologic lesions associated with the hypoplastic left heart syndrome. *Pediatrics.* 1990;85(6):991–1000.
11. Du Plessis AJ. Neurologic complications of cardiac disease in the newborn. *Clin Perinatol.* 1997;24(4):807–826.
12. Mahle WT, Clancy RR, Moss EM, et al. Neurodevelopmental outcome and lifestyle assessment in school-aged and adolescent children with hypoplastic left heart syndrome. *Pediatrics.* 2000;105(5):1082–1089.
13. Miller G, Mamourian AC, Tesman JR, et al. Long-term MRI changes in brain after pediatric open heart surgery. *J Child Neurol.* 1994;9(4):390–397.
14. Van Houten JP, Rothman A, Bejar R. High incidence of cranial ultrasound abnormalities in full-term infants with congenital heart disease. *Am J Perinatol.* 1996;13(1):47–53.
15. Limperopoulos C, Majnemer A, Shevell MI, et al. Neurodevelopmental status of newborns and infants with congenital heart defects before and after open heart surgery. *J Pediatr.* 2000;137(5):638–645.
16. Ferry PC. Neurologic sequelae of cardiac surgery in children. *Am J Dis Child.* 1987;141(3):309–312.
17. Ferry PC. Neurologic sequelae of open-heart surgery in children. An 'irritating question.' *Am J Dis Child.* 1990;144(3):369–373.
18. Bellinger DC, Wernovsky G, Rappaport LA, et al. Cognitive development of children following early repair of transposition of the great arteries using deep hypothermic circulatory arrest. *Pediatrics.* 1991;87(5):701–707.
19. Newburger JW, Jonas RA, Wernovsky G, et al. A comparison of the perioperative neurologic effects of hypothermic circulatory arrest versus low-flow cardiopulmonary bypass in infant heart surgery. *N Engl J Med.* 1993;329:1057–1064.
20. Oates RK, Simpson JM, Cartmill TB, et al. Intellectual function and age of repair in cyanotic congenital heart disease. *Arch Dis Child.* 1995;72(4):298–301.
21. Oates RK, Simpson JM, Turnbull JA, et al. The relationship between intelligence and duration of circulatory arrest with deep hypothermia. *J Thorac Cardiovasc Surg.* 1995;110(3):786–792.
22. Walsh AZ, Morrow DF, Jonas RA. Neurologic and developmental outcomes following pediatric cardiac surgery. *Nurs Clin North Am.* 1995;30(2):347–364.
23. Bellinger DC, Jonas RA, Rappaport LA, et al. Developmental and neurologic status of children after heart surgery with hypothermic circulatory arrest or low-flow cardiopulmonary bypass. *N Engl J Med.* 1995 2;332(9):549–555.
24. Fallon P, Aparicio JM, Elliott MJ, et al. Incidence of neurological complications of surgery for congenital heart disease. *Arch Dis Child.* 1995;72(5):418–422.
25. Miller G, Tesman JR, Ramer JC, et al. Outcome after open-heart surgery in infants and children. *J Child Neurol.* 1996;11(1):49–53.
26. Bellinger DC, Rappaport LA, Wypij D, et al. Patterns of developmental dysfunction after surgery during infancy to correct transposition of the great arteries. *Developmental and Behavioral Pediatrics.* 1997;18(2):75–83.
27. Hovels-Gurich HH, Seghaye MC, Dabritz S, et al. Cognitive and motor development in preschool and school-aged children after neonatal arterial switch operation. *J Thorac Cardiovasc Surg.* 1997;114(4):578–585.
28. Utens EM, Verhulst FC, Duivenvoorden HJ, et al. Prediction of behavioural and emotional problems in children and adolescents with operated congenital heart disease. *Eur Heart J.* 1998;19(5):801–807.
29. Ellerbeck KA, Smith MA, Holden EW, et al. Neurodevelopmental outcomes in children surviving d-transposition of the great arteries. *Developmental and Behavioral Pediatrics.* 1998;19(5):335–341.
30. Stieh J, Kramer HH, Harding P, et al. Gross and fine motor development is impaired in children with cyanotic congenital heart disease. *Neuropediatrics.* 1999;30(2):77–82.
31. Bellinger DC, Wypij D, Kuban KCK, et al. Developmental and neurological status of children at 4 years of age after heart surgery with hypothermic circulatory arrest or low-flow cardiopulmonary bypass. *Circulation.* 1999;100:526–532.
32. Forbes JM, Visconti KJ, Bellinger DC, et al. Neurodevelopmental outcomes in children after the Fontan operation. *Circulation.* 2001; 104[Suppl 1]:I127–I132.
33. Limperopoulos C, Majnemer A, Shevell MI, et al. Predictors of developmental disabilities after open heart surgery in young children with congenital heart defects. *J Pediatr.* 2002;141(1):51–58.
34. Bellinger DC, Wypij D, duDuplessis AJ, et al. Neurodevelopmental status at eight years in children with dextro-transposition of the great arteries: The Boston Circulatory Arrest Trial. *J Thorac Cardiovasc Surg.* 2003;126(5):1385–1396.
35. Galli KK, Zimmerman RA, Jarvik GP, et al. Periventricular leukomalacia is common after neonatal cardiac surgery. *J Thorac Cardiovasc Surg.* 2004;127:692–704.
36. Karl TR, Hall S, Ford G, et al. Arterial switch with full-flow cardiopulmonary bypass and limited circulatory arrest: Neurodevelopmental outcome. *J Thorac Cardiovasc Surg.* 2004;127(1):213–222.
37. Newburger JW, Bellinger DC. Brain injury in congenital heart disease [Editorial]. *Circulation.* 2006;113:183–185.
38. Park SC, Neches WH. The neurologic complications of congenital heart disease. *Neurol Clin.* 1993;11(2):441–462.
39. Berthrong M, Sabiston DC, Jr. Cerebral lesions in congenital heart disease: A review of autopsies on 162 cases. *Bull Johns Hopkins Hosp.* 1951;89(5):384–406.
40. Cottrill CM, Kaplan S. Cerebral vascular accidents in cyanotic congenital heart disease. *Am J Dis Child.* 1973;125(4):484–487.
41. Amitai Y, Blieden L, Shemtov A, et al. Cerebrovascular accidents in infants and children with congenital cyanotic heart disease. *Isr J Med Sci.* 1984;20(12):1143–1145.
42. Kurlan R, Krall RL, Deweese JA. Vertebrobasilar ischemia after total repair of tetralogy of Fallot: Significance of subclavian steal created by Blalock-Taussig anastomosis. *Stroke.* 1984;15(2):359–362.
43. Barker PC, Nowak C, King K, et al. Risk factors for cerebrovascular events following Fontan palliation in patients with a functional single ventricle. *Am J Cardiol.* 2005;96(4):587–591.
44. Oechslin EN, Harrison DA, Connelly MS, et al. Mode of death in adults with congenital heart disease. *Am J Cardiol.* 2000;86(11):1111–1116.
45. Perloff JK, Marelli AJ, Miner PD. Risk of stroke in adults with cyanotic congenital heart disease. *Circulation.* 1993;87(6):1954–1959.
46. Ammash N, Warnes CA. Cerebrovascular events in adult patients with cyanotic congenital heart disease. *J Am Coll Cardiol.* 1996;28(3):768–772.
47. Di Tullio M, Sacco RL, Gopal A, et al. Patent foramen ovale as a risk factor for cryptogenic stroke. *Ann Intern Med.* 1992;117(3):461–465.
48. Homma S, Sacco RL, Di Tullio MR, et al. Effect of medical treatment in stroke patients with patent foramen ovale: Patent foramen ovale in Cryptogenic Stroke Study. *Circulation.* 2002;105(24):2625–2631.
49. Mas JL, Arquizan C, Lamy C, et al. Recurrent cerebrovascular events associated with patent foramen ovale, atrial septal aneurysm, or both. *N Engl J Med.* 2001;345(24):1740–1746.
50. Stone DA, Godard J, Corretti MC, et al. Patent foramen ovale: Association between the degree of shunt by contrast transesophageal echocardiography and the risk of future ischemic neurologic events. *Am Heart J.* 1996;131(2):158–161.
51. Windecker S, Wahl A, Nedeltchev K, et al. Comparison of medical treatment with percutaneous closure of patent foramen ovale in patients with cryptogenic stroke. *J Am Coll Cardiol.* 2004;44(4):750–758.
52. Perloff JK, Child JS. *Congenital Heart Disease in Adults.* Philadelphia: WB Saunders; 1997.
53. Rosove MH, Perloff JK, Hocking WG, et al. Chronic hypoxaemia and decompensated erythrocytosis in cyanotic congenital heart disease. *Lancet.* 1986;I313–I316.

54. Broberg CS, Bax BE, Okonko DO, et al. Blood viscosity and its relationship to iron deficiency, symptoms, and exercise capacity in adults with cyanotic congenital heart disease. *J Am Coll Cardiol.* 2006;48(2):356–365.
55. Addour LM. Infective endocarditis: Diagnosis, antimicrobial therapy, and management of complications: A statement for healthcare professionals from the Committee on Rheumatic Fever, Endocarditis, and Kawasaki Disease, Council on Cardiovascular Disease in the Young, and the Councils on Clinical Cardiology, Stroke, and Cardiovascular Surgery and Anesthesia, American Heart Association. *Circulation.* 2005;111(23):3167–3184.
56. Gluck R, Hall JW, Stevenson LD. Brain abscess associated with congenital heart disease. *Pediatrics.* 1952;9(2):192–203.
57. Cohen M, Fuster V, Steele PM, et al. Coarctation of the aorta: Long-term follow-up and prediction of outcome after surgical correction. *Circulation.* 1989;80(8):840–845.
58. Atkinson JL, Sundt TM, Houser OW, et al. Angiographic frequency of anterior circulation intracranial aneurysms. *J Neurosurg.* 1989;70(6):551–555.
59. Connolly HM, Huston J, Brown RD, Jr., et al. Intracranial aneurysms in patients with coarctation of the aorta: A prospective magnetic resonance angiographic study of 100 patients. *Mayo Clin Proc.* 2003;78(12):1491–1499.
60. Fukuda H, Sako K, Yonemasu Y. Coarctation of the descending aorta with aneurysm of the anterior communicating artery. *Surg Neurol.* 1985;23(3):380–382.
61. Petty GW, Khandheria BK, Meissner I, et al. Population-based study of the relationship between patent foramen ovale and cerebrovascular ischemic events. *Mayo Clin Proc.* 2006;81(5):602–608.
62. Windecker S, Wahl A, Nedeltchev K, et al. Comparison of medical treatment with percutaneous closure of patent foramen ovale in patients with cryptogenic stroke. *J Am Coll Cardiol.* 2004;44(4):750–758.
63. Blackshear JL. Closure of patent foramen ovale in cryptogenic stroke. *J Am Coll Cardiol.* 2004;44(4):759–761.
64. Homma S, Sacco RL, Di Tullio MR, et al. Effect of medical treatment in stroke patients with patent foramen ovale. Patent Foramen Ovale in Cryptogenic Stroke Study. *Circulation.* 2002;105(11):2625–2631.
65. Hong TE, Thaler D, Brorson J, et al. Transcatheter closure of patent foramen ovale associated with paradoxical embolism using the Amplatzer PFO occluder: Initial and intermediate-term results of the U.S. multicenter clinical trial. *Catheter Cardiovasc Interv.* 2003;60(5): 524–528.

CHAPTER 3

Acquired Valvular Heart Disease

Fred Leya

OBJECTIVES

- To review the pathophysiology of acquired valvular heart disease
- To discuss the hemodynamic principles governing acquired valvular heart disease
- To review the auscultatory findings of acquired valvular heart disease
- To describe the diagnostic approach, prophylaxis, risk stratification, and management of cases of acquired valvular heart disease

CASE VIGNETTE

A 19-year-old Mexican man recently immigrated to the United States where he joined the US Army. He was sent for 6 months of basic military training. Because he had excellent hand–eye coordination, his superiors selected him to become a sharpshooter. At the end of his basic military training, he and three of his friends developed a sore throat secondary to pharyngitis. His pharyngitis subsided in 3 days. Three weeks later, he developed bilateral elbow and knee pain and stiffness that resolved within 1 week. He recalls having frequent sore throats while growing up in rural Mexico.

After successfully completing his basic military training, he was sent to the Middle East for a military tour of duty, where he soon found himself in the midst of the chaos of war. He was seriously wounded, but promptly recovered. Three months later, he became emotionally labile, and lost all his sharp-shooting and superior hand–eye coordination skills. His speech became more "explosive" and halting, and his handwriting became nearly illegible, prompting his superior officer to arrange for psychiatric counseling to evaluate for a possible "posttraumatic stress syndrome."

DEFINITION

The most common forms of acquired valvular heart disease include mitral valve stenosis (MVS), mitral valve regurgitation (MVR), aortic valve stenosis (AVS), and aortic valve insufficiency (AVI).

EPIDEMIOLOGY

The predominant cause of MVS is rheumatic fever (RF). Approximately 25% of all patients with rheumatic heart disease (RHD) have pure MVS; 40% have combined MVS and MVR and 60% of patients with RF are women.

Anatomic changes of rheumatic mitral stenosis (RMS) result from a smoldering inflammatory process and constant trauma produced by turbulent transvalvular blood flow, leading to progressive valve fibrosis, scarring, and calcification.

PATHOPHYSIOLOGY

The normal cross-sectional area of the mitral valve orifice of 4 to 6 cm^2 allows the flow of blood from the left atrium (LA) through the normal MV into the left ventricle (LV), without any resistance or pressure gradient. When the MV orifice is mildly reduced to approximately 2 cm^2 or half of the normal size, blood no longer flows freely across the MV, but instead needs to be forcefully propelled by the atrium, creating a small, but abnormal pressure gradient between the LA and the LV during diastole (Fig. 3-1).

When the MV opening becomes critically narrowed and the MV orifice is reduced to 1 cm^2 or, one fourth the normal size, a substantial, approximately 20 mm Hg pressure gradient develop between the LA and the LV during diastole to propel blood from the LA into the LV to maintain a normal cardiac output. This gradient elevates the mean LA pressure, backing up blood within the lungs, and triggering lung congestion. Lung congestion, in turn, raises the pulmonary venous and capillary pressures causing exertional dyspnea, usually made worse by tachycardia.

To assess the severity of obstruction of a given heart valve, the transvalvular pressure gradients and blood flow must be measured. The transvalvular blood flow is a function of cardiac output and heart rate. An increase in heart rate shortens mostly diastole, thereby shortening the predominantly diastolic time available for blood to flow across the MV.

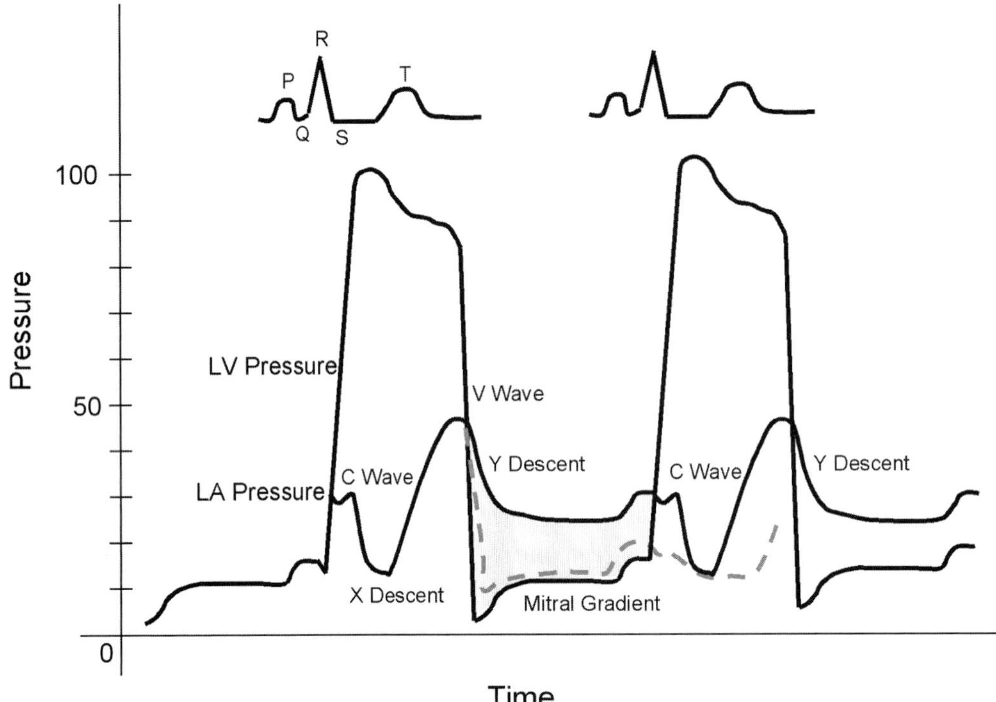

FIGURE 3-1. Demonstrates greatly elevated LA pressure, and a large LA-LV transmitral pressure gradient during LV diastole (*solid line*). The *dashed line* depicts a normal LA pressure, and no LA-LV pressure gradient during diastole. LA, left atrium; LV, left ventricle.

The MV area (MVA) is calculated using the Gorlin formula as follows:

$$\text{MVA} = \frac{\text{Cardiac Output}}{37.7\ (\text{DFP})\ (\text{HR})\ \sqrt{\text{Mean Gradient}}}$$

MVA = Mitral Valve Area
CO = Cardiac Output
DFP = Diastolic Filling Period
HR = Heart Rate

Hydraulic considerations of the Gorlin formula indicate that at any given orifice size (MVA), the transvalvular pressure gradient is a function of the square of the transvalvular flow rate. Thus, doubling the flow rate, quadruples the pressure gradient.

CLINICAL MANIFESTATION

HISTORY

Exertional dyspnea, cough, wheezing, orthopnea, and hemoptysis are primary symptoms of rheumatic MS. Chest pain may be a presenting symptom when advanced MS causes severe pulmonary and right ventricular hypertension.

Systemic embolization is a common sequel of rheumatic mitral valvular heart disease (RMVHD). Before the anticoagulant era, approximately 25% of all RMVHD fatalities were caused by systemic embolism. The risk of systemic embolism directly correlates with a patient's age and LA appendage size, and inversely with the cardiac output. No correlation exists between risk of systemic embolism and severity of MS. Embolism may be the first presenting symptom of mild, or even nearly asymptomatic MS. Approximately half of all clinically apparent emboli travel to the brain. Emboli are often recurrent and multiple. Infective endocarditis, a rare but serious complication of RHD, is mostly encountered in patients with mild MS rather than among those with severe MS. Hoarseness results from compression of the left recurrent laryngeal nerve (Ortner syndrome) by a distended LA, enlarged tracheobronchial lymph nodes, or a dilated pulmonary artery.

PHYSICAL EXAMINATION

Patients with severe MS have a low cardiac output, significant systemic vasoconstriction, and often exhibit a *mitral facies* characterized by pinkish-purple patches of both cheeks. Classic auscultatory signs include an opening snap, a long diastolic rumble, and a loud (P_2) pulmonic component of the second heart sound (Fig. 3-2).

DIAGNOSTIC APPROACH

Electrocardiography in cases of moderate to severe MS demonstrate LA enlargement with P-wave duration in lead II ≥0.12 second and P-wave axis +45° to 30° in 90% of patients. Atrial fibrillation relates to LA size, extent of LA wall fibrosis, patient's age, and duration of RHD.

Echocardiography demonstrates a thickened, calcified, stenotic valve with poor leaflet separation in diastole. The chordae tendineae are frequently scarred and fused. The LA is usually enlarged, and the LA appendage may contain thrombi. The MV annulus is usually calcified. Doppler echocardiography

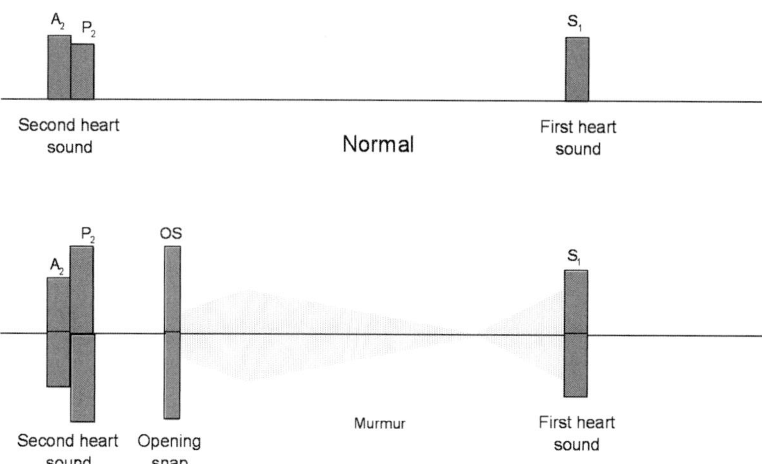

FIGURE 3-2. Demonstrates auscultatory findings of mitral stenosis (MS) as compared with normal. Note the accentuated P_2 opening snap of the mitral valve (MV) and a soft diastolic rumble.

provides accurate and noninvasive measurement of the severity of MS, MR, and pulmonary artery (PA) pressure.

TREATMENT

Patients with RMVHD require penicillin prophylaxis for β-hemolytic streptococcal infections and endocarditis prophylaxis. Patients who are symptomatic benefit from oral diuretics and digitalis when atrial fibrillation is present. Beta-blocking agents and rate-slowing calcium antagonists may increase exercise capacity by reducing the heart rate among patients with normal sinus rhythm, and especially for those with atrial fibrillation.

Warfarin anticoagulation (international normalized ratio [INR] between 2.0 to 3.0) is helpful in preventing venous thrombosis in patients at high risk for systemic embolization, such as those ≥70 years of age with atrial fibrillation, and those with prior systemic emoblization. Percutaneous balloon mitral valvuloplasty (BMV) or surgical commisurotomy should be offered to patients who are symptomatic with moderate to severe MS, MVA ≤1.5 cm^2 in normal-sized adults (Fig. 3-3). It is also indicated in cases of mild MS, MVA ≥1.5 cm^2 for symptomatic patients during ordinary activity who develop PA-systolic blood pressure (BP) ≥60 mm Hg or a mean pulmonary capillary wedge pressure (PCWP) ≥25 mm Hg during exercise.

Mitral Regurgitation

The MV apparatus consists of mitral leaflets per se, chordae tendineae, papillary muscles, and mitral annulus. Abnormali-

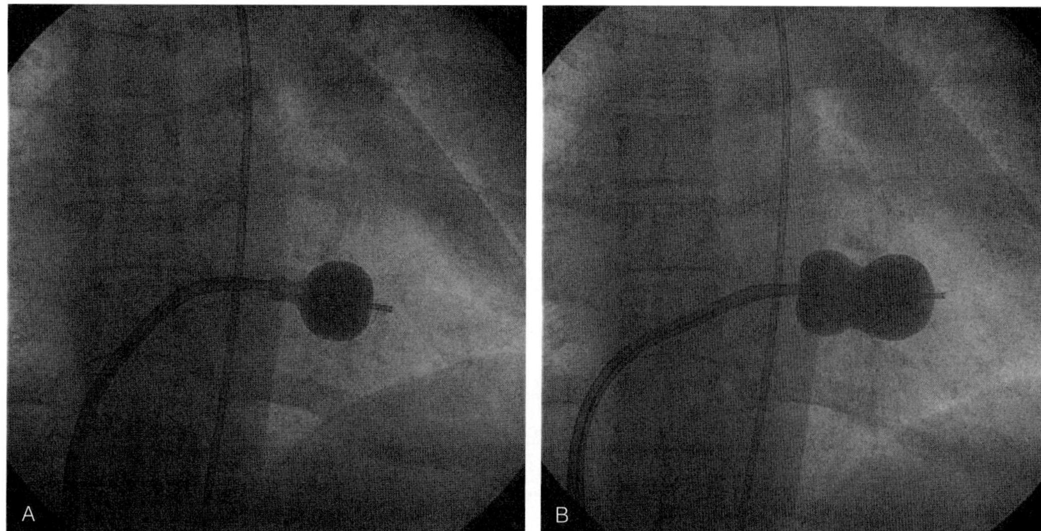

FIGURE 3-3. (**A**) Demonstrates percutaneous balloon mitral valvuloplasty (BMV) using Inoue balloon, partially inflated inside the left ventricle (LV). (**B**) Shows completely inflated balloon across the MV. Note calcification of the MV annulus seen in the middle waist of the balloon.

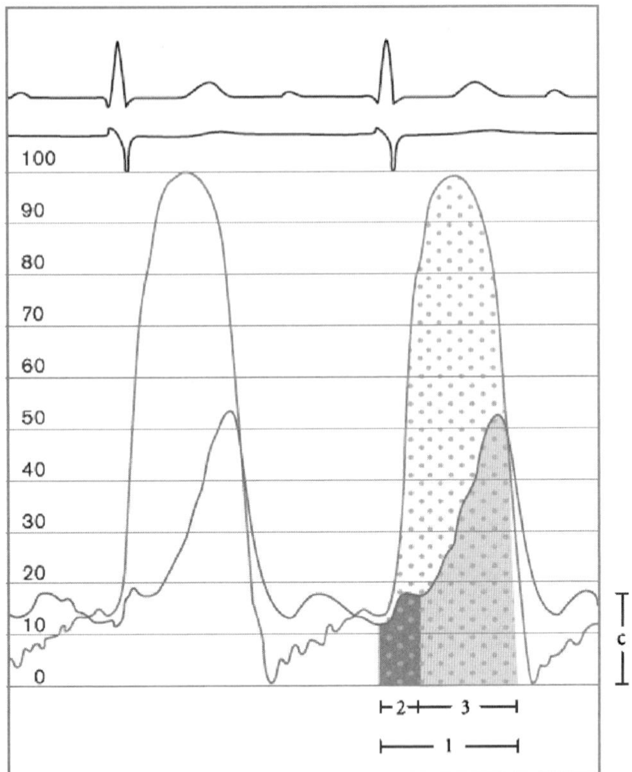

FIGURE 3-4. Simultaneous left atrium (LA) and left ventricle (LV) pressure recordings. *Dotted area* represents area under the curve of LV systole. Dark gray shading represents area under the curve of the C-wave. Light gray shading represents area under the curve of the V-wave. Dark gray and light gray shaded area represent total LA area during LV systole. **1.** Duration of LV systole. **2.** Time to onset of the V-wave from the beginning or LV systole. **3.** Duration of the V-wave during LV systole c, height of C-wave; V, height of V-wave.

ties in any of these components can result in MV leaking. Major causes of acquired MVR include mitral valve prolapse (MVP), RHD, infective endocarditis, mitral annular calcification (MAC), cardiomyopathy, and ischemic heart disease. MVP is the most important cause of significant MR in the United States.

HEMODYNAMICS

Effective or forward cardiac output is markedly depressed among highly symptomatic patients with severe MR, whereas total LV output, the sum of forward and regurgitant flow, remains elevated until late into the natural course of the disease.

In healthy conditions, the area under the LV pressure-time curve (LVa) during LV systole represents the total amount of potential force generated by the LV. In MR, the LV loses its potential energy (force) backward to the LA, because the MV is no longer competent. Because during LV systole, the LA is in diastole, the regurgitant blood flow escaping from the LV into the LA should be considered as lost forward cardiac output or LV flow, because this regurgitant portion of the total LV cardiac output does not contribute to the forward cardiac output.

With increasing severity of MR, the area under the LA pressure-time curve (LAa) increases, while the area under the LV pressure-time curve (LVa) declines. Thus, forward or useful LV force gradually declines with increasing duration and increasing severity of MR. During this process, onset of V wave occurs earlier in systole, encroaching upon the X-descent until it obliterates it nearly completely (1) (Figs. 3-4, 3-5).

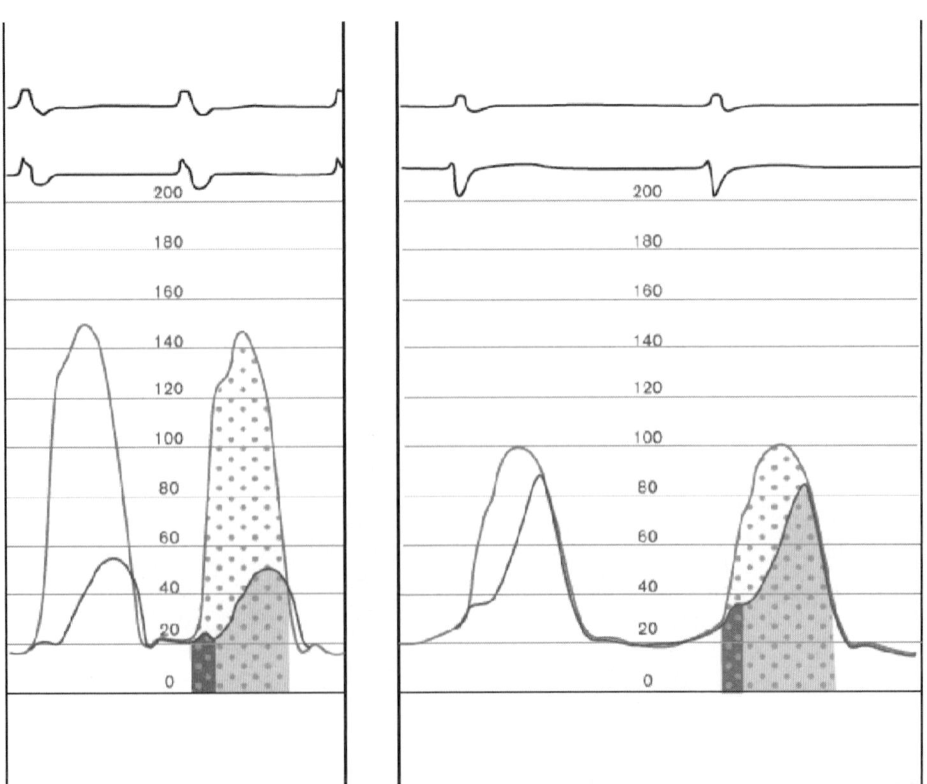

FIGURE 3-5. Simultaneous left atrium (LA) and left ventricle (LV) pressure recordings in the same patient from 2002 (**left**) and 2006 (**right**). In 2002, this patient had 2+ mitral regurgitation (MR) according to the Sellers classification, whereas he had 4+ MR in 2006. Notice that as the severity of MR increased with time, the area under the LA pressure curve increased at the expense of a proportional decrease of the LV pressure–time area, reflecting a significant loss of LV forward blood pumping ability or loss of useful LV work.

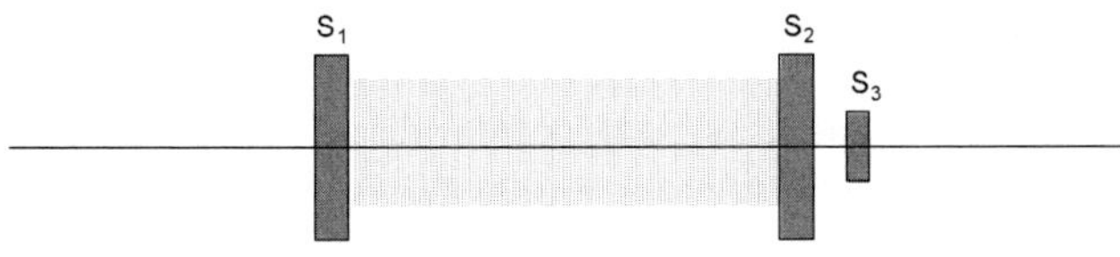

FIGURE 3-6. S_1, first heart sound. S_2, second heart sound. S_3, third heart sound.

CLINICAL MANIFESTATIONS

The nature and severity of symptoms in patients with chronic MVR reflect a function of multiple interrelated factors, including severity of MR, level of LA, PCWP, and PA pressures, as well as presence of atrial fibrillation or other associated cardiac diseases. Most patients with MR have only mild clinical disability. The indolent course of MR can be deceptive, however, and by the time symptoms of reduced cardiac output and/or pulmonary congestion become apparent, serious, and sometimes irreversible, LV dysfunction may have already taken place.

Depressed cardiac output symptoms, such as fatigue or exhaustion, symptoms of pulmonary hypertension, and right ventricular failure with congestive hepatomegaly, leg edema, and ascites, are common in patients with moderate to severe MR.

PHYSICAL EXAMINATION

During auscultation of chronic MVR , the first heart sound (S_1) is usually diminished, the systolic murmur commences immediately after S_1, and continues beyond the aortic component (A_2) of the second heart sound (S_2). The holosystolic murmur of chronic MR is usually constant and blowing, loudest at the apex, and radiating to the axilla (Fig. 3-6).

Mitral Valve Prolapse

Mitral valve prolapse, billowing mitral cusp syndrome, or floppy MV syndrome, is one of the most prevalent cardiac valvular abnormalities occurring in 2% to 3% of the population. MVP syndrome is twice as frequent in women as in men. MVR occurs when the MV leaflet edges fail to coapt. In MVP, the murmur of MR differs substantially from the murmur of chronic MR. The MVP murmur usually has a mid to late systolic click and a mid to late systolic murmur of "whoop" (Fig. 3-7).

DIAGNOSTIC APPROACH

Echocardiography remains the best qualitative and quantitative tool to estimate the severity of MR. Quantitative methods to measure the regurgitant fraction, volume, and the orifice area, have great accuracy in comparison with angiography.

MANAGEMENT

The role of vasodilators for chronic MVR remain controversial. Afterload in most patients with chronic MR is not excessive.

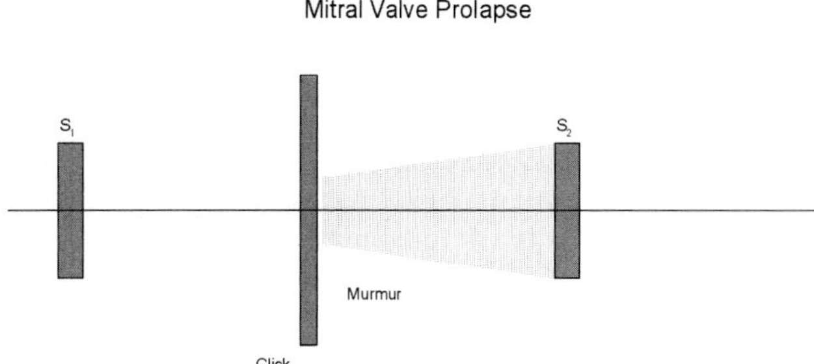

FIGURE 3-7. Mid systolic click. S_1, first heart sound. S_2, second heart sound.

The LV systolic shortening during MR is already facilitated by a reduced systolic LV wall stress because emptying of the LV is already easier into the low pressure LA. Therefore, systemic vasodilator therapy to reduce the afterload further may not be beneficial. All patients with MR require prophylactic antibiotics to prevent endocarditis. All patients with atrial fibrillation should receive warfarin therapy aiming for an INR value of 2.0 to 3.0. Surgical treatment is considered for symptomatic patients, or for asymptomatic patients with evidence of LV dysfunction as documented by noninvasive studies.

Acquired Aortic Stenosis

DEFINITIONS

Rheumatic AS results from adhesion and fusion of the commisures of the aortic cusps, and vascularization of the leaflets leading to retraction, scarring, and stiffening of the edges of the cusps with time. Calcific nodules appear on both the aortic and ventricular valve surfaces. Gradually, the valve orifice is reduced to a small opening that is both stenotic and regurgitant. Degenerative AS represents an age-related "wear and tear" process of the aortic valve, with proliferative inflammation leading to AS.

EPIDEMIOLOGY

Degenerative or age-related senile calcific AS is the most common cause of AVS in adults. Of people above 65 years of age, 2% have calcific AS, and 30% have aortic valve sclerosis without stenosis.

PATHOPHYSIOLOGY

Degenerative processes affecting the aortic valve represent proliferative and inflammatory changes, with lipid accumulation, infiltration of macrophages and T-lymphocytes, ultimately leading to bone formation (2–4), similar to the process of calcific atherosclerosis.

Progressive calcification leads to immobilization of the aortic cusps with resulting AS, and only rarely to aortic regurgitation (AR). Frequently, degenerative AS shares common cardiovascular risk factors with MAC and with vascular calcific atherosclerosis. Not infrequently, these three processes coexist clinically. Commonly shared cardiovascular risks include elevated low-density lipoprotein (LDL) and Lp(a), diabetes mellitus, cigarette smoking, and arterial hypertension. Degenerative calcific AS shares many pathologic features with atherosclerosis. As an example, children with homozygous type II hyperlipidemia have calcific AS. Calcific AS is also observed in Paget disease of bone, end-stage renal disease, and alkaptonuria (5,6).

HEMODYNAMICS

The aortic valve area is calculated using the simplified Gorlin formula:

$$\text{AVR} = \frac{\text{Cardiac Output}}{\sqrt{\text{Mean Gradient}}}$$

Because the square root of the gradient used in the Gorlin formula, the aortic valve area calculation is predominantly influenced by the cardiac output rather than by the pressure gradient. Especially in low cardiac output states (i.e., LV ejection fraction [EF] $\leq$20%), the Gorlin formula may significantly underestimate the actual aortic valve area. Calculating aortic valve resistance using Ohm's law instead, may be helpful in distinguishing severe from mild AS in patients with borderline aortic stenosis (aortic valve area [AVA] 0.8 to 1 cm^2) (7–9).

$$\text{Aortic Valve Resistance} = \frac{\text{Mean Gradient}}{\text{Flow}}$$

Normal AVA measures	3.0 to 4.0 cm^2
Mild aortic stenosis has orifice area of	1.5 to 2.0 cm^2
Moderate aortic stenosis has orifice area	1.0 to 1.5 cm^2

Critical AS has an orifice area 0.8 cm^2 or less than one fourth of the normal aortic orifice with a peak systolic pressure frequently exceeding 50 mm Hg.

CLINICAL MANIFESTATIONS

Patients with severe AS tend to be asymptomatic until relatively late in the natural course of their disease. AS is a progressive and insidious disease, however, with the AVA decreasing gradually by 0.2 to 0.3 cm annually. Echo Doppler studies show that the aortic jet velocity gradually increases by 0.3 m/sec/year, and the mean transvalvular gradient increases by 7 mm Hg annually. Most patients with peak echo Doppler aortic valve velocity >4 m/sec become symptomatic within 3 to 4 years (10,11).

Cardinal signs of severe AS include

1. *Angina pectoris* occurs in 60% of patients with severe AS; about half of them also have associated significant coronary artery disease (CAD). Angina is usually the harbinger of progressive clinical symptoms, with an expected overall survival of 3 to 5 years from onset of angina.
2. *Syncope* is most commonly caused by reduced cerebral perfusion, when the arterial blood pressure declines with exertion, secondary to vasodilatation in the context of a limited and fixed cardiac output. Exertional syncope has been attributed to baroreceptor malfunction in cases of severe AS, as well as to a vasodepressor response to a greatly increased LV systolic pressure during exercise. Presyncopal symptoms are common, described as *graying out* spells or dizziness on effort, are common. Syncope at rest can be caused by atrial fibrillation, ventricular tachycardia, other ventricular arrhythmias, or heart block, owing to extension of the aortic valve calcification into the cardiac conduction system. Syncope is usually the second cardinal manifestation of AS, predicting 2 to 3 years of expected survival.
3. *Congestive heart failure (CHF)* reflects varying degrees of pulmonary hypertension. CHF is relatively late in the course of AS, with an expected survival of <2 years. Clinical manifestations of a low cardiac output state are usually not prominent until late in the course of AS (12,13).

Asymptomatic patients often have excellent prognosis. Death, even sudden death, usually occurs among symptomatic patients. Once clinical symptoms develop, mortality risk with severe AS accelerates exponentially, and prognosis becomes poor, unless the aortic valve obstruction is relieved.

Gastrointestinal bleeding can also develop with severe AS, often caused by an associated angiodysplasia of the right colon. The angiodysplasia, and other AS-induced vascular malformations, correlate with the severity of AS, and are correctable by aortic valve replacement (AVR) (14,15).

Infective endocarditis mostly affects younger patients with a milder degree of aortic valvular deformity, rather than older patients, with "rock-like" calcific aortic deformities. Cerebral emboli can result in stroke or transient ischemic attacks (TIA). Embolism of calcified debris to the brain or other organs is mostly a feature of degenerative and calcified AS (12).

PHYSICAL EXAMINATION

The arterial pulse in patient with advanced AS rises slowly, and is weak and sustained (pulsus parvus et tardus). The anacrotic notch and coarse systolic vibration is felt readily in both carotid arteries as a carotid shudder. On auscultation, the S_1 is normal, the S_4 is usually prominent, and the S_2 might be single as the A_2 might be inaudible. An aortic ejection sound is rarely heard in adults with calcific AS. The systolic murmur of AS is usually late peaking, and radiates to both carotid arteries (Figs. 3-8, 3-9).

LABORATORY EXAMINATION

Electrocardiogram (ECG): The main ECG change in AS is LV hypertrophy (LVH), found in 85% of patients with severe AS. T-wave inversion and ST-segment depression in leads with upright QRS complexes are common. ST-segment depression >0.2 mV indicates LV strain, and suggest the presence of severe AS.

ECHOCARDIOGRAPHY

The normal echocardiographic opening of the aortic valve is 1.6 cm to 2.6 cm. Three-dimensional echocardiography holds promise for assessing aortic valve structure and mobility of leaflets and for quantifying the severity of AS. Using a modified Bernoulli equation:

$$P = 4V^2$$

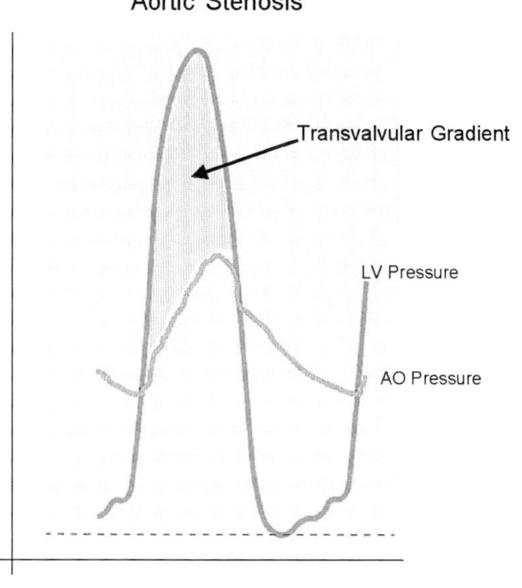

FIGURE 3-8. Demonstrates simultaneous blood pressure recordings obtained in the left ventricle (LV pressure) and in the ascending aorta (AO pressure) in a patient with severe aortic stenosis. Notice a transvalvular pressure gradient, a significant difference exists between the high pressure in the LV and lower pressure in the aorta.

Doppler echocardiography can also calculate the LV-Ao pressure gradient from the systolic aortic valve blood velocity signal. These gradients correlate well with those obtained in the cardiac catheterization laboratory. Also, color flow Doppler is helpful in detecting AR that often coexists in nearly 75% of patients with calcific AS.

MANAGEMENT

Patients with known severe AS who are asymptomatic, have a 1% to 2% annual risk of death. These patients should be advised to report promptly if they develop any symptoms attributable to AS. Patients with mild AS do not have to limit their physical activity significantly. Patients with severe AS, however, should be cautioned to avoid rigorous physical activity. Patients with AS require endocarditis prophylaxis. Exercise testing may be helpful in apparently asymptomatic patients to detect covert symptoms, limited exercise capacity, and abnormal blood pressure responses (11,16,17). Exercise stress testing is contraindicated in patients with AS symptoms. Symptomatic patients with severe AS should have surgery, because medical therapy has little to offer under these circumstances.

Aortic Regurgitation

DEFINITION

Aortic regurgitation can be caused by primary disease of the aortic valve leaflets or the wall of the aortic root.

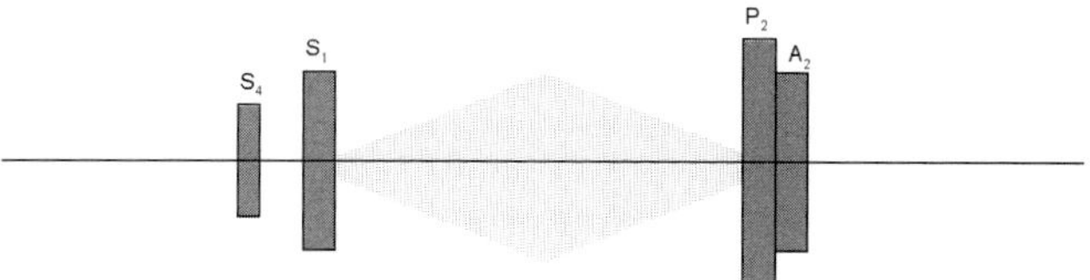

FIGURE 3-9. S_1, first heart sound. S_2, second heart sound. P_2, pulmonary component. A_2, aortic component. S_4, fourth heart sound.

EPIDEMIOLOGY

Common causes of AR include RF, calcific AS, infective endocarditis, trauma, bicuspid aortic valve, and myxomatous proliferation of the aortic valve. Less common causes of AR include congenital aortic valve defects, connective tissue disorders, systemic lupus erythematosus (SLE), ankylosing spondylitis, Takayasu disease, and Whipple disease. Other conditions responsible for aortic root disease include age-related degenerative aortic dilatation, cystic medial necrosis, Marfan syndrome, and systemic arterial hypertension. When the ascending aorta becomes greatly dilated, the aortic leaflets separate, and AR may ensue. Regardless of cause, AR produces LV dilatation and LV hypertrophy (18).

CLINICAL MANIFESTATIONS

In patients with chronic, severe AR, the LV gradually enlarges while patients remain asymptomatic. Exertional dyspnea, orthopnea, and paroxysmal nocturnal dyspnea usually appear late and only after considerable cardiomyopathy and myocardial dysfunction have occurred.

PHYSICAL EXAMINATION

Patients with severe chronic AR have the following clinical signs:

- De Musset sign: Head bobbing prominent with each heartbeat
- Water-Hammer pulse or collapsing type with abrupt distention and quick collapse (Corrigan pulse)
- Traube sign: A pistol shot sound auscultated over the femoral artery
- Duroziez sign: Systolic murmur auscultated over the femoral artery when compressed proximally, and a diastolic murmur over the femoral artery when compressed distally
- Quincke sign: Capillary pulsations

In cases of significant chronic AR, the systolic blood pressure is elevated, and the diastolic blood pressure is very low.

AUSCULTATION

An AR murmur is a high frequency murmur that begins after A_2. A mild AR murmur is heard in early diastole. Severe AR is associated with a characteristic holodiastolic murmur. When the murmur is musical, "cooing dove," it often implies that a perforation of the aortic cusp took place. The Austin-Flint mur-

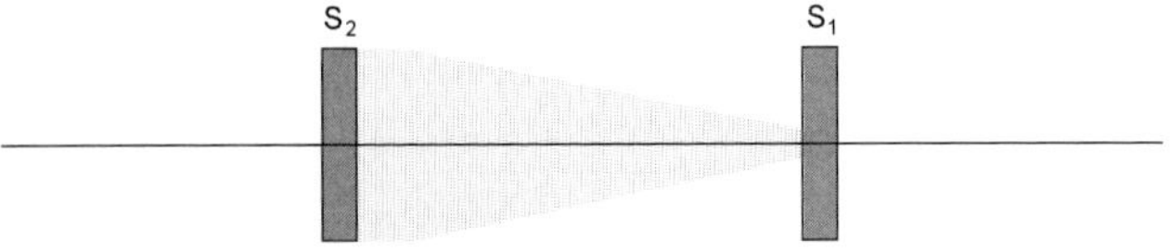

FIGURE 3-10. S_2, second heart sound. S_1, first heart sound.

mur is a mid to late diastolic apical rumble when severe AR is present (Fig. 3-10).

LABORATORY EXAMINATION

Doppler echocardiography and color flow Doppler imaging are the most sensitive and accurate techniques in diagnosing and evaluating AR.

MANAGEMENT

All patients with AR should receive endocarditis prophylaxis. Asymptomatic patients with mild to moderate AR with normal or near normal LV require no treatment, and no restriction of their physical activity. Asymptomatic patients with chronic severe AR who have good exercise tolerance, and have an EF ≥50% without severe LV dilatation, a left ventricular end systolic dimension (LVESD) ≤70 mm, and an LVESD ≤50 mm, do not require surgery. Surgical treatment is advisable for symptomatic patients with severe AR, and for asymptomatic patients with an EF ≤50%, LVESD ≥70 mm Hg, and LVESD ≥50 mm. All symptomatic patients, besides having AVR, require appropriate management of heart failure (19,20).

CLINICAL RECOMMENDATIONS OF THE VIGNETTE

The patient was a military recruit living in crowded conditions. He grew up in rural Mexico, having frequent sore throats probably related to streptococcal pharyngitis. A causal relationship exists between RF and group A streptococcus pharyngitis. The prevalence of RF, especially in developing countries, is high, approaching 100 per 100,000, in contrast to 2 per 100,000 in the United States. The acute phase of RF is characterized by proliferative inflammation involving connective or collagen tissues, affecting primarily the heart, joints, brain, and skin.

Major clinical manifestations of RF include carditis, polyarthritis, chorea, erythema marginatum, and subcutaneous nodules. The patient presented with clinical manifestations consistent with Sydenham chorea. Sydenham chorea (rheumatic chorea, chorea minor, St. Vitus dance, or St. Johannes chorea) is related to group A-beta hemolytic streptococcal infections, and often occurs in childhood and adolescence. Sydenham chorea is predominantly or exclusively unilateral (hemichorea) in approximately half of the cases. Sydenham chorea is reported in approximately 20% of patients with RF and is thought to result from molecular mimicry, with streptococcus-induced antibodies targeting basal ganglia neurons (21). The rheumatic inflammatory process specifically involves the basal ganglia and caudate nuclei. Chorea usually develops a few months after onset of a precipitating streptococcal infection.

Sydenham chorea is characterized by chorea, hypotonia, and emotional lability. Chorea is clinically characterized by sudden, brief involuntary, purposeless, and unpredictable movements. Clinical manifestations are more evident under stress. Distal appendicular involvement is predominant with Sydenham chorea. Speech can also be affected, becoming explosive and halting. The handwriting deteriorates and patients often become uncoordinated and frustrated. Sydenham chorea is a delayed manifestation of RF and, as such, it may be the only manifestation of RF.

Patients with group A streptococcus pharyngitis are also at higher risk of PANDAS (pediatric autoimmune neuropsychiatric disorder associated with group A streptococci), and characterized by obsessive compulsive disorder, choreiform movements, tics, and other neuropsychiatric manifestations (22).

SUMMARY

Acquired valvular heart diseases in the aging population play an increasingly important pathophysiologic role in neurologic disorders. Nearly 85% of all strokes are ischemic in nature. Many ischemic strokes are brought about by cardiac emboli. These emboli usually originate either from diseased cardiac valves or from intracavitary thrombi. Occasionally, syncope, dizziness, and TIA might be the first sign of severe valvular heart disease. Therefore, the diagnostic workup of patients with any serious valvular heart disease must incorporate also a careful neurologic evaluation of the patient.

REFERENCES

1. Freihage JH, Joyal D, Leya, F, et al. Invasive assessment of mitral regurgitation: Comparison of hemodynamic parameters. *Catheter Cardiovasc Interv.* In press.
2. Rajamannan NM, Gersh B, Bonow RO. Calcific aortic stenosis: From bench to bedside—Emerging clinical and cellular concepts. *Heart.* 2003;89:801–805.
3. Mohler ER, Gannon F, Reynolds C, et al. Bone formation and inflammation in cardiac valves. *Circulation.* 2001;103:1522–1528.
4. Rajamannan NM, Subramaniam M, Richard D, et al. Human aortic valve calcification is associated with an osteoblast phenotype. *Circulation.* 2003;107:2181–2184.
5. Peltier M, Trojette F, Enriquez-Sarano M, et al. Relation between cardiovascular risk factors and nonrheumatic severe calcific aortic stenosis among patients with a three cuspid aortic valve. *Am J Cardiol.* 2003;91:97–99.
6. Novaro GM, Iong IY, Pearce GL, et al. Effect of hydoxymethylglutaryl coenzyme A reductase inhibitors on the progression of calcific aortic stenosis. *Circulation.* 2001;104:2205–2209.
7. Connolly HM, Oh JK, Schaff HV, et al. Severe aortic stenosis with low transvalvular gradient and severe left ventricular dysfunction: Result of aortic valve replacement in 52 patients. *Circulation.* 2000;101:1940–1946.
8. Rahimtoola SH. Severe aortic stenosis with low systolic gradient: The good and bad news. *Circulation.* 2000;101:1892–1894.
9. Pereira JJ, Lauer MS, Bashir M, et al. Survival after aortic valve replacement for severe aortic stenosis with low transvalvular gradients and severe left ventricular dysfunction. *J Am Coll Cardiol.* 2002;39:1356–1363.
10. Carabello BA Evaluation and management of patients with aortic stenosis. *Circulation* 2002;105:1746–1750.
11. Otto CM, Burwarsh IG, Legget ME, et al. A prospective study of asymptomatic valvular aortic stenosis: Clinical, echocardiographic, and exercise predictors of outcome. *Circulation.* 1997;95:2262–2270.
12. Levinson GE, Alpert JS. Aortic stenosis. In: Alpert JS, Dalen JE, Rahimtoola SH, eds. *Valvular Heart Disease,* 3rd ed. Philadelphia: Lippincott Williams & Wilkins; 2000:183–211.
13. Carabello BA. Aortic stenosis. *N Engl J Med.* 2002;346:677–682.
14. Pareti FI, Lattuada A, Bressi C, et al. Proteolysis of von Willebrand factor and shear stress-induced platelet aggregation in patients with aortic stenosis. *Circulation.* 2000;102:1290–1295.

15. Vincentelli A, Susen S, Le Tourneau T, et al. Acquired von Willebrand syndrome in aortic stenosis. *N Engl J Med.* 2003;343–349.
16. Rosenhek R, Porenta G, Lang I, et al. Predictors of outcome in severe, asymptomatic aortic stenosis. *N Engl J Med.* 2000;343:611–617.
17. Amato MCM, Moffa PJ, Ramires JAF. Treatment decision in asymptomatic aortic valve stenosis: Role of exercise testing. *Heart.* 2001;86:381–386.
18. Rahimtoola SH. Aortic regurgitation. In: Rahimtoola SH, ed. *Valvular Heart Disease. Atlas of Heart Diseases.* Vol. 11. Philadelphia: Current Medicine; 1997:7–9.
19. Borer JS. Aortic valve replacement for the asymptomatic patient with aortic regurgitation: A new piece of the strategic puzzle. *Circulation.* 2002;106:2637–2639.
20. Tornos MO, Olona M, Permanyer-Miralda G, et al. Heart failure after aortic valve replacement for aortic regurgitation: Prospective 20-year study. *Am Heart J.* 1998;136:681–687.
21. Ryan M, Anthony JH, Grattan-Smith PJ. Sydenham's chorea: A resurgence of the 1990's. *J Pediatr Child Health.* 2000;36:95–96.
22. Swedo SE. Pediatric autoimmune neuropsychiatric disorders associated with streptococcal infections (PANDAS). *Mol Psychiatry.* 2002;7[Suppl l2]:S24–S25.

CHAPTER 4

Infective Endocarditis

Minerva A. Galang • J. Paul O'Keefe

OBJECTIVES

- To review the epidemiology and pathogenesis of infective endocarditis
- To identify microorganisms commonly involved in infective endocarditis
- To recognize the clinical manifestations and complications of infective endocarditis
- To be familiar with the diagnostic approach in patients with infective endocarditis
- To review treatment options and patient management in patients with infective endocarditis

CASE VIGNETTE

A previously healthy 34-year-old man was brought to the emergency room because of unresponsiveness. He had been complaining of generalized malaise, fatigue, and fevers for the past 3 to 4 weeks and had lost 10 pounds. He was seen in the clinic 2 weeks before admission and viral illness was the diagnosis. A few hours before being admitted, he was noted to have slurred speech and right-sided weakness. On examination, he barely grimaced on painful stimuli. Temperature was 38.9°C, blood pressure was 116/89, heart rate was 110/min and respiration was 16/min. He had bilateral conjunctival petechiae. Neck was supple without any lymphadenopathy. Chest examination finding was unremarkable, but he had a diastolic rumble at the apex. Besides a palpable spleen tip, the rest of the abdominal examination was unremarkable. Neurological examination was pertinent for mild, nonfluent aphasia and right-sided hemiparesis. Laboratory evaluation disclosed a white blood cell (WBC) count of 13,000/mm^3. Multiple sets of blood cultures were drawn. A transthoracic echocardiogram (TTE) demonstrated an enlarged left atrium and mitral regurgitation. Cranial computed tomography (CT) scan showed left middle cerebral artery territory infarct. He was admitted to the intensive care unit with a diagnosis of embolic cerebral infarction secondary to presumptive infective endocarditis, and he was empirically started on nafcillin, ampicillin, and gentamicin.

DEFINITION

Infective endocarditis (IE) is a microbial infection of the endocardial surface of the heart, involving the valves and adjacent structures. It is characterized by microbial colonization or invasion of the heart valves leading to accumulation of thrombotic debris and organisms that forms bulky, friable vegetations and can lead to cardiac tissue destruction (1). IE is often classified into four categories: native-valve IE, prosthetic valve IE (PVE), IE in intravenous drug users, and nosocomial IE. PVE is further classified as either early or late infection, depending on whether the onset occurs within or 60 days after the operation. Endocarditis is most commonly caused by various types of bacteria, but fungi and atypical bacteria also account for a few cases. IE has been traditionally classified as either "acute" or "subacute-chronic," based on severity and timing of clinical presentation. Acute bacterial endocarditis (ABE) usually presents with rapidly developing symptoms and has an onset of several days. It can be fatal within weeks without treatment. Subacute bacterial endocarditis (SBE) has an insidious onset that develops over several weeks to months. Hospital-acquired IE has been defined as IE with an onset of symptoms ≥72 hours after hospitalization or IE occurring within 4 to 8 weeks of a hospital discharge in which an invasive procedure was performed (2).

EPIDEMIOLOGY

The precise incidence of IE is difficult to establish because case definition in published articles varies and IE is not a reportable disease. In the developed countries, the incidence is between 1.7 to as high as 9.2 cases per 100,000 person-years with a male-to-female ratio of 1.7:1 (3,4). The highest incidence is in those over 65 years of age: more than 15 per 100,000 person-years (5). Age of patients with IE is increasing, from a median age of 30 to 40 in the preantibiotic era to the current 47 to 69 years (3,4). This shift is mainly attributed to increased longevity, which has given rise to more degenerative heart disease, increased placement of prosthetic valves, increased exposure to nosocomial bacteremia, and long-term hemodialysis. The incidence of PVE is also increasing, accounting for 30% of cases in some series. The risk of PVE is 1% at 12 months and 2% to 3% at 60 months (6). The annual incidence among injection drug users, which is 150 to 200 cases per 100,000 population, is seen in younger patients (7). Rates of nosocomial IE are also increasing, accounting for 28% in one series with most from intravenous catheter-related infections (8). Overall mortality rate in patients with IE is about 20%.

Rheumatic heart disease continues to be the most common underlying cardiac condition in developing nations, but degenerative valvular diseases (e.g., calcified aortic stenosis, calcified mitral annulus) and mitral valve prolapse are the leading underlying conditions in the United States and most industrialized countries 9 (1,3–6). Other conditions associated with increased risk of IE include poor oral hygiene, long-term hemodialysis, diabetes mellitus, and human immunodeficiency virus (HIV) infection.

ETIOLOGY AND PATHOGENESIS

ETIOLOGY

The microbiology of IE depends on whether it occurs on a native or prosthetic valve, and on whether parenteral drug use is a major risk factor (Table 4-1). Viridans streptococci were the most common causative agents until the mid 1990s when most series reported *Staphylococcus aureus* as the predominant pathogen (8–11). Coagulase-negative staphylococci (CoNS), once considered pathogens in PVE, only are now known to cause infection in native valves as well. A particular species of CoNS, *Staphylococcus lugdunensis*, a perianal skin commensal, is known to cause severe valvular destruction and fulminant clinical disease in otherwise healthy hosts (12,13). The most commonly encountered of the viridans or α-hemolytic streptococci include *S. sangius, S. oralis (mitis), S. salivarus, S. mutans, Gemella morbillorum* (formerly *S. morbillorum*), and the *S. anginosus* group, also known as the *S. milleri* group (*S. intermedius, anginosus,* and *constellatus*). The latter group is noted for its tendency to form abscesses and cause metastatic infection (e.g., myocarditis, vertebral osteomyelitis, septic arthritis, and visceral abscesses) (14). *Streptococcus bovis,* a nonenterococcal group D streptococcus commonly causes IE in the elderly and is associated with intestinal neoplastic diseases (6). Other streptococci causing IE include *S. pneumoniae, S. pyogenes, S. agalactiae* (group B streptococcus), and the nutritionally deficient streptococcal species *Abiotrophia defectiva, Granulicatella* spp.

Enterococci (*E. faecalis* and *E. faecium*) originating from the gastrointestinal and genitourinary tracts are also important causes of IE and are notoriously difficult to treat. Fastidious gram-negative bacilli of the HACEK group (*Haemophillus* spp., *Actinobacillus actinomycetemcomitans, Cardiobaterium hominis, Eikinella correodens,* and *Kingella kingae*) account for about 4% of native-valve IE in nonintravenous drug users (5). Less commonly identified bacterial species causing IE include *Neisseria gonorrhoeae, Salmonella, Legionella, Coxiella burnetti, Chlamydia psittaci, Corynebacterium species, Listeria, Tropheryma whipplei,* and *Bartonella species.* Also not common, fungi—both yeast and mold—can cause endocarditis. *Candida,* usually as a complication of prosthetic valve placement, parenteral drug use, or presence of intravascular device (e.g., pacemaker) are the leading cause of fungal IE (15). Endocarditis caused by mycelial or dimorphic fungi is rare, with most cases caused by *Aspergillus spp.* Between 5% and 31% of patients with IE have negative blood cultures with etiologic diagnosis established by other means (16).

PATHOGENESIS

The steps in the pathogenesis of endocarditis are (*a*) valvular endothelial damage, (*b*) platelet-fibrin thrombus formation, (*c*) adherence of bacteria to platelet thrombus plaque, and (*d*) local bacterial proliferation with hematogenous seeding (5,7,17). The intact endothelial surface is resistant to invasion by bacteria or to thrombus formation. Excoriations of the endothelium result in direct contact between the blood and the subendothelial host components, including proteins of the extracellular matrix, thromboplastin, and tissue factor, which trigger blood coagulation. Turbulent blood flow occurring in preexisting valvular disease (e.g., rheumatic heart disease or degenerative valvular disease) damages the endothelium. In intravenous drug use, talc-induced valvular granulomas, diluent-related damage, and

TABLE 4-1. Microbiology of Infective Endocarditis (IE) in the General Population and in Specific At-Risk Groups (5)

Pathogen	*Native Valve IE (N = 280)*	*IE in Intravenous Drug Users (N = 87)*	*Prosthetic-Valve IE*	
			Early (*N* = 15)	Late (*N* = 72)
Staphylococci	124 (44%)	60 (69%)	10 (67%)	33 (46%)
Staphylococcus aureus	106 (38%)	60 (69%)	3 (20%)	15 (21%)
Coagulase negative	16 (6%)	0	7 (47%)	18 (25%)
Streptococci	86 (31%)	7 (8%)	0	25 (35%)
Oral streptococci	59 (21%)	3 (3%)	0	19 (26%)
Others (nonenterococcal)	27 (10%)[a]	4 (5%)	0	6 (8%)
Enterococcus spp[b]	21 (8%)	2(2%)	1 (7%)	5 (7%)
HACEK group[c]	12 (4%)	0	0	1 (1%)
Polymicrobial	6 (2%)	8 (9%)	0	1 (1%)
Other bacteria[d]	12 (4%)	4 (5%)	0	2 (3%)
Fungi	3 (1%)	4 (5%)	4 (27%)	5 (7%)
Negative blood cultures	16 (6%)	4 (5%)	4 (27%)	5 (7%)

[a]Includes *S. agalactiae* (9), *S. bovis* (6), *S. pneumoniae* (3), *S. pyogenes* (2), group B streptococcus (1), *Abiotrophia* spp. (1)
[b]>80% *Enterococcus faecalis*
[c]*Haemophillus* spp., *Actinobacillus actinomycetemcomitans, Cardiobaterium hominis, Eikinella correodens,* and *Kingella kingae*
[d]Includes *Escherichia coli* (4), *Corynebacterium spp.* (2), *Proteus mirabilis* (2), *Mycobacterium tuberculosis* (1), *Bacteroides fragilis* (1).

drug-induced pulmonary hypertension all contribute to disrupt the normal endothelial surface (7). The damaged endothelium permits deposition of platelets and fibrin forming the so-called *sterile platelet aggregate*—the lesion of nonbacterial thrombotic endocarditis. This lesion contains large quantities of fibrinogen, fibrin, fibronectin, plasma proteins, and platelets to which passing microorganism during transient bacteremia avidly bind. As an example, viridans streptococci, with their ability to produce dextrans and other "sticky molecules," readily adhere to the platelet thrombus (18). Successful colonization is promoted by the higher oxygen saturation content of the left side of heart (for left-sided cases). Infecting microorganisms survive and avoid host defenses by a variety of mechanisms. Subsequent bacterial proliferation promotes formation of dense colonies and results in release of cytokines and procoagulant factors, leading to more thrombosis resulting in expanding the infected coagulum.

PATHOLOGY

The classic vegetation of IE usually is located along the line of the closure of a valve leaflet, either on the atrial surface of atrioventricular valves or the ventricular surface of the semilunar valves. Vegetations can be single or multiple and vary in size, consistency, and gross appearance; typically, they are friable and bulky. The vegetation can erode through the valve, causing incompetence, or into underlying myocardium, producing an abscess. Histologically, the lesion consists primarily of fibrin, platelet aggregates, and an intense inflammatory response. Gram stain often demonstrates masses of bacteria. Myocarditis, myocardial infarction, and pericarditis are frequently noted at autopsy. Because of the friable nature of the vegetation, systemic emboli can occur at any time and cause infarcts in the brain, kidneys, myocardium, spleen, lung, and other tissues. The risk of major systemic emboli is reduced after 2 weeks of effective antimicrobial therapy. Abscesses can develop at the infarcted sites because the embolic fragments contain many viable organisms (17,19).

CLINICAL MANIFESTATIONS

Fever is the most common symptom and sign of IE, although it might be absent in severely debilitated patients and the elderly or in those who have received prior antibiotics. The fever is often intermittent, rarely high grade, and associated with nonspecific symptoms of anorexia, weight loss, generalized malaise, fatigue, and night sweats. Most patients with IE have a heart murmur (most commonly preexisting). Other cardiac manifestations include congestive heart failure, and any degree of atrioventricular block. In right-sided endocarditis, the initial symptoms can be predominantly pulmonary. IE can present initially with extracardiac manifestations, which include musculoskeletal complaints (myalgias, arthralgias, back pain); cutaneous manifestations, such as splinter hemorrhages, conjunctival petechiae, Osler nodes (tender, subcutaneous nodules, often in the pulp of digits or the thenar eminence), and Janeway lesions (nontender erythematous, hemorrhagic, or pustular lesions, often on the palms and soles); splenomegaly; and neurological manifestations as a consequence of embolism (20). Prosthetic valve endocarditis can present either as an indolent illness or acutely with high fever, systemic toxicity, and leukocytosis as might be seen in patients with *S. aureus* IE. Unexplained fever in a patient with a prosthetic valve should prompt evaluation for PVE. Nosocomial endocarditis usually presents acutely without the stigmata of peripheral lesions and is the suggested diagnosis if patients with intravascular devices have bacteremia that persists after removal of the device. Hematologic parameters are often abnormal in IE, none of which is diagnostic. Anemia is seen in more than 70% of patients and can worsen with the duration of illness. The erythrocyte sedimentation rate (ESR) is almost always elevated. Routine urinalysis is frequently abnormal; microscopic hematuria and proteinuria can be seen in more than half of patients. Other sequelae of IE are related to bacteremic seeding: splenic abscesses, vertebral abscess or osteomyelitis, and renal or psoas abscess.

Patients with IE can present with any number of neurological manifestations. About 25% to 40% of patients develop these complications. Embolism most commonly involving the middle cerebral artery territory is the most frequent neurological manifestation and can be the initial manifestation. Thus, IE should be suspected in a patient with fever, underlying valvular heart disease, and a stroke syndrome. Cerebral hemorrhage is less common and could be caused by rupture of a mycotic aneurysm or bleeding into an infarcted area. Mycotic aneurysms develop from septic embolization of vegetations to the arterial vasa vasorum with subsequent spread of infection through the intima and outward through the vessel wall. They develop most commonly at sites of bifurcation and occur frequently in the distal segment of intracranial arteries (secondary or tertiary branches), but can be extracranial as well (visceral and lower extremity circulation) (14). Despite the original description of mycotic aneurysms meaning *fresh fungus vegetations*, most cases are bacterial. Patients who develop intracranial mycotic aneurysm can present with severe headache, altered sensorium, or focal neurologic deficits, which suggest a mass lesion or an embolic event. Mycotic aneurysms can be detected by CT or magnetic resonance angiography (MRA), but conventional catheter cerebral angiography is the diagnostic gold standard (20). More uncommon neurologic complications of IE include acute encephalopathy, brain abscess or cerebritis, meningitis, meningoencephalitis, or seizures. Mental status alteration at presentation is a poor prognostic sign (21).

DIAGNOSTIC APPROACH

The diagnosis of IE is sometimes obvious in a patient who presents with a constellation of symptoms including a new murmur and the presence of a major risk factor (e.g., intravenous drug use). Definitive diagnosis of IE, however, relies on two major tests: blood cultures and echocardiography. Blood cultures are positive in about 90% of cases, but can be negative in cases of patients who have had prior antibiotic therapy or infection with fastidious organisms. Because diagnostic yield is increased, performing three sets of blood cultures before initiation of antibiotic therapy is mandatory when IE is suspected. All patients should have echocardiography to identify vegetations, abscesses, or new prosthetic dehiscence, as well as to assess the severity of valve damage and heart function. Whether TTE or transesophageal echocardiogram (TEE) should be performed first, depends on individual patients (14). A TTE is reasonable to perform where suspicion for IE is low, in children, and when TEE is not immediately available. In situations in

TABLE 4-2. Modified Duke Criteria for Diagnosis of Infective Endocarditis (IE)

MAJOR CRITERIA

Blood culture positive for IE
- Typical microorganisms consistent with IE from two separate blood cultures:
  - Viridans streptococci, *Streptococcus bovis,* HACEK group, *Staphylococcus aureus;* or community-acquired enterococci in the absence of primary focus; or
- Microorganisms consistent with IE from persistently positive blood cultures defined as follows:
  - At least two positive cultures of blood samples drawn >12 h apart; or
  - All three or most of four or more separate cultures of blood (with first and last sample drawn at least 1 h apart)
- Single positive culture for *Coxiella burnetti* or antibody titer against phase I >1 in 800
- Evidence of endocardial involvement
- Echocardiogram positive for IE (TEE recommended in patients with prosthetic valves, patients rated as possible IE by clinical criteria, or complicated IE (paravalvular abscess); TTE as first test in other patients) defined as follows:
  - Oscillating intracardiac mass on valve or supporting structure, or in the path of regurgitant jets, or on implanted material, in the absence of an alternative anatomical explanation, *or*
  - Abscess, *or*
  - New partial dehiscence of prosthetic valve
- New valvular regurgitation (worsening or changing of preexisting murmur not sufficient)

MINOR CRITERIA

- Predisposing cardiac condition or intravenous drug use
- Fever (temperature ≥38°C or 100.4°F)
- Vascular phenomena, major arterial emboli, septic pulmonary infarct, mycotic aneurysms, intracranial hemorrhage, conjunctival hemorrhage, Janeway's lesions
- Immunologic phenomena: glomerulonephritis, Osler's nodes, Roth's spots and rheumatoid factor
- Microbiological evidence: positive blood culture, but does not meet major criteria or serological evidence of active infection with plausible microorganism

DIAGNOSIS

Definite IE
- Pathologic criteria
  - (1) Microorganism demonstrated by culture or histologic examination of a vegetation, a vegetation that has embolized, or an intracardiac abscess specimen; or
  - (2) Pathologic lesions; vegetation or intracardiac abscess confirmed by histologic examination showing active endocarditis
- Clinical criteria
  - (1) Two major criteria, *or*
  - (2) One major and three minor criteria *or*
  - (3) Five minor criteria

Possible IE
- (1) One major and one minor criterion, *or*
- (2) Three minor criteria

Rejected
- (1) Firm alternative diagnosis, *or*
- (2) Resolution of syndrome after ≤4 days of antibiotic therapy, *or*
- (3) No pathological evidence at surgery or autopsy after ≤4 days of antibiotic therapy
- (4) Does not meet criteria for possible IE

TEE, transesophageal echocardiogram; TTE, transthoracic echocardiogram.
(From Habib G. Management of infective endocarditis. *Heart.* 2006; 92(1):124–130, with permission.)

which initial clinical suspicion is high, TEE has been found to be more sensitive in detecting vegetations and abscesses. It also proves to be more cost effective, especially in the setting of *S. aureus bacteremia* (22,23). Also, keep in mind that both echocardiography and blood cultures can be negative in some patients. In 1994, the Duke Endocarditis service published the Duke criteria for diagnosis of endocarditis. The Duke criteria have been validated in several studies and have become the clinical standard for diagnosing IE (24,25). In 2000, the Duke criteria were modified (Table 4-2) to address situations with negative blood culture and in the setting of bacteremia with *S. aureus* (26).

TREATMENT

Treatment of IE requires a multidisciplinary approach with infectious disease specialists, cardiologists, neurologists, and cardiothoracic surgeons. The American Heart Association (AHA) and Infectious Disease Society of America (IDSA) have published standards for antibiotic treatment. Table 4-3 shows these recommendations for most causes of IE. Appropriate parenteral antimicrobial therapy should be initiated in the hospital. When the patient has clinically stabilized and blood cultures have converted to negative, therapy can be completed on an out-patient basis. By the second week of therapy, fever has resolved in 90% of patients. Persistent fever can indicate extension of the infection beyond the valve or formation of perivalvular abscess. Other causes of persistent fever after 2 weeks of therapy include a metastatic focus of infection, such as a splenic or renal abscess, reaction to a drug, or nosocomial infections with particular attention to the intravascular catheter devices.

Cardiac valve surgery may be necessary in some patients. Congestive heart failure (CHF) occurring more frequently with aortic valve infection is the most common indication. Other valve lesions requiring surgery include perforation of a native or bioprosthetic valve leaflet, rupture of infected mitral chordae, valve obstruction, or bulky vegetations (27). Echocardiographic indications for surgical intervention include evidence of valve dehiscense, perforation, rupture, fistula, or a large perivalvular abscess (14). Other echocardiographic findings that highlight the possible need for surgery are large anterior mitral leaflet vegetations (>10 mm) or persistent vegetation after systemic embolization. Prosthetic valve IE, particularly the early PVE caused by S. *aureus,* is more severe and more commonly associated with perivalvular abscess, thus often necessitating surgical intervention. Failure of medical therapy is the rule with fungal endocarditis; therefore, surgery is recommended. For the same reason, gram-negative endocarditis, especially if caused by *Pseudomonas aeruginosa,* often requires surgery for reliable cure. Optimal timing of valve surgery in patients with IE with cerebral embolism is still debated. Some experts recommend delaying for at least 2 weeks after cerebral infarction (up to 1 month after cerebral hemorrhage) because of the high risk of neurologic deterioration associated with early surgery. Limited data exist on how to approach a patient with a mycotic aneurysm that needs both aneurysm clipping or ligation and valve replacement. Anticoagulation in IE is controversial. Although not of benefit in native valve disease, cautiously continuing anticoagulation is appropriate for patients with PVE. In patients who experience recent cerebral emboli, particularly those with *S. aureus* IE, withholding

TABLE 4-3. Antimicrobial Therapy for Common Causes of Endocarditis

	Native-Valve Endocarditis		*Prosthetic-Valve Endocarditis*	
Pathogen	Antimicrobial Therapy	Comments	Antimicrobial Therapy	Comments
Penicillin-susceptible viridans streptococci, *Streptococcus bovis,* and other streptococci (MIC of penicillin ≤0.12 μg/mL)	Penicillin G or ceftriaxone for 4 wk[a]	Preferred in most patients >65 y or patients with impairment of cranial nerve VIII function or renal function	Penicillin G or ceftriaxone **with or without** gentamicin for 6 wk[a]	Penicillin or ceftriaxone together with gentamicin has not demonstrated superior cure rates compared with monotherapy with penicillin or ceftriaxone for patients with highly susceptible strain; gentamicin should not be administered to patients with creatinine clearance of <30 mL/min
	Penicillin G or ceftriaxone **plus** gentamicin for 2 wk	2-wk regimen not intended for patients with known cardiac or extracardiac abscess or for those with creatinine clearance of <20 mL/min, impaired cranial nerve VIII function, or *Abiotrophia, Granulicatella,* or *Gemella* spp. infection; gentamicin dosage should be adjusted to achieve peak serum concentration of <1 μg/mL when three divided doses are used		
Relatively penicillin-resistant streptococci strains (MIC >0.12 to ≤0.5 μg/mL)	Penicillin G or ceftriaxone for 4 wk **plus** gentamicin for 2 wk		Penicillin G or ceftriaxone with gentamicin for 6 wk	
Penicillin resistant streptococcal strains (MIC >0.5 μg/mL)	See therapy for penicillin-resistant enterococci		See therapy for penicillin-resistant enterococci	
Enterococci susceptible to penicillin, vancomycin, and aminoglycosides	Ampicillin or penicillin G[a] **plus** gentamicin[b] for 4 to 6 wk	4-wk therapy recommended for patients with symptoms of illness ≤3 mo; 6-wk therapy recommended for patients with symptoms >3 mo	Ampicillin or penicillin G[a] **plus** gentamicin[b] for 6 wk	Minimum of 6 wk combined therapy is recommended
Enterococci susceptible to penicillin, vancomycin, but resistant to gentamicin	Ampicillin or penicillin G[a] **plus** streptomycin for 4 to 6 wk		Ampicillin or penicillin G[a] **plus** streptomycin for 4 to 6 wk	Minimum of 6 wk combined therapy is recommended
β-lactamase producing enterococci resistant to penicillin and susceptible to aminoglycoside and vancomycin	Ampicillin-sulbactam[a] plus gentamicin for 6 wk		Ampicillin-sulbactam[a] plus gentamicin for 6 wk	Unlikely that the strain will be susceptible to gentamicin; if strain is gentamicin resistant, then >6 wk of ampicillin-sulbactam therapy will be needed
Enterococci with intrinsic penicillin resistance	Vancomycin plus gentamicin for 6 wk		Vancomycin plus gentamicin for 6 wk	
Enterococci with resistance to penicillin, aminoglycosides and vancomycin	Linezolid or quinipristin-dalfopristin ≥8 wk for *E. faecium* Imipenem/cilastin plus ampicillin or ceftriaxone plus ampicillin ≥8 wk for *E. faecalis*	Limited data on treatment options; cure with antimicrobials alone may be <50% and cardiac valve replacement may be necessary	Linezolid or quinipristin-dalfopristin ≥8 wk for *E. faecium* Imipenem/cilastin plus ampicillin or ceftriaxone plus ampicillin ≥8 wk for *E. faecalis*	Limited data on treatment options; cure with antimicrobials alone may be <50% and cardiac valve replacement may be necessary
Methicillin-susceptible staphylococci	Nafcillin or cefazolin for 6 wk with optional 3 to 5 d of gentamicin	Cefazolin recommended for patients with nonanaphylactoid type penicillin allergy; clinical benefit of aminoglycosides has not been established	Nafcillin **plus** rifampin for ≥6 wk **plus** gentamicin in first 2 wk	Cardiac surgical intervention may play a role in maximizing outcome

(*continued*)

TABLE 4-3. (*Continued*)

	Native-Valve Endocarditis		*Prosthetic-Valve Endocarditis*	
Pathogen	Antimicrobial Therapy	Comments	Antimicrobial Therapy	Comments
Methicillin-resistant staphylococci	Vancomycin for 6 wk		Vancomycin **plus** rifampin for ≥6 wk **plus** gentamicin in first 2 wk	If organism is resistant to gentamicin, then an aminoglycoside to which it is susceptible should be used; aminoglycoside should be omitted if the organism is resistant to all available aminoglycosides
HACEK[c]	Ceftriaxone for 4 wk		Ceftriaxone 4 wk	Ampicillin-sulbactam is the alternative

MIC, minimum inhibitory concentration.
[a]Vancomycin therapy recommended only for patients unable to tolerate penicillin or ceftriaxone; vancomycin dosage should be adjusted to obtain peak (1 h after infusion completed) serum concentration of 30 to 45 μg/mL and a trough concentration range of 10 to 15 μg/mL.
[b]For enterococci resistant to gentamicin but susceptible to streptomycin, then streptomycin is used.
[c]*Haemophilus parainfluenzae, H. aphrophilus, Actinobacillus actinomycetemcomitans, Cardiobactrium hominis, Eikenella corrodens, Kingella kingae.*
(From Baddour LM, Wilson WR, Bayer AS, et al. Infective endocarditis: Diagnosis, antimicrobial therapy, and management of complications. A statement for healthcare professionals from the Committee on Rheumatic Fever, Endocarditis, and Kawasaki Disease, Council on Cardiovascular Disease in the Young, and the Councils on Clinical Cardiology, Stroke, and Cardiovascular Surgery and Anesthesia, American Heart Association: Endorsed by the Infectious Diseases Society of America. *Circulation.* 2005;111(23):e394–e434, with permission.)

anticoagulation for at least the first 2 weeks of antibiotic therapy prevents hemorrhagic transformation of embolic lesions (28).

CLINICAL RECOMMENDATIONS OF THE VIGNETTE

Infective endocarditis continues to have significant morbidity and mortality even in the antibiotic era. It is important for clinicians to suspect IE, especially when major risk factors are present. In our patient, the negative TTE does not rule out endocarditis and the clinician should proceed to a transesophageal echocardiogram to assess definitively for vegetations. Our patient's TEE showed a mitral valve vegetation, and he had had a valve replacement. Blood cultures grew S. *mitis* with a minimum inhibitory concentration (MIC) to penicillin of less than 0.12 μg/mL; therefore, 2 weeks of penicillin and gentamicin combination or 4 weeks of penicillin is the treatment of choice (Table 4-3). Patients in whom IE is suspected, especially those with significant risk factors, such as parenteral drug use, indwelling intravenous devices, and underlying cardiac valve abnormalities, should have three sets of blood cultures drawn. If possible, antibiotics are not started until the cultures are positive. After blood cultures are drawn, antibiotics should be started empirically only in patients who are critically ill or septic. Decision on whether to start with a TTE depends on the strength of the suspicion for IE. Patients with positive blood cultures and a positive TTE do not require a TEE unless exists clinical change or suspected complication, such as perivalvular extension of the infection. Notify the cardiothoracic surgeon early, particularly when the vegetation measures >10 mm. Patients need not stay in the hospital for the duration of the IE treatment. Documentation of clearing of bacteremia and resolution of fever, however, are important key features that may signal response to antimicrobial therapy. Most patients can be successfully followed up as outpatients to complete the recommended course of therapy. Patients should be evaluated for clinical signs and symptoms of recurrent illness or side effects from the antimicrobials. Blood cultures should be repeated 1 or 2 weeks after completion of antibiotic therapy to ensure cure. A good dental evaluation may be necessary, especially for those whose infecting organisms are oral flora.

SUMMARY

Infective endocarditis remains a common problem, and even a slight increase is seen in its incidence, owing to the increased life expectancy and prevalence of degenerative valvular heart diseases. Despite good antimicrobial availability, morbidity and mortality from IE remain significant. Multiple blood cultures and echocardiography are the mainstay in the work-up of a patient suspected with IE. A prolonged, parenteral antibiotic course is necessary to achieve cure. For complicated cases surgical intervention is warranted.

REFERENCES

1. Mylonakis E, Calderwood SB. Infective endocarditis in adults. *N Engl J Med.* 2001; 345:1318–1330.
2. Ben-Ami R, Giladi M, Carmeli Y, et al. Hospital-acquired infective endocarditis: Should the definition be broadened? *Clin Infect Dis.* 2004;38(6):843–850.
3. Hogevik H, Olaison L, Andersson R, et al. Epidemiologic aspects of infective endocarditis in an urban population. A 5-year prospective study. *Medicine* (Baltimore). 1995;74:324–339.
4. Walpot J, Blok W, van Zwienen J, et al. Incidence and complication rate of infective endocarditis in the Dutch region of Walcheren: A 3-year retrospective study. *Acta Cardiol.* 2006;61(2):175–181.
5. Moreillon P, Que YA. Infective endocarditis. *Lancet.* 2004;363:139–149.

6. Hill EE, Herijgers P, Herregods MC, et al. Evolving trends in infective endocarditis. *Clin Microbiol Infect.* 2006;12(1):5–12.
7. Frontera JA, Gradon JD. Right-sided endocarditis in injection drug users: Review of proposed mechanism of pathogenesis. *Clin Infect Dis.* 2000;30:374–379.
8. Cheng A, Athan E, Appelbe A, et al. The changing profile of bacterial endocarditis as seen at an Australian provincial centre. *Heart Lung Circ.* 2002;11:26–31.
9. Hoen B, Alla F, Selton-Suty C, et al. Changing profile of infective endocarditis: Results of a 1-year survey in France. *JAMA.* 2002;288(1):75–81.
10. Heiro M, Helenius H, Makila S, et al. Infective endocarditis in a Finnish teaching hospital: A study on 326 episodes treated during 1980–2004. *Heart.* 2006;Apr 27:Epub.
11. Hsu CN, Wang JY, Tseng CD, et al. Clinical features and predictors for mortality in patients with infective endocarditis at a university hospital in Taiwan from 1995 to 2003. *Epidemiol Infect.* 2006;134(3):589–597.
12. Patel R, Piper KE, Rouse MS, et al. Frequency of isolation of *Staphylococcus lugunensis* among staphylococcal isolates causing endocarditis: A 20-year experience. *J Clin Microbiol.* 2000;38:4262–4263.
13. Van Hoovels L, De Munter P, Colaert J, et al. Three cases of destructive native valve endocarditis caused by *Staphylococcus lugdunensis. Eur J Clin Microbiol Infect Dis.* 2005;24: 149–152.
14. Baddour LM, Wilson WR, Bayer AS, et al. Infective endocarditis: Diagnosis, antimicrobial therapy, and management of complications. A statement for healthcare professionals from the Committee on Rheumatic Fever, Endocarditis, and Kawasaki Disease, Council on Cardiovascular Disease in the Young, and the Councils on Clinical Cardiology, Stroke, and Cardiovascular Surgery and Anesthesia, American Heart Association: Endorsed by the Infectious Diseases Society of America. *Circulation.* 2005;111(23): e394–e434.
15. Ellis ME, Al-Abdely H, Sandridge A, et al. Fungal endocarditis: Evidence in the world literature, 1965–1995. *Clin Infect Dis.* 2001;32(1):50–62.
16. Houpikian P, Raoult D. Blood culture-negative endocarditis in a reference center: Etiologic diagnosis of 348 cases. *Medicine* (Baltimore). 2005;84(3):162–173.
17. Mandell GL, Bennett JE, Dolin R, eds. *Principles and Practice of Infectious Diseases,* 6th ed. Philadelphia: Elsevier Churchill Livingstone; 2005.
18. Moreillon P, Que YA, Bayer AS. Pathogenesis of streptococcal and staphylococcal endocarditis. *Infect Dis Clin North Am.* 2002;16:297–318.
19. Kumar V, Abbas AK, Fausto N. *Robbins and Cotran, Pathologic Basis of Disease,* 7th ed. Philadelphia: WB Saunders; 2005.
20. Hasbun R, Vikram HR, Barakat LA, et al. Complicated left-sided native valve endocarditis in adults: Risk classification for mortality. *JAMA.* 2003;289:1933–1940.
21. Habib G. Management of infective endocarditis. *Heart.* 2006;92(1):124–130.
22. Heidenreich, PA, Masoudi FA, Maini B, et al. Echocardiography in patients with suspected endocarditis: A cost-effective analysis. *Am J Med.* 1999;107(3):198–208.
23. Rosen AB, Fowler VG, Corey R, et al. Cost-effectiveness of transesophageal echocardiography to determine duration of therapy for intravascular catheter-associated *Staphylococcus aureus* bacteremia. *Ann Intern Med.* 1999;130:810–820.
24. Gagliardi JP, Nettles RE, McCarthy DE, et al. Native valve infective endocarditis in elderly and younger adult patients: Comparison of clinical features and outcomes with the use of the Duke criteria and the Duke endocarditis database. *Clin Infect Dis.* 1998;26:1165–1168.
25. Perez-Vazquez A, Farinas MC, Garcia-Palomo JD, et al. Evaluation of the Duke criteria in 93 episodes of prosthetic valve endocarditis: Could sensitivity be improved? *Arch Intern Med.* 2000;160:1185–1191.
26. Li JS, Sexton DJ, Mick N, et al. Proposed modifications to the Duke criteria for the diagnosis of infective endocarditis. *Clin Infect Dis.* 2000;30:633–638.
27. Sexton DJ, Spelman D. Current best practices and guidelines: Assessment and management of complications in infective endocarditis. *Cardiol Clin.* 2003;21:273–282.
28. Tornos P, Almirante B, Mirabet S, et al. Infective endocarditis due to *Staphylococcus aureus*: Deleterious effect of anticoagulant therapy. *Arch Intern Med.* 1999;159:473–475.

CHAPTER **5**

Coronary Artery Disease

Fred Leya

OBJECTIVES

- To review the anatomy and physiology of the coronary circulation
- To describe the pathophysiology of coronary atherothrombosis
- To discuss endothelial function in health and disease
- To describe the vulnerable plaque and its role in the acute coronary syndrome
- To review the clinical manifestation of myocardial ischemia
- To discuss the diagnostic approach, risk stratification, and treatment of patients with coronary artery disease

CASE VIGNETTE

A 52-year-old man was admitted to the hospital after his left arm and leg were paralyzed. He waited 10 hours before coming to the hospital. This was his second hospitalization. A month earlier, he had an extensive anterior wall myocardial infarction (MI) that resulted in extensive left ventricular (LV) damage, and a large LV aneurysm. After initial hospitalization, the patient complained of frequent, recurrent, episodes of palpitations and lightheadedness.

DEFINITION

Coronary artery disease (CAD) is most commonly caused by atheromatous obstruction of the coronary arteries by a plaque that might limit the adequate coronary blood supply to meet the metabolic demands of the heart. Angina pectoris or severe suffocating chest pain results from insufficient blood oxygen supply to the heart. Chest discomfort is usually the predominant symptom. Syndromes of CAD also occur, however, when chest discomfort is absent, such as diabetic silent myocardial ischemia, ischemic cardiomyopathy with congestive heart failure (CHF), cardiac arrhythmia, and sudden death.

EPIDEMIOLOGY

Coronary artery disease (ischemic heart disease) is the dominant cause of death in the world. In the developed world, CAD accounts for nearly 50% of all deaths. It is estimated that nearly 14 million Americans have CAD, nearly 7 million of whom have angina pectoris (AP), and 7 million have had an MI; 5 million have ischemic stroke and 8 million have peripheral vascular disease. The lifetime risk of developing symptomatic CAD after the age of 40 years is nearly 50% for men, and 33% for women (1).

The economic cost of CAD in the United States in 2006 was estimated at $250 billion (1). It is expected that the rate of CAD will accelerate with the aging of the baby boomers, aided by alarming increases in the prevalence of obesity, type II diabetes, the metabolic syndrome, as well as by the increasing prevalence of cardiovascular (CV) risk factors among younger generations.

ANATOMY AND PHYSIOLOGY OF CORONARY CIRCULATION

The coronary arteries are made up of three distinct anatomic layers. The inner most layer of tightly woven endothelial cells is called the *intima*, the thicker middle muscular layer is called the *tunica media*, and the most outer thin layer of connective tissue is called the *adventitia*. The left main (LM) coronary artery branches into the left anterior descending (LAD) coronary artery and the circumflex coronary artery. The LM coronary artery and its branches provide most of the blood supply to the LV, and to the two thirds of the anterior interventricular septum. The right coronary artery (RCA) provides most of the blood supply to the right ventricle (RV), and to one third of the inferior part of the septum.

Blood flow through the coronary arteries is pulsatile, with phasic systolic and diastolic flow components. During systole, muscle of the thick LV wall compresses the lumen of the intramural coronary vessels, restricting their arterial blood flow during systole to a fraction (about one-fourth) relative to a nonrestrictive diastolic coronary blood flow. On average, about 70% to 80% of blood flow to the heart takes place during diastole, and only about 20% to 30% during systole. Coronary venous flow is out of phase with the coronary arterial flow, occurring predominantly in systole. The coronary arteries continuously supply the heart muscle with oxygen and nutrients to maintain good cardiac function (2–4).

The human heart is an aerobic organ that relies almost entirely on the oxidation of substrates, mostly fatty acids for energy generation. The heart can develop only a small oxygen debt. Even at rest, the heart nearly maximally extracts its oxygen from the arterial blood, leaving its venous blood nearly completely desaturated. Coronary sinus venous blood oxygen saturation is 30% ± 5%, which is among the lowest venous blood saturation in the body.

Because the heart cannot extract additional oxygen from its blood, any additional increase in the heart oxygen demand (heart MV O_2) can only be met by a proportional increase in the coronary blood flow. Increase in coronary blood flow is chiefly mediated by a reduction in the coronary arteriolar resistance vessels. The so-called *arteriolar resistors*, in turn, are controlled by a complex interplay of neural, hormonal, and metabolic factors (4).

The resting human heart consumes 6 to 8 mL/min/100 g of oxygen (heart MV O_2) at rest. Heart rate (HR), myocardial contractility, and ventricular wall tension (the larger the heart chamber, the greater the wall tension) are the primary determinants of cardiac oxygen requirements, being responsible for more than 60% of the total heart oxygen needs. Myocardial relaxation and the electrical activity of the heart consume 20% of MV O_2, and the remaining 20% of heart MV O_2 goes to support the basal cellular metabolism of the living heart. The total metabolism of the resting heart is only a very small fraction of that of the working heart. Myocardial oxygen supply comes through the coronary arteries in the form of coronary blood flow. Coronary blood flow, in turn, is a product of perfusion pressure, mean diastolic aortic blood pressure (BP), and the diastolic time (4).

Myocardial oxygen supply rises and falls in response to the oxygen needs of the myocardium. Any sudden alterations in systemic hemodynamics are promptly matched with appropriate adjustment of the coronary blood flow to meet the changing metabolic needs, only to return to baseline when the demands have ceased. This ability of the heart to maintain its coronary perfusion at a constant level in the face of changing perfusion pressure is known as *coronary blood flow auto regulation* (5,6).

Coronary autoregulation is able to maintain a steady coronary blood flow of about 100 mL/min/100 g over a wide range (40 to 130 mm Hg) of mean aortic perfusion pressure. When mean aortic BP falls outside the boundaries of the autoregulatory capability, steady coronary blood flow is no longer maintained. It can either become dangerously low when the mean aortic perfusion pressure falls below 40 mm Hg, or it can rise when aortic perfusion pressure is excessively elevated above the mean aortic BP of 130 mm Hg. Potent coronary vasodilatory agents, such as nitric oxide (NO), adenosine, and dipyridamole, can both relax vascular resistance vessels and attenuate the autoregulation, increasing the coronary flow to its maximum of about 300 to 400 mL/min. The difference between the highest, hyperemic 400 mL/min coronary blood flow during maximal vasodilatation and the baseline coronary blood flow of 100 mL/min, is called the *coronary flow reserve* (CFR) (7–10).

The CFR or hyperemic blood flow remains unaltered, even by a moderate coronary artery blockage. A coronary artery lesion causing 50% to 60% of luminal narrowing will not impede maximal hyperemic coronary artery blood flow. It is important, therefore, to realize that any diagnostic test relying on the assessment of hyperemic coronary blood flow (e.g., treadmill test) will remain normal, despite a moderate (50% to 60%) coronary artery blockage. Because most (about two thirds) of first time heart attacks or episodes of acute coronary syndromes (ACS) occur when coronary artery blockages are ≤50%, it seems obvious why treadmill testing could occasionally be falsely reassuring.

When progressive expansion of an atherothrombotic plaque narrows 60% of the coronary lumen or more, the CFR gradually begins to decline. The beginning of CFR decline correlates with the start of exertional AP and, at that stage, the stress test begins to become increasingly abnormal. When the coronary blockage reaches 80% of luminal narrowing, the CFR nearly completely disappears as the hyperemic coronary flow can no longer be increased over the baseline (80 to 100 mL) flow. This results in patients having AP with minimal effort, or even chest pain at rest (Fig. 5-1)

Any further progression of a coronary lesion above 80% to 90% ultimately produces hypoperfusion of the myocardium, triggering resting myocardial ischemia. Resting myocardial ischemia is marked by a constellation of clinical signs and symptoms known as the ACS. The ACS is characterized by resting chest pain, abnormal resting electrocardiogram (ECG), ST-T segment depression, and subendocardial myocardial necrosis and positive cardiac enzymes (i.e., creatine kinase MB [CK-MB] and troponins). Further complete coronary lumen obliteration

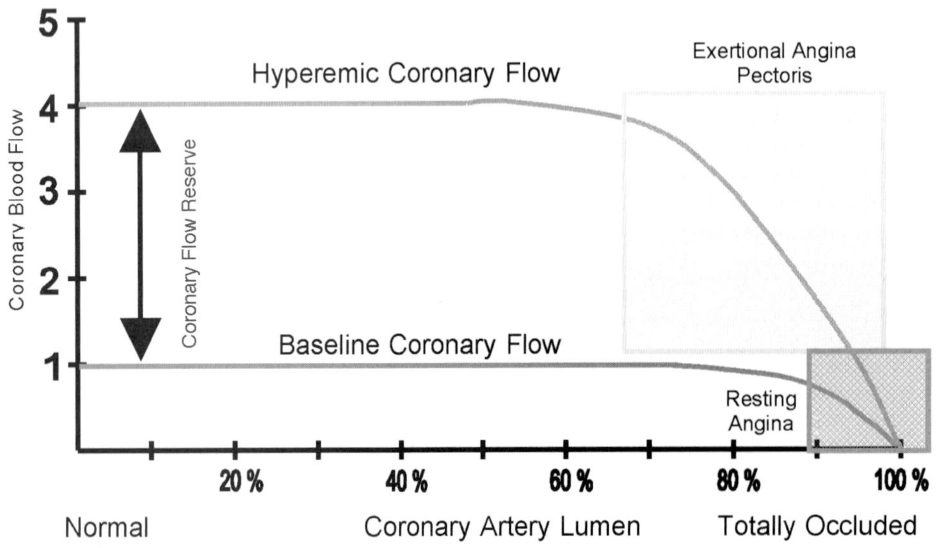

FIGURE 5-1. Represents the relationship between coronary blood flow Y-AXIS at rest and after maximum vasodilatation-hyperemic flow—as a function of increasing severity of coronary blockage on X-AXIS. Notice that resting coronary flow remains normal until the coronary lesion becomes quite severe 85% or greater. Severe lesion 85% or greater will restrict resting coronary flow causing resting angina pectoris. Hyperemic flow remains normal up to coronary lesion of 50% or less. If coronary blockage accedes 50% of the hypermic coronary flow or coronary flow reserve begins to decline, triggering even increasing exertional angina. Until the lesion becomes severe 85% or greater, at that level coronary flow severe is no longer present and the heart relies on coronary blood flow only.

or thrombosis inevitably triggers myocardial cell death that begins within 15 to 30 minutes of termination of blood flow, starting deep in the subendocardium, and then progressively expanding toward the epicardium (11–16).

PATHOPHYSIOLOGY OF ATHEROTHROMBOSIS

Atherosclerotic CAD is the most common cause of myocardial ischemia. Not infrequently, its pathophysiology begins in the second or third decade of life with early endothelial dysfunction. Normally, a monolayer of healthy endothelial cells lines the intimal surface of the entire circulatory tree, creating an enormous endothelial surface area equivalent to about six tennis courts. The endothelium is a dynamic organ with complex metabolic capabilities, including, among others, angiogenesis, control of vascular tone and blood flow, thrombotic and antithrombotic vascular activity, and the inflammatory vascular response to injury. In response to repeated injury, the endothelium, while visually appearing normal, becomes functionally abnormal. Normally, the muscular vascular wall relaxes in response to NO or acetylcholine (ACH), when its endothelium functions normally. The opposite is true: The vessel goes into spasm in response to ACH when its endothelium functions abnormally (17,18). It demonstrates severe spasm of the mid left anterior descending (LAD) coronary artery in response to ACH (Fig. 5-2), and widely opened mid LAD segment in response to intracoronary nitroglycerine (Fig. 5-3).

Normal endothelium maintains a vascular thrombotic balance promoting anticoagulant activity to counter-balance vascular procoagulant mechanisms. The anticoagulant, profibrinolytic function of the normal endothelium includes production of prostacyclin (PGI_2); thombomodulin; heparin sulfate; and tissue plasminogen activator (t-PA) to oppose the procoagulant factors plasminogen activator inhibitor (PAI-1); tissue factor (TF), and von Willebrand factor (VWF) (19,20).

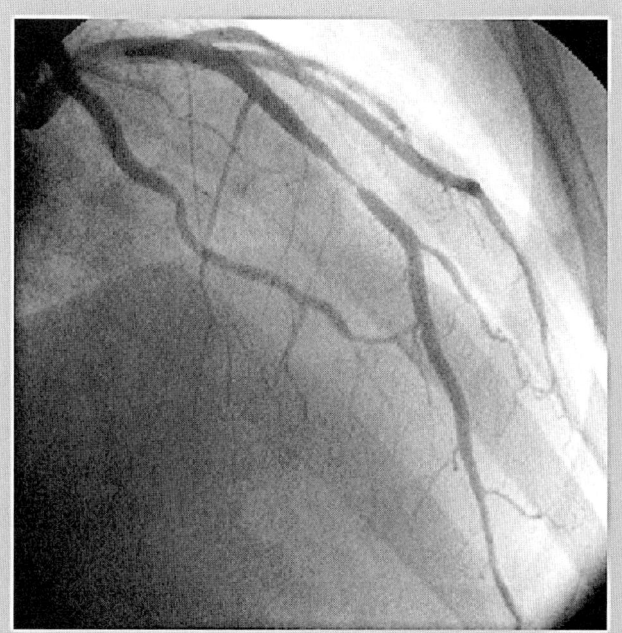

FIGURE 5-2. Demonstrates lesion narrowing of the left anterior descending (LAD) coronary artery lumen, caused by coronary artery spasm in response to acetylcholine challenge.

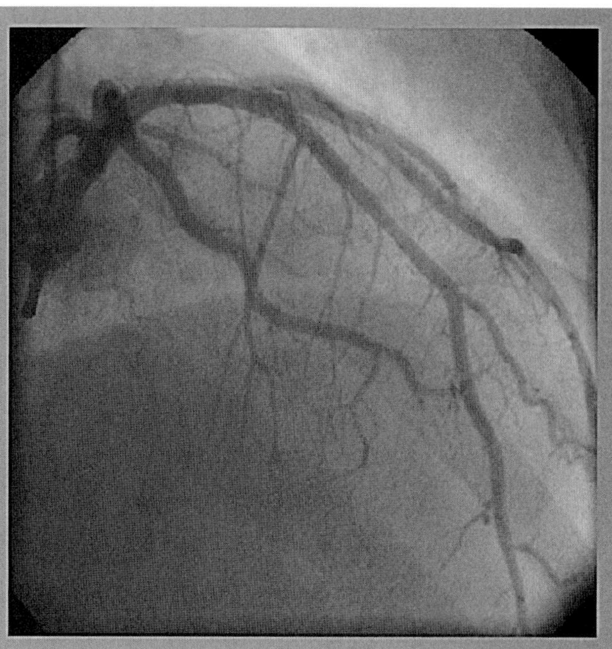

FIGURE 5-3. Demonstrates widely open mid left anterior descending (LAD) segment—coronary artery relaxation—after intracoronary nitroglycerine challenge.

The endothelium can become abnormal in response to sustained insults from elevated blood lipoprotein particles and other proinflammatory stimuli. Normal endothelium resists leukocyte adhesion, but when abnormal, the endothelium expresses on its surface vascular adhesion molecules (VCAM-1) and chemokines, such as MCP-1 monocyte chemotactic protein-1, which attracts inflammatory monocytes to attach themselves to the endothelial cells. The leukocytes begin to adhere to the endothelial surface and then they begin to diapedese between endothelial cell junctions, where they enter the deeper intimal medial layers and accumulate lipids turning into vascular foam cells. Usually, atherosclerosis begins in the local vascular areas, where the greatest local flow disturbances occur, such as at the arterial bifurcating points.

Within the atherosclerotic plaques, the macrophage foam cells provide a rich source of proinflammatory and procoagulant factors (i.e., tissue factor [TF]). Thus, they contribute to the progression of atherothrombotic lesions. The subsequent evolution of the atheromatous plaque into more complex coronary artery lesions involves smooth muscle migration from the media into the intima. There, smooth muscle cells, produce extracellular matrix, replicate, and die by programmed cell death or apoptosis. With time, the plaque expands and begins to mineralize. As the plaque grows in size and volume, the artery remodels expanding outward in a process known as *positive remodeling*. Eventually, the pace of this arterial remodeling process fails to keep up with the ever-expanding atheromatous plaques, leading to the critical loss of the arterial lumen, thus leading to myocardial ischemia. Frequently, however, the atherosclerotic process, although silent for many decades, strikes without warning. The plaque can rupture suddenly, exposing its highly thrombogenic content to the circulating blood, thereby triggering instant arterial thrombosis. In many cases of ACS or myocardial infarction, no history exists of prior stable angina to precede the acute event.

Instead of slow, gradually progressive, predictable growth of atherosclerotic lesions, the cap of the plaque unexpectedly may develop cracks and fissures that precipitate the formation of nonocclusive arterial thrombi. These small thrombi may organize and accumulate on the top of the old lesion, further accelerating the lumen narrowing process. Usually, noncritical, 50% to 60% lesions, far outnumber the more advanced 80% to 90% focal lesions in a given coronary artery tree, which is why the lesser coronary artery stenoses cause more MI even though high-grade coronary artery stenosis has greater individual probability of causing ACS or MI (21–23).

Frequently, patients with diffuse atherosclerosis have multiple lesions throughout their vascular tree that are likely to rupture. These plaques, called *vulnerable plaques* are made up of a large lipid pool containing cholesterol and cellular debris, numerous macrophages, and foam cells with large amounts of TF. These vulnerable vascular plaques are covered by thin, fragile, and inflamed fibrous caps devoid of smooth muscle cells. When the inflamed cap of the vascular plaque ruptures, it releases intraluminally a large amount of highly thrombogenic procoagulants (i.e., TF or platelet-activating factors). When that occurs, rapid activation and degranulation of circulating platelets take place. Initially, platelets adhere to the injured wall binding to collagen and von Willebrand receptors. Then, rapid activation of numerous platelet surface IIb/IIIa receptors occurs, allowing platelets to "pile up" or to aggregate to form intravascular platelet thrombi. Activated IIb/IIIa surface platelet receptors bind fibrinogen to aggregate platelets forming small intra-arterial *white platelet thrombi.* Emerging occlusive or nonocclusive intra-arterial thrombi constitute a critical pathophysiologic mechanism of transition from chronic stable AP to the ACS (24–32).

CLINICAL MANIFESTATIONS

Historically, ischemia has been defined as tissue anemia (lack of red blood cells) caused by obstruction of arterial inflow, underscoring the importance of the abnormal supply component of the myocardial ischemic equation. Yet, myocardial ischemia reflects an imbalance between myocardial oxygen supply and demand, irrespective of any abnormality in coronary artery blood flow. Myocardial ischemia can result from hypoxemia (e.g., asphyxiation, carbon monoxide [CO] poisoning, severe anemia), even if coronary artery blood flow remains normal.

The oxygen demand component of the ischemic equation is predominantly determined by the HR, LV contractility, and the ventricular wall stress according to Laplace's law:

$$\text{Wall Stress} = \frac{\text{LV Pressure} \times \text{LV Radius}}{2\ (\text{Wall Thickness})}$$

This equation emphasizes two points: First, the larger the LV size, the greater its radius; therefore, the greater the wall stress. Second, at any LV radius, the greater the LV pressure, the greater the wall stress. An increased LV wall thickness, during the compensatory phase of LV hypertrophy, balances the increased LV pressure and the LV radius to reduce existing LV wall stress. A thickened LV wall, in turn, increases the total oxygen consumption of the heart (heart MV O_2). Occasionally, severe LV hypertrophy outstrips the ability of even normal coronary arteries to supply adequate quantities of blood, especially to the subendocardium where myocardial ischemia may develop.

When myocardial ischemia develops, it produces a typical cascade of clinical events beginning with metabolic alterations leading to impaired ventricular relaxation, diastolic dysfunction, impaired systolic function, ECG abnormalities, anginal pain, and, lastly, myocardial cell death (Fig. 5-4).

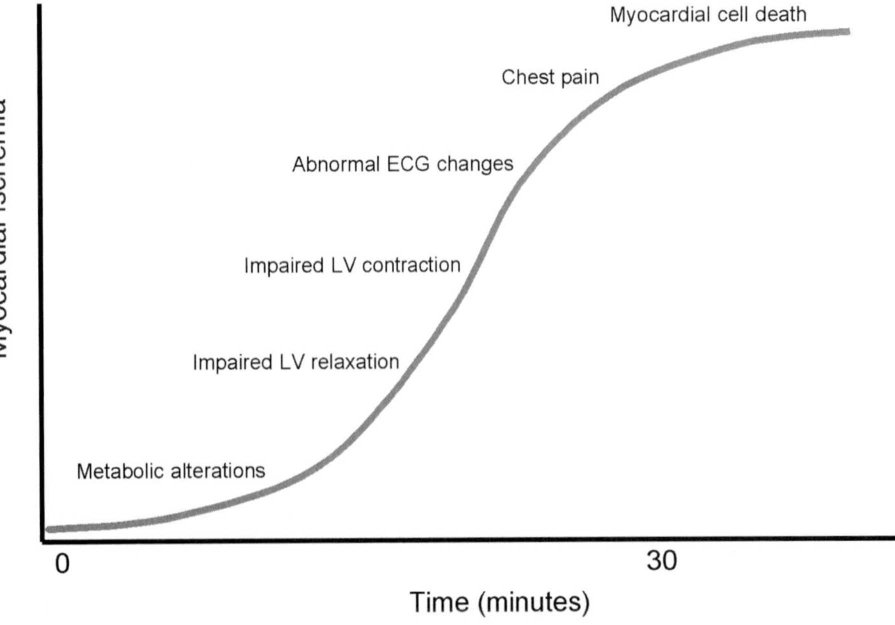

FIGURE 5-4. Illustrates myocardial ischemia time-dependent cascade of events starting with metabolic alteration at the onset of ischemia and ending with myocardial cell death.

MYOCARDIAL STUNNING

Severe acute myocardial ischemia can produce prolonged myocardial dysfunction known as *myocardial stunning*. The myocardium is still alive, but it fails to contract and appears dead (i.e., during MI, a stunned zone of myocardium surrounds the necrotic myocardium). The alive, but not contracting myocardium, will slowly begin to contract again after adequate reperfusion therapy. Improvement in LV function usually occurs gradually over the course of weeks and months.

MYOCARDIAL HYBERNATION

Chronic myocardial ischemia leads to impaired resting LV function also known as *myocardial hibernation*. During hibernation, the myocardial muscle reduces its contractility and its MV O_2 to match reduced perfusion and to preserve cellular viability. Hibernating myocardium is found in nearly one third of patients with chronic CAD and LV dysfunction. The impaired LV function will gradually improve in such patients after revascularization.

MYOCARDIAL NECROSIS

Myocardial necrosis or cell death results from unrelieved ischemia. The subendocardium is the most susceptible region to ischemic injury. Myocardial cell death starts deep in the subendocardium beginning as early as 15 to 20 minutes after complete coronary artery occlusion. The ensuing wave front of necrosis gradually progresses in a transmural direction toward the epicardium over the subsequent 4 to 6 hours. The recognition of this time-dependent progressive necrotic wave front constitutes the basis for timely reperfusion therapy during hyperacute MI (33–36).

Clinical presentations of myocardial ischemia include the following:

I. Chronic stable angina or variant angina pectoris (AP)
   Stable (AP) is characterized by deep, poorly localized chest pain or arm discomfort that is reproducibly associated with physical exertion or emotional stress, and relieved within 5 to 15 minutes by rest, administration of sublingual nitroglycerin (NTG), or both.

II. Acute coronary syndrome (ACS)
   A. Unstable angina pectoris
      Unstable AP is defined as AP or equivalent type of ischemic discomfort with at least one of three features:
      1. Occurring at rest or with minimal exertion, lasting at least 20 minutes
      2. Usually severe and described as a frank pain of recent onset, (i.e., within 1 month)
      3. Occurring with a crescendo pattern
   B. Non-ST-elevation MI (NSTMI)
      The NSTMI is present when cardiac enzymes are positive, indicating myocardial cell death. Yet, the ECG does not show ST segment elevation; rather, it usually shows ST-segment depression or nonspecific T-wave abnormalities. Patients may or may not have chest pain.

III. ST-ELEVATION MI (STMI)
   STMI is present when the ECG shows ST-segment elevation in at least two consecutive ECG leads and cardiac markers (i.e., CK–MB or troponins) are positive. Patients may present with or without chest discomfort.

DIAGNOSTIC APPROACH

Most patients who have chest pain do not necessarily have significant CAD. Differential diagnoses of chest pain, besides CAD, include noncardiac causes of chest pain, such as

A. Gastrointestinal disorders: Gastroesophageal reflux disease (GERD); esophageal motility disorders; biliary colic
B. Costosternal syndrome characterized by local chest wall pain and tenderness; other musculoskeletal disorders; cervical radiculopathies; compression of brachial plexus by cervical ribs; tendonitis or bursitis of the left shoulder
C. Aortic dissection
D. Severe pulmonary hypertension
E. Pulmonary embolus
F. Pericarditis

PHYSICAL EXAMINATION AND ANCILLARY EVALUATION

Most patients with significant CAD have normal or nearly normal physical examination findings.

Clinical testing of patients with CAD include the following:

1. Blood tests: Fasting total cholesterol; low-density lipoprotein (LDL); triglycerides (TG); high-density lipoprotein (HDL); lipoprotein a [Lp(a)]; apolipoprotein [Apo(B)]; small dense LDL; glycated hemoglobin (HbA1 C); and high sensitivity C-reactive protein, especially for patients with intermediate cardiovascular risk
   For patients presenting with ACS, resting ECG changes, or resting chest pain, blood tests for cardiac markers are recommended.
2. ECG
3. Stress test
   The stress test may identify patients at high cardiovascular risk who need cardiac catheterization. Stress test parameters associated with high cardiovascular risk and multivessel CAD include the following:
   a. Exercise duration <5 metabolic equivalents (MET)
   b. Failure to increase systolic BP >120 mm Hg, sustained decrease in systolic BP >10 mm Hg, or sustained decrease in systolic BP below rest level
   c. Abnormal ST-segment: Depression >2 mm; downsloping ST-segment; starting <5 METS; involving more than five leads; persisting for more than 5 minutes.
   d. Abnormal ST-elevation
   e. Abnormal symptoms of chest pain at short (<5 minutes) exercise level
   f. Abnormal arrhythmia: Sustained ventricular tachycardia >30 seconds (37).
4. Computed tomography (CT), including 64-slice CT scan, can detect coronary artery calcifications with high (90%) sensitivity. Finding coronary artery calcifications is an accurate marker of coronary atherosclerosis. The specificity of this finding for identifying patients with significant obstructive CAD is low, however. The utility of 64-slice CT scan as a diagnostic tool to assess the severity of CAD remains investigational.

Medical history and diagnostic testing are used to identify patients with moderate to severe CAD. It is especially important to identify those patients at high risk who have >3% annual mortality rate.

The high risk group includes patients with severe LV dysfunction (LV ejection factor [EF] ≤35%), high risk treadmill score, stress-induced large perfusion defect or multiple perfusion defects of moderate size, large fixed perfusion defect with LV dilatation or lung uptake of thallium 201 during stress test, or ECG wall motion abnormality involving more than two LV wall segments.

The intermediate risk group (1% to 3% expected annual mortality rate) include patients who have mild or moderate LV dysfunction (LVEF 35% to 50%), intermediate risk treadmill, stress-induced moderate defect or limited stress echo—ischemia.

The low cardiovascular risk group (≤1% annual mortality rate) include patients who have low risk treadmill score, normal or small myocardial perfusion defect, or normal stress echocardiography.

Regardless of severity of symptoms, patients with high risk, noninvasive test results have a high likelihood of CAD, and should have coronary arteriography and coronary revascularization, if needed.

In contrast, patients with exercise test results that are clearly negative for CAD, regardless of symptoms, have an excellent prognosis. Such patients usually do not need coronary arteriography.

Although clinical examination and noninvasive testing are extremely valuable in establishing the diagnoses of CAD, currently, the precise assessment of the severity of CAD requires cardiac catheterization (38).

TREATMENT OF ATHEROTHROMBOTIC CORNARY ARTERY DISEASE

Comprehensive management of patients with CAD is based of five principles:

1. Identification and treatment of associated diseases precipitating angina
2. Reduction of cardiovascular risk factors
3. Dietary and lifestyle modification
4. Pharmacologic therapy
   - Therapies proved to reduce mortality and morbidity in patients with chronic stable CAD and normal LV include statins, antiplatelet agents, such as aspirin and clopidogrel, and angiotensin-converting enzyme (ACE) inhibitors.
   - Other therapies, such as nitrates, β-blockers, and calcium-channel blockers, have been shown to improve symptoms.
5. Revascularization therapy in the form of percutaneous coronary interventions or coronary bypass surgery is reserved for patients in the higher cardiovascular risk group not responding to medical therapy.

Treatment to block the activation of the surface IIb/IIIa platelet receptors constitutes the primary mode of antiplatelet therapy to prevent atherothrombotic complications. The aggregation of activated platelets is inhibited, if not stopped, by blocking the platelet surface active glycoprotein Gp IIb/IIIa receptors. Gp IIb/IIIa intravenous antagonists belong to one of the following classes:

1. Monoclonal antibody against Gp IIb/IIIa receptor: abciximab (ReoPro)
2. Peptidomimetic antagonist: eptifibatide (Integrilin)
3. Nonpeptidomimetic antagonist: tirofiban (Aggrastat)

Because Gp IIa/IIIb antagonists do not block thromboxane (TXA_2) production by activated platelets, concomitant use of aspirin enhances their antithrombotic efficacy. These drugs are currently available to treat patients with ACS at high risk ACS during coronary angioplasty procedure or to treat patients during elective coronary angioplasty procedures.

Antiplatelet agents, such as aspirin, clopidogrel, low-dose aspirin in combination with modified release dipyridamole (Aggrenox), and cilostazol inhibit the intermediate platelet activation steps and, as such, are expected to be less potent, if they were to block either the initial (adhesion) or final (aggregation) points of the platelet activation process. After initial adhesion, platelets bind several specific agonists to activate intracellular pathways (e.g., adenosine diphosphate [ADP] release, TXA_2 synthesis) that act in concert to induce the final step of platelets aggregation. Pharmacologic interruption of only one of these intermediate steps (e.g., with aspirin, clopidogrel, or antithrombins) may permit platelet activation through alternative, uninhibited pathways.

Aspirin, through its free acetyl groups, irreversibly acetylates cyclooxygenase (COX) leading to its irreversible inactivation. Inactive COX cannot catalyze the oxygenation of arachidonic acid to prostaglandin G_2, thereby blocking the formation of TXA_2. The inhibitory effects of aspirin on platelet (TXA_2) is rapid, occurring within 15 to 30 minutes. Aspirin also inhibits COX in vascular endothelial cells, leading to the suppression of endothelium-derived prostacyclin (PGI_2).

Clopidogrel and ticlopidine, both thienopyridine derivatives, inhibit ADP-induced platelet aggregation.

Phosphodiesterase inhibitors, such as dipyridamole, do not prolong the bleeding time or inhibit platelet aggregation.

Cilostazol, a quinolone derivative and a potent inhibitor of platelet phosphodiesterase-3 with vasodilatory effects, is used to treat intermittent claudication in patients with peripheral vascular disease (PVD).

Two classes of anticoagulants are available: Indirect thrombin inhibitors such as heparin, and direct thrombin inhibitors, such as bivalirudin (Angiomax or Hirulog).

Anticoagulants are used to block active thrombin in its free and clot-bound form. Heparin interacts with antithrombin, preventing antithrombin from binding to thrombin. When antithrombin binds to thrombin, it neutralizes thrombin as well as other activated clotting factors. Standard unfractionated heparin has equal inhibitory power to block thrombin, factor II and factor X_a.

Low molecular weight heparins (LMWH) are manufactured from unfractionated heparin by the fractionation of heparin to smaller fragments of about one third the size of standard heparin. Shorter heparin chains selectively inhibit only factor X_a in the coagulation cascade. Therefore, LMWH have more antithrombotic properties and have little or no anticoagulant or antithrombin properties, because LMWH do not bind thrombin (27).

Warfarin is the most frequently used oral anticoagulant, exerting its anticoagulant actions as a vitamin K antagonist. Warfarin has no direct role in treating coronary artery thrombotic events caused by atherothrombosis. Its primary role is in the prevention of stroke in patients with atrial fibrillation.

The thrombolytic–fibrinolytic drugs, streptokinase, urokinase, and tPA, convert plasminogen to plasmin. Plasmin indiscriminately lyses both fibrin and fibrinogen, thereby enhancing the tendency toward systemic bleeding. Fibrinolytic agents are currently used to treat patients with hyperacute MI when angioplasty cannot be accomplished (28–32).

Percutaneous coronary angioplasty or open heart surgery is reserved for patients who remain symptomatic, despite maximal medical therapy, or for those who have the clinical features of high cardiovascular risks of morbidity and mortality.

CLINICAL RECOMMENDATIONS OF THE VIGNETTE

The patient described in the vignette had had an extensive MI. He developed a large LV aneurysm and most likely had recurrent episodes of cardiac arrhythmias (A-Fib). CAD and cerebrovascular disease often coexist because they share same cardiovascular risks and often the same pathophysiology. Most probably, our patient had had a cardioembolic ischemic stroke. Stroke affects approximately 15 million people worldwide. It is the third leading cause of death in most industrialized nations and the leading cause of long-term disability among adults. Ischemic strokes account for approximately 85% of all strokes. We believe the embolus most likely originated either in the LA appendage (A-Fib) or in the LV aneurysm. Nearly 50% of all systemic emboli arising from the heart lodge in the brain and predominately involve the middle cerebral artery territory. It is less likely that the patient had an atheroembolic stroke arising from the right internal carotid artery. The patient, however, presented too late into his stroke to quality for thrombolytic treatment. His case was managed with medical therapy and an extensive diagnostic search was made to identify the source of his presumptive cardioembolic brain infarct. When a high embolic risk cardiac source such as atrial fibrillation is identified, careful anticoagulation to prevent further recurrences of stroke should be considered unless contraindicated.

SUMMARY

Atherosclerosis is a diffuse systemic vascular disorder affecting the heart and also the brain and peripheral arteries. Presenting clinical symptoms result from local tissue ischemia, progressive arterial lumen loss, arterial inflammation, and arterial thrombosis. All these factors play a pivotal role in the pathogenesis of coronary syndromes and ischemic strokes. Diagnostic evaluation of ischemic stroke requires a complete cardiovascular evaluation and comprehensive review and modification of all cardiovascular risk factors. Treatment plans must be based on the recognition that atherothrombosis is a systemic and progressive vascular disorder.

REFERENCES

1. American Heart Association. Heart Disease and Stroke Statistics—2006 Update. Dallas: American Heart Association; 2006.
2. Spaan JAE. *Coronary Blood Flow: Mechanics, Distribution, and Control.* Dordrecht, Netherlands: Kluwer; 1991.
3. Chilian WM. Coronary microcirculation in health and disease: Summary of an NHLBI workshop. *Circulation.* 1997;95:522–528.
4. Braunwald E. Myocardial oxygen consumption: The quest for its determinants and some clinical fallout. *J Am Coll Cardiol.*. 2000;35:45B.
5. Pijls NHJ, De Bruyne B. *Coronary Pressure.* Dordrecht, Netherlands: Kluwer; 1997:12–13.
6. Yada T, Richmond KN, Van Bibber R, et al. Role of adenosine in local metabolic coronary vasodilation. *Am J Physiol.* 1999;276:H1425–H1433.
7. Siebes M, Campbell CS, D'Argenio DZ. Fluid dynamics of a partially collapsible stenosis in a flow model of the coronary circulation. *ASME J Biomech Eng.* 1996;118:489–497.
8. Kern M. Curriculum in interventional cardiology: Coronary pressure and flow measurements in the cardiac catheterization laboratory. *Cathet Cardiovasc Intervent.* 2002; 54:378–400.
9. Baumgart D, Haude M, Liu F, et al. Current concepts of coronary flow reserve for clinical decision making during cardiac catheterization. *Am Heart J.* 1998;136:136–149.
10. Akasaka T, Yoshida K, Hozumi T, et al. Retinopathy identifies marked restriction of coronary flow reserve in patients with diabetes mellitus. *J Am Coll Cardiol.* 1997;30:935–941.
11. Kloner RA, Bolli R, Marban E, et al. Medical and cellular implications of stunning, hibernation, and preconditioning: An NHLBI workshop. *Circulation.* 1998;97:1848–1867.
12. Bolli R, Marban E. Molecular and cellular mechanisms of myocardial stunning. *Physiol Rev.* 1999;79:609–634.
13. Gerber BL, Wijns W, Vanoverschelde JL, et al. Myocardial perfusion and oxygen consumption in reperfused noninfarcted dysfunctional myocardium after unstable angina: Direct evidence for myocardial stunning in humans. *J Am Coll Cardiol.* 1999;34:1939–1946.
14. Elsasser A, Schlepper M, Klovekorn WP, et al. Hibernating myocardium: An incomplete adaptation to ischemia. *Circulation.* 1997;96:2920–2931.
15. Bogaert J, Maes A, Van de Werf F, et al. Functional recovery of subepicardial myocardial tissue in transmural myocardial infarction after successful reperfusion: An important contribution to the improvement of regional and global left ventricular function. *Circulation.* 1999;99:36–43.
16. Jennings RB, Steenbergen C, Jr., Reimer KA. Myocardial ischemia and reperfusion. *Monographs in Pathology.* 1995;37:47–80.
17. Libby P, Aikawa M, Schonbeck U. Cholesterol and atherosclerosis. *Biochim Biophys Acta.* 2000;1529:299.
18. Gimbrone MA, Jr., Nagel T, Topper JN. Biomechanical activation: An emerging paradigm in endothelial adhesion biology. *J Clin Invest.* 1997;100:S61.
19. Pasterkamp G, de Kleijn DP, Borst C. Arterial remodeling in atherosclerosis, restenosis and after alteration of blood flow: Potential mechanisms and clinical implications. *Cardiovasc Res.* 2000;45:843.
20. Rong JX, Rangaswamy S, Shen L, et al. Arterial injury by cholesterol oxidation products causes endothelial dysfunction and arterial wall cholesterol accumulation. *Arterioscler Thromb Vasc Biol.* 1998;18:1885.
21. Iiyama K, Hajra L, Iiyama M, et al. Patterns of vascular cell adhesion molecule-1 and intercellular adhesion molecule-1 expression in rabbit and mouse atherosclerotic lesions and at sites predisposed to lesion formation. *Circ Res.* 1999;85:199.
22. Cybulski MI, Iiyama K, Li H, et al. A major role for VCAM-1, but not ICAM-1, in early atherosclerosis. *J Clin Invest.* 107:1255.
23. Luster AD. Chemokines: Chemotactic cytokines that mediate inflammation. *N Engl J Med.* 1998;338:436.
24. Nakamura T, Kambayashi J, Okuma M. Activation of the Gp IIb/IIIa complex induced by platelet adhesion to collagen is mediated by both alpha$_2$–beta$_1$ integrin and Gp VI. *J Biol Chem.* 1999;274:11897.
25. Ruggeri ZM. Platelets in atherothrombosis. *Nat Med.* 2002;8:1227.
26. Mann KG, Butenas S, Brummel K. The dynamics of thrombin formation. *Arterioscler Thromb Vasc Biol.* 2003;23:17.
27. Hirsh J, Warkentin TE, Shaughnessy S, et al. Heparin and low-molecular-weight heparin: Mechanisms of action, pharmacokinetics, dosing, monitoring, efficacy and safety. *Chest,* 2001;119:64S.
28. Bennett JS, Mousa S. Platelet function inhibitors in the year 2000. *Thromb Haemost.* 2001;85:395.
29. Bennett JS. Novel platelet inhibitors. *Annu Rev Med.* 2001;52:161.
30. Mehta P. Aspirin in the prophylaxis of coronary artery disease. *Curr Opin Cardiol.* 2002;17:552.
31. Schafer AI. Effects of nonsteroidal anti-inflammatory therapy on platelets. *Am J Med.* 1999;106:25S.
32. Kloner RA, Bolli R, Marban E, et al. Medical and cellular implications of stunning, hibernation, and preconditioning: An NHLBI workshop. *Circulation.* 1998;97:1848–1867.
33. Gerber BL, Wijns W, Vanoverschelde JL, et al. Myocardial perfusion and oxygen consumption in reperfused noninfarcted dysfunctional myocardium after unstable angina: Direct evidence for myocardial stunning in humans. *J Am Coll Cardiol.* 1999;34:1939–1946.
34. Elsasser A, Schlepper M, Klovekorn WP, et al. Hibernating myocardium: An incomplete adaptation to ischemia. *Circulation.* 1997;96:2920–2931.
35. Jennings RB, Steenbergen C, Jr., Reimer KA. Myocardial ischemia and reperfusion. *Monographs in Pathology.* 1995;37:47–80.
36. Gibbons RJ, Balady GJ, Bricker JT, et al. ACC/AHA 2002 guideline update for exercise testing-summary article: A report of the American College of Cardiology/American Heart Association Task Force on Practice Guidelines (Committee to Update the 1997 Exercise Testing Guidelines). *Circulation.* 2002;106:1883–1892.
37. Gibbons RJ, Abrams J, Chatterjee K, et al. ACC/AHA 2002 guideline update for the management of patients with chronic stable angina: A report of the American College of Cardiology/American Heart Association Task Force on Practice Guidelines (Committee to Update the 1999 Guidelines for the Management of Patients with Chronic Stable Angina), 2002. (Available at www.acc.org/clinical/guidelines/stable/stable.pdf).

CHAPTER **6**

Heart Failure

Candice K. Sech • Alain Heroux • José Biller

OBJECTIVES

- To define the syndrome and classification of heart failure
- To discuss the pathophysiology and clinical manifestations of heart failure
- To discuss the diagnostic approach to heart failure
- To discuss the current treatment recommendations
- To discuss neurologic complications that can be seen in patients with heart failure

CASE VIGNETTE

A 55-year-old man with a long-standing history of uncontrolled arterial hypertension presents to the emergency department with acute onset of right-sided weakness and difficulty speaking. On examination, blood pressure is 180/100 mm Hg. Neurologic examination demonstrates a nonfluent aphasia and right hemiparesis. Cardiac examination is remarkable for an irregularly, irregular rhythm and systolic murmur consistent with mitral regurgitation. Computed tomography (CT) of the head shows an area of decreased attenuation on the left frontoparietal cortex. Electrocardiogram (ECG) shows atrial fibrillation, evidence of left ventricular hypertrophy (LVH), and left atrial enlargement. On further questioning, the patient states he has had gradual worsening of dyspnea on exertion for the last 6 months. A transthoracic echocardiogram (TTE) shows left atrial enlargement, left ventricular hypertrophy, an ejection fraction of 30%, and a transesophageal echocardiogram (TEE) demonstrates a left atrial thrombus.

DEFINITION

The understanding of heart failure (HF) has undergone much evolution since the 5th century BC, when initially ascribed to the passage of excess phlegm from the brain into the chest (cold humor). Description of the circulation by William Harvey in the 17th century, along with clinicopathologic correlation by astute physicians, eventually led to the discovery of a hemodynamic explanation of HF (1). Currently, HF is most concisely defined as a complex clinical syndrome resulting from either a structural or functional cardiac disease impairing the heart's capacity to eject blood at a rate appropriate for metabolizing tissue, or does so at an abnormally elevated ventricular diastolic pressure. This definition, however, does not emphasize the likely summation of anatomic, functional, and biologic alterations that contribute to the syndrome of HF, nor its progressive nature.

EPIDEMIOLOGY

HF is an important and growing public health problem in the United States. Approximately 550,000 new cases are diagnosed each year, and an estimated 5 million people in the United States have HF (2). It occurs both in men and women of all age groups, and by age 40, the lifetime risk of developing HF for both men and women is one in five (3). The prevalence of HF in patients aged 55 to 64 years is 6.2% for men, and 3.4% for women, and nears 10% in both sexes for those 75 years or older (4). In 2003, the prevalence of HF in white, African American, and Mexican-American men was 2.5%, 3.1%, and 2.7%, respectively, and 1.9%, 3.5%, and 1.6% in women (3). From 1990 to 2004, hospitalizations have increased from approximately 810,000 to 1.1 million with HF as a primary diagnosis (5). HF accounts for 12 to 15 million office visits and 6.5 million hospital days each year (6). The number of deaths attributed to HF has continued to increase, despite medical and device-based advances in treatment, with nearly 58,000 patients dying of HF as a primary cause in 2003. From 1993 to 2003, deaths attributed to HF increased 20.5%, with the all-cause death rate declining 2% during that same period (3). Some suggest this paradox exists because of improved treatment of patients with coronary artery disease (CAD) earlier in life (7).

A study looking at trends in survival of patients in the Framingham Heart study found that the 5-year mortality rate in patients diagnosed with HF was 59% in men, and 45% in women (8). Trends in the survival of patients with HF in a community-based study found that 5-year mortality rate in those patients with HF was 50% in men, and 46% in women (9).

HF is an expensive disease to treat, with an estimated direct cost of $25.6 billion in the United States for the year 2006 (2). An admission for HF costs approximately $5,500 per hospitalization, and the number of discharges from hospitals of patients with this diagnosis has nearly doubled from 1982 to 2002. HF is also the most common Medicare hospital discharge diagnosis, and more Medicare dollars are spent for the diagnosis and treatment of HF than for any other diagnosis (10).

CLASSIFICATION AND STAGING

Several classifications of HF exist. This chapter focuses on left ventricular HF. One classification distinguishes HF with systolic dysfunction and HF with preserved systolic function, also referred to as *diastolic dysfunction*. Systolic and diastolic dysfunctions are not mutually exclusive, and most patients with systolic dysfunction will exhibit evidence of both. Systolic dysfunction refers to a decreased LV ejection fraction, and resultant elevated left ventricular end diastolic pressures (LVEDP). HF with preserved systolic function refers to a left ventricle that is *stiff* or unable to relax fully to allow adequate filling, and the development of elevated LVEDP. Most patients with HF with preserved systolic function have nonobstructive LVH and a history of arterial hypertension. Less frequent causes of HF with preserved systolic function include hypertrophic obstructive cardiomyopathy (HCM), idiopathic restrictive cardiomyopathy, and infiltrative cardiomyopathies (amyloidosis, hemochromatosis). HF with preserved systolic function accounts for half of all patients with HF. Advanced age and female sex are associated more frequently with HF with preserved systolic function (11,12). Guidelines on the treatment of patients with HF with preserved systolic function are not well defined, because most clinical trials have exclusively included patients with systolic dysfunction. A recent study done at the Mayo Clinic looked at approximately 5,000 admissions for HF, and found that the average prevalence of HF with preserved systolic function has increased from 38% to 54% over the 15-year study period, again emphasizing the importance of future research in this area (13).

Another classification includes the four stages involved in the development of. These stages have been defined to aid clinicians in the recognition of HF risk factors and emphasize stage-focused treatment; they are presented in the 2005 American College of Cardiology/American Heart Association Heart Failure guidelines (ACC/AHA) (Table 6-1). The staging classification is an objective aid for the clinician to recognize the established risk factors for HF, and to focus on prevention before left ventricular (LV) dysfunction and HF symptoms develop. Patients in stage A are at high risk for HF, but without structural heart disease or symptoms of HF (e.g., hypertension, atherosclerotic disease, diabetes, obesity, metabolic syndrome, or other known risks). Unlike stage A, patients in stage B have structural heart disease, but lack signs or symptoms of HF (e.g., previous myocardial infarction [MI], asymptomatic valvular disease). Stage C includes patients with structural heart disease, with prior or current symptoms of HF. Patients in stage D have marked symptoms, despite maximal medical therapy, and are often referred to as having *refractory HF*. This staging classifica-

TABLE 6-1. Stages of Heart Failure Development

At Risk for Heart Failure *Heart Failure*

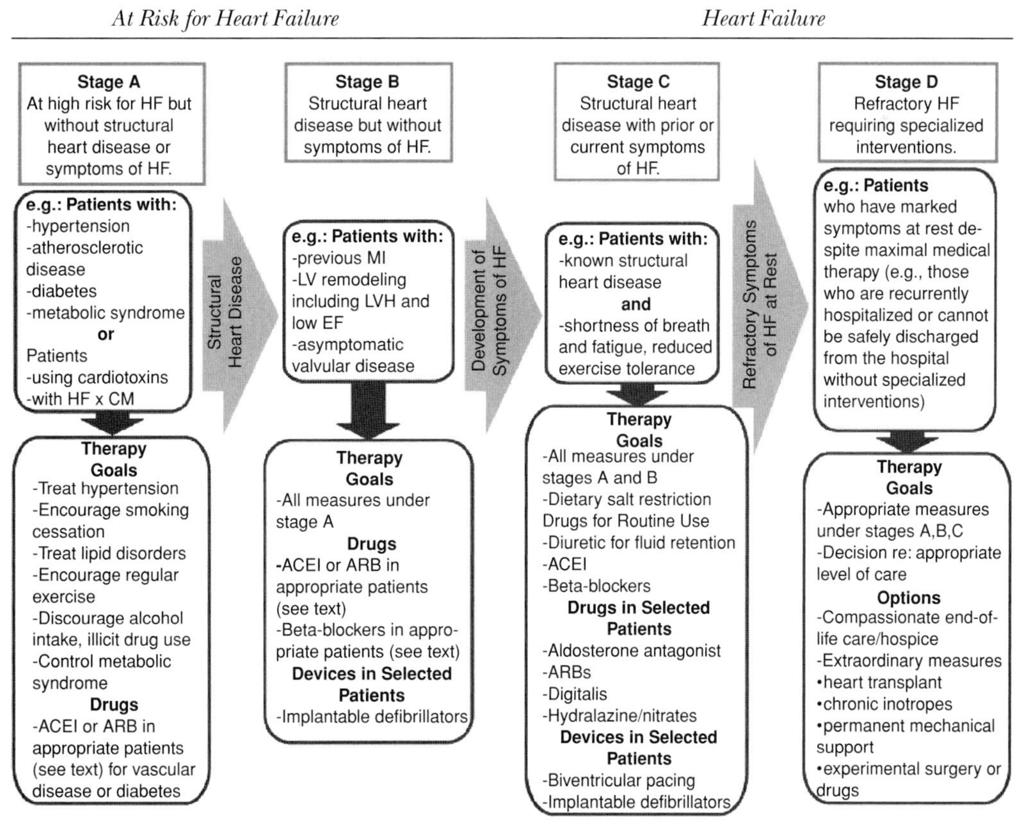

From Hunt SA, Abraham WT, Chin MH, et al. ACC/AHA 2005 Guideline Update for the Diagnosis and Management of Chronic HF: A report of the ACC/AHA Task Force on Practice Guidelines (Writing Committee to Update the 2001 Guidelines for the Evaluation and Management of HF). American College of Cardiology Website. Available at: http://www.acc.org/clinical/statements.htm. *J Am Coll Cardiol.* 2005;46:1116–1143, with permission.

TABLE 6-2. New York Heart Association (NYHA) Classification of Heart Failure (HF)

Class I	Patients with cardiac disease but without resulting limitation of physical activity. Ordinary physical activity does not cause undue fatigue, palpitations, dyspnea, or anginal pain
Class II	Patients with cardiac disease resulting in slight limitation of physical activity. They are comfortable at rest. Ordinary physical activity results in fatigue, palpitations, dyspnea or anginal pain
Class III	Patients with cardiac disease resulting in marked limitation of physical activity. They are comfortable at rest. Less than ordinary activity causes fatigue, palpitations, dyspnea, or anginal pain
Class IV	Patients with cardiac disease resulting in inability to carry on any physical activity without discomfort. Symptoms of HF or the anginal syndrome may be present even at rest. If any physical activity is undertaken, discomfort is increased.

(From The Criteria Committee of the New York Heart Association: *Nomenclature and Criteria for Diagnosis of Diseases of the Heart and Great Vessels*, 9th ed. Boston: Little, Brown; 1994, with permission.)

TABLE 6-3. Primary Cardiomyopathies

Genetic
HCM (hypertrophic cardiomyopathy)
AVRC/D (arrhythmogenic right ventricular cardiomyopathy
LVNC (left ventricular concompaction cardiomyopathy)
Glycogen storage diseases
Mitochondrial myopathies
Conduction defects
Ion channel defects
Mixed
Dilated cardiomyopathy (DCM)
Restrictive (non-hypertrophied and nondilated)
Acquired
Stress provoked
Inflammatory
Peripartum
Tachycardia induced

(Adapted from Maron BJ, Towbin JA, Thiene G, et al. Contemporary definitions and classification of the cardiomyopathies. *Circulation.* 2006;113:1807–1816, with permission).

tion divides patients by those that are *at risk* of HF (stage A and B), and those *with* HF (stage C and D). These staging guidelines should not be confused with the New York Heart Association (NYHA) classes, a subjective classification used to determine functional status (Table 6-2). Whereas the patient can fluctuate among different NYHA classes, depending on degree of compensation and disease progression, succession through the stages in the development of HF is expected with the natural progression of it.

ETIOLOGY AND PRECIPITANTS OF HEART FAILURE

The most common cause of HF no longer is valvular heart disease or hypertension (HTN), as in the past, but CAD (14). About 22% of men and 46% of women will develop HF within 6 years of having a heart attack (2,15). CAD, which is thought to be the underlying cause of HF in about two thirds of patients with systolic dysfunction, contributes to the progression of HF (16). Factors in CAD that lead to HF include LV remodeling after MI, with eventual development of chamber dilatation and neurohormonal activation and ischemia of viable myocardium with resultant transient LV dysfunction.

The etiologic classification of HF has become somewhat complex as the understanding of the genetics involved has evolved. The AHA expert consensus panel agreed on the following definition for cardiomyopathy:

> Cardiomyopathies are a heterogeneous group of diseases of the myocardium associated with mechanical and/or electrical dysfunction that usually (but not invariably) exhibit inappropriate ventricular hypertrophy or dilatation and are due to a variety of causes that frequently are genetic. Cardiomyopathies either are confined to the heart or are part of generalized systemic disorders, often leading to cardiovascular death or progressive HF–related disability (17).

Nonischemic cardiomyopathies can be divided into primary (genetic, nongenetic, acquired), which affect solely the myocardium, and secondary, which have evidence of pathologic involvement of the myocardium as part of a systemic disease (Tables 6-3 and 6-4). Frequently, the cause of HF cannot be identified, and the term *idiopathic dilated cardiomyopathy* (IDCM) is used. Perhaps, in the future, the etiology of IDCM will be better understood when genetics or viral causes are better defined.

Several noncardiac drugs can exacerbate symptoms of HF and cause cardiomyopathy by various mechanisms. Medications that are known to be cardiotoxic include anticancer agents (anthracyclines, such as doxorubicin, cyclophosphamide, fluorouracil, trastuzumab, capecitabine, mitoxantrone), immunomodulating agents (infliximab, interleukin-2, etanercept, interferon-α_2), clozapine, and amphotericin B. Some commonly used medications known to exacerbate symptoms of HF by various mechanisms include the thiazolidinedione class of antihyperglycemic agents (rosiglitazone, pioglitazone and troglitazone), appetite suppressants (fenfluramine, dexfenfluramine), nonsteroidal anti-inflammatory drugs (NSAID), medications used in migraine treatment (ergotamines, methylsergide, phentermine), medications used in treatment of neurologic disorders (cabergoline, pergolide), antifungal agents (itraconazole, amphotericin B), and cyclooxygenase (COX)-2 inhibitors (18).

Several cardiac medications are known to precipitate and worsen HF, including negative inotropes, such as diltiazem and verapamil, and antiarrhythmics, such as propafenone.

PATHOPHYSIOLOGY AND DISEASE PROGRESSION

HF initially was viewed in terms of a *cardiorenal* model, and seen as an edematous state resulting from excessive salt and water, with therapy directed at reducing the edema. As time progressed, clinicians turned focus to the hemodynamic assessment of patients with HF and determined that reduced cardiac output and peripheral vasoconstriction were apparent. This became known as the *hemodynamic* model of HF, and focused on the abnormal pumping function of the heart. Both the cardiorenal and hemodynamic models of HF became the basis for treatment with diuretics and inotropes to control the volume status and augment cardiac output, respectively.

TABLE 6-4. Secondary Cardiomyopathies

Infiltrative	**Storage**
Amyloidosis	Fabry's disease
Gaucher disease	Glycogen storage disease (type II, Pompe)
Hurler disease	Niemann-Pick disease
Hunter disease	
Toxicity	**Endomyocardial**
Drugs, heavy metals, chemical agents	Endomyocardial fibrosis
	Hypereosinophilic syndrome (Loeffler's endocarditis)
Neuromuscular/neurological	**Endocrine**
Friedreich ataxia	Diabetes mellitus
Duchenne-Becker muscular dystrophy	Hyperthyroidism
Emery-Dreifuss muscular dystrophy	Hypothyroidism
Myotonic dystrophy	Hyperparathyroidism
Neurofibromatosis	Pheochromocytoma
Tuberous sclerosis complex	Acromegaly
Inflammatory (granulomatous)	**Cardiofacial**
Sarcoidosis	Noonan syndrome
	Lentiginosis
Autoimmune/collagen	**Consequence of cancer therapy**
Systemic lupus erythematosus (SLE)	Anthracyclines: doxorubicin (adriamycin) daunorubicin
Dermatomyositis	Cyclophosphamide
Rheumatoid arthritis	Radiation
Scleroderma	
Nutritional deficiencies	**Electrolyte imbalances**
Beriberi, pellagra, scurvy, selenium carnitine, kwashiorkor	
Polyarteritis nodosa (PAN)	

(From Maron BJ, Towbin JA, Thiene G, et al. Contemporary definitions and classification of the cardiomyopathies. *Circulation.* 2006;113:1807–1816, with permission.)

Treatment based on either of these models, however, was not sufficient to halt the continued progression of HF (19).

More recently, a *neurohormonal* model has been developed as a link between the cardiorenal and hemodynamic models of HF. In the neurohormonal model, several factors, including angiotensin II, endothelin, aldosterone, vasopressin, various cytokines, and norepinephrine, are believed to play a role in the progression of HF. Some of these factors contribute to LV remodeling, and may have deleterious effects on both the heart and circulation. Remodeling has been defined as the "genome expression, molecular, cellular, and interstitial changes that are manifested clinically as changes in size, shape, and function of the heart after cardiac injury" (20). Simply stated, the diseased heart undergoes compensatory hypertrophy, dilatation, or both in response to various stimuli, changing from the normal elliptical shape, to a more spherical shape. These changes are associated with increased hemodynamic stress on the heart walls, decreased performance, and mitral regurgitation. Remodeling usually precedes the development of symptoms by months or years, and continues after symptoms develop (21). Treatment, to be discussed below, focuses on blocking these neurohormones, in an attempt to prevent the progression of HF and reverse LV remodeling. More recent studies have suggested, however, that neurohormone blockade alone may not be sufficient to prevent further progression of HF, suggesting that other factors may be involved.

SPECIAL POPULATIONS

Women make up a large proportion of patients with HF, and a large percentage of patients with HF with preserved systolic function are elderly women. Although treatment of HF is the same in women and men, most large trials have not included sufficient women to make conclusions about treatment for their HF. The Digitalis Investigation Group (DIG) trial evaluated the use of digoxin in patients with systolic HF, and found that its use reduced symptoms and decreased hospitalizations in all patients. Increased mortality rate was found among women, however (22). More recent retrospective analysis of the DIG trial data found that no significant increase in mortality rate was found among women with lower serum digoxin levels, but was increased in those with higher digoxin concentrations (23).

HF is common among African Americans, affecting 3% of that population. African American patients are more likely to have HF resulting from hypertension, rather than CAD, as do their white counterparts. HF with preserved systolic function also occurs commonly in African Americans. Very limited data exist regarding the etiologic differences and natural history of HF in African Americans. The African American HF Trial (A-HeFT) found that the addition of a fixed-dose combination of hydralazine and isosorbide dinitrate, in addition to standard therapy, improves survival in NYHA class III/IV patients (24).

CLINICAL MANIFESTATIONS OF HEART FAILURE

The diagnosis of HF is clinical. The initial evaluation should focus on the history and physical examination. Ancillary investigations, chest x-ray studies, or an echocardiogram can confirm the bedside diagnosis, and be used in determining disease severity or prognosis. The Framingham criteria for the diagnosis of HF, which focuses on the clinical presentation, can help guide the diagnosis (Table 6-5).

TABLE 6-5. Framingham Criteria for Diagnosis of Heart Failure[a]

Major Criteria	*Minor Criteria*	*Major or Minor Criteria*
Paroxysmal nocturnal dyspnea (PND) or orthopnea	Ankle edema, night cough, dyspnea on exertion	Weight loss >4.5 kg in 5 days in response to treatment
Neck-vein distension	Hepatomegaly	
Rales	Pleural effusion	
Cardiomegaly	Vital capacity decreased 50% from maximal capacity	
Acute pulmonary edema	Tachycardia (>120/min)	
S_3 gallop		
Increased venous pressure >6 cm H_20		
Circulation time >25 sec		
Hepatojugular reflux		

[a]Diagnosis: two major, or one major and two minor criteria.
(From McKee PA, Castelli WP, McNamara PM, et al. The natural history of congestive heart failure: The Framingham Study. *N Engl J Med.* 1971;285(26):1441–1446, with permission.)

Symptoms of HF include shortness of breath and fatigue occurring at rest or on exertion. Patients can have a range of presentations, from gradual worsening in exercise tolerance, to acute shortness of breath consistent with pulmonary edema. Obviously, several other etiologic causes could explain such presentations, and questions and further testing should be directed to differentiate between pulmonary and cardiac causes of shortness of breath. When diagnosis is uncertain, serum levels of B-type natriuretic peptide (BNP) can be considered in patients with dyspnea and symptoms of HF.

Atypical presentations of HF can be seen, with symptoms initially attributed to noncardiac causes. For example, tender hepatomegaly can initially be attributed to gallbladder disease. Nonspecific gastrointestinal complaints, such as early satiety, can predominate the clinical picture of advanced HF. Elderly patients may present with somnolence. HF-related encephalopathy, because of low cardiac output, can be confused with *metabolic encephalopathy*. Cognitive impairments resulting from HF can result in forgetfulness, poor disease understanding by patients, and ultimately, poor treatment compliance (25,26). Additionally, studies have shown that cognitive impairment is common among patients with HF and seems to be causally related to disease severity (27). On rare occasion, some patients with HF present with stroke as the first manifestation of long-standing disease (case vignette).

Patients with HF should have their volume status evaluated at initial and follow-up examinations. Prior studies evaluating the usefulness of the bedside cardiac examination in the diagnosis of HF found that jugular venous distension at rest, or inducible by the hepatojugular reflex, had the highest sensitivity and specificity on clinical examination for identifying hypervolemia (28). Patients with peripheral edema can be considered to have volume overload. Noncardiac causes should be considered also, however. Peripheral edema in patients with HF tends to accumulate in dependant areas first. Thus, in ambulatory patients, fluid will first accumulate in the lower extremities, although anasarca may be seen in advanced disease. It should be noted, that most patients with chronic HF do not have rales or pulmonary edema, which generally reflects the rapidity of HF onset, rather than the degree of volume overload. The absence of pulmonary edema is postulated to result from the development of increased lymphatic drainage of pulmonary alveolar fluid. Clinical evidence of hypoperfusion (e.g., cool extremities, narrow pulse pressure, altered mentation, resting tachycardia, and disproportionate elevation of blood urea nitrogen [BUN] relative to serum creatinine, or frank worsening of BUN and serum creatinine levels) can develop when cardiac output declines. Cardiac examination may demonstrate an S_3, indicative of elevated filling pressures. Other examination findings consistent with increased volume include an enlarged, pulsatile liver.

Once the clinical diagnosis of HF is made, patients should have a two-dimensional echocardiogram (2-D echo) with Doppler to determine the LV ejection fraction (LVEF), systolic and diastolic LV dimension, and presence of valvular abnormalities. The 2-D echo is the single most useful diagnostic test for the evaluation of patients with HF. It is common for patients to have more than one cardiac abnormality contributing to the development of HF, and echocardiographic evaluation may identify several cardiac abnormalities.

DIAGNOSTIC APPROACH

Diagnosis of HF can be approached by addressing its initiating cause, as well as recognizing precipitating factors. Once the patient is diagnosed with HF, the predisposing cause should be determined. Disorders commonly associated include arterial hypertension, CAD, diabetes mellitus, tachyarrhythmias and valvular heart disease, all of which must be further investigated with appropriate diagnostic testing, and aggressively treated when appropriate. Recognition of the precipitating cause of acute HF, as well as avoidance of these factors, can assist in prevention of decompensated HF. It is important to realize that several precipitating causes can coincide. Inappropriate reduction of therapy by the patient or physician, as well as dietary sodium and fluid indiscretions, and failure to monitor fluid intake, are all major factors contributing to HF decompensation. A study evaluating acute precipitants of HF found that dietary sodium indiscretion was the leading cause of worsening HF (29). In appropriate settings, cardiac ischemia or infarction and cardiac arrhythmias are common precipitating causes as well. For example, atrial fibrillation or atrial flutter in a patient with underlying CAD can increase oxygen demands and precipitate HF. Avoid the use of cardiac depressant drugs and medications or toxins known to precipitate or worsen HF. Other important precipitants of HF include systemic infections, pulmonary embolism, and physical, emotional or environmental stress.

Cessation of behaviors that can increase the risk of HF, such as cigarette smoking, alcohol consumption, and use of cocaine, amphetamines, and other illicit drugs should not be overlooked. Also, history of therapeutic drugs or interventions, such as ionizing radiation to the mediastinum, and use of medications known to cause cardiomyopathy should be carefully sought.

The usefulness of endomyocardial biopsy in patients with cardiomyopathy of unknown cause is not clear. Biopsies from patients with nonischemic cardiomyopathy show nonspecific changes, and it has not been established how endomyocardial biopsy findings affect patient management. Current ACC/AHA guidelines do not recommend routine endomyocardial biopsy in the evaluation of patients with HF.

TREATMENT

Treatment for HF, as discussed below, is summarized from the 2005 ACC/AHA guidelines, and focuses on the treatment at the different developmental stages of HF. As in the diagnosis of HF, clinicians should first consider the patient's risk factors, the underlying cause of the disease, and the precipitating factors. Continued reassessment of cardiac function and treatment adjustments are important.

STAGE A

Treatment of patients in stage A HF focuses on the management of risk factors known to contribute to its development. Appropriate treatment of hypertension, diabetes, hyperlipidemia, and CAD, according to current guidelines, is important in the prevention and treatment of HF. Additionally, patients should be counseled on risk factors that can increase the risk of HF, such as cigarette smoking, excessive use of alcohol, and use of cocaine, amphetamines, and other illicit drugs. If the patient is found to have a supraventricular tachyarrhythmia, ventricular rate should be controlled, or sinus rhythm restored to prevent induced-induced cardiomyopathy.

STAGE B

In addition to the above, treatment of patients in stage B focuses on prevention of further remodeling of the heart and reducing the risk of additional myocardial injury. Preventative management of risk factors, as described above for patients who are stage A, should be continued, and medications known to prevent further progression of remodeling should be used.

Both beta-blockers and angiotensin-converting enzyme inhibitors (ACEI) have been shown to decrease mortality in patients with HF, and should be titrated to doses used in clinical studies (Table 6-6). Angiotensin II receptor blockers (ARB) can be used in patients intolerant to ACEI. Valve replacement and coronary revascularization should be recommended in appropriate candidates, according to current guidelines.

TABLE 6-6. Inhibitors of the Renin-Angiotensin-Aldosterone System and Beta-Blockers Commonly Used for the Treatment of Heart Failure

Drug	*Initial Daily Dose*	*Maximum Dose*
ACE inhibitors		
Captopril	6.25 mg 3 times	50 mg 3 times
Enalapril	2.5 mg twice	10 to 20 mg twice
Fosinopril	5 to 10 mg once	40 mg once
Lisinopril	2.5 to 5 mg once	20 to 40 mg once
Perindopril	2 mg once	8 to 16 mg twice
Quinapril	5 mg twice	20 mg twice
Ramipril	1.25 to 2.5 mg once	10 mg once
Trandolapril	1 mg once	4 mg once
ARBs		
Candesartan	4 to 8 mg once	32 mg once
Losartan	25 to 50 mg once	50 to 100 mg once
Valsartan	20 to 40 mg twice	160 mg twice
Aldosterone antagonists		
Spironolactone	12.5 to 25 mg once	25 mg once or twice
Eplerenone	25 mg once	50 mg once
Beta-blockers		
Bisoprolol	1.25 mg once	10 mg once
Carvedilol	3.125 mg twice	25 mg twice 50 mg twice for weight >85 kg
Metoprolol succinate	12.5 to 25 mg once	200 mg once

ACE, angiotension-converting enzyme; ARBs, angiotensin II receptor blockers.
(From Hunt SA, Abraham WT, Chin MH, et al. ACC/AHA 2005 Guideline Update for the Diagnosis and Management of Chronic HF: A report of the ACC/AHA Task Force on Practice Guidelines (Writing Committee to Update the 2001 Guidelines for the Evaluation and Management of HF). American College of Cardiology Website. Available at: http://www.acc.org/clinical/statements.htm. *J Am Coll Cardiol.* 2005;46:1116–1143, with permission.)

STAGE C

Stage C continues to focus on treatment of risk factors, prevention of further cardiac remodeling, and neurohormonal blockade, with the addition of symptomatic treatment. Again, medications known to decrease mortality in HF should be used. Specifically, ACEI, beta-blockers, and aldosterone antagonists are recommended for all stable patients with current or prior symptoms of HF, unless contraindicated. ACEI and beta-blockers shown in clinical trials to reduce mortality should be used (Table 6-7). Patients on aldosterone antagonists should have their serum potassium levels monitored closely, especially while taking an ACEI, or if suspicion of underlying renal dysfunction exists. Digitalis can be considered, and it has been shown to improve symptoms and reduce the need for hospitalizations. Digoxin, however, has not been shown to decrease mortality, and higher serum digoxin levels were associated with increased mortality in women. Anticoagulation with warfarin for low ejection fraction (EF) is controversial; currently, studies are underway to determine its potential value. Also, attempts to maintain euvolemia with use of diuretics and patient monitoring of sodium and fluid intake, is important. The Candesartan in HF: Assessment of Reduction in Mortality and Morbidity (CHARM) trial found that the addition of the ARB candesartan, in NYHA class II-IV, in addition to standard medical therapy, had decreased mortality caused by cardiovascular deaths or nonfatal MI (30).

TABLE 6-7. Medications Used in the Treatment in Stages of Development of Heart Failure (HF)

Drug	*Stage A*	*Stage B*	*Stage C*
ACE Inhibitors			
Benazepril	H	—	—
Captopril	H, DN	Post MI	HF
Enalapril	H, DN	HF	HF
Fosinopril	H	—	HF
Lisinopril	H, DN	Post MI	HF
Moexipril	H	—	—
Perindopril	H, CV risk	—	—
Quinapril	H	—	HF
Ramipril	H, CV risk	Post MI	Post MI
Trandolapril	H	Post MI	Post MI
ARBs			
Candesartan	H	—	HF
Eprosartan	H	—	—
Irbesartan	H, DN	—	—
Losartan	H, DN	CV risk	—
Olmesartan	H	—	—
Telmisartan	H	—	—
Valsartan	H, DN	Post MI	Post MI, HF
Aldosterone Antagonists			
Eplerenone	H	Post MI	Post MI
Spironolactone	H	—	HF
Beta blockers			
Acebutolol	H	—	—
Atenolol	H	Post MI	—
Betaxolol	H	—	—
Bisoprolol	H	—	HF
Carteolol	H	—	—
Carvedilol	H	Post MI	HF, Post MI
Labetalol	H	—	—
Metoprolol succinate	H	—	HF
Metoprolol tartarate	H	Post MI	—
Nadolol	H	—	—
Penbutolol	H	—	—
Pindolol	H	—	—
Propranolol	H	Post MI	—
Timolol	H	Post MI	—
Cardiac glycoside			
Digoxin	—	—	HF

ACE, angiotensin-converting enzyme; ARBs, angiotensin II receptor blockers. Cardiovascular (CV) risk indicates reduction in future cardiovascular events; DN, diabetic nephropathy; H, hypertension; HF, heart failure and asymptomatic LV dysfunction; post MI, reduction in HF or other cardiac events following MI.

(From Hunt SA, Abraham WT, Chin MH, et al. ACC/AHA 2005 Guideline Update for the Diagnosis and Management of Chronic Heart Failure: a report of the ACC/AHA Task Force on Practice Guidelines (Writing Committee to Update the 2001 Guidelines for the Evaluation and Management of Heart Failure). American College of Cardiology, with permission.)

STAGE D

Patients in stage D are considered to have end-stage HF, refractory to treatment. Meticulous control of fluid retention is recommended in patients in stage D. Referral of potentially eligible patients for cardiac transplantation or to a program with expertise in management of end-stage HF is recommended. Consideration of a LV assist device (LVAD) as permanent or "destination" therapy is reasonable in highly selected patients with estimated 1-year mortality over 50% with medical therapy. Sufficient emphasis cannot be placed on end-of-life discussions with patients in end-stage HF.

TREATMENT OF HEART FAILURE WITH PRESERVED SYSTOLIC FUNCTION

Guidelines for treatment of HF with preserved systolic function are not well defined. The goal is meticulous blood pressure control and maintenance of euvolemia. Overdiuresis should be avoided, however, because patients with HF with preserved systolic function rely on elevated preload to maintain cardiac output, and hence, are very sensitive to preload reduction. Patients with HF with preserved systolic function rely on atrial contraction for LV filling.

DEVICE-BASED AND SURGICAL TREATMENTS

The risk of sudden cardiac death (SCD) from ventricular arrhythmias is increased in patients with HF compared with the general population. The Multicenter Automatic Defibrillator Implantation Trial (MADIT), published in 1991, randomized patients with known CAD, nonsustained ventricular tachycardia (NSVT), and an EF ≤35%, to an implantable cardioverto defibrillator (ICD) group, versus conventional therapy (74% amiodarone). The study found a 54% reduction in mortality in the defibrillator group as compared with the group on standard therapy (31). The Multicenter Automatic Defibrillator Implantation Trial II (MADIT-II) was similar, except that inclusion criteria did not include a history of NSVT, and EF ≤30%. MADIT-II was stopped early after reaching the prespecified efficacy boundary, and found a 31% reduction in risk of death in patients post-MI compared with the group on standard therapy alone. Placement of an ICD is reasonable in patients with ischemic cardiomyopathy, at least 40 days post-MI, who have an EF ≤30%, who are on optimal medical treatment, and with a reasonable expectation for survival (32).

The Sudden Cardiac Death in Heart Failure Trial (SCD-Heft) compared the use of amiodarone to placement of an ICD in HF with NYHA class II/III, and LVEF ≤35%. The ICD reduced overall mortality by 23% (33). Similarly, the multicenter, randomized Defibrillators in Non-Ischemic Cardiomyopathy Treatment Evaluation (DEFINITE) trial found that implantation of an ICD significantly reduced the risk of death from arrhythmias in patients with EF ≤35%, nonischemic dilated cardiomyopathy, and treated with ACE-I and beta-blockers (34,35).

Almost 15% to 30% of patients with HF have an intraventricular conduction delay that causes the ventricles to contract in an asynchronous fashion. Ventricular dyssynchrony causes suboptimal ventricular filling and greater severity of mitral regurgitation, and has been associated with increased death rate in patients with HF. A specific type of pacemaker, called a bi-ventricular (Bi-V) pacemaker, can re-coordinate ventricular contraction by pacing both ventricles simultaneously. The re-coordination of ventricular contraction provided by Bi-V pacemakers is known as *cardiac resynchronization therapy* (CRT). The Comparison of Medical Therapy, Pacing, and Defibrillation in Heart Failure (COMPANION) trial, compared patients on optimal medical therapy with NYHA class III/IV, EF ≤35%, both ischemic and nonischemic, with QRS >120 milliseconds and PR >150 milliseconds, to receive either a cardiac resynchronization therapy pacemaker (CRT-P) or a cardiac resynchronization therapy defibrillator (CRT-D). Both the CRT-P and CRT-D, in combination with optimal medical therapy, reduced the risk of all-cause mortality or first hospitalization by 19% and 20%, respectively, versus optimal medical therapy alone. One third of deaths in the CRT-P group were sudden, suggesting the benefit of adding an implantable cardiac defibrillator to CRT (36). Additionally, the Cardiac Resynchronization-Heart Failure (CARE-HF) trial found that CRT reverses ventricular remodeling and improves myocardial performance progressively for at least 18 months, and also reduces symptoms and improves the quality of life (37). Current indications for CRT include patients with symptomatic HF (NYHA III or IV) despite optimal medical therapy, with a prolonged QRS duration (>120 milliseconds), and LVEF ≤35%. Indications for CRT are evolving, and may be expanded as other categories of patients found to benefit are identified.

Several surgical approaches have emerged, and may be potentially useful for treatment of ischemic HF. Most target reduction of mitral regurgitation, and restoration of a more normal LV geometry. The surgical ventricular restoration (SVR) procedure has been studied for reshaping the LV and excluding areas with asynergy, and has been shown to improve both LV function and functional status for patients with advanced HF (38,39). The Dor procedure removes akinetic or dyskinetic portions of the septum and anterior wall, reshapes the LV, and uses a patch to re-establish ventricular wall continuity (40).

Several wrapping devices that resist further ventricular dilatation, which may potentially improve performance, are undergoing clinical studies.

NEUROLOGIC COMPLICATIONS SEEN IN PATIENTS WITH HEART FAILURE

Cerebrovascular events are common among patients with HF. Review of several large HF trials show that the rate of clinically obvious stroke in patients with HF is about 2% per year (41). This number is believed to be an underestimate, because many cerebral infarctions may go unnoticed clinically, manifesting only as cognitive impairment. Sudden death is also more likely to occur among patients with HF with cerebrovascular events. Sympathetic activation and provoked arrhythmias, with resultant myocardial ischemia, may explain the increased numbers of sudden death in this population of patients.

In patients with sinus rhythm and decreased EF, LV thrombus can form because of generalized hypokinesis, or because of prior MI with resultant aneurysm. TTE can identify LV thrombus, with or without the use of contrast. In patients with atrial fibrillation, thrombus forms most commonly in the left atrial (LA) appendage, and TEE is the test of choice for diagnosis of a LA clot. Anticoagulation remains important therapy in prevention of embolic cerebrovascular events, and patients with documented intraatrial or intraventricular thrombus, should be evaluated for anticoagulation treatment.

Hemorrhagic strokes can also occur in patients with HF, possibly as a result of use of warfarin in patients with atrial fibrillation, left ventricular or atrial thrombus, and more controversially, in patients with low EF.

CLINICAL RECOMMENDATIONS OF THE VIGNETTE

Our vignette illustrates the presentation of an embolic brain infarct in a patient with previously undiagnosed HF. The patient also had atrial fibrillation and evidence of structural heart disease on ECG and echocardiogram (LVH, left atrial enlargement). The source of the embolus in a patient with atrial fibrillation is most commonly thrombus in the LA. If this patient had prior undiagnosed MI with apical aneurysm, thrombus could have formed in the aneurysm.

At presentation, the patient had no signs or symptoms of acute HF. On questioning, however, symptoms possibly attributable to HF were present. Patients with HF with systolic dysfunction eventually will undergo LV remodeling with dilatation. The resulting mitral regurgitation can lead to elevated left atrial pressures and may eventually develop left atrial enlargement. The increased left atrial pressure can increase the risk of atrial fibrillation. Atrial fibrillation, which is the most common supraventricular arrhythmia in HF, occurring in 15% to 30% of patients, is known to be a poor prognostic indicator (42–44). Nonvalvular atrial fibrillation is an independent risk factor for stroke, increasing the risk about fivefold (45).

The patient presented in the vignette is considered stage C, and stage-appropriate treatments would include medications that decrease mortality (beta-blocker, ACEI, aldosterone antagonist), diuretics to maintain euvolemia, and device therapy, if indicated after additional studies. Restoration of normal sinus rhythm should be considered in this patient, according to current treatment of atrial fibrillation or flutter. If normal sinus rhythm cannot be maintained, rate control should be maintained to augment ventricular filling.

SUMMARY

HF is a complex clinical syndrome resulting from multiple causes, and it affects a large proportion of the population. Diagnosis and management of HF should always involve consideration of its underlying cause, as well as precipitating causes. Adverse cardiac remodeling has been found to be associated with increased mortality, and medications used to target various neurohormones involved in LV remodeling are used in the treatment of HF. Other nonpharmacologic treatments, including ICD and CRT, are beneficial because they decrease sudden cardiac death and improved functional status in patients with HF. Stroke is the most severe neurologic complication of HF and atrial fibrillation, because these cardiac conditions are associated with intracardiac thrombi. Anticoagulation is the main therapy in preventing embolic strokes.

REFERENCES

1. Katz AM. Evolving concept of HF: Cooling furnace, malfunctioning pump, enlarging muscle—Part I. *J Card Fail.* 1997;3(4):319–334.
2. American Heart Association. *Heart Disease and Stroke Facts, 2006.* Dallas, TX: American Heart Association; 2006.
3. Lloyd-Jones DM, Larson MG, Leip EP, et al. for the Framingham Heart Study. Lifetime risk for developing congestive HF: The Framingham Heart Study. *Circulation.* 2002;106:3068–3072.
4. CDC/NCHS, http://www.cdc.gov; and NHLBI, http://www.nhlbi.nih.gov.
5. National Hospital Discharge Summary, http://www.cdc.gov/nchs.
6. O'Connell JB, Bristow MR. Economic impact of HF in the United States: Time for a different approach. *J Heart Lung Transplant.* 1994;13:S107–S112.
7. *American Heart Association Heart Disease and Stroke Statistics: 2005 Update.* Dallas, TX: American Heart Association; 2005.
8. Levy D, Kenchaiah S, Larson MG, et al. Long-term trends in the incidence of and survival with HF. *N Engl J Med.* 2002;347(18):1397–1402.
9. Roger VL, Weston SA, Redfield MM, et al. Trends in HF incidence and survival in a community-based population. *JAMA.* 2004;292:344–350.
10. Massie BM, Shah NB. Evolving trends in the epidemiologic factors of HF: Rationale for preventative strategies and comprehensive disease management. *Am Heart J.* 1997;133:703–712.
11. Vasan RS, Larson MG, Benjamin EJ, et al. Congestive HF in subjects with normal versus reduced left ventricular ejection fraction: Prevalence and mortality in a population-based cohort. *J Am Coll Cardiol.* 1999;33:1948–1955.
12. Kitzman DW, Gardin JM, Gottdiener JS, et al. Importance of HF with preserved systolic function in patients ≥ 65 years of age. CHS Research Group. Cardiovascular Health Study. *Am J Cardiol.* 2001;87:413–419.
13. Owan TE, Hodge DO, Herges RM, et al. Trends in prevalence and outcome of HF with preserved ejection fraction. *N Engl J Med.* 2006;355(3):251–259.
14. Bourassa MG, Gurne O, Bangdiwala SI, et al. Natural history and patterns of current practice in HF. *J Am Coll Cardiol.* 1993;22[Suppl A]:14A–19A.
15. *National Heart, Lung and Blood Institute, Disease and Conditions Index, HF.* Bethesda, MD.
16. Gheorghiade M, Bonow RO. Chronic HF in the United States: A manifestation of coronary artery disease. *Circulation.* 1998;97:282–289.
17. Maron BJ, Towbin JA, Thiene G, et al. Contemporary definitions and classification of the cardiomyopathies. *Circulation.* 2006;113:1807–1816.
18. Slordal L, Spigset O. HF induced by non-cardiac drugs. *Drug Saf.* 2006;29(7):567–586.
19. Mann DL. *Heart Failure. A Companion to Braunwald's Heart Disease.* Philadelphia: WB Saunders; 2004.
20. Cohn JN, Ferrari R, Sharpe N. Cardiac remodeling—Concepts and clinical implications: A consensus paper from an international forum on cardiac remodeling. Behalf of an International Forum on Cardiac Remodeling. *J Am Coll Cardiol.* 2000;35(3):569–582.
21. Hunt SA, Abraham WT, Chin MH, et al. ACC/AHA 2005 Guideline Update for the Diagnosis and Management of Chronic HF: A report of the ACC/AHA Task Force on Practice Guidelines (Writing Committee to Update the 2001 Guidelines for the Evaluation and Management of HF). American College of Cardiology Website. Available at: http://www.acc.org/clinical/statements.htm. *J Am Coll Cardiol.* 2005;46:1116–1143.
22. The effect of digoxin on mortality and morbidity in patients with HF. The Digitalis Investigation Group. *N Eng J Med.* 1997;336(8):525–533.
23. Adams KF Jr, Patterson JH, Gattis WA, et al. Relationship of serum digoxin concentration to mortality and morbidity in women in the digitalis investigation group trial: A retrospective analysis. *J Am Coll Cardiol.* 2005;46(3):497–504.
24. Taylor AL, Ziesche S, Yancy C, et al. African-American HF Investigators. Combination of isosorbide dinitrate and hydralazine in blacks with HF. *N Engl J Med.* 2004;351(20):2049–2057.
25. Wolfe R, Worrall-Carter L, Foister K, et al. Assessment of cognitive function in HF patients. European Journal of Cardiovascular Nursing. 2006;5(2):158–164.
26. Almeida OP, Flicker L. The mind of a failing heart: A systematic review of the association between congestive HF and cognitive functioning. *Intern Med J.* 2001;31(5):290–295.
27. Trojano L, Antonelli Incalzi R, Acanfora D, et al; Congestive HF Italian Study Investigators. Cognitive impairment: A key feature of congestive HF in the elderly. *J Neurol.* 2003;250(12):1456–1463.
28. Butman SM, Ewy GA, Standen JR, et al. Bedside cardiovascular examination in patients with severe, chronic HF: Importance of rest or inducible jugular venous distension. *J Am Coll Cardiol.* 1993 Oct;22(4):968–974.
29. Tsuyuki RT, McKelvie RS, Arnold JM, et al. Acute precipitants of congestive HF exacerbations. *Arch Intern Med.* 2001;161(19):2337–2342.
30. Demers C, McMurray JJ, Swedberg K, et al.; CHARM Investigators. Impact of candesartan on nonfatal myocardial infarction and cardiovascular death in patients with HF. *JAMA.* 2005;294(14):1794–1798.
31. Moss AJ, Hall WJ, Cannom DS et al. Improved survival with an implanted defibrillator in patients with coronary disease at high risk for ventricular arrhythmia. Multicenter Automatic Defibrillator Implantation Trial Investigators. *N Engl J Med.* 1996;335:1933–1940.
32. Moss AJ, Zareba W, Hall WJ, et al, for the Multicenter Automatic Defibrillator Implantation Trial II Investigators. Prophylactic implantation of a defibrillator in patients with myocardial infarction and reduced ejection fraction. *N Engl J Med.* 2002;346:877–883.
33. Bardy GH, Lee KL, Mark DB, et al. Sudden Cardiac Death in Heart Failure (SCD-HeFT) Investigators. Amiodarone or an implantable cardioverter-defibrillator for congestive heart failure. *N Engl J Med.* 2005;352(3):225–237.
34. Kadish A, Dyer A, Daubert JP, et al. Defibrillators in Non-Ischemic Cardiomyopathy Treatment Evaluation (DEFINITE) Investigators. Prophylactic defibrillator implantation in patients with nonischemic dilated cardiomyopathy. *N Engl J Med.* 2004;350(21):2151–2158.
35. Schaechter A, Kadish AH. Defibrillators in non-ischemic cardiomyopathy treatment evaluation. DEFibrillators in Non-Ischemic Cardiomyopathy Treatment Evaluation (DEFINITE). *Card Electrophysiol Rev.* 2003;7(4):457–462.
36. Bristow MR, Saxon LA, Boehmer J, et al. Cardiac resynchronization therapy with or without an implantable defibrillator in advanced chronic heart failure. *N Engl J Med.* 2004;350:2140–2150.

37. Cleland JG, Daubert JC, Erdmann E, et al. Cardiac Resynchronization-Heart Failure (CARE-HF) Study Investigators. The effect of cardiac resynchronization on morbidity and mortality in heart failure. *N Engl J Med.* 2005;352(15):1539–1549.
38. Patel ND, Barreiro CJ, Williams JA, et al. Surgical ventricular remodeling for patients with clinically advanced congestive HF and severe left ventricular dysfunction. *J Heart Lung Transplant.* 2005;24(12):2202–2210.
39. Athanasuleas CL, Buckberg GD, Stanley AW, et al. RESTORE Group. Surgical ventricular restoration: The RESTORE group experience. *Heart Fail Rev.* 2004;9(4):287–297.
40. Dor V, Saab M, Coste P, et al. Left ventricular aneurysm: A new surgical approach. *Thorac Cardiovasc Surg.* 1989;1:11–19.
41. Cleland JGF. Anticoagulant and antiplatelet therapy in HF. *Curr Opinion Cardiol.* 1997;12:276–287.
42. Middlekauff HR, Stevenson WG, Stevenson LW. Prognostic significance of atrial fibrillation in advanced HF: A study of 390 patients. *Circulation.* 1991;84:40.
43. Stevenson WG, Stevenson LW, Middlekauff HR, et al. Improving survival for patients with atrial fibrillation and advanced HF. *J Am Coll Cardiol.* 1996;28:1458.
44. Carson PE, Johnson GR, Dunkman WB, et al. The influence of atrial fibrillation on prognosis in mild to moderate HF. The V-HeFT Studies. The V-HeFT VA Cooperative Studies Group. *Circulation.* 1993;87:VI102.
45. Wolf PA, Abbott RD, Kannel WB. Atrial fibrillation as an independent risk factor for stroke: The Framingham study. *Stroke.* 1991;22:983–988.
46. The Criteria Committee of the New York Heart Association. *Nomenclature and Criteria for Diagnosis of Diseases of the Heart and Great Vessels,* 9th ed. Boston: Little, Brown; 1994.
47. McKee PA, Castelli WP, McNamara PM, et al. The natural history of congestive heart failure: The Framingham Study. *N Engl J Med.* 1971;285(26):1441–1446.

CHAPTER **7**

Cardiomyopathies and Other Myocardial Diseases

Amytis Towfighi • Latisha K. Ali • Alain Heroux • Jeffrey L. Saver

OBJECTIVES

- To describe the presentation, diagnosis, and management of neurologic manifestations of structural cardiomyopathies in clinical practice
- To highlight that cardioembolism, syncope, and presyncope can signal the presence of structural heart disease
- To survey the neurologic features of the following specific cardiomyopathies: Hypertrophic cardiomyopathy, arrhythmogenic right ventricular cardiomyopathy, restrictive cardiomyopathy, myocarditis, and Chagasic cardiomyopathy

CASE VIGNETTE

A 58-year-old man presents with sudden onset of right hemiparesis. On examination, his heart rate is 155 beats per minute and blood pressure is 120/70 mm Hg. Cardiac examination reveals an irregularly irregular rhythm. Neurologic examination shows diminished hearing in the right ear, and right face, arm, and leg weakness. Magnetic resonance discloses a left pontine infarction. Atrial fibrillation with rapid ventricular response is demonstrated on electrocardiogram (ECG). Transthoracic echocardiogram shows symmetric left and right ventricular hypertrophy, and an estimated ejection fraction of 40%. Laboratory analysis is notable for normal creatinine level, elevated urine protein, and elevated urine microalbumin.

His medical history dates back to the age of 10 years, when he developed pain in his hands and feet, often triggered by cold weather. He also developed postprandial diarrhea. In his twenties, he noticed that he did not sweat, even after running marathons. At age 32, he had an episode of vertigo and hearing loss. At age 45, he presented to his primary care physician with flulike symptoms and was documented to be in atrial fibrillation. Over the years, he has had 26 cardioversions and 4 radiofrequency ablations without success in maintaining sinus rhythm. He currently takes only warfarin. Family history is remarkable for a brother with a history of strokes in his forties, a cousin with a diagnosis of Fabry disease, and two daughters with decreased sweating. Given the patient's presentation and family history, Fabry disease was suspected and laboratory analysis confirmed α-galactosidase deficiency.

Hypertrophic Cardiomyopathy

DEFINITION

Hypertrophic cardiomyopathy (HCM), previously referred to as *idiopathic hypertrophic subaortic stenosis* or *muscular subaortic stenosis*, is a unique cardiomyopathy of diastolic dysfunction where inappropriate myocardial hypertrophy occurs in the absence of an obvious cause for hypertrophy (1).

EPIDEMIOLOGY

The prevalence of unexplained left ventricular hypertrophy (LVH) is 1 in 500 patients in the general population. HCM may account for up to 60% of unexplained LVH and is the most common genetic cardiovascular disorder (2). The disorder has a variable presentation; some children with HCM are completely asymptomatic, whereas others have a high incidence of sudden death. Most commonly identified in adults in their fourth and fifth decades, HCM has an annual mortality rate of 1% to 3% (3). In children, the risk of sudden death is much higher at 6% (3,4). HCM is the leading cause of sudden cardiac death during exertion in adolescent children (3). The incidence of cerebral and system embolism is 0.4% to 2.4% yearly (5).

ETIOLOGY AND PATHOGENESIS

HCM was described over 100 years ago and remains a complex disease. It may be inherited as an autosomal dominant trait or sporadic and is caused by sarcomere mutations (6). HCM can also mimic other diseases, such as hypertensive heart disease and, rarely, cardiac amyloidosis. The prevalence of systemic hypertension can be as high as 30% in patients with HCM and it can be difficult to determine if the hypertrophy is primary or is caused by the hypertension (7). Metabolic cardiomyopathies, identified as part of the spectrum of Danon disease (LAMP-2 gene) and Noonan syndrome are new causes of inherited HCM (2).

Syncope and cardioembolic infarction are the most common neurologic manifestations of HCM. Presyncope and syncope reflect transient global cerebral ischemia arising from ventricular outflow tract obstruction, supraventricular tachyarrhythmias, or both (8). Strokes are primarily related to the supraventricular tachyarrhythmias, which are found in up to one half of patients (8,9). Atrial fibrillation (AF) is the most common sustained rhythm, more common with older age, and occurring in 25% of patients (10,11). AF predisposes to embolic stroke by promoting clot precipitation in static or slowly moving blood within the atrium, especially within the left atrial appendage. An additional cause of cardioembolic stroke in HCM is myocardial infarction and segmental wall dyskinesis. Myocardial infarction in HCM is caused by various factors, such as small intramural coronary arteries, increased oxygen demand, and elevated filling pressures with subendocardial ischemia (1).

Ventricular tachycardia or fibrillation results in sudden death (4). The generation of ventricular tachyarrhythmias is related to left atrial enlargement and fibrosis developing in the context of chronically elevated filling pressures as a consequence of obstruction, diastolic dysfunction, or mitral valve dysfunction. Depending on its duration, ventricular fibrillation can cause irreversible anoxic-ischemic brain damage (12).

PATHOLOGY

The disease is characterized macroscopically by myocardial hypertrophy, which can be asymmetric or symmetric (13). It typically involves the left ventricle (LV) more than the right and, in most patients, the interventricular septum and the anterolateral wall are more involved than the posterior segment of the free wall of the LV (13). The atria may also be dilated and are often hypertrophied. Although any region of the LV can be involved, when the hypertrophy involves the interventricular septum, it can result in the distinctive feature of an obstruction in the LV outflow tract.

CLINICAL MANIFESTATIONS

Although the first manifestation of HCM may be sudden cardiac death (1,13), typically, patients with HCM are asymptomatic or have mild complaints, such as fatigue, dizziness, presyncope, syncope, palpitations, paroxysmal nocturnal dyspnea, and congestive heart failure. Presyncope and syncope, reflecting global cerebral ischemia, can be preceded by nonspecific premonitory symptoms such as paresthesias, lightheadedness, palpitations, and a graying-out of vision. Syncope is associated with pallor and loss of muscle tone, but prolonged ischemia results in tonic posturing, sometimes accompanied by irregular jerking movements that resemble seizures. In elderly patients, syncope can present simply as unexplained falls (14). Paroxysmal episodes of AF often cause rapid clinical deterioration by reducing diastolic filling and cardiac output, usually as a consequence of the high ventricular rate. Cardioembolic cerebral infarctions tend to be abrupt and maximal at onset, with symptoms dependent on the neurologic functions supported by the recipient cerebral artery (15).

The physical examination is usually normal in asymptomatic patients or in those with mild disease. Patients who are symptomatic, however, may have a laterally displaced apical precordial impulse, a prominent presystolic impulse, and occasionally, a triple apical beat. A hallmark finding of HCM associated with an outflow gradient is a harsh systolic crescendo-decrescendo murmur heard best at the apex or left sternal border (1,16).

DIAGNOSTIC APPROACH

In the patient presenting with syncope or cardioembolic stroke, clues to underlying HCM will generally come from the history, including a detailed family history, physical examination, and echocardiography. A chest roentgenogram will have variable findings, ranging from normal to marked cardiac cardiomegaly (17). Two-dimensional transthoracic echocardiography detects almost all cases and quantifies morphologic features. The classic finding of LVH usually involves the septum and anterolateral free wall (13). The appearance of an outflow tract obstruction, hypercontractility, and systolic function can also be determined on echocardiogram (16,17). Treadmill or bicycle testing may expose arrhythmias not present at rest, but continuous ambulatory monitoring is better at detecting repetitive ventricular arrhythmias. Cardiac magnetic resonance imaging (MRI) may also be useful in identifying patients with HCM, and can distinguish between different causes of hypertrophy. In addition, in gadolinium-enhanced MRI, a pattern of hyperenhancement may be seen, perhaps reflecting the myocardial disarray or fibrosis. This is clinically useful because patients with this pattern can be at higher risk for premature death. In patients with syncope and presyncope, cardiac telemetry may disclose an underlying dysrhythmia. An early decrease in cardiac output is noted on tilt table testing in patients with HCM and a history of syncope (18). Genetic testing can be specific and allow for accurate diagnosis in certain populations; however, a negative analysis does not exclude a genetic origin (2).

TREATMENT

Patients with cardioembolic stroke are treated acutely with recanalization therapies, including intravenous tissue plasminogen activator and mechanical embolectomy, if they present early. In patients presenting later, aspirin is employed initially. For patients with AF and a cerebral ischemic episode, anticoagulation is the optimal long-term secondary prevention strategy. Once HCM is documented, management of the underlying disease is targeted to symptomatic relief and reducing the risk of death (1). Diuretics are used to reduce symptoms of pulmonary congestion, often used in combination with β-adrenergic blockers or calcium channel blockers (19). Vasodilators, used to treat hypertension, are contraindicated in obstructive HCM because they can worsen the obstruction and symptoms (7). Invasive interventions are required in 5% to 10% of patients who are symptomatic, despite optimal medical therapy. These include insertion of a dual-chamber pacemaker, defibrillator implantation, and alcohol septal ablation (13,20). Surgical therapy is used in symptomatic patients who are medically refractory (1,13). The most widely used operation is a myotomy-myectomy; rarely, mitral valve replacement is performed (13). Cardiac transplantation is considered in patients who have failed both medical and surgical management. Prophylactic antiplatelet therapy is also a consideration (5). In competitive sports, guidelines have been developed for patients with HCM. In both asymptomatic and symptomatic patients, strenuous exercise is generally avoided (6). Those with marked disease are at higher risk (4,6). Women with HCM may experience an increase in the relative risk of maternal mortality during pregnancy.

Arrhythmogenic Right Ventricular Cardiomyopathy

DEFINITION

Arrhythmogenic right ventricular cardiomyopathy or arrhythmogenic right ventricular dysplasia (ARVC/D) is a heritable disorder characterized by progressive degeneration and fibrofatty replacement of the right ventricular myocardium causing ventricular tachyarrhythmias and right-sided heart failure.

EPIDEMIOLOGY

Although first described in 1977, ARVC is still not well understood despite the relative frequency of the disorder. The estimated prevalence of ARVC ranges from 6 per 10,000 in the general population to as high as 44 per 10,000 in certain Mediterranean and southern US populations. After hypertrophic heart disease, ARVC is the most common cause of sudden cardiac death in young persons, especially athletes. ARVC is demonstrated in 5% of sudden cardiac deaths in persons younger than 65 years of age and 3% to 4% of deaths occurring in sports (21,22). Familial occurrence appears in 30% to 50% of individuals and inheritance as an autosomal dominant trait with reduced penetrance has been described (22a).

ETIOLOGY AND PATHOGENESIS

The most frequent presenting finding is recurrent, sustained ventricular tachycardia with left bundle branch configuration in the QRS complex. Other arrhythmias can occur (23). Syncope and presyncope caused by transient global cerebral ischemia are the major neurologic manifestations (23). Rarely, sudden death from ventricular fibrillation can occur. AF is an uncommon manifestation of ARVC, occurring in the late stages of the disease. Cardioembolic stroke related to AF in ARVC is a rare event.

PATHOLOGY

The disease process is characterized by a progressive loss of myocytes caused by either total or partial replacement of the myocardium by adipose and fibrous tissue. The process primarily affects the epicardium and mid-myocardium, with relative sparing of the trabeculae (1,24). The residual islands or strands of myocytes are surrounded by fat or fibrous tissue, providing a substrate for electrical instability leading to sustained ventricular arrhythmias and sudden death.

CLINICAL MANIFESTATIONS

ARVC is an important cause of ventricular tachycardia in children as well as older adults. Clinical manifestations typically appear in childhood or early adulthood (33 ± 14 years); a male predominance (3:1) is seen, and generally the physical examination is normal. Palpitations, fatigue, and syncope are common, but nonspecific complaints, such as abdominal pain and mental confusion, are also possible. Cardiac arrest after physical exertion while participating in sports may be the initial presentation (12). If ARVC is suspected, a thorough history, including family history, is important. Often, the diagnosis is made after a patient has had extensive diagnostic workup for tachycardia.

DIAGNOSTIC APPROACH

The diagnosis of ARVC is based on a combination of clinical, ECG, echocardiographic, computed tomographic, magnetic resonance imaging (MRI), right ventricular angiography studies, and histologic documentation of localized or widespread structural and dynamic abnormalities involving mainly or exclusively the right ventricle, in the absence of valvular disease, shunts, active myocarditis, and coronary artery disease (25). Myocardial biopsy can be useful in difficult cases, but lacks sensitivity because of the segmental nature of the disease (24).

TREATMENT

Automatic implantable cardioverter defibrillators (ICD) are recommended to cover the risk of sudden cardiac death in ARVC. Patients can also be treated with antiarrhythmic therapy, especially β-adrenoceptor blockers, sotalol, and amiodarone to decrease the number of shocks (1). Cryo- or catheter-based radiofrequency ablation can be used for patients with recurrent, sustained ventricular tachycardias while on optimal medical therapy. In addition, for refractory cases, ventriculotomy or cardiac transplant are also considered (1).

Restrictive Cardiomyopathy

DEFINITION

Restrictive cardiomyopathy (RCM) is an uncommon condition of diverse cause, characterized by rigid ventricular walls, elevated filling pressures, restrictive filling, diastolic dysfunction, dilated atria, normal or mildly reduced systolic function, and normal ventricular wall thickness.

EPIDEMIOLOGY

Epidemiologic studies of RCM are sparse. In one population-based, retrospective cohort study in Australia, RCM accounted for 2.5% of the cases of cardiomyopathy in children <10 years of age (26). RCM is responsible for 15% to 25% of cardiac deaths in equatorial Africa (27).

ETIOLOGY AND PATHOGENESIS

RCM is caused by processes that stiffen the ventricles, via infiltration or fibrosis of the myocardium or endocardium (28). Underlying causes can be subdivided into noninfiltrative (including idiopathic cardiomyopathy, familial cardiomyopathy, hypertrophic cardiomyopathy, scleroderma, pseudoxanthoma elasticum, and diabetic cardiomyopathy), infiltrative (including amyloidosis, sarcoidosis, Gaucher disease, Hurler disease, and fatty infiltration), and storage disorders (including hemochromatosis, Fabry disease, and glycogen storage disorders). Endomyocardial diseases include endomyocardial fibrosis (EMF), carcinoid heart disease, metastatic cancer, radiation, and toxic effects of drugs, such as anthracycline, chloroquine, and methysergide. This chapter covers those processes that most commonly have neurologic manifestations.

Idiopathic RCM has been described in three families and is associated with distal skeletal myopathy (29–31). Patients typically develop atrial enlargement, which predisposes them to atrial thrombus formation and cardioembolism (27).

Amyloidosis is a multisystem disease involving amyloid protein fibril deposition in the interstitium or vessel walls of various tissues, including the heart, kidney, liver, and nervous system. Primary amyloidosis (AL amyloidosis) is caused by plasma cell production of immunoglobulin light chains and can be associated with multiple myeloma, B-cell lymphoma, and Waldenstrom macroglobulinemia. Secondary amyloidosis, which includes hereditary amyloidosis, senile amyloidosis, and amyloidosis caused by chronic inflammatory processes, is caused by deposition of proteins other than immunoglobulins. Hereditary amyloidosis is caused by an autosomal dominant mutation, most frequently in the transthyretin (TTR) gene. Senile systemic amyloidosis is caused by wild-type TTR deposition. Chronic inflammatory diseases, such as tuberculosis and other chronic infections, rheumatoid arthritis, and inflammatory bowel disease, cause production of acute phase reactants, such as reactive amyloid fibrils, that can deposit in cardiac muscle, causing amyloidosis. In cardiac amyloidosis, amyloid deposits in sinoatrial and atrioventricular nodes and bundle branches result in a variety of cardiac arrhythmias, including AF, predisposing patients to development of atrial thrombi, and subsequent ischemic stroke. Other neurologic manifestations are caused by amyloid deposition in meninges, nerve trunks, plexuses, sensory and autonomic ganglia, peripheral nerves, cranial nerves, and brain parenchyma (see Table 7-1) (32).

Sarcoidosis is a multisystem inflammatory disease of unknown etiology in which noncaseating granulomas develop in affected organs. Sarcoidosis has multiple systemic and neurologic manifestations (Table 7-1). Sarcoidosis can rarely involve the sinoatrial and atrioventricular nodes, bundle of His, and myocardium, leading to intraventricular conduction defects, ventricular arrhythmias, and supraventricular arrhythmias, including atrial flutter and AF, predisposing patients to development of atrial thrombi and subsequent ischemic stroke. Sarcoidosis directly affects the nervous system in 5% of cases, with granulomatous infiltration of the meninges, cranial nerves, brain parenchyma, and cerebral vasculature (33–35).

Several diseases caused by enzyme deficiencies associated with RCM also produce developmental derangements of the central and peripheral nervous system (Table 7-2) (36–38). Neurologic manifestations typically result from product accumulation in skeletal muscles, brain, and meninges. In Fabry disease, glycosphingolipid deposition results in dilatation, angiectasia, and dolichoectasia of the cerebral vasculature (39). The vertebrobasilar arteries are particularly susceptible. Cerebral infarcts result from direct vascular occlusion and from distention of branches of the dolichoectatic parent vessels. Dolichoectatic intracranial arteries can also cause compressive complications (39).

EMF is characterized by fibrotic thickening of endocardium and development of mural thrombi in the apices of both ventricles, with partial cavity obliteration and involvement of both atrioventricular valves (40). The two types of EMF are Loeffler endocarditis and tropical EMF, or Davies' disease. Loeffler endocarditis occurs in temperate climates; tropical EMF was originally described in Uganda and is most prevalent in tropical and subtropical countries in Africa, Asia, and South America. EMF is associated with hypereosinophilia and evidence suggests that eosinophils may be responsible for cardiac damage. Patients with hypereosinophilic syndrome can present with encephalopathy, neuropathy, and ischemic stroke secondary to cardioembolism (41,42).

Radiation-induced myocardial and endocardial fibrosis can cause RCM several years after treatment. Many drugs, including anthracyclines and methysergide, can cause endomyocardial fibrosis. Long-term chloroquine therapy has been associated with RCM, encephalopathy, neuropathy, myopathy, retinopa-

TABLE 7-1. Neurologic and Systemic Manifestations of Sarcoidosis and Amyloidosis

	Systemic Manifestations	*Neurologic Manifestations*
AMYLOIDOSIS	Renal insufficiency	Peripheral neuropathy
	Gastric ulcers	Autonomic dysfunction
	Corneal lattice dystrophy	Cranial neuropathy
		Central nervous system findings: Dementia, ataxia, spasticity, seizures, visual disturbances, intraparenchymal, or subarachnoid hemorrhage
SARCOIDOSIS	Fatigue	Transient ischemic attack, stroke
	Malaise	Encephalopathy
	Weight loss	Seizures
	Hilar lymphadenopathy	Cranial neuropathy
	Erythema nodosum	Peripheral neuropathy
	Anterior and posterior uveitis	Mass lesion
	Retinal vasculitis	Meningitis
	Keratoconjunctivitis	Brainstem encephalitis
	Conjunctival follicles	Intracerebral hemorrhage
	Cataracts	Myositis and myopathy
	Glaucoma	Optic neuritis
	Hepatosplenomegaly	Intramedullary and extramedullary spinal cord lesions
	Renal insufficiency	
	Arthritis	

TABLE 7-2. Systemic and Neurologic Manifestations of Enzyme Deficiencies Associated with Restrictive Cardiomyopathy

Disease	*Enzyme Deficiency*	*Systemic Manifestations*	*Neurologic Manifestations*
Gaucher disease	Glucocerebrosidase	Bone pain Osteopenia and pathologic fractures Hepatosplenomegaly Hepatic failure Thrombocytopenia Anemia Ichthyosis Corneal opacities Growth retardation Interstitial lung disease	Developmental delay Supranuclear gaze palsy Pyramidal tract involvement with spasm, opisthotonus, head retroflexion Dementia Ataxia Myoclonus Parkinsonism Myoclonic and tonic-clonic seizures
Hurler syndrome	α-L-iduronidase	Coarse facial features, wide nasal bridge, and flattened midface Hepatosplenomegaly Inguinal and umbilical hernias Dysostosis multiplex Chronic ear, sinus, and pulmonary infections Corneal clouding	Developmental delay Communicating hydrocephalus Sensorineural hearing loss Anterior C1-C2 subluxation with cord compression
Pompe disease	Acid maltase	Macroglossia Hepatomegaly	Hypotonia Motor delay Skeletal myopathy, primarily limb-girdle and respiratory
Andersen disease	Transglucosidase	Failure to thrive Hepatosplenomegaly Hepatic failure Hepatocellular carcinoma	Myopathy
Fabry disease	α-galactosidase A	Telangiectasias Angiokeratomas Corneal deposits Renal failure	Acroparesthesias Peripheral neuropathy Autonomic neuropathy Ischemic stroke Intraparenchymal hemorrhage Nonischemic complications of dolichoectatic vessels (hydrocephalus, optic atrophy, cranial nerve palsies, trigeminal neuralgia)

thy, blood dyscrasias, corneal deposits, and impairment of auditory function (43).

PATHOLOGY

Histology in RCM typically depicts myocyte hypertrophy, interstitial fibrosis, myocytolysis, and endocardial sclerosis. In idiopathic RCM, myocardial interstitial fibrosis ranges in its extent; it is usually patchy and can involve the sinoatrial and atrioventricular nodes (30). In some patients with idiopathic RCM, endomyocardial and skeletal muscle biopsy reveals granulofilamentous desmin-immunoreactive subsarcolemmal deposits (44). Necropsy studies of cardiac amyloidosis typically demonstrate a thickened myocardium with enlarged chambers. Gross inspection may also reveal a rubbery consistency and the presence of intracardiac thrombi (45). Microscopically, amyloid fibril deposits can be found in the myocardial interstitium and cardiac valves and within the media of intramyocardial coronary arteries (27,28). The deposits surround individual myocytes, forming a *honeycomb* pattern (28). In sarcoidosis, peripheral nerve biopsy can reveal segmental demyelination, degenerating nerve roots with inflammatory cells, and granulomatous destruction of nerves; muscle biopsy can reveal granulomas surrounded by normal muscle, noncaseous granulomatous myositis, or chronic myopathic changes; blood vessel biopsy can show involvement of the vessel wall; and brain biopsy can show granulomas (46). Muscle biopsy in Pompe disease reveals vacuolar myopathy with glycogen storage within lysosomes, and free glycogen in the cytoplasm by electron microscopy. The vacuoles are periodic acid-Schiff (PAS) positive and positive for acid phosphatase. Muscle biopsy in Andersen disease reveals the storage of PAS-positive material.

CLINICAL MANIFESTATIONS

RCM can affect either or both ventricles; therefore, it can manifest with signs and symptoms of either left or right ventricular failure (27). Patients can present with dyspnea, paroxysmal nocturnal dyspnea, orthopnea, peripheral edema, ascites, general fatigue, and weakness. Cardiac conduction disturbances are typically seen in amyloidosis (47,48) and sarcoidosis (49). AF is common in idiopathic RCM and cardiac amyloidosis (50).

Physical findings in RCM include Kussmaul sign (rise in venous pulse during inspiration), crackles, ascites, enlarged pulsatile liver, peripheral edema, presence of a third and possibly fourth heart sound, sinus tachycardia, low pulse volume, and pulsus paradoxus.

RCM can directly cause neurologic complications and can be associated with neurologic manifestations in the setting of multisystem disease. Patients with RCM frequently develop atrial arrhythmias, and atrial and ventricular thrombi, making them susceptible to cardioembolic stroke. In one series of 94 patients with idiopathic RCM, 74% of patients evaluated had AF at the time of examination and an additional 4% had a history of paroxysmal AF (51). Over 68 months of follow-up, 50% of patients died; 47% from congestive heart failure, 17% from sudden death, 11% from arrhythmias, 4% from ischemic stroke; the remaining died of causes unrelated to RCM (51). In a small retrospective analysis of children with RCM, 17% of patients had embolic strokes (52). Up to one third of patients with idiopathic RCM present with thromboembolic complications (53). Systemic diseases that cause RCM often have neurologic manifestations (Tables 7-1 and 7-2), involving both the central and peripheral nervous system (32,38,45,54,55).

DIAGNOSTIC APPROACH

In RCM, ECG can show nonspecific ST- and T-wave abnormalities, ventricular hypertrophy, or abnormalities in conduction. Chest film typically shows normal cardiac size, pulmonary congestion, pleural effusions, and interstitial edema. Doppler echocardiography typically demonstrates increased diastolic filling velocity, decreased isovolumic relaxation time, normal to symmetrically thickened walls, normal or slightly reduced ventricular volume and systolic function, minimal respiratory variation in Doppler flow velocities, and no pericardial thickening. In amyloidosis, the echocardiogram often shows a diagnostic gray, glittery appearance of the myocardium. During cardiac catheterization, the characteristic hemodynamic feature is a deep and rapid early decline in ventricular pressure at the onset of diastole, with a rapid rise to a plateau in early diastole (dip and plateau or square-root sign). Cardiac CT or MRI can be useful in differentiating RCM from constrictive pericarditis, because most cases of the latter demonstrate a thickened pericardium. Endomyocardial biopsy should be considered for patients in whom the diagnosis is not clear by other methods of evaluation. Detailed history and physical examination are critical to detect nervous system and other extracardiac manifestations of diseases that cause RCM (Tables 7-1 and 7-2). In patients with systemic disease with peripheral nervous system involvement, muscle and nerve biopsy can often provide a diagnosis.

TREATMENT

Treatment of RCM includes both symptomatic therapy and therapy for the underlying disorder. Symptomatic therapy includes use of diuretics to treat venous congestion in the pulmonary and systemic circulation, pacemaker or automatic ICD for conduction abnormalities, rate control for AF, and warfarin to prevent thromboembolism in patients with AF or LV thrombus.

Patients with systemic disease may benefit from treatment of the underlying disease. Chemotherapy has shown benefit in primary systemic amyloidosis. Orthotopic liver transplantation stops amyloidosis progression and can improve neurologic outcome by removing the main production site of the amyloidogenic protein (32,56). Neurosarcoidosis can be treated with steroids and immunosuppression. Several small series suggest that radiotherapy might be useful in patients whose disease is refractory to conventional treatment (57). Corticosteroid and cytotoxic drugs improve both symptoms and survival in Loeffler endocarditis. Surgical therapy, with excision of fibrotic endocardium and replacement of involved valves, is palliative in the fibrotic stage of the disease, but has a 15% to 25% operative mortality rate. Hemochromatosis can be treated with phlebotomy or iron-chelation therapy. Lysosomal storage disorders, such as Gaucher, Hurler, and Fabry diseases, can be treated with enzyme replacement therapy (38). Recently, imaging-guided direct convective delivery of glucocerebrosidase has been performed in a patient with neuronopathic Gaucher disease while monitoring enzyme distribution with MRI (58). Hurler disease has been treated with bone marrow transplantation with variable success (38,59). Antiplatelet agents and anticoagulants have been used for secondary stroke prevention in Fabry disease, but their effectiveness in this setting is uncertain (39).

Cardiac transplantation is an option for patients with severe RCM, but in patients who have an underlying systemic illness, the illness often affects the transplanted heart.

Myocarditis

DEFINITION

Myocarditis is a collection of diseases of infectious, toxic, and autoimmune causes characterized by inflammation of the heart.

EPIDEMIOLOGY

The actual incidence of myocarditis is unknown because many cases are asymptomatic and myocarditis may be responsible for a significant number of unexplained sudden deaths. In the United States, most cases are caused by viral illness, whereas, in Central and South America, Chagas disease is the most frequent cause.

ETIOLOGY AND PATHOGENESIS

Myocarditis can be caused by infection, autoimmune processes, and toxins. The major cause of acute myocarditis is presumed to be viral, predominantly Coxsackie B and adenovirus. Coxsackie genomic material is found in about one third of acute myocarditis cases using polymerase chain reaction (PCR) on myocardial tissue (60). Other viruses responsible for myocarditis include influenza virus, echovirus, herpes simplex virus, varicella-zoster virus, hepatitis, Epstein-Barr virus, cytomegalovirus, and human immunodeficiency virus (HIV). Other organisms responsible for causing myocarditis include diphtheria, streptococcal and staphylococcal species, *Borrelia burgdorferi*, *Bartonella*, *Brucella*, *Leptospira*, *Salmonella*, trypanosomiasis, trichinosis, and, in the immunocompromised host, toxoplasmosis.

Immunologic causes of myocarditis include connective tissue, inflammatory and infiltrative disorders, such as systemic lupus erythematosus (SLE), rheumatoid arthritis, dermatomyositis, Kawasaki disease, sarcoidosis, and idiopathic giant cell myocarditis (61,62).

The most common drugs that cause hypersensitivity reactions are penicillin, ampicillin, hydrochlorothiazide, methyldopa, and sulfonamide drugs. Numerous drugs such as lithium, doxorubicin, cocaine, catecholamines, acetaminophen, and zidovudine, cause a direct cytotoxic effect on the heart. Environmental toxins responsible for myocarditis include lead, arsenic, and carbon monoxide. Radiation therapy can cause a myocarditis with subsequent development of dilated cardiomyopathy.

Cardioembolic infarcts in myocarditis are secondary to atrial thrombus formation in the setting of atrial formation and ventricular thrombus formation in the setting of heart failure.

PATHOLOGY

In severe cases, myocardial biopsy reveals multifocal or regional myocyte necrosis and a lymphocytic interstitial infiltrate (described by the Dallas criteria). Given the patchy nature of the disease, less than 30% of patients with a clinical presentation of acute myocarditis have a positive biopsy. Other potential biopsy findings include mild or absent myocyte damage with a florid interstitial inflammatory cell infiltrate (60,63), giant cell granulomas and fibrosis in cardiac sarcoid, and irregular areas of myocardial necrosis with margins of large giant cells in idiopathic giant cell myocarditis.

CLINICAL MANIFESTATIONS

Most cases of myocarditis are subclinical. When patients are symptomatic, they typically develop a viral syndrome characterized by fever, fatigue, arthralgias, myalgias, and malaise, followed approximately 2 weeks later with cardiopulmonary symptoms including chest pain, dyspnea on exertion, orthopnea, paroxysmal nocturnal dyspnea, palpitations, and syncope. Idiopathic giant cell myocarditis typically presents with sudden onset of severe cardiac failure, leading to death within days unless cardiac transplant is available. Chronic myocarditis, characterized by an inflammatory infiltrate on pathology, typically presents with ventricular arrhythmias.

Physical examination findings include fever, tachypnea, tachycardia, hypotension, signs of heart failure (jugular venous distention, peripheral edema, crackles, ascites), diminished S_1, presence of an S_3 or a summation gallop, pericardial friction rub, murmurs of mitral and tricuspid regurgitation, and cyanosis.

Survival from myocarditis is approximately 80% (64). Fulminant myocarditis has a better prognosis than nonfulminant myocarditis (65). If patients survive the acute phase, recovery tends to be complete, although some cases progress to chronic dilated cardiomyopathy.

The principal neurologic manifestation of myocarditis is ischemic stroke secondary to cardioembolism.

DIAGNOSTIC APPROACH

Helpful tests include erythrocyte sedimentation rate, a tracheal aspirate for viral PCR, paired serology (including Coxsackie, respiratory syncytial virus, rubella, cytomegalovirus, Epstein-Barr virus, HIV, parvovirus, mycoplasma, and endemic infections, depending on geography), blood count for lymphocytosis, toxins if suggested by history, autoimmune markers, cardiac troponin, and immunocytology. The ECG is rarely normal, but it is not specific. Findings on ECG include sinus tachycardia, reduced voltage, transitory Q-wave development, arrhythmias, conduction delay or block, bundle branch block, and ST changes. Chest radiography generally reveals a normal cardiac silhouette, vascular redistribution, interstitial and alveolar edema, and pleural effusions. Echocardiography typically shows impairment in systolic and diastolic function, segmental wall motion abnormalities, and occasionally a pericardial effusion. Ventricular thrombi are present in up to 15% of patients with myocarditis. Cardiac catheterization usually reveals normal coronary vessels and depressed ejection fraction. Cardiac MRI can reveal late epicardial gadolinium enhancement (66). Definitive diagnosis can be made with endomyocardial biopsy, but usually yield a high rate of false negative findings.

TREATMENT

The treatment of heart failure caused by myocarditis is supportive. Because patients are at risk for mural thrombus formation, anticoagulation with warfarin is often indicated to prevent embolic stroke. Randomized studies have failed to show benefit with immunosuppression or immunoglobulin therapy, except in cases of giant cell myocarditis and autoimmune myocarditis, which respond to immunosuppression (62,64,67). Patients with fulminant myocarditis can be supported through the course of the illness using biventricular assist devices (68). In young children, extracorporeal membrane oxygenation can be used, whereas older children are typically supported with pneumatic external assist devices (69). Patients with acute or nonfulminant myocarditis are more likely to have a progressive course, necessitating cardiac transplant for survival (69). Recurrence of sarcoidosis and giant cell myocarditis in donor hearts can occur.

Chagasic Cardiomyopathy

DEFINITION

Chagas disease (CD), also known as *American trypanosomiasis*, is one of the most common causes of nonischemic cardiomyopathy (Chagasic cardiomyopathy). It is caused by the protozoan *Trypanosoma cruzi* and leads to extensive myocarditis that typically becomes evident years after the initial infection.

EPIDEMIOLOGY

The disease is mostly prevalent in Central and South America, particularly in Brazil, Argentina, and Chile. At least 20 million people (8% of the population) are thought to be infected with the parasite and an estimated 100 million are at risk of infection (70). In the United States, rare cases have been reported in immigrants, but the prevalence is likely underestimated because screening for the disease, especially in patients who have had stroke, is not routinely performed in clinical practice (71). Chagasic cardiomyopathy (CCM) usually affects 10% to 30% of patients with CD. In endemic areas, CCM and hypertensive cardiomyopathy are the leading causes of chronic heart failure and sudden cardiac death (72,73). The 10-year mortality in patients at high risk is 84% and 10% or less in those patients at low risk. The overall mortality rate is 3.9% per year and the rate of sudden death is 2.4% per year (74).

ETIOLOGY AND PATHOGENESIS

The disease was first described by the Brazilian physician Carlos Chagas a century ago. The basis for CCM is unknown, but may be immunologic, involving antibodies generated against *T. cruzi* cross-reacting with cardiac myocyte antigens, including myosin. A variety of antibodies against myocyte sarcoplasmic reticulum, laminin, and other constituents (most recently the cardiac beta receptor) have also been implicated in the pathogenesis of Chagas myocarditis (70). Another hypothesis suggests that cardiac parasympathetic denervation leads to eventual chronic CD (1).

The natural history of the disease is characterized by three phases: Acute, latent, and chronic. During the acute phase, the disease is transmitted to humans (usually <20 years of age) through the bite of a reduviid bug (subfamily *Triatominae*), which harbors the parasite in its gastrointestinal tract (70). The bug bites the human host around the eyes, and infection occurs when the trypanosomes in the animal's feces gain entry through abraded skin or through the conjunctivae. Nonvectorial mechanisms include blood transfusions. In nonendemic areas, such as the United States, where the vector *Triatoma* is found only in the southwest, individuals who have emigrated from endemic countries may serve as sources of transmission (75). The acute myocardial infection of childhood is usually a mild illness with a case fatality rate of less than 5%. A latent period follows during which the number of parasites is nearly undetectable, and 10 to 30 years later it may be reactivated, leading to irreversible heart damage. Death in CD is usually caused by arrhythmia, although congestive failure and systemic thromboembolism are serious complications (76). The greatest risk of mortality is observed in patients with LV enlargement and impaired LV function.

The leading neurologic manifestations of CD are neuropathy, meningoencepalitis, cardioembolic stroke, and syncope. The involvement of the peripheral and autonomic nervous systems, especially of autonomic nerves supplying the cardiovascular and gastrointestinal systems, is felt to be caused by autoimmune destruction. The existence of circulating antibodies in CD bind to β-adrenergic and muscarinic cholinergic receptor (mAChR). The neurotransmitter receptor-autoantibody interaction triggers in the cells intracellular signal transductions that alter the physiologic behavior of the target organs, leading to tissue damage (77–79). Between 10% and 12% of patients with intermediate or chronic stage disease show signs and symptoms of peripheral nervous system involvement in the form of sensory impairment and diminished tendon jerks, suggesting the presence of a mild sensory-motor peripheral neuropathy (80). Although a small percentage of patients develop fulminant meningoencephalitis or myocarditis at the time of initial infection, late meningoencephaliitis in individuals with acquired immune compromise is more common. CD can reactivate in patients with acquired immunodeficiency syndrome (AIDS) and present as a brain mass lesion or an acute diffuse meningoencephalitis indistinguishable from other opportunistic infections or neoplastic processes, such as toxoplasma encephalitis or central nervous system (CNS) primary lymphoma. Lesions appear on MRI as single or multiple hypodense ring enhancing lesions mainly in the subcortical areas. The CNS tumorlike lesion is the most common manifestation of CD reactivation in patients with AIDS (81,82).

Chagasic cardiomyopathy has been identified as an independent risk factor for ischemic stroke (71,83). Cardioembolism can arise from ventricular sources because of direct injury to the ventricular wall or from atrial fibrillation. Postmortem studies have shown cerebral infarction in 9.4% to 36% of patients with chronic disease. At least 56.3% of strokes are caused by cardioembolism and 25.53% by an undetermined cause (83). The apical region of the LV is a critical location where aneurysm, thrombus, or both occur with high frequency (83). AF is a common sustained rhythm, which can predispose patients to embolic stroke by promoting clot precipitation in static or slowly moving blood with the atrium, especially within the left atrial appendage.

Syncope most often occurs as a result of ventricular arrhythmias, sinus bradycardia related to cardiac autonomic dysfunction, or AF. Uncommonly, fainting appears as a manifestation of sudden inappropriate vasodilation caused by autonomic dysfunction in the absence of an arrhythmia.

PATHOLOGY

CD affects the neurons of the parasympathetic ganglia and produces megaesophagus, megacolon, and myocardiopathy. Inflammatory lesions occur in the muscle, nerve, and autonomic ganglia. There is denervation of the intrinsic enteric neurons of submucosal (Meissner) and myenteric (Auerbach) plexuses. Dilation of the stomach, duodenum, ureter, and bronchi can also occur. Lesions of the cardiac nerves are routinely found in patients with chronic CD, with evidence of cardiac parasympathetic denervation. Pathologic cardiac findings include cardiac enlargement with dilation and hypertrophy of all cardiac chambers. In more than half the patients, the left (and occasionally right) ventricular apex is thin and bulging, resembling an aneurysm. Thrombus formation is frequent and may fill much of the apex. This may be a result of intravascular platelet aggregation leading to focal myocardial necrosis. The microscopic findings are principally those of extensive fibrosis, particularly of the LV. A chronic cellular infiltrate composed of lymphocytes, plasma cells, and macrophages often is present. also seen is involvement of the right bundle branch and the anterior fascicle of the left bundle branch by inflammatory and fibrotic changes that can explain the frequent occurrence of right bundle branch and left anterior fascicular block. It is unusual to find parasites in the myofibers of patients at autopsy.

CLINICAL MANIFESTATIONS

Clinical manifestations include unilateral periorbital edema and swelling of the eyelid (Romaña sign), and entry through the skin can result in a nodular area of local edema and redness (75% of cases) called a *chagoma*. In the early stage, the systemic spread of the parasites from the site of entry and their initial multiplication can be accompanied by fever, malaise, and edema of the face and lower extremities, as well as generalized lymphadenopathy and hepatosplenomegaly (75). The disease can present with fever, vomiting, seizures, and focal neurologic signs in immunosuppressed patients with meningoencephalitis. Other cardiac manifestations include chest pain, symptomatic conducting system disease, sudden death, and chronic progressive heart failure, often predominantly right-sided. Fatigue because of diminished cardiac output, peripheral edema, ascites, and hepatic congestion can also occur. Tricuspid regurgitation and mitral regurgitation are frequently present. Autonomic dysfunction is common, with marked abnormalities in the expected reflex changes in heart rate produced by various maneuvers. Patients can die as a result of pump failure or present with sudden death, especially if apical aneurysms and LV dilation are present. Syncope as a result of ventricular arrhythmias is especially common during and after exercise. Syncope can also reflect sinus bradycardia, atrial fibrillation, or dysautonomic vasodilation. Atrial arrhythmias, including atrial fibrillation, can also occur and thromboembolic phenomena are a frequent complication, occurring in more than 50% of the patients.

Several authors have observed a higher frequency of stroke in Chagasic women (75,84). One study suggested the mechanism may be longer survival of women with Chagasic heart failure, exposing them to greater risk of embolic stroke (83).

The most frequent neurologic findings in patients with CD are distal extremity sensory loss and impairment of the muscle stretch reflexes, owing to polyneuropathy.

DIAGNOSTIC APPROACH

Chest radiography may demonstrate severe cardiomegaly, with or without pulmonary venous hypertension. Serum aldolase level is usually elevated. Abnormalities on ECG, such as right bundle branch block, left anterior hemiblock, AF, and ventricular premature depolarizations, are observed later in the course of the disease. Administration of the antiarrhythmic agent ajmaline may precipitate the appearance of ECG abnormalities and, thus, identify patients with as yet clinically silent cardiac involvement (70). Electrophysiologic testing of patients who are asymptomatic may demonstrate abnormalities of the conducting system. The echocardiographic findings in advanced cases are those of a dilated cardiomyopathy with increased end-diastolic and end-systolic volumes and reduced ejection fraction, often with enlargement of the left atrium and right ventricle. There is LV posterior wall hypokinesis and relatively preserved interventricular septal motion; an apical aneurysm is often seen on two-dimensional echocardiography (75,83). Radionuclide ventriculography demonstrates right or left ventricular wall motion abnormalities in the absence of an overall depression of global ventricular function. Perfusion scanning with thallium-201 may show fixed defects and evidence of reversible ischemia. Cardiac MRI with the use of gadolinium can identify cardiac involvement. Cineangiography in advanced cases shows a dilated, hypokinetic LV with one large or several apical aneurysms. Serodiagnosis using the complement-fixation test (Machado-Guerreiro test) is useful with a high sensitivity, but evidence of prior infection may be detected more frequently by the much more sensitive PCR technique (85). In endemic areas, xenodiagnosis can detect parasites in the blood of patients with chronic CD. Only one test for antibodies to *T. cruzi* (Chagas' IgG ELISA, Gull Laboratories, Salt Lake City) is available in the United States. It is available for clinical testing, but not for screening in blood banks (75).

Electromyography and nerve conduction studies may be useful in determining the presence of a peripheral neuropathy and the findings are typically fragmented or polyphasic motor unit potentials and reduced sensory and motor conduction velocities with diminished amplitude of the sensory action potential (80).

TREATMENT

No definitive treatment for CD exists. Patients may respond to β-blockade, and some evidence suggests that captopril, early in the course of disease, may alleviate disease in animal models (86). Vector control methods have also been successful at preventing both the initial infection and reinfection that may play a role in determining the severity of the cardiomyopathy. Amiodarone has been used to control the ventricular arrhythmias. ICD may also be useful. Antiparasitic agents, such as nifurtimox, benzimidazole, and itraconazole, are effective in reducing parasitemia and are useful in acute disease, but it is uncertain whether they alter the course of later disease. Immunoprophylaxis is currently in development. Heart transplantations have been performed in a few patients, but episodes of parasitemia and recurrent CD can be a problem. Anticoagulation may be beneficial in preventing thromboembolic episodes in patients with atrial fibrillation and patients with apical aneurysms (83).

CLINICAL RECOMMENDATIONS OF THE VIGNETTE

The patient presents with many classic findings of Fabry disease. He describes acroparesthesias and hypohydrosis, reflecting peripheral and autonomic neuropathy. Renal involvement is evident, with proteinuria and albuminuria. The postprandial diarrhea suggests gastrointestinal dysmotility. His hearing loss is likely caused by sphingolipid accumulation in vascular endothelial and ganglion cells of the auditory system. Characteristic cardiac involvement is noted, with atrial arrhythmia and heart failure predisposing him to thrombus formation and subsequent cardioembolism. He presented with a lacunar stroke, most likely caused by sphingolipid accumulation in the basilar perforator vessels and less likely by cardioembolism.

This patient requires enzyme replacement therapy with agalsidase-α or agalsidase-β for Fabry disease, rate control medications for atrial fibrillation, and warfarin for stroke prevention.

SUMMARY

Cardiomyopathies and myocarditis have a variety of associated neurologic findings. Neurologic manifestations of HCM include presyncope, syncope, and ischemic stroke. Neurologic manifestations of ARVC are typically limited to presyncope and syncope, but rarely, ischemic strokes can occur. Patients with RCM frequently present with ischemic stroke. In addition, RCM can be associated with a multitude of systemic conditions that have central and peripheral nervous system involvement, including, amyloidosis, sarcoidosis, and Gaucher, Hurler, Fabry, Pompe, and Andersen diseases. The most frequent neurologic complication of infectious, autoimmune, and toxic myocarditis is cardioembolic stroke. Neurologic involvement in Chagas cardiomyopathy includes embolic stroke, autonomic dysfunction, and meningoencephalitis.

REFERENCES

1. Braunwald E, Zipes DP, MD Consult LLC. Braunwald's Heart Disease: *A Textbook of Cardiovascular Medicine*, 7th ed. St. Louis: MO Consult; 2005.
2. Ho CY, Seidman CE. A contemporary approach to hypertrophic cardiomyopathy. *Circulation.* 2006;113(24):e858–e862.
3. Pelliccia A, Di Paolo FM, Maron BJ. The athlete's heart: Remodeling, electrocardiogram and preparticipation screening. *Cardiol Rev.* 2002;10(2):85–90.
4. Maron BJ, Shen WK, Link MS, et al. Efficacy of implantable cardioverter-defibrillators for the prevention of sudden death in patients with hypertrophic cardiomyopathy. *N Engl J Med.* 2000;342(6):365–373.
5. Russell JW, Biller J, Hajduczok ZD, et al. Ischemic cerebrovascular complications and risk factors in idiopathic hypertrophic subaortic stenosis. *Stroke.* 1991;22(9):1143–1147.
6. Maron BJ, Carney KP, Lever HM, et al. Relationship of race to sudden cardiac death in competitive athletes with hypertrophic cardiomyopathy. *J Am Coll Cardiol.* 2003;41(6):974–980.
7. Sherrid MV. Pathophysiology and treatment of hypertrophic cardiomyopathy. *Prog Cardiovasc Dis.* 2006;49(2):123–151.
8. Furlan AJ, Craciun AR, Raju NR, et al. Cerebrovascular complications associated with idiopathic hypertrophic subaortic stenosis. *Stroke.* 1984;15(2):282–284.
9. Inoue H, Nozawa T, Hirai T, et al. Accumulation of risk factors increases risk of thromboembolic events in patients with nonvalvular atrial fibrillation. *Circ J.* 2006;70(6):651–656.
10. Olivotto I, Cecchi F, Casey SA, et al. Impact of atrial fibrillation on the clinical course of hypertrophic cardiomyopathy. *Circulation.* 2001;104(21):2517–2524.
11. Norris JW, Froggatt GM, Hachinski VC. Cardiac arrhythmias in acute stroke. *Stroke.* 1978;9(4):392–396.
12. Nava A, Thiene G, Canciani B, et al. Clinical profile of concealed form of arrhythmogenic right ventricular cardiomyopathy presenting with apparently idiopathic ventricular arrhythmias. *Int J Cardiol.* 1992;35(2):195–206; discussion 207–209.
13. Maron BJ. Hypertrophic cardiomyopathy. *Lancet.* 1997;350(9071):127–133.
14. Hadjikoutis S, O'Callaghan P, Smith PE. The investigation of syncope. *Seizure.* 2004; 13(8):537–548.
15. Segal JB, McNamara RL, Miller MR, et al. Anticoagulants or antiplatelet therapy for non-rheumatic atrial fibrillation and flutter. *Cochrane Database Syst Rev.* 2001(1):CD001938.
16. Yu EH, Omran AS, Wigle ED, et al. Mitral regurgitation in hypertrophic obstructive cardiomyopathy: Relationship to obstruction and relief with myectomy. *J Am Coll Cardiol.* 2000; 36(7):2219–2225.
17. Wigle ED. Cardiomyopathy: The diagnosis of hypertrophic cardiomyopathy. *Heart.* 2001;86(6):709–714.
18. Manganelli F, Betocchi S, Ciampi Q, et al. Comparison of hemodynamic adaptation to orthostatic stress in patients with hypertrophic cardiomyopathy with or without syncope and in vasovagal syncope. *Am J Cardiol.* 2002;89(12):1405–1410.
19. McKenna WJ, Behr ER. Hypertrophic cardiomyopathy: Management, risk stratification, and prevention of sudden death. *Heart.* 2002;87(2):169–176.
20. Elliott PM, Sharma S, Varnava A, et al. Survival after cardiac arrest or sustained ventricular tachycardia in patients with hypertrophic cardiomyopathy. *J Am Coll Cardiol.* 1999;33(6): 1596–1601.
21. Peters S, Peters H, Thierfelder L. Risk stratification of sudden cardiac death and malignant ventricular arrhythmias in right ventricular dysplasia-cardiomyopathy. *Int J Cardiol.* 1999;71(3):243–250.
22. Thiene G, Nava A, Corrado D, et al. Right ventricular cardiomyopathy and sudden death in young people. *N Engl J Med.* 1988;318(3):129–133.

22a. Corrado D, Basso C, Thiene G. Arrhythmogenic right ventricular cardiomyopathy: diagnosis, prognosis, and treatment. *Heart.* 2000;83:588–595.

23. Gemayel C, Pelliccia A, Thompson PD. Arrhythmogenic right ventricular cardiomyopathy. *J Am Coll Cardiol.* 2001;38(7):1773–1781.
24. Marcus FI, Fontaine G. Arrhythmogenic right ventricular dysplasia/cardiomyopathy: A review. *Pacing Clin Electrophysiol.* 1995;18(6):1298–1314.
25. Naccarella F, Naccarelli G, Fattori R, et al. Arrhythmogenic right ventricular dysplasia: Cardiomyopathy current opinions on diagnostic and therapeutic aspects. *Curr Opin Cardiol.* 2001;16(1):8–16.
26. Nugent AW, Daubeney PE, Chondros P, et al. The epidemiology of childhood cardiomyopathy in Australia. *N Engl J Med.* 2003;348(17):1639–1646.
27. Kushwaha SS, Fallon JT, Fuster V. Restrictive cardiomyopathy. *N Engl J Med.* 1997;336(4): 267–276.
28. Hughes SE, McKenna WJ. New insights into the pathology of inherited cardiomyopathy. *Heart.* 2005;91(2):257–264.
29. Angelini A, Calzolari V, Thiene G, et al. Morphologic spectrum of primary restrictive cardiomyopathy. *Am J Cardiol.* 1997;80(8):1046–1050.
30. Fitzpatrick AP, Shapiro LM, Rickards AF, et al. Familial restrictive cardiomyopathy with atrioventricular block and skeletal myopathy. *Br Heart J.* 1990;63(2):114–118.
31. Mogensen J, Klausen IC, Pedersen AK, et al. Alpha-cardiac actin is a novel disease gene in familial hypertrophic cardiomyopathy. *J Clin Invest.* 1999;103(10):R39–R43.
32. Hund E, Linke RP, Willig F, et al. Transthyretin-associated neuropathic amyloidosis. Pathogenesis and treatment. *Neurology.* 2001;56(4):431–435.
33. Oksanen V. Neurosarcoidosis. *Sarcoidosis.* 1994;11(1):76–79.
34. Delaney P. Neurologic manifestations in sarcoidosis: Review of the literature, with a report of 23 cases. *Ann Intern Med.* 1977;87(3):336–345.
35. Marcus F, Towbin JA, Zareba W, et al. Arrhythmogenic right ventricular dysplasia/ cardiomyopathy (ARVD/C). A multidisciplinary study: Design and protocol. *Circulation.* 2003;107(23):2975–2978.
36. Smith RL, Hutchins GM, Sack GH, Jr., et al. Unusual cardiac, renal and pulmonary involvement in Gaucher's disease. Intersitial glucocerebroside accumulation, pulmonary hypertension and fatal bone marrow embolization. *Am J Med.* 1978;65(2):352–360.
37. Renteria VG, Ferrans VJ, Roberts WC. The heart in the Hurler syndrome: Gross, histologic and ultrastructural observations in five necropsy cases. *Am J Cardiol.* 1976;38(4): 487–501.
38. Hoffmann B, Mayatepek E. Neurological manifestations in lysosomal storage disorders—From pathology to first therapeutic possibilities. *Neuropediatrics.* 2005;36(5):285–289.
39. Mitsias P, Levine SR. Cerebrovascular complications of Fabry's disease. *Ann Neurol.* 1996; 40(1):8–17.
40. Zubenko GS, Stiffler S, Stabler S, et al. Association of the apolipoprotein E epsilon 4 allele with clinical subtypes of autopsy-confirmed Alzheimer's disease. *Am J Med Genet.* 1994;54(3):199–205.
41. Sarazin M, Caumes E, Cohen A, et al. Multiple microembolic borderzone brain infarctions and endomyocardial fibrosis in idiopathic hypereosinophilic syndrome and in Schistosoma mansoni infestation. *J Neurol Neurosurg Psychiatry.* 2004;75(2):305–307.
42. Moore PM, Harley JB, Fauci AS. Neurologic dysfunction in the idiopathic hypereosinophilic syndrome. *Ann Intern Med.* 1985;102(1):109–114.
43. Ochsendorf FR, Runne U. [Chloroquine and hydroxychloroquine: Side effect profile of important therapeutic drugs]. *Hautarzt.* 1991;42(3):140–146.
44. Arbustini E, Morbini P, Grasso M, et al. Restrictive cardiomyopathy, atrioventricular block and mild to subclinical myopathy in patients with desmin-immunoreactive material deposits. *J Am Coll Cardiol.* 1998;31(3):645–653.
45. Nagueh SF, Bachinski LL, Meyer D, et al. Tissue Doppler imaging consistently detects myocardial abnormalities in patients with hypertrophic cardiomyopathy and provides a novel means for an early diagnosis before and independently of hypertrophy. *Circulation.* 2001;104(2):128–130.
46. Nishie M, Mori F, Suzuki C, et al. Disseminated intraparenchymal microgranulomas in the brainstem in central nervous system sarcoidosis. *Neuropathology.* 2005;25(4): 361–364.
47. Eriksson P, Boman K, Jacobsson B, et al. Cardiac arrhythmias in familial amyloid polyneuropathy during anaesthesia. *Acta Anaesthesiol Scand.* 1986;30(4):317–320.
48. Nakata T, Shimamoto K, Yonekura S, et al. Cardiac sympathetic denervation in transthyretin-related familial amyloidotic polyneuropathy: Detection with iodine-123-MIBG. *J Nucl Med.* 1995;36(6):1040–1042.
49. Winters SL, Cohen M, Greenberg S, et al. Sustained ventricular tachycardia associated with sarcoidosis: Assessment of the underlying cardiac anatomy and the prospective utility of programmed ventricular stimulation, drug therapy and an implantable antitachycardia device. *J Am Coll Cardiol.* 1991;18(4):937–943.
50. Child JS, Perloff JK. The restrictive cardiomyopathies. *Cardiol Clin.* 1988;6(2):289–316.
51. Ammash NM, Seward JB, Bailey KR, et al. Clinical profile and outcome of idiopathic restrictive cardiomyopathy. *Circulation.* 2000;101(21):2490–2496.
52. Yang Z, McMahon CJ, Smith LR, et al. Danon disease as an underrecognized cause of hypertrophic cardiomyopathy in children. *Circulation.* 2005;112(11):1612–1617.
53. Hirota Y, Shimizu G, Kita Y, et al. Spectrum of restrictive cardiomyopathy: Report of the national survey in Japan. *Am Heart J.* 1990;120(1):188–194.
54. Camp WA, Frierson JG. Sarcoidosis of the central nervous system. A case with postmortem studies. *Arch Neurol.* 1962;7:432–441.
55. Burns T. Neurosarcoidosis. *Arch Neurol.* 2003(60):1166–1168.
56. Bergethon PR, Sabin TD, Lewis D, et al. Improvement in the polyneuropathy associated with familial amyloid polyneuropathy after liver transplantation. *Neurology.* 1996; 47(4):944–951.
57. Menninger MD, Amdur RJ, Marcus RB, Jr. Role of radiotherapy in the treatment of neurosarcoidosis. *Am J Clin Oncol.* 2003;26(4):e115–e118.
58. Lonser RR, Schiffman R, Robison RA, et al. Image-guided, direct convective delivery of glucocerebrosidase for neuronopathic Gaucher disease. *Neurology.* 2007;68:254–261.
59. Grigull L, Beilken A, Schrappe M, et al. Transplantation of allogeneic CD34-selected stem cells after fludarabine-based conditioning regimen for children with mucopolysaccharidosis 1H (M. Hurler). *Bone Marrow Transplant.* 2005;35(3):265–269.
60. Varnava AM, Elliott PM, Sharma S, et al. Hypertrophic cardiomyopathy: The interrelation of disarray, fibrosis, and small vessel disease. *Heart.* 2000;84(5):476–482.
61. Silverman KJ, Hutchins GM, Bulkley BH. Cardiac sarcoid: A clinicopathologic study of 84 unselected patients with systemic sarcoidosis. *Circulation.* 1978;58(6):1204–1211.
62. Cooper LT, Jr., Berry GJ, Shabetai R. Idiopathic giant-cell myocarditis—Natural history and treatment. Multicenter Giant Cell Myocarditis Study Group Investigators. *N Engl J Med.* 1997;336(26):1860–1866.
63. Mason JW. Endomyocardial biopsy: The balance of success and failure. *Circulation.* 1985;71(2):185–188.
64. Mason JW, O'Connell JB, Herskowitz A, et al. A clinical trial of immunosuppressive therapy for myocarditis. The Myocarditis Treatment Trial Investigators. *N Engl J Med.* 1995;333(5): 269–275.
65. McCarthy RE, 3rd, Boehmer JP, Hruban RH, et al. Long-term outcome of fulminant myocarditis as compared with acute (nonfulminant) myocarditis. *N Engl J Med.* 2000; 342(10):690–695.
66. Varghese A, Davies S, Pennell DJ. Diagnosis of myocarditis by cardiovascular magnetic resonance. *Heart.* 2005;91(5):567.
67. Fuster V, Ryden LE, Asinger RW, et al. ACC/AHA/ESC Guidelines for the Management of Patients with Atrial Fibrillation: Executive Summary: A Report of the American College of Cardiology/American Heart Association Task Force on Practice Guidelines and the European Society of Cardiology Committee for Practice Guidelines and Policy Conferences (Committee to Develop Guidelines for the Management of Patients With Atrial Fibrillation) Developed in Collaboration With the North American Society of Pacing and Electrophysiology. *Circulation.* 2001;104(17):2118–2150.
68. Stiller B, Dahnert I, Weng YG, et al. Children may survive severe myocarditis with prolonged use of biventricular assist devices. *Heart.* 1999;82(2):237–240.
69. Burch M. Heart failure in the young. *Heart.* 2002;88(2):198–202.
70. Rassi A, Jr., Rassi A, Little WC. Chagas' heart disease. *Clin Cardiol.* 2000;23(12):883–889.

71. Oliveira-Filho J, Viana LC, Vieira-de-Melo RM, et al. Chagas disease is an independent risk factor for stroke: Baseline characteristics of a Chagas disease cohort. *Stroke.* 2005;36(9): 2015–2017.
72. Bestetti RB, Rossi MA. A rationale approach for mortality risk stratification in Chagas' heart disease. *Int J Cardiol.* 1997;58(3):199–209.
73. Rossi MA, Ramos SG, Bestetti RB. Chagas' heart disease: Clinical-pathological correlation. *Front Biosci.* 2003;8:e94–e109.
74. Rassi A, Jr., Rassi A, Little WC, et al. Development and validation of a risk score for predicting death in Chagas' heart disease. *N Engl J Med.* 2006;355(8):799–808.
75. Kirchhoff LV. American trypanosomiasis (Chagas' disease)—A tropical disease now in the United States. *N Engl J Med.* 1993;329(9):639–644.
76. Nunes Mdo C, Barbosa MM, Rocha MO. Peculiar aspects of cardiogenic embolism in patients with Chagas' cardiomyopathy: A transthoracic and transesophageal echocardiographic study. *J Am Soc Echocardiogr.* 2005;18(7):761–767.
77. Sterin-Borda L, Borda E. Role of neurotransmitter autoantibodies in the pathogenesis of chagasic peripheral dysautonomia. *Ann N Y Acad Sci.* 2000;917:273–280.
78. Sica RE, Genovese OM, Gargia Erro M. Peripheral motor nerve conduction studies in patients with chronic Chagas' disease. *Arq Neuropsiquiatr.* 1991;49(4):405–408.
79. Gonzalez Cappa SM, Sanz OP, Muller LA, et al. Peripheral nervous system damage in experimental chronic Chagas' disease. *Am J Trop Med Hyg.* 1987;36(1):41–45.
80. Genovese O, Ballario C, Storino R, et al. Clinical manifestations of peripheral nervous system involvement in human chronic Chagas disease. *Arq Neuropsiquiatr.* 1996;54(2): 190–196.
81. Lazo J, Meneses AC, Rocha A, et al. Chagasic meningoencephalitis in the immunodeficient. *Arq Neuropsiquiatr.* 1998;56(1):93–97.
82. Rocha A, de Meneses AC, da Silva AM, et al. Pathology of patients with Chagas' disease and acquired immunodeficiency syndrome. *Am J Trop Med Hyg.* 1994;50(3):261–268.
83. Carod-Artal FJ, Vargas AP, Horan TA, et al. Chagasic cardiomyopathy is independently associated with ischemic stroke in Chagas disease. *Stroke.* 2005;36(5):965–970.
84. Leon-Sarmiento FE, Mendoza E, Torres-Hillera M, et al. Trypanosoma cruzi-associated cerebrovascular disease: A case-control study in Eastern Colombia. *J Neurol Sci.* 2004; 217(1):61–64.
85. Bellotti G, Bocchi EA, de Moraes AV, et al. In vivo detection of Trypanosoma cruzi antigens in hearts of patients with chronic Chagas' heart disease. *Am Heart J.* 1996;131(2):301–307.
86. Leon JS, Wang K, Engman DM. Captopril ameliorates myocarditis in acute experimental Chagas disease. *Circulation.* 2003;107(17):2264–2269.

CHAPTER **8**

Cardiac Arrhythmias

William H. Spear • David J. Wilber

OBJECTIVES

- To understand how specific neurological disorders can produce electrocardiographic (ECG) abnormalities and cardiac arrhythmias
- To understand the neurological disorders associated with an increased risk of serious arrhythmias or sudden cardiac death
- To understand how cardiac arrhythmias can mimic or produce neurological syndromes

CASE VIGNETTE

A 35-year-old man with a history of mildly symptomatic myotonic dystrophy, confirmed by electromyogram (EMG) and genetic testing, presents with two syncopal episodes. He had no previous cardiac symptoms. Electrocardiogram demonstrated a normal PR interval and a right bundle branch block. Echocardiography demonstrated normal right and left ventricular (LV) size and function. Because of his known neurological disease, and the occurrence of syncope with a right bundle branch block on the ECG, he had electrophysiological testing.

Atrial studies were normal. The HV interval was 60 milliseconds. During programmed ventricular stimulation, a sustained wide complex tachycardia was induced. Electrophysiologic findings and pacing maneuvers confirmed the diagnosis of bundle branch reentry of the unusual variety with antegrade conduction down the left bundle branch, and retrograde conduction up the right bundle branch. Ablation of the right bundle branch eliminated the tachycardia and was not associated with a change in the HV interval. No other inducible ventricular arrhythmias were found. He has done well over the subsequent 3 years, without recurrent tachycardia or symptoms, and with no evidence of progression of his cardiac disease.

DEFINITION

Cardiac arrhythmias result from altered electrical activation of the heart. Supraventricular arrhythmias originate from the atria or the atrioventricular (AV) junction, whereas ventricular rhythms originate from the ventricles or the His-Purkinje system. Arrhythmias can be caused by reentry, altered automaticity or triggered activity. The autonomic nervous system exerts a significant influence on cardiac electrical activity; central or peripheral alterations in sympathetic or parasympathetic activity can predispose patients to both cardiac arrhythmias and abnormalities of the surface ECG.

EPIDEMIOLOGY

Cardiac arrhythmias are relatively common in neurological diseases. Stroke may produce or be a consequence of cardiac arrhythmias. Cardiac arrhythmias and neurological disorders often share common pathophysiologic defects in ion channels or muscle proteins, coexisting as specific syndrome with both neurological and cardiac manifestations. More than 200,000 people will die each year in the United States from stroke. It is estimated that 15% of all ischemic strokes emanate from a cardiac source of embolism secondary to atrial fibrillation (1). The incidence of atrial fibrillation increases with age. It is present in less than 1% of patients under the age of 55 and up to 9% of patients aged 80 or over. The presence of nonvalvular atrial fibrillation increases the risk of stroke fivefold or more. Major risk factors for stroke associated with atrial fibrillation include a history of thromboembolic events and rheumatic mitral stenosis. Moderate risk factors include age >75 years, hypertension, impaired systolic function or heart failure, and diabetes. Anticoagulation with Coumadin is recommended for all patients at high risk, and for those with two or more moderate risk factors (2).

ETIOLOGY, PATHOLOGY, AND CLINICAL MANIFESTATIONS

CEREBROVASCULAR DISEASE

Acute Ischemic Stroke

Up to 90% of patients presenting with acute ischemic stroke have ECG abnormalities (3). These include LV hypertrophy, prolonged QT interval, ST segment depression, T-wave inversion, peaked T-waves, U-waves, conduction defects, atrial fibrillation, and premature atrial and ventricular beats. Hemispheric strokes appear more likely to be associated with cardiac arrhythmias than brainstem strokes. Although it is often difficult to distinguish preexisting from secondary arrhythmias, Norris et al. (3) found a statistically significant increase in arrhythmias in patients presenting with acute stroke compared with age-matched controls. The incidence of chronic or paroxysmal atrial fibrillation was more common in the subgroup with hemispheric strokes, pointing to a potential cardioembolic source.

More recent studies have focused on sudden cardiac death risk associated with acute ischemic stroke, reported to be as high as 6% (4). Pathophysiologic mechanisms most likely involve autonomic dysfunction associated with acute stroke. Hemispheric lesions involving the right insular cortex are more likely to cause autonomic dysfunction as evidenced by decreased heart rate variability (5). Other risk factors for sudden death in stroke are nonsustained ventricular tachycardia, advanced age, T-wave alternans, and stroke severity (6,7).

Hemorrhagic Stroke

Hemorrhagic stroke increases both sympathetic and parasympathetic stimulation of the heart and circulating catecholamines, resulting in both resting ECG abnormalities and arrhythmias (8). Resting ECG abnormalities including prolonged QT interval, deeply inverted or peaked T-waves, ST segment elevation and depression, and prominent U-waves. In experimental preparations, these abnormalities can be reproduced by hypothalamic stimulation and blood in the subarachnoid space, and are blocked or diminished by spinal transection, vagolytic agents, and adrenergic blockade (8). In a series of 120 patients admitted with subarachnoid hemorrhage, 81% had resting ECG abnormalities of which ST segment abnormalities were the most common (9). Of patients, 90% had arrhythmias during the acute 48-hour phase of monitoring. Most were relatively minor, consisting of premature ventricular contractions (PVC) (34%), sinus tachycardia (29%), sinus bradycardia (19%), and premature atrial contractions (PAC) (14%). Potentially more serious arrhythmias occurred in 14%: asystole, sinoatrial arrest, ventricular flutter, ventricular fibrillation, and torsades de pointes. The QT interval was prolonged in 43% of patients. A significantly longer QT interval was noted in patients with malignant ventricular arrhythmias. Serum potassium concentration was significantly lower in patients with ventricular arrhythmias. These results demonstrate the importance of continuous ECG monitoring during the acute phase of intracranial hemorrhage. Most life-threatening arrhythmias occur within the first 24 hours, and the risk increases with the severity of neurological injury.

Cerebral Trauma

Cerebral trauma can mimic intracranial hemorrhage as a result of increased intracranial pressure and blood in the central nervous system, resulting in similar degrees of autonomic stimulation. In addition, patients often have severe electrolyte disturbances that can lead to QT prolongation torsades des pointes. Patients with head trauma are more likely to have increased QTc intervals relative to other trauma victims (10). Depressed heart rate variability, a measure of autonomic dysfunction, is associated with higher mortality rates in head trauma victims (11).

EPILEPSY

Cardiac arrhythmias, usually benign, are relatively common during epileptic activity (12). Sinus tachycardia is the most common, and precedes the episode. Rarely, more severe arrhythmias have been documented, including asystole, AV block, and ventricular fibrillation. Similar to ischemic stroke, the seizure activity involving the insular area of the temporal lobes is more likely to be associated with either a bradycardia or tachycardia response.

Sudden unexpected death in epileptic patients (SUDEP) is uncommon, occurring in 0.35 to 9.3 per 1,000 patient-years, depending on the severity of epilepsy, but is a significant cause of death in patients with epilepsy (13,14). Epileptic patients have a 24 times increase in mortality compared with age-matched controls (13). Deaths often occur during sleep. Several hypotheses have been advanced, including cardiac arrhythmias (mediated by myocardial ischemia or autonomic dysfunction), neurogenic pulmonary edema, and central or obstructive apnea. In a retrospective review, Nei et al. (15) found several risk factors: young age, seizures during sleep, clustered seizures, higher maximal heart rates during seizure activity, and generalized tonic-clonic seizure activity. These patients also demonstrated a greater incidence of autonomic disturbances and arrhythmias during seizure episodes.

Some characteristics of SUDEP are strikingly similar to the long QT syndrome. LQTS is an ion channelopathy associated with heterogenous lengthening of cardiac repolarization, manifested on the surface ECG as a prolonged QT interval. At least seven different ion channel defects have been implicated to date. Patients are predisposed to episodes of polymorphic ventricular tachycardia (VT) and sudden cardiac death. Akalin et al. (16) studied the QT intervals of children with newly diagnosed epilepsy and compared them with age-matched controls. They found no difference in the QT or QTc interval, but they found that patients with epilepsy had more QT dispersion (16). This latter finding is a marker for heterogeneous ventricular repolarization and has been implicated as a risk factor for sudden death. Tavernor et al. (17) found that patients with epilepsy who died suddenly were more likely to have prolonged QT intervals. It is important to emphasize that initial presentation with the long QT syndrome can mimic epilepsy. An ECG should be obtained for all patients initially presenting with seizure disorder, and cardiac consultation and genetic analysis obtained if the QT interval is prolonged. Finally, any prolonged, but self-terminating cardiac arrhythmia associated with cerebral hypoperfusion can result in seizure activity, and should be considered in the differential diagnosis of new onset of seizures.

PERIPHERAL NERVOUS SYSTEM DISORDERS

Guillain-Barré Syndrome (GBS)

GBS is an acute autoimmune polyneuropathy characterized by cranial, peripheral, and autonomic nerve dysfunction. The primary cardiac manifestation is arrhythmias, mediated by autonomic dysfunction. Sir William Osler first described the cardiac involvement of GBS when he described patients with GBS who died of "paralysis of the heart." In a series of 16 patients with GBS, nine had evidence of autonomic dysfunction, primarily bradyarrhythmias (18). Two patients required pacemaker insertion because of prolonged periods of sinus arrest. Other arrhythmias include sinus tachycardia, atrial fibrillation or flutter, atrial tachycardia, and ventricular tachycardia. More recently, Flacheneker et al. (19) identified heart rate variability as a surrogate marker of autonomic dysfunction predicting serious bradyarrhythmias. In a prospective study of 100 consecutive patients with GBS, *life-threatening* arrhythmias occurred only in 11 of 33 patients who required assisted ventilation (20). These included asystole or severe bradycardia in seven, rapid atrial arrhythmias in two, and ventricular tachycardia or fibrillation in two. Death was attributed to arrhythmias in four patients.

Friedreich Ataxia (FA)

FA is the most common autosomal recessive spinocerebellar ataxia, and commonly involves the heart (21,22). The incidence is approximately 1 in 50,000, and neurological symptoms usually manifest by the third decade. Most patients have minor ECG abnormalities (commonly ST and T-wave changes). Cardiac involvement is primarily LV hypertrophy (either concentric or asymmetric); ventricular dilation and systolic dysfunction are uncommon and late findings. The extent of cardiac involvement does not correlate well with neurological impairment. Life-threatening ventricular arrhythmias and sudden death are rare, and limited to the small subgroup of patients with dilated cardiomyopathy.

Hereditary Motor and Sensory Polyneuropathies (HSMP)

HSMP involves a rare and heterogenous group of disorders that results from mutations in genes encoding myelin proteins (23). HSMP is not associated with cardiomyopathy, but individual cases of intraventricular conduction defects and complete heart block have been reported (24).

NEUROMUSCULAR DISORDERS

Myasthenia Gravis

Electrocardiographic abnormalities and minor cardiac arrhythmias are common in myasthenia gravis and they include prolonged QT interval, sinus tachycardia, sinus arrhythmia, right bundle branch block, and nonspecific T-wave abnormalities (25,26). These abnormalities appear more common in patients with malignant thymoma. The association may be nonspecific, because the coexistence of unrelated cardiac disease is frequently seen in this patient population. Heart block and sudden death, however, have been reported, with postmortem pathology consistent with myocarditis (27). Anticholinesterase medications can aggravate preexisiting sinus node or AV node dysfunction, or potentiate the effects of other cardiac drugs that depress conduction (28).

Familial Periodic Paralysis

This clinical syndrome manifests as episodic weakness, often precipitated by cold temperature or after exercise. The syndrome can result from one of several different mutations in the genes encoding sodium, potassium, and calcium channel proteins usually specific to skeletal muscle, and has diverse phenotypic expression (29). Both hypo- and hyperkalemic forms of the disorder exist, with ventricular arrhythmias being more severe in the latter. The arrhythmias include frequent PVC and bidirectional tachycardia, which may not correlate well with potassium levels. QT prolongation and sudden death have been reported.

Andersen syndrome is a distinct form of periodic paralysis associated with a long QT interval, and episodes of polymorphic ventricular tachycardia. It is considered a variant of the long QT syndrome. It is inherited in an autosomal dominant fashion. Multiple sites of mutation exist, all of which lead ultimately to a loss of function of the Kir2.1 inward rectifier potassium channel, present in both skeletal and cardiac muscle (30). This abnormality prolongs cardiac repolarization and predisposes to ventricular arrhythmias and torsades de pointes.

MUSCULAR DYSTROPHY

Myotonic Dystrophy Type 1

Myotonic dystrophy type 1 (DM1) is caused by an expansion mutation (CTG) in the 19q13 chromosome (31–36). It is the most common inherited muscle disorder of adults, with an incidence of 1 of 8,000. DM is inherited in an autosomal dominant fashion and muscle dysfunction begins in the distal limbs and cranium. Cardiac involvement is common and primarily involves fibrofatty replacement of cardiac conduction tissue (sinus node, AV node, and Purkinje fibers). Degenerative changes can also be observed elsewhere in the atrium and ventricles, but LV systolic dysfunction and clinical heart failure are very uncommon (33–35). Median survival is 50 to 60 years of age, and can be longer in patients with mild neurological symptoms. Conduction disturbances and cardiac arrhythmias are the most common clinical manifestations. First-degree AV block is seen in 40% of patients, and intraventricular conduction defects in 20% (33,35). Complete heart block of the infranodal variety is often observed, requiring permanent pacing. The reported risk of sudden death during long-term follow-up has ranged from 2% in populations with many asymptomatic family members (33) to 20% to 30% in more symptomatic populations (31–33). The severity of the cardiac conduction involvement and arrhythmias increases with a higher number of CTG expansion repeats and age in some (35,36). Ventricular arrhythmias appear to be caused by reentry. Given the high frequency of His-Purkinje system disease, bundle branch reentry is a common cause, and it is treatable with radiofrequency catheter ablation (37). Reentry, however, can also occur in ventricular myocardium in areas of fibrofatty infiltration (38). Given the relatively prolonged survival in this disease, prophylactic pacemaker or defibrillator implantation has been advocated in patients at high risk. Appropriate criteria for risk stratification, including the utility of electrophysiologic testing, remain uncertain, however.

Myotonic Dystrophy Type 2 (DM2)

DM2, also known as PROMM (proximal myotonic myopathy), is a disorder with a similar phenotype to that of DM1. DM2 is caused by a repeat tetranucleotide (CCTG) expansion defect on chromosome 3q. DM2 resembles adult onset DM1 with a similar clinical picture and similar cardiac manifestations (39). Schoser et al. (40) examined 297 patients with genetically proved DM2. They found four cases of sudden cardiac death before the age of 45. They concluded that patients with DM2 are at risk for similar fibrofatty replacement in the ventricles and conduction system, and susceptible to sudden death (40).

Dystrophinopathies

Duchene muscular dystrophy (DMD) and Becker muscular dystrophy (BMD) are degenerative muscular diseases characterized by mutations in the dystrophin gene (41).

Both typically manifest cardiac involvement, characterized by fibrofatty replacement of the myocardium and Purkinje fibers. Typically, the atria and right ventricle are spared or have minor involvement. DMD is the more common and severe disorder, occurring in 1 of 3,500 live-born males and reflecting near complete absence of dystrophin. Symptom onset is in early childhood with most deaths from respiratory failure in the second and third decades. Subclinical ECG abnormalities may be present in the first decade, and nearly all patients ultimately develop cardiomyopathy. BMD has a milder and more heterogenous course, with slower onset of neurological symptoms delayed to the third or fourth decade of life. Cardiac involvement is more variable and may precede, coincide, or follow neurological manifestations, and severity is unrelated to neurological manifestations. Although progression of cardiac disease is slower in BMD, because of longer survival, heart failure can be the terminal event in up to 50% of patients.

Electrocardiographic abnormalities reflect the predominant involvement of the posterolateral left ventricle, resulting in tall right precordial R waves, an increased R/S amplitude ratio, and Q waves in leads 1, V6, and aVL, and less commonly in II, III, and aVF (41,42). Prolonged QTc intervals are common. Conduction disturbances (bundle branch block, fascicular block, first degree AV block) and asymptomatic arrhythmias (atrial tachycardia, flutter, fibrillation, sinus tachycardia, PVC, and nonsustained ventricular tachycardia) are also frequent (43). Complete heart block is uncommon. Patients with both forms appear to be at risk for cardiac arrest during general anesthesia, and avoidance of succinylcholine and volatile anesthetics has been recommended (44). The risk of life-threatening ventricular arrhythmias appears related to the degree of LV dysfunction, similar to patients with other cardiac disease (45).

Emery-Dreifuss Muscular Dystrophy (EDMD)

EDMD results from one of several mutations in cardiac nuclear membrane proteins, including emerin, and lamin A and C (46,47). The disease is characterized by progressive skeletal muscle weakness and atrophy, early contractures, and cardiomyopathy with conduction abnormalities. Cardiac arrhythmias can be an early and primary feature, with relatively mild neurologic manifestations, leading to clinical underdiagnosis. Patients with EDMD are at high risk for developing atrial fibrillation, complete heart block, sinus node dysfunction, and sudden cardiac death, despite the institution of pacing. The atria tend to be involved early in the disease, with later ventricular involvement. Pacing is typically required by the fourth decade of life. The development of a typical dilated cardiomyopathy is common, but can occur later in the disease. A rare entity called *persistent atrial standstill*, characterized by the absence of atrial electrograms, atrial mechanical activity, and the inability to stimulate the atrium on pacing, has been described.

Facioscapulohumeral Muscular Dystrophy

This slowly progressive muscular dystrophy has an incidence of 1 of 20,000. Cardiac involvement in facioscapulohumeral dystrophy is extremely uncommon. Arrhythmias have been reported in <5% of patients, and most were asymptomatic (48).

Scapuloperoneal Syndrome

Scapuloperoneal syndrome is a myopathy that localizes to the shoulder girdle and distal lower extremities. It is characterized by muscle fibers with hyaline desmin containing cytoplasmic inclusions in combination with focal myopathic changes. Cardiac manifestations include progression to severe cardiac failure, complete heart block, and sudden cardiac death. The genetics of this disorder are not completely understood, and it appears subsets of patients exist who are more likely to have cardiac manifestations (49,50).

MITOCHONDRIAL ENCEPHALOMYOPATHIES

Kearns-Sayre Syndrome

This mitochondrial disorder is characterized by progressive external opthalmoplegia, pigmentary retinopathy, and heart block. The disease is associated with fibrofatty replacement of the infranodal conduction system, leading progressively to intraventricular conduction defects and complete heart block (51,52). Pacing may improve survival, and is recommended prophylactically in patients with evidence of infranodal conduction disease. The disease has also been associated less commonly with a dilated cardiomyopathy, ventricular tachycardia, and sudden death (53).

DIAGNOSTIC APPROACH

Continuous ECG monitoring should be undertaken during the first 48 hours in most patients with acute cerebrovascular disease to permit prompt detection and treatment of serious arrhythmias, which can occur during this high risk period. Because of the persistence of autonomic instability for several months after the acute event, patients with known or suspected underlying structural heart disease might be at increased risk of sudden death, and may benefit from additional cardiac evaluation. New or recent onset seizures should prompt a search for a potential cardiac cause, including an ECG, and in older patients with risk factors, assessment of myocardial function and assessment of cardiac function. In patients with known or suspected muscular dystrophy, long-term periodic assessment for potential arrhythmia-related symptoms (dizziness, syncope, fatigue), ECG evidence of conduction disease, and alterations in ventricular function is mandatory. The intensity of monitoring can vary, depending on the risk and severity of cardiac manifestations associated with specific syndromes as discussed in previous sections.

TREATMENT

Acute management of cardiac arrhythmias in patients with neurological disease is similar to that in other settings. Cardiac and noncardiac drugs known to cause QT prolongation should be used with caution in patients with acute cerebrovascular disease, and potentially those with epilepsy at risk for SUDEP. Continuously updated lists of such drugs are available from several online sources (e.g., www.long-QT-syndrome.com or www.arizonacert.org). Drugs with anticholinergic properties or those producing bradycardia should be used with caution in patients with myasthenia gravis. As discussed, patients with dystrophinopathies may require special precautions in anesthetic management.

Use of implantable cardiac devices (pacemakers, defibrillators, and resynchronization therapy) for neurologic patients with symptomatic cardiac disease should follow standard indications and guidelines. Prophylactic pacemaker or defibrillator therapy may be considered for some patients at unusually high risk of heart block or sudden death (myotonic and Emery-Dreifus forms of muscular dystrophy), although limited data exist to guide patient selection.

CLINICAL RECOMMENDATIONS OF THE VIGNETTE

The case vignette represents a typical cardiac manifestation of myotonic dystrophy, with an intraventricular conduction defect and ventricular tachycardia caused by bundle branch reentry. Unlike other muscular dystrophies, cardiac function in this disorder is commonly well preserved, as in this patient. Because the patient's arrhythmia was successfully treated by catheter ablation, other ventricular tachycardias could not be induced, and the HV interval was not prolonged after ablation, we elected not to implant a pacemaker or defibrillator. Had infranodal conduction disease been more extensive, or ablation unsuccessful, however, device therapy represents reasonable alternative therapy.

SUMMARY

Cardiac arrhythmias are associated with a heterogeneous group of acquired and genetic neurological disorders. These disorders can produce multiple ECG abnormalities, which typically are benign, but some can produce malignant arrhythmias. It is critical to recognize when an arrhythmia may have malignant potential and to initiate proper treatment (i.e., atrial fibrillation and warfarin). Proper intensive care monitoring is an integral part of acute cerebral insult to quickly identify those patients who may have life-threatening arrhythmias. Many inherited and acquired syndromes present with cardiac involvement that could potentially be life threatening if associated with sudden cardiac death. Therefore, when evaluating patients with epilepsy or muscular dystrophy, it is important to recognize cardiac involvement and search for cardiac causes for symptoms such as palpitations or syncope. Arrhythmias can be treated pharmacologically, with implantable devices, or with catheter ablation. If the clinical arrhythmia can be discerned by ECG, Holter monitoring, or electrophysiologic testing, it can often be ablated with radiofrequency energy, thus obviating a need for an implantable defibrillator. Sufficiently strong data do not exist for the implantation of cardiac defibrillators for the primary prevention of sudden cardiac death in patients with neurological disease. Similar guidelines for patients with nonischemic heart failure should be followed for primary prevention (i.e., ejection fraction less than 35%). A role exists for implantable defibrillators in the secondary prevention of sudden cardiac death from different neurological diseases. Without question, those at highest risk should receive these devices.

REFERENCES

1. Go AS, Hylek EM, Phillips KA, et al. Prevalence of diagnosed atrial fibrillation in adults. *JAMA.* 2001;285:2370–2375.
2. Fuster V, Ryden LE, Cannom DS, et al. ACC/AHA/ESC 2006 guidelines for the management of patients with atrial fibrillation. *J Am Coll Cardiol.* 2006;48:854–906.
3. Norris JW, Froggatt MB, Hachinski VC. Cardiac arrhythmias in acute stroke. *Stroke.* 1978;9:392–396.
4. Silver FI, Norris JW. Early mortality following stroke: A prospective review. *Stroke.* 1984;15:492–496.
5. Tokgozoglu SL, Batur MK, Topcuoglu MA, et al. Effects of stroke localization on cardiac autonomic balance and sudden death. *Stroke.* 1999;30:1307–1311.
6. Colivicchi F, Bassi A, Santini, M, et al. Prognostic implications of right-sided insular damage, cardiac autonomic derangement, and arrhythmias after acute ischemic stroke. *Stroke.* 2005;36:1710–1715.
7. Ananthasubramaniam K, Karthikeyan V. T wave alternans: An electrocardiographic sign of instability. *Heart.* 2001;85(4):389.
8. Sakr YL, Ghosn I, Vincent JL. Cardiac manifestations after subarachnoid hemorrhage: a systematic review of the literature. *Prog Cardiovasc Dis.* 2002;45:67–80.
9. Di Pasquale G, Pinelli G, Andreoli Alvaro. Holter detection of cardiac arrhythmias in intracranial subarachnoid hemorrhage. *Am J Cardiol.* 1987;59:596–600.
10. Hersch C. Electrocardiographic changes in head injuries. *Circulation.* 1961;23: 853–860.
11. Winchell RJ, Hoyt DB. Analysis of heart rate variability: a noninvasive predictor of death and poor outcome in patients with severe head injury. *J Trauma.* 1997;43(6): 927–933.
12. Zijlmans M, Flanagan D, Gotman J. Heart rate changes and ECG abnormalities during epileptic seizures: Prevalence and definition of an objective clinical sign. *Epilepsia.* 2002;43:847–854.
13. Walczak TS, Leppik IE, D'Amelio M, et al. Incidence and risk factors in sudden unexpected death in epilepsy: A prospective cohort study. *Neurology.* 2001:42:667–673.
14. Stollberger C, Finsterer J. Cardiorespiratory findings in sudden unexplained/unexpected death in epilepsy (SUDEP). *Epilepsy Res.* 2004;59:51–60.
15. Nei M, Ho RT, Abou-khalil BW. EEG and ECG in sudden unexplained death in epilepsy. *Epilepsia.* 2004;45(4)338–345.
16. Akalin F, Tirtir A, Yilmaz Y. Increased QT dispersion in epileptic children. *Acta Paediatr.* 2003;92:916–920.
17. Tavernor SJ, Brown SW, Tavernor RM, et al. Electrocardiograph QT lengthening associated with epileptiform EEG discharges—A role in sudden unexplained death in epilepsy? *Seizure.* 1996;5(1):79–83.
18. Greenland P, Griggs RC. Arrhythmic complications in the Guillain-Barré syndrome. *Arch Intern Med.* 1980;140:1053–1055.
19. Flachenker P, Lem K, Mullges W. Detection of serious bradyarrhythmias in Guillain-Barré syndrome: Sensitivity and specificity of the 24 hour heart rate power spectrum. *Clin Auton Res.* 2000;10(4):185–191.
20. Zochodne DW. Autonomic involvement in Guillain-Barré syndrome: A review. *Muscle Nerve.* 1994;17:1145–1155.
21. Child JS, Perloff JK, Bach PM, et al. Cardiac involvement in Friedreich's ataxia: A clinical study of 75 patients. *J Am Coll Cardiol.* 1986; 7:1370–1378
22. Dutka DP, Donnelly JE, Nihoyannopoulos P, et al. Marked variation in the cardiomyopathy associated with Friedreich's ataxia. *Heart.* 1999;81:141–147.
23. Harding AE. From the syndrome of Charcot, Marie and Tooth to disorders of peripheral myelin proteins. *Brain.* 1995;118:809–818.
24. Isner JM, Hawley RJ, Weintraub AM, et al. Cardiac findings in Charcot Marie-Tooth disease. A prospective study of 68 patients. *Arch Intern Med.* 1979;139(10): 1161–1165.
25. Buyukozturk K, Ozdemir C, Kohen D. Electrocardiographic findings in 24 patients with myasthenia gravis. Acta Cardiol 1976;31(4):301–305.
26. Gibson TC. The heart in myasthenia gravis. *Am Heart J.* 1975;90(3):389–396.
27. Hofstad H, Ohm OJ, Mork SJ, et al. Heart disease in myasthenia gravis. *Acta Neurol Scand.* 1984;176–184.
28. Asura EL, Brunner NG, Namba T, et al. Adverse cardiovascular effects of anticholinesterase medications. *Am J Med Sci.* 1987; 293:18–23.
29. Ptacek L, Fu YH. Channels and disease: past, present and future. *Arch Neurol.* 2004;61:1665–1668.
30. Tristani-Firouzi M, Jensen JL, Donaldson MR. Functional and clinical characterization of KCNJ2 mutations associated with LQT7 (Andersen Syndrome). *J Clin Invest.* 2002;110: 381–388.
31. Bassez G, Lazarus A, Desguerre I, et al. Severe cardiac arrhythmias in young patients with myotonic dystrophy type 1. *Neurology.* 2004;63:1939–1941.
32. Lazarus A, Varin J, Babuty D. Long term follow up of arrhythmias in patients with myotonic dystrophy treated by pacing. *J Am Coll Cardiol.* 2002;40(9):1645–1652.
33. Mathieu J, Allard P, Potvin L, et al. A 10 year study of mortality in a cohort of patients with myotonic dystrophy. *Neurology.* 1999;52:1658–1662.
34. Bhakta D, Lowe MR, Groh WJ. Prevalence of structural cardiac abnormalities in patients with myotonic dystrophy type I. *Am Heart J.* 2004;147:224–227.
35. Groh WJ, Lowe MR, Zipes DP. Severity of cardiac conduction involvement and arrhythmias in myotonic dystrophy type 1 correlates with age and CTG repeat length. *J Cariovasc Electrophysiol.* 2002;13(5):444–448.
36. Clarke NR, Kelion AD, Nixon J, et al. Does cytosine-thymine-guanine(CTG) expansion size predict cardiac events and ECG progression in myotonic dystrophy. *Heart.* 2001;86(4): 411–416.

37. Merino JL, Carmona JR, Fernandez-Lozano I, et al. Mechanisms of sustained ventricular tachycardia in myotonic dystrophy: implications for catheter ablation. *Circulation.* 1998;98(6):541–546.
38. Muraoka H, Negoro N, Terasaki F, et al. Re-entry circuit in ventricular tachycardia due to focal fatty-fibrosis in a patient with myotonic dystrophy. *Intern Med.* 2005;44(2):122–135.
39. Day JW, Ricker K, Jacobsen JF. Myotonic dystrophy type 2: Molecular, diagnostic and clinical spectrum. *Neurology.* 2003;60:657–664.
40. Schoser BG, Ricker K, Schneider-Gold C, et al. Sudden cardiac death in myotonic dystrophy type 2. *Neurology.* 2004;63:2402–2404.
41. Finsterer J, Stollberger C. The heart in human dystrophinopathies. *Cardiology.* 2003;99:1–19.
42. Bhatttacharyya KB, Basu N, Ray TN, et al. Profile of electrocardiographic changes in Duchenne's muscular dystrophy. *J Indian Med Assoc.* 1997;95(2):40–42.
43. Perloff JK. Cardiac rhythm and conduction in Duchenne's muscular dystrophy: a prospective study of 20 patients. *J Am Coll Cardiol.* 1984;3(5)1263–1268.
44. Breucking E, Reimnitz P, Schara U, et al. Anesthetic complications. The incidence of severe anesthetic complications in patients and families with progressive muscular dystrophy of the Duchenne and Becker types. *Anaesthsist.* 2000;49:187–195.
45. Kirchman C, Kececioglu D, Korinthenberg R, et al. Echocardiographic and electrocardiographic findings of cardiomyopathy in Duschenne and Becker-Keiner muscular dystrophies. *Pediatr Cardiol.* 2005;26:66–72.
46. Sakata K, Shimizu M, Ino H, et al. High incidence of sudden cardiac death with conduction disturbances and atrial cardiomyopathy caused by a nonsense mutation in the STA gene. *Circulation.* 2005;111:3352–3358.
47. van Berlo JH, de Voogt WE, van der Kooi AJ, et al. Meta analysis of clinical characteristics of 299 carries of the LMNA gene mutation: do lamin A/C mutations portend a high risk of sudden death? *J Mol Med.* 2005;83:79–83.
48. Laforet P, de Toma C, Eymard B, et al. Cardiac involvement in confirmed facioscapulohumeral muscular dystrophy. *Neurology.* 1998;51:1454–1456.
49. Wilhelmsen KC, Blake DM, Lynch T, et al. Chromosome 12-linked autosomal dominant scapuloperoneal syndrome muscular dystrophy. *Ann Neurol.* 1996;39(4):507–520.
50. Chakrabarti A, Pearce JM. Scapuloperoneal syndrome with cardiomyopathy: A report of a family with autosomal dominant inheritance and unusual features. *J Neurol Neurosurg Psychiatry.* 1981;44(12):1146–1152.
51. Gallastegi J, Hariman RJ, Handler B, et al. Cardiac involvement in the Kearns-Sayre syndrome. *Am J Cardiol.* 1987;60:385–388
52. Anan R, Nakagawa N, Miyata M, et al. Cardiac involvement in the mitochondrial diseases. *Circulation.* 1995;955–961.
53. Oginosawa Y, Abe H, Nagatomo T. Sustained polymorphic ventricular tachycardia unassociated with QT prolongation or bradycardia in the Kearns-Sayre syndrome. *Pacing Clin Electrophysiol.* 2003;26(9):1911–1912.

CHAPTER 9

Hypertension and Hypertensive Encephalopathy

David C. Bonovich

OBJECTIVES

- To define the relationship between blood pressure and brain blood flow
- To define hypertensive emergency and the neurologic manifestations of hypertensive emergency
- To describe the approach to the diagnosis of hypertensive urgency and its treatment

CASE VIGNETTE

A 35-year-old, right-handed woman presented with altered mental status. On examination she was sleepy but arousable, and answered only in "yes," and "no" responses, and did not cooperate with the examination. Pupils were equally round and reactive to light. Ocular motility was intact, but she had horizontal nystagmus on primary gaze. She moved all four extremities symmetrically but did not follow commands. Blood pressure was 180/110 mm Hg and heart rate was 80 beats per minute. Respiratory rate was 12 per minute with an oxygen saturation of 98%. She was afebrile. Laboratory examinations showed a normal complete blood cell count and normal electrolytes. Blood urea nitrogen (BUN) was 45 mg/dL and serum creatinine was 2.1 mg/dL. Electrocardiogram was normal as was the chest radiographic study. Computed tomography (CT) showed a small fourth ventricle and evidence of edema in the cerebellum.

DEFINITIONS

The Joint National Committee on Prevention, Detection, Evaluation, and Treatment of High Blood Pressure (JNC-7) classifies hypertension into four stages: (i) Prehypertension: systolic blood pressures (SBP) ranging from 120 to 139 mm Hg or a diastolic blood pressure (DBP) ranging from 80 to 89 mm Hg; (ii) Stage 1: SBP 140 to 159 mm Hg or DBP 90 to 99 mm Hg; (iii) Stage 2: SBP 160 to 179 mm Hg or DBP 100 to 109 mm Hg; and (iv) Stage 3: Also called severe or accelerated hypertension, SBP >180 mm Hg or diastolic >110 mm Hg (1).

Hypertensive crisis or emergency is defined as sudden increases in either DBP or SBP with associated end-organ damage of the brain, kidneys, or the heart. Hypertensive urgency is defined as sudden increases in SBP and DBP without associated end-organ damage (2–4). Postoperative hypertension is defined as a SBP >190 mm Hg or a DBP >100 mm Hg on two consecutive measurements following surgery (5,6). Hypertension in pregnant women just before or just after delivery is defined as a SBP >169 mm Hg or a DBP >109 mm Hg is considered a hypertensive emergency (7,8).

Hypertensive encephalopathy is defined as an acute encephalopathy resulting from failure of the upper limits of cerebral autoregulation. It is characterized by headaches and focal neurologic signs associated with subcortical edema, usually involving the occipital, temporal, parietal, and posterior fossa structures (9).

EPIDEMIOLOGY

Arterial hypertension affects approximately 1 billion people worldwide and, in approximately 30%, it is undiagnosed (4,10). Approximately 7.1 millions deaths each year can be blamed on hypertension (1). Recent data suggest that the risk of death from heart disease and stroke increases linearly as SBP rises above 115 mm Hg and DBP above 75 mm Hg (11). For every 20 mm Hg systolic and each 10 mm Hg diastolic increase in pressure a doubling occurs of mortality for both heart disease and stroke.

The association between systolic hypertension and stroke, both ischemic and hemorrhagic, appears to be stronger than that seen with DBP. Approximately 40% of all strokes can be attributed to a SBP of 140 mm Hg. 'Isolated' systolic hypertension, increased SBP with normal DBP, has been associated with increased risk especially in the elderly (12). At least two studies have shown that lowering blood pressure is associated with at least a 40% reduction in stroke risk (13,14).

Approximately 1% of patients with arterial hypertension will develop hypertensive crisis at some point in their life (15). The incidence is 1 to 2 per 100,000 (16) and, in the United States, has a higher incidence in African-Americans and the elderly, with men being affected two times a frequently as women (17). Despite advances in the treatment of hypertension, the overall incidence of hypertensive emergencies has increased with hospital admissions for hypertensive emergency tripling between the years 1983 and 1991 (4).

The incidence of postoperative hypertension varies, depending on the study, from 4% to 35% (5,18). Preeclampsia occurs in about 7% of women and is more often seen during a first pregnancy (19).

ETIOLOGY, PATHOGENESIS, AND PATHOPHYSIOLOGY

In the white population, essential hypertension accounts for about 20% to 30% of severe or malignant hypertension, whereas in blacks it may account for up to 80% of cases. Secondary causes include renal parenchymal disease, renovascular disease, and endocrine abnormalities, such as pheochromocytoma, primary hyperaldosteronism, or Cushing's syndrome. Drugs associated with severe hypertension include sympathomimetic agents, such as cocaine and methamphetamine, phencyclidine, and abrupt clonidine withdrawal (4,20).

The factors leading to the development of hypertensive urgency or emergency are not well understood. It is felt to be related to the release of humoral vasoconstrictors, such as norepinephrine, angiotensin II, vasopressin, or endothelin (4,21). Some evidence indicates that angiotensin II exerts toxic effects on vessel walls and some of these effects may be responsible for the end-organ damage seen in hypertensive emergency (4,23). The initial response of the endothelium is to release vasodilator substances such as nitric oxide; however, with sustained hypertension, these compensatory mechanisms can become exhausted, promoting further increases in blood pressure and endothelial damage, thereby setting up a vicious cycle (21).

The exact molecular mechanisms leading to endothelial failure are poorly understood. They appear, however, to involve proinflammatory responses such as mechanical stress, increased endothelial calcium concentrations, monocyte chemotactic factor, and the upregulation of endothelial adhesion molecules (24–27). Ultimately, these events lead to increased permeability, inhibition of fibrinolytic activity promoting coagulation, platelet aggregation, and further vasoconstriction.

In normotensive subjects, blood flow to the brain remains the same between mean arterial pressures of about 60 to 160 mm Hg and is referred to as *cerebral pressure autoregulation.* This occurs through vasoconstriction and vasodilation as pressure increases or decreases respectively (Fig. 9-1). When blood pressure exceeds the limits of autoregulation, autoregulatory failure occurs, resulting in perfusion breakthrough. As vasoconstrictor ability is overwhelmed, vessels dilate, and cerebral edema develops.

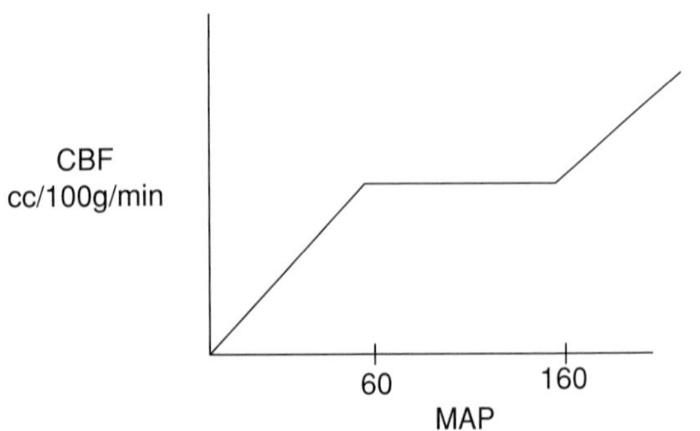

FIGURE 9-1. Pressure autoregulation of blood flow to the brain showing that over a wide range of pressures, blood flow remains constant. This is accomplished by vasoconstriction or vasodilation in response to blood pressure changes.

The edema is typically more prominent in the subcortical areas of the occipital lobes, parietal lobes, the frontoparietal junction, and the temporal lobes, as noted on neuroimaging studies (28,29). A similar condition can also occur with only mild elevations in blood pressure. As a result, a series of terms have been proposed for similar clinical and radiographic features but without significant changes in blood pressure. These terms include (a) reversible posterior leukoencephalopathy (30); (b) reversible posterior cerebral edema syndrome (31); (c) occipital-parietal encephalopathy (32); (d) vasculature autoregulatory dysfunction (33); and (e) hyperperfusion encephalopathy (34).

DIAGNOSTIC APPROACH

The first key in evaluating patients presenting with increased blood pressure should be to distinguish between hypertensive urgency and hypertensive crises. Patients should be assessed for specific symptoms suggestive of end-organ involvement: Chest pain suggestive of aortic dissection or myocardial infarction; shortness of breath or evidence of decreased oxygen saturation, suggestive of pulmonary edema; and neurologic symptoms, such as seizures or encephalopathy. The history should also include determining any prior hypertensive urgency or crisis; recreational drug use, especially sympathomimetic agents, phencyclidine, or monamine oxidase inhibitors.

The examination should include funduscopic evaluation assessing for evidence of papilledema or retinal hemorrhages. Cardiovascular evaluation should assess for evidence of jugular distension and crackles on pulmonary evaluation. Urinalysis and serologic tests should be done to investigate for possible evidence of renal damage, such as increases in BUN and creatinine, and the presence of protein. Signs of encephalopathy include lethargy, confusion, headache, visual difficulties including blindness, and either focal or generalized seizures.

Cranial CT may demonstrate edema in the posterior brain regions and evidence of hemorrhage. These findings are even better demonstrated on T2 weighted magnetic resonance imaging (MRI) of the brain. Edema can also be seen in the brainstem and the cerebellum. Diffusion weighted MRI demonstrates that the edema is vasogenic as opposed to cytotoxic (29). One reason given for why the cerebral edema is predominately in the posterior regions of the brain is because this region has a relative paucity of vascular sympathetic innervation to the basilar artery and the vessels arising from it (35). Hypertensive encephalopathy with imaging changes isolated to, or predominately in, the brainstem has also been reported (36). Neuroimaging abnormalities typically resolve with treatment.

Electroencephalogram (EEG) shows evidence of generalized slowing and epileptiform discharges and loss of posterior dominant alpha rhythm, correlating with neuroimaging findings (37,38). These EEG findings, as with the neuroimaging findings, typically resolve with treatment.

TREATMENT

Because no large clinical trials have been conducted on the treatment of hypertensive urgency and emergency, no evidence-based guidelines exist. Instead, treatment recommendations are largely made by consensus (39). Management should be tailored to the patient, individualized blood pressure goals, and the presence or absence of end-organ damage.

Many different agents are available for the treatment of hypertensive urgency and hypertensive emergency. In general, treatment aim to (a) reduce systemic vascular resistance (Blood Pressure = SVR × Cardiac Output) through vasodilation and sympatholysis and (b) reduce cardiac output by decreasing myocardial contractility and decreasing venous tone, thereby decreasing ventricular filling (40). Patients with hypertensive urgency can have their blood pressure lowered gradually, often with oral agents. Patients with hypertensive crises need to have blood pressure controlled in an intensive care unit (ICU) setting.

The choice of agent in hypertensive emergency should be targeted to the goal desired. In general, blood pressure should be lowered by about 10% to 15% or to a mean arterial pressure (MAP) of 110 mm Hg. Patients with aortic dissection need rapid blood pressure control (within 5 to 10 minutes); in other conditions, bringing blood pressure to the desired end-point within an hour is reasonable (4). One exception is in patients who have had an ischemic cerebrovascular event where it is not advisable to lower blood pressure unless SBP >220 mm Hg or DBP >110 mm Hg (41). In hypertensive crises, the agent chosen should be rapid acting and titratable to desired goals. In addition, effects on cerebral autoregulation and intracranial pressure should be kept in mind, especially in those patients who are manifesting signs and symptoms of encephalopathy.

VASODILATORS

Nitroprusside is a balanced venous and arterial dilator that will decrease both afterload and preload on the heart. The problem in patients with hypertensive encephalopathy is that it may increase intracranial pressure (42,43). It has an onset of action within seconds and its effect lasts several minutes (44). Its mechanism of action is by donating nitric oxide, resulting stimulating the formation of cyclic guanasine monophosphate, which relaxes smooth muscle. Nitroprusside is eventually converted to thiocyanate in the liver. Thiocyanate is much less toxic than cyanide and is excreted through the kidneys. Nitroprusside can cause toxicity through the release of the cyanide molecule, interfering with cellular respiration; it can also cause toxicity through the release of nitric oxide and subsequent free radical formation (45). Nitroprusside should be used only when other agents are not available, and only in patients with normal renal and liver function (46).

Nitroglycerin, a strong venodilator, is an arterial dilator only at high doses. Its effect is also through nitric oxide, but it requires an enzymatic reaction for its release. Nitroglycerin reduces preload and cardiac output. Because of its effect on cardiac output, it may not be desirable in those patients where cerebral perfusion is already compromised.

Hydralazine is an arterial dilator. A brief latent period occurs between its administration and onset of action. Blood pressure drop can be dramatic and prolonged (up to 12 hours). The unpredictability of this agent makes it less suitable for acute treatment. Hydralazine has complex effects on the brain. Studies suggest that it raises intracranial pressure and can create an uneven distribution of blood flow, resulting in the development of ischemic areas in the brain (47,48).

Angiotensin-converting enzymes (ACE) inhibitors, such as enalaprilat, have been used for >20 years (49–51). Angiotensin II is felt to play an important role in hypertensive crisis and so ACE inhibitors can have an important role in treatment. Enalaprilat has an onset of action within 15 minutes and its effects last up to 24 hours, thus the onset and offset time might be too long to be used for rapid titration of blood pressure. No adverse side effects have been reported with this agent; however, it is contraindicated in pregnancy (52).

Calcium channel blockers clinically have three primary effects: (i) negative inotropic effects; (ii) atrioventricular (AV) blockade; and (iii) vasodilation. Of the calcium channel blockers, the dihydropyridines are predominately vasodilators. Nifedipine and nicardipine are both dihydropyridine calcium channel blockers. The difference between the two is that nicardipine is much more water soluble so that it can be administered intravenously (IV) (53,54). Nicardipine has an onset of action within 5 minutes and has been found to compare favorably with nitroprusside, but with fewer side effects (55). It has also been shown to reduce both cardiac and cerebral ischemia (56).

BETA BLOCKERS

Beta blockers are separated into long-, intermediate-, and short-acting agents. Esmolol has an onset of action of 60 seconds, and its duration of action is about 10 minutes. It has been used in both supraventricular tachycardia and more recently in the treatment of hypertensive crisis (57). The usual dose is 0.5 mg/kg followed by 25 to 300 mg/kg/min.

Labetalol is a combined α- and β-blocker in a ratio of 1:7 (58). Labetalol maintains cardiac output, unlike other (pure) β-blockers. It also reduces peripheral vascular resistance without affecting blood flow and it maintains renal and cerebral perfusion (59). Labetalol has its onset of action within 5 minutes and can last several hours. It has been shown to be effective in hypertensive crisis, myocardial infarction, and in treating severe hypertension (59,60).

DOPAMINERGIC AGENTS

Fenoldopam is a short-acting dopamine-1 (DA1) agonist that increases both blood flow to the kidneys and sodium excretion. Fenoldopam acts only on DA1 receptors and has no interaction with α- and β-receptors. The onset is within 5 minutes and its effect lasts up to an hour (61). The initial starting dose is 0.1 μ/kg/min. Because of its effects on the kidneys, it is a good agent to treat patients with hypertensive crisis and renal manifestations (62).

TREATMENT

HYPERTENSIVE ENCEPHALOPATHY

Patients with hypertensive encephalopathy should be immediately admitted to an intensive care unit and immediately have their blood pressure lowered. The choice of agent to reduce blood pressure is important. Nitroprusside is an effective agent in lowering blood pressure; however, its effect on venodilation has been associated with increases in intracranial pressure in addition to its toxic effects (42,43).

Hydralazine is an effective agent to lower blood pressure. Its unpredictability and its variable effects on intracranial pressure and circulation, however, make it less desirable than other drugs.

Nicardipine is a potent vasodilator that has no adverse effects on intracranial pressure (63). It has also been shown to reduce cerebral ischemia (40,56).

Labetalol has also been shown to be an effective agent in lowering blood pressure in hypertensive encephalopathy, owing to its ability to lower blood pressure while preserving cerebral perfusion. Esmolol is also felt to be effective in lowering blood pressure without significant effects on cerebral blood flow or intracranial pressure (64).

Fenoldopam has been associated with reduced regional and global cerebral blood flow (65).

Seizures should be managed with antiepileptic medication as soon as possible so that seizures can be rapidly brought under control. Fosphenytoin can be given as an IV loading dose (10 to 20 mg/kg) and is effective in treating seizures (66). Valproic acid is also effective in treating seizures associated with hypertensive encephalopathy. The loading dose for valproic acid is 10 to 15 mg/kg (67). Both agents can be administered IV.

CLINICAL RECOMMENDATIONS OF THE VIGNETTE

The patient in the vignette presented with hypertensive crisis with evidence of end-organ damage in her kidneys (increased creatinine), and her brain: Edema in the posterior fossa is reported as part of the radiographic appearance of hypertensive encephalopathy. As noted, edema posteriorly can reflect the relative paucity of sympathetic vascular efferents compared with those seen more anteriorly. Subsequent MRI demonstrated white matter edema in the posterior fossa causing compression of the fourth ventricle. The patient was urgently admitted to the intensive care unit and a nicardipine drip was started with the target of lowering blood pressure by 20% during the first 8 hours. Nicardipine was selected because of its easy titratability and its ability to reduce both cardiac and cerebral ischemia. Other antihypertensive choices would be esmolol or labetalol. Neurosurgical consultation was obtained to evaluate the need for ventricular drainage. After resolution of the patient's symptoms, it is important to emphasize the need for tight blood pressure control to avoid further episodes of hypertensive urgency or emergency and to avoid the long-term sequelae of hypertension.

SUMMARY

Arterial hypertension, a major health concern worldwide, is responsible for more than 7 millions deaths per year worldwide. Hypertensive emergency is life-threatening, manifesting as increased blood pressure with evidence of end-organ injury. Encephalopathy related to hypertension manifests as headache, lethargy, altered mental status, and seizures related to the effects of perfusion breakthrough because of autoregulatory failure. The key to treatment of hypertensive encephalopathy is to lower blood pressure. In choosing which agent is most appropriate, keep in mind the potential effects on intracranial pressure and cerebral blood flow. Nicardipine, esmolol, and labetalol are excellent choices because these agents will effectively lower blood pressure without risk of adverse effects on intracranial pressure or cerebral blood flow. Other agents, such as nitroprusside and hydralazine, should be avoided because of their potential adverse effects on intracranial pressure, in the case of nitroprusside, and unpredictable cerebral effects associated with hydralazine.

REFERENCES

1. Chobanian AV, Bakris GL, Black HR, et al. Seventh report of the Joint National Committee on Prevention, Detection, Evaluation, and Treatment of High Blood Pressure. *Hypertension.* 2003;42(6): 1206–1252.
2. Ferguson RK, Vlasses PH. Hypertensive emergencies and urgencies. *JAMA.* 1986;255(12): 1607–1613.
3. Reuler JB, Magarian GJ. Hypertensive emergencies and urgencies: Definition, recognition, and management. *J Gen Intern Med.* 1988;3(1):64–74.
4. Varon J, Marik PE. Clinical review: The management of hypertensive crises. *Crit Care.* 2003;7(5):374–384.
5. Halpern NA, et al. Postoperative hypertension: A multicenter, prospective, randomized comparison between intravenous nicardipine and sodium nitroprusside. *Crit Care Med.* 1992;20(12):1637–1643.
6. Gal TJ, Cooperman LH. Hypertension in the immediate postoperative period. *Br J Anaesth.* 1975;47(1):70–74.
7. Rey E, et al. Report of the Canadian Hypertension Society Consensus Conference: 3. Pharmacologic treatment of hypertensive disorders in pregnancy. *CMAJ.* 1997;157(9): 1245–1254.
8. Gifford RW, Jr. Management of hypertensive crises. *JAMA.* 1991;266(6):829–835.
9. Schwartz RB. Hyperperfusion encephalopathies: Hypertensive encephalopathy and related conditions. *Neurologist.* 2002;8(1):22–34.
10. Burt VL, et al. Prevalence of hypertension in the US adult population. Results from the Third National Health and Nutrition Examination Survey, 1988–1991. *Hypertension.* 1995;25(3):305–313.
11. Lewington S, et al. Age-specific relevance of usual blood pressure to vascular mortality: A meta-analysis of individual data for one million adults in 61 prospective studies. *Lancet.* 2002;360(9349):1903–1913.
12. Vokonas PS, Kannel WB, Cupples LA. Epidemiology and risk of hypertension in the elderly: The Framingham Study. *J Hypertens Suppl.* 1988;6(1):S3–S9.
13. Collins R, et al. Blood pressure, stroke, and coronary heart disease. Part 2, Short-term reductions in blood pressure: Overview of randomised drug trials in their epidemiological context. *Lancet.* 1990;335(8693):827–838.
14. Lawes CM, et al. Blood pressure and stroke: An overview of published reviews. *Stroke.* 2004;35(4):1024.
15. Vidt DG. Current concepts in treatment of hypertensive emergencies. *Am Heart J.* 1986;111(1):220–225.
16. Elliott WJ. Management of hypertension emergencies. *Curr Hypertens Rep.* 2003;5(6):486–492.
17. Kaplan NM. Treatment of hypertensive emergencies and urgencies. *Heart Dis Stroke.* 1992;1(6):373–378.
18. Prys-Rroberts C. Anaesthesia and hypertension. *Br J Anaesth.* 1984;56(7):711–724.
19. Coppage KH, Sibai BM. Treatment of hypertensive complications in pregnancy. *Curr Pharm Des.* 2005;11(6):749–757.
20. Milne FJ, James SH, Veriava Y. Malignant hypertension and its renal complications in black South Africans. *S Afr Med J.* 1989;76(4):164–167.
21. Vaughan CJ, Delanty N Hypertensive emergencies. *Lancet.* 2000;356(9227):411–417.
22. Funakoshi Y, et al., Induction of interleukin-6 expression by angiotensin II in rat vascular smooth muscle cells. *Hypertension.* 1999;34(1):118–125.
23. Muller DN, et al. NF-kappaB inhibition ameliorates angiotensin II-induced inflammatory damage in rats. *Hypertension.* 2000;35(1 Pt 2):193–201.
24. Okada M, et al. Cyclic stretch upregulates production of interleukin-8 and monocyte chemotactic and activating factor/monocyte chemoattractant protein-1 in human endothelial cells. *Arterioscler Thromb Vasc Biol.* 1998;18(6):894–901.
25. Wung BS, et al. Cyclical strain increases monocyte chemotactic protein-1 secretion in human endothelial cells. *Am J Physiol.* 1996;270(4 Pt 2):H1462–H468.
26. Touyz RM, Milne FJ. Alterations in intracellular cations and cell membrane ATPase activity in patients with malignant hypertension. *J Hypertens.* 1995;13(8):867–874.
27. Verhaar MC, et al. Progressive vascular damage in hypertension is associated with increased levels of circulating P-selectin. *J Hypertens.* 1998;16(1):45–50.
28. Schwartz RB, et al. Hypertensive encephalopathy: Findings on CT, MR imaging, and SPECT imaging in 14 cases. *AJR Am J Roentgenol.* 1992;159(2):379–383.
29. Schwartz RB, et al. Diffusion-weighted MR imaging in hypertensive encephalopathy: Clues to pathogenesis. *AJNR Am J Neuroradiol.* 1998;19(5):859–862.
30. Hinchey J, et al. A reversible posterior leukoencephalopathy syndrome. *N Engl J Med.* 1996;334(8):494–500.
31. Dillon WP, Rowley H. The reversible posterior cerebral edema syndrome. *AJNR Am J Neuroradiol.* 1998;19(3):591.

32. Casey SO, Truwit CL. Pontine reversible edema: A newly recognized imaging variant of hypertensive encephalopathy? *AJNR Am J Neuroradiol.* 2000;21(2):243–245.
33. Port JD, Beauchamp NJ, Jr. Reversible intracerebral pathologic entities mediated by vascular autoregulatory dysfunction. *Radiographics.* 1998;18(2):353–367.
34. Schwartz RB. A reversible posterior leukoencephalopathy syndrome. *N Engl J Med.* 1996;334(26):1743; author reply 1746.
35. Beausang-Linder M, Bill A. Cerebral circulation in acute arterial hypertension—Protective effects of sympathetic nervous activity. *Acta Physiol Scand.* 1981;111(2):193–199.
36. Wang MC, Escott EJ, Breeze RE. Posterior fossa swelling and hydrocephalus resulting from hypertensive encephalopathy: Case report and review of the literature. *Neurosurgery.* 1999;44(6):1325–1327.
37. Bakshi R, et al. Thrombotic thrombocytopenic purpura: Brain CT and MRI findings in 12 patients. *Neurology.* 1999;52(6):1285–1288.
38. Manfredi M, et al. Eclampic encephalopathy: Imaging and pathogenetic considerations. *Acta Neurol Scand.* 1997;96(5):277–282.
39. Calhoun DA, Oparil S. Treatment of hypertensive crisis. *N Engl J Med.* 1990;323(17): 1177–1183.
40. Oates JA, Brown NJ. Chapter 33 in Hardman JG and Limbird LE. (Eds.), *Goodman and Gilman's The Pharmacological Basis of Therapeutics,* 10 ed. New York: McGraw-Hill; 2001.
41. Adams H, et al. Guidelines for the early management of patients with ischemic stroke: 2005 guidelines update a scientific statement from the Stroke Council of the American Heart Association/American Stroke Association. *Stroke.* 2005;36(4):916–923.
42. Hartmann A, et al. Alteration of intracranial pressure, cerebral blood flow, autoregulation and carbondioxide-reactivity by hypotensive agents in baboons with intracranial hypertension. *Neurochirurgia (Stuttg).* 1989;32(2):37–43.
43. Griswold WR, Reznik V, Mendoza SA. Nitroprusside-induced intracranial hypertension. *JAMA.* 1981;246(23):2679–2680.
44. Francis GS. Vasodilators in the intensive care unit. *Am Heart J.* 1991;121(6 Pt 1): 1875–1878.
45. Gobbel GT, Chan TY, Chan PH. Nitric oxide- and superoxide-mediated toxicity in cerebral endothelial cells. *J Pharmacol Exp Ther.* 1997;282(3):1600–1607.
46. Robin ED, McCauley R. Nitroprusside-related cyanide poisoning. Time (long past due) for urgent, effective interventions. *Chest.* 199;102(6):1842–1845.
47. Barry DI, et al. Cerebral blood flow during dihydralazine-induced hypotension in hypertensive rats. *Stroke.* 1984;15(1):102–108.
48. Overgaard J, Skinhoj E. A paradoxical cerebral hemodynamic effect of hydralazine. *Stroke.* 1975;6(4):402–410.
49. Rutledge J, et al. Effect of intravenous enalaprilat in moderate and severe systemic hypertension. *Am J Cardiol.* 1988;62(16):1062–1067.
50. Hirschl MM, et al. Impact of the renin-angiotensin-aldosterone system on blood pressure response to intravenous enalaprilat in patients with hypertensive crises. *J Hum Hypertens.* 1997;11(3):177–183.
51. Tsuchihashi T, et al. Comparison of effects of enalapril and captopril on serum potassium concentration in the treatment of malignant hypertension. *Cardiovasc Drugs Ther.* 1992;6(5):495–498.
52. DiPette DJ, et al. Enalaprilat, an intravenous angiotensin-converting enzyme inhibitor, in hypertensive crises. *Clin Pharmacol Ther.* 1985;38(2):199–204.
53. Turlapaty P, Vary R, Kaplan JA. Nicardipine, a new intravenous calcium antagonist: A review of its pharmacology, pharmacokinetics, and perioperative applications. *J Cardiothorac Anesth.* 1989;3(3):344–355.
54. Efficacy and safety of intravenous nicardipine in the control of postoperative hypertension. IV Nicardipine Study Group. *Chest.* 1991;99(2):393–398.
55. Halpern NA, et al. Nicardipine infusion for postoperative hypertension after surgery of the head and neck. *Crit Care Med.* 1990;18(9):950–955.
56. Schillinger D. Nifedipine in hypertensive emergencies: A prospective study. *J Emerg Med.* 1987;5(6):463–473.
57. Balser JR, et al. Beta-adrenergic blockade accelerates conversion of postoperative supraventricular tachyarrhythmias. *Anesthesiology.* 1998;89(5):1052–1059.
58. Lund-Johansen P. Pharmacology of combined alpha-beta-blockade. II. Haemodynamic effects of labetalol. *Drugs.* 1984;28[Suppl 2]:35–50.
59. Pearce CJ, Wallin JD. Labetalol and other agents that block both alpha- and beta-adrenergic receptors. *Cleve Clin J Med.* 1994;61(1):59–69; quiz 80–82.
60. Wilson DJ, et al. Intravenous labetalol in the treatment of severe hypertension and hypertensive emergencies. *Am J Med.* 1983;75(4A):95–102.
61. Bodmann KF, et al. Hemodynamic profile of intravenous fenoldopam in patients with hypertensive crisis. *Clin Invest.* 1993;72(1):60–64.
62. Reisin E, et al. Intravenous fenoldopam versus sodium nitroprusside in patients with severe hypertension. *Hypertension.* 1990;15[2 Supp]:I59–I62.
63. Nishiyama T, et al. Continuous nicardipine infusion to control blood pressure after evacuation of acute cerebral hemorrhage. *Can J Anaesth.* 2000;47(12):1196–1201.
64. Rose JC, Mayer SA. Optimizing blood pressure in neurological emergencies. *Neurocrit Care.* 2004;1(3):287–299.
65. Prielipp RC, et al. Reduced regional and global cerebral blood flow during fenoldopam-induced hypotension in volunteers. *Anesth Analg.* 2001;93(1):45–52.
66. Uthman BM, Wilde BJ. Emergency management of seizures: An overview. *Epilepsia.* 1989;30[Suppl 2]:S33–S37.
67. Misra UK, Kalita J, Patel R. Sodium valproate vs phenytoin in status epilepticus: A pilot study. *Neurology.* 2006;67(2):340–342.

CHAPTER 10

Orthostatic and Postprandial Hypotension

Eduardo E. Benarroch

OBJECTIVES

- To recognize the clinical symptoms associated with orthostatic hypotension (OH)
- To recognize the most common causes of OH and postprandial hypotension
- To emphasize the main points on the evaluation of patients with OH
- To understand the basic management principles for OH

CASE VIGNETTE

A 65-year-old man with a 10-year-history of non–insulin-dependent diabetes mellitus is evaluated for increasingly frequent episodes of dizziness on getting up from bed in the morning. These episodes started approximately 3 months ago. They also occur approximately 30 minutes after a meal, or when he works outdoors on a hot and humid day. He describes this sensation as lightheadedness, occasionally associated with blurred vision, pain in the occiput and shoulders, or both. He cannot stand up for more than 5 minutes before having to sit down to avoid fainting. He has a 10-year history of symmetric numbness in the toes bilaterally, a 4-year history of urinary urgency, erectile dysfunction, and constipation. Medications include glyburide, aspirin, and terazosin. He has no family history of neurologic disease.

Examination revealed a normal mental status and cranial nerve functions. He had some difficulties walking on heels and he complained of lightheadedness and neck tightness during examination of posture and gait. These symptoms resolved immediately after sitting down. Motor strength, tone, and alternate motor rate, and coordination were normal in the upper and lower limbs. He had absent ankle jerks. Plantar responses were flexors. Except for absent vibration sense in the toes, sensory examination finding was normal. In supine position, arterial blood pressure (ABP) was 140/90 mm Hg and heart rate (HR) was 90 beats per minute. When standing for 1 minute, ABP was 80/50 mm Hg and HR 94 beats per minute, and this was associated with an impending sensation of fainting.

DEFINITION

Orthostatic hypotension has been defined as a reduction of systolic ABP of at least 20 mm Hg or diastolic ABP of at least 10 mm Hg within 3 minutes after standing or during head-up tilt (HUT) of at least 60 degrees (1). OH can be either symptomatic or asymptomatic. The severity of OH can be graded on the basis of the frequency of orthostatic symptoms, standing time before onset of symptoms or presyncope, influence on the ability to perform activities of daily living, and indices of adrenergic failure on laboratory testing (2). Postprandial hypotension is the development or exacerbation of hypotension after a meal, in general between 30 minutes to 2 hours following a meal (3,4).

EPIDEMIOLOGY

The exact prevalence of OH is not known, but it occurs in approximately 14% to 26% of persons >70 years of age (5). Orthostatic hypotension was found to be the cause of 24% of syncopal events evaluated in an emergency department (6). For adults with diabetes mellitus, the prevalence of symptomatic OH has been estimated to be approximately 10% (2). OOH is the most disabling manifestation of central and peripheral autonomic disorders, such as nondiabetic autonomic neuropathies, which have a prevalence of 10 to 50 per 100,000 and multiple system atrophy (MSA), which has a prevalence of 5 to 15 per 100,000.

ETIOLOGY AND PATHOGENESIS

Orthostatic hypotension is a manifestation of central and peripheral disorders affecting the baroreflex-mediated sympathetic vasoconstriction of limb muscle and splanchnic vessels on standing. When OH is pronounced and cerebral blood flow decreases below a critical level (~25 mL/min/100 g), syncope occurs.

The main causes of OH include central neurodegenerative disorders, autonomic neuropathies, and drug effects. Neurodegenerative disorders with OH include synucleinopathies, such as multiple system atrophy (MSA) (7); and Lewy body disorders, such as Parkinson disease (PD) (8); dementia with Lewy bodies (DLB) (9); and pure autonomic failure (PAF) (3,10). Other central causes associated with OH include high spinal cord lesions above T-5, medullary lesions, such as vascular malformations or syringobulbia. Many autonomic neuropathies are found in which OH is a prominent finding (11). These include acute autoimmune autonomic neuropathies associated (or not) with nicotinic ganglionic acetylcholine antibodies (12–14) paraneoplastic neuropathies, Guillain-Barré syndrome (15), and porphyria. Chronic autonomic neuropathies include diabetic autonomic neuropathy (11), amyloidosis, and sensory neuronopathy associated with Sjögren syndrome (16). Other disorders include some hereditary neuropathies, such as familial dysautonomia and familial amyloidosis (11). OH can also be a prominent manifestation of specific biochemical disorders, such as dopamine β-hydroxylase (DBH) deficiency, systemic mastocytosis (17), and rare cases of pheochromocytoma (18).

Several drugs have been associated with OH. These include antihypertensive agents (diuretics, angiotensin-converting enzyme (ACE) inhibitors, α_1-blockers, β-blockers, and calcium channel blockers), nitrates, tamsulosin, and other α_1-receptor antagonists for treatment of benign prostatic hypertrophy; dopaminergic agonists for treatment of PD (including levodopa, direct dopaminergic agonists, and entacapone), antidepressants (particularly amitriptyline and trazodone), and antipsychotic drugs (e.g., chlorpromazine and clozapine). The elderly population is at the highest risk of drug-induced hypotension (19–21).

On assuming the upright position, a pooling of 500 to 1,000 mL of blood occurs in the lower limbs and splanchnic circulation. This leads to a decrease in venous return to the heart, which reduces cardiac filling pressure and, thus, cardiac output and ABP (22). These hemodynamic changes are sensed by the carotid and aortic arch baroreceptors which, via inputs to the nucleus tractus solitarius (NTS) in the medulla, initiate compensatory responses, mediated by sympathoexcitatory neurons of the rostral ventrolateral medulla, vagal cardioinhibitory neurons in the nucleus ambiguus and dorsal vagal nucleus, and magnocellular hypothalamic neurons secreting arginine vasopressin (AVP) (23). In response to orthostatic stress, a baroreflex-triggered increase occurs in sympathetic outflow, as measured by increase in muscle sympathetic activity and at least a twofold increase in circulating plasma norepinephrine. This leads to α_1-adrenergic receptor-mediated vasoconstriction of resistance limb and splanchnic vessels, resulting in an increase in total peripheral resistance. In addition, withdrawal of vagal cardioinhibitory output ensues, leading to tachycardia. Baroreflex-mediated vasoconstriction is the primary mechanism protecting against OH. In normal subjects, the normal response to standing is a fall in systolic ABP (5 to 10 mm Hg), an increase in diastolic ABP (5 to 10 mm Hg), and an increase in heart rate (10 to 25 beats/min). The exacerbation of hypotension following meals (postprandial hypotension) is thought to reflect the effects of splanchnic vasodilatation mediated by vasoactive peptides, adenosine, or other mediators released by endocrine cells of the enteropancreatic axis in response to meals, particularly those rich in carbohydrates. Most, if not all patients with neurogenic OH also have supine hypertension (24), and this is commonly associated with nocturia and nocturnal natriuresis. This likely reflects both an increased renal blood flow and glomerular filtration rate and inhibition of the renin-angiotensin-aldosterone system in response to increase in arterial pressure in the supine position. This not only results in increased urinary frequency at night, but leads to worsening of OH in early morning hours.

PATHOLOGY

Central, peripheral, and pharmacologic causes of OH primarily affect the baroreflex circuits at various levels. OH in MSA reflects loss of both sympathetic preganglionic neurons and sympathoexcitatory neurons in the rostral ventrolateral medulla (VLM). In this disorder, a blunted reflex increase in plasma AVP is also seen, because of interruption of medullary inputs to the hypothalamus. Evidence indicates that a residual sympathetic tone exists, as manifested by the normal resting levels of plasma norepinephrine and the reduction in ABP elicited by sympathetic ganglion blockade. In Lewy body disorders, including PD, DLB, and pure autonomic failure, OH may reflect primary involvement of the sympathetic ganglia. Positron emission tomography and single photon computer emission tomography studies show reduced uptake of norepinephrine precursors in cardiac sympathetic terminals in PD, DLB, and pure autonomic failure, but not in MSA. OH in autoimmune autonomic neuropathies may reflect impairment of sympathetic ganglion function caused by autoantibodies directed against the α_3 subunit of the ganglionic nicotinic receptor. Some autoimmune neuropathies are associated with inflammatory changes in the postganglionic sympathetic axons. In Guillain-Barré syndrome is found demyelination of baroreceptor afferents and preganglionic sympathetic axons.

CLINICAL MANIFESTATIONS AND SPECIAL SITUATIONS

Orthostatic hypotension can manifest with the typical symptoms of cerebral hypoperfusion, such as lightheadedness, visual disturbances (e.g., blurring, tunneling, or darkening of vision), and presyncope. It can also manifest with atypical symptoms of orthostatic intolerance, including generalized fatigue, head and neck ("coat-hanger") pain caused by ischemia of neck and occiput muscles, intermittent claudication, restless legs syndrome while sitting, or dyspnea (25). In a study of 100 consecutive patients having ambulatory blood pressure recordings for OH, coexisting neurologic diseases were found in 38%, and the most common symptoms were lightheadedness and weakness (26).

Neurogenic OH caused by autonomic failure is characterized by inability to increase heart rate, forearm plasma norepinephrine, and muscle sympathetic nerve activity in response to standing or HUT. Also seen are impaired compensatory sympathoexcitation in response to vasodilatation of the skin (e.g., on exposure to heat), splanchnic bed (e.g., after meals), and muscle (e.g., during strenuous exercise) or in response to reduced cardiac output elicited by valsalva-type maneuvers (e.g., straining at stools).

Orthostatic hypotension is a common finding in the elderly, particularly in early morning hours (27). In this population, OH is an important cause of falls. Several factors, including use of antihypertensive drugs, low sodium diet, decreased water intake because of a reduced thirst mechanism, anemia, and arterial stiffness (28) can contribute to OH in these patients.

Several drugs produce OH in the elderly, among the most common are hydrochlorothiazide, lisinopril, trazodone, furosemide, and terazosin (29). Prolonged (>24 h) bedrest can produce seated postural hypotension in the elderly (30). In elderly patients with syncope, the presence of comorbidity should always be considered. For example, OH may be present in patients with aortic stenosis and contribute to syncope (31). In the elderly, OH can be associated with vitamin B_{12} deficiency, and vitamin replacement has been associated with improved orthostatic tolerance to HUT in these patients (32). OH can increase the risk of myocardial infarction (33) and could lead to cerebral hypoperfusion that has been associated with cognitive decline in these patients (34).

DIAGNOSTIC APPROACH

The evaluation of patients with OH requires a careful history and physical examination, selected laboratory tests, and laboratory assessment of autonomic functions. Neuroimaging, electromyogram and special studies, such as polysomnography, and urodynamic and gastrointestinal motility tests, may be helpful in specific conditions. Some studies, such as measurement of plasma catecholamines and cardiac imaging to assess sympathetic innervation, can be helpful in very special circumstances.

CLINICAL HISTORY

The clinical history is a crucial component of the assessment of patients with OH and is very important to guide therapeutic recommendations. Important data include the time that the patient is able to remain in standing position before developing presyncopal symptoms; special circumstances in which OH is more likely to occur or is more severe; associated symptoms of autonomic failure; symptoms suggesting parkinsonism or peripheral neuropathy; and dietary habits or drug treatments that can cause, trigger, or exacerbate OH.

Typically, OH is more severe on getting up from bed in the morning, within 1 to 2 hours after meals; on exposure to hot and humid environment; during heavy exercise or straining at stools. In general, patients with OH caused by autonomic failure do not have pallor, diaphoresis, or complain of palpitations or chest pain in association with lightheadedness. These presyncopal manifestations commonly occur in patients with other forms of orthostatic intolerance, such as those with predisposition to neurally mediated syncope, postural tachycardia syndrome (POTS), hypovolemia, or, rarely, baroreflex failure or hyperadrenergic states, such as anxiety disorders or pheochromocytoma. Neurally mediated (also to as referred to as *vasovagal, vasodepressor*, or *reflex*) syncope is caused by a paroxysmal cessation of sympathetic vasomotor activity (leading to hypotension) and cardiac vagal activation (leading to bradycardia), which can be triggered by standing. In contrast to patients with chronic autonomic failure in whom syncope appears as a gradual fading of vision and loss of awareness, patients with neurally mediated syncope often have signs and symptoms of autonomic overactivity, such as diaphoresis and nausea, before the event. This distinction and the episodic nature of neurally mediated syncope should be part of a thorough clinical history.

Neurogenic OH is commonly associated with other manifestations of sympathetic or parasympathetic failure. Impaired sympathetic-mediated sweating may first manifest seen only by the presence of dry socks and a lack of skin moisture. When abnormalities are severe, the patient can develop heat intolerance, flushing, or even heat-stroke symptoms. Impaired vagal modulation of enteric neurons manifests with delayed gastric emptying and constipation, whereas impaired sympathetic inhibition of enteric reflexes manifests with diarrhea. Impaired sacral parasympathetic control manifests with urinary retention and erectile dysfunction. Other manifestations of autonomic failure include intolerance to light (because of impaired sympathetically mediated pupil constriction), or dry mouth and dry eyes (Sicca syndrome) caused by impaired cranial parasympathetic outflow to lacrimal and salivary glands.

Pure autonomic failure with no other neurologic deficits is rare. More often, autonomic failure occurs in combination with other neurologic disorders, such as MSA, PD, DLB, or peripheral neuropathies. With suspected central neurodegenerative disorders, it is important to inquire about abnormalities in gait or balance, changes in facial expression, dysarthria or dysphagia, cognitive impairment, or sleep disturbances, including enacting of dreams (which suggests rapid eye movement ([REM] sleep behavior disorder), or snoring with or without sleep apnea. The history should also assess symptoms related to peripheral neuropathies, particularly painful feet and hand and foot numbness or weakness, as well as of diabetes mellitus, antecedent viral infections, rheumatologic or other autoimmune disease, risk factors for lung and other neoplasms, and family history of OH or peripheral neuropathy.

Because the most frequent type of autonomic dysfunction encountered in medical practice is pharmacologic, a thorough review of medication use, especially antihypertensives and psychotropic drugs, should always be undertaken.

PHYSICAL EXAMINATION

Autonomic function should be assessed during examination of the pupil (size, symmetry, and reactivity), skin (temperature, moisture, color, and trophic changes), and cardiovascular system (arterial pressure and rather, both in supine and standing position). Pupil examination may reveal an Adie's pupil or Horner syndrome. Sudomotor failure can be recognized by the localized or generalized absence of sweating. Changes in skin temperature or color should also be noted. Skin examination may reveal angiokeratomas in the trunk and lower limbs in patients with Fabry disease, and the tongue may be enlarged in those with amyloidosis. Absence of fungiform papillae may also be demonstrated in children with familial dysautonomia (Riley-Day syndrome).

Blood pressure and HR should be measured after 2 minutes in the supine position and at 1 and 2 minutes after standing. In normal conditions, on changing from the supine to standing position, a 5 to 20 mm Hg drop occurs in systolic blood pressure accompanied by no change or a slight rise in diastolic pressure and a 5 to 25 beats per minute increase in HR. In some cases, it may be useful to have the patient do 12 squats before repeating the blood pressure recordings. The presence of OH without reflex tachycardia is evidence of baroreflex or sympathetic failure. If reflex tachycardia is present, hypovolemia has to be excluded. An increase of HR >30 beats per minute above basal or >120 beats per minute on standing erect, if associated with symptoms, define the postural tachycardia syndrome. This syndrome has multiple possible causes, including hypovolemia, deconditioning, hyperadrenergic states (including anxiety) or, in some cases, restricted adrenergic neuropathies affecting the lower limbs.

The main elements on neurologic examination are the evaluation of the motor and peripheral sensory systems. Abnormal cognitive functions, particularly in the visuospatial domain, suggest DLB. Parkinsonism occurs in DLB, PD, and MSA. The presence of early postural instability, antecollis, and cerebellar, pyramidal, or both signs raises the possibility of MSA. Proximal muscle weakness and areflexia are typical of prejunctional neuromuscular transmission defects associated with cholinergic autonomic failure, such as botulism and the Lambert-Eaton myasthenic syndrome. Distal, symmetric loss of sensation to pinprick and temperature indicates a small fiber peripheral autonomic neuropathy, such as diabetes or amyloidosis, whereas loss of vibration and joint position sense, sensory ataxia, and pseudoathetosis can occur in sensory ganglionopathies, such as those associated with occult neoplasms or Sjögren syndrome.

ANCILLARY STUDIES

Blood tests useful in the initial evaluation of patients with OH and suspect autonomic failure include determinations of blood glucose and glycosylated hemoglobin protein immunoelectrophoresis, vitamin B_{12} and folate, sedimentation rate, antinuclear antibody, extractable nuclear antigen, paraneoplastic panel (including antineuronal nuclear antibodies), and human immunodeficiency virus (HIV) serology. Some tests are indicated in selected cases. They include determination of antibodies against the α_3 subunit of the ganglionic nicotinic acetylcholine receptor in acute or subacute autoimmune autonomic neuropathy; porphobilinogen and urinary heavy metals; α-galactosidase for suspected Fabry disease, or genetic tests for the transthyretin mutations in patients in whom familial amyloidosis is suspected.

Determinations of forearm venous plasma catecholamines for assessment of sympathoadrenal function have important limitations and sources of variability, including failure to standardize conditions of sampling and assay. Circulating norepinephrine (NE) originates primarily in the sympathetic nerves innervating the blood vessels of muscles. Plasma NE constitutes approximately 10% of NE released into the synaptic cleft that escapes neuronal reuptake and "spills over" into the bloodstream. Patients with postganglionic autonomic disorders, such as pure autonomic failure or diabetic neuropathy, frequently have reduced plasma NE levels at rest in the supine position. In normal subjects, plasma NE levels double when assuming the upright posture. In contrast, this response is absent in patients with both pre- and postganglionic sympathetic failure. Determination of plasma and urinary levels of NE metabolites, such as dihydroxyphenylglycol (DHPG) and normetanephrine, may also be useful for separating preganglionic from postganglionic causes of autonomic failure. In patients who lack dopamine β-hydroxylase, the enzyme that converts dopamine to NE, NE in plasma is virtually undetectable, whereas dopamine is high and increases further with maneuvers that increase sympathetic neural discharge.

In general, neuroimaging is of low yield in the evaluation of patients with generalized autonomic failure. Magnetic resonance imaging (MRI) of the head may show atrophy of the putamen or cerebellum and increased signal in the pons in patients with MSA. Rarely, it may be useful to identify hypothalamic or brainstem lesions that can produce OH. The MRI of the spine is performed in patients with traumatic, vascular, and inflammatory (particularly demyelinating) disorders; acute lesions above the T5 spinal level produce OH.

Electromyography (EMG) is indicated for evaluation of all peripheral neuropathies, sensory ganglionopathies, and prejunctional neuromuscular transmission disorders associated with autonomic failure (e.g., botulism, Lambert-Eaton myasthenic syndrome). The anal sphincter EMG may show denervation in patients with MSA. Polysomnogram is indicated in patients with parkinsonism and autonomic failure to detect REM sleep behavior disorder (RBD), which is typical of all synucleinopathies. Abdominal fat aspirate, rectal biopsy, or sural nerve biopsy should be considered in patients in whom amyloid neuropathy or Fabry disease is suspected. Salivary or lacrimal gland biopsy is indicated in patients suspected of having Sjögren syndrome.

AUTONOMIC LABORATORY TESTING

Laboratory autonomic evaluation of OH is indicated in patients with parkinsonism and in whom autonomic failure, distal small fiber neuropathy, and other peripheral neuropathies are suspected, and patients with symptoms of orthostatic intolerance. Although the autonomic test batteries vary among different laboratories, they typically include assessment of sudomotor, cardiovagal, and sympathetic vasoconstrictor reflexes.

Sympathetic sudomotor function can be assessed with a thermoregulatory sweat test (TST), which assesses the entire thermoregulatory axis from the hypothalamus to the sweat gland; the quantitative sudomotor axon reflex test (Q-SART, which assesses the peripheral innervation of the sweat gland, by stimulating a cholinergic axon reflex); and other pertinent tests.

Several tests are done to evaluate the integrity of the vagal innervation of the heart. In normal subjects are seen spontaneous fluctuations of the HR that reflect the level of autonomic activity modulating sinus node discharge. At rest, the vagal inhibitory influence on the sinus node provides a beat-to-beat control of HR. This vagal influence is inhibited during inspiration and maximal at the end of inspiration. This is the basis of the respiratory sinus arrhythmia (tachycardia during inspiration and bradycardia during in expiration). This HR response to deep breathing is the most commonly used test of cardiovagal function. Amplitude of response is progressively reduced with increasing age. Other less commonly utilized tests of cardiovagal function exist. Spectral analysis, using the fast Fourier transform algorithm, is used to assess HR variability. Power in the high frequency band (0.15 to 0.4 Hz) reflects vagal influences on the sinus node and power in the low frequency band (0.02 to 0.15 Hz) reflects mainly sympathetic activity. This technique is used primarily for clinical research.

The integrity of the sympathetic vasoconstrictor outflow can be assessed by different noninvasive techniques, including determination of the increase in diastolic blood pressure (normally >15 mm Hg) in response to immersion of a hand in cold water for 1 minute (cold pressor test); isometric exercise (handgrip maneuver), and emotional stress (mental arithmetic). These tests, however, are of limited sensitivity and specificity.

The most commonly used indicators of the integrity of reflex sympathetic vasoconstriction function are the beat-to-beat blood pressure responses to the valsalva maneuver (VM) and orthostatic stress, including standing or HUT, using noninvasive methods. Together with continuous electrocardiographic (ECG) recordings, these also allow the determination of reflex changes in the HR and provide a noninvasive way to assess baroreceptor function.

The VM consists of an abrupt, transient elevation of intrathoracic and intraabdominal pressures, induced by blowing against a pneumatic resistance while maintaining a predetermined pressure, in general 40 mm Hg for 15 seconds. This impairs venous return to the heart and the resulting decrease in cardiac output triggers reflex compensatory tachycardia and vasoconstriction. The responses to the VM have been divided into four phases (I-IV). Phase II occurs during the strain and consists of an initial fall (early phase II) followed by recovery (late phase II) of ABP because of sympathetic vasoconstriction. The magnitude of the ABP fall and later partial recovery during phase II are useful indicators of sympathetic vasoconstrictor function. Throughout phase II, there is a continuous increase of heart rate, first due to inhibition of vagal output, and later to sympathetically mediated cardioacceleration. Phase IV, which occurs after release of the strain, is characterized by an elevation of systolic and diastolic ABP above control levels; this is referred to as *overshoot* and is accompanied by baroreflex-induced, vagally mediated bradycardia. The valsalva ratio (VR) is defined as the ratio of the longest R-R interval after the maneuver (phase IV) to the shortest R-R interval during the maneuver (phase II) and it assesses cardiovagal as well as sympathetic function.

Determination of the changes in ABP and HR induced by standing or passive HUT is one of the most useful tests of autonomic cardiovascular reflexes. During upright tilt at 60 degrees or more, normal subjects undergo a transient reduction of systolic pressure and maintenance of mild increase in diastolic pressure, followed by a recovery within 1 minute. These changes are associated with an increase of HR of 10 to 20 beats per minute. Patients with adrenergic failure have a marked reduction in pulse pressure with no recovery and insufficient compensatory tachycardia. Ambulatory 24-hour blood pressure recordings (5) may be helpful to detect OH in patients with orthostatic symptoms in whom routine autonomic testing is normal.

Many other autonomic tests are used in the clinical research setting. These include microneurography, which allows recording of postganglionic sympathetic nerve activity in muscle or skin; pharmacologic stimulation of NE release; determination of sensitivity of adrenergic receptors by measuring responses to norepinephrine or isoproterenol; and determination of reflex release of arginine vasopressin (AVP) in response to hypotension induced by HUT.

TREATMENT

GENERAL PRINCIPLES

The management of OH should be individualized. The main goal is (*a*) to improve the patient's functional capacity and sense of well-being rather than reaching a fixed value of arterial pressure and (*b*) to prevent supine hypertension (35). Treatment success of OH is reflected by the increase in the time that the patient can stand motionless without symptoms. The basis for management includes avoidance of precipitating factors, measures to increase intravascular volume, drugs that promote vasoconstriction, and prevention of postprandial hypotension and supine hypertension. The principles of management of OH are composed of patient education, adjustments in the diet, physical maneuvers, and drug therapy. The first step in management of OH is always nonpharmacologic.

PATIENT EDUCATION

Patient education is the single most important step for successful management of neurogenic OH. The patients should be instructed about the mechanisms of maintenance of postural normotension, orthostatic stress, blood pressure fluctuations that occur throughout the day according to activities, and effect of diet and posture on OH symptoms. They should be able to recognize even "atypical" symptoms of orthostatic intolerance, such as fatigue or head and neck (*coat-hanger*) pain, to prevent syncope (36). Patients are instructed to keep a symptom and arterial pressure diary for about 2 weeks and after any change in drug regimen. Also discuss avoidance of exposure during hot weather, straining, and vigorous exercise, and benefits of mild isotonic exercise with the patient. Potentially reversible causes of OH, particularly the use of drugs such as diuretics, antihypertensive agents, antianginal agents, α-adrenoreceptor antagonists (e.g., terazosin) used to treat symptoms of prostatic hypertrophy;, antidepressants (particularly tricyclics), clozapine, dopaminergic agonists, and catechol-O-methyltransferase (COMT) inhibitors, should be recognized and avoided if possible. The patient should be instructed to keep a blood pressure log. This is particularly useful when symptoms worsen or when case management changes. The patient or, preferably, the spouse or another caregiver should use an automated sphygmomanometer to measure ABP when the patient is supine and after standing for 1 to 2 minutes. Recordings should be obtained on awakening, after a meal, during a time of maximal orthostatic tolerance or of poor orthostatic tolerance, and before and 1 hour after taking medication.

POSTURAL AND OTHER PHYSICAL MANEUVERS

Patients with OH should move from supine to standing position in gradual stages, particularly in the morning when orthostatic tolerance is lowest. They should be encouraged to maintain physical activity, including isotonic aerobic exercises in supine and sitting positions. Patients with autonomic failure can use a variety of physical maneuvers to increase orthostatic tolerance and prevent dizziness while standing. These include leg-crossing, lowering the head in stooped position, bending forward, muscle-pumping, placing a foot on a chair, or squatting. These maneuvers have been shown to increase stroke volume, arterial pressure, cerebral perfusion, and tolerance to standing from 1 to 3 to 5 minutes. Physical counter maneuvers can have a marked positive effect on the patient's ability to perform activities of daily living. A home-based training program using elastic bands have been shown to improve functional ability in elderly patients with OH, despite a lack of objective changes in arterial pressure (37). Male patients should be advised to urinate in the sitting position, particularly at night, to reduce the risk of syncope.

Most patients with neurogenic OH have supine hypertension even before treatment of the OH. Supine hypertension likely reflects a combination of factors, including baroreflex dysfunction and the presence of residual sympathetic outflow, particularly in patients with central disorders, such as MSA. Although most patients tolerate sustained supine hypertension without end-organ damage, ventricular hypertrophy has been documented echocardiographically in some cases. One important consequence of supine hypertension is pressure diuresis during the night, which leads to nocturnal volume depletion. This is responsible for the more severe symptoms of OH observed in the morning. All patients, therefore, are advised to sleep with the head of the bed elevated by 10 to 20 degrees in reverse Trendelenburg position. This prevents supine hypertension, activates the renin-angiotensin system, reduces nocturnal natriuresis, and improves orthostatic tolerance in early morning hours.

VOLUME EXPANSION

Plasma volume expansion is critical to increase orthostatic tolerance. Patients should have a daily intake of sodium of at least 10 g, accompanied with an increase of fluid intake to at least 2 to 2.5 L (5 cups or glasses) daily. Salt tablets (available as 0.5- and 1-g tablets) can be used as a supplement, but patients may experience undesirable gastrointestinal side effects. Some foods with high-sodium content, including canned soups, chili, bacon, ham, and additives, such as soy sauce. Many patients who have inadequate control of OH despite medications have an inadequate sodium intake. This can be verified by checking the 24-hour urinary concentration of sodium. A value of less than 170 mmol per 24 hours indicates the need of supplementary sodium (1 to 2 g three times daily). The patient's weight, symptoms, and urinary sodium concentration should be checked again 1 to 2 weeks later. Patients also need to have a high potassium diet, including fruits (especially banana) and vegetables, particularly if they are also receiving mineralocorticoids. Patients with autonomic failure may show a marked pressor response and improvement in symptoms for approximately 1 hour following the ingestion of approximately 500 mL of water (38). The beneficial effect of drinking tap water, however, may reflect a transient sympathoexcitatory effect more than volume expansion per se.

A classic approach to increase venous return in standing position is the use of custom fitted elasticized thigh-high stockings (Jobst or Barton-Carey leotard), lower abdominal compression binder, or both. This permits the application of graded pressure to the lower limbs and abdomen, thus reducing blood pooling in the lower limbs and splanchnic circulation, and improving orthostatic tolerance (39). Elderly patients or patients with severe parkinsonism may have some difficulty to put them on, however, and the garment is poorly tolerated in hot days (40).

FIRST-LINE DRUG THERAPY: FLUDROCORTISONE AND MIDODRINE

In general, the first step in drug-therapy of OH is either 9-α-fludrocortisone acetate (Florinef) or a sympathomimetic drug, commonly midodrine. Fludrocortisone is a mineralocorticoid with a long duration of action that enhances sensitivity of blood vessels to catecholamines and increases blood volume. The full pressor action of fludrocortisone depends on its mineralocorticoid effect, which usually is seen after 1 to 2 weeks of treatment. Treatment is started with a 0.1-mg tablet taken before noon and then increased slowly, at 0.1-mg increments, at 1- to 2-week intervals. In general, little benefit is obtained by increasing beyond 0.5 mg daily. Side effects include supine hypertension, ankle edema, hypokalemia, (which develops in almost 50% of patients within 2 to weeks of treatment), hypomagnesemia (in about 5% of patients), headache (particularly in young patients), rarely congestive heart failure, and reduced effects of warfarin.

Sympathomimetic drugs can be used in combination or after fludrocortisone therapy or as initial therapy in patients who are able to replete intravascular volume adequately with salt and fluid ingestion. In the United States, the only US Food and Drug Administration (FDA)-approved treatment for OH is midodrine. Midodrine is an α_1-adrenoreceptor selective agonist that has several advantages over other sympathomimetic drugs, such as the direct agonist, ephedrine, or indirect sympathomimetic agents, methylphenidate, and dextroamphetamine. The efficacy of midodrine has been demonstrated in many double-blind, placebo-controlled studies.

Midodrine is absorbed almost completely after oral administration, with a peak plasma concentration at 20 to 40 minutes after ingestion and a half-life of 30 minutes. Midodrine is a prodrug that is transformed in the liver to desglymidodrine, a potent α_1-adrenoreceptor agonist in arteries and veins. Desglymidodrine is 15 times more potent than midodrine and has an elimination half-life of 2 to 4 hours. Midodrine is usually started at a dose of 2.5 mg at breakfast and lunch and increased at 2.5-mg steps daily until a satisfactory response occurs or a dose of 30 to 40 mg daily is achieved. Almost all patients experience piloerection, paresthesia in the scalp, and pruritus, which are in general mild and rarely lead to discontinuation of the drug. The most important adverse side effect of midodrine, as with all other sympathomimetic agents, is supine hypertension. Patients, therefore, should not take this drug for 4 hours before recumbency and should avoid taking the drug in the evening.

CHOLINESTERASE INHIBITORS AND NOREPINEPHRINE PRECURSORS

Two new approaches to vasoconstrictor management of OH include the use of anticholinesterase drugs and norepinephrine precursors. Cholinesterase inhibitors, such as pyridostigmine, increase the efficacy of cholinergic transmission at the sympathetic ganglia and potentiate the effects of the increased preganglionic input that normally occurs on standing. This could improve orthostatic tolerance without the risk of supine hypertension. In a prospective, open-label, single dose trial, 15 patients with neurogenic OH of different causes received an oral dose of 60 mg pyridostigmine. This drug produced only a modest and nonsignificant increase in supine blood pressure, but significantly reduced the degree of orthostatic fall of blood pressure and of orthostatic symptoms (41,42).

The synthetic amino acid, L-threo-3,4-dihydroxyphenylserine (L-DOPS), which is decarboxylated by the L-amino acid decarboxylase to norepinephrine. This drug, which acts through its peripheral but not central conversion to norepinephrine, is extremely useful for treatment of OH in patients with dopamine-β-hydroxylase deficiency. In a double-blind, placebo-controlled, cross-over trial, L-DOPS significantly raised plasma norepinephrine levels and mean blood pressure, both in supine and standing position, for several hours and improved orthostatic tolerance in all 19 patients with severe OH included in the study (43).

SECONDARY THERAPY

In patients who continue to show symptoms despite adequate dosing of fludrocortisone and midodrine, secondary therapy may be helpful. Erythropoietin corrects the normocytic normochromic anemia that frequently accompanies autonomic failure and improves standing blood pressure and orthostatic intolerance in these patients (44,45). Recombinant human erythropoietin-α is administered subcutaneously or intravenously at doses between 25 and 75 U/kg three times a week until the hematocrit level approaches normal (in general, within 3 weeks); lower maintenance doses (25 mg/kg three times a week) can then be used. Iron supplementation is usually required, particularly during the period when the hematocrit is increasing. The mechanism of the pressor effect of this drug is still unresolved, but it may include an increase in blood volume and regulation of vascular tone via interaction of hemoglobin with nitric oxide. Supine hypertension can occur with the use of this drug.

The potent, synthetic vasopressin analogue desmopressin acetate (DDAVP) acts on V_2 receptors in the collecting ducts of the kidney leading to water reabsorption; it has minimal V_1 receptor-mediated vasoconstrictor effect. DDAVP is used to prevent nocturia and weight loss and it reduces the morning postural fall of AP. It can be administered as a nasal spray (5 to 40 μg), orally (100 to 800 μg), or intramuscularly (2 to 4 μg) in a single dose at night. Because of the risk of water intoxication and hyponatremia developing, DDAVP therapy should always started with the patient in the hospital.

PREVENTION OF POSTPRANDIAL HYPOTENSION

To prevent postprandial hypotension, the patients should avoid ingestion of large, carbohydrate-rich meals (which trigger the release of vasodilator substance from the gut and pancreas) and the use of alcohol (which produces vasodilatation). Caffeine, which blocks vasodilating adenosine receptors, may also be used to attenuate postprandial hypotension in patients with autonomic failure. Typical doses are 100 to 250 mg three times a day, either as tablets or caffeinated beverages (one cup of coffee contains approximately 85 mg and one cup of tea 50 mg of caffeine). Continued use of caffeine leads to tachyphylaxis. Cyclooxygenase inhibitors, such as ibuprofen (400 to 800 mg), decrease production of vasodilating prostaglandins and other arachidonic acid derivatives. They can be used as an adjuvant in patients with postprandial hypotension, but are rarely effective as monotherapy. Octreotide is an analogue of somatostatin that inhibits release of vasodilator gastrointestinal peptides; its main indication is treatment of severe postprandial hypotension in patients with autonomic failure. It is administered subcutaneously at a dose of 25 to 200 μg. Side effects include nausea and abdominal cramps.

PREVENTION OF SUPINE HYPERTENSION

Spine hypertension is a common problem presenting in patients with OH (46,47). In patients with neurogenic OH, midodrine should not be given after 5 PM. The patients should avoid lying flat. Sleeping with the head of the bed elevated by 15 to 30 cm (reverse Trendelenburg position) or in the sitting position not only prevents nocturnal polyuria (and thus worsening of OH on in the morning), but also reduces the risk of supine hypertension. Ingestion of a bedtime snack or drinking small amounts of alcohol before bedtime may be of benefit in reducing supine hypertension during the night. If needed, a short-acting vasodilator agent, such as nifedipine, transdermal nitroglycerin or captopril can also be used at night. Clonidine reduces sympathetic activity and may prevent supine hypertension and excessive natriuresis at night (46).

OTHER THERAPIES

In extreme and refractory cases, other vasoconstrictor drugs can be tried. These include clonidine (an agonist of α_2-adrenergic and I_1 imidazoline receptors), yohimbine (α_2-adrenoreceptor antagonist), nonselective β-blockers (particularly those with intrinsic sympathomimetic activity), and dihydroergotamine (an ergot that act on α-receptors and has selective vasoconstrictor effect). In general, these drugs are of limited benefit in the management of OH, and exert only modest or inconsistent pressor effects. The patients should be closely monitored, however, for their potentially serious side effects.

CLINICAL RECOMMENDATIONS OF THE VIGNETTE

The patient had an autonomic reflex screen to asses the extent and severity of autonomic failure. The thermoregulatory sweat test revealed anhidrosis in the feet, and sudomotor axon reflex responses were reduced in the distal leg and absent in the foot. The HR response to deep breathing and the VM were markedly impaired, which is consistent with cardiovagal failure. The beat-to-beat blood pressure responses to the VM revealed an impaired recovery during late phase II and impaired overshoot during phase IV, which indicates sympathetic adrenergic vasomotor and cardiomotor failure. In supine position, ABP was 140/90 with a HR of 90 beats per minute. Within 2 minutes of HUT, ABP was 80/50 mm Hg and HR 92 beats per minute. In summary, the autonomic laboratory evaluation revealed distal postganglionic sudomotor, severe cardiovagal, and severe adrenergic failure. This is consistent with a diabetic autonomic neuropathy.

The patient was first informed of the results of the tests, the presence of OH as the cause of his dizziness, and the multiple factors that can trigger his symptoms. In this patient, the use of terazosin, an α-blocker, is likely to have contributed to OH, and it should be discontinued. He was also instructed to recognize that others symptoms, such as his neck and occiput pain, may also be caused by OH. He was instructed to learn to monitor his blood pressure, particularly before and immediately after getting out of bed in the morning, within 1 hour of meals, and at bedtime in a supine position, as well as whenever he was symptomatic. It was emphasized that there is not a value of low ABP that is too low or life-threatening, that the most serious consequence is syncope, and that the aim of the treatment is to prevent this symptom and increase the sense of well-being and standing time and not to achieve a particular value of ABP. He was instructed to sit at the edge of the bed before standing in the morning, to urinate sitting in a toilet, and to perform postural maneuvers, such as squatting or crossing his legs, to increase orthostatic tolerance. He was also instructed to sleep with the head elevated approximately 4 inches (15 to 30 cm)to reduce the risk of nocturnal hypertension and nocturia and to improve orthostatic tolerance on getting up from bed in the morning. He was encouraged increase his salt intake by adding salt to his food or to eat salty foods, such as pickles, drink at least 5 cups or glasses of water daily, and to eat smaller, more frequent meals to avoid postprandial hypotension. The option to wear custom-fitted elasticized high-thigh stockings and, if tolerated, a compression binder was also discussed. On returning a week later, his symptoms had improved after following all these recommendation. He continued to experience episodes of dizziness, particularly in the morning, and was still reluctant to start exercising or going shopping with his wife. Potential options for pharmacologic treatment, including midodrine and fludrocortisone, and potential side effects of these drugs were discussed. The patient opted for fludrocortisone, and was stared on a dose of 0.1 mg orally in the morning. A blood test 2 weeks later revealed no evidence of hypokalemia or hypomagnesemia. At that time, he had developed mild ankle edema. On examination, his supine blood pressure was 160/90 mm Hg and his standing ABP 120/70 mm Hg. He could now stand for 1 hour without symptoms. Three months later, he returned because of worsening of his orthostatic dizziness. He could not tolerate more than 0.1 mg of fludrocortisone because with higher dose he developed shortness of breath and increased ankle edema. A trial dose of midodrine (0.25 mg) was given at the office and his supine and standing blood pressure was measured at 30, 60, and 120 minutes. At approximately 30 minutes after this dose, the patient developed mild scalp itching. He was reassured that this is an expected effect of the drug that is transient and, in general, becomes less frequent over time. One hour after 2.5 mg of midodrine, his supine ABP was 160/90 mm Hg and standing ABP 110/70 mm Hg. He was asymptomatic. He was started on midodrine: 2.5 mg to be taken 30 to 60 minutes before getting up from bed, 30 to 60 minutes before lunch, and 2.5 mg at 4 PM before supper. He was told that the dose can be increased by 2.5-mg steps to a maximum of 10 mg four times daily. He was strongly instructed not to take midodrine after 5 PM and was reminded of the importance of avoiding lying flat and to sleep with the head of the bed elevated to avoid supine hypertension.

SUMMARY

- OH and prostprandial hypotension (PPH) can be manifestation of central or peripheral autonomic disorders.
- A frequent cause of OH is effect of medications, particularly in the elderly.
- OH is an important cause of fall in the elderly.
- OH can manifest with atypical symptoms.
- Patient education is the mainstay of treatment of OH.
- Treatment of OH should include first nonpharmacologic measures, such as increased sodium and water intake, postural maneuvers, mild exercise, smaller, frequent meals; and avoidance of precipitating factors.
- Fludrocortisone, midodrine, or both constitute the most efficacious drugs for management of OH.
- Pyridostigmine may be considered as an adjuvant treatment in patients with risk of supine hypertension.
- Erythropoietin improves orthostatic tolerance in patients with OH and anemia; octreotide may be considered in patients with severe PPH.
- Supine hypertension may be prevented by sleeping with the head of the bed elevated, avoiding vasoconstrictor drugs in the evening hours, eating a snack at night, or taking short-acting antihypertensive drugs on retiring.

REFERENCES

1. Consensus statement on the definition of orthostatic hypotension, pure autonomic failure, and multiple system atrophy. *J Neurol Sci.* 1996;144:218–219.
2. Low PA. Laboratory evaluation of autonomic function. In: Low PA, ed. *Clinical Autonomic Disorders: Evaluation and Management,* 2 ed. Philadelphia: Lippincott-Raven; 1997:179–208.
3. Trofimiuk M, Huszno B, Golkowski F, et al. Postprandial hypotension and gastric emptying in longstanding diabetes mellitus. *Przeglad Lek.* 2003;60(2):107–110.
4. O'Mara G, Lyons D. Postprandial hypotension. *Clin Geriatr Med.* 2002;18(2):307–321.
5. Gardner SF, Schneider EF. 24-Hour ambulatory blood pressure monitoring in primary care. *J Am Board Fam Pract.* 2001;14(3):166–171.
6. Sarasin FP, Louis-Simonet M, Carballo D, et al. Prevalence of orthostatic hypotension among patients presenting with syncope in the ED. *Am J Emerg Med.* 2002;20(6):497–501.
7. Wenning GK, Colosimo C, Geser F, et al. Multiple system atrophy. *Lancet Neurology.* 2004;3(2):93–103.
8. Allcock LM, Ullyart K, Kenny RA, et al. Frequency of orthostatic hypotension in a community based cohort of patients with Parkinson's disease. *J Neurol Neurosurg Psychiatry.* 2004;75(10):1470–1471.
9. Thaisetthawatkul P, Boeve BF, Benarroch EE, et al. Autonomic dysfunction in dementia with Lewy bodies. *Neurology.* 2004;62:1804–1809.
10. Kaufmann H, Biaggioni I. Autonomic failure in neurodegenerative disorders. *Semin Neurol.* 2003;23(4):351–363.
11. Low PA, Vernino S, Suarez G. Autonomic dysfunction in peripheral nerve disease. *Muscle Nerve.* 2003;27(6):646–661.
12. Suarez GA, Fealey RD, Camilleri M, et al. Idiopathic autonomic neuropathy: Clinical, neurophysiologic, and follow-up studies on 27 patients. *Neurology.* 1994;44(9):1675–1682.
13. Klein CM, Vernino S, Lennon VA, et al. The spectrum of autoimmune autonomic neuropathies. *Ann Neurol.* 2003;53(6):752–758.
14. Vernino S, Adamski J, Kryzer TJ, et al. Neuronal nicotinic ACh receptor antibody in subacute autonomic neuropathy and cancer-related syndromes. *Neurology.* 1998;50:1806–1813.
15. Zochodne DW. Autonomic involvement in Guillain-Barre syndrome: A review. *Muscle Nerve.* 1994;17(10):1145–1155.
16. Etienne M, Weimer LH. Immune-mediated autonomic neuropathies. *Curr Neurol Neurosci Rep.* 2006;6(1):57–64.
17. Boncoraglio GB, Brucato A, Carriero MR, et al. Systemic mastocytosis: A potential neurologic emergency. *Neurology.* 2005;65(2):332–333.
18. Tagle R, Acosta P, Valdes G. Orthostatic hypotension: An unusual manifestation of pheochromocytoma. *Revista Medica de Chile.* 2003;131(12):1429–1433.
19. Verhaeverbeke I, Mets T. Drug-induced orthostatic hypotension in the elderly: Avoiding its onset. *Drug Saf.* 1997;17(2):105–118.
20. Duplantier C, Courtat-Bailly B, Moreau C, et al. Iatrogenic syncopes and malaises. *Ann Cardiol Angeiol* (Paris). 2004;53(6):320–324.
21. Lagi A, Rossi A, Comelli A, et al. Postural hypotension in hypertensive patients. *Blood Press.* 2003;12(5–6):340–344.
22. Smit AA, Halliwill JR, Low PA, et al. Pathophysiological basis of orthostatic hypotension in autonomic failure. *J Physiol.* 1999;519:1–10.
23. Spyer KM. Annual Review Prize Lecture: Central nervous mechanisms contributing to cardiovascular control. *J Physiol.* 1994;474:1–19.
24. Goldstein DS, Pechnik S, Holmes C, et al. Association between supine hypertension and orthostatic hypotension in autonomic failure. *Hypertension.* 2003;42(2):136–142.
25. Gibbons CH, Freeman R. Orthostatic dyspnea: A neglected symptom of orthostatic hypotension. *Clin Auton Res.* 2005;15(1):40–44.
26. Ejaz AA, Haley WE, Wasiluk A, et al. Characteristics of 100 consecutive patients presenting with orthostatic hypotension. *Mayo Clin Proc.* 2004;79(7):890–894.
27. Weiss A, Chagnac A, Beloosesky Y, et al. Orthostatic hypotension in the elderly: Are the diagnostic criteria adequate? *J Hum Hypertens.* 2004;18(5):301–305.
28. Boddaert J, Tamim H, Verny M, et al. Arterial stiffness is associated with orthostatic hypotension in elderly subjects with history of falls. *J Am Geriatr Soc.* 2004;52(4):568–572.
29. Poon IO, Braun U. High prevalence of orthostatic hypotension and its correlation with potentially causative medications among elderly veterans. *J Clin Pharm Ther.* 2005;30(2):173–178.
30. Cohen N, Gorelik O, Fishlev G, et al. Seated postural hypotension is common among older inpatients. *Clin Auton Res.* 2003;13(6):447–449.
31. Taneja I, Marney A, Robertson D. Aortic stenosis and autonomic dysfunction: Co-conspirators in syncope. *Am J Med Sci.* 2004;327(5):281–283.
32. Moore A, Ryan J, Watts M, et al. Orthostatic tolerance in older patients with vitamin B12 deficiency before and after vitamin B12 replacement. *Clin Auton Res.* 2004;14(2):67–71.

33. Luukinen H, Koski K, Laippala P, et al. Orthostatic hypotension and the risk of myocardial infarction in the home-dwelling elderly. *J Intern Med.* 2004;255(4): 486–493.
34. Viramo P, Luukinen H, Koski K, et al. Orthostatic hypotension and cognitive decline in older people. *J Am Geriatr Soc.* 1999;47(5):600–604.
35. Gibbons CH, Freeman R. Treatment options for autonomic neuropathies. *Current Treatment Options in Neurology.* 2006;8(2):119–132.
36. Low PA. Neurogenic orthostatic hypotension. In: Johnson R, ed. *Current Therapy in Neurologic Disease*, 4 ed. Philadelphia: Mosby Year Book; 1994.
37. Zion AS, De Meersman R, Diamond BE, et al. A home-based resistance-training program using elastic bands for elderly patients with orthostatic hypotension. *Clin Auton Res.* 2003;13(4):286–292.
38. Jordan J. Acute effect of water on blood pressure. What do we know? *Clin Auton Res.* 2002;12(4):250–255.
39. Smit AA, Wieling W, Fujimura J, et al. Use of lower abdominal compression to combat orthostatic hypotension in patients with autonomic dysfunction. *Clin Auton Res.* 2004;14(3):167–175.
40. Fealey RD, Robertson D. Management of orthostatic hypotension. In: Low PA, ed. *Clinical Autonomic Disorders: Evaluation and Management.* 1st ed. Boston: Little, Brown; 1993:731–743.
41. Singer W, Opfer-Gehrking TL, McPhee BR, et al. Acetylcholinesterase inhibition: A novel approach in the treatment of neurogenic orthostatic hypotension. *J Neurol Neurosurg Psychiatry.* 2003;74(9):1294–1298.
42. Sandroni P, Opfer-Gehrking TL, Singer W, et al. Pyridostigmine for treatment of neurogenic orthostatic hypotension [correction of hypertension]—A follow-up survey study. *Clin Auton Res.* 2005;15(1):51–53.
43. Kaufmann H, Saadia D, Voustianiouk A, et al. Norepinephrine precursor therapy in neurogenic orthostatic hypotension. *Circulation.* 2003;108(6):724–728.
44. Freeman R. Treatment of orthostatic hypotension. *Semin Neurol.* 2003;23(4):435–442.
45. Rao SV, Stamler JS. Erythropoietin, anemia, and orthostatic hypotension: The evidence mounts. *Clin Auton Res.* 2002;12(3):141–143.
46. Shibao C, Gamboa A, Diedrich A, et al. Management of hypertension in the setting of autonomic dysfunction. *Current Treatment Options in Cardiovascular Medicine.* 2006;8(2):105–109.
47. Jordan J, Biaggioni I. Diagnosis and treatment of supine hypertension in autonomic failure patients with orthostatic hypotension. *J Clin Hypertens.* 2002;4(2):139–145.

CHAPTER **11**

Coronary Artery Bypass Surgery

James D. Fleck • José Biller

OBJECTIVES

- To discuss the neurologic complications of coronary artery bypass graft (CABG)
- To state the risk of stroke associated with CABG
- To discuss the risk of cognitive decline associated with CABG
- To discuss the treatment options for patients with stroke associated with CABG

CASE VIGNETTE

A 70-year-old right-handed woman is admitted with interscapular back pain radiating to her jaw. She has a history of hypertension, diabetes mellitus, and hypercholesterolemia. She is diagnosed with an acute non-ST elevation myocardial infarction. Coronary angiography shows multivessel coronary artery disease and she has coronary artery bypass surgery. The day after surgery she is noted to be moving the left side of her body less than the right side. Examination is notable for left arm and leg plegia and decreased sensation in the left arm and leg. A head computed tomographic (CT) scan shows findings consistent with acute ischemic lesions involving the right frontal and parietal lobes.

DEFINITION

In discussions of stroke in the setting of a CABG, assume it is a reference to ischemic stroke or brain infarcts unless otherwise specified.

EPIDEMIOLOGY

Coronary artery disease (CAD) is an exceedingly prevalent disease. It is estimated that 700,000 Americans this year will have a new coronary attack and about 500,000 will have a recurrent attack (1). As one of the treatment options for patients with CAD, coronary artery bypass graft (CABG) is a common procedure. It is estimated that 467,000 inpatient bypass procedures were performed in the United States in 2003 (1). Neurologic complications, especially those affecting the brain, are certainly a significant fear factor for patients and physicians following this procedure. Cerebral injury in the form of stroke and cognitive dysfunction is not uncommon.

ETIOLOGY AND PATHOGENESIS

To understand the potential mechanisms of morbidity in patients having CABG using cardiopulmonary bypass (CPB), it is helpful also to understand the basic setup of the machine. Blood is taken away from the right atrium of the heart and driven through the machine via a mechanical pump. The second major component of the circuit is the oxygenator, which adds oxygen and removes carbon dioxide from the blood. After flowing through filters and air bubble detectors blood is returned to the aorta via a cannula placed distal to the aortic cross-clamping site. The heart is immobilized by temporary interruption of coronary blood flow with the aortic cross-clamp. The myocardium is preserved with infusion of a high-potassium cardioplegic solution into the aorta proximal to the cross-clamp. A cardiotomy suction line returns blood from the surgical field to the bypass machine. This procedure allows a bloodless and motionless surgical field for the surgeon to make the necessary vascular bypasses of diseased coronary vessels. Although this is certainly an oversimplification of the process, it does make it easier to see the many sources of potential emboli from the heart. In hope of decreasing potential morbidity associated with the use of CPB and its attendant significant manipulation of the aorta, increasing interest and use has arisen of CABG techniques that do not use the CPB machine, so-called *off-pump CABG* (OPCABG). The introduction of cardiac stabilization techniques has allowed surgeons to operate on the beating heart.

PATHOLOGY

The mechanisms by which brain injury can occur in the setting of a CABG procedure are multiple. Many types of embolism can occur, including thromboembolism of blood constituents such as fibrin, platelets, leukocytes, cholesterol, air or gas, fat, foreign objects, or combinations of these. Thousands of small capillary and arteriolar dilatations (SCAD) have been reported to occur in patients who died shortly after CPB, which are thought to represent fat emboli (2,3). Transcranial Doppler (TCD) monitoring of both middle cerebral arteries has been used to detect high-intensity transient signals (HITS) thought to represent emboli in patients having open-heart valve operations or CABG using CPB (4,5). Although emboli were observed at the time of aortic cannulation and at the start of CPB, it appeared that more emboli were detected at the time of cross-clamp release, especially with the heart beating while empty (4). CPB machines allow for cardioplegia, but can lead to low flow rates or arterial hypotension. Hypoperfusion and arterial hypotension can also lead to focal, multifocal, or global areas of brain ischemia. Cerebrovascular occlusive disease and poor collateral flow within the circle of Willis can predispose patients to more severe effects of brain hypoperfusion.

CLINICAL MANIFESTATIONS

Because of the multiple areas of the brain that can be affected, the clinical presentation of patients with cerebrovascular events associated with CABG will vary. The location and extent of neuronal injury will also play a significant role in the clinical presentation. Cerebral infarcts are often multiple and frequently involve posterior parts of the brain (6). Focal motor or sensory deficits most often occur with focal brain ischemia. Behavioral or cognitive abnormalities can occur with focal ischemic lesions of the temporal, parietal, or frontal lobes. Encephalopathy or cognitive decline can be a manifestation of smaller areas of multifocal brain ischemia in patients who do not show obvious focal motor or sensory deficits. Coma can occur in patients with brainstem or notable bihemispheric ischemia. Bilateral ischemia between the anterior and middle cerebral arteries can result in bilateral arm sensory and motor impairments, the "man-in-a-barrel" syndrome. Pituitary apoplexy has also been described as a complication of cardiac surgery (7). Spinal cord infarction is also possible during CABG and can also occur with placement of an intraaortic balloon pump. Peripheral nervous system complications can also occur with CABG (8). The most common is a brachial plexopathy, usually in the distribution of the C8-T1 roots or lower trunk or medial cord of the plexus. Other nerves can be injured or irritated during CABG surgery, including the saphenous, peroneal, phrenic, ulnar, and recurrent laryngeal nerves. Most of these peripheral nervous system difficulties are transient with only rare occurrence of lasting deficits.

The range of perioperative stroke rates in several case series published after 1990 ranges from 1.4% to 5.7%, typically around 2% to 4% (9–19). These numbers reflect stroke rates in patients having only CABG and not combined procedures, such as CABG and cardiac valve surgery, repair of other cardiac abnormalities, or carotid endarterectomy. In these patients, the risk of stroke is greater (20,21). All patients were placed on CBP machines and most surgeries were elective, if specified. As would be expected, patients who had strokes had higher mortality rates, longer hospitalizations, and a higher rate of discharge to facilities for intermediate- or long-term care (9,11).

It should be taken into account, however, that in later time periods patients referred for isolated CABG were significantly older, sicker, and had a higher predicted operative risk as the decade passed. Despite this, the observed operative mortality in the 1,154,486 charts reviewed declined from 3.9% in 1990 to 3.0% in 1999 (22). Several studies identified risk factors for stroke associated with CABG and these are listed in Table 11-1 (9–19). Many of these seem intuitive because they are risk factors for stroke itself. Interestingly, female gender appears to be a risk factor for stroke. In a large study reviewing clinical information on 416,347 patients, the risk of new neurologic events was significantly greater in women having several types of cardiac surgery requiring CPB, including CABG surgery alone (men 2.4% vs. women 3.8%) (18). This association remained after multivariable analysis adjusting for many traditional risk factors. Atrial fibrillation is a common complication of cardiac surgery and can be associated with thromboembolic stroke. The likelihood of developing atrial fibrillation after CABG is increased by advancing age, male gender, and the presence of severe right CAD (23).

TABLE 11-1. Risk Factors for Stroke Associated with Coronary Artery Bypass Graft

PATIENT RELATED
Increasing age
Female gender
Previous transient ischemic attack (TIA), stroke, or cerebrovascular disease
Carotid artery disease or carotid bruit
History of neurologic disease
Proximal aortic atherosclerosis or calcified aorta
Previous cardiac surgery
Preoperative infection
Recent myocardial infarction (MI)
Poor left ventricular ejection fraction
Cardiac mural thrombus
Peripheral vascular disease
Arterial hypertension
Diabetes mellitus
Renal failure
Chronic obstructive pulmonary disease (COPD)
Cigarette smoking
PROCEDURE RELATED
Urgent operation
Longer duration of cardiopulmonary bypass
Use of α-adrenergic drugs after bypass
High transfusion requirement
Need for intraoperative hemofiltration
Intraaortic balloon pump
Postoperative arrhythmias

Aortic atherosclerosis also appears to be a significant risk factor for stroke associated with CABG. Measures to evaluate the degree of aortic atherosclerosis include gentle manual palpation of the aorta by the surgeon, epiaortic ultrasound, and intraoperative transesophageal echocardiograpy (TEE) (24,25). Severe aortic arch disease discovered by TEE does correlate with a significantly increased risk of stroke. Based on the results of testing, changes in operative technique can be attempted, such as using alternative sites for aortic cross-clamping, aortic cannulation, infusion of cardioplegic solutions, and proximal attachments of vein grafts. The ascending aorta has been replaced by some surgeons to reduce the risk of stroke in those with severe aortic atherosclerosis (24).

A number of retrospective case series have been published with stroke rates in OPCABG and also comparison of stroke rate in on-pump and OPCABG (26–37). The percentage of patients having a perioperative stroke was lower in the off-pump group (0% to 3.3%) than in the on-pump group (1.6% to 9.3%). This trend also seems to hold for elderly patients. It is important to realize that all of these case series were retrospective and obviously not randomized, which brings up the potential for multiple types of bias. Results from a randomized study showing early outcomes after on-pump versus off-pump CABG has been published (38). The number of strokes measured after 1 month was low in both groups with only one stroke noted in the off-pump group (142 patients; 0.7%) and two strokes noted in the on-pump group (139 patients; 1.4%), one of which occurred before surgery. This study may have been underpowered to show differences in complication rates (39). These patients were then followed to 1 year and no further strokes occurred in this patient population after the first month (40). In general, it appears that patients having OPCABG have a lower risk of stroke, but this has yet to be definitively proved in a large-scale, randomized study.

Neuropsychologic decline or cognitive decline certainly does occur after CABG, especially early after surgery. It is likely a multifactorial process with several potential risk factors that are patient related, exacerbated by the pathophysiologic stress of a major operation, metabolic derangements, and microemboli from the CABG surgery itself likely play some role. The incidence of cognitive dysfunction reported has varied widely from 3% to more than 50% (9,41). Much of this variation comes from patient selection, the definition of the neuropsychologic decline, the timing and type of the neuropsychologic assessment, and likely multiple other factors. Assessing the longitudinal impact of any decline in cognitive dysfunction has been a more difficult task, however. Newman et al. (41) evaluated 261 patients who had had CABG using CPB using a battery of cognitive tests before surgery, and at intervals up to 5 years after surgery (41). The incidence of cognitive decline at discharge, 6 weeks, 6 months, and 5 years was 53%, 36%, 24%, and 42%, respectively. Cognitive function at discharge was a significant predictor of long-term function. Interestingly, the incidence seems to decline over time except at the 5-year mark where a jump in the incidence is noted. The exact mechanism related to this finding is not known. Others have noted a late cognitive decline at 1 year after CABG with CPB in some patients (42). On the other hand, not all have found a significant decline in neuropsychologic test performance in those having CABG with CPB (43). If the number of microemboli reaching the brain during CABG with CPB is in some way related to postoperative neuropsychologic performance, it would seem reasonable to consider OPCABG to be an alternative to decrease the embolic load. The results in this area of study, however, have been conflicting also. Diegeler et al. (44) assessed the neurocognitive status preoperatively and postoperatively in patients undergoing CABG either on-pump or off-pump. The median value of HITS noted on intraoperative TCD was higher in the on-pump group and cognitive impairment was strongly associated with CPB and the occurrence of microemboli. A randomized trial of cognitive outcome after off-pump and on-pump CABG was performed by Van Dijk et al (45). Cognitive outcome was assessed at 3 months and 12 months with a set of 12 tests. The off-pump group of patients had improved cognitive outcomes 3 months after the procedure, but the differences became negligible by 12 months. Protein S-100 is found in high concentrations in glial and Schwann cells. The appearance of this protein in serum is thought to represent both neuronal damage and increased permeability of the blood–brain barrier. In a prospective study of patients having on-pump or off-pump CABG, S-100 was measured at intervals up to 24 hours postoperatively and neuropsychologic performance was assessed preoperatively and at 12 weeks after CABG (46). Significantly higher levels of serum S-100 were noted in the on-pump group 30 minutes after the surgery, but no significant difference was seen in neuropsychologic performance between the two groups at 12 weeks. If patients having CABG with CPB are compared with a control group of patients with comparable risk factors for CAD who did not have surgery, it does not appear that their long-term psychological performance differed much (47). At 12 months postoperatively, significant consistent differences do not appear in cognitive decline comparing those having CABG with CPB and off-pump (48). It may be that whereas both short-term and long-term cognitive changes have been associated with CABG, only the transient changes are related to CPB (49).

DIAGNOSTIC APPROACH

When evaluating patients postoperatively with suspected stroke, a careful preoperative history, especially regarding vascular risk factors, is helpful. Also useful is a review of the intraoperative record and postoperative course looking at the duration of CPB and also looking for complications such as periods of hypotension or cardiac rhythm disturbance. A thorough general and neurologic examination is necessary. A review of pertinent laboratory data is done looking for metabolic derangements that can mimic subtle focal deficits or cause delirium or encephalopathy. If a strong suspicion for brain ischemia remains, the next step in the evaluation process is typically a brain imaging study. Although a head CT without intravenous contrast is typically easier and quicker to perform and is sensitive for acute intracranial bleeding, its sensitivity for acute ischemia is somewhat limited. A magnetic resonance image (MRI) of the brain, including diffusion-weighted images, is a much more sensitive tool when looking for ischemic lesions, especially smaller ones and those located in the brainstem or posterior fossa.

TREATMENT

Next, some treatment approaches for ischemic stroke after CABG are discussed. Obviously, prevention of stroke would be the ideal treatment. Minimizing sources of air or particulate emboli, minimizing aortic manipulation, and prevention of arterial hypotension and hypoperfusion will lessen the chances of intraoperative strokes. It would also seem reasonable to protect the brain from the effects of ischemia, no medications yet have been proved to do so in the setting of CABG. Hyperbaric oxygen therapy is a potential treatment option for those with proved air emboli. Intravenous thrombolysis with tissue plasminogen activator (tPA) has been proved to be beneficial if given to patients with acute ischemic stroke within 3 hours of the onset of symptoms. Major surgery such as CABG is a contraindication to intravenous tPA, however. Intraarterial thrombolysis typically uses a lower dose of a thromoblytic agent with direct local delivery of the agent to the vascular occlusion via an endovascular approach. It has been attempted with some success in a few selected patients who have had an ischemic stroke after CABG without excessive severe bleeding risks (50). The Merci retrieval device is designed to mechanically remove thrombus and restore blood flow in the neurovasculature of patients experiencing ischemic stroke. It has been approved for that indication by the US Food and Drug Administration. For those patients with concomitant need for CABG and severe extracranial carotid artery disease indicating a potential need for carotid endarterectomy (CEA), a clear consensus of opinion on how to surgically deal with these patients has not been reached (21). Depending on the patient and the surgeon, the CEA and CABG can be performed separately or concurrently. With regard to the general care of patients who have had an ischemic stroke, it is optimal to do the following: maintain normal body temperature and adequate oxygenation, avoid hypotension or brain hypoperfusion, maintain normal serum glucose, avoid hypotonic intravenous fluids, prevent deep venous thrombosis, and avoid aspiration pneumonia by carefully evaluating the swallowing capabilities of those considered for oral feeding.

CLINICAL RECOMMENDATIONS OF THE VIGNETTE

The patient in the vignette above did have a cerebral infarct likely related to her CABG. As is often the case, her stroke was not clinically suspected until too much time had passed and she is not a candidate for any acute stroke intervention as outlined above. Maintenance of antiplatelet therapy, most often with aspirin, and appropriate postoperative and poststroke care should be delivered. Her swallowing capabilities should be evaluated by a speech therapist. Physical and occupational therapists should see the patient as soon as possible to start a rehabilitation program.

SUMMARY

CABG is a relatively common surgical procedure. Despite more operations on patients who are older and with more potential risk factors, the rate of strokes has not increased. Improved operative procedures and care delivered by the teams performing the operations, as well as improved postoperative care, are factors contributing to keeping the risk of stroke low. Given the recognition that neurologic complications can occur and can be devastating, continued interest exists in decreasing the complication rate of this potentially life-saving procedure.

REFERENCES

1. Heart Disease and Stroke Statistics—2006 Update. [cited; Available from: American Heart Association.
2. Challa VR, Moody DM, Troost BT. Brain embolic phenomena associated with cardiopulmonary bypass. *J Neurol Sci.* 1993;117(1–2):224–231.
3. Moody DM, Bell MA, Challa VR, et al. Brain microemboli during cardiac surgery or aortography [Comment]. *Ann Neurol.* 1990;28(4):477–486.
4. Van der Linden J, Casimir-Ahn H. When do cerebral emboli appear during open heart operations? A transcranial Doppler study [Comment]. *Ann Thorac Surg.* 1991;51(2):237–241.
5. Sylivris S, Levi C, Matalanis G, et al. Pattern and significance of cerebral microemboli during coronary artery bypass grafting. *Ann Thorac Surg.* 1998;66(5):1674–1678.
6. Barbut D, Grassineau D, Lis E, et al. Posterior distribution of infarcts in strokes related to cardiac operations. *Ann Thorac Surg.* 1998;65(6):1656–1659.
7. Cooper DM, Bazaral MG, Furlan AJ, et al. Pituitary apoplexy: A complication of cardiac surgery. *Ann Thorac Surg.* 1986;41(5):547–550.
8. Lederman RJ, Breuer AC, Hanson MR, et al. Peripheral nervous system complications of coronary artery bypass graft surgery. *Ann Neurol.* 1982;12(3):297–301.
9. Roach GW, Kanchuger M, Mangano CM, et al. Adverse cerebral outcomes after coronary bypass surgery. Multicenter Study of Perioperative Ischemia Research Group and the Ischemia Research and Education Foundation Investigators [Comment]. *N Engl J Med.* 1996;335(25):1857–1863.
10. Puskas JD, Winston AD, Wright CE, et al. Stroke after coronary artery operation: Incidence, correlates, outcome, and cost. *Ann Thorac Surg.* 2000;69(4):1053–1056.
11. McKhann GM, Grega MA, Borowicz LM, Jr., et al. Encephalopathy and stroke after coronary artery bypass grafting: Incidence, consequences, and prediction. *Arch Neurol.* 2002;59(9):1422–1428.
12. Frye RL, Kronmal R, Schaff HV, et al. Stroke in coronary artery bypass graft surgery: An analysis of the CASS experience. The participants in the Coronary Artery Surgery Study. *Int J Cardiol.* 1992;36(2):213–221.
13. Tuman KJ, McCarthy RJ, Najafi H, et al. Differential effects of advanced age on neurologic and cardiac risks of coronary artery operations. *J Thorac Cardiovasc Surg.* 1992;104(6): 1510–1517.
14. Borger MA, Ivanov J, Weisel RD, et al. Stroke during coronary bypass surgery: Principal role of cerebral macroemboli. *Eur J Cardiothorac Surg.* 2001;19(5):627–632.
15. Lynn GM, Stefanko K, Reed JF, 3rd, et al. Risk factors for stroke after coronary artery bypass. *J Thorac Cardiovasc Surg.* 1992;104(6):1518–1523.
16. McKhann GM, Goldsborough MA, Borowicz LM, Jr., et al. Predictors of stroke risk in coronary artery bypass patients.[comment]. *Ann Thorac Surg.* 1997;63(2):516–521.
17. Ricotta JJ, Faggioli GL, Castilone A, et al. Risk factors for stroke after cardiac surgery: Buffalo Cardiac-Cerebral Study Group. *J Vasc Surg.* 1995;21(2):359–363; discussion 64.
18. Hogue CWJMD, Barzilai BMD, Pieper KSMS, et al. Sex differences in neurological outcomes and mortality after cardiac surgery: A Society of Thoracic Surgery National Database Report. *Circulation.* 2001;103(17):2133–2137.
19. John R, Choudhri AF, Weinberg AD, et al. Multicenter review of preoperative risk factors for stroke after coronary artery bypass grafting [Comment]. *Ann Thorac Surg.* 2000;69(1): 30–35; discussion 5–6.
20. Wolman RL, Nussmeier NA, Aggarwal A, et al. Cerebral injury after cardiac surgery: Identification of a group at extraordinary risk. Multicenter Study of Perioperative Ischemia Research Group (McSPI) and the Ischemia Research Education Foundation (IREF) Investigators. *Stroke.* 1999;30(3):514–522.
21. Fleck JD, O'Donnell JA, Biller J. Cardiac evaluation of patients with carotid artery stenosis and treatment strategies for coexisting disease. In: TFLCK ed. *Carotid Artery Surgery.* New York: Thieme 2000:121–129.
22. Ferguson TB, Jr., Hammill BG, Peterson ED, et al.; Committee STSND. A decade of change—Risk profiles and outcomes for isolated coronary artery bypass grafting procedures, 1990–1999: A report from the STS National Database Committee and the Duke Clinical Research Institute. Society of Thoracic Surgeons. *Ann Thorac Surg.* 2002;73(2):480–489; discussion 9–90.
23. Mendes LA, Connelly GP, McKenney PA, et al. Right coronary artery stenosis: An independent predictor of atrial fibrillation after coronary artery bypass surgery. *J Am Coll Cardiol.* 1995;25(1):198–202.
24. Wareing TH, Davila-Roman VG, Daily BB, et al. Strategy for the reduction of stroke incidence in cardiac surgical patients [Comment]. *Ann Thorac Surg.* 1993;55(6):1400–1407; discussion 7–8.
25. Marschall K, Kanchuger M, Kessler K, et al. Superiority of transesophageal echocardiography in detecting aortic arch atheromatous disease: Identification of patients at increased risk of stroke during cardiac surgery. *J Cardiothorac Vasc Anesth.* 1994;8(1):5–13.
26. Ricci M, Karamanoukian HL, Abraham R, et al. Stroke in octogenarians undergoing coronary artery surgery with and without cardiopulmonary bypass. *Ann Thorac Surg.* 2000;69(5):1471–1475.
27. Yokoyama T, Baumgartner FJ, Gheissari A, et al. Off-pump versus on-pump coronary bypass in high-risk subgroups. *Ann Thorac Surg.* 2000;70(5):1546–1550.
28. Bucerius J, Gummert JF, Borger MA, et al. Stroke after cardiac surgery: A risk factor analysis of 16,184 consecutive adult patients. *Ann Thorac Surg.* 2003;75(2):472–478.
29. Hoff SJ, Ball SK, Coltharp WH, et al. Coronary artery bypass in patients 80 years and over: Is off-pump the operation of choice? *Ann Thorac Surg.* 2002;74(4):S1340–S1343.
30. Demaria RG, Carrier M, Fortier S, et al. Reduced mortality and strokes with off-pump coronary artery bypass grafting surgery in octogenarians. *Circulation.* 2002;106[12 Suppl 1]:I5–I10.
31. Anyanwu AC, Al-Ruzzeh S, George SJ, et al. Conversion to off-pump coronary bypass without increased morbidity or change in practice. *Ann Thorac Surg.* 2002;73(3):798–802.
32. Hernandez F, Cohn WE, Baribeau YR, et al. In-hospital outcomes of off-pump versus on-pump coronary artery bypass procedures: A multicenter experience. *Ann Thorac Surg.* 2001;72(5):1528–1533; discussion 1533–1534.
33. Puskas JD, Thourani VH, Marshall JJ, et al. Clinical outcomes, angiographic patency, and resource utilization in 200 consecutive off-pump coronary bypass patients. *Ann Thorac Surg.* 2001;71(5):1477–1483; discussion 83–84.
34. Hart JC, Spooner TH, Pym J, et al. A review of 1,582 consecutive Octopus off-pump coronary bypass patients. *Ann Thorac Surg.* 2000;70(3):1017–1020.
35. Cleveland JC, Jr., Shroyer AL, Chen AY, et al. Off-pump coronary artery bypass grafting decreases risk-adjusted mortality and morbidity. *Ann Thorac Surg.* 2001;72(4):1282–1288; discussion 8–9.
36. Patel NC, Deodhar AP, Grayson AD, et al. Neurological outcomes in coronary surgery: Independent effect of avoiding cardiopulmonary bypass. *Ann Thorac Surg.* 2002;74(2):400–405; discussion 5–6.
37. Stamou SC, Jablonski KA, Pfister AJ, et al. Stroke after conventional versus minimally invasive coronary artery bypass [Comment]. *Ann Thorac Surg.* 2002;74(2):394–399.
38. Van Dijk D, Nierich AP, Jansen EW, et al. Early outcome after off-pump versus on-pump coronary bypass surgery: Results from a randomized study [Comment]. *Circulation.* 2001;104(15):1761–1766.
39. Rose EA. Off-pump coronary-artery bypass surgery [Comment]. *N Engl J Med.* 2003;348(5): 379–380.
40. Nathoe HM, van Dijk D, Jansen EW, et al. A comparison of on-pump and off-pump coronary bypass surgery in low-risk patients [Comment]. *N Engl J Med.* 2003;348(5):394–402.
41. Newman MF, Kirchner JL, Phillips-Bute B, et al. Longitudinal assessment of neurocognitive function after coronary-artery bypass surgery [Comment]. [Erratum appears in *N Engl J Med.* 2001;344(24):1876]. *N Engl J Med.* 2001;344(6):395–402.
42. McKhann GM, Goldsborough MA, Borowicz LM, Jr., et al. Cognitive outcome after coronary artery bypass: A one-year prospective study [Comment]. *Ann Thorac Surg.* 1997;63(2): 510–515.

43. Mullges W, Babin-Ebell J, Reents W, et al. Cognitive performance after coronary artery bypass grafting: A follow-up study [Comment]. *Neurology.* 2002;59(5):741–743.
44. Diegeler A, Hirsch R, Schneider F, et al. Neuromonitoring and neurocognitive outcome in off-pump versus conventional coronary bypass operation. *Ann Thorac Surg.* 2000;69(4):1162–1166.
45. Van Dijk D, Jansen EW, Hijman R, et al. Cognitive outcome after off-pump and on-pump coronary artery bypass graft surgery: A randomized trial [Comment]. *JAMA.* 2002;287(11): 1405–1412.
46. Lloyd CT, Ascione R, Underwood MJ, et al. Serum S-100 protein release and neuropsychologic outcome during coronary revascularization on the beating heart: A prospective randomized study. *J Thorac Cardiovasc Surg.* 2000;119(1):148–154.
47. Selnes OA, Grega MA, Borowicz LM, Jr., et al. Cognitive changes with coronary artery disease: A prospective study of coronary artery bypass graft patients and nonsurgical controls. *Ann Thorac Surg.* 2003;75(5):1377–1384; discussion 84–86.
48. McKhann GM, Grega MA, Borowicz LM, Jr., et al. Is there cognitive decline 1 year after CABG? Comparison with surgical and nonsurgical controls [Comment]. *Neurology.* 2005;65(7):991–999.
49. Selnes OA, McKhann GM. Neurocognitive complications after coronary artery bypass surgery [Review; 51 refs]. *Ann Neurol* 2005;57(5):615–621.
50. Chalela JA, Katzan I, Liebeskind DS, et al. Safety of intra-arterial thrombolysis in the postoperative period. *Stroke.* 2001;32(6):1365–1369.

CHAPTER **12**

Other Cardiovascular Surgical/Endovascular Procedures

Richard A. Bernstein • Michael J. Schneck

OBJECTIVES

- To identify the indications for carotid artery angioplasty and stenting
- To consider the evidence comparing carotid angioplasty and stenting with carotid endarterectomy
- To discuss the role of carotid artery angioplasty and stenting for symptomatic and asymptomatic stenoses

CASE VIGNETTE

An 83-year-old woman had been seen in follow-up evaluation 1 year following angioplasty and stenting of her left anterior descending and right coronary arteries. The patient was asymptomatic except for reports of presyncope; she had no history of retinal or hemispheric transient ischemic attack (TIA) or stroke. A cervical bruit was identified and the patient had carotid ultrasonography, which disclosed a 70% to 80% stenosis of the right carotid bifurcation and a 50% to 60% stenosis of the left carotid bifurcation. Her physician considered methods of carotid revascularization and sought neurologic consultation regarding the choice between carotid endarterectomy or angioplasty and stenting.

DEFINITION

The management of atherosclerotic stenosis of the cervical internal carotid artery (ICA) entered the realm of evidence-based medicine with the publication of landmark trials showing the benefit of carotid endarterectomy (CEA) compared with medical therapy alone in selected patients with symptomatic (1,2) or asymptomatic (3,4) stenosis. Although CEA is an effective and safe operation, continuous improvements in endovascular technology have made revascularization via catheter-based methods an attractive theoretic alternative. Endovascular carotid revascularization generally involves the balloon dilation of an atherosclerotic or nonatherosclerotic stenosis at the carotid bifurcation or elsewhere in the course of the cervical ICA (angioplasty), followed by the placement of an intravascular metal stent at the site of the angioplasty. Many theoretic advantages exist to carotid angioplasty and stenting (CAS). No skin incision or neck dissection is required, which decreases the risk of injury to cranial nerves, and results in a lower risk of perioperative wound infection. The procedure can be performed without general anesthesia and endotracheal intubation, perhaps with less risk of myocardial infarction (MI). Patients with unfavorable anatomy for surgery (short necks, high cervical bifurcations, previous neck surgery or irradiation) may be amenable to CAS. Some have suggested that recovery may be faster, hospital stays shorter, and overall financial expenditures lower, with endovascular therapy (5).

Despite these theoretic advantages, CEA remains the most rigorously studied and validated method for carotid revascularization, and CAS remains an unproved substitute for CEA (6). This chapter explores the clinical decision-making process for choosing between CEA and endovascular therapy in patients with asymptomatic (as in our case vignette) and symptomatic carotid stenosis.

EPIDEMIOLOGY

Carotid artery stenosis can be symptomatic or asymptomatic. The risks and benefits of carotid revascularization differ, depending on the symptomatic status of a carotid stenosis. Symptomatic and asymptomatic stenoses are considered separately below.

Symptomatic carotid artery stenosis refers to any narrowing of the internal carotid artery that is ipsilateral to a stroke or TIA in the central nervous system (CNS) area supplied by that carotid artery. Strokes and TIA can be in the anterior or middle cerebral artery territory or retinal circulation. In some cases, the posterior cerebral artery (PCA) is supplied by the ICA ("fetal" configuration), in which case a PCA territory stroke or TIA would mark an ipsilateral carotid artery stenosis as *symptomatic*. Approximately 10% to 20% of all strokes are attributed to cervical carotid artery stenosis. Large randomized trials have shown the benefit of CEA in patients with symptomatic carotid artery stenosis measured >70% by catheter angiography (1,2), and in selected patients with stenosis 50% to 69% (7), compared with medical therapy alone. The magnitude of the benefit of CEA in symptomatic carotid artery stenosis is high, with an absolute annual risk reduction of ipsilateral stroke of 11%, assuming a risk of surgical mortality and major morbidity of about 6%. The number needed to treat (NNT) to prevent one stroke per year is low, about nine patients (1). For moderate carotid artery stenoses (50% to 69%), the NNT is higher, about 75%, but benefit remains of surgery over medical therapy alone in selected patients (7). The risk of ipsilateral stroke from a symptomatic carotid stenosis is highest in the first 2 weeks after the onset of symptoms (8). Therefore, a strong impetus exists to revascularize a symptomatic carotid artery stenosis of >50% soon after symptoms.

CAS is often considered as an alternative to CEA in patients, such as the ones randomized into the trials described above, who are good surgical candidates (patients with average risk). This decision requires consideration of the risks and benefits of CAS to be compared with the risks and benefits of CEA, in patients who are good surgical candidates. Recent large randomized trials have addressed this issue and the data from these trials can be used to help make this decision (see *Treatment* below).

The trials comparing CEA with medical therapy alone described above *excluded* patients who were not ideal surgical candidates because of unfavorable cervical anatomy or severe medical comorbidity (patients at high risk). Typical reasons patients are considered "high risk" include clinically significant cardiac disease (congestive heart failure, recent MI, abnormal stress test, or a need for open heart surgery), severe pulmonary disease, contralateral carotid occlusion, contralateral laryngeal nerve palsy, previous radical neck surgery or radiation therapy directed at the neck, recurrent carotid stenosis after endarterectomy, or age >80 years. Trial data pertaining to the management of symptomatic carotid stenosis in patients at high risk exist and can help guide clinical decision-making.

Some patients are ineligible for CEA because of unfavorable anatomy, such as patients with diffuse atherosclerotic lesions or lesions that are surgically inaccessible. In these patients not eligible for surgery, CAS is the only option for carotid revascularization.

The risk-to-benefit calculation in patients with asymptomatic carotid artery stenosis is less clear. Two large randomized trials have shown that CEA in patients with asymptomatic carotid artery stenosis prevents stroke (3,4). An asymptomatic stenosis, however, poses a much lower risk of stroke than a symptomatic stenosis. With medical therapy, the risk of ipsilateral stroke from an asymptomatic stenosis is approximately 11% over 5 years. In ideal surgical candidates with a combined surgical and angiographic stroke risk is <3%, CEA can reduce that risk to approximately 5% over 5 years (3,4). This yields a NNT to prevent one ipsilateral stroke per year of about 90 patients; the NNT may be lower (e.g., the benefit greater) in patients diagnosed without catheter angiography, because half of the procedural risk in the earlier trial (3) resulted from the *diagnostic* angiogram itself. Many patients, such as the patient in the *vignette,* with asymptomatic stenosis are less than ideal candidates for CEA because of severe medical comorbidity or advanced age (generally considered >75 to 80 years). In such patients, carotid revascularization, *by any method,* is of unproved benefit when compared with medical therapy.

ETIOLOGY AND PATHOGENESIS

Carotid artery stenosis is usually caused by atherosclerosis. Risk factors for atherosclerotic carotid artery stenosis include arterial hypertension, diabetes mellitus, elevated cholesterol, cigarette smoking, and family history (9). Atherosclerotic carotid artery stenosis can result in stroke when thrombi form on the surface of the plaque and then embolize to distal vessels in the brain. Alternatively, severe stenoses can lead to low-flow states and *border-zone* infarction. Rarely, an acute carotid artery occlusion can lead to the formation of a column of stagnant blood in the cervical ICA that extends anterograde and then embolizes (*stump embolism*), although this stroke mechanism is likely rare. Nonatherosclerotic causes of carotid stenosis are rare and include intimal dissection, fibromuscular dysplasia, and intravascular webs and tumors.

CLINICAL MANIFESTATIONS

The symptoms of carotid artery stenosis include retinal and cerebral TIA and stroke. Retinal TIA lead to transient loss of or blurring of vision in the ipsilateral eye; retinal *stroke* leads to infarction of all or a part of the retina, with a corresponding loss of monocular vision. Hemispheric TIA can manifest as transient mono- or hemiparesis or hemiplegia, transient aphasia (dominant hemisphere), or spatial disorientation or neglect (nondominant hemisphere); rare patients with severe carotid stenosis will manifest transient nonepileptic *limb-shaking* TIA (10). Strokes manifest similar to TIA, except that the deficits persist. Although any anterior circulation stroke or TIA can result from carotid artery stenosis, the syndrome of *fractional* weakness of the arm (weakness of the hand with sparing of the shoulder, or *vice versa*) is highly suggestive of carotid stenosis as stroke mechanism (11,12). Occasional patients will present with *crescendo* TIA, in which one episode follows rapidly after another with an accelerating pace.

Asymptomatic carotid artery stenoses have no clinical manifestations by definition, and may be detected when a physician hears a bruit in the neck or by routine carotid duplex screening. In general, fatigue, syncope, light-headedness, and vertigo are not manifestations of carotid stenosis.

TREATMENT OF CAROTID STENOSIS BY ENDOVASCULAR METHODS: ASSESSING THE EVIDENCE

Here, is considered the role of carotid artery stenting in four patient populations. First, in symptomatic patients who are average risk surgical candidates (defined above); second, in symptomatic patients who are high risk surgical candidates; third, in symptomatic patients who are not surgical candidates. Finally, CAS consideration in patients with asymptomatic stenoses.

Average-Risk Symptomatic Patients

CAS has been compared with CEA in patients with average surgical risks in several recent, large, carefully conducted trials. The results of these trials were remarkably concordant.

In the Stent-Supported Percutaneous Angioplasty of the Carotid Artery versus Endarterectomy (SPACE) trial, 1,183 patients with symptomatic carotid artery stenosis who were good candidates for either surgical CEA or CAS were randomized between these two treatments (13). The primary endpoint was ipsilateral stroke or death within 30 days of the procedure. The trial set a low bar for CAS; it was designed to show that CAS was not inferior to CEA in a population known to benefit from CEA. This endpoint was **not** reached. A 0.5% increase was seen in periprocedural stroke or death in the CAS compared with CEA group, and the 95% confidence interval (CI) for this endpoint suggested that CAS could be >2.5% inferior to CEA (13). In addition, for secondary endpoints (disabling ipsilateral stroke or death, disabling ipsilateral stroke alone, any stroke, any stroke or death, and procedural failure, no significant trends favored CEA over CAS (13). *Overall, the SPACE trial failed to show that CAS was as safe as CEA, and may have shown that it is inferior.*

Another recent trial compared CEA with CAS in symptomatic patients judged good candidates for both procedures. The Endarterectomy versus Angioplasty in Patients with Symptomatic Severe Carotid Stenosis (EVA-3S) study had nearly the same design as the SPACE trial (14). Patients with symptomatic severe carotid stenosis who were eligible for either treatment were randomly assigned to CAS or CEA, and followed for a primary endpoint of stroke or death within 30 days. As with SPACE, EVA-3S was designed to test for noninferiority of CAS compared with CEA, but *failed* to show this. The risk of stroke or death with CAS was 9.6%, compared with 3.6% in the CEA group (OR 2.5, $p = 0.01$) (14). In addition, CAS was associated with more than two times as many nonfatal strokes (2.7% for CEA vs. 8.8% for CAS, $p = 0.004$) and nearly three times as many strokes and deaths in follow up (3.6% for CEA vs. 9.6% for CAS), compared with CEA (14). Not unexpectedly, seven times fewer cranial nerve injuries occurred in the CAS group than in the CEA group ($p < 0.001$) and considerably more episodes of bradycardia in the CAS group (0.0% vs. 4.2%, $p < 0.001$). In this trial, the results of CAS were clearly *worse* than with CEA. Importantly, in both trials, an effort was made to ensure rigorous credentialing of both surgeons and endovascular operators, and apparently no difference was seen in outcome between the more and less experienced operators, suggesting that the credentialing process was effective.

CAS has not been shown to be as safe or effective as CEA for the treatment of symptomatic carotid stenosis in patients who are *average* surgical risks. In each trial, CEA was superior to CAS. *Based on these data, as well as prior trials* (6), *we cannot recommend CAS for symptomatic patients who are judged favorable candidates for CEA.*

High-Risk Symptomatic Patients

The Stenting and Angioplasty with Protection in Patients at High Risk for Endarterectomy (SAPPHIRE) trial compared CAS with CEA in patients with carotid stenosis judged to be high surgical risk (15). A total of 334 patients were randomized between CAS and CEA. Patients were included if they had a symptomatic carotid stenosis of at least 50%, or an asymptomatic stenosis of at least 80%, plus at least one coexisting condition that marked them as high risk. These conditions included clinically significant cardiac disease (congestive heart failure [CHF], abnormal stress test, or a need for open heart surgery), severe pulmonary disease, contralateral carotid artery occlusion, contralateral laryngeal nerve palsy, previous radical neck surgery or radiation therapy directed at the neck, recurrent carotid artery stenosis after endarterectomy, or age >80 years. The primary endpoint was stroke, MI, or death within 30 days of the procedure plus ipsilateral stroke or death from neurologic causes between 31 days and 1 year from the procedure. In this section are analyzed the results in the 96 symptomatic patients included in this trial.

In SAPPHIRE, the primary endpoint (periprocedural stroke, MI, or death, plus ipsilateral stroke or neurologic death from 1 to 12 months postprocedure) was reached in 16.8% of patients treated with stenting, and 16.5% in patients treated with CEA ($p = 0.95$). Interestingly, a trend favored CAS when the risk of stroke, MI, and death was compared at 30 days (2.1% for CAS, 9.3% for CEA ($p = 0.18$). This single trial suggests that in patients at high risk in whom both CAS and CEA are technically feasible, either procedure may be acceptable, and there *might* be more short-term safety with CAS. The results of this single trial have not been replicated, however, and the above analysis represents a subgroup of this single trial with <100 patients. *Both CEA and CAS are reasonable procedures for revascularization of symptomatic carotid stenoses in patients at high risk in whom both procedures are feasible.* The decision about which procedure to choose should be based on local expertise and patient preference.

Symptomatic Patients in Whom CEA Is Not Feasible

A subgroup of patients who are symptomatic and in whom CEA is not feasible represents a dilemma, because no randomized clinical trial data have directly compared the only two options open to such patients, namely CAS versus medical therapy. A general approach is to favor revascularization by CAS if it is technically feasible. The risk of recurrent stroke from a symptomatic carotid stenosis is extremely high on medical therapy alone, and the benefit of carotid revascularization (by CEA) is highest in the first 2 weeks after initial symptoms (8,16). Patients with TIA are especially high risk for early recurrent stroke despite medical therapy (17). In one analysis, pf patients who had a TIA preceding a stroke (23% of all strokes), 17% of strokes occurred on the same day as the TIA, the strokes occurred the next day in 9%, and within a week of the TIA in 43% (16). Several registries have documented complication rates from CAS between 2% and 8% (5). These registries may underestimate the true risks of the procedure, and hidden biases in registries can result in underestimates of the risk of the procedure when implemented in routine clinical practice. Nevertheless, the risks of recurrent stroke with medical therapy alone, particularly early after symptom onset, likely outweigh the risks of endovascular therapy. *In these patients, CAS can be offered as an option.*

Asymptomatic Carotid Artery Stenosis

Two large randomized trials have shown that CEA reduces the risk of stroke in patients with asymptomatic carotid artery stenosis, when compared with medical therapy alone (3,4). It must be emphasized that both of these trials enrolled only patients who were ideal surgical risks, and the 30-day complication rate from surgery and angiography was extremely low (2.3%); in the earlier trial, half of the procedural risk came from angiography alone (3). No analogous data have compared CAS with *medical therapy* alone in patients who are asymptomatic. One trial

(SAPPHIRE) compared CAS with CEA in 238 patients who were high risk and asymptomatic (15). As discussed, the primary endpoint was the risk of stroke, MI, and death within 30 days, plus ipsilateral stroke or neurologic death within 1 year. In SAPPHIRE, patients who were asymptomatic and who had carotid stenting had a 9.9% risk of reaching this endpoint, compared with a 21.5% risk with CEA ($p = 0.02$), suggesting that CAS may be a better option than CEA for these patients (15). The 1-year risk of stroke, MI, and death in the CAS group, although lower than the risk with CEA, was *higher* than the risk in patients treated *medically* in the Asymptomatic Carotid Atherosclerosis Study (ACAS) and the Asymptomatic Carotid Surgery Trial (ACST) (3,4). Therefore, although CAS may be safer than CEA in those who are high risk and asymptomatic, it is not at all clear that *either* CAS or CEA is appropriate for these patients. *Therefore, CAS (or CEA) cannot be recommended for patients with asymptomatic stenoses who are less than ideal surgical candidates. This includes most patients > 75 to 80 years of age, because they are unlikely to survive sufficiently long to accrue the modest benefit offered by revascularization of an asymptomatic carotid artery stenosis.*

CLINICAL RECOMMENDATIONS OF THE VIGNETTE

The patient in the vignette had an asymptomatic carotid artery stenosis and is 83 years of age. Given her advanced age, she is unlikely to benefit from carotid revascularization by any method, including CAS, and the suggestion is medical reduction of vascular risk factors with antiplatelet agents, antihypertensive agents, and statins. Should she develop symptoms of stroke or TIA ipsilateral to her high-grade carotid stenosis, however, a medical assessment of her fitness for surgery should be initiated. If she is judged too high risk for general anesthesia and CEA, CAS is a reasonable therapeutic option. If her coronary disease is stable and she is cleared for surgery, CEA would be preferred over CAS.

SUMMARY

Endovascular therapy of carotid artery atherosclerotic stenosis represents a treatment modality in which the technology is rapidly evolving. This therapy has not yet been proved superior, or even non-inferior, to CEA, however, in most situations in which it is considered. Most patients who require carotid revascularization should have CEA if it is technically feasible and the patients represent average surgical risks (18). Currently no evidence supports CAS in patients who are asymptomatic.

REFERENCES

1. Anonymous. Beneficial effect of carotid endarterectomy in symptomatic patients with high-grade carotid stenosis. North American Symptomatic Carotid Endarterectomy Trial Collaborators [see comment]. *N Engl J Med.* 1991;325(7):445–453.
2. Anonymous. MRC European Carotid Surgery Trial: Interim results for symptomatic patients with severe (70-99%) or with mild (0-29%) carotid stenosis. European Carotid Surgery Trialists' Collaborative Group [see comment]. *Lancet.* 1991;337(8752):1235–1243.
3. Anonymous. Endarterectomy for asymptomatic carotid artery stenosis. Executive Committee for the Asymptomatic Carotid Atherosclerosis Study [see comment]. *JAMA.* 1995;273(18):1421–1428.
4. Halliday A, Mansfield A, Marro J, et al. Prevention of disabling and fatal strokes by successful carotid endarterectomy in patients without recent neurological symptoms: Randomised controlled trial [see comment][erratum appears in *Lancet.* 2004;364(9432):416]. *Lancet.* 2004;363(9420):1491–1502.
5. Brott TG, Brown RD, Jr., Meyer FB, et al. Carotid revascularization for prevention of stroke: Carotid endarterectomy and carotid artery stenting. *Mayo Clinic Proc.* 2004;79(9):1197–1208.
6. Chaturvedi S, Bruno A, Feasby T, et al. Carotid endarterectomy—An evidence-based review: Report of the Therapeutics and Technology Assessment Subcommittee of the American Academy of Neurology. *Neurology.* 2005;65(6):794–801.
7. Barnett HJ, Taylor DW, Eliasziw M, et al. Benefit of carotid endarterectomy in patients with symptomatic moderate or severe stenosis. North American Symptomatic Carotid Endarterectomy Trial Collaborators. *N Engl J Med.* 1998;339(20):1415–1425.
8. Rothwell PM, Eliasziw M, Gutnikov SA, et al. Carotid Endarterectomy Trialists C. Endarterectomy for symptomatic carotid stenosis in relation to clinical subgroups and timing of surgery. *Lancet.* 2004;363(9413):915–924.
9. Ionita CC, Xavier AR, Kirmani JF, et al. What proportion of stroke is not explained by classic risk factors? *Prev Cardiol.* 2005;8(1):41–46.
10. Baquis GD, Pessin MS, Scott RM. Limb shaking—A carotid TIA. *Stroke.* 1985;16(3):444–448.
11. Timsit SG, Sacco RL, Mohr JP, et al. Early clinical differentiation of cerebral infarction from severe atherosclerotic stenosis and cardioembolism. *Stroke.* 1992;23(4):486–491.
12. Timsit SG, Sacco RL, Mohr JP, et al. Brain infarction severity differs according to cardiac or arterial embolic source. *Neurology.* 1993;43(4):728–733.
13. Group SC, Ringleb PA, Allenberg J, et al. 30 day results from the SPACE trial of stent-protected angioplasty versus carotid endarterectomy in symptomatic patients: A randomised non-inferiority trial. *Lancet.* 2006;368(9543):1239–1247.
14. Mas JL, Chatellier G, Beyssen B, et al. Endarterectomy versus stenting in patients with symptomatic severe carotid stenosis [see comment]. *N Engl J Med.* 2006;355(16):1660–1671.
15. Yadav JS, Wholey MH, Kuntz RE, et al. Protected carotid-artery stenting versus endarterectomy in high-risk patients [see comment]. *N Engl J Med.* 2004;351(15):1493–1501.
16. Rothwell PM, Warlow CP. Timing of TIAs preceding stroke: Time window for prevention is very short. *Neurology.* 2005;64(5):817–820.
17. Johnston SC, Gress DR, Browner WS, et al. Short-term prognosis after emergency department diagnosis of TIA. *JAMA.* 2000;284(22):2901–2906.
18. Coward LJ, Featherstone RL, Brown MM. Percutaneous transluminal angioplasty and stenting for vertebral artery stenosis [update of *Cochrane Database Syst Rev.* 2000;(2):CD000516; PMID: 10796383]. *Cochrane Database Syst Rev.* 2005(2):CD000516.

CHAPTER 13

Atrial Myxomas

Laurie E. Knepper • William Levy

OBJECTIVES

- To identify a rare, but treatable cause of stroke in the young
- To discuss the epidemiology of atrial myxomas
- To elucidate the clinical presentation—systemic, obstructive, and embolic
- To describe how to diagnose atrial myxomas
- To discuss the treatment and prognosis in patients with atrial myxomas

CASE VIGNETTE

A 57-year-old man had an acute onset of diplopia and ataxia. Two weeks previously he had a 1-hour episode of binocular vertical diplopia. On the night of admission, he began to snore with periods of apnea, according to his wife. She was unable to awaken him and called the ambulance. In the hospital he was intubated and remained lethargic for 3 days. After extubation, he complained of binocular diplopia and had difficulty finding words and recalling recent events. Medical history was notable only for an emergent and unrevealing evaluation for chest pain 3 months previously with a normal electrocardiogram (ECG) and stress test.

General examination findings, including cardiac auscultation, were normal. Neurologic examination was notable for slow vertical saccades and a right pronator drift. On laboratory evaluation, the erythrocyte sedimentation rate (ESR) was 50 mm/h, ECG showed nonspecific ST wave changes. A right thalamic hypodensity was seen on cranial computed tomography (CT). Magnetic resonance imaging (MRI) of his brain showed bilateral medial thalamic infarcts. A left atrial mass was visualized on echocardiogram, as well as left atrial enlargement. The mass was successfully resected and pathology was consistent with an atrial myxoma. No postoperative complications and no residual neurologic sequelae occurred.

DEFINITION

Primary cardiac tumors are rare, found in 0.001% to 0.035% of autopsy series (1,2). Three fourths of cardiac tumors are benign. Of benign cardiac tumors, 50% are myxomas; lipomas, papillary fibroelastomas, and rhabdomyomas comprise the remainder. One quarter of cardiac tumors are malignant, 95% of these are sarcomas, with lymphomas accounting for only 5% (2).

EPIDEMIOLOGY

This chapter concentrates on the most common type of cardiac tumor, atrial myxomas. Cardiac myxomas are an uncommon, although overlooked cause of stroke. Of atrial myxomas, 75% occur in the left atrium. The annual incidence is 0.5 per million population (3). There is a female predominance, ranging from 2:1 to 3:1. The average age of diagnosis is 43 years (4), although the reported age range is 3 to 84 years. The first antemortem diagnosis of atrial myxoma was a 3-year-old boy with stroke reported in 1952 by Goldberg et al. (5). Before this report, atrial myxomas had been diagnosed only at autopsy. About half of patients diagnosed with atrial myxoma are younger than 50 years of age. The delay from symptom onset to diagnosis ranges from 0 to 10 years, with an average delay of 4 months (6). This delay has decreased significantly since the advent of echocardiography.

ETIOLOGY AND PATHOGENESIS

Most cases of atrial myxomas are sporadic; 7% to 12% are hereditary (7). The most common familial form is the autosomal dominant, Carney complex, characterized by skin hyperpigmentation and lentiginosis, cutaneous, and cardiac myxomas; extracardiac (nonmyxomatous) tumors; and endocrinopathies (8). The Carney complex disease gene has been localized to chromosome 17q2.

In 1954, the first atrial myxoma was successfully removed surgically (6), and the first report of an atrial myxoma diagnosed by echocardiography was in 1959. Now, with the advent of improved diagnostic imaging techniques, atrial myxomas are detected much earlier, allowing intervention before recurrent systemic and neurologic events.

PATHOLOGY

The reported size of atrial myxomas during gross pathologic examination ranges from 1 to 15 cm, with a weight range of 15 to 180 g, in one series (6). Myxomas are most often pedunculated with a short stalk. Eighty percent arise from the septal fossa ovalis margin, 5% from the posterior atrium, and less commonly the external, superior and inferomedial walls, the left auricle base, posterior commissure, and occasionally the mitral valve. Most often, the myxoma is compact and has a smooth surface with little tendency toward fragmentation. The less common villous, papillary myxomas have a surface of "fine villous, gelatinous and fragile extensions" which can fragment spontaneously (6). Histopathology includes characteristic myxoma cells in an amorphous myxoid matrix. The myxoma cells are spindle or stellate shaped, and have an ovoid nucleus and pink eosinophilic cytoplasm. The tumor surface is covered by a layer of flat endothelial cells. Of myxomas, 90% are calcified in Pinede's series (6). Histology varies from normal to poor differentiation, which correlates with tumor recurrence. Large myxomas, greater than 5 cm, have been significantly associated with an increase in cardiac symptoms. A villous surface significantly increases the risk of neurologic symptoms and embolic complications.

CLINICAL MANIFESTATIONS

The clinical presentation of atrial myxomas is determined by their size, location, mobility, and pathologic features. Symptoms include constitutional, obstructive, and embolic events. Constitutional symptoms occur in 30% to 90% of patients (9). Myalgias, arthralgias, diffuse weakness, fever, weight loss, fatigue, livedo reticularis, and Raynaud syndrome can all occur. These systemic symptoms may be mistaken as secondary to a collagen vascular disorder (3). Psychiatric presentations have also been reported in 23% (4). Women are more likely to have systemic symptoms.

In a recent series of 112 consecutive cases (6), the most frequent presenting symptoms were related to mitral valve obstruction. They included dizziness, palpitations, syncope, dyspnea, cough, congestive heart failure, and pulmonary edema in 67% of patients. Paroxysmal symptoms, which also occurred, included chest pain, hemoptysis, limb claudication, thoracic noise, dyspnea, and syncope, sometimes only occurring when reclining. Positional symptoms are unusual, but pathognomonic for atrial myxoma. A ball valve mitral valve obstruction from the tumor can precipitate cardiac arrest.

Cerebral and peripheral embolism can occur with atrial myxomas. Emboli can either be composed of tumor fragments or thrombus adherent to the tumor. Tumors can also become infected and result in septic emboli (10). Atrial mxyomas occur in the right atrium in 15% to 20% of cases. Pulmonary embolism, which can be recurrent, has been reported (11,12). Cyanosis and hypoxia can occur with tricuspid valve obstruction resulting in a high right atrial pressure (1). Left atrial myxomas can embolize to the coronary arteries and cause acute myocardial infarction (13). Peripheral embolization has been reported to the spleen, adrenals, intestine, kidneys, abdominal aorta, and mesentery and limb (upper and lower) arteries in 10% to 45% of cases (9,14). Emboli from atrial myxomas have been reported to cause cerebral infarction in 27% to 83% (3,6) of cases. Strokes often occur before the onset of constitutional and obstructive symptoms, and are more common in young men. Strokes are often recurrent, multiple, and may be embolic or hemorrhagic (3). The range of cerebrovascular sequelae includes death from large embolic infarction to multi infarct dementia from recurrent stroke. Spinal cord embolism with paraplegia has also been reported (9). Retinal infarction can occur from tumor emboli, often with ipsilateral middle cerebral artery infarction. Because emboli can be caused by tumor fragments, anticoagulation may not prevent recurrent stroke. Myxomas can become infected and result in septic embolic infarction. The organisms involved are similar to those causing infective endocarditis (10).

Other neurologic sequelae can occur from myxomatous emboli and can result in the formation of intracranial aneurysms, which can cause intracerebral hemorrhage (15). These aneurysms can be multiple and bilateral and most often occur in peripheral intracranial, arterial branches. The aneurysms may, but do not always, resolve after tumor resection (4). Seizures, vertigo, and intracranial mass lesions can occur in patients with atrial myxoma, but they are rare.

DIAGNOSTIC APPROACH

On cardiac auscultation, a variety of abnormalities can be present in up to 64% of patients with diagnosed atrial myxoma. Most commonly, the murmurs resemble mitral stenosis and include an apical diastolic or presystolic murmur. A tumor plop can be heard, as can a gallop, or a split first heart sound (6). Abnormal auscultation was more common in patients with systemic symptoms and cardiac failure.

Two thirds of patients have nonspecific ECG findings, including left atrial hypertrophy, ST segment abnormalities, ventricular hypertrophy, atrial arrhythmias (atrial fibrillation or flutter), and conduction abnormalities. Chest x-ray studies are abnormal in 50% of cases. Findings were most often nonspecific, including congestive heart failure, cardiomegaly, and left atrial enlargement. Tumor calcifications occurred, but they were uncommon.

The ability to diagnose atrial myxomas has improved greatly since the advent of transthoracic echocardiography (TTE) in 1977. More recently, transesophageal echocardiography (TEE) has further improved the detection of cardiac tumors. The Canadian Task Force reported that intracardiac masses were detected by TTE in 4%, and by TEE in 11% of patients presenting with stroke (16). The yield is higher if clinical signs of cardiac disease are present. TEE has been reported to have almost 100% sensitivity for detecting cardiac myxoma and is preferred to TTC because it may help to detect other associated conditions, including patent foramen ovale, atrial septal aneurysm, and intracardiac thrombus (16). Occasionally, large pedunculated masses may have the ECG appearance of a myxoma, but are found to be thrombus at surgery (17). On occasion, large cardiac myxomas are discovered incidentally on echocardiogram. In one reported case, a giant left atrial mass was detected in a 73-year-old man who had never had cardiac or neurologic symptoms (18). Alternatively, echocardiogram has been unable to differentiate between a biatrial mobile mass in a patent foramen ovale, which was felt to be a clot in transit and in fact was a biatrial myxoma (19). Other methods used to detect intracardiac masses include gated, ultrafast cardiac CT scan and MRI of the heart (3,9). Cardiac MRI can clarify tumor size, attachment, and mobility, which may help to guide surgical resection. Occasionally, atrial masses are found incidentally on cardiac catheterization.

Atrial myxoma can be associated with an elevated ESR and C-reactive protein, hyperglobulinemia, and anemia. Constitutional symptoms are felt to be caused by interleukin-6 produced by the tumor, and resolve with myxoma resection.

Because secondary infection can result in sepsis and, in rare cases, meningitis, blood cultures should be considered as well.

TREATMENT

Optimal treatment of atrial myxoma is surgical excision. The most common postoperative complications have been transient arrhythmias. In a large series, postoperative death occurred in 3.5% of patients, one death was a second operation for a recurrent atrial myxoma. If an embolic stroke or hemorrhage has occurred, the timing of surgery needs to be considered, and may need to be delayed. Constitutional symptoms and laboratory abnormalities most often resolve with tumor resection. The recurrence rate, excepting the Carney complex (25%), is low 1% to 5% (3), but periodic echocardiography following resection should be considered for the first 4 years, when the recurrence rate is highest.

CLINICAL RECOMMENDATIONS OF THE VIGNETTE

This patient recovered completely and did not have any further neurologic events. Serial echocardiography was done to evaluate for tumor recurrence, but the finding was negative.

SUMMARY

Atrial myxomas are a rare, but treatable cause of peripheral, pulmonary, and cerebrovascular ischemic events, and most commonly occur in young patients. Cerebral infarction can be multiple and recurrent if these tumors are undetected. Constitutional symptoms and signs of cardiac obstruction can lead to misdiagnosis. With newer imaging techniques, these tumors are more readily detected, and when removed can prevent stroke.

REFERENCES

1. Guhathakurta S, Riordan JP. Surgical treatment of right atrial myxoma. *Tex Heart Inst J.* 2000;27(1):61–63
2. Butany J, Nair V, Naseemuddin A, et al. Cardiac tumors: Diagnosis and management. *Lancet Oncol.* 2005;6:219–228.
3. O'Rourke F, Dean N, Mouradian MS, et al. Atrial myxoma as a cause of stroke: Case report and discussion. *Canadian Medical Association Journal.* 2003;169:1049–1051.
4. Ekinci EI, Donnan GA. Neurological manifestations of cardiac myxoma: A review of the literature and report of cases. *Intern Med J.* 2004;34(5):243–249.
5. Goldberg HP, Glenn F, Dotter CT, et al. Myxoma of the left atrium: Diagnosis made during life with operative and post-mortem findings. *Circulation.* 1952;6:762–767.
6. Pinede L, Duhaut P, Loire R. Clinical presentation of left atrial cardiac myxoma: A series of 112 consecutive cases. *Medicine.* 2001;80(3):159–172.
7. McCarthy PM, Piehler JM, Schaff HV, et al. The significance of multiple, recurrent and "complex" cardiac myxomas. *J Thorac Cardiovasc Surg.* 1986;91:389–396.
8. Casey M, Mah C, Merliss AD, et al. Identification of a novel genetic locus for familial cardiac myxomas and Carney complex. *Circulation.* 1998;98:2560–2566.
9. Knepper LE, Biller J, Adams HP, et al. Neurologic manifestations of atrial myxoma. *Stroke.* 1988;19:1434–1440.
10. Revankar SG, Clark RA. Infected cardiac myxoma. Case report and literature review. *Medicine.* 1998;77(5):337–344.
11. Jardine DL, Lamont DL. Right atrial myxoma mistaken for recurrent pulmonary thromboembolism. *Heart.* 1997;78(5):512–514.
12. McCoskey EH, Mehta JB, Krishnan K, et al. Right atrial myxoma with extracardiac manifestations. *Chest.* 2000;118:547–549.
13. Demir M, Akpinar O, Acarturk E. Atrial myxoma: An unusual cause of myocardial infarction. *Tex Heart Inst J.* 2005;32:445–447.
14. Coley C, Lee K, Steiner M, et al. Complete embolization of a left atrial myxoma resulting in acute lower extremity ischemia. *Tex Heart Inst J.* 2005;32:238–240.
15. Herbst M, Wattjes MP, Urbach H, et al. Cerebral embolism from left atrial myxoma leading to cerebral and retinal aneurysms: A case report. *American Journal of Neuroradiology.* 2005;26:666–669.
16. Kapral MK, Silver F, and Canadian Task Force on Preventive Health Care. Preventive health care, 199 update:2. Echocardiography for the detection of a cardiac source of embolus in patients with stroke. *Canadian Medical Association Journal.* 1999;161:989–996.
17. Mottram PM, Gelman JS. Mitral valve thrombus mimicking a primary tumor in the antiphospholipid syndrome. *J Am Soc Echocardiogr.* 2002;15:746–748.
18. Lamparter S, Moosdorf R, Maisch B. Giant left atrial mass in an asymptomatic patient. *Heart.* 2004;90:e:24.
19. Umana E, Alpert MA, Massey CV, et al. Bi-atrial myxoma resembling an interatrial clot in transit on echocardiogram. *South Med J.* 1999;92:1019–1022.

CHAPTER **14**

Neurologic Sequelae of Cardiac Transplantation

Beth K. Rush • Daniel S. Yip • James F. Meschia

OBJECTIVES

- To review the early neurologic complications of heart transplantation
- To review the long-term neurologic complications following heart transplantation
- To define the incidence and prevalence of neurologic sequelae following heart transplantation
- To review clinical warning signs of posttransplantation neurologic compromise

CASE VIGNETTE

A 56-year-old man with a history of severe end-stage ischemic cardiomyopathy caused by multiple myocardial infarctions had had a ventricular assist device implanted 2 months before having heart transplantation. He experienced a seizure within the first 24 hours following transplantation. Examination shows the patient to be febrile, agitated, and poorly oriented to person, place, time, and setting. Hypotonic paresis is noted of the left upper and lower extremities, with left facial droop. Why is this patient showing neurologic deficits? What are the implications of his symptoms for the subacute and long-term transplant outcome?

DEFINITION

Neurologic sequelae of cardiac transplantation can be defined as any peripheral or central neurologic disorder, whether fixed or transient, that arises *de novo* following transplantation of a heart and that can reasonably be attributed to anesthesia, surgical transplantation of the heart, functioning of the transplanted heart, or reaction to medications required as a result of receiving a transplanted heart.

EPIDEMIOLOGY

The American Heart Association reported that 2,016 heart transplants were performed in the United States in 2004. Of these, 72% were men, and 70% were white. Forty-six percent were ages 50 to 65 years, and 20% were ages 35 to 49 years. Coronary artery disease is the most common cause of end-stage heart failure leading to transplantation. According to the 2005 US Organ and Procurement Transplant Network/Scientific Registry of Transplant Recipients (OPTN/SRTR) annual report, coronary artery disease exists in about 45% of the heart transplant recipients, followed by cardiomyopathy (43%) and congenital heart disease (6%). Survival following transplantation has remained steady since the modern period of immunosuppression. In 2003, the adjusted patient survival rates are 88% at 1 year, 80% at 3 years, and 73% 5 years (1). The average length of survival of heart transplant recipients is approximately 9 years (2).

The incidence of neurologic complications following transplantation has not been well studied. The data consist of a limited number of single center reports. The reports range from 13.7% to 60% (3,4). In one review of 205 orthotopic heart transplantation recipients, 46% (95/205) presented with neurologic complications; the most common manifestations were encephalopathy, seizure, neuromuscular disorder, and ischemic stroke (5). In a separate review of 322 orthotopic heart transplantation recipients, 13.7% (44/322) presented with neurologic complications; the most common manifestations were encephalopathy, seizures, and neuromuscular disorders (3).

A study that reviewed separate series of adult and child heart transplant cases reported a neurologic complication rate of 30% in adults, with peripheral neuropathies representing the most common manifestation; and a neurologic complication rate of 22% in children, with seizures representing the most common manifestation (6).

PATHOGENESIS

Cerebrovascular events result from ischemic-anoxic changes that occur perioperatively or are caused by cardioembolism. Cardiopulmonary bypass for cardiac surgery carries the risk of embolization from platelet aggregation, fibrin, or air. Pretransplant atrial fibrillation, left ventricular thrombus, and the presence of a ventricular assist device increases the risk of thromboembolic stroke. Inoue et al. (7) reported the incidence of perioperative cerebrovascular complications as being 19.8% in heart transplant recipients, compared with 3.1% in patients having elective coronary artery bypass grafting, and 10.3% in patients having elective valve surgery (7). In contrast, the incidence of perioperative cerebrovascular complications is 10.3% for those having emergency coronary artery bypass grafting, and 51.3% for those having emergency valve surgery.

The *2006 International Society for Heart and Lung Transplantation Registry* reports that 6.4% of deaths within the first 30 days following heart transplant are caused by cerebrovascular disease. Cerebrovascular disease is responsible of 4.3% of the deaths between 31 days and 1 year following transplant, 3.4% between years 1 and 3, 3.3% between years 3 and 5, and 4.1% >5 years after heart transplantation (2).

The incidence of cerebrovascular lesions found in autopsy series has been described as being 16% to 43% (8). Clinical series report the incidence of cerebrovascular events as being 4% to 20% (7). These events manifest clinically as strokes, seizures, confusion, or encephalopathy. Most of the symptoms are self-limited; however, some are left with mild-to-moderate permanent disabilities. Improvements in surgical technique may decrease the frequency of perioperative cerebrovascular events, such as from the classic biatrial anastomosis to a bicaval anastomosis.

Belvis et al. (9) describe a single center experience where 22 of 314 heart transplant recipients developed cerebrovascular disease (9). Six recipients developed a transient ischemic attack (TIA), 13 developed an ischemic stroke, and 3 developed a hemorrhagic stroke. Prior stroke was a significant risk factor for development of cerebrovascular disease following transplant. The onset of cerebrovascular disease occurred within 2 weeks in 20% of the recipients.

The most common cause of ischemic stroke in patients who have had cardiac transplantation is cardioembolism. Patients are at risk for stasis thrombosis within the left atrium, which can then embolize to the intracranial circulation. The classic biatrial anastomosis, where the anastomosis of donor to recipient atrium, leads to left atrial enlargement. The recipient atrium is noncontractile, and asynchrony occurs between the donor and recipient atrium. Intracardiac thrombi and spontaneous echo contrast have long been recognized in the transplanted heart (10–12). The incidence of cardiac thrombi and the risk of stroke associated with them are not known, however. Specific surgical techniques for performing cardiac transplantation have a bearing on risk of systemic embolism. Riberi et al. (13) performed a comparative echocardiographic study of patients who had classic biatrial anastomosis cardiac transplantation versus modified cardiac transplantation with bicaval anastomosis. Bicaval anastomosis minimizes the recipient left atrium to a cuff of tissue surrounding the pulmonary veins, thus minimizing the left atrial size enlargement following transplantation. The standard transplantation group had a systemic embolism rate of 15.3% (11/72) versus no instance of systemic embolism in the modified group (0/106). Left atrial surface area and rate of spontaneous echo contrast were significantly greater in the group having the classic biatrial anastomosis.

Although cardioembolic ischemic stroke appears to be the most common type of stroke encountered in the posttransplantation population, some hemorrhagic stroke has been seen (13). Hemorrhagic stroke typically occurs in the setting of anticoagulation while on cardiopulmonary bypass during surgery. In addition, a previous ischemic stroke can be transformed to a hemorrhagic stroke while having cardiopulmonary bypass.

The incidence of seizures ranges from 1.9% to 18% (3,14). Seizures in the early postoperative period are typically isolated events generally not requiring long-term antiepileptic drug therapy. Early seizures are usually associated with acute cerebrovascular events, whereas focal or generalized seizures occurring outside the early postoperative period may signal an intracranial opportunistic infection. Severe metabolic disturbances, such as hypomagnesemia related to cyclosporine use, have been associated with seizures (15). Elevated levels of cyclosporine in the absence of hypomagnesemia have been associated with seizures, which improve by lowering the cyclosporine dose (4). Seizures, however, have also occurred in heart transplant recipients with low or therapeutic levels of cyclosporine (16). Seizures have also been reported in recipients treated with tacrolimus (17). Seizures typically resolve with removal of the offending drug. Switching calcineurin inhibitors usually does not result in the return of seizures.

Grigg et al. (16) report a 15% incidence of seizures in their single center experience. Half of the seizures were associated with postoperatively acquired focal cerebral infarctions. Of the recipients who had strokes within 24 hours after transplantation, 80% had also developed seizures at the time of infarction. One third of the seizures occurred within 24 hours after transplantation. Half of the seizures occurred within the first 9 months. Headache and sudden rise in blood pressure were associated with 25% of the seizures. Of the seizures, 25% were associated with severe infections or organ rejection.

Some degree of encephalopathy is perhaps the most common central nervous system (CNS) complication seen in the recipients after heart transplantation. Although global cerebral hypoperfusion may be the proximate cause of encephalopathy in some cases, the most common cause of encephalopathy is side effects of medications (18).

The incidence of heart transplant-associated CNS infections has decreased from 14% to 5% with the use of modern immunosuppressive and antibiotic prophylaxis regimens. The dose of corticosteroids has significantly decreased with widespread use of cyclosporine. Many heart transplant programs withdraw corticosteroids after a period of time in stable patients, with the result being a reduction of CNS infections. The peak incidence of CNS infections occurs between 1 and 6 months following transplantation. After 6 months, at least half of the CNS infections are associated with increased immunosuppression.

Aspergillus fumigatus is the most common cause of focal meningoencephalitis or brain abscesses, accounting for about 25% of intracranial infections (19). It causes solitary or multiple brain abscesses, most commonly in the cerebral and cerebellar hemispheres. Ring enhancement is often not seen on computed tomographic (CT) scanning. Magnetic resonance imaging (MRI) can detect small areas of hemorrhage in the abscesses. The clinical presentation may be acute focal neurologic deficits, encephalopathy, or seizures. Meningeal infection may be present in up to 50% of cases (8). CNS *Aspergillus* infection is almost always a result of disseminated pulmonary infection. Early antifungal therapy can successfully contain the infection, but mortality remains high with disseminated disease (19). Diagnosis is made by brain imaging studies and the presence of pulmonary *Aspergillus*, or by direct needle aspiration or biopsy of the brain lesion. A serological test for *Aspergillus* antigen is available. Voriconazole is currently the antifungal agent of choice. Other antifungal agents, such as amphotericin B (previous drug of choice), itraconazole, and caspofungin have been used.

Toxoplasma gondii is the second most common cause of focal meningoencephalitis or brain abscesses, accounting for about 12% of intracranial infections (4). Disseminated toxoplasmosis produces characteristic multiple brain abscesses (8). *Toxoplasma* abscesses differ from *Aspergillus* by often having ring contrast enhancement, even early in the course of the infection. Radiographic findings, rising serum antibody titers, and improvement with empiric treatment allow a presumptive diagnosis, but stereotaxic brain biopsy or aspiration provides the only definitive means of diagnosis. Recipients who are *toxoplasma* antibody-negative who receive an organ from a *toxoplasma* antibody-positive donor should have close observation for signs of *Toxoplasma* infection and prophylaxis treatment with trimethoprim-sulfamethoxazole.

Cryptococcus accounts for 10% of intracranial infections (4). It typically presents as chronic meningitis with headaches and fever, but not meningeal signs. Cerebrospinal fluid (CSF) examination demonstrates lymphocytic pleocytosis with encapsulated yeast demonstrated by India ink staining. Detection of cryptococcal antigen in the CSF is the most sensitive method of diagnosis. Titers <1:250 are associated with good clinical outcomes. Amphotericin B is the treatment of choice, although itraconazole has been used successfully.

Listeria monocytogenes also accounts for 10% of intracranial infections (4). It presents as acute or subacute meningitis, usually lasting <10 days. Symptoms include fever and headache with variable meningeal irritation. CSF examination reveals prominent polymorphonuclear and mononuclear pleocytosis (8). Gram stain of the CSF fluid may fail to show gram-negative bacilli, but the organism readily grows in culture. Penicillin is the drug of choice.

Other opportunistic CNS infections include *Candida, Phycomycosis, Nocardia, Coccidiodomycosis, and Pseudallescheria boydii* (8). As with *Aspergillus*, CNS *Nocardia* is associated with pulmonary infection, but with a more chronic progression of symptoms. CNS seeding with Candida is usually associated with subacute or chronic meningitis, or multiple cerebral abscesses.

Diffuse viral encephalitis is caused by the herpes group viruses: cytomegalovirus (CMV), herpes simplex, herpes zoster, and Epstein-Barr (4,8). CMV is usually associated with a disseminated infection involving lung, gastrointestinal tract, or retina, as well as brain. Diagnosis can be made by isolating DNA from serum or CSF. Titers are not as sensitive. Valganciclovir is now the antiviral agents of choice. Other antiviral agents, such as ganciclovir and acyclovir, are not as effective because of drug resistance.

Herpes simplex encephalitis also occurs with a disseminated viremia and can be cultured from accompanied skin or mucosal lesions, tracheal aspirates, or urine. Occasionally, the virus can be cultured from CSF. Treatment with acyclovir has been effective.

Herpes zoster infection usually occurs after dissemination from a localized dermatologic infection. It usually involves the spinal roots and cord at that level, but can extend further into the brain, resulting in segmental polyradiculopathy or myelopathy combined with confusion. Treatment is typically with acyclovir.

Rhinocerebral involvement with mucormyosis accounts for 4% of intracranial infections and tends to occur in diabetics (4). Infection begins in the sinuses and spreads contiguously to involve orbits, cranial nerves, and, ultimately, brain. The organism may gain access to the carotid artery and embolize distally to cause lesions in the anterior and middle cerebral artery distributions (8). The presence of blackish purulent drainage, or a black eschar on the palate or nasal mucosa, is characteristic. Treatment may include surgical debridement combined with amphotericin B.

Primary CNS lymphoma occurs in about 2% of all transplant recipients (4). Epstein-Barr virus infection impairs modulation of B-lymphocytes and is felt to be an important determinant in the development of monoclonal lymphoma or posttransplant lymphoproliferative disease (PTLD). Clinical presentation depends on the location of the tumor (8). Encephalopathy and neurobehavioral changes are the most common presentations. Focal neurologic deficits are less common. Biopsy may be necessary for diagnosis. At times, the presence of PTLD can be seen concomitantly in the gastrointestinal tract or the pulmonary system. Treatment includes reduction of immunosuppression, use of antiviral agents, and radiotherapy.

Calcineurin inhibitors (cyclosporine and tacrolimus) have various neurotoxic effects. Although neurotoxicity with cyclosporine has been described in greater detail, similar neurotoxic effects can be seen with tacrolimus. Drachman et al. (20) reported that 20% to 39% of patients developed tremor with cyclosporine. In addition, 11% reported paresthesias, and 1.5% to 5% reported seizure activity. Other symptoms include psychosis, confusion, coma, aphasia, severe ataxia, hemiparesis, quadraparesis, paraparesis, visual hallucinations, and cortical blindness. Cortical blindness has also been reported with tacrolimus-based immunosuppression (17). CT scanning shows nonenhancing areas of low attenuation, and MRI shows focal areas of increased signal on T2-weighted images in both cyclosporine (21) and tacrolimus (22) treated recipients. Hypocholesterolemia may be a risk factor for CNS toxicity in those receiving cyclosporine (23). Toxic symptoms typically ameliorate with reduction of the calcineurin dose.

Acute administration of high-dose corticosteroids can cause delirium, psychosis, hallucinations, and mood alterations, such as euphoria, dysphoria, and mild agitation. Symptoms abate as high doses of corticosteroids used in the first postoperative days are reduced quickly to modest levels. Acute quadriplegic myopathy with loss of thick (myosin) filaments has been observed in critically ill patients (24). It is characterized by proximal or diffuse weakness of the extremities and can complicate weaning from mechanical ventilation.

Adair et al. (25) reported a series of recipients who developed aseptic meningitis associated with the use of the monoclonal anti-CD3 antibody (OKT3). This occurred in 6% of those treated with OKT3. Symptoms included mental status change, generalized seizures, headache, photophobia, and fever. Meningeal signs were not reported, but CSF fluid examination revealed pleocytosis in all those affected. The degree of pleocytosis correlated positively with the fever severity, and correlated inversely with the interval between exposure to OKT3 and onset of neurologic symptoms. Most had normal CSF protein and glucose concentrations.

Cyclosporine and related medications that are used to prevent organ rejection can cause polyneuropathy. Terrovitis et al. (26) reported a case of a 47-year-old woman who developed a subacute symmetric sensory motor polyneuropathy with cyclosporine at levels of 397 to 430 ng/mL. Electromyography showed fibrillation potentials and reduced recruitment patterns with only mild reduction in motor conduction velocities consistent with axonal neuropathy. Symptoms resolved with dose reduction.

Peripheral nerve injuries following heart transplantation are similar to those seen following cardiac surgery. These are focal and typically reversible, with a reported incidence of 6% (4,8,14). The most common injury is a lower trunk brachial plexopathy from sternal retraction (8), resulting in weakness and numbness in the forearm and hand (Klumpke palsy).

Other peripheral nerve injuries include recurrent laryngeal and phrenic nerve injury occurring intraoperatively. Neuropathies of the peroneal and ulnar nerves are related to compression from either intraoperative positioning or prolonged periods of bed rest (4).

Reduced cardiac output with cerebral hypoperfusion is hypothesized to be a key contributing factor for cognitive impairment associated with cardiac transplantation (27,28). Advanced heart failure commonly results in general cognitive decline. In a cross-sectional study that compared patient groups of varying stages of advanced heart failure, cognitive impairment progressed with increasing severity of heart failure; motor functions were affected at the earliest stages, followed by additional impairments in visual memory, verbal memory, and cognitive processing speed (29). The most common cognitive impairments in the context of heart failure and heart transplantation involve attention, but executive functions, processing speed, and memory are also affected (30,31).

Cognitive impairment in the context of heart failure may be related to the acute reduction of cerebral perfusion (ischemia), dips in oxygen saturation (anoxia), or the cumulative effects of microemboli from the diseased heart (27,32–34). Whereas some studies suggest that cognitive function does not improve after cardiac transplantation (35), others suggest that it does (30,36). One study demonstrated that an exercise program may reverse cognitive impairment in patients with advanced heart failure who do not have transplantation or any mechanical intervention (37).

Cerebrovascular insults can result from disturbances in cardiac output or hypotension during transplantation, or via the dislodgement of emboli within the diseased heart to the cerebrovascular supply during the transplantation. Embolic ischemic strokes may be particularly common after thromboses form in left ventricular assist devices that are implanted to maximize systemic circulation during heart transplantation (38). If patients develop thromboses secondary to the derangements of blood flow generated by mechanical assist devices, cognitive impairment may evolve, even without clinical signs of stroke.

A different source of cognitive impairment in heart transplantation stems from metabolic or toxic encephalopathies. In the context of significant renal or hepatic dysfunction, transplantation recipients can demonstrate deficits in attention, memory, cognitive processing speed, and executive functions.

Few studies have focused on cognitive and academic outcomes after heart transplantation in infants and children. In a study of 39 children who had cardiac transplantation in the first year of life, delays in motor development were consistently observed along with delays in speech and language acquisition and in abstract reasoning and goal-directed behaviors for those cases with long-term follow-up (39). These data suggest that heart transplantation in infants carries risk. Similarly, children ages 1 to 3 years having heart transplantation may also experience significant cognitive impairment leading to developmental delay and limitations in academic achievement. A cross-sectional study of cognitive outcomes in pediatric cardiac transplantation demonstrated that 46% of cases fell >2 standard deviations below average on tests across cognitive domains of memory, processing speed, attention, and motor skills (40).

PATHOLOGY

The pathologic processes of neurologic impairment are diverse, including toxic, metabolic, ischemic, embolic, and infectious disorders. No specific pathology is unique to the cardiac transplantation recipient population.

CLINICAL MANIFESTATIONS

Careful monitoring and thorough examination of the cardiac transplantation recipient during the perioperative and postoperative periods is essential for early detection of neurologic complications. Whereas a seizure may immediately direct the clinician's attention to the importance of a neurologic examination, it is important to conduct proactively a comprehensive neurologic examination of the patient immediately following the surgical procedure and at regularly scheduled intervals thereafter. Confusion, disorientation, and other signs of delirium should raise suspicion of encephalopathy, drug toxicity, acute renal or hepatic dysfunction, or the possibility of a sudden ischemic infarct.

DIAGNOSTIC APPROACH

Diagnosis begins with taking a detailed history and a physical and neurologic examination. Timely head imaging is essential for the patient with a focal neurologic deficit that localizes to the CNS. It may be impractical or impossible to obtain emergent MRI, especially in patients on ventricular assist devices. Noncontrasted head CT usually suffices, however, for detecting the offending lesion, which is usually an infarct.

Neuropsychological testing in heart transplant candidates pre- and posttransplantation can be helpful in identifying who will have the most difficulty complying to the complicated posttransplantation treatment regimen, or identifying those who will have the greatest difficulty in returning to active life within their community or workplace (41). Formal evaluation of cognitive impairment can be useful in designing individually tailored education regarding transplantation. Addressing individual educational needs increaseses the probability of compliance with the complicated posttransplant treatment regimen.

TREATMENT

Patients with acute ischemic stroke who have had a recent (within 30 days) cardiac transplantation or have a ventricular assist device would not be candidates for reperfusion therapy with intravenous tissue plasminogen activator (tPA). The risk of systemic or intracranial hemorrhage likely outweighs the benefits of attempted cerebral reperfusion with tPA. In a patient with an acute (<3 hours) large thrombus stroke syndrome (NIH Stroke Scale >10 to 15 points), consider CT with concurrent CT angiography and CT perfusion as the diagnostic head imaging protocol of choice.

Many patients who present with a first-ever seizure are *observed* rather than started on an anticonvulsant. If the patient has had a first-ever seizure concurrent with toxicity of epileptogenic drugs, then tapering or eliminating the offending agent may be sufficient to avoid recurrent seizures. If on head imaging, a patient with a first-ever seizure is found to have a predisposing epileptogenic lesion, such as a cortical abscess, infarct, or hemorrhage, then coverage with an anticonvulsant is reasonable. Because of the polypharmacy that necessarily accompanies cardiac transplantation, an anticonvulsant such as levetiracetam that has minimal effects on drug levels should be considered.

CLINICAL RECOMMENDATIONS OF THE VIGNETTE

The patient described in the vignette has most likely sustained an ischemic stroke during the perioperative or postoperative transplantation period. An immediate noncontrast CT scan of the brain should be done to rule out the presence of an acute hemorrhagic stroke. Calcineurin inhibitor neurotoxicity is not likely, because this drug is not usually begun within the first 24 hours following transplantation. It is unlikely that an opportunistic infection is the cause of these symptoms, because its peak onset is 1 to 6 months following transplantation. Frequent neurologic assessments, continuous ECG, and dynamic blood pressure monitoring may be helpful to ensure adequate perfusion of the penumbra. MRI or magnetic resonance angiography (MRA) will be useful in determining the extent of the infarct, and the boundaries of the ischemic penumbra after the acute phase. Once the patient has recovered from surgery, neuropsychological testing may be useful in terms of identifying and understanding the effects of transplantation on cognition. If significant cognitive impairment is found, the patient may have difficulty complying with the posttransplantation care regimen that is essential for increasing the probability of long-term graft acceptance.

SUMMARY

The functional integrity of the brain requires strong and consistent cardiac output. In cases of severe congestive heart failure, a substantial risk exists of neurologic sequelae. Although cardiac transplantation can be life-saving, the process of transplantation carries risk of neurologic injury. Risk of cerebrovascular complications is greatest during the perioperative and postoperative periods of transplantation, and remains elevated thereafter. Risk of CNS infection is greatest between the first and sixth months after transplantation, and falls as the intensity of immunosuppression decreases. Late CNS infections typically occur as a consequence of increasing the intensity of immunosuppression to treat acute rejection. Neurologic side effects from chronic immunosuppressant medications can be ameliorated by using lowest effective doses. Proper assessment of cerebral dysfunction after cardiac transplantation may guide patient education and improve short- and long-term rates of compliance with posttransplantation treatment recommendations.

REFERENCES

1. 2005 OPTN / SRTR Annual Report. The US Organ Procurement and Transplantation Network and the Scientific Registry of Transplant Recipients. http://www.ustransplant.org/annual_Reports/current/default.htm. Accessed November 21, 2006.
2. Taylor DO, Edwards LB, Boucek MM, et al. Registry of the International Society for Heart and Lung Transplantation: Twenty-third official adult heart transplantation report—2006. *J Heart Lung Transplant.* 2006;25:869–879.
3. Perez-Miralles F, Sanchez-Manso JC, Almenar-Bonet L, et al. Incidence of and risk factors for neurologic complications after heart transplantation. *Transplant Proc.* 2005;37:4067–4070.
4. Sila CA. Spectrum of neurologic events following cardiac transplantation. *Stroke.* 1989;20:1586–1589.
5. Cemillan CA, Alonso-Pulpon L, Burgos-Lazaro R, et al. Neurological complications in a series of 205 orthotopic heart transplant patients. *Rev Neurol.* 2004;38:906–912.
6. Mayer TO, Biller J, O'Donnell J, et al. Contrasting the neurologic complications of cardiac transplantation in adults and children. *J Child Neurol.* 2002;17:195–199.
7. Inoue K, Luth JU, Pottkamper D, et al. Incidence and risk factors of perioperative cerebral complications. Heart transplantation compared to coronary artery bypass grafting and valve surgery. *J Cardiovasc Surg (Torino).* 1998;39:201–208.
8. Hotson JR, Enzmann DR. Neurologic complications of cardiac transplantation. *Neurol Clin.* 1988;6:349–365.
9. Belvis R, Marti-Fabregas J, Cocho D, et al. Cerebrovascular disease as a complication of cardiac transplantation. *Cerebrovasc Dis.* 2005;19:267–271.
10. Derumeaux G, Habib G, Schleifer DM, et al. Standard orthotopic heart transplantation versus total orthotopic heart transplantation. A transesophageal echocardiography study of the incidence of left atrial thrombosis. *Circulation.* 1995;92:196–201.
11. Fernandez-Gonzalez AL, Llorens R, Herreros JM, et al. Intracardiac thrombi after orthotopic heart transplantation: clinical significance and etiologic factors. *J Heart Lung Transplant.* 1994;13:236–240.
12. Polanco G, Jafri SM, Alam M, et al. Transesophageal echocardiographic findings in patients with orthotopic heart transplantation. *Chest.* 1992;101:599–602.
13. Riberi A, Ambrosi P, Habib G, et al. Systemic embolism: A serious complication after cardiac transplantation avoidable by bicaval technique. *Eur J Cardiothorac Surg.* 2001;19:307–311; discussion 311–302.
14. Malheiros SM, Almeida DR, Massaro AR, et al. Neurologic complications after heart transplantation. *Arq Neuropsiquiatr.* 2002;60:192–197.
15. Walker RW, Brochstein JA. Neurologic complications of immunosuppressive agents. *Neurol Clin.* 1988;6:261–278.
16. Grigg MM, Costanzo-Nordin MR, Celesia GG, et al. The etiology of seizures after cardiac transplantation. *Transplant Proc.* 1988;20:937–944.
17. Steg RE, Kessinger A, Wszolek ZK. Cortical blindness and seizures in a patient receiving FK506 after bone marrow transplantation. *Bone Marrow Transplant.* 1999;23:959–962.
18. Hughes RL. Cyclosporine-related central nervous system toxicity in cardiac transplantation. *N Engl J Med.* 1990;323:420–421.
19. Rueter F, Hirsch HH, Kunz F, et al. Late Aspergillus fumigatus endomyocarditis with brain abscess as a lethal complication after heart transplantation. *J Heart Lung Transplant.* 2002;21:1242–1245.
20. Drachman BM, DeNofrio D, Acker MA, et al. Cortical blindness secondary to cyclosporine after orthotopic heart transplantation: A case report and review of the literature. *J Heart Lung Transplant.* 1996;15:1158–1164.
21. Lanzino G, Cloft H, Hemstreet MK, et al. Reversible posterior leukoencephalopathy following organ transplantation. Description of two cases. *Clin Neurol Neurosurg.* 1997;99:222–226.
22. Lavigne CM, Shrier DA, Ketkar M, et al. Tacrolimus leukoencephalopathy: A neuropathologic confirmation. *Neurology.* 2004;63:1132–1133.
23. Cooper DK, Novitzky D, Davis L, et al. Does central nervous system toxicity occur in transplant patients with hypocholesterolemia receiving cyclosporine? *J Heart Transplant.* 1989;8:221–224.
24. Perea M, Picon M, Miro O, et al. Acute quadriplegic myopathy with loss of thick (myosin) filaments following heart transplantation. *J Heart Lung Transplant.* 2001;20:1136–1141.
25. Adair JC, Woodley SL, O'Connell JB, et al. Aseptic meningitis following cardiac transplantation: clinical characteristics and relationship to immunosuppressive regimen. *Neurology.* 1991;41:249–252.
26. Terrovitis IV, Nanas SN, Rombos AK, et al. Reversible symmetric polyneuropathy with paraplegia after heart transplantation. *Transplantation.* 1998;65:1394–1395.
27. Bornstein RA, Starling RC, Myerowitz PD, et al. Neuropsychological function in patients with end-stage heart failure before and after cardiac transplantation. *Acta Neurol Scand.* 1995;91:260–265.
28. Sulkava R, Erkinjuntti T. Vascular dementia due to cardiac arrhythmias and systemic hypotension. *Acta Neurol Scand.* 1987;76:123–128.
29. Petrucci RJ, Truesdell KC, Carter A, et al. Cognitive dysfunction in advanced heart failure and prospective cardiac assist device patients. *Ann Thorac Surg.* 2006;81:1738–1744.
30. Deshields TL, McDonough EM, Mannen RK, et al. Psychological and cognitive status before and after heart transplantation. *Gen Hosp Psychiatry.* 1996;18:62S–69S.
31. Temple RO, Putzke JD, Boll TJ. Neuropsychological performance as a function of cardiac status among heart transplant candidates: A replication. *Perceptions on Motor Skills.* 2000;91:821–825.

32. Newman MF, Croughwell ND, Blumenthal JA, et al. Predictors of cognitive decline after cardiac operation. *Ann Thorac Surg.* 1995;59:1326–1330.
33. Pugsley W, Klinger L, Paschalis C, et al. The impact of microemboli during cardiopulmonary bypass on neuropsychological functioning. *Stroke.* 1994;25:1393–1399.
34. Putzke JD, Williams MA, Rayburn BK, et al. The relationship between cardiac function and neuropsychological status among heart transplant candidates. *J Card Fail.* 1998;4:295–303.
35. Schall RR, Petrucci RJ, Brozena SC, et al. Cognitive function in patients with symptomatic dilated cardiomyopathy before and after cardiac transplantation. *J Am Coll Cardiol.* 1989;14:1666–1672.
36. Roman DD, Kubo SH, Ormaza S, et al. Memory improvement following cardiac transplantation. *J Clin Exp Neuropsychol.* 1997;19:692–697.
37. Tanne D, Freimark D, Poreh A, et al. Cognitive functions in severe congestive heart failure before and after an exercise training program. *Int J Cardiol.* 2005;103:145–149.
38. Komoda T, Drews T, Sakuraba S, et al. Executive cognitive dysfunction without stroke after long-term mechanical circulatory support. *ASAIO J.* 2005;51:764–768.
39. Freier MC, Babikian T, Pivonka J, et al. A longitudinal perspective on neurodevelopmental outcome after infant cardiac transplantation. *J Heart Lung Transplant.* 2004;23:857–864.
40. Brosig C, Hintermeyer M, Zlotocha J, et al. An exploratory study of the cognitive, academic, and behavioral functioning of pediatric cardiothoracic transplant recipients. *Prog Transplant.* 2006;16:38–45.
41. Putzke JD, Williams MA, Daniel FJ, et al. Activities of daily living among heart transplant candidates: Neuropsychological and cardiac function predictors. *J Heart Lung Transplant.* 2000;19:995–1006.

CHAPTER 15

Aortic Diseases

Candice K. Sech • José Biller • Alain Heroux • Jeffrey Schwartz

OBJECTIVES

- To define various aortic diseases
  - Aortic dissection
  - Atheroma of the aortic arch
  - Collagen vascular disease and aortic involvement
  - Aortic aneurysm: Thoracic and abdominal
  - Noninfectious aortitis
- To describe the pathophysiology of aortic disease
- To discuss the diagnostic approach to aortic disease
- To discuss current treatment recommendations
- To discuss neurologic complications that can be seen in patients with aortic disease, and after aortic surgery

CASE VIGNETTE

A 55-year-old right-handed woman with a long-standing history of hypertension and hyperlipidemia; a 20 pack-year history of tobacco use; and a history of aortic valve replacement 1 year ago presents to the emergency department with complaints of transient dizziness, slurred speech, and difficulty walking. Neurologic examination was unremarkable. Nonenhanced cranial computed tomography (CT) scan was normal. Carotid ultrasonography was unremarkable. CT of her thorax showed aortic dissection extending from the ascending aorta to the left subclavian and to the origin of the left vertebral artery.

INTRODUCTION

Aortic diseases cause significant morbidity and mortality, and predispose patients to a multitude of symptoms. The phrase "acute thoracic aortic syndromes" includes aortic dissection, traumatic aortic dissection and rupture, contained rupture (pseudoaneurysm), and acute expansion of aortic dissection. Additionally, atypical presentations of aortic dissection can occur, including intramural hematoma of the aorta, and penetrating atherosclerotic ulcer of the aorta. Other aortic diseases include aortic aneurysm, atheroma of the aortic arch, collagen vascular diseases affecting the aorta, and noninfectious aortitis. Infectious causes of aortic disease, such as syphilitic aortitis and aortic root abscess, are covered elsewhere in this book.

Acute Thoracic Aortic Syndromes

Classic Aortic Dissection

DEFINITION/EPIDEMIOLOGY

Morgagni first described aortic dissection more than 200 years ago (1). Classic aortic dissection is defined as an intimal tear that causes blood to move from a true lumen to false lumen within the middle or outer layer of the aortic media (2). The aortic wall may be split <1 mm or involve the entire diameter of the aorta, causing complete occlusion of the true lumen by the false lumen. Aortic dissection is relatively uncommon, with an incidence between 5 to 30 cases per million persons per year, and is largely dependent on the prevalence of risk factors in the population (3–6). Aortic dissection can have devastating consequences when not diagnosed or adequately treated. When ruptured, the false lumen may undergo retrograde dissection, thrombotic occlusion, and pseudoaneurysm formation (7). Left untreated, fewer than 10% of patients with proximal aortic dissection survive a year. Most die within the first 3 months, usually of acute aortic insufficiency, major branch vessel occlusion, or rupture into the pericardium, mediastinum, or left hemithorax (8). Aortic rupture is also a late complication of aortic dissection. In one study of 20 years of follow-up of 527 patients with aortic dissection, nearly 30% of deaths were caused by ruptured aortic aneurysm (9).

CLASSIFICATION

Aortic dissection is classified as either acute or chronic, depending on the time of onset. An onset of <2 weeks is defined as acute, and it has been found that 74% of deaths occur within this 2-week period, when untreated (10).

Aortic dissection can be classified using the Stanford or DeBakey classification scheme. In the Stanford (most widely used system) classification, type A dissections include the ascending aorta, and type B are dissections excluding the ascending aorta. The DeBakey classification subdivides aortic dissections, with type I involving the entire aorta, type II involving only the ascending aorta, and type III excluding the ascending aorta and arch (see Fig. 15-1).

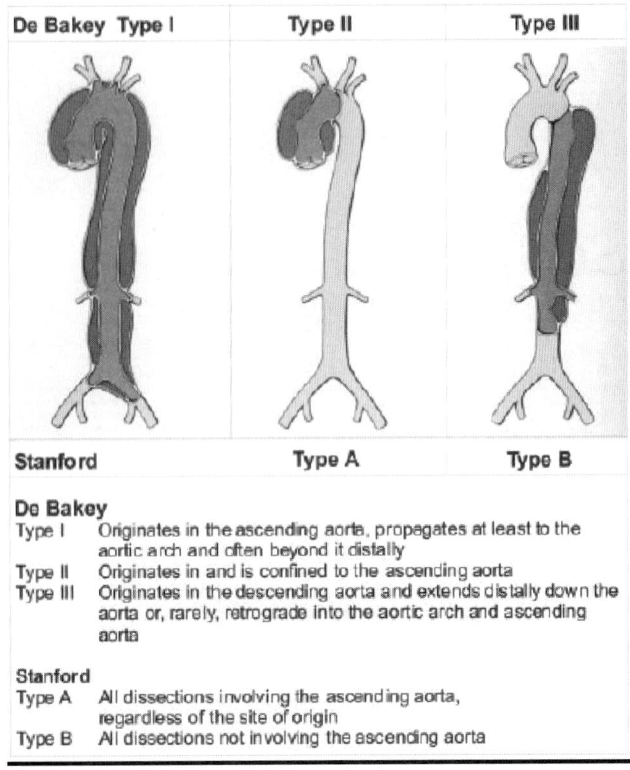

FIGURE 15-1. DeBakey and Stanford classification schemes for aortic dissection. (From Nienaber CA, Eagle KA. Aortic dissection: New frontiers in diagnosis and management. Part I: From etiology to diagnostic strategies. *Circulation.* 2003;108:628–635, with permission.)

Further discussion of aortic dissections within this chapter will be based on the Stanford classification of aortic dissection.

TYPE A (PROXIMAL) DISSECTION

Type A (proximal) dissections are usually fatal, with a mortality rate of 1% to 2% per hour after symptoms begin (3,10). Presenting symptoms can include abrupt onset of chest pain (85%) or back pain (47%), but stroke (6%) and syncope (12.7%) are also common. Complications associated with type A dissections include aortic valve disruption with resulting acute heart failure, cardiac tamponade, and coronary artery dissection, leading to myocardial ischemia or infarction.

TYPE B (DISTAL) DISSECTION

Type B acute aortic dissection affecting the distal aorta is less lethal than proximal aortic dissection. Presentation is similar to proximal dissection, with severe pain in back, chest, or abdomen being common. Spinal cord ischemia and ischemic peripheral neuropathy occasionally is encountered. The 30-day mortality rate in uncomplicated distal aortic dissections is 10% (3).

PATHOPHYSIOLOGY

Several proposed views exist on why aortic dissection occurs. One thought is that dissection begins with an intimal tear, which exposes the underlying diseased media to the pressure of intraluminal blood. The dissection may progress forward from the tear, along the length of the aorta (antegrade), or undergo dissection retrograde to the tear. An additional explanation involves the rupture of the vasovasorum in the media, and subsequent development of an intramural hematoma. Local hemorrhage then occurs, with subsequent rupture through the intimal layer, causing an intimal tear and dissection. Additionally, some recognize that aortic dissection can occur as a consequence of smooth muscle contraction, especially when there is cystic degeneration occurs in the media (11).

RISK FACTORS

Risk factors for aortic dissection can be divided into inherited and acquired. Inherited risk factors include fibrillinopathies, such as Marfan syndrome (MFS) and Ehler-Danlos syndrome (EDS), Turner syndrome, and vascular disorders, such as bicuspid aortic valve and coarctation of the aorta. A postmortem study of 186 autopsies of patients who died of aortic dissection, found that the aortic valve was five times as likely to be congenitally malformed in adults who died of aortic dissection (12).

Chronic hypertension causes arterial wall intimal thickening and fibrosis, and degradation of the extracellular matrix. These changes result in vulnerability to forces, and the potential for dissection and aneurysm formation. Additionally, smoking, dyslipidemia, and use of crack cocaine are potential risk factors for formation of aortic dissection (13–17).

Clinical Manifestations

The clinical presentation of aortic dissection is nonspecific and can mimic many other diseases, including myocardial ischemia or infarction. The diagnosis of aortic dissection is missed in 38% of initial evaluations, and is diagnosed for the first time postmortem in 28% of patients. Thus, maintaining a high index of suspicion is critically important (3–5).

Pain is the most frequent presenting symptom of aortic dissection, the location of which depends on the area involved. Patients with dissections of the ascending aorta typically experience anterior chest pain, whereas dissections of the descending aorta may have posterior chest, back, and abdominal pain (7). Abrupt onset of pain that reaches a maximal level quickly is typical of aortic dissection. A report from the International Registry of Acute Aortic Dissection (IRAD) looked at 464 cases of aortic dissection, and found that 95% of patients presented with pain, and 85% had pain abrupt in onset. The quality of pain of aortic dissection is typically thought of as *tearing.* In the IRAD registry, the quality of pain was described as sharp in 64% of the patients, and tearing or ripping in 51% (3). In a population-based study evaluating aortic dissection, 42% of patients had frequent neurologic symptoms and 3% had paraplegia (8). Approximately 15% to 20% of patients with aortic dissection will develop a neurologic deficit. Syncope can also be the initial presentation of patients with aortic dissection.

Physical examination findings in aortic dissection include a diastolic murmur of aortic insufficiency found in 40% to 50% of proximal dissections. Pulse deficits, an ominous finding, are more common in type A aortic dissection and likely indicative of complications and poor outcomes. Evidence of cardiac tamponade on physical examination should prompt the physician to rapidly obtain diagnostic confirmation. Neurologic complications, including stroke and syncope, may be the initial presentation of aortic dissection as well. Other complications include the presence of Horner syndrome (oculosympathetic dysfunction) caused by compression of the superior cervical ganglion, and vocal cord paralysis because of involvement of the left recurrent laryngeal nerve.

DIAGNOSTIC APPROACH

Several diagnostic tests exist for aortic dissection evaluation, including transthoracic echocardiogram (TTE), transesophageal echocardiogram (TEE), magnetic resonance imaging (MRI), contrast-enhanced CT, and aortography. The clinical situation, patient stability, preferred use, accuracy, and availability should have an impact on the choice of testing modality.

AORTOGRAPHY

Aortography was used routinely beginning in the 1960s as the standard tool for diagnosis of clinically suspected aortic dissection. Aortography involves injecting a variable amount of contrast material at different levels and using several views to best visualize the thoracic aortic anatomy. Several criteria are used in the diagnosis of dissection, including *direct* angiographic signs, such as visualization of the intimal flap or two separate lumens, and *indirect* angiographic signs, such as lumen irregularities, compression, branch vessel abnormalities, and aortic regurgitation. Aortography accurately visualizes branch vessel abnormalities. Because of its invasive nature, use of potentially nephrotoxic contrast material, and current availability of less-invasive testing, aortography is used less commonly today. Aortography was once thought to be highly sensitive and specific in detection of suspected aortic dissection. However, studies have found the diagnostic sensitivity to be less than initially thought, ranging from 81 to 91 percent (17,18).

TRANSESOPHAGEAL ECHOCARDIOGRAM

TEE is often used for diagnosis of aortic dissection in cases of time constraints, or when the patient has hemodynamic compromise. TEE diagnoses aortic dissection when an intimal flap within the aorta separates two lumina. Color flow Doppler TEE is advantageous in confirming the diagnosis of aortic valve insufficiency related to aortic dissection. The distal portion of the ascending aorta and branches of the aortic arch are not adequately seen with TEE. Sensitivity and specificity for diagnosis of dissection in the ascending aorta range from 77% to 80%, and 93% to 96%, respectively (20–22).

COMPUTED TOMOGRAPHY (CT)

CT is the most commonly used modality for diagnosis of suspected aortic dissection. Criteria used for diagnosis include visualization of an intimal flap separating the true and false lumen, which is identified as a low attenuation linear structure in the aortic lumen (Fig. 15-2). Other findings can include delayed enhancement of the aortic lumen, aortic widening, and displacement of intimal calcifications. CT may detect involvement of the visceral or iliac arteries as well. In contrast to conventional CT, helical CT has been found to be more beneficial in the diagnosis of aortic dissection. Although not as many studies exist looking at helical CT, specificity and sensitivity are reported to be 100% and 98%, respectively. Overall, the sensitivity of conventional CT for detection of aortic dissection is 83% to 94%, with a specificity of >87% to 100% (23,24). The limitation of CT in diagnosis of aortic dissection includes both poor localization of the intimal tear and diagnosis of subtle aortic dissection. Additionally, potential nephrotoxicity related to contrast use, and poor evaluation of aortic regurgitation may limit the use of CT in certain circumstances.

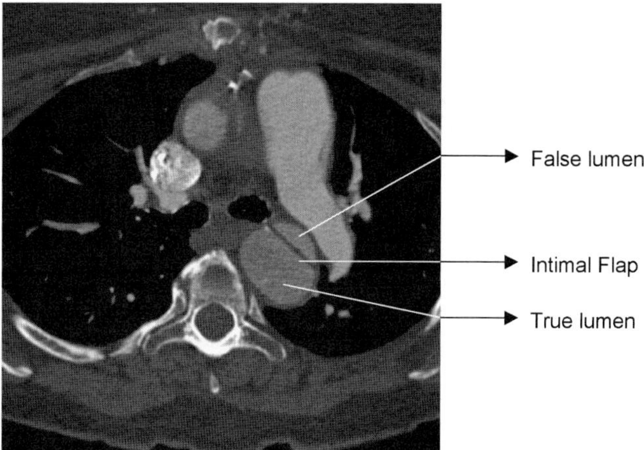

FIGURE 15-2. Aortic dissection diagnosed on computed tomography (CT).

MAGNETIC RESONANCE IMAGING

Use of MRI in diagnostic evaluation of aortic dissection largely relies on availability in emergent situations and evaluation of hemodynamically stable patients. A newer contrast MR aortography, in combination with MRI, may more clearly elucidate the involved area. MRI has the highest sensitivity and specificity, nearing 100% for diagnosis of aortic dissection, except for discrete dissection. MRI clearly visualizes both the entry and re-entry area of dissection, branch vessel involvement, and associated complications. MRI is most often used in hemodynamically stable patients, and for follow-up of chronic aortic dissection (25).

In a large meta-analysis evaluating the accuracy of MRI, TEE, and helical CT in the diagnosis of aortic dissection, all three modalities yielded reliable diagnostic values in confirming or excluding dissection. In this review, for patients with low pretest probability (5%) of aortic dissection, CT was best for excluding aortic dissection. In patients with high (50%) pretest probability for aortic dissection, MRI was best for confirming aortic dissection (26). Because all three testing modalities have high performance in confirmation or exclusion of aortic dissection, other criteria, including the availability of test, expertise in conducting and interpretating the test, and hemodynamic stability of the patient should help guide the decision (26).

ADDITIONAL TESTING

Electrocardiogram

Chest pain may be the presenting complaint in both aortic dissection and myocardial infarction (MI), and an electrocardiogram (ECG) should be obtained to help differentiate, because thrombolytic therapy is potentially life saving in MI, but could be detrimental in dissection. As mentioned, both MI and aortic dissection can coincide if dissection propagates into the coronary ostium. In this situation, myocardial ischemia and resultant ECG changes can incite thrombolytic use, with potentially catastrophic results. A normal ECG is present in one third of patients with coronary involvement in aortic dissection, and many patients have nonspecific ST-T segment changes. Approximately 20% of patients with type A dissection have evidence of acute myocardial ischemia or infarction on ECG. Attention should be taken to perform diagnostic imaging to exclude aortic dissection in patients with suspected aortic dissection, and ECG changes indicative of MI before instituting thrombolytic therapy (27).

Chest X-ray

Evidence is unclear on the benefit of chest X-ray (CXR) studies in patients presenting with suspected aortic dissection. A CXR will be abnormal (mediastinal or aortic widening) in 60% to 90% of cases of suspected aortic dissection, which may make the diagnosis more likely (3,28). Acute dissection may have a normal CXR, however, especially type A dissection. Patients with hemodynamic instability should have no further diagnostic testing or therapy not withheld in order for a CXR to be completed.

TREATMENT

Initial medical management of aortic dissection focuses on prevention of additional propagation of the dissected aorta. Both elevated blood pressure and the velocity of left ventricular contraction enhance further dissection (29).

Although vasodilators are sufficient to lower blood pressure, vasodilator use alone may actually increase the velocity of blood across the area and potentially increase the risk of further dissection. A β-blocker should be used in addition to a vasodilator to decrease this velocity. Sodium nitroprusside is the classic drug used to control blood pressure in aortic dissection, and is a potent arterial and venous vasodilator. It is appealing as a drug of choice in aortic dissection, because it has a rapid onset of action and short half-life; however, it has been shown to cause coronary steal and reflex tachycardia, and it has the potential for causing cyanide toxicity.

Fenoldopam, a selective arterial or renal vasodilator, with a rapid onset of action and short half-life, which improves renal blood flow, and may be of use in patients with impaired renal blood flow. Unlike sodium nitroprusside, fenoldopam does not cause coronary steal, but is associated with reflex tachycardia and a potential for ventricular extra systoles or ST-T changes.

Nicardipine, a nondihydropyridine calcium channel blocker, with vasodilatory effects, can be considered for decreasing blood pressure.

Medical management focuses on rapid, adequate blood pressure control. A target systolic blood pressure goal of 110 to 120 mm Hg (mean, 60 to 75 mm Hg), or the lowest tolerated blood pressure with adequate flow to vital organs, should be attained within 20 minutes.

Overall prognosis for patients with type A versus type B aortic dissection, dictates whether surgical treatment is used.

TYPE A

Surgical treatment is the management key for type A aortic dissections. The goal of surgery in type A aortic dissection is to prevent aortic rupture and possible complications (the development of pericardial effusion that can lead to cardiac tamponade, myocardial ischemia, aortic regurgitation). The appropriate surgical technique used depends on the aortic root size and the condition of the aortic valve. When the ascending and aortic arch diameters are within normal limits and no aortic valvular commissural detachment or evidence of pathologic aortic valvular disease exists, a tubular graft is used. If, however, aortic valvular disease is present or the aorta is ectatic, the aortic valve is replaced in addition to a tubular graft aortic replacement (composite aortic graft).

TYPE B

Surgical repair of type B aortic dissection is limited to prevention or relief of life-threatening complications, intractable pain, rapidly expanding aortic diameter, or periaortic or mediastinal hematoma. Dissection occurring in a previously aneurysmal aorta may also be an indication for surgery. In patients with complications, including ischemia of legs, kidney, or gut, a consideration is catheter-guided therapies aimed at decompressing the true lumen, allowing for increased blood flow to affected areas. If this technique does not resolve symptoms promptly, surgical intervention is warranted. Otherwise, uncomplicated type B aortic dissections are usually managed conservatively.

ATYPICAL PRESENTATIONS OF AORTIC DISSECTION

Penetrating atherosclerotic ulcer (PAU) and intramural hematoma (IMH) are atypical presentations of aortic dissection. They are more readily defined radiologically since high-resolution, three-dimensional imaging has become available. It is now recognized that PAU and IMH may have a distinct natural history that differ from classic aortic dissection, and hence, should be managed differently.

IMH involves a spontaneous hemorrhage collection in the medial layer of the aortic wall; unlike aortic dissection, however, it does not have any evidence of a tear in the intima or communication between the hematoma and aortic lumen. IMH cannot be distinguished from aortic dissection clinically; IMH accounts for 10% to 30% of acute aortic syndromes. Atherosclerosis and older age are risk factors associated with IMH as compared with aortic dissection. It is located in the descending aorta in 60% to 70% of cases. Many hypotheses exist to explain the pathophysiology of intramural hematoma formation. Some believe that a microintimal tear, too small to be visualized, incites the hematoma formation, with eventual thrombosis versus dissection formation. Additionally, rupture of the vasovasorum within the aortic wall has been postulated as explaining the formation of intramural hematomas. Mortality of patients with IMH depends on the location of the hematoma. IMH may eventually convert to classic aortic dissection, and the hematoma may resolve or become an aneurysm or pseudoaneurysm.

PAU involve atheromatous plaques that ulcerate and disrupt the internal elastic lamina, into the aortic media. The ulcer can precipitate a local intramedial dissection, form a hematoma or pseudoaneurysm, or may rupture. Diagnosis is made by CT, which demonstrates a contrast filled outpouching in the aorta with absence of an intimal flap. Clinical presentation of PAU is similar to classic aortic dissection, with chest and abdominal pain being the frequent symptoms. Hypertension is a common risk factor for PAU, as with classic aortic dissection; however, patients with PAU tend to be older. Initial management of PAU, as with dissection, involves prompt blood pressure control (30).

Atheroma of the Aortic Arch

DEFINITION/EPIDEMIOLOGY

Stroke was initially thought to be secondary to cerebral vasospasm in the 1940s. Carotid artery atherosclerosis was subsequently found to be a major cause of cerebral infarction (31). Later, both atrial fibrillation and atrial thrombus were discovered to be causes of stroke as well (32,33). Despite the importance of atrial fibrillation and carotid atherosclerosis in cerebral infarction, nearly 40% of strokes in the Stroke Data Bank of the National Institute of Neurological and Communicative Disorders and Stroke (NINCDS) were from undetermined causes (34).

Known to be a source of emboli since the early 20th century, atheroma of the aortic arch was not recognized as a cause of stroke until the use of TEE. Atheromatous material in the ascending aorta and arch has been found to be an independent risk factor for cerebral ischemia (35). In 1990, severe atherosclerotic disease in the aortic arch was identified as a third cause of embolic cerebral infarction in a report that identified aortic arch atheroma on TEE in three patients (36). In 1992, a postmortem study to evaluate the prevalence of atheroma of the aorta found that the prevalence in patients with cerebrovascular disease was 28%, as compared with 5% in patients with neurologic disease (37).

Aortic arch atheroma has long been postulated to cause cerebral infarction, but until use of TEE and other imaging modalities, such as CT and MRI, that are better able to image the aorta, has atheroma more definitively been linked to infarction.

In the Stroke Prevention: Assessment of Risk in a Community (SPARC) study, patients were randomized and, of 588 patients who had a TEE, aortic plaques were found in the aortic arch in 31% (38). The French Aortic Plaque in Stroke (FAPS) study evaluated patients with aortic arch atheroma and found that increasing plaque thickness imparts a greater risk of stroke. In the FAPS study, the incidence of recurrent stroke was 12% per year in patients with aortic atheroma >4 mm, compared with 3% per year in patients with atheroma <1 mm (39). Additionally, aortic arch plaque thickness >4 mm is a strong and independent risk factor for ischemic stroke in patients over the age of 60 (40).

RISK FACTORS/CLINICAL MANIFESTATIONS

Traditional atherosclerotic risk factors—hypertension, hyperlipidemia, and tobacco use—are associated with aortic arch atheroma formation (41–43). Aortic arch atheroma is associated with two types of embolic phenomenon: Thrombus embolization, and cholesterol crystal embolization. Cholesterol crystal embolization is less common, and may result in acute renal failure, ischemic digits, or skin lesions. More common is dislodgment of aortic plaque thrombus, resulting in vessel occlusion. Atheromas that are large and ulcerated are more likely to form thrombi, which are visualized as mobile masses on TEE (44).

Embolization can occur spontaneously, or as result of mechanical manipulation of the aorta during procedures such as cardiac catheterization, cardiac surgery, or balloon pump placement. Studies have shown that stroke occurs six times more frequently with protruding atheromas (12%), and 12 times more frequently in patients with mobile components (25%) (45).

TREATMENT

Treatment of aortic arch atheroma is not clear. Currently, a prospective, randomized trial comparing warfarin with antiplatelet use in aortic arch atheroma is underway. Although statins were shown to reduce stroke in the Cholesterol and Recurrent Events (CARE) trial, no randomized trial looking specifically at statin effect on stroke in patients with aortic arch atheroma has been done (46). Although randomized trials to evaluate surgical removal of aortic atheromas have not been conducted, prophylactic aortic arch endarterectomy before coronary bypass or valve surgery is not indicated, and may be dangerous (47,48).

Connective Tissue Disorders Affecting the Aorta

Patients with Marfan syndrome (MFS) and Ehlers-Danlos Syndrome (EDS) have a genetic predilection to develop vascular complications, including aortic dissection and rupture. The most common inherited connective tissue disorder is MFS, with a prevalence of 4 to 6 per 100,000 persons. EDS and pseudoxanthoma elasticum are encountered less frequently (49).

Marfan Syndrome

DEFINITION/EPIDEMIOLOGY

MFS is an inherited disorder of the connective tissue, involving a mutation on the fibrillin-1 gene (FBN 1) located at chromosome 15q-21.1. MFS is genetically transmitted in an autosomal-dominant fashion with variable penetrance, and also can occur spontaneously by mutation. Approximately 70% to 80% have a family history of MFS, with the remainder being either a result of new spontaneous mutations or heterogenous disease (50).

CLINICAL MANIFESTATIONS

Patients with MFS may have ocular, musculoskeletal, and cardiovascular abnormalities. Musculoskeletal deformities include arm span greater than height, reduced upper body to lower body segment ratio (dolichostenomelia), arachnodactyly of the fingers and toes, joint hypermobility, recurrent dislocations, pectus excavatum or carinatum, and scoliosis. A displaced or subluxated lens, known as *ectopia lentis*, is the most common ocular abnormality, and is present in 87% of patients (51). Dural ectasia involves progressive dilation of the dural sac from cerebrospinal fluid (CSF) pulsation, as a result of altered elastin composition of the dura mater. Dural ectasia is found only in MFS, EDS, and neurofibramatosis. A study evaluated dural ectasia by MRI in 83 patients with MFS, and found that dural ectasia is present in >90% of the study population. Dural ectasia is the most prevalent disorder of MFS, and may be a sensitive sign in the diagnosis of MFS (52).

Cardiovascular abnormalities include mitral and aortic valve disease. Mitral valve prolapse occurs in 90% of patients, and mitral regurgitation is present in one third to one half of patients. Aortic disease is common in MFS, and includes aortic valve regurgitation, dilated aortic root, aortic ectasia, and aortic dissection or aneurysmal disease. Dilated aortic root occurs in about 80% of patients with MFS (51). Studies have demonstrated that ascending aortic dilation occurs more frequently and rapidly in males as compared to females (53). The typical progression of aortic dilation is dilation of the sinuses of Valsalva, followed by dilation of the sinotubular ridge, and eventual dilation of the ascending aorta and arch. The distal ascending aorta, abdominal aorta, and descending thoracic aorta are rarely involved first by aneurysmal formation. Patients are at risk for aortic dissection, particularly in those with a family history of aortic dissection. Occasionally, dissection occurs in patients with no aortic dilation (50). Aortic dissection is often painless, and patients may have no history of hemodynamic compromise (54).

DIAGNOSES

Diagnosis of MFS is primarily clinical. Criteria for the diagnosis of MFS were most recently revised in 1996 at the Ghent Nosology meeting, and are based on previous criteria established by McKusick and Pyeritz (55,56). Diagnosis involves various major and minor criteria of abnormalities in the skeletal, ocular, cardiovascular, dura, skin, and pulmonary systems, and considers whether the patient has a family history of MFS. Diagnosis usually involves an ophthalmologic examination, echocardiogram, and CT scan with contrast of the chest and abdomen.

TREATMENT

Death of patients with MFS usually occurs from progression of cardiovascular complications, and prolongation of life relies on early diagnosis and prevention of complications (50,57). Studies have suggested that therapy with β-blockers may retard the rate of dilation of the aorta, possibly secondary to the negative inotropic effect and increased cross-linking of collagen fibers (54,58,59). Surgical aortic repair is indicated when aortic dilation $\geq$5 to 7 mm per year. In general, aneurysms >4.7 cm to 5 cm in diameter are at high risk of rupture, and surgery is recommended in such cases.

Ehlers-Danlos Syndrome

EDS is a group of heritable connective tissue disorders related to defects in type III collagen; it is characterized by joint hypermobility, skin hyperextensibility, and tissue fragility. The exact incidence of EDS is unknown, and eleven types have been described. Aortic involvement is mostly seen in EDS autosomal-dominant type IV. Treatment of patients with EDS is similar to that of patients with MFS.

Aortic Aneurysm

DEFINITION/EPIDEMIOLOGY

Aortic aneurysm is the 13th most common cause of death in the United States (60). With improvement in imaging techniques, the prevalence of aortic aneurysms has increased. Approximately 0.6% of all women and 1.2% of all men die of aortic aneurysms (61). Patients who die because of a ruptured aneurysm are more likely to be over the age of 65 (83%) (62). The mortality rate for elective repair of thoracoabdominal aneurysms ranges from 4% to 21%. Important risk factors in predicting mortality at 30 days are advanced age, renal failure, and postoperative paraplegia (63).

CLASSIFICATION

Thoracoabdominal aneurysms are classified by the Crawford classification system, which ranges from I to IV, depending on the area affected. Type I originates in the proximal descending thoracic aorta and ends above the renal arteries; type II begins in the proximal descending thoracic aorta and ends below the renal arteries; type III begins in the distal descending aorta; and type IV involves most of the abdominal aorta (Fig. 15-3). The ratio of thoracic aneurysm to abdominal aortic aneurysms is approximately 1:3.

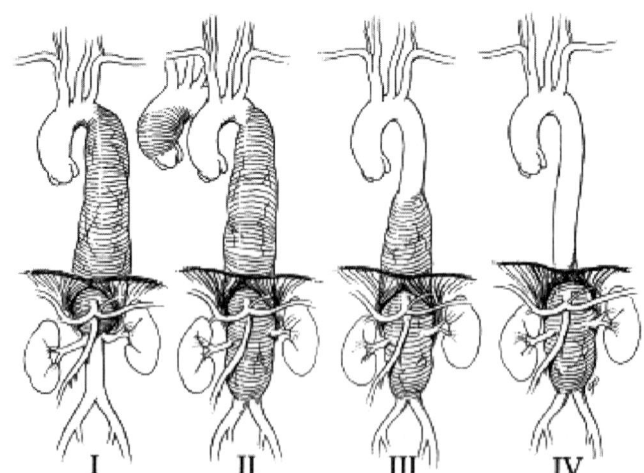

FIGURE 15-3. Crawford classification of thoracoabdominal aneurysms. Type I originates in the proximal descending thoracic aorta and ends above the renal arteries. Type II begins in the proximal descending thoracic aorta and terminates below the renal arteries. Type III originates in the distal descending aorta, below the sixth intercostals space. Type IV involves most of the abdominal aorta, generally from the diaphragm to the level of bifurcation. (From the Society of Thoracic Surgeons. *Ann Thorac Surg.* 2001;71:1233–1238, with permission.)

CLINICAL MANIFESTATIONS

Approximately 75% of aneurysms are asymptomatic, and are detected incidentally by physicians. Heart failure, MI, aortic rupture, cardiac tamponade, superior vena cava syndrome, arrhythmias, murmurs, fever, brain ischemia or neurologic events, seizures, stroke, vertebrobasilar symptoms, nonischemic atypical chest pain, backache, shortness of breath, dysphagia, hoarseness, hemoptysis, palpitations, and neck fullness may all be signs and symptoms that may alert the physician to aortic aneurysm as the diagnosis. Additionally, patients with descending thoracic aneurysms may have chest pain, paraplegia or paraparesis, renal failure, and shoulder pain. Abdominal aneurysms can cause symptoms of backache or tenderness in the flank, abdomen, shoulder, or groin. Nonspecific symptoms, including nausea, vomiting, weight loss, melena, hematemesis, fever, leg weakness, and leg pain, are less common, but possible (64). Einstein sign refers to patients with ruptured aneurysm and manifestations typical of acute cholecystitis (65).

Thoracic Aortic Aneurysm

EPIDEMIOLOGY

The incidence of thoracic aortic aneurysm (TAA) is estimated at 4.5 cases per 100,000. Patients with supravalvular TAA tend to be older and more likely men, with the mean age at time of diagnosis of 59 to 69 years with a sex ratio of 3:1, as compared to 30 to 50 years with aortic root aneurysms and a 1:1 sex ratio. One study looking at 72 patients with TAA, found that 51% involved the ascending aorta, 11% the aortic arch, and 38% the descending thoracic aorta (66). Approximately 25% of arteriosclerotic aortic aneurysms involve the thoracic aorta.

CLASSIFICATION

Thoracic aortic aneurysm is classified by location involved. One type involves the aortic root, and includes the sinuses of Valsalva. Additionally, the aneurysm may be *supravalvular,* without involvement of the sinuses of Valsalva, and may extend down the brachiocephalic trunk.

RISK FACTORS

The etiology of supravalvular aortic aneurysms includes atherosclerosis and hypertension, whereas aortic root aneurysms are more likely to be as a result of diseases causing cystic medial necrosis (i.e., MFS, EDS, bicuspid aortic valve).

Syphilis used to be a major cause of ascending aortic aneurysms, but is now less common with adequate antibiotic treatment. Arteritis is also a cause of TAA, and includes both Takayasu disease and giant cell arteritis, which will be discussed later in this chapter.

MANAGEMENT

Timing of surgical repair of TAA takes into account the surgical risk, as well as the risk of morbidity and mortality of nonrepaired aneurysms. Complications of TAA include aortic rupture and dissection, which can lead to arterial occlusion and organ ischemia. Studies have shown that as aneurysms increase in size, the risk of dissection, and rupture increases. Rupture rates of surgically nonrepaired TAA have been estimated from 21% to 74%. Mortality of elective surgical repair of TAA ranges from 5% to 9%, and increases to 59% in emergency repair. In addition to mortality risk, morbidity associated with surgical repair, including stroke, and risk of spinal cord injury should be considered. Patients with surgically nonrepaired TAA have poor outcomes, with an estimated 46% of patients with large aneurysms dead at 5 years. A patient with an aneurysm >6 cm, can expect a yearly rate of rupture or dissection of about 6.9%. A retrospective review of surgically nonrepaired TAA found that increasing aneurysm size is associated with an increased risk of rupture, with a 3.7% average yearly rate of rupture in aneurysms >6 cm.

Abdominal Aortic Aneurysm

DEFINITION/EPIDEMIOLOGY

Approximately 75% of aortic aneurysms involve the abdominal aorta distal to the renal arteries. The normal abdominal aorta diameter depends on which area of the aorta is measured, and it also increases with age, gender, or body surface area. Some believe that abdominal aortic aneurysm (AAA) should be diagnosed after using formulas that adjust for age and body surface, or by calculating the ratio between normal and diseased areas of the aorta (67–71). A diameter of 2.9 cm exceeds the upper level of normal, irrespective of age, gender, or body surface area, so that, in general, an AAA is considered to be present when the anteroposterior diameter of the abdominal aorta reaches 3 cm.

RISK FACTORS

Various risk factors, including tobacco use, age, family history, male gender, and established atherosclerosis, are involved in the prevalence of AAA. The prevalence of AAA >2.9 cm to 4.9 cm in diameter ranges from 1.3% for men aged 45 to 54 years, and 0% for women of the same age bracket, and up to 12.5% for men aged 75 to 84 years, with a prevalence of 5.2% for women (72).

Long thought to represent aortic medial degeneration, data now suggests that AAA form in response to altered matrix metalloproteinases that decrease the integrity of the aortic wall.

It appears that genetic predisposition can influence a patient's likelihood of developing an AAA. A family history of AAA is particularly important for male siblings of patients with AAA, in whom the relative risk for development of AAA is up to 18% (72). Additionally, polycystic kidney disease, and use of chronic hemodialysis have been associated with AAA (73–75).

MANAGEMENT

Patients with AAA should have their blood pressure and fasting lipid profile monitored and controlled as is done for patients with atherosclerotic disease. Also, patients with AAA or family history should be counseled to cease smoking. Patients with infrarenal or juxtarenal AAAs measuring ≥5.5 cm should have repair to eliminate the risk of rupture. AAAs measuring 4.0 to

5.4 cm should be monitored by ultrasound or CT every 6 to 12 months to detect expansion, and those <4.0 cm every 2 to 3 years. Guidelines state that repair is probably indicated in patients with suprarenal AAA >5.5 to 6.0 cm (72).

Noninfectious Aortitis

The presence of inflammatory cells in the aortic media or adventitia is indicative of aortitis. The aortic wall is typically thickened macroscopically, appearing edematous during the acute phase of aortitis to a scarred, white appearance later in the disease process. Aortitis can have both infectious and noninfectious causes. Noninfectous aortitis is typically separated into those diseases involving predominately the aorta and those that occasionally have aortic involvement. Aortitis involving predominately the aorta include Takayasu disease and isolated aortitis. Diseases that can have aortitis include giant cell arteritis (GCA), rheumatoid aortitis, relapsing polychondritis, ankylosing spondylitis, Behçet disease, Sjögren disease, systemic lupus erythematosus (SLE), Kawasaki disease, Crohn disease, ulcerative colitis, sarcoidosis, and polymyalgia rheumatica. The two most common causes of noninfectious aortitis—Takayasu Disease and giant cell arteritis—are discussed below.

Takayasu Disease

DEFINITION/EPIDEMIOLOGY

Takayasu, a Japanese ophthalmologist, initially described changes of retinal artery arteriovenous anastomoses and microaneurysms in 1908 (76). Eventual discovery of involvement of other vasculature led to the disease description. Takayasu arteritis is a chronic panarteritis localized to the aorta and its proximal branches (aortic arch or its branches, the ascending thoracic aorta, the abdominal aorta, or the entire aorta.) Takayasu aortitis tends to affect women predominately, with a ratio of 4 to 1, although 7 to 1 has been reported. The disease is more common in the Orient and India, with an incidence of 1% to 2%, whereas in the United States, the incidence is thought to be around 0.11%. This difference in incidence is thought result from a genetic hereditary predisposition related to HLA antigen haplotypes. Patients in the United States tend to have more extensive diffuse disease of the aorta, as compared with patients in Japan, where aortic arch disease is more common. In Africa, South Korea, and Singapore, midaortic disease is more frequent, suggesting environmental factors, in addition to genetics, may be involved.

Pathologic evaluation of surgically resected aortas has discovered that aortitis is an important factor in ascending aortic aneurysms in the elderly. A recent retrospective clinicopathologic review of active noninfectious aortitis revealed that 47% has isolated aortitis and, of those, only 10% went on to develop aortic aneurysm. Isolated aortitis tended to affect women and patients >50 years of age (77).

CLINICAL MANIFESTATIONS

Takayasu arteritis has two distinctive phases: A prepulseless or systemic phase, and a pulseless phase. Transient monocular blindness (amaurosis fugax), transient ischemic attacks (TIA), and strokes are relatively common. Other ischemic-related symptoms include decreased visual acuity, ischemic optic neuropathy, vertigo when looking upward, syncope, convulsions, dementia, headaches, claudication in one arm or leg, intermittent claudication of the jaw muscles, or ischemia of the extremities. Differences in blood pressure between both arms, a diminished or absent radial pulse, and widespread bruits, are helpful diagnostic clues.

Giant Cell Arteritis

DEFINITION/EPIDEMIOLOGY

Giant cell arteritis, also known as temporal arteritis, cranial arteritis, and Horton disease, is an autoimmune disease involving large- and medium-size vessels, and occasionally the aorta. The condition can also involve the temporal arteries, "temporal arteritis," with symptoms of severe headache and a predisposition for blindness. Histologic findings include intimal thickening by inflammatory cells and infiltration of the aortic media by granulomas, multinucleated giant cells, and various white cells.

The incidence of GCA is 17.4 patients per 100,000 persons per annum. The prevalence increases with age, with an incidence of 30 cases per 100,000 per annum in patients >50 years of age. Females are more affected at a ratio of 2:1. The disease is more common in people of northern (Scandinavian descent) European countries. The demographics for GCA is the same as for polymyalgia rheumatica, and 30% to 50% of patients with GCA may concurrently have features of polymyalgia rheumatica.

CLINICAL MANIFESTATIONS

The characteristic features of GCA are often atypical. Occasionally, patients have severe headache, scalp and temporal tenderness, acute vision loss, polymyalgia rheumatica, and pain and weakness in the muscles of mastication (jaw claudication). Visual loss is most often secondary to reduced blood flow to the short posterior ciliary arteries, causing infarction of the optic nerve head (arteritic anterior ischemic optic neuropathy) or, less frequently, secondary to infarction of the retina caused by central retinal artery occlusion. Stenosis or occlusion of the carotid or vertebral arteries can cause TIA or strokes. Occipital lobe infarctions can cause cortical blindness. Aortic manifestations of GCA occur in approximately 15% of patients, often several years after the initial acute illness (78,79). Consistent with the pattern of aortic arch involvement is the presentation of lower limb ischemia, resulting from involvement of aortic branches. Also, the abdominal visceral arteries, vertebral arteries, coronary arteries, and the intracranial branches of the carotid arteries may be involved. Patients with GCA are 17 times more likely than aged-matched control subjects to have thoracic aortic aneurysms, and about 2.5 more times likely to have AAA (78,79). Aortic rupture can occur infrequently as can acute dissection with aortic valve regurgitation.

MANAGEMENT

High-dose, long-term corticosteroids are the mainstay of treatment of GCA, usually relieving symptoms in 1 to 2 days, and often eliminating them within a week. Headaches are usually relieved and blindness may be prevented. Aortic lesions in the chronic phase should be treated surgically. In some patients, once aneurysms have occurred in one location, a progressive dilation of the rest of the aorta occurs.

Neurologic Complications and Aortic Surgery

Stroke and spinal cord ischemia will result in paraplegia and are important complications when having any type of thoracoabdominal aortic surgery. Initially described with syphilitic arteritis, spinal cord infarction can result from aortic dissection, atherosclerosis of the aorta and its branches, acute aortic thrombosis, repair of coarctation of aorta, and following surgery of the abdominal aorta. Several techniques and measures are taken to decrease the risk of postoperative neurologic complications, including CSF drainage, and distal aortic or visceral perfusion. One study looked at 1,004 patients having aortic surgery, and found that postoperative neurologic deficits occurred in 6.8% of patients who had not had adjunctive measures (CSF drainage, distal aortic perfusion), whereas neurologic deficits occurred in only 2.4% of those patients who had these measures (80).

Several studies looking at neurologic complications after endovascular treatment of thoracic aortic disease showed paraplegia or parapareis in 0% to 12.5%, and stroke in 0% to 18.6%. Several patients who developed stroke postoperatively had surgery on proximal aneurysmal disease, potentially implicating emboli arising from the aortic arch. To help alleviate this problem, some centers opt to do intraoperative echocardiogram of the aorta once the chest is open, to evaluate for atheroma or thrombi (81).

CLINICAL RECOMMENDATIONS OF THE VIGNETTE

The patient illustrates the presentation of vertebrobasilar ischemia with ascending aortic dissection extending to the left subclavian and origin of the left vertebral artery. The recognition of TIA is important, because approximately 10% to 30% of patients with ischemic stroke, some of which may have been preventable, have a history of earlier TIA. Approximately 6% of patients with ascending aortic dissection will present with stroke. Under the Stanford classification scheme, this patient would have a type A dissection, and surgery would be the recommendation for management.

SUMMARY

Significant morbidity and mortality are associated with a wide spectrum of aortic diseases. Neurologic complications associated with aortic diseases are protean and include, among others, TIA, stroke, spinal cord ischemia, ischemic peripheral neuropathies, Horner syndrome, vagal or recurrent laryngeal nerve palsies, and phrenic nerve paralysis. In patients presenting with transient or permanent ischemic neurologic symptoms, aortic disease is a consideration.

REFERENCES

1. Acierno LJ. *The History of Cardiology.* New York: Parthenon Publishing Group; 1994.
2. DeSanctis RW, Doroghazi RM, Austen WG, et al. Aortic dissection. *N Engl J Med.* 1990;317:1060–1067.
3. Hagan PG, Nienaber CA, Isselbacher EM, et al. The International Registry of Acute Aortic Dissection (IRAD): New insights into an old disease. *JAMA.* 2000;283:897–903.
4. Spittell PC, Spittell JA, Jr., Joyce JW, et al. Clinical features and differential diagnosis of aortic dissection: Experience with 236 cases (1980 through 1990). *Mayo Clin Proc.* 1993; 68:642–651.
5. Bickerstaff LK, Pairolero PC, Hollier LH, et al. Thoracic aortic aneurysms: A population-based study. *Surgery.* 1982;92:1103–1108.
6. Eisenberg MJ, Rice SA, Paraschos A, et al. The clinical spectrum of patients with aneurysms of the ascending aorta. *Am Heart J.* 1993;125:1380–1385.
7. Coplan JL, Goldman B, Mechanic G, et al. Sudden hemodynamic collapse following relief of cardiac tamponade in a patient with aortic dissection. *Am Heart J.* 1986;111:405–406.
8. Meszaros I, Morocz J, Szlavi J, et al: Epidemiology and clinicopathology of aortic dissection: A population-based longitudinal study over 27 years. *Chest.* 2000;117:1271.
9. DeBakey ME, McCollum CH, Crawford ES, et al. Dissection and dissecting aneurysms of the aorta: Twenty-year follow up of five hundred twenty-seven patients treated surgically. *Surgery.* 1982;92:1118–1134.
10. Hirst AE, Jr., Johns VJ, Jr., Klime SW, Sr. Dissecting aneurysm of the aorta: A review of 505 cases. *Medicine (Baltimore).* 1958;37:217–279.
11. Mikich B. Dissection of the aorta: A new approach. *Heart.* 2003;89(1):6–8.
12. Roberts C, Roberts W. Dissection of the aorta associated with congenital malformation of the aortic valve. *J Am Coll Cardiol.* 1991;17:712–716.
13. von Kodilitsch Y, Aydin MA, Loose R, et al. Predictors of aneurysm formation after surgery of aortic coarctation. *J Am Coll Cardiol.* 2002;39:617–624.
14. Ward C. Clinical significance of the bicuspid aortic valve. *Heart.* 2000;83:81–85.
15. Reed D, Reed C, Stemmermann G, et al. Are aortic aneurysms caused by atherosclerosis? *Circulation.* 1992;85:205–211.
16. Stefanadis CI, Karayannacos PE, Doudoulas HK, et al. Medial necrosis and acute alterations in aortic distensibility following removal of the vasa vasorum of canine ascending aorta. *Cardiovasc Res.* 1993;27:951–956.
17. Wilbers CRH, Carrol CL, Hnilica MA. Optimal diagnostic imaging of aortic dissection. *Tex Heart Inst J.* 1990;17:271–278.
18. Shuford WH, Sybers RG, Weens HS. Problems in the aortographic diagnosis of dissecting aneurysm of the aorta. *N Engl J Med.* 1969;280:225–231.
19. Larson EW, Edwards WD. Risk factors for aortic dissection: A necropsy study of 161 cases. *Am J Cardiol.* 1984;53:849–855.
20. Mintz GS, Kotler MN, Segal BL, et al. Two-dimensional echocardiograpic recognition of the descending thoracic aorta. *Am J Cardiol.* 1979;44:232–238.
21. Khandheria BK, Tajik AJ, Taylor CL, et al. Aortic dissection: Review of value and limitations of two-dimensional echocardiography in a six-year experience. *J Am Soc Echocardiogr.* 1989;2:17–24.
22. Illiceto S, Ettore G, Francisco G, et al. Diagnosis of aneurysm of the thoracic aorta. Comparison between two non invasive techniques: Two-dimensional echocardiography and computed tomography. *Eur Heart J.* 1984;5:545–555.
23. Erbel R, Engberding R, Daniel W, et al. Echocardiography in diagnosis of aortic dissection. *Lancet.* 1989;1:457–461.
24. Sommer T, Fehske W, Holzknecht N, et al. Aortic dissection: A comparative study of diagnosis with spiral CT, multiplanar transesophageal echocardiography, and MR imaging. *Radiology.* 1996;199:347–352.
25. Erbel R, Alfonso F, Boileau C, et al. Diagnosis and management of aortic dissection. *Eur Heart J.* 2001;22(18):1642–1681.
26. Shiga T, Wajima Z, Apfel C, et al. Diagnostic accuracy of transesophageal echocardiography, helical computed tomography, and magnetic resonance imaging for suspected thoracic aortic dissection. *Arch Intern Med.* 2006;166:1350–1356.
27. Kamp TJ, Goldschmidt-Clermont PJ, Brinker JA, et al. Myocardial infarction, aortic dissection, and thrombolytic therapy. *Am Heart J.* 1994;128:1234–1237.
28. Slater EE, DeSanctis RW. The clinical recognition of dissecting aortic aneurysm. *Am J Med.* 1976;60:625–633.
29. Varon J, Marik PE. The diagnosis and management of hypertensive crises. *Chest.* 2000;118:214–227.
30. Coady MA, Rizzo JA, Hammond GL, et al. Penetrating ulcer of the thoracic aorta: What is it? How do we recognize it? How do we manage it? *J Vasc Surg.* 1998;27(6):1006–1015.
31. Fisher CM. Occlusion of the internal carotid artery. *Arch Neurol Psychiatry.* 1951; 65:346–377.
32. Weintraub G, Sprecace G. Paroxysmal atrial fibrillation and cerebral embolism with apparently normal heart. *N Engl J Med.* 1958;259:875–876.
33. Lewis KB, Criley JM, Ross RS. Detection of left atrial thrombus by cineangiocardiography. *Am Heart J.* 1965;70:612–619.
34. Sacco RL, Ellenberg JH, Mohr JP, et al. Infarcts of undetermined cause: The NINCDS stroke data bank. *Ann Neurol.* 1989;25:382–390.
35. Jones EF, Kalman JM, Calafiore P, et al. Proximal aortic atheroma. An independent risk factor for cerebral ischemia. *Stroke.* 1995;26(2):218–224.
36. Tunick PA, Kronzon I. Protruding atherosclerotic plaque in the aortic arch of patients with systemic embolization: A new finding seen by transesophageal echocardiography. *Am Heart J.* 1990;120:658–660.
37. Amarenco P, Duyckaerts C, Tzourio C, et al. The prevalence of ulcerated plaques in the aortic arch in patients with stroke. *N Engl J Med.* 1992;326(4):221–225.
38. Meissner I, Khandheria BK, Sheps SG, et al. Atherosclerosis of the aorta: Risk factor, risk marker, or innocent bystander? A prospective population-based transesophageal echocardiography study. *J Am Coll Cardiol.* 2004;44:1018–1024.
39. The French Study of Aortic Plaques in Stroke Group. Atherosclerotic disease of the aortic arch as a risk factor for recurrent ischemic stroke. *N Engl J Med.* 1996;334(19): 1216–1221.
40. Amarenco P, Cohen A, Tzourio C, et al. Atherosclerotic disease of the aortic arch and the risk of ischemic stroke. *N Engl J Med.* 1994;331:1474–1479.

41. Agmon Y, Khandheria BK, Meissner I, et al. Independent association of high blood pressure and aortic atherosclerosis: A population-based study. *Circulation.* 2000;102(17): 2087–2093.
42. Agmon Y, Khandheria BK, Meissner I, et al. Relation of coronary artery disease and cerebrovascular disease with atherosclerosis of the thoracic aorta in the general population. *Am J Cardiol.* 2002;89(3):262–267.
43. Tribouilloy CM, Peltier M, Iannetta Peltier MC, et al. Plasma homocysteine and severity of thoracic aortic atherosclerosis. *Chest.* 2000;118(6):1685–1689.
44. Vaduganathan P, Ewton A, Nahueh SF, et al. Pathologic correlates of aortic plaques, thrombi and mobile "aortic debris" imaged in vivo with transesophageal echocardiography. *J Am Coll Cardiol.* 1997;30:357–363.
45. Stern A, Tunick PA, Culliford AT, et al. Protruding aortic arch atheromas: Risk of stroke during heart surgery with and without aortic arch endarterectomy. *Am Heart J.* 1999;138(4 Pt 1):746–752.
46. Lewis SJ, Moye LA, Sacks FM, et al. Effect of pravastatin on cardiovascular events in older patients with myocardial infarction and cholesterol levels in the average range: Results of the Cholesterol and Recurrent Events (CARE) trial. *Ann Intern Med.* 1998;129:681–689.
47. Stern A, Tunick PA, Culliford AT, et al. Protruding aortic arch atheromas: Risk of stroke during heart surgery with and without aortic arch endarterectomy. *Am Heart J.* 1999;138:746–752.
48. Kronzon I, Tunick PA. Aortic atherosclerotic disease and stroke. *Circulation.* 2006; 114(1):63–75
49. McKusick VA. The cardiovascular aspects of Marfan syndrome: A heritable disorder of connective tissue. *Circulation.* 1955;2:321–341.
50. Svensson LG, Crawford ES, Coselli JS, et al. Impact of cardiovascular operation on survival in the Marfan patient. *Circulation.* 1989;80(3 Pt1):i233–i242.
51. Sun QB, Zhang KZ, Cheng TO, et al. Marfan syndrome in China: A collective review of 564 cases among 98 families. *Am Heart J.* 1990;120:934–948.
52. Fattori R, Nienaber CA, Descovich B, et al. Importance of dural ectasia in phenotypic assessment of Marfan's syndrome. *Lancet.* 1999;354(9182):910–913.
53. Roman MJ, Rosen SE, Kramer-Fox R, et al. Prognostic significance of the pattern of aortic root dilation in the Marfan syndrome. *J Am Coll Cardiol.* 1993;22:1470–1476.
54. Svensson LG, Crawford ES. Aortic dissection and aortic aneurysm surgery: Clinical observations, experimental investigations, and statistical analyses. Part III. *Curr Probl Surg.* 1993;30:1–163.
55. De Paepe A, Devereux RB, Dietz HC, et al. Revised diagnostic criteria for the Marfan syndrome. *Am J Med Genet.* 1996;62:417–426.
56. Pyeritz RE, McKusick VA. The Marfan syndrome: Diagnosis and management. *N Engl J Med.* 1979;300:772–777.
57. Pyeritz RE. Marfan syndrome [Editorial]. *N Engl J Med.* 1990;323:987–989.
58. Gott VL, Pyeritz RE, Cameraon DE, et al. Composite graft repair of Marfan aneurysm of the ascending aorta: Results in 100 patients. *Ann Thorac Surg.* 1991;52:38–44.
59. Taherina AC. Cardiovascular anomalies in Marfan's syndrome: The role of echocardiography and beta-blockers. *South Med J.* 1993;86:305–310.
60. Majumber PP, St. Jeah PL, Ferrell RE, et al. On the inheritance of abdominal aortic aneurysm. *Am J Hum Genet.* 1991;48:164–170.
61. National Center for Health Statistics: Data Line. *Public Health Rep.* 1987;102(5):563–565.
62. Amundsen S, Trippestad A, Viste A, et al. Abdominal aortic aneurysms—A national multicenter study. *Eur J Vasc Surg.* 1987;1:239–243.
63. Coselli JS, LeMaire SA, Conklin LD, et al. Left heart bypass during descending thoracic aortic aneurysm repair does not reduce the incidence of paraplegia. *Ann Thorac Surg.* 2004;77:1298–1303.
64. Svensson LG, Crawford ES. *Cardiovascular and Vascular Disease of the Aorta,* Svensson and Crawford. Philadelphia: WB Saunders; 1997.
65. Chandler JJ. The Einstein sign: The clinical picture of acute cholecystitis cause by ruptured abdominal aortic aneurysm [Letter]. *N Engl J Med.* 1984;310:1538.
66. Bickerstaff LK, Pairolero PC, Hollier LH, et al. Thoracic aortic aneurysms: A population based study. *Surgery.* 1982;92:1103–1109.
67. Ebaugh JL, Garcia ND, Matsumura JS. Screening and surveillance for abdominal aortic aneurysms: Who needs it and when. *Semin Vasc Surg.* 2001;14:193–199.
68. Alcom HG, Wolfson SK, Jr., Sutton-Tyrrell K, et al. Risk factors for abdominal aortic aneurysms in older adults enrolled in The Cardiovascular Health Study. *Arterioscler Thromb Vasc Biol.* 1996;16:963–970.
69. Pedersen OM, Aslaksen A, Vik-Mo H. Ultrasound measurement of the luminal diameter of the abdominal aorta and iliac arteries in patients without vascular disease. *J Vasc Surg.* 1993;17:596–601.
70. Lanne T, Sandgren T, Sonesson B. A dynamic view on the diameter of abdominal aortic aneurysms. *Eur J Vasc Endovasc Surg.* 1998;15:308–312.
71. Johnston KW, Rutherford RB, Tilson MD, et al. Suggested standards for reporting on arterial aneurysms. Subcommittee on Reporting Standards for Arterial Aneurysms, Ad Hoc Committee on Reporting Standards, Society for Vascular Surgery and North American Chapter, International Society for Cardiovascular Surgery. *J Vasc Surg.* 1991;13: 452–458.
72. Hirsch AT, Haskal ZJ, Hertzer NR, et al. ACC/AHA 2005 Guidelines for the Management of Patients With Peripheral Arterial Disease (Lower Extremity, Renal, Mesenteric, and Abdominal Aortic): A Collaborative Report from the American Association for Vascular Surgery/Society for Vascular Surgery, Society for Cardiovascular Angiography and Interventions, Society for Vascular Medicine and Biology, Society of Interventional Radiology, and the ACC/AHA Task Force on Practice Guidelines (Writing Committee to Develop Guidelines for the Management of Patients With Peripheral Arterial Disease). *J Am Coll Cardiol.* 2006;47:1–192.
73. Verloes A, Sakalihasan N, Koulischer L, et al. Aneurysms of the abdominal aorta: Familial and genetic aspects in three hundred thirteen pedigrees. *J Vasc Surg.* 1995; 21:646–655.
74. Leier CV, Baker PB, Kilman JW, et al. Cardiovascular abnormalities associated with adult polycystic kidney disease. *Ann Intern Med.* 1984;100:683–688.
75. Torra R, Nicolau C, Badenas C, et al. Abdominal aortic aneurysms and autosomal dominant polycystic kidney disease. *J Am Soc Nephrol.* 1996;7:2483–2486.
76. Takayasu M. A case with unusual changes of the central vessels in the retina. *Acta Soc Ophthalmol J.* 1908;12:554–555.
77. Miller DV, Isotalo PA, Weyand CM, et al. Surgical pathology of noninfectious ascending aortitis: A study of 45 cases with emphasis on an isolated variant. *Am J Surg Pathol.* 2006;30(9): 1150–1158.
78. Evans J, Hunder GG. The implications of recognizing large-vessel involvement in elderly patients with giant cell arteritis. *Curr Opin Rheumatol.* 1997;9:37.
79. Evans JM, O'Fallon WM, Hunder GG. Increased incidence of aortic aneurysm and dissection in giant cell (temporal) arteritis. *Ann Intern Med.* 1995;122:502.
80. Safi HJ, Barroli S, Hess KR, et al. Neurologic deficit in patients at high risk with thoracoabdominal aortic aneurysms: The role of cerebral spinal fluid drainage and distal aortic perfusion. *J Vasc Surg.* 1994;20:434–444.
81. Sullivan TM, Sundt TM. Complications of thoracic aortic endografts: Spinal cord ischemia and stroke. *J Vasc Surg.* 2006;43[Suppl A]:85A–88A.

CHAPTER 16

Commonly Used Cardiovascular Drugs

Lisa M. Hurst • Mark A. Ross

OBJECTIVES

- To review the neurologic complications of commonly used cardiovascular drugs
- To review the spectrum of neuromuscular complications of statin therapy
- To identify characteristics of patients at high risk for statin-induced myopathy
- To discuss potential mechanisms for statin-induced myopathy
- To review care recommendations for statin-induced myopathy

CASE VIGNETTE

A 78-year-old man presented with a 10-day history of progressive generalized weakness. He had difficulty walking and raising his arms above his head. He had no bulbar or visual symptoms. He denied new sensory complaints. One month earlier, when hospitalized for an acute myocardial infarction, simvastatin was increased from 20 to 40 mg daily. Medical history was remarkable for type 2 diabetes mellitus, hyperlipidemia, coronary artery disease, polycystic kidney disease with two cadaveric kidney transplants, and disseminated coccidioidomycosis. Pertinent medications were fluconazole, cyclosporine, and simvastatin.

Neurologic examination demonstrated normal mental status and cranial nerves. He had proximal and distal weakness of all limbs. Muscle stretch reflexes were reduced in the arms and absent in the legs. Sensory examination showed decreased pin sensation in a stocking-glove distribution, which was unchanged from prior records. Laboratory assessment showed elevated creatine kinase (CK) of 1,048 U/L, with normal troponin T. Magnetic resonance imaging (MRI) studies of the entire spine showed chronic degenerative changes with no abnormality of the spinal cord or nerve roots. An electromyogram showed evidence of a myopathic process.

He was diagnosed with a statin-induced myopathy, precipitated by the recent increase in simvastatin. In addition, he had an underlying sensorimotor poyneuropathy attributed to diabetes. Therapy consisted of hydration and discontinuation of simvastatin. Over several days, the CK level decreased and his strength improved. He was discharged on no lipid-lowering therapy with plans to review cholesterol management further with his primary physician.

DEFINITION

The most effective therapeutic agents for the treatment of elevated low-density lipoprotein (LDL) cholesterol are the 3-hydroxy-3-methylglutaryl coenzyme A (HMG-CoA) reductase inhibitors, better known as "statins" (1). Despite an exceptional safety profile (2), muscle toxicity or *myopathy* occurs in approximately 0.5% of treated individuals (3), with a wide spectrum of clinical manifestations.

In 2002, the American College of Cardiology, the American Heart Association, and the National Heart, Lung and Blood Institute defined the following terms in the spectrum of myopathy:

> *myalgia*—muscle pain or weakness without CK elevation; *myositis*—pain or weakness with CK elevation; *rhabdomyolysis*—muscle pain or weakness with CK elevation typically >10 times the upper limit of normal, usually associated with creatinine elevation (4).

In clinical trials of statins for treatment of elevated cholesterol, the most widely used definition of *myopathy* is a CK level >10 times the upper limit of normal with associated muscle symptoms that are not attributable to other causes (5).

Rare reports have been made of polyneuropathy associated with statin therapy (6), but the evidence of this association has been questioned (7). Other cardiovascular agents that have been associated with polyneuropathy are summarized in Table 16-1.

EPIDEMIOLOGY

Statins have been shown to reduce cardiac mortality and adverse cardiac events and are recommended for primary and secondary prevention of coronary artery disease (8–11). Myopathy is the most common adverse effect of statin drugs; however, the occurrence of serious muscle toxicity with statins is rare. According to findings from 21 clinical trials providing 180,000 person years of follow-up in patients treated with statin or placebo, myopathy occurred in 5 patients per 100,000 person-years and rhabdomyolysis in 1.6 patients per 100,000 person-years (12).

TABLE 16-1. Cardiovascular Drugs Causing Polyneuropathy

Medication	*Clinical Use*	*Pathophysiology*	*Fiber Type*	*Clinical Features*	*Weakness*
Amiodarone	Arrhythmia	Demyelination	S, M	Myopathy may occur	D, ± P
Perhexiline	Angina pectoris	Demyelination	S, M, A	Papilledema, facial weakness	P and D
Hydralazine	Hypertension	Axon loss	S, ± M	Distal sensory symptoms	Uncommon

S, sensory; M, motor; A, autonomic; D, distal; P, proximal.

The risk of myotoxicity from statins is increased by specific patient characteristics, including increased age, small stature, renal or hepatic insufficiency, hypothyroidism, diabetes, and excessive alcohol use (13). The risk of myotoxicity from statin use is also influenced by statin type and dose, and concurrent drug therapy (14). Myotoxicity has been reported with all statins; however, a higher risk of myotoxicity is found in some statins. Statin properties that increase the risk of myotoxicity include high systemic exposure (not necessarily dose related), lipophilicity, high bioavailability, and limited protein binding (15). Statins metabolized by cytochrome P450 3A4, such as lovastatin, simvastatin, and atorvastatin, have a higher incidence of rhabdomyolysis than statins metabolized by the cytochrome P450 A29, such as fluvastatin, or hydrophilic statins such as pravastatin. Theoretically, the low lipid solubility of pravastatin limits passage across the muscle cell membrane, and reduces the risk of muscle injury (1). In a systemic review of 21 randomized trials, no cases of rhabdomyolysis occurred in the treated or placebo groups in trials of pravastatin or fluvastatin (12).

Concurrent medications are also strong predictors of the risk of statin-induced myopathy. Concurrent use of a statin drug with other medications that inhibit the cytochrome P450 3A4 pathway results in increased statin drug levels and an increased potential for an adverse reaction. Medications that inhibit the cytochrome P450 3A4 pathway include macrolides, azole antifungals, non-dihydropyridine calcium-channel blockers, protease inhibitors, and cyclosporine. Grapefruit juice also inhibits the cytochrome P450 3A4 system (12). Fibrates, principally gemfibrozil, can independently cause myopathy through a mechanism other than inhibiting the cytochrome P450 pathway. The combination of fibrates and statin therapy leads to a substantially higher risk of rhabdomyolysis compared with the sum of the two independently (12). The mechanism behind this is poorly understood, although it could be related to the inhibition of glucuronidation of statins by gemfibrozil (1).

ETIOLOGY AND PATHOGENESIS

Pathologic findings in statin-induced myopathy are characterized by muscle fiber necrosis and fragmentation with inflammatory cell infiltration in the perivascular and endomysial areas (16). The pathophysiologic mechanisms underlying statin-induced myopathy are poorly understood, largely because of the multiple complicated biochemical pathways related to cholesterol synthesis. Statins reversibly inhibit HMG-CoA reductase, the enzyme that converts HMG-CoA to mevalonate. Mevalonate is a precursor to multiple metabolic pathways upstream to cholesterol synthesis. Muscle membrane instability from reduction of cholesterol was an attractive early hypothesis for statin myotoxicity. Current thinking is that the inhibition of multiple biochemical pathways related to mevalonate metabolism, particularly the isoprenoids, are the more likely cause of statin myopathy (17). The isoprenoids are involved in modification of numerous critical proteins including co-enzyme Q10, lamins, α-dystroglycan, and selenoproteins (17). Another pathophysiologic consideration is that individuals with subclinical muscle disease may develop overt muscle disease when treated with statins (18).

CLINICAL MANIFESTATIONS

The clinical manifestations of statin-induced myopathy range from mild myalgia to overt rhabdomyolysis. Although muscle symptoms can occur at any time during the use of statins, these usually begin within weeks to months of initiation. The most common symptoms include muscle pain, weakness, and muscle cramping. Muscle involvement is usually symmetric and predominantly affects the large proximal muscle groups.

Depending on the severity of the myopathy, the CK level can range from normal to >50 times the upper limit of normal. Some patients receiving statin therapy have developed muscle weakness with histopathologic evidence of myopathy, despite normal CK levels (2). In severe cases of myopathy, individuals develop weakness associated with markedly increased CK levels and myoglobinuria leading to acute tubular necrosis and renal failure. Associated metabolic consequences include hyperkalemia, hypocalcemia, hyperphosphatemia, hyperuricemia, and metabolic acidosis.

Management of statin-induced myopathy is supportive. Typically, myalgias and weakness resolve and serum CK concentrations return toward normal within a month after discontinuation of the statin (3). The authors, however, have seen many cases in which the CK level does not completely normalize many months after muscle symptoms have resolved.

DIAGNOSTIC APPROACH AND TREATMENT

Prevention is the best approach to managing statin-related myopathy. When initiating statin therapy, select a low dose, and adjust it as necessary to achieve therapeutic goals. Other efforts to lower cholesterol, including diet and exercise, should be considered. A careful review of medications must be made to avoid concomitant therapy with fibrates or medications that inhibit the cytochrome P450 pathway. Patients should be cautioned to avoid concurrent use of grapefruit juice. When initiating statin therapy, the patient should be warned about the possibility of muscle symptoms and encouraged to seek medical attention if muscle pain, weakness, or dark colored urine occur.

A baseline CK is not always necessary according to the National Lipid Association's Muscle Safety Expert Panel (5). A baseline CK is recommended, however, in those individuals with renal or hepatic dysfunction or those on medications that can affect statin metabolism. A thytropin test should also be considered because hypothyroidism can cause hypercholesterolemia and is a risk factor for statin-induced myopathy.

If a patient presents with symptoms consistent with statin-induced myopathy, a thorough history and physical examination should be performed and a CK obtained. Assess for contributing factors, such as the addition of new medications inhibiting the cytochrome P450 pathway, an increase in statin dose, or extreme physical exertion. When statin-induced myopathy is suspected, the statin should be withheld until the evaluation is complete and myopathy resolves. If a patient has a significant CK elevation or describes dark colored urine, obtain laboratory studies to evaluate renal function and urine myoglobin.

In a patient with complaints of myalgia with no, or mild to moderate elevation in CK, consider stopping the statin and observing the patient. After symptoms resolve, an alternative statin can be tried or the same statin could be tried again at a lower dose.

If the patient has renal failure and a significantly elevated CK (10 times upper limit of normal), hospitalization is recommended for intravenous hydration and close observation. After an episode of rhabdomyolysis, strong consideration should be given to using alternative lipid lowering agents, although successful restarting a lower dose of the offending statin or switching to a different statin has been reported (1).

CLINICAL RECOMMENDATIONS OF THE VIGNETTE

The patient presented had a complicated medical history and took three medications that inhibit the cytochrome P450 pathway: fluconazole, cyclosporine, and simvastatin. It was imperative to continue fluconazole for treatment of disseminated coccidiomycosis and cyclosporine to prevent transplant rejection. Continued therapy of hyperlipidemia was necessary in this patient with diabetes and recent myocardial infarction (8–11).

A therapeutic option for this patient could be a trial of pravastatin, which does not interfere with the cytochrome P450 pathway, and therefore, there is less risk of myopathy. Pravastatin is the only statin approved by the US Food and Drug Administration for combination therapy in patients treated with cyclosporine. Following resolution of the patient's symptoms and normalization of the CK levels, we recommended initiation of pravastatin at a low dose and titrating to achieve target cholesterol levels with close monitoring for recurrence of muscle symptoms or elevated CK levels.

SUMMARY

Statins are effective at decreasing mortality and cardiovascular event rates and are the most widely prescribed treatment for hypercholesterolemia. Although uncommon, muscle toxicity is the most frequent adverse effect of statin therapy. The spectrum of statin-induced myopathy ranges from mild myalgia to overt rhabdomyolysis. The myotoxic risk of statins can be increased by specific patient characteristics, statin type and dose, and concurrent drug therapy. The precise mechanism of statin-induced myopathy remains unclear, but is likely related to inhibition of mevalonate metabolism, particularly isoprenoids, leading to loss of critical proteins involved with membrane structure and energy production. Treatment is primarily conservative, with discontinuation of the statin and close follow-up. The decision to restart statin therapy following resolution of the symptoms depends on the risk and benefits of statin therapy for the particular patient.

REFERENCES

1. Thompson PD, Clarkson P, Karas RH. Statin-associated myopathy. *JAMA*. 2003;289(13):1681–1690.
2. Phillips PS, Haas RH, Bannykh S, et al. Statin-associated myopathy with normal creatine kinase levels. *Ann Intern Med*. 2002;137(7):581–585.
3. Hansen KE, Hildebrand JP, Ferguson EE, et al. Outcomes in 45 patients with statin-associated myopathy. *Arch Intern Med*. 2005;165(22):2671–2676.
4. Pasternak RC, Smith SC, Jr., Bairey-Merz CN, et al. ACC/AHA/NHLBI Clinical Advisory on the Use and Safety of Statins. *Circulation*. 2002;106(8):1024–1028.
5. Thompson PD, Clarkson PM, Rosenson RS. An assessment of statin safety by muscle experts. *Am J Cardiol*. 2006;97(8A):69C–76C.
6. Gaist D, Jeppesen U, Anderson M, et al. Statins and risk of polyneuropathy: A case control study. *Neurology*. 2002;58:1333–1337.
7. Leis AA, Stokic DS, Oliveir J. Statins and polyneuropathy: setting the record straight. *Muscle Nerve*. 2005;32:428–430.
8. Sacks FM, Pfeffer MA, Moye LA, et al. The effect of pravastatin on coronary events after myocardial infarction in patients with average cholesterol levels. Cholesterol and Recurrent Events Trial investigators. *N Engl J Med*. 1996;335(14):1001–1999.
9. Prevention of cardiovascular events and death with pravastatin in patients with coronary heart disease and a broad range of initial cholesterol levels. The Long-Term Intervention with Pravastatin in Ischaemic Disease (LIPID) Study Group. *N Engl J Med*. 1998;339(19):1349–1357.
10. Randomized trial of cholesterol lowering in 4444 patients with coronary heart disease: The Scandinavian Simvastatin Survival Study (4S). *Lancet*. 1994;344(8934):1383–1389.
11. Downs JR, Clearfield M, Weis S, et al. Primary prevention of acute coronary events with lovastatin in men and women with average cholesterol levels: results of AFCAPS/TexCAPS. Air Force/Texas Coronary Atherosclerosis Prevention Study. *JAMA*. 1998;279(20):1615–1622.
12. Law M, Rudnicka AR. Statin safety: A systematic review. *Am J Cardiol*. 2006;97(8A):52C–60C.
13. Seehusen DA, Asplund CA, Johnson DR, et al. Primary evaluation and management of statin therapy complications. *South Med J*. 2006;99(3):250–256.
14. Bays H. Statin safety: An overview and assessment of the data—2005. *Am J Cardiol*. 2006;97(8A):6C–26C.
15. Rosenson RS. Current overview of statin-induced myopathy. *Am J Med*. 2004;116(6):408–416.
16. Ucar M, Mjorndal T, Dahlqvist R. HMG-CoA reductase inhibitors and myotoxicity. *Drug Saf*. 2000;22(6):441–457.
17. Baker SK. Molecular clues into the pathogenesis of statin-induced muscle toxicity. *Muscle Nerve*. 2005;31:572–580.
18. Miller JAL. Statins—Challenges and provocations. *Curr Opin Neurol*. 2005;18:494–496.

CHAPTER 17

Acute and Chronic Respiratory Failure

Lisa F. Wolfe • Senda Ajroud-Driss

OBJECTIVES

- To identify neurologic causes for acute and chronic respiratory failure
- To recognize clinical manifestations of acute and chronic respiratory failure
- To order and interpret clinical and laboratory tests that will aid the diagnosis of acute and chronic respiratory failure
- To be comfortable with the different treatment methods of acute and chronic respiratory failure

CASE VIGNETTES

CASE VIGNETTE 1

A 20-year-old-man with Duchenne muscular dystrophy (DMD) presented for evaluation of dyspnea. He was diagnosed with DMD at the age of 5 years. His symptoms started at the age of 3 with falls and difficulties running, and he became wheelchair-bound at the age of 12. He currently has significant kyphoscoliosis as well and complains of weak cough and increased sputum. He was having early morning headaches and gasping arousals for several weeks before the onset of daytime dyspnea. His dyspnea had recently become worse in association with fever, sputum, and chest congestion. The chest x-ray studies before and after treatment are shown in Figure 17-1.

CASE VIGNETTE 2

A 65-year-old, 80 kg man, with history of myasthenia gravis, presents to the emergency room (ER) complaining of worsening double vision, difficulties swallowing, and shortness of breath with exertion. On examination, he complained of diplopia in all direction of gaze and had bilateral, asymmetric eyelid ptosis. Speech was slightly nasal and dysarthric. He also had bifacial weakness, and neck flexors were weak. Upper extremities strength was 4/5 proximally, and 5/5 distally. While in the ER waiting to be admitted to the hospital, he became anxious and tachypneic. Speech became more nasal and he had considerable difficulties completing his sentences. Forced vital capacity (FVC) was 1.4 L.

DEFINITION

"Neurological dysfunction can lead to respiratory complications, and respiratory dysfunction may adversely affect the nervous system and lead to neurological consultation" (1).

In the setting of neurologic impairment, respiratory failure occurs either from an inability to execute central control over ventilation or, in the setting of an intact respiratory drive, ongoing impairment of the muscles of respiration (diaphragm and accessory muscles). Sudden shift in respiratory performance, those occurring over minutes to a few weeks, are associated with an acute respiratory acidosis. This *acute respiratory failure* is noted to cause large shifts in serum pH, in association with insufficient time for metabolic compensation. *Chronic respiratory failure*, on the other hand, may progress over long periods of time from months to even years. In this setting, bicarbonate elevation prevents large swings in serum pH, and blood gas testing reveals chronic respiratory acidosis with metabolic compensation (2).

EPIDEMIOLOGY

Although the incidence of acute respiratory failure in association with neurologic illness is unknown overall, the use of mechanical ventilation rose in the US population to 314 of 100,000 in 2002 (3). The overall use of noninvasive ventilation (NIV) may also be on the rise. The use of NIV for chronic neuromuscular disease remains limited, however. For example, in the setting of amyotrophic lateral sclerosis (ALS), the use of NIV is estimated to be limited to 15.6% (4).

ETIOLOGY AND PATHOGENESIS

NEUROLOGY OF BREATHING

Spontaneous ventilation is the result of rhythmic neural activity in respiratory centers located in the lower brainstem. The dorsal respiratory group located in the dorsal medulla primarily acts during inspiration, and the ventral respiratory group in the ventral medulla, mainly acts during expiration. Two pontine areas influence the dorsal medullary center. A lower pontine (apneustic) center is excitatory, whereas an upper pontine

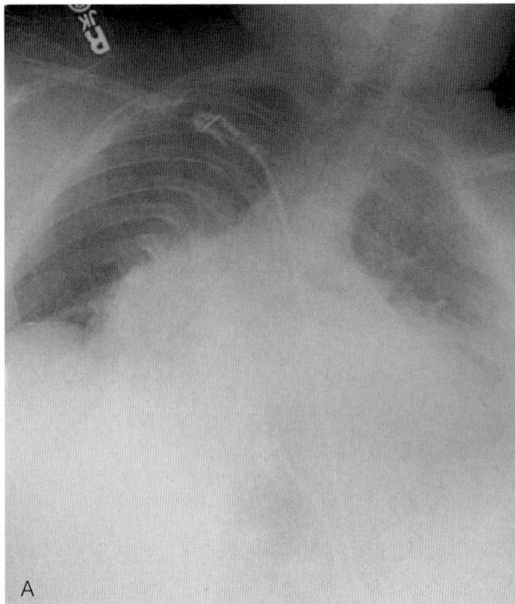

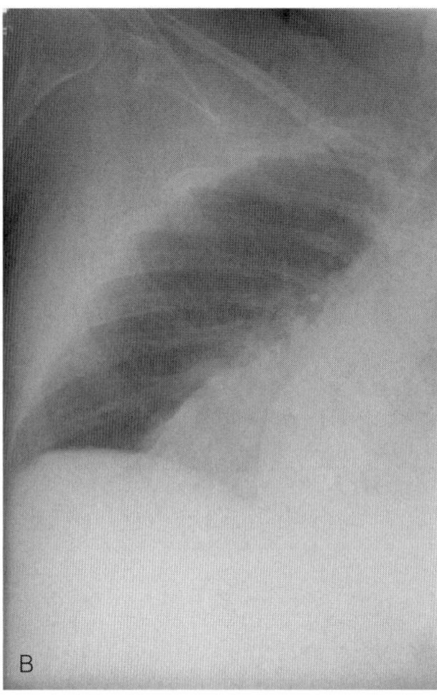

FIGURE 17-1. **(A)** Chest x-ray study before treatment. **(B)** Chest x-ray study after treatment.

(pneumotaxic) center is inhibitory. These two clusters of cells in the dorsolateral pons appear to act as on/off switches in the transition between inspiration and expiration. Descending fibers arise in the respiratory nuclei and terminate on the motor neurons of the phrenic nerve, innervating the diaphragm, the crucial muscle of respiration. These fibers lie just lateral to the anterior horn of the upper three cervical cord segments. The motor neurons of the phrenic nerve extend from the 3rd to the 5th cervical cord segments. The sternocleidomastoids, trapezii, scalenes, and intercostal muscles are accessory muscles of respiration. Their motor neurons lay in the nucleus of CN XI and C1-C2 segments of the spinal cord for the sternocleidomastoids and trapezii muscles, the C4-C8 segments for the scalenes muscles, and the T1-T12 segments for the intercostal muscles.

Any change in $Pa{CO_2}$ will result in a linear change in the concentration of hydrogen ions in the cerebrospinal fluid (CSF). Hydrogen ion concentration in the CSF will either activate or inhibit the central chemoreceptors and modulate the action of the respiratory medullary centers to increase or decrease alveolar ventilation and return the $Pa{CO_2}$ back to normal levels (5–7).

Respiratory failure occurs when the lung is either unable to supply oxygen to the blood for delivery to tissues (hypoxemic respiratory failure) or to clear the blood of carbon dioxide produced during tissue metabolism (ventilatory failure) (7).

Because ventilation is a harmonized action of the brainstem generator of the central respiratory drive and the effectors of the act of breathing, anterior horn cells, efferent nerves, neuromuscular junction, muscles of respiration, the lung and chest wall, any disturbance of any component of this pathway will lead to ventilatory failure.

Ventilatory Failure

FAILURE OF THE CENTRAL RESPIRATORY DRIVE. Acute central respiratory drive failure occurs mainly in states of a depressed level of consciousness or coma. Narcotics, substance abuse, structural brainstem lesions (e.g., tumor), ischemic or hemorrhagic stroke, traumatic brain injury, increased intracranial pressure, as well as any metabolic or toxic encephalopathy will decrease central respiratory drive because of either depressed level of consciousness or a direct effect on the brainstem respiratory centers, leading to acute respiratory failure (7).

Central hypoventilation syndrome generally causes chronic central respiratory drive failure and will be discussed in Chapter 22.

SPINAL CORD. Acute spinal cord injury above the level of C5 will cause acute respiratory failure (8). Chiari type I malformation can rarely present with acute respiratory failure (9). Chronic cervical compressive myelopathy above the level of C4 can cause a drop in FVC that may improve with decompressive surgery (10).

ANTERIOR HORN CELL

Acute anterior poliomyelitis. Although the last epidemics in the United States were in the 1940s and 1950s, poliomyelitis can still be encountered as a vaccine-associated illness from the attenuated virus or in the immunocompromised host. Acute polio infection can cause acute respiratory failure from destruction of the anterior horn cells, leading to respiratory muscle weakness or paralysis. In countries where poliomyelitis has been eradicated, other enteroviruses, such as Coxsackie A and B, enterovirus type 70, Japanese encephalitis virus, and West Nile virus, are found in a small percentage of cases, associated with a lower motor neuron paralytic syndrome resembling poliomyelitis (6).

Post-polio syndrome. Many years after recovering from acute poliomyelitis, some patients experience progressive muscle weakness, called *progressive post-poliomyelitis muscular atrophy*, defined as progressive muscle weakness developing in a patient who has recovered from acute poliomyelitis and has remained stable for at least 15 years after the initial recovery (11). Patients with history of polio may have asymptomatic lung function compromise, but risk factors, such as history of ventilation during the acute episode of polio or onset of polio before the age of 10 years, can help predict those at risk of respiratory failure. Patients not ventilated who were then ventilated during the acute episode of poliomyelitis have significantly weaker respiratory muscle strength than patients who were never on ventilation.

Spinal muscular atrophy. Spinal muscular atrophies (SMA) are a group of autosomal recessive neuromuscular disorders characterized by degeneration of the anterior horn cells of the brainstem and the spinal cord, leading to symmetric muscle weakness and restrictive respiratory insufficiency. Depending on age of onset and severity of symptoms, four main types of SMA are recognized: Type I, Werdnig-Hoffman disease with onset of symptoms before 6 months and death from respiratory insufficiency and severe bulbar dysfunction within 2 years; type II or intermediate SMA with onset of symptoms between 6 and 18 months; type III, juvenile SMA, or Wohlfart-Kugelberg-Welander disease with onset of symptoms after the age of 18 months; and type IV or adult-onset SMA. Recessive mutations in the survival motor neuron1 gene (SMN1) are found in more than 95% of patients with SMA. In patients with SMA, respiratory muscle weakness involves mainly intercostal muscles with relative sparing of the diaphragm (12,13). The intercostal muscle weakness is responsible for a triangular chest deformity with falling ribs, and results in recurrent atelectasis and bronchopulmonary infections. In spinal muscular atrophy with respiratory distress 1 or SMARD1, there is early involvement of the diaphragm and predominance of distal muscle weakness, which clearly distinguishes it from SMA1. SMARD1 is caused by mutations of the gene encoding immunoglobulin μ-binding protein 2 (*IGHMBP2*) (14).

Amyotrophic lateral sclerosis. ALS is a progressive paralytic disorder caused by degeneration of the upper motor neurons of the motor cortex in the brain and lower motor neurons in brainstem and spinal cord, resulting in progressive wasting and paralysis of voluntary muscles. The progressive paralysis in ALS usually affects respiratory muscles, leading to ventilatory failure and death within 3 to 5 years. In a few cases, acute respiratory failure can be the initial manifestation of the disease. ALS is most often sporadic, but 10% of patients have affected relatives. The disease can be either autosomal dominant, recessive, or X-linked. To date, only two genes have been associated with this disease: The SOD1 gene on chromosome 21 causing the autosomal dominant adult form of ALS, and the Alsin gene on chromosome 2 causing recessive juvenile ALS. Several families unlinked to these loci are under investigation (15).

EFFERENT NERVES

Bilateral phrenic nerve dysfunction. Respiratory failure with diaphragmatic paralysis can result from bilateral phrenic nerve dysfunction. Thoracic surgery, especially of the heart or the mediastinum, or surgical manipulations of the neck, can cause traumatic phrenic nerve injury. Furthermore, neoplastic lesions of the neck or chest can compress or infiltrate the phrenic nerve(s) and lead to diaphragmatic weakness (16).

Bilateral phrenic nerve involvement can also be seen in patients with idiopathic brachial neuritis or neuralgic amyotrophy (Parsonage Turner syndrome) (17). Phrenic nerve neuropathy has also been reported as a complication of diabetes (18), herpes virus infection, Lyme disease (19), and neurosarcoidosis (20). Many cases of unilateral phrenic nerve dysfunction are idiopathic.

Guillain-Barré syndrome. Guillain-Barré syndrome (GBS), or acute inflammatory demyelinating polyradiculoneuropathy (AIDP), is an acute immune-mediated polyradiculoneuropathy characterized by acute or subacute progressive symmetric ascending limb weakness with distal paresthesias and limb hyporeflexia or areflexia in a previously healthy patient. In the western countries, GBS is the most common cause of acute generalized muscle weakness since the eradication of polio. A mild respiratory or gastrointestinal infection usually precedes the disease, but other systemic illnesses, surgery, or a recent trauma can trigger it too. The preceding infection, often campylobacter species can trigger an autoimmune response through molecular mimicry or cross-reactivity between a microbial antigen and a myelin component setting off the demyelination. In its severe form, AIDP can cause quadriplegia and cranial and phrenic nerve paralysis, resulting an acute ventilatory failure (21).

Chronic inflammatory demyelinating polyneuropathy. Also an immune-mediated disease, chronic inflammatory demyelinating polyneuropathy (CIDP) has many similarities to AIDP, but has a more protracted course and is responsive to corticosteroid treatment. There are case reports of phrenic nerve involvement in CIDP (22) and a prospective evaluation of a phrenic nerve conduction study showed subclinical phrenic nerve involvement in patients with CIDP (23).

NEUROMUSCULAR JUNCTION. Myasthenia gravis is an autoimmune disease caused by the presence of autoantibodies directed against a postsynaptic endplate component, either acetylcholine receptors (85%) or muscle specific kinase (MuSK) (5% to 10%) with the rest an unknown antigen(s). This causes impairment of neuromuscular transmission that results in muscle weakness. Common areas of weakness include eyelid and extraocular movements, but involvement of pharyngeal, laryngeal, or respiratory muscles can cause ventilatory failure. Infection, thyroid dysfunction, and certain medications can worsen myasthenia gravis and lead to myasthenic crisis (6).

Congenital myasthenic syndrome is composed of a group of rare genetic neuromuscular disorders caused by architectural abnormalities of the neuromuscular junction, resulting in either a pre- or postsynaptic defect of neuromuscular transmission. These abnormalities generally present in the neonatal period or early childhood with hypotonia and ocular, severe bulbar, and respiratory weakness requiring ventilatory support. Some can have a milder course with fluctuating weakness into adulthood (24).

Lambert-Eaton myasthenic syndrome is a rare condition in which muscle weakness results from presynaptic abnormality of acetylcholine release, Lambert-Eaton myasthenic syndrome is caused by the presence of voltage-gated calcium channels (VGCC) auto-antibodies usually triggered by an associated tumor, a small cell cancer of the lung in most cases. Respiratory failure is rare, but has been reported at the onset of the disease (25).

Botulism is a paralyzing disease caused by the toxins of *Clostridium botulinum,* most commonly serotype A. The toxin produces skeletal muscle paralysis by lysing or interfering with any of several so-called SNARE proteins. These proteins, such as SNAP-25, are necessary for acetylcholine vesicle fusion with the presynaptic membrane. Until these proteins are replaced (many weeks), weakness will persist. Severe involvement of the bulbar and respiratory musculature will lead to respiratory failure requiring mechanical ventilation (26).

Organophosphate intoxication can be caused by organophosphates that are used as insecticides worldwide. They are well absorbed by all routes of exposure. They inhibit the acetylcholinesterases and cause acetylcholine to accumulate at the synapse, leading to an excess cholinergic stimulation or cholinergic crisis. Increased parasympathetic muscarinic activity causes bronchorrhea that can be so severe to result in life-threatening pulmonary edema. Increased nicotinic stimulation at the neuromuscular junction is responsible for rapid depolarization with muscle fasciculations followed by receptor blockade manifesting as muscle weakness or paralysis that can affect the respiratory muscles causing ventilatory failure (27).

MUSCLES. Congenital myopathies are a heterogeneous group of hereditary muscle disorders that present usually in the neonatal period with hypotonia or "floppy infant syndrome," or in early childhood with dysmorphic features and delayed motor milestones. Occasionally, they may not become manifest until later in childhood or adulthood. The most severe congenital myopathy is X-linked centronuclear or myotubular myopathy. Affected boys die in the neonatal period of respiratory failure. Nemaline myopathy is complicated with respiratory failure in about 50% of the cases (28). The disease has a severe course in infants, with early death from respiratory failure. When presenting in childhood, it has a more benign, nonprogressive course. Adult onset nemaline myopathy is rare, but respiratory failure has been reported as a presenting feature of the disease (29).

Muscular dystrophies are a group of genetically determined progressive disorders primarily affecting the skeletal muscle. The inheritance can vary from X-linked, such as Duchenne or Becker muscular dystrophy, to autosomal recessive or dominant, such as in congenital or limb-girdle muscular dystrophies. Because of respiratory muscle weakness, patients develop a progressive restrictive syndrome with chronic hypercapnic respiratory failure. The development and progression of scoliosis will further worsen the respiratory failure.

Myotonic muscular dystrophy is an autosomal-dominant, multisystem disease characterized by muscle weakness, myotonia, cataract, frontal balding, cardiac conduction defects, and endocrine abnormalities. Respiratory failure in patients with myotonic dystrophy seems to be more related to a decreased central response to both alveolar hypercapnic and hypoxic stimulation rather than to weakness of the respiratory muscle. Pharyngeal muscle weakness will cause obstructive sleep apnea worsening nocturnal hypoventilation.

Pompe disease (glycogen storage disease type II, acid maltase deficiency) is a progressive metabolic myopathy caused by deficiency of the lysosomal enzyme acid α-glucosidase. This leads to an accumulation of glycogen in various tissues of the body, most notably in skeletal muscle. The classic neonatal form is characterized by generalized hypotonia, failure to thrive, and cardiorespiratory failure. Patients usually die within the first year of life. The late-onset form of the disease can occur at any age in childhood or adulthood. It presents predominantly as a slowly progressive proximal myopathy. About half of the patients will develop diaphragmatic weakness manifested initially as nocturnal hypoventilation, eventually leading to daytime respiratory failure requiring the use of invasive or noninvasive mechanical ventilation (30).

Inflammatory myopathies include polymyositis, dermatopolymyositis, and inclusion body myositis. Respiratory involvement can be multifactorial and consist of aspiration pneumonia, interstitial pneumonitis, or respiratory muscle myositis. In patients with dermatomyositis or polymyositis, interstitial lung disease leading to pulmonary fibrosis seems to be more frequent than previously reported. It is associated with anti-Jo1 antibodies in more than 70% of the cases, and it is considered a major risk factor of premature death in these patients (31).

CLINICAL MANIFESTATIONS

ACUTE RESPIRATORY FAILURE, CLINICAL MANIFESTATIONS

Clinical manifestations of respiratory distress reflect signs and symptoms of hypoxemia, hypercapnia, or the increased work of breathing that is necessary. Dyspnea and anxiety are near-universal symptoms if mental status is not depressed, but soon patients become agitated or somnolent and show autonomic hyperactivity, such as tachycardia and diaphoresis.

In loss of central drive, lethargy or coma is typical. In this case, the history will be taken from family or friends, mainly asking about medications and substances of abuse, previous medical history for stroke risk factors, history of trauma, or recent illness.

Detailed pupillary examination is crucial, because small, constricted pupils that are reactive to light will point to opiate overdose. Pinpoint pupils (reactive to light with a magnifying glass) will suggest a pontine infarct. A unilateral dilated pupil will suggest either a midbrain structural lesion or an impeding transtentorial herniation. Asymmetric limb withdrawal to nociceptive stimuli can be a clue to a structural brain lesion. Identifying aberrant respiratory patterns in a comatose patient can sometime help localize the level of the lesion in the central nervous system (CNS).

Cheyne-Stokes respiration, characterized by oscillating cycles of hyperpnea alternating with periods of apnea, is seen in bilateral widespread cortical lesions, but is more likely to be associated with bilateral thalamic dysfunction and has also been described with lesions of the descending pathways anywhere from the cerebral hemispheres to the level of the upper pons. Some elderly patients have Cheyne-Stokes respiration without known disease. Patients with heart failure can also have Cheyne-Stokes respiration, presumably caused by a time lag from slowed circulation. Central neurogenic hyperventilation with rapid deep breathing can be seen in a lesion between the diencephalon and pons. Apneustic breathing characterized by a long inspiratory pause, after which the air is retained for several seconds and then released, is seen with lower pontine lesions. Cluster breathing is seen in low pontine or high medullary lesions, and is recognized when the patient is breathing with a cluster of breaths following each other in an irregular sequence. Ataxic breathing is a completely irregular pattern of breathing in which inspiratory gasps of diverse amplitude and lengths are intermingled with periods of apnea. This respiratory abnormality often present in agonal patients; it is a precursor to complete respiratory failure and follows damage to the dorsomedial medulla (5).

Patients with decreased level of alertness cannot protect their airways to prevent aspiration of gastric content and aspiration pneumonia will complicate the picture. In acute or worsening neuromuscular weakness, respiratory failure usually evolves rapidly. In a matter of hours, patients become anxious, tachycardic, and diaphoretic. The clinical hallmark of advanced diaphragmatic weakness is paradoxical breathing with simultaneous outward movements of the chest and inward movements of the abdomen during inspiration. Associated retraction of the intercostal muscles is usually seen. Neck flexion weakness correlates closely with diaphragmatic weakness. At this point, patients are dyspneic and distressed, specially when supine (32). If intervention is delayed, hypercapnia ensues and will lead to frank respiratory collapse.

In GBS and in myasthenia gravis, weakness of bulbar muscles often contributes to ventilatory insufficiency. The presence of jaw muscle and tongue weakness, bifacial weakness, and nasal quality to the speech are signs of bulbar dysfunction, and should alert the physician to the increased risk of aspiration.

Acute respiratory failure can be precipitated in neuromuscular conditions causing chronic respiratory failure by pulmonary complications such as pneumonia, pulmonary embolism, or large atelectasis.

CHRONIC RESPIRATORY MUSCLE WEAKNESS, CLINICAL MANIFESTATIONS

In patients with stable weakness of the respiratory muscles, chronic CO_2 retention causes daytime somnolence, headaches on awakening, nightmares, and, in extreme cases, papilledema. The accessory muscles of respiration tend to maximize tidal volume and a tendency exists for the patient to gulp or assume a rounded "fish mouth" appearance in an effort to inhale additional air.

Patients with chronic respiratory difficulties tolerate lower tidal volumes without dyspnea than can patients with acute disease, and symptoms in the former may occur only at night when respiratory drive is diminished and compensatory mechanisms for obtaining additional air are not available, causing nocturnal hypoventilation. Sleeping in an upright position may help improve diaphragmatic efficiency and minimize nocturnal hypoxemia. At times, patients may do this spontaneously, so it is worth asking during the history whether they sleep with more than one pillow or whether they sleep in a recliner. In patients with profound bulbar weakness, obstructive apnea may aggravate the ventilatory problem.

DIAGNOSTIC APPROACH

Available tools for the diagnosis of acute and chronic respiratory failure consist in:

Pulmonary function tests
Blood gas
Overnight oxymetry
Polysomnography or Sleep study
Chest x-ray study

The FVC is the amount of air exhaled as forcefully as possible after a deep inhalation. Maximal inspiratory pressure (MIP) and maximal expiratory pressure (MEP) can help assess respiratory muscle strength (normal >100cm H_2O). If overnight oxymetry shows multiple 4% desaturation even with normal O_2 saturation, a sleep study is needed. On a polysomnography, look for elevated apnea-hypopnea index or central apnea and hypopnea that are rapid eye movement (REM) related. Finally, a blood gas will help determine the presence and the severity of hypercapnea and a chest x-ray study will be of value in the diagnosis of pneumonia, posterior atelectasis, or elevation of a hemidiaphragm.

DIAGNOSTIC APPROACH TO ACUTE RESPIRATORY FAILURE

In the setting of acute neurologic injury, such as AIDP, spirometry and respiratory pressure measurements assist in screening for the need to initiate therapy for respiratory failure. A vital capacity (VC) <20 mL/kg or >30% reductions in VC from baseline, an MIP ≤30 cm H_2O, and an MEP <40 cm H_2O were associated with progression to respiratory failure. Bulbar dysfunction and associated aspiration has been shown to be an independent risk factor for respiratory failure in adults with GBS (21). These are late findings, however; early findings suggest a high risk of respiratory failure. These early findings include time from onset to admission of <7 days; inability to cough, to stand, and to lift the elbows or head; and increases in liver enzyme (33). Changes in blood gas are late and should not be used to determine the need to initiate mechanical ventilation.

DIAGNOSTIC APPROACH TO CHRONIC RESPIRATORY FAILURE

In the setting of chronic respiratory failure, such as ALS, screening lung function using routine spirometry, respiratory pressure measurements, polysomnography, and blood gases can be helpful and should be performed when the patient is asymptomatic, because nocturnal hypoventilation occurs earlier than daytime symptoms and early introduction of NIV is key to extending survival and quality of life in patients with ALS (Fig. 17-2) (34,35).

An FVC of <50% should trigger a discussion about respiratory management and initiation of NIV. In addition, an MIP of ≥60, oxygen saturation of ≤88% for 5 continuous minutes or a PCO_2 >45 can be used as sufficient markers for the initiation of NIV (36). To increase awareness of occult diaphragm weakness, measure spirometry in the supine position. A drop in FVC from the upright to supine position of 25% or more is consistent with diaphragm weakness (37).

TREATMENT

Although mechanisms and time course for acute and chronic neurologically associated respiratory failure differ, treatment strategies are similar. These therapies fall into two large categories—direct support for hypoventilation and assistance in airway clearance.

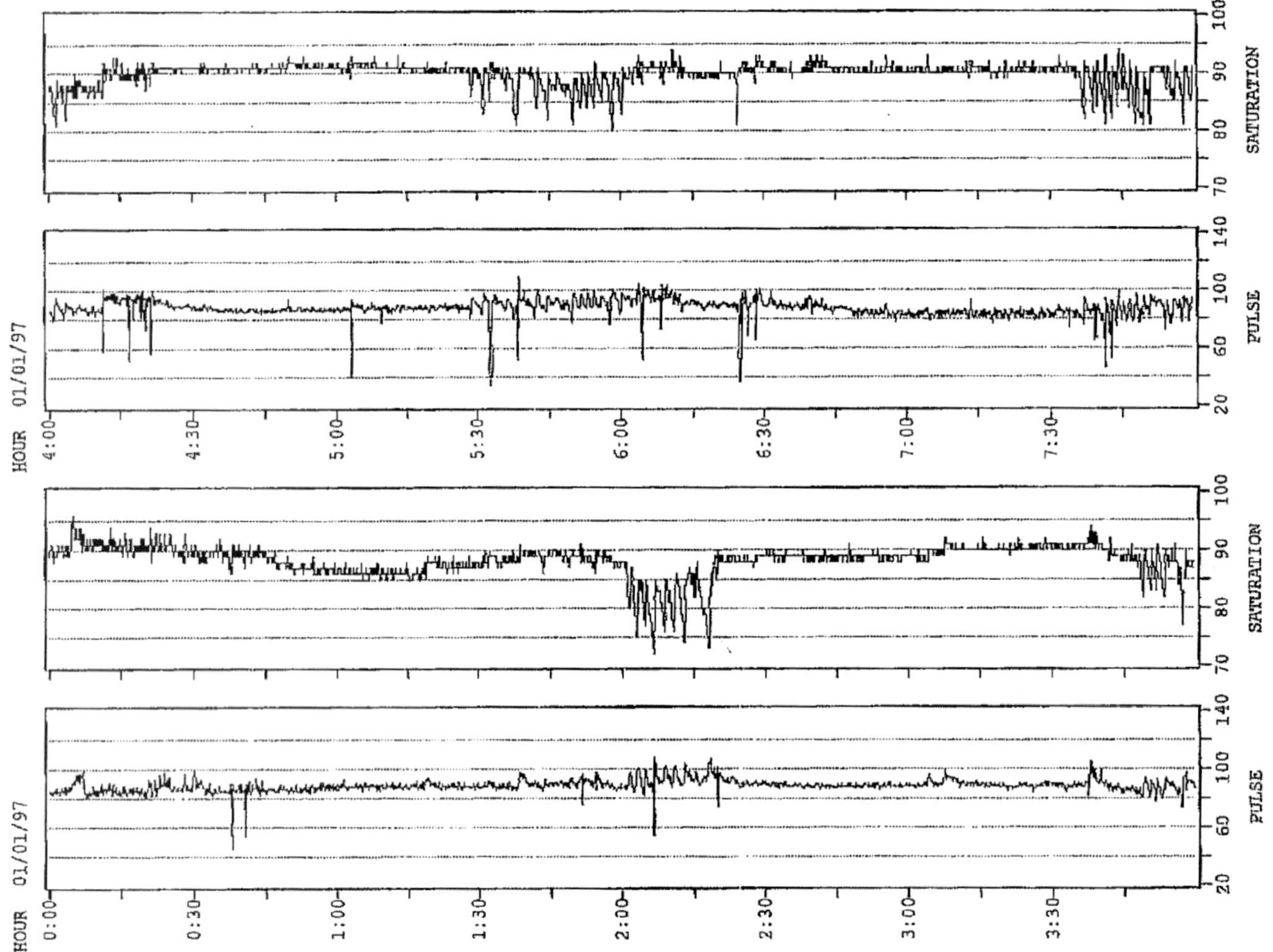

FIGURE 17-2: Overnight oximetry in the setting of amyotrophic lateral sclerosis (ALS) shows desaturation in clumps. This is likely caused by the rapid movement (REM)-related central hypoventilation or apnea.

Historically, ventilatory support was only available or offered utilizing tracheostomy with mechanical ventilation (see Chapter 130). Although this remains an available option, the high burden of care, complications, and cost have shifted the focus of initial ventilatory care of patients with neuromuscular disorder to noninvasive ventilation (NIV).The use of nasal bi-level positive pressure therapy in acute respiratory failure should be initiated in the intensive care unit (ICU) setting, because respiratory weakness may be rapidly changing. Although no large clinical trials have studied the use of NIV in the setting of acute respiratory failure caused by neuromuscular disease, NIV has been successfully used for the acute management of respiratory failure caused by pulmonary processes (38). Much more data exist regarding the use of NIV in the setting of chronic respiratory failure caused by neuromuscular diseases, including DMD, ALS, post-polio syndrome, and so forth (39,40). Although the benefit of early intervention of NIV has been well studied in the setting of chronic neuromuscular disease, strategies to manage the device itself have not been well standardized or documented. On average, recommendations are typically as follows (41):

1. First, the patient should be desensitized to the mask and device during the daytime, while the device is set at very low pressures, and mask changes can be instituted until the fit is optimized.
2. Once the patient can take a short daytime nap with the device in place, then adjust the pressures. This can either be done at a sleep laboratory or in the home, using remote monitoring techniques, such as overnight oxymetry or NIV devices with built-in self-monitoring or recording devices that can report data from home use.
3. The goals of titration are twofold—to optimize comfort in breathing and assisting in the work of breathing while augmenting ventilation. Adjustments in rise time and humidification can help improve comfort. Increasing inspiratory time and inspiratory positive airway pressure (IPAP) can help drive up tidal volumes. This will both improve lung compliance and reduce the work of breathing (42,43). Expiratory positive airway pressure (EPAP) should be minimized to improve comfort, set at the minimal value needed to keep the upper airway patent during sleep. Use of a spontaneous timed (ST) mode will allow the addition of a back-up rate. This will compensate for

diaphragmatic weakness that may be preventing the patient from spontaneously triggering ventilatory support from the bi-level device.

Airway clearance is a goal for pulmonary management in both acute and chronic neuromuscular conditions, because of an ineffective or weak cough as well as high risk of aspiration seen in association with potential bulbar weakness (44). Modes of respiratory clearance either reduce the production of secretions or improve the mobilization and removal of secretions. Reduction in the formation of pulmonary secretion should focus on reducing the risk of aspiration from the upper airway and the production of mucus from the lower respiratory tract. Drying of the airway should be performed with caution because overdrying can cause insipated secretions, which would be more difficult to liberate from the airway. Helpful strategies include the following:

1. Sialorrhea is frequently seen in bulbar dysfunction and can be associated with cough and infection caused by aspiration. Treatment with anticholinergics, such as scopolamine or amitriptyline, may be helpful (45).
2. Obstructive airway disease: Because of the frequent finding of asthma or tobacco-related lung disease, patients with neuromuscular disorders can also have obstructive airway conditions with increased mucus production. The use of the nebulized β-agonist, ipratropium, steroid, or both may be helpful (46).

Removing secretions from the airway should focus on the both the upper and lower airway. To achieve this goal, assistive techniques are required to increase both lung volume and flow rate. Options include the following:

1. Mechanical chest wall oscillation generates shear stress at the air mucus interface and increases mucus flow rates. A pneumatic vest delivers a constant pressure with secondary air pressure oscillations. Oscillations drive air movements within the lungs, including small peripheral airways, and reduce mucous viscosity, by reducing cross-linkages (47). Although typically used in the setting of cystic fibrosis, this device has been used in patients with neuromuscular disorder, such as those with ALS (48); even with no parenchymal lung disease, the presence of atelectasis and thickened secretions requires the additional shear force provided by the pneumatic vest to encourage secretion liberation.
2. A mechanical cough assist device aids in the cough process by applying pressurized air through a mask over the nose and mouth or through a tracheostomy tube. Both inhalation and exhalation are assisted as the volume, force, and flow of the cough efforts are improved. Pressure is delivered between +70 and −70 cm of water. This device has been shown to improve secretion clearance in ALS (49) and reduce the need for mechanical ventilation in acutely ill patients with neuromuscular disorders (50).
3. Manual cough assist is a device that can help in improving cough by adding pressure to the abdomen by pressing the hands and forearms to the abdomen during the exhalatory portion of the cough effort. This has been shown to increase cough flow in ALS and DMD (51,52).
4. Although no specific data about the use of the suction or resuscitation devices, they can commonly help to clear secretions in weak patients and are available for use in both hospital and at home.

CLINICAL RECOMMENDATIONS OF THE VIGNETTES

CASE VIGNETTE 1

The routine use of spirometry is recommended in the setting of DMD. Once patients are wheelchair-bound, the addition of yearly polysomnography is suggested (53). This may help anticipate the need for early intervention with NIV and airway clearance techniques, to avoid the development of difficult-to-manage secretions and pneumonia. Once a patient presents to the hospital with pneumonia, NIV, with the use of a heated humidifier to improve comfort, should be started as soon as possible to help avert the need for mechanical ventilation. The addition of aggressive airway clearance, using nebulizer, suction, mechanical cough assist, and high-frequency chest wall oscillations would be an important foundation of acute therapy. It is important to have a high suspicion for a possible aspiration as the mechanism for the development of pneumonia. As such, a swallowing evaluation and antibiotic coverage broadened to include a likely polymicrobial infection is appropriate.

CASE VIGNETTE 2

The patient presented with myasthenic crisis on the verge of acute respiratory failure. Early spirometry testing revealed a VC of 17.5 mL/kg. This value suggests that NIV should be initiated in a monitored setting, such as the ICU. The addition of a back-up rate of 10 to 14 may be helpful as well as assuring an effective inspiratory time of approximately 1.0 seconds, which will help to relive atalectasis. Heated humidity, rise time adjustments, and multiple mask fittings may also be necessary. IPAP should be set low to start and increased, as needed, to achieve a goal of comfortable breathing with adequate size tidal volumes. (Ex: Start at IPAP = 8 and increase, as needed, to achieve a tidal volume of at least 5 mL/kg). After stabilization of the patient's respiratory status, plasmapheresis or intravenous immunoglobulin will be initiated to treat his myasthenic crisis.

SUMMARY

Noninvasive ventilation has made a significant impact in the management of acute and chronic respiratory failure caused by neurologic diseases. Emphasis on aggressive therapy to address secretion clearance and early use of pulmonary screening before symptoms of dyspnea appear will help improve medical care and quality of life.

REFERENCES

1. Aminoff MJ. *Neurology and General Medicine*, 3rd ed. New York: Churchill Livingstone; 2001.
2. West JB. *Pulmonary Pathophysiology. The Essentials*, 6th ed. Baltimore: Lippincott Williams & Wilkins; 2003.
3. Carson SS, Cox CE, Holmes GM, et al. The changing epidemiology of mechanical ventilation: A population-based study. *Journal of Intensive Care Medicine*. 2006;21:173–182.
4. Bourke SC, McColl E, Shaw PJ, et al. Validation of quality of life instruments in ALS. *Amyotroph Lateral Scler Other Motor Neuron Disord*. 2004;5:55–60.
5. Brazis PW, Masdeu JC, Biller J. *Localization in Clinical Neurology*, 5th ed. Philadelphia: Lippincott Williams & Wilkins; 2007.

6. Adams RD, Victor M, Ropper AH, et al. *Adams and Victor's Principles of Neurology*, 8th ed. New York: McGraw-Hill; 2005.
7. Hanley ME, Welsh CH. *Current Diagnosis & Treatment in Pulmonary Medicine.* New York: Lange Medical Books/McGraw-Hill; 2003.
8. Ball PA. Critical care of spinal cord injury. *Spine.* 2001;26:S27–S30.
9. Tsara V, Serasli E, Kimiskidis V, et al. Acute respiratory failure and sleep-disordered breathing in Arnold-Chiari malformation. *Clin Neurol Neurosurg.* 2005;107:521–524.
10. Toyoda H, Nakamura H, Konishi S, et al. Does chronic cervical myelopathy affect respiratory function? *J Neurosurg Spine.* 2004;1:175–178.
11. Farbu E, Gilhus NE, Barnes MP, et al. EFNS guideline on diagnosis and management of post-polio syndrome. Report of an EFNS task force. *Eur J Neurol.* 2006;13:795–801.
12. Kuzuhara S, Chou SM. Preservation of the phrenic motoneurons in Werdnig-Hoffmann disease. *Ann Neurol.* 1981;9:506–510.
13. Ioos C, Leclair-Richard D, Mrad S, et al. Respiratory capacity course in patients with infantile spinal muscular atrophy. *Chest.* 2004;126:831–837.
14. Grohmann K, Varon R, Stolz P, et al. Infantile spinal muscular atrophy with respiratory distress type 1 (SMARD1). *Ann Neurol.* 2003;54:719–724.
15. Mitsumoto H, Przedborski S, Gordon PH. *Amyotrophic Lateral Sclerosis.* Marcel Dekker, Inc. 2005.
16. Fuhrman BP, Zimmerman JJ. *Pediatric Critical Care*, 2nd ed. St. Louis: Mosby-Year Book; 1998.
17. Tsao BE, Ostrovskiy DA, Wilbourn AJ, et al. Phrenic neuropathy due to neuralgic amyotro phy. *Neurology.* 2006;66:1582–1584.
18. White JE, Bullock RE, Hudgson P, et al. Phrenic neuropathy in association with diabetes. *Diabet Med.* 1992;9:954–956.
19. Ishaq S, Quinet R, Saba J. Phrenic nerve paralysis secondary to Lyme neuroborreliosis. *Neurology.* 2002;59:1810–1811.
20. Robinson LR, Brownsberger R, Raghu G. Respiratory failure and hypoventilation secondary to neurosarcoidosis. *Am J Respir Crit Care Med.* 1998;157:1316–1318.
21. Lawn ND, Fletcher DD, Henderson RD, et al. Anticipating mechanical ventilation in Guillain-Barré syndrome. *Arch Neurol.* 2001;58:893–898.
22. Henderson RD, Sandroni P, Wijdicks EF. Chronic inflammatory demyelinating polyneuropathy and respiratory failure. *J Neurol.* 2005;252:1235–1237.
23. Cocito D, Ciaramitaro P, Rota E, et al. Subclinical electrophysiological alterations of phrenic nerve in chronic inflammatory demyelinating polyneuropathy. *J Neurol.* 2005;252:916–920.
24. Engel AG, Ohno K, Sine SM. Congenital myasthenic syndromes: Progress over the past decade. *Muscle Nerve.* 2003;27:4–25.
25. Brueck M, Vogel S, Waeger S, et al. [Lambert-Eaton myasthenic syndrome with acute respiratory failure associated with small cell lung cancer]. *Dtsch Med Wochenschr.* 2004;129: 193–196.
26. Gilchrist JM. Overview of neuromuscular disorders affecting respiratory function. *Seminars in Respiratory Critical Care Medicine.* 2002;23:191–200.
27. Rusyniak DE, Nanagas KA. Organophosphate poisoning. *Semin Neurol.* 2004;24:197–204.
28. Ryan MM, Schnell C, Strickland CD, et al. Nemaline myopathy: A clinical study of 143 cases. *Ann Neurol.* 2001;50:312–320.
29. Falga-Tirado C, Perez-Peman P, Ordi-Ros J, et al. Adult onset of nemaline myopathy presenting as respiratory insufficiency. *Respiration.* 1995;62:353–354.
30. Mellies U, Ragette R, Schwake C, et al. Sleep-disordered breathing and respiratory failure in acid maltase deficiency. *Neurology.* 2001;57:1290–1295.
31. Fathi M, Lundberg IE. Interstitial lung disease in polymyositis and dermatomyositis. *Curr Opin Rheumatol.* 2005;17:701–706.
32. Rabinstein AA, Wijdicks EF. Warning signs of imminent respiratory failure in neurological patients. *Semin Neurol.* 2003;23:97–104.
33. Sharshar T, Chevret S, Bourdain F, et al. Early predictors of mechanical ventilation in Guillain-Barré syndrome. *Crit Care Med.* 2003;31:278–283.
34. Clinical indications for noninvasive positive pressure ventilation in chronic respiratory failure due to restrictive lung disease, COPD, and nocturnal hypoventilation—A consensus conference report. *Chest.* 1999;116:521–534.
35. Bourke SC, Tomlinson M, Williams TL, et al. Effects of non-invasive ventilation on survival and quality of life in patients with amyotrophic lateral sclerosis: A randomised controlled trial. *Lancet Neurol.* 2006;5:140–147.
36. Miller RG, Rosenberg JA, Gelinas DF, et al. Practice parameter: The care of the patient with amyotrophic lateral sclerosis (an evidence-based review): Report of the Quality Standards Subcommittee of the American Academy of Neurology: ALS Practice Parameters Task Force. *Neurology.* 1999;52:1311–1323.
37. Fromageot C, Lofaso F, Annane D, et al. Supine fall in lung volumes in the assessment of diaphragmatic weakness in neuromuscular disorders. *Arch Phys Med Rehabil.* 2001;82:123–128.
38. Brochard L, Mancebo J, Wysocki M, et al. Noninvasive ventilation for acute exacerbations of chronic obstructive pulmonary disease. *N Engl J Med.* 1995;333:817–822.
39. Simonds AK, Muntoni F, Heather S, et al. Impact of nasal ventilation on survival in hypercapnic Duchenne muscular dystrophy. *Thorax.* 1998;53:949–952.
40. Bach JR. Management of post-polio respiratory sequelae. *Ann N Y Acad Sci.* 1995;753:96–102.
41. Bourke SC, Bullock RE, Williams TL, et al. Noninvasive ventilation in ALS: Indications and effect on quality of life. *Neurology.* 2003;61:171–177.
42. Aliverti A, Carlesso E, Dellaca R, et al. Chest wall mechanics during pressure support ventilation. *Crit Care.* 2006;10:R54.
43. Lechtzin N, Shade D, Clawson L, et al. Supramaximal inflation improves lung compliance in subjects with amyotrophic lateral sclerosis. *Chest.* 2006;129:1322–1329.
44. Trebbia G, Lacombe M, Fermanian C, et al. Cough determinants in patients with neuromuscular disease. *Respir Physiol Neurobiol.* 2005;146:291–300.
45. Boyce HW, Bakheet MR. Sialorrhea: A review of a vexing, often unrecognized sign of oropharyngeal and esophageal disease. *J Clin Gastroenterol.* 2005;39:89–97.
46. Fabbri LM, Hurd SS. Global strategy for the diagnosis, management and prevention of COPD: 2003 update. *Eur Respir J.* 2003;22:1–2.
47. Dosman CF, Jones RL. High-frequency chest compression: A summary of the literature. *Can Respir J.* 2005;12:37–41.
48. Lange DJ, Lechtzin N, Davey C, et al. High-frequency chest wall oscillation in ALS: An exploratory randomized, controlled trial. *Neurology.* 2006;67:991–997.
49. Sancho J, Servera E, Vergara P, et al. Mechanical insufflation-exsufflation vs. tracheal suctioning via tracheostomy tubes for patients with amyotrophic lateral sclerosis: A pilot study. *Am J Phys Med Rehabil.* 2003;82:750–753.
50. Vianello A, Corrado A, Arcaro G, et al. Mechanical insufflation-exsufflation improves outcomes for neuromuscular disease patients with respiratory tract infections. *Am J Phys Med Rehabil.* 2005;84:83–88; discussion 89–91.
51. Mustfa N, Aiello M, Lyall RA, et al. Cough augmentation in amyotrophic lateral sclerosis. *Neurology.* 2003;61:1285–1287.
52. Kang SW, Kang YS, Sohn HS, et al. Respiratory muscle strength and cough capacity in patients with Duchenne muscular dystrophy. *Yonsei Med J.* 2006;47:184–190.
53. Finder JD, Birnkrant D, Carl J, et al. Respiratory care of the patient with Duchenne muscular dystrophy: ATS consensus statement. *Am J Respir Crit Care Med.* 2004;170:456–465.

CHAPTER 18

Chronic Obstructive Pulmonary Disease

Thomas C. Corbridge • Richard A. Bernstein

OBJECTIVES

- To review the definition of chronic obstructive pulmonary disease (COPD)
- To examine the pathogenesis of COPD
- To consider the clinical manifestations of COPD
- To review pharmacologic and nonpharmacologic therapy of COPD

CASE VIGNETTE

A 65-year-old woman with an 80 pack per year history of cigarette smoking and severe COPD presented for evaluation of weight loss, weakness, and fatigue. An extensive evaluation for smoking-related malignancy was negative. Sertraline was started for depression and the patient was referred to neurology for further evaluation. Medications at the time of evaluation included albuterol combined with ipratropium bromide, a long-acting β-agonist combined with an inhaled corticosteroid and supplemental oxygen by nasal cannula.

On examination the patient was cachectic with a body mass index of 19 kg/m^2. She had a flat affect, temporal wasting, decreased air entry on lung auscultation, expiratory phase prolongation, a hyperresonant pulmonary percussion note, and diffuse skeletal muscle wasting.

Laboratory values were notable for mild normochromic, normocytic anemia, low normal serum potassium, and a normal creatine phosphokinase (CPK).

DEFINITION

Chronic obstructive pulmonary disease is a disease of chronic airflow limitation caused by variable mixtures of chronic bronchitis and emphysema (1,2). Chronic bronchitis refers to the inflammatory and structural changes that occur in affected airways resulting in cough, phlegm, wheeze, and breathlessness. Strictly speaking, the diagnosis requires cough and sputum to be present on most days for at least 3 months in each of two consecutive years (without another cause). *Emphysema* is the term used to describe the presence of parenchymal destruction and loss of alveolar attachments and gas exchanging alveolar-capillary units. In simple terms, emphysema is considered a "hole" in parenchymal lung tissue. Pure emphysema causes breathlessness without cough or phlegm.

Although the relative contributions vary, most patients have bronchitis and emphysema resulting in expiratory airflow obstruction and abnormal spirometry (see below) (1). Airflow limitation typically abates after bronchodilator use, but does not fully reverse (1); complete reversibility (i.e., normal spirometry after bronchodilator administration) is more consistent with asthma. Although predominately a disease of the lung, COPD has a number of recognized systemic features (see below).

COPD most commonly results from the inhalation of a noxious stimulus (e.g., tobacco smoke) in susceptible hosts. When the stimulus continues, the disease invariably progresses. When the stimulus is removed (i.e., the patient quits smoking), pulmonary function can stabilize (except for expected declines in lung function explained by aging), but it never returns to normal. Some patient's condition continues to deteriorate despite smoking cessation.

With these concepts in mind, expert members of the Global Initiative for Obstructive Lung Disease (GOLD) put forth the following definition of COPD in their 2006 update (1):

> "Chronic obstructive lung disease (COPD) is a preventable and treatable disease with some extra pulmonary effects that may contribute to the severity in individual patients. Its pulmonary component is characterized by airflow limitation that is not fully reversible. The airflow limitation is usually progressive and associated with an abnormal inflammatory response of the lung to noxious particles or gases."

EPIDEMIOLOGY

COPD is a leading cause of morbidity and mortality worldwide. In the United States alone, COPD affects 6% to 7% of the population, which translates to approximately 20 million patients. Each year in the United States, COPD results in 1.5 million emergency department visits, nearly 700,000 admissions to hospital, and 120,000 deaths (which makes COPD the fourth leading cause of death in adults in the United States) (3). Mortality trends have been particularly alarming in women; recently the number of deaths in women has surpassed the number of deaths in men (3).

ETIOLOGY AND PATHOGENESIS

Most patients with COPD are current or exsmokers. The greater the lifetime burden of smoking, the greater is the likelihood of developing disease (4). Most patients with clinically apparent disease have smoked for more than 20 pack-years, but the disease should be considered in all patients 40 years of age or older with >10 pack-years of smoking (5).

Not all patients with COPD have smoked. Exposure to secondhand smoke, occupational dusts and chemicals, and indoor and outdoor air pollution are additional recognized risk factors (6–8). Also a readily testable genetic risk factor known for emphysema: α_1-antitrypsin deficiency. Patients with homozygous α_1-antitrypsin deficiency states (corresponding to serum levels <20% of normal) are susceptible to emphysema (even if they have never smoked) because they lose the lung protective effects of α_1-antitrypsin, leading to a harmful imbalance between proteases and antiproteases (see below) (9).

Interestingly, most cigarette smokers do not develop clinically apparent COPD (1).This suggests that tobacco smoke alone is not sufficient for disease development and that an additional genetic predisposition is required. Again, α_1-antitrypsin deficiency is the best described genetic predisposition, but a number of other susceptibility genes have been identified as well (1).

Tobacco smoke causes lung inflammation. Inflammatory cells consisting mainly of neutrophils, macrophages and CD8 lymphocytes are present in greater numbers in smokers than in nonsmokers, leading to the release of toxic oxygen species (10). Toxic oxygen species, in turn, activate nuclear factor kappa beta (NF-kB) and increase tumor necrosis factor-α_1 (TNF-α) leukotriene B4, IL-6, and IL-8, causing additional neutrophil recruitment (11,12). The result is neutrophilic bronchitis, mucus hypersecretion, bronhcospasm, air-trapping, and destruction of alveolar walls. Toxic oxygen species further decrease antiproteases (such as α_1-antitrypsin and leukoprotease inhibitor), leading to protease or antiprotease imbalance and lung injury (even in patients without α_1-antitrypsin deficiency).

PATHOLOGY

Chronic airway wall inflammation with repeated cycles of injury and attempted repair can result in permanent structural changes contributing to airflow limitation. Classic histopathologic findings include squamous metaplasia, mucus gland hypertrophy, goblet cell hyperplasia, intraluminal mucus, airway smooth muscle proliferation, and neutrophilic bronchitis (13). The result is airway narrowing and elevated airway resistance.

Alveolar destruction, decreased alveolar elastin, and loss of parenchymal tissue are the hallmarks of emphysema (13). Decreased lung elasticity is a major determinant of hyperinflation and decreased expiratory flow rates (see below); it further interferes with the ability of the lung to tether or "pull open" airways, causing their collapse. Further evidence suggests that alveolar collagen deposition causes fibrosis of remaining alveolar tissue (13). Pulmonary vascular remodeling consisting of intimal hyperplasia and medial hypertrophy may develop in hypoxemic patients from hypoxia-induced vasoconstriction (1).

CLINICAL MANIFESTATIONS

Clinical features of chronic bronchitis include cough, phlegm, wheeze, and breathlessness (14). Because narrowed airways lower ventilation to perfused lung units early in the course of the disease, hypoxemia develops (and so patients may have a bluish tint to skin and lips and be referred to as *BLUE*) (15). Hypoxic pulmonary vasoscontriction contributes to the development of mild to moderate pulmonary hypertension and the potential for right-sided heart strain and peripheral edema (thus, the descriptive term *BLOATER*) (16). The term *BLUE BLOATER*, thus, describes the subset of patients with severe forms of chronic bronchitis.

In more pure cases of emphysema, airways are not inflamed. They can collapse from the loss of tethering during exhalation, but they are likely pulled open during inspiration. Ventilation, therefore, is maintained to perfused lung units and hypoxemia is less likely to occur. Indeed, patients with emphysema may have adequate values for resting oxygen saturation on room air. They may be *PINK* even when breathless and breathing through pursed lips, a maneuver that might pressure stent open collapsing airways, leading to the historical descriptive term *PINK PUFFER*. Right-sided heart failure is less common in patients with pure emphysema, occurring later in the course of the disease from drop out of alveolar-capillary units (16). Patients with emphysema can also lose weight and skeletal muscle mass (a condition referred to as *pulmonary cachexia*). Proposed explanations for weight loss are increased work of breathing (a chronic state of exercise), malnutrition, and release of proinflammatory mediators such as TNF-α (1). Beyond cachexia, other systemic manifestations of COPD are seen. These include osteoporosis, depression and anxiety, anemia, and increased risk for cardiovascular disease associated with increased levels of C-reactive protein (CRP) (17–20).

DIAGNOSTIC APPROACH

The diagnosis of COPD typically relies on spirometric documentation of expiratory airflow obstruction in a patient with a significant smoking history (21). Spirometry demonstrates delayed emptying of alveolar gas (from loss of elastic recoil and increased airway resistance) as signaled by a fall in FEV_1. FEV_1 is the amount of gas that is exhaled from total lung capacity (TLC) in the first second of trying forcefully during a forced vital capacity (FVC) maneuver. The FVC is the total amount of air exhaled from full lung inflation (TLC) to full exhalation or residual volume (RV). Although the FVC falls in COPD, it generally falls less than the FEV_1 because motivated patients can "time compensate" (i.e., exhale longer to remove more alveolar gas). In health, the FVC maneuver takes 3 to 5 seconds; in COPD, it takes longer. Because the FEV_1 falls more than the FVC in patients with expiratory airflow obstruction, the ratio of FEV_1 to FVC (FEV_1:FVC) falls from a normal value of 75% to 80% to <70%.

The FEV_1 correlates with disease severity (i.e., the lower the FEV_1, the sicker the patient). Considerable variability is seen, however, in exercise capacity dyspnea and quality of life at any value of FEV_1 (22). Thus, many investigators and clinicians have gone beyond the FEV_1 when assessing severity or measuring therapeutic responses. Additional measures include the use of validated assessments of dyspnea, 6-minute hall walk distances, and body mass index (23).

Other hallmarks of obstruction are lung hyperinflation and air-trapping that worsens with exercise (24). In emphysema, a drop in the diffusing capacity for carbon monoxide (DLCO) reflects loss of alveolar capillary units.

Other diagnostic tests of interest include the chest radiograph, which may show signs of lung hyperinflation (e.g., flattening of the diaphragms) and hyperlucency. Chest radiographs are generally not diagnostic of COPD; rather, they provide support for the diagnosis and help exclude other conditions. CT imaging (particularly with high resolution cuts) is more sensitive and specific in patients with emphysema, although costly and generally not recommended in routine cases. Classic CT findings include enlargement of alveolar spaces (the "holes" of emphysema), with apical predominance, airway wall thickening, and air-trapping (25,26).

Measurement of oxygen saturation by pulse oximetry detects patients with hypoxemia. Resting values on ambient air of ≤88% identify patients eligible for continuous oxygen supplementation. Not uncommonly, COPD causes exercise-induced hypoxemia, possibly on the grounds of decreased (faster) red cell transit time through pulmonary vessels, a rise in arterial PCO_2 or a fall in venous O_2 reflecting inadequate cardiac output or increased oxygen consumption (27).

Arterial blood gas measurements should be considered in patient with FEV_1 <50%, particularly with evidence for right-sided heart strain (1). Arterial blood gases (ABG) define hypoxemia severity and help establish acid-base status. Chronic ventilatory failure (chronic hypercapnia) signifies severe disease and inadequate alveolar ventilation.

TREATMENT

Treatment of COPD starts with avoidance of risk factors. For smokers, smoking cessation helps prevent disease progression and prolongs survival (28). A comprehensive review of smoking cessation is beyond the scope of this chapter. Suffice it to say that positive reinforcement of benefits, individual or group counseling, and use of pharmacologic agents, such as nicotine replacement, bupropion, and varenicline are core recommendations.

Bronchodilators are the mainstay of pharmacotherapy in COPD. Most patients respond to bronchodilators, which is defined as an improvement in FEV_1 of ≥12% and ≥200 mL. By decreasing lung hyperinflation, bronchodilators also improve inspiratory capacity and exercise tolerance, and reduce breathlessness (29,30). Commonly used drugs include inhaled β_2-agonists (short and long acting), inhaled anticholigergics (short and long acting), and combinations of short-acting β-agonists and short-acting anticholinergics (Table 18-1).

Short-acting bronchodilators are recommended for intermittent use. When symptoms warrant repeated use of short-acting preparations, a long-acting bronchodilator with or without an inhaled steroid should be considered (see below), along with *as needed* use of a short-acting preparation (1). Included in the list of long-acting bronchodilators is theophylline. Theophylline can be effective in COPD, but inhaled agents are preferred because of fewer side effects.

Inhaled corticosteroids (ICS) can be added to long-acting bronchodilators when disease severity is moderate to severe with increasing the risk of acute exacerbation. Inhaled corticosteroids decrease the risk of exacerbation in moderate and severe illness, but not in patients with mild disease (31,32). Inhaled corticosteroids can also decrease COPD mortality (33). This may stem from exacerbation protection in sicker patients; ICS also lower CRP levels and, theoretically, may lower the risk of death from cardiovascular disease (34).

Patients with moderate to severe disease receiving bronchodilator therapy benefit from adding a second bronchodilator with a different mechanism of action. For example, data demonstrate that the combination of a long-acting β-agonist and a long-acting anticholingeric is more effective than either drug used alone (35). Thus, in common clinical practice, patients with severe COPD may receive a short-acting β-agonist for rescue therapy, a daily long-acting β-agonist combined with an ICS, and a long-acting anticholinergic (with or without theophylline).

Supplemental oxygen is indicated for oxygen saturations ≤88% on ambient air (or PaO_2 ≤55 mm Hg). If measured at rest, patients meeting this cut-off value are candidates for continuous supplemental oxygen aimed at elevating oxygen saturations >90%. Importantly, the use of supplemental oxygen in this situation prolongs survival (36). Oxygen saturation should also be assessed during exercise and sleep, and supplemental oxygen should be titrated accordingly to achieve saturations >90%. Supplemental oxygen is approved for patients with an oxygen saturation of 89% (corresponding to a PaO_2 of 56 to 59 mm Hg) with evidence for right-sided heart strain. Supplemental oxygen is not indicated for saturations >90% or PaO_2 values >60 mm Hg.

Nonpharmacologic therapy for COPD includes vaccinations and pulmonary rehabilitation. Yearly influenza vaccination reduces serious complications and mortality during the flu and pneumonia season and is highly recommended (37). Pneumococcal vaccination is also recommended.

TABLE 18-1. Inhaled Bronchodilators Commonly Used in COPD

Short-Acting β-Agonists	*Long-Acting Bronchodilators*	*Short-Acting Anticholinergics*	*Long-Acting Anticholinergics*
Albuterol (Ventolin, Proventil)	Salmeterol (Serevent)	Ipratropium bromide (Atrovent)	Tiotropium (Spiriva)
Levalbuterol (Xopenex)	Formoterol (Foradil)	Ipratoropium bromide plus albuterol (Combivent)	
	Salmeterol plus fluticasone (Advair)		
	Formoterol plus budesonide (Symbicort)		

Symptomatic patients are candidates for pulmonary rehabilitation. Benefits of pulmonary rehabilitation have been evaluated in a number of clinical trials (38). They include improved exercise tolerance, decreased dyspnea, improved quality of life, and decreased anxiety and depression. Pulmonary rehabilitation decreases the number, and length, of hospitalizations. In patients recently discharged from the hospital after treatment of COPD exacerbation, pulmonary rehabilitation may reduce mortality (39). Benefits of rehabilitation generally wane with time. Home exercise, however, maintains patients above prerehabilitation levels (1).

Treatment of COPD exacerbation consists of increased use of inhaled albuterol and ipratropium bromide and supplemental oxygen in hypoxemic patients (40). It is important to titrate supplemental oxygen to a saturation of 90% to 91%; overshooting this target runs the risk of acute hypercapnia and acidemia. Systemic corticosteroids are indicated for moderate to severe COPD exacerbations, but should be used for no more than 2 weeks (41). Antibiotics are generally reserved for patients with increased mucus amount and purulence (42). Hospitalized patients are candidates for noninvasive ventilation, which decreases the risk of intubation and improves mortality attributable to COPD (43).

CLINICAL RECOMMENDATIONS OF THE VIGNETTE

It is increasingly recognized that COPD, particularly when severe, has systemic manifestations, including cachexia and skeletal muscle wasting, apoptosis, and disuse muscle atrophy (1). Other extrapulmonary manifestations include depression and anemia (also present in this case), along with osteoporosis and increased risk of cardiovascular disease. It is suspected that increased concentrations of inflammatory mediators, such as TNF-α and CRP are responsible for many of the systemic features. In this case, after excluding other possibilities, depression, anemia, weakness, and weight loss were all attributed to COPD. Low normal serum potassium was attributed to use of β-agonists. Treatment recommendations included increased caloric intake using small, frequent meals, and pulmonary rehabilitation (44).

SUMMARY

COPD is a preventable and treatable disease affecting millions of Americans. It has components of chronic bronchitis (a neutrophil predominant process) and emphysema (characterized by alveolar destruction and loss of elasticity) that cause usual symptoms of cough, phlegm, wheeze, and breathlessness. Extrapulmonary manifestations occur. COPD is invariably related to cigarette smoking, but not all smokers develop COPD, underscoring the importance of host genetics. A testable genetic risk factor is α_1-antitrypsin deficiency; others have been described. Not all patients with COPD have themselves smoked; some have been exposed to secondhand smoke, air pollution, or occupational dusts or chemicals; others have a genetic predisposition, such as α_1-antitrypsin deficiency. The diagnosis of COPD should be considered in patients 40 years of age or older who have smoked ≥10 pack-years. The diagnostic test of choice is spriometry, which classically reveals a low FEV_1:FVC. Treatment of COPD consists of smoking cessation, bronchodilators, inhaled corticosteroids, vaccinations, and pulmonary rehabilitation.

REFERENCES

1. Pauwells RA, Buist AS, Calverley PMA, et al. Global strategy for the diagnosis, management and prevention of chronic obstructive lung disease. NHLBI/WHO Global Initiative for Chronic Obstructive Lung Disease (GOLD) Workshop Summary. *Am J Respir Crit Care Med.* 2001;163:1256; with 2006 update available at http://www.goldcopd.com.
2. Hogg JC. Pathophysiology of airflow limitation in chronic obstructive pulmonary disease. *Lancet.* 2004;364:709–721.
3. Mannino DM, Homa DM, Akinbami LJ, et al. Chronic obstructive pulmonary disease surveillance—United States. 1971–2000. *MMWR Surveill Summ.* 2002;51:1–16.
4. Burrows B, Knudson RJ, Cline MG, et al. Quantitative relationships between cigarette smoking and ventilatory function. *Am Rev Respir Dis.* 1977;115:195–205.
5. Zielinski J, Bednarek M. Know the age of your lung study group. Early detection of COPD in a high-risk population using spirometric screening. *Chest.* 2001;119:731–736.
6. Hnizdo E, Sullivan PA, Bang KM, et al. Airflow obstruction attributable to work in industry and occupation among U.S. race/ethnic groups. A study of NHANES III data. *Am J Ind Med.* 2004;46:126–135.
7. Ezzati M. Indoor air pollution and health in developing countries. *Lancet.* 2005;366: 104–106.
8. Eisner MD, Balmes J, Katz, BP, et al. Lifetime environmental tobacco smoke exposure and the risk of chronic obstructive pulmonary disease. *Environ Health Perspect.* 2005;4:7–15.
9. Stoller JK, Aboussouan LS. Alpha-one antitrypsin deficiency. *Lancet.* 2005;365:2225–2236.
10. Bowler RP, Barnes PF, Crapo JD. The role of oxidative stress in chronic obstructive lung disease. *Chronic Obstructive Pulmonary Disease.* 2004;1:255–277.
11. Barnes P. Chronic obstructive lung disease. *N Engl J Med.* 2000;343:269–280.
12. Barnes PJ. Mediators of chronic obstructive lung disease. *Pharmacol Rev.* 2004;56:515.
13. Rodriquez-Roisin, R. The airway pathology of COPD: Implications for treatment. Journal of Chronic Obstructive Pulmonary Disease. 2005;2:253–256.
14. Georgopoulas D, Anthonisen NR. Symptoms and signs of COPD. In: Cherniack NS, ed. *Chronic Obstructive Pulmonary Disease.* Toronto: WB Saunders; 1991:357–363.
15. Wagner PD, Dantzker DR, Dueck R, et al. Ventilation-perfusion inequality in chronic obstructive pulmonary disease. *J Clin Invest.* 1977;59:203–216.
16. Barbera PR, Peinado VI, Santos S. Pulmonary hypertension in chronic obstructive pulmonary disease. *Am J Respir Crit Care Med.* 2001;164:770–777.
17. Wouters EF, Creutzberg EC, Schols AM. Systemic effects in COPD. *Chest.* 2002;121 [Suppl]:127–130.
18. Agusti AG, Noguera A, Sauleda J, et al. Systemic effects of chronic obstructive pulmonary disease. *Eur Respir J.* 2003;21:347–360.
19. Gan WQ, Man SF, Senthilselvan A, et al. Association between chronic obstructive pulmonary disease and systemic inflammation: A systematic review and meta-analysis. *Thorax.* 2004;59:574–580.
20. Similowski T, Agusti AG, MacNee W, et al. The potential impact of anemia of chronic disease in COPD. *Eur Respir J.* 2006;27:390–396.
21. Poels PF, Schermer TR, van Weel C, et al. Spirometry in chronic obstructive pulmonary disease. *BMJ.* 2006;333:870–871.
22. Jones PW. Issues concerning health-related quality of life in COPD. *Chest.* 1995;107 [Suppl]:187–193.
23. Celli BR, Cote CG, Marin JM, et al. The body-mass index, airflow obstruction, dyspnea and exercise capacity index in chronic obstructive pulmonary disease. *N Engl J Med.* 2004;350:1005–1012.
24. O'Donnell DE, Revill SM, Webb KA. Dynamic hyperinflation and exercise intolerance in chronic obstructive pulmonary disease. *Am J Respir Crit Care Med.* 2001;164:770–777.
25. Reilly J. Using computed tomography scanning to advance understanding of chronic obstructive lung disease. *Proc Am Thorac Soc.* 2006;3:450–455.
26. Newel JD Jr. CT of emphysema. *Radiol Clin North Am.* 2002;40:31–42.
27. Dantzker DR, D'Alonzo GE. The effect of exercise on pulmonary gas exchange in patients with severe chronic obstructive lung disease. *Am Rev Respir Dis.* 1986;134: 1135–1139.
28. Anthonisen NR, Skeans MA, Wise RA, et al. The effects of smoking cessation intervention on 14.5 year mortality: A randomized clinical trial. *Ann Intern Med.* 2005;142:233–239.
29. O'Donnell DE, Fluge T, Gerken F, et al. Effects of tiotropium on lung hyperinflation, dyspnea and exercise tolerance in COPD. *Eur Respir J.* 2004;23:832–840.
30. O'Donnell DE, Sciurba F, Celli B, et al. Effect of fluticasone propionate/salmeterol on lung hyperinflation and exercise endurance in COPD. *Chest.* 2006;130:647–656.
31. Burge PS, Calverley PM, Jones PW, et al. Randomized, double blind, placebo controlled study of fluticasone propionate in patients with moderate to severe chronic obstructive pulmonary disease: The ISOLDE trial. *BMJ.* 2000;320:1297–1303.
32. Burge PS. EUROSCOP, ISOLDE and the Copenhagen city lung study. *Thorax.* 1999;54: 1535–1544.
33. Sin DD, Wu L, Anderson JA, et al. Inhaled corticosteroids and mortality in chronic obstructive pulmonary disease. *Thorax.* 2005;60:992–997.
34. Man SF, Sin DD. Effects of corticosteroids on systemic inflammation in chronic obstructive pulmonary disease. *Proc Am Thorac Soc.* 2005;2:78–82.
35. van Noord JA, Aumann JL, Janssens E, et al. Effects of tiotropium with and without formoterol on airflow obstruction and resting hyperinflation in patients with COPD. *Chest.* 2006;129:509–517.
36. Heaton RK, Grant I, McSweeny AJ. Physiologic effects of continuous and nocturnal oxygen therapy in hypoxemic patients with chronic obstructive pulmonary disease. *Arch Intern Med.* 1983;143:1941–1947.
37. Nichol KL, Margolis KL, Wuorenma J, et al. The efficacy and cost effectiveness of vaccination against influenza among elderly persons living in the community. *N Engl J Med.* 1994;331:778–784.

38. Troosters T, Casaburi R, Gosselink R, et al. Pulmonary rehabilitation in chronic obstructive pulmonary disease. *Am J Respir Crit Care Med.* 2005;172:19–38.
39. Puhan MA, Scharplatz M, Troosters T, et al. Respiratory rehabilitation after an acute exacerbation of COPD may reduce risk for readmission and mortality—A systematic review. *Respir Res.* 2005;6:54.
40. Snow V, Lascher S, Mottur-Pilson C; Joint Expert Panel ACCP-ASIM. Evidence base for management of acute exacerbations of chronic obstructive pulmonary disease. *Ann Intern Med.* 2001;134:595–599.
41. Niewoehner DE, Erbland ML, Deupree RH, et al. Effect of systemic glucocorticoids on exacerbations of chronic obstructive pulmonary disease. Department of Veterans Affairs Cooperative Study Group. *N Engl J Med.* 1999;54:422–426.
42. Anthonisen NR, Manfreda J, Warren CP, et al. Antibiotic therapy in exacerbations of chronic obstructive pulmonary disease. *Ann Intern Med.* 1987;62:1179–1185.
43. Brochard L, Mancebo J, Wysocki M, et al. Noninvasive ventilation for acute exacerbations of chronic obstructive pulmonary disease. *N Engl J Med.* 1995;333:817–822.
44. Steiner MC, Barton RL, Singh S, et al. Nutritional enhancement of exercise performance in chronic obstructive pulmonary disease: A randomized trial. *Thorax.* 2003;58:745.

CHAPTER 19

Pulmonary/Pleural Infections

Richard G. Wunderink • Andrew M. Naidech

OBJECTIVES

- To emphasize that mental status changes in patients with pneumonia or other severe infections are more likely to be secondary to septic encephalopathy than concomitant meningitis
- To reinforce the concept that the pneumococcus is the most likely cause of concomitant meningitis in nonimmunocompromised patients with pneumonia
- To highlight that septic encephalopathy is not associated with focal neurologic findings; presence of these should suggest alternative diagnoses

CASE VIGNETTE

A 74-year-old man is brought to the emergency department by his family because of cough, fever, and confusion. The patient had been functioning as a freelance accountant until 3 days before presentation. He continued to smoke one pack of cigarettes per day as he had for the last 35 years.

Physical examination was remarkable for an oral temperature of 102°F, respiratory rate of 28, heart rate 114, and blood pressure of 105/62 mm Hg. His arterial saturation was 91%. He was lethargic and needed physical stimulation to answer questions. He was disoriented to name, place, and date, and could not identify his daughter. His optic discs were flat and he had no neck stiffness or jugular venous distension. Pulmonary examination was remarkable for coarse rales in the lower left posterior chest with egophony. He had no cardiac murmur. Neurologic examination was limited by lethargy, but did not demonstrate focal findings. The rest of his examination revealed nothing contributory.

Chest radiograph demonstrated an infiltrate with air bronchogram in the left lower lobe. He had leukocytosis, platelet count of $120{,}000/mm^3$, and mild increases in both blood urea nitrogen (BUN) and activated partial thromboplastin time (aPTT). Blood cultures were drawn. As the patient was being positioned for a lumbar puncture (LP), the systolic blood pressure was noted to be 65 mm Hg. The procedure was aborted and empiric antibiotics started. Once stabilized in the medical intensive care unit (ICU), a discussion regarding the need for the LP or other diagnostic procedures ensued.

DEFINITION

Encephalopathy is a deterioration of mental status or consciousness initiated by a disease process extrinsic to the brain (1). Sepsis is now defined as the systemic inflammatory response syndrome (SIRS) secondary to an infection (2). Severe sepsis is defined as sepsis that has induced organ dysfunction. The definitions for specific organ dysfunctions are not clear. Encephalopathy, however, would be considered one of the organ dysfunctions qualifying for the severe sepsis designation. The concept of a systemic response is important. If pneumonia only induces a localized pulmonary response, altered mental status likely stems from other causes.

An earlier definition included the concept of the presence of microorganisms or their toxins in the blood. Septic encephalopathy can clearly occur, however, without any detectable toxin or cultured microorganism. The present concept is that septic encephalopathy is the central neurologic organ dysfunction associated with the diffuse mediator activation seen in SIRS (1).

EPIDEMIOLOGY

The incidence of septic encephalopathy is in the 40% to 50% range, depending on the definition used. At least in some studies, septic encephalopathy appears to be less common with pneumonia as the cause of sepsis than other sources such as peritonitis.

The incidence of confusion in all patients admitted with community-acquired pneumonia (CAP) is 4% to 17% (3–6). The incidence of septic encephalopathy progressively increases with increased age (Fig. 19-1) (7,8). Therefore, encephalopathy in a young person is more significant. For patients deemed sufficiently stable to be treated as outpatients, the incidence of altered mental status is <1% (6). For patients admitted to the ICU, the incidence may be as high as 24% (5). The incidence of septic encephalopathy in patients with hospital-acquired pneumonia or ventilator-associated pneumonia (VAP) is not known. Determining the incidence in VAP is particularly problematic with the use of sedation in most ventilated patients.

One of the most consistent findings is the excess mortality associated with altered mental status in sepsis and pneumonia. The presence of septic encephalopathy was found to increase the mortality rate from 26% to 49% (9). The greatest increase was when altered mental status occurred in a patient whose

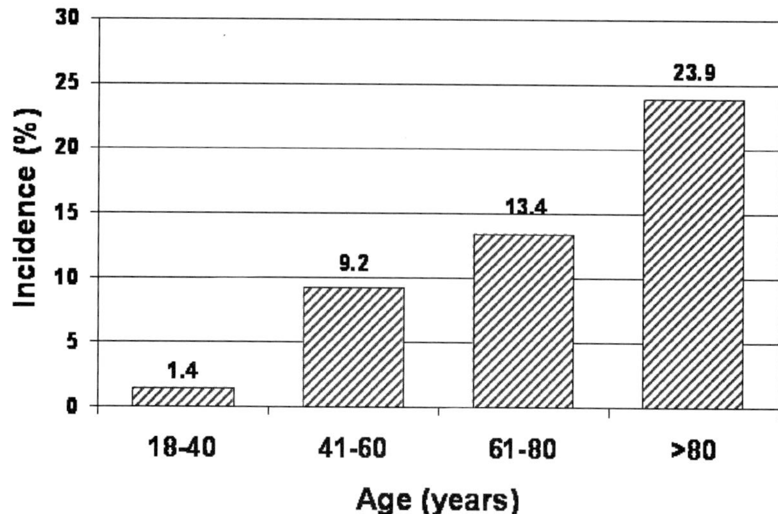

FIGURE 19-1. Increasing incidence of septic encephalopathy in community-acquired pneumonia with increasing age. (Data from Waterer GW, Kessler LA, Wunderink RG. Delayed administration of antibiotics and atypical presentation in community-acquired pneumonia. *Chest.* 2006;130(1):11–15, with permission.)

mental status was normal before developing sepsis; a change from an abnormal baseline mental status carried less prognostic significance.

The adverse effect of altered mental status in CAP is demonstrated by its inclusion in both of the most commonly used criteria for risk of death in CAP—the Pneumonia Severity Index (PSI) (6) and the CURB (**C**onfusion, **U**remia, elevated **R**espiratory rate, and low **B**lood pressure) score (3). A meta-analysis suggests that the odds ratio for excess mortality of altered mental status in CAP is approximately 2.5 times greater risk, with an absolute risk increase that is almost equivalent to presence of shock (10). Altered mental status, one explanation for a delay in the time to first antibiotic dose in CAP (11), has been associated with excess mortality (12). Interestingly, abnormal mental status in association with CAP is not only independently associated with hospital mortality but also with a higher death rate in the subsequent few years (8).

ETIOLOGY AND PATHOGENESIS

Multiple possible etiologies exist for septic encephalopathy (Table 19-1). The etiology and pathogenesis are likely multifactorial and interrelated. The most commonly cited mechanisms include the following.

TABLE 19-1. Potential Causes of Septic Encephalopathy

Reduced cerebral blood flow
Global hypoperfusion
Ischemia reperfusion injury
Microthrombi
Increased cytokine levels (tumor necrosis factor [TNF], IL-6, IL-1)
Disruption of the blood–brain barrier
Elevated catecholamine levels, both endogenous and exogenous
Altered levels of amino acids (>neutral aromatic, <branched chain)
Increased false transmitter levels
Altered cerebral metabolism
Impaired oxygen utilization
Impaired glucose metabolism
Disseminated cerebral microabscesses

DECREASED CEREBRAL PERFUSION

The easiest mechanism to understand is simply decreased perfusion. Obviously, if the patient has refractory shock, cerebral perfusion will be decreased just as it is in all tissue beds. Although cerebral circulation is relatively protected, sometimes at the expense of other tissue beds, adequate flow is usually maintained to prevent overt cerebral ischemia. Even relatively short periods of severe hypoperfusion, however, can result in a reperfusion injury via activation of toxic oxygen and nitrogen radicals, just as in many other vascular beds.

In contrast to other organ failure in sepsis, the evidence for microthrombi is less with septic encephalopathy, nor does treatment based on ameliorating the coagulopathy of sepsis lead to better outcome. Use of drotrecogin alfa (activated) was not predicted by presence of mental status changes (13).

Cerebral blood flow is reduced by 40% in sepsis, however, even without overt hypotension (14). The central hyperventilation of SIRS may contribute to this decreased flow. Abnormal cerebral metabolism is also a possibility because central venous oxygen saturations (which are disproportionately influenced by cerebral venous saturations) and specific jugular bulb oximetry are high in sepsis. This decrease in cerebral oxygen consumption can be as low as 33% of normal (14). More importantly, it does not consistently decrease with measures that increase cerebral blood flow, but rather correlate best with resolution of SIRS.

INCREASED CYTOKINE LEVELS

Cytokine storm can also cause altered mental status. In particular, levels of tumor necrosis factor (TNF) can influence the lethargy noted with sepsis. TNF has been shown to be associated with more septic encephalopathy in patients with nosocomial pneumonia. This effect seems to peak after the first dose of cell wall active agents, such as cephalosporins, a phenomenon well known in meningitis. Patient with septic encephalopathy appear to have a more prolonged peak in TNF and less counterregulatory neurotransmitter production (15). Interleukin-6, IL-1, and other cytokines are also increased in sepsis and have been linked to changes in central nervous system (CNS) function.

BREAKDOWN IN BLOOD–BRAIN BARRIER

A common theme in the pathogenesis of septic encephalopathy is a breakdown in the blood–brain barrier. Many different animal studies have documented high protein flux into brain parenchyma associated with sepsis. This breakdown may allow both endogenous and exogenous catecholamines to influence cerebral vascular resistance directly, resulting in localized areas of hypoperfusion.

ALTERED NEUROTRANSMITTER LEVELS

Levels of neurotransmitters can be altered by sepsis, especially with a breakdown in the blood–brain barrier. Increased diffusion of its precursor tryptophan can lead to the higher intracerebral levels of serotonin. Similarly, increased diffusion of tyrosine and phenylalanine can lead to an increased level of their breakdown products, which are *false* neurotransmitters that inhibit normal central noradrenergic pathways and manifest clinically as lethargy.

An altered blood–brain barrier is not necessarily required for increased intracerebral levels of these neutral or aromatic amino acids. Severe sepsis is characterized by a catabolic state as muscle is broken down to release branched chain amino acids, which can be used as an energy source (16). The increase in cerebral aromatic amino acid levels can result from decreased competition with branched-chain amino acids for transport across the blood–brain barrier because of their lower circulating levels. The parallel with hepatic encephalopathy has led to clinical studies of supplementation of branched-chain amino acids, the benefit of which on septic encephalopathy is not clear.

GLUCOSE HOMEOSTASIS

Hyperglycemia is well known to be associated both with poorer outcome in sepsis and possibly with altered neuronal injury. The greatest evidence comes from clinical trials of tight glycemic control, which suggested that the incidence of critical illness polyneuropathy could be decreased with tighter glycemic control (17). Altered glucose metabolism in the reticular activation system has also been found in animal models of sepsis.

PATHOLOGY

The pathology of septic encephalopathy is complicated by the complex interactions occurring in critically ill patients. The findings probably vary significantly, depending on whether the patients die from florid septic shock or from multiorgan system failure after a prolonged ICU course. Patients with profound shock or postcardiopulmonary arrest associated with sepsis will routinely have evidence of widespread ischemia (18).

Interestingly, neuronal apoptosis was more pronounced in the autonomic nuclei of patients who were septic than in patients dying of nonseptic shock. Neuron-specific enolase, a marker of neurons and neuroendocrine cell death, is elevated in 50% of patients with septic shock, especially cases with early death (19). This predominance of neuroendocrine involvement may be a partial explanation for the refractory shock and high mortality rate found in some patients with encephalopathic sepsis.

In a small minority (<10%) of patients, microabscesses can be detected (18). Hemorrhages can be present in as many as 25% of patients dying of septic shock.

CLINICAL MANIFESTATIONS/ SPECIAL SITUATIONS

Generally, two types of encephalopathy can be differentiated. The first is characterized as agitation, disorientation, confusion, and irritability; the second by somnolence, stupor, and coma (19). The two types appear to have approximately equal frequency in a group of patients with sepsis. The latter may be more common in later stages of sepsis-induced multiorgan system failure. A significant percent of patients with the somnolent or coma pattern will exhibit structural abnormalities on computed tomographic (CT) scan or magnetic resonance imaging (MRI), whereas no patient with the agitated or disoriented pattern exhibit structural abnormalities.

The confusion of pneumonia sepsis can be somewhat subtle. The British Thoracic Society (BTS) study of patients with pneumonia used a specific, relatively complex test to detect subtle abnormalities (20). Subsequent studies have used only a subjective abnormal in any way from baseline and found similar prognostic significance (4). Querying the family may be more clinically relevant and accurate.

DIAGNOSTIC APPROACH

The diagnosis of septic encephalopathy is essentially a diagnosis of exclusion. Even electroencephalograms and evoked potentials, while clearly appearing abnormal in septic encephalopathy, are not specific, especially in differentiating from other causes of encephalopathy.

The diagnostic approach, therefore, aims at excluding alternative diagnoses. The major alternative diagnoses are listed in Table 19-2. History and physical examination findings are critical in the differential diagnosis of septic encephalopathy. By definition, encephalopathy is not associated with localizing signs on neurologic examination. Presence of localizing signs of any sort would suggest the need for diagnostic radiology to exclude cerebral hemorrhage or infarct, septic emboli, or brain abscesses.

One of the major issues in the diagnostic approach when mental status changes are seen in a patient with pneumonia is

TABLE 19-2. Differential Diagnosis of Mental Status Changes in Patients with Pneumonia

Septic encephalopathy
Septic shock with hypoperfusion
Alcohol and other drug withdrawal
Exaggerated response to sedatives or narcotics
Secondary meningitis
Cerebral hemorrhage/thrombosis in association with septic coagulopathy
Pneumonia mimics
Systemic lupus erythematosis
Septic emboli from endocarditis
Hypercarbia or hypoxemia from respiratory failure
Hepatic encephalopathy
Concomitant central nervous system (CNS) infection (severely immunocompromised)

differentiation from concomitant meningitis. Despite the frequency of abnormal mental status in patients with CAP, the incidence of concomitant meningitis is low (<5%). Conversely, pneumonia is present in 12% of adult patients with meningitis (21). Altered mental status is present in 69% of patients, whereas neck stiffness was present in 83% of patients of all ages. The classic triad of fever, neck stiffness, and altered mental status was only present in 44% overall. Interestingly, the classic triad is more common in patients with pneumococcal meningitis (58%), therefore more likely to have concomitant pneumonia, than with meningococcal meningitis (27%) (21). Focal neurologic signs at the time of admission also have occurred with relatively high frequency (33%).

For these reasons, the need for a lumbar puncture to rule out meningitis in an adult patient with pneumonia is very low unless physical examination reveals neck stiffness or focal neurologic signs. A lower threshold may be needed in pediatric cases. Nosocomial pneumonia is never complicated by meningitis unless the patient has had recent neurologic surgery or CNS catheters. In these situations, it is unclear whether the pneumonia and meningitis are caused by the same microorganisms or even related in any way.

A history of alcohol abuse is critical to obtain. Alcohol withdrawal is often confused with the agitated form of septic encephalopathy. Occasionally, patients are admitted to the hospital with a primary diagnosis of delirium tremens and when fever occurs because of pneumonia, benzodiazepines are prescribed rather than antibiotics—with disastrous results. The pneumonia can be either true CAP—pneumococcus and enteric Gram-negatives being the major etiologic concerns, an episode of aspiration pneumonitis—or true nosocomial pneumonia. A history of alcohol abuse is also a trigger of concern about a pleural effusion in a patient who presents with altered mental status. A previous episode of loss of consciousness and aspiration may predispose to an anaerobic pleuropulmonary infection.

Other drug withdrawal is also a cause of altered mental status. Benzodiazepine withdrawal after having oral medications held for a surgical procedure may only be detected by careful questioning of family regarding daily use of sedatives.

For nosocomial pneumonia, distinguishing between pneumonia as the cause of altered mental status and altered mental status as the cause of pneumonia is often difficult. Aspiration, especially in the elderly, is often exacerbated by acute illnesses and their treatment. Aspiration and altered mental status are commonly found in a variety of neurologic conditions, especially acute stroke. Patients with many neurologic diseases can also have decreased mental status in association with acute hypercarbic respiratory failure. Many of these patients also have an increased incidence of aspiration, either because of the hypercarbic narcosis or from bulbar involvement with the primary disorder. Conversely, acute noninfectious illness may already predispose to altered mental status, especially agitation. Subsequent sedation may then predispose to aspiration and pneumonia.

Laboratory tests can also narrow the diagnosis. Evidence of end-stage renal or hepatic disease would increase the likelihood that encephalopathy is caused or exacerbated by these organ failures. Pneumonia and other infections are often precipitating causes of worsened mental or functional status leading the patient or, more typically, the family member to seek medical care.

Thrombocytopenia is frequently associated with poor outcome in sepsis in general and increases the possibility of concomitant intracerebral hemorrhage. Use of an agent that increases the risk of bleeding, such as drotrecogin alfa (activated), will also increase the risk of CNS bleeds (22). The threshold for diagnostic radiology in these settings should be lower.

One of the major issues in evaluation of abnormal mental status in patients with pneumonia is the use of sedatives and narcotics. CAP occurs disproportionately in the elderly and any sedative or narcotic can have a prolonged or more pronounced effect. The most critically ill patients with pneumonia are the most likely to have septic encephalopathy, but they are also the most likely to require intubation and mechanical ventilation. Sedation administered at the time of intubation or subsequently to allow better ventilatory support frequently interferes with assessment of neurologic status and concern regarding the presence of other causes of altered mental status. Regular sedation holidays or titrating sedation to minimal levels will help clarify the true neurologic status.

In a patient with an episode of severe hypotension or who is on prolonged vasopressors, the issue is the presence of anoxic encephalopathy. While the patient's infection is still not under control, separation of anoxic from septic encephalopathy may be nearly impossible. Persistence after control of the infection, such that fever, hyperventilation, and leukocytosis are resolved, would tend to favor an anoxic problem. Head CT scan may still appear normal in these cases, but MRI may occasionally demonstrate small multifocal lesions.

TREATMENT

The treatment of septic encephalopathy is essentially the treatment of the underlying disease. This includes both appropriate antibiotics and hemodynamic support. The increasing emphasis on hemodynamic support goals, more than on just adequate blood pressure, may be even more pertinent to patients with septic encephalopathy, given that altered cerebral perfusion is one of the major factors regarding pathogenesis. Manipulations to increase the central venous saturation to >70% has now become the standard of care for patients with sepsis and pneumonia (23).

Tight glycemic control also appears to be more highly warranted in the population with septic encephalopathy. This may be a slight extension of the observed benefit on the peripheral neuropathy of critical illness (17), but several retrospective studies also suggest that worse outcome of infections, including meningitis (21), are associated with increased glucose levels.

The benefit of other metabolic manipulations is also not clear. Use of parenteral or enteral nutrition with increased branched chain and fewer aromatic amino acids has not demonstrated improved mortality (24).

Specific treatment for septic shock with drotrecogin alfa (activated) (22) has an unclear effect on septic encephalopathy. Several experimental therapies, which have not been approved for routine treatment of septic shock may have benefit, including anti-TNF strategies and plasmapheresis. Clearly, further research is needed regarding pathogenesis to design better therapeutic options.

CLINICAL RECOMMENDATIONS OF THE VIGNETTE

The most likely explanation for the patient's abnormal mental status was felt to be septic encephalopathy. The differential diagnosis of abnormal mental status in a patient with pneumonia is listed in Table 19-2. Central venous saturation was initially found to be 54% with a central venous pressure of 4 cm H_2O and a rapid urinary antigen test was positive for *Staphylococcus pneumoniae.* For these reasons and the fact that examinations done before intubation and sedation had not demonstrated neck stiffness, a repeat attempt at a lumbar puncture was not felt to be indicated. High dose ceftriaxone and azithromycin were continued, but empiric meningitis therapy was also not felt to be indicated.

Hypotension resolved overnight with aggressive volume resuscitation. Sedation was withheld the next morning and the patient awakened quickly and was responsive to commands. After successful extubation, his family was able to communicate with him without problems and he appeared to be at his baseline mental functioning. He was discharged after 5 days in the hospital.

SUMMARY

Septic encephalopathy is a common manifestation of severe sepsis in patients with pneumonia. Its presence should alert the clinician to the increased acute and median term mortality. Although septic encephalopathy is a diagnosis of exclusion, the alternative diagnoses can usually be ruled out by history, clinical examination with special focus on the presence of localizing neurologic signs, and laboratory tests routinely available in patients with sepsis patients.

REFERENCES

1. Papadopoulos MC, Davies DC, Moss RF, et al. Pathophysiology of septic encephalopathy: A review. *Crit Care Med.* 2000;28(8):3019–3024.
2. American College of Chest Physicians/Society of Critical Care Medicine Consensus Conference: Definitions for sepsis and organ failure and guidelines for the use of innovative therapies in sepsis. *Crit Care Med.* 1992;20(6):864–874.
3. Lim WS, Lewis S, Macfarlane JT. Severity prediction rules in community acquired pneumonia: A validation study. *Thorax.* 2000;55(3):219–223.
4. Lim WS, van der Eerden MM, Laing R, et al. Defining community acquired pneumonia severity on presentation to hospital: An international derivation and validation study. *Thorax.* 2003;58(5):377–382.
5. Angus DC, Marrie TJ, Obrosky DS, et al. Severe community-acquired pneumonia: Use of intensive care services and evaluation of American and British Thoracic Society Diagnostic criteria. *American Journal of Respiratory and Critical Care Medicine (AJRCCM)* 2002;166(5): 717–723.
6. Fine MJ, Auble TE, Yealy DM, et al. A prediction rule to identify low-risk patients with community-acquired pneumonia. *N Engl J Med.* 1997;336:243–250.
7. Meehan TP, Fine MJ, Krumholz HM, et al. Quality of care, process, and outcomes in elderly patients with pneumonia. *JAMA.* 1997;278:2080–2084.
8. Waterer GW, Kessler LA, Wunderink RG. Medium-term survival after hospitalization with community-acquired pneumonia. *Am J Respir Crit Care Med.* 2004;169(8):910–914.
9. Sprung CL, Peduzzi PN, Shatney CH, et al. Impact of encephalopathy on mortality in the sepsis syndrome. The Veterans Administration Systemic Sepsis Cooperative Study Group. *Crit Care Med.* 1990;18(8):801–806.
10. Fine MJ, Smith MA, Carson CA, et al. Prognosis and outcomes of patients with community-acquired pneumonia. A meta-analysis. *JAMA.* 1996;275(2):134–141.
11. Waterer GW, Kessler LA, Wunderink RG. Delayed administration of antibiotics and atypical presentation in community-acquired pneumonia. *Chest.* 2006;130(1):11–15.
12. Houck PM, Bratzler DW, Nsa W, et al. Timing of antibiotic administration and outcomes for Medicare patients hospitalized with community-acquired pneumonia. *Arch Intern Med.* 2004;164(6):637–644.
13. Ely EW, Laterre PF, Angus DC, et al. Drotrecogin alfa (activated) administration across clinically important subgroups of patients with severe sepsis. *Crit Care Med.* 2003;31(1): 12–19.
14. Bowton DL, Bertels NH, Prough DS, et al. Cerebral blood flow is reduced in patients with sepsis syndrome. *Crit Care Med.* 1989;17(5):399–403.
15. Eggers V, Fugener K, Hein OV, et al. Antibiotic-mediated release of tumour necrosis factor alpha and norharman in patients with hospital-acquired pneumonia and septic encephalopathy. *Intensive Care Med.* 2004;30(8):1544–1551.
16. Basler T, Meier-Hellmann A, Bredle D, et al. Amino acid imbalance early in septic encephalopathy. *Intensive Care Med.* 2002;28(3):293–298.
17. Van den Berghe G, Wouters P, Weekers F, et al. Intensive insulin therapy in the critically ill patients. *N Engl J Med.* 2001;345(19):1359–1367.
18. Sharshar T, Annane D, de la Grandmaison GL, et al. The neuropathology of septic shock. *Brain Pathol.* 2004;14(1):21–33.
19. Nguyen DN, Spapen H, Su F, et al. Elevated serum levels of S-100 beta protein and neuron-specific enolase are associated with brain injury in patients with severe sepsis and septic shock. *Crit Care Med.* 2006;34(7):1967–1974.
20. Neill AM, Martin IR, Weir R, et al. Community acquired pneumonia: Aetiology and usefulness of severity criteria on admission. *Thorax.* 1996;51(10):1010–1016.
21. van de Beek D, de Gans J, Spanjaard L, et al. Clinical features and prognostic factors in adults with bacterial meningitis. *N Engl J Med.* 2004;351(18):1849–1859.
22. Bernard GR, Vincent JL, Laterre PF, et al. Efficacy and safety of recombinant human activated protein C for severe sepsis. *N Engl J Med.* 2001;344(10):699–709.
23. Rivers E, Nguyen B, Havstad S, et al. Early goal-directed therapy in the treatment of severe sepsis and septic shock. *N Engl J Med.* 2001;345(19):1368–1377.
24. Bower RH, Muggia-Sullam M, Vallgren S, et al. Branched chain amino acid-enriched solutions in the septic patient. A randomized, prospective trial. *Ann Surg.* 1986;203(1):13–20.

CHAPTER 20

Venous Thromboembolism

Kenneth V. Leeper, Jr.

OBJECTIVES

- To review the incidence and risk factors of venous thromboembolism
- To highlight the pathophysiology of venous thromboembolism
- To describe the diagnostic approach, risk stratification, and management of patient with venous thromboembolism

CASE VIGNETTE

A 72-year-old man presents to the emergency room (ER) with a 2-day history of acute dyspnea. He has a history of prostate cancer diagnosed 2 years ago and has completed chemotherapy. In the ER, he appeared to be in moderate respiratory distress with a respiratory rate of 26 breaths per minute. Heart rate was 116, temperature 38.4°C, and oxygen saturation on room air was 85%. Physical examination was remarkable for mild right ventricular (RV) heave. Chest radiography was normal. Electrocardiogram (ECG) was unremarkable except for sinus tachycardia. The brain natriuretic peptide (BNP) and cardiac troponins were elevated. A spiral computed tomographic (CT) scan with contrast showed bilateral large pulmonary emboli (Fig. 20-1). The patient was given a bolus of unfractionated heparin (UFH) and then started on UFH infusion. ECG showed severe RV dysfunction with RV dilatation. Lower extremity venous Doppler ultrasound showed a right-sided proximal thrombus. The patient was transferred to the medical intensive care unit (MICU) for further evaluation.

DEFINITION

Venous thromboembolic (VTE) disease is associated with considerable morbidity in terms of suffering, cost, and mortality. The sequelae of VTE are venous insufficiency with chronic swelling in the lower extremities as a result of deep venous thrombosis (DVT), potential for fatal pulmonary embolism (PE), and development of pulmonary hypertension. Despite newer diagnostic techniques, VTE remains underdiagnosed. The reason for this is that the signs and symptoms are relatively nonspecific and often overlap with a variety of common cardiopulmonary diseases.

VTE represents a spectrum of two disease process: DVT and the subsequent development of acute PE. In patients who have proximal DVT, nearly 60% will have concomitant PE (1). Furthermore, in patients with DVT without clinical evidence of acute PE, nearly 40% will have imaged-documented PE (2).

Reducing the burden of VTE requires effective primary prevention, prompt diagnosis, appropriate treatment of acute thrombosis, and effective long-term secondary prevention.

EPIDEMIOLOGY

Pulmonary embolism is the fourth most common cause of cardiovascular death. Based on population studies, the incidence of VTE increases from 1 of 10,000 for those younger than 40 years, and 1 of 100 for individuals older than 60 years (3,4). Recurrent disease may be responsible for one third of the cases. The national incidence of VTE from these data suggest that >250,000 cases are diagnosed annually, and at least 50,000 of these cases result in death (4,5).

In the International Cooperative Pulmonary Embolism Registry, the 3-month mortality rate after PE diagnosis was 15.5% The overall 3-month mortality rate in the Prospective-Investigation of Pulmonary Embolism Diagnosis (PIOPED) study was 15%, but only 10% of deaths in the 1-year follow-up were associated with PE (6). The age-adjusted rate of death from pulmonary thromboembolism, however, decreased by 56% for men and 46% for women from 1979 to 1998. During this period, however, the age-adjusted mortality rates for blacks were 50% higher than for whites. Mortality rates were consistently 20% to 30% higher among men than women (7).

RISKS FACTORS

Nearly 150 years ago, the triad of stasis, endothelial injury, and alterations in blood coagulability was proposed by Virchow as the pathophysiologic mechanisms for increased risk for the development of VTE. Still valid today, these factors can identify potential risks for thrombosis in a number of clinical situations (Table 20-1). Thrombophilia can be inherited, acquired, or both. Before 1993, a heritable cause of thrombophilia was identified in <20% of affected patients. Now, since the discovery of factor V Leiden (Arg 506Gln mutation) and the prothrombin gene mutation G20210A, this percentage has risen dramatically (8). Acquired risk factors, such as prolonged immobilization, malignancy, obesity, pregnancy, stroke, myocardial infarction, fracture, and repair of the femur, hip and pelvis, inflammatory bowel disease, and indwelling femoral catheters must be considered. Recently, acute infections, such as urinary tract

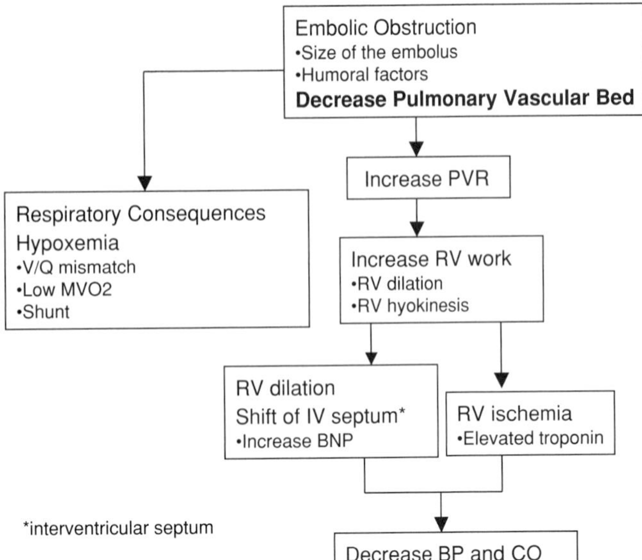

FIGURE 20-1. Pathophysiology of acute pulmonary embolism (PE).

infections, have been associated with transient increases in VTE risk in the community (9). Activation of the coagulation system can contribute to the increased risk of VTE in long-distance air travel (10,11). Still, many cases of VTE remain idiopathic. Extensive testing for the presence of a thrombophilic state is not cost effective. Screening should be reserved for patients who sustain their first event before 50 years of age, have a history of recurrent events, or who have a first-degree relative with a venous thromboembolic event that also occurred before the age of 50 (8). The most common thrombophilic conditions are not affected by the commencement of antithrombotic therapy. These conditions are factor V Leiden deficiency, prothrombin gene mutation, antiphospholipid syndrome, and hyperhomocysteinemia (12).

PATHOPHYSIOLOGY AND CLINICAL PRESENTATION OF DEEP VEIN THROMBOSIS

Thrombi of the lower extremities develop as a result of trauma to the vein or reduced or sluggish blood flow usually originating in the venous cusps. This results in the accumulation of fibrin and platelets forming the nidus for the developing thrombus. This process is usually controlled by endogenous fibrinolysis. The embolic potential is much greater when proximal lower extremities thrombi develop (13,14).

The signs and symptoms of DVT in the lower extremities are not specific. The most common symptoms of DVT include leg pain, edema, erythema, and warmth in the involved area. On physical examination may be seen swelling of the leg and a palpable cord in cases of an associated superficial vein thrombosis. Homans' sign (calf pain on sudden dorsiflexion of the foot), and Lowenberg sign (calf pain in response to lower pressure than expected on inflation of a sphygmomanometer cuff) are insensitive and non-specific findings. The differential diagnosis of lower extremity DVT includes, nonspecific edema, Baker cyst, or cellulites (15,16).

Although the clinical signs and symptoms of DVT are not specific, using a clinical model in a patient who is symptomatic can help the clinician estimate the pretest probability of DVT (Table 20-2) (17).

Among patients in whom DVT and PE are suspected, evaluation for the D-dimer is a good screening test that has an excellent negative predictive probability in excluding VTE. Plasmin degrades cross-linked fibrin-forming D-dimers. Measured by enzyme-linked immunosorbent assay (ELISA), a whole-blood agglutination test (e.g., SimpliRED) or a latex agglutination test, D-dimers are nearly always elevated in all patients with venous thromboembolic disease as well as in patients with active cardiopulmonary disease or malignancy, and in those who have experienced recent surgery or trauma. Hence, the D-dimer measurement is most useful in excluding a diagnosis of VTE disease and more suited in the outpatient evaluation of VTE. In patients who are clinically suspected of having DVT, a D-dimer level of <500 ng/mL on ELISA testing has a negative predictive value of 95% (18,19).

DIAGNOSIS OF DVT

DUPLEX ULTRASOUND

B-mode imaging (brightness modulation) and color Doppler techniques of duplex ultrasonography have truly revolutionized the establishment of DVT for both the upper and lower extremities. The duality of detecting the presence of an intraluminal echo, which is the visual representation of a thrombus, and the assessment of the blood-flow characteristics enhance the diagnostic accuracy of this test, establishing it as the most

TABLE 20-1. Risk factors for Venous Thromboembolism (VTE)

Stasis	*Endothelial Injury*	*Hypercoagulable State*
Immobility	Sepsis	***Acquired***
Congestive heart failure (CHF)	Intravascular catheters	Malignancy
Pregnancy	Trauma	Oral contraceptives
Previous deep venous thrombosis (DVT)	Orthopedic procedures	Polycythemia vera
Cor pulmonale		Homocystinuria
Paralysis		***Genetic***
Obesity		Factor V Leiden
Age		Prothrombin gene mutation
		Antithrombin deficiency
		Protein C and S deficiency

TABLE 20-2. Clinical Prediction Model for Deep Venous Thrombosis (DVT)

Clinical Feature	*Score (points)*
• Active cancer	1
• Paralysis, paresis, or recent plaster immobilization of the lower extremities	1
• Recently bedridden for 3 wk, or major surgery within the previous 4 wk	1
• Localized tenderness along the distribution of the deep venous system	1
• Entire swollen leg	1
• Calf swelling >3 cm when compared with asymptomatic leg (at 10 cm below tibial tuberosity)	1
• Pitting edema (greater in symptomatic leg)	1
• Collateral superficial veins (non-varicose)	1
• Alternative diagnosis as likely or greater than that of DVT	–2

In patients with symptoms in both legs, the more symptomatic leg is used. A low pretest probability exists if the score is ≤0, moderate if 1–2, and high if ≥3.

common ancillary method for diagnosing DVT. In a patient who is symptomatic, an inability to fully compress a vein and thereby obliterate its lumen is a demonstrable sign (>95% sensitivity and specificity) of proximal DVT. Diagnostic vulnerability occurs when trying to establish the presence of calf DVT. Major advantages of duplex ultrasonography are its noninvasive nature and wide availability. Limitations include that this technique is highly operator dependent, besides the difficulties in performing it on obese patients, patients with significant tenderness or edema, and patients whose limbs are in a cast or other immobilizing device. Moreover, duplex ultrasonography cannot always accurately distinguish between an acute and chronic thrombus (20). In asymptomatic patients, venous ultrasonography is very insensitive for diagnosing DVT (21,22).

CONTRAST VENOGRAPHY

Contrast venography is considered the gold standard for diagnosing DVT. This technique, however, has major limitations as a diagnostic test. Because patients are exposed to the administration of contrast dye and the discomfort encountered with the test, the widespread use of this test is limited. A DVT is confirmed when an intraluminal defect or an abrupt cut-off is present. Unlike duplex ultrasonography, contrast venography is more sensitive in confirming calf vein thrombosis.

CT magnetic resonance venography has a sensitivity and specificity approaching that of contrast venography, but it is cost-prohibitive as a screening test (23,24).

Clinical Presentation for Acute Pulmonary Embolism

PATHOPHYSIOLOGY

Approximately 60% of patients with documented PE have a DVT (1). It is these lower extremity thrombi, especially proximal in location, that potentially will embolize to the lung. The PE can vary in size and lodge in the main, segmental, and subsegmental pulmonary arteries. These emboli can also straddle the pulmonary artery bifurcation, giving rise to a saddle embolus. A PE has both respiratory and hemodynamic consequences. The respiratory consequences are the development of hypoxemia and a widen A-a gradient. Hyperventilation occurs with resultant hypocapnia and respiratory alkalosis. The mechanisms for impaired gas exchange that occurs with acute PE are multifactorial. Ventilation-perfusion mismatch occurs, ranging from impaired perfusion with adequate ventilation-dead space ventilation to intrapulmonary shunting occurring as a result surfactant loss distal to the clot resulting in atelectasis and edema. Right-to-left shunting can occur in the event of the development of a patent foramen ovale (PFO) a result of a sudden increase in pulmonary artery pressures. Hypercapnia can also occur in patients with massive PE (25).

The size of the embolus, underlying cardiopulmonary reserve, and the more elusive humoral mediator release are the factors that determine the hemodynamic response to the embolism (Fig. 20-1). Mechanical obstruction of the pulmonary vascular bed (PVB) directly corresponds to the degree of reduction of pulmonary vascular cross-sectional area and subsequent pulmonary hypertension. The decrease in cross-section of the PVB can transiently be affected by humoral factors, such as platelet-released serotonin and thromboxane. The release of these mediators causes pulmonary vasoconstriction and an increase in pulmonary vascular resistance. Both these mechanical and humoral factors increase RV work characterized by RV volume overload with resultant RV dilation and RV wall motion abnormalities (hypokinesis). This RV pressure overload leads to RV wall stress and the development of RV ischemia with elevation of brain natriuretic peptide (BNP) and troponin levels. If the embolic event is sufficiently large, severe RV dilation will occur, shifting the interventricular septum into the LV, reducing LV chamber size, and decreasing RV stroke volume and cardiac output, leading to shock, cardiac failure, and death (25,26).

CLINICAL MANIFESTATIONS

The signs and symptoms of acute PE are not specific and share many of the features with other common cardiopulmonary diseases (e.g., pneumonia, congestive heart failure [CHF]). The most common symptoms in individuals without preexisting cardiopulmonary disease are dyspnea, pleuritic chest pain, cough, leg edema, leg pain, hemoptysis, and palpitations. The most common findings on physical examination are tachypnea, rales (crackles), tachycardia, a fourth heart sound, accentuation of the second heart sound (closure of the pulmonic valve), DVT, and diaphoresis. Nearly 50% of patients with DVT have an asymptomatic PE at diagnosis (27,28).

The hemodynamic presentation of acute PE allows for risk stratification of these patients and leads to earlier consideration of more definitive therapy. Risk stratification of acute PE describes the spectrum of the initial clinical presentation. The range can be from small, peripheral emboli causing pleuritic chest pain and dyspnea, to massive PE with circulatory collapse and shock. The degree of RV dysfunction appears to play a key role in determining the risk of an embolic event. Elevated biomarkers, such as cardiac troponins and BNP, have correlated well with RV dysfunction and are a significant predictor for early mortality. Echocardiographic abnormalities of RV function and RV enlargement on CT scan have been associated with increased risk of adverse outcomes.

DIAGNOSIS

A diagnostic algorithm for acute pulmonary embolism is proposed in Figure 20-2. The clinical diagnosis of acute PE is often not specific. The clinical presentation will differ from patient to patient. Therefore, a high clinical suspicion for acute PE must be maintained when faced with an unknown subacute or acute cardiopulmonary process. Several clinical predictive models for acute PE diagnosis exist. An often used model is the Wells score, which categorizes patients as low, intermediate, or high clinical probability of PE with a D-dimer test. A normal D-dimer test finding with a low clinical probability may exclude 20% to 40% of patients suspected of PE with no further imaging or commencement of treatment (29).

A recent study assessed a clinical evaluation consisting of a dichotomized clinical decision rule from the Wells score (PE unlikely or likely), D-dimer testing, and CT scan in patients in whom PE is suspected. The main outcome measure was the occurrence of symptomatic or fatal thromboembolism during a 3-month follow-up. The investigators found that if PE was unlikely by the decision rule combined with a normal D-dimer, a 0.5% incidence was seen of nonfatal VTE when anticoagulation was held. Further, when the spiral CT scan was negative, the incidence of VTE in patients not treated was 1.3% (30).

ELECTROCARDIOGRAPHY

The ECG in the diagnosis of PE plays a role in determining the degree of RV work and also suggests alternative diagnosis, such as myocardial infarction and cardiac tamponade. In patients with pulmonary embolism, the ECG might appear normal, especially in young people. Sinus tachycardia is common along with nonspecific ST-T wave changes (27). In patients with an embolus sufficiently large to increase RV work patterns consistent with right-sided heart strain are often seen. Patterns include right-axis deviation, right bundle branch block, P-wave pulmonale, an $S_1Q_3T_3$ pattern (a prominence of S waves in lead I, Q waves in lead III, and T-wave inversion in lead III), nonspecific ST-T-wave changes, and arrhythmias (31).

CHEST RADIOGRAPHY

Findings on chest radiographs are also nonspecific and abnormal in most cases of PE. The PIOPED study showed that, among patients with angiographically proved pulmonary embolism, only 12% had chest radiograph films interpreted as normal. Pleural effusions, atelectasis, elevation of a hemidiaphragm, and pulmonary infiltrates are often seen in patients with a PE. Hampton hump (a wedge-shaped opacity along the pleural surface), Westermark sign (decreased vascularity), and Palla sign (an enlarged right descending pulmonary artery) are classic radiographic findings, but infrequently observed (27). In one study, the most common radiographic abnormality was cardiomegaly (32).

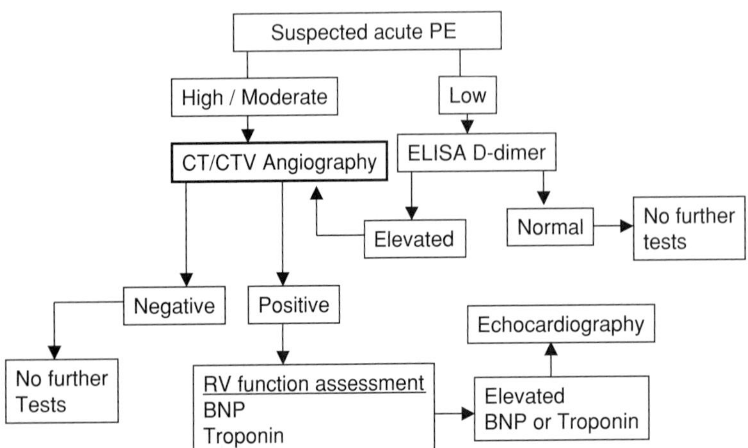

FIGURE 20-2. Diagnostic algorithm for acute pulmonary embolism (PE).

ARTERIAL BLOOD GAS

Results of arterial blood gas analysis can be normal in patients with a small PE as well as in younger individuals who have a larger embolus without preexisting cardiopulmonary disease. A low PaO_2 level, a normal or low Pa CO_2 level, and an elevated alveolar-arterial oxygen gradient (>20 mm Hg) are findings consistent with the diagnosis of a pulmonary embolism (27).

IMAGING STUDIES

Ventilation Perfusion Lung Scan

The PIOPED study demonstrated that results from a ventilation/perfusion (V/Q) scan have limited value. The diagnostic accuracy of this test was estimated to be 27% (33). A recent chest radiograph is necessary for the proper interpretation of a lung scintigram because many other cardiopulmonary diseases also cause ventilation or perfusion defects. The ventilation lung scan should be considered in patients who have renal disease and have contraindication to contrast dye or in pregnant patients.

Pulmonary Angiography

Pulmonary angiography has been considered the gold standard test for acute PE. As with venography, this is an invasive test requiring a considerable amount of contrast dye. The morbidity from pulmonary angiography is approximately 3% and mortality is 0.3% (34,35). A negative pulmonary angiogram result essentially excludes clinically relevant PE.

Spiral Computed Tomography Scan

Currently, most US hospitals have spiral CT scan capability to utilize in the diagnosis of VTE (Fig 20-3). The major advantage of spiral CT scanning is that it allows for direct visualization of the embolus. Depending on the number of multislice detectors, thrombi can be visualized to the subsegmental level. In addition, if PE is not found on spiral CT scan, alternative diagnoses can include cardiac tamponade, aortic dissection, pneumonia, pleural effusion, and pneumothorax. Recently, the PIOPED II study evaluated the diagnostic accuracy of multidetector spiral CT scan technology and found that the sensitivity and specificity of CT scan alone is 83% and 96%, respectively. With the combination of CT scan of the chest and CT venography of the lower extremities (CTV) the sensitivity and specificity was 93% and 95% respectively (36-37). CT scanning can also be used to assess RV function. With two-dimensional reconstructed images, the ratio of RV:LV >0.9 was associated with RV dysfunction and increase in hospital morbidity (38). Finally, a normal CT scan of the chest has an excellent negative predictive value and anticoagulation can be held (39–41).

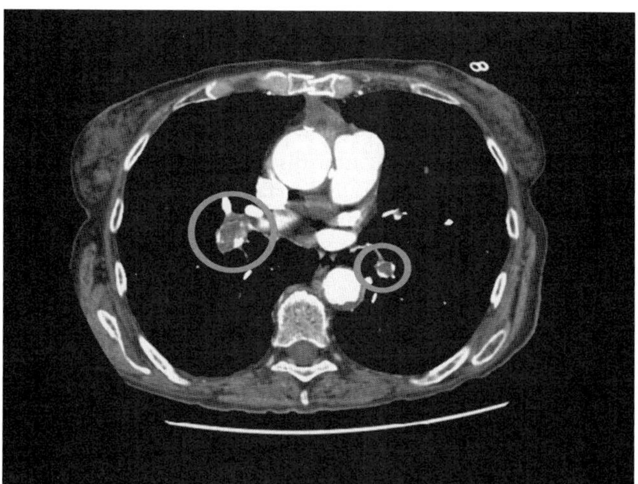

FIGURE 20-3. Multidetector spiral computed tomographic (CT) scan demonstrating bilateral pulmonary emboli.

Contrast–Enhanced Magnetic Resonance Angiography

The PIOPED II study showed that nearly 24% of patients suspected of PE had some sort of contraindication to spiral CT scanning (37). One of the major contraindications involved patients who had renal insufficiency. Potentially, this can be overcome by using gadolinium-enhanced magnetic resonance angiography (MRA) to diagnose PE when iodinated contrast dye is to be avoided. Contrast-enhanced MRA has been shown to have comparable sensitivity and specificity with that of pulmonary angiography (43–45). Although this modality looks promising, its lack of widespread availability and long examination times limits its application for PE diagnosis.

Echocardiography

The echocardiogram is not used to establish the diagnosis of PE, but it demonstrates the degree of RV dysfunction that has occurred as result of the embolic event. Therefore, the echocardiogram is useful in risk stratification and prognostication after the PE diagnosis has been confirmed. RV wall motion abnormalities, RV enlargement and dilation, tricuspid regurgitation, and estimated elevation of pulmonary artery pressures are some of the echocardiographic features of acute PE (30).

PHARMACOLOGIC TREATMENT

Pulmonary embolism and DVT are treated using similar drugs (Table 20-3). The Seventh ACCP Guidelines of Antithrombotic Therapy and Thrombolysis provide an extensive review of the pharmacologic management of VTE (47).

Heparin

Unfractionated heparin (UHF), administered by continuous infusion or subcutaneous injections adjusted to achieve an activated partial thromboplastin time (aPTT) >1.5, is effective as initial treatment of VTE. Weight-based dosing (an 80 U/kg bolus followed by 18 U/kg/h) is associated with a lower risk of recurrent thromboembolism. The target value is 1.5 to 2.5 times the mean control value (which corresponds to 0.3 to 0.6 U/mL on the amidolytic anti-factor Xa assay) and should be checked 6 hours after a dose adjustment. aPTT ratios of <1.5 during the first few days of heparin therapy increase the long-term risk of VTE recurrence. Adverse drug reactions include bleeding, heparin-induced thrombocytopenia, and osteoporosis with prolonged use. Initial heparinization should be

TABLE 20-3. Initial Antithrombotic Therapy for Venous Thromboembolism (VTE) (DVT and PE)

	Unfractionated Heparin	*LMWH Enoxaparin*	*Fondaparinux*
Dose	Loading dose 80 IU/kg, infusion 18 IU/kg/hr	1 mg/kg twice a day or 1.5 mg/kg once a day	5.0 mg subcutaneously
Monitoring	Measure APTT 6 hr after bolus and adjust infusion. Check platelet count every 72 hr	Renal failure, obesity or pregnancy	
Target	APTT level corresponding to anti-Xa 0.3–0.7 U/mL	Anti-Xa 0.6–1.0 U/mL twice daily dosing Anti-Xa 1.0–2.0 U/mL once a day	

DVT, deep venous thrombosis; PE, pulmonary embolism; LMWH, low-molecular-weight heparin; APTT, activated partial thromboplast time.

followed by long-term anticoagulation with oral anticoagulants (48–50).

Low-Molecular-Weight Heparin (LMWH)

A low-molecular-weight heparin (LMWH) is a small heparin fragment whose mechanism of action is similar to that of UFH. LMWH has a more predictable relation between dose and response than UFH and does not need monitoring or adjustments if the dose is based on patient body weight. LMWH, however, has less nonspecific binding to proteins, which results in a longer plasma half-life (4 hours) and a more predictable dose-response relationship. Laboratory monitoring is usually not necessary, but it must be performed with a chromogenic anti-Xa assay (rather than the aPTT measurement) 4 hours after a dose has been given (therapeutic range: 0.6 to 1.0 IU/mL in most laboratories). LMWH is also associated with a lower risk of thrombocytopenia. Its use in DVT and PE is now firmly established: Many trials and meta-analyses have confirmed its superior efficacy, safer profile, and greater cost-effectiveness over UFH (51,52). The introduction of LMWH has advanced antithrombotic therapy by providing effective anticoagulation without the need for monitoring or adjustments. It also allows patients with uncomplicated DVT to be treated in the community, saving an average of 4 to 5 days' admission per patient (48,49).

Fondaparinux

Fondaparinus, antithrombotic agent, is a synthetic pentasaccharide possessing anti-Xa activity. Fondaparinux has been approved by the US Food and Drug Administration (FDA) for the treatment of VTE. It has been found to be as effective as UFH in patients with acute PE who are stable (53). This drug is administered subcutaneously once a day in fixed doses. It does not require dose adjustments. Because this drug is cleared renally, it is contraindicated in patients with severe renal impairment. In addition, in contrast to heparins, fondaparinux is not associated with heparin-induced thrombocytopenia (HIT).

Warfarin

Warfarin is the most widely used oral anticoagulant for treating VTE. Inhibition of γ-carboxylation of the vitamin K-dependent coagulation factors II, VII, IX, and X is the major mode of action for warfarin. Warfarin has excellent gastrointestinal absorption; it is metabolized in the liver and excreted in urine. Prothrombin time (PT) prolongation can begin in 5 to 7 hours after drug administration as a result of the short half-life of factor VII. The full warfarin anticoagulant effect can take as long as 72 hours, which is the half-life of factor II. Warfarin and heparin should be started on the same day, with concomitant administration of these drugs for 4 or 5 days. A target INR range of 2.0 to 3.0 is standard for treatment of VTE. Higher levels tend to increase the risk of bleeding without reducing recurrent thromboembolism. The exception to this is for patients with the antiphospholipid antibody syndrome, where the risk of recurrent VTE is high. In this condition, an INR of 3 to 4.5 is recommended. Warfarin interacts with many other drugs and alcohol. It is also teratogenic and can induce spontaneous abortion (54,55).

HEPARIN-INDUCED THROMBOCYTOPENIA

Patients who have been exposed to UFH and to a much less extent LMWH can develop HIT. This occurs as a result of heparin-dependent immunoglobulin G antibodies directed against heparin platelet factor 4, potentially leading to the development of both arterial and venous thrombosis. This is becoming a very common cause of VTE development postoperatively in critically ill patients, usually after coronary artery bypass grafting and orthopedic surgery. If HIT is suspected, all heparins should be stopped and clinicians have the option to use a direct thrombin inhibitor (DTI), such as lepirudin or argatroban (56).

LONG-TERM ANTICOAGULATION

Warfarin (target INR, 2.0 to 3.0) is the anticoagulant of choice for long-term treatment of most patients with VTE. Oral administration of warfarin results in significant reduction in the risk of recurrent VTE (57). In patients with provoked DVT, the risk of recurrent VTE after discontinuation of warfarin is 1% to 4% per year. Generally, warfarin treatment should be continued for 3 months, some evidence indicates that 6 weeks of treatment is as effective as 3 months in patients with a provoked distal DVT (58).

In patients with unprovoked DVT, major chronic predispositions, or active malignancy, the risk of recurrent VTE after discontinuation of warfarin is substantially higher (at least 5% to 10% per year) than for provoked events (≤4% per year). Decisions regarding the duration of anticoagulant treatment should be individualized by balancing the absolute risk of recurrent VTE with the potential absolute benefits (80% to 90% relative risk reduction) and cumulative risks of bleeding associated with anticoagulation (57).

Most patients with unprovoked DVT should be treated for at least 6 months, and long-term LMWH therapy is more effective than warfarin to prevent recurrent VTE in patients with cancer (59).

Thrombolytic Therapy

Thrombolytic therapy is usually second line therapy for the treatment of VTE. For DVT, thrombolytic therapy has been shown to reduce the incidence of venous insufficiency and seems to be effective in clot dissolution when given locally. Although it is recommended to give thrombolytic therapy in patients with massive PE with hemodynamic compromise (i.e., shock), considerable controversy is seen to extend thrombolytic therapy to patients with hemodynamic stability and various degrees of RV function. The major concern with thrombolytic therapy is the potential for intracranial bleeding, with a reported rate as high as 3% (60). Various multicenter registries and one underpowered prospective study suggest that thrombolytic therapy in submassive PE with RV dysfunction may reduce mortality and the need for escalation of therapy (61–63).

INFERIOR VENA CAVA FILTERS

The role of inferior vena cava (IVC) filters in the management of VTE is simply to prevent the next embolic event from thrombi originating from the lower extremities. Contraindications from antithrombotic therapy, adverse events from anticoagulant therapy, or recurrent embolic events on anticoagulant therapy are the main reasons for IVC filter usage (64). IVC filters are placed prophylactically in patients having pulmonary embolectomy. An analysis from a PE multicenter registry demonstrated a reduced 90-day mortality associated with IVC filter placement (60). Also, IVC filters have been associated with an increased frequency of DVT (65). Complications include central migration of the filter, filter fracture, IVC perforation, and vena cava thrombosis. Numerous types of filters are available, but recently temporary placement or retrievable IVC filters are increasingly being used.

SURGICAL MANAGEMENT

Pulmonary embolectomy is indicated in patients with life-threatening PE. Usually, thrombolytic therapy has failed or the patients have such severe RV function that if another embolic event occurred, it would most likely be fatal. In centers that have developed a multidisciplinary approach to the management of life-threatening PE, pulmonary embolectomy has been shown to be a viable, safe, and effective therapy for these patients (66). Catheter-directed pulmonary embolectomy is an emerging modality for massive PE. This technique uses local mechanical disruption of the clot, usually with local infusion of thrombolytic agent. This is primarily indicated in patients who cannot undergo open surgical embolectomy (25,26).

TREATMENT DURING PREGNANCY

Pulmonary embolism is the most common cause of death during pregnancy. Once PE is diagnosed, heparin should be used. UFU and LMWH do not cross the placenta and have little, if any, effect on the fetus. In contrast, oral anticoagulants cross the placenta and cause fetal hemorrhage and malformations. Pregnant women can be treated with UFH or LMWH until at least 6 weeks postpartum and then warfarin can be started (67).

Clinical Vignette

In the MICU, the patient received intravenous t-PA at 100 mg infused over 2 hours. The patient had a dramatic improvement in oxygenation and a reduction in heart rate. The patient was subsequently treated with LMWH and continued on prolonged anticoagulation therapy.

CLINICAL RECOMMENDATIONS OF THE VIGNETTE

The patient demonstrated severe RV dysfunction. Even with hemodynamic stability, the patient is at risk for early mortality from the embolic event. Therefore, thrombolytic therapy or IVC filter placement in conjunction with adequate anticoagulation should be considered. In addition, this patient will need to be evaluated for possible recurrence of his prostate cancer because this will influence his duration of long-term anticoagulation.

SUMMARY

VTE is common disorder that is encountered in various clinical settings. Awareness of the risk factors for the development of VTE and clinical presentation allow clinicians to risk-stratify these patients, based on laboratory and imaging studies assessing RV function. Based on these findings, appropriate initial therapy can start. Long-term antithrombotic therapy is based on risk of recurrent disease balanced by risk of bleeding. Clinicians must be mindful of the following caveats: (a) Clinical diagnosis of DVT is unreliable and must be confirmed by compression ultrasonography; (b) a low clinical pretest probability of DVT and PE and negative D-dimer result reliably exclude the diagnosis, with no need for further diagnostic imaging; (c) risk-stratification based on the state of RV function is important in PE prognosis; (d) initial treatment of VTE is with LMWH, UFH, or fondaparinux for at least 5 days, followed by warfarin (target INR, 2.0 to 3.0) for at least 3 months; and (e) an IVC filter is indicated in patients ineligible for anticoagulant therapy or who experience embolism despite therapeutic anticoagulation.

REFERENCES

1. Girard P, Sanchez O, Leroyer C, et al.; for the evaluation du scanner spirale dans l'embolie pulmonaire study group. Deep venous thrombosis in patients with acute pulmonary embolism: Prevalence, risk factors, and clinical significance. *Chest.* 2005:128;1593–1600.
2. Meignan M, Rosso J, Gauthier H, et al. Systematic lung scans reveal a high frequency of silent pulmonary embolism in patients with proximal deep venous thrombosis. *Arch Intern Med.* 2000;160:159–164.
3. Anderson FA, Jr., Wheeler HB, Goldberg RJ, et al. A population-based perspective of the hospital incidence and case-fatality rates of deep vein thrombosis and pulmonary embolism. The Worcester DVT Study. *Arch Intern Med.* 1991;151:933–938.
4. Silverstein MD, Heit JA, Mohr DN, et al. Trends in the incidence of deep vein thrombosis and pulmonary embolism: A 25-year population-based study. *Arch Intern Med.* 1998;158: 585–593.

5. Heit JA. The epidemiology of venous thromboembolism in the community: Implications for prevention and management. *J Thromb Thrombolysis.* 2006;21:23–29.
6. Goldhaber SZ. Pulmonary embolism. *N Engl J Med.* 1998;339:93–104.
7. Horlander KT, Leeper KV, Mannino D. Pulmonary embolism mortality in the United States, 1979–1998: An analysis using multiple-cause mortality data. *Arch Intern Med.* 2003;163:1711–1717.
8. Bauer KA. The thrombophilias: Well-defined risk factors with uncertain therapeutic implications. *Ann Intern Med.* 2001;135:367–373.
9. Smeeth L, Cook C, Thomas S, et al. Risk of deep vein thrombosis and pulmonary embolism after acute infection in a community setting. *Lancet.* 2006;367:1075–1079.
10. Lapostolle F, Surget V, Borron SW, et al. Severe pulmonary embolism associated with air travel. *N Engl J Med.* 2001;345:779–783.
11. Schreijer AJ, Cannegieter SC, Meijers JC, et al. Activation of coagulation system during air travel: A crossover study. *Lancet.* 2006;367:832–838.
12. Piazza G, Goldhaber SZ. Acute pulmonary embolism: Epidemiology and diagnosis. *Circulation.* 2006;114;e28–e32.
13. Kearon C. Natural history of venous thromboembolism. *Circulation.* 2003;107:122–130.
14. Hyers TM. Venous thromboembolism. *Am J Respir Crit Care Med.* 1999;159:1–14.
15. Haeger K. Problems of acute deep venous thrombosis. I. The interpretation of signs and symptoms. *Angiology.* 1969;20:219–223.
16. Prandoni P, Lensing AW, Cogo A, et al. The long-term clinical course of acute deep venous thrombosis. *Ann Intern Med.* 1996;125:1–7.
17. Wells PS, Anderson DR, Bormanis J, et al. Value of assessment of pretest probability of deep-vein thrombosis in clinical management. *Lancet.* 1997;350:1795–1798.
18. Bounameaux H, de Moerloose P, Perrier A, et al. Plasma measurement of D-dimer as diagnostic aid in suspected venous thromboembolism: An overview. *Thromb Haemost.* 1994;71:1–6.
19. Stein PD, Hull RD, Patel KC, et al. D-dimer for the exclusion of acute venous thrombosis and pulmonary embolism: A systematic review. *Ann Intern Med.* 2004;140:589–602.
20. Lensing AW, Prandoni P, Brandjes D, et al. Detection of deep-vein thrombosis by real-time B-mode ultrasonography. *N Engl J Med.* 1989;320:342–345.
21. Wells PS, Lensing AW, Davidson BL, et al. Accuracy of ultrasound for the diagnosis of deep venous thrombosis in asymptomatic patients after orthopedic surgery: A meta-analysis. *Ann Intern Med.*. 1995;122:47–53.
22. Turkstra F, Kuijer PM, van Beek EJ, et al. Diagnostic utility of ultrasound of the leg veins in patients suspected of having pulmonary embolism. *Ann Intern Med.* 1997;126:775–781.
23. Carpenter JP, Holland GA, Baum RA, et al. Magnetic resonance venography for the detection of deep venous thrombosis: Comparison with contrast venography and duplex Doppler ultrasonography. *J Vasc Surg.* 1993;18:734–741.
24. Fraser DGW, Moody AR, Morgan PS, et al. Diagnosis of lower-limb deep venous thrombosis: A prospective blinded study of magnetic reasonance direct thrombus imaging. *Ann Intern Med.* 2002;136:89–98.
25. Kucher N, Rossi E, DeRosa M, et al. Massive pulmonary embolism. *Circulation.* 2006; 113:1143–1150.
26. Wood KE. Major pulmonary embolism—Review of a pathophysiologic approach to the golden hour of hemodynamically significant pulmonary embolism. *Chest.* 2002;121:877–905.
27. Stein PD, Terrin ML, Hales CA, et al. Clinical, laboratory, roentgenographic, and electrocardiographic findings in patients with acute pulmonary embolism and no pre-existing cardiac or pulmonary disease. *Chest.* 1991;100:598–603.
28. Piazza G, Goldhaber SZ. Acute pulmonary embolism: Epidemiology and diagnosis. *Circulation.* 2006;114;e28–e32.
29. Wells PS, Anderson Dr, Rodger M, et al. Derivation of a simple clinical model to categorize patients' probability of pulmonary embolism: Increasing the model's utility with SimpliRED D-dimer. *Thromb Haemost.* 2000;83;416–420.
30. Goldhaber SZ. Echocardiography in the management of pulmonary embolism. *Ann Intern Med.* 2002;136:691–700.
31. Daniel KR, Courtney DM, Kline JA. Assessment of cardiac stress from massive pulmonary embolism with 12-lead ECG. *Chest.* 2001;120:474–481.
32. Elliot CG, Goldhaber SZ, Visani L, et al. Chest radiographs in acute pulmonary embolism: Results from the International Cooperative Pulmonary Embolism Registry. *Chest.* 2000:118:33–38.
33. PIOPED investigators. Value of the ventilation/perfusion scan in acute pulmonary embolism. *JAMA.* 1990;95:498–502.
34. Mills SR, Jackson DC, Older RA, et al. The incidence, etiologies and avoidance of complications of pulmonary angiography in a large series. *Radiology.* 1980:136;295–299.
35. Stein, P, Athanasoulis C, Alavi A, et al. Complications and validity of pulmonary angiography in acute pulmonary embolus. *Circulation.* 1992;85:462–468.
36. Garg K, Wesh CH, Feyerabend AJ, et al. Pulmonary embolism: Diagnosis and spiral CT and ventilation-perfusion scanning: Correlation with pulmonary angiographic results or clinical outcome. *Radiology.* 1998;208:201–208.
37. Stein PD and the PIOPED II Investigators. Multi detector computed tomography for acute pulmonary embolism. *N Engl J Med.* 2006;354:2317–2327.
38. Schoeph UJ, Goldhaber SZ, Constello P. Spiral computed tomography for acute pulmonary embolism. *Circulation.* 2004;109:2160–2167.
39. Ost D, Rozenshtein A, Saffran L, et al. The negative predictive value of spiral computed tomography for the diagnosis of pulmonary embolism in patients with nondiagnostic ventilation-perfusion scans. *Am J Med.* 2001;110:16–21.
40. Henry JW, Relya B, Stein PD. Continuing risk of thromboemboli among patients with normal pulmonary angiograms. *Chest.* 1995;107:1375–1378.
41. Tillie-Leblond I, Mastora I, Radenne F, et al. Risk of pulmonary embolism after a negative spiral CT angiogram in patients with pulmonary disease: 1-year clinical followup study. *Radiology.* 2002;223:461–467.
42. Quiroz R, Kucher N, Zou KH, et al. Clinical validity of a negative computed tomography scan in patients with suspected pulmonary embolism: A systemic review. *JAMA.* 2005; 293:2012–2017.
43. Meaney J, Weg JG, Chenevert TL, et al. Diagnosis of pulmonary embolism with magnetic resonance angiography. *N Engl J Med.* 1997;336:1422–1427.
44. Gupta A, Frazer CK, Ferguson JM, et al. Acute pulmonary embolism: Diagnosis with MR angiography. *Radiology.* 1999;210:353–359.
45. Oudkerk M, van Beek EJ, Wielolski P, et al. Comparison of contrast enhanced magnetic resonance angiography and conventional pulmonary angiography for the diagnosis of pulmonary embolism: A prospective study. *Lancet.* 2002;359:1643–1647.
46. Writing Group for the Christopher Study Investigators. Effectiveness of managing suspected pulmonary embolism using an algorithm combining clinical probability, d-dimer testing and computed tomography. *JAMA.* 2006;295:172–179.
47. Buller HR, Agnelli G, Hull RD, et al. Antithrombotic therapy for venous thromboembolic disease; the Seventh ACCP Conference on Antithrombotic and Thrombolytic Therapy. *Chest.* 2004;126[Suppl];411S–428S.
48. Hyers TM, Agnelli G, Hull RD, et al. Antithrombotic therapy for venous thromboembolic disease. *Chest.* 2001;119[Suppl]:176S–193S.
49. Raschke RA, Reilly BM, Guidry JR, et al. The weight-based heparin dosing nomogram compared with a "standard care" nomogram. A randomized controlled trial. *Ann Intern Med.* 1993;119:874–881.
50. Hull RD, Raskob GE, Rosenbloom D, et al. Heparin for 5 days as compared with 10 days in the initial treatment of proximal venous thrombosis. *N Engl J Med.* 1990;322:1260–1264.
51. The Columbus Investigators. Low-molecular-weight heparin in the treatment of patients with venous thromboembolism. *N Engl J Med.* 1997;337:657–662.
52. Simonneau G, Sors H, Charbonnier B, et al. A comparison of low-molecular-weight heparin with unfractionated heparin for acute pulmonary embolism. The THESEE Study Group. Tinzaparine ou Heparine Standard: Evaluations dans l'Embolie Pulmonaire. *N Engl J Med.* 1997;337:663–669.
53. Buller HR, Davidson BL, Decousus H, et al. Subcutaneous fondaparinux versus intravenous unfractionated heparin in the initial treatment of pulmonary embolism. *N Engl J Med.* 2003;349;1695–1702.
54. Hirsh J, Dalen J, Anderson DR, et al. Oral anticoagulants: Mechanism of action, clinical effectiveness, and optimal therapeutic range. *Chest.* 2001;119[Suppl]:8S–21S.
55. Ansell J, Hirsh J, Poller L, et al. The pharmacology and management of the vitamin K antagonist. The Seventh ACCP Conference on Antithrombotic and Thrombolytic Therapy. *Chest.* 2004;126:287S–310S.
56. Warkentin TE, Levine MN, Hirsh J, et al. Heparin-induced thrombocytopenia in patients treated with low-molecular-weight heparin or unfractionated heparin. *N Engl J Med.* 1995;332(20):1330–1335
57. Kearon C. Long term management of patients after venous thromboembolism. *Chest.* 2004;110[Suppl 1]:110–118.
58. Pinede L, Ninet J, Duhaul P, et al. Comparison of 3 and 6 months of oral anticoagulant therapy after a first episode of proximal deep venous thrombosis or pulmonary embolism and comparison 6 and 12 weeks of therapy after isolated calk deep vein thrombosis. *Circulation.* 2001;103:2453–2460.
59. Lee AY, Levine MN, Baker RI, et al. Low-molecular weight heparin versus a coumarin for the prevention of recurrent venous thromboembolism in patients with cancer. *N Engl J Med.* 2003;349:146–153.
60. Goldhaber SZ, Visani L, De Rosa M. Acute pulmonary embolism: Clinical outcomes in the International Cooperative Pulmonary embolism Registry (ICOPER). *Lancet.* 1999;353: 1386–1389.
61. Ribeiro A, Lindmarker P, Juhlin-Dannfelt A, et al. Echocardiography Doppler in pulmonary embolism: Right ventricular dysfunction as a predictor of mortality rate. *Am Heart J.* 1997;134:479–487.
62. Konstantinides S, Geibel A, Olschewski M, et al. Association between thrombolytic treatment and the prognosis of hemodynamically stable patients with major pulmonary embolism: Results of a multicenter registry. *Circulation.* 1997;96:882–888.
63. Konstantinides S, Geibel A, Heusel G, et al. Heparin plus alteplace compared with heparin alone in patients with submassive pulmonary embolism. *N Engl J Med.* 2002;347:1143–1150.
64. Streiff MB. Vena caval filters: A comprehensive review. *Blood.* 2000;95:3669–3677.
65. Decousus H, Leizorovicz A, Parent F, et al. A clinical trial of vena caval filters in the prevention of pulmonary embolism in patients with proximal deep-vein thrombosis. Prevention du Risque d'Embolie Pulmonaire par Interruption Cave Study Group. *N Engl J Med.* 1998;338:409–415.
66. Leacche M, Unic D, Goldhaber SZ, et al. Modern surgical treatment of massive pulmonary embolism: Results in 47 consecutive patients after rapid diagnosis and aggressive surgical approach. *J Thorac Cardiovasc Surg.* 2005;129(5):1018–1023.
67. Bates SM, Greer IA, Hirsh J, et al. Use of antithrombotic agents during pregnancy: The Seventh ACCP Conference on Antithrombotic and Thrombolytic Therapy. *Chest.* 2004;126: 627S–644S.

CHAPTER **21**

Lung Cancer

Peter I. Mazzone • Samuel T. Chao • John H. Suh

Paraneoplastic Neurologic Syndromes

OBJECTIVES

- To discuss what is meant by a paraneoplastic neurologic syndrome
- To list a few of the most common paraneoplastic neurologic syndromes
- To explain the proposed pathogenesis of the most common paraneoplastic neurologic syndromes
- To describe the presentation of the most common paraneoplastic neurologic syndromes
- To outline an approach to the diagnosis of a paraneoplastic neurologic syndrome
- To discuss the principles of treatment of paraneoplastic neurologic syndromes

CASE VIGNETTE

A 64-year-old man presents for evaluation of progressive neurologic symptoms. Two months ago, he noted minor changes in the sensation of his right leg, which has become more pronounced over time. Over the past 1 to 2 weeks, he has noticed unsteadiness and occasional double vision. His family comments that he has become irritable and forgetful. He does not describe other cardiopulmonary or systemic symptoms. His medical history is significant for mild chronic obstructive pulmonary disease (COPD). He is an active smoker.

On examination, a sensory deficit is noted over the lateral lower right leg. He has mild muscle weakness of the leg as well. He is ataxic and has nystagmus. The rest of his general examination is unremarkable.

DEFINITION

Paraneoplastic neurologic syndromes (PNS) are neurologic disorders caused by the presence of malignancy, but not by the direct effects of the tumor or its metastases. A PNS can affect any part of the nervous system, from the central nervous system (CNS) through the neuromuscular junction (NMJ) and muscles.

Many PNS exist. All are relatively uncommon. Following will be outlined the most common PNS associated with lung cancer, including the spectrum of paraneoplastic encephalomyelitis syndromes, cancer-associated retinopathy (CAR), and the Lambert-Eaton myasthenic syndrome (LEMS).

EPIDEMIOLOGY

Individuals with lung cancer who develop a PNS most likely have small cell lung cancer (SCLC). An estimated 174,770 new lung cancer cases was diagnosed in the United States in 2006 (1). Of these, approximately 20% or 35,000 cases will be small cell carcinomas. Most of these individuals are active or former smokers.

The incidence of PNS in lung cancer is difficult to specify because it varies, based on the definition of the syndrome and the population studied. For example, individuals with lung cancer may have a measurable autoantibody known to be associated with a PNS yet not have clinical manifestations of the syndrome (2,3). Thus, if the incidence was reported based on the presence of the clinical syndrome, it would be much lower than if it was reported based on the presence of the autoantibody. With this in mind, the incidence of PNS in small cell carcinoma of the lung has been reported to be approximately 4% (4).

The paraneoplastic encephalomyelitis syndromes (sensory neuropathy, limbic encephalitis, cerebellar degeneration, and opsoclonus-myoclonus [OM]) are very uncommon (5). Paraneoplastic encephalomyelitis or sensory motor neuropathy (the "anti-Hu" syndrome) was identified in 73 of 3,500 individuals who had specimens submitted with the clinical suspicion of a PNS (2.1%) (6). Of these, 56 had lung cancer. CAR is also very rare. The LEMS has variably been reported to be the most common PNS, with an incidence of up to 3% in SCLC when studies systematically searched for it (7,8). In population-based studies, the incidence of LEMS has been reported to be as low as 0.4% (9). Many of these neurologic syndromes can occur in individuals without an underlying tumor as well (i.e., an idiopathic form).

ETIOLOGY AND PATHOGENESIS

Paraneoplastic neurologic syndromes appear to be mediated by autoimmune mechanisms. Tumor-related antigens share similarities with antigens throughout the central and peripheral nervous systems. Antibodies directed against the tumor antigens cross-react with their counterparts in the nervous system, which can result in dysfunction by producing inflammatory changes, or blocking key neural activities. The manifestations

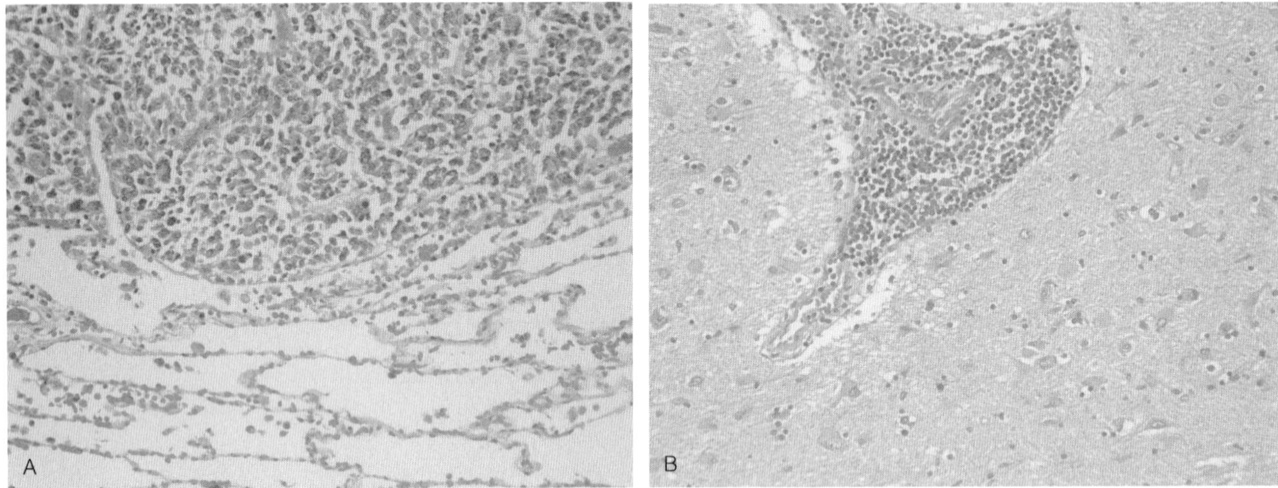

FIGURE 21-1. Pathology from the autopsy of a 69-year-old who presented with seizures. **(A)** A lung cancer was found. The picture demonstrates a mixed small cell–large cell carcinoma (H+E staining at 200 × magnification). **(B)** A section through the temporal lobe is marked by chronic perivascular inflammation consisting mostly of lymphocytes with surrounding reactive astrocytosis consistent with a paraneoplastic encephalomyelitis (H+E staining at 200× magnification). Courtesy of Dr. Richard Prayson.

of these syndromes vary depending on the location of the cross-reacting neural antigens (10). Many different onconeural antibodies have been identified (see Section VIII). Some are directed against neural nuclear targets, others neural cytoplasmic targets, and others at nerve terminals (11,12). Each antibody has different tissue sensitivity (12). In some syndromes, the pathogenic role of the antibody is well defined. For example, in LEMS IgG antibodies against P/Q type voltage-gated calcium channels are found. These antibodies block channels responsible for the influx of calcium into cells, which is required for the release of acetylcholine. Thus, the presence of these antibodies can result in a depletion of neurotransmitters at the neuromuscular junction (13–15). On the other hand, the pathogenic role of the antinuclear antibodies is less well defined. They are felt to trigger a cytotoxic T-cell response in the reacting tissues, but immunotherapies have not been consistently effective in treating these syndromes (6,16). The rapidity of production, persistence of immune stimulation, and production of antibodies directly within the CNS have been described as explanations for the lack of response to immunotherapies.

PATHOLOGY

PARANEOPLASTIC ENCEPHALOMYELITIS SYNDROMES

Pathology is not typically obtained outside of postmortem examinations in individuals with a paraneoplastic encephalomyelitis syndrome. In paraneoplastic limbic encephalitis (PLE), pathology has been reported to show lymphocytic interstitial infiltrates, microglial proliferation, gliosis, and neuronal degeneration (5,17,18). In paraneoplastic cerebellar degeneration (PCD), the cerebellum is macroscopically atrophic. Inflammatory infiltrates and perivascular lymphocytic cuffing occur, usually with sparing of the cerebellar cortex. Severe and sometimes total loss of Purkinje cells is seen (19,20). In OM, mild patchy or diffuse perivascular lymphocytic infiltrates have been reported. Loss of Purkinje cells and olivary neurons is also reported (20,21). In the encephalomyelitis or sensory motor neuropathy syndrome neuronal loss, reactive gliosis, hyperplasia of the microglia, and lymphocytic infiltration is seen. The location of these changes within the CNS and PNS varies from patient to patient. Other findings include dorsal root ganglionitis with destruction of ganglion cells and anterior horn myelitis with destruction of alpha motor neurons. Both B and T cells are involved, with CD4 cells predominating around the vessels and CD8 cytotoxic T-lymphocytes within the parenchyma (20,22) (Fig. 21-1).

CANCER-ASSOCIATED RETINOPATHY

Pathologic findings in CAR include photoreceptor degeneration with loss, predominantly of rods, relative sparing of cones, and scattered melanin laden macrophages in the outer retinal layers. Other retinal layers, the optic nerve, and vasculature are not affected. A large inflammatory component has not been recognized (20,23).

LAMBERT-EATON MYASTHENIC SYNDROME

Little has been reported about the pathology of the LEMS. Elongation of the postsynaptic membrane of the NMJ and an increase in the number of acetylcholine receptors have been reported (24). Type II muscle fiber atrophy is noted (25). In individuals with combined cerebellar degeneration and LEMS, a reduction in P/Q-type voltage-gated calcium channels in the cerebellar molecular layer has been described (26).

CLINICAL MANIFESTATIONS

The clinical manifestations of PNS often develop before the identification of the tumor (4,27). Symptoms and signs vary,

TABLE 21-1. Presentation of the Most Common Paraneoplastic Neurologic Syndromes

Paraneoplastic Neurologic Syndrome	*Symptoms*
PARANEOPLASTIC ENCEPHALOMYELITIS SYNDROMES	
Paraneoplastic limbic encephalitis	Mood and behavior changes Memory problems Seizures
Paraneoplastic cerebellar degeneration	Ataxia, nystagmus, dysarthria, diplopia
Opsoclonus-myoclonus	Involuntary rapid conjugate eye movements Myoclonus, truncal ataxia, dysarthria Encephalopathy
Encephalomyelitis subacute sensory or motor neuropathy syndrome	Sensory and motor neuropathies Symptoms of any of the above syndromes
CANCER-ASSOCIATE RETINOPATHY	Rapid vision loss, night blindness, color loss, central or ring scotomas
LAMBERT-EATON MYASTHENIC SYNDROME	Proximal muscle weakness (lower extremities > upper), increased strength with exercise, fatigue, slurred speech, difficulty chewing and swallowing Autonomic manifestations

depending on the location of the cross-reacting antigen and the function of its target (Table 21-1).

PARANEOPLASTIC ENCEPHALOMYELITIS SYNDROMES

Paraneoplastic Limbic Encephalitis

Individuals with PLE present with subacute changes in their mood and behavior, memory problems that progress to dementia, and occasionally seizures. These manifestations progress over the course of weeks to months (5,18,28). Individuals with PLE and high titer type-1 antineuronal nuclear antibody (ANNA-1) are more likely to develop additional neurologic manifestations (see below) over time than those without detectable ANNA-1 (29,30).

Paraneoplastic Cerebellar Degeneration

The presentation of PCD includes ataxia, nystagmus, dysarthria, and diplopia. Symptoms typically progress over the course of weeks to months, ultimately limiting a person's ability to ambulate. If ANNA-1 is present, the patient is more likely to be female, develop extracerebellar manifestations, and have severe disability and progressive manifestations (19).

Opsoclonus-Myoclonus

Involuntary rapid conjugate eye movements, myoclonus, truncal ataxia, dysarthria, and encephalopathy are the predominant clinical features of OM (31). The course tends to be monophasic. Those with the paraneoplastic form tend to be older than those with idiopathic OM (31).

Encephalomyelitis Subacute Sensory or Motor Neuropathy Syndrome (the Anti-Hu Antibody Syndrome)

Individuals with the encephalomyelitis subacute sensory or motor neuropathy syndrome present with a sensory neuropathy or one of the above manifestations of encephalomyelitis. The most frequent signs and symptoms at presentation include sensory neuropathy (55% to 74%), cerebellar degeneration (15% to 22%), limbic encephalitis (15% to 20%), and brainstem encephalitis (14% to 16%) (6,30). They typically progress to a diffuse encephalomyelopathy with peripheral nervous system deficits (4,27). Autonomic dysfunction occurs in 10% to 23% of afflicted individuals with gastrointestinal motility disorders in 14% (6,30). Sensory neuropathies are more common than mixed somatic and autonomic neuropathies. Motor peripheral neuropathies manifest in up to 20% of those affected (30).

CANCER-ASSOCIATED RETINOPATHY

Clinical features of the CAR syndrome include rapid loss of vision, night blindness, color loss, and central or ring scotomas. The loss of visual acuity can be asymmetric. Vitreous cells, disc pallor, and arteriole narrowing are noted on examination (32).

LAMBERT-EATON MYASTHENIC SYNDROME

The LEMS is characterized by proximal muscle weakness. The weakness affects the lower extremities more than the upper. A transient increase in strength with exercise can be seen. Autonomic features, such as dry mouth, dry eyes, blurred vision, constipation, orthostasis, erectile dysfunction, and ptosis, are common. Fatigue, decreased deep muscle stretch reflexes, slurred speech, and difficulty chewing and swallowing are other frequent findings (25,33,34). Those with LEMS related to a tumor are more likely to be male, older, and have a more progressive course than individuals with idiopathic LEMS (33). No differences are seen in the clinical presentation of those with LEMS and the anti-P/Q-type voltage gated calcium channel (VGCC) antibody and those without (35).

DIAGNOSTIC APPROACH

Recognizing the clinical manifestations outlined above is the first step in the diagnostic approach to all of the PNS. Further testing can help to confirm the clinical suspicion. While confirming the presence of a PNS, a search for an underlying tumor is frequently required because the PNS is often the first manifestation of the tumor. Chest computed tomography (CT) has been used with more success than chest x-ray studies (CXR) (36). [^{18}F]Fluorodeoxyglucose positron emission tomography (FDG-PET) imaging has also been successful in uncovering a hidden malignancy (37). In individuals with compatible symptoms, the presence of an onconeural antibody and negative conventional imaging, FDG-PET imaging has been reported to be 83% sensitive and 25% specific in identifying an underlying tumor (38).

PARANEOPLASTIC ENCEPHALOMYELITIS SYNDROMES

Paraneoplastic Limbic Encephalitis

Computed tomography imaging of the brain is often unrevealing in PLE. Magnetic resonance imaging (MRI) frequently shows increased T2 signal in the limbic system (6) (Fig. 21-2). FDG-PET has shown hypermetabolism in the medial temporal lobe (39). The cerebrospinal fluid (CSF) can be normal or demonstrate a mononuclear pleocytosis, elevated protein level, increased IgG synthesis, and oligoclonal bands (5,18,28). An electroencephalogram (EEG) often demonstrates generalized slowing, a temporal epileptic focus, or periodic lateralized epileptiform discharges (5,18,28). An ANNA may be found in the serum in 50% to 80% of the patients (5,29).

Paraneoplastic Cerebellar Degeneration

Abnormal imaging studies are found in fewer than 50% of patients with PCD. Periventricular white matter changes and abnormal T2 signal on MRI have been noted. The CSF will often appear inflammatory (19). High titer ANNA can be found in up to half of the individuals diagnosed (19).

Opsoclonus-Myoclonus

Neuroimaging can show areas of increased T2 signal on the MRI. The CSF can reveal a mild pleocytosis, elevated protein, and, occasionally, oligoclonal bands. The EEG can be normal or reveal diffuse, severe, background slowing (21). It is uncommon to identify immune markers in the blood in OM, but ANNA-1 and antiamphiphysin antibodies have been reported (31).

Encephalomyelitis Subacute Sensory or Motor Neuropathy Syndrome (the Anti-Hu Antibody Syndrome)

Neuroimaging, CSF analysis, and EEG findings in encephalomyelitis subacute sensory or motor neuropathy syndrome (anti-Hu antibody syndrome) can be similar to the paraneoplastic encephalomyelitis syndromes detailed above. Any one or all of these syndromes can be present in addition to peripheral sensory and motor neuropathies. The most common immune marker is the ANNA-1 (anti-Hu antibody). Low-titer ANNA-1 has been found in 16% of patients with small cell carcinoma who do not have a PNS (40). The ANNA-1 titer is considered high or positive when it is above 1:10,000 serum dilutions by immunoblot of recombinant Hu proteins (4,41). Following the ANNA-1 titers over time has not been found to be useful for predicting outcomes (42).

Other antibodies have been identified with lower frequency in these syndromes, typically associated with small cell carcinoma. The presence of a particular antibody is not specific for a given presentation. Symptoms can include any or all of those described above, depending on the area of the nervous system

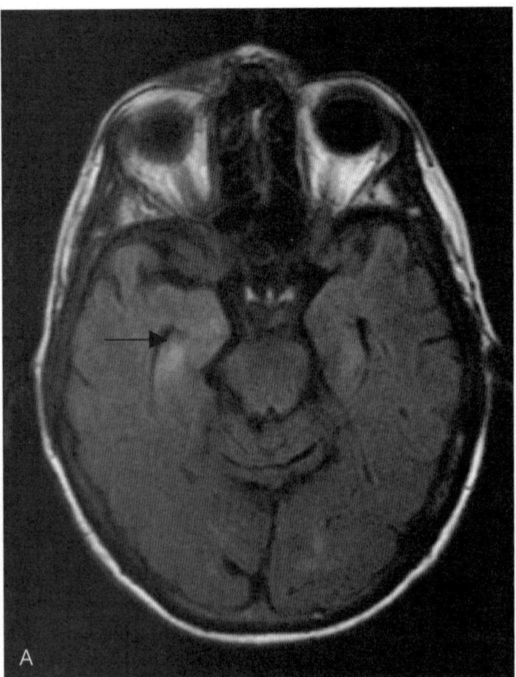

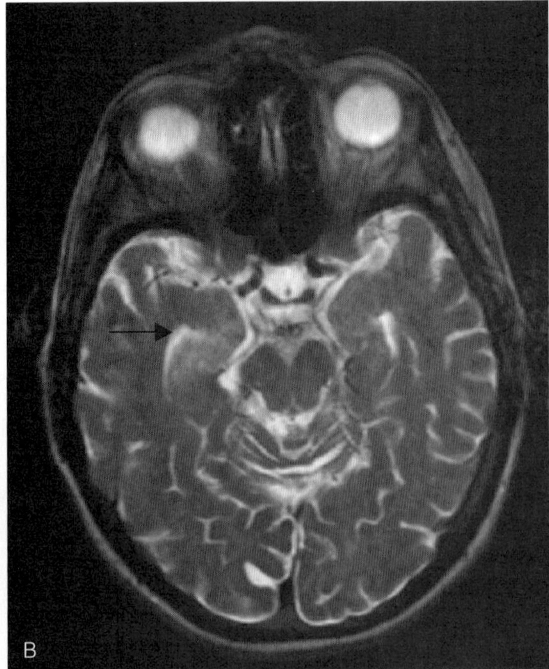

FIGURE 21-2. Increased signal (*arrow*) in the right hippocampal area on FLAIR (**A**) and T2 (**B**) images compatible with limbic encephalitis.

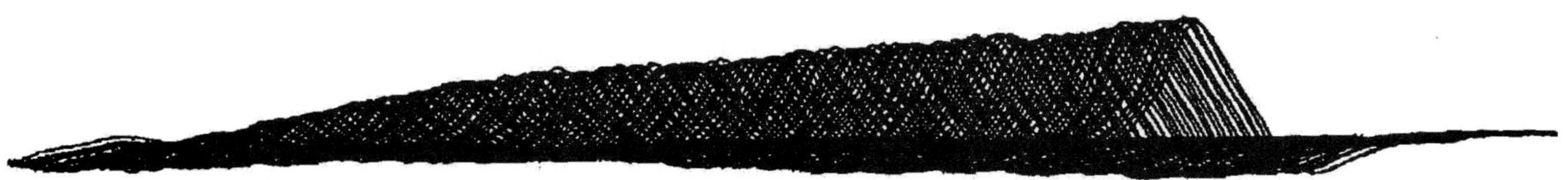

FIGURE 21-3. Repetitive stimulation at 40 Hz of the right abductor digiti minimi during electromyography showing a decrease in baseline muscle action potential (0.2 mV) with an increase in action potential with repeated stimulation (1.3 mV at stimulus 200). There was a 471% increase in amplitude, which is compatible with a severe Lambert-Eaton myasthenic syndrome. Courtesy of Dr. Kamal Chemali.

most affected. Symptoms, in addition to those listed above, such as movement disorders and sleep disorders, have been reported with other onconeural antibodies. Examples of antibodies reported include ANNA-2, ANNA-3, anti-Ma2, collapsing response-mediator protein-5, amphiphysin, Purkinje cell cytoplasmic antibody-2, anti-CV2, and anti-BR serine or threonine kinase 2 (6,12,43–45). Thus, if screening for a paraneoplastic encephalomyelitis syndrome, measuring a panel of antibodies may be more useful than focusing on ANNA-1 alone.

CANCER-ASSOCIATED RETINOPATHY

The triad of ring scotomata, photosensitivity, and decreased retinal arteriole caliber suggests the presence of CAR. An electroretinogram will show flat or greatly reduced amplitudes. Fluorescein angiography will reveal leakage from retinal vessels, mottling of retinal pigment epithelium, and a window defect through altered retinal pigment epithelium or along the retinal vessels (46). Autoantibodies to retinal proteins can be detected in the serum. The most common is the antirecoverin antibody, which is directed against the photoreceptor-specific 23-kd protein recoverin (23,47). This antibody has been detected in low titer in up to 10% of individuals with small cell carcinoma who do not have other features of CAR (2,3). Other antibodies have been reported in case reports of patients with CAR (48).

LAMBERT-EATON MYASTHENIC SYNDROME

Testing with electromyography will show a decrease in baseline muscle action potential with an increase in action potential with repeated stimulation in patients with LEMS (Fig. 21-3). MRI may show an increased T2 signal in scattered regions (49). Measurement of IgG antibodies against P/Q type VGCC in the serum is a very sensitive test in paraneoplastic LEMS. Elevated levels have been found in individuals with small cell carcinoma without manifestations of LEMS (50,51). An inverse relationship has been reported between the antibody titer and disease severity (50). The edrophonium test may be minimally positive in LEMS. The response is weaker than seen in myasthenia gravis (8). An association between non–tumor-related LEMS and HLAB8 has been found. A history of smoking and testing that suggests the patient is HLAB8 negative should lead to a search for a tumor (52). Additional onconeural antibodies have been identified in paraneoplastic LEMS, such as the antiglial nuclear antibody (53).

TREATMENT AND PROGNOSIS

Treatment of the patient with PNS focuses on removing the immune stimulus by treating the underlying tumor and attempting to suppress the immune response felt to be driving the syndrome. These strategies are variably effective.

PARANEOPLASTIC ENCEPHALOMYELITIS SYNDROMES

Little is reported about treatment responses in patients with PLE. Individuals with PLE who are ANNA-1 positive are less likely to respond to therapy and more likely to die because of their neurologic syndrome than of the cancer itself (29,30). For PCD, neither treatment of the tumor nor the use of immune-modulating therapy has been shown to alter the course of the illness. Those with PCD have a shorter survival than those who do not have the syndrome. Those with PCD who are ANNA-1 positive are more likely to die of progressive neurologic dysfunction than those with PCD who are ANNA-1 negative (19). In OM, treatment of the underlying tumor leads to a partial or complete recovery from the neurologic syndrome. Treatment with corticosteroids, plasmapheresis, and intravenous immunoglobulins has been tried without success (21,31). The paraneoplastic manifestations of the encephalomyelitis or sensory motor neuropathy syndrome can stabilize with a complete response of the tumor to therapy. Treatment directed at modulation of the immune response has not been successful (5,54). The tumors in these patients appear to be more indolent than in those without the syndrome (4,54). Death can result from progression of the neurologic dysfunction. Survival has been reported to be 64% at 3 months and 22% at 3 years (6). Those with low-titer antibodies and no neurologic manifestations are more likely to have limited stage disease, a complete response to therapy, and a longer survival (40).

CANCER-ASSOCIATED RETINOPATHY

Treatment of the primary tumor appears to have little effect on the progression of CAR. Immune-modulating therapy with corticosteroids has been modestly effective (23,32). The prognosis is poor, with most cases progressing to blindness over several months.

LAMBERT-EATON MYASTHENIC SYNDROME

Treatment of the primary tumor usually leads to improvement in patients with the LEMS. Other therapies that have proved beneficial include immunosuppression with corticosteroids and azathioprine, plasma exchange, and intravenous immunoglobulin. In addition, 3,4-diaminopyridine, a drug known to promote the release of acetylcholine from presynaptic terminals, has been helpful (55–58). Anticholinesterase drugs do not have much effect on the symptoms of LEMS (8).

The prognosis for patients with the LEMS and small cell carcinoma has been reported to be better than in those without

LEMS. The autoimmune response may be able to retard tumor growth (59). The prognosis is better in those who are HLAB8 positive (52).

CLINICAL RECOMMENDATIONS OF THE VIGNETTE

The patient's clinical presentation is suggestive of a systemic syndrome, particularly a PNS. Testing should include brain imaging with an MRI scan, an EEG, a lumbar puncture, and an electromyography/nerve conduction study (EMG/NCS). Laboratory evaluation could include sending serum for a panel of antibodies, particularly ANNA-1. At the same time, chest imaging with a CT scan should be performed to look for an underlying malignancy. If this is negative, a PET scan could be considered.

If testing confirms the presence of the paraneoplastic encephalomyelitis or sensory motor neuropathy syndrome, the primary treatment will be directed at the underlying tumor (likely, a small cell carcinoma of the lung).

SUMMARY

Paraneoplastic neurologic syndromes are uncommon manifestations of lung cancer. They result from the body's immune response to a tumor antigen that resembles a neurologic antigen. The manifestations depend on the site of the cross-reacting antigen within the nervous system. By recognizing the clinical presentation of these syndromes, direct diagnostic testing can be done to confirm their presence while uncovering the underlying malignancy. In general, treatment of the primary tumor tends to be the best treatment of the PNS.

Brain Metastases

OBJECTIVES

- To define brain metastases
- To describe the clinical manifestations and necessary workup for brain metastases, particularly from lung cancer
- To explain the factors that can affect prognosis, such as age, control of primary disease, no extracranial disease, and performance status
- To discuss treatment options available, especially for patients with brain metastases from lung cancer
- To describe the role of prophylactic cranial irradiation in the preventing brain metastases from lung cancer

CASE VIGNETTE

A 57-year-old woman was found in her car confused. She was brought to the local emergency room. MRI showed a ring-enhancing lesion in the right parietal lobe measuring 2.5 cm in diameter. She was admitted to the hospital. A CT scan of the chest, abdomen, and pelvis showed a 2.6-cm spiculated mass in the right upper lobe, with mediastinal and hilar adenopathy. She had no other evidence of metastatic disease. She had bronchoscopy with fine-needle aspiration of a lymph node, revealing adenocarcinoma. She was started on dexamethasone (4 mg twice a day). During her hospitalization, her confusion resolved. Her Karnofsky performance status is currently 80. Her physical examination is negative for any neurologic deficits. How should this patient's brain metastasis be handled?

DEFINITION

Brain metastasis is spread to the brain from a primary malignancy outside of the CNS.

EPIDEMIOLOGY

Brain metastasis is the most common neurologic complication of cancer, afflicting 170,000 patients in the United States yearly (60), and it accounts for 10% of the annual cancer diagnoses (61). Recently, the incidence has been on the rise because of better imaging techniques with MRI and CT, greater awareness among physicians, and improved survival from the primary cancer because of advances in cancer treatment (62).

In non-small cell lung cancer (NSCLS), the brain is the first site of metastases in 30% of individuals, with 50% eventually developing brain metastases (63). Stage has an impact on the incidence of brain metastases. In NSCLC, the incidence of brain metastasis detected by MRI was 0% in patients with N0, 5.2% in N1, and 4.7% in N2 disease, according to one study (64). Adenocarcinoma metastasizes more frequently than squamous cell carcinoma (65). The first failure rate in patients with squamous cell carcinoma was 8% and 16% in patients with adenocarcinoma (66). In SCLC, approximately 60% of patients develop metastases to the brain (67).

ETIOLOGY AND PATHOGENESIS

These tumors tend to arise from hematogenous spread to watershed areas in the brain and the gray–white matter junction. The distribution tends to coincide with the size and blood supply in these areas. Approximately 85% form in the cerebral hemispheres, whereas 10% to 15% form in the cerebellum (68). Less commonly, they involve the brainstem. They are often spherical and well-demarcated. Symptoms develop from displacement of normal brain parenchyma and associated edema.

PATHOLOGY

The most common primary tumors responsible for brain metastasis are lung cancers, breast cancers, and melanomas. Less commonly, brain metastasis can also arise from renal cell carcinomas, gynecologic cancers, sarcomas, and cancers of the gastrointestinal (GI) tract. It is estimated that 40.5% of all brain metastases arise from lung cancers, 18.6% from breast cancers, and 9.5% from melanomas (61).

CLINICAL MANIFESTATIONS

Because of staging a workup, which may include a CT or MRI of the brain, some brain metastases are found asymptomatically. For instance, in one series, 13.6% of patients evaluated with NSCLC were found to have an abnormal brain scan on staging CT (69). When symptoms do develop, they include headaches, nausea and vomiting, sensory changes, focal weakness, mental changes, cranial nerve dysfunction, seizures, ataxia, and aphasia (70). Table 21-2 summarizes data presented by Le Chevalier et al. (71) and lists the percentages of patients presenting

TABLE 21-2. Presentation of Individuals with Brain Metastases

Symptoms	*% of cases*
Headache/vomiting	64
Focal weakness/motor deficit	58
Behavioral and mental changes	42
Seizures	30
Sensory deficit	24
Aphasia	18
Cranial nerve dysfunction	16
Cerebellar syndrome	14

(From Le Chevalier T, Smith FP, Caille P, et al. Sites of primary malignancies in patients presenting with cerebral metastases: A review of 120 cases. *Cancer.* 1985;56(4):880–882, with permission.)

with these symptoms. Cerebellar lesions, which are highly symptomatic, may manifest in a wide and staggering gait, poor coordination, and nystagmus (70).

Metastatic brain tumors can also hemorrhage and present with the symptoms of stroke. Brain metastases from renal cell carcinoma, choriocarcinoma, melanoma, and bronchogenic carcinoma are those most likely to hemorrhage. Symptoms of hemorrhage include headache, obtundation, and confusion (70).

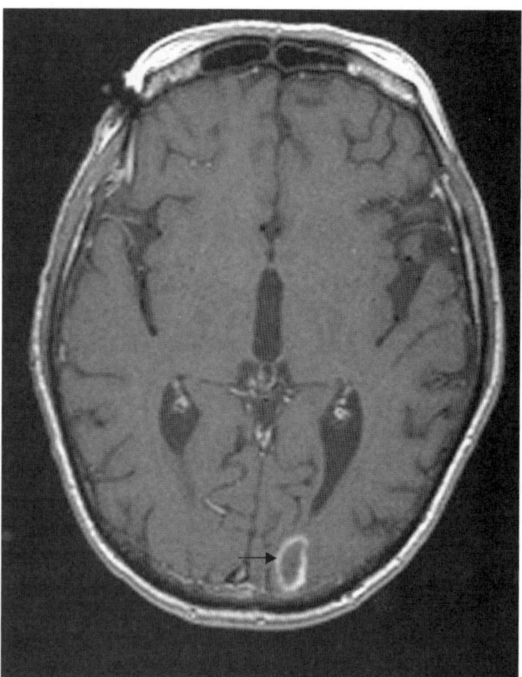

FIGURE 21-4. Magnetic resonance image (MRI) of the brain showing a metastases from a non-small cell carcinoma of the lung (*arrow*).

DIAGNOSTIC APPROACH

Differential diagnoses include primary brain tumors, granulomas, demyelinating lesions, infarction, paraneoplastic syndromes, and encephalitis (70). A diagnosis of brain metastasis can be made by MRI, which demonstrates a ring-enhancing lesion (Fig. 21-4) in addition to the presence of a primary tumor. In up to one third of the cases (72), no primary tumor was found and a diagnosis was made only with a biopsy or resection of the brain tumor.

TREATMENT

Prognostic factors have implications on treatment decision-making. They include the histology of the primary cancer, control of the primary cancer, extent of extracranial disease, medical comorbidity, age, and performance status. For brain metastases, the Karnofsky performance status (KPS) is often used to measure performance status (Table 21-3) (73). Gaspar et al. (74) grouped patients in order to predict survival and performed recursive partitioning analysis (RPA) using data from three randomized Radiation Therapy Oncology Group (RTOG) studies. RPA class I patients have a KPS of $\geq$70, age $<$65 years, controlled primary cancer, and no extracranial metastases. In that group, median survival was 7.1 months. RPA class III patients have a KPS $<$70 and they had a median survival of 2.3 months. All other patients are grouped into RPA class II and had a median survival of 4.2 months. These factors were consistent, despite histology, including NSCLC and SCLC (75). Gender as a prognostic factor in brain metastases was studied specifically in those patients with NSCLC, showing better survival in females (76).

TABLE 21-3. Karnofsky Performance Status

KPS	*Description*
100	Normal, no complaints; no evidence of disease
90	Able to carry on normal activity; minor symptoms of disease
80	Normal activity with effort; some signs or symptoms of disease
70	Cares for self; unable to carry on normal activity or do active work
60	Requires occasional assistance, but is able to care for most needs
50	Requires considerable assistance and frequent medical care
40	Disabled; requires special care and assistance
30	Severely disabled; hospitalization is indicated, although death not imminent
20	Very sick; hospitalization necessary; active supportive treatment is necessary
10	Moribund; fatal processes progressing rapidly
0	Dead

(From Karnofsky D, Abelman W, Craver L, et al. The use of nitrogen mustards in the palliative treatment of carcinoma. *Cancer.* 1948;1:634–656, with permission.)

These prognostic factors are useful to those treating brain metastases; patients expected to do well may benefit with more aggressive treatment, but those expected to do poorly may be treated more conservatively.

MEDICAL MANAGEMENT

Medical management of brain metastasis involves controlling brain edema and seizures. Brain edema from brain metastasis is usually vasogenic in origin and results from a disruption in the blood–brain barrier by the tumor. Brain edema increases intracranial pressure, and can result in herniation and disruption of the local blood supply (77). Because of these effects, brain edema is responsible for most of the signs and symptoms of brain metastases. Treatment for intracranial edema involves steroids, commonly dexamethasone. The typical dose is 16 mg in four divided doses. Average life expectancy is extended from 1 to 2 months without any treatment, to between 2 and 2.5 months with steroids alone (78).

Adverse effects from steroids include Cushingoid face, weight gain, hirsutism, acne, steroid myopathy, psychotic reactions, neuropsychologic impairment, ulceration and perforation of the GI tract, opportunistic infections, osteoporosis, and visual problems, including blurring, glaucoma, and cataract formation (79). As such, only the minimally effective dose should be used for the shortest period of time. Although controversial, some physicians prescribe histamine receptor antagonists (H2-blockers), proton pump inhibitors, or other antiulcer medications as prophylaxis for gastritis and gastrointestinal ulceration. Some patients develop withdrawal symptoms after discontinuing steroid treatment. Withdrawal symptoms include headaches, lethargy, weakness, shortness of breath, orthostatic hypotension, dizziness, anorexia, and diffuse arthralgias and myalgias (79,80). Many of these symptoms mimic worsening brain metastasis, and workup is often necessary to rule out progressive disease. Although rare, emergency therapy for edema includes hyperventilation to induce cerebral vasoconstriction and osmotherapy with mannitol to drive the movement of fluid back into the blood vessels.

Seizure is another common manifestation of brain metastasis and is the presenting symptom in 30% of patients with brain metastasis (71). Treatment for seizures involves anticonvulsants, such as levetiracetam, phenytoin, carbamazepine, phenobarbital, and valproic acid. It is important to note that phenytoin induces the cytochrome P450 system and increases the clearance of dexamethasone. Likewise, dexamethasone increases the clearance of phenytoin by the same mechanism (80). Prophylactic treatment with anticonvulsants is controversial because of their potential adverse effects. In addition, published data suggest no benefit to prophylaxis with anticonvulsants (79).

WHOLE BRAIN RADIOTHERAPY

Whole brain radiotherapy (WBRT) is the most common treatment for brain metastasis. WBRT delivers fractionated radiation to the entire brain and treats not only the known brain tumor, but also any micrometastases or other metastases not detected on imaging. Radiation is from a linear accelerator or, less frequently, cobalt-60 source. A typical dosage scheme delivers a total of 37.5 Gy in 15 fractions over 3 weeks or 30 Gy in 10 fractions over 2 weeks, although other schemes can be used (81). The acute adverse effects of radiotherapy can include mild fatigue, alopecia, and erythema. More chronic effects can include dementia and short-term memory loss (82). Radiation necrosis, focal necrosis of tissue from radiation, is a very rare complication of WBRT. WBRT alone has been shown to increase average life expectancy to between 3 and 6 months (82).

To increase the effectiveness of radiation in the treatment of brain metastases, radiation sensitizers, agents that potentiate the therapeutic effects of radiation (83), are being developed and researched. Typically, effectiveness is achieved in one of two ways. One approach is to increase the oxygenation of the tumor cells, which promotes fixation of DNA damage caused by radiation. Second is to have an agent that is preferentially incorporated into tumor cells, making them more sensitive to radiation.

Two radiosensitizers have shown promise in the treatment of brain metastasis. Efaproxiral, known previously as RSR13, is an allosteric modifier of hemoglobin. This facilitates the release of oxygen, especially in hypoxic tissues such as tumor. The main toxicity is hypoxemia. In a phase II study, patients were found to have a median survival of 6.4 months (84). This was greater than patients in the RTOG database with a median survival of 4.1 months. These encouraging results led to a phase III study, which compared WBRT and supplemental oxygen with efaproxiral with WBRT and supplemental oxygen (85). The median survival of patients receiving efaproxiral was 5.26 months compared with 4.47 months in patients not receiving the drug ($p = 0.17$). Although this was not significant, subgroup analysis showed that patients with breast cancer with brain metastasis had a significant improvement in survival. The patients with breast cancer who received efaproxiral had a median survival of 8.67 months, which was greater than the control which had a median survival of 4.57 months ($p = 0.006$). A confirmatory study has been completed [ENRICH (ENhancing whole brain Radiation In patients with breast Cancer and Hypoxic brain metastases)].

In patients with lung cancer, the lack of pulmonary reserve that characterizes them has implications on the dose of efaproxiral that can be given. Hypoxemia, to which patients with lung cancer patients are sensitive, necessitated dose reductions in the phase III study. This dose reduction may be responsible for its lack of efficacy in patients with brain metastases from lung cancer (86).

Motexafin gadolinium is another radiosensitizer being investigated. This agent is a redox modulator that preferentially localizes to tumor cells. It oxidizes reducing metabolites, thus increasing reactive oxygen species, allowing for greater fixation of radiation damage. The main toxicities are reversible liver toxicity and green skin discoloration. This was studied in a phase III trial of 401 patients where patients were randomized to WBRT with motexafin gadolinium or WBRT alone (87). Patients receiving motexafin gadolinium had a median survival of 5.2 months and those receiving WBRT alone had a median survival of 4.9 months ($p = 0.48$). For those receiving motexafin gadolinium, the rate of neurologic death was 48.6% versus 51.6% for the WBRT alone arm. This difference was not significant ($p = 0.60$). In a subgroup analysis of patients with brain metastases from NSCLC, however, the difference was significant with a rate of 36.4% for the motexafin gadolinium arm

TABLE 21-4. Characteristics of a Brain Metastasis Ideal for Stereotactic Radiosurgery

Spherical
Radiographically distinct
<3 cm at presentation
Minimally invasive
Displaces normal brain parenchyma circumferentially. This decreases the risk for injury of normal brain tissue during treatment.

and 51.5% for the WBRT alone arm ($p = 0.037$). Careful neurologic testing and follow-up showed a longer time to neurocognitive progression for memory and executive function in patients with brain metastases from NSCLC receiving motexafin gadolinium ($p = 0.062$) (88). A confirmatory study phase III study, Study of Neurological Progression with Motexafin Gadolinium and Radiation Therapy (SMART) assessed neurologic progression in patients with brain metastases from NSCLS. This study recently completed accrual.

SURGICAL RESECTION

The advantage of surgery is that it provides pathology and leads to immediate local control and decompression. This is particularly beneficial for patients with a single or a large brain metastasis and for those without a diagnosis. Only half of the cases are single metastasis that can be resected (89). Complications from surgery include intracerebral hematoma, infections, postsurgical neurologic deficits, deep venous thrombosis, and postoperative fever (90,91). Surgical resection improves survival over radiotherapy alone. A prospective study randomized 48 patients to resection of their single metastasis followed by WBRT or biopsy followed by WBRT. Those receiving resection had a median survival of 40 weeks and those who had only a biopsy had a median survival of 15 weeks ($p < 0.01$) (89). Resection also decreased local recurrence from 52% with biopsy and WBRT to 20% with resection and WBRT ($p < 0.02$). Factors improving survival following resection include young age and controlled extracranial disease (92).

Adjuvant radiotherapy is essential to maintaining both local and distant control. In one study, intracranial failure was found in 85% of the resection only group compared with 21% in the resection with WBRT group (93). This study group also found that those treated with WBRT after resection lived an average of 21 months, 9.5 months longer than those who had had resection only or resection with WBRT after recurrence. A prospective study randomized patients to adjuvant WBRT or no WBRT after resection for a single metastasis (94). The addition of WBRT decreased intracranial failure from 70% to 18% ($p < 0.001$). It also decreased local recurrence from 46% to 10% ($p < 0.001$). In this study, no difference was seen in survival, but it is important to note that the study was powered for local control and not survival. As such, WBRT is often recommended as adjuvant therapy following surgery.

STEREOTACTIC RADIOSURGERY

Stereotactic radiosurgery (SRS) involves the delivery of high-dose radiation focally to the tumor. SRS can be linear accelerator (LINAC)-based or accomplished through the gamma knife. Unlike surgery, these procedures are often minimally invasive, do not require general anesthesia, and are offered on an outpatient basis. SRS is also less expensive and more cost-effective (95). SRS, however, does not provide histology and is not ideal for metastases >4 cm. Ideal brain metastasis characteristics for radiosurgery are listed in Table 21-4 (96).

Regardless of the SRS modality (LINAC or gamma knife), the concept is the same. Head frames are used in both, similar to the stereotactic head frames used in neurosurgery. The tumor is localized in reference to the head frame using MRI, CT, or both. Using a computer, the treatment is planned. The patient's head is fixed in regard to the machine and treatment is delivered.

The difference between the two modalities is how the treatment is delivered. In LINAC radiosurgery, treatment is delivered using multiple arcs over different angles. High-dose radiation is delivered at the intersection of the arcs. In gamma knife surgery, 201 beams of Cobalt-60 radiation intersect and target a precise point (shot) using a collimator helmet. By varying the size of the collimator, the size of the shots can be adjusted. Several shots are often used to cover the tumor target and minimize the dose to normal brain.

Some acute adverse effects of stereotactic radiosurgery are transient motor weakness, nausea, seizures, and headaches. Neurologic deterioration and a need for steroids are some subacute effects of radiosurgery and present within 6 months following therapy. Chronic adverse effects include radiation necrosis and steroid dependence (97).

The best candidates for radiosurgery are those patients who have fewer than three brain metastases, high KPS scores, and controlled extracranial disease (97). Based on retrospective studies, the median survival after radiosurgery with WBRT is 13 months (99) in selected cases and is comparable to surgery with WBRT. Similar to surgery, local control with radiosurgery combined with WBRT is 86% (98), which is better than the 48% local control rate with WBRT alone (89).

The RTOG performed a prospective, randomized trial comparing WBRT alone with WBRT with SRS boost for patients with one to three brain metastases (99). No survival difference was seen between the two arms for all patients. For patients with a single brain metastasis, survival improved, however, from a mean of 4.9 months to 6.5 months with the addition of upfront SRS ($p = 0.0390$). Note: This survival is less than previously described above because of the selection bias in retrospective studies. For patients who are RPA class I, mean survival was 11.6 months for patients with upfront SRS versus 9.6 months for those without ($p = 0.0453$). Local control at 1 year improved from 71% to 82% with SRS ($p = 0.01$). On multivariate analysis, RPA class I and NSCLC histology were found to be prognostic for survival. Thus, in selected patients, SRS can improve survival.

Prospective SRS studies on patients with NSCLC brain metastases are underway, given the results of the RTOG study. This includes using MGd in a phase II setting for patients having WBRT and SRS. Also, a randomized RTOG study is currently assessing the use of temozolomide or erlotinib with WBRT and SRS.

It is controversial whether WBRT is beneficial after SRS, given the strong opinion regarding potential side effects of WBRT versus the effect of neurologic disease progression. In a Japanese study, patients were randomized to SRS with WBRT or SRS alone (100). No difference in survival was seen between the two arms, but a 46.8% recurrence rate was found in the SRS with WBRT arm versus 76.4% for SRS alone ($p < 0.001$), which is currently being studied.

CHEMOTHERAPY

The use of chemotherapy for brain metastases is a subject of active research. Traditionally, the thought was that the blood–brain barrier prevented an efficacious dose of chemotherapy from entering the brain parenchyma. Tumors resected at autopsy, however, were found to have significant concentrations of chemotherapy (101).

Temozolomide is an alkylating agent that can penetrate through the blood–brain barrier, making it ideal for treating brain tumors. This was studied in a phase III setting in Greece as a concurrent and adjuvant agent (102). This study randomized 134 patients to WBRT alone versus WBRT with temozolomide and found that the addition of temozolomide improved response rates. The improvement in response rates was more significant for patients <60 years of age and patients with a KPS of 90 or 100. The median survival for patients receiving temozolomide was 8.3 months versus 6.3 months for those who had radiation alone ($p = 0.179$). Based on this study, additional investigation of temozolomide and radiation are planned.

Chemotherapy does have use in patients previously treated with whole brain radiation, but who now have too many lesions to be treated with either surgery or SRS. Agents under study include vinorelbine and intraarterial carboplatin for metastases from lung (103,104).

PROPHYLACTIC CRANIAL IRRADIATION

Given the high rates of brain metastases in NSCLC and SCLC, prophylactic cranial irradiation (PCI) to prevent brain metastases has been investigated. In SCLC, for patients who had a complete response (CR) to therapy, the use of PCI reduced brain relapse from 67% to 40% in 2 years ($p < 0.0001$), but no difference was found in overall survival (67). Using the data from seven prospective randomized trials, a meta-analysis was performed (105). In patients with a CR to therapy, PCI for SCLC decreased the 3-year incidence of brain metastasis from 58.6% to 33.3% ($p < 0.001$) and improved the 3-year of survival from 15.3% to 20.7% ($p = 0.01$). The typical dose of PCI is 25 Gy in 10 fractions. Given the survival benefit, it is standard to treat patients with PCI after a CR to SCLC therapy. The optimal dose for PCI is being studied in the latest RTOG study, which will randomize patients to 25 Gy in 10 fractions, 36 Gy in 18 fractions, and 36 Gy in 24 fractions twice a day.

The role of PCI in NSCLC has been investigated. A Veterans Administration (VA) study showed that PCI for locally advanced NSCLC reduced brain relapse from 13% to 6% ($p = 0.038$), but did not affect overall survival (106). Other studies resulted in similar conclusions. Many of these studies are older, and with recent improvements in the treatment of locally advanced NSCLC, the conclusions of these studies may be outdated. As such, the role of PCI is being reinvestigated in an RTOG study. The dose in this study is 30 Gy in 15 fractions.

CLINICAL RECOMMENDATIONS OF THE VIGNETTE

The treatment of brain metastases is complicated by the variety of treatment options, all of which are complementary to each other. Surgery is often used for large tumors with symptomatic mass effect, single lesions, and lesions without a primary cancer diagnosis or histology. Patients who do well with surgery include RPA class I and some RPA class II patients. SRS is often used in patients with few lesions (usually fewer than four) within the brain and small lesions <4 cm in size, and in patients who are expected to do well (RPA class I and some RPA class II patients). SRS is also used in patients who are not surgical candidates or who do not want to have surgery. For patients with one to three brain metastases having SRS boost after WBRT, NSCLC is prognostic for survival. WBRT is used alone in patients with a poor prognosis, poor functional status, radiosensitive histologies (germinomas, lymphomas, or small cell tumor) or numerous brain metastases. WBRT is added to surgery and SRS to prevent local and distant brain recurrence.

For the patient described in the vignette, surgery and SRS are options for treatment. The risks and benefits of both treatments should be presented so that the patient can make an informed choice. In addition, WBRT should also be presented as an option to complement the surgery or SRS. The physician and the patient should weigh the risk of distant brain recurrence (and local recurrence in the case of surgery), which can have an impact on neurologic status, versus the potential toxicities of WBRT. These are active controversies in the treatment of brain metastases and further research will help better define optimal treatment in these patients.

SUMMARY

Brain metastasis is the most common neurologic complication of cancer. Lung cancer, either non-small cell or small cell histology, has a propensity to spread to the brain. Although PCI is proved to benefit patients with SCLC with a CR to treatment, the benefit is less clear in patients with NSCLC. For patients who have brain metastases, surgery, stereotactic radiosurgery, and whole-brain radiation therapy are the main treatment options. The role of chemotherapy and radiation sensitizers is being investigated, especially in NSCLC brain metastases. With more research, optimal treatment strategies will be better defined.

REFERENCES

1. Jemal A, Siegel R, Ward E, et al. Cancer Statistics, 2006. *CA Cancer J Clin.* 2006;56(2):106–130.
2. Bazhin A, Shifrina ON, Savchenko MS, et al. Low titre autoantibodies against recoverin in sera of patients with small cell lung cancer but without a loss of vision. *Lung Cancer.* 2001;34(1):99–104.
3. Savchenko MS, Bazhin AV, Shifrina ON, et al. Antirecoverin autoantibodies in the patient with non-small cell lung cancer but without cancer-associated retinopathy. *Lung Cancer.* 2003;41(3):363–367.
4. Voltz RD, Posner JB, Dalmau J, et al. Paraneoplastic encephalomyelitis: An update of the effects of the anti-Hu immune response on the nervous system and tumour. *J Neurol Neurosurg Psychiatry.* 1997;63(2):133–136.
5. Gultekin SH, Rosenfeld MR, Voltz R, et al. Paraneoplastic limbic encephalitis: Neurological symptoms, immunological findings and tumour association in 50 patients. *Brain.* 2000;123(7):1481–1494.
6. Smitt PS, Grefkens J, de Leeuw B, et al. Survival and outcome in 73 anti-Hu positive patients with paraneoplastic encephalomyelitis/sensory neuronopathy. *J Neurol.* 2002;249 (6):745–753.
7. Elrington GM, Murray NMF, Spiro SG, et al. Neurological paraneoplastic syndromes in patients with small cell lung cancer. A prospective survey of 150 patients. *J Neurol Neurosurg Psychiatry.* 1991;54(9):764–767.
8. Seneviratne U, de Silva R. Lambert-Eaton myasthenic syndrome. *Postgrad Med J.* 1999;75(887):516–520.
9. Wirtz PW, Nijnuis MG, Sotodeh M, et al. The epidemiology of myasthenia gravis, Lambert-Eaton myasthenic syndrome and their associated tumours in the northern part of the province of South Holland. *J Neurol.* 2003;250(6):698–701.
10. Posner JB, Dalmau J. Paraneoplastic syndromes. *Curr Opin Immunol.* 1997;9(5):723–729.
11. Inuzuka T. Autoantibodies in paraneoplastic neurological syndrome. *Am J Med Sci.* 2000; 319(4):217–226.

12. Chan KH, Vernino S, Lennon VA. ANNA-3 anti-neuronal nuclear antibody: Marker of lung cancer-related autoimmunity. *Ann Neurol.*. 2001;50(3):301–311.
13. Lennon VA, Kryzer TJ, Griesmann GE, et al. Calcium-channel antibodies in the Lambert-Eaton syndrome and other paraneoplastic syndromes. *N Engl J Med.* 1995;332(22):1467–1474.
14. Morris CS, Esiri MM, Marx A, et al. Immunocytochemical characteristics of small cell lung carcinoma associated with the Lambert-Eaton myasthenic syndrome. *Am J Pathol.* 1992; 140(4):839–845.
15. Viglione MP, O'Shaughnessy TJ, Kim YI. Inhibition of calcium currents and exocytosis by Lambert-Eaton syndrome antibodies in human lung cancer cells. *J Physiol.* 1995;488(2): 303–317.
16. Voltz R, Dalmau J, Posner JB, et al. T-cell receptor analysis in anti-Hu associated paraneoplastic encephalomyelitis. *Neurology.* 1998;51(4):1146–1150.
17. Bakheit AMO, Kennedy PGE, Behan PO. Paraneoplastic limbic encephalitis: Clinicopathological correlations. *J Neurol Neurosurg Psychiatry.* 1990;53(12):1084–1088.
18. Newman NJ, Bell IR, McKee AC. Paraneoplastic limbic encephalitis: Neuropsychiatric presentation. *Biol Psychiatry.* 1990;27(5):529–542.
19. Mason WP, Graus F, Lang B, et al. Small-cell lung cancer, paraneoplastic cerebellar degeneration and the Lambert-Eaton myasthenic syndrome. *Brain.* 1997;120(8):1279–1300.
20. Scaravilli F, An SF, Groves M, et al. The neuropathology of paraneoplastic syndromes. *Brain Pathol.* 1999;9(2):251–260.
21. Anderson NE, Budde-Steffen C, Rosenblum MK, et al. Opsoclonus, myoclonus, ataxia, and encephalopathy in adults with cancer: A distinct paraneoplastic syndrome. *Medicine.* 1988; 67(2):100–109.
22. Gazic B, Pizem J, Dolenc-Groselj L, et al. Paraneoplastic encephalomyelitis/sensory motor peripheral neuropathy—An autopsy case study. *Folia Neuropathol.* 2005;43(2):113–117.
23. Murphy MA, Thirkill CE, Hart WM. Paraneoplastic retinopathy: A novel autoantibody reaction associated with small-cell lung carcinoma. *J Neuroophthalmol.* 1997;17(2):77–83.
24. Song D, Shi J, Lu Q. Ultrastructural study on neuromuscular junction of patients with Lambert-Eaton myasthenia syndrome or mitochondrial encephalomyopathy. *Chinese Med J.* 1998;78(7):512–514.
25. O'Neill JH, Murray NM, Newsom-Davis J. The Lambert-Eaton myasthenic syndrome. A review of 50 cases. *Brain.* 1988;111(3):577–596.
26. Fukuda T, Motomura M, Yoko N, et al. Reduction of P/Q-type calcium channels in the postmortem cerebellum of paraneoplastic cerebellar degeneration with Lambert-Eaton myasthenic syndrome. *Ann Neurol.* 2003;53(1):21–28.
27. Lucchinetti CF, Kimmel DW, Lennon VA. Paraneoplastic and oncologic profiles of patients seropositive for type 1 antineuronal nuclear autoantibodies. *Neurology.* 1998;50(3):652–657.
28. Bakheit AMO, Kennedy PGE, Behan PO. Paraneoplastic limbic encephalitis: Clinicopathological correlations. *J Neurol Neurosurg Psychiatry.* 1990;53(12):1084–1088.
29. Alanowitch S, Graus F, Uchuya M. Limbic encephalitis and small cell lung cancer. Clinical and immunological features. *Brain.* 1997;120(6):923–928.
30. Dalmau J, Graus F, Rosenblum MK, et al. Anti-Hu-associated paraneoplastic encephalomyelitis/sensory neuronopathy. A clinical study of 71 patients. *Medicine.* 1992;71(2):59–72.
31. Bataller L, Graus F, Saiz A, et al. Clinical outcome in adult onset idiopathic or paraneoplastic opsoclonus-myoclonus. *Brain.* 2001;124(2):437–443.
32. Thirkill CE, Keltner JL, Tyler NK, et al. Antibody reactions with retina and cancer-associated antigens in 10 patients with cancer-associated retinopathy. *Arch Ophthalmol.* 1993;111(7):931–937.
33. Wirtz PW, Wintzen AR, Verschuuren JJ. Lambert-Eaton myasthenic syndrome has a more progressive course in patients with lung cancer. *Muscle Nerve.* 2005;32(2):226–229.
34. Wirtz PW, Smallegange TM, Wintzen AR, et al. Differences in clinical features between the Lambert-Eaton myasthenic syndrome with and without cancer: An analysis of 227 published cases. *Clin Neurol Neurosurg.* 2002;104(4):359–363.
35. Nakao YK, Motomura M, Fukudome T, et al. Seronegative Lambert-Eaton myasthenic syndrome. Study of 110 Japanese patients. *Neurology.* 2002;59(11):1773–1775.
36. Chartrand-Lefebvre C, Howarth N, Grenier P, et al. Association of small cell lung cancer and the anti-Hu paraneoplastic syndrome: Radiographic and CT findings. *AJR Am J Roentgenol.* 1998;170(6):1513–1517.
37. Antoine JC, Cinotti L, Tilikete C, et al. [^{18}F]Fluorodeoxyglucose positron emission tomography in the diagnosis of cancer in patients with paraneoplastic neurological syndrome and anti-Hu antibodies. *Ann Neurol.* 2000;48(1):105–108.
38. Younes-Mhenni S, Janier MF, Cinotti L, et al. FDG-PET improves tumour detection in patients with paraneoplastic neurological syndromes. *Brain.* 2004;127(10):2331–2338.
39. Na DL, Hahm DS, Park JM, et al. Hypermetabolism of the medial temporal lobe in limbic encephalitis on ^{18}FDG-PET scan: A case report. *Eur Neurol.* 2001;45(3):187–189.
40. Graus F, Dalmau J, Rene R, et al. Anti-Hu antibodies in patients with small-cell lung cancer: Association with complete response to therapy and improved survival. *J Clin Oncol.*. 1997;15(8):2866–2872.
41. Sillevis-Smitt P, Manley G, Moll JWB, et al. Pitfalls in the diagnosis of autoantibodies associated with paraneoplastic neurologic disease. *Neurology.* 1996;46(6):1739–1741.
42. Llado A, Mannucci P, Carpentier AF, et al. Value of Hu antibody determinations in the follow-up of paraneoplastic neurologic syndromes. *Neurology.* 2004;63(10):1947–1949.
43. Dalmau J, Graus F, Villarejo A, et al. Clinical analysis of anti-Ma2-associated encephalitis. *Brain.* 2004;127(8):1831–1844.
44. Overeem S, Dalmau J, Bataller L, et al. Hypocretin-1 CSF levels in anti-Ma2 associated encephalitis. *Neurology.* 2004;62(1):138–140.
45. Sabater L, Gomez-Choco M, Saiz A, et al. BR serine/threonine kinase 2: A new autoantigen in paraneoplastic limbic encephalitis. *J Neuroimmunol.*. 2005;170(1–2):186–190.
46. Masaoka N, Emoto Y, Sasaoka A, et al. Fluorescein angiographic findings in a case of cancer-associated retinopathy. *Retina.* 1999;19(5):462–464.
47. Thirkill CE, Fitzgerald P, Sergott RC, et al. Cancer-associated retinopathy (CAR syndrome) with antibodies reacting with retinal, optic-nerve, and cancer cells. *N Engl J Med.* 1989;321 (23):1589–1594.
48. Dot C, Guigay J, Adamus G. Anti-alpha-enolase antibodies in cancer-associated retinopathy with small cell carcinoma of the lung. *Am J Ophthalmol.* 2005;139(4):746–747.
49. Glantz MJ, Biran H, Myers ME, et al. The radiographic diagnosis and treatment of paraneoplastic central nervous system disease. *Cancer.* 1994;73(1):168–175.
50. Motomura M, Lang B, Johnston I, et al. Incidence of serum anti-P/Q-type and anti-N-type calcium channel autoantibodies in the Lambert-Eaton myasthenic syndrome. *J Neurol Sci.* 1997;147(1):35–42.
51. Pelucchi A, Ciceri E, Clementi F, et al. Calcium channel autoantibodies in myasthenic syndrome and small cell lung cancer. *Am Rev Respir Dis.* 1993;147(5):1229–1232.
52. Wirtz PW, Willcox N, van der Slik AR, et al. HLA and smoking in prediction and prognosis of small cell lung cancer in autoimmune Lambert-Eaton myasthenic syndrome. *J Neuroimmunol.* 2005;159(1–2):230–237.
53. Graus F, Vincent A, Pozo-Rosich P, et al. Anti-glial nuclear antibody: Marker of lung cancer-related paraneoplastic neurological syndromes. *J Neuroimmunol.* 2005;165(1–2):166–171.
54. Keime-Guibert F, Graus F, Broet P, et al. Clinical outcome of patients with anti-Hu-associated encephalomyelitis after treatment of the tumor. *Neurology.* 1999;53(8):1719–1723.
55. McEvoy KM, Windebanck AJ, Daube JR, et al. 3,4-Diaminopyridine in the treatment of Lambert-Eaton myasthenic syndrome. *N Engl J Med.* 1989;321(23):1567–1571.
56. Sanders DB, Massey JM, Sanders LL, et al. A randomized trial of 3,4-diaminopyridine in Lambert-Eaton myasthenic syndrome. *Neurology.* 2000;54(3):603–607.
57. Takano H, Tanaka M, Koike R, et al. Effect of intravenous immunoglobulin in Lambert-Eaton myasthenic syndrome with small-cell lung cancer: Correlation with the titer of anti-voltage-gated calcium channel antibody. *Muscle Nerve.* 1994;17(9):1073–1075.
58. Tim RW, Massey JM, Sanders DB. Lambert-Eaton myasthenic syndrome: Electrodiagnostic findings and response to treatment. *Neurology.* 2000;54(11):2176–2178.
59. Maddison P, Newsom-Davis J, Mills KR, et al. Favourable prognosis in Lambert-Eaton myasthenic syndrome and small-cell lung carcinoma. *Lancet.* 1999;353(9147):117–118.
60. Langer CJ, Mehta MP. Current management of brain metastases, with a focus on systemic options. *J Clin Oncol.* 2005;23(25):6207–6219.
61. Posner JB. *Neurologic Complications of Cancer.* Contemporary Neurology Series. Vol. 45. Philadelphia: FA Davis; 1995:3–14, 77–110.
62. Johnson JD, Young B. Demographics of brain metastasis. *Neurosurg Clin N Am.* 1996;7 (3):337–344.
63. Stuschke M, Eberhardt W, Pottgen C, et al. Prophylactic cranial irradiation in locally advanced non-small-cell lung cancer after multimodality treatment: Long-term follow-up and investigations of late neuropsychologic effects. *J Clin Oncol.* 1999;17(9):2700–2709.
64. Yohena T, Yoshino I, Kitajima M, et al. Necessity of preoperative screening for brain metastasis in non-small cell lung cancer patients without lymph node metastasis. *Ann Thorac Cardiovasc Surg.* 2004;10(6):347–349.
65. Madej PJ, Bitran JD, Golomb HM, et al. Combined modality therapy for Stage IIIMO non-small cell lung cancer. A five-year experience. *Cancer.* 1984;54(1):5–12.
66. Cox JD, Scott CB, Byhardt RW, et al. Addition of chemotherapy to radiation therapy alters failure patterns by cell type within non-small cell carcinoma of lung (NSCCL): Analysis of radiation therapy oncology group (RTOG) trials. *Int J Radiat Oncol Biol Phys.* 1999;43 (3):505–509.
67. Arriagada R, Le Chevalier T, Borie F, et al. Prophylactic cranial irradiation for patients with small-cell lung cancer in complete remission. *J Natl Cancer Inst.* 1995;87(3):183–190.
68. Delattre JY, Krol G, Thaler HT, et al. Distribution of brain metastases. *Arch Neurol.* 1988;45(7):741–744.
69. Ferrigno D, Buccheri G. Cranial computed tomography as a part of the initial staging procedures for patients with non-small-cell lung cancer. *Chest.* 1994;106(4):1025–1029.
70. Das A, Hochberg FH. Clinical presentation of intracranial metastases. *Neurosurg Clin N Am.* 1996;7(3):377–391.
71. Le Chevalier T, Smith FP, Caille P, et al. Sites of primary malignancies in patients presenting with cerebral metastases: A review of 120 cases. *Cancer.* 1985;56(4):880–882.
72. Dhopesh VP, Yagnik PM. Brain metastasis: Analysis of patients without known cancer. *South Med J.* 1985;78(2):171–172.
73. Karnofsky D, Abelman W, Craver L, et al. The use of nitrogen mustards in the palliative treatment of carcinoma. *Cancer.* 1948;1:634–656.
74. Gaspar L, Scott C, Rotman M, et al. Recursive partitioning analysis (RPA) of prognostic factors in three Radiation Therapy Oncology Group (RTOG) brain metastasis trials. *Int J Radiat Oncol Biol Phys.* 1997;37(4):745–751.
75. Videtic GM, Adelstein DJ, Mekhail T, et al. Validation of the RTOG recursive partitioning analysis (RPA) classification for small cell lung cancer-only brain metastases: A single institution experience. *J Clin Oncol.* 2004;22(14s):1557(abst).
76. Videtic GMM, Reddy CA, Chao ST, et al. Women with brain metastases from non-small cell lung cancer live longer than men: An outcomes study utilizing the RTOG RPA class stratification. *Eur J Cancer.* 2005;3[Suppl]:138(abst).
77. Weaver DD, Winn HR, Jane JA. Differential intracranial pressure in patients with unilateral mass lesions. *J Neurosurg.* 1982;56(5):660–665.
78. Horton J, Baxter DH, Olson KB. The management of metastases to the brain by irradiation and corticosteroids. *Am J Roentgenol Radium Ther Nucl Med.* 1971;111(2):334–336.
79. Batchelor T, DeAngelis LM. Medical management of cerebral metastases. *Neurosurg Clin N Am.* 1996;7(3):435–446.
80. Vecht CJ. Clinical management of brain metastasis. *J Neurol.* 1998;245(3):127–131.
81. Borgelt B, Gelber R, Kramer S, et al. The palliation of brain metastases: Final results of the first two studies by the Radiation Therapy Oncology Group. *Int J Radiat Oncol Biol Phys.* 1980;6(1):1–9.
82. Sneed PK, Larson DA, Wara WM. Radiotherapy for Cerebral Metastases. *Neurosurg Clin N Am.* 1996;7(3):505–515.
83. Hall EJ. *Radiobiology for the Radiologist.* Philadelphia: Lippincott Williams & Wilkins; 2000.
84. Shaw E, Scott C, Suh J, et al. RSR13 plus cranial radiation therapy in patients with brain metastases: Comparison with the radiation therapy oncology group recursive partitioning analysis brain metastases database. *J Clin Oncol.* 2003;21(12):2364–2371.

85. Suh JH, Stea BD, Kresl JJ, et al. RT-13. A phase 3, randomized open-label, comparative study of standard whole brain radiation therapy (WBRT) with supplemental oxygen (O_2), with or without RSR13, in patients with brain metastases. *Neurooncology.* 2003;5:279–359.
86. Stea B, Shaw E, Pinter T, et al. Efaproxiral red blood cell concentration predicts efficacy in patients with brain metastases. *Br J Cancer.* 2006;94(12):1777–1784.
87. Mehta MP, Rodrigus P, Terhaard CH, et al. Survival and neurologic outcomes in a randomized trial of motexafin gadolinium and whole-brain radiation therapy in brain metastases. *J Clin Oncol.* 2003;21(13):2529–2536.
88. Meyers CA, Smith JA, Bezjak A, et al. Neurocognitive function and progression in patients with brain metastases treated with whole-brain radiation and motexafin gadolinium: Results of a randomized phase III trial. *J Clin Oncol.* 2004;22(1):157–165.
89. Patchell RA, Tibbs PA, Walsh JW, et al. A randomized trial of surgery in the treatment of single metastases to the brain. *N Engl J Med.* 1990;322(8):494–500.
90. Sundaresan N, Galicich JH. Surgical treatment of brain metastases. *Cancer.* 1995;55(6): 1382–1388.
91. Vecht CJ, Haaxma-Reiche H, Noordijk EM, et al. Treatment of single brain metastasis: Radiotherapy alone or combined with neurosurgery? *Ann Neurol.* 1993;33(6):583–590.
92. Noordijk EM, Vecht CJ, Haaxma-Reiche H, et al. The choice of treatment of single brain metastasis should be based on extracranial tumor activity and age. *Int J Radiat Oncol Biol Phys.* 1994;29(4):711–717.
93. Smalley SR, Schray MF, Laws ER, Jr., et al. Adjuvant radiation therapy after surgical resection of solitary brain metastasis: Association with pattern of failure and survival. *Int J Radiat Oncol Biol Phys.* 1987;13(11):1611–1616.
94. Patchell RA, Tibbs PA, Regine WF, et al. Postoperative radiotherapy in the treatment of single metastases to the brain. *JAMA.* 1998;280(17):1485–1489.
95. Rutigliano MJ, Lunsford LD, Kondziolka D, et al. The cost effectiveness of stereotactic radiosurgery versus surgical resection in the treatment of solitary metastatic brain tumors. Neurosurgery. 1995;37(3):445–453.
96. Loeffler JS, Shrieve DC, Wen PY, et al. Radiosurgery for intracranial malignancies. *Semin Radiat Oncol.* 1995;5:225–234.
97. Mehta MP, Boyd TS, Sinha P. The status of stereotactic radiosurgery for cerebral metastases in 1998. *J Radiosurg.* 1998;1:17–30.
98. Auchter RM, Lamond JP, Alexander E, et al. A multi-institutional outcome and prognostic factor analysis of radiosurgery for resectable single brain metastasis. *Int J Radiat Oncol Biol Phys.* 1996;35(1):27–35.
99. Andrews DW, Scott CB, Sperduto PW, et al. Whole brain radiation therapy with or without stereotactic radiosurgery boost for patients with one to three brain metastases: Phase III results of the RTOG 9508 randomised trial. *Lancet.* 2004;363(9422):1665–1672.
100. Aoyama H, Shirato H, Tago M, et al. Stereotactic radiosurgery plus whole-brain radiation therapy vs stereotactic radiosurgery alone for treatment of brain metastases: A randomized controlled trial. *JAMA.* 2006;295(21):2483–2491.
101. Hasegawa H, Ushio Y, Hayakawa T, et al. Changes of the blood–brain barrier in experimental metastatic brain tumors. *J Neurosurg.* 1983;59(2):304–310.
102. Antonadou D, Coliarakis N, Paraskevaidis M, et al. Whole brain radiotherapy alone or in combination with temozolomide for brain metastases. A phase III study. *Int J Radiat Oncol Biol Phys.* 2002;54(2S):93.
103. Omuro AM, Raizer JJ, Demopoulos A, et al. Vinorelbine combined with a protracted course of temozolomide for recurrent brain metastases: A phase I trial. *Journal of Neurooncology.* 2006;78(3):277–280.
104. Newton HB, Slivka MA, Volpi C, et al. Intra-arterial carboplatin and intravenous etoposide for the treatment of metastatic brain tumors. *Journal of Neurooncology.* 2003;61(1):35–44.
105. Auperin A, Arriagada R, Pignon JP, et al. Prophylactic cranial irradiation for patients with small-cell lung cancer in complete remission. Prophylactic Cranial Irradiation Overview Collaborative Group. *N Engl J Med.* 1999;341(7):476–484.
106. Cox JD, Stanley K, Petrovich Z, et al. Cranial irradiation in cancer of the lung of all cell types. *JAMA* 1981;245(5):469–472.

CHAPTER **22**

Sleep Apnea and Other Sleep-Related Breathing Disorders

Gökhan M. Mutlu • Phyllis C. Zee

OBJECTIVES

- To summarize the clinical characteristics of obstructive sleep apnea and other sleep-related breathing disorders
- To review the incidence and risk factors of sleep-related breathing disorders
- To understand the pathogenesis of sleep-related breathing disorders
- To review the diagnostic workup for sleep-related breathing disorders
- To summarize the approach to treatment of sleep-related breathing disorders

CASE VIGNETTE

A 61-year-old woman, morbidly obese and with hypertension was brought to the emergency room after she was noted to be less responsive than usual and sleeping all day. In addition to hypersomnolence, the patient also snored loudly, which was more prominent in the supine position. Also witnessed were apneas, gasping arousals, and unrefreshing sleep.

Physical examination showed a morbidly obese woman with a body mass index of 48 kg/m^2. She was somnolent, but arousable. She had episodes of obstructive apneas evidenced by cessation of audible breathing and thoracoabdominal paradoxical movement. Her SpO_2 was 87% while she was awake and decreased to 70% during apneas. An arterial blood gas revealed a pH of 7.22, $PaCO_2$ of 72 mm Hg and PaO_2 of 51 mm Hg.

The patient was subsequently admitted to the medical intensive care unit for further management of respiratory failure. She was placed on bilevel positive airway pressure (PAP) with an inspiratory PAP of 16 cm H_2O and expiratory PAP of 12 cm H_2O. Her mental status improved paralleling the improvement in $PaCO_2$, which decreased to 47 mm Hg. She had an inpatient polysomnography that was consistent with severe obstructive sleep apnea (apnea-hypopnea index [AHI] of 83 events per hour with an SpO_2 nadir of 68%, In addition, evidence was seen of sleep-related hypoventilation.

INTRODUCTION

Transition from wakefulness to sleep is associated with a myriad of cardiorespiratory changes that predispose to sleep-related breathing disorders. First will be reviewed the effects of sleep on cardiorespiratory function and then discussion of current approaches to the evaluation and management of common sleep-related breathing disorders with emphasis on obstructive sleep apnea (OSA).

Sleep is associated with relative hypoventilation because of a reduction in both tidal volume and respiratory rate leading to a 4- to 6-mm Hg rise in $PaCO_2$ levels compared with wakefulness (1,2). As sleep becomes more consolidated and advances from stage II to stage III and IV (slow wave or deep sleep), ventilation is controlled primarily by metabolic changes resulting in a regular pattern of breathing (1–3). Transition from non-rapid eye movement NREM sleep to REM sleep is associated with a further reduction in minute ventilation, in part because of skeletal muscle atonia (2). During REM sleep, respiration also becomes irregular, with breath-by-breath changes in tidal volume (1). During REM sleep, control of ventilation becomes less dependent on metabolic drive and more on behavioral factors (1,2). Furthermore, the threshold for ventilatory responses increases as a result of decreased response to chemostimulation (2,4).

Normal cardiovascular response to sleep is characterized by an increase in parasympathetic tone and a reduction in sympathetic nervous system activity, which is evident by reduced epinephrine level, reduced heart rate and blood pressure ("nocturnal dip"), decreased evening to early morning cortisol level, and arrhythmogenicity (2). Decreased heart rate and stroke volume lead to diminished cardiac output. Although the cardiovascular system is relatively stable during NREM sleep with decreased baroreflex sensitivity compared with wakefulness, K-complexes and spontaneous arousals intermittently alter this quiescent state (5). Arousals are also associated with augmented ventilation caused by abrupt increase in chemosensitivity (2). Transition into REM sleep is associated with increased sympathetic nervous system activity and relative increase in heart rate and blood pressure with irregular surges being linked to phasic REM (2).

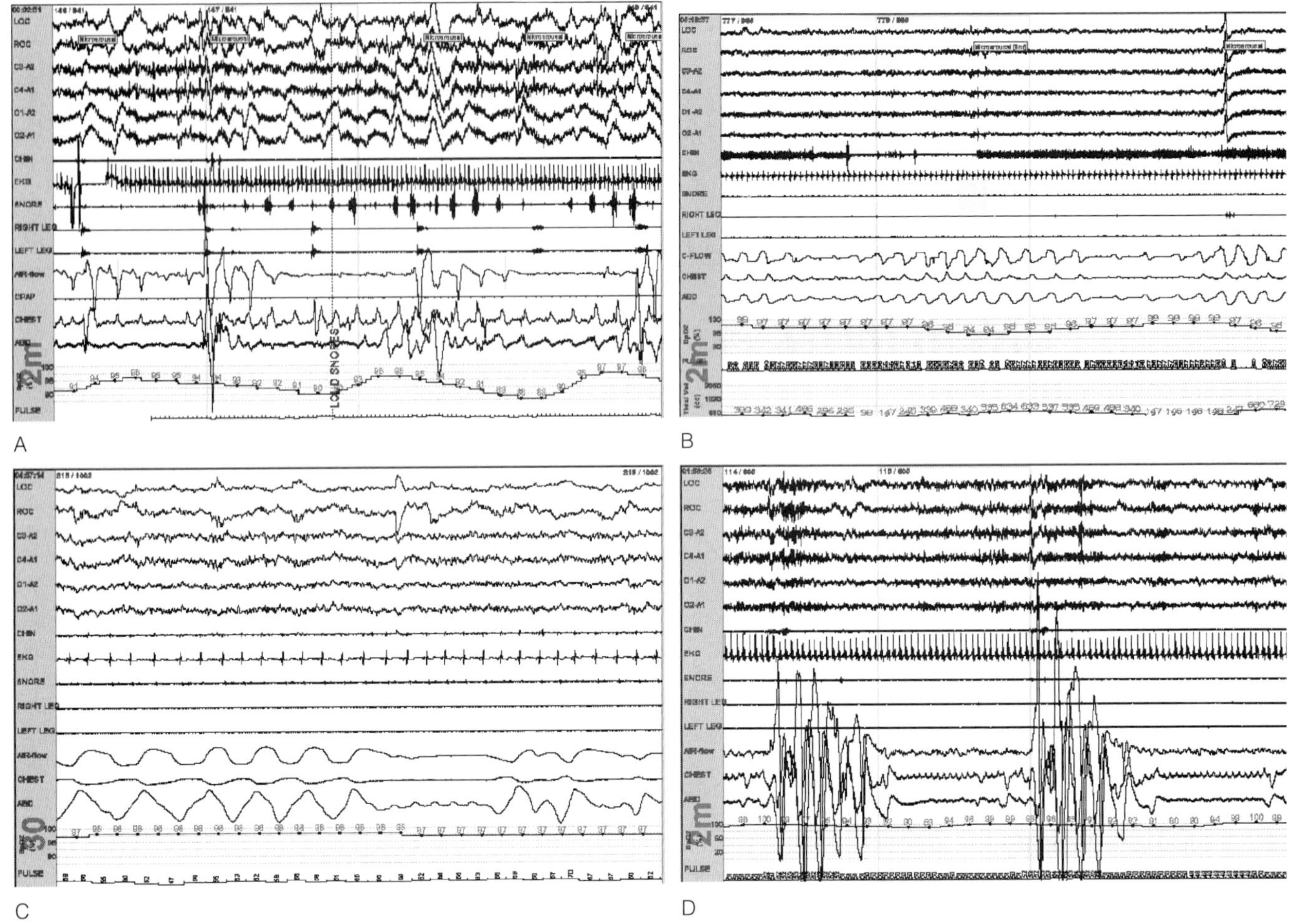

FIGURE 22-1. **(A)** Obstructive apnea. There is continued respiratory effort, despite complete cessation of airflow associated with subsequent O_2 desaturation. **(B) Obstructive hypopnea.** There is a reduction in airflow, with a >4% reduction in O_2 saturation. Hypopneas were associated with a reduction in tidal volume (*arrow*). **(C) Central apnea.** There is complete cessation of airflow paralleled by loss of respiratory effort. Cardiac oscillations are seen on the tracing from abdominal belt (*arrow*). **(D) Mixed apnea.** The apnea initially is central (without respiratory effort) and followed by a period of obstructive apnea.

DEFINITION

Apnea is defined as temporary cessation of airflow that lasts for 10 seconds or longer. Respiratory events are considered obstructive when respiratory efforts are constant or increasing, and central when respiratory efforts are absent. Mixed apneas begin as central events and terminate as obstructive, usually associated with crescendo respiratory efforts. Although the definition of hypopnea is variable, the American Academy of Sleep Medicine and the Centers for Medicare and Medicaid Services define hypopnea as airflow reduction of at least 30% that lasts for 10 seconds or longer and results in at least 4% oxygen desaturation (6) (Fig. 22-1). Cheyne-Stokes respiration (CSR) is a type of periodic breathing characterized by the presence of central apneas that alternate with periods of hyperventilation, which have a crescendo-decrescendo pattern (7).

Sleep-disordered breathing has classically been defined as OSA or central sleep apnea (CSA). OSA is a disorder characterized by a repetitive collapse of the upper airway during sleep that results in oxygen desaturation and arousals from sleep. *OSA hypopnea syndrome* is a term used to describe OSA when it is associated with hypersomnia. CSA is characterized by repetitive central apneas associated with oxygen desaturations that are typically less severe than in OSA and improve during REM sleep.

More recent data suggested the limitation of this simplified classification and has led to the development of the term, *complex sleep-disordered breathing* (8). Gilmartin et al. (8) proposed another type of breathing disorder, *complex sleep apnea* (CompSA), which does not have a predominant type (obstructive vs. central) breathing disorder. The pattern of breathing is rather mixed, characterized by mixed apneas, periodic breathing, position- (obstructive in supine, central in nonsupine position) and stage-dependent (periodic breathing during NREM and severe OSA during REM) variability in the apnea and timing of nightly variability (obstructive in the beginning of the night and central at the end) (8).

Respiratory effort-related arousal occurs as a result of increasingly vigorous respiratory efforts made against a narrowed airway (9). Although not officially recognized in the new

International Classification of Sleep Disorders-2, it can be associated with hypersomnolence (9,10).

EPIDEMIOLOGY

OBSTRUCTIVE SLEEP APNEA

OSA with hypersomnia is a common disorder with an estimated prevalence of 2% in women and 4% in men in the United States (11,12). The prevalence of OSA elsewhere varies from 0.3% to 25%. OSA is often overlooked and it is estimated that 80% to 90% of cases are undiagnosed because of the high prevalence of snoring, (~50% of adults) and paucity of symptoms in as many as 20% of adults with an AHI >5 (13).

Estimated prevalence of OSA with at least mild disease (AHI ≥5) is 20% and at least moderate disease (AHI ≥15) is about 6% to 7% (11,12,14–17). AHI is a measure of the frequency of obstructive events, but does not provide information about the degree of oxygen desaturation. Respiratory disturbance index, which includes number of arousals in addition to AHI, may a better marker of sleep fragmentation and predictor of daytime sleepiness (18).

CENTRAL SLEEP APNEA

Most central apneas reflect the instability of breathing control. CSA is commonly seen in patients with underlying neurologic (i.e., stroke) and cardiac disease, particularly congestive heart failure (CHF). In patients with stroke, OSA is the most common (43% to 91%) type of sleep-disordered breathing and CSA is seen in <10% (19,20). CSR is uncommon in patients with stroke. CSA with CSR is present in about 25% to 40% of patients with left-sided heart failure, particularly those with New York Heart Association class III to IV (21–24).

COMPLEX SLEEP APNEA

Because CompSA is a newly proposed category of sleep-related breathing disorder, the diagnostic criteria are not well established. Therefore, the data on the epidemiology are limited. A recent study showed a prevalence of 15% (25).

ETIOLOGY AND PATHOGENESIS

OBSTRUCTIVE SLEEP APNEA

The upper airway is a compliant tube and, therefore, subjected to collapse when the negative airway pressure from inspiratory activity of the diaphragm and the other respiratory muscles exceeds the force generated by the upper airway dilating muscles. During transition from wakefulness to sleep, upper airway diameter decreases because of a reduction in tonic pharyngeal muscle activity and attenuation of the compensatory reflex dilator (9). These alterations in upper airway diameter can be exaggerated in the presence of upper airway abnormalities and clinical risk factors for OSA, such as obesity, nasal congestions, smoking, and sleeping in a supine position, as well as anatomic factors (i.e., macroglossia and retrognathia) (26,27). Upper airway obstruction occurs at two major sites: One at the level of the soft palate (retropalatal area) and another at the level of the tongue (retrolingual area). Occlusion of the upper airway results in oxygen desaturation, hypercapnia, and pronounced swings in intrathoracic pressure.

Central breathing instability can also contribute to the development of obstructive respiratory events suggested by the presence of upper airway obstruction in the absence of ventilatory motor output (28), reduction in pharyngeal dilator activity associated with periodic breathing (29,30), and hypocapnia in patients with evidence of inspiratory flow limitation (31).

CENTRAL SLEEP APNEA

Central breathing instability is also important in the pathogenesis of CSA (2,32,33). The pathogenesis of CSA is complex, but it can be simplified based on the status of the respiratory drive (decreased vs. increased) and, consequently, $PaCO_2$ (hypercapnia vs. hypocapnia), respectively. Hypercapnic CSA occurs in patients with decreased respiratory drive or ability to breathe, such as neuromuscular disease or medication overdose (i.e., narcotic analgesics). Hypocapnic CSA occurs in conditions that are associated high respiratory drive, such as pain, anxiety, high altitude, and CHF, which can lead to cyclic hyperventilation resulting in relative hypocapnia (34,35).

COMPLEX SLEEP APNEA

Both obstructive and respiratory control factors are present in the pathogenesis of CompSA. Dysregulation of CO_2 hemostasis is the dominant mechanism in the pathophysiology of CompSA (8). Nasal continuous positive airway pressure (CPAP) therapy is successful in the treatment of obstructive events but the patients continue to have high residual sleep-disordered breathing, mostly from central apneas (25).

PATHOLOGY

The acute physiologic effects of obstructive apnea include marked intrathoracic pressure changes, oxyhemoglobin desaturation, hypercapnia, arousal, and sympathoexcitation, all of which have significant consequences, particularly for those with underlying cardiorespiratory diseases (Table 22-1). Intrathoracic pressure swings are hallmark of obstructive apneas. When intrathoracic pressure becomes more negative, left ventricle (LV) afterload increases, because of increased LV transmural pressure, and LV preload decreases, because of impaired LV diastolic filling and impaired LV relaxation (2). Experimental evidence suggests that oxidative stress caused by intermittent hypoxia can lead to LV dysfunction itself (36).

Animal studies suggest that OSA can increase systemic blood pressure as a result of intermittent hypoxia and arousal (37). OSA also causes endothelial dysfunction evident by a reduction in flow-mediated dilation correlating with AHI (38). Both of these effects are reversible with resolution of apnea or arousal and nasal CPAP therapy, respectively. OSA also has an impact on blood/coagulation profile such as increased hemoglobin, viscosity, P-selectin, factor levels, and platelet aggregation (39).

Patients with OSA often exhibit impaired neuropsychological function (40) and residual hypersomnolence despite compliance with nasal CPAP, which is attributed to oxidative stress caused by intermittent hypoxia (41). OSA is associated with increases in C-reactive protein and proinflammatory cytokines, such as interleukin-6, an effect that is independent of body weight and correlates with the severity of OSA and improves with nasal CPAP therapy (42). Interleukin-6 and C-reactive protein

TABLE 22-1. Proposed Mechanisms of Obstructive Sleep Apnea (OSA)-Related Adverse Effects on Cardiovascular System

IMMEDIATE CONSEQUENCES OF AN OBSTRUCTIVE APNEA

Intrathoracic pressure swings
Intermittent hypoxemia
Sympathoexcitation
Electroencephalogram (EEG) arousals

EFFECTS ON OXIDATIVE STRESS/INFLAMMATION

↑ Oxidative stress
↑ Proinflammatory cytokines

EFFECTS ON BLOOD/COAGULATION PROFILE

↑ Hematocrit
↑ Whole blood viscosity
↑ Fibrinogen
↑ Platelet aggregation
↑ FXIIa and FVIIa levels
↑ Thrombin-antithrombin complex levels
↑ Soluble P-selectin

EFFECTS ON ENDOCRINE FUNCTION

Insulin resistance
↓ Growth hormone
↑ AM cortisol
↓ Thyroid-stimulating hormone

OTHER EFFECTS

Endothelial dysfunction
↓ Production of nitric oxide

TABLE 22-2. Clinical Features of Obstructive Sleep Apnea

SYMPTOMS

Snoring
Witnessed apneas
Choking arousals
Gasping arousals
Unrefreshing sleep
Excessive daytime sleepiness

PHYSICAL EXAMINATION

Male gender
Obesity
Age >40 years
Hypertension
Increased neck size (>17 inches)
Crowded oropharynx
Low-lying soft palate
Cobblestoning (in patients with gastroesophageal reflex disease [GERD])
Craniofacial abnormalities

CONSEQUENCES

Neurocognitive
- Excessive daytime sleepiness
- Motor vehicle accidents
- Poor work performance
- Disrupted social interaction

Cardiovascular
- Systemic hypertension
- Pulmonary hypertension
- Ischemic cardiovascular events
- Arrhythmias

are independently associated with risk of ischemic cardiovascular disease. OSA and sleep deprivation can cause many changes in endocrine function, including impaired glucose tolerance associated with hyperinsulinemia, increased insulinlike growth factor-1, elevated AM cortisol, and decreased thyroid-stimulating hormone and growth hormone (43,44).

CLINICAL MANIFESTATIONS

SIGNS AND SYMPTOMS

OSA is a major health issue that has both acute physiologic effects (as described above) and chronic neurobehavioral and cardiovascular consequences (Table 22-2). Patients with OSA frequently present with complaints of loud snoring, unrefreshing sleep, excessive daytime sleepiness, fatigue, and lack of energy as a result of OSA-related sleep deprivation and chronic sleep loss. Other symptoms include witnessed apneas, dry mouth, morning headaches, poor attention, difficulty concentrating, and memory loss. Neuropsychologic dysfunction associated with OSA occurs with even mild disease, although significant individual variability is seen (45). Persons who have OSA are at risk for motor vehicle accidents (46).

Common findings on physical examination include obesity and hypertension (47,48). Inspection of the upper airway may show nasal obstruction caused by rhinitis, septal deviation, nasal polyps, low-lying soft palate, enlarged uvula, prominent, hypertrophied tongue (macroglossia), tonsillar hypertrophy, and jaw abnormalities (i.e., retrognathia). Neck circumference >17 inches in men and >16 inches in women is highly predictive of OSA (49).

Clinical features of patients with CompSA are indistinguishable from those with OSA (25). Patients with CSA clinically differ from those with OSA and do not have the classic clinical features of OSA (i.e., snoring, hypersomnia) and may have symptoms and signs of underlying causes (i.e., CHF, neuromuscular diseases) that lead to CSA.

CONSEQUENCES OF OSA

OSA is independently associated with cardiovascular disease. OSA is associated with increased risk of sudden death between the hours of midnight and 6 AM as compared with the general population (sudden death is more common between 6 AM and noon) (50). Retrospective data indicate that mortality from OSA correlates with AHI. It has been difficult, however, to study the independent effect of OSA on cardiovascular disease because of the overlap between the risk factors for cardiovascular disease and OSA, such as obesity, male gender, and older age. In the Sleep Heart Health Study, a cross-sectional evaluation of more than 6,000 patients, those with the highest AHI had an adjusted odd ratio of self-reported cardiovascular disease of 1.42 (51) with a plateau in the odds ratio of an AHI >11. Interestingly, among the cardiovascular events, the strongest link appears to be with CHF.

Systemic hypertension is seen up to two thirds of patients with OSA. A severity dependent link is found between AHI and hypertension (17,52,53). Both Wisconsin Cohort and Sleep

Heart Health Study have shown that this risk is independent of obesity, age, alcohol intake, and smoking (54–56). The risk of hypertension is even more prominent in Native Americans, those <65 years of age, and those who are obese (52).

Sleep Heart Health Study showed OSA (AHI >11) as being an independent risk for ischemic heart disease (52). Ischemic events that are triggered by OSA are linked to both oxygen desaturation and postapneic surges in the sympathetic nervous system. Diseased myocardium is more susceptible to the adverse effects of OSA than healthy myocardium. Both brady- and tachyarrhythmias are also associated with OSA. Atrial fibrillation is twice as likely to recur after cardioversion, if OSA is left untreated (57).

The incidence of apnea in stroke patients is high, with the predominant type being obstructive. Although OSA is not independent risk for stroke (52,58), it is not clear whether OSA is a consequence of stroke rather than a preexisting condition. Patients with the highest AHI appear to have the highest risk for stroke (58).

More recent evidence suggests an association between OSA and impaired glucose tolerance, independent of obesity (43,59–61). Other clinical consequences of OSA include nocturia, erectile dysfunction, gastroesophageal reflux, and morning headaches.

DIAGNOSTIC APPROACH

Recognition of the typical signs and symptoms listed above is the key step in the diagnosis of OSA. High incidence of these symptoms in the general population also makes the diagnosis of OSA more complicated, however. In the United States, almost half of men and one quarter of women are habitual snorers. Furthermore, about two thirds of adults are overweight and >30% of the population report excessive daytime sleepiness, yet only 1 in 20 middle-aged adults has OSA (14,62).

Patients often seek medical attention independently or at the request of a bed partner for further evaluation of snoring and excessive daytime somnolence (63). Questions that should be asked include the quality of sleep, presence of witnessed breathing disturbances, snoring and its intensity and changes with position, and choking or gasping arousals. It is important to exclude sleep curtailment caused by social circumstances.

POLYSOMNOGRAPHY

Polysomnography (PSG) is the definitive diagnostic test used for OSA and indicated for individuals who have intermediate to high probability of having OSA. PSG evaluates sleep and cardiorespiratory function using electoencephalography, electrooculography, chin electromyography, airflow, chin electromyography, thoracoabdominal movement, oxygen, and electrocardiography.

Although most patients can be referred directly to sleep center for PSG without a prior consultation, a referral to a sleep specialist for preliminary assessment should be considered in patients with underlying cardiopulmonary disorders, severe obesity, neuromuscular disease or chest wall disorders, or suspected concomitant sleep disorders, such as insomnia and narcolepsy.

The "traditional" approach in diagnosis and management of OSA is to obtain a full-night diagnostic PSG, followed by a full-night titration of CPAP. An alternative is the split-night PSG, which combines an initial diagnostic part that is usually concluded within 2 to 3 hours, followed by titration of CPAP during the rest of the night. The patient, however, needs to meet the following criteria, including an AHI of at least 40 during a minimum of 2 hours of diagnostic portion of PSG: CPAP titration can be carried out for >3 hours and PSG shows elimination of obstructive respiratory events during REM sleep in the supine position (64). Although a *negative* PSG excludes the possibility of a significant OSA, a repeat testing should be considered if OSA is strongly suspected. Approximately 10% of patients with an AHI <5 may have an AHI >5 during a second night PSG (65).

Although portable PSG has become available for use and has eliminated the need to perform the study at sleep centers, its precise role continues to be debated. Not sufficient evidence exists to support the use of portable monitoring devices in an unattended setting, neither for confirmation nor for exclusion of OSA (66). Similarly, overnight pulse oximetry should not be used as a screening diagnostic study for OSA.

OTHER DIAGNOSTIC WORKUP

Routine workup for pulmonary hypertension is not recommended for patients with OSA (67). Significant pulmonary hypertension in a patient with obstructive sleep apnea (OSA) is usually indicative of the presence of concurrent or preexisting cardiorespiratory conditions, such as left-sided heart failure, valvular heart disease, pulmonary disease (i.e., chronic obstructive pulmonary disease, pulmonary fibrosis), or pulmonary vascular disease (i.e., venous thromboembolic disease). Although hypercapnia is seen in a small percentage of patients, an arterial blood gas should be considered to measure $PaCO_2$ in patients with low or low normal SpO_2 at rest and those with concomitant cardiopulmonary or neuromuscular diseases or chest wall deformities. Those with CSA should have a transthoracic echocardiography to assess LV function. Further neurologic workup should be done as clinically indicated.

TREATMENT

OBSTRUCTIVE SEEP APNEA

Positive Airway Pressure Therapy

Treatment of OSA depends on the severity of OSA. Based on current Medicare guidelines specifying the criteria for ordering nasal CPAP, all patients with at least moderate disease (AHI >15 events per hour) are eligible for CPAP regardless of their daytime symptoms. Patients with mild OSA (AHI of 5 to 14) may be candidates for CPAP if they are symptomatic (i.e., hypersomnolence or cardiovascular disease).

Nasal CPAP is the most effective therapy for OSA and, thus, is the standard of care. It treats OSA by splinting the upper airway and preventing its collapse. A full-night, attended, in-laboratory CPAP titration is usually done before initiation of therapy at home. Auto-CPAP, newer equipment that automatically changes pressure based on the quality of flow and the presence of respiratory events, are also available for use (68,69). Nonetheless, the precise role of these devices is still being studied (69).

Nasal CPAP improves neurocognitive function in patients with hypersomnia, but not in those without daytime symptoms (70–72). Nasal CPAP can also provide several benefits for the cardiovascular system (73). Nasal CPAP therapy decreases blood pressure (68,71,74) and improves LV ejection fraction in patients with CHF and OSA (75).

Bilevel PAP works similarly by splinting the upper airway and preventing its collapse. In contrast to a fixed pressure during inhalation and exhalation, bilevel PAP delivers two different levels of pressure: Higher during inhalation and lower during exhalation. Bilevel PAP is usually reserved for those with concomitant hypoventilation, significant aerophagia, and intolerance to CPAP.

Compliance with nasal CPAP is a major hurdle in treatment of OSA. About half the patients who are prescribed nasal CPAP are compliant with therapy. Adherence to therapy and compliance can be improved with the use of a heated humidifier, pressure ramp, better mask fitting, and pressure relief CPAP, which allows the lowering of the pressure at the beginning of expiration with return to set pressure before the end of expiration without compromising the upper airway (76). The most common side effects of CPAP are dry mouth, rhinitis, and sinus congestion, which can be minimized with routine use of humidification as well as nasal or systemic antihistamines and nasal steroids, as needed.

Oral Appliances

Oral devices work by moving the tongue and jaw forward in an attempt to improve the size of posterior airspace. Oral appliances decrease AHI in most patients, but are recommended as an alternative therapy to nasal CPAP in mild disease, particularly in patients who prefer alternative therapies to nasal CPAP (77).

Surgery

Although the role of surgical intervention in an attempt to reconfigure upper airway remains controversial, it may still be an option for some patients, particularly for those who cannot tolerate nasal CPAP, for whom nasal CPAP was unsuccessful, and those with mild OSA (AHI <10) (17). Common surgical procedures for OSA include tonsillectomy, adenoidectomy, nasal surgery, and uvulopalatopharyngoplasty. Other surgical interventions are mandibular advancement and tracheostomy. The latter is considered for patients with severe OSA and underlying cardiopulmonary disease who cannot tolerate, or are not compliant with, nasal CPAP.

CENTRAL SLEEP APNEA

CPAP may eliminate CSA in some patients; however, its clinical effectiveness is less well documented. Although initial studies have shown beneficial effects of nasal CPAP on CSA and CSR in CHF, the Canadian Positive Airway Pressure study (CANPAP) trial testing the use of nasal CPAP for patients with CHF who were medically optimized, found that nasal CPAP attenuated central sleep apnea, improved nocturnal oxygenation, increased LV ejection fraction, lowered sympathetic nervous system activity, and increased the 6-minute walk test distance, but failed to improve survival (35). Thus, routine use of nasal CPAP is not recommended for patients with CHF to treat CSR or CSA.

Adaptive servoventilation (ASV) is newer mode of ventilatory support in which a small but varying amount of ventilatory support is provided (78). ASV provides a 4- to 5-cm H_2O expiratory and 8 cm H_2O end-inspiratory support during regular breathing (78). Inspiratory pressure support is increased up to 15 cm H_2O if a central apnea is detected to maintain minute ventilation at 90% of the average ventilation of the patient. ASV has been shown to alleviate CSA, and improve daytime sleepiness and sleep structure with increases in slow-wave and REM sleep (78–80).

COMPLEX SLEEP APNEA

Nasal CPAP is successful in the treatment of obstructive events in CompSA, but it also unmasks the CSA and CSR, which continue to disrupt breathing and sleep despite CPAP. The optimal treatment strategy for these patients is not known. Supplemental oxygen or low-concentration CO_2 used to prevent hypocapnia and, consequently, central events may be an effective adjunct therapy in the management; however, is yet to be studied (81). Similar to CSA, ASV may be useful in treatment of CompSA.

CLINICAL RECOMMENDATIONS OF THE VIGNETTE

The patient was discharged home on bilevel PAP of 16/12 cm H_2O without any supplemental oxygen. Her final diagnoses were OSA and obesity hypoventilation syndrome.

History and physical examination findings can provide important clues for sleep-related breathing disorders. Neurocognitive and cardiovascular consequences of OSA warrant the need to have a low suspicion for OSA. Polysomnography is the diagnostic method of choice for further evaluation of sleep-related breathing disorders. Nasal CPAP is the most effective treatment for OSA. The optimal treatment modality for CSA and CompSA is still unknown.

SUMMARY

Sleep-related breathing disorders are common, but often underdiagnosed, partly because of limited knowledge about these disorders. Better understanding of OSA, as well as other sleep-related breathing disorders, is warranted to improve the rate of diagnosis as well as the treatment of these disorders, which may be associated with serious neurocognitive and cardiovascular consequences.

REFERENCES

1. Phillipson EA. Control of breathing during sleep. *Am Rev Respir Dis.* 1978;118:909–939.
2. Leung RS, Bradley TD. Sleep apnea and cardiovascular disease. *Am J Respir Crit Care Med.* 2001;164:2147–2165.
3. Orem J, Osorio I, Brooks E, et al. Activity of respiratory neurons during NREM sleep. *J Neurophysiol.* 1985;54:1144–1156.
4. Chandler SH, Chase MH, Nakamura Y. Intracellular analysis of synaptic mechanisms controlling trigeminal motoneuron activity during sleep and wakefulness. *J Neurophysiol.* 1980;44:359–371.
5. Hornyak M, Cejnar M, Elam M, et al. Sympathetic muscle nerve activity during sleep in man. *Brain.* 1991;114(Pt 3):1281–1295.
6. Meoli AL, Casey KR, Clark RW, et al. Hypopnea in sleep-disordered breathing in adults. *Sleep.* 2001;24:469–470.
7. Dowdell WT, Javaheri S, McGinnis W. Cheyne-Stokes respiration presenting as sleep apnea syndrome. Clinical and polysomnographic features. *Am Rev Respir Dis.* 1990;141:871–879.
8. Gilmartin GS, Daly RW, Thomas RJ. Recognition and management of complex sleep-disordered breathing. *Curr Opin Pulm Med.* 2005;11:485–493.
9. Wiegand L, Zwillich CW, White DP. Collapsibility of the human upper airway during normal sleep. *J Appl Physiol.* 1989;66:1800–1808.
10. Guilleminault C, Stoohs R, Clerk A, et al. A cause of excessive daytime sleepiness. The upper airway resistance syndrome. *Chest.* 1993;104:781–787.
11. Bixler EO, Vgontzas AN, Lin HM, et al. Prevalence of sleep-disordered breathing in women: Effects of gender. *Am J Respir Crit Care Med.* 2001;163:608–613.

12. Bixler EO, Vgontzas AN, Ten Have T, et al. Effects of age on sleep apnea in men: I. Prevalence and severity. *Am J Respir Crit Care Med.* 1998;157:144–148.
13. Young T, Evans L, Finn L, et al. Estimation of the clinically diagnosed proportion of sleep apnea syndrome in middle-aged men and women. *Sleep.* 1997;20:705–706.
14. Young T, Palta M, Dempsey J, et al. The occurrence of sleep-disordered breathing among middle-aged adults. *N Engl J Med.* 1993;328:1230–1235.
15. Young T, Peppard PE, Gottlieb DJ. Epidemiology of obstructive sleep apnea: A population health perspective. *Am J Respir Crit Care Med.* 2002;165:1217–1239.
16. Duran J, Esnaola S, Rubio R, et al. Obstructive sleep apnea-hypopnea and related clinical features in a population-based sample of subjects aged 30 to 70 yr. *Am J Respir Crit Care Med.* 2001;163:685–689.
17. Caples SM, Gami AS, Somers VK. Obstructive sleep apnea. *Ann Intern Med.* 2005;142: 187–197.
18. Hosselet J, Ayappa I, Norman RG, et al. Classification of sleep-disordered breathing. *Am J Respir Crit Care Med.* 2001;163:398–405.
19. Good DC, Henkle JQ, Gelber D, et al. Sleep-disordered breathing and poor functional outcome after stroke. *Stroke.* 1996;27:252–259.
20. Bassetti C, Aldrich MS. Sleep apnea in acute cerebrovascular diseases: Final report on 128 patients. *Sleep.* 1999;22:217–223.
21. Lofaso F, Verschueren P, Rande JL, et al. Prevalence of sleep-disordered breathing in patients on a heart transplant waiting list. *Chest.* 1994;106:1689–1694.
22. Hanly PJ, Millar TW, Steljes DG, et al. Respiration and abnormal sleep in patients with congestive heart failure. *Chest.* 1989;96:480–488.
23. Javaheri S, Parker TJ, Liming JD, et al. Sleep apnea in 81 ambulatory male patients with stable heart failure. Types and their prevalences, consequences, and presentations. *Circulation.* 1998;97:2154–2159.
24. Sin DD, Fitzgerald F, Parker JD, et al. Risk factors for central and obstructive sleep apnea in 450 men and women with congestive heart failure. *Am J Respir Crit Care Med.* 1999;160: 1101–1106.
25. Morgenthaler TI, Kagramanov V, Hanak V, et al. Complex sleep apnea syndrome: Is it a unique clinical syndrome? *Sleep.* 2006;29:1203–1209.
26. Young T, Skatrud J, Peppard PE. Risk factors for obstructive sleep apnea in adults. *JAMA.* 2004;291:2013–2016.
27. Fogel RB, Malhotra A, White DP. Sleep. 2: Pathophysiology of obstructive sleep apnoea/hypopnoea syndrome. *Thorax.* 2004;59:159–163.
28. Badr MS, Toiber F, Skatrud JB, et al. Pharyngeal narrowing/occlusion during central sleep apnea. *J Appl Physiol.* 1995;78:1806–1815.
29. Hudgel DW, Chapman KR, Faulks C, et al. Changes in inspiratory muscle electrical activity and upper airway resistance during periodic breathing induced by hypoxia during sleep. *Am Rev Respir Dis.* 1987;135:899–906.
30. Onal E, Burrows DL, Hart RH, et al. Induction of periodic breathing during sleep causes upper airway obstruction in humans. *J Appl Physiol.* 1986;61:1438–1443.
31. Badr MS, Kawak A, Skatrud JB, et al. Effect of induced hypocapnic hypopnea on upper airway patency in humans during NREM sleep. *Respir Physiol.* 1997;110:33–45.
32. Xie A, Rutherford R, Rankin F, et al. Hypocapnia and increased ventilatory responsiveness in patients with idiopathic central sleep apnea. *Am J Respir Crit Care Med.* 1995;152:1950–1955.
33. Xie A, Skatrud JB, Puleo DS, et al. Apnea-hypopnea threshold for CO_2 in patients with congestive heart failure. *Am J Respir Crit Care Med.* 2002;165:1245–1250.
34. Naughton MT, Benard DC, Liu PP, et al. Effects of nasal CPAP on sympathetic activity in patients with heart failure and central sleep apnea. *Am J Respir Crit Care Med.* 1995;152:473–479.
35. Bradley TD, Logan AG, Kimoff RJ, et al. Continuous positive airway pressure for central sleep apnea and heart failure. *N Engl J Med.* 2005;353:2025–2033.
36. Chen L, Einbinder E, Zhang Q, et al. Oxidative stress and left ventricular function with chronic intermittent hypoxia in rats. *Am J Respir Crit Care Med.* 2005;172:915–920.
37. Brooks D, Horner RL, Kozar LF, et al. Obstructive sleep apnea as a cause of systemic hypertension. Evidence from a canine model. *J Clin Invest.* 1997;99:106–109.
38. Ip MS, Tse HF, Lam B, et al. Endothelial function in obstructive sleep apnea and response to treatment. *Am J Respir Crit Care Med.* 2004;169:348–353.
39. Robinson GV, Pepperell JC, Segal HC, et al. Circulating cardiovascular risk factors in obstructive sleep apnoea: Data from randomised controlled trials. *Thorax.* 2004;59:777–782.
40. O'Donoghue FJ, Briellmann RS, Rochford PD, et al. Cerebral structural changes in severe obstructive sleep apnea. *Am J Respir Crit Care Med.* 2005;171:1185–1190.
41. Zhan G, Fenik P, Pratico D, et al. Inducible nitric oxide synthase in long-term intermittent hypoxia: Hypersomnolence and brain injury. *Am J Respir Crit Care Med.* 2005;171:1414–1420.
42. Yokoe T, Minoguchi K, Matsuo H, et al. Elevated levels of C-reactive protein and interleukin-6 in patients with obstructive sleep apnea syndrome are decreased by nasal continuous positive airway pressure. *Circulation.* 2003;107:1129–1134.
43. Spiegel K, Leproult R, Van Cauter E. Impact of sleep debt on metabolic and endocrine function. *Lancet.* 1999;354:1435–1439.
44. Punjabi NM, Sorkin JD, Katzel LI, et al. Sleep-disordered breathing and insulin resistance in middle-aged and overweight men. *Am J Respir Crit Care Med.* 2002;165:677–682.
45. Kim HC, Young T, Matthews CG, et al. Sleep-disordered breathing and neuropsychological deficits. A population-based study. *Am J Respir Crit Care Med.* 1997;156:1813–1819.
46. Sassani A, Findley LJ, Kryger M, et al. Reducing motor-vehicle collisions, costs, and fatalities by treating obstructive sleep apnea syndrome. *Sleep.* 2004;27:453–458.
47. Tsai WH, Remmers JE, Brant R, et al. A decision rule for diagnostic testing in obstructive sleep apnea. *Am J Respir Crit Care Med.* 2003;167:1427–1432.
48. Netzer NC, Stoohs RA, Netzer CM, et al. Using the Berlin Questionnaire to identify patients at risk for the sleep apnea syndrome. *Ann Intern Med.* 1999;131:485–491.
49. Schellenberg JB, Maislin G, Schwab RJ. Physical findings and the risk for obstructive sleep apnea. The importance of oropharyngeal structures. *Am J Respir Crit Care Med.* 2000;162: 740–748.
50. Gami AS, Howard DE, Olson EJ, et al. Day-night pattern of sudden death in obstructive sleep apnea. *N Engl J Med.* 2005;352:1206–1214.
51. Shahar E, Whitney CW, Redline S, et al. Sleep-disordered breathing and cardiovascular disease: Cross-sectional results of the Sleep Heart Health Study. *Am J Respir Crit Care Med.* 2001;163:19–25.
52. Nieto FJ, Young TB, Lind BK, et al. Association of sleep-disordered breathing, sleep apnea, and hypertension in a large community-based study. Sleep Heart Health Study. *JAMA.* 2000;283:1829–1836.
53. Peppard PE, Young T, Palta M, et al. Prospective study of the association between sleep-disordered breathing and hypertension. *N Engl J Med.* 2000;342:1378–1384.
54. Hla KM, Young TB, Bidwell T, et al. Sleep apnea and hypertension. A population-based study. *Ann Intern Med.* 1994;120:382–388.
55. Nieto FJ, Herrington DM, Redline S, et al. Sleep apnea and markers of vascular endothelial function in a large community sample of older adults. *Am J Respir Crit Care Med.* 2004;169:354–360.
56. Young T, Peppard P, Palta M, et al. Population-based study of sleep-disordered breathing as a risk factor for hypertension. *Arch Intern Med.* 1997;157:1746–1752.
57. Kanagala R, Murali NS, Friedman PA, et al. Obstructive sleep apnea and the recurrence of atrial fibrillation. *Circulation.* 2003;107:2589–2594.
58. Yaggi HK, Concato J, Kernan WN, et al. Obstructive sleep apnea as a risk factor for stroke and death. *N Engl J Med.* 2005;353:2034–2041.
59. Punjabi NM, Ahmed MM, Polotsky VY, et al. Sleep-disordered breathing, glucose intolerance, and insulin resistance. *Respir Physiol Neurobiol.* 2003;136:167–178.
60. Punjabi NM, Shahar E, Redline S, et al. Sleep-disordered breathing, glucose intolerance, and insulin resistance: The Sleep Heart Health Study. *Am J Epidemiol.* 2004;160:521–530.
61. Spiegel K, Tasali E, Penev P, et al. Brief communication: Sleep curtailment in healthy young men is associated with decreased leptin levels, elevated ghrelin levels, and increased hunger and appetite. *Ann Intern Med.* 2004;141:846–850.
62. Flegal KM, Carroll MD, Ogden CL, et al. Prevalence and trends in obesity among US adults, 1999–2000. *JAMA.* 2002;288:1723–1727.
63. Beninati W, Harris CD, Herold DL, et al. The effect of snoring and obstructive sleep apnea on the sleep quality of bed partners. *Mayo Clin Proc.* 1999;74:955–958.
64. Kushida CA, Littner MR, Morgenthaler T, et al. Practice parameters for the indications for polysomnography and related procedures: An update for 2005. *Sleep.* 2005;28:499–521.
65. Le Bon O, Hoffmann G, Tecco J, et al. Mild to moderate sleep respiratory events: One negative night may not be enough. *Chest.* 2000;118:353–359.
66. Chesson AL, Jr., Berry RB, Pack A. Practice parameters for the use of portable monitoring devices in the investigation of suspected obstructive sleep apnea in adults. *Sleep.* 2003;26:907–913.
67. Atwood CW, Jr., McCrory D, Garcia JG, et al. Pulmonary artery hypertension and sleep-disordered breathing: ACCP evidence-based clinical practice guidelines. *Chest.* 2004;126:72S–77S.
68. Becker HF, Jerrentrup A, Ploch T, et al. Effect of nasal continuous positive airway pressure treatment on blood pressure in patients with obstructive sleep apnea. *Circulation.* 2003; 107:68–73.
69. Littner M, Hirshkowitz M, Davila D, et al. Practice parameters for the use of auto-titrating continuous positive airway pressure devices for titrating pressures and treating adult patients with obstructive sleep apnea syndrome. An American Academy of Sleep Medicine report. *Sleep.* 2002;25:143–147.
70. Engleman HM, Martin SE, Deary IJ, et al. Effect of continuous positive airway pressure treatment on daytime function in sleep apnoea/hypopnoea syndrome. *Lancet.* 1994;343: 572–575.
71. Pepperell JC, Ramdassingh-Dow S, Crosthwaite N, et al. Ambulatory blood pressure after therapeutic and subtherapeutic nasal continuous positive airway pressure for obstructive sleep apnoea: A randomised parallel trial. *Lancet.* 2002;359:204–210.
72. Barbe F, Mayoralas LR, Duran J, et al. Treatment with continuous positive airway pressure is not effective in patients with sleep apnea but no daytime sleepiness. A randomized, controlled trial. *Ann Intern Med.* 2001;134:1015–1023.
73. Bradley TD, Floras JS. Sleep apnea and heart failure: Part I: Obstructive sleep apnea. *Circulation.* 2003;107:1671–1678.
74. Faccenda JF, Mackay TW, Boon NA, et al. Randomized placebo-controlled trial of continuous positive airway pressure on blood pressure in the sleep apnea-hypopnea syndrome. *Am J Respir Crit Care Med.* 2001;163:344–348.
75. Kaneko Y, Floras JS, Usui K, et al. Cardiovascular effects of continuous positive airway pressure in patients with heart failure and obstructive sleep apnea. *N Engl J Med.* 2003;348: 1233–1241.
76. Nilius G, Happel A, Domanski U, et al. Pressure-relief continuous positive airway pressure vs constant continuous positive airway pressure: A comparison of efficacy and compliance. *Chest.* 2006;130:1018–1024.
77. Kushida CA, Morgenthaler TI, Littner MR, et al. Practice parameters for the treatment of snoring and obstructive sleep apnea with oral appliances: An update for 2005. *Sleep.* 2006;29:240–243.
78. Teschler H, Dohring J, Wang YM, et al. Adaptive pressure support servo-ventilation: A novel treatment for Cheyne-Stokes respiration in heart failure. *Am J Respir Crit Care Med.* 2001;164:614–619.
79. Pepperell JC, Maskell NA, Jones DR, et al. A randomized controlled trial of adaptive ventilation for Cheyne-Stokes breathing in heart failure. *Am J Respir Crit Care Med.* 2003;168: 1109–1114.
80. Philippe C, Stoica-Herman M, Drouot X, et al. Compliance with and effectiveness of adaptive servoventilation versus continuous positive airway pressure in the treatment of Cheyne-Stokes respiration in heart failure over a six month period. *Heart.* 2006;92: 337–342.
81. Thomas RJ, Daly RW, Weiss JW. Low-concentration carbon dioxide is an effective adjunct to positive airway pressure in the treatment of refractory mixed central and obstructive sleep-disordered breathing. *Sleep.* 2005;28:69–77.

CHAPTER 23

Neurologic Manifestations of Interstitial Lung Disease

Robert P. Baughman • Istvan Pirko

OBJECTIVES

- To understand that sarcoidosis can present with just neurologic disease; however, careful evaluation will often discover other organ involvement
- To emphasize that cranial nerve involvement, especially seventh nerve paralysis, is the most common form of neurosarcoidosis
- To understand that neurosarcoidosis and multiple sclerosis (MS) can share several features; however, the major distinguishing feature is the extracranial manifestations of sarcoidosis
- To understand that neurosarcoidosis initially responds to corticosteroid therapy. With time, over half of the patients may require steroid-sparing agents to control the disease.

CASE VIGNETTE

The patient is a 39-year-old black woman who initially noted headache. She saw her primary care physician, who ordered a magnetic resonance imaging (MRI) study of her head. This demonstrated several areas of increased signal intensity in the brain. She was referred to a neurosurgeon. In the week before she saw the neurosurgeon, she developed paresthesias in both her arms and legs. An MRI of her cervical spine showed multiple lesions (Fig. 23-1) as well as adenopathy in the neck. A chest computed tomography (CT) scan demonstrated mediastinal adenopathy.

DEFINITION

Sarcoidosis is a multisystem disease of unknown etiology (1,2). It is characterized by the presence of noncaseating granulomas in one or more organs. The diagnosis requires the exclusion of all known causes of granulomatous disease. The diagnosis of neurosarcoidosis can be made when granulomatous involvement is proved by biopsy of neurologic tissue. The diagnosis of neurosarcoidosis is also felt to be definite in a patient with sarcoidosis confirmed from a non-neurologic area who has typical MRI findings, a lymphocytic meningitis, or diabetes insipidus in the absence of alternative causes. A patient with sarcoidosis has probable neurosarcoidosis in cases of findings of nonspecific MRI changes or a peripheral neuropathy which could not be explained by other diseases.

EPIDEMIOLOGY

Sarcoidosis is a worldwide disease, with increased incidence in some areas, such as nordic countries. It has also been reported as more frequent in blacks than in whites in the United States. In one study of patients seen in a large health care system in Detroit, the lifetime risk for sarcoidosis was about 1% for whites and 4% for blacks.

The incidence of neurologic involvement in patients with sarcoidosis has been reported as 5% to 25%, with higher numbers having been reported from referral centers (3–5). In a prospective epidemiologic study of 736 patients newly diagnosed with sarcoidosis in the United States, 34 (4.6%) had definite or probable neurosarcoidosis. No difference was found in the frequency of the disease in regard to race or gender. Of the 215 patients reevaluated 2 years later, 5 (2.3%) new cases of neurosarcoidosis were found.

ETIOLOGY AND PATHOGENESIS

The cause of sarcoidosis remains unknown. A common hypothesis is that sarcoidosis is an abnormal immune response to an environmental or infectious agent in a genetically susceptible host. Environmental studies have detected an increased risk for those exposed to certain environmental agents, such as mold, and in certain occupations, such as health care workers and firemen. Recent studies have suggested a possible role for infections, such as mycobacteria and *Propiniobacter acnes.* The granulomatous response of sarcoidosis may be triggered by more than one antigen.

Whatever the inciting event, the initial granulomatous response of sarcoidosis is felt to be a characteristic Th-1 response. The putative agent(s) seems to be presented by antigen-presenting cells to a T-helper cell. This interaction triggers an initial inflammatory cascade, which includes the cytokines IL-2, IL-12, γ-interferon, and tumor necrosis factor-α (TNF-α). The initial granuloma is characterized by CD4 lymphocytes and mononuclear giant cells.

The granulomas of sarcoidosis are usually well formed, compact lesions. Occasional areas of necrosis can be found, but caseation should not be present. The pathologist must look for evidence of other causes of granulomatous diseases, such as tuberculosis or fungal infections.

CLINICAL MANIFESTATIONS/ SPECIAL SITUATIONS

The clinician needs to consider neurosarcoidosis in three situations. The first is the patient with known sarcoidosis who presents with possible neurologic involvement. The second is the patient who presents with granulomatous disease of the nervous system in whom sarcoidosis may be the cause. The third is the patient who presents with a neurologic complaint that could be caused by sarcoidosis or another condition, such as multiple sclerosis (MS).

The clinical presentation of neurosarcoidosis varies. Some patterns of common involvement are seen, however, in patients with neurosarcoidosis. Cranial nerve involvement is the most common manifestation. Whereas VII nerve paralysis is most commonly reported by some, optic nerve involvement was the most common feature noted by others. In some cases, the cranial nerve involvement can occur before the diagnosis of sarcoidosis and resolve either spontaneously or with short-term corticosteroid therapy. The differential diagnosis of VII cranial nerve paralysis should include sarcoidosis. The presence of bilateral VII nerve paralysis makes sarcoidosis even more likely.

Hypothalamic involvement, including diabetes insipidus, can be the initial presentation of sarcoidosis. Although the hypothalamic lesion may respond to corticosteroid therapy, patients are often left with chronic diabetes insipidus. This is easily managed with desmopressin.

Leptomeningeal disease, which can be the only manifestation of neurosarcoidosis, can lead to chronic meningitis. The long-term consequence of this inflammation can be hydrocephalus. This is one of the few surgically treatable forms of sarcoidosis. Because the shunt itself can lead to a granulomatous reaction, a patient often still requires chronic systemic therapy.

Spinal cord disease can also occur as a result of sarcoidosis (Fig. 23-1). This unusual form of neurosarcoidosis can be difficult to diagnose. The differential diagnosis includes intervertebral disc disease, intramedullary or spinal cord tumors, tuberculosis infection, and MS. The presenting symptoms are usually paresthesias followed by paralysis. Regardless of the level of the lesion, symptoms usually start in the lower extremities. Onset of symptoms can be relatively slow and it is not uncommon for patients to have symptoms for several months before a specific diagnosis is made.

Peripheral neuropathy as either a mononeuritis or polyneuropathy has been described with neurosarcoidosis. One difficulty is the presence of diabetes mellitus, which can cause a similar peripheral neuropathy. In this situation, the management of such cases can be challenging, because the clinician can not be sure whether corticosteroids will make the symptoms worse or better.

MULTIPLE SCLEROSIS VERSUS SARCOIDOSIS

Multiple sclerosis and neurosarcoidosis can be similar in appearance and presentation. Both of these can be associated with nonspecific white matter changes in the brain. Table 23-1 lists some of the differentiating features between neurosarcoidosis and MS. Sarcoidosis is more common in women, whereas neurosarcoidosis does not differ between male and female patients. The age of onset appears similar for both diseases.

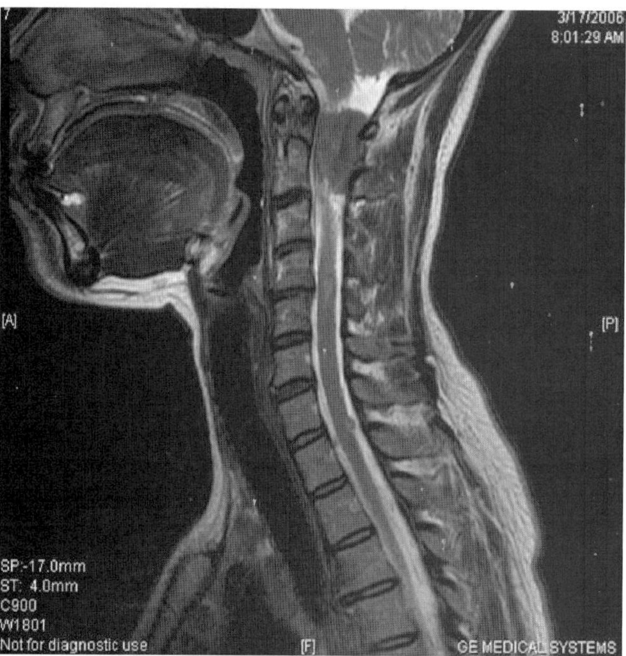

FIGURE 23-1. Cervical spine magnetic resonance image (MRI) showing areas of abnormal signal intensity within the high cervical cord that are compatible with a neurosarcoidosis lesion.

Ocular involvement, including optic neuritis and uveitis, is seen with both conditions (6). In MS, uveitis is seen in approximately 1% of cases. Patients with sarcoidosis have uveitis in 20% to 70% of cases, with the higher percentage in Japanese patients. In the United States, uveitis is more common in blacks. Intermediate uveitis with pars planitis is usually caused by only one of three conditions: MS, sarcoidosis, and idiopathic. Patients with pars planitis can eventually develop other evidence for MS. Treatment for uveitis is often glucocorticoids. For intermediate and posterior uveitis, topical steroid therapy is not sufficient. Periocular steroid injections and systemic glucocorticoids are often needed in this situation. Both diseases will respond to this regimen. Additional agents include methotrexate and infliximab.

A major difference between MS and sarcoidosis is the presence of thoracic disease. More than 90% of patients with sarcoidosis have thoracic disease. This includes parenchymal lung disease as well as adenopathy. In cases where some doubt exists about chest involvement, CT scan can be useful. Also positron emission tomography (PET) scan and gallium scan may detect mediastinal and hilar activity in patients with sarcoidosis. Such scanning should prove negative in patients with MS.

DIAGNOSTIC APPROACH

A focused history and physical examination comprise the first step in evaluating any case of potential neurosarcoidosis. As

TABLE 23-1. Comparison Between Neurosarcoidosis and Multiple Sclerosis

	Neurosarcoidosis	*Multiple Sclerosis*
Female predominance	No	Yes
Classic MRI findings	Gadolinium uptake in lesion	Demyelinating plaques
Most common MRI findings	Nonspecific white matter changes	Nonspecific white matter changes
Self-limited disease	Cranial facial nerve	Most aspects
Spinal fluid findings	Increased lymphocytes Moderate elevation protein No oligoclonal bands	Normal cells Mild elevation protein Oligoclonal bands
Ocular disease	Anterior uveitis Panuveitis Pars planitis Optic neuritis	Anterior uveitis Panuveitis Pars planitis Optic neuritis
Thoracic disease	Extremely common	Does not occur

MRI, magnetic resonance imaging.

noted, the condition may be considered in patients with known sarcoidosis. In conditions where either a specific granulomatous lesion of the nervous system has been identified or the patient has the potential for neurosarcoidosis, a standard evaluation for potential extra-neurologic systems is advised, Table 23-2 lists the recommended testing that should be considered in patients with potential or known sarcoidosis.

Testing for neurologic disease includes a detailed history and physical examination. Many of the manifestations of neurosarcoidosis can be slowly progressive, so that a patient may describe gradual onset of symptoms, such as headache or peripheral neuropathy. Other symptoms, such as seizures or paralysis, can be sudden. The history of VII nerve cranial paralysis may not have been associated with sarcoidosis by the patient or previous physician.

Of imaging studies, the MRI with gadolinium appears to be the more sensitive than CT scan (Figs. 23-1 and 23-2) (7–9). Although gadolinium enhancement may detect some lesions, the most common lesions in the brain parenchyma are multiple nonenhancing periventricular white matter lesions seen as high signal intensity on T2-weighted images. Others have found MRI enhancement a useful method to detect neurosarcoidosis. In one study of 22 patients with neurosarcoidosis, a range of MRI findings was described, including periventricular and white matter lesions on T2W spin echo images, mimicking MS (46%); multiple supratentorial and infratentorial brain lesions, mimicking metastases (36%); solitary intraaxial mass, mimicking high-grade astrocytoma (9%); solitary extra-axial mass, mimicking meningioma (5%); and leptomeningeal enhancement (36%).

TABLE 23-2. Recommended Initial Evaluation of Patients with Known or Suspected Sarcoidosis

1. History (including symptoms and occupational exposures)
2. Physical examination
3. Posterior anterior chest roentgenogram
4. Pulmonary function studies: Spirometry and Diffusion in Lung of Carbon Monoxide (DLCO)
5. Peripheral blood counts
6. Serum chemistries: Calcium, liver function testing (alkaline phosphatase, alanine aminotransferase, aspirate aminotransferase, total bilirubin), creatinine, glucose
7. Routine ophthalmologic examination
8. Electrocardiogram*
9. Urine analysis*
10. Tuberculin skin test*

* Suggested if clinically indicated.

Spinal cord involvement can also be detected by MRI scanning. Among the lesions detected are intramedullary lesions and leptomeningeal disease. Serial studies have shown improvement in MRI lesions of the spine in some, but not all, cases.

Radiologic imaging of the chest remains an important part of assessing possible cases of neurologic sarcoidosis. Traditionally, the chest roentgenogram of sarcoidosis is characterized by four patterns: Stage 1, hilar adenopathy alone; stage 2, hilar adenopathy plus infiltrates; stage 3, infiltrates alone; and stage 4, fibrosis.

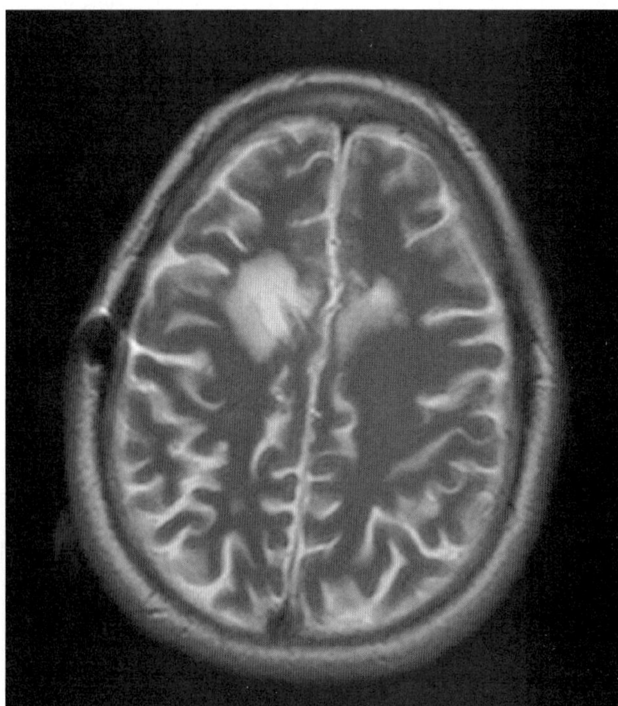

FIGURE 23-2. Magnetic resonance image (MRI) of brain showing increased signal intensities involving the frontal white matter bilaterally.

TABLE 23-3. Comparison of Cerebrospinal Fluid (CSF) Findings in Chronic Inflammatory Diseases of the Central Nervous System (CNS)

Disease	*Cells*	*Increased Protein*	*IgG Index*	*Low Glucose*	*Oligoclonal Bands*	*Other Features*
Sarcoidosis	Lymphocytes common	Common	Increased	Unusual	Rare	Elevated ACE
Multiple sclerosis	Mild increase lymphocytes	Normal	Almost always	Rare	Very common	
Neuro lupus erythematosis	Usually no cells	Rare	Commonly increased	Rare	Common	
Neurologic Behçet disease	Neutrophils, lymphocytes	Common	Commonly increased		Common	
Sjögren syndrome	Common lymphocytes, monocytes	Common	Commonly increased	Common	Very common	
Tuberculous meningitis	Common lymphocytes	Common	N.A.	Common		PCR for *Mycobacterium tuberculosis*
Cryptococcal meningitis	Common lymphocytes	Common	N.A.	Common		Cryptococcal antigen
Leptomeningeal carcinomatosis	Common lymphocytes	Common	N.A.	Common		Cytology

N.A., not available.
ACE, angiotensin-converting enzyme; PCR, polymerase chain reaction.

More than 80% of patients with sarcoidosis will have lung involvement that can be characterized into these four stages. CT scan can be more sensitive for lung involvement than plain chest roentgenogram in sarcoidosis. The CT scan features include hilar adenopathy, peribronchial thickening, ground glass opacities, and subpleural nodularity.

Cerebrospinal fluid (CSF) analysis is also useful in detecting neurosarcoidosis (10). The usual findings are increased protein and lymphocytes, and less frequently, reduced glucose. Increased protein, increased lymphocytes, or both have been reported in 73% and 81% of patients studied in two large studies of neurosarcoidosis. An increased IgG index can be seen, but oligoclonal bands are rare. Table 23-3 summarizes the CSF patterns of the most commonly encountered chronic inflammatory diseases in the CSF. Infectious granulomatous diseases, such as tuberculosis and cryptococcus, should also be sought with appropriate cultures.

Special studies of the CSF have been proposed as helpful in the diagnosis of neurosarcoidosis. An increase in the CD4:CD8 ratio of the lymphocytes in the CSF has been reported in neurosarcoidosis. The usual method of determining T-lymphocyte subsets, however, is with flow cytometry. That technique requires a large number of viable lymphocytes and, therefore, is usually not suitable for routine analysis.

Increased angiotensin-converting enzyme (ACE) in the CSF has been reported. Increased levels, however, have been reported in other conditions, including schizophrenia. Elevation of CSF ACE seems to occur when diffuse enhancing lesions are seen on MRI. Overall, increased CSF ACE appears to occur in about half of the cases of neurosarcoidosis.

Elevation in serum ACE is fairly specific for sarcoidosis. During acute disease, about two thirds of patients with sarcoidosis will have an elevated ACE level. Analysis of ACE polymorphisms will enhance the diagnostic yield of the serum ACE level. The effect, however, is relatively small and, therefore, not commonly performed. ACE levels can be normal in neurosarcoidosis, and a normal level does not rule out sarcoidosis. Elevation of ACE levels in the serum is also seen with Gaucher disease, leprosy, tuberculosis, histoplasmosis, coccidiomycosis, and hyperthyroidism. The ACE test is a biological test and, therefore, patients taking ACE inhibitors will have very low levels.

TREATMENT

Corticosteroids remain the drug of choice for initial manifestations of serious pulmonary and extrapulmonary disease. Convincing evidence indicates a role for corticosteroids for symptomatic pulmonary disease. Less convincing data exist for neurologic disease. In two large series looking at therapy for chronic neurosarcoidosis, corticosteroids alone were the final treatment in only 29% and 38%, respectively. The dose to control chronic neurosarcoidosis was usually between 10 and 20 mg per day. Patients often require years of therapy.

Because of the high dosage and the toxicity of prolonged corticosteroid use, alternatives have been sought. These have included the antimalarial agents chloroquine and hydroxychloroquine, which were reported as useful in a series of selected cases of neurosarcoidosis.

The cytotoxic drugs have been used for refractory neurosarcoidosis. In one series of 28 patients with neurosarcoidosis, methotrexate was effective 65% of the time, The dose to control neurosarcoidosis was usually between 10 and 20 mg of prednisone per day. Patients with neurosarcoidosis are usually cotreated with corticosteroids for the first 6 months while waiting to see if the drug will be effective. Monitoring includes at least bimonthly complete blood counts, and liver and renal function. The major toxicities of methotrexate include nausea, mouth sores, and leucopenia, which can be minimized by dose

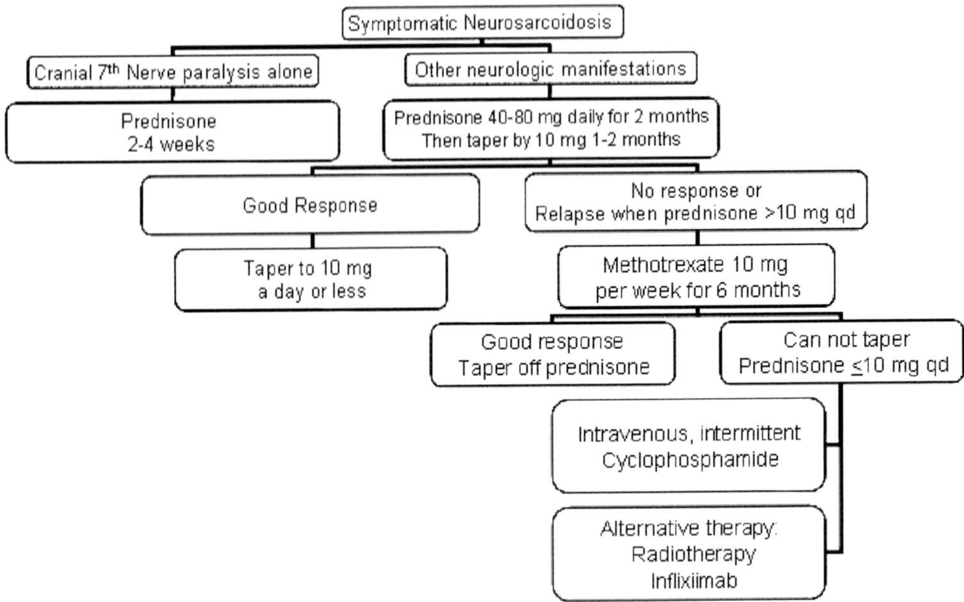

FIGURE 23-3. Algorithm of therapeutic approach of symptomatic neurosarcoidosis.

adjustment and use of folic acid (1 mg/day). Long-term use has been associated with pulmonary fibrosis and liver damage. The latter can be screened for by liver biopsies after every 1 to 1.5 gm of cumulative dose.

Cyclophosphamide has been also reported as useful in treating neurosarcoidosis. The use of intermittent, intravenous cyclophosphamide is associated with less toxicity. Response rates of 90% or more have been reported in several series. Toxicities include nausea, leucopenia, and bladder irritation. Long-term risk includes an increased risk for cancer, especially bladder cancer. This appears to be lower in patients receiving intravenous dosing.

Cyclosporine has also been reported as useful in selected cases of neurosarcoidosis. It was reported as useful when other agents, including cytotoxic drugs, were unsuccessful. For pulmonary sarcoidosis, cyclosporine was not found to be steroid sparing in a randomized, controlled trial.

Figure 23-3 shows a treatment algorithm that can be used for treating neurosarcoidosis. This algorithm emphasizes the chronic nature of most cases of neurosarcoidosis. It balances the different response rates versus toxicities.

CLINICAL RECOMMENDATIONS OF THE VIGNETTE

The patient was started on prednisone (80 mg/day) and within a week her headaches and paresthesias resolved. She denied any respiratory symptoms, rash, weight loss, or night sweats. She had a bronchoscopy, whicht was nondiagnostic. A mediastinoscopy was performed. It showed a large number of compact, well-formed granulomas. Subsequent cultures were negative for fungus or mycobacteria.

After the confirmation of the diagnosis of sarcoidosis by mediastinoscopy, the patient was continued on prednisone, and methotrexate was added (10 mg/week). Her prednisone was tapered from her initial dose of 80 mg a day to 20 mg over the first 6 month, and she is now taking methotrexate and prednisone (5 mg/day) 1 year after initial presentation of symptoms.

SUMMARY

Neurosarcoidosis can be difficult to diagnose and treat. For most cases, however, sarcoidosis can be diagnosed because of its multisystem involvement. Treatment for neurosarcoidosis has not been standardized. Corticosteroids represent the usual first choice, but steroid-sparing agents are often useful in controlling the disease with minimal toxicity.

REFERENCES

1. Hunninghake GW, Costabel U, Ando M, et al. ATS/ERS/WASOG statement on sarcoidosis. American Thoracic Society/European Respiratory Society/World Association of Sarcoidosis and other Granulomatous Disorders. *Sarcoidosis Vasc Diffuse Lung Dis.* 1999;16:149–173.
2. Baughman RP, du Bois RM, Lower EE. Sarcoidosis. *Lancet.* 2003;361:1111–1118.
3. Lower EE, Broderick JP, Brott TG, et al. Diagnosis and management of neurologic sarcoidosis. *Arch Intern Med.* 1997;157:1864–1868.
4. Zajicek JP, Scolding NJ, Foster O, et al. Central nervous system sarcoidosis—Diagnosis and management. *QJ Med.* 1999;92:103–117.
5. Maca SM, Scharitzer M, Barisani-Asenbauer T. Uveitis and neurologic diseases: An often overlooked relationship. *Wien Klin Wochenschr.* 2006;118:273–279.
6. Allen RK, Sellars RE, Sandstrom PA. A prospective study of 32 patients with neurosarcoidosis. *Sarcoidosis Vasc Diffuse Lung Dis.* 2003;20:118–125.
7. Pickuth D, Heywang-Kobrunner SH. Neurosarcoidosis: Evaluation with MRI. *J Neuroradiol.* 2000;27:185–188.
8. Smith JK, Matheus MG, Castillo M. Imaging manifestations of neurosarcoidosis. *AJR Am J Roentgenol.* 2004;182:289–295.
9. Nowak DA, Widenka DC. Neurosarcoidosis: A review of its intracranial manifestation. *J Neurol.* 2001;248:363–372.
10. Reske D, Petereit HF, Heiss WD. Difficulties in the differentiation of chronic inflammatory diseases of the central nervous system—Value of cerebrospinal fluid analysis and immunological abnormalities in the diagnosis. *Acta Neurol Scand.* 2005;112:207–213.

CHAPTER **24**

Lung Transplantation

William D. Schweickert • Gregory Gruener • Edward R. Garrity, Jr

OBJECTIVES

- To describe the five main categories of neuromuscular complications in lung transplant recipients: (i) injuries associated with the transplant; (ii) medication effects; (iii) infection; (iv) malignancy; and (v) impaired posttransplant neuromuscular function
- To review the approach to distinguish between traumatic, vascular, infectious, neoplastic, and metabolic causes of neurologic symptoms in transplant recipients
- To emphasize the commonality of neurotoxicity from immunosuppressive agents and how drug interactions and altered renal or hepatic function can exacerbate them

CASE VIGNETTE

A 28-year-old man with cystic fibrosis status after bilateral sequential lung transplant presents in the emergency room with new-onset seizures. He reports feeling well until 3 days previously when he began experiencing dull, bitemporal headaches. He had been taking intermittent ibuprofen to control the pain. The morning of admission, he was witnessed to have a generalized tonic-clonic seizure. He denies persistent neurologic deficits.

He has been followed closely by his lung transplant team who report no significant complications to date, including stable lung function. During the last evaluation, his transplant physician suspected gastroesophageal reflux, based on symptoms of increased cough during recumbency, and prescribed lansoprazole.

On examination, he is fatigued, but in no distress. He is afebrile; his blood pressure is 160/110 mm Hg, heart rate is 90, and respiratory rate is not labored at 16. Neck is supple, and he has no lymphadenopathy. Cardiopulmonary examination findings are normal. Neurologic examination demonstrates normal cranial nerve function and no motor or sensory deficits. Muscle stretch reflexes are 1+ symmetrically. Plantar responses are flexor bilaterally.

A nonenhanced brain computed tomography (CT) scan is normal. The lung transplant and neurology teams evaluate the patient and the merits of further testing are discussed.

DEFINITION

Lung transplantation, one of the most dynamic fields in medicine, has evolved into a life-saving option for thousands of patients with previously fatal pulmonary disease. Any ambulatory patient less than 65 years of age with end-stage pulmonary disease in the absence of other significant organ dysfunction should be considered for referral for lung transplant evaluation. The indications for lung and heart–lung transplantation span the spectrum of lung diseases, but the most common diagnoses have been chronic obstructive pulmonary disease (COPD), emphysema caused by α_1-antitrypsin deficiency, idiopathic pulmonary fibrosis (IPF), cystic fibrosis (CF), idiopathic pulmonary arterial hypertension (IPAH), and Eisenmenger syndrome (1).

End-stage lung disease with concomitant uncorrectable cardiac pathology warrants en bloc replacement of the heart and lungs. Bilateral, sequential ("double") lung transplantation, however, has largely replaced heart–lung transplant as the preferred approach for pulmonary arterial hypertension and those patients in whom chronic suppuration mandates replacement of both lungs. The optimal procedure for the remaining (majority) of patients with end-stage lung failure remains controversial. For most candidates, either a single or bilateral, sequential procedure provides symptomatic relief, independence from supplemental oxygen, and similar 1-year mortality and quality of life. On the other hand, 5-year survival, time to onset of chronic rejection, exercise tolerance, objective measures of lung function, and quality of life tend to favor double-lung recipients.

Quality of life is the prime motivation for transplantation in many patients, but prognosis should be the main determinant of timing. Survival rates after transplantation can be compared with the prognosis of the underlying disease, but the patient's clinical course must be incorporated into the decision. Despite the improving outcomes for lung transplant recipients, neurologic complications can limit quality of life and survival.

EPIDEMIOLOGY

Successful clinical heart–lung transplantation was first achieved in the early 1980s after nearly 20 years of instructive failures. Improved donor management, lung preservation, immunosuppression, and antimicrobial therapy have contributed to a 1-year survival rate of >80%. New changes in lung allocation policy, emphasizing survival benefit and urgency rather than waiting time, have culminated in a more efficient transplant process. In 2005, >1,400 patients had lung transplantation in the United States, with an active waiting list of approximately 1,000 patients.

Neurologic complications are common in transplantation, affecting as many as 30% to 80% of solid organ or bone marrow allograft recipients (2). Complications seen with all transplanted organs include seizures, opportunistic central nervous system (CNS) infections, stroke, and encephalopathy. Lung transplantation follows suit-limited; retrospective data evaluating global neurologic complications document event rates between 26% and 45% (3,4).

ETIOLOGY AND PATHOGENESIS

The common neurologic complications of lung transplant recipients can be subdivided into five main categories. These include (i) injuries associated with the lung transplant procedure and perioperative period; (ii) complications of commonly employed medications; (iii) infections; (iv) malignancy; and (v) posttransplant neuromuscular dysfunction.

INJURIES ASSOCIATED WITH THE TRANSPLANT PROCEDURE

Intraoperative nerve injury is one of the best described neurologic complications of the transplant procedure. In lung transplantation, mechanical injury from intraoperative retraction of the sternum and mediastinal dissection can result in phrenic and vagus nerve injury. Two prospective studies of lung transplant recipients have reported phrenic nerve injury in 7% and 30%, respectively, of the study cohorts (5,6). The varied frequencies reported may result from the diagnostic modality used—radiographic evidence of diaphragmatic dysfunction versus the more sensitive phrenic nerve conduction studies. Such phrenic nerve injury has been associated with increased morbidity, increased length of stay in the intensive care unit, prolonged mechanical ventilation, and greater need for tracheostomy (7).

Surgical manipulation of the posterior mediastinum can injure the vagus nerve, leading to gastroparesis. Consequences of gastroparesis include an increased risk of aspiration, gastroesophageal reflux disease (GERD), malnutrition, and poor absorption of medications. Recurrent aspiration can result in lung injury leading to graft dysfunction, especially in the early posttransplant period, and GERD has been implicated in the development of bronchiolitis obliterans syndrome, the clinical manifestation of chronic allograft dysfunction (8–10).

Postthoracotomy neuralgia affects up to 55% of patients having thoracotomy followed for more than 1 year (11). Chronic pain can result from the disarticulation of the costovertebral junction and injury to the intercostal nerves during chest wall manipulation. Other focal neuropathies (radial, ulnar, and peroneal nerve) are most frequently associated with traction, compression, positioning, ischemia, or internal mechanical complications of invasive procedures. Risk factors for development of a persistent neuropathy of a lower extremity include slender body shape, prolonged operative time, and diabetes (12).

Brain ischemia is most commonly associated with cardiopulmonary bypass used to accomplish the transplantation operation. The implementation of isolated lung transplantation (without bypass) has lessened this problem; however, complications of the vascular anastomoses can have devastating effects. Thrombus formation at the left atrial-pulmonary venous anastomotic suture line increases the risk of systemic embolization and stroke. In one prospective study, 15% had evidence of anastomotic clot within 48 hours of the transplant, and this subset of patients had an increased risk of death (13). Otherwise, patients experience the usual risk of intraoperative stroke caused by cerebral hypoperfusion (intraoperative hypotension or diminished cardiac output) and embolization. Three major types of emboli occur during cardiac operations: thromboemboli, atheroemboli, and air emboli.

INJURIES ASSOCIATED WITH MEDICATIONS

Neurologic complications have been well described in medications commonly used in lung transplantation—particularly calcineurin inhibitors, corticosteroids, and statins. These side effects can occur in dose-dependent fashion; therefore, drug–drug interactions must be sought and minimized, while disturbances of hepatic and renal metabolism mandate careful investigation.

The immunosuppressive, and possibly neurotoxic action, of both cyclosporine A (CSA) and tacrolimus are exerted through inhibition of the calcium calmodulin-dependent protein phosphatase, calcineurin. Both bind to the group of proteins called *immunophilins*—divided into CSA-binding cyclophilins and FK-binding proteins. Calcineurin and immunophilins have a widespread expression in the central and peripheral nervous systems, but the exact mechanism of CSA- or tacrolimus-induced neurotoxicity is not yet well understood. Edema and demyelination have been observed with special magnetic resonance techniques and probably play a major role (14). Increased permeability of brain endothelial cells may be responsible of these abnormalities (15). Initial reports suggested hypocholesterolemia and hypomagnesemia as possible precipitating factors for CSA neurotoxicity, yet neurotoxicity can be seen in their absence.

Neurologic complications, which occur in 25% of patients treated with CSA, include tremor, headache, seizures, and less frequently, encephalopathy. Tacrolimus, another calcineurin inhibitor, has a similar neurologic spectrum of complications, but with significantly decreased frequency (5.4% with tacrolimus vs. 25% with CSA) (16). Complications typically occur in the early posttransplant period, when higher doses and intravenous formulations are used. Paradoxically, tacrolimus has demonstrated neuroprotective properties in some experimental models of peripheral nerve injury (17,18).

Corticosteroid therapy is one of the cornerstones of immunosuppression protocols, used for maintenance therapy as well as for treatment of acute rejection. Direct neurologic complications include behavioral changes, myopathy, and epidural lipomatosis. Behavioral changes can manifest as emotional lability or excitability. Severe psychosis can occur in rare cases, particularly in patients with known psychological difficulties. High doses of glucocorticoids can induce significant myopathy, with the loss of thick myofilament from the muscle (19). The incidence of steroid myopathy has varied from 7% to 60%; interestingly, no proof exists of a relationship between the duration or dose and occurrence of myopathy (20). Epidural lipomatosis is a rare complication of steroid therapy; spinal cord compression and radiculopathy have been reported (21). Finally, rare instances of pseudotumor cerebri have been reported (more commonly in children), characterized by intracranial hypertension and papilledema, when corticosteroid doses are rapidly decreased (22).

In addition to the specific neurotoxicities of calcineurin inhibitors and glucocorticoids, immunosuppressive regimens can impart complications via the increased risk of infection or through acceleration of malignancy and atherogenesis.

The increasing use of 3-hydroxy-3-methylglutaryl coenzyme A reductase inhibitors (statins) in transplant recipients introduces additional potential for muscle injury, ranging in scope from myalgias to myositis to overt rhabdomyolysis. This class of drugs is most commonly prescribed in the event of dyslipidemia, either the result of a chronic medical condition or precipitated by the immunosuppressive regimen (especially, sirolimus and corticosteroids). Recent data have suggested that these antilipidemic agents may be immunomodulatory (23,24), including a case-control study of 39 lung allograft recipients demonstrating reduced rates of acute rejection and obliterative bronchiolitis coupled with a 6-year mortality benefit (25). Given these findings, increasing numbers of lung transplant recipients may be prescribed statins.

Other medications used in routine practice, such as antibiotics and analgesics, may cause neurologic complications in transplant recipients similar to the general population.

INFECTION

Despite improvements in diagnostic techniques and antimicrobial therapies, infection remains a leading cause of morbidity and mortality after lung transplantation. Bacterial pneumonia and cytomegalovirus (CMV) pneumonitis are the most common infections, although fungi, protozoa, mycobacteria, and other viruses can also be problematic.

According to Fishman and Rubin (26), CNS infection in transplant recipients has four distinct patterns: acute meningitis, subacute or chronic meningitis, focal brain infections, and progressive dementia. *Listeria monocytogenes, Cryptocccus neoformans,* and *Aspergillus fumigatus* account for most CNS infections in transplant recipients (27), but some linkage of pathogen to presentation can be described (26). Acute meningitis is usually caused by *L. monocytogenes.* Subacute or chronic meningitis, characterized by fever and headache evolving over a several days to weeks, is usually caused by *C. neoformans,* although systemic infection with *Mycobacterium tuberculosis, L. monocytogenes, Histoplasma capsulatum, Nocardia asteroides, Strongyloides stercoralis,* or *Coccidioides immitis* can also lead to a similar subacute neurologic presentation. Focal brain infection, presenting with seizures or focal neurologic abnormalities, can be caused by *L. monocytogenes, Toxoplama gondii,* or *N. asteroides,* and occasionally by Epstein-Barr Virus (EBV)-associated posttransplantation lymphoproliferative disease, but it is most commonly the result of metastatic aspergillus infection. Finally, progressive dementia, with or without focal abnormalities or seizures, can be related to progressive multifocal leukoencephalopathy (PML) caused by JC virus, or infections with other viruses, including herpes simplex virus, CMV, and EBV (26).

MALIGNANCY

Solid organ transplant recipients have an increased risk for developing malignancy. The cumulative incidence of cancer following kidney and heart transplantation is approximately 6% (28,29); however, the frequency of malignancy after lung transplantation has not been described. In the Cincinnati Transplant Tumor Registry, the predominant neoplasms have been lymphomas, skin and lip carcinomas, vulvar or perineal carcinomas, in situ cervical cancer, and Kaposi sarcoma (28,29). Several factors have been implicated in the increased incidence of secondary malignancies among transplant recipients, including sun exposure, extent and duration of immunosuppression, concomitant viral infection, and in rare cases, malignancy transplanted from the donor (30).

CNS malignancy in lung transplant recipients is most commonly from metastatic lung cancer or posttransplant lymphoproliferative disease (PTLD). PTLD, which includes lymphoma, is a morphologically and clonally heterogeneous group closely associated with EBV infection. The risk of PTLD is markedly increased in transplant recipients who were EBV-seronegative before transplantation and then acquired a primary EBV infection in the posttransplant setting (31).

Although controversial, the degree of overall immunosuppression is postulated to be a determinant of the development of a lymphoproliferative disorder (32,33). Immunosuppression may act by impairing EBV-specific T cell-mediated immunity.

PTLD tends to present at an advanced stage and often involves the transplanted lung. The allograft frequently has single or multiple well-defined nodules, and involvement of other sites, including the CNS, is common. For example, in the Cincinnati Registry of solid organ transplants, CNS involvement occurred in 22% of patients with posttransplant non-Hodgkins lymphoma. Lesions were confined to the CNS in 55% of patients, and 88% of those had brain involvement. All patient whose only involvement of the CNS was with the meninges or cerebrospinal fluid (CSF) had lymphomas involving multiple organs (34).

POSTTRANSPLANT NEUROMUSCULAR DYSFUNCTION

Although lung transplant can lead to significant improvements in pulmonary function and exercise capacity, patients may still report muscle weakness and suboptimal exercise performance. Cardiopulmonary exercise testing in lung transplant recipients demonstrates reduced anaerobic threshold and reduced maximal oxygen consumption, despite the absence of significant cardiac or ventilatory limitation (35–37). Phosphorus magnetic resonance spectroscopy shows that transplant recipients undergoing extension exercises to exhaustion had a lower resting pH in the quadriceps muscle and an earlier drop in pH than observed in healthy volunteers; impaired peripheral muscle oxidative capacity is an important contributing factor (38). This result, reinforcing patient's subjective reports of leg fatigue, implicates peripheral skeletal muscle tissue as the cause of the exercise limitation (36). Notably, most patients with end-stage lung disease often have pretransplant, concomitant muscle weakness, reduced muscle mass, and deconditioning.

CLINICAL MANIFESTATIONS

Given the range of insults that can occur to lung transplant recipients, clinical manifestations are quite variable. Focal neurologic deficits, stemming from vascular injury, peripheral nerve trauma, or medication effect, are generally self-evident, occurring most commonly in the early postoperative period. Global neurologic symptoms range from headache to seizures to lethargy and mental status changes. As described above, these nonspecific symptoms most commonly stem from medication effects (particularly, the calcineurin inhibitors) and infection.

Neurotoxicity from calcineurin inhibitors can manifest isolated symptoms of severe headaches, seizures, and visual abnormalities. In rare instances, the pattern of all three can occur, mimicking hypertensive encephalopathy both clinically and radiographically (39). Patients are noted to have marked systemic hypertension, and may manifest microscopic hemolytic anemia and thrombocytopenia. CT and MRI studies may show extensive bilateral white-matter abnormalities suggestive of edema without infarction (40). Although best described in the posterior regions of the cerebral hemispheres, prompting the term "posterior leukoencephalopathy," the changes can involve other cerebral areas, the brainstem, or the cerebellum. Although this presentation has been noted to be reversible with antihypertensive medications and cessation of the immunosuppressive, cases can result in severe, and sometime fatal, intracranial hemorrhage (41).

Mild tremor is a much more common sequela of calcineurin inhibitors. Studies have demonstrated incidence rates of 35% to 55%; however, symptoms may improve despite continued therapy (42,43). Other, less-common neurologic features of calcineurin toxicity can include akinetic mutism, and rarely, psychosis, speech apraxia, dysesthesias, anxiety, and sleep disturbances (44).

In contrast, mental status changes can reflect primary CNS infection or, more commonly, septic encephalopathy. Meningeal signs of inflammation can be masked by immunosuppressive therapy, and changes in the level of consciousness can be subtle. The most reliable constellation of symptoms that suggests CNS infection includes unexplained fever and headache.

Patients with dyspnea generally have a comprehensive workup of lung function and structure by the transplant team. Suspicions for phrenic nerve dysfunction arise in patients unable to be liberated from the ventilator, patients with unilateral diaphragm elevation, and patients with dyspnea that worsens within minutes of adopting the recumbent position—frequently misinterpreted as a sign of heart failure. Symptoms are generally universal in patients with bilateral diaphragm paralysis; unilateral phrenic nerve dysfunction is clinically evident when the contralateral lung function remains impaired or weakening of the accessory muscles of respiration occur. Close observation of the breathing pattern may reveal paradoxical abdominal wall retraction during inspiration, best appreciated when the patient is supine.

DIAGNOSTIC APPROACH

Patients in the early postoperative period exhibiting focal neurologic deficits need complete examination to delineate central versus peripheral nerve injury. Given the high risk for embolization, the default should be a conclusive imaging study of the CNS. Most focal deficits in the later course demand structural evaluation for evidence of space-occupying lesions.

As a result of the myriad of effects attributed to calcineurin inhibitors, all diagnostic evaluations should include early review of blood levels of such agents. Although no specific threshold exists at which toxicity occurs, usual levels are titrated based on time since transplantation and previous evidence of rejection. Although elevated levels can incriminate drug toxicity as responsible for presentations such as seizures, most clinicians still perform imaging studies to exclude structural pathology.

Infection is evaluated in usual fashion, using blood counts and cultures (blood, urine, respiratory, CSF) as appropriate. Patients in whom concern exists for CNS infection should receive an MRI with gadolinium. This modality permits evaluation of posterior fossa abscesses and can demonstrate cerebritis, surrounding edema, the extent of mass effect, or associated thrombosis. In many cases, lumbar puncture should be performed only after brain imaging excludes the presence of a brain abscess or other intracranial mass lesion with impending herniation. Ideally, CSF examination will identify the causative agent.

The diagnosis of CNS malignancy may be evident when it stems from metastatic lung cancer, but diagnosing (limited) PTLD can be difficult. Nonspecific symptoms—mental status changes or new neurologic findings—precipitate brain imaging. MRI with gadolinium-enhancing lesions, a positive CSF analysis for EBV by polymerase chain reaction, and an increased EBV load in the peripheral blood are highly suggestive of this diagnosis. Confirmation requires the presence of malignant lymphocytes in the CSF or direct biopsy of the lesion.

Neurologists may become involved in cases of dyspnea in which phrenic nerve dysfunction is suspected—usually after full functional and imaging studies of the lung have been completed. The chest radiograph may demonstrate an elevated hemidiaphragm(s), small lung volume, and atelectasis. Pulmonary function testing may show loss of vital capacity in assuming the recumbent position.

Unilateral diaphragmatic paralysis can be confirmed with a fluoroscopic sniff test, which evaluates for paradoxical elevation of the paralyzed hemidiaphragm with inspiration. In bilateral disease, fluoroscopy can be misleading; cephalad movement of the ribs as the accessory muscles contract can be misinterpreted as caudad displacement of the diaphragm. The test of choice is generally diaphragmatic electromyography (EMG), recorded with either esophageal or surface electrodes. The EMG may show either a neuropathic or a myopathic pattern, depending on the cause of the paralysis. In some cases, absence of a signal may indicate complete transection of the phrenic nerves. EMG may be complemented by phrenic nerve stimulation at the neck. Prolongation of nerve conduction time helps differentiate neuropathy from myopathy.

TREATMENT

Injuries associated with the transplant procedure have varied therapies, but all are generally supportive. Patients experiencing phrenic neuropathy require early and aggressive physical therapy to promote strengthening of the accessory muscles of respiration. The remaining modalities, including upright posture and intermittent (usually nocturnal), noninvasive ventilation, provide the best opportunity for functional recovery.

Vagal nerve injuries with associated GERD or gastroparesis are treated with proton pump inhibition; the role of gastric fundoplication continues to be investigated. In the event of vascular injury or embolization, the transplant procedure precludes thrombolytic therapies, and makes anticoagulation hazardous. Care is generally supportive. Finally, patients with postthoracotomy neuralgia may experience relief with anticonvulsants or tricyclic antidepressants.

Neurotoxicity associated with medications is most easily remedied when attributed to supratherapeutic levels (most commonly, stemming from drug–drug interactions or acquired renal or hepatic dysfunction); dose reduction alone suffices. As mentioned, however, tacrolimus and CSA neurotoxicity is intermittently and idiosyncratically observed in the setting of *therapeutic* serum levels. If the symptoms persist in affecting quality of life, limited data exist that sirolimus can be a reasonable substitution for patients experiencing calcineurin inhibitor toxicity (45).

Toxicity from corticosteroids is universally recognized; all ailments requiring prolonged immunosuppression have sought to reduce corticosteroid use. Steroids, however, are currently peerless in the acute management of allograft rejection; therefore, management is directed at the secondary illness. In contrast, patients experiencing statin toxicity can be transitioned (if not already) to those not blocking CYP-3A4. Pravastatin and fluvastatin are not extensively metabolized by CYP3A4, and can be considered the drugs of choice (46–49). If symptoms persist, the statin should be discontinued until the merits of the drug class are fully understood in the pathogenesis of rejection.

In patients with suspected infection, broad antimicrobial and antiviral coverage can be initiated. All efforts should be directed at pathogen isolation to tailor the drug regimen. The individual antimicrobial therapies for isolated pathogens will be discussed in detail elsewhere. Patients with CNS malignancy can be treated with chemotherapy. In localized disease, particularly CNS involvement, field radiation therapy may be beneficial.

CLINICAL RECOMMENDATIONS OF THE VIGNETTE

In the case described above, routine blood work demonstrated that the patient had impaired renal function and elevated levels of tacrolimus. MRI with gadolinium demonstrated no structural disease. This finding, combined with the absence of evidence for infection, incriminate calcineurin inhibitor toxicity as the precipitant of the patient's new seizures and hypertension. The increased tacrolimus level stemmed from (*a*) lansoprazole administration, and (*b*) impaired renal function—the byproduct of nonsteroidal anti-inflammatory drug (NSAID) use and poor oral intake. The patient was given a brief course of antihypertensive medications and phenytoin until therapeutic levels of tacrolimus were reachieved. Renal function improved with hydration, and he was counseled to avoid further NSAID use without prior physician discussion. His proton pump inhibitor was changed to pantoprazole, known for less influence on tacrolimus levels. The case highlights the neurotoxicity of calcineurin inhibitors and the challenges of the necessary polypharmacy in lung transplantation.

SUMMARY

Lung transplant recipients commonly experience neurologic complications. A systematic approach incorporating clinical features, timing, and appropriate investigation can guide the clinician toward the most likely culprit. As immunosuppressive treatment protocols evolve and more patients experience prolonged survival, recognition and early diagnosis of these complications will be necessary to ensure a good quality of life.

REFERENCES

1. Trulock EP, Edwards LB, Taylor DO, et al. Registry of the International Society for Heart and Lung Transplantation: Twenty-third official adult lung and heart-lung transplantation report—2006. *J Heart Lung Transplant.* 2006;25:880–892.
2. Pless M, Zivkovic SA. Neurologic complications of transplantation. *Neurologist.* 2002;8: 107–120.
3. Goldstein LS, Haug MT, 3rd, Perl J, 2nd, et al. Central nervous system complications after lung transplantation. *J Heart Lung Transplant.* 1998;17:185–191.
4. Wong M, Mallory GB, Jr., Goldstein J, et al. Neurologic complications of pediatric lung transplantation. *Neurology.* 1999;53:1542–1549.
5. Maziak DE, Maurer JR, Kesten S. Diaphragmatic paralysis: A complication of lung transplantation. *Ann Thorac Surg.* 1996;61:170–173.
6. Sheridan PH, Jr., Cheriyan A, Doud J, et al. Incidence of phrenic neuropathy after isolated lung transplantation. The Loyola University Lung Transplant Group. *J Heart Lung Transplant.* 1995;14:684–691.
7. Ferdinande P, Bruyninckx F, Van Raemdonck D, et al. Phrenic nerve dysfunction after heart–lung and lung transplantation. *J Heart Lung Transplant.* 2004;23:105–109.
8. Davis RD, Jr., Lau CL, Eubanks S, et al. Improved lung allograft function after fundoplication in patients with gastroesophageal reflux disease undergoing lung transplantation. *J Thorac Cardiovasc Surg.* 2003;125:533–542.
9. Young LR, Hadjiliadis D, Davis RD, et al. Lung transplantation exacerbates gastroesophageal reflux disease. *Chest.* 2003;124:1689–1693.
10. Hadjiliadis D, Duane Davis R, Steele MP, et al. Gastroesophageal reflux disease in lung transplant recipients. *Clin Transpl.* 2003;17:363–368.
11. Dajczman E, Gordon A, Kreisman H, et al. Long-term postthoracotomy pain. *Chest.* 1991; 99:270–274.
12. Nonthasoot B, Sirichindakul B, Nivatvongs S, et al. Common peroneal nerve palsy: An unexpected complication of liver surgery. *Transplant Proc.* 2006;38:1396–1397.
13. Schulman LL, Anandarangam T, Leibowitz DW, et al. Four-year prospective study of pulmonary venous thrombosis after lung transplantation. *J Am Soc Echocardiogr.* 2001;14: 806–812.
14. Lacaille F, Hertz-Pannier L, Nassogne MC. Magnetic resonance imaging for the diagnosis of acute leukoencephalopathy in children treated with tacrolimus. *Neuropediatrics.* 2004;35: 130–133.
15. Dohgu S, Kataoka Y, Ikesue H, et al. Involvement of glial cells in cyclosporine-increased permeability of brain endothelial cells. *Cell Mol Neurobiol.* 2000;20:781–786.
16. Eidelman BH, Abu-Elmagd K, Wilson J, et al. Neurologic complications of FK 506. *Transplant Proc.* 1991;23:3175–3178.
17. Doolabh VB, Mackinnon SE. FK506 accelerates functional recovery following nerve grafting in a rat model. *Plast Reconstr Surg.* 1999;103:1928–1936.
18. Lee M, Doolabh VB, Mackinnon SE, et al. FK506 promotes functional recovery in crushed rat sciatic nerve. *Muscle Nerve.* 2000;23:633–640.
19. Owczarek J, Jasinska M, Orszulak-Michalak D. Drug-induced myopathies. An overview of the possible mechanisms. *Pharmacol Rep.* 2005;57:23–34.
20. Batchelor TT, Taylor LP, Thaler HT, et al. Steroid myopathy in cancer patients. *Neurology.* 1997;48:1234–1238.
21. Fogel GR, Cunningham PY, 3rd, Esses SI. Spinal epidural lipomatosis: Case reports, literature review and meta-analysis. *Spine.* 2005;5:202–211.
22. Lorrot M, Bader-Meunier B, Sebire G, et al. [Benign intracranial hypertension: An unrecognized complication of corticosteroid therapy]. *Arch Pediatr.* 1999;6:40–42.
23. Li Y, Koster T, Morike C, et al. Pravastatin prolongs graft survival in an allogeneic rat model of orthotopic single lung transplantation. *Eur J Cardiothorac Surg.* 2006;30:515–524.
24. Kobashigawa JA. Statins in solid organ transplantation: Is there an immunosuppressive effect? *Am J Transplant.* 2004;4:1013–1018.
25. Johnson BA, Iacono AT, Zeevi A, et al. Statin use is associated with improved function and survival of lung allografts. *Am J Respir Crit Care Med.* 2003;167:1271–1278.
26. Fishman JA, Rubin RH. Infection in organ-transplant recipients. *N Engl J Med.* 1998;338: 1741–1751.
27. Hooper DC, Pruitt AA, Rubin RH. Central nervous system infection in the chronically immunosuppressed. *Medicine (Baltimore).* 1982;61:166–188.
28. Penn I. Incidence and treatment of neoplasia after transplantation. *J Heart Lung Transplant.* 1993;12:S328–S336.
29. Penn I. Neoplastic complications of transplantation. *Semin Respir Infect.* 1993;8:233–239.
30. Buell JF, Trofe J, Hanaway MJ, et al. Transmission of donor cancer into cardiothoracic transplant recipients. *Surgery.* 2001;130:660–666; discussion 666–668.
31. Walker RC, Marshall WF, Strickler JG, et al. Pretransplantation assessment of the risk of lymphoproliferative disorder. *Clin Infect Dis.* 1995;20:1346–1353.
32. Opelz G, Henderson R. Incidence of non-Hodgkin lymphoma in kidney and heart transplant recipients. Lancet 1993; 342:1514–1516.
33. Swinnen LJ, Costanzo-Nordin MR, Fisher SG, et al. Increased incidence of lymphoproliferative disorder after immunosuppression with the monoclonal antibody OKT3 in cardiac-transplant recipients. *N Engl J Med.* 1990;323:1723–1728.
34. Penn I, Porat G. Central nervous system lymphomas in organ allograft recipients. *Transplantation.* 1995;59:240–244.
35. Levy RD, Ernst P, Levine SM, et al. Exercise performance after lung transplantation. *J Heart Lung Transplant.* 1993;12:27–33.
36. Williams TJ, Patterson GA, McClean PA, et al. Maximal exercise testing in single and double lung transplant recipients. *Am Rev Respir Dis.* 1992;145:101–105.
37. Schwaiblmair M, Reichenspurner H, Muller C, et al. Cardiopulmonary exercise testing before and after lung and heart-lung transplantation. *Am J Respir Crit Care Med.* 1999;159: 1277–1283.
38. Evans AB, Al-Himyary AJ, Hrovat MI, et al. Abnormal skeletal muscle oxidative capacity after lung transplantation by 31P-MRS. *Am J Respir Crit Care Med.* 1997;155:615–621.

39. Schwartz RB, Bravo SM, Klufas RA, et al. Cyclosporine neurotoxicity and its relationship to hypertensive encephalopathy: CT and MR findings in 16 cases. *AJR Am J Roentgenol.* 1995;165:627–631.
40. Hinchey J, Chaves C, Appignani B, et al. A reversible posterior leukoencephalopathy syndrome. *N Engl J Med.* 1996;334:494–500.
41. Schwartz RB. A reversible posterior leukoencephalopathy syndrome. *N Engl J Med.* 1996;334:1743; author reply 1746.
42. Randomised trial comparing tacrolimus (FK506) and cyclosporin in prevention of liver allograft rejection. European FK506 Multicentre Liver Study Group. *Lancet.* 1994;344:423–428.
43. A comparison of tacrolimus (FK 506) and cyclosporine for immunosuppression in liver transplantation. The U.S. Multicenter FK506 Liver Study Group. *N Engl J Med.* 1994;331:1110–1115.
44. Wijdicks EF, Wiesner RH, Krom RA. Neurotoxicity in liver transplant recipients with cyclosporine immunosuppression. *Neurology.* 1995;45:1962–1964.
45. Maramattom BV, Wijdicks EF. Sirolimus may not cause neurotoxicity in kidney and liver transplant recipients. *Neurology.* 2004;63:1958–1959.
46. Keogh A, Macdonald P, Kaan A, et al. Efficacy and safety of pravastatin vs simvastatin after cardiac transplantation. *J Heart Lung Transplant.* 2000;19:529–537.
47. Kobashigawa JA, Katznelson S, Laks H, et al. Effect of pravastatin on outcomes after cardiac transplantation. *N Engl J Med.* 1995; 333:621–627.
48. Schrama YC, Hene RJ, de Jonge N, et al. Efficacy and muscle safety of fluvastatin in cyclosporine-treated cardiac and renal transplant recipients: An exercise provocation test. *Transplantation.* 1998;66:1175–1181.
49. Yoshimura N, Oka T, Okamoto M, et al. The effects of pravastatin on hyperlipidemia in renal transplant recipients. *Transplantation.* 1992;53:94–99.

CHAPTER **25**

Pharmacology of Respiratory Diseases

Thomas C. Corbridge • Richard A. Bernstein

OBJECTIVES

- To describe the mechanism of action of drugs commonly used in the management of pulmonary diseases
- To review clinical indications for commonly prescribed medications
- To examine common side effects from medications used in pulmonary disease states

CASE VIGNETTE

A 55-year-old woman with a 40 pack-year history of cigarette smoking (and a current smoker of 1 pack of cigarettes per day) developed chronic obstructive pulmonary disease (COPD). Smoking cessation had been repeatedly recommended, to no avail, and albuterol and tiotropium had been prescribed for symptomatic breathlessness. The patient was unable to afford tiotropium and theophylline was prescribed as a less-expensive alternative.

Subsequently, the patient was referred to neurology for lower extremity paraesthesias. She was diagnosed with peripheral vascular disease. Pentoxifylline was prescribed and smoking cessation was once again strongly recommended. On return to her primary care physician, smoking cessation was again discussed and the patient was started on varenicline. The patient successfully quit smoking 2 weeks later, at which time she also developed an acute exacerbation of COPD quickly followed by headache, tremor, and a generalized tonic-clonic seizure. She was brought to an emergency department and a neurology consult was requested.

INTRODUCTION

Pharmacotherapy is integral to the treatment of respiratory diseases, yet surprisingly few drugs are used in common day pulmonary practice. Central among these are inhalation remedies that date back to Pedanius Dioscorides, a first-century Greek physician and pharmacologist, who recommended inhalation of herbs for a number of ailments in his pharmacopeia, *De Materia Medica* (1). Indians of Madras further promoted fumigations of datura leaves to treat asthma; even Sir William Osler promoted the anticholinergic properties of belladonna, through smoking no less (2).

Inhalation therapy has evolved extensively with the introduction of selective β_2-adrenergic agonists in the 1960s and 1970s and selective anticholinergics and inhaled corticosteroids in the 1970s. Inhalation of these agents allowed for the use of smaller drug dosages, quick onset of action, and minimal side-effects; in the years that followed, these medications have helped millions of patients with asthma and COPD.

Steeped in the roots of pulmonary medicine is orally administered theophylline. Theophylline is a naturally occurring alkaloid found in tea and coffee that has effects similar to caffeine. Primarily viewed as a bronchodilator, theophylline also has important nonbronchodilating effects. Although the use of theophylline has waned with the emergence of safer and more potent inhaled agents, it remains an important member of the pulmonary armamentarium. Oral agents that affect the leukotriene pathway, such as montelukast and zileuton, are more recent additions to the field of pulmonary pharmacology. These agents have been particularly helpful in the management of select cases of asthma.

β_2-ADRENERGIC AGONISTS

The β_2-adrenergic agonists bind to transmembrane receptor proteins. These receptors are linked to Gs-proteins which, in turn, are linked to adenylate cyclase. Activation of adenylate cyclase induces cyclic adenosine monophosphate (cAMP), phosphorylation of muscle regulatory proteins, and changes in cellular calcium concentrations, ultimately relaxing airway smooth muscle (3). When inhaled, short-acting β_2 agonists (SABA) act within minutes and provide clinically apparent bronchodilation for 4 to 6 hours (Table 25-1).

SABA are used for rescue and before activities anticipated to cause bronchospasm. Albuterol is the most widely prescribed drug in this category. It is usually delivered by metered dose inhaler (MDI) at a dose of two puffs (90 μg/puff) every 4 to 6 hours, as needed. Handheld nebulizers are equally effective, but more cumbersome (approximately 4 to 10 puffs of albuterol by MDI using a spacing device is equivalent to one 2.5 mg nebulizer treatment) (4,5).

Albuterol is a racemate consisting of equal parts of R- and S-albuterol. The R isomer confers bronchodilator effects, whereas

TABLE 25-1. Short Acting Inhaled Beta 2 Agonists: Monotherapies

Brand Names	*Generic Names*
SHORT-ACTING INHALED β_2 AGONISTS	
Ventolin, Proventil	Albuterol sulfate
Xopenex	Levalbuterol hydrochloride solution
	Levalbuterol tartrate HFA
Alupent	Metaproterenol sulfate
Maxair	Pirbuterol acetate
Tornalate	Bitolterol mesylate
Brethine, Bricanyl, Brethaire	Terbutaline

the S isomer has been viewed as either inert or proinflammatory (6,7). Emerging preclinical and now clinical data suggest that levalbuterol, the R isomer alone, is at least as good, if not better, than racemic albuterol in children and adults with stable disease (8,9).

Failure of a previously effective dosing regimen to relieve symptoms indicates deterioration in airway function and likely exacerbation increasing the risk of hospitalization. Furthermore, excessive SABA use is a marker of poor asthma control, mortality risk, and the need for additional therapeutic considerations (10). Important in this regard is the use of a daily controller agent targeting the inflammatory component of asthma, preferably an inhaled corticosteroid (ICS) with or without a long-acting β_2 agonist (LABA) (11). In COPD, frequent use of a SABA is an indication for a long-acting anticholinergic agent or LABA, again with or without an ICS. Note: LABA are approved in both asthma and COPD, but in asthma, LABA should always be combined with an anti-inflammatory controller medication because monotherapy with a LABA is associated with deterioration in asthma control and more frequent exacerbations (12).

Salmeterol and formoterol are the two most commonly prescribed LABA (Table 25-2). Both are available alone or in combination with an ICS in a single inhaler. These agents provide clinically apparent bronchodilation for up to 12 hours. Formoterol has acute bronchodilator properties similar to that of albuterol, whereas significant bronchodilation does not occur for 30 to 60 minutes after salmeterol administration.

Long-acting β_2 agonists are more effective than multiple doses of SABA for maintenance therapy in asthma and COPD. Numerous clinical trials in asthmatics have demonstrated that the combination of an LABA and an ICS significantly improves pulmonary function, asthma symptom scores, nighttime awakenings, and quality of life (13). LABA lower requirements for rescue medications during the day and night (14). In COPD, LABA are more effective than frequent doses of SABA, and they provide an additional benefit of lowering lung volume, thereby reducing dyspnea and improving exercise tolerance (15).

TABLE 25-2. Long Acting Inhaled Beta 2 Agonists: Combination Agents with Inhaled Corticosteroids

Brand Names	*Generic Names*
LONG-ACTING INHALED β_2 AGONISTS	
Serevent	Salmeterol xinafoate
Foradil	Formoterol fumarate
LONG-ACTING INHALED β_2 AGONISTS COMBINED WITH AN INHALED CORTICOSTEROID	
Advair	Salmeterol/fluticasone
Symbicort	Formoterol/budesonide

Hospitalized patients with asthma and COPD typically demonstrate a lackluster response to SABA, thus requiring high doses by repetitive or continuous delivery (16–20). For acutely ill patients, the recommended dose of albuterol is 2.5 mg by nebulization every 20 minutes during the first hour of treatment, depending on clinical response and side effects (15). Levalbuterol, which is also effective, may lower hospitalization rates in adults and children (21,22). LABA are not recommended in the initial treatment of acute asthma or COPD, although formoterol has been shown to be as effective as albuterol (23). LABA added to standard therapies in hospitalized patients improves airflow rates better than albuterol alone (24).

Beta agonists are generally well tolerated. Common adverse reactions are similar to those occurring with other sympathomimetics agents (Table 25-3). In general, toxicity is limited by the lower dosages allowed through inhalation therapy. Oral preparations increase side effects without additional benefit; subcutaneous injections of epinephrine or terbutaline are reserved for critically ill asthmatics who are unable to comply with inhaled therapy or have fail inhaled therapy. These agents must be used with extreme caution in patients with coronary artery disease (25). Intravenous β agonist administration confers no additional benefit and is significantly more toxic (26,27).

Results of a large, randomized trial of salmeterol or placebo added to usual asthma therapies have raised concerns about LABA safety (28). In this trial, 13 asthma-related deaths occurred in >13,000 patients receiving salmeterol compared with 3 deaths in >13,000 patients in the placebo arm. Although this study was not designed to determine the reason for increased deaths in the salmeterol arm, two points are worth considering. First, black patients were at greatest risk of asthma-related death. These patients were sicker at baseline than their white counterparts and less likely to be taking an ICS. Only 38% of black patients were taking an ICS—which is not in keeping with current recommendations that all asthmatics treated with a LABA for maintenance therapy receive an ICS (12,13). Second, blacks have a greater prevalence of the Arg-Arg genotype at position 16 of the β agonist adrenergic receptor (instead of the usual Gly-Gly genotype). Patients with the Arg-Arg genotype may have an impaired therapeutic response to salmeterol regardless of ICS use (29). Interestingly, these patients may respond favorably to anticholinergic medications (which are reserved for patients with COPD) (30).

TABLE 25-3. Adverse Reactions to β_2 Agonists

Tremor	Paradoxical bronchospasm
Nervousness	Hypokalemia
Tachyarrhythmias	Dizziness
Hypertension	Gastroesophageal reflux
ECG changes	Nausea

ANTICHOLINERGICS

Two anticholinergic medications are used in common pulmonary practice: Ipratropium bromide (Atrovent) and tiotropium bromide (Spiriva). Ipratropium bromide is a synthetic quaternary amine that is poorly absorbed through the lung and gastrointestinal tract and much less likely than atropine to cause systemic anticholinergic effects. Anticholinergic bronchodilators prevent the increase in cyclic guanosine monophosphate (cGMP) caused by cholinergic binding to muscarinic receptors on airway smooth muscle cells. Significant improvement in pulmonary function occurs within 15 minutes of inhalation of ipratropium bromide by MDI. Peak effect is reached in 1 to 2 hours and clinically apparent bronchodilation lasts 4 to 6 hours. The usual starting dose of ipratropium bromide is two puffs (18 μg/puff) four times daily, although some patients take 12 to 16 puffs daily as planned therapy for COPD. Use of a long-acting anticholinergic agent (e.g., LABA), with or without an ICS, is preferred, however, over frequent doses of a short-acting preparation.

Ipratropium bromide can be administered alone or in combination with an SABA in COPD. Combinations of ipratropium bromide and SABA are more effective than either agent alone in improving lung function, and combination therapy increases the percent of bronchodilator responders in comparison to single drug use (31,32).

Tiotropium bromide is a long-acting anticholinergic agent indicated for once-daily maintenance therapy in COPD. As with ipratropium bromide, tiotropium bromide is a quaternary amine that binds to M1, M2, and M3 muscarinic receptor subtypes. Tiotropium bromide, however, is highly selective for M1 and M3 receptors (favoring bronchodilation) and dissociates quickly from M2 receptors (also favoring bronchodilation because M2 receptors are feedback inhibitory receptors at cholinergic nerve endings that inhibit the release of acetycholine) (33). Clinically significant bronchodilation occurs 30 minutes after administration and the effects last for 24 hours (34–36). Similar to LABA in COPD, tiotropium decreases lung volume, reduces dyspnea, increases quality of life and exercise tolerance, and decreases the risk of an acute exacerbation (37). In patients with severe COPD, combinations of an LABA and tiotropium provide additional benefits (38).

Bronchodilating properties of anticholinergics in asthma are generally modest, precluding their routine use in this patient population. One exception may be the patient with the Arg-Arg β-receptor genotype and β_2 agonist unresponsiveness. Another possible role for ipratropium bromide in asthma is in the treatment of acutely ill patients. Here the data generally support repetitive doses of ipratropium bromide combined with albuterol are more effective than albuterol alone (39–43).

Anticholinergic preparations generally have a safe track record (Table 25-4). Care must be taken not to spray the eye—mydriasis can confuse the neurologic picture.

TABLE 25-4. Selected Anticholinergic Side Effects

Dry mouth
Cough
Blurred vision
Worsening of narrow-angle glaucoma
Urinary retention

CORTICOSTEROIDS

The precise mechanisms of ICS action in asthma and COPD are unknown. Inhaled corticosteroids inhibit a number of cell types responsible for airway wall inflammation and decrease production of inflammatory mediators. They play a dominant role in the management of asthmatic inflammation characterized by CD4 lymphocytes and eosinophils and a lesser role in COPD where there is a preponderance of CD8 lymphocytes and neutrophils. In asthma, ICS use improves pulmonary function, asthma symptom scores, and need for SABA rescue. ICS use also decreases the risk of hospitalization and asthma-related death (44,45). Indeed, most acutely ill asthmatics requiring emergency department treatment have not been taking an ICS (46). Reflecting the importance of ICS in asthma, the Expert Panel Report of the National Asthma Education and Prevention Program positioned them as preferred therapy for persistent asthma (13).

In COPD, however, ICS are not in and of themselves approved by the US Food and Drug Administration, even though they have been shown to decrease the risk of acute exacerbations, reduce dyspnea, and enhance quality of life (47,48). Inhaled corticosteroids combined with a LABA are approved for use in both asthma and COPD.

A number of ICS preparations are available for clinical use (Table 25-5).

These preparations are generally used twice daily for maintenance therapy. Usual instructions include rinsing and spitting after use to decrease oropharyngeal deposition and the chance for oral absorption, localized candidal infection, and dysphonia. Side effects from the long-term use of ICS are listed in Table 25-6.

THEOPHYLLINE

Theophylline is a methylxanthine with bronchodilator and nonbronchodilator properties. Among its nonbronchodilator actions are an increase in diaphragm force generation, diuresis, respiratory center stimulation, and steroid sparing/anti-inflammatory effects (49). Although precise mechanism(s) of action of theophylline is unclear, it appears that inhibition of phosphodiesterase III and phosphodiesterase IV and increased intracellular cAMP are responsible for bronchodilation (50).

TABLE 25-5. Commonly Used Inhaled Corticosteroids

Brand Names	*Generic Names*
Vanceril, Beclovent, Qvar	Beclomethasone dipropionate
Flovent	Fluticasone propionate
Pulmicort	Budesonide
Asmanex	Mometasone furoate
Azmacort	Triamcinolone acetonide
Aerobid	Flunisolide

TABLE 25-6. Inhaled Corticosteroid Side Effects

Dysphonia
Oropharyngeal candidiasis
Osteopenia/osteoporosis
Cataracts
Glaucoma

Use of sustained-release theophylline has waned with the introduction of safer, more potent, and less toxic inhaled agents. Reservations about the high incidence of side effects at the upper limit of its therapeutic range has led many pulmonologists to prescribe lower drug doses, a strategy that still provides clinical benefit while minimizing toxicity, and to pay particular attention to drug–drug interactions (Table 25-7) (51). Nevertheless, theophylline's low cost, ease of administration, and proved efficacy continue to fuel its use.

In asthma, theophylline is primarily used as an additive maintenance drug in patients whose asthma is not adequately controlled by an ICS, or rarely as the primary maintenance drug in patients intolerant of ICS preparations. Several studies have demonstrated that adding theophylline to ICS provides additional clinical benefit to the patient, even when theophylline concentrations fall below the usually stated therapeutic range, allowing for lower ICS dosages and cost (52). Sustained-release theophylline is useful in controlling nocturnal symptoms (51).

Theophylline has a modest effect on pulmonary function, arterial blood gases, dyspnea, and exercise tolerance in patients with COPD, without affecting cognitive function (53–55). Theophylline is generally reserved for cases not adequately managed on a short-acting rescue bronchodilator and either tiotropium or the combination of a long-acting bronchodilator and an ICS.

Theophylline has a number of clinically relevant side effects that are listed in Table 25-8.

Methylxanthines are generally not recommended in the management of acute exacerbations of asthma or COPD because they generally to not add to the efficacy of β_2 agonists used properly. They do, however, increase the risk of side effects (56,57).

LEUKOTRIENE MODIFIERS

Arachidonic acid is a polyunsaturated fatty acid that is present in phospholipids of cell membranes. It is transformed by way of the 5-lipoxygenase (5-LO) pathway into leukotrienes, which act by binding to, and activating, specific receptors (58). Leukotrienes induce many of the abnormalities seen in asthma, including bronchospasm, vascular leak, mucous gland secretion, proliferation of airway smooth muscle, and cellular infiltration (59). Leukotrienes C_4, D_4, and E_4 are referred to as *cysteinyl leukotrienes* because they contain the amino acid cysteine. Leukotriene B_4 is a noncysteinyl leukotriene that chemoattracts neutrophils.

TABLE 25-7. Drug Interactions

Decrease Theophylline Clearance	*Increase Theophylline Clearance*
Allopurinol	Carbamazepine
Cimetidine	Phenobarbital
Ciprofloxacin	Rifampin
Clarithromycin	Phenytoin
Erythromycin	
Estrogen	
Methotrexate	
Disulfiram	
Verapamil	
Ticlodipine	
Pentoxifylline	

TABLE 25-8. Selected Adverse Reactions to Theophylline

Tremor	Disrupted sleep
Nausea	Hypokalemia
Tachyarrhythmias	Hypercalcemia
Headache	Gastroesophageal reflux
Diarrhea	Muscle cramps

Montelukast and zafirlukast are cysteinyl leukotriene receptor antagonists, whereas zileuton is a 5-LO inhibitor that decreases formation of cysteinyl leukotrienes and leukotriene B_4 (Table 25-9). Thus, zileuton has broader actions than cysteinyl receptor antagonists. This broader action has not convincingly translated to greater clinical efficacy. The importance of leukotriene B_4 in the neutrophilic inflammation of COPD, however, raises a possible role for zileuton beyond its use in asthma (51). In current practice, zileuton prescriptions have been hampered by the need to monitor serum transaminases, drug–drug interactions, and four times daily dosing.

Leukotriene modifiers inhibit allergen-induced early and late responses, exercise-induced bronchospasm, and airway hyperresponsiveness (51). They are bronchodilators, but their effects are not as marked as those of β_2 agonists and they are not indicated for rescue. Rather, leukotriene modifiers should be considered alternatives to low-dose ICS in mild persistent asthma, although ICS are generally viewed as superior agents (60). More commonly, leukotriene modifiers are added to ICS to improve asthma control or reduce ICS dosage requirements (61). Interestingly, genetic factors leading to changes in 5-LO expression appear to account for failure to respond to leukotriene modifier treatment (62).

Limited data support the use of leukotriene receptor antagonists in acute asthma. In one study, two orally administered doses of zafirlukast (20 mg and 160 mg) were compared with placebo in 641 asthmatics after 30 minutes of standard treatment (63). The group receiving zafirlukast (160 mg) had fewer hospital admissions, relapses, and treatment failures. Another prospective study of 20 patients showed that oral montelukast (10 mg) resulted in a nonstatistical trend toward shorter lengths of hospitalization and higher peak flows, and fewer patients requiring subsequent treatment with aminophylline or steroids (64). More recently, Camargo et al. (65) conducted a randomized, double-blinded, parallel group trial

TABLE 25-9. Commonly Prescribed Leukotriene Modifiers

Brand Names	*Generic Names*
Singulair	Montelukast
Accolate	Zafirlukast
Zyflo	Zileuton

with 201 acute asthmatics receiving standard therapy plus montelukast (7 mg or 14 mg) intravenous or placebo. Montelukast improved FEV_1 over the first 20 minutes (14.8% vs. 3.6% with placebo). Effects were seen within 10 minutes and lasted for 2 hours. The two doses were equally effective. Montelukast is not available for intravenous administration in the United States.

CLINICAL RECOMMENDATIONS OF THE VIGNETTE

This case illustrates the potential for drug–drug and drug–disease interactions causing clinically important side effects. Theophylline, which can be effective in asthma and COPD, is generally not preferred over inhaled long-acting bronchodilators because of its potential for such toxicity. In this case, theophylline toxicity developed for several reasons. First, a drug–drug interaction occurred between theophylline and pentoxifylline, resulting in decreased theophylline metabolism. Second, smoking cessation elevates theophylline levels (and smoking decreases theophylline levels). Finally, viral infections and hypoxemia associated with COPD exacerbation have the potential to decrease theophylline metabolism. This patient developed toxic levels of theophylline with clinical manifestations of headache, tremor, and seizures. Other manifestations of theophylline toxicity include atrial and ventricular arrhythmias, insomnia, nausea, and heartburn.

SUMMARY

A limited number of drugs are commonly used in pulmonary practice. Central among these are inhalational agents, including short- and long-acting bronchodilators and inhaled corticosteroids. These drugs are essential in the management of asthma and COPD and can be used in most cases with minimal toxicity. Oral medications include theophylline and leukotriene modifiers. These have bronchodilating and anti-inflammatory properties. Theophylline is indicated for patients with asthma and COPD, but has a narrow therapeutic range. Leukotriene modifiers are primarily asthma medications. They are generally well tolerated and normally considered to be add-on agents to an inhaled corticosteroid-based regimen.

REFERENCES

1. Dessanges J. A history of nebulizaton. *Journal of Aerosol Medicine.* 2001;14:65–71.
2. Chu EK, Drazen JM. Asthma: One hundred years of treatment and onward. *Am J Respir Crit Care Med.* 2005;171:1202–1208.
3. Johnson M. Beta2-adrenoceptors: Mechanisms of action of beta2-agonists. Pediatric Respiratory Review. 2001;2:57–62.
4. Colacone A, Afilalo M, Wolkove N, et al. A comparison of albuterol administered by metered dose inhaler (and holding chamber) or wet nebulizer in acute asthma. *Chest.* 1993;104:835–841.
5. Rodrigo C, Rodrigo G. Salbutamol treatment of acute severe asthma in the ED: MDI vs hand-held nebulizer. *Am J Med.* 1998;16:637.
6. Baramki D, Koester J, Anderson AJ, et al. Modulation of T-cell function by R and S-isomers of albuterol: Anti-inflammatory influences of R-isomers are negated by the presence of the S-isomer. *J Allergy Clin Immunol.* 2002;109:449.
7. Dhand R, Goode M, Reid R, et al. Preferential pulmonary retention of S-albuterol after inhalation of racemic albuterol. *Am J Respir Crit Care Med.* 1999;160:1136.
8. Milgrom H. Levosalbutamol in the treatment of asthma. *Expert Opin Pharmacother.* 2006;12:1659–1668.
9. Milgrom H, Skoner DP, Bensch G, et al.; Levalbuterol Pediatric Study Group. Low-dose levalbuterol in children with asthma: Safety and efficacy in comparison with placebo and racemic albuterol. *J Allergy Clin Immunol.* 2001;108:938–945.
10. Suissa S, Ernst P, Boivin JF, et al. A cohort analysis of excess mortality in asthma and the use of inhaled beta-agonists. *Am J Respir Crit Care Med.* 1994;149:604–610.
11. National Asthma Education and Prevention Program: Clinical Practice Guidelines. Expert Panel 2 Report. Guidelines for the Diagnosis and Management of Asthma. NIH Publication 97-4051, 1997.
12. Lazarus SC, Boushey HA, Fahy JV, et al.; for the Asthma Clinical Research Network for the National Heart, Lung, and Blood Institute. Long-acting β_2-agonist monotherapy vs continued therapy with inhaled corticosteroids in patients with persistent asthma: A randomized controlled trial. *JAMA.* 2001;285:2583–2593.
13. National Asthma Education and Prevention Program. Expert Panel Report. Guidelines for the Diagnosis and Management of Asthma. Update on Selected Topics—2002. *J Allergy Clin Immunol.* 2002;110:S141.
14. Walters EH, Walters JAE, Gibson, PW. Regular treatment with long acting beta agonists versus daily regular treatment with short acting beta agonists in adults and children with stable asthma. *Cochrane Database Syst Rev.* 2006 Issue 1. The Cochrane Collaboration. Published by John Wiley and Sons, Ltd.
15. O'Donnell DE, Sciurba F, Celli B, et al. Effect of fluticasone propionate/salmeterol on lung hyperinflation and exercise endurance in COPD. *Chest.* 2006;130:647–656.
16. Camargo CA, Jr., Spooner CH, Rowe BH. Continuous versus intermittent beta-agonists for acute asthma. *Cochrane Database Syst Rev.* 2006 Issue 1. The Cochrane Collaboration. Published by John Wiley and Sons, Ltd.
17. Reisner C, Kotch A, Dworkin G. Continuous versus intermittent nebulization of albuterol in acute asthma: A randomized, prospective study. *Ann Allergy Asthma Immunol.* 1995;75:41–47.
18. Rudnitsky GS, Eberlein RS, Schoffstall JM, et al. Comparison of intermittent and continuously nebulized albuterol for treatment of asthma in an urban emergency department. *Ann Emerg Med.* 1993;22:1842.
19. Lin RY, Astiz ME, Saxon JC, et al. Continuous versus intermittent albuterol nebulization in the treatment of acute asthma. *Ann Emerg Med.* 1993;22:1847.
20. Besbes-Ouanes L, Nouira S, Elatrous S, et al. Continuous versus intermittent nebulization of salbutamol in acute severe asthma: A randomized, controlled trial. *Ann Emerg Med.* 200;36:198.
21. Nowak R, Emerman C, Hanrahan JP, et al. A comparison of levalbuterol with racemic albuterol in the treatment of acute severe asthma exacerbations in adults. *Am J Emerg Med.* 2006;24:259–267.
22. Carl JC, Myers TR, Kirchner L, et al.; Comparison of racemic albuterol and levalbuterol for treatment of acute asthma. *J Pediatr.* 2003;143:731–736.
23. Rubinfeld AR, Scicchitano R, Hunt A, et al. Formoterol Turbuhaler as reliever medication in acute asthma. *Eur Respir J.* 2006;27:735–741.
24. Peters JI, Shelledy DC, Jones AP, et al. A randomized, placebo-controlled study to evaluate the role of salmeterol in the in-hospital management of asthma. *Chest.* 2000;118:313.
25. Cydulka R, Davison R, Grammer L, et al. The use of epinephrine in the treatment of older adult asthmatics. *Ann Emerg Med.* 1990;17:322.
26. Travers A, Jones AP, Kelly K, et al. Intravenous beta2-agonists for acute asthma in the emergency department. *Cochrane Database Syst Rev.* 2006 Issue 1. The Cochrane Collaboration. Published by John Wiley and Sons, Ltd.
27. Salmeron S, Brochard L, Mal H, et al. Nebulized versus intravenous albuterol in hypercapnic acute asthma: A multicenter, double-blind, randomized study. *Am J Respir Crit Care Med.* 1994;149:1466.
28. Nelson H, Weiss ST, Bleecher ER, et al. The Salmeterol Multicenter Asthma Research Trial: A comparison of usual pharmacotherapy for asthma or usual pharmacotherapy plus salmeterol. SMART. *Chest.* 2006;129:12–26.
29. Wechsler ME, Lehman E, Lazarus SC, et al. Beta-adrenergic receptor polymorphisms and response to salmeterol. *Am J Respir Crit Care Med.* 2006;173:519–526.
30. Glassroth J. The role of long-acting beta-agonists in the management of asthma: Analysis, meta-analysis, and more analysis. *Ann Intern Med.* 2006;144:904–912.
31. Combivent Inhalation Study Group. In chronic obstructive pulmonary disease, a combination of ipratropium and albuterol is more effective than either agent alone. An 85-day multicenter trial. *Chest.* 1994;105:1411–1419.
32. Dorinsky PM, Reisner C, Ferguson GT, et al. The combination of ipratropium and albuterol optimizes pulmonary function reversibility testing in patients with COPD. *Chest.* 1999;115:966–971.
33. Barnes PJ. The pharmacological properties of tiotropium. *Chest.* 2000;117:63S.
34. Calverley PM, Lee A, Towse L, et al. Effect of tiotropium bromide on circadian variation in airflow limitation in chronic obstructive pulmonary disease. *Thorax.* 2003;58: 855–860.
35. Vincken W, van Noord JA, Greefhorst AP. Improved health outcomes in patients with COPD during 1 year's treatment with tiotropium. *Eur Respir J.* 2002;19:209–216.
36. Casaburi R, Mahler DA, Jones PW, et al. A long-term evaluation of once-daily inhaled tiotropium in chronic obstructive pulmonary disease. *Eur Respir J.* 2002;19:217–224.
37. O'Donnell DE, Fluge T, Gerken F, et al. Effects of tiotropium on lung hyperinflation, dyspnea and exercise tolerance in COPD. *Eur Respir J.* 2004;23:832–840.
38. Cazzola M, Ando F, Santus P, et al. A pilot study to assess the effects of combining fluticasone propionate/salmeterol and tiotropium on the airflow obstruction of patients with severe-to-very severe COPD. *Pulm Pharmacol Ther.* 2006. Epub ahead of print.
39. Stoodley RG, Aaron SD, Dales RE. The role of ipratropium bromide in the emergency management of acute asthma exacerbation: A meta-analysis of randomized clinical trials. *Ann Emerg Med.* 1999;34:8.
40. Lanes SF, Garrett JE, Wentworth CE, 3rd, et al. The effect of adding ipratropium bromide to salbutamol in the treatment of acute asthma: A pooled analysis of three trials. *Chest.* 1998;114:365.
41. Plotnick LH, Ducharme FM. Combined inhaled anticholinergics and beta2-agonists for initial treatment of acute asthma in children. *Cochrane Database Syst Rev.* The Cochrane Library 2000, Issue 2.
42. Rodrigo GJ, Rodrigo C. First-line therapy for adult patients with acute severe asthma receiving a multiple-dose protocol of ipratropium bromide plus albuterol in the emergency department. *Am J Respir Crit Care Med.* 2000;161:1862–1868.

43. Plotnick LH, Ducharme FM. Combined inhaled anticholinergics and beta 2-agonists for initial treatment of acute asthma in children. *Cochrane Database Syst Rev.* 2006, Issue 1. The Cochrane Collaboration. Published by John Wiley and Sons, Ltd.
44. Suissa S, Ernst P, Benayoun S, et al. Low-dose inhaled corticosteroids and the prevention of death from asthma. *N Engl J Med.* 2000;343:332–336.
45. Suissa S, Ernst P, Kezouh A. Regular use of inhaled corticosteroids and the long term prevention of hospitalization for asthma. *Thorax.* 2002;57:880–884.
46. Marks GB, Heslop W, Yates DH. Prehospital management of exacerbations of asthma: Relation to patient and disease characteristics. *Respirology.* 2000;5:45–50.
47. Fabbri L, Pauwels RA, Hurd SS; GOLD Scientific Committee. Global strategy for the diagnosis, management and prevention of chronic obstructive pulmonary disease: GOLD executive summary updated 2003. *Chronic Obstructive Pulmonary Disease.* 2004;1:105–141.
48. Burge PS, Calverley PM, Jones PW, et al. Randomised, double blind, placebo controlled study of fluticasone propionate in patients with moderate to severe chronic obstructive pulmonary disease: The ISOLDE trial. *BMJ.* 2000;320:1297–1303.
49. Markham A, Faulds D. Theophylline. A review of its potential steroid sparing effects in asthma. *Drugs.* 1998;56:1081–1091.
50. Rabe KF, Magnussen H, Dent G. Theophylline and selective PDE inhibitors as bronchodilators and smooth muscle relaxants. *Eur Respir J.* 1995;8:637–642.
51. Donohue JF. Therapeutic responses in asthma and COPD. *Chest.* 2004;126:125S–137S.
52. Evans DJ, Taylor DA, Zetterstrom O, et al. A comparison of low-dose inhaled budesonide plus theophylline and high-dose inhaled budesonide for moderate asthma. *N Engl J Med.* 1997;337:1412–1418.
53. Ram FSF, Jones PW, Castro AA, et al. Oral theophylline for chronic obstructive pulmonary disease. *Cochrane Database Syst Rev.* 2004 Issue 4. The Cochrane Collaboration. Published by John Wiley and Sons, Ltd.
54. Newman D, Tamir J, Speedy L, et al. Physiological and neuropsychological effects of theophylline in chronic obstructive pulmonary disease. *Isr J Med Sci.* 1994;30:811–816.
55. Vaz Fragoso CA, Miller MA. Review of the clinical efficacy of theophylline in the treatment of chronic obstructive pulmonary disease. *Am Rev Respir Dis.* 1993;147:S40–S47.
56. Parameswaran K, Belda J, Rowe BH. Addition of intravenous aminophylline to beta2-agonists in adults with acute asthma. *Cochrane Database Syst Rev.* 2006 Issue 1. The Cochrane Collaboration. Published by John Wiley and Sons, Ltd.
57. Snow V, Lascher S, Mottur-Pilson C. Evidence base for management of acute exacerbations of chronic obstructive pulmonary disease. *Ann Intern Med.* 2001;134:595–599.
58. Drazen JM, Israel E, O'Byrne PM. Treatment of asthma with drugs modifying the leukotriene pathway. *N Engl J Med.* 1999;340:197–206.
59. Piper PJ. Leukotrienes and the airways. *Eur J Anaesthesiol.* 1989;6:241–255.
60. Malmstrom K, Rodriguez-Gomez G, Guerra J. Oral montelukast, inhaled beclomethasone, and placebo for chronic asthma. A randomized, controlled trial. Montelukast/Beclomethasone Study Group. *Ann Intern Med.* 1999;130:487–495.
61. Vaquerizo MJ, Casan P, Castillo J, et al. Effect of montelukast added to inhaled budesonide on control of mild to moderate asthma. *Thorax.* 2003;58:204–210.
62. Lima JJ, Zhang S, Grant A. Influence of leukotriene pathway polymorphisms on response to montelukast in asthma. *Am J Respir Crit Care Med.* 2006;173:379–385.
63. Silverman R, Miller C, Chen Y, et al. Zafirlukast reduces relapses and treatment failures after an acute asthma episode. *Chest.* 1999:116:296S
64. Ferreira MB, Santos AS, Pregal AL, et al. Leukotriene receptor antagonists (Montelukast) in the treatment of asthma crisis: Preliminary results of a double-blind placebo controlled randomized study. *Allergy Immunol* (Paris). 2001;33:315.
65. Camargo CA, Jr., Smithline HA, Malice MP, et al. A randomized controlled trial of intravenous montelukast in acute asthma. *Am J Respir Crit Care Med.* 2003;167:528.

CHAPTER 26

Acute Renal Failure

Vinod K. Bansal

OBJECTIVES

- To define and classify acute renal failure and its prevalence in hospitalized patients
- To outline the pathophysiologic processes that result in acute renal failure
- To describe the clinical signs, laboratory abnormalities, and neurologic manifestations of acute renal failure
- To review the current management of acute renal failure

CASE VIGNETTE

A 40-year-old man was airlifted after a motor vehicle accident and after onsite resuscitation of copious amount of fluid. General course during hospitalization showed him to be alert with adequate urine output, blood pressure (BP) of 100/70 mm Hg, pulse 72. Admission laboratory tests were blood urea nitrogen (BUN) of 27 mg/dL, serum creatinine of 1.3 mg/dL, and hemoglobin of 8.7 g/dL.

During evaluation, multiple organ injury was identified. Emergency abdominal surgery showed liver laceration, gut perforation, and right-sided hemothorax. Surgery lasted 4 hours during which time he received 10 U of blood and 15 U of crystalloid fluids. Intraoperative BP recording showed significant periods of 80 to 90 mm Hg range. Postoperatively, BP was supported by norepinephrine (Levophed) and intravenous (IV) fluid and was hovering at a level of 90 to 100 mm Hg. No urine was recorded during the first 4 hours postoperative. Multiple injections of IV furosemide were given, but without response. The patient was intubated and heavily sedated. His laboratory values were as follows: BUN 80 mg/dL, serum creatinine 4.5 mg/dL, serum potassium 5.6 mEq/L, and serum bicarbonate 14 mEq/L. Progress during the next 24 hours showed continuation of no urine output, with laboratory BUN of 90 mg/dL and serum creatinine of 5.6 mg/L. Oxygen saturation was maintained at 50%. Despite no further sedation, the patient remained obtunded A renal consult was ordered because of mental state changes and fluid overload.

DEFINITION

Acute renal failure (ARF) is defined as a rapid decline in glomerular filtration rate (GFR) leading to accumulation of nitrogenous waste products, BUN, creatinine (Cr), and disturbances in fluids and electrolytes and acid-base state. It can be accompanied by a decrease in urine output, but this may not be present in all cases. The injury to the kidneys occurs much earlier than the traditional definition of rise in BUN or serum Cr and *acute kidney injury* has been suggested as a better term. No clear consensus exists on the definition of ARF.

Recently the Acute Dialysis Quality Initiative has proposed a new definition and classification:

Mild:	Decrease in calculated GFR of 25% or urine output <0.5 mL/kg/6 h
Moderate:	Decrease in calculated GFR of 50% or urine output <0.5 mL/kg/12 h
Severe:	Decrease in calculated GFR of 75% or urine output of 0.3 mL/kg/h for 24 h or anuria for >12 h (1)

EPIDEMIOLOGY

The incidence of ARF varies, depending on the definition used. The overall incidence in hospitalized patients is reported to be 4.9% to 15.9% when elevation of serum Cr of 0.5 mg/dL is used as a determinant. The overall mortality varies between 19.4% and 51.0%, with the highest mortality reported (76%) in sepsis-associated ARF (2–5).

ETIOLOGY AND PATHOGENESIS

ARF is classified into three major categories, based on pathogenesis, as shown in Table 26-1.

Prerenal is the most common form of ARF seen hospitalized patients. It results from decreased renal perfusion resulting in hemodynamically mediated reduction of glomerular perfusion. By definition, the kidney parenchyma is believed to be intact and functional. The manifestations seen are the result of hypoperfusion and, if promptly restored, the renal function returns to normal. Any persistent low perfusion, however, leads to the cellular injury and development of established or intrinsic ARF. Prerenal failure or azotemia can complicate any disease characterized by hypovolemia, low cardiac output, vasodilatation, or intrarenal vasoconstriction. True or effective hypovolemia leads to a fall in mean systemic arterial pressure, resulting in decreased perfusion of the kidneys. The concept of true effective circulating volume is an important one to emphasize. In face of low cardiac output or conditions in which fluid is sequestered in interstitial space (i.e., ascites), an overall

TABLE 26-1. Classification of Acute Renal Failure

Disease Category	*Patients (%)*
PRERENAL AZOTEMIA	**55–60**
Renal hypoperfusion Intravascular volume depletion (excess diuresis, hypoalbuminemia) Decreased cardiac output (renal vasoconstriction, disruption of renal autoregulation)	
INTRINSIC ACUTE RENAL FAILURE (ACUTE TUBULAR NECROSIS)	**35–40**
Ischemic* Nephrotoxic* Acute interstitial nephritis Atherothrombotic disease Diseases involving large and small vessels Glomerular disease	
POSTRENAL FAILURE (OBSTRUCTIVE UROPATHY)	**<5**
Acute obstruction of urinary tract collecting system (must be bilateral or single functioning kidney)	

*Accounts for 90% of intrinsic acute renal failure.
(Adapted from Brady HR, Clarkson MR, Lieberthal W. Acute renal failure. In: Brenner BA, ed. *The Kidney*, 7th ed. Philadelphia: WB Saunders; 2004:1216, with permission.)

increase in the total body fluid may occur, but the effective circulating volume is low (Table 26-2). The baroreceptors are activated, which further causes both neural and hormonal changes to preserve blood pressure. Therefore, prerenal failure and ARF (acute tubular necrosis [ATN]) are part of the same spectrum.

Intrinsic or ATN is the disease state in which the renal parenchyma is injured, either owing to ischemia (poor perfusion) or nephrotoxic agents. These changes affect tubular cells leading to cell death, alteration of cellular polarity, and shedding of tubular cells in the tubular lumen. This results in tubular obstruction and back diffusion of the glomerular filtrate resulting in oliguria or anuria. The two major causes of ARF are ischemic and nephrotoxic injury to renal parenchyma. The ischemic insult is the continuation of a more severe prerenal state. If the perfusion of the kidneys is compromised more severely or is prolonged, ARF develops. Restoration of perfusion may not lead to recovery. The major causes of acute intrinsic renal failure are summarized in Table 26-3. Rarely does pure volume depletion in otherwise normal kidneys lead to ARF. The predisposing factors are preexisting renal failure, advanced age with presence of other comorbidity, loss of fluid during surgery, postoperatively owing to trauma, burns, and nephrotoxic injury. The cause for nephrotoxic injury may be linked to the use of radiocontrast dye, prolonged perioperative course, use of sedatives, or presence of sepsis itself. In cardiac surgery, the duration of bypass time has been linked to the development of ARF. Sepsis causes hypoperfusion by vasodilatation or intracranial vasoconstriction and endotoxins that sensitize renal tissue to the deleterious effects (6). Postsurgically, 50% of patients with ARF may not have any documented hypotension. ARF is reported in 20% of burn victims and depends on the extent of burn injury and the fluid resuscitation immediate response. It is usually multifactorial: A combination of hypotension, rhabdomyolysis, sepsis, and nephrotoxic antibiotics.

Nephrotoxic ATN is caused by either intrinsic or extrinsic agents, such as rhabdomolysis or pigment injury, and hemoglobinuria. The major pathologic pathway in this injury may be ischemic in nature. The extrinsic toxins responsible for ARF are a diverse group of pharmacologic agents, including antibiotics. Most nephrotoxic agents are antibiotics or chemotherapeutic agents. Some drugs contribute to ARF, but mainly cause acute interstitial nephritis rather than ATN. Such an injury can be a mixture of many drugs; the diagnostic picture may be confusing; and these conditions have been

TABLE 26-2. Common Causes of Prerenal Azotemia

(Key Disorder: Kidney Hypoperfusion)

INTRAVASCULAR VOLUME DEPLETION

Hemorrhage: Traumatic, surgical, gastrointestinal, postpartum
Gastrointestinal losses: Vomiting, nasogastric suction, diarrhea
Kidney losses: Diuresis, adrenal insufficiency, diabetes insipidus, induced osmotic diuresis after brain surgery
Skin and mucous membrane losses: Burns
"Third-space" losses: Pancreatitis, crush syndrome, hypoalbuminemia

DECREASED CARDIAC OUTPUT FROM ANY CAUSE

RENAL VASOCONSTRICTION

Norepinephrine, ergotamine liver disease, sepsis, hypercalcemia

DRUGS THAT IMPAIR RENAL AUTOREGULATION OR GLOMERULAR FILTRATION

Angiotensin-converting enzyme inhibitors, angiotensin receptor blockers, nonsteroidal anti-inflammatory agents

(Adapted from Brady HR, Clarkson MR, Lieberthal W. Acute renal failure. In: Brenner BA, ed. *The Kidney*, 7th ed. Philadelphia: WB Saunders; 2004:1216, with permission.)

TABLE 26-3. Major Causes of Acute Nephrotoxic Intrinsic Renal Failure

ENDOGENOUS NEPHROTOXINS

RHABDOMYOLYSIS WITH MYOGLOBINURIA

Muscle injury, extreme muscle exertion, muscle ischemia
Infections, immunologic diseases (polymyositis, dermatomyositis)
Drugs: Cocaine, HMG CoA (3-hydroxyl-3-methylglutayl coenzyme A) reductase inhibitors, heroin

HEMOLYSIS WITH HEMOGLOBINURIA

Tranfusion reaction, infections and venoms, drugs, chemicals, mechanical (microangiopathic hemoytic anemia)

INCREASED URIC ACID PRODUCTION WITH HYPERURICOSURIA

MISCELLANEOUS

Tumor lysis syndrome, myeloma light chains

(Adapted from Fraser CL, Arieff AI. Brain abnormalities and peripheral neuropathy. In: Brenner BA, ed. *The Kidney*, 7th ed. Philadelphia: WB Saunders; 2004:1283, with permission.)

described as acute tubulointerstitial nephritis (AIN). This list of possible damaging agents continues to increase and it is advisable to review possible nephrotoxic side effects of all drugs before using them in a patient with kidney injury.

Radiocontrast nephropathy (RCN) is a common occurrence in hospital settings with frequent use of diagnostic and therapeutic procedures. The typical course is a slow rise in serum Cr within 24 to 48 hours of contrast administration, peaking in 3 to 7 days, and then returning to baseline, usually within a week. The overall incidence of RCN is low. Risk factors associated with RCN are initial Cr clearance <60 mL/min, intraaortic balloon pump, emergency procedure where no prior preparation for prevention was possible, diabetes mellitus, congestive heart failure, peripheral vascular disease, hypertension, and contrast volume of >260 mL (7,8). The pathogenesis of RCN is a mixture of ischemia, direct tubular toxicity, and oxidative stress.

Postrenal injury results from an obstruction to the urinary tract that can occur at any level between the renal pelvis to the urethra. Bladder neck obstruction in men because of prostate enlargement is the most common cause for postrenal failure, also known as *obstructive uropathy*. Proximal lesions to urinary bladder obstruction, unless bilateral, would not result in ARF unless the obstruction is present either in a solitary kidney or the other kidney is nonfunctional.

A few of the specific forms of ARF are as follows:

1. Hepatorenal syndrome. ARF, characterized by decreasing urine volume, hyponatremia, and prerenal azotemia in the presence of advanced chronic liver disease and portal hypertension. This is an avid sodium retentive state and fractional excretion of sodium (FE_{NA}) is low. The cause is unknown, but intense renal circulation vasoconstriction is noted. The ARF reverses after liver transplantation or improvement of liver function (9).
2. ARF in human immunodeficiency virus (HIV) or acquired immunodeficiency syndrome (AIDS). The ARF in patients with HIV may result from the antiviral therapy used. The protease inhibitor, indinavir, causes nephrolithiasis and crystal-induced renal failure. Another protease inhibitor, ritonavir, has also been associated with ARF. The nucleotide reverse transcriptase inhibitors, such as tenofovir, adefovir, and cidofovir, can produce a proximal tubular injury manifested by a Fanconi-like syndrome and ARF (10,11).
3. Rhabdomyolysis. A frequent cause of ARF, rhabdomyolysis can occur with either traumatic or nontraumatic injury to muscles, most commonly in the setting of volume depletion and hypotension. Although the mechanism of renal failure is unknown, it is associated with intrarenal vasoconstriction, intratubal obstruction, and direct tubular injury caused by myoglobin.
4. Drug-induced ARF. This form of ARF can result from an allergic reaction, in which case the picture is one of AIN. The patients are rarely severely oliguric and, on withdrawal of the incriminating drug, renal function is restored. Other drugs, such as the aminoglycosides, are directly tubular toxic and the toxicity is related to the cumulative amount of medication.

PATHOLOGY

The pathologic changes in ATN are subtle, with poor correlation between structure and function in ARF. Prominent changes are seen at the corticomedullary junction, but scattered foci of injury may be present in the cortex involving both proximal and distal segments. Found are necrosis of tubules, damage to the brush border of proximal tubules, and loss of microvilli and of individual or cluster of cells. These changes cause exposure of denuded basement membrane of tubules. The sloughed off cells are shed in the tubular lumen and may be trapped by Tamm-Horsfell glycoproteins, resulting in casts as well as obstruction of the tubular lumen. Almost simultaneously, evidence is seen of cellular regeneration with basophilic cytoplasm and occasionally mitosis.

CLINICAL MANIFESTATIONS

In hospitalized patients, ARF generally occurs in association with other diseases and multiple organ failure. Clinical manifestations are a decrease in urine output, and retention of metabolic waste products manifested by rising serum BUN and Cr. The ARF may be oliguric (urine output <500 mL/d) or nonoliguric. The electrolyte abnormalities seen are hyperkalemia and metabolic acidosis. Fluid retention soon follows. In many settings, overall total body fluid may be increased, but effective circulating arterial volume is low.

Patients with renal failure often manifest a variety of neurologic disorders that can occur before, during, or after initiation of dialysis. Symptoms could be mild or sensorial cloudiness to coma and death. Because of routine blood workup, patients with renal failure are often identified before overt symptoms appear. Patients may manifest subtle nervous system dysfunctions, such as impaired mentation, generalized weakness, or peripheral neuropathy. Dialysis is associated with dialysis disequilibrium syndrome, dialysis dementia, and progressive intellectual dysfunction.

Uremic encephalopathy is a central neurologic state seen in patients with rapidly developing renal failure. Usually seen when GFR falls <10 mL/min, this is defined as a variable disorder of consciousness that can affect psychomotor behavior, thinking, memory, speech, perception, and emotion. The diagnosis of uremic encephalopathy is difficult. Most of the symptoms are also present in other types of metabolic encephalopathy caused by drugs with potential central nervous system (CNS) toxicity affected by renal excretion or metabolism. In patients with liver failure, it may be difficult to differentiate uremic encephalopathy from hepatic encephalopathy. BUN and serum Cr may not always adequately reflect the degree of renal impairment. The most common clinical neurologic manifestations are listed in Table 26-4 (12,13).

DIAGNOSTIC APPROACH

The diagnosis depends on a meticulous history—chronologic documentation of events that may have contributed to the development of ARF: History of nephrotoxic agents, including antibiotics, over-the-counter drugs, such as nonsteroidal anti-inflammatory agents (NSAID), or any other prescription medications, such as converting enzyme inhibitors or angiotensin II antagonists which are known to be associated with ARF.

Urinalysis, including urine sediment, should be done. The major findings seen in urinary sediment are listed in Table 26-5. In ATN, the sediment is characterized by brownish dirty casts, although the absence of casts does not rule out ARF diagnosis. Urinary indices provide a good clue to diagnosis. The

TABLE 26-4. Common Clinical Neurologic Manifestations in Acute Renal Failure

Insomnia and sleep inversion
Restlessness
Decreased attention span
Drowsiness
Decreased cognitive function
Disorientation
Confusion
Bizarre behavior
Slurring of speech
Myoclonus
Asterixis
Convulsions
Stupor
Coma

most common urinary indices are FE_{NA} and fractional excretion of urea nitrogen (FE_{UNA}). FE_{NA} <1.0 indicates prerenal azotemia and >1.0 indicates ATN. When urine sodium is unreliable, such as with use of diuretics, FE_{UNA} is a better marker. A FE_{UNA} of <35% indicates prerenal azotemia.

TREATMENT

Preventive measures for ARF are important because they forestall the development of ARF. The most important factor is volume. A well-hydrated state, with appropriate effective circulating volume, is the most important preventive measure. When volume state cannot be adequately assessed, central venous pressure (CVP) or Swan-Ganz catheter may be required to judge the volume status. For renal volume expansion, either normal saline or isotonic bicarbonate presents the best option.

Several pharmacologic agents have been used to either prevent or to abrogate ARF development. Many are used when ARF is well established. Almost none of the pharmaceutical agents uniformly have stood the vigorous scientific proof. Most data are weak or sporadic to support or recommend their routine use in ARF.

Low-dose dopamine to prevent ARF is not effective and its use is not recommended. Fenoldopam, another dopamine agnostic, is also not effective. Loop diuretics are extensively used in ARF, as both preventive and therapeutic measures. Extensive literature has failed, however, to show any consistent results and the data remain inconclusive. In some instances, such as dye-induced ARF, it can worsen the nephrotoxic effect of dye. Mannitol use is also not beneficial and can be associated with direct tubular injury. *N*-acetylcysteine (NAC) reduces oxidative stress and has been postulated to potentially reduce risk of ARF, particularly in RCN. The effect of NAC is inconsistent, however, and most of the studies have failed to show any benefit from NAC to prevent ARF (14–16).

Therapy for ARF is aimed at maintaining a euhydrated state, restoring normal electrolyte and acid-base status, and removing retained products of metabolism as measured by BUN and serum Cr. Dialysis provides the means to achieve these goals.

Peritoneal dialysis is a very slow process and is not the preferred method. Hemodialysis is the method of choice. It can be used either (*a*) on an intermittent basis (three to five times per week 3 to 4 hours per session) or, more recently, (*b*) as a continuous renal replacement therapy (CRRT) using low flow hemodialysis. The advantage of CRRT is that it is more physiologic, removes fluid slowly, and, therefore, can be used in a patient whose condition is unstable. A hybrid form of intermittent hemodialysis known as *slow low efficiency dialysis* (SLED) is also used in the same setting. It consists of low blood flow, but for 8 to 12 hours a day, and is easier to maintain. Regardless of the technique used, no difference is found in the overall outcome. It should be emphasized that dialysis is only a supportive measure until the kidney injury heals and renal function improves.

TABLE 26-5. Urine Indices Used in the Differential Diagnosis of Prerenal and Intrinsic Renal Azotemia

Diagnostic Index	*Prerenal Azotemia*	*Intrinsic Azotemia*
Fractional excretion of sodium ($FE_{Na}\%$)	<1	>1
Urinary Na+ concentration (mEq/L)	<10	>20
Urinary creatinine:plasma creatinine ratio	>40	>20
Urinary urea nitrogen:plasma nitrogen ratio	>8	<3
Urine specific gravity	>1.018	<1.012
Urine osmolality (mOsm/kg/H_2O)	>500	<250
Blood urea nitrogen: creatinine ratio	>20	<10–15
Renal failure index (UNa/Ucr/Pcr)	<1	>1
Urine sediment	Hyaline casts	Muddy brown granular casts

*The most sensitive indices are fractional excretion of Na+ and the renal failure index.
PNa, plasma Na concentration; Pcr, plasma creatinine concentration; UNa, urine Na concentration; Ucr, urine creatinine concentration.
(From Brady HR, Clarkson MR, Lieberthal W. Acute renal failure. In: Brenner BA, ed. *The kidney*. 7th ed. Philadelphia: WB Saunders; 2004:1253, with permission.)

The indications for dialysis are not clear cut or absolute. The decision depends on the overall assessment of the patient. Dialysis is done on an emergency basis in the presence of hyperkalemia, pericarditis, marked acidosis, or pulmonary edema. Dialysis has no effect on the overall recovery from renal failure.

CLINICAL RECOMMENDATIONS OF THE VIGNETTE

The patient had well established ARF. The cause is multifactorial, with both hemodynamic injury and nephrotoxic injury secondary to rhabdomyolysis. The nephrology consult recommended placement of a central line to monitor CVP or pulmonary capillary wedge (PCW) pressure. Because of pulmonary edema, an emergency dialysis was started. After several dialysis treatments, the neurologic conditions remained unchanged and a neurology consult suggested hypoxic encephalopathy.

SUMMARY

The mortality rate in ARF in a critical setting is high, most commonly in an aggressive dialysis approach, with mortality associated with the number of organs failure. A meticulous attention to fluids, acidosis, and sepsis is vital to reduce this excessive mortality.

REFERENCES

1. Acute dialysis quality initiative. www.adqi.net. Accessed: July 20, 2006.
2. Simmons EM, Himmelfarb J, Sezer MT, et al. PICARD Study Group. Plasma cytokine levels predict mortality in patients with acute renal failure. *Kidney Int.* 2004;65:1357–1365.
3. Hou SH, Bushinsky DA, Wish JB, et al. Hospital-acquired renal insufficiency: A prospective study. *Am J Med.* 1983;74:243–248.
4. Nash K, Hafeez A, Hou S. Hospital-acquired renal insufficiency. *Am J Kidney Dis.* 2002; 39:930–936.
5. Liano F, Pascual J. Epidemiology of acute renal failure: A prospective, multicenter, community-based study. Madrid Acute Renal Failure Study Group. *Kidney Int.* 1996;50:811–818.
6. Zager RA. Escherichia coli endotoxin injections potentiate experimental ischemic renal injury. *Am J Physiol.* 1986;251:F988–F994.
7. Bartholomew BA, Harjai KJ, Dukkipati S, et al. Impact of nephropathy after percutaneous intervention and a method for risk stratification. *Am J Cardiol.* 2004;93:1515–1519.
8. Marenzi G, Lauri G, Assanelli E, et al. Contrast-induced nephropathy in patients undergoing primary angioplasty for acute myocardial infarction. *J Am Coll Cardiol.* 2004;44:1780–1785.
9. Cardenas A. Hepatorenal syndrome: A dreaded complication of end-stage liver disease. *Am J Gastroenterol.* 2005;100:460–467.
10. Daugas E, Rougier JP, Hill G. HAART-related nephropathies in HIV-infected patients. *Kidney Int.* 2005;67:393–404.
11. Franceschini N, Napravnik S, Eron JJ, et al. Incidence and etiology of acute renal failure among ambulatory HIV-infected patients. Kidney Int. 2005;67:1526–1531.
12. Fraser CL, Arieff AI. Nervous system manifestations of renal failure. In: Schrier RW, ed. *Diseases of the Kidney and Urinary Tract,* 7th ed. Philadelphia: Lippincott Williams & Wilkins; 2001:2769–2794.
13. Fraser CL, Arieff AI. Nervous system complications in uremia. *Ann Intern Med.* 1988; 109:143–153.
14. Friedrich JO, Adhikari N, Herridge MS, et al. Meta-analysis: Low-dose dopamine increases urine output but does not prevent renal dysfunction or death. *Ann Intern Med.* 2005; 142:510–524.
15. Tumlin JA, Finkel KW, Murray PT, et al. Fenoldopam mesylate in early acute tubular necrosis: A randomized, double-blind, placebo-controlled clinical trial. *Am J Kidney Dis.* 2005; 46:26–34.
16. Gomes VO, Poli de Figueredo CE, Caramori P, et al. N-acetylcysteine does not prevent contrast induced nephropathy after cardiac catheterization with an ionic low osmolality contrast medium: A multicentre clinical trial. *Heart.* 2005;91:774–778.

CHAPTER **27**

Chronic Renal Failure

Joseph Mattana

OBJECTIVES

- To review the clinical burden of chronic kidney disease
- To discuss the clinical features of the major forms of central nervous system (CNS) and peripheral nervous system (PNS) dysfunction among these patients
- To review recent literature on the mechanisms of neurologic dysfunction in chronic kidney disease
- To review current therapy for neurologic disorders in chronic kidney disease and emphasize the importance of considering alternative causes and contributory factors

CASE VIGNETTE

A 66-year-old hypertensive man with polycystic kidney disease had an arteriovenous fistula created in anticipation of starting hemodialysis within the next year. He moved out of state and failed to seek medical follow up until now. He had no chest pain, dyspnea, or nausea, but reported mild anorexia. What disturbed him most, however, was that he was suffering from unexpected and unprovoked episodes of crying. He was also frustrated by a progressive loss of memory function. On examination, blood pressure was 160/100 mm Hg and mild bilateral asterixis was present. A well-developed arteriovenous fistula was present in the left arm. Laboratory data showed a serum creatinine of 12.5 mg/dL, potassium 5.6 mEq/L, and hemoglobin of 8.4 g/dL.

The patient was started on hemodialysis using a cellulose acetate dialyzer and received erythropoietin (4,000) intravenously three times per week. Treatments were uneventful and, with time, his emotional lability resolved and his memory improved substantially. Five years later he had a cadaveric renal transplant and displayed no evidence of neurologic abnormality.

DEFINITION AND EPIDEMIOLOGY

Chronic kidney disease, defined as kidney damage or a glomerular filtration rate of <60 mL/min/1.73 m^2 body surface area for at least 3 months, afflicts close to 20 million individuals in the United States and is a significant worldwide health problem (1). Despite our success in improving the care of these patients, they often have multiple pathophysiologic derangements secondary to the loss of kidney function. With the decline in the glomerular filtration rate, various known and as yet unidentified substances normally kept at low levels accumulate in blood and other body tissues. In addition, the kidney's ability to regulate erythropoiesis and calcium and phosphorus metabolism declines. The kidney's impact on the control of extracellular volume and blood pressure is also impaired. Anemia, abnormal calcium, phosphorus, vitamin D, and parathyroid hormone metabolism, accelerated atherogenesis, a propensity to infections, increased risk of malignancies, infertility, and highly constrained and complex pharmacokinetic parameters resulting in a predisposition to drug toxicity. These disturbances account for substantial morbidity and mortality in many of these patients and pose vexing therapeutic challenges.

Millions of patients worldwide with chronic kidney disease are also susceptible to a variety of neurologic disorders that can result in substantially altered CNS and PNS function. Although patients with end-stage kidney disease requiring renal replacement therapy are well known to suffer from neurologic dysfunction, neurologic abnormalities can also afflict patients with lesser degrees of impairment of renal function. Recognition of these subtle abnormalities may not be readily apparent to patients, their family members, and their physicians when the development is gradual as often is the case when the decline in the glomerular filtration rate is protracted. Physicians caring for these patients should be vigilant in screening for neurologic disorders because various interventions may be beneficial. Equally important, although neurologic abnormalities may be attributed to the underlying chronic kidney disease, other causes must always be considered in the differential diagnosis, including primary neurologic diseases unrelated to renal failure, drug toxicity, endocrine dysfunction, infection, malignancy (including paraneoplastic syndromes), nutritional deficiencies, and psychiatric disorders among others.

Central Nervous System

Uremic Encephalopathy

ETIOLOGY AND PATHOGENESIS

CLINICAL FEATURES

Uremic encephalopathy can present with an altered level of consciousness, behavioral and cognitive dysfunction, slurred speech, impaired abstract thinking, emotional lability, limited attention span, restlessness, myoclonus, asterixis, and hallucinations progressing to seizures and coma (2–4). Patients may also have nausea, vomiting, hiccoughs, neuropathic complaints, and weakness. Although these findings may be attributed to the retention of various substances as a consequence of a decreased glomerular filtration rate, alternative causes must always be considered in these patients with frequent and substantial comorbidity. Drug toxicity resulting from altered pharmacokinetics, including decreased drug clearance; cerebrovascular disease in these stroke-susceptible patients; infection; and liver disease, among others, all must be considered in the differential diagnosis of patients with chronic kidney disease with evidence of CNS dysfunction.

Cognitive Impairment

Cognitive impairment is an important and incompletely understood CNS manifestation of chronic kidney disease. Using standardized cognitive function tests, 15% of patients with advanced chronic kidney disease and 27% of patients with end-stage renal disease were found to have evidence of globally impaired cognitive function (5). When executive functions were examined more specifically, they were found to be impaired in 38% of patients with end-stage renal disease, in 23% of patients with advanced chronic kidney disease, and in 5% of those with mild to moderate chronic kidney disease (5). Evidence of cognitive impairment remained after adjusting for age, sex, race, education, and comorbidity. Hence, it appears that a gradation of cognitive impairment exists in patients with chronic kidney disease, although the mechanisms are unknown. Although it may be speculated that this results from elevated levels of one or more uremic toxins, therefore it would be expected this would be attenuated in patients with end-stage renal disease on dialysis. In contrast to the effects of dialysis on other neurologic disorders, however, the prevalence of cognitive impairment among these patients is higher. Perhaps extensive and irreversible neurologic damage has already taken place by the time renal replacement therapy is undertaken or the actions of hemodialysis may be disconnected from the pathophysiologic disturbances contributing to cognitive impairment.

CLINICAL FINDINGS AND DIAGNOSTIC STUDIES

Variable imaging abnormalities have been reported in patients with encephalopathies with chronic kidney disease, including cerebral atrophy (3,6), as seen on cranial computed tomography (CT) or brain magnetic resonance imaging (MRI). MRI may also show signal changes in various CNS anatomic regions, including basal ganglia, internal capsule, and periventricular white matter (3). Neuroimaging studies, however, do not provide specific findings diagnostic of uremic encephalopathy as opposed to other encephalopathic processes. Nevertheless, CT or MRI can be invaluable in excluding other causes of altered CNS function. Electroencephalographic (EEG) abnormalities are most pronounced among patients with acute renal failure, although patients with chronic kidney disease also manifest EEG abnormalities such as slowing as evidenced by an increased percentage of EEG frequencies below 7 Hz (7).

INVESTIGATIONAL FINDINGS IN UREMIC ENCEPHALOPATHY

Multiple brain abnormalities have been described in patients with kidney disease (8,9). Brain calcium content is increased in uremia and thought to play a pathophysiologic role in causing CNS dysfunction. Although calcium levels have been reported to be normal in the subcortical white matter, pons, medulla, cerebellum, thalami, and caudate nuclei, they are 60% above control in the cortical gray matter and the hypothalamus (10). Plasma osmolality increases in uremia are caused by the retention of various solutes and with a corresponding increase in brain osmolality, half of this accounted for by urea and the other half by idiogenic osmoles (10). Acid-base balance is also altered in uremia with an initial nonanion gap metabolic acidosis evolving into an anion gap metabolic acidosis. Despite the presence of a metabolic acidosis, intracellular brain pH remains within the normal range (10). In uremia, the brain metabolic rate is also diminished (11) in association with decreased adenosine triphosphate (ATP) consumption, and the sodium-potassium adenosine triphosphatase (ATPase) activity appears to be decreased as well (12).

Potential Neurotoxins in Uremic Encephalopathy

Although CNS changes in uremia are thought to result from the indirect effects of increased levels of one or more agents, no such substances have been definitively linked to these abnormalities. A role for several candidate molecules exists, however. These include low molecular weight water-soluble compounds, such as guanidinosuccinic acid (13), whose concentration in uremic brain is increased up to 100 times, including in patients not on dialysis (14) and lower the seizure threshold, and other guanidines that can act as arginine analogs and thereby inhibit nitric oxide synthase, causing changes in vascular tone which can contribute to neurologic abnormalities.

Many molecules are suspected to play a role in uremic encephalopathy. Advanced glycation endproducts (AGE), parathyroid hormone (PTH), spermine (protein bound molecule that reacts with the *N*-methyl-D-aspartate [NMDA] receptor, which affects calcium and sodium permeability in brain cells), and others have been investigated. As mentioned, brain calcium content is increased in kidney disease. PTH levels are typically elevated because of several factors, including elevated serum phosphorus levels and impaired synthesis of 1,25-dihydroxy vitamin D by the kidney. PTH has been suspected to play a role in CNS changes seen in kidney disease via an effect on brain calcium levels. For example, it has been shown that experimental parathyroidectomy can prevent the EEG changes associated with kidney failure and can also attenuate the increased levels of brain calcium (15). In addition, patients with kidney failure who had parathyroidectomy often show improvements in both their EEG findings and neuropsychologic measures (16).

To evaluate abnormal neuroexcitation in uremia, D'Hooge et al. (17) recently reported the effects of 17 suspected uremic neurotoxins in in vitro and in vivo studies. Using cultured murine spinal cord neurons, 3-indoxyl sulfate, guanidinosuccinate, spermine, and phenol were found to cause significant currents using a whole-cell recording method. Interaction with voltage- and ligand-gated calcium channels was found to account for inward whole-cell currents resulting from incubation with guanidinosuccinate and spermine. Guanidinosuccinate's effect takes place via activation of NMDA receptor-associated channels. High-dose spermine had a direct effect on voltage-gated calcium channels, whereas low doses exert their action via the NMDA receptor complex. In vivo studies in Swiss mice showed that intraperitoneal injections of guanidinosuccinate induced seizures. When mice were pretreated with an intraventricular injection of spermine before administration of guanidinosuccinate, this effect was enhanced (17). These data suggest that these and other compounds may partly account for the CNS dysfunction in chronic kidney disease, and given their action via ligand- and voltage-gated calcium channels provide further support for the hypothesis that calcium plays a role in uremic encephalopathy.

Other Potential Contributors to Uremic Encephalopathy

ANEMIA. Anemia has long been thought to play a role in CNS dysfunction among patients with advanced chronic kidney disease, and its correction appears to have a favorable impact on uremic encephalopathy (18). Previously managed through blood transfusions with the attendant risk of iron overload, HLA antigen sensitization, and infection, anemia of chronic kidney disease has now become relatively straightforward to control with the use of erythropoiesis-stimulating agents.

ALUMINUM. A relationship between aluminum and CNS dysfunction in kidney failure has been long suspected (19). This typically occurred in patients on dialysis using aluminum hydroxide as a dietary phosphate binder, or through the exposure to aluminum-containing dialysate, which predisposed them to increased aluminum deposition in the brain and other organs, including bone. Over the past several decades, replacement of aluminum hydroxide with non–aluminum-containing phosphate binders as well as dialysate water treatments have led to the virtual disappearance of aluminum brain deposition as a major clinical problem. As illustrated, however, by a recent case of fatal aluminum encephalopathy in a patient with chronic kidney disease not on dialysis (20), despite the lack of use of aluminum hydroxide as a phosphate binder, patients may ingest aluminum from over-the-counter as well as prescribed medications containing aluminum, such as sucralfate (21). Although patients on dialysis have routine blood testing for aluminum, this is generally not the case for patients with chronic kidney disease, although this might be worthwhile to consider in patients displaying CNS abnormalities unaccounted by the degree of renal failure or other factors.

THERAPY

Hemodialysis, peritoneal dialysis, and transplantation exert a favorable impact on uremic encephalopathy. At times, the CNS changes seen with uremia are subtle and may be recognized only retrospectively by patients and or family members after patients have been on renal replacement therapy and the abnormalities have remitted.

Peripheral Nervous System
Peripheral Neuropathy

Although patients with chronic kidney disease are susceptible mononeuropathies such as the carpal tunnel syndrome (3), this section mainly focuses on polyneuropathies that appear to be associated with systemic abnormalities seen in the uremic state. Analogous to the evaluation of patients with suspected uremic encephalopathy, it is important to consider other causes of polyneuropathy, such as diabetes mellitus, multiple myeloma and other malignancies, collagen vascular disease, and drug toxicity.

CLINICAL FEATURES

Patients with advanced chronic kidney disease are susceptible to peripheral neuropathy occurring in approximately two thirds of patients with end-stage renal disease beginning renal replacement therapy (22). The polyneuropathy is often symmetric, length-dependent, and associated with abnormalities of motor, sensory, and autonomic function (2). Patients often report paresthesias and pain, as well as loss of sensation, classically in a "stocking-glove" distribution. Weakness, restless legs, and loss of reflexes occur as well (2,23). Patients with autonomic nervous system involvement can develop orthostatic hypotension (24). Cranial nerve dysfunction, manifesting as hearing loss or visual impairment, has been reported as well (25,26).

DIAGNOSTIC APPROACH

Neurophysiologic testing may show several abnormalities helpful in the assessment of uremic peripheral neuropathy. F-wave abnormalities, vibration detection thresholds in the feet, and sensory action potential amplitude in the sural nerves have been shown to be the most sensitive measures of uremic polyneuropathy correlating with the degree of symptoms (27).

INVESTIGATIONAL FINDINGS IN UREMIC PERIPHERAL NEUROPATHY

Typical pathologic findings in uremic peripheral neuropathy include predominantly distal axonal changes with demyelination (28). Patients with uremic peripheral neuropathy have been reported to have diminished sensory and motor amplitudes (29), which is consistent with an axonal process. In a recent study, predialysis nerve excitability changes consistent with axonal hyperpolarization were found and these changes were attenuated by dialysis (30). Recently (31), sodium-potassium ATPase function in patients with end-stage renal disease was found not to be diminished, a finding against the hypothesis of a possible uremic substance impairing sodium-potassium ATPase activity, thus suggesting that elevated serum potassium levels might play a significant role instead.

Various other substances have been proposed as potential uremic neurotoxins to account for the peripheral neuropathy in chronic kidney disease. Robles et al (32) demonstrated that dialysis treatment using a synthetic membrane (polyacrylonitrile) capable of achieving better removal of middle-sized molecules improved both sensory and motor nerve conduction velocities, whereas dialysis using a cellulose-based membrane (cellulose acetate), which is less effective at removing middle molecules, did not have an observable effect. These data suggest that one or more middle-sized molecules might play a role in uremic peripheral neuropathy.

Central Sensory and Motor Pathways

Peripheral nerve changes are well known with chronic kidney disease, but much less is known regarding central sensory and motor pathway changes. Kalita et al. (33) carried out nerve conduction studies on 19 patients with end-stage renal disease on hemodialysis. Abnormalities (sural nerve conduction and peroneal nerve conduction) were found in 12 of them. In contrast, central conduction was modestly abnormal in only 5 of these patients. These findings suggest that peripheral nerve changes occur more commonly and to a greater extent than central pathway changes.

ADENOSINE DEAMINASE ACTIVITY AND NEUROPATHY. Speculation has been that elevated levels of various substances may contribute directly or indirectly to the development of uremic neuropathy via myelin sheath degeneration. Decreased adenosine deaminase activity has been described among patients on hemodialysis (34). In vitro studies using plasma from patients before and after dialysis show that adenosine deaminase activity was inhibited by predialysis plasma, but not by postdialysis plasma. Of note, the plasma of 3 of these 20 patients who had no evidence of neuropathy, demonstrated no inhibitory effect on adenosine deaminase activity, suggesting that one or more uremic toxins may contribute to the neuropathy through direct effects on nerve function, but also indirect effects may be exerted via enzymes and other proteins playing a role in normal peripheral nerve structure and function (34).

ROLE OF ERYTHROPOIETIN IN UREMIC NEUROPATHY. Neurons have erythropoietin receptors and, given the reduction in erythropoietin synthesis in chronic kidney disease, its potential role in peripheral neuropathy has been recently investigated. In a group of 22 patients with advanced chronic kidney disease not yet on dialysis, nerve conduction studies were carried out before and after 5 months of erythropoietin treatment (35). Improvements in motor nerve conduction velocities of median, peroneal, and tibial nerves were noted, and compound muscle action potentials of the median nerve increased as well. Conversely, sensory nerve function was not affected. Although hemoglobin levels increased, no correlation was found between the increase in hemoglobin levels and the improvement in motor nerve function, suggesting that the erythropoietin effect on nerve function may be related to interaction with erythropoietin receptors rather than to an indirect effect via treatment of the underlying anemia.

THERAPY

The sensory changes often seen in uremic peripheral neuropathy tend to favorably respond to dialysis (hemodialysis and peritoneal dialysis) and are the earliest to improve in the course of renal replacement therapy. Motor function improvement is seen subsequently. Transplantation may have a favorable impact on autonomic and cranial nerve abnormalities (3,25). In general, the likelihood of clinical improvement is greatest among those patients with mild symptoms at the time of starting renal replacement therapy with lesser degrees of recovery seen among those with more advanced abnormalities (22). Pharmacologic strategies aimed at alleviating pain and paresthesias from peripheral neuropathy may be useful; the impact of the decreased glomerular filtration rate on drug pharmacokinetics and the potential for drug toxicity must always be considered.

CLINICAL RECOMMENDATIONS OF THE VIGNETTE

The patient displayed some of the features often seen with uremic encephalopathy. During the time he had not received clinical follow up, his glomerular filtration rate further declined and reached a threshold such that CNS abnormalities became obvious, particularly in the form of emotional lability and cognitive impairment. These disturbances, however, responded well to hemodialysis and erythropoietin therapy.

SUMMARY

Chronic kidney disease affects both the CNS and PNS and often presents clinical problems before and after the institution of renal replacement therapy. Renal replacement therapy, however, can ameliorate both the CNS and PNS dysfunction. Neurologic abnormalities associated with chronic kidney disease may serve as markers for the consequences of a decreased glomerular filtration rate, but alternative causes of neurologic dysfunction must always be considered and carefully excluded.

REFERENCES

1. Levey AS. Clinical practice. Nondiabetic kidney disease. *N Engl J Med.* 2002;347:1505–1511.
2. Brouns R, De Deyn PP. Neurological complications in renal failure: A review. *Clin Neurol Neurosurg.* 2004;107:1–16.
3. Burn DJ, Bates D. Neurology and the kidney. *J Neurol Neurosurg Psychiatry.* 1998;65:810–821.
4. Smogorzewski MJ. Central nervous dysfunction in uremia. *Am J Kidney Dis.* 2001;38[4 Suppl 1]:S122–S128.
5. Kurella M, Chertow GM, Luan J, et al. Cognitive impairment in chronic kidney disease. *J Am Geriatr Soc.* 2004;52:1863–1869.
6. Savazzi GM, Cusmano F, Musini S. Cerebral imaging changes in patients with chronic renal failure treated conservatively or in hemodialysis. *Nephron.* 2001;89:31–36.
7. Teschan PE, Bourne JR, Reed RB. Electrophysiological and neurobehavioral responses to therapy: The National Cooperative Dialysis Study. *Kidney Int Suppl.* 1983;S58–S65.
8. Fraser CL. Neurologic manifestations of the uremic state. In: Arieff AI, Griggs RG, eds. *Metabolic Brain Dysfunction. Systemic Disorders.* Boston: Little, Brown; 1992:139–166.
9. Kamata T, Hishida A, Takita T, et al. Morphologic abnormality in the brain of chronically hemodialyzed patients without cerebrovascular disease. *Am J Nephrol.* 2000; 20:27–31.
10. Mahoney LA, Arieff IA. Central and peripheral nervous system effects of chronic renal failure. *Kidney Int.* 1983;24:170–177.
11. Mahoney CA, Sarnacki P, Arieff AI. Uremic encephalopathy: Role of brain energy metabolism. *Am J Physiol.* 1984;247:F527.
12. Minkoff L, Gaertner G, Darab C, et al. Inhibition of brain sodium-potassium ATPase in uremic rats. *J Lab Clin Med.* 1972;80:71–78.
13. De Deyn PP, D'Hooge R, Van Bogaert PP, et al. Endogenous guanidine compounds as uremic neurotoxins. *Kidney Int Suppl.* 2001;78:S77–S83.
14. De Deyn PP, Marescau B, D'Hooge R, et al. Guanidino compound levels in brain regions of non-dialyzed uremic patients. *Neurochem Int.* 1995;27:227–237.
15. Guisado R, Arieff AI, Massry SG, et al. Changes in the electroencephalogram in acute uremia. Effects of parathyroid hormone and brain electrolytes. *J Clin Invest.* 1975;55:738–745.
16. Cogan MG, Covey CM, Arieff AI, et al. Central nervous system manifestations of hyperparathyroidism. *Am J Med.* 1978;65:963–970.
17. D'Hooge R, Van de Vijver G, Van Bogaert PP, et al. Involvement of voltage- and ligand-gated $Ca2+$ channels in the neuroexcitatory and synergistic effects of putative uremic neurotoxins. *Kidney Int.* 2003;63:1764–1775.

18. Singh NP, Sahni V, Wadhwa A, et al. Effect of improvement in anemia on electroneurophysiological markers (P300) of cognitive dysfunction in chronic kidney disease. *Hemodialysis International.* 2006;10:267–273.
19. Wills MR, Savory J. Aluminum and chronic renal failure: Sources, absorption, transport, and toxicity. *Crit Rev Clin Lab Sci.* 1989;27:59–107.
20. Zatta P, Zambenedetti P, Reusche E, et al. A fatal case of aluminum encephalopathy in a patient with severe chronic renal failure not on dialysis. *Nephrol Dial Transplant.* 2004;19:2929–2931.
21. Robertson JA, Salusky IB, Goodman WG, et al. Sucralfate, intestinal aluminum absorption, and aluminum toxicity in a patient on dialysis. *Ann Intern Med.* 1989;111:179–181.
22. Raskin NH, Fishman RA. Neurologic disorders in renal failure. *N Engl J Med.* 1976;294:143–148.
23. Kavanagh, D, Siddiqui, S, Geddes, CC. Restless legs syndrome in patients on dialysis. *Am J Kidney Dis.* 2004;43:763–771.
24. Robinson TG, Carr SJ. Cardiovascular autonomic dysfunction in uremia. *Kidney Int.* 2002;62:1921–1932.
25. Anteunis LJ, Mooy JM. Hearing loss in a uraemic patient: Indications of involvement of the VIIIth nerve. *J Laryngol Otol.* 1987;101:492–496.
26. Winkelmayer WC, Eigner M, Berger O, et al. Optic neuropathy in uremia: An interdisciplinary emergency. *Am J Kidney Dis.* 2001;37:E23.
27. Laaksonen S, Metsarinne K, Voipio-Pulkki LM, et al. Neurophysiologic parameters and symptoms in chronic renal failure. *Muscle Nerve.* 2002;25:884–890.
28. Galassi G, Ferrari S, Cobelli M, et al. Neuromuscular complications of kidney diseases. *Nephrol Dial Transplant.* 1998;13[Suppl 7]:41–47.
29. Angus-Leppan H, Burke D. The function of large and small nerve fibers in renal failure. *Muscle Nerve.* 1992;15:288–294.
30. Krishnan AV, Phoon RK, Pussell BA, et al. Sensory nerve excitability and neuropathy in end stage kidney disease. *J Neurol Neurosurg Psychiatry.* 2006;77:548–551.
31. Krishnan AV, Phoon RK, Pussell BA, et al. Neuropathy, axonal Na+/K+ pump function and activity-dependent excitability changes in end-stage kidney disease. *Clin Neurophysiol.* 2006;117:992–999.
32. Robles NR, Cancho B, Pizarro J, et al. Acute effect of hemodialysis with polyacrylonitrile membrane on nerve conduction velocities. *Ren Fail.* 2001;23:251–257.
33. Kalita J, Misra UK, Rajani M, et al. Central sensory motor pathways are less affected than peripheral in chronic renal failure. *Electromyogr Clin Neurophysiol.* 2004;44:7–10.
34. Severini G. Uremic toxins and adenosine deaminase activity. *Clin Biochem.* 1994;27:273–276.
35. Hassan K, Simri W, Rubenchik I, et al. Effect of erythropoietin therapy on polyneuropathy in predialytic patients. *J Nephrol.* 2003;16:121–125.

CHAPTER 28

Glomerular Diseases

Subhash Popli

OBJECTIVES

- To define the various glomerulonephritidies
- To describe the classification, clinical features, and diagnosis of acute nephritis
- To define primary and secondary glomerular diseases
- To describe clinical features, diagnostic approaches, and treatment guidelines for primary and secondary glomerular diseases
- To define the pathogenesis of the nephrotic syndrome and its complications
- To review treatment of various glomerular diseases, both primary and secondary

CASE VIGNETTES

PATIENT 1

A 55-year-old man with a long-standing history of intravenous drug abuse was evaluated for a right foot drop of 4 hours duration. Five days earlier, he had skin rash on his legs. He had seen a physician for aches and pains a year ago; acetaminophen was given for pain relief. On examination, he appeared cachectic. His blood pressure (BP) was 158/96 mm Hg. Liver span was 14 cm. A palpable purpura was noted on his back and legs along with a lower motor neuron type of foot drop. Laboratory tests showed a serum creatinine of 3.0 mg/dL (previously was 1 mg/dL); blood urea nitrogen (BUN) was 30 mg/dL. Urine sediment was remarkable for the presence of red blood cells (RBC) and RBC casts. Urine protein:creatinine ratio was 3, (normal <0.1). Hemoglobin was 11 g/dL. Serum C4 was 8 mg/dL (normal 10 to 50). Serum C3 was 100 mg/dL (normal 90 to 150). Rheumatoid factor was positive.

PATIENT 2

A 60-year-old black woman was evaluated for vague abdominal discomfort and dizziness. Remarkable physical findings were a BP 120/70 mm Hg supine and 100/60 mm Hg standing. Hepatomegaly and 2+ lower extremity edema were noted. Hemoglobin was 11 gm/dL. Serum calcium was 11 mg/dL. BUN was 28 mg/dL. Serum creatinine was 1.8 mg/dL. Anion gap was 5 mEq/L. Serum albumin was 2 g/dL. Urine analysis showed 4+ protein, and fatty casts. A 24-hour urine collection showed 5 g of protein, and spot urine protein to creatinine ratio of 5. Antinuclear antibody (ANA) test was negative. Serum C3 and C4 were normal.

INTRODUCTION

Glomerular disease can present as asymptomatic urinary abnormalities, acute glomerulonephritis, nephrotic syndrome, a mixed picture of nephritis and nephrosis, a rapidly progressive glomerulonephritis (RPGN), or as a chronic glomerulonephritis.

Acute Glomerulonephritis

DEFINITION

Glomerulonephritis is an inflammatory disease involving the glomeruli.

EPIDEMIOLOGY

Patients with glomerulonephritis account for approximately 6% of patients in an outpatient nephrology practice. In patients treated for end-stage renal disease (ESRD), nondiabetic glomerular disease accounts for 5% of cases of chronic renal failure. This represents a considerable decrease from 11% reported in 1990 (1).

ETIOLOGY AND PATHOGENESIS OF NEPHRITIS

Glomerular injury results in decreased renal function. Humoral immune mechanisms predominate in glomerular injury. Antibody can react with structural or planted antigen. Examples include antiglomerular basement membrane antibody (anti-GMB) in Goodpasture disease; circulating immune complex deposition (DNA and anti-DNA) in systemic lupus erythematosus (SLE); or soluble mediators (complement and cytokines) (2).

PATHOLOGY

The diagnosis of glomerulonephritis depends on identifying the specific histologic patterns of glomerular injury as determined

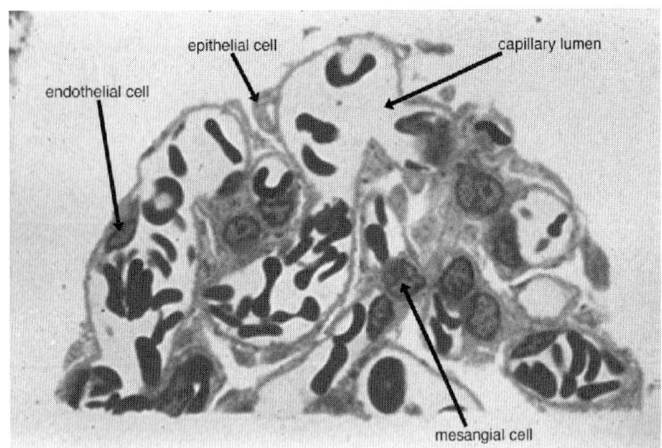

FIGURE 28-1. High power view of a glomerulus showing various cells.

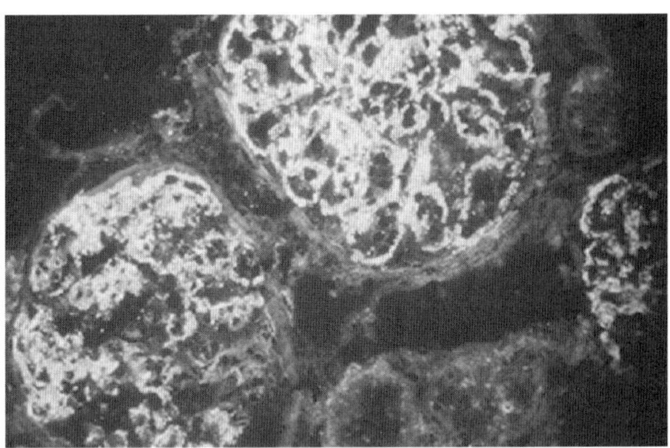

FIGURE 28-3. Granular pattern of immunofluorescence.

by renal biopsy. Renal tissue is examined under light microscopy (LM), electron microscopy (EM), and immunofluorescence (IF). The disease process can be *diffuse*, involving most of the glomeruli, *focal* with few tufts involved, or *segmental* with part of the tuft being involved. It can also show cellular crescents. In addition, the lesion may show proliferation of cells and thickening of capillary wall. Cellular infiltrates, both in the glomeruli or interstitial tissues, may be found. The extent and type of cellular infiltrate determines the activity and severity of the disease process. EM may show the presence of electron-dense deposits and IF stain determines the immune complex process. Figure 28-1 shows a glomerulus with various types of cells. Staining with an antihuman IgG IgM, IgA, or light chains tagged with IF is critical in establishing the correct diagnosis. Two patterns of fluorescence may be seen: A linear, ribbonlike pattern suggestive of anti-GBM, as seen on Figure 28-2, or a granular or *lumpy-bumpy* pattern as seen with immune complex glomerulonephritis (Fig. 28-3). If no deposits are seen on IF, this would be suggestive of pauci-immune diseases such as in cases of Wegener granulomatosis or other vasculitides. EM may demonstrate fusion of foot processes, basement membrane abnormalities, and the nature and site of electron-dense deposits that may be diagnostic of the underlying disease process (Fig. 28-4).

CLINICAL MANIFESTATIONS OF ACUTE GLOMERULONEPHRITIS

Patients with acute glomerulonephritis may present with nausea, headaches, flank pain, malaise, anorexia, or weakness. Rarely, the presentation of acute glomerulonephritis is with neurologic manifestations. Many patients have no symptoms whatsoever at presentation. Examination may demonstrate arterial hypertension, edema, hematuria, anemia with dysmorphic RBC, proteinuria, pyuria, and RBC or WBC casts. RBC casts in the urine sediment are pathognomonic for glomerulonephritis. In cases of a nephritic syndrome, the proteinuria is generally <3.5 g/24 h. The clinical evolution of glomerulonephritis often depends on the type of disease. Poststreptococcal glomerulonephritis (PSGN) and Henoch-Schonlein purpura (HSP) are usually self-limited. Anti-GBM disease, antineutrophil cytoplasmic antibodies (ANCA)-associated vasculitis, or hepatitis C-related vasculitis with cryoglobulinemia and SLE may have a rapid onset, and progress rapidly if untreated, to ESRD.

CLASSIFICATION OF GLOMERULONEPHRITIS

Classification is based on the histology and the predominance of cells involved.

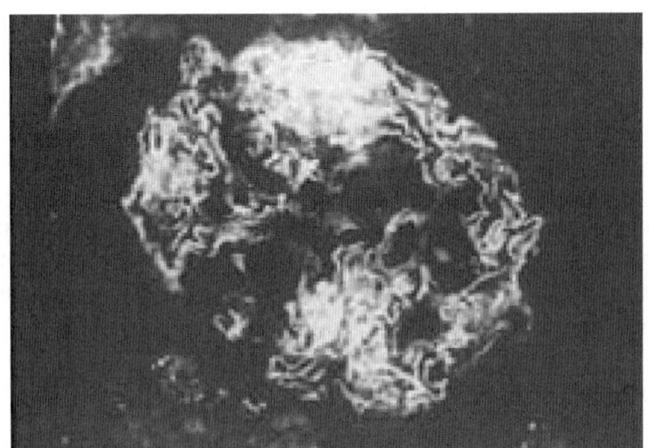

FIGURE 28-2. Linear IgG deposition in glomerular capillary wall.

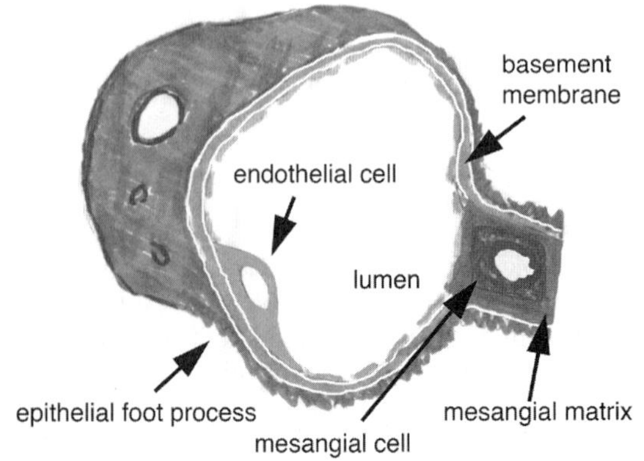

FIGURE 28-4. Cartoon diagram of normal capillary loop under electron microscope.

Endothelial Cell Proliferative Glomerulonephritis

The classic example of endothelial cell proliferative glomerulonephritis is acute PSGN, but other infectious causes of glomerulonephritis can also present with a similar picture. PSGN often occurs 1 to 3 weeks following a throat or skin infection with group A β-hemolytic streptococci. PSGN is immune-complex mediated. Clinical manifestations include acute oliguria, edema, and arterial hypertension. Neurologic manifestations, which are generally seen among children, can include headaches, somnolence, encephalopathy, or convulsions.

The serum C3 is low and the serum C4 is normal. Antistreptolysin O titers (ASO) are elevated. High titers of anti-hyaluronidase or anti-deoxyribonuclease (DNase) B may be seen in cases of streptococcal impetigo. Renal histology is remarkable for excessive endothelial cell proliferation in the glomerular capillaries associated with polymorphonuclear cell infiltration. EM shows classic subepithelial *humps*. Prognosis is excellent, with full recovery, especially among children (3).

Streptococcal infections have also been implicated in a pediatric neuropsychiatry disease known as PANDAS. PANDAS is the acronym for pediatric autoimmune neuropsychiatric disorders associated with streptococcal infections. This controversial disorder can be characterized by an abrupt or episodic onset, during prepubertal age, of obsessive–compulsive behaviors, Tourette syndrome or other tic disorders, and Sydenham chorea. PANDAS is presumed to be caused by an immune-mediated injury to basal ganglia antigens following a streptococcal infection. Elevated antitrypsin O (ASO) and anti DNase B titers have been noted. Contrary to PSGN, administrating penicillin and azithromycin therapy have been shown in preliminary study to be effective in preventing poststreptococcal neuropsychiatric exacerbations (4).

Epithelial Proliferative Glomerulonephritis

Also called RPGN or crescentic glomerulonephritis, epithelial proliferative glomerulonephritis is a clinicopathologic entity characterized by a rapidly progressive renal failure with crescents involving >50% of the glomeruli (Fig. 28-5). RPGN can be primary (idiopathic) or secondary to systemic diseases. In idiopathic RPGN, 15% are anti-GBM antibody related, 25% immune complex mediated, and 60% are pauci-immune. Pauci-immune means absence of any immunologic deposits or staining of the glomeruli on kidney biopsy. The pauci-immune variety is usually perinuclear ANCA (p-ANCA) positive (5).

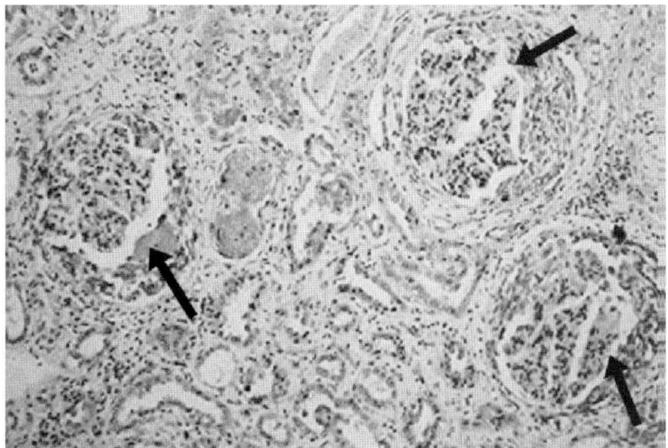

FIGURE 28-5. Light microscopy of renal biopsy showing three glomeruli with crescents (*arrows*).

Secondary RPGN can be seen following infections, such as infective endocarditis, hepatitis B and C, SLE, systemic vasculitidies, such as Wegener granulomatosis; polyarteritis nodosa, hypersensitivity vasculitis, IgA nephropathy, or HSP. Urgent diagnosis of RPGN is extremely important, because prognosis is considerably better if therapy is implemented early.

Goodpasture Syndrome

Goodpasture syndrome is a rare disorder occurring in approximately 0.9 cases/million/year. Pathogenesis is caused by antibody directed against the noncollagen domain of α_3 chain of type IV collagen in the glomerular capillary, which also cross-reacts with the alveolar wall. Iron deficiency anemia is common because of bleeding into the lungs. Exposure to smoke, hydrocarbons, and viral respiratory infections can unmask the antigen and induce antibody formation. Hypertension is uncommon. Diffuse necrotizing proliferative nephritis with crescents and rapidly progressive renal failure occur along with pulmonary hemorrhage. Serum complement levels are often normal. About 70% of patients have anti-GBM antibody in serum and 30% also have p-ANCA). Linear IgG and C3 deposition along GBM is pathognomonic (Fig. 28-3). An early aggressive therapy combining intravenous corticosteroids along with plasmapheresis and cyclophosphamide are key therapeutic strategies in reversing the disease.

Systemic Lupus Erythematosus

SLE is a chronic, relapsing-remitting systemic autoimmune disease predominantly affecting young black women. Widespread inflammation occurs because of circulating immune complexes of DNA and anti-DNA antibodies. ANA are present in 95% of cases. Low serum C3 and C4 levels, anemia, leucopenia, and other serologic markers indicate disease activity. A renal biopsy is necessary to assess the true renal lesion (Table 28-1) and determine treatment options and prognosis (6,7). The neuropsychiatry manifestations of SLE (NPSLE) encompass a wide array of clinical manifestations affecting 20% to 75% of patients with SLE (see Chapter 87).

Wagener Granulomatosis

Wagener granulomatosis is a disease of middle-aged individual, characterized by chronic upper and lower respiratory tract disease and nephritis with systemic necrotizing granulomatous vasculitis. The nephritic syndrome can lead to acute or rapidly progressive glomerulonephritis. Cytoplasmic ANCA are positive in most cases with active Wegener granulomatosis. Complement levels are normal. LM of renal biopsy shows diffuse or segmental necrotizing nephritis with crescents. No immune deposits are seen on IF or EM (pauci-immune). Treatment is a combination of steroids and cyclophosphamide. Untreated, the 2-year mortality rate for this condition is 80% to 90% (8).

TABLE 28-1. World Health Organization (WHO) Histologic Classification of Systemic Lupus Erythematosus with Reference to Glomerulonephritis

Class I	Normal LM, IF and EM
Class II	Mesangial: Mild clinical renal disease
Class III	Focal proliferative
Class IV	Diffuse proliferative: Most severe, active serology and active urine sediment
Class V	Membranous nephropathy.

LM, light microscopy; IF, immunofluorescence; EM, electron microscopy.

Mesangial Proliferative Glomerulonephritis

Mesangial proliferative glomerulonephritis is the classic form of IgA nephropathy or Berger disease. It is the most common cause of idiopathic nephritis in young men. It may be associated with alcoholic cirrhosis or HLA antigen B27-associated disorders. Patients present with asymptomatic microscopic or intermittent gross hematuria, with or without proteinuria after an upper respiratory tract infection (URI). Approximately 30% to 50% of patients may progress to ESRD over 2 decades. The pathogenesis and antigen are unknown; however, the antibody is mucosal IgA. A focal segmental glomerulonephritis is seen on LM. IF and EM show IgA and C3 deposits in the mesangium. Treatment options include steroids, fish oil, and angiotensin-converting enzyme inhibitors (ACEI), which may slow the progression of renal disease (9).

Henoch-Schonlein Purpura

HSP is common in children who often present with abdominal pains, arthralgias, purpura, and nephritis (see Chapter 157). Histology of HSP is similar to IgA nephropathy. Most patients recover without treatment.

Membranoproliferative Glomerulonephritis

In patients with membranoproliferative glomerulonephritis (MPGN), the capillary basement membrane is thickened and a proliferation of cells is noted. MPGN can rarely be idiopathic affecting young adults. In cases of the idiopathic variety MPGN, two histologic types are seen. Type 1, characterized by subendothelial deposits with mesangial interposition of capillary wall, low serum C4, C3, and C1q; and a type 2, characterized by dense deposit disease where electron-dense material is seen in basement membrane. The serum C3 is low in 90% of cases, with normal serum C4 and C1q levels. The C3 nephritic factor is present in half of the cases. These patients may also have partial lipodystrophy. No treatment is of proved benefit, although corticosteroids are often used. Secondary MPGN has been more commonly reported in association with hepatitis C, with or without mixed cryoglobulinemia, hepatitis B, SLE, Lyme disease, other systemic infections, and neoplasms.

HEPATITIS C VIRUS RELATED RENAL DISEASE

Hepatitis C, on occasions, can present with a clinical picture of a nephritic syndrome or non-nephrotic proteinuria. The usual histologic lesion is a MPGN, although membranous nephropathy may also be present in a few patients. A more florid course is seen among those in whom cyroglobinuria is present (10). These patients may present with palpable purpura, arthralgias, neuropathy, or abdominal pain caused by an underlying vasculitis. Arterial hypertension is common. Chronic nephritis or nephrotic syndrome may be seen. The total hemolytic complement CH50 is low in approximately 90% of cases; Ciq and C4 are low in 75% of cases; and the C3 low in about 50% of cases. Severe cryglobulinemic vasculitis, with rapidly progressive lesions, may respond to the administration of corticosteroids, cyclophosphamide, and plasmapheresis. After 2 to 4 months interferon-α (INF-α) with ribavirin should be attempted. In less severe acute disease, INF-α and ribavirin are the treatments of choice. This combined treatment may reduce proteinuria and improve the glomerular filtration rate (GFR), but relapses are common on cessation of treatment (10).

Nephrotic Syndrome

The nephrotic syndrome is defined when proteinuria is >3.5 g/day or urine protein:urine creatinine ratio is >3 or higher. Hypoalbuminemia, edema, hyperlipidemia, and lipiduria with fatty casts are the consequences of the severity of the proteinuria. A hypercoagulable state may be present (11). The causes of nephrotic syndrome are summarized in Table 28-2.

Minimal Change Disease

The pathogenesis of minimal change disease (MCD) remains unknown. This is a primary disorder of podocytes and may be linked to T-cell mediated immunity. It is the main cause of nephrotic syndrome in children. In adults, it accounts for 10% to 15% of idiopathic nephrotic syndrome. Renal function and BP are usually normal; adults may have arterial hypertension. MCD can also be seen in patients treated with nonsteroidal anti-inflammatory drugs (NSAID), lithium, and among those

TABLE 28-2. Causes of Nephrotic Syndrome in Adults

PRIMARY	Minimal change
	Focal and segmental glomerulosclerosis (FSGS)
	Membranous nephropathy
	Membranoproliferative GN
	Mesangialproliferative glomerulonephritis (IgA nephropathy)
SECONDARY	Systemic
	Diabetes mellitus
	Systemic lupus erythematosus (SLE)
	Amyloidosis
	Henoch-Schonlein purpura (HSP)
	Drugs
	Nonsteroidal anti-inflammatory drugs (NSAID)
	Heroin
	Gold
	Penicillamine
	Interferon-α_{1a} (INF-α_{1a})
	Lithium
	Neoplasms
	Lung adenocarcinoma
	Colon adenocarcinoma
	Stomach adenocarcinoma
	Hodgkin lymphoma

with Hodgkin lymphoma and chronic lymphatic leukemia (CLL). On renal biopsy, the glomeruli are normal on LM, negative IF staining, and fusion of foot processes on EM. Remissions and relapses are common. More than 80% of patients respond to high-dose corticosteroids or immunosuppressive drugs. Renal failure is seen in <2%. Relapse can occur in 50% within a year. Cyclophosphamide or chlorambucil is effective in corticosteroid-dependent and, frequently, relapsing cases.

Membranous Nephropathy

Membranous nephropathy is the most common cause of idiopathic nephrotic syndrome in adults, usually seen in the fourth and sixth decades. Nephrotic proteinuria is seen in >90% of cases who have normal GFR at presentation. Hypertension and microhematuria may be present. A high incidence is seen of thrombotic events, especially deep venous thrombosis and renal vein thrombosis. Serologic tests are normal. Secondary membranous nephropathy may also be seen with infections (hepatitis B and C, syphilis), SLE, medications (gold, penicillamine and IFN-β_{1a}), solid tumors, and lymphomas. Thickened capillary loops are seen on LM. No cellular proliferation is seen. IF shows granular deposits if IgG and C3 in the glomerular capillary walls. Subepithelial electron-dense deposits are seen on EM.

Approximately one third of patients have spontaneous remissions, one third progress to ESRD, and the other third remain stable with proteinuria. Treatment with immunosuppressive drugs is controversial, especially among those with low risk of progression. Greater remissions and better GFR is maintained in those patients at high risk when treated with steroids and chlorambucil or cyclophosphamide (12).

Focal and Segmental Glomerulosclerosis

Idiopathic focal and segmental glomerulosclerosis (FSGS) is the most common form of primary nephrotic syndrome in all races, leading to ESRD. Primary FSGS is more common among blacks. FSGS presents with massive proteinuria, arterial hypertension, and rapid progression to ESRD. Half of the patients with FSGS develop ESRD in 10 years if they have a nephrotic range proteinuria. Secondary causes of FSGS include intravenous drug use, reflux nephropathy, sickle cell disease, morbid obesity, infestation with the human immune deficiency virus (HIV), parvovirus infection, and administration of pamidronate. FSGS was initially felt to be corticosteroid resistant, but 20% to 40% of patients respond to 3 to 6 months of high-dose corticosteroids. In corticosteroid-resistant cases, 6 to 12 months of prednisone with cytotoxic drugs or cyclosporine A may also induce a remission in the degree of proteinuria.

Diabetic Nephropathy

Diabetic nephropathy is the leading cause of nephrotic syndrome and ESRD. Proteinuria develops in >30% over 25 years, in both insulin-dependent and non–insulin-dependent diabetes mellitus. No biopsy is needed in patients with typical presentation, especially if the patient also has diabetic retinopathy. Aggressive BP reduction to a target of 120/80 mm Hg and strict glucose control is effective to slow the progression of renal failure.

Amyloid Nephropathy

Renal involvement is common in both primary (AL) and secondary (AA) amyloidosis. AL amyloid seen in systemic idiopathic amyloidosis or multiple myeloma is caused by overproduction of monoclonal immunoglobulin or immunoglobulin light chains by a clone of B cells; in 80% of cases, the light chains these are lambda type (13). Clinical features are albuminuria, nephrotic syndrome, and renal insufficiency. In the elderly, AL amyloidosis accounts for 10% of cases of nephrotic syndrome. The treatment is that of the amyloidosis. The 5-year survival is estimated to be <20%. Documenting abnormal protein in the serum or urine, abdominal fat pad, rectal or renal biopsy showing Congo red positive, and extracellular nonbranching fibrils on EM, makes diagnosis. Melphalan and prednisone or vincristine and/or autologus stem cell transplant may induce remission in AL amyloidosis.

Complications of Nephrotic Syndrome

Hypoalbuminemia, edema, hyperlipidemia, and a hypercoagulable state are common in patients with nephrotic syndrome (14) (Table 28-3). Approximately 10% to 40% of patients with nephrotic syndrome may present with lower extremity, pulmonary, or renal vein thrombosis caused by the hypercoagulable state. Renal vein thrombosis is common in patients with membranous nephropathy. Patients may present with sudden increase in serum creatinine, flank pain, hematuria, or systemic emboli. Diagnosis is established by Doppler sonography of the renal veins, CT angiography, or MR angiography. Cerebral venous thrombosis involving the sagittal, transverse, and sigmoid sinuses have been described in children, as well as in adults (15). In contrast to venous thrombosis, arterial thrombosis is relatively infrequent in patients with nephrotic syndrome. Rarely, transient ischemic attacks or stroke can be the initial manifestation of nephrotic syndrome (16–18).

DIAGNOSTIC APPROACH

Preliminary tests include urine analysis, urine protein:urine creatinine ratio, or 24-hour urine for protein and creatinine collection; and serum creatinine and creatinine clearance. Although the value of multiple tests is uncertain, serum complement, ANA, urine and serum protein electrophoresis, antistreptolysin O, antihyaluronidase, anti-DNase B, cryoglobulins, syphilis serology, hepatitis serology, ANCA, and rheumatoid factor are often evaluated. Depending on the clinical suspicion, renal ultrasound is obtained to evaluate renal size. Renal biopsy is indicated for definite diagnosis, prognosis, and potential response to therapy in patients with glomerular diseases.

TREATMENT

Therapy of glomerular diseases involves managing the specific primary disease or the underlying cause, whenever possible, as well as treatment of any complications (Table 28-4). Definitive therapy is directed toward the specific histologic type of glomerulonephritis, as previously discussed. The major treatment is symptomatic. Rigid blood pressure control to a target level of 120/80 mm Hg is required. Hyperlipidemia should be normalized; during remission, the lipid profile may improve.

TABLE 28-3. Complications of Nephrotic Syndrome

Complication	*Clinical Consequences*
Hypovolemia	Postural hypotension Circulatory collapse Acute renal failure
Loss of IgG, complement factor B and D	Diminished resistance to infection Cellulitis, sepsis
Protein depletion	Muscle wasting
Altered blood coagulation from: ↓ Anti-thrombin III, antiplasmin ↑ factor V, VIII, fibrinogen and platelets	Venous and arterial thrombosis Pulmonary embolism
Electrolyte disturbances	Hyponatremia Hypokalemia
Reduced renal function	Uremia, ESRD hypertension
Hyperlipidemia ↑ VLDL, LDL	Accelerated atherosclerosis
Miscellaneous Loss of binding proteins:	
Calciferol	Osteomalacia
Transferrin	Refractory iron-deficiency anemia
Thyroid-binding globulin	Abnormal thyroid function tests

VLDL, very low-density lipoprotein; ESRD, end-stage renal disease.

In the presence of edema, administration of diuretics is essential. No specific antihypertensive agent is considered more renal protective in the absence of adequate blood pressure control. Blockade of the renin angiotensin system with either ACEI, or angiotensin receptor blockers (ARB) reduces the degree of proteinuria, and may also have a beneficial effect on slowing down the progression of the underlying renal disease.

CLINICAL RECOMMENDATION OF THE VIGNETTES

The patients described above had nephritis (case 1), and nephrosis (case 2). In the first patient, the etiology was related to hepatitis C. Cryoglobulins were positive. Renal biopsy showed MPGN with deposition of cryoglobulins in the glomeruli. Liver biopsy showed stage 2 hepatitis. Plasmapheresis and high-dose corticosteroids were initially recommended for the cryoglobulinemia. Subsequently, the patient was treated with pegylated interferon and ribavirin (at reduced dose for his renal function) for a total of 9 months. Serum complement levels returned to normal, and the serum creatinine improved to 1.4 mg/dL. His right foot drop improved. Six month after stopping treatment, he had recurrence of the proteinuria and an increase in the serum creatinine levels.

The second patient was presumed to have focal segmental FSGS causing nephrotic syndrome. Because FSGS is the common cause of idiopathic nephrotic syndrome among blacks, membranous nephropathy, MCD, and amyloidosis were also initially considered in the differential diagnosis. The serum protein electrophoresis showed low IgM and IgA, with an IgG monoclonal peak. The urine protein electrophoresis showed albumin and monoclonal peaks in the gamma region. Immunofixation studies showed IgG lambda. A bone marrow biopsy demonstrated 80% plasma cells with staining for lambda light chains. The patient was diagnosed to have a nephrotic syndrome caused by AL amyloid. She developed lower extremity deep venous thrombosis and pulmonary embolism 5 days after admission. A renal biopsy was not performed. An abdominal fat pad biopsy showed AL amyloid. She was treated with chemotherapy and later received an autologus stem cell transplant. Her serum creatinine improved to 1.5 mg/dL.

TABLE 28-4. Treatment of Nephrotic Syndrome

1. Specific therapy of the underlying lesion with steroids and immunosuppressive agents
2. Diet: 2 g sodium, low fat, soy-protein (0.7 to 1 g/kg/d)
3. Diuretics, water restriction if hyponatremic
4. Antihypertensives: Angiotensin-converting enzyme inhibitor (ACE-I) and angiotensin receptor blockers (ARB)
   Target blood pressure (BP) 120/75 mm Hg
5. Lipid-lowering agents
6. Multivitamins, vitamin D, iron supplementation

SUMMARY

Timely diagnosis and treatment of glomerular diseases can reduce mortality and morbidity, and delay progression to ESRD.

REFERENCES

1. United States Renal Data System (USRDS). USRDS 2004 Annual Data Report: Atlas of End-Stage Renal Disease in the United States. Bethesda MD, National Institute of Health, National Institute of Diabetes and Digestive and Kidney Diseases; 2005.
2. Hricik DE, Chung-Park M, Sedor JR. Glomerulonephritis. *N Engl J Med.* 1998;339:888–899.
3. Tejani A, Ingulli E. Post streptococcal glomerulonephritis: Current clinical and pathologic concepts. *Nephron.* 1990;55:1–5.
4. Snider LA, Swedo SE. PANDAS: Current status and directions for research. *Mol Psychiatry.* 2004;9(10):900–907.
5. Jenette JC. Rapidly progressive crescentic glomerulonephritis. *Kidney Int.* 2003;63: 1164–1177.

6. Houssiau F. Management of lupus nephritis: An update. *J Am Soc Nephrology.* 2004;5: 2694–2704.
7. Bansal VK, Beto JA. Treatment of lupus nephritis: A meta-analysis of clinical trials. *Am J Kidney Dis.* 1997;29:193–199.
8. Seo P, Stone JH. The antineutrophil cytoplasmic antibody-associated vasculitides. *Am J Med.* 2004;117:39–50.
9. Haas M. IgA nephropathy. *Semin Nephrol.* 2004;24:177–295.
10. D'Amico G. Renal involvement in hepatitis C infection: Cryoglobulinemic glomerulonephritis. *Kidney Int.* 1998;54:650–671.
11. Orth SR, Ritz R. The nephrotic syndrome. *N Engl J Med.* 1998; 338:1202–1211.
12. Bolton CK. Treatment of membranous nephropathy. *Semin Nephrol.* 2003;28:323–400.
13. Gertz MA, Lacy MQ, Dispenzier A. Immunoglobulin light chain amyloidosis and kidney. *Kidney Int.* 2002;61:1–9.
14. Bernard DB. Extrarenal complications of the nephrotic syndrome. *Kidney Int.* 1988;33:1184–1202.
15. Nishi H, Abe A, Kita A, et al. Cerebral venous thrombosis in adult nephrotic syndrome due to amyloidosis. *Clin Nephrol.* 2006;65:161–164.
16. Marsh EE, Biller J, Adams HP, Jr., et al. Cerebral infarction in patients with nephrotic syndrome. *Stroke.* 1991;22:91–93.
17. Yunez A, Biller J. Nephrotic syndrome and stroke. In: Bogousslavsky J, Caplan LR, eds. *Uncommon Causes of Stroke.* New York: Cambridge University Press 2001:280–289.
18. Dafer R, Biller J. Nephrotic syndrome and stroke. In: Bogousslavsky J, Caplan LR, eds. *Uncommon Causes of Stroke,* 3rd ed. New York: Cambridge University Press. In press.

CHAPTER **29**

Vascular Diseases of the Kidney

Hitesh H. Shah • Brian Silver

Renal Artery Stenosis

OBJECTIVES

- To review the clinical significance of renal artery stenosis
- To review the approach and current management of renal artery stenosis

CASE VIGNETTE

A 72-year-old man with diabetes mellitus and arterial hypertension was evaluated because of an elevated serum creatinine level. His medical history was also noteworthy for coronary artery disease, peripheral arterial disease, hyperlipidemia, right carotid endarterectomy for symptomatic right carotid artery stenosis, and coronary artery bypass. He recently quit smoking cigarettes; however, he smoked one pack of cigarettes per day for the last 40 years. Current medications included insulin, furosemide, carvedilol, amlodipine, losartan, clopidogrel, and atorvastatin. Physical examination showed a blood pressure (BP) of 140/88 mm Hg, abdominal bruit, weak pedal pulses, and 1+ edema of both legs. Laboratory studies showed elevated blood urea nitrogen (BUN) (30 mg/dL) and serum creatinine (1.6 mg/dL) level. Fasting lipid profile demonstrated elevated levels of both total cholesterol (252 mg/dL) and triglyceride (410 mg/dL). Glycosylated hemoglobin was 8.3 mg/dL. Urinalysis showed trace proteinuria. Renal ultrasound demonstrated small left kidney. Magnetic resonance angiography (MRA) showed left renal artery stenosis.

DEFINITION

Renal artery stenosis (RAS) defined as the presence of an obstructive lesion in the renal artery, may or may not be functionally significant. Two major types of RAS are recognized: The most common atherosclerotic RAS accounts for more than two thirds of all cases and the less common fibromuscular dysplasia (FMD) accounts for less than one third of the remaining cases. Rarely, renal artery narrowing is caused by neurofibromatosis, extrinsic compression, radiation fibrosis, embolism, and Takayasu arteritis (TA).

EPIDEMIOLOGY

Although the prevalence of atherosclerotic RAS in the general population is unknown, one large autopsy study found RAS in 4.3% of all their cases (1). In this study, patients with diabetes had an increase incidence (8.3%) of RAS as compared with those without diabetes. Another autopsy study found RAS among 12% of their patients with myocardial infarction (2). Men are more commonly affected with atherosclerotic RAS than are women.

FMD involving the renal arteries accounts for approximately 60% to 75% of cases (3). Involvement of other arterial system, including the cervicocephalic vessels, brachial, mesenteric, and rarely the coronary arteries, has also been described. FMD is most commonly diagnosed in women <50 years of age, except for cervicocephalic FMD (4).

The true prevalence of renal artery disease as a result of TA is unknown, although it remains an important cause of renal artery stenosis and renovascular hypertension in young women.

ETIOLOGY AND PATHOGENESIS

Cigarette smoking and hyperlipidemia are commonly associated with atherosclerotic RAS. Hence, it is commonly seen in patients with vascular diseases involving other systems, namely coronary artery disease, peripheral vascular disease, and aortic disease (5).

The etiology of FMD remains elusive. A variety of factors are implicated, however, including genetic predisposition (6), hormonal influence; mechanical factors, such as stretching of smooth muscle cells; and ischemia of blood vessel walls as a result of fibrotic occlusion of the vasa vasorum.

Arterial hypertension and ischemic nephropathy leading to progressive kidney failure develop when RAS compromises the blood flow to the functioning renal parenchyma. This usually develops when the obstruction >70%. This degree of stenosis would usually cause a reduction of renal perfusion pressure below the range of effective autoregulation, leading to decrease in renal blood flow and glomerular filtration rate (GFR) (7). This, in turn, would activate the renin-angiotensin system and lead to arterial hypertension and further scarring of the kidney.

Chronic kidney ischemia ultimately leads to glomerulosclerosis, tubular atrophy, and interstitial fibrosis. Several factors, including endothelial cell dysfunction, release of various cytokines, and inflammatory mediators such as angiotensin 2, endothelin-1, and transforming growth factor alpha, have been implicated (8). This, in turn, would lead to progressive chronic kidney disease and end-stage renal disease (ESRD) in some patients. Interestingly, FMD rarely leads to ischemic nephropathy despite similar degrees of arterial stenosis.

Large vessel vasculitis, such as TA, can narrow the abdominal aorta or renal arteries, resulting in renal ischemia and renovascular hypertension.

PATHOLOGY

Atherosclerotic renal artery disease, which is most commonly seen proximally, is often ostial and involves the aorta. Atherosclerotic RAS results in renal scarring and kidney atrophy leading to the decrease in size of the kidneys. Renal atrophy is associated with irreversible patchy areas of cortical scarring, sclerotic glomeruli, and interstitial fibrosis.

FMD most often affects the mid and distal segments of the renal arteries or branches, and is bilateral in 60% of cases. Fibrous lesions are classified based on the arterial layer involved (intima, media, or adventitia) and the composition of the lesion (9). Medial fibroplasia represents the most common type of FMD, accounting for 75% to 80% of FMD lesions. Radiologically, medial fibroplasia is characterized by the classic "string of beads" appearance. Internal elastic lamina is lacking in areas of aneurysmal dilatation. Vessel occlusion, thrombosis, and dissection are uncommon. Other categories of fibrous lesions are less common.

Takayasu arteritis is characterized by focal granulomatous inflammation of the aorta and its major branches. The ongoing inflammatory injury evolves into fibrosis and frequently leads to vascular narrowing. This chronic injury leads to renovascular hypertension when a renal artery is involved.

CLINICAL MANIFESTATIONS

RAS occurs in approximately 0.5% to 5% of all patients with arterial hypertension. The clinical picture suggesting RAS includes age (<30 years and >55 years), recent worsening of blood pressure control that had previously been controlled in a hypertensive patient, and accelerated, malignant, or refractory hypertension. Recurrent flash pulmonary edema, worsening renal failure after initiation of medications blocking the renin-angiotensin system, or the presence of an abdominal bruit suggest RAS, particularly among patients with compromise of other vascular beds. Rarely, hypertensive encephalopathy has been described as a presenting manifestation of renal artery stenosis.

DIAGNOSTIC APPROACH

Laboratory tests may reveal a normal urinalysis. Despite renal failure, there may be absence of proteinuria. Mild to moderate proteinuria may be seen secondary to hypertensive nephrosclerosis. Rarely, a nephrotic range proteinuria has been described with RAS. Hypokalemia with metabolic alkalosis occasionally is seen as a result of elevated renin-angiotensin-aldosterone system. The presence of an asymmetric kidney size, atrophic kidney, or bilateral small kidneys in the right clinical setting should increase the suggestion of RAS.

Several radiologic tests are available to screen for RAS. These include duplex ultrasound, computed tomography angiography (CTA), and MRA. Although ultrasound with Doppler flow studies of the renal arteries is an excellent noninvasive test for diagnosing RAS, it is highly operator dependent. MRA has rapidly become a highly sensitive and specific test for both screening and diagnosing RAS. MRA is contraindicated, however, in patients with metallic implants, including pacemakers, ferromagnetic intracranial aneurysm clips, cochlear implants, and recently placed stent. MRA also overestimates the degree of stenosis as often as 21% of the time, more commonly in distal lesions. Conversely, MRA may also underestimate RAS in approximately 14% as compared with conventional angiography (10). CTA is also a highly sensitive and specific test. CTA, however, carries the risk of contrast nephropathy in patients with abnormal renal function. Both MRA and CTA were found to have better diagnostic accuracy than ultrasound in a recent meta-analysis that evaluated studies to identify patients with RAS (11).

Functional testing with angiotensin-converting enzyme inhibitor (ACEI) renography may be warranted in patients in whom MRA or CTA cannot be performed. This test, however, may not be completely accurate among patients with moderate to severe renal failure (12), and among those on chronic ACEI. This test has a high rate of false-negative findings.

Finally, conventional renal angiography remains the gold standard for diagnosis RAS. It is expensive, invasive, and can worsen renal function as a result of radiocontrast nephropathy. Renal angiography can also increase the risk of cholesterol atheroembolic renal disease, especially among patients with atherosclerotic RAS. Intraarterial digital subtraction angiography offers high diagnostic advantage over conventional angiography with smaller amounts of contrast. Carbon dioxide angiography may avoid contrast use; however, it is not available in all centers.

TREATMENT

The primary goals of therapy in atherosclerotic RAS include better blood pressure control and improvement or preservation of renal function. These goals can be achieved with aggressive medical management with or without renal revascularization.

Although percutaneous transluminal renal angioplasty (PTRA) has replaced surgery as the revascularization procedure of choice in patients with FMD, it is not clear whether primary angioplasty improves both renal and patient outcomes in patients with atherosclerotic RAS. Several small, randomized, controlled trials have failed to demonstrate a significant long-term benefit of PTRA with or without stent placement (13–15). Hence, PTRA should be considered in patients with atherosclerotic RAS who have somewhat rapid progressive renal failure or resistant arterial hypertension despite aggressive medical management. Surgical revascularization is rarely considered when PTRA cannot be performed.

Aggressive medical therapy to control blood pressure and other traditional atherosclerosis risk factors is recommended. Most patients will require multiple medications to lower the blood pressure. Smoking cessation may also be beneficial by preventing progression of RAS. Antiplatelet therapy is also likely to be beneficial in patients with RAS. The use of ACEI should be considered because they have been shown to improve survival in patients with atherosclerotic RAS (16).

CLINICAL RECOMMENDATIONS OF THE VIGNETTE

The patient had a clinical picture highly suggestive of underlying RAS; MRA confirmed atherosclerotic RAS.

Aggressive medical management and revascularization of the left renal artery were reviewed with the patient. Because his renal function remained stable and blood pressure was subsequently better controlled with adjustment in his antihypertensive medications, the decision was regular follow-up of the patient with medical therapy. He was also advised to continue with smoking cessation. The dose of lipid-lowering medication was increased, and the patient was referred back to his endocrinologist for tighter glucose control.

Results from the on-going National Institutes of Health (NIH)-funded multicenter, prospective randomized trial comparing PTRA and stenting with medical therapy versus medical therapy alone in patients with atherosclerotic RAS should provide better information in the management of RAS (17).

SUMMARY

Atherosclerotic RAS is likely to be a common cause of chronic kidney disease and secondary arterial hypertension in the increasingly surviving elderly population worldwide. Atherosclerotic RAS must be considered as a potential cause of kidney disease in patients who have vascular disease in other beds.

RAS is an anatomic abnormality that often tends to progress. The mere presence of RAS may not be functionally significant, however.

Treatment of RAS is individualized, based on clinical and laboratory testing. PTRA remains the treatment of choice for most patients with FMD and it is usually successful. In patients with atherosclerotic RAS, however, no definite evidence indicates that PTRA improves long-term clinical outcomes as compared with medical therapy. Hence, revascularization seems reasonable in patients with resistant hypertension, rapidly worsening renal function, or recurrent episodes of pulmonary edema. Aggressive medical therapy should be considered in all patients with atherosclerotic RAS.

Antineutrophil Cytoplasmic Antibodies-Positive Small-Vessel Vasculitis

OBJECTIVES

- To describe both the clinical findings in patients with systemic vasculitis and the concurrent renal and neurologic findings in patients with antineutrophil cytoplasmic antibodies (ANCA)-positive small-vessel vasculitis
- To review treatment options for patients with ANCA-positive small-vessel vasculitis

CASE VIGNETTE

A 65-year-old woman with arterial hypertension presented with diplopia, drooling while eating, and a right wrist drop, which developed stepwise over 2 weeks. Her recent history includes fever, bloody nasal discharge, and cough, which did not respond to oral antibiotics. Physical examination showed right sixth and seventh nerve palsy, and right radial neuropathy. Nasal ulcers were also seen. Urine examination showed moderate proteinuria, microscopic hematuria, and red blood cell casts. Laboratory testing showed significant elevation of erythrocyte sedimentation rate, serum creatinine, and cytoplasmic ANCA (C-ANCA) titer. Chest x-ray study showed multiple lung nodules. A renal biopsy done subsequently showed a necrotizing crescentic glomerulonephritis. A diagnosis of Wegener granulomatosis (WG) was made.

DEFINITION

The primary systemic vasculitides is composed of a group of idiopathic inflammatory diseases distinguished by clinical, serologic, and pathologic findings (18). In general, vasculitides are divided into three broad categories according to the size of vessel involvement (small, medium, and large). Some disease entities involve vessels of different sizes, but the primary vessel size affected is the designation for a particular process. Further distinction, particularly in the small vessel vasculitides, is based on the presence of C-ANCA. A further distinction is whether the disease is primary (i.e., idiopathic) or secondary (i.e., caused by medications, systemic lupus erythematosus [SLE], and infections).

Neurologic and renal involvements are most often seen with small-vessel vasculitides. The most common small-vessel vasculitides associated with ANCA include WG, Churg-Strauss syndrome (CSS), microscopic polyangiitis (MPA), and renal-limited vasculitis (RLV). ANCA-negative, small-vessel vasculitides include Henoch-Schonlein purpura and essential cryoglobulinemia. Polyarteritis nodosa and Kawasaki disease affect medium-sized vessels whereas giant cell arteritis (GCA), TA, and primary central nervous system (CNS) vasculitis affect large-sized vessels.

EPIDEMIOLOGY

The annual incidence of primary systemic vasculitis in Europe is approximately 10 to 20/million/year (19). A considerably greater incidence is seen among individuals aged 65 to 74 years (annual incidence 60.1/million/year) and a slightly greater incidence is seen in men (annual incidence 23.5/million/year) (20). WG may be more common at higher latitudes, whereas MPA is more common at lower latitudes (19). A Japanese study found an annual incidence of ANCA-positive renal vasculitis of approximately 14.8/million/year, which increased to 44.8/million/year for individuals over the age of 65 years (21). WG and CSS were much less commonly found in this study than in those conducted in Europe. The annual incidence of Kawasaki disease is greatest in Japan (108 to 111/100,000 children/year). Reported rates of Kawasaki disease in China, the United Kingdom, and United States range from 2.4 to 27.8/100,000 children/year (19). The incidence of Kawasaki disease appears to be increasing (19).

ETIOLOGY AND PATHOGENESIS

Although the etiology of primary systemic vasculitis remains unknown, it is believed to be multifactorial. Suspected triggers include environmental exposures (infection, silica) and genetic factors (22). Certain drugs, such as propylthiouracil, hydralazine, and penicillamine, can induce ANCA concurrent with small vessel vasculitis. Infectious causes include putative pathogens, such as hepatitis (B and C), human immunodeficiency virus (HIV), *Mycoplasma pneumoniae*, chlamydia, and parvovirus B19. Other viruses, such as parainfluenza virus, herpes simplex 1 and 2, herpes varicellae, cytomegalovirus, and Epstein-Barr virus have also been implicated. In Denmark and in Olmsted County, Minnesota, peaks of GCA occur approximately every 5 to 7 years (23,24) and are temporally associated with outbreaks in *M. pneumoniae*, chlamydia, and parvovirus B19 (25). In one case report, a varicella infection in a 7-year-old girl was associated with the simultaneous occurrence of ischemic infarctions in the kidneys, brain, and spinal cord affecting medium- to large-sized vessels (26). Treatment with acyclovir and methylprednisolone was associated with rapid recovery. The genetics of the primary vasculitides also remain to be clarified. No association has been found with any of the HLA class II antigens in WG, although HLA-DR13DR6 may be protective (23).

PATHOLOGY

The typical acute vascular lesion of ANCA-associated pauci-immune small vessel vasculitides is segmental fibrinoid necrosis, often accompanied by leukocyte infiltration. These necrotizing lesions subsequently develop into sclerotic lesions. These focal necrotizing lesions can affect different blood vessels, thus causing various signs and symptoms; for example, involvement of glomerular capillaries causing nephritis, and epidural arteries causing mononeurtitis multiplex.

The typical appearance of an ANCA-associated renal vasculitis is a pauci-immune necrotizing, crescentic glomerulonephritis (27). Early mild disease may have segmental fibrinoid necrosis, with or without adjacent small crescent formation. Severe acute glomerular lesions may show global necrosis with large circumferential crescent. Patients with WG and CSS also will have necrotizing granulomatous inflammation seen mainly in the respiratory tract.

Most kidney biopsy specimens on immunfluorescence demonstrate little or no glomerular staining for immunoglobulin. Approximately 15% of patients, however, have evidence of immune complex deposition, which is of unclear significance.

CLINICAL MANIFESTATIONS/SPECIAL SITUATIONS

Patients with large vessel and medium-sized vasculitis are rarely seen in a nephrology practice. Small vessel vasculitis (particularly those that are ANCA-positive) most typically have kidney involvement. Patients usually present with rapidly progressive glomerulonephritis and renal failure. Hematuria with varying degree of proteinuria is also seen.

Most patients with small vessel vasculitis, however, present with generalized nonspecific complaints, such as fever, malaise, anorexia, weight loss, myalgias, and arthralgias.

Upper and lower respiratory tract involvement, although, more commonly seen with WG and CSS, can occur in patients with MPA. Sinusitis, rhinitis, otitis media, and ocular inflammation are some manifestations seen predominately in WG, but they may also occur in CSS and MPA. Cutaneous manifestations, such as purpura, are commonly seen in ANCA-positive small-vessel vasculitis. Cutaneous nodular lesions are more commonly seen in WG and CSS, however.

Nervous system involvement is seen in approximately one third of patients with WG (28). Approximately half of these patients have a peripheral neuropathy. Eighty percent have mononeuritis multiplex, whereas approximately 10% have a distal symmetric polyneuropathy. Mononeuritis multiplex is a major presenting feature in approximately 2% of patients. Cranial neuropathies (II, VI, VII) may be present. The presence of a peripheral neuropathy is more likely to be associated with renal involvement. Ischemic stroke (4%), cerebritis (2%), and seizures (3%) are relatively infrequent findings compared with peripheral nervous system involvement.

The triad of small vessel vasculitis, asthma, and peripheral blood eosinophilia characterizes CSS. Peripheral neuropathy, typically a mononeuritis multiplex, may also be seen (29).

When considering large vessel arteridites, important clinical clues, which help distinguish TA from GCA, include patient age (<50 years in TA vs. >50 years in GCA) and presence of kidney disease (more typical, although unusual, for TA). Renovascular hypertension, which results from renal ischemia that is caused by RAS or aortic coarctation, can be seen in patients with TA. Other clinical clues helpful in suggesting a diagnosis are the presence of diminished pulses in TA, and temporal artery tenderness or jaw claudication in cases of GCA.

Kawasaki disease, which typically affects children, has a predilection for involvement of mucocutaneous areas, lymph nodes, and coronary arteries. Clinically significant kidney disease is uncommon.

DIAGNOSTIC APPROACH

When a patient presents with neurologic symptoms consistent with a mononeuritis multiplex and renal dysfunction, a vasculitic process should be strongly considered. Detailed skin inspection may help uncover previously undetected purpura and petechiae. Laboratory testing should include a complete blood count with differential (with attention to the presence of eosinophilia); electrolytes, including BUN, creatinine, calcium, phosphorous, and magnesium; total protein, albumin; liver function tests; and erythrocyte sedimentation rate. Urinalysis is useful to evaluate for proteinuria and hematuria. Serologic testing should include antinuclear antibody (ANA), rheumatoid factor, cryoglobulin, complements (C3 and C4), and ANCA.

Laboratory testing for ANCA should include both indirect immunofluorescence assay (screening test) and enzyme immunoassay (confirmatory test). Two major patterns of staining are seen on indirect immunofluorescence assay, which include C-ANCA, and perinuclear (P-ANCA). By enzyme immunoassay, most C-ANCA has specificity for proteinase 3 (PR3-ANCA), whereas most P-ANCA has specificity for myeloperioxidase (MPO-ANCA). PR3-ANCA is more commonly seen in WG, whereas MPO-ANCA is most prevalent in RLV and CSS. Patients with MPA can have either pattern of ANCA.

Testing of thyroid function, folate, vitamin B_{12}, methylmalonic acid, homocysteine, and monoclonal protein evaluation may be useful to exclude other causes of neuropathy.

Electromyography (EMG) and nerve conduction velocities (NCV) help establish the presence and nature of a neuropathy. Neuroimaging (CT or MRI; preferably the latter) may be indicated with evidence of CNS dysfunction. A chest x-ray study, CT scan, or both of the chest are indicated when respiratory symptoms are present. CT scanning of the sinuses may be useful to evaluate for opacification of the sinuses, which can occur on WG and CSS.

A kidney biopsy (typically percutaneous with ultrasound guidance) or nerve biopsy (typically of the sural nerve) may be ultimately helpful in establishing the pathologic diagnosis.

TREATMENT

Untreated, patients with ANCA-associated small-vessel vasculitides have a 1-year mortality rate of approximately 80%. With the introduction of corticosteroids, azathioprine, and cyclophosphamide, survival rates are approximately 75% at 5 years based on retrospective studies in the late 1990s (30). Older patients remain at particularly high risk for death. Combination therapy with cyclophosphamide and prednisolone is the common practice for active vasculitis, although dosing, route of administration, duration, and adjuvant role of plasma exchange have not been subjected to adequately powered, rigorous clinical trials (31).

Three major randomized trials in WG have been reported between 2003 and 2005. The Cyclophosphamide versus Azathioprine as Remission Maintenance Therapy for ANCA-Associated Vasculitis Study found that the withdrawal of cyclophosphamide and the substitution of azathioprine after remission did not increase the rate of relapse, thus shortening the duration of exposure to cyclophosphamide (32). Further, the European Vasculitis Study Group found that methotrexate can replace cyclophosphamide for initial treatment of early ANCA-associated systemic vaculitis (33). The methotrexate regimen used in this study was less effective than cyclophosphamide to produce remission in cases of extensive disease and pulmonary involvement and it was associated with more relapses after termination of treatment. High relapse rates were noted in both groups, which supports the practice of continuation of immunosuppressive treatment beyond 12 months.

Current consensus is that cyclophosphamide remains the drug of choice for patients with generalized vasculitis to induce a remission period of 3 to 6 months (34). A meta-analysis of smaller clinical trials found that intravenous pulsed cyclophosphamide was as effective as daily oral cyclophosphamide to induce remission, but it was associated with fewer severe infections. Relapse rates were higher, however, in the intravenous pulsed group (35). Whether pulsed cyclophosphamide is superior to daily oral treatment is being studied in a large randomized trial. For induction of remission in patients without renal insufficiency, vital organ failure, or pronounced respiratory granulomatous changes, methotrexate can be used in place of cyclophosphamide.

The Wegener's Granulomatosis Etanercept Trial found that etanercept, a soluble tumor necrosis factor-alpha inhibitor, is not effective to maintain remission in patients with WG and its use had a high rate of treatment-related complications (36). Other candidate drugs considered include antithymocyte globulin, rituximab, mycophenolate mofetil, and deoxyspergualin.

CLINICAL RECOMMENDATIONS OF THE VIGNETTE

The patient had clinical and laboratory findings highly suggestive of systemic vasculitis, namely WG.

The patient initially received pulse intravenous corticosteroid therapy for 3 days, followed by oral corticosteroid and cyclophosphamide. Complete clinical remission was achieved by 4 months, after which oral azathioprine was substituted for cyclophosphamide to reduce long-term exposure to cyclophosphamide and to decrease the likelihood of relapse. Azathioprine was continued for 1 year after complete remission. Oral corticosteroid therapy was gradually tapered over a period of 6 months.

SUMMARY

The primary systemic vasculitides, particularly those that preferentially affect small vessels and are associated with ANCA (i.e., WG, CSS, MPA, and RLV), are frequently associated with concurrent renal and neurologic involvement. Although these diseases are rare, they are important to recognize because of the high mortality rate that occurs without treatment. Kidney or sural nerve biopsy may be helpful. In the last decade, significant advances have been made in treatment with the introduction of steroids and immunosuppressive agents. Large randomized trials have been completed and others are ongoing, which will further refine therapy.

REFERENCES

1. Sawicki PT, Kaiser S, Heinemann L, et al. Prevalence of renal artery stenosis in diabetes mellitus-An autopsy study. *J Intern Med.* 1991;229(6):489–492.
2. Uzu T, Inoue T, Fuji T, et al. Prevalence and predictors of renal artery stenosis in patients with myocardial infarction. *Am J Kidney Dis.* 1997;29(5):733–738.
3. Luscher TF, Keller HM, Imhof HG, et al. Fibromuscular hyperplasia: Extension of the disease and therapeutic outcome. Results of the University Hospital Zurich Cooperative Study on Fibromuscular Hyperplasia. *Nephron.* 1986;44[Suppl 1]:109–114.
4. Chiche L, Bahnini A, Koskas F, et al. Occlusive fibromuscular disease of arteries supplying the brain: Results of surgical treatment. *Ann Vasc Surg.* 1997;11(5):496–504.
5. Olin JW, Melia M, Young JR, et al. Prevalence of atherosclerotic renal artery stenosis in patients with atherosclerosis elsewhere. *Am J Med.* 1990;88(1N):46N–51N.
6. Schievink WI, Bjornsson J. Fibromuscular dysplasia of the internal carotid artery: A clinicopathological study. *Clin Neuropathol.* 1996;15(1):2–6.
7. Lewis J, Barbara G. *Atheromatous Renovascular Disease.* Mosby; 2003.
8. Lerman L, Textor SC. Pathophysiology of ischemic nephropathy. *Urol Clin North Am.* 2001;28(4):793–803.
9. Begelman SM, Olin JW. Fibromuscular dysplasia. *Curr Opin Rheumatol.* 2000;2(1):41–47.
10. Gilfeather M, Yoon HC, Siegelman ES, et al. Renal artery stenosis: Evaluation with conventional angiography versus gadolinium-enhanced MR angiography. *Radiology.* 1999;210(2):367–372.
11. Vasbinder GB, Nelemans PJ, Kessels AG, et al. Diagnostic tests for renal artery stenosis in patients suspected of having renovascular hypertension: A meta-analysis. *Ann Intern Med.* 2001;135(6):401–411.
12. Taylor A. Functional testing: ACEI renography. *Semin Nephrol.* 2000;20(5):437–444.
13. Webster J, Marshall F, Abdalla M, et al. Randomised comparison of percutaneous angioplasty vs continued medical therapy for hypertensive patients with atheromatous renal artery stenosis. Scottish and Newcastle Renal Artery Stenosis Collaborative Group. *J Hum Hypertens.* 1998;12(5):329–335.
14. Plouin PF, Chatellier G, Darne B, et al. Blood pressure outcome of angioplasty in atherosclerotic renal artery stenosis: A randomized trial. Essai Multicentrique Medicaments vs Angioplastie (EMMA) Study Group. *Hypertension.* 1998;31(3):823–829.
15. van Jaarsveld BC, Krijnen P, Pieterman H, et al. The effect of balloon angioplasty on hypertension in atherosclerotic renal-artery stenosis. Dutch Renal Artery Stenosis Intervention Cooperative Study Group. *N Engl J Med.* 2000;342(14):1007–1014.
16. Losito A, Gaburri M, Errico R, et al. Survival of patients with renovascular disease and ACE inhibition. *Clin Nephrol.* 1999;52(6):339–343.
17. Cooper CJ, Murphy TP, Matsumoto A, et al. Stent revascularization for the prevention of cardiovascular and renal events among patients with renal artery stenosis and systolic hypertension: Rationale and design of the CORAL trial. *Am Heart J.* 2006;152(1):59–66.
18. Jennette JC, Falk RJ, Andrassy K, et al. Nomenclature of systemic vasculitides. Proposal of an international consensus conference. *Arthritis Rheum.* 1994;37(2):187–192.
19. Watts RA, Scott DG. Epidemiology of the vasculitides. *Curr Opin Rheumatol.* 2003;15(1):11–16.
20. Watts RA, Lane SE, Bentham G, et al. Epidemiology of systemic vasculitis: A ten-year study in the United Kingdom. *Arthritis Rheum.* 2000;43(2):414–419.
21. Fujimoto S, Uezono S, Hisanaga S, et al. Incidence of ANCA-associated primary renal vasculitis in the Miyazaki prefecture: The first population-based, retrospective, epidemiologic survey in Japan. *Clinical Journal of the American Society of Nephrology.* 2006;1(5):1016–1022.

22. Hogan SL, Satterly KK, Dooley MA, et al. Silica exposure in anti-neutrophil cytoplasmic autoantibody-associated glomerulonephritis and lupus nephritis. *J Am Soc Nephrol.* 2001;12(1):134–142.
23. Hagen EC, Stegeman CA, D'Amaro J, et al. Decreased frequency of HLA-DR13DR6 in Wegener's granulomatosis. *Kidney Int.* 1995;48(3):801–805.
24. Salvarani C, Gabriel SE, O'Fallon WM, et al. The incidence of giant cell arteritis in Olmsted County, Minnesota: Apparent fluctuations in a cyclic pattern. *Ann Intern Med.* 1995;123(3):192–194.
25. Elling P, Olsson AT, Elling H. Synchronous variations of the incidence of temporal arteritis and polymyalgia rheumatica in different regions of Denmark: Association with epidemics of Mycoplasma pneumoniae infection. *J Rheumatol.* 1996;23(1):112–119.
26. Caruso JM, Tung GA, Brown WD. Central nervous system and renal vasculitis associated with primary varicella infection in a child. Pediatrics. 2001;107(1):E9.
27. Jennette JC, Wilkman AS, Falk RJ. Anti-neutrophil cytoplasmic autoantibody-associated glomerulonephritis and vasculitis. *Am J Pathol.* 1989;135(5):921–930.
28. Nishino H, Rubino FA, DeRemee RA, et al. Neurological involvement in Wegener's granulomatosis: An analysis of 324 consecutive patients at the Mayo Clinic. *Ann Neurol.* 1993;33(1):4–9.
29. Noth I, Strek ME, Leff AR. Churg-Strauss syndrome. *Lancet.* 2003;361(9357):587–594.
30. Booth AD, Almond MK, Burns A, et al. Outcome of ANCA-associated renal vasculitis: A 5-year retrospective study. *Am J Kidney Dis.* 2003;41(4):776–784.
31. Booth AD, Pusey CD, Jayne DR. Renal vasculitis—An update in 2004. *Nephrol Dial Transplant.* 2004;19(8):1964–1968.
32. Jayne D, Rasmussen N, Andrassy K, et al. A randomized trial of maintenance therapy for vasculitis associated with antineutrophil cytoplasmic autoantibodies. *N Engl J Med.* 2003;349(1):36–44.
33. De Groot K, Rasmussen N, Bacon PA, et al. Randomized trial of cyclophosphamide versus methotrexate for induction of remission in early systemic antineutrophil cytoplasmic antibody-associated vasculitis. *Arthritis Rheum.* 2005;52(8):2461–2469.
34. de Groot K, Jayne D. What is new in the therapy of ANCA-associated vasculitides? Take home messages from the 12th workshop on ANCA and systemic vasculitides. *Clin Nephrol.* 2005;64(6):480–484.
35. de Groot K, Adu D, Savage CO. The value of pulse cyclophosphamide in ANCA-associated vasculitis: Meta-analysis and critical review. *Nephrol Dial Transplant.* 2001;16(10):2018–2027.
36. Etanercept plus standard therapy for Wegener's granulomatosis. Wegener's Granulomatosis Etanercept Trial (WGET) Research Group. *N Engl J Med.* 2005;352(4):351–361.

CHAPTER 30

Dialysis

John D. Wagner • Isabelle Korn-Lubetzki

OBJECTIVES

- To describe the types of renal replacement therapy
- To review the neurologic complications that appear to be linked to the patient status as a recipient of dialysis therapy
- To highlight that some of the neurologic complications in a patient on dialysis are not easy to diagnose and a high index of suspicion is important
- To provide an overview of diagnosis and treatment of some of these entities

CASE VIGNETTE

A 65-year-old hypertensive man with advanced chronic renal failure presented with progressive confusion and forgetfulness, generalized weakness, a serum creatinine of 12 mg/dL, and a hemoglobin of 8 g/dL. After initially resisting the idea, he agreed to initiate maintenance hemodialysis therapy through a previously placed left forearm fistula. Rather than improving his situation, his first treatment resulted in the onset of nausea and headache, which subsided over a 24-hour period. Over the course of several weeks of three times weekly dialysis and the administration of erythropoietic agents, the patient felt he regained his strength and his ability to concentrate, although he was not able to function as he had 5 years earlier. Five years later, he once again experienced periods of forgetfulness and confusion over the course of several weeks associated with headaches. He developed difficulty walking, tending to fall to his right. Physical examination revealed mild right-sided weakness, distal as well as proximal.

DEFINITION

End-stage renal disease (ESRD) refers to a phase of chronic renal failure expected to be irreversible, mandating renal replacement therapy to maintain life. Dialytic therapy can be offered to patients with either acute or chronic renal disease associated with a severe reduction in glomerular filtration rate (<15 mL/min typically) (1). Its purpose is to prevent complications from accumulation of uremic toxins and to treat medically unmanageable electrolyte acid-base disturbances or volume excess states. In addition, dialytic therapy is an incomplete substitute for renal function and long-term therapy is associated with neurologic syndromes, which can reflect (*a*) the accumulation and long-term exposure to substances normally eliminated via the renal route, and (*b*) the stress on the neurologic system imposed by the chronic inflammatory state that characterizes the patient on maintenance dialysis.

DIALYSIS TECHNIQUES: HEMODIALYSIS AND PERITONEAL DIALYSIS

HEMODIALYSIS

The most common form of dialysis is hemodialysis, which involves the withdrawal of blood from a patient using a suitable vascular conduit (surgically created arteriovenous fistula or graft, or catheter inserted in a large vein) and which then is infused into a dialyzer that confines the blood to a membrane-bound space that is surrounded by dialysate flowing in a direction that is counter to blood flow. The arteriovenous conduit (fistula or graft) is usually situated in the forearm or upper arm (2,3). The dialysis membrane is porous to small molecular weight solutes and water. Hence, substances will diffuse along their chemical gradient and an ultrafiltrate of plasma water will result from convective forces. A hemodialysis session is commonly offered for a 3- to 4-hour period three times weekly. Uremic toxins, which can pass through the dialyzer membrane, diffuse into the dialysis fluid (dialysate) and are thereby eliminated. Similarly permeable substances, such as urea nitrogen, considered a surrogate marker of these toxins, or potassium, will escape into the dialysate at a rate dependent on membrane characteristics, concentration gradients, and blood and dialysate flows. Removal of excess amounts may be feasible. Less permeable substances, such as a β_2-microglobulin, a major histocompatibility locus (MHC) cell surface molecule, accumulate because hemodialysis is an inefficient means of removal (4).

Patients will gain variable amounts of fluid during the intradialytic interval, depending on residual urine output (often negligible after 6 months of hemodialysis), dietary salt and water intake, and insensible losses. Patients can remain asymptomatic despite the gain of several liters of volume, although vascular congestion can provoke dyspnea and hypertension responsive to the dialytic treatment. The dialysis machine is programmed to eliminate a certain volume of fluid during the course of the treatment, achieved by altering the transmembrane pressure gradient in the dialyzer such that an ultrafiltrate of plasma passes through the membrane and escapes into the dialysate. The dialysis prescriber exercises judgment to how much fluid to remove during a treatment, a value that can be modified during the treatment, depending on the patient's tolerance. Hypotension, with or without symptoms or muscle cramps, can limit achievable fluid removal (5).

Because blood travels through an extracorporeal circuit composed of nonbiological materials, patients usually receive anticoagulants during hemodialysis treatments to prevent clotting within the blood pathways. Heparin is commonly used for this purpose, although it is feasible to offer dialysis treatments without anticoagulation or, less frequently, using other anticoagulants.

PERITONEAL DIALYSIS

The principles of removal of toxins, solute, and accumulated fluid via a dialysate are similar (3). The membrane used for transfer, however, is the peritoneum, accessed by a chronically indwelling peritoneal cavity catheter. The blood flow on one side of this membrane is the result of the patient's own perfusion rather than a blood pump, and the dialysate flow results from the manual or automated infusion of small volumes of dialysate (~2 to 3 L in adults) left to dwell over several hours during which time a slow equilibration occurs. Fluid removal is driven by an osmotic gradient, the result of a high concentration of dextrose or other osmotically active substance in the dialysate. The process is less efficient compared with hemodialysis and patients generally have fluid within the peritoneal cavity for the purpose of dialysis for 12 or more hours of the day, and this fluid is periodically exchanged for fresh solution.

EPIDEMIOLOGY

At the end of 2003, approximately 325,000 patients in the United States and 1,129,000 patients worldwide received dialysis (6). The most common form of dialysis is hemodialysis (~92% of patients in the United States). A few patients in the United States have peritoneal dialysis rather than hemodialysis as renal replacement therapy. Commonly, acute renal failure necessitating renal replacement therapy is managed by hemodialysis, although peritoneal dialysis is an option. For critically ill patients, continuous renal replacement therapies, variations on venovenous hemofiltration, can be offered as a way of achieving more precise control of fluid balance, particularly in hemodynamically unstable patients (7).

NEUROLOGIC COMPLICATIONS

Dialysis Disequilibrium

The effects of uremic toxins on the central nervous system (CNS) have already been reviewed. Dialysis removes these toxins, and symptoms and signs of uremic encephalopathy improve. The reduction of high levels of accumulated solute, paradoxically, can worsen symptoms, however, provoking headache, nausea, weakness, cramps, twitching, delirium, visual disturbances, seizures, and coma. These symptoms more likely occur as the result of rapid reduction in the level of azotemia via dialysis in patients with advanced, symptomatic renal failure. For uncertain reasons, cerebral edema develops. Barring evolution into life-threatening manifestations, symptoms tend to resolve over several days (8).

One explanation of this phenomenon is the *reverse urea hypothesis* in which the efficient removal of extracellular versus intracellular urea creates an osmotic gradient favoring water movement inside of brain cells. The *idiogenic osmole hypothesis* claims that intracellular substances created at the time of dialysis generate the brain swelling osmotic gradient (9). To minimize the risk of the disequilibrium syndrome, patients with advanced azotemia typically receive shorter, relatively inefficient dialysis treatments when commencing dialysis therapy over the course of several treatments before being offered the dialysis prescription deemed to suffice as *maintenance*. Hence, life-threatening disequilibrium is a rare event. Nonetheless, some patients will experience headache, fatigue, and cramps in association with dialysis, raising the possibility that some form of disequilibrium may be present. Patients who skip dialysis treatments may also be placing themselves at risk for the syndrome, because the level of uremic toxins is necessarily higher in patients who are under dialyzed. A single case report speculated that reversible posterior leukoencephalopathy syndrome shared features in common with the dialysis disequilibrium syndrome. Severe arterial hypertension and a history of taking certain medications accompany the radiographic findings in this latter entity, but in this report, the symptoms seemed to have been related temporally to dialysis treatments (10).

Headache

Headache is commonly reported. In one study, exclusion of other headache disorders left 30% of patients fulfilling criteria for dialysis headache (headache during at least half of dialysis sessions, resolving within 72 hours of dialysis). The mean duration of headache was slightly more than 5 hours. Statistical analysis suggested subtle differences in serum sodium and magnesium levels of uncertain clinical significance between those patients who had headache and those who did not (11). The differential diagnosis of headache includes rare instances of intracranial hypertension caused by cerebral edema (causing headache, transient visual obscuration, and diplopia). Acute onset of headache may herald stroke, usually hemorrhagic, or subdural hematoma.

Muscle Symptoms

Limited exercise capacity and easy fatigability are common in the dialysis population. Muscle weakness, particularly proximal muscle weakness, may be evident. Investigators have tried to tease out the potential components of this, inasmuch as deconditioning, and inadequate vascular supply and oxygen delivery, rather than a primary muscle disorder, might explain these findings. Johansen et al. (12) studied incremental isometric contraction of the dorsiflexor muscles of the foot in patients on hemodialysis, reasoning that such muscles are in constant use and less likely to be deconditioned. When comparing patients with controls, they found greater fatigue in patients in association with central activation failure on neurodiagnostic testing of the peroneal nerve, impaired oxidative metabolism, and accumulation of metabolic by-products. Only half of the patients could complete the protocol, whereas all controls did. Recovery of maximal voluntary contraction force was delayed in the patients compared with the controls.

Kemp et al. (13) performed ^{31}P-magnetic resonance spectroscopy (MRS) and near infrared spectroscopy (NIRS) studies on the lateral gastrocnemius during isometric contraction in 23 men on hemodialysis and 18 controls. Exercise duration was 30% lower, cross-sectional areas of the muscle were significantly smaller, but contractile efficiency was normal in patients compared with controls. The finding of slow postexercise phosphocreatinine recovery relative to NIRS recovery in the patients suggested an intrinsic mitochondrial, rather than an oxygen supply, problem (13).

Why patients on dialysis would have such a defect is unclear. Oxidative stress and carnitine metabolism (see below) have received some attention with respect to muscle symptoms in this population. Patients receiving hemodialysis appear to have a different pattern of gene activation compared with normal controls (83 genes reported upregulated and 8 genes downregulated). The affected genes include those involved with early response, inflammation, muscle wasting, and apoptosis (14). In addition, speculation regarding the toxic effects of elevated parathyroid hormone levels in ESRD includes one paper that noted the decrease in symptoms and signs of an undefined myopathy from 89% to 15% of subjects after subtotal parathyroidectomy (15).

Cramps are said to occur in 20% of patients receiving dialysis treatments, and may reflect salt and water shifts (5). L-carnitine plays a variety of roles in intracellular or mitochondrial metabolism, particularly with respect to fatty acids, and a variety of studies have suggested a potential etiologic role of carnitine in ESRD muscle disorders. Patients having hemodialysis are at risk for carnitine deficiency, the basis of which is multifactorial, including dietary changes, effects of hemodialysis, metabolic defects associated with uremia, and the loss of renal effects on balancing free versus acyl-L-carnitine. Selected patients with no other apparent cause for muscle fatigue and weakness may respond to carnitine supplementation (16), but high-quality clinical studies are lacking (17). Other proposed therapies for dialysis-associated cramps include quinine, hypertonic saline, vitamins E and C, and oral creatine monohydrate administered before dialysis (18,19).

Cognitive Impairment and Dementia

Cognitive impairment is discussed in Chapter 26, *Acute Renal Failure*, and its persistence despite dialysis therapy has been noted. This section presents data regarding the epidemiology of cognitive impairment and dementia, and highlights recent findings. Murray et al. (20) conducted neuropsychologic testing in 374 urban hemodialysis patients age ≥55 years and classified cognitive impairment according to a four-strata algorithm, ranging from normal to severe. Of the 338 evaluable patients, mean age was 71.2 years, mean educational attainment was 12.8 years, 47.9% were diabetic, 45.9% were female, and 11.2% were black. Hypertension was present in 91.7%. Study subjects were age matched to a cohort recruited from various clinics and the community. The comparison group had slightly higher educational attainment (14.3 years), and fewer diabetes (22.6% vs. 47.9%), hypertension (22.6% vs. 91.7%), and depression (4.9% vs. 25%). About 73.4% of patients had moderate to severe cognitive impairment, despite that only 2.9% had a history of cognitive impairment. Bivariate analysis indicated ($p \leq 0.1$) that duration of dialysis >24 months, higher levels of urea removal (a measure of dialysis adequacy), hemoglobin values less than the guideline target of 11 g/dL, vascular-related causes of the ESRD, and prior stroke were related to severe impairment. Furthermore, white race and more years of education were less likely to accompany severe impairment. The adjusted logistic regression model linked a history of stroke, urea removal (dialysis dose), and lower educational attainment to severe impairment. When adjusted for age, sex, race or ethnicity, education, depression, diabetes, arterial hypertension, and stroke, the odds ratio for severe cognitive impairment 3.54 compared with the comparison group not having dialysis. The authors speculated that the dialysis process itself contributed to the cognitive impairment beyond the possible role that traditional risk factors and chronic kidney disease might play. The paradoxical link between a greater dialysis dose and impairment was possibly evidence of this, although the reason why was not clear. The authors cited published evidence of altered cerebral blood flow in dialysis as one way that hemodialysis might contribute to chronic brain injury.

A recent report continues to support the hypothesis that at least some of the cognitive dysfunction of the patient with ESRD stems from the inadequacy of standard three times weekly renal replacement therapy. Jassal et al. (21) performed neuropsychologic testing on 12 patients before converting to nocturnal quotidian hemodialysis (a more intensive dialysis regimen) and again after 6 months. Psychomotor efficiency and processing improved by 7%, and attention and working memory improved by 32%. Learning efficiency did not manifest a statistically significant improvement (21).

According to the *US Renal Data System* (USRDS) *2005 Annual Data Report*, risk factors for dementia are age, history

TABLE 30-1. Odds Ratios of Incident Dementias

	Hemodialysis					*Peritoneal dialysis*					*Transplant*			
	OR	LL	UL	p-value		OR	LL	UL	p-value		OR	LL	UL	p-value
45–64	*Reference*				45–64	*Reference*				45–64	*Reference*			
65–74	2.59	2.39	2.81	0.00	65–74	3.73	2.34	5.94	0.00	65+	3.72	2.47	5.61	0.00
75–84	3.93	3.63	4.26	0.00	75+	5.76	3.55	9.35	0.00					
85+	6.20	5.55	6.91	0.00										
Female	*Reference*				Female	*Reference*				Female	*Reference*			
Male	0.92	0.87	0.97	0.00	Male	1.07	0.75	1.52	0.73	Male	1.38	0.89	2.13	0.15
White	*Reference*				White	*Reference*				White	*Reference*			
Black	1.30	1.22	1.38	0.00	Black	1.49	0.98	2.27	0.06	Black	1.62	1.04	2.52	0.03
Other Race	0.86	0.75	0.98	0.03	Other Race	1.06	0.53	2.14	0.86	Other Race	0.78	0.28	2.15	0.63
DM	1.46	1.36	1.58	0.00	DM	1.78	1.14	2.79	0.01	DM	2.29	1.43	3.66	0.00
HTN	1.24	1.14	1.34	0.00	HTN	1.39	0.87	2.21	0.17	HTN	0.82	0.43	1.56	0.54
Other Cause	*Reference*				Other Cause	*Reference*				Other Cause	*Reference*			
Stroke	2.31	2.16	2.47	0.00	Stroke	2.51	1.59	3.97	0.00	Stroke	3.59	2.10	6.13	0.00

(From 2005 Annual Data Report, US Renal Data System [USnRDS].)

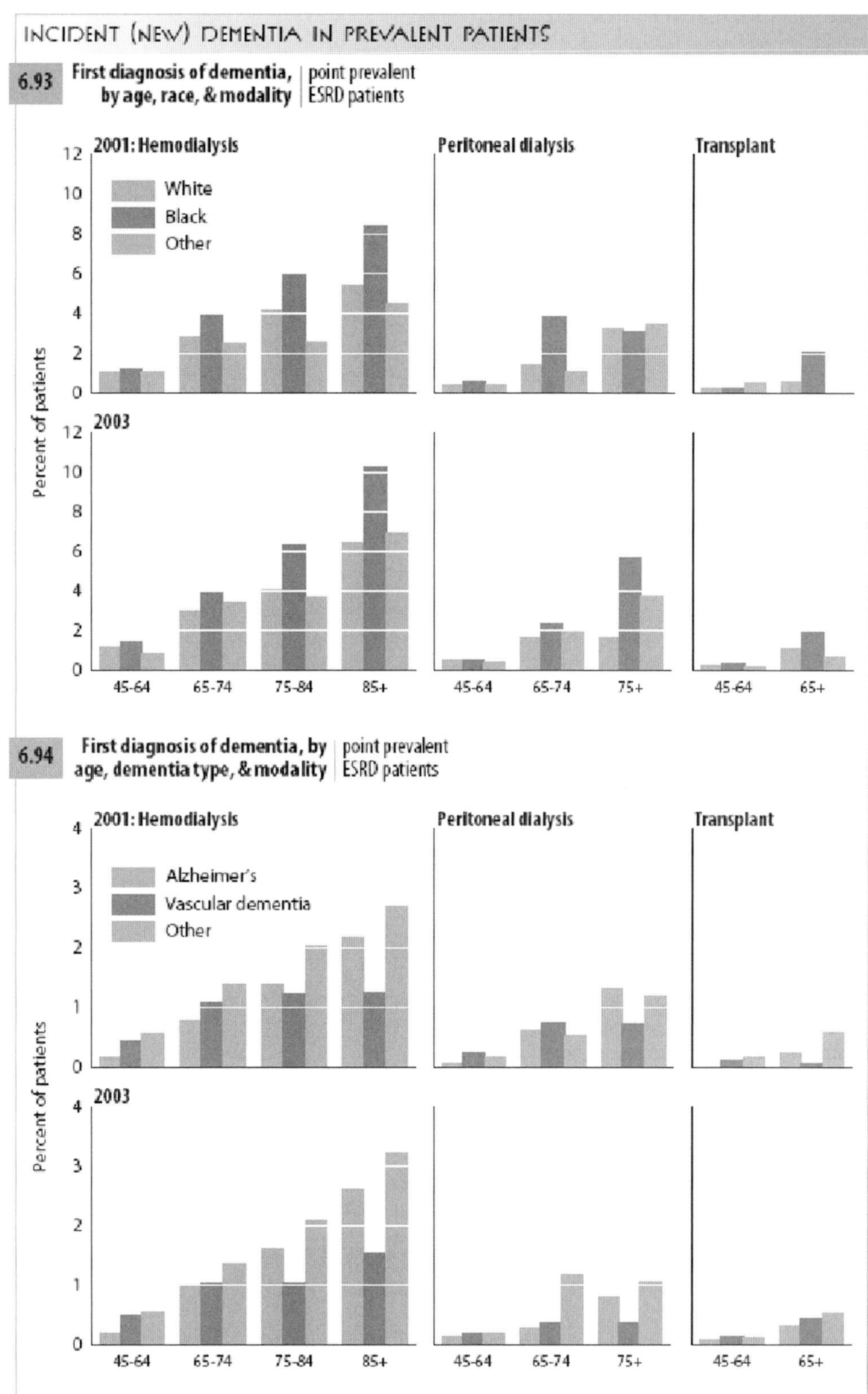

FIGURE 30-1. US Renal Data System, USRDS 2005 Annual Data Report: *Atlas of End-Stage Renal Disease in the United States.* Bethesda: National Institutes of Health, National Institutes of Diabetes and Digestive and Kidney Diseases; 2005. The data reported here have been supplied by the United States Renal Data System (USRDS). The interpretation and reporting of these data are the responsibility of the author(s) and in no way should be seen as an official policy or interpretation by the US government.

of stroke, diabetes, black race, and arterial hypertension (Table 30-1 and Fig. 30-1) (6). Data from the international The Dialysis Outcomes and Practice Patterns Study (DOPPS) (22) added fewer years of educational attainment, cancer, depression, absence of residual renal function, markers of malnutrition, and low hemoglobin values as correlates to dementia diagnoses among patients on dialysis. The odds ratios (OR) for risk factors for patients diagnosed with dementia varied by country as well. In Japan, older age compared with those younger than 60 years of age had an OR of 9.45 versus 2.68 in the United States and Europe. Depression was more strongly associated with an OR of 12.99 in Japan versus 2.36. No significant associations for smoking status, blood pressure values, cholesterol levels, parathyroid hormone levels, dialysis dose, or aluminum concentration were evident. The prevalence of dementia in the ESRD population was 4% overall, a figure comparable to studies in the general population utilizing objective criteria for diagnosis (which was not necessarily the case for the DOPPS data). The authors speculated that under diagnosis, therefore, was likely, suggesting a higher rate of dementia than in the general population. The relative risk of death in patients diagnosed with dementia was 1.48 and these patients exhibited a higher risk for withdrawal from dialysis.

Dialysis dementia has been referred to as a progressive fatal neurologic disorder associated in its early phases with dysarthria and dysphasia, and later with myoclonic jerks. The recognition that aluminum intoxication has given rise to this disorder led to measures that have markedly reduced the exposure of patients on dialysis to this metal and relegated the appearance of dialysis dementia to rare sporadic cases (8).

OTHER METABOLIC CNS DISORDERS

Clinicians have diagnosed Wernicke encephalopathy in patients on dialysis on rare occasions, which is a fatal complication if untreated. The relationship to dialysis status is uncertain: Poor nutritional status and dialytic losses are possible causes. In ESRD, however, the renal route of thiamine losses found in normal subjects is substantially reduced if not eliminated. Hung et al. (23) reported 10 patients in a cohort of 30 who were chronically dialyzed and who developed encephalopathy attributed to thiamine deficiency. Nine recovered, but one patient failed to respond in the setting of delayed treatment (23). The complete Wernicke encephalopathy triad (confusion, ataxia, ophthalmoplegia) is rare, and in particular, ophthalmoplegia may not be present. Given its similarities to uremic encephalopathy, the disorder may not be recognized (8), but a good outcome can be obtained if thiamine is administered early after presentation.

The osmotic demyelination syndrome related to rapid correction of hyponatremia via hemodialysis has been reported rarely. The rarity of this event suggests that the hemodialysis urea disequilibrium described previously might actually prove protective in this situation (24).

Certain commonly used medications have potential neurologic side effects when used in patients with ESRD. Accumulation can occur in the absence of the normal renal route of excretion of drug or metabolites. Examples include penicillin and β-lactam antibiotics, nucleoside analogue antivirals (e.g., acyclovir), aminoglycosides, and opioids. Dose adjustment or avoidance may be necessary.

Subdural Hematoma

Uremic platelet dysfunction and hemodialysis-related episodic anticoagulation might predispose to chronic subdural hematoma, an entity which can manifest with a disturbance in mentation and consciousness, focal signs and ataxia, and headaches. Recent incidence figures and OR for the dialyzed versus not dialyzed populations are lacking (8). Diagnosis can be easily made by noncontrast brain computed tomography (CT).

Stroke

Despite the increase (estimated at four- to tenfold) in stroke risk that characterizes the patient with ESRD (25), data are sparse compared with the information gathered on cardiovascular disease. According to USRDS data, most incident strokes are ischemic, with a tenfold higher incidence rate than hemorrhagic strokes, and twice the rate of transient ischemic attacks (TIA) (6). Diabetes, arterial hypertension, and increasing age are associated with an increasing incidence rates. Highest rates are found in those with diabetes who are ≥75 years of age and in hypertensive patient receiving peritoneal dialysis (6). Strokes are associated with a markedly diminished survival in the subsequent 2 years compared with patients who had not had stroke (approximately two thirds are dead at 2 years versus one half in the hemodialysis group).

Toyoda et al. (26) reported their findings on stroke in patients on hemodialysis presenting to a single institution in Fukuoka, Japan over a 22-year period. The institution created a stroke center in 1996, and the authors analyzed and compared patient data in the prestroke center with data from 1997 to 2002. The frequency of hemorrhagic stroke declined form 52% to 29%, a decline comparable to that seen in a normal renal function comparison group. Brain infarction events increased from 41% to 68%, again similar to those with normal renal function. The frequency of brain infarction increased from 41% to 68% between the two time periods, again similar to the increase in those with normal renal function, whereas subarachnoid hemorrhage events were lower in the hemodialysis group than among the patients without kidney failure (3% vs. 10%, $p < 0.07$).

In the Toyoda et al. analysis, patients on hemodialysis admitted after 1996 (the HD-B group) were slightly younger, and more frequently hypertensive and diabetic than those admitted before 1997. Vertebrobasilar territory infarctions were more prevalent (48% vs. 33%). By multivariate analysis of the HD-B group compared with those patients not on dialysis admitted to the stroke center, diabetes was an independent risk factor for a vertebrobasilar territory infarct (OR, 1.53), whereas atrial fibrillation was a risk factor for carotid artery distribution territorial infarcts (OR, 2.78). In this analysis, hemodialysis status alone did not explain the territory of infarction. Toyoda et al. (27), however, had reported previously that the frequency of vertebrobasilar infarction in peritoneal dialysis patients was similar to those not on dialysis. The authors speculated that differences in territory of infarction between patients on peritoneal dialysis and those on hemodialysis might be related to the effects of the arteriovenous shunt on the vertebrobasilar circulation. Patients with infarction were older, more likely to be diabetic, have atrial fibrillation, and have lower blood pressures than patients with hemorrhage.

This same group reported that 34% of the ischemic strokes occurred during or within one-half hour of the conclusion of dialysis compared with 19% of hemorrhagic strokes (27). They felt this suggested a possible link to the procedure itself and the stroke event. As an example, Wells and Foroozan (28) reported a case of a patient who had several premonitory episodes of transient visual loss during hypotensive episodes in dialysis that ultimately culminated in a fixed right homonymous superior quadrantic defect. Severe arterial hypotension can result in cerebral hypoperfusion and eventually ischemic strokes in watershed areas between two vascular territories.

Silent cerebral infarctions are more prevalent in hemodialysis than in normal controls, and these patients may have a greatly increased risk of symptomatic events (29,30). Although arterial hypertension, evidence of poor nutrition, age, diabetes, and ethnicity have been linked to stroke risk, attention has focused on the role of potential nontraditional cardiovascular risk factors in patients on dialysis, such as serum homocysteine levels, elevated levels of markers of inflammation and oxidative stress; the influence of calcium, phosphorus, and parathyroid hormone on vascular pathology; and studies of carotid anatomy and flow via ultrasound. Given the limited understanding of distinctive characteristics for stroke risk in the dialysis population and the paucity of outcomes data, it is difficult to draw conclusions with respect to unique approaches to screening, preventing, and treating cerebrovascular disease in the dialysis population. The Kidney Disease Outcomes Quality Initiative (K/DOQI) workgroup addressed this by modifying the *American Heart Association Guidelines* with a view toward instilling caution regarding the use of anticoagulant therapy, and highlighting the uncertainty over optimal targets for blood pressure control (31).

Restless Legs Syndrome

Although the idiopathic form of restless legs syndrome (RLS) occurs in the general population, a range of 6.6% to 62% of patients on dialysis exhibit the secondary form (32). A predilection may exist for patients of European descent compared with African Americans (33). Symptoms tend to worsen during inactivity and may be particularly problematic at night. The familial tendency is much less evident in patients with the uremic as compared with the idiopathic form (34). Although the relationship to dialysis is not clear, the forced confinement of a hemodialysis session affords an opportunity for symptoms to develop.

The pathophysiology of RLS has been reviewed (35). Dopaminergic pathways appear to be involved, given the relationship of symptoms to therapy influencing them. Spinal cord dysfunction may play a role. Removal of aggravating agents, such as selective serotonin uptake inhibitors, lithium, dopamine antagonists, and tricyclic antidepressants, may alleviate symptoms. Using a lower temperature dialysate may also be helpful. Correction of iron deficiency and treatment of anemia may prove useful. Dopamine agonists, such ropinirole, pergolide, and pramipexole, may bring relief and may offer an advantage over levodopa in that augmentation of symptoms may occur with levodopa. Other treatments include opioids, carbamazepine, clonazepam, and clonidine. Transplantation is typically curative.

Dialysis-Associated Neuropathy

Dialysis is an inefficient means of eliminating β_2-microglobulin, a light chain component of the major histocompatibility locus class I molecule found on, and shed from, cell surfaces. Over time, it can form amyloid fibrils, which are found in periarticular tissue and bone. Carpal tunnel syndrome is one sequela of this deposition (4,36). It typically occurs after many years of dialytic therapy, and one group has suggested that current patient management has reduced the incidence of symptomatic disease (37). Receipt of a functioning transplant will normalize β_2-microglobulin excretion, but will not reverse the deposits (4,36). Destructive cervical spondylopathy is another disorder that has been linked to β_2-microglobulin amyloidosis, in rare instances leading to spinal pain, nerve root pain, or spinal cord compression by unstable vertebral bodies (38).

Placement of arteriovenous fistulae and grafts for hemodialysis access is associated with several types of neuropathy. The surgical procedure itself can result in direct nerve injury or ischemia-related neuropathy via a steal mechanism. Thermann et al. (39) described their experience in cephalic arteriovenous fistula banding with restoration of hand function affected by an ischemic median nerve.

Patients can also develop compression injury related to arm positioning during the hemodialysis treatment. Patients may feel constrained from moving the limb with the dialysis needles inserted into a high-flow arteriovenous conduit, because needle dislodgement might interfere with blood flow or lead to disastrous blood loss. A typical position is pronation with the cubital tunnel in contact with the arm rest. Nardin et al. (40) reviewed the prevalence of ulnar neuropathy in 102 patients in a single dialysis facility. They confirmed via electrodiagnostic studies ulnar neuropathy in 51% of patients tested, and suspected it in 17 more, yielding a possible range of 41% to 60% of patients. Diabetes did not correlate with isolated neuropathy. Subjects with ulnar neuropathy tended to have been on dialysis treatment for a shorter number of months (39.9 vs. 62.8). Sensory symptoms were not prominent features. The investigators suggested that dialysis providers should strive to institute preventive measures, given the high prevalence rate.

In addition to neuropathy from ischemia and compression from positioning or amyloid, tumoral calcinosis has also been described as a mechanism of nerve injury in patients on dialysis (41). Tumoral calcinosis may reflect deranged calcium-phosphate metabolism, with resultant deposition of calcium salts in vulnerable areas. Garcia et al. (41) described a case of ulnar neuropathy related to calcific deposits in Guyon's canal.

Spinal epidural abscess is a rare condition that needs adequate treatment to prevent permanent neurologic deficit or death. Kovalik et al. (42) and Obrador et al. (43) reported a series of patients receiving chronic hemodialysis who developed spinal epidural abscesses. Patients on hemodialyis via a long-term indwelling catheter may be at particular risk for such metastatic infections related to bacterial seeding from the catheter. The only presenting symptom might be back pain. If fever, local tenderness, and radicular or cord compression signs are added, the diagnosis is easier. Magnetic resonance imaging (MRI) should be done if the diagnosis is suspected. Early intervention provides a higher likelihood of a good outcome.

CLINICAL RECOMMENDATIONS OF THE VIGNETTE

The patient with advanced renal failure had evidence of a metabolic encephalopathy related to uremia and anemia that improved with the initiation of dialysis and administration of erythropoietic agents. Despite achieving the targets of therapy, three times weekly hemodialysis is not a substitute for normal renal function, and the patient continued to have cognitive and exercise limitations. A further deterioration of his neurologic status over the course of weeks mimicked some of the symptoms that persuaded the patient to start dialysis in the first place. The focal findings suggested, however, a structural, not metabolic brain lesion. A noncontrast CT revealed a left subdural hematoma, which the neurosurgeon evacuated. After a period of some weeks, the patient made a good neurologic recovery.

SUMMARY

Patients on renal replacement therapy may experience a progression of uremic complications secondary to inadequate restoration of the internal milieu present in those with normal renal function, by progressive accumulation of toxins and exposure to inflammatory mediators associated with dialysis, and by adverse effects of the dialysis procedure itself. Given the significant morbidity and mortality attached to these neurologic complications, a greater understanding regarding differences in therapeutic options and responses to the patient on dialysis in particular is paramount.

REFERENCES

1. Korevaar JC, van Manen JG, Boeschoten EW, et al; NECOSAD Study Group. When to start dialysis treatment: Where do we stand? *Perit Dial Int.* 2005;25[Suppl 3]:S69–S72.
2. Ikizler TA, Schulman G. Hemodialysis: Techniques and prescription. *Am J Kidney Dis.* 2005;46:976–981.
3. Pastan S, Bailey J. Dialysis therapy. *N Engl J Med.* 1998;338:1428–1437.
4. Dember LM, Jaber BL. Dialysis-related amyloidosis: Late finding or hidden epidemic? *Semin Dial.* 2006;19:105–109.
5. Himmelfarb J. Hemodialysis complications. *Am J Kidney Dis.* 2005;45:1122–1131.
6. U.S. Renal Data System. USRDS 2005 Annual Data Report. Bethesda (MD): National Institutes of Health, National Institute of Diabetes and Digestive and Kidney Diseases; 2006.
7. O'Reilly P, Tolwani A. Renal replacement therapy III: IHD, CRRT, SLED. *Crit Care Clin.* 2005;21:367–378.
8. Burn DJ, Bates D. Neurology and the kidney. *J Neurol Neurosurg Psychiatry.* 1998;65:810–821.
9. Silver SM, Sterns RH, Halperin ML. Brain swelling after dialysis: Old urea or new osmoles? *Am J Kidney Dis.* 1996;28:1–13.
10. Sheth KN, Wu GF, Messé SR, et al. Dialysis disequilibrium: Another reversible posterior leukoencephalopathy syndrome? *Clin Neurol Neurosurg.* 2003;105:249–252.
11. Goksel BK, Torun D, Karaca S, et al. Is low blood magnesium level associated with hemodialysis headache? *Headache.* 2006;46:40–45.
12. Johansen KL, Doyle J, Sakkas GK, et al. Neural and metabolic mechanisms of excessive muscle fatigue in maintenance hemodialysis patients. *Am J Physiol Regul Integr Comp Physiol.* 2005;289:R805–R813.
13. Kemp GJ, Crowe AV, Anijeet HK, et al. Abnormal mitochondrial function and muscle wasting, but normal contractile efficiency, in haemodialysed patients studied non-invasively in vivo. *Nephrol Dial Transplant.* 2004;19:1520–1527.
14. Shah VO, Dominic EA, Moseley P, et al. Hemodialysis modulates gene expression profile in skeletal muscle. *Am J Kidney Dis.* 2006;48:616–628.
15. Jovanovic DB, Pejanovic S, Vukovic L, et al. Ten years' experience in subtotal parathyroidectomy of hemodialysis patients. *Ren Fail.* 2005;17:19–24.
16. Savica V, Calvani M, Benatti P, et al. Newer aspects of carnitine metabolism in uremia. *Semin Nephrol.* 2006;26:52–55.
17. Hedayati SS. Dialysis-related carnitine disorder. *Semin Dial.* 2006;19:323–328.
18. Khajehdehi P, Mojerlou M, Behzadi S, et al. A randomized double-blind, placebo-controlled trial of supplementary vitamins E, C and their combination for treatment of haemodialysis cramps. *Nephrol Dial Transplant.* 2001;16:1448–1451.
19. Chang CT, Wu CH, Yang CW, et al. Creatine monohydrate treatment alleviates muscle cramps associated with haemodialysis. *Nephrol Dial Transplant.* 2002;17:1978–1981.
20. Murray AM, Tupper DE, Knopman DS, et al. Cognitive impairment in hemodialysis patients is common. *Neurology.* 2006;67:216–223.
21. Jassal SV, Devins GM, Chan CT, et al. Improvements in cognition in patients converting from thrice weekly hemodialysis to nocturnal hemodialysis: A longitudinal pilot study. *Kidney Int.* 2006;70:956–962.
22. Kurella M, Mapes DL, Port FK, et al. Correlates and outcomes of dementia among dialysis patients: The Dialysis Outcomes and Practice Patterns Study. *Nephrol Dial Transplant.* 2006;21:2543–2548.
23. Hung SC, Hung SH, Tarng DC, et al. Thiamine deficiency and unexplained encephalopathy in hemodialysis and peritoneal dialysis patients. *Am J Kidney Dis.* 2001;38:941–947.
24. Oo TN, Smith, CL, Swan SK. Does uremia protect against the demyelination associated with correction of hyponatremia during hemodialysis? A case report and literature review. *Semin Dial.* 2003;16:68–71.
25. Seliger SL, Gillen DL, Longstreth WT, Jr., et al. Elevated risk of stroke among patients with end-stage renal disease. *Kidney Int.* 2003;64:603–609.
26. Toyoda K, Fujii K, Fujimi S, et al. Stroke in patients on maintenance hemodialysis: A 22-year single-center study. *Am J Kidney Dis.* 2005;45:1058–1066.
27. Toyoda K, Fujii K, Ando T, et al. Incidence, etiology, and outcome of stroke in patients on continuous ambulatory peritoneal dialysis. *Cerebrovasc Dis.* 2004;17:98–105.
28. Wells M, Foroozan R. Transient visual loss may anticipate occipital infarction from hemodialysis. *Am J Kidney Dis.* 2004;43(5):e29–e33.
29. Vermeer SE, den Heijer T, Koudstaal PJ, et al. Incidence and risk factors of silent brain infarcts in the population-based Rotterdam Scan Study. *Stroke.* 2003;34:392–396.
30. Nakatani T, Naganuma T, Uchida J, et al. Silent cerebral infarction in hemodialysis patients. *Am J Nephrol.* 2003;23:86–90.
31. National Kidney Foundation. K/DOQI clinical practice guidelines on cardiovascular disease in dialysis patients. *Am J Kidney Dis.* 2005;45[Suppl 3]:S39–S42.
32. Kavanagh D, Siddiqui S, Geddes CC. Restless legs syndrome in patients on dialysis. *Am J Kidney Dis.* 2004;43:763–771.
33. Kutner N, Bliwise D. Restless legs complaint in African-American and Caucasian hemodialysis patients. *Sleep Medicine.* 2002;3:497–500.
34. Winkelmann J, Wetter TC, Collado-Seidel V, et al. Clinical characteristics and frequency of the hereditary restless legs syndrome in a population of 300 patients. *Sleep.* 2000;23:597–602.
35. Walters AS. Toward a better definition of the restless legs syndrome. The International Restless Legs Syndrome Study Group. *Mov Disord.* 1995;10:634–642.
36. Saito A, Gejyo F. Current clinical aspects of dialysis-related amyloidosis in chronic dialysis patients. *Therapeutic Apheresis Dialysis.* 2006;10:316–320.
37. Schwalbe S, Holzhauer M, Schaeffer J, et al. Beta 2-microglobulin associated amyloidosis: A vanishing complication of long term hemodialysis? *Kidney Int.* 1997;52:1077–1083.
38. Van Driessche S, Goutallier D, Odent T, et al. Surgical treatment of destructive cervical spondyloarthropathy with neurologic impairment in hemodialysis patients. *Spine.* 2006;31:705–711.
39. Thermann F, Brauckhoff M, Kornhuber M. Dialysis shunt-associated ischaemic monomelic neuropathy: Neurological recovery preserving the dialysis access [Letter]. *Nephrol Dial Transplant.* Epub 2006 July 19.
40. Nardin R, Chapman K, Raynor EM. Prevalence of ulnar neuropathy in patients receiving hemodialysis. *Arch Neurol.* 2005;62:271–325.
41. Garcia S, Cofan F, Combalia A, et al. Compression of the ulnar nerve in Guyon's canal by uremic tumoral calcinosis. *Arch Orthop Trauma Surg.* 2000;120:228–230.
42. Kovalik EC, Raymond JR, Albers FJ, et al. A clustering of epidural abscesses in chronic hemodialysis patients: Risks of salvaging access catheters in cases of infection. *J Am Soc Nephrol.* 1996;7:2264–2267.
43. Obrador GT, Levenson DJ. Spinal epidural abscess in hemodialysis patients: Report of three cases and review of the literature. *Am J Kidney Dis.* 1996;27:75–83.

CHAPTER 31

Renal Transplantation

Susan H. Hou

OBJECTIVES

- To recognize the neurologic effects of immunosuppressive drugs
- To distinguish between infectious, metabolic, vascular, and neoplastic causes of neurologic symptoms in transplant recipients
- To explain the difference in presentation and severity of infectious agents in transplant recipients compared with the general population
- To describe the effect of immunosuppressive drugs on susceptibility to tumors that are unusual in the general population

CASE VIGNETTE

A 64-year-old man with end-stage renal disease (ESRD) secondary to membranoproliferative glomerulonephritis was admitted to the hospital with a 2-day history of fever and chills 2 years after receiving a kidney transplant from his son. He had no localizing signs, except an increase in right hip pain where he had known avascular necrosis. Medications on admission included levothyroxine, tacrolimus, mycophenolate mofetil, prednisone, atorvastatin, and felodipine. On examination, his blood pressure was 94/60 mm Hg, temperature was 103°F, pulse was 126 beats per minute, and respiratory rate was 24 breaths per minute. He was alert and oriented. The remainder of his physical examination was remarkable only for decreased range of motion of the right hip. Laboratory findings: Blood urea nitrogen (BUN) 18 mg/dL, serum creatinine 1.6 mg/dL, white blood cell (WBC) count 9,000, Hb 13.6, and glucose 162 mg/dL. Tacrolimus level was 12.5. He was started on vancomycin, ceftriaxone, acyclovir, zolpidem (Ambien), salicylate, and doxycycline. Two days after admission, he became confused and agitated. On examination, his temperature was 104°F, pulse was 108 beats per minute, blood pressure was 139/71 mm Hg, and respiratory rate was 24 breaths per minute. He was oriented only to person. The remainder of neurologic examination as far as he could cooperate was normal. Magnetic resonance imaging (MRI) of the brain showed increased signal intensity in the left periventricular white matter. Cerebrospinal fluid (CSF) examination showed 130 WBC (51% neutrophils, 46% lymphocytes), 8 red blood cells (RBC). Protein was 107 mg/dL, glucose 42 mg/dL (serum glucose of 156 mg/dL). India ink preparation showed no yeast. Cultures were negative for bacteria and fungi. CSF was negative for cryptococcal antigen, histoplasmosis, blastomycosis, coccidiodes, aspergillus, and herpes simplex. Serum tests for cytomegalovirus (CMV), Epstein-Barr virus (EBV), measles, and mumps showed elevated IgG and negative IgM. He became unresponsive for 6 days and, when he began to respond, he had marked dysarthria and severe quadriparesis. Titers for West Nile virus on lumbar puncture (LP) done on day 3 of hospitalization were equivocal. Repeat CSF examination on day 9 of hospitalization was positive for IgM for West Nile virus. He continued to have slow improvement in both speech and strength 2 years after the illness, but dysarthria and limb weakness remained.

DEFINITION

Neurologic complications following kidney transplantation include changes in mentation and focal abnormalities of both central and peripheral origin. It is most useful to divide them according to etiology because the cause is the most important determinant of prognosis and treatment.

EPIDEMIOLOGY

Kidney transplant has become the preferred treatment for ESRD. In 2005, 16,481 kidney transplants were done in the United States. Increasingly, patients with kidney failure and other vascular and metabolic diseases receive kidney transplants, including many with diabetes. Life can be sustained by dialysis in patients with renal failure, allowing many to live years while awaiting a transplant, but during that time they suffer from the long-term consequences of kidney failure and these sometimes result in neurologic problems. All are treated with immunosuppressive drugs, which put them at risk for opportunistic infection and have neurologic side effects.

ETIOLOGY AND PATHOGENESIS

Transplant recipients are at risk for a wide variety of illnesses that give rise to diverse neurologic symptoms. In many of these illnesses, the prognosis is markedly improved by prompt treatment. Every effort should be made to establish the etiology of symptoms because empiric treatment would require the use of a wide variety of potentially toxic drugs.

CLINICAL MANIFESTATIONS

INFECTIOUS CAUSES OF NEUROLOGIC SYMPTOMS IN TRANSPLANT RECIPIENTS

In renal transplant recipients, mental status changes can occur as a result of CNS infection or as a response to generalized infection. Bacteremia, without meningitis or encephalitis, can cause confusion and blood cultures should be part of the workup of any transplant recipient with mental status changes.

Although bacterial infections remain the most common infections in transplant recipients, unusual infections figure prominently in the differential diagnosis of CNS infections. In the early posttransplant period, infection acquired from the donor, as well as infection acquired from the environment or reactivation of a latent infection in the recipient, should be considered. The likelihood of a donor infection transplanted with the kidney is particularly high in the recipients of kidneys purchased in countries with a thriving black market in kidneys (1).

West Nile Virus

Some of the first deaths from West Nile virus were described among transplant recipients from a single infected donor (2). The Organ Procurement and Transplant Network does not routinely test deceased donors for West Nile virus because testing has a high false–positive rate, which would lead to a failure to use good organs and a net loss of life (3). The practice may change when more accurate tests for active infection are developed. The infection may be asymptomatic in healthy people. Living donors who reside in endemic areas can be questioned about exposure to mosquitoes in the immediate pretransplant period if West Nile virus is occurring in the area. The donor can then be tested and transplant delayed with any suspicion of acute infection, without losing the organ for transplant. The problem is somewhat limited because the disease is seasonal and the period of infectiousness is short. Because the disease has a wide distribution, the possibility of acquiring the disease long after transplant is present. Transplant recipients generally present with symptoms similar to nonimmunosuppressed patients with clinical illness. Encephalitis, flaccid paralysis, and movement disorders are common presenting symptoms (4). CSF examination shows atypical lymphocytes. MRI shows hyperintense lesions usually involving the white matter. Most patients survive, but sequelae are common, and may be severe.

Cryptococcal Meningitis

Cryptococcal meningitis is among the most common subacute meningitides seen in transplant recipients and is universally fatal without treatment. As with other fungal infections, cryptococci usually enter the body through the respiratory tract, but have a predilection for the CNS (5). Patients present with headache, fever, lethargy or coma, and personality changes or memory loss, with symptoms often waxing and waning over time. Lumbar puncture is needed for diagnosis. Opening pressures are often high, and CSF examination shows an increased number of white cells, usually mononuclear cells, whereas changes in glucose and protein may be minimal. India ink examination of the CSF will show encapsulated yeast forms in 50% of cases, and cultures will be positive in 90% of cases. Cryptococcal antigen can be obtained immediately with nearly 90% of patients having positive results. Brain imaging should be done before lumbar puncture because 10% of patients will have mass lesions and hydrocephalus may also be present. Treatment is with amphotericin B and flucytosine.

OTHER FUNGAL MENINGITIS. The route of entry for fungal infections is generally through the lungs, but infection often occurs through reactivation of remote infection. Unlike crypotococcal meningitis, other fungal CNS infections are usually accompanied by pulmonary or systemic manifestations.

Tuberculosis

Although tuberculosis (TB) is one of the infections that can be transmitted with the transplanted kidney, most CNS TB is the result of activation of dormant disease. It is minimized by treating patients with positive purified protein derivative (PPD) with isoniazid (INH) before or at the time of transplant. Tuberculosis can cause meningitis, CNS tuberculomas, or arachnoiditis (6). The presentation of TB meningitis varies from an acute course suggestive of bacterial meningitis to a very indolent course suggestive of progressive dementia. Typically, a febrile prodrome occurs before onset of meningeal signs. Tuberculous meningitis frequently occurs without active pulmonary lesions. In immunosuppressed patients, the PPD is frequently negative. CSF analysis typically shows low glucose (<45 mg/dL), high protein content (100 to 500 mg/dL), and a mononuclear pleocytosis. Repeated LPs with examination of acid-fast bacilli (AFB) smears may be necessary to establish the diagnosis. The diagnostic yield can be increased by polymerase chain reaction (PCR) performed on CSF, but the sensitivity is still too low to warrant delaying treatment when the test finding is negative. Neuroradiologic imaging should be done to identify tuberculomas, arachnoiditis, or hydrocephalus. Tuberculomas may be asymptomatic or present with focal neurologic signs or signs of increased intracranial pressure. Rachnoiditis may present with symptoms of nerve root and cord compression. Treatment has to be initiated before cultures grow out Mycobacterium tuberculosis. Treatment requires a four-drug regimen and, in some instances, corticosteroids are used (7). The use of rifampin speeds the metabolism of cyclosporine and complicates dosing. One center attributes a high rate of graft loss to this interaction (8).

Toxoplasmosis

The widespread use of trimethoprim sulfamethoxazole to prevent *Pneumocystis carnii* pneumonia (PCP) infections has lowered the risk of toxoplasmosis. Most clinical disease occurs through reactivation of latent disease with reactivation occurring preferentially in the CNS (9). Although toxoplasmosis can be acquired from a donor, such patients usually present with systemic disease rather than with neurologic symptoms 10). The diagnosis is suggested on the basis of ring-enhancing lesions on MRI or CT scan. CSF findings are normal or nonspecific.

Nocardia

Nocardia is an uncommon cause of infection among transplant recipients, particularly since prophylaxis with trimethoprim sulfamethoxazole has been widely adopted, but 15% to 16% of infections involve the CNS (11). Diagnosis is facilitated by the common involvement of lung and skin. Brain abscess is the most common CNS manifestation of *Nocardia* infection, with meningitis being rare.

Herpes Encephalitis

Although herpes infections are extremely common in transplant recipients, the frequency of encephalitis is not significantly increased over the normal population. Patients usually present with fever, change in level of consciousness, and focal neurologic symptoms. CSF findings are not specific, but PCR is positive in >95% of cases (12,13). MRI frequently shows temporal lobe lesions. Mortality and long-term disability are reduced by acyclovir treatment but still remain high. Remember, the drug itself can cause mental status changes, especially if renal function is changing and precise dose adjustment is difficult. Drug toxicity should be considered in patients whose symptoms are not abating.

Listeria Meningitis

Transplant recipients can develop any type of bacterial meningitis, but 69% of *Listeria* infection in nonpregnant adults occurs among immunosuppressed patients. The infection presents with fever and mental status changes, with or without meningeal signs. It may be accompanied by seizures or focal neurologic signs (14). CSF protein concentration is usually increased, but glucose is low in only about half of patients. Gram stain is usually negative and when the Gram stain is positive, the gram-positive rods can be confused with pneumococcal or diptheroids. Although granulocytes frequently predominate, pure lymphocyosis can occur and the absence of polymorphonuclear cells should not automatically lead to the assumption that viral, fungal, or tuberculous meningitis is present. Treatment is with ampicillin, penicillin, or trimethoprim-sulfamethoxazole. *Listeria* is not sensitive to cephalosporins.

Malaria

Malaria can cause CNS symptoms, but it generally presents as a systemic disease with incidental CNS involvement. The diagnosis is generally suggested on the basis of travel history, including travel for transplant. One report found malaria among 11% of recipients of kidneys purchased in India (15).

NEUROLOGIC TOXICITY FROM TRANSPLANT MEDICATIONS

Calcineurin Inhibitors

The most commonly used immunosuppressive medications, the calcineurin inhibitors, can be associated with neurotoxicity, with mild neurologic symptoms occurring in as many as 20% to 40% of patients receiving calcineurin inhibitors (Table 31-1). Both tacrolimus and cyclosporine cause tremor in a substantial percentage of patients.

Much less common is a reversible posterior leukoencephalopathy that has been associated with tacrolimus (16–18). Patients can present with mental status changes, seizures, paralysis, dystonia, abulia, and visual and speech abnormalities. About 10% of the time, leukoencephalopathy is associated with fever, sometimes as high as 40% of the time, making it necessary to rule out infectious causes of neurologic symptoms. More than 80% of renal transplant recipients with posterior leukoencephalopathy have hypertension. CT scans and MRI show edema of the white matter, primarily in the posterior cerebral hemispheres, findings that can also be seen in malignant hypertension. CSF examination is unremarkable. It generally has its onset during the first month after transplant, but has been described as late as 4 years after transplant. No specific serum level precipitates the syndrome and it has been seen with levels as low as 5 ng/mL, but it usually improves with lowering serum drug levels. It does not necessarily mean that the drug needs to be stopped, although many centers switch to a different calcineurin inhibitor. Symptoms usually resolve within 2 weeks, but can take up to a month, and resolution of neuroimaging abnormalities generally takes much longer.

TABLE 31-1. Neurologic Side Effects of Calcineurin Inhibitors

Tremors
Sleep disturbances
Paresthesias
Mood disturbances
Leukoencephalopathy
Mental status changes: Confusion, disorientation, lethargy, irritability, hallucinations
Seizures
Visual disturbances: Hemianopsia, cortical blindness, blurred vision
Motor symptoms: Paraplegia, quadriplegia, paresis, dystonia
Speech or language disturbances: Aphasia, akinetic mutism, slurred speech
Other movement disorders: Asterixis

OKT3

OKT3 has been associated with aseptic meningitis that has its onset within 72 hours of drug administration. It is generally benign and self-limited (19).

Steroids

Steroid psychosis, once a relatively common occurrence in transplant recipients, is now rare with steroid-free and low-dose steroid regimens, but it may still be seen in patients treated for rejection with high-dose steroids.

Nonimmunosuppressive Drugs That Cause Neurologic Symptoms

Many of the neurologic effects of drugs other than immunosuppressive drugs in transplant recipients are the result of renal insufficiency. These are covered elsewhere in this book. Only a few of the drugs that are frequently used in transplant recipients are briefly discussed. The propensity for changing renal function increases the risk of CNS side effects from common antimicrobial drugs, sometimes resulting in new neurologic symptoms during treatment of a CNS infection.

PENICILLIN. Penicillin is notable for a high toxic therapeutic ratio such that no hesitation should exist to its use in patients with renal insufficiency. When high doses of penicillin are used to treat patients with meningitis, a decline in renal function combined with increased permeability of the meninges can result in seizures.

ACYCLOVIR. Because transplant recipients are at risk for herpetic infections, treatment with acyclovir is common. Acute renal failure can occur with both acyclovir and valacyclovir. The drug can cause acute renal failure through precipitation of crystals in the tubules. Levels of the drug rise as a result and lead to neurologic symptoms, most commonly confusion or coma.

NEOPLASTIC DISEASES

Lymphoma

Transplant recipients have a risk of malignant lymphoma that is 11.8 times greater than age-matched individuals in the non-transplant population. A predilection exists for extra nodal disease with 24% of extra nodal disease being CNS disease (20). CNS involvement was described in the earliest cases of post-transplant lymphoma (21). The most common presentation for CNS lymphomas include focal neurologic symptoms, such as hemiparesis or aphasia, seizures, symptoms of increased intracranial pressure, or a combination of these. Most tumors test positive for B-cell markers, and EBV can be identified in the tumors (22). Patients with negative serologies for EBV before transplant are at high risk for lymphoma, particularly if they receive a kidney from an EBV-positive donor, but EBV-related CNS lymphomas can occur in patients who are EBV positive before transplant. Because patients who are EBV seronegative are rare, most patients with CNS lymphomas are seropositive before transplant. Because most donors are also seropositive for EBV, requiring an EBV-negative donor for a negative recipient would often preclude transplant. Cyclosporine, antithymocyte globulin, and OKT3 have been associated with higher frequencies of lymphoma, but the risk is more likely related to the total amount of immunosuppression than to a specific drug. The diagnosis is usually made by the discovery of enhancing lesions on either CT scan or MRI. Almost three fourths of tumors are multifocal. The radiologic appearance can be confused with intracerebral abscess or toxoplasmosis, and biopsy may be necessary to confirm the diagnosis. The CSF is generally remarkable only for slightly increased protein content. The lymphoma may be either monoclonal or polyclonal. Reduction of immunosuppression or immunotherapy alone is rarely sufficient treatment. The best outcomes usually require a combination of radiation and chemotherapy.

OTHER CENTRAL NERVOUS SYSTEM TUMORS

The risk of Kaposi sarcoma is increased among transplant recipients, but CNS involvement is rare. The increased risk of lymphoma and Kaposi sarcoma in transplant recipients has been explained on the basis of decreased immune surveillance resulting in cancers associated with identified viruses, either latent in the recipient or introduced from the donor. Glioblastomas have also been described in transplant recipients, and generally appears years after transplant (23). Glioblastomas present with the usual variety of symptoms of an intracranial mass, including headache, seizures, focal neurologic deficits, and coma. The prognosis for patients described to date has been poor. Cadaveric donors with glioblastomas confined to the brain are accepted because of the low rate of metastases. In the rare cases of tumor transmission, the tumor has been seen in the transplanted organ and other sites outside the CNS rather than in the brain (24).

The Usual Suspects

Despite the long list of esoteric neurologic problems see in transplant recipients, the most common problems are similar to those that occur in the general population. Many of the metabolic problems discussed below are not diagnostic dilemmas because transplant recipients are constantly monitored for such changes.

METABOLIC CAUSES OF NEUROLOGIC SYMPTOMS

Patients with renal disease are at risk for a wide range of metabolic abnormalities and generally have a more profound response to them than those without renal disease. (The one exception is a less profound response to severe hyperglycemia in patients on dialysis with no urine output who are spared the volume contraction associated with osmotic diuresis.) Although uremia certainly causes neurologic symptoms, the elevated BUN and creatinine levels are rarely the cause of lethargy and mental status changes. It is more common to see myoclonus and muscle twitching associated with high levels of BUN and creatinine. These symptoms have to be distinguished from effects induced by medication.

Hyperglycemia is common, and most transplant recipients do have an osmotic diuresis. They may develop posttransplant diabetes mellitus and are routinely monitored for elevations in blood sugar. More commonly, in the immediate posttransplant period, patients with diabetes pretransplant have deterioration in glucose control because of medications and the restoration of normal kidney function. Accordingly, transplant recipients with diabetes are instructed to increase their glucose monitoring at discharge even if they have been requiring no medication while on dialysis.

Hypercalcemia can occur when hypertrophied parathyroid glands continue parathyroid hormone (PTH) production in the setting near normal kidney function. Although PTH levels generally drop, they frequently remain above normal and occasionally symptomatic hypercalcemia occurs.

Hypomagnesemia associated with calcineurin inhibitors and hypocalcemia can lead to hyperreflexia.

With good renal function, hypo- and hypernatremia are rare, but are always considered in patients with mental status changes. Muscle weakness can result from profound hyperkalemia or hypokalemia, but is rare because these conditions are generally detected and treated before potassium levels become so profoundly abnormal.

Liver failure is rare, but can occur when hepatotoxic drugs are used in patients with underlying liver disease. Close monitoring of liver function tests make this unlikely.

Profound muscle weakness may be seen in the rare patient who develops rhabdomyolysis from the combination of calcineurin inhibitors and 3-hydroxy-3-methylglutaryl coenzyme A (HMG-CoA) reductase inhibitors. The muscle weakness may take longer to resolve than the patient's renal function abnormalities.

Thyroid disease does not appear to be increased in transplant recipients, but is common. Some vigilance is needed to avoid attributing all tremors and all tachycardia to drugs.

CEREBROVASCULAR DISEASE

Cerebrovascular disease is more common in transplant recipients than in the general population. The strongest predictors of stroke are diabetes, diabetic nephropathy, and peripheral vascular disease (25). Patients with polycystic kidney disease are at increased risk for bleeding from cerebral aneurysms. They are at no higher risk for death from cerebrovascular disease than other transplant recipients, however, and they are still more susceptible to ischemic strokes than intracranial hemorrhage from ruptured aneurysm. Efforts to prevent stroke include aggressive control of hypertension and treatment of other cardiovascular risk factors. No contraindication exists to low dose aspirin, even in transplant recipients with renal insufficiency.

DIAGNOSTIC APPROACH

The history should include a review of the patient's place of birth as well as recent and remote travel. The patient and family should be questioned about exposure to mosquitoes and other insects, and to animals, including cats and birds. Home remodeling projects can result in exposure to fungal pathogens and bird and rodent droppings. The history also includes a careful review of occupational hazards and gardening and agricultural contact.

The pretransplant evaluation generally includes serology for EBV, varicella, herpes simplex, and rapid plasma reagin (RPR). PPD status and treatment are also known. Donor serologies may not be available in the case of purchased kidneys, but at least living donors evaluated in US transplant centers will have known EVB status. Medication history should be reviewed for any drugs known to cause neurologic symptoms, with the recognition that sedatives and narcotics can have an exaggerated effect in patients with renal insufficiency.

Many different illnesses given rise to similar neurologic symptoms and the neurologic examination may not clarify the cause of symptoms. A careful search for evidence of systemic disease or focal disease outside the CNS may be helpful in making a diagnosis or may at least provide a source of tissue or cultures outside the CNS.

CT scan or MRI of the head (and sometimes spine and sinuses) is indicated in most patients with neurologic symptoms unless their cause is apparent on screening laboratory studies for metabolic abnormalities. MRI is usually more sensitive and avoids exposure to nephrotoxic contrast agents. Neuroradiologic studies may be indicated in asymptomatic patients with systemic illnesses, such as fungal infections which have a high frequency of CNS involvement (Table 31-2).

CSF examination is essential in determining the nature of an infectious process.

Brain biopsy may be necessary to make the diagnosis of malignancy and, less commonly, infection. In some infections, drainage of a cerebral abscess may be necessary. Brain biopsy carries a substantial risk of morbidity and sometimes even mortality so that every effort should be made to establish a diagnosis with other tests.

TABLE 31-2. Diagnostic Findings in Central Nervous System (CNS) Infections and Other Disorders

Cerebrospinal Fluid	*Neuroradiologic Studies*
TUBERCULOSIS	
Protein: 100–500 mg/dL Glucose: <45 mg/dL (80%) Lymphocytes (PMN early) PCR: 30%–60% AFB smear: 1 smear <40% + 4 smears >80% +	Tuberculomas 5%–10% Hydrocephalus Basilar meningeal enhancement Cerebral infarcts
CRYPTOCOCCUS	
Protein: Mild abnormality Glucose: Mild abnormality Mononuclear cells: 50%–75% Cryptococcal antigen: 90% Culture: 90%–100%	Mass lesion 10%
TOXOPLASMOSIS	
Protein elevated Mononuclear pleocytosis	Ring-enhancing lesions
LISTERIA	
Protein elevated Glucose: Low in 50% WBC: 9–3,300 PMN: (2%–100%)	
WEST NILE VIRUS	
Protein: 60–140 mg/dL Glucose: Normal WBC: Mixed differential	White matter hyperintensities
HERPES SIMPLEX ENCEPHALITIS	
Protein: Elevated Glucose: Normal Lymphocytic pleocytosis PCR >95% positive	Temporal lobe lesions
NOCARDIA	
Usually unremarkable	Single or multiple loculated abscesses
LYMPHOMA	
Unremarkable	Enhancing lesions 75% multifocal
CNI-ASSOCIATED LEUKOENCEPHALOPATHY	
Unremarkable	White matter hyperintensities

PMN, polymorphonuclears; PCR, polymerase chain reaction; AFB, acid-fast bacilli; WBC, white blood cells; CNI, calcineurin inhibitors

TREATMENT

Most of the infectious problems respond to specific antimicrobial therapy, but in life-threatening infection, reduction of immunosuppression may be necessary. Drugs toxicity can be addressed by reducing levels or changing drugs. Other diagnostic possibilities and treatments may need to be pursued when resolution of drug-related symptoms is slow. Correction of metabolic abnormalities is done along the same lines as in other patients. Reduction of immunosuppression is almost always a part of treating malignancy. Further surgery, immunotherapy, and chemotherapy are determined by the type and aggressiveness of the tumor. Treatment of cerebrovascular disease is similar to treatment in the general population, with the recognition that aggressive treatment of risk factors is needed.

CLINICAL RECOMMENDATIONS OF THE VIGNETTE

The patient had West Nile virus, for which no specific treatment is available. His illness highlights the importance of prevention, which is the use of insect repellent in areas where West Nile virus and other arthropod-borne diseases are endemic.

His presentation with fever makes infection the most likely cause of his symptoms, but he initially had no neurologic symptoms. On admission, he was started on acyclovir and zolpidem (Ambien), both of which can cause neurologic symptoms, broadening the differential diagnosis of his confusion and agitation. With a persistent high fever, infection still remains the most likely problem. The acute onset of symptoms makes it essential to rule out bacterial meningitis, fungal infections, and tuberculosis. The first CSF examination provided good evidence against cryptococcal meningitis, eliminating the need to start amphotericin, but did not exclude either *Listeria* or tuberculosis, although his symptoms became more consistent with an encephalitis than with pure meningitis. At this point, it would have been reasonable to broaden the antibiotic coverage because *Listeria* would not be susceptible to the cephalosporin he was given. Ampicillin could have been given until the bacterial culture results were reported. Repeated CSF examinations are needed to rule out tuberculosis until the diagnosis of West Nile virus could be made.

Because no specific treatment for West Nile virus exists, reduction of immunosuppression can be considered.

SUMMARY

Renal transplant recipients are at risk for a wide range of conditions that lead to neurologic symptoms. Decreased cellular immunity, accelerated vascular disease, the need for multiple drugs, and the frequency of metabolic abnormalities are the most common factors predisposing to neurologic symptoms. Effective treatment of the patient requires distinguishing between the multitude of problems that are easily treated or self-limited and life-threatening infections requiring early specific treatment. The time frame for diagnosis and treatment is often hours to a few days. The time frame is slightly longer for tumors, but early diagnosis is important for posttransplant lymphomas because successful treatment rate is high in the early stages. Neuroradiologic imaging and testing of CSF fluid are central to making a diagnosis in those life-threatening conditions. Although the array of tests that can be done on CSF has increased, the low technologic lumbar (or rarely cisternal) tap is still necessary to obtain a CSF sample. Often, repeat CSF examinations are needed. The range of metabolic abnormalities is slightly different from the general population. Unique neurologic syndromes are associated with some of the drugs used to prevent rejection. Only heightened vigilance and a thorough familiarity with these problems make timely diagnosis and treatment possible.

REFERENCES

1. Salahudeen AK, Woods HF, Pingle A, et al. High mortality among recipients of bought living unrelated donor transplants. *Lancet.* 1990;336:725–728.
2. Iwamoto M, Jernigan DB, Guasch A, et al. Transmission of west Nile virus from an organ donor to four transplant recipients. *N Engl J Med.* 2003;348:196–203.
3. Kiberd D, Forward K. Screening for West Nile virus in organ transplantation: A medical decision analysis. *Am J Transplant.* 2004;4:1296–1301.
4. Kleinschmidt-DeMasters BK, Marder BA, Levi ME, et al. Naturally acquired west Nile virus encephalomyelitis in transplant recipients: Clinical, laboratory, diagnostic and neuropathological features. *Arch Neurol.* 2004;61:1210–1220.
5. Vilchez RA, Fung J, Kusne S. Cryptococcus in organ transplant recipients: An overview. *Am J Transplant.* 2002;2:575–580.
6. Mrowka C, Heintz B, Reul J, et al. Cerebral tuberculoma 11 years after renal transplantation. *Am J Nephrol.* 1998;18:557–559.
7. Thwaites GE, Bang ND, Dung NH, et al. Dexamethasone for the treatment of tuberculous meningitis in adolescents and adults. *N Engl J Med.* 2004;351:1741–1751.
8. El-Agroudy AE, Refaie AF, Moussa OM, et al. Tuberculosis in Egyptian transplant recipients: Study of clinical course and outcome. *Nephrology.* 2003;16:404–411.
9. Ferreira MS, Borges AS. Some aspects of protozoan infection in immunocompromised patients—A review. *Mem Inst Oswaldo Cruz.* 2002;97:443–477.
10. Renoult E, Biava MF, Hulin C, et al Transmission of toxoplasmosis by renal transplant: A report of four cases. *Transplant Proc.* 1996;28:181–183.
11. Wilson JP, Turner HR, Kirchner KA, et al. Nocardia infections in renal transplant recipients. *Medicine.* 1989;68:38–57.
12. Lewis P, Glaser CA. Encephalitis. *Pediatr Rev.* 2005;26:353–363.
13. Kennedy PGE. Viral encephalitis. *J Neurol.* 2005;252:268–272.
14. Mylonakis E, Hohmann EL, Calderwood SB. Central nervous system infection with Listeria monocytogenes. *Medicine.* 1998;77:313–336.
15. Türkmen A, Sever MS, Ecder T, et al. Post transplant malaria. *Transplantation.* 1996;62:1521–1523.
16. Parvex P, Pinsk M, Bell LE, et al. Reversible encephalopathy associated with tacrolimus in pediatric renal transplants. *Pediatr Nephrol.* 2001;16:537–542.
17. Hinchey J, Chaves C, Appignani B, et al. A reversible posterior leukoencephalopathy. *N Engl J Med.* 1996;334:494–500.
18. Singh N, Bonham A, Fukui M. Immunosuppressive associated leukoencephalopathy in organ transplant recipients. *Transplantation.* 2000;69:467–472.
19. Martin MA, Massanari RM, Nghiem DD, et al. Nosocomial aseptic meningitis associated with administration of OKT3. *JAMA.* 1988;259:2002–2005.
20. Snanoudj R, Durrbach A, Leblond V, et al. Primary brain lymphomas after kidney transplantation: Presentation and outcome. *Transplantation.* 2003;76:930–937.
21. Penn I, Hammond W, Brettschneider L, et al. Malignant lymphomas in transplantation patients. *Transplant Proc.* 1969;50:106–112.
22. Opelz G, Dohler B. Lymphomas after solid organ transplantation: A collaborative transplant study report. *Am J Transplant.* 2003;4:222–230.
23. Salvati M, Frati A, Caroli E, et al. Glioblastoma in kidney transplant recipients. *J Neurooncol.* 2003;63:33–37.
24. Colquhoun SD, Robert ME, Shaked A, et al. Transmission of CNS malignancy by organ transplantation. *Transplant.* 1994;57:970–974.
25. Oliveras A, Roquer J, Puig JM, et al. Stroke in renal transplant recipients: Epidemiology, predictive risk factors and outcome. *Clin Transplant.* 2003;17:1–8.
26. Perrone RD, Ruthazer R, Terrin NC. Survival after end stage renal disease in autosomal dominant polycystic kidney disease: Contribution of extrarenal complications to mortality. *Am J Kidney Dis.* 2001;38:777–784.

CHAPTER **32**

Commonly Used Renal Drugs

Vivekanand Jha

OBJECTIVES

- To explain the mechanisms of renal vulnerability to drugs
- To discuss the nephrotoxic effect of commonly used drugs
- To explain the changes in drug handling, metabolism, and excretion in chronic kidney disease (CKD)
- To describe the clinical implications of the altered drug kinetics in CKD
- To discuss modification of the drug dosage in CKD, with emphasis on drugs acting on the central nervous system
- To explain how drug use can interfere with common kidney function tests

CASE VIGNETTE

A 62-year-old-man with hypertension of several years' duration presented to a nephrologist with uncontrolled hypertension. His serum creatinine level was 4.4 mg/dL; urinalysis showed 2+ protein; and ultrasound and Doppler studies showed small kidneys, no evidence of renovascular disease, and gallstones. His antihypertensive medications were increased. Addition of ramipril was followed by a rise in creatinine to 5.4 mg/dL. A rise in serum potassium to 5.5 mEq/L was managed with dietary modification and oral potassium binding resins.

Four months later, he developed severe pain in the right hypochondrium and recurrent vomiting. Intravenous meperidine was administered (75 mg) three times over the next 24 hours at a local health facility. Serum creatinine was 5.8 mg/dL. The abdominal pain gradually abated, but 1 day later, he developed multiple episodes of generalized tonic-clonic seizures and became unresponsive. Seizures were controlled with intravenous diazepam and phenytoin. Magnetic resonance image (MRI) of the brain was normal. In view of the likelihood of an accumulation of neuroexcitatory metabolites of meperidine, this drug was stopped. His level of alertness improved, and he was discharged home after 4 days.

DEFINITION AND EPIDEMIOLOGY

An ever-expanding therapeutic armamentarium has been paralleled by increasing awareness of the potential of drugs to cause adverse effects on the kidneys. The true incidence of drug-induced kidney disease is difficult to ascertain. Diagnosis is often delayed until kidney damage is sufficiently advanced to produce an elevation in serum creatinine value, implying a >50% decline in the glomerular filtration rate (GFR).

The kidneys play an important role in the disposal of most drugs. Alteration in kidney function results in accumulation of many drugs or their metabolites, increasing the potential of toxicities, especially for drugs with narrow therapeutic windows, which necessitates modification in dose or frequency of administration. Therefore, access to appropriate dose modification tables is critical. Such tables are available in nephrology textbooks, handbooks, and in electronic format.

In addition, some commonly used drugs can interfere with renal function tests, and awareness of this knowledge helps in interpreting these tests.

ETIOLOGY AND PATHOGENESIS

RENAL SUSCEPTIBILITY TO TOXIC INSULTS

The kidneys are uniquely susceptible to toxic insults. A number of anatomic and functional characteristics account for this vulnerability, including the following:

1. A high renal blood flow (20% to 35% of the cardiac output supplies 0.4% of total body weight) ensures prompt delivery of toxic solute to the renal cortex.
2. A high metabolic activity of the renal tubular cells makes the kidney highly vulnerable to metabolic inhibitors.
3. Countercurrent multiplier mechanisms raise drug concentrations in the renal medulla to levels higher than elsewhere in the body, increasing the risk of toxic exposure.
4. Urinary concentration mechanisms enhance increase solute concentrations in the tubular lumen, exposing the epithelium to high toxic concentration.
5. Changes in urinary pH alter solubility of excreted drugs, leading to their intratubular precipitation.
6. Specific cell-surface receptors and elaborate tubular ion transport mechanisms facilitate drug binding and entry into cells.
7. The large endothelial cell surface area accounts for the kidneys' vulnerability to damage by vasoactive drugs or immune complexes.

Kidney damage can result from either a result of direct reactivity of nephrotoxic drugs with cellular macromolecules and membrane components, (e.g., aminoglycosides and amphotericin B),

TABLE 32-1. Clinical Syndromes of Drug-Induced Renal Disease*

Hypertension	Hyperkalemia
Acute nephritis	Hyponatremia
Nephrotic syndrome	Fanconi syndrome
Acute renal failure	Renal tubular acidosis
Chronic renal failure	Renal salt wasting
Obstructive uropathy	Nephrogenic diabetes insipidus
Prerenal azotemia	Sterile pyuria

*A combination of syndromes can be encountered (e.g., nephrotic syndrome and acute renal failure as with nonsteroidal anti-inflammatory drugs [NSAID]).

or from their metabolism within cells to toxic products (e.g., cisplatinum, cephalosporins, and acetaminophen). The time frame depends on the amount of toxin exposure and the insult mechanisms. The interval between exposure and onset of manifestations could be hours (some cephalosporins and anesthetic agents), days (aminoglycosides and cis-platinum), or weeks to months (nonsteroidal anti-inflammatory drugs [NSAID]); or even several years (analgesic nephropathy and lithium) (1).

Awareness of the clinical syndromes of drug-induced renal disease and the factors that place patients at a heightened risk for such problems is of utmost importance. These are listed in Tables 32-1–32-3.

EFFECT OF ABNORMAL KIDNEY FUNCTION ON DRUG DISPOSITION

The kidneys are the major organs responsible for the metabolism and elimination of most drugs. Reduced kidney function causes accumulation of the parent drug or its metabolites, resulting in an increase in the frequency and severity of adverse reactions. An altered milieu of renal dysfunction also has a significant impact on other pharmacokinetic aspects, such as absorption, distribution, protein binding, and metabolism (2). Understanding the basic principles and processes controlling drug clearance under normal conditions and during renal failure is therefore extremely important.

TABLE 32-2. Drugs Causing Acute Interstitial Nephritis*

PENICILLINS:

Methicillin, ampicillin, carbenicillin, penicillin, nafcillin, oxacillin, amoxicillin

OTHER ANTIBIOTICS:

Sulfonamides, polymixin, cephalosporins, rifampicin, erythromycin, cotrimoxazole, lincomycin, PAS, quinolones, indianavir, nitrofurantoin, vancomycin, teicoplanin.

NSAID:

Aspirin, fenoprofen, benoxaprofen, glafenine, ibuprofen, indomethacin, ketoprofen, mefenamic acid, naproxen, phenylbutazone, sulfinpyrazone, tolmetin, zomepirac.

DIURETICS:

Thiazides, furosemide, ethacrynic acid, triamterene, indapamide

HEAVY METALS:

Gold, bismuth

MISCELLANEOUS:

Allopurinol, amphetamine, azathioprine, captopril, cimetidine, clofibrate, phenindione, phenobarbital, phenytoin, propranolol, carbamazepine, valproate, omeprazole, ranitidine, warfarin.

*This list will continue to expand.
NSAID, nonsteroidal anti-inflammatory drugs.

Absorption

Diffusion of ammonia across the gastric epithelium buffers the gastric acid and raises the pH. This affects the pH-dependent absorption of drugs, such as ferrous sulfate, folic acid, pindolol, ketoconazole, and cloxacillin. Coadministration of ascorbic acid may partly offset this effect on gastric acidity.

Distribution

After absorption, the parent drug or its active metabolite is distributed throughout various body compartments. The volume of distribution depends on its water or lipid solubility, and binding to carrier molecules, such as plasma proteins. A number of cationic compounds accumulate in renal failure and compete for binding with negatively charged albumin (3). This competitively inhibits the protein binding of a number of drugs. Hypoalbuminemia, a frequent finding in renal failure, also limits the number of available binding sites. Both these factors serve to raise the free drug concentration in the circulation. Another important factor altering drug distribution is the hydration status. Fluid retention increases the volume of distribution, especially of water-soluble drugs. Alteration in the fat-to-muscle ratio, such as with age, can also affect the volume of distribution (4).

Metabolism

Pharmacokinetic studies demonstrate that the nonrenal clearance of several drugs is reduced in chronic renal failure (CRF). Although the mechanism is unclear, studies have shown that CRF affects drug metabolism by inhibiting key enzymatic systems in the liver, intestine, and kidney. CRF also affects intestinal absorption secondary to altered activity of important transporter proteins encoded by the CYP and MDR1 genes. The repercussions of such alterations on the systemic clearance of drugs are still poorly defined for most drugs. Drugs whose clearance is reduced include acyclovir, aztreonam, moxalactam, cefotaxime, captopril, cimetidine, allopurinol, and metoclopramide. In contrast, the clearance of phenytoin is enhanced.

Elimination

The kidneys play a central role in drug elimination via glomerular filtration, active tubular secretion, and passive diffusion. After filtration, polar compounds are concentrated in the urine and some are secreted in the tubules by active ion transport mechanisms. Some examples are penicillins, cephalosporins, salicylates, furosemide, thiazides, amiloride, procainamide, and quinidine. Drugs that are handled by the same transport system compete for excretion, and may inhibit each other's tubular secretion (e.g., probenecid, penicillins,

TABLE 32-3. Drugs Causing Dyselectrolytemias

1. Hypokalemia or hypomagnesemia: Gentamicin, cisplatin, diuretics, carboplatin, steroids, amphotericin B, β-adrenergic agonists.
2. Metabolic alkalosis: Thiazide or loop diuretics
3. Hyperkalemia
   a. ACE inhibitors: Antialdosterone effect. Risk factors are ↓ Renal blood flow and ↑ K
   b. Beta-blockade: Antiadrenergic effect
   c. Digitalis overdose: Inhibition of the Na-K ATPase
   d. Succinylcholine: Reduction of membrane potential
   e. Alcohol, statins, fibrates: By causing rhabdomyolysis
4. Hyponatremia:
   a. ↑ ADH secretion, ↓ water excretion (SIADH): IV cyclophosphamide, vinca alkaloids, thiothixene, thioridazine, haloperidol, amitriptyline, MAOI, bromocriptine
   b. ↑ ADH sensitivity: Chlorpropamide, carbamazepine, tolbutamide, IV cyclophosphamide
   c. Exogenous ADH administration: Vasopressin, oxytocin
5. Hypernatremia caused by ↓ ADH response in collecting tubules → polyuria (nephrogenic diabetes insipidus): Lithium, demeclocycline, ifosfamide, propoxyphene, methoxyflurane
6. Renal tubular acidosis (RTA):
   a. Type I (distal) RTA: Amphotericin B, lithium, analgesic abuse, ifosfamide, toluene, vitamin D overdose
   b. Type II (proximal) RTA: Acetazolamide, outdated tetracycline, lead, cadmium, mercurials, ifosfamide

ACE, angiotensin-converting enzymes; ATPase, adenosine triphosphatase; ADH, antidiuretic hormone; SIADH, syndrome of inappropriate secretion of antidiuretic hormone; IV, intravenous; MAOI, monoamine oxidase inhibitor.

cephalosporins, and furosemide). As nonpolar compounds are passively reabsorbed from the lumen down the concentration gradient, their elimination is less efficient. Hepatic metabolism converts many nonpolar compounds to more polar ones, suitable for excretion by the kidneys.

EFFECT OF DRUGS ON COMMON KIDNEY FUNCTION TESTS

In addition to their effect on the structure and function of the kidneys, several drugs interfere with commonly used assays for testing kidney function, even when the kidneys are structurally and functionally healthy. Awareness of such interactions prevents unnecessary search for kidney disease and allows use of appropriate drugs. A list of these is provided in Table 32-4. Further, cimetidine blocks the tubular secretion of creatinine. Because secretion contributes significantly to creatinine excretion in states with reduced GFR, interference may elevate the serum creatinine, producing an erroneous impression of reduced kidney function.

CLINICAL MANIFESTATIONS AND PATHOLOGY

NONSTEROIDAL ANTI-INFLAMMATORY DRUGS (NSAID)

Adverse renal consequences of NSAID, which are mediated by inhibition of the cyclo-oxygenase (COX) (5), can take several forms. These are hemodynamic acute renal failure, water retention manifesting as hyponatremia, blunting of diuresis induced by loop diuretics, and hyperkalemia. Some NSAID (sulindac, low-dose aspirin, and ibuprofen) may have a lower nephrotoxic potential, possibly because of their relative sparing of renal prostaglandin synthesis (6). Even the selective COX-2 inhibitors have been shown to produce acute renal failure (ARF).

A unique syndrome encountered with long-term NSAID use is a combination of acute tubulointerstitial nephritis and minimal change nephrotic syndrome. Usually seen after months to years of NSAID use, this syndrome resolves when therapy is discontinued. Prolonged NSAID use has also been implicated in renal papillary necrosis and CRF, but the cause-and-effect relationship remains unproved (7,8).

DRUGS ACTING ON RENIN-ANGIOTENSIN SYSTEM

Agents acting on the rennin-angiotensin system (angiotensin-converting-enzyme inhibitors and angiotensin receptor blockers) have emerged as powerful drugs for cardiovascular and renal protection in patients with diabetes mellitus, hypertension, and other vascular diseases. They can produce a syndrome of functional acute renal insufficiency in patients with bilateral renal artery stenosis or stenosis in a solitary kidney, and in those with reduced effective intravascular volume and preexisting chronic renal disease (9). An approximate 30% reduction in GFR is expected on initiation of angiotensin-converting enzyme inhibitors or angiotensin II receptor blockers (ACEI/ARB) and should not prompt discontinuation of the drug in view of the long-term benefits that accrue with the use of these agents (10). Hyperkalemia is another potentially serious side effect. ACE inhibitors should not be used during pregnancy. Women in the reproductive age group should be counseled and switched to alternate drugs before a planned pregnancy. In case pregnancy occurs while on these drugs, they should be stopped in the first trimester.

TABLE 32-4. Effect of Drugs on Common Kidney Function Tests

1. Semiquantitative exaimination of proteinuria
   a. False–positive dipstick test: Alkalizers, phenazopyridine, contamination with antiseptics
   b. False–positive turbidimetric test: Tolbutamide, penicilline, cephalosporins (large doses), sulfisoxazole, contrast media
2. Serum creatinine
   a. Elevate creatinine value by interfering with tubular secretion: Cimetidine, trimethoprim, triamterene, amiloride, probenecid.
   b. Elevate creatinine value by interfering with chromogenic reac tion in Jaffe's method: vitamin C, cephalosporins

AMINOGLYCOSIDE ANTIBIOTICS

Aminoglycoside antibiotics are excreted by glomerular filtration; a small portion is reabsorbed and stored in the proximal tubular cells. After entry into the tubular cells, aminoglycosides are sequestered in lysosomes, where they interfere with the enzymatic action of phospholipases and sphingomyelinases (11). Toxicity often presents as acute tubular necrosis. Major risk factors include drug dose and duration, concurrent administration of other nephrotoxins, renal ischemia, and liver failure. Toxic potential is highest for neomycin, followed by gentamicin, tobramycin, netilmicin, amikacin, and streptomycin.

Experimental studies and human clinical trials have confirmed the effect of dose schedule on renal uptake of aminoglycosides (12–14). Compared with split dosing, consolidated administration of the drug once every 24 to 48 hours reduces the incidence of ARF, without compromising drug efficacy.

RADIOCONTRAST MEDIA

Use of water-soluble iodinated contrast media is associated with the risk of ARF and it is directly related to the osmolality of the contrast solution. Pre-existing renal insufficiency, diabetes, heart failure, and high contrast dose increase the risk of this complication. The risk can be minimized by using low or iso-osmolar contrast agents or the lowest possible dose, avoiding closely spaced repetitive studies and using adequate hydration. Although not universally accepted, administration of N-acetylcysteine on the day before and the day of the procedure, or sodium bicarbonate before contrast injection and for 6 hours afterwards can further reduce the risk (15,16). Alternative use of imaging procedures, such as ultrasound or MRI, should be done wherever possible. Gadolinium, the contrast agent used in MRI, carries low, or no, risk of nephrotoxicity in those with normal renal function, but can precipitate ARF in stage 3 to 4 CKD patients.

CIS-PLATINUM

Cis-platinum use carries a substantial (25% to 40%) risk of ARF. The prevalence of this complication increases during subsequent chemotherapeutic cycles, and renal failure may become irreversible with prolonged use. The vulnerability is almost certainly linked to the primary role of the kidney in its excretion. The drug is toxic to the S3 segment of the proximal tubule, especially in low-chloride states (17). Other abnormalities noted with cis-platinum use are hypomagnesemia, hypocalcaemia, hypokalemia, impaired concentrating ability, and incomplete distal tubular acidosis. Hydration with hypertonic saline before administration is protective. Dose fractionation or infusion over 3 to 5 days and administration of sodium thiosulfate or amifostine reduces the risk of renal toxicity.

LITHIUM

Long-term lithium use can give rise to renal injury. The most common clinical manifestations are nephrogenic diabetes insipidus and chronic interstitial nephritis; but acute renal failure, renal tubular acidosis, nephrotic syndrome, and focal segmental glomerulosclerosis have also been described (18). Some degree of concentrating defect must be accepted along with the therapeutic effect of this drug. The mechanism is reduction of water channels and interference with the H^+-adenosine triphosphatase (ATPase) pump activity in cells of collecting tubule. A progressive tubulointerstitial nephropathy characterized by interstitial fibrosis and tubular dilatation has been described in 15% to 20% of patients on long-term lithium therapy, especially among those on high dosage and those with decreased effective circulating volume or low sodium intake (19). Careful monitoring of serum lithium concentration and maintenance of volume status are helpful in preventing this complication. Monitoring of serum creatinine and early withdrawal at the first indication of a rise can prevent progressive disease. Once the creatinine level exceeds 2 mg/dL, withdrawal may not halt disease progression.

CHINESE HERBAL NEPHROPATHY

A unique rapidly progressive renal failure characterized by a bland interstitial nephritis was described in the early 1990s among young European women on a slimming cocktail containing the appetite suppressants fenfluramine and diethylpropion and some Chinese herbs. A few went on to develop urothelial malignancies. Subsequent research showed a plant nephrotoxin, aristolochic acid (AA), to be the chief etiologic agent. Animal models of disease demonstrate renal hypocellular interstitial fibrosis, and atypical and malignant uroepithelial cells (20). Disease progression is related to duration of exposure and can be slowed down if detected early (serum creatinine <2 mg/dL). No effective treatment exists for this condition. In view of the high likelihood of urothelial malignancy, prophylactic bilateral nephroureterectomy has been advocated.

MANAGEMENT

DRUG-INDUCED NEPHROTOXICITY

Certain guiding principles are useful in the management of all types of drug-related nephrotoxicities. These include the following:

1. Prompt withdrawal of the offending agent, especially in acute insults
2. Assessment of intravascular volume and proper replacement, wherever necessary
3. Correction of metabolic abnormalities (e.g., acidosis, hypercalcemia, hyperuricemia)
4. Identification and correction of confounding factors (e.g., arterial and venous insufficiency)

Except for N-acetylcysteine, specific pharmacologic agents have not been found to be useful in the prevention or management of drug-induced kidney diseases. Corticosteroids may be of use in some cases of drug-induced tubulointerstitial nephritis (AIN), especially caused by use of penicillins and cephalosporins.

DRUG DOSE ADJUSTMENT IN RENAL FAILURE

Accurate prediction of pharmacokinetic parameters of a given drug in an individual patient is difficult. Periodic estimation of drug concentration in plasma or other tissues is suggested as a method for dose adjustment, which is not always practical. Moreover, the site of drug action is often not in immediate contact with the tissue or fluid being sampled. Assuming that nonrenal clearance is unaffected by renal disease and that renal clearance is proportional to the GFR, an estimate of the plasma clearance can be made if drug clearances in normal renal function are known.

In practice, serum creatinine is used as a predictor of GFR. A reciprocal relationship exists between serum creatinine and the GFR when the endogenous production and metabolism of creatinine are constant. These, however, are dependent on gender, age, and muscle mass. It is important, therefore, to calculate the creatinine clearance, rather than to rely only on serum creatinine for dose modification. Several formulae and nomograms are available for predicting the creatinine clearance from serum creatinine concentrations without the necessity of collecting urine. Because extreme accuracy is not essential, the Cockroft-Gault formula works well in this situation and is appropriate for calculating dose modifications (21).

$$Cr_{Cl} = \frac{(140 - age) \times Weight\ (kg)}{Screat\ (mg/dL) \times 72} (\times 0.85\ for\ women)$$

The goal of dose modification is to achieve the minimum, maximum, and steady-state drug concentrations as close to those with normal kidney function as possible. This can be achieved either by lowering the individual dose, increasing the dose interval, or combining the two strategies. In practice, the decision whether to reduce the dose or prolong the dose interval is not always equivalent (22,23). Adjustments should be kept simple because unfamiliar dosages at odd times of administration can result in errors (24).

All these estimates are valid only for patients with stable renal function, and may not hold true in case of ARF or unstable renal function, among patients receiving dialysis, and among

TABLE 32-5. Drugs Acting on the Central Nervous System Affected By Altered Kidney Function Along With Recommended Appropriate Dose Modifications

Drug	*Effect and Dose Modification*
Atracurium	Removed by dialysis and hemofiltration, dose adjustment needed for therapeutic effect
Chlordiazepoxide	Clcr <10 mL/min: Administer 50% of dose.
Codeine, dihydrocodeine	Clcr 10–50: Administer 75% of normal dose. Clcr <10 : Administer 50% of normal dose.
Diazepam	Accumulation can cause prolonged drowsiness in Clcr <10. Short-acting agents preferred.
Felbamate	Reduce loading and maintenance dose by 50% if Cl_{Cr} <50
Fentanyl, alfentanil	Contraindicated in severe renal failure
Gabapentin	Cl_{Cr} 30–60: 200–700 mg bid Cl_{Cr} 15–30: 25–150 mg qd Cl_{Cr} <15: 100–300 mg qd Supplement after hemodialysis
Levetiracetam	Cl_{Cr} 50–80: 500–1,000 mg bid Cl_{Cr} 30–50: 250–750 mg bid Cl_{Cr}<30: 250–500 mg bid Supplement after hemodialysis
Lithium	Clcr 10–50: Administer 50% to 75% of normal dose. Clcr <10: Administer 25% to 50% of normal dose. Hemodialysis useful in removal in cases of overdose, HD four to seven times more efficient than PD
Meperidine	Clcr 10–50: Administer 75% of normal dose. Clcr <10: Administer 50% of normal dose.
Morphine	Clcr 10–50: Administer 75% of normal dose. Clcr<10: Administer 50% of normal dose.
Morphine	Metabolite (morphine-6-glucuronide) accumulates, can cause prolonged narcosis
Oxcarbazepine	Decrease dose if Clcr <10
Phenobarbital	Clcr <10: Accumulation may occur, reduce dose frequency.
Phenytoin, valproic acid	Protein binding reduced. Free drug concentration monitoring recommended for dose adjustment.
Pregabalin	Cl_{Cr} 30–60: 75–300 mg/d in two to three doses Cl_{Cr} 15–30: 25–150 mg/d in one to two doses Cl_{Cr} <15: 25–75 mg/d Supplement after hemodialysis
Terfenadine	Can cause QT prolongation. Avoid if Clcr <10
Thiopentone	Potency increased in uremia
Topiramate	Cl_{Cr} 10–70: Decrease dose by 50% Cl_{Cr} <10: Decrease dose by 75% Supplement after hemodialysis
Tramadol	Clcr <30: 50–100 mg bid (maximum: 200 mg/d). Extended release forms should not be used if Clcr <30.
Tubocurarine, gallamine, alcuronium, pancuronium, vecuronium	Avoid in renal failure
Vigabatrin	Clcr <60: Initiate in reduced dosage. Monitor closely for sedation and confusion
Zonisamide	Contraindicated if Cl_{Cr} <50

HD, hemodialysis; PD, peritoneal dialysis; Cl_{Cr}, creatinine clearance; bid, twice daily.

patients with altered muscle mass (e.g., extreme emaciation, muscular dystrophies, and rhabdomyolysis). The GFR should be considered to be <10 mL/min in any patient with oliguric ARF, irrespective of serum creatinine values. Wherever possible, these estimates should be fine tuned on the basis of information obtained from monitoring plasma drug concentration and from assessment of the clinical response. Whether to measure steady state or peak or trough concentrations varies, and should be verified for each drug (22).

Drugs that can be cleared by hemodialysis need supplemental postdialysis dosing. Clearance during dialysis is related inversely to the degree of plasma protein binding and volume of distribution, and directly to the pore size and surface area of the filter and the blood and dialysate flows. In general, drugs with a molecular weight of >500 D, and the ones that are poorly water soluble, highly plasma protein bound, and have large volume of distribution are eliminated poorly by hemodialysis. Only drugs that have a fractional removal of >20% need postdialysis dosing. Removal of drugs is poor in continuous ambulatory peritoneal dialysis, and dosage modifications should be made assuming that the patient has a removal rate comparable with a GFR of 10 mL/min (25).

The metabolism of many commonly used drugs acting on the central nervous system (CNS) is affected in renal failure. Table 32-5 depicts the effect and appropriate dose modifications for such drugs at different levels of kidney function. A more complete list can be found in nephrology texts and drug formularies.

CLINICAL RECOMMENDATIONS OF THE VIGNETTE

The patient illustrates the effect of a drug (ramipril) on kidney function and the potentiation of toxic effect of another (meperidine) in CKD. The rise in serum creatinine and serum potassium was secondary to the hemodynamic and antialdosterone effects of ramipril. The second event highlights the need to recognize the increase in extrarenal toxic potential as a result of altered drug pharmacokinetics in CKD. In this case, the accumulation of neuroexcitatory metabolites (normeperidine) of meperidine, as a result of reduced renal excretion, led to seizures. Appropriate dose modification for the level of GFR and avoiding repeated dosing could have prevented this complication.

SUMMARY

Drugs have an intimate relationship with the kidney, a major metabolically active organ. Each one influences how the other functions. The relationship is a dynamic and complex one and has important clinical consequences. This awareness is important for optimal drug use, especially in those with pre-existing kidney disease.

REFERENCES

1. De Broe ME. Drug induced nephropathies. In: Davison AM, Ed. *Oxford Textbook of Clinical Nephrology*, 3rd ed. Oxford: Oxford University Press; 2005:2581–2598.
2. Carmichael DJS. Handling of drugs in kidney disease. In: Davison AM, ed. *Oxford Textbook of Clinical Nephrology*, 3rd ed. Oxford: Oxford University Press; 2005:2599–2618.
3. Brunner F, Zini R, Tillement JP. Dependence of drug-protein binding parameters on human serum and albumin concentration. *J Pharm Pharmacol.* 1983;35:526–528.
4. Herman RJ, McAllister CB, Branch RA, et al. Effects of age on meperidine disposition. *Clin Pharmacol Ther.* 1985;37:19–24.
5. Whelton A. Renal and related cardiovascular effects of conventional and COX-2-specific NSAIDs and non-NSAID analgesics. *Am J Ther.* 2000;7:63–74.
6. Whelton A, Stout RL, Spilman PS, et al. Renal effects of ibuprofen, piroxicam, and sulindac in patients with asymptomatic renal failure. A prospective, randomized, crossover comparison. *Ann Intern Med.* 1990;112:568–576.
7. Nuyts GD, Van Vlem E, Thys J, et al. New occupational risk factors for chronic renal failure. *Lancet.* 1995;346:7–11.
8. Sandler DP, Burr FR, Weinberg CR. Nonsteroidal anti-inflammatory drugs and the risk for chronic renal disease. *Ann Intern Med.* 1991;115:165–172.
9. Hricik DE, Browning PJ, Kopelman R, et al. Captopril-induced functional renal insufficiency in patients with bilateral renal-artery stenoses or renal-artery stenosis in a solitary kidney. *N Engl J Med.* 1983;308:373–376.
10. Opie LH, Przybojewski JZ. Angiotensin-converting enzyme inhibitor therapy. *S Afr Med J.* 1992;81:183–185.
11. Sandoval RM, Dunn KW, Molitoris BA. Gentamicin traffics rapidly and directly to the Golgi complex in LLC-PK(1) cells. *Am J Physiol Renal Physiol.* 2000;279:F884–F890.
12. Bennett WM, Plamp CE, Gilbert DN, et al. The influence of dosage regimen on experimental gentamicin nephrotoxicity: Dissociation of peak serum levels from renal failure. *J Infect Dis.* 1979;140:576–580.
13. Verpooten GA, Giuliano RA, Verbist L, et al. Once-daily dosing decreases renal accumulation of gentamicin and netilmicin. *Clin Pharmacol Ther.* 1989;45:22–27.
14. De Broe ME, Verbist L, Verpooten GA. Influence of dosage schedule on renal cortical accumulation of amikacin and tobramycin in man. *J Antimicrob Chemother.* 1991;27[Suppl C]: 41–47.
15. Sanaei-Ardekani M, Movahed MR, Movafagh S, et al. Contrast-induced nephropathy: A review. *Cardiovasc Revasc Med.* 2005;6:82–88.
16. Bagshaw SM, McAlister FA, Manns BJ, et al. Acetylcysteine in the prevention of contrast-induced nephropathy: A case study of the pitfalls in the evolution of evidence. *Arch Intern Med.* 2006;166:161–166.
17. Agarwal A, Balla J, Alam J, et al. Induction of heme oxygenase in toxic renal injury: A protective role in cisplatin nephrotoxicity in the rat. *Kidney Int.* 1995;48:1298–1307.
18. Peet M, Pratt JP. Lithium. Current status in psychiatric disorders. *Drugs.* 1993;46:7–17.
19. Markowitz GS, Radhakrishnan J, Kambham N, et al. Lithium nephrotoxicity: A progressive combined glomerular and tubulointerstitial nephropathy. *J Am Soc Nephrol.* 2000;11:1439–1448.
20. Cosyns JP. Aristolochic acid and 'Chinese herbs nephropathy': A review of the evidence to date. *Drug Saf.* 2003;26:33–48.
21. Aronoff GR, Brier ME. Use of drugs in renal failure. In: Massry SA, Glassock RW, eds. *Massry and Glassock's Textbook of Nephrology.* Philadelphia: Lippincott Williams & Wilkins; 2001:1583–1598
22. Preston SL, Briceland LL, Lomaestro BM, et al. Dosing adjustment of 10 antimicrobials for patients with renal impairment. *Ann Pharmacother.* 1995;29:1202–1207.
23. Preston SL, Briceland LL. Single daily dosing of aminoglycosides. *Pharmacotherapy.* 1995;15:297–316.
24. Swan SK, Bennett WM. Drug dosing guidelines in patients with renal failure. *West J Med.* 1992;156:633–638.
25. Lam YW, Banerji S, Hatfield C, et al. Principles of drug administration in renal insufficiency. *Clin Pharmacokinet.* 1997;32:30–57.

PART IV Gastrointestinal Diseases

CHAPTER **33**

Esophageal Disorders and Surgery

Joel M. Trugman • Colin C. Quinn • Hubert A. Shaffer, Jr.

OBJECTIVES

- To describe the clinical features of achalasia in a patient with Parkinson disease
- To explain the neuropathology and pathophysiology of achalasia
- To discuss the tests required to diagnose achalasia
- To describe the treatment options for patients with achalasia

CASE VIGNETTE

A 74-year-old woman with a 7-year history of Parkinson disease (PD) presented with 6 months of dysphagia and a 40-lb weight loss. The PD was typical in onset (asymmetric rest tremor in the hands) and mild in severity with a stable response to amantadine and low-dose carbidopa or levodopa without motor fluctuation. The patient had a 10-year history of intermittent, atypical retrosternal and upper abdominal pain for which she received a cholecystectomy without relief of symptoms. She then developed dysphagia for liquids and solids and complained of food getting caught in her throat. At night, she noted coughing and choking, particularly if she had eaten within several hours of going to bed. In the 2 months before hospital admission eating had become nearly impossible with regurgitation after each meal resulting in a 40-lb weight loss.

Esophagogastroduodenoscopy (EGD) showed no structural lesions, although it was difficult to pass the scope through the lower esophageal sphincter (LES). Barium swallow with fluoroscopy and thoracic esophagography demonstrated a dilated aperistaltic thoracic esophagus with a smooth tapering to a very narrow lumen at the LES, with only a thin line of contrast agent crossing the junction between the esophagus and stomach (Fig. 33-1). Esophageal manometry showed an aperistaltic esophagus and a nonrelaxing LES.

Based on the clinical findings and studies, the patient was diagnosed with primary achalasia. Initial treatments, including mechanical dilation and botulinum toxin injection into the LES, were minimally effective. The patient was then treated surgically with a Heller myotomy and Toupet fundoplication. Her ability to eat and drink improved, but with time she still noted significant dysphagia and regurgitation. She has required several balloon dilations of the LES. Her weight has stabilized, but the dysphagia and regurgitation persist; the swallowing problem remains much more troublesome than the motor features of parkinsonism.

DEFINITION

Achalasia is a disorder of esophageal motility characterized by failure of the LES to relax completely following swallowing and impaired peristalsis in the smooth muscle esophagus (1). Achalasia is a syndrome diagnosis with multiple causes. Achalasia is termed *primary* if no underlying cause can be found. If an underlying cause can be found (e.g., Chagas disease, carcinoma, lymphoma), achalasia is termed *secondary*. Most cases of achalasia in the United States are primary or idiopathic.

EPIDEMIOLOGY

Achalasia is a rare disease with an incidence of about 0.5 cases per 100,000 population per year and a prevalence of about 8 per 100,000 population per year (2). Males and females are affected equally and no clear racial differences are found. Achalasia is seen in children under the age of 15 years, although it is much less common than in adults, with an incidence of <0.1 per 100,000 population per year in mainland Britain.

To look for epidemiologic patterns, Sonnenberg et al. (3) analyzed the records of 15,000 achalasia hospital discharges using Medicare data on patients aged 65 years and older. Achalasia discharge rates increased fivefold in a linear fashion from the seventh to the ninth decade. In a comparable study of hospital discharge records in Great Britain, a similar and marked increase was seen in age-specific incidence of achalasia, from <1 per 100,000 population per year in the second decade to 7 per 100,000 population per year in the ninth decade (4). Interestingly, these hospital discharge data detected the concordant occurrence of achalasia in patients with PD and other *myoneural disorders*, suggesting a possible causative relationship: PD increased the risk for achalasia by twofold.

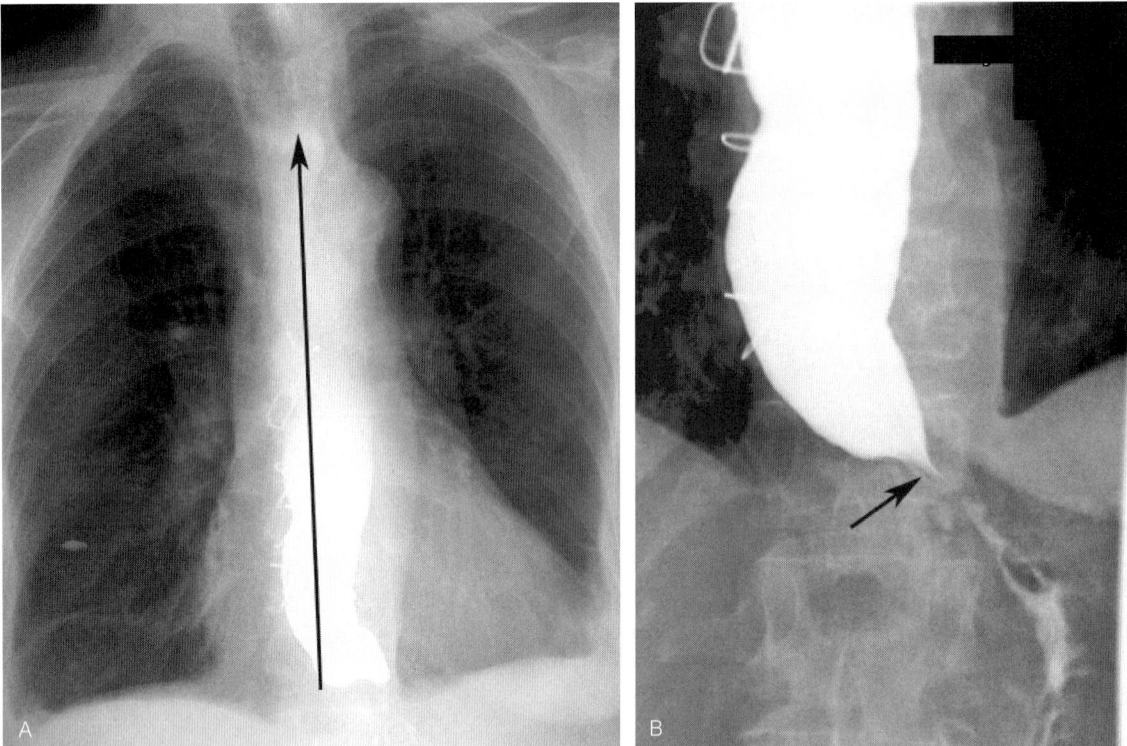

FIGURE 33-1. Achalasia. (**A**) Dilated esophagus filled with a column of barium in the standing patient 5 minutes after a barium swallow. (**B**) Dilated esophagus with a classic "bird's beak" appearance representing failure of lower esophageal sphincter (LES) relaxation.

ETIOLOGY AND PATHOGENESIS

Swallowing initiates esophageal peristalsis and triggers relaxation of the LES, the combination of which allows food to enter the stomach. Peristalsis and deglutative inhibition are mediated by neural reflexes; the motor neurons of the myenteric plexus, lying between the circular and longitudinal layers of muscle, are a critical component of these reflexes. These enteric motor neurons are either excitatory (using acetylcholine as a transmitter) or inhibitory (using nitric oxide [NO] and vasoactive polypeptide [VIP]) on esophageal smooth muscle (5).

In achalasia, the fundamental problem is a failure of deglutative inhibition with impaired relaxation of the LES after swallowing. The pathology that underlies this dysfunction is a loss of ganglion cells, particularly in the lower esophagus. Evidence suggests that the loss of inhibitory enteric motor neurons is the key feature of achalasia pathophysiology.

In the early 1990s NO was discovered as the transmitter that mediates inhibition (relaxation) of the LES. This prompted the investigation of NO in achalasia. Mearin et al. (6) studied surgical specimens from eight patients with achalasia and six controls. NO synthase enzyme activity in esophageal muscle was present in controls and not detectable in the patients with achalasia. Similarly, NO synthase was present immunohistochemically in the myenteric plexus of the gastroesophageal junction in controls, but was absent in the achalasia specimens. This evidence for the loss of NO-utilizing inhibitory myenteric neurons provides a basis for the failure of LES relaxation in achalasia and is consistent with the observation that nitrates relax the LES and are therapeutically useful in this disorder.

The cause of the ganglion cell loss in primary achalasia is unknown. Two main theories have been proposed, an immune-mediated pathogenesis and a neurodegenerative cell loss. Evidence supporting an immune-mediated pathogenesis includes the inflammatory infiltrate seen pathologically with cytotoxic T cells and the presence of serum antibodies against myenteric neurons in some patients with achalasia. Evidence supporting a neurodegenerative basis for the myenteric cell loss is the pathologic report of Lewy bodies in degenerating ganglion cells in patients with achalasia.

Cancer, usually gastric or esophageal carcinoma or lymphoma, is an important cause of secondary achalasia. These tumors can cause an achalasia phenotype by mechanical obstruction, invasion of the myenteric plexus, or by paraneoplastic ganglion cell loss. In Chagas disease, the esophageal infection with the parasite *Trypanosoma cruzi* leads to destruction of the myenteric ganglion cells. Other secondary causes of achalasia include amyloidosis, eosinophilic gastroenteritis, and sarcoidosis.

PATHOLOGY

The main pathologic abnormality in achalasia is loss of ganglion cells in the myenteric (Auerbach) plexus, resulting in denervation of the smooth muscle esophagus, including the LES. Therefore, achalasia is a neurologic disorder, a primary disorder of the enteric nervous system. Although not as well documented, evidence also exists for cell loss in the dorsal motor nucleus of the vagus (DMNX) in the medulla, which provides the preganglionic parasympathetic innervation to the esophagus, as well as degeneration of the vagus nerve.

The pathology of both early and late-stage achalasia has been studied (7,8). In 42 patients who had total thoracic esophagectomy for end-stage achalasia, findings at gross examination included tapering of the gastroesophageal junction, dilatation of the esophageal body, and hypertrophy of the muscular layer. The main histologic finding was a near-total loss of ganglion cells and destruction of the myenteric nerves. Inflammation was present in the myenteric plexus in all cases and the infiltrate was a mixture of lympocytes and eosinophils with a few plasma cells and mast cells. The inflammatory infiltrate was in and around the myenteric nerves, which were focally replaced with collagen. Other pathologic features, likely secondary to the physiologic obstruction, included hypertrophy of the circular layer of the muscularis propria and stasis-related changes in the mucosa. The histopathologic features of earlier-stage achalasia were studied by examining deep muscle strips taken at the time of esophagomyotomy in 11 patients with mild to moderate esophageal dilatation. Ganglion cells were markedly diminished in number or absent in 8 of 11 cases. Myenteric inflammation, which was present in all cases, ranged from slight to severe. Infiltration of the ganglion cell cytoplasm by lymphocytes (ganglionitis) was observed in 2 of 11 cases. Myenteric inflammation may be the earliest pathologic feature of achalasia. The authors concluded that achalasia results from a primary inflammatory process with a secondary destruction of ganglion cells and nerves. In the earlier stage of the disease, the myenteric infiltrate is composed mainly of CD3-positive T cells. In the patients with end-stage disease, the myenteric infiltrate is T cells or a mixture of T and B cells. The extent of inflammation appears to decrease with disease progression. The immunologic characteristics of the myenteric infiltrate are consistent with an immune-mediated cause of achalasia (9).

A different line of evidence suggests that a primary neurodegenerative process may underlie achalasia in a subset of patients. Cassella et al. (10) studied 34 patients with achalasia at autopsy and demonstrated wallerian degeneration in the vagus nerve branches in the lower esophagus, and approximately 40% neuronal loss in the DMNX, in addition to a marked loss of ganglion cells in the myenteric plexus. In another autopsy study, Qualman et al. (11) reported Lewy bodies, intracytoplasmic inclusions which are the histological hallmark of PD, in degenerating ganglion cells in the esophageal myenteric plexus in two of eight patients with achalasia. They also reported esophageal Lewy bodies in patients with PD and dysphagia. One patient with achalasia also had Lewy bodies in both the DMNX and the substantia nigra, clearly meeting pathologic criteria for PD. Lewy bodies were absent in patients with long-standing achalasia and near-total ganglion cell loss. In another study of seven patients with PD, Lewy bodies were found in Auerbach and Meissner plexuses, more frequently in the myenteric plexus (Auerbach) than in the submucosal plexus (Meissner) (12). Lewy bodies were found throughout the gastrointestinal tract, but were most abundant in the lower esophagus. Wakabayashi et al. (12) showed that Lewy bodies in PD are observed mainly in vasoactive intestinal peptide (VIP) inhibitory neurons of the enteric nervous system, the same neurons preferentially affected in achalasia. Braak et al. (13) recently demonstrated alpha-synuclein immunoreactivity in the nerve cells and processes of both Auerbach and Meissner plexuses in PD. These interesting studies spanning 40 years suggest that, in a subset of patients, the enteric pathology of PD, with a preferential loss of VIP inhibitory neurons, may cause achalasia. These studies may be particularly relevant to the patient presented in the case vignette.

CLINICAL MANIFESTATIONS

Dysphagia, a common symptom in patients with PD, is often attributed to oropharyngeal dysfunction. Using simultaneous videoradiography and pharyngeal manometry, Ali et al. (14) documented impaired upper esophageal sphincter relaxation and weak pharyngeal contraction in patients with PD. Dysphagia caused by esophageal dysfunction in PD has received less systematic study.

The common presenting features of achalasia are dysphagia, regurgitation, chest pain, and weight loss. Dysphagia is for both solids and liquids and results from functional obstruction at the gastroesophageal junction. This is in contrast to patients with obstructing mass lesions, such as esophageal carcinoma, who experience more dysphagia for solids than liquids. Patients with achalasia typically can swallow without difficulty but note that food gets stuck in the substernal region; the site of obstruction is at or below the level that the patient identifies.

Some symptoms can be attributed to retained food in the esophagus. Regurgitation of undigested food and saliva is common; aspiration of esophageal contents can lead to cough and pulmonary complications. Chest pain may be caused by esophageal dilatation or spasm. Difficulty with belching, caused by an impaired upper esophageal sphincter belch reflex, occurs and may contribute to chest pain. Heartburn, which is surprisingly common, is caused by esophageal acidification because of fermentation of retained food rather than gastroesophageal reflux. Weight loss has been reported in 65% of patients and can range from mild to severe. For the patient presented in the clinical vignette, weight loss was profound and life-threatening.

The symptoms of achalasia can be atypical and insidious in onset. Patients often do not realize the degree to which their swallow has been impaired and their eating habits altered. In a prospective study, dysphagia was the initial symptom in only 39% of patients; slow eating, regurgitation, and stereotyped movements during meals (e.g., arching of the neck and shoulders or raising the arms) were common symptoms at the time of diagnosis (15). The average time from first symptom to diagnosis is 4 to 5 years and this delay mainly results from misinterpretation of symptoms and misdiagnosis (15,16). Dysphagia is not the most frequently reported symptom over time and no clear correlation exists between symptom severity and radiographic findings (15).

DIAGNOSTIC APPROACH

The diagnosis of achalasia is established with barium swallow radiography and esophageal manometry. Findings on thoracic esophagography include a dilated esophagus with an air–fluid level and a nonrelaxing LES giving the distal esophagus a classic "bird's beak" appearance. The esophagus can be tortuous and sigmoidal and the gastric air bubble may be absent. Fluoroscopy reveals the absence of peristalsis in the middle and lower esophagus; the nonperistaltic and uncoordinated contractions of "vigorous achalasia" can also be seen. Esophageal dilatation and air–fluid level can occasionally be seen on plain chest x-ray film. Barium swallow radiography has limited sensitivity, however; the diagnosis of achalasia is suggested in only 65% of cases by radiography alone (17,18).

Manometry is the most sensitive test for the diagnosis of achalasia. The defining features of achalasia are absence of peristalsis in the distal esophagus and absent or incomplete LES relaxation; using these criteria, the diagnostic sensitivity of manometry is 90% (19). Supportive features include an elevated resting LES pressure and low amplitude esophageal body contractions. Variants have been described, including high amplitude esophageal body contractions (vigorous achalasia) and the presence of transient LES relaxation (19). These variants have expanded the spectrum of manometric findings seen in achalasia and emphasize that manometry must be considered in the context of other clinical data to detect atypical cases. Endoscopy is used mainly to exclude structural pathology, such as strictures and tumors. Endoscopic findings consistent with achalasia include dilatation, atony of the esophageal body, and a pinpoint appearance of the LES (1). Endoscopy is not a sensitive screening test for the diagnosis of achalasia; less than a third of endoscopies in appropriately diagnosed patients are consistent with achalasia and 44% are normal (17).

TREATMENT

Because the basic mechanism underlying myenteric ganglion cell degeneration is unknown, no treatment is aimed at preventing cell death. Rather, the treatment of achalasia aims to reduce the LES pressure to correct the functional obstruction. LES pressure can be reduced by drugs, dilation, or surgical myotomy. The definitive treatment is disruption of the LES surgically or with pneumatic balloon dilation.

Several drugs, including nitrates (isosorbide dinitrate), calcium channel blockers (nifedipine), and phosphodiesterase type 5 inhibitors (sildenafil), reduce LES pressure. They can be given before meals and have benefit in achalasia (20). Medical therapy is generally ineffective over the long term, however, and is used as a temporary measure before definitive treatment.

The intrasphincteric injection of botulinum toxin, introduced in the 1990s, reduces LES pressure and improves dysphagia (21). Botulinum toxin inhibits the release of acetylcholine from the nerve terminals of excitatory enteric motor neurons. The clinical benefit is short lived, similar to its effect in skeletal muscle, and it is not considered definitive treatment.

Therapeutic balloon dilation of the LES to a diameter of about 3 cm disrupts the circular muscle of the sphincter and lowers LES pressure. Reducing the pressure to <10 mm Hg is predictive of a good outcome and repeat dilations are not unusual. Esophageal perforation is a rare complication.

Laparoscopic esophagomyotomy, combined with a partial fundoplication, is the surgical procedure of choice for achalasia. Dysphagia is improved in >90% of patients and the complication rate is low (22). Postmyotomy reflux is treated with proton pump inhibitors. Laparoscopic myotomy and pneumatic dilation are both considered effective and debate exists to which is the optimal initial therapy. The patient presented in the vignette was treated surgically and has required repeat pneumatic dilations.

CLINICAL RECOMMENDATIONS OF THE VIGNETTE

The patient with PD developed dysphagia and weight loss. Dysphagia is common in PD and is most often attributed to oropharyngeal dysfunction. The modified barium swallow with videofluoroscopy is often used to evaluate dysphagia, but this test examines only the oropharyngeal and upper esophageal swallowing function. This case illustrates that lower esophageal causes of dysphagia should not be overlooked in patients with PD; thoracic esophagography, endoscopy, and manometry are needed to evaluate such cases thoroughly.

SUMMARY

We presented a patient with mild PD who developed severe dysphagia and weight loss caused by achalasia. Achalasia is a disorder of esophageal motility characterized by failure of the LES to relax with swallowing and impaired peristalsis in the smooth muscle esophagus. Pathologically, there is loss of ganglion cells in the myenteric plexus, resulting in denervation of the smooth muscle esophagus. Therefore, achalasia is a neurologic disorder, a primary disorder of the enteric nervous system. Evidence suggests achalasia is caused by inflammation in the myenteric ganglia, other evidence also suggest that a primary neurodegenerative process with Lewy body formation may underlie achalasia in some patients. Physiologically, the loss of NO-utilizing inhibitory enteric neurons accounts for the failure of LES relaxation. The common clinical symptoms of achalasia are dysphagia, regurgitation, chest pain, and weight loss. Esophageal manometry and barium swallow esophagography are needed to establish the diagnosis. Pneumatic balloon dilation and surgical esophagomyotomy are the best treatments to reduce LES pressure and correct the physiologic obstruction.

REFERENCES

1. Kahrilas PJ, Pandolfino JE. Motility disorders of the esophagus. In: Yamada T, ed. *Textbook of Gastroenterology*, 4th ed. Philadelphia: Lippincott William & Wilkins; 2003:1165–1195.
2. Mayberry JF. Epidemiology and demographics of achalasia. *Gastrointest Endosc Clin N Am.* 2001;11(2):235–248.
3. Sonnenberg A, Massey BT, McCarty DJ, et al. Epidemiology of hospitalization for achalasia in the United States. *Dig Dis Sci.* 1993;38(2):233–244.
4. Mayberry JF, Atkinson M. Variations in the prevalence of achalasia in Great Britain and Ireland: An epidemiological study based on hospital admissions. *Q J Med.* 1987;62(237):67–74.
5. Goyal RK, Hirano I. The enteric nervous system. *N Engl J Med.* 1996;334(17):1106–1115.
6. Mearin F, Mourelle M, Guarner F, et al. Patients with achalasia lack nitric oxide synthase in the gastro-oesophageal junction. *Eur J Clin Invest.* 1993;23(11):724–728.
7. Goldblum JR, Whyte RI, Orringer MB, et al. Achalasia: A morphologic study of 42 resected specimens. *Am J Surg Pathol.* 1994;18(4):327–337.
8. Goldblum JR, Rice TW, Richter JE. Histopathologic features in esophagomyotomy specimens from patients with achalasia. *Gastroenterology.* 1996;111(3):648–654.
9. Clark SB, Rice TW, Tubbs RR, et al. The nature of the myenteric infiltrate in achalasia: An immunohistochemical analysis. *Am J Surg Pathol.* 2000;24(8):1153–1158.
10. Cassella RR, Brown AL, Jr., Sayre GP, et al. Achalasia of the esophagus: Pathologic and etiologic considerations. *Ann Surg.* 1964;160:474–487.
11. Qualman SJ, Haupt HM, Yang P, et al. Esophageal Lewy bodies associated with ganglion cell loss in achalasia. Similarity to Parkinson's disease. *Gastroenterology.* 1984;87(4):848–856.
12. Wakabayashi K, Takahashi H, Takeda S, et al. Parkinson's disease: The presence of Lewy bodies in Auerbach's and Meissner's plexuses. *Acta Neuropathol (Berl).* 1988;76(3):217–221.
13. Braak H, de Vos RA, Bohl J, et al. Gastric alpha-synuclein immunoreactive inclusions in Meissner's and Auerbach's plexuses in cases staged for Parkinson's disease-related brain pathology. *Neurosci Lett.* 2006;396(1):67–72.
14. Ali GN, Wallace KL, Schwartz R, et al. Mechanisms of oral-pharyngeal dysphagia in patients with Parkinson's disease. *Gastroenterology.* 1996;110(2):383–392.
15. Blam ME, Delfyett W, Levine MS, et al. Achalasia: A disease of varied and subtle symptoms that do not correlate with radiographic findings. *Am J Gastroenterol.* 2002;97(8):1916–1923.
16. Eckardt VF, Kohne U, Junginger T, et al. Risk factors for diagnostic delay in achalasia. *Dig Dis Sci.* 1997;42(3):580–585.

17. Howard PJ, Maher L, Pryde A, et al. Five year prospective study of the incidence, clinical features, and diagnosis of achalasia in Edinburgh. *Gut.* 1992;33(8):1011–1015.
18. El Takli I, O'Brien P, Paterson WG. Clinical diagnosis of achalasia: How reliable is the barium x-ray? *Can J Gastroenterol.* 2006;20(5):335–337.
19. Hirano I, Tatum RP, Shi G, et al. Manometric heterogeneity in patients with idiopathic achalasia. *Gastroenterology.* 2001;120(4):789–798.
20. Annese V, Bassotti G. Non-surgical treatment of esophageal achalasia. *World J Gastroenterol.* 2006;12(36):5763–5766.
21. Kolbasnik J, Waterfall WE, Fachnie B, et al. Long-term efficacy of Botulinum toxin in classical achalasia: A prospective study. *Am J Gastroenterol.* 1999;94(12):3434–3439.
22. Patti MG, Pellegrini CA, Horgan S, et al. Minimally invasive surgery for achalasia: An 8-year experience with 168 patients. *Ann Surg.* 1999;230(4):587–593.

CHAPTER **34**

Diseases of the Stomach and Duodenum

Wolfgang H. Jost • Volker F. Eckardt

OBJECTIVES

- To define the neuroanatomic and neuropathologic causes of gastroduodenal emptying disorders
- To describe neurologic disorders that can affect upper gastrointestinal function
- To discuss the interdisciplinary relations between gastroenterology and neurology in the evaluation of patients with upper gastrointestinal motility disorders
- To suggest therapeutic alternatives from both neurologic and gastroenterologic view points

CASE VIGNETTE

A 64-year-old man presents with the chief complaint of epigastric fullness, heartburn, and nausea occurring especially on intake of fatty food. He also had two recent episodes of vomiting. He is known to have type 2 diabetes mellitus that is managed by dietary measures alone. He is a nonsmoker who rarely drinks alcohol. More recently, he has noted difficulties in buttoning his shirts as well as a disturbance of smell. Examination demonstrates an overweight man (BMI 27.5 kg/m^2) with prominent muscle stretch reflexes and increased muscle tone on his right side. Laboratory tests show a fasting serum glucose of 142 mg% and HbA1c of 7.2%. Other abnormalities were not observed. Magnetic resonance image (MRI) of the brain was normal.

DEFINITION

Gastroduodenal motor function is complex and requires the undisturbed coordination between cerebral cortex, hypothalamus, brainstem nuclei, extrinsic parasympathetic and sympathetic nerves, enteric nervous system, interstitial cells of Cajal, and the longitudinal and circular smooth muscles. Neurologic disorders involving either the central nervous system (CNS) or the peripheral nervous system (PNS) can also affect gastrointestinal motor function. The stomach and duodenum receive input from the CNS by means of sympathetic and parasympathetic nerve fibers. These nerves can modulate the activity of the enteric nervous system (*little brain of the gut*), which provides the most important control of gastrointestinal function. A wide variety of CNS disorders involving the autonomic nervous system (i.e., the nucleus of the dorsal motor vagus [DMV]) may thus lead to significantly impaired gastrointestinal motor function. Similar alterations can be caused by diseases mainly affecting the peripheral autonomic nervous system (e.g., diabetes mellitus) or the release of neurotransmitters (e.g., myasthenia gravis). On rare occasions, myopathies can involve the tunica muscularis propria of the upper gastrointestinal tract and thereby lead to significantly delayed gastroduodenal emptying (e.g., amyloidosis, muscular dystrophies, familial visceral myopathies) (Tables 34-1–34-3).

EPIDEMIOLOGY

A study reviewing the etiology of gastroparesis in 143 patients treated at a single institution, found diabetes mellitus to be the most frequent cause (1), found in 29% of all patients. This was followed by idiopathic gastroparesis, the cause of which could not be identified (28%), surgical procedures (14%), and Parkinson disease (10%). Cross-sectional studies in patients with diabetes mellitus have shown that gastric emptying is delayed in up to 50% of all patients with long-standing disease (2–5). Such finding poorly correlates with symptoms (6), but may significantly interfere with glycemic control. It is traditionally believed that gastrointestinal motor dysfunction more commonly occurs in type 1 than type 2 diabetes, but more recent studies suggest that patients with type 2 diabetes may be more frequently affected. Among several risk factors for the development of gastroparesis, the presence of cardiovascular autonomic dysfunction is the most likely clinical feature that may be associated with a motility disorder of the upper gastrointestinal tract (3,7,8).

Patients with Parkinson disease frequently complain about a variety of nonspecific gastrointestinal symptoms (9,10). Central degenerations originating at the DMV and postganglionic disturbance are possibly responsible. If carefully investigated by radioscintigraphy or 13C-octanoate breath tests, up to 88% of all patients present with significantly delayed gastric emptying for solids and liquids (11,12). Reduced gastric motility is of considerable clinical relevance because it has an impact on drug action.

TABLE 34-1. Myopathies and Neuromuscular Junction Disorders Accounting for Impaired Motility of Stomach and Duodenum

- Myopathies with gastrointestinal tract (GIT) involvement
  - Myotonic dystrophy
  - Duchene muscular dystrophy
  - Mitochondrial myopathy
  - Myasthenia gravis
- Primary myopathies of the GIT (rare)
- Secondary GIT myopathies
  - Amyloidosis
  - Scleroderma
  - Dermatomyositis

A similar alteration in gastric motor function has been described in patients with multiple system atrophy (13); a purely central cause is assumed here. Rare pathologies of the CNS resulting in abnormalities of gastroduodenal motor function are brainstem lesions, such as inflammatory diseases, tumors, arteriovenous malformations, syringomyelia, or ischemic events.

Multisystem disorders, such as scleroderma and amyloidosis, can affect gastric motor function by injuring the myenteric neurons and the different layers of gastrointestinal smooth muscle. In scleroderma, collagen replacement of vascular and enteric smooth muscle occurs in approximately 90% of all cases (14). In patients studied by either electrogastrography or gastric emptying analysis, the prevalence of motor disturbances was found to be high and could exceed 80% (15,16). These alterations almost always correlate with the presence of esophageal motor abnormalities. Amyloidosis much less frequently accounts for gastrointestinal motor dysfunction. Gastrointestinal involvement ascertained by biopsy is seen in <10% of all patients with primary amyloidosis, and only a tenth of these have symptomatic gastric disease (17). It has been suggested that gastrointestinal motor abnormalities in amyloidosis are secondary to amyloid infiltration of the myenteric plexus rather than to muscular involvement (18).

Muscular dystrophies are mainly characterized by wasting of the skeletal muscle. Involvement of gastrointestinal structures is common in myotonic muscular dystrophy, however; it is also observed in those parts of the gastrointestinal tract that consist of striated muscle (19,20). Symptoms related to the stomach are rare in these patients, but on careful investigation by scintigraphic methods, >90% exhibit impaired gastric emptying for solids and two thirds will have a delay in liquid emptying (21). The morphologic correlate to these findings remains obscure. No abnormalities were detected on light microscopy studies on esophageal smooth muscle in patients with myotonic dystrophy (19). A single investigation, however, showed dystrophic changes and fatty infiltration in the smooth muscle of the gastric wall (22).

TABLE 34-2. Neuropathies and Neuromuscular Junction Disorders Accounting for Impaired Motility of Stomach and Duodenum

- Acute peripheral neuropathies:
  - Viral infections
  - Guillain-Barré syndrome
  - Botulism
- Chronic peripheral neuropathies:
  - Chronic peripheral neuropathies (polyneuropathies as a rule)
  - Paraneoplastic neuropathies
  - Drug-induced neuropathies
  - Neurofibromatosis
  - Chronic autonomic neuropathy with inclusion bodies
  - Postvagotomy syndrome
- Autonomic neuropathies:
  - Idiopathic orthostatic hypotension
  - Pandysautonomias
  - Failure of muscarinic cholinergic receptors

TABLE 34-3. Spinal Cord and Cerebral Causes of Gastroduodenal Motility Disorder

- Spinal cord
  - Inflammatory diseases of the spinal cord
  - Vascular lesions of the spinal cord
- Cerebral
- Acute
  - Epilepsy
  - Migraine
  - Infarction
  - Encephalitides, meningitides
  - Vestibular disorders
  - Mental and emotional stress
- Chronic
  - Neurodegenerative diseases
  - Parkinson disease
  - Multisystem atrophies
  - Alzheimer disease
  - Other neurodegenerative disorders
  - Brainstem lesions
  - Vestibular deficits
  - Space-occupying lesions
  - Normal pressure hydrocephalus
  - Psychiatric diseases

ETIOLOGY AND PATHOGENESIS

Causes of gastroduodenal motor dysfunction are manifold. First, it is necessary to differentiate with regard to the organ involved (i.e., CNS, PNS, or muscle) and second, with respect to the etiology. In many disturbances of the upper gastrointestinal tract (GIT), the causes cannot be elicited.

Disorders of autonomic innervation of the upper gastrointestinal tract can be congenital, neurogenerative, or secondary in nature. Congenital disorders are felt to be rare; neuronal intestinal dysplasia would pertain to this group. Neurodegenerative disorders are much more common. A parkinsonian syndrome is an outstanding example here (see above), associated not only with ascending degeneration (23), but also with postganglionic impairment. Involvement of the CNS or PNS within the context of systemic illness (e.g., inflammatory disorders) is, however, the most common cause of dysfunction. Additional causes are a severance of a nerve or other damage to the CNS.

PATHOLOGY

The stomach and small intestine, as well as the entire gastrointestinal tract, are innervated by the sympathetic and parasympathetic nerves, with the latter being responsible for motility enhancement. The vagus nerve plays a substantial role in parasympathetic innervation because its realm of action does not only cover the upper GIT down to the left colonic flexure,

TABLE 34-4. Autonomic Innervation of the Stomach and Small Intestine

Organ	*Preganglionic Neuron, Parasympathetic*	*Postganglionic Neuron, Parasympathetic*	*Preganglionic Neuron, Sympathetic*	*Postganglionic Neuron, Sympathetic*
Stomach	Dorsal motor nucleus of the vagus	Gastric plexus	T_6 to T_{10} (greater splanchnic nerve)	Celiac ganglion
Small intestine	Dorsal motor nucleus of the vagus	Myenteric and submucous plexus (ganglion)	T_6 to T_{10} (greater splanchnic nerve)	Celiac ganglion plus superior and inferior mesenteric ganglia

but also it affects the heart, lungs, liver, and gallbladder. Sympathetic innervation is effected via the sympathetic nerve trunk (T_6 to T_{10}) and the greater splanchnic nerve. The gastric plexus and the enteric nervous system serve as the postganglionic neuron of the parasympathetic nerve. The celiac ganglion and the superior and inferior mesenteric ganglia (Table 34-4) support the sympathetic nervous system. Moreover, gastroduodenal function is significantly and autonomously steered via the intrinsic nervous system (see Chapter 33).

The causes of impaired gastroduodenal function, thus, are found on various levels, and can originate in the cerebral, spinal, peripheral, intramural, or myogenic area (Fig. 34-1). Selective perception is not a rare phenomenon among different medical specialists. Whereas neurologists tend to focus on central lesions, gastroenterologists look for a primary lesion of the intestine or of the PNS. In peripheral lesions, the classification of cause and clinical findings is relatively simple. The classification of central lesions is considerably more demanding (Table 34-3).

In the latter situation, symptoms and findings are determined by the localization of the lesion. The DMV is apparently the most critical one, because it contributes substantially to the parasympathetic activity of the stomach and duodenum. Any lesion, either acute (e.g., stroke) or chronic (e.g., parkinsonism), will lead to reduced motility. Involvement of multiple central structures makes the clinical situation more complicated. Gastric motility is notably reduced in migraines, for instance. Cyclic vomiting is a prominent feature, even in a subgroup of patients with migraine—particularly children (24). Emotional strain can also either reduce motility or accelerate it (nucleus tractus solitarius, area postrema).

The clinical identification of peripheral lesions is somewhat easier. Neuropathies usually result in impaired motility of the entire GIT. Neuropathies can involve the entire nervous system (polyneuropathy), or it can develop focally with the stomach being the site of predilection. Autonomic neuropathy within the framework of diabetes mellitus is likely to be the most common cause of gastroparesis.

In some instances, the morphologic lesion only involves the gastrointestinal smooth muscle. Classic examples are primary and secondary myopathies as listed in Table 34-1. Most are easily recognized by the obvious systemic neuromuscular manifestations. Only rarely do patients present with gastrointestinal symptoms being the sole primary clinical manifestation. Primary myopathies limited to gastroduodenal symptoms are believed to be extremely uncommon; intestinal pseudo-obstruction can be included in that group. Some diseases affect both the intramural ganglia and the muscular system (e.g., systemic sclerosis).

CLINICAL MANIFESTATIONS

Leading symptoms in patients with gastroparesis are epigastric fullness, early satiety, nausea, vomiting, and—to a lesser extent—abdominal pain. To avoid such discomfort, these patients may have been subjecting themselves to severe dietary restrictions with resultant significant weight loss. With gastroparesis unrelated to acute viral illnesses, symptoms have usually

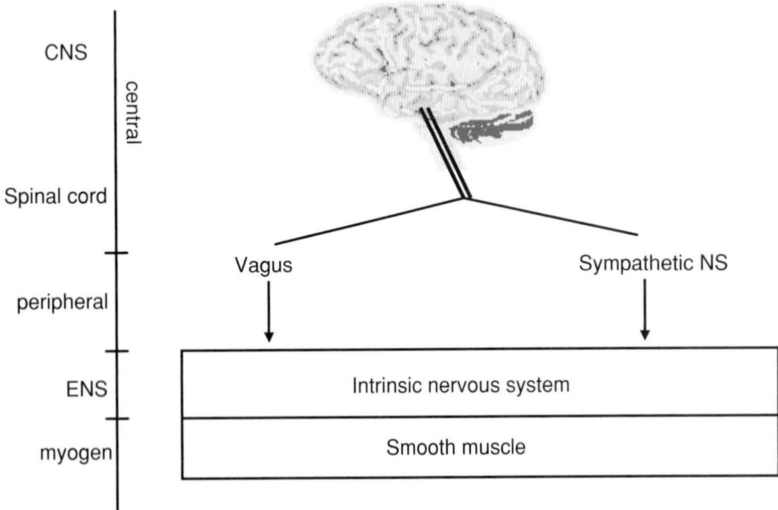

FIGURE 34-1. Efferent autonomic innervation of stomach and duodenum.

been present for several months before the patients seek medical advice, and a diagnosis can be established.

Symptoms of gastroparesis must not be confused with those of the rumination syndrome that is predominantly seen in children and young adults (25). These patients do not complain about nausea, but mainly of involuntary and gentle regurgitation of recently ingested food that is then chewed and swallowed again. In a few patients gastric emptying studies may turn out abnormal, and such results are likely to be artifactitious, owing to the frequent regurgitations encountered.

Nausea and vomiting are also an integral part of the cyclic vomiting syndrome (CVS), which is more commonly observed in children than in adults. It is characterized by recurrent episodes of nausea and vomiting lasting for hours or days, interrupted by asymptomatic intervals typically lasting weeks or months (26,27). Because all features resemble those of migraine, CVS has often been referred to as "abdominal migraine" (and been entered accordingly into the classification of the International Headache Society). Vomiting is also a frequent symptom in cerebral processes, especially with increased intracranial pressure. In infants, this symptom may give a clue to specific neurologic disorders (24).

Nausea affects up to 85% of women during their early pregnancy and about half of them will have recurrent episodes of vomiting. The precise cause of these symptoms remains unclear. Hormonal and psychological factors are most likely playing a causative part. Anorexia and early satiety are more frequently present in elderly persons than in the young (28). Studies on gastric emptying, however, have not revealed significant changes with regard to liquid and solid emptying (29).

In the early stage of Parkinson disease, patients merely indicate nonspecific gastrointestinal symptoms, such as epigastric fullness, early satiety, and heartburn (9,10). Dysphagia and relative hypersalivation are often the first symptoms (the patient produces a normal amount of saliva, but fails in swallowing it properly). The further course is characterized by notably delayed gastric emptying and substantial slow transit constipation. Delayed gastric emptying can lead to partly protracted or incalculable drug action (30).

DIAGNOSTIC APPROACH

The initial, and perhaps most important, step in evaluating patients with symptoms of disturbed gastric emptying consists in taking a careful history. This should focus on the duration of symptoms and their association with previous surgical procedures or with earlier illnesses and neurologic disturbances. A patient with recent onset of nausea, vomiting, and abdominal bloating may either have an acute viral infection, drug-induced motility disturbance, or a mechanical obstruction. In elderly patients, the differential diagnosis also includes a malignancy with ensuing obstruction or inhibition of myenteric plexus activity (e.g., paraneoplastic syndrome). In contrast, the history of patients presenting with rumination syndrome and cyclic vomiting may be so typical that further investigation need not go beyond a few noninvasive tests. On diligent review of the list of administered drugs, special attention should be paid to narcotics, anticholinergics, antihistaminics (diphenhydramine), tricyclic antidepressants, and neuroleptics that might have been used. All of these drugs are potential inhibitors of gastric emptying.

Although physical examination is rarely helpful in demonstrating the causes of gastroparesis, it is important to pay attention to possible manifestations of underlying collagen vascular diseases (Raynaud syndrome) or to signs of neurologic disorders that can potentially affect gastrointestinal motor function. A detailed neurologic examination will exclude most of the central and peripheral neurogenic causes. Cranial nerve function impairment, changes in muscle tone, paralyses and muscle stretch reflex differences, for example, are highly suggestive of neurologic disease. Ancillary laboratory investigations are aimed at detecting underlying hormonal and metabolic abnormalities, and usually can be limited to just a few parameters, such as complete blood count (CBC), erythrocyte sedimentation rate (ESR), electrolytes, calcium, serum glucose, thyrotropin, and serum cortisol levels.

Upper gastrointestinal endoscopy will be required for most patients to rule out organic obstruction. Such invasive procedures are not usually necessary in young patients with a typical history of anorexia, rumination, or cyclic vomiting. In these patients, the likelihood of detecting a mucosal disease is so low that further investigation should concentrate on gastric emptying studies. These tests are carried out for two reasons: (*a*) to avoid confusion with dyspepsia or rapid gastric emptying (31) and (*b*) to obtain quantitative information on the degree of motor disturbance, which may contribute to an objective definition of therapeutic effects.

Gastric scintigraphy is the gold standard for measuring gastric emptying abnormalities. It can be performed by either a liquid or solid meal, the latter being more informative and conclusive in terms of quantifying the clinically most important motor abnormalities. Following the intake of a 99-technetium-labeled low-fat meal, radioactivity is measured at 1, 2, and 4 hours. Retention of more than 10% after 4 hours is considered the most reliable marker for delayed gastric emptying (32).

An alternative gastric emptying test that is safe to use in children and pregnant women is the newly developed stable isotope breath test. This test is based on a meal containing $^{13}CO_2$-labeled octanoic acid, a medium-chain fatty acid that is readily absorbed in the proximal intestine, metabolized by the liver and exhaled as $^{13}CO_2$ by the lungs (33). Possible limitations of this test include unknown performance in patients with malabsorptive, hepatic and chronic pulmonary disorders.

Further methods of investigating gastric motor function are real-time ultrasonography, MRI, and gastric marker application. All of these methods are interesting investigative tools albeit of little value in daily clinical practice. Real-time ultrasonography can only be used with liquid meals; it is operator dependant, time consuming, and fails when intragastric gas is present (34). Similarly, the value of MRI-gastric emptying studies (35) is limited because they are expensive, have only been validated for liquids, and are performed in an unphysiologic supine position. The most simple, least costly, and noninvasive approach to investigate gastroduodenal motor function consists in measuring the emptying of radiopaque markers (36) from the stomach with a single upper abdominal x-ray study. These markers, however, are only expelled during phase III of the interdigestive motor complex, thus providing no reliable answer to the question of impaired emptying.

No neurophysiologic studies on gastrointestinal disorders are available in the field of neurology, however. Evoked potentials can detect and even localize spinal cord lesions, and sympathetic skin response may be a sign indicating damage to the sympathetic nervous system.

TREATMENT

In any therapy of gastrointestinal motility disorders, it is of the utmost importance to cure or improve any associated or underlying neurologic disorder. It is important to always be aware that many drugs used in the management of other diseases can also affect gastrointestinal motility (see below).

Parenteral nutrition may be required in patients presenting with the most severe forms of gastroparesis. Such therapeutic intervention should be restricted, however, to brief hospitalizations only, after which a gradual return to oral feeding is advisable. To avoid dehydration, an electrolyte solution should be given first. If this is tolerated, soft meals including soups, noodles, and rice should be offered next. The third step of oral feeding includes meals containing starches and white meat, whereas vegetables and red meat should only be offered if step 2 is tolerated without consecutive nausea or vomiting. Fatty meals will impede gastric emptying and must thus be avoided.

As stated, it is important to check for pharmaceuticals with possible or known negative effects on gastrointestinal motor function and, whenever possible, they should be withdrawn. This would pertain, for instance, to the anticholinergic action of tricyclic and tetracyclic antidepressants and many urologic agents. Table 34-5 lists substances known to interfere with normal gastric emptying (37). Every attempt should be made in diabetic patients to achieve euglycemia. Serum glucose levels between 16 and 20 mmol/L can delay gastric emptying in diabetic patients (38).

A number of prokinetic drugs shown to improve gastroparesis are now available. The first drug to be introduced into the market was the dopamine and serotonin antagonist metoclopramide (39), which possesses both antiemetic and prokinetic properties. To reduce nausea and vomiting, it has to be administered in doses of 10 to 15 mg four times daily, either orally or intravenously. It does cross the blood–brain barrier, however, and this frequently leads to CNS side effects, such as extrapyramidal symptoms, depression, and tardive dyskinesia. For this reason, it is contraindicated in neurologic disorders, such as depression and Parkinson disease. Domperidone is an alternative dopamine (D2) receptor antagonist widely available in all of Europe, but not in the United States. The prokinetic action of this drug is similar to metoclopramide (40,41), but it does not readily cross the blood–brain barrier and rarely causes adverse CNS effects. The recommended oral dose is 10 mg before meals and at bedtime, and should not exceed 20 mg three times a day. It, therefore, is the treatment of choice in Parkinson disease associated with motility problems of the upper gastrointestinal tract.

TABLE 34-5. Selection of Drugs and Substances Known to Have an Influence on Gastrointestinal Motility

Alcohol
Aluminium hydroxide antacids
Anticholinergic agents
Antidepressants, tricyclic
β-adrenergic receptor agonists
Calcium channel blockers
Calcitonin
Dexfenfluramine
Diphenhydramine
Dopamine agonists
Dopamine antagonists
Fibers
Glucagon
H_2-receptor antagonists
Interferon-α
Levodopa
Neuroleptics
Nicotine
Octreotide
Opioid analgesics
Progesterone
Proton pump inhibitors
5-hydroxytryptamine (5HT)-agonists
5HT-antagonists
Sucralfate
Tetrahydrocannabinol

The macrolide antibiotic erythromycin should be tried in those who do not respond to metoclopramide or domperidone. Erythromycin acts on the gastrointestinal receptors of motilin, thereby stimulating phase III of the migrating motor complex. It is more efficient when given intravenously (200 mg every 6 hours) than orally. If administered orally, it should be applied as a liquid suspension at doses between 250 and 500 mg 20 minutes before each meal (41). Shortcomings in the treatment with erythromycin include decreasing efficacy with long-term use, and the potential development of antibiotic resistance. Currently, intensive research is underway for a macrolide compound that would activate motilin receptors without antimicrobial effects.

Good results had been obtained when using cisapride for dysfunction of the upper gastrointestinal tract (41). This agent was taken off the market, however, because of its considerable side effects (cardiac conduction defects). It was hoped that the newer 5-hydroxytryptamine-4 (5-HT4) receptor agonists would be added to the therapeutic armamentarium in patients with gastric emptying disorders. A recent double-blind study evaluating the effectiveness of tegaserod on gastric motor and sensory function has come up with disappointing results, however (42). A more promising therapy for patients, who are not responding to any of the above treatment modalities, has been injection of botulinum toxin into the pyloric region. Botulinum toxin inhibits the cholinergic neuromuscular transmission, which may attenuate isolated pyloric pressure waves and normalize antroduodenal peristaltic activity (43). It also has been found to improve emptying of solids in patients with gastroparesis (44). The duration of a single treatment with up to 200 U of botulinum toxin has rarely exceeded 6 months (43), however, and it remains uncertain whether repeat injections would bring about the same or an even more lasting effect.

In patients refractory to any type of medical treatment, the eventual options are gastric electrostimulation or surgical procedures in the form of gastrostomy, jejunostomy, or even near-total gastrectomy. In a double-blind trial, low-energy high-frequency electrical stimulation with surgically placed electrodes at the greater curvature of the gastric antrum was shown to reduce gastroparetic symptoms in patients refractory to prokinetic drugs (45). Response to this therapy, however, is not alike in all patients, and some will develop infections requiring the removal of that device. A venting gastrostomy or feeding jejunostomy, surgically or endoscopically placed, may reduce symptoms in most severely afflicted patients refractory to any of the above measures, and thereby reduce their rate of hospitalizations (46). A near-total gastrectomy might be the last therapeutic resort when everything else has failed. Only very few patients with diabetic or idiopathic gastroparesis have had surgery so far. Therefore, no valid conclusions can be drawn yet regarding the effectiveness and safety of this approach (47).

CLINICAL RECOMMENDATIONS OF THE VIGNETTE

Two causes are related to the complaints given by the patient. It is possible that the gastroparesis was the result of improperly controlled diabetes mellitus, meaning a peripheral, autonomic cause might exist (48). Second, early parkinsonism may also be present in the patient. Parkinsonism is characterized by ascending degeneration, with degeneration of the substantia nigra being grade 3 of degeneration (23). Grade 1 presents with degeneration of the dorsal vagal nucleus and of the bulbus olfactorius (impaired smell). Abnormal gastrointestinal motility, which is frequently encountered before the onset of motor deficits, is seen in the course of this disease in approximately 80% of the patients (9), and it is responsible for some of the therapeutic complications incurred (unpredictable on-off). Optimal control of the patient's diabetes mellitus would be the primary invention in this case, along with treatment of his parkinsonism. Domperidone should be used only in case of inadequate effect. Metoclopramide would be contraindicated.

SUMMARY

Neuromuscular dysfunction of the stomach and duodenum is frequently encountered in a variety of neurologic diseases involving the autonomic nervous system. The morphologic lesions can be localized to the cerebrum, spinal cord, peripheral nervous system, neuromuscular junction, or the smooth musculature. Despite the increasing availability of elaborate ancillary diagnostic methods and therapeutic advances, an exact definition of the underlying cause may not always be possible, rendering treatment a medical challenge. If gastroenterologists and neurologists are simultaneously involved in the care of patients with disorder gastroduodenal motor function, however, a significant improvement in outcome can be anticipated.

REFERENCES

1. Bizyutskiy LP, Soykan I, McCallum RW. Viral gastroparesis: A subgroup of idiopathic gastroparesis—Clinical characteristics and long-term outcomes. *Am J Gastroenterol.* 1997;92: 1501–1509.
2. Keshavarzian A, Iber FL, Vaeth J. Gastric emptying in patients with insulin-requiring diabetes mellitus. *Am J Gastroenterol.* 1987;82:29–35.
3. Horowitz M, Maddox AF, Wishart JM, et al. Relationships between esophageal transit and solid and liquid gastric emptying in diabetes mellitus. *Eur J Nucl Med.* 1991;18:229–234.
4. Iber FL, Parveen S, Vandrunen M, et al. Relation of symptoms to impaired stomach, small bowel, and colon motility in long-standing diabetes. *Dig Dis Sci.* 1993;38:45–50.
5. Horowitz M, Fraser R. Disordered gastric motor function in diabetes mellitus. *Diabetologia* 1994;37:543–551.
6. Samsom M, Vermeijden JR, Smout AJPM, et al. Prevalence of delayed gastric emptying in diabetic patients and relationship to dyspeptic symptoms. *Diabetes Care.* 2003;26:3116–3122.
7. Ziegler D, Schadewaldt P, Pour Mirza A, et al. [13C]octanoic acid breath test for non-invasive assessment of gastric emptying in diabetic patients: Validation and relationship to gastric symptoms and cardiovascular autonomic function. *Diabetologia.* 1996;39:823–830.
8. Buysschart M, Moulart M, Urban JL, et al. Impaired gastric emptying in diabetic patients with cardiac autonomic neuropathy. *Diabetes Care.* 1987;10:448–452.
9. Edwards LL, Quigley EMM, Pfeiffer RF. Gastrointestinal dysfunction in Parkinson's disease: Frequency and pathophysiology. *Neurology.* 1992;42:726–732.
10. Jost WH. Gastrointestinal motility problems in patients with Parkinson's disease. Effects of antiparkinsonian treatment and guidelines for management. *Drugs Aging.* 1997;10:249–258.
11. Goetze O, Wieczorek J, Mueller T, et al. Impaired gastric emptying of a solid test meal in patients with Parkinson's disease using 13-C sodium octanate breath test. *Neuroscience Lett.* 2005;375:170–173.
12. Goetze O, Nikodem AB, Wieczorek J, et al. Predictors of gastric emptying in Parkinson's disease. *Neurogastroenterol Motil.* 2006;18:369–375.
13. Thomaides T, Karapanyiotides T, Zoukos Y, et al. Gastric emptying after semi-solid food in multiple system atrophy and Parkinson's disease. *J Neurol.* 2005;252:1055–1059.
14. Sallam H, McNearny TA, Chen JD. Systemic review: Pathophysiology and management of gastrointestinal motility in systemic sclerosis (scleroderma). *Aliment Pharmacol Ther.* 2006;23:691–712.
15. Sridar KR, Lange RC, Magyar L, et al. Prevalence of impaired gastric emptying of solids in systemic sclerosis: Diagnostic and therapeutic implications. *J Lab Clin Med.* 1998;132:541–546.
16. Marie I, Levesque H, Ducrotte P, et al. Gastric involvement in systemic sclerosis: A prospective study. *Am J Gastroenterol.* 2001;96:77–83.
17. Menke DM, Kyle RA, Fleming CR, et al. Symptomatic gastric amyloidosis in patients with primary amyloidosis. *Mayo Clin Proc.* 1993;68:763–767.
18. Battle WM, Rubin MR, Cohen S, et al. Gastrointestinal-motility dysfunction in amyloidosis. *N Engl J Med.* 1979;301:24–25.
19. Eckardt VF, Nix W, Kraus W, et al. Esophageal motor function in patients with muscular dystrophy. *Gastroenterology.* 1986;90:628–635.
20. Eckardt VF, Nix W. The anal sphincter in patients with myotonic muscular dystrophy. *Gastroenterology.* 1991;100:424–430.
21. Pruzanski W, Huvos AG. Smooth muscle involvement in primary muscle disease. *Arch Pathol.* 1967;83:229–233.
22. Horowitz M, Maddox A, Maddern GJ, et al. Gastric and esophageal emptying in dystrophica myotonica. Effect of metoclopramide. *Gastroenterology.* 1987;92:570–577.
23. Braak H, Del Tredici K, Bratzke H, et al. Staging of the intracerebral inclusion body pathology associated with idiopathic Parkinson's disease (preclinical and clinical stages). *J Neurol.* 2003;249[Suppl 3]:III1–III5.
24. Johns DW. Disorders of the central and autonomic nervous systems as a cause of emesis in infants. *Semin Pediatr Surg.* 1995;4:152–156.
25. Chial HJ, Camilleri M, Williams DE, et al. Rumination syndrome in children and adolescents: Diagnosis, treatment, and prognosis. *Pediatrics.* 2003;111:158–162.
26. Fleisher D, Gornowicz B, Adams K, et al. Cyclic vomiting syndrome in 41 adults: The illness, the patients, and problems of management. *BMC Medicine.* 2005;3:1–12.
27. Prakash C, Clouse RE. Cyclic vomiting syndrome in adults: Clinical features and response to trycyclic antidepressants. *Am J Gastroenterol.* 1999;94:2855–2860.
28. Firth M, Prather CM. Gastrointestinal motility problems in the elderly patient. *Gastroenterology.* 2002;122:1688–1700.
29. Madsen JL, Graff JL. Effects of ageing on gastrointestinal motor function. *Age Ageing.* 2004;33:154–159.
30. Pfeiffer RF. Gastrointestinal dysfunction in Parkinson's disease. *Lancet Neurol.* 2003;2: 107–116.
31. Delgado-Aros S, Camilleri M, Cremonini F, et al. Contributions of gastric volumes and gastric emptying to meal size and postmeal symptoms in functional dyspepsia. *Gastroenterology.* 2004;127:1685–1694.
32. Guo JP, Maurer AH, Fisher RS, et al. Extending gastric emptying scintigraphy from two to four hours detects more patients with gastroparesis. *Dig Dis Sci.* 2001;46:24–29.
33. Ghoos YF, Maes BD, Geypens BJ, et al. Measurement of gastric emptying rate of solids by means of a carbon-labeled octanoic acid breath test. *Gastroenterology.* 1993;104:1640–1647.
34. Holt S, Cervantes J, Wilkinson AA, et al. Measurement of gastric emptying rate in humans by real-time ultrasound. *Gastroenterology.* 1986;90:918–923.
35. Schwizer W, Maecke H, Fried M. Measurement of gastric emptying by magnetic resonance imaging in humans. *Gastroenterology.* 1992;103:369–376.
36. Feldman M, Smith HJ, Simon TR. Gastric emptying of solid radiopaque markers: Studies in healthy subjects and diabetic patients. *Gastroenterology.* 1984;87:895–902.
37. Parkman HP, Hasler WL, Fisher RS. American Gastroenterological Association technical review on the diagnosis and treatment of gastroparesis. *Gastroenterology.* 2004;127:1592–1622.
38. Fraser RJ, Horowitz M, Maddox AF, et al. Hyperglycaemia slows gastric emptying in type 1 (insulin-dependant) diabetes mellitus. *Diabetologia.* 1990;33:675–680.
39. Longstreth GF, Malagelada J-R, Kell KA. Metoclopramide stimulation of gastric motility and emptying in diabetic gastroparesis. *Ann Intern Med.* 1977;86:195–196.
40. Horowitz M, Harding PE, Chatterton BE, et al. Acute and chronic effects of domperidone on gastric emptying in diabetic autonomic neuropathy. *Dig Dis Sci.* 1985;30:1–9.
41. Richards RD, Davenport K, McCallum RW. The treatment of idiopathic and diabetic gastroparesis with acute intravenous and chronic oral erythromycin. *Am J Gastroenterol.* 1993;88:203–207.
42. Talley NJ, Camilleri M, Burton D, et al. Double-blind, randomized, placebo-controlled study to evaluate the effects of tegaserod on gastric motor, sensory and myoelectric function in healthy volunteers. *Aliment Pharmacol Ther.* 2006;24:859–867.
43. Gupta P, Rao SS. Attenuation of isolated pyloric pressure waves in gastroparesis in response to botulinum toxin injection: A case report. *Gastrointest Endosc.* 2002;56:770–772.
44. Arts J, van Gool S, Caenepeel P, et al. Influence of intrapyloric botulinum toxin injection on gastric emptying and meal-related symptoms in gastroparesis symptoms. *Aliment Pharmacol Ther.* 2006;24:661–667.
45. Abell T, McCallum R, Hocking M, et al. Gastric electrical stimulation for medically refractory gastroparesis. *Gastroenterology.* 2003;125:421–428.
46. Maple JT, Petersen BT, Baron TH, et al. Direct percutaneous endoscopic jejunostomy: Outcomes in 307 consecutive attempts. *Am J Gastroenterol.* 2005;100:2681–2688.
47. Jones MP, Maganti K. A systematic review of surgical therapy for gastroparesis. *Am J Gastroenterol.* 2003;98:2122–2129.
48. Kong MF, Horowitz M. Diabetic gastroparesis. *Diabet Med.* 2005;22[Suppl 4]:13–18.

CHAPTER **35**

Inflammatory Bowel Disease

Ronald F. Pfeiffer • Fergus Shanahan

OBJECTIVES

- To briefly characterize the clinical characteristics and pathophysiologic basis of Crohn disease and ulcerative colitis
- To delineate the neurologic complications that can occur in individuals with Crohn disease and ulcerative colitis
- To illuminate the mechanisms by which neurologic complications can develop in the setting of Crohn disease and ulcerative colitis

CASE VIGNETTE

A 28-year-old man began to experience abdominal and back pain, along with intermittent diarrhea while attending graduate school. His medical history was unremarkable except for psoriasis that had first appeared at about age 16. Irritable bowel syndrome was diagnosed, but his symptoms persisted despite symptomatic treatment. He progressively lost weight (>40 pounds) and began to experience recurrent leg and foot cramping. Colonoscopy was performed and, at age 29, a diagnosis of Crohn disease (CrD) was confirmed. Shortly thereafter, flulike symptoms with fever (up to 104°F) developed and he began to cough up blood-tinged sputum. He then experienced an episode of transient right hemiparesis and hemisensory deficit that prompted hospitalization. Magnetic resonance imaging (MRI) of the brain was normal, but lung scan demonstrated multiple pulmonary emboli. Further workup demonstrated the presence of deep venous thrombosis in the legs, whereas laboratory studies were remarkable for the presence of antiphospholipid antibodies.

DEFINITION

Two similar but distinct disease entities, ulcerative colitis and CrD (also known as regional enteritis or granulomatous colitis) are the most widely recognized members of a group of conditions collectively labeled *inflammatory bowel disease* (IBD). Despite many similarities, the clinical features and pathologic profiles of the two conditions demonstrate distinct differences (Table 35-1). Neurologic dysfunction may occur in both.

In 1932 Crohn et al. (1) pooled their experiences and described a condition they termed *terminal ileitis.* Colonic involvement was later recognized, prompting a renaming of the process as regional enteritis or granulomatous enterocolitis. More recently, however, it has become customary to use the eponymous designation, Crohn disease. Earlier descriptions of what probably was CrD exist. In fact, some speculate that Alfred the Great, the first king of England, may have had this condition in the 9th century.

Recognition of ulcerative colitis (UC) as a distinct disease process preceded that of CrD. Initially labeled as *idiopathic colitis,* UC was first described by Wilks in 1859 (2). By 1909, however, the disease had been more clearly recognized and it had received its current name (3).

EPIDEMIOLOGY

The incidence of CrD has considerable geographic variation. In Europe and North America, a distinct north-south gradient is present, with a higher incidence in northern latitudes. In northern Europe, for example, incidence rates of 6 to 10 per 100,000 have been noted compared with 0.9 to 3.4 per 100,000 in Spain and Italy. A significant rise in the incidence of CrD occurred in the latter half of the 20th century; the rate has now stabilized, but the reason for the increase remains uncertain (4). The incidence of CrD disease in Japan is low, and the disease is rare in much of Africa and South America. CrD occurs slightly more frequently in women than men. Median age of diagnosis is approximately 30 years.

The incidence of UC also has geographic variation. In higher incidence regions, such as Europe and North America, rates range from 3 to 15 per 100,000. Women may be at higher risk than men to develop UC, but this is less clear than with CrD. Unlike CrD, the incidence of UC has remained stable during the latter portion of the 20th century. In general, however, IBD is increasing in all developing countries and in places where it was previously rare.

One epidemiologic feature that polarizes the two conditions is smoking. Smoking is more common in CrD and it adversely affects the clinical course, whereas the cessation of smoking is often linked with the onset or exacerbation of UC. Another feature that differs between the two conditions is the apparent protective effect of early appendectomy on risk of UC with no impact on CrD.

Extraintestinal manifestations are common in both UC and CrD; reported frequencies range from approximately 25% to >50% (5–8). Some extraintestinal complications, such as involvement of joints, skin, mouth, and eyes, correlate with the presence of active colonic inflammation. Others, such as

TABLE 35-1. Gastrointestinal Features of Inflammatory Bowel Disease

Feature	*Ulcerative Colitis*	*Crohn Disease*
CLINICAL		
Malaise, fever	Only in severe cases	Common
Abdominal pain	Uncommon	Common
Diarrhea	Common	Common
Rectal bleeding	Very common	Occasionally occurs
Weight loss	Uncommon	Common
Signs of malnutrition	Uncommon	Common with small bowel involvement
Perianal disease	Rare	Common
Abdominal mass	No	Common
BOWEL COMPLICATIONS		
Stricture	Rare	Common
Fistulas	Very Rare	Common
Sepsis	Uncommon	Common
Toxic megacolon	A common cause	Can occur
Perforation	Uncommon	Uncommon
Risk of malignancy	Increased	Somewhat increased
ENDOSCOPIC		
Friability	Characteristic	Can occur
Aphthous and linear ulcers	Rare	Common
Cobblestone appearance	Never	Common
Pseudopolyps	Common	Can occur
Distribution	Continuous	Discontinuous (skip lesions)
Rectal involvement	Characteristic	Occasionally occurs
RADIOLOGIC		
Mucosal detail	Fine superficial ulcers	Deep ulceration
Fissures	Never	Characteristic
Strictures or fistulas	Rare	Common
Ileal involvement	Dilated (backwash ileitis)	Narrowed
Distribution	Continuous, symmetric	Discontinuous, asymmetric

gallstones and renal calculi, reflect small intestinal involvement and are seen primarily in CrD (9).

Complications involving the nervous system are relatively infrequent in the setting of IBD. Lossos et al. (10) reported the presence of neurologic involvement in 3% of 638 individuals they studied who had either UC or CrD. They segregated neurologic dysfunction into four categories: Peripheral neuropathy, myopathy or myoneural junction dysfunction, myelopathy, and cerebrovascular disease. Seizures, encephalopathy, and demyelinating processes have been described by other investigators. Although neurologic impairment often becomes evident during periods of disease activity, it can also emerge when the disease process appears to be quiescent. Medications used in the treatment of IBD can also cause neurologic complications to develop, but will not be addressed in detail in this chapter.

ETIOLOGY AND PATHOGENESIS

A complex interplay of an array of genetic, environmental, immunologic, and microbial factors appears to be operative in the genesis of IBD (11). Genetic factors are probably active in both CrD and UC, but have been most clearly delineated in CrD, where the CARD15 gene, which is involved in the immune detection of bacterial products, has been identified as a susceptibility gene (12,13). Mutations of this gene are present in 25% to 35% of patients of European ancestry (14). Mutations in three additional genes in CrD (PPARG, DLG5, SLC22A4/SLC22A5) and one in UC (MDR1) have also been associated with IBD. Environmental factors implicated in the pathogenesis of IBD include infection, stress, nonsteroidal anti-inflammatory drugs (NSAID) and antibiotics. Smoking is another triggering factor in CrD, but is protective in UC. How these factors incite the pathologic process is not certain, but they may increase susceptibility to inflammation by altering mucosal barrier integrity, stimulating immune responses, or changing the bacterial microenvironment within the gut lumen (11). Individuals with IBD have impaired ability to downregulate inflammatory responses to these environmental triggers, with consequent activation of both macrophage and T-cell immune responses that is persistent and destructive (11,15).

PATHOLOGY

The pathologic hallmark of CrD is focal intestinal inflammation that can develop at any level of the gastrointestinal tract, although it has a distinct predilection for the distal small intestine and proximal colon. This leads to formation of aphthous ulcers, which represent focal areas of immune activation (16). Over time, the ulcers enlarge and coalesce, producing the classic *cobblestone* appearance of the intestinal mucosa. Noncaseating granuloma formation is also characteristic of CrD, although it is neither pathognomonic for, nor universally present in, the disease. With disease progression, the inflammatory process extends transmurally, with consequent formation of sinus tracts and fistulas. Fibrosis with stricture formation is also common.

In contrast to CrD, UC is characterized by diffuse inflammation of the colonic mucosa and submucosa. Small, punctuate ulcers form and the mucosa becomes hyperemic and hemorrhagic (17). Transmural extension typically does not develop and the inflammatory process remains confined to the colon (18).

The pathophysiology of neurologic dysfunction in IBD is primarily autoimmune in character. Nutritional deficiency, coagulation abnormalities, infectious processes, such as abscess formation, and perhaps other processes may also be responsible. When known, the pathophysiology of specific neurologic complications of IBD will be noted in the discussion of their clinical manifestations.

CLINICAL MANIFESTATIONS

PERIPHERAL NEUROPATHY

Peripheral neuropathy is the most common neurologic complication of UC and CrD, accounting for 31.5% of neurologically affected patients (10). A striking array of peripheral neuropathic processes has been identified. Acute inflammatory demyelinating neuropathy (Guillain-Barré syndrome), axonal sensorimotor neuropathy, mononeuropathy, brachial plexopathy, mononeuritis multiplex, and cranial neuropathies have all been described (10,19–21). In individuals with peripheral neuropathy, axonal involvement is evident in approximately 70%, whereas the neuropathy is demyelinating in slightly less than 30% (22).

Cranial nerve involvement can also develop in IBD. Melkersson-Rosenthal syndrome, characterized by recurrent facial nerve palsy along with intermittent orofacial swelling and fissuring of the tongue, has been described in the setting of CrD. That its pathologic hallmark, formation of noncaseating granulomas, also occurs in CrD has prompted some investigators to propose that the two disorders are part of the same pathologic spectrum (23). Auditory nerve involvement, with either acute sensorineural hearing loss or chronic subclinical hearing impairment, has been reported in individuals with UC (24–28). An autoimmune basis for the auditory nerve involvement is presumed but has not yet proved.

The genesis of peripheral neuropathic involvement in IBD has not been clearly explained, and it may be multifactorial. Some investigators (29,30) have suggested nutritional deficiencies, such as vitamin B_{12} or folate. Others favor an autoimmune basis (31).

MUSCLE AND MYONEURAL JUNCTION DISEASE

Myopathic involvement was the basis for 16% of the cases of neurologic dysfunction in IBD in the experience of Lossos et al. (10). It occurs in both CrD and UC, but more frequently in CrD. A variety of myopathic processes has been described.

Inflammatory myopathies, such as dermatomyositis, polymyositis, granulomatous myositis, and rimmed vacuole myopathy, have been described in individuals with IBD. The myositic symptoms most often correlate with colonic disease activity, but occasionally may precede the development of gastrointestinal dysfunction (32). Focal myositis can also occur in CrD; involvement of the gastrocnemius has been specifically described (33).

Psoas abscess formation is a potentially dangerous complication of CrD that can lead to significant morbidity and even death (34–38). It is characterized by flank, pelvic, or abdominal pain and typically associated with fever and leukocytosis. Flexion contracture of the hip and gait impairment can be consequences of the abscess formation. Abscesses in other muscles, such as the obturator or hamstrings, can also occur. Diagnosis is confirmed by ultrasound or abdominal computed tomography (CT).

Myoneural junction dysfunction in the form of myasthenia gravis has been noted, albeit rarely, in both CrD and UC. Rhabdomyolysis, sometimes secondary to electrolyte depletion and sometimes without obvious provocation, has also been described in CrD (39).

SPINAL CORD DISEASE (MYELOPATHY AND MOTOR NEURON DISEASE)

Chronic, slowly progressive myelopathy accounted for 26% of the patients with neurologic involvement reported by Lossos et al. (10). Most individuals had CrD. The presence of oligoclonal banding in one individual prompted speculation of an inflammatory basis for the myelopathy in this setting. In patients with CrD who have had resection of the terminal ileum, subacute combined degeneration caused by vitamin B_{12} deficiency has also been reported to produce myelopathy (40,41). Transverse myelitis was reported in an individual with UC who also was found to have Jo-1 antibody (antisynthetase) syndrome (42).

Extension of fistulas to involve the epidural or subdural space can lead to epidural or subdural empyema in persons with CrD. Individuals may present with back and leg pain; progressive leg weakness can also develop (43–45).

DEMYELINATING DISEASE

Retrospective studies have suggested an association between some demyelinating diseases and IBD (46,47). Multiple sclerosis occurs more frequently in individuals with IBD than in control subjects; the association is most evident for UC (48,49). Demyelinating disease can either precede or follow the onset of gastrointestinal symptoms. The mechanism of the concurrence of the two disease processes is uncertain. In some instances, the onset of the demyelinating disease has correlated with antitumor necrosis-α therapy, such as infliximab (50,51), but this is certainly not always the case.

CEREBROVASCULAR DISEASE

Vascular complications have been well documented in the setting of both CrD and UC (52,53). In a large study involving 7,199 patients, vascular complications were evident in 1.3% (52). Deep venous thrombosis and pulmonary embolus were the most frequent sites of involvement. Cerebrovascular complications also occurred, but accounted for only 9.8% of the cases of vascular involvement. Individuals with CrD are more likely to be affected than those with UC, although cerebrovascular complications can develop in both.

Cerebrovascular complications can present in many guises in individuals with IBD. Large artery disease, with stroke caused by carotid artery stenosis, has been reported (54), as has small vessel involvement with lacunar infarction (55). Spinal cord ischemia has also been described (56). Cerebral vasculitis, presumably autoimmune in origin, can develop in the setting of both CrD and UC (57,58). Cerebrovascular complications in IBD are not confined to the arterial circulation. Venous involvement in the form of venous sinus thrombosis can occur in both CrD and UC, but predominantly in UC (59–61). Both dural and cortical venous sinus involvement have been documented, perhaps most frequently involving the superior sagittal sinus.

A unitary etiologic explanation for cerebrovascular events in IBD is unlikely. Hypercoagulability may be responsible in some instances. Elevations of factors V, VIII, and fibrinogen, along with decreased antithrombin III, have been noted in some individuals (62,63). Anticardiolipin antibodies and lupus anticoagulant antibodies may be present in others (64), although their presence does not necessarily correlate with the presence of cerebrovascular disease (65). A role has also been proposed for hyperhomocysteinemia (66,67) and both vitamin B_{12} (68) and pyridoxine deficiency (54).

ENCEPHALOPATHY AND SEIZURES

Nutritional deficiencies emerging consequent to faulty parenteral nutrition can lead to the development of diffuse encephalopathy in individuals with IBD. Both Wernicke encephalopathy (69) and possibly selenium-induced encephalopathy (70) have been described in this setting. Wernicke encephalopathy, however, has also been reported in an individual with clinically quiescent CrD (71). Other processes, such as cerebral vasculitis, can also produce diffuse encephalopathy in persons with IBD.

Seizures can occur as complications of the surgical or medical treatment of IBD, but only rarely develop as an extraintestinal component of the disease process itself (72). Fluid overload, electrolyte imbalance, and even hypoxia can trigger seizures in the surgical or postsurgical setting, whereas seizures can also be precipitated by immunosuppressant medications, such as cyclosporine, and either administration or withdrawal of steroids (73–76). Status epilepticus has also been described in the setting of UC (77).

DIAGNOSTIC APPROACH

For the most part, diagnostic evaluation of neurologic complications in the setting of IBD is accomplished via the same diagnostic testing measures that are used when these processes occur in other circumstances. Neuroimaging and neurophysiologic studies are used frequently, as are appropriate laboratory tests.

TREATMENT

The primary treatment of CrD and UC is aimed at altering the aberrant immunologic responses present in IBD (78). Glucocorticoids (e.g., prednisone) and aminosalicylate compounds (e.g., sulfasalazine and mesalamine) are widely used. Immunosuppressive agents, including azathioprine, 6-mercaptopurine, methotrexate, and cyclosporine, are also frequently utilized. In recent years, the immunomodulating agent, infliximab, has been used extensively in the treatment of CrD; its effectiveness in UC has also recently been documented (79). Antibiotics are necessary for treating pyogenic complications in CrD, but are rarely needed in UC. Surgical treatment, which can consist of resection or other procedures, often becomes necessary for patients with CrD and UC.

Treatment for the neurologic complications of IBD depends on the specific nature of the complication. Identified nutritional deficiencies must be corrected. Infections and abscesses mandate antibiotic therapy and surgical correction. Hypercoagulable states may necessitate chronic anticoagulation. Seizures may require temporary or sometimes chronic treatment with anticonvulsant medications. Use of steroids and immunosuppressive agents is frequently necessary if the basis for the neurologic complication is inflammatory.

CLINICAL RECOMMENDATIONS OF THE VIGNETTE

The presence of deep venous thrombosis with multiple pulmonary emboli prompted placement of a Greenfield filter in the patient presented in the case vignette. The concurrent presence of antiphospholipid antibodies, however, prompted additional treatment with institution of long-term warfarin anticoagulation. No further peripheral or cerebrovascular events have occurred. The CrD itself has been treated with a combination of azathioprine, low-dose prednisone, and intermittent infliximab infusions, with reasonably adequate, although not complete, control of bowel symptomatology.

SUMMARY

Although neurologic complications are relatively infrequent in IBD, they do occur. The spectrum of complications encompasses a broad array of neurologic processes. Peripheral nervous system involvement can consist of peripheral neuropathy, myoneural junction dysfunction, or myopathy, whereas involvement of the central nervous system can also become evident because of cerebrovascular, demyelinating, diffuse encephalopathic, or epileptiform processes. Diagnostic evaluation and treatment approaches depend on the specific problem that is present, and usually mirror what would be done if the same problem presented outside of the context of IBD.

REFERENCES

1. Crohn BB, Ginzburg K, Oppenheimer GD. Regional ileitis: A pathological and clinical entity. *JAMA*. 1932;99:1323–1328.
2. Wilks S. *Lectures on Pathological Anatomy*. London: Longmans; 1859.
3. Hurst AF. Ulcerative colitis. *Guy's Hospital Report*. 1909;71:26.
4. Loftus EV, Jr. Clinical epidemiology of inflammatory bowel disease: Incidence, prevalence, and environmental influences. *Gastroenterology*. 2004;126:1504–1517.
5. Veloso FT, Carvalho J, Magro F. Immune-related systemic manifestations of inflammatory bowel disease. A prospective study of 792 patients. *J Clin Gastroenterol*. 1996;23:29–34.
6. Christodoulou DK, Katsanos KH, Kitsanou M, et al. Frequency of extraintestinal manifestations in patients with inflammatory bowel disease in Northwest Greece and review of the literature. *Dig Liver Dis*. 2002;34:781–786.
7. Novotny DA, Rubin RJ, Slezak FA, et al. Arterial thromboembolic complications of inflammatory bowel disease. Report of three cases. *Dis Colon Rectum*. 1992;35:193–196.
8. Rogler G, Scholmerich J. Extraintestinal manifestations of inflammatory bowel disease [in German]. *Med Klin (Munich)*. 2004;99:123–130.
9. Greenstein AJ, Janowitz HD, Sachar DB. The extra-intestinal complications of Crohn's disease and ulcerative colitis: A study of 700 patients. *Medicine*. 1976;55:401–412.
10. Lossos A, River Y, Eliakim A, et al. Neurologic aspects of inflammatory bowel disease. *Neurology*. 1995;45:416–421.
11. Sartor RB. Mechanisms of disease: Pathogenesis of Crohn's disease and ulcerative colitis. *Nature Clinical Practice Gastroenterology & Hepatology*. 2006;3:390–407.
12. Philpott DJ, Viala J. Towards an understanding of the role of NOD2/CARD15 in the pathogenesis of Crohn's disease. *Best Pract Res Clin Gastroenterol*. 2004;18:555–568.
13. Mathew CG, Lewis CM. Genetics of inflammatory bowel disease: Progress and prospects. *Hum Mol Genet*. 2004;13:161–168.

14. Newman B, Siminovitch KA. Recent advances in the genetics of inflammatory bowel disease. *Current Opinion in Gastroenterology.* 2005;21:401–407.
15. Shanahan F. Crohn's disease. *Lancet.* 2002;359:62–69.
16. Sands BE. Crohn's disease. In: Feldman M, Friedman LS, Sleisenger MH, eds. *Sleisenger and Fordtran's Gastrointestinal and Liver Disease,* 7th ed. Philadelphia: WB Saunders; 2002: 2005–2038.
17. Jewell DP. Ulcerative colitis. In: Feldman M, Friedman LS, Sleisenger MH, eds. *Sleisenger and Fordtran's Gastrointestinal and Liver Disease,* 7th ed. Philadelphia: WB Saunders; 2002:2039–2067.
18. Podolsky DK. Inflammatory bowel disease (1). *N Engl J Med.* 1991;325:928–937.
19. Coert JH, Dellon AL. Neuropathy related to Crohn's disease treated by peripheral nerve decompression. *Scand J Plast Recontr Surg Hand Surg.* 2003;37:243–244.
20. Demarquay JF, Caroli-Bosc FX, Buckley M, et al. Right-sided sciatalgia complicating Crohn's disease. *Am J Gastroenterol.* 1998;93:2296–2298.
21. Greco F, Pavone P, Falsaperla R, et al. Peripheral neuropathy as first sign of ulcerative colitis in a child. *J Clin Gastroenterol.* 2004;38:115–117.
22. Gondim FA, Brannagan TH, 3rd, Sander HW, et al. Peripheral neuropathy in patients with inflammatory bowel disease. *Brain.* 2005;128:867–879.
23. Lloyd DA, Payton KB, Guenther L, et al. Melkersson-Rosenthal syndrome and Crohn's disease: One disease or two? Report of a case and discussion of the literature. *J Clin Gastroenterol.* 1994;18:213–217.
24. Summers RW, Harker L. Ulcerative colitis and sensorineural hearing loss: Is there a relationship? *J Clin Gastroenterol.* 1982;4:251–252.
25. Kumar BN, Walsh RM, Wilson PS, et al. Sensorineural hearing loss and ulcerative colitis. *J Laryngol Otol.* 1997;111:277–278.
26. Weber RS, Jenkins HA, Coker NJ. Sensorineural hearing loss associated with ulcerative colitis. A case report. *Arch Otolaryngol.* 1984;110:810–812.
27. Hollanders D. Sensorineural deafness—A new complication of ulcerative colitis? *Postgrad Med J.* 1986;753–755.
28. Kumar BN, Smith MS, Walsh RM, et al. Sensorineural hearing loss in ulcerative colitis. *Clin Otolaryngol.* 2000;25:143–145.
29. Contamin F, Ollat H, Levy VG, et al. Involvement of the peripheral and pyramidal nervous system in Crohn disease. Determining the role of folic acid deficiency [in French]. *La semaine des hôpitaux.* 1983;59:1381–1385.
30. Lossos A, Argov Z, Ackerman Z, et al. Peripheral neuropathy and folate deficiency as the first sign of Crohn's disease. *J Clin Gastroenterol.* 1991;13:442–444.
31. Humbert P, Monnier G, Billerey C, et al. Polyneuropathy: An unusual extraintestinal manifestation of Crohn's disease. *Acta Neurol Scand.* 1989;80:301–306.
32. Al-Kawas FH. Myositis associated with Crohn's colitis. *Am J Gastroenterol.* 1986;81:583–585.
33. Christopoulos C, Savva S, Pylarinou S, et al. Localised gastrocnemius myositis in Crohn's disease. *Clin Rheumatol.* 2003;22:143–145.
34. Burul CJ, Ritchie JK, Hawley PR, et al. Psoas abscess: A complication of Crohn's disease. *Br J Surg.* 1980;67:355–356.
35. Leu SY, Leonard MB, Beart RW, Jr., et al. Psoas abscess: Changing patterns of diagnosis and etiology. *Dis Colon Rectum.* 1986;29:694–698.
36. Shokouh-Amiri MH, Palnaes Hansen C, Moesgaard F, et al. Psoas abscess complicating Crohn's disease. *Acta Chirugica Scandinavica.* 1989;155:409–412.
37. Van Dongen LM, Lubbers EJ. Psoas abscess in Crohn's disease. *Br J Surg.* 1982;69:589–590.
38. Bartolo DC, Ebbs SR, Cooper MJ. Psoas abscess in Bristol: A 10-year review. *Int J Colorectal Dis.* 1987;2:72–76.
39. Chiba M, Igarashi K, Ohta H, et al. Rhabdomyolysis associated with Crohn's disease. *Jpn J Med.* 1987;26:255–260.
40. Best CN. Subacute combined degeneration of the spinal cord after extensive resection of ileum in Crohn's disease: Report of a case. *Br Med J.* 1959;2:862–864.
41. Baker SM, Bogoch A. Subacute combined degeneration of the spinal cord after ileal resection and folic acid administration in Crohn's disease. *Neurology.* 1973;23:40–41.
42. Ray DW, Bridger J, Hawnaur J, et al. Transverse myelitis as the presentation of Jo-1 antibody syndrome (myositis and fibrosing alveolitis) in long-standing ulcerative colitis. *British Journal of Rheumatology.* 1993;32:1105–1108.
43. Hershkowitz S, Link R, Ravden M, et al. Spinal empyema in Crohn's disease. *J Clin Gastroenterol.* 1990;12:67–69.
44. Sacher M, Gopfrich H, Hochberger O. Crohn's disease penetrating into the spinal canal. *Acta Paediatr Scand.* 1989;78:647–649.
45. Gelfenbeyn M, Goodkin R, Kliot M. Sterile recurrent spinal epidural abscess in a patient with Crohn's disease: A case report. *Surg Neurol.* 2006;65:178–184.
46. Gupta G, Gelfand JM, Lewis JD. Increased risk for demyelinating diseases in patients with inflammatory bowel disease. *Gastroenterology.* 2005;129:819–826.
47. Kimura K, Hunter SF, Thollander MS, et al. Concurrence of inflammatory bowel disease and multiple sclerosis. *Mayo Clin Proc..* 2000;75:802–806.
48. Rang EH, Brooke BN, Hermon-Taylor J. Association of ulcerative colitis with multiple sclerosis. *Lancet.* 1982;2:555.
49. Bernstein CN, Wajda A, Blanchard JF. The clustering of other inflammatory diseases in inflammatory bowel disease: A population-based study. *Gastroenterology.* 2005;129:827–836.
50. Freeman HJ, Flak B. Demyelination-like syndrome in Crohn's disease after infliximab therapy. *Can J Gastroenterol.* 2005;19:313–316.
51. Thomas CW, Jr., Weinshenker BG, Sandborn WJ. Demyelination during anti-tumor necrosis factor alpha therapy with infliximab for Crohn's disease. *Inflamm Bowel Dis.* 2004;10:28–31.
52. Talbot RW, Heppell J, Dozois RR, et al. Vascular complications of inflammatory bowel disease. *Mayo Clin Proc.* 1986;61:140–145.
53. Quera R, Shanahan F. Thromboembolism—An important manifestation of inflammatory bowel disease. *Am J Gastroenterol.* 2004;99:1971–1973.
54. Younes-Mhenni S, Derex L, Berruyer M, et al. Large-artery stroke in a young patient with Crohn's disease. Role of vitamin B_6 deficiency-induced hyperhomocysteinemia. *J Neurol Sci.* 2004;221:113–115.
55. Fukuhara T, Tsuchida S, Kinugasa K, et al. A case of pontine lacunar infarction with ulcerative colitis. *Clin Neurol Neurosurg.* 1993;95:159–162.
56. Slot WB, van Kasteel V, Coerkamp EG, et al. Severe thrombotic complications in a postpartum patient with active Crohn's disease resulting in ischemic spinal cord injury. *Dig Dis Sci.* 1995;40:1395–1399.
57. Gobbele R, Reith W, Block F. Cerebral vasculitis as a concomitant neurological illness in Crohn's disease [in German]. *Nervenarzt.* 2000;71:299–304.
58. Pandian JD, Henderson RD, O'Sullivan JD, et al. Cerebral vasculitis in ulcerative colitis. *Arch Neurol.* 2006;63:780.
59. Johns DR. Cerebrovascular complications of inflammatory bowel disease. *Am J Gastroenterol.* 1991;86:367–370.
60. Garcia-Monco JC, Gomez Beldarrain M. Superior sagittal sinus thrombosis complicating Crohn's disease. *Neurology.* 1991;41:1324–1325.
61. Samal SC, Patra S, Reddy DC, et al. Cerebral venous sinus thrombosis as a presenting feature of Crohn's disease. *Indian J Gastroenterol.* 2004;23:148–149.
62. Musio F, Older SA, Jenkins T, et al. Case report: Cerebral venous thrombosis as a manifestation of acute ulcerative colitis. *Am J Med Sci.* 1993;305:28–35.
63. Danese S, Papa A, Saibeni S, et al. Inflammation and coagulation in inflammatory bowel disease: The clot thickens. *Am J Gastroenterology* 2007; 102(1): 174–186.
64. Mevorach D, Goldberg Y, Gomori JM, et al. Antiphospholipid syndrome manifested by ischemic stroke in a patient with Crohn's disease. *J Clin Gastroenterol.* 1996;22:141–143.
65. Aichbichler BW, Petritsch W, Reicht GA, et al. Anti-cardiolipin antibodies in patients with inflammatory bowel disease. *Dig Dis Sci.* 1999;44:852–856.
66. Mahmood A, Needham J, Prosser J, et al. Prevalence of hyperhomocysteinaemia, activated protein C resistance and prothrombin gene mutation in inflammatory bowel disease. *Eur J Gastroenterol Hepatol.* 2005;17:739–744.
67. Oldenburg B, Van Tuyl BA, van der Griend R, et al. Risk factors for thromboembolic complications in inflammatory bowel disease: The role of hyperhomocysteinaemia. *Dig Dis Sci.* 2005;50:235–240.
68. Penix LP. Ischemic strokes secondary to vitamin B_{12} deficiency-induced hyperhomocysteinemia. *Neurology.* 1998;51:622–624.
69. Hahn JS, Berquist W, Alcorn DM, et al. Wernicke encephalopathy and beriberi during total parenteral nutrition attributable to multivitamin infusion shortage. *Pediatrics.* 1998;101: E10.
70. Kawakubo K, Iida M, Matsumoto T, et al. Progressive encephalopathy in a Crohn's disease patient on long-term total parenteral nutrition: Possible relationship to selenium deficiency. *Postgrad Med J.* 1994;70:215–219.
71. Eggspühler AW, Bauerfeind P, Dorn T, et al. Wernicke encephalopathy—A severe neurological complication in a clinically inactive Crohn's disease. *Eur J Neurol.* 2003;50:184–185.
72. Elsehety A, Bertorini TE. Neurologic and neuropsychiatric complications of Crohn's disease. *South Med J.* 1997;90:606–610.
73. Schulak JA, Moossa R, Block GE, et al. Convulsions complicating colectomy in inflammatory bowel disease. *JAMA.* 1977;237:1456–1458.
74. Fagan C, Phelan D. Severe convulsant hypomagnesaemia and short bowel syndrome. *Anaesth Intensive Care.* 2001;29:281–283.
75. Barabino A, Castellano E, Gandullia P, et al. A girl with severe fistulizing Crohn's disease. *Dig Liver Dis.* 2000;32:792–794.
76. Rosencrantz R, Moon A, Raynes H, et al. Cyclosporine-induced neurotoxicity during treatment of Crohn's disease: Lack of correlation with previously reported risk factors. *Am J Gastroenterol.* 2001;96:2778–2782.
77. Akhan G, Andermann F, Gotman MJ. Ulcerative colitis, status epilepticus and intractable temporal seizures. *Epileptic Disord.* 2002;4:135–137.
78. Shanahan F. Inflammatory bowel disease: Immunodiagnostics, immunotherapeutics, and ecotherapeutics. *Gastroenterology.* 2001;120:622–635.
79. Thukral C, Cheifetz A, Peppercorn MA. Anti-tumor necrosis factor therapy for ulcerative colitis: Evidence to date. *Drugs.* 2006;66:2059–2065.

CHAPTER **36**

Neurologic Manifestations of Gluten Sensitivity

Marios Hadjivassiliou • David S. Sanders

OBJECTIVES

- To discuss the gluten sensitivity that can result in an autoimmune systemic disease with a spectrum of diverse manifestations
- To discuss the common neurologic manifestations of gluten sensitivity
- To describe the neurologic manifestations that can occur even in the absence of gluten sensitive enteropathy
- To describe the neurologic manifestations that are a result of immune-mediated pathogenic mechanisms and rarely result from deficiency states
- To explain the need for early diagnosis to achieve best response to treatment with a gluten-free diet

CASE VIGNETTE

A 32-year-old woman presented with a rapidly progressive neuropathy and ataxia, the onset of which coincided with the diagnosis of gluten sensitivity. Gastrointestinal symptoms were absent, but she had serologic evidence of gluten sensitivity (positive antigliadin antibodies). A duodenal biopsy showed evidence of gluten sensitive enteropathy. She was unable to adhere to a strict gluten-free diet and her neurologic problems worsened. She was treated with steroids and other immunosuppressive medication but continued to deteriorate neurologically and eventually died of bronchopneumonia 18 months after the neurologic presentation. There was no family history of celiac disease, but her mother had hypothyroidism and one sister had type 1 diabetes. Autopsy examination showed inflammatory changes in both the central and the peripheral nervous systems. Capillaries within the brain appeared prominent in some areas, with hypertrophic endothelial cells. These vascular changes were most conspicuous in white matter, including cerebral, cerebellar, and brainstem white matter. Similar changes were seen focally in gray matter areas including hippocampus and inferior olivary nucleus. The capillary changes were associated with a vascular and perivascular inflammatory cell infiltrate. No tissue necrosis or microinfarction was seen, and only mild focal myelin loss noted. Similar changes were also seen in the spinal cord. The cerebellum showed marked loss of Purkinje cells, with increased Bergmann glia, and mild patchy loss of neurons was noted in the inferior olivary nucleus. Spinal roots of peripheral nerve showed inflammatory cell infiltrate of both lymphocytes and macrophages. Muscle histology also showed inflammation with lymphocytic infiltrates. No evidence was seen of malignancy or vasculitis.

This case illustrates the typical distribution of neuropathologic abnormalities encountered in cases of gluten sensitivity-related neurologic dysfunction. The unusual features here are the rapidity of progression and the widespread involvement of the nervous system. Such severe cases are rare, however, and most cases with neurologic manifestations present with a gradual onset and gradual progression of ataxia or peripheral neuropathy, with less frequent manifestations of myopathy, myelopathy, and encephalopathy (white matter abnormalities on magnetic resonance imaging [MRI] with episodic headaches).

DEFINITION

Celiac disease (CD), also known as *gluten sensitive enteropathy*, was first described by Aretaeus the Cappadocian, one of the most distinguished ancient Greek doctors of the first century AD. CD remained obscure until 1887 when Samuel Gee gave a lecture entitled "On the celiac affection" at the Hospital for Sick Children, Great Ormond Street, London. This was an accurate description of CD in children, based on his own clinical observations. With clinical manifestations primarily confined to the gastrointestinal tract or attributable to malabsorption, it was logical to assume that the target organ and, hence, the key to the pathogenesis of this disease was the gut.

The treatment of CD remained empiric until 1953 when the Dutch pediatrician Willem Dicke noted the deleterious effect of wheat flour on children with CD (1). Removal of dietary products containing wheat was shown to result in complete resolution of the gastrointestinal symptoms and a resumption of normal health.

The introduction of the small bowel biopsy in 1954 confirmed the gut as a target organ showing the characteristic features of villous atrophy, crypt hyperplasia, and increase in intraepithelial lymphocytes, with subsequent improvement while on a gluten-free diet.

In 1966, Marks et al. (2) demonstrated an enteropathy in 9 of 12 patients with dermatitis herpetiformis, an itchy vesicular skin rash mainly occurring over the extensor aspect of the elbows and knees. The enteropathy was strikingly similar to that seen in CD (2). It was later shown that the enteropathy and the skin rash were gluten dependent, but skin involvement could occur even without histologic evidence of gut involvement. This was the first evidence that the gut may not be the sole protagonist in this disease.

The immunology of CD has been pursued with renewed interest in the last 20 years or so, because of the work of a number of visionaries who were prepared to abandon dogma and suggest that the definition of gluten sensitivity based solely on bowel involvement was outmoded. This is what led to the modern definition of gluten sensitivity as "a state of heightened immunologic responsiveness in genetically susceptible individuals," a definition that does not imply gut involvement as a prerequisite for the diagnosis (3). By altering the gluten load, a range of bowel mucosal abnormalities in patients with gluten sensitivity was demonstrated, ranging from histologically normal (also known as marsh type 0) to the flat destructive lesion (4). This observation suggested that some patients with gluten sensitivity can have a histologically normal mucosa, with the only marker of the disease being the presence of circulating antibodies against the etiologic agent. More recent work has suggested that the presence of IgA deposits against tissue transglutaminases in the small bowel can be one of the earliest markers of the whole spectrum of gluten sensitivity, including those cases with potential CD where the small bowel mucosa is otherwise histologically normal (5). The term CD is best reserved for those patients with evidence of enteropathy on small bowel biopsy. Gluten sensitivity is best considered a systemic disease with diverse manifestations of which enteropathy (CD), dermatopathy (dermatitis herpetiformis), and neurologic dysfunction are examples.

EPIDEMIOLOGY

Studies of CD in many European countries and North America, based on healthy individuals, have come up with a prevalence figure of 1%. This observation led to the realization that for every one patient with CD presenting with gastrointestinal symptoms there are eight patients without such symptoms (silent CD). Based on data from a long established gastrointestinal clinic with an interest in CD, 6% of patients with CD seem to develop otherwise unexplained neurologic dysfunction (6). This, however, may well be an underestimate, because a neurophysiologic study looking specifically at the presence of peripheral neuropathy in patients with CD found evidence of neuropathy in 23% of cases (7). Approaching the neurologic manifestations of gluten sensitivity from a neurologic perspective, led to the study of the prevalence of antigliadin antibodies (a sensitive marker of the whole spectrum of gluten sensitivity) in patients with neurologic dysfunction of unknown cause. This study showed the prevalence of antigliadin antibodies in patients with unexplained neurologic dysfunction to be 57%, compared with 12% in a large cohort of the healthy population. The same study showed the prevalence of the enteropathy to be 16% in the neurology group compared with 1% in the healthy population (8,9). Such neurologic manifestations have since been shown to occur even without the presence of enteropathy. Prevalence figures for specific types of manifestations include a range of 11% to 40% for gluten ataxia (among patients with otherwise sporadic idiopathic ataxia) and 34% for gluten neuropathy (among patients with idiopathic sporadic neuropathy) (10–12). A recent study has found the prevalence of antigliadin antibodies in patients with inflammatory myopathy to be 37% (13).

ETIOLOGY AND PATHOGENESIS

Gluten sensitivity is an autoimmune disease with a known external trigger factor (gluten). The cause of the neurologic manifestations has an immunologic basis and is not related to vitamin deficiencies. Up to 50% of patients with gluten ataxia have been shown to have oligoclonal bands present on examination of the cerebrospinal fluid (CSF) (14). Pathologic data obtained from sural nerve biopsies, as well as post mortem examinations, are also suggestive of an inflammatory pathogenesis with evidence of perivascular inflammation that has a predilection for the cerebellum, brainstem, and the peripheral nerves (12). Other parts of the nervous system can also be affected less frequently (muscle, dorsal root ganglia, spinal cord, cerebrum). Patients with gluten ataxia have evidence of IgA deposits against tissue transglutaminase within the small bowel mucosa (15). This finding, which has been shown to be a reliable marker of the whole spectrum of gluten sensitivity, has been described in patients with dermatitis herpetiformis and patients with CD before the development of enteropathy (5). Of particular interest is also the finding of such deposits on vessels within the cerebellum and brainstem in a patient with gluten ataxia (15). This suggests that transglutaminases may play an important role in the pathogenesis of a vascular-based inflammation contributing to the breakdown of the blood–brain barrier, allowing the entry of gluten sensitivity-related antibodies. A cross-reactivity between antigliadin antibodies and Purkinje cell antigens has already been shown to exist (16). Intraventricular injection of serum from a patient with gluten ataxia induces ataxia in mice. Ataxia can also be induced by the injection of tissue transglutaminase antibodies produced using a phage display library from duodenal biopsy tissue. This finding favors an antibody-mediated response in the production of ataxia. Cell-mediated responses are also important in the production of the enteropathy, but their role in the neurologic manifestations remains unclear.

PATHOLOGY

A landmark paper on 16 patients with neurologic disorders associated with adult CD, published in 1966, provided the first neuropathologic data from postmortem examinations (17), which showed extensive perivascular inflammatory changes affecting both central and peripheral nervous systems. A striking feature was the loss of Purkinje cells, with atrophy and gliosis of the cerebellum. More recent data confirm similar findings, with perivascular inflammatory changes that have a predilection for the cerebellum and brainstem but at times can be found elsewhere (12,18). Involvement of muscle is in the form of an inflammatory myopathy that can be indistinguishable from idiopathic polymyositis, but a few cases of inclusion body myositis have also been described (19,20). In cases of slowly progressive gluten sensitivity-related peripheral neuropathy, the most common neuropathologic findings on sural nerve biopsy are those of axonal degeneration—not always with evidence of active inflammation.

CLINICAL MANIFESTATIONS

A review of all case reports (with biopsy-proved CD) from 1964 to date reveals that ataxia and peripheral neuropathy are the commonest neurologic manifestations (21). Less common manifestations included myopathy, myoclonic ataxia, and myelopathy. A number of patients with epilepsy, associated with occipital calcifications on computed tomography (CT), having CD have also been described, mainly in Italy (22). Based on data collected in a dedicated gluten sensitivity–neurology clinic on patients presenting with neurologic dysfunction, as a result of which the diagnosis of gluten sensitivity with or without enteropathy is made, the most frequent neurologic manifestations appear to be ataxia and peripheral neuropathy (Table 36-1).

GLUTEN ATAXIA

Gluten ataxia is defined as sporadic, otherwise idiopathic, ataxia with serologic evidence of gluten sensitivity. The clinical characteristics of patients with gluten ataxia, based on 100 patients, have been documented. The mean age at onset of the ataxia was 54 years, with equal male-to-female ratio. All patients had gait ataxia and most (80%) also had limb ataxia and ocular signs. Up to 60% had evidence of cerebellar atrophy on brain MRI scans. Some patients had additional white matter abnormalities; 30% had evidence of enteropathy, despite the absence of gastrointestinal symptoms (11,18). As in CD, often evidence is seen of a coexistence of additional autoimmune diseases, such as hypothyroidism, pernicious anemia, vitiligo, and type 1 diabetes. Although the ataxia usually is slowly progressive, some cases follow a rapidly progressive course similar to that seen in paraneoplastic cerebellar degeneration, but which can also respond to a strict gluten-free diet. Contrary to previous case reports, myoclonic ataxia is a rare manifestation (only three patients in this cohort). Additional findings encountered in some of these patients with gluten ataxia included palatal myoclonus (two patients), chorea (three patients), and opsoclonus myoclonus (one patient).

TABLE 36-1. Patients ($N = 312$) Seen in the Gluten Sensitivity–Neurology Clinic (1994 to November 2006)

Ataxia (total)	147
with myoclonus	3
with palatal tremor	32
with opsoclonus myoclonus	1
Peripheral neuropathy	
Sensorimotor axonal neuropathy	116
Mononeuropathy multiplex	25
Motor neuropathy	10
Small fiber neuropathy	5
Sensory neuronopathy	2
Encephalopathy	28
Myopathies	13
Myelopathy	8
Stiff-man syndrome	6
Chorea	3
Neuromyotonia	2
Epilepsy and occipital calcifications	1

GLUTEN NEUROPATHY

The most frequent type of gluten neuropathy is symmetric axonal peripheral neuropathy, but other types of neuropathies have also been reported (12). It is a slowly progressive disease. The mean age at onset of the neuropathy, based on 100 patients, was 55 years (range 24 to 77) with a mean duration of 9 years (range 1 to 33). A total of 66 patients had a symmetric generalized sensorimotor axonal neuropathy, 16 had mononeuropathy multiplex, 9 had a pure motor neuropathy, 7 had a small fiber neuropathy, and 2 had sensory neuronopathy. Gluten-sensitive enteropathy was present in 26 of 89 (29%) of those patients who had duodenal biopsy. The HLA antigen types associated with CD were present in 80% of these patients.

GLUTEN MYOPATHY

Myopathy is a less common neurologic manifestation of gluten sensitivity. The following data are based on 13 cases encountered over the last 12 years (19). The male-to-female ratio was 5:8. The mean age at onset of the myopathic symptoms was 54 years. Eight patients (62%) had predominantly proximal weakness, four patients (31%) had both proximal and distal weakness, and one patient had primarily distal weakness. Two patients had ataxia and neuropathy in addition to the myopathy, and one patient had just neuropathy in addition to the myopathy. Serum creatine kinase (CK) level ranged between normal to 4,380 IU/L at presentation (normal, 25 to 190 IU/L). Enteropathy was identified following duodenal biopsy in six patients.

GLUTEN ENCEPHALOPATHY

The term *gluten encephalopathy* is used to describe a subgroup of patients with gluten sensitivity who have episodic, often severe, headaches that may resemble migraine and are sometimes associated with focal neurologic deficits (23). MRI often shows white matter abnormalities, sometimes patchy and, on other occasions, confluent. A gluten-free diet usually results in complete resolution of the headaches. The white matter abnormalities usually do not resolve but do not progress as long as the patient remains on a strict gluten-free diet.

OTHER MANIFESTATIONS

Myelopathy can be seen in the context of gluten sensitivity. Some patients develop spinal cord atrophy. Postmortem examination shows a predilection for damage affecting the posterior columns. Inflammatory lesions of the cord can also be seen, sometimes in association with peripheral neuropathies. The authors have identified a high prevalence of antigliadin antibodies in patients with stiff person syndrome. This may be explained on the basis of autoimmune association and, at present, it is unclear if a gluten-free diet has a role to play with regard to the neurologic symptoms of the condition. Some old reports have suggested an association of CD with epilepsy, whereas more recent large studies have not confirmed this. The entity of epilepsy with occipital calcifications and CD has been well characterized in Italy (22). Such cases are uncommon in other countries. The authors have encountered two patients with Isaac syndrome and gluten sensitivity. Again, an association on an autoimmune basis is likely here.

DIAGNOSTIC APPROACH

The choice of serologic markers for the diagnosis of gluten sensitivity-related neurologic dysfunction is clearly of significance. Antigliadin antibodies can be found in the healthy population (5% to 12%) and, thus, it is possible that, in a proportion of patients with neurologic problems and positive antigliadin antibodies, these antibodies are coincidental rather than being etiologically linked to the neurologic dysfunction. No marker currently exists that is 100% specific to the neurologic manifestations of gluten sensitivity. Antigliadin antibodies, however, (particularly of the IgG class) remain the most sensitive marker of the whole spectrum of gluten sensitivity. Antiendomysium antibodies are specific to the presence of enteropathy. Antitissue transglutaminase antibodies are also said to be specific for the presence of enteropathy, but in the authors' experience they are found to be positive in >50% of patients with gluten ataxia at various titers, despite that the prevalence of enteropathy in these patients is about 30%. In practice, it is best to perform all of the gluten-related antibodies (antigliadin IgG and IgA, endomysium, transglutaminase) as well as the HLA antigen typing. Positive endomysium antibodies imply the presence of enteropathy. The HLA DQ2 or DQ8 have a strong association with CD and have also been found in at least 80% of patients with neurologic manifestations. The remaining patients have the HLA DQ1. Small bowel biopsy is advisable in all patients in whom one or more of the antibody titers is positive. In those patients with enteropathy on biopsy who only have one of the two classes of antigliadin antibodies at baseline (IgG or IgA), the type of antibody is reflected in the type of presentation. Individuals with neurologic manifestations at presentation tend to display IgG antibody positivity, whereas those with gastrointestinal manifestations tend to demonstrate IgA. It is extremely rare, in the authors' experience, to have endomysium or transglutaminase antibody positivity without positive antigliadin antibodies. This is why antigliadin antibodies remain the best marker of the whole spectrum of gluten sensitivity.

TREATMENT

Strict gluten-free diet is the main treatment for these conditions. Previous case reports on patients with CD and neurologic dysfunction suggested variable response to the diet. No documentation of strict adherence to the gluten-free diet was provided, however. Such monitoring can be undertaken with the use of antigliadin antibodies on a 6-month basis. The antibody titers fall within the first 6 months and complete elimination is usually seen by 1 year, assuming a strict diet is followed. Neurologic improvement usually manifests by 1 year. It has been shown that gluten ataxia, gluten neuropathy, and gluten sensitivity-associated myopathy improve with a gluten-free diet and that the improvement is independent of the presence or absence of enteropathy (19,24,25). Improvement is more likely to be observed when the diagnosis has been made early and the treatment instigated immediately. This is particularly important for patients with gluten ataxia, where the loss of Purkinje cells in the cerebellum is irreversible. Intravenous immunoglobulins have also been shown to be beneficial in a small, uncontrolled trial of patients with gluten ataxia (26). In cases where neurologic complications progress despite what appears to be a strict gluten-free diet, recommendation is that a wheat-free diet be followed to ensure elimination of the antibodies. If the complications continue to progress despite a wheat-free diet, immunosuppressive treatment can be initiated in the form of cyclosporine or mycophenolate. It is important to emphasize, however, that such cases are rare and that most patients will respond to a strict gluten-free diet.

CLINICAL RECOMMENDATIONS OF THE VIGNETTE

All patients with sporadic idiopathic ataxia or peripheral neuropathy should be screened for gluten sensitivity. If positive, the patient should be referred for small bowel biopsy. If available, in addition to histologic examination, the presence of IgA deposits against TG2 should be sought on the biopsy because this appears to be the most sensitive marker of the whole spectrum of gluten sensitivity (5). Irrespective of the findings on biopsy, a strict gluten-free diet should be recommended, with close monitoring of the response to the diet and the evidence of elimination of all gluten-related antibodies in the serum. The case described above illustrates the spectrum of neurologic involvement, but also emphasizes the important issue of strictness of the gluten-free diet as a means of treatment. Unlike the enteropathy, where some patients experience significant benefit in terms of gastrointestinal symptoms even with partial adherence to the diet, in the neurologic spectrum, partial adherence to the diet is not sufficient to allow recovery or stabilization of the neurologic problem. In the authors' experience, this is the most frequent cause of lack of response to the diet.

SUMMARY

Gluten sensitivity is an autoimmune systemic disease with diverse manifestations. Neurologic manifestations, which can be seen in the absence of an enteropathy, are common. Gluten sensitivity accounts for a substantial number of patients with sporadic idiopathic ataxias and sporadic idiopathic axonal neuropathies, but can also be responsible for involvement of other parts of the peripheral and central nervous systems. The pathophysiology has an immunologic basis. Diagnosis and treatment in the form of a strict gluten-free diet should be considered early before permanent damage occurs. Immunosuppressive treatment should be used only if adherence to a strict gluten-free diet with evidence of elimination of gluten-related antibodies is not associated with stabilization or improvement of the neurologic dysfunction. The search for a specific marker for the neurologic spectrum is ongoing; until this becomes available, antigliadin antibodies and IgA deposits against TG2 in the small bowel appear to be the most sensitive markers of the whole spectrum of gluten sensitivity.

REFERENCES

1. Dicke WK, Weijers HA, Van De Kamer JH. Coeliac disease II: The presence in wheat of a factor having a deleterious effect in cases of coeliac disease. *Acta Paediatr.* 1953;42:34–42.
2. Marks J, Shuster S, Watson AJ. Small bowel changes in dermatitis herpetiformis. *Lancet.* 1966;ii:1280–1282.
3. Marsh MN. The natural history of gluten sensitivity: Defining, refining and re-defining. *QJ Med.* 1995;85:9–13.
4. Marsh MN. Gluten major histocompatibility complex, and the small intestine: A molecular and immunobiologic approach to the spectrum of gluten sensitivity. *Gastroenterology.* 1992;102:330.
5. Korponay-Szabo IR, Halttunen T, Szalai Z, et al. In vivo targeting of intestinal and extraintestinal transglutaminase 2 by celiac autoantibodies. *Gut.* 2004 53:641–648.
6. Holmes GKT. Neurological and psychiatric complications in coeliac disease. In: Gobbi G, Anderman F, Naccarato S, et al., ed. *Epilepsy and Other Neurological Disorders in Coeliac Disease.* London: John Libbey; 1997:251–264.
7. Luostarinen L, Himanen SL, Luostarinen M, et al. Neuromuscular and sensory disturbances in patients with well treated coeliac disease. *J Neurol Neurosurg Psychiatry.* 2003; 74:490–494.
8. Hadjivassiliou M, Gibson A, Davies-Jones GAB, et al. Is cryptic gluten sensitivity an important cause of neurological illness? *Lancet.* 1996;347:369–371.
9. Sanders DS, Patel D, Stephenson TJ, et al. A primary care cross-sectional study of undiagnosed adult celiac disease. *Eur J Gastroenterol Hepatol.* 2003;15:407–413.
10. Bürk K, Bösch S, Müller CA, et al. Sporadic cerebellar ataxia associated with gluten sensitivity. *Brain.* 2001;124:1013–1019.
11. Hadjivassiliou M, Grünewald RA, Sharrack B, et al. Gluten ataxia in perspective: Epidemiology, genetic susceptibility and clinical characteristics. *Brain.* 2003;126:685–691.
12. Hadjivassiliou M, Grunewald RA, Kandler RH, et al. Neuropathy associated with gluten sensitivity. *J Neurol Neurosurg Psychiatry.* 2006;77:1262–1266.
13. Selva-O'Callaghan A, Casellas F, De Torres I, et al. Celiac disease and antibodies associated with celiac disease in patients with inflammatory myopathy. *Muscle Nerve.* 2007;35: 49–54.
14. Hadjivassiliou M, Williamson CA, Woodroofe NM. The humoral response in the pathogenesis of gluten ataxia: Reply from authors. *Neurology.* 2003;60:1397–1399.
15. Hadjivassiliou M, Maki M, Sanders DS, et al. Autoantibody targeting of brain and intestinal transglutaminase in gluten ataxia *Neurology.* 2006;66:373–377.
16. Hadjivassiliou M, Boscolo S, Davies-Jones A, et al. The humoral response in the pathogenesis of gluten ataxia. *Neurology.* 2002;58:1221–1226.
17. Cooke WT, Thomas-Smith W. Neurological disorders associated with adult coeliac disease. *Brain.* 1966;89:683–722.
18. Hadjivassiliou M, Grünewald RA, Chattopadhyay AK, et al. Clinical, radiological, neurophysiological and neuropathological characteristics of gluten ataxia. *Lancet.* 1998;352:1582–1585.
19. Hadjivassiliou M, Chattopadhyay AK, Grünewald RA, et al. Myopathy associated with gluten sensitivity. *Muscle Nerve* 2006 Dec. 1 [Epub ahead of print].
20. Kleopa AK, Kyriacou K, Papanicolaou ZE, et al. Reversible inflammatory and vacuolar myopathy with vitamin E deficiency in coeliac disease. *Muscle Nerve.* 2005;31:260–265.
21. Hadjivassiliou M, Grünewald RA, Davies-Jones GAB. Gluten sensitivity as a neurological illness. *J Neurol Neurosurg Psychiatry.* 2002;72:560–563.
22. Gobbi G, Bouquet F, Greco L, et al. Coeliac disease, epilepsy, and cerebral calcifications. *Lancet.* 1992;340:439–443.
23. Hadjivassiliou M, Grünewald RAG, Lawden M, et al. Headache and CNS white matter abnormalities associated with gluten sensitivity. *Neurology.* 2001;56:385–388.
24. Hadjivassiliou M, Davies-Jones GAB, Sanders DS, et al. Dietary treatment of gluten ataxia. *J Neurol Neurosurg Psychiatry.* 2003;74(9):1221–1224.
25. Hadjivassiliou M, Kandler RH, Chattopadhyay AK, et al. Dietary treatment of gluten neuropathy. *Muscle Nerve.* 2006; epub. 10.1002/mus.20642.
26. Burk K, Melms A, Schulz JB, et al. Effectiveness of intravenous immunoglobulin therapy in cerebellar ataxia associated with gluten sensitivity. *Ann Neurol.* 2001;50:827–828.

CHAPTER 37

Diseases of the Pancreas

Michael Jacewicz • Christopher R. Marino

INTRODUCTION

The pancreas has both exocrine and endocrine functions. Disease of the endocrine pancreas, specifically diabetes mellitus, is responsible for most of the neurologic complications associated with pancreatic disease. Neurologic aspects of diabetes are beyond the scope of this chapter, but are addressed elsewhere in this textbook. In this chapter, is examined how disorders of the exocrine pancreas (pancreatitis) and pancreatic tumors can affect the nervous system. Although nondiabetic neurologic complications of pancreatic disease are uncommon, clinicians need to be cognizant of several associations between these two organ systems. These include pancreatic encephalopathy, hypoglycemia from insulinoma, and nonbacterial thrombotic endocarditis (NBTE) in pancreatic adenocarcinoma.

Pancreatic Encephalopathy

OBJECTIVES

- To describe the complications associated with acute pancreatitis
- To explain why pancreatic encephalopathy is a rare and controversial entity

CASE VIGNETTE

A 43-year-old man with known gallbladder stones developed acute pancreatitis. He recovered in 1 month, but relapsed after stopping a low-fat diet. A pancreatic abscess was excised, and his condition improved again. After stopping total intravenous nutrition, a third episode of increased blood amylase (590 IU/L; normal 100 to 300 IU/L) was accompanied with disorientation, auditory hallucinations, and a gradual deterioration into coma. A cranial computed tomography (CT) scan, complete blood count (CBC), electrolytes, and other metabolic parameters were normal. The patient recovered from coma over 2 days and was transferred to a university hospital. There he demonstrated dysphonia, dysarthria, facial paresis, auditory and visual impairment, vertical nystagmus, right-sided paresis, bilateral dysmetria, and severe cerebellar ataxia. A small hemorrhage was found along the edge of the left retinal macula. He was disoriented and inattentive, and had impaired memory and language. The Mini-Mental State Examination (MMSE) score was 19 of 30. Cerebrospinal fluid (CSF) was normal, except for an elevated glucose (250 mg/dL), which it was felt was unrelated to the pancreatitis. An electroencephalogram (EEG) disclosed nonspecific slowing. Cranial CT and magnetic resonance imaging (MRI) were normal.

He was treated with intravenous corticosteroids, somatostatin, an H_2 antagonist and a low-fat diet. Within 1 week, blood amylase reverted to normal. After 10 days of treatment, the dysarthria, nystagmus, and auditory hallucinations disappeared. During a gradual steroid reduction, however, the blood amylase increased (510 IU/L), and he had a coincident neurologic worsening. Six months later, the neurologic deficits had improved, but he still could not walk because of cerebellar ataxia and right-sided weakness. He still had hearing loss.

Neuropsychologic testing showed improvement, including an MMSE score of 25. He was apathetic, socially impaired, and could not work, however. Visual evoked potentials were normal, but auditory, somatosensory, and motor evoked potentials were abnormal. MRI showed moderate cortical and subcortical atrophy. Five years later, the patient walked with a cane. Mild cerebellar ataxia was present, but the right-sided weakness had resolved. Residual right-sided hyperreflexia remained. Hearing was now normal. Cognition testing was normal, except for a persistent decrease in verbal fluency. The MMSE was 29. The patient could not work because of an "abulic-apathetic" state. The evoked potentials remained altered. Six years later, he could walk independently. He remained apathetic and absent minded. Seven years later, he had a recurrence of abdominal pain. The amylase was elevated (460 IU/L), and he could not walk because of cerebellar ataxia, right hemiparesis, and vertical nystagmus. These deficits resolved over 2 days. The third brain MRI showed no new abnormality. The MMSE was 29 and neuropsychologic testing was unchanged from previous examinations. Blood testing was unremarkable, and 2 weeks later, the blood amylase level was normal as well (1).

DEFINITION

Pancreatic encephalopathy refers to a variety of neuropsychiatric symptoms that can complicate acute pancreatitis. The signs and symptoms are indistinguishable from metabolic encephalopathy of any other cause, and because so many metabolic disorders can affect the central nervous system (CNS) in the setting of acute pancreatitis, the diagnosis of pancreatic encephalopathy is problematic. As a nosological entity, pancreatic encephalopathy is considered rare and controversial.

EPIDEMIOLOGY

Acute pancreatitis occurs with an incidence of about 240 new cases per 1 million per year (2,3) and may be increasing over time (4). In acute pancreatitis, encephalopathy has been reported in 9% to 35% of subjects without an alcoholic history (5). Clinical documentation has often been less than complete, however, and other causes of metabolic encephalopathy may not have been rigorously excluded. Hence, the true incidence of pancreatic encephalopathy is likely to be much less than quoted.

ETIOLOGY AND PATHOGENESIS

More than 80% of acute pancreatitis cases are caused by alcoholism or biliary tract disease (6). Other causes, include infection (mumps virus, cytomegalovirus [CMV], coxsackie B, human immunodeficiency virus [HIV]), ischemia, metabolic derangement (hyperlipidemia, hypercalcemia), drug toxicity (e.g., valproate, azathioprine, thiazides, sulfa drugs), trauma, autoimmune, and genetics (hereditary pancreatitis). Common to all is the activation of pancreatic enzymes within the pancreas that results in tissue damage, inflammation, edema, and, in severe cases, hemorrhage and necrosis. Mortality approaches 30% in patients with infected pancreatic necrosis. Enzymes that enter the systemic circulation and overwhelm normal protective mechanisms produce a systemic inflammatory response syndrome (SIRS) that can cause multiple organ dysfunction syndrome (circulatory collapse, renal failure, acute respiratory distress syndrome, and disseminated intravascular coagulation). likely, SIRS plays an important role in the pathophysiology of CNS dysfunction in acute pancreatitis, but the concept that the CNS might be directly injured by pancreatic enzymes has been a source of speculation since the 1930s. In the early 1950s, Vogel (7,8) performed several experiments to advance this notion. He injected pancreatic lipase into rabbit brain and found focal areas of demyelination without other notable inflammatory changes. Demyelination did not occur if the lipase was inactivated by heat. Incubating the spinal cord in a solution containing lipase damaged the myelin sheaths. In comparison, trypsin and chymotrypsin were without effect. If trypsin or chymotrypsin were injected directly into the brain, however, axons as well as myelin underwent necrosis. Vogel (9) published a single report of a 44-year-old woman who had an acute hemorrhagic pancreatitis and massive cerebral edema after failing to awaken from anesthesia for thoracolumbar sympathectomy. The pathology showed patchy areas of myelin pallor, but no myelin breakdown, and variable neuronal changes. The author interpreted the changes as caused by the action of lipase; in retrospect, however, the pathology could be just as readily explained by cerebral anoxia. In 1979, Estrada et al. (10) performed a prospective study of 17 patients with nonalcoholic acute pancreatitis. Six patients developed neuropsychiatric changes (disorientation, hallucinations, or agitation) without metabolic cause and all six had elevated lipase activity in their CSF. They also had nonspecific abnormalities on EEG. None of the 11 patients with pancreatitis without neuropsychiatric changes had elevated CSF lipase, nor did any of 41 control subjects. The neuropsychiatric symptoms, as well as the CSF and EEG changes, resolved within several days of illness onset. Interestingly, the severity of pancreatitis did not correlate with development of encephalopathy. No further clinical trials have been performed confirming a direct role for pancreatic enzymes in the pathophysiology of pancreatic encephalopathy. Elevated CSF amino acid levels have also been implicated in pancreatic encephalopathy (11), but these findings have not been substantiated either. It is possible that the elevated CSF pancreatic enzyme or amino acid levels simply represent markers of a compromised blood–brain barrier in the setting of SIRS. Also unknown is the role of cytokines in the pathophysiology of CNS function in acute pancreatitis.

PATHOLOGY

A variety of neuropathologic changes have been reported in patients who developed neurologic complications during acute pancreatitis. They include patchy myelin pallor (9), pontine myelinolysis (12), acute hemorrhagic leukoencephalitis (13), and fat embolism (14–16).

CLINICAL MANIFESTATIONS

Pancreatitis presents with a steady, boring pain in the upper abdomen, often radiating to the back. It can develop over a few days in alcoholics or suddenly with gallstone obstruction. It is typically accompanied by nausea and vomiting and abdominal tenderness. Low-grade fever and mild leukocytosis can accompany the inflammatory process. In severe disease, systemic complications include electrolyte abnormalities, hypotension or shock, renal failure, acute respiratory distress syndrome, disseminated intravascular coagulation, subcutaneous fat necrosis with hypocalcemia, hyperglycemia, and encephalopathy (17). Hypocalcemia can cause neuromuscular irritability. In alcoholics, hypomagnesemia can trigger seizures, whereas thiamine deficiency can cause Wernicke encephalopathy. True *pancreatic encephalopathy* is said to manifest itself between the second and fifth day after the onset of pancreatitis and typically fluctuates over time. The sensorium may be blunted and a wide variety of global clinical signs and symptoms may be noted, including fluctuating mental status, disorientation, confusion, dysarthria, hallucinations, delirium, akinetic mutism, seizures, stupor, and coma (18).

DIAGNOSTIC APPROACH

Pancreatitis should be suspected in any patient with severe abdominal pain and elevated levels of serum amylase and lipase (over twice the upper limit of normal). Mimics include perforated gastric or duodenal ulcer, mesenteric infarction, intestinal obstruction, ectopic pregnancy, and pelvic inflammatory disease. Abdominal ultrasound can detect gallstones and biliary tract obstruction. Abdominal CT with contrast can identify pancreatic edema, fluid collections, and necrosis. The differential diagnosis for altered mental status in a patient with pancreatitis is long and pancreatic encephalopathy should be considered only when testing or treatment has exhausted the more likely possibilities (e.g., ischemia, uremia, hypoxemia, electrolyte abnormalities, thiamine deficiency). Particularly challenging is eliminating the diagnosis of delirium tremens, because alcohol consumption is a common cause of pancreatitis and an accurate history of alcohol use can be difficult to obtain. Tachycardia, hypertension, and delirium in acute alcoholic pancreatitis should be managed as delirium tremens, whereas the focus of altered mental status in nonalcoholic pancreatitis should initially be on metabolic causes. In pancreatic encephalopathy, cranial MRI studies have disclosed small, nonspecific lesions scattered in the subcortical white matter (19), pontine and extrapontine myelinolysis (13) and extensive white matter lesions (20), and isolated cerebral atrophy (1). CSF examination generally shows normal pressure, cell count, and chemistries. Occasionally, a mild lymphocytosis or mild protein elevation is detected. In general, CSF examination is more helpful in excluding other diagnoses than in establishing a diagnosis of pancreatic encephalopathy. Although CSF lipase levels may be elevated in this disorder (7–10), no apparent correlation exists between serum and CSF lipase values (10) and *normal* CSF levels by current methodologies have not been established. Thus, CSF lipase determination is not a practical clinical tool at this time.

TREATMENT

The neurologic deficits clear once the pancreatitis starts to subside. Treatment for pancreatitis involves withholding oral intake for 1 to 2 days, nasogastric suctioning for vomiting, intensive fluid replacement, correction of electrolyte abnormalities, and administration of parenteral opioids and antiemetics for pain and vomiting. For severe and prolonged cases, enteral feeding by jejunal tube or total parental nutrition can be used for nutritional support. Drugs that suppress pancreatic secretion are of unproved benefit. Some patients need to be in an intensive care unit (ICU) for treatment of systemic complications, such as hypotension, hypoxemia, electrolyte derangements, renal failure, sepsis, and multiorgan failure.

CLINICAL RECOMMENDATIONS OF THE VIGNETTE

The case vignette (1) is exceptional among published reports in that the appearance of encephalopathy was not complicated by any other systemic illnesses, at least not overtly. The details of the metabolic testing were not provided, however, and it is conceivable that a metabolic disorder affecting both the pancreas and CNS was missed. Importantly, three spaced MRI studies did not disclose any lesion other than cerebral atrophy, despite persisting neurologic deficits. Similarly the CSF appeared benign in the single instance that it was examined, but lipase activity was not tested. This patient may qualify as a genuine case of *pancreatic encephalopathy*, but whether it has any bearing on what Vogel originally described is uncertain. White matter lesions were not demonstrated. It seems likely that more than a single pathophysiologic process is responsible for pancreatic encephalopathy.

SUMMARY

Pancreatic encephalopathy is a rare disorder associated with acute pancreatitis. Its existence as a distinct pathophysiologic entity is uncertain, because most case reports have not excluded coexistent medical disorders that very likely contributed to the encephalopathic process and, in fact, might account for all of it. The now quarter century old report by Estrada (10) that CSF lipase activity is increased selectively and transiently in pancreatic encephalopathy is provocative; to our knowledge, however, the findings have not been re-examined. Future investigations on how the systemic inflammatory response syndrome in acute pancreatitis affects the CNS are warranted.

Insulinoma and Hypoglycemia

OBJECTIVES

- To describe the neurologic complications of hypoglycemia caused by insulinomas
- To discuss the management of hypoglycemia associated with insulinomas

CASE VIGNETTE

An 82-year-old woman presented with a 10-year history of episodic confusion and somnolence. Episodes occurred about twice a year, usually just after waking, and were relieved with breakfast. In the past year, the episodes increased in frequency and occurred throughout the day. Normal physical and neurological examination findings were noted by her doctor who attributed her symptoms to anxiety and reassured her. At checkout, however, she became confused, and her blood glucose was 28 mg/dL. She was hospitalized and placed on a fasting protocol. Blood testing showed persistently low blood glucose (low 30s), inappropriately high levels of insulin and C-peptide, and the absence of sulfonylurea agents. An abdominal CT disclosed a contrast-enhancing mass in the pancreatic head consistent with an insulinoma. With intraoperative ultrasound, a 1-cm discrete, firm pancreatic nodule was identified and excised. Afterwards, her blood sugars normalized, and she became asymptomatic (21).

DEFINITION

Hypoglycemia refers to low blood glucose levels (<40 mg/dL) that produce symptoms by stimulating the sympathetic nervous system and causing dysfunction of the CNS. Most commonly, hypoglycemia occurs in diabetics from therapeutic misadventure (excessive insulin or oral hypoglycemic agent administration). Rarely, hypoglycemia is provoked by abnormal endogenous insulin secretion. If it does occur, most often it is caused by a rare pancreatic islet cell tumor called an *insulinoma*.

EPIDEMIOLOGY

Insulinomas are rare. About four new cases per 1 million occur annually (22). Most are solitary and pathologically benign but approximately 10% are malignant and approximately 10% occur in the context of multiple endocrine neoplasia type 1 (MEN-1). The median age is 50 years, except in MEN-1, where the median age is in the 20s.

ETIOLOGY AND PATHOGENESIS

Insulinomas secrete excessive insulin, resulting in hypoglycemia (blood sugar <40 mg/dL), which triggers a sympathetic nervous system response. The CNS uses glucose almost exclusively as a source of metabolic fuel. When blood sugar drops sharply (blood sugar <30 mg/dL), cerebral function deteriorates to produce global and, occasionally, focal neurologic deficits (23). Thus, the neurologic consequences of insulinoma result entirely from insulin hypersecretion and subsequent hypoglycemia. What induces islet cells to neoplastic transformation and insulin hypersecretion is unknown. The gene implicated in MEN-1, an autosomal-dominant disease, is believed to function as a tumor suppressor gene and may play a role in MEN-1 and in sporadic neuroendocrine tumors in general.

PATHOLOGY

About 80% of islet cell tumors are small (<2 cm), solitary benign adenomas in the pancreas that can be surgically removed. In MEN-1, multiple microinsulinomas and macroinsulinomas appear throughout the pancreas and their removal is difficult. Malignant transformation, which occurs in approximately 10% of cases, produces larger tumors that metastasize to the liver in about one third of cases. Tumor cells can be histologically distinguished from normal islet cells by higher levels of proinsulin, lower levels of insulin, and fewer secretory granules than the normal islet cells. Insulin is initially synthesized as proinsulin, a single polypeptide chain containing disulfide-linked A and B chains (insulin) and a connecting peptide (C-peptide). Proteolytic cleavage of the C-peptide within the secretion granule liberates the double chain insulin molecule and both insulin and C-peptide are exocytosed in equimolar quantities from the islet cells in response to hyperglycemia. Insulinomas are relatively insensitive to serum glucose levels, so insulin secretion proceeds even when blood glucose levels are low. When hypoglycemia is severe or prolonged, CNS damage primarily involves neurons in the cerebral cortex, with resultant laminar necrosis and a special predilection for the dentate gyrus of the hippocampus (24). Demyelination can occasionally be pronounced.

CLINICAL MANIFESTATIONS

Insulinomas are characterized by episodic hypoglycemia (25). Hypoglycemia produces CNS signs and symptoms that vary in severity and duration (23,26). Symptoms can be insidious and mimic a variety of neuropsychiatric disorders. When a person's blood glucose falls to <40 mg/dL, the sympathetic nervous system is stimulated, which result in anxiety, trembling, hunger, sweating, pallor, and palpitations. All symptoms resolve rapidly with timely glucose administration or a snack. Not uncommonly, patients with insulinoma manage their symptoms with frequent small meals, which can lead to a delay in diagnosis. More profound hypoglycemia (<30 mg/dL) causes mental confusion, headache, muscle spasms or myoclonic twitching that can progress to seizures, focal strokelike deficits, coma, depression of cardiovascular and respiratory functions, and ultimately death.

DIAGNOSTIC APPROACH

The symptoms of hypoglycemia are variable (23,25,26), and the differential diagnosis includes many other causes (e.g., delirium tremens, opiate withdrawal, hypertensive encephalopathy, thyrotoxicosis, brain hemorrhage) that can produce sympathetic overdrive with mental confusion, stupor, coma, seizures or strokelike deficits. The blood glucose should be checked immediately and glucose administered empirically. Hypoglycemia can occur with diseases of the liver, pituitary or adrenal, but these can usually be identified by other organ signs and symptoms. When hypoglycemia is episodic and blood glucose measurements are <40 mg/dL, serum proinsulin, insulin, and C-peptide levels should be quantified from a concurrent blood sample. The finding of an elevated insulin level (normal <6 uIU/mL) with normal C-peptide (<2 ng/mL) and proinsulin levels suggests an exogenous insulin cause for the hypoglycemia (surreptitious or factitious). The presence of low insulin, C-peptide, and proinsulin levels justifies determination of serum sulfonylurea (oral hypoglycemic) agent levels. In contrast, elevation of serum proinsulin, insulin, and C-peptide levels in the setting of hypoglycemia suggest inappropriate, endogenous insulin secretion from an insulinoma.

Most patients harboring an insulinoma are asymptomatic (euglycemic) at the time of evaluation. Induction of hypoglycemia with a 2- to 3-day fast under close hospital observation may be required to obtain the proinsulin, insulin, and C-peptide levels. About three quarters of the patients become symptomatic from hypoglycemia within 24 hours and virtually all do so after 3 days of fasting. Failure of insulin to be suppressed by hypoglycemia in a prolonged fast is characteristic of an insulinoma. MEN-1 must be excluded by measuring serum calcium (hyperparathyroidism from parathyroid adenoma) and prolactin levels (pituitary tumor). Confirmation of MEN-1 reduces the likelihood for curative surgical resection. Absence of MEN-1 warrants a search to localize the insulinoma for curative resection. Because most (~80%) of insulinomas are <2 cm in size, imaging by contrast CT, MRI, transabdominal ultrasound, and arteriography will detect only 40% to 80% of the tumors. Endoscopic ultrasound is much more sensitive than CT for the localization of insulinomas (27,28) and should be the next procedure of choice if CT or MRI imaging is not diagnostic. Selective arteriography, with or without selective venous sampling for insulin measurements, should be reserved for only the most challenging cases. Although octreotide scintigraphy scanning is useful to localize the primary and metastatic neuroendocrine tumors in general, its sensitivity for the detection of insulinomas is less than for other lesions.

TREATMENT

Acute hypoglycemia, whatever its cause, must be treated aggressively with glucose to prevent CNS damage. For solitary insulinomas, surgical resection for cure is the treatment of choice (cure rate ~90%). For insulinomas associated with MEN-1, surgical cure is more difficult to achieve and cases must be individualized. In patients who cannot undergo surgery or who have metastatic disease, measures are taken to prevent hypoglycemia. Diazoxide inhibits insulin secretion by the tumor, but promotes sodium retention and edema, with an increased risk for congestive heart failure. Hence, hydrocholothiazide should be coadministered to reduce edema and to enhance the hyperglycemic effect. If hypoglycemia proves refractory to diazoxide, the somatostatin analogue, octreotide, may be of benefit. About half of insulinomas exhibit the somatostatin receptor type 2 and will be responsive to octreotide. Other medications with modest and less predictable inhibition of insulin secretion include phenytoin, verapamil, and diltiazem. Other palliative treatment modalities include embolization or radiofrequency ablation of liver metastases and chemotherapy for stage IV disease.

CLINICAL RECOMMENDATIONS OF THE VIGNETTE

Missing the diagnosis of insulinoma as the cause for neuropsychiatric dysfunction is common. As many as 20% of patients may be diagnosed with a psychiatric, seizure, or other neurologic disorder before the insulinoma is recognized (29).

SUMMARY

Hypoglycemia should always be considered in the differential diagnosis of altered consciousness and a rapid clinical response to glucose replacement establishes cause and effect. Insulinoma is a rare but potentially curable cause of hypoglycemia. Measuring serum proinsulin, insulin, and C-peptide levels during episodes of hypoglycemia is the first step in diagnosing insulinoma, followed by CT or endoscopic ultrasonography for localization. Although medical treatments to control symptoms are available, surgical resection for cure is the treatment modality of choice.

Pancreatic Adenocarcinoma and Cerebral Thromboembolism due to Nonbacterial Thrombotic Endocarditis

OBJECTIVES

- To describe nonbacterial thrombotic endocarditis (NBTE) in patients with pancreatic adenocarcinoma
- To discuss treatment options of NBTE in patients with pancreatic adenpocarcinoma

CASE VIGNETTE

A 62-year-old man awoke with slurred speech, visual blurring, and left-sided weakness after 4 months of progressive malaise, weight loss, and epigastric discomfort. He was cachectic and had mild epigastric and right upper quadrant abdominal tenderness and a massively enlarged liver. He was depressed, had a mild short term memory deficit, but was otherwise coherent. He had bilateral internuclear ophthalmoplegia, dysarthria, left lower facial weakness, left hemiparesis, and peripheral sensory loss in both legs. Serum amylase and liver enzymes were modestly elevated. Chest x-ray study and head CT scan findings were normal. He was treated with thiamine, insulin, and intravenous fluids. On the following day, he became febrile and confused and his focal deficits worsened. CSF examination was unremarkable. Antibiotics were given for a urinary tract infection, and 3 days later, he became alert and oriented. Blood cultures were negative. His left-sided weakness improved. An abdominal CT revealed ascites and an enlarged liver with multiple nodules and lymphadenopathy in the right pelvis. The pancreas appeared normal. Liver biopsy disclosed a poorly differentiated metastatic adenocarcinoma with signet ring cells. He declined chemotherapy and died 3 weeks later. Autopsy disclosed a poorly differentiated mucin-secreting adenocarcinoma in the body of the pancreas, with ascites and widespread metastasis to the peritoneum, liver, and lung. Both legs showed deep venous thrombosis (DVT). The mitral valve had friable vegetations with a denuded area from which vegetations were recently dislodged. Multiple platelet-fibrin emboli were found in the end arterioles of the cerebral gray matter producing multiple small infarcts with occasional hemorrhage. The largest infarcts (1 to 1.5 cm) were found in the right precentral gyrus and the right occipital cortex. No pontine lesion was found. The pathology was characteristic for NBTE with cerebral embolism in the setting of a pancreatic adenocarcinoma.

DEFINITION

NBTE, also called *marantic endocarditis*, refers to sterile platelet-fibrin thrombi that occur as vegetations on cardiac valves in association with several disease processes, including hypercoagulable states and advanced malignancy. It is most commonly associated with adenocarcinomas of the pancreas, lung, and stomach. Symptoms are caused by arterial embolism, primarily to the brain.

EPIDEMIOLOGY

NBTE is relatively uncommon, found in approximately 4% of autopsies (30). In the absence of stroke, the prevalence of NBTE in cancer patients is about 1% (31). In patients with cancer who have had a stroke, however, the prevalence of NBTE is between 20% and 30% (32,33). Adenocarcinoma of the pancreas, lung, and stomach accounts for 60% to 80% of all cases of NBTE. NBTE appears to be most common in patients with pancreatic cancer. In one autopsy series, 17 of 41 cases of NBTE were caused by cancer of the pancreas (34).

ETIOLOGY AND PATHOGENESIS

NBTE is part of a hypercoagulable spectrum that includes disseminated intravascular coagulation (DIC) and venous thrombosis. It occurs in patients with cancer and other debilitating systemic diseases. Cancer can promote a hypercoagulable state through a variety of mechanisms, including fibrinolytic activation, neovascularization of tumor with abnormal endothelial lining, and procoagulant (e.g., mucin) release into the systemic circulation (35). An underlying valvular abnormality predisposes to the deposition of platelets and fibrin under these conditions. Vegetations are typically multiverrucous, <3 mm in size, and are most commonly found on the mitral and aortic valves (36). Arterial embolism is responsible for cerebral symptoms, but brain hemorrhages occur as well, when thrombocytopenia, liver failure, or sepsis aggravates the coagulopathy (33). These patients are at greater risk for DVT, paradoxic embolism, and cerebral venous thrombosis.

PATHOLOGY

Autopsy typically shows widespread platelet-fibrin emboli affecting many organs. Vegetations are most commonly found on the flow surfaces of the mitral or aortic valves, with one third of patients having more than one valve affected (37). In only 5% of cases do vegetations affect the valves of the right side of the heart. Microscopically, the vegetations consist of bland, eosinophilic platelet-fibrin thrombi, and these thrombi can also be found lodged in end arterioles of the cerebral and cerebellar cortices. In about 50% of cases, fibrin thrombi can also be detected in the venous circulation, indicating the presence of DIC (38). Hemorrhages, which are caused by the coagulopathy, are usually located in the cerebral white matter and are often a solitary occurrence. Although rare, CNS symptoms from mucin-secreting pancreatic adenocarcinomas can also arise from metastases to the dura that produce subdural effusions (39).

CLINICAL MANIFESTATIONS

Patients with adenocarcinoma of the pancreas typically complain of weight loss and abdominal pain that radiates to the back. Unless the lesion is in the head of the pancreas, where early biliary obstruction and jaundice can lead to early diagnosis, most patients have advanced local disease or metastases to the liver or lung at the time of diagnosis. Diabetes occurs in up to 50% of cases and new onset diabetes in a nonobese elderly patient should alert to the possibility of pancreatic cancer.

Because of their small size, the vegetations of NBTE do not typically cause valvular dysfunction. Consequently, cardiac symptoms (murmurs or clinically significant stenosis or regurgitation) are infrequent. More commonly, NBTE presents with symptoms from arterial embolism, and the CNS is the most sensitive target. Focal, strokelike symptoms appear suddenly, but because embolic events and symptoms are often multifocal, NBTE can present as a global encephalopathy with or without focal cerebral deficits (40). Occasionally, stroke can be the presenting sign of cancer. DIC, unaccompanied by NBTE, commonly produces encephalopathy, but it too can present with transient focal signs (41). Clinical signs can fluctuate, but the overall clinical course of these coagulation disorders is progressive. Cerebral vein thrombosis can produce seizures or present with focal or global neurologic deficits. The superior sagittal sinus is the most common cerebral vein involved (42,43).

DIAGNOSTIC APPROACH

NBTE should be suspected in any patient with cancer who has a stroke, especially if the cancer is a mucin-secreting adenocarcinoma. Because the valvular vegetations are small, a new or changing heart murmur is seldom detected by auscultation. In the setting of negative blood cultures, NBTE can be diagnosed by echocardiography, with the transesophageal approach being more sensitive that the transthoracic one (30,32). Routine laboratory tests may show abnormalities of coagulation, but changes may be mild or confused with the effects of chemotherapy or liver disease on clotting (44). D-dimer is a measure of the hypercoagulable state, but it can be influenced by tumor volume and by stroke itself (45). Abdominal imaging with CT or ultrasound is helpful in the diagnosis of pancreatic or other intraabdominal cancers. In the presence of a pancreatic lesion, an elevation in the tumor marker CA19-9 further supports the diagnosis. Frequently, cytologic examination of the mass following CT or endoscopic ultrasound-guided tissue sampling is necessary to firmly establish the diagnosis.

Cranial MRI is important to exclude metastases, cerebral venous thrombosis, subdural effusion, and hemorrhage, as well as to confirm the diagnosis of acute ischemic stroke with diffusion-weighted imaging. Rarely, neurologic signs can arise from thrombotic thrombocytopenic purpura (TTP) associated with pancreatic adenocarcinoma (46).

TREATMENT

The best hope for survival is control of the underlying disease and reduction in tumor burden (47). Only 20% of pancreatic adenocarcinomas are preoperatively considered resectable for cure and only half of these actually are resectable in the operating room. Thus, most pancreatic cancers are incurable, with palliative surgery, chemotherapy, or both forming the basis for treatment. How to manage the hypercoagulable state is controversial, but heparin is generally administered and considered to be more effective than warfarin. In one randomized study, low–molecular-weight heparin suppressed recurrent thromboembolism in patients with cancer twice as frequently as did warfarin (48). Heparin can attenuate cerebral symptoms in some, but not all patients, with NBTE (40). Disease spread is often extensive by the time that NBTE is suspected, however, so prognosis is poor and treatment is palliative.

CLINICAL RECOMMENDATIONS OF THE VIGNETTE

The case vignette illustrates the characteristic multifocal neurologic manifestations of NBTE coinciding with classic signs and symptoms of advanced pancreatic cancer and a hypercoagulable state.

SUMMARY

NBTE is a common cause of ischemic stroke in patients with cancer. It is most often associated with adenocarcinomas of the pancreas, stomach, or lung. The release of mucin into the systemic circulation may contribute to the associated hypercoagulable state and DIC. Vegetations are most commonly found on valves on the left side of the heart and murmurs are typically not heard. Blood cultures are negative. Transesophageal echocardiography is the most sensitive study for the detection of NBTE vegetations. Heparin may be helpful when the tumor is treatable, but all too often, disease is advanced and life expectancy can be measured in weeks to months.

REFERENCES

1. Ruggieri RM, Lupo I, Piccoli F. Pancreatic encephalopathy: A 7-year follow-up case report and review of the literature. *Neurol Sci.* 2002;23(4):203–205.
2. Appelros S, Borgstrom A. Incidence, aetiology and mortality rate of acute pancreatitis over 10 years in a defined urban population in Sweden. *Br J Surg.* 1999;86(4):465–470.
3. Thomson SR, Hendry WS, McFarlane GA, et al. Epidemiology and outcome of acute pancreatitis. *Br J Surg.* 1987;74(5):398–401.
4. Yadav D, Lowenfels AB. Trends in the epidemiology of the first attack of acute pancreatitis: A systematic review. *Pancreas.* 2006;33(4):323–330.
5. De Falco FA, Sollazzo D, Campanella G. Pancreatic encephalopathy. A case report with multifocal neurological signs. *Acta Neurol (Napoli).* 1980;2(6):482–487.
6. Whitcomb DC. Clinical practice. Acute pancreatitis. *N Engl J Med.* 2006;354(20):2142–2150.
7. Vogel FA. Demyelination induced experimentally by means of lipase. *Fed Proc.* 1950;9:347.
8. Vogel FS. Demyelinization induced in living rabbits by means of a lipolytic enzyme preparation. *J Exp Med.* 1951;93(4):297–304.
9. Vogel FS. Cerebral demyelination and focal visceral lesions in a case of acute hemorrhagic pancreatitis, with a consideration of the possible role of circulating enzymes in the causation of the lesions. *AMA Arch Pathol.* 1951;52(4):355–362.

10. Estrada RV, Moreno J, Martinez E, et al. Pancreatic encephalopathy. *Acta Neurol Scand.* 1979;59(2–3):135–139.
11. Sjaastad O, Gjessing L, Ritland S, et al. Chronic relapsing pancreatitis, encephalopathy with disturbances of consciousness and CSF amino acid aberration. *J Neurol.* 1979;220(2):83–94.
12. Sherins RJ, Verity MA. Central pontine myelinolysis associated with acute haemorrhagic pancreatitis. *J Neurol Neurosurg Psychiatry.* 1968;31(6):583–588.
13. Chan C, Fryer J, Herkes G, et al. Fatal brain stem event complicating acute pancreatitis. *J Clin Neurosci.* 2003;10(3):351–358.
14. Bhalla A, Sachdev A, Lehl SS, et al. Cerebral fat embolism as a rare possible complication of traumatic pancreatitis. *JOP.* 2003;4(4):155–157.
15. Guardia SN, Bilbao JM, Murray D, et al. Fat embolism in acute pancreatitis. *Arch Pathol Lab Med.* 1989;113(5):503–506.
16. Johnson DA, Tong NT. Pancreatic encephalopathy. *South Med J.* 1977;70(2):165–167.
17. Pitchumoni CS, Agarwal N, Jain NK. Systemic complications of acute pancreatitis. *Am J Gastroenterol.* 1988;83(6):597–606.
18. Sharf B, Levy N. Pancreatic encephalopathy. In: Vinken PJ, Bruyn GW, Klawans H, eds. *Handbook of Clinical Neurology Metabolic and Deficiency Diseases of the Nervous System.* Amsterdam: North Holland; 1976:449–458.
19. Boon P, de Reuck J, Achten E, et al. Pancreatic encephalopathy. A case report and review of the literature. *Clin Neurol Neurosurg.* 1991;93(2):137–141.
20. Ohkubo T, Shiojiri T, Matsunaga T. Severe diffuse white matter lesions in a patient with pancreatic encephalopathy. *J Neurol.* 2004;251(4):476–478.
21. Fahmi Ya PR. Case Study: An 82-year-old woman presents with severe hypoglycemia induced by an insulinoma. *Clinical Diabetes.* 2004;22(2):102–104.
22. Service FJ, McMahon MM, O'Brien PC, et al. Functioning insulinoma—Incidence, recurrence, and long-term survival of patients: A 60-year study. *Mayo Clin Proc.* 1991;66(7):711–719.
23. Chang G. Hypoglycemia. *www.medlink.com* 2006.
24. Auer RN, Sutherland GR. Hypoxic brain damage. In: Graham DI, Lantos P, eds. *Greenfield's Neuropathology,* 7th ed. New York: Oxford University Press; 2002:260–262.
25. Dizon AM, Kowalyk S, Hoogwerf BJ. Neuroglycopenic and other symptoms in patients with insulinomas. *Am J Med.* 1999;106(3):307–310.
26. Malouf R, Brust JC. Hypoglycemia: Causes, neurological manifestations, and outcome. *Ann Neurol.* 1985;17(5):421–430.
27. Anderson MA, Carpenter S, Thompson NW, et al. Endoscopic ultrasound is highly accurate and directs management in patients with neuroendocrine tumors of the pancreas. *Am J Gastroenterol.* 2000 Sep;95(9):2271–2277.
28. Tamerisa R, Irisawa A, Bhutani MS. Endoscopic ultrasound in the diagnosis, staging, and management of gastrointestinal and adjacent malignancies. *Med Clin North Am.* 2005;89(1):139–158, viii.
29. Service FJ, Dale AJ, Elveback LR, et al. Insulinoma: Clinical and diagnostic features of 60 consecutive cases. *Mayo Clin Proc.* 1976;51(7):417–429.
30. Lopez JA, Ross RS, Fishbein MC, et al. Nonbacterial thrombotic endocarditis: A review. *Am Heart J.* 1987;113(3):773–784.
31. Macdonell RA, Kalnins RM, Donnan GA. Non-bacterial thrombotic endocarditis and stroke. *Clin Exp Neurol.* 1986;22:123–132.
32. Dutta T, Karas MG, Segal AZ, et al. Yield of transesophageal echocardiography for nonbacterial thrombotic endocarditis and other cardiac sources of embolism in cancer patients with cerebral ischemia. *Am J Cardiol.* 2006;97(6):894–898.
33. Graus F, Rogers LR, Posner JB. Cerebrovascular complications in patients with cancer. *Medicine (Baltimore).* 1985;64(1):16–35.
34. Sack GH, Jr., Levin J, Bell WR. Trousseau's syndrome and other manifestations of chronic disseminated coagulopathy in patients with neoplasms: Clinical, pathophysiologic, and therapeutic features. *Medicine (Baltimore).* 1977;56(1):1–37.
35. Khorana AA, Fine RL. Pancreatic cancer and thromboembolic disease. *Lancet Oncol.* 2004;5(11):655–663.
36. Biller J, Challa VR, Toole JF, et al. Nonbacterial thrombotic endocarditis. A neurologic perspective of clinicopathologic correlations of 99 patients. *Arch Neurol.* 1982;39(2):95–98.
37. Bryan CS. Nonbacterial thrombotic endocarditis with malignant tumors. *Am J Med.* 1969;46(5):787–793.
38. Kim HS, Suzuki M, Lie JT, et al. Nonbacterial thrombotic endocarditis (NBTE) and disseminated intravascular coagulation (DIC): Autopsy study of 36 patients. *Arch Pathol Lab Med.* 1977;101(2):65–68.
39. Castleman B. MGH CPC Case 12-1972. *N Engl J Med.* 1972;286(12):650–656.
40. Rogers LR, Cho ES, Kempin S, et al. Cerebral infarction from non-bacterial thrombotic endocarditis. Clinical and pathological study including the effects of anticoagulation. *Am J Med.* 1987;83(4):746–756.
41. Collins RC, Al-Mondhiry H, Chernik NL, et al. Neurologic manifestations of intravascular coagulation in patients with cancer. A clinicopathologic analysis of 12 cases. *Neurology.* 1975;25(9):795–806.
42. Raizer JJ, DeAngelis LM. Cerebral sinus thrombosis diagnosed by MRI and MR venography in cancer patients. *Neurology.* 2000;54(6):1222–1226.
43. Sigsbee B, Deck MD, Posner JB. Nonmetastatic superior sagittal sinus thrombosis complicating systemic cancer. *Neurology.* 1979;29(2):139–146.
44. Rogers LR. Cerebrovascular complications in cancer patients. *Neurol Clin.* 2003;21(1):167–192.
45. Cestari DM, Weine DM, Panageas KS, et al. Stroke in patients with cancer: Incidence and etiology. *Neurology.* 2004;62(11):2025–2030.
46. Wolff D, Brinkmann B, Emmrich J, et al. Metastatic pancreatic carcinoma presenting as thrombotic thrombocytopenic purpura. *Pancreas.* 2003;26(3):314.
47. Rogers L. Cerebrovascular complications of cancer. *www.medlink.com* 2006.
48. Lee AY, Levine MN, Baker RI, et al. Low-molecular-weight heparin versus a coumarin for the prevention of recurrent venous thromboembolism in patients with cancer. *N Engl J Med.* 2003;349(2):146–153.

CHAPTER **38**

Neurologic Complications of Gastrointestinal Malignancies

Mervat Wahba • John K. DiBaise

INTRODUCTION

The gastrointestinal tract is the third most common area affected by cancer; malignancies within the gut comprise approximately 20% of new cancer diagnoses. This chapter reviews the major gastrointestinal tract and pancreaticobiliary cancers and the neurologic complications, both metastatic and nonmetastatic, of these tumors and their treatments. A detailed discussion of diseases of the pancreas, including pancreatic adenocarcinomas and insulinomas, is available in Chapter 37. An extensive discussion of paraneoplastic disorders of the central and peripheral nervous systems is covered in Chapters 57 and 58, and the neurologic side effects of chemotherapy are covered in Chapter 60.

OBJECTIVES

- To review the neurologic complications of gastrointestinal malignancies
- To discuss corresponding chemotherapeutic complications

CASE VIGNETTE

A 55-year-old man consulted a neurologist for subacute onset of generalized headaches and episodic confusion. Two days earlier, he was found to have right-sided facial weakness, abduction weakness of the right eye, and an unsteady gait. His medical history was remarkable for a recent change in bowel habits, a deep vein thrombosis (DVT) of his right lower extremity below the popliteal vein, and 20-pound weight loss over the last 4 months. Magnetic resonance imaging (MRI) of the brain showed diffuse leptomeningeal enhancement with scattered nodular deposits in the subarachnoid space. Cerebrospinal fluid (CSF) analysis showed elevated opening pressure, and a mild lymphocytic pleocytosis. CSF protein concentration was high and glucose content was low. Cytology was positive for malignant cells. A computed tomographic (CT) scan of the pelvis showed a malignant growth in the ascending colon.

DEFINITION

Various gastrointestinal tract malignancies can affect the central nervous system (CNS) or peripheral nervous system (PNS) by direct spread or through paraneoplastic mechanisms. Chemotherapy given for treatment of these cancers can also cause adverse effects on the nervous system.

Esophageal Cancer

EPIDEMIOLOGY

Esophageal cancer is the seventh leading cause of cancer deaths in men. For the past two decades, the incidence of esophageal adenocarcinoma has increased dramatically in Western countries so that the two tumor types currently occur with almost the same frequency. The overall male-to-female ratio is about 3:1, with a higher prevalence of squamous cell cancer among black men and a higher prevalence of adenocarcinoma among white men.

ETIOLOGY, PATHOGENESIS, AND PATHOPHYSIOLOGY

Ethanol consumption and smoking are major risk factors for squamous cell tumors, whereas Barrett's esophagus and gastroesophageal reflux disease increase the risk of esophageal adenocarcinoma.

PATHOLOGY

Squamous cell cancer and adenocarcinoma account for 95% of all malignant esophageal tumors. Squamous cell carcinoma originates in squamous cells lining the esophagus and most often develops in the upper or middle portion of the esophagus. Adenocarcinoma develops in glandular cells, usually within the lower esophageal region.

NEUROLOGIC COMPLICATIONS

Brain Metastases

Brain metastases secondary to esophageal cancer are relatively rare. A review of 334 esophagectomy cases demonstrated only 10 patients with esophageal adenocarcinoma and

2 patients with squamous cell carcinoma who developed brain metastases (1).

Paraneoplastic Syndromes

Paraneoplastic vasculitis has been reported in a man with concurrent esophageal and gastric cancers presenting with fever and leg numbness 3 months before the cancer diagnosis was made. The esophageal cancer was a well-differentiated squamous cell carcinoma with lymph node involvement (2). Paraneoplastic cerebellar degeneration with anti-Yo antibodies has also been reported in a man with esophageal adenocarcinoma (3).

TREATMENT

The 5-year survival remains very poor despite improvements in the staging evaluation, primarily because of the late tumor stage at the time of diagnosis. Although surgery may increase survival in early cases, these cases represent the minority. For most patients, palliative therapies, including chemotherapy, radiation therapy, combined chemoradiation therapy, photodynamic therapy, or esophageal stenting are more commonly used. The 5-year survival rates for curatively resectable disease are about 20% to 25%. In more advanced cases, median survival with radiation therapy is up to 12 months. There is improved 2- and 5-year survival with chemoradiation compared with radiation alone (4). The role of neoadjuvant therapy to downstage tumors before surgical resection appears promising.

Gastric Cancer

EPIDEMIOLOGY

Gastric cancer, which is rare in the United States, is the second most common cancer worldwide. The mortality rate from gastric cancer has significantly declined in the United States compared with other countries such as Japan, Chile, and Iceland, presumably because of a decreased use of nitrites, which leads to the formation of nitrosamines, which are proved carcinogens.

ETIOLOGY, PATHOGENESIS, AND PATHOPHYSIOLOGY

In addition to nitrites, *Helicobacter pylori* infection and atrophic gastritis are also associated with gastric cancer. Overall, environmental factors appear to be more important than genetic factors in the causation of gastric cancer (5).

PATHOLOGY

Most gastric cancers are adenocarcinoma and they generally affect the distal portion of the stomach. Nevertheless, in recent years, an increase has been seen in gastroesophageal junction or cardia tumors.

NEUROLOGIC COMPLICATIONS

Brain Metastases

In a group of 210 patients with brain metastases, Posner and Chernik (6) found that only 14 had primary tumors of the gastrointestinal system (8 colon, 4 esophagus, and 1 each of gastric and pancreatic origin).

Lumbosacral Plexopathy and Epidural Spinal Cord Compression

In a review of 85 patients with lumbosacral plexopathy, investigators from the Memorial Sloan-Kettering Cancer Center (MSKCC) identified 17 who had colorectal cancer and 2 who had gastric cancer. The mean survival was only 5.5 months from the time of diagnosis (7). Lumbosacral epidural metastases typically present with back or leg pain. Epidural spinal compression has been reported in a few patients with gastric cancer. In another report from MSKCC involving 235 patients with metastatic epidural spinal cord involvement, only 9 cases were caused by a primary gastrointestinal tumor (8,9).

Leptomeningeal Metastases

Leptomeningeal carcinomatosis is rare in gastric cancer and is associated with poor survival (10).

Paraneoplastic Syndromes

Paraneoplastic syndromes are also rather uncommon among patients with gastric cancers. Paraneoplastic cerebellar degeneration has been reported in a patient with a mixed adenocarcinoma and neuroendocrine carcinoma of the stomach presenting with ataxia without opsoclonus and anti-Ri antibodies (11).

Neurologic Sequelae of Gastrectomy

Both total and partial gastrectomy can result in a dumping syndrome whereby the loss of the physiologic delay of food transport to the small intestine results in rapid gastric emptying followed by characteristic symptoms such as diaphoresis, lethargy, presyncope, and diarrhea. These symptoms correlate with rapid fluctuations in blood glucose levels and the precipitous release of certain gut hormones.

Anemia can develop after gastrectomy secondary to altered iron and vitamin B_{12} absorption; subacute combined degeneration can develop because of the latter (12). Vitamin B_{12} replacement should be initiated once the deficiency is identified, followed by monthly supplementation thereafter. Recovery of the gait disturbance is anticipated if the condition is treated within a few weeks of symptom onset (13).

TREATMENT

As with esophageal cancer, survival remains poor, with a 5-year survival rate of only 10% to 15%. Improved 5-year survival rates of 90% have been reported for earlier stage gastric cancer limited to the mucosa and submucosa.

Surgical resection might be curative in early stage disease. This, however, is not the situation in many patients whose cancer is often diagnosed late. Improved survival has been reported when surgery is followed by combined chemotherapy (e.g., leucovorin-modulated 5-fluorourcil [5-FU]) and radiation. In a review of 603 patients with gastric and gastroesophageal junction adenocarcinoma, 85% of those with lymph node spread demonstrated improved survival rate following this adjuvant combined modality approach (14).

Colorectal Cancer

EPIDEMIOLOGY

Colorectal cancer is the third most common form of newly diagnosed cancers in both genders. Colorectal cancer also has the third highest cancer mortality rate, following cancers of the lung and prostate in men and cancers of the lung and breast in women. The survival rates are stage dependent. Overall, 1- and 5-year survival rates for patients with colorectal cancer are 82% and 61%, respectively; however, the 5-year survival rate drops to 8% when distant metastases are present (15,16).

ETIOLOGY, PATHOGENESIS, AND PATHOPHYSIOLOGY

The development of colorectal cancer has been associated with a diet high in red meat and fat intake and low in fiber intake. A personal or family history of colorectal cancer or polyps is another common risk factor. Hereditary colorectal cancer syndromes, such as familial adenomatous polyposis and hereditary nonpolyposis colorectal cancer syndrome, although rare, greatly increase the risk of both colonic and extracolonic tumors. Turcot syndrome is worth special note because of its status as a familial polyposis syndrome with associated CNS neoplasms, such as glioblastoma multiforme, astrocytoma, medulloblastoma, and ependymoma (17). Idiopathic inflammatory bowel diseases, such as Crohn disease and ulcerative colitis of long-standing duration (i.e., >8 years if pancolonic involvement and >12 years if left-sided involvement only) are also associated with an increased risk of colon cancer. Indeed, patients with ulcerative colitis have a 1% annual risk of developing colon cancer.

PATHOLOGY

Most colorectal cancers go through a recognizable premalignant adenoma phase. The adenoma is considered equivalent to a low-grade epithelial dysplasia. Adenocarcinomas and mucinous adenocarcinomas account for most colorectal malignancies (5).

NEUROLOGIC COMPLICATIONS

Cerebral Metastases

Cerebral metastases occur in 0.3% to 6% of patients with colon cancer and comprise about 8% of all brain metastases (18). In a study of patients with brain metastases from MSKCC, an incidence of 4% was seen with colon cancer. The median survival was 24.5 months since the original diagnosis and all patients had concurrent systemic spread (15). Another study involving 20 patients with colon cancer demonstrated that in 25% of patients, the brain was the first site of metastasis. The overall median survival was 51 days with a 1-year survival rate of 6% (19). Surgical resection appears to be an important factor correlating with increased survival (20).

Skeletal Metastases

Skeletal metastases are uncommon among patients with colorectal cancer. A 25-year retrospective review from the Saskatchewan Cancer Registry reported 355 patients with skeletal metastases of 5,352 individuals with colorectal cancer (21). Most of the patients had concurrent brain, lung, or liver metastases.

Lumbosacral Plexopathy and Epidural Spinal Cord Compression

Colorectal cancer is a relatively common cause of lumbosacral plexopathy. A study from MSKCC demonstrated a total of 17 patients with primary colorectal cancer of 85 patients presenting with lumbosacral plexopathy (7). Rectal tumors can also present with coccygeal plexus involvement causing perineal sensory loss and sphincter weakness (7). Radiation lumbosacral plexopathy can occur months to years following pelvic radiation; differentiation from neoplastic involvement may be challenging. The presence of painless weakness and myokimic discharges on electromyography favor the diagnosis of radiation plexopathy (22).

Epidural spinal cord compression is relatively uncommon among patients with gastrointestinal cancers. A retrospective review from the MSKCC found that only 9 of 235 patients with metastatic epidural spinal cord involvement had a primary gastrointestinal tumor (8,9). Another study of 34 patients with colorectal cancer and spinal cord compression determined that 55% of the cases involved the lumbar area; treatment consisting of external beam radiation resulted in a median survival of 7.9 months for patients with rectal cancer and 2.7 months for patients with colon cancer (23).

Leptomeningeal Carcinomatosis

Leptomeningeal carcinomatosis was found in only 1% of autopsies performed on 311 patients with colorectal cancer (24).

Paraneoplastic Syndromes

Colon cancer has been found in 6% to 35% of patients previously diagnosed with dermatomyositis (25). Paraneoplastic antineutrophil cytoplasmic antibodies (ANCA)-associated vasculitis with peripheral nerve involvement (26) and paraneoplastic limbic encephalitis (27) have also been reported in the setting of colon cancer. Paraneoplastic cerebellar degeneration is less frequently reported in patients with gastrointestinal malignancies than in individuals with carcinomas of the lung, ovaries, and breast, and in those with lymphoma (24).

Neurologic Complications of Chemotherapy

Acute neurotoxicity secondary to 5-FU can present as a cerebellar syndrome and encephalopathy, and is dose related. Seizures can also occur. Treatment with thiamine has been recommended (28). Multifocal inflammatory leukoencephalopathy has been reported with levamisole treatment of adenocarcinoma of the colon (29).

TREATMENT

Colorectal cancer is preventable in most instances if proper screening is undertaken. Multiple screening options are available for the person at average risk of colon cancer, starting at age 50 years and include annual home fecal occult blood testing, flexible sigmoidoscopy with or without barium enema every 5 years, or colonoscopy every 10 years. Individuals at higher risk of colon cancer, such as those with first-degree relatives with colon cancer or adenomatous polyps, should have screening beginning at the age of 40 or 10 years before the age the relative developed cancer, whichever is earlier. Colonoscopy is recommended every 5 years in those individuals.

Surgical resection is the primary treatment of localized adenocarcinoma of the colon and rectum. Improved survival rates for patients with stage III colon cancer (lymph-node positive) have been demonstrated when adjuvant treatment with either leucovorin- or levamisole-modulated 5-FU chemotherapy is administered when compared with surgery alone (30,31). Adjuvant therapy in patients with negative lymph nodes (stage II) remains controversial. In contrast to colon cancer, rectal cancer appears to be best approached with neoadjuvant combined radiation and 5-FU-based chemotherapy in hopes of preserving the anal sphincter and preventing the need for a permanent colostomy (32). Of colon and rectal adenocarcinoma, metastases occur within 2 to 3 years of the cancer diagnosis in 80% to 90% of patients. Liver and lung are the most common sites of metastasis, with bone and brain less often affected. Isolated lung or liver metastases occasionally can be cured by surgical resection (5). Newer chemotherapeutic agents, irinotecan and oxaliplatin, have shown benefit in patients with metastatic colorectal cancer when used in combination with leucovorin-modulated 5-FU (33,34).

Pancreatic Cancer

Pancreatic cancer is covered in Chapter 37: *Diseases of the Pancreas.*

Gallbladder Carcinoma

EPIDEMIOLOGY

Gallbladder cancer, which is rare in the United States, is the fourth most common gastrointestinal cancer worldwide, comprising 0.5% of all malignancies. Women are more commonly affected.

ETIOLOGY, PATHOGENESIS, AND PATHOPHYSIOLOGY

The finding of a "porcelain" gallbladder, characterized by calcification of the gallbladder wall, on abdominal radiograph has been associated with gallbladder cancer. Of cases, 70% to 80% are associated with chronic gallstone disease; 3.5% of patients having cholecystectomy are found to have gallbladder carcinoma *in situ.*

PATHOLOGY

Dysplastic intraepithelial proliferation is present in 1% to 34% of cholecystectomy specimens. Gallbladder carcinomas are often adenocarcinoma, papillary carcinoma, poorly differentiated adenocarcinoma, or clear cell adenocarcinoma (5).

NEUROLOGIC COMPLICATIONS

Leptomeningeal carcinomatosis has been reported in a few cases. Signet cell carcinoma has an increased tendency for leptomeningeal spread (35,36).

TREATMENT

Radical cholecystectomy is the only potentially curative treatment. As with most of the other gastrointestinal malignancies describe previously, the diagnosis, however, is often made late, precluding resection. No established effective treatment exists for advanced disease (5). Palliation of symptoms is often preferred.

Cholangiocarcinoma (Bile Duct Carcinoma)

EPIDEMIOLOGY

Cholangiocarcinoma is rare in the United States. It, however, is the most frequent cause of malignant cholestasis in Southeast Asia. The prognosis is extremely poor, with a 5-year survival of only 5% to 10%.

ETIOLOGY, PATHOGENESIS, AND PATHOPHYSIOLOGY

The etiology of bile duct cancers remains undetermined. Chronic viral hepatitis and cirrhosis do not appear to be established risk factors. Chronic infections with the liver flukes, *Clonorchis sinensis,* and *Opisthorcis viverrini* have been causally related to cholangiocarcinoma. *Ascaris lumbricoides* is another of the implicated parasites. A strong causal relationship exists between primary sclerosing cholangitis, which generally occurs in the setting of long-standing ulcerative colitis and cholangiocarcinoma (37).

PATHOLOGY

More than 90% of cholangiocarcinomas are adenocarcinomas; the remainder are squamous cell tumors (37).

NEUROLOGIC COMPLICATIONS

A single case has been reported of cholangiocarcinoma metastatic to the cerebellum and another case with leptomeningeal carcinomatosis (38,39).

TREATMENT

Surgery is the only potential cure, but it is infrequently appropriate because of advanced stage of the cancer at the time of diagnosis. The benefit of any adjuvant therapy remains unproved in advanced, unresectable cases. Palliation of symptoms, generally with either internal or external biliary drainage, is often preferred.

CLINICAL RECOMMENDATIONS OF THE VIGNETTE

The patient had subacute onset of headaches, confusion, and cranial neuropathies. He had a CSF pattern highly suggestive of neoplastic invasion of the leptomeninges. Typical CSF abnormalities included an elevated opening pressure, mild pleocytosis, usually lymphocytic, elevated CSF protein concentration, and decreased CSF glucose concentration (CSF: serum ratio <0.6).

Leptomeningeal carcinomatosis occurs in less than 1% of patients with colorectal cancers. Communicating hydrocephalus can occur as a complication. Treatment consists of spinal radiation combined with intrathecal chemotherapy delivered by an Ommaya reservoir. Treatment of the primary tumor may help ameliorate the neurologic symptoms.

SUMMARY

Clinical neurologists occasionally encounter patients with gastrointestinal malignancies requiring neurologic investigation and management. Neurologists should have a high index of suspicion for subtle neurologic complications among patients receiving active treatment for gastrointestinal malignancies.

REFERENCES

1. Gabrielsen TO, Eldevik OP, Orringer MB, et al. Esophageal carcinoma metastatic to the brain: Clinical value and cost-effectiveness of routine enhanced head CT before esophagectomy. *AJNR Am J Neuroradiol.* 1995;16(9):1915–1921.
2. Mita T, Nakanishi Y, Ochiai A, et al. Paraneoplastic vasculitis associated with esophageal carcinoma. *Pathol Int.* 1999;49(7):643–647.
3. Sutton IJ, Fursdon Davis CJ, Esiri MM, et al. Anti-Yo antibodies and cerebellar degeneration in a man with adenocarcinoma of the esophagus. *Ann Neurol.* 2001;49(2):253–257.
4. Smith TJ, Ryan LM, Douglas HO, Jr., et al. Combined chemoradiotherapy vs radiotherapy alone for early stage squamous cell carcinoma of the esophagus: A study of the Eastern Cooperative Oncology Group. *Int J Radiat Oncol Biol Phys.* 1998;42(2):269–276.
5. Blumenthal DT, Wheeler RH. Neurologic complications of gastrointestinal malignancies. In: Schiff D, Wen PY, eds. *Cancer Neurology in Clinical Practice.* Totowa, NJ: Humana Press; 2003:411.
6. Posner JB, Chernik NL. Intracranial metastases from systemic cancer. *Adv Neurol.* 1978; 19:575–587.
7. Jackle KA, Young DF, Foley KM. The natural history of lumbosacral plexopathy in cancer. *Neurology.* 1985;35(1):8–15.
8. Chamberlain MC, Kormanik PA. Epidural spinal cord compression: A single institution's retrospective experience. *Neurooncology.* 1999;1:120–123.
9. Gilbert RW, Kim J-H, Posner JB. Epidural spinal cord compression from metastatic tumor: Diagnosis and treatment. *Ann Neurol.* 1978;3:40–51.
10. Fisher MA, Weiss RB. Carcinomatous meningitis in gastrointestinal malignancies. *South Med J.* 1979;72(8):930–932.
11. Batallar L, Graus F, Saiz A, et al. Clinical outcome in adult onset idiopathic or paraneoplastic opsoclonus-myoclonus. *Brain.* 2001;124(Pt 2):437–443.
12. Williams JA, Hall GS, Thompson AG, et al. Neurological disease after gastrectomy. *BJM.* 1969;3:210–212.
13. Asbury AK, McKhann GM, McDonald IW. *Diseases of the Nervous System. Clinical Neurobiology,* Vol II. Philadelphia: WB Saunders; 1992:1450.
14. Macdonald JS, Smalley S, Benedetti J, et al. Postoperative combined radiation and chemotherapy improves disease-free survival and overall survival in resected adenocarcinoma of the stomach and G.E junction. Results of intergroup study INT-0116 (SWOG 9008). *Proceedings of the American Society of Clinical Oncology.* 2000;1.
15. *Cancer Facts and Figures 2001.* Atlanta, GA: American Cancer Society.
16. Boring CC, Squires TS, Tong T, et al. Cancer statistics, 1994. *CA Cancer J Clin.* 1994;44:7–26.
17. Newton HB, Rosenblum MK, Malkin MG. Turcot's syndrome flow cytometric analysis. *Cancer.* 1991;68(7):1633–1639.
18. Rovirosa A, Bodi R, Vicente P, et al. Cerebral metastases in adenocarcinoma of the colon. *Rev Esp Enferm Dig.* 1991;79(4):281–283.
19. Nieder C, Niewald M, Schnabel K. Brain metastases of colon and rectal carcinomas. *Wein Klin Wochenschr.* 1997;109(7):239–243.
20. Wronski M, Arbit E. Resection of brain metastases from colorectal carcinoma in 73 patients. *Cancer.* 1999;85(8):1677–1685.
21. Kanthan R, Loewy J, Kanthan SC. Skeletal metastases in colorectal carcinomas: A Saskatchewan profile. *Dis Colon Rectum.* 1999;42(12):1592–1597.
22. Aho I, Saino K. Late radiation-induced lesions of the lumbosacral plexus in cancer. *Neurology.* 1983;33:953–955.
23. Brown PD, Stafford SL, Schild SE, et al. Metastatic spinal cord compression in patients with colorectal cancer. *Journal of Neurooncology.* 1999;44(2):175–180
24. Posner JB. *Neurologic Complications of Cancer.* Philadelphia: FA Davis; 1995.
25. Triboulet JP, Piette F, Bergoend H, et al. Dermatomyosistis and colonic cancer. *Sem Hop.* 1983;59(4):255–260.
26. Diez-Porrs L, Rios-Blanco JJ, Robles-Marhuenda A, et al. ANCA-associated vasculitis as paraneoplastic syndrome with colon cancer: A case report. *Lupus.* 2005;14(8):632–634.
27. Gultekin SH, Rosenfeld RM, Voltz R, et al. Paraneoplastic limbic encephalitis: Neurological symptoms, immunological findings and tumor association in 50 patients. *Brain.* 2000;123:1481–1494.
28. Pirzada NA, Ali II, Dafer RM. Fluorouracil-induced neurotoxicity. *Ann Pharmacother.* 2000;34(1):35–38.
29. Chen TC, Hinton R, Leichman L, et al. Multifocal inflammatory leukoencephalopathy associated with levamisole and 5-fluorouracil: Case report. *Neurosurgery.* 1994;35: 1138–1142.
30. Laurie JA, Moetrel CG, Fleming TR, et al. Surgical adjuvant therapy of large bowel carcinoma: An evaluation of levamisole and the combination of levamisole and fluorouracil. *J Clin Oncol.* 1989;7:1447–1456.
31. O'Connell MJ. North Central Cancer Treatment Group-Mayo Clinic trials in colon cancer. *Semin Oncol.* 2001;28:[1 Suppl 1]:4–8.
32. Krook JE, Moertel CG, Gunderson LL, et al. Effective surgical adjuvant therapy for high risk rectal carcinoma. *N Engl J Med.* 1991;324:709–715.
33. Saltz LB, Locker PK, Pirotta N, et al. Weekly irinotecan (CPT-11), leucovorin (LV), and fluorouracil (FU) is superior to daily to daily × 5 LV /FU in patients with previously untreated metastatic colorectal cancer. *Proceedings of the American Society of Clinical Oncology.* 1999;18:233a;898.
34. Knight RD, Langdon LM, Pirotta N, et al. First-line irinotecan (C) fluorouracil (F), leucovorin (L), especially improves survival in metastatic colorectal cancer (MCRC) patients with favorable prognostic indicators. *Proceedings of the American Society of Clinical Oncology ASCO.* 2000;991.
35. Gaumann A, Marx J, Bohl J, et al. Leptomeningeal carcinomatosis and cranial nerve palsy as presenting symptoms of a clinically inapparent gallbladder carcinoma. *Pathol Res Pract.* 1999;195(7):495–499.
36. Higes-Pascual F, Beroiz-Groh P, Bravo-Guillen AI, et al. Leptomeningeal carcinomatosis and cranial nerve palsy as presenting symptoms of a gallbladder carcinoma. *Rev Neurol.* 2000;30(9):841–844.
37. Darwin P, Kennedy A. Cholangiocarcinoma. *Emedicine.* October 10, 2006.
38. Gudesblatt MS, Sencer W, Song SK, et al. Cholangiocarcinoma presenting as a cerebellar metastasis: Case report and review of the literature. *J Comput Tomogr.* 1984;8(3):191–195.
39. Huffman JL, Yeatman TJ, Smith JB. Leptomeningeal carcinomatosis: A sequela of cholangiocarcinoma. *Am Surg.* 1997;63(4):310–313.

CHAPTER 39

Bariatric Surgery

Boyd M. Koffman • Isam Daboul

OBJECTIVES

- To describe the neurologic lesions following bariatric surgeries
- To describe the symptoms that constitute neurologic emergencies after bariatric surgeries
- To list potential metabolic derangements or nutritional deficiencies resulting in neurologic problems after bariatric surgeries
- To discuss potential diagnostic modalities available for evaluation of patients with neurologic lesions following bariatric surgeries
- To list potential strategies to monitor and prevent metabolic disorders following bariatric surgeries or among the newborn of female patients

CASE VIGNETTE

A 43-year-old woman presented to the emergency department 3 weeks after Roux-en-Y gastric bypass with a 10-day history of emesis. She lost 8 kg (~18 lb) body weight since surgery. She began to develop numbness and a "prickling" sensation in both legs, and fell twice at home. Confusion was noted on admission. On examination, she was drowsy, although arousable to vocal and tactile stimuli, followed commands intermittently, and demonstrated normal speech, except mild dysarthria. Neurologic examination was also remarkable for nystagmus, hypoactive muscle stretch reflexes, ataxic gait, and sensory gradient affecting the legs for cold and pin-prick with preserved power and coordination. Lower extremities were tender to touch. No skin rash or edema was noted. Electrolyte analysis revealed mild hypokalemia, normal serum glucose, normal complete blood count with differential cell count, creatine kinase (CK), and urinalysis. Noncontrast brain computed tomographic (CT) scan was unremarkable.

DEFINITION

Body mass index (BMI) is calculated as the mass (kg) divided by the square of the height (meters). BMI is used to categorize weight as normal (BMI of 18.5 to 24.9), overweight (BMI of 25 to 29.9), obese (BMI ≥30), or extreme obesity (BMI ≥40) (1).

If, after having attempted and failed diet or medical management for weight loss, surgical treatment of obesity (bariatric surgery) is an option considered for persons with a BMI ≥35 (with an obesity-related comorbidity) or BMI >40 in the absence of an obesity-related comorbidity (1).

Several types of surgery have been performed over time (Fig. 39-1), and it is important to know which type of procedure a patient had because some surgical procedures are more susceptible to complications from malabsorption than others. Initial global malabsorption procedures, such as the jejunocolic shunt (2) and jejunoileal bypass (3), have been abandoned because of severe metabolic complications (4–7). Gastric restriction procedures (gastric partitioning, gastroplasty, vertical banded gastroplasty, gastric stapling) separate the stomach into a restricted upper pouch that empties through a narrow channel into the rest of the stomach (4,5,8). Weight loss with these procedures is not sustained and they are less satisfactory than gastric bypass.

Gastric bypass restricts the volume ingested, induces a dumping syndrome if a high-carbohydrate meal is ingested, and yields sustained weight loss (5). Roux-en-Y gastric bypass combines gastric restriction and dumping physiology. It is a first-line procedure for many surgeons (5), and is increasingly done laparoscopically (9).

For persons with a BMI >50, partial biliopancreatic bypass, distal gastric bypass (10), very, very long-limb gastric bypass (11), and biliopancreatic bypass with duodenal switch modification (12) are considered.

Neurologic complications of bariatric surgery can include compartment syndromes, acute or chronic compression mononeuropathies, or neurologic injury caused by acute or chronic malabsorption affecting virtually any level of the neuroaxis.

EPIDEMIOLOGY

Different surgical approaches and sporadic and anecdotal case reports of complications make characterization of the incidence of such complications difficult to calculate. Two studies have provided an estimate of the incidence of neurologic complications of bariatric surgeries. Among 500 patients who had gastric restriction surgery, 18 (3.6%) developed neurologic complications by 14 months (13), and increased to 23 (4.6%) when observations were extended to 20 months (14).

In a controlled, retrospective study of peripheral neuropathy complicating bariatric surgery, 71 (16%) developed peripheral neuropathy. Of these, 27 had polyneuropathy, 39 had mononeuropathy, and 5 had radiculoplexopathy (15).

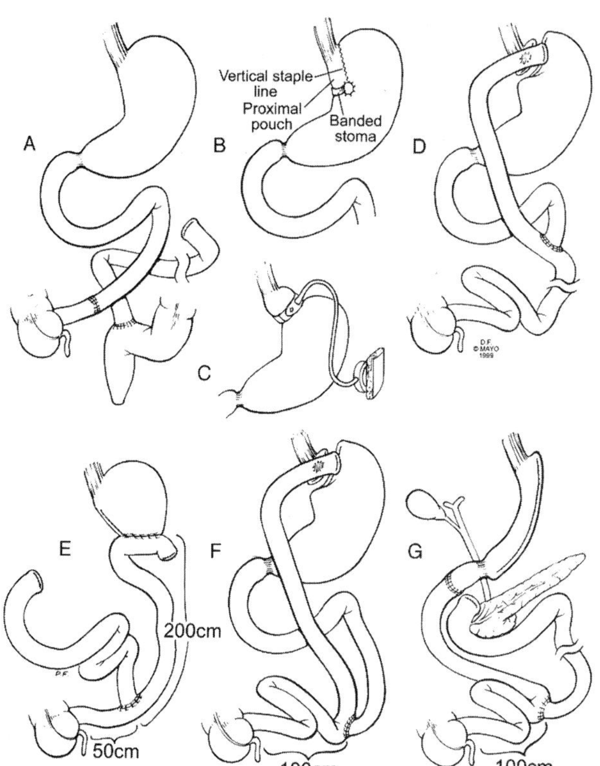

FIGURE 39-1. Various bariatric surgical procedures. (**A**) Jejunoileal bypass. (**B**) Vertical banded gastroplasty. (**C**) Gastric banding. (**D**) Roux-en-Y gastric bypass. (**E**) Partial biliopancreatic bypass. (**F**) Very, very long-limb Roux-en-Y gastric bypass. (**G**) Partial biliopancreatic bypass with duodenal switch. (From Balsiger BM, Murr MM, Poggio JL, et al. Bariatric surgery. Surgery for weight control in patients with morbid obesity. *Med Clin North Am.* 2000;84(2):477–489, with permission.)

ETIOLOGY AND PATHOGENESIS

Compartment syndromes (e.g., rhabdomyolysis) or compression mononeuropathies (e.g., meralgia paresthetica) can present as acute neurologic complications following bariatric surgery. Malabsorption syndromes, which potentially result in dysfunction at numerous levels of the neuraxis, can occur months to years after the procedure.

Among eight studies evaluating micronutrient levels following bariatric surgery in 957 patients (16–23), 236 (25%) had vitamin B_{12} deficiency, 195 (20%) had serum folate deficiency, and 11 (1%) had thiamine deficiency. Neurologic complications of such deficiencies are predictable and are related to their biochemical functions (24).

PATHOLOGY

VITAMIN B_{12}

Surgical series have identified vitamin B_{12} deficiency in 24% to 70% of patients followed for 1 to 9 years after surgery (18–20,25). Low vitamin B_{12} levels were found in 30% of patients who had gastric bypass patients 1 year after surgery, despite theoretically adequate oral supplementation (21).

Eukaryotes are unable to synthesize vitamin B_{12}. Vitamin B_{12} in animals is primarily a product of bacterial synthesis. Potential causes of vitamin B_{12} deficiency following gastric bypass include inadequate intake (18,19), impaired hydrolysis of vitamin B_{12} from dietary protein (18,19,26), or impairment in the availability or interaction of intrinsic factor with vitamin B_{12} (18,22).

Gastric parietal cells produce an intrinsic factor that binds vitamin B_{12} in the stomach and facilitates absorption at receptors in the ileum. Vitamin B_{12} transfers across the intestinal mucosa to transcobalamin II, a plasma transport protein that mediates systemic distribution (27). Because of large stores of vitamin B_{12} and an enterohepatic circulation, symptoms of deficiency may not present for months to years after surgery (27,28).

Vitamin B_{12} catalyzes two enzymatic reactions in humans: conversion of L-methylmalonyl coenzyme A into succinyl coenzyme A, and methylation of homocysteine to methionine (29). Succinyl coenzyme A participates in gluconeogenesis once it enters the citric acid cycle, and links carbohydrate and fat metabolism, thus playing a role in myelin synthesis (30). Methyl-B_{12} methylates animal RNA (31), which slows messenger RNA (mRNA) degradation. Impaired RNA methylation may explain "dying back" or involvement of long axons in vitamin B_{12} deficiency (30), because RNA turnover in axons is very high, and rapid mRNA degradation would result in limitation of proteins necessary for axon maintenance.

FOLATE

Folate deficiency following gastric bypass approaches 10% (16,32). The neurologic complications of folate deficiency are not well-characterized and are even debatable. Older literature suggests that affective disorders are more closely associated with folate deficiency than vitamin B_{12} deficiency (33), although some case reports link folate deficiency to peripheral neuropathy (34), myelopathy (34), or restless legs syndrome (35). Lindenbaum et al. (36) found that 40 of 141 patients with neuropsychiatric abnormalities caused by vitamin B_{12} deficiency did not have anemia, and subsequently found no correlation between the severity of neurologic deficit and serum folate (37).

PYRIDOXINE (VITAMIN B_6)

Pyridoxine and its related forms (pyridoxal and pyridoxamine) are converted to pyrodoxal phosphate by the liver and red blood cells and other tissues for use as a cofactor in transamination reactions, decarboxylation, and racemization of amino acids; metabolism of lipids and nucleic acids; and as a coenzyme for glycogen phosphorylase (27). Reduced serum pyridoxine levels have been noted, despite pyridoxine supplementation following gastric bypass (16). Signs of deficiency include seizures, dermatitis, and anemia. Peripheral polyneuropathy and subacute combined degeneration attributed to pyridoxine deficiency have been reported (16).

THIAMINE

Thiamine is found in both plant and animal sources, and is likely absorbed in the proximal small intestine by a carrier-mediated process when lumenal concentrations are low, and also by passive diffusion with pharmacologic doses (27,38). Thiamine can be depleted from the human body in 18 days (39).

Thiamine pyrophosphate participates in oxidative decarboxylation of carbohydrates in three enzymatic reactions. Thiamine pyrophosphate serves as a cofactor for pyrvate dehydrogenase and α–keoglutarate dehydrogenase catalyzing conversion of pyruvate to acetyl coenzyme A and α–ketoglutarate to succinyl coenzyme A, respectively, and as a cofactor for transketolase in the transfer to activated aldehydes in the hexose monophosphate shunt to generate the reduced form of nicotinamide adenine dinucleotide phosphate (NADPH) for reductive biosynthesis (40).

Thiamine deficiency results in lactic acidosis, reduced oxygen uptake, and depression of brainstem transketolase activity (41), correlating with the clinical presentation of Wernicke encephalopathy. Thiamine deficiency can be precipitated by malnutrition, administration of carbohydrates, and intake of thiaminase from tea and fish (42,43). Among case reports (44), the most common reason for thiamine deficiency following bariatric surgery is protracted emesis.

VITAMIN D

Fortified foods and conversion of inactive to active vitamin D by ultraviolet radiation or sunlight exposure to the skin serve as sources of vitamin D (45). Apart from classic manifestations of vitamin D deficiency (rickets, hypocalcemia, and osteopenia), syndromes that have been described with vitamin D deficiency include osteomalacic myopathy (46) with features of myopathy (47,48) and diffuse pain (49–51). Although no literature has yet reported vitamin D deficiency following gastric bypass, myopathy has been attributed to vitamin D deficiency following gastrectomy (52) and improved with treatment. Biliopancreatic diversion can place patients at risk for this potential complication.

VITAMIN E

Vitamin E is derived from vegetable oils or their products, leafy vegetables, nuts, and wheat germ. Although no case reports of vitamin E deficiency following gastric bypass surgery are found, a potentially treatable human vitamin E deficiency has been associated with both myopathy (53) and neuropathy (54,55), and should be considered in the differential diagnosis of neuropathy or myopathic complications of bariatric surgeries.

OTHER MICRONUTRIENTS

Little data exist on the effects of gastric bypass on minerals or trace elements. Calcium and phosphorous intake have both been noted to be reduced in most patients after bariatric surgeries (18). New or worsening pains more than a year after gastric bypass occurred in 26 of 41 (65%) patients, and has been referred to as "bypass bone disease," which is thought to result from bone demineralization because of impaired calcium absorption (18). Magnesium deficiency has also been noted following bariatric procedures (56).

CLINICAL MANIFESTATIONS/SPECIAL SITUATIONS

BRAIN

Wernicke encephalopathy complicated 24 of 96 patients (25%) among retrospective reviews (44). Among the prospective series of Abarbanel et al. (14), 2 of 500 patients (0.4%) had Wernicke encephalopathy. Malnutrition—most often from prolonged emesis—preceded onset of Wernicke encephalopathy after bariatric surgeries. Emesis was occasionally caused by mechanical obstruction (57), increased alcohol consumption, or noncompliance with vitamin supplementation. Weight loss >7 kg (~14 lb) per month in the first few months may herald intake restriction (58).

OPTIC NERVES

Optic nerve lesions complicated eight cases in retrospect (59–66). Cranial nerve lesions were reported more for global or selective malabsorption procedures than for more recent bypass procedures (44). Findings included central scotoma, nyctalopia, optic neuropathy, nutritional amblyopia, and carotene deficiency.

SPINAL CORD

Two cases of myelopathy after gastric bypass have been reported (14). The cause remained uncertain. Potentially treatable causes to consider include deficiencies of serum copper, vitamin B_{12}, pyridoxine, and folate. Copper deficiency has been implicated in development of myelopathy following both partial gastrectomy (67,68) and intestinal bypass (67).

Subacute combined degeneration is classically associated with vitamin B_{12} deficiency (33,36), and been reported following partial (30,69) or complete (52) gastrectomy, but not gastric bypass.

PERIPHERAL NERVE

Peripheral neuropathy was identified in 60 of 96 patients (63%) among 50 case reports (44). In a controlled retrospective study (15), 71 of 435 patients (16%) developed peripheral polyneuropathy.

POLYNEUROPATHY

Of the patients with peripheral neuropathy in the series by Thaisetthawatkul et al. (15), 27 had polyneuropathy. Most cases presented as chronic conditions, likely related to micronutrient deficiency, although Guillain-Barré syndrome was reported among some cases (44) and in surgical series (70,71), although several of these case reports acknowledge findings atypical for Guillain-Barré syndrome. Patients with a generalized polyneuropathy were predominantly sensory in one series (15). Most presented with a slow onset with a chronic course. Wernicke encephalopathy can also be associated with polyneuropathy (dry beriberi), although it remains unclear whether the neuropathy results from thiamine deficiency or multiple vitamin deficiencies (72).

Potentially treatable malabsorption syndromes that can affect peripheral nerves after gastric bypass include deficiencies of vitamin B_{12} (36), thiamine (41), and vitamin E (73). Vitamin D deficiency can affect peripheral nerves, although this is not confirmed (46). Although vitamin E deficiency is associated with neuropathy, no reports are found in the literature. The possibility of an immunologic mechanism in polyneuropathy has also been cited (15) based on sural nerve biopsy data.

FOCAL MONONEUROPATHIES

Of the 71 patients with peripheral neuropathy following gastric bypass in the retrospective case-control series by Thaisetthawatkul et al. (15), 39 (55%) had mononeuropathy. The most frequent mononeuropathy in these 39 patients was carpal tunnel syndrome in 31 (79%). Other syndromes included ulnar neuropathy at the elbow (2), peroneal mononeuropathy at the fibular head (2), radial mononeuropathy (1), superficial radial sensory neuropathy (1), sciatic neuropathy (1).

Lateral femoral cutaneous neuropathy (meralgia paresthetica) is reported with an incidence of 0.5% to 1.4% following gastric bypass (14,15,74). The cause is unknown, although some speculate for (75) and some against (74) compression by the Gomez retractor during the procedure, or predisposition to compression of the lateral femoral cutaneous nerve because of certain anatomical variants (74,76). Macgregor and Thoburn (74) noted acute onset of most of their 11 cases of meralgia paresthetica following either Roux-en-Y gastric bypass or silicon ring vertical gastroplasty (74).

MUSCLE

Primary muscle disease is reported as a cause of weakness among 7 of 96 (7%) case reports (44). One report attributed myopathy following Roux-en-Y gastric bypass to global malnutrition (77). Surgical series additionally noted myotonic syndrome in one case (14) and hypokalemic paralysis in one case (71). Rhabdomyolysis also occurs acutely after surgery and is reported in 1.4% of cases (78).

SPECIAL SITUATIONS

One prospective study evaluated birth outcomes of 79 obese women after laparascopic adjustable gastric banding (79). No significant difference in measured outcomes (stillbirths, preterm deliveries, low birth weight, high birth weight, vitamin B_{12} levels, and folate levels) were found, except that six women who had surgery had an elevated homocysteine level at the annual visit closest to delivery.

Two cases were reported of vitamin B_{12} deficiency in infants born to mothers who had bariatric surgery. One case was attributed to maternal subclinical vitamin B_{12} deficiency, likely caused by a decrease in available intrinsic factor 2 years after gastric bypass; her 10-month-old male infant was breastfed exclusively and developed symptomatic vitamin B_{12} deficiency (80). A second case documented vitamin B_{12} deficiency identified in the first 2 weeks of life in a newborn whose mother had gastric bypass surgery 3.5 years before delivery and who discontinued prenatal vitamins because of side effects (81).

DIAGNOSTIC APPROACH

Careful clinical, neuroimaging (as appropriate), and electrodiagnostic evaluations are warranted, and appropriate biopsy of nerve or muscle may be indicated. Electromyography and nerve conduction studies are traditionally underutilized in the diagnosis of neurologic complications of bariatric surgeries, and histologic evaluation was virtually nonexistent in literature reported between 1976 and 2004 (44).

Electrodiagnostic evaluation may be critical for localization, diagnosis, and exclusion of alternative pathologies, such as Guillain-Barré syndrome. Tissue diagnosis of either muscle or nerve should also be considered; many of these patients are at risk for neuropathy, myopathy, or both. Alternate causes of weakness, such as idiopathic inflammatory myopathy or critical illness polyneuropathy or myopathy, should be excluded. Skin biopsy may be helpful in confirming a small-fiber neuropathy (82).

TREATMENT

Treatment begins with prevention. Cognizance of prolonged immobility and protective padding at pressure points may help prevent development of compartment syndromes and rhabdomyolysis. Checking CK in the immediate postoperative period may also help detect rhabdomyolysis when symptoms of pain, weakness, skeletal muscle swelling, and myglobinuria exist (78). Brolin (83) recommends monitoring complete blood count, serum iron, total iron-binding capacity, and serum vitamin B_{12} following Roux-en-Y gastric bypass (83).

Crowley et al. (18) recommend long-term follow-up, dietary counseling, clinical and laboratory evaluations every 6 months to include complete blood count, urinalysis, serum iron, total iron-binding capacity, serum vitamin B_{12}, folic acid, and a chemistry profile (including calcium, phosphorous, and alkaline phosphatase), and indefinite use of supplementation with a multivitamin-mineral containing vitamin B_{12}, folic acid, and iron, an additional iron tablet with vitamin C, and additional 50 to 100 μg vitamin B_{12} tablet, and a calcium supplement of 1,000 to 1,200 mg daily (18).

Although some disagreement exists regarding oral vitamin B_{12} supplementation following surgery, there is a consensus about most of these recommendations (84).

CLINICAL RECOMMENDATIONS OF THE VIGNETTE

Electrolyte analysis showed mild hypokalemia, normal glucose, normal complete blood count with differential cell count, CK, and urinalysis. Noncontrast brain CT was unremarkable. Surgical consultation and evaluation failed to demonstrate a mechanical obstruction to account for emesis. Electromyelogram (EMG) and nerve conduction studies (NCS) demonstrated a normal study. Laboratory studies for vitamins B_{12} and E were drawn and subsequently returned normal. Because a history of either prolonged emesis or weight loss >7 kg (~14 lb) per month may predispose to thiamine deficiency, empiric treatment with thiamine was instituted and the encephalopathy, nystagmus, gait ataxia, and sensory symptoms rapidly resolved over the next 24 hours. The patient was counseled regarding the size of the gastric pouch to help to prevent overeating that could result in emesis and thiamine deficiency.

SUMMARY

Neurologic complications following bariatric surgical procedures can affect nearly every level of the neuraxis. Most complications are caused by metabolic alterations or nutritional deficiencies, which are predictable, delayed in onset, and may be monitored and prevented. A few complications (e.g., rhabdomyolysis, meralgia paresthetica) are acute. Accurate diagnosis is essential to exclude alternative causes of symptoms, such as Guillain-Barré syndrome, critical illness myopathy, or polyneuropathy. Thorough neurologic and electrodiagnostic evaluations and tissue studies, when appropriate, are indicated to help localize, diagnose, and guide therapy. Follow-up should include multivitamin and micronutrient supplementation, with concurrent postsurgical laboratory monitoring.

REFERENCES

1. Clinical Guidelines on the Identification, Evaluation, and Treatment of Overweight and Obesity in Adults—The Evidence Report. National Institutes of Health. *Obes Res.* 1998; [6 Suppl 2]:51S-209S.
2. Payne JH, DeWind LT. Surgical treatment of obesity. *Am J Surg.* 1969;118(2):141–147.
3. Scott HW, Jr., Sandstead HH, Brill AB, et al. Experience with a new technic of intestinal bypass in the treatment of morbid obesity. *Ann Surg.* 1971;174(4):560–572.
4. Alden JF. Gastric and jejunoileal bypass. A comparison in the treatment of morbid obesity. *Arch Surg.* 1977;112(7):799–806.
5. Balsiger BM, Murr MM, Poggio JL, et al. Bariatric surgery. Surgery for weight control in patients with morbid obesity. *Med Clin North Am.* 2000;84(2):477–489.
6. Griffen WO, Jr., Young VL, Stevenson CC. A prospective comparison of gastric and jejunoileal bypass procedures for morbid obesity. *Ann Surg.* 1977;186(4):500–509.
7. Sjostrom L. Surgical intervention as a strategy for treatment of obesity. *Endocrine.* 2000;13(2):213–230.
8. Mason EE. Vertical banded gastroplasty for obesity. *Arch Surg.* 1982;117(5):701–706.
9. Higa KD, Boone KB, Ho T, et al. Laparoscopic Roux-en-Y gastric bypass for morbid obesity: Technique and preliminary results of our first 400 patients. *Arch Surg.* 2000;135(9): 1029–1033.
10. Sugerman HJ, Kellum JM, DeMaria EJ. Conversion of proximal to distal gastric bypass for failed gastric bypass for superobesity. *J Gastrointest Surg.* 1997;1(6):517–525.
11. Murr MM, Balsiger BM, Kennedy FP, et al. Malabsorptive procedures for severe obesity: Comparison of pancreaticobiliary bypass and very very long limb Roux-en-Y gastric bypass. *J Gastrointest Surg.* 1999;3(6):607–612.
12. Marceau P, Hould FS, Simard S, et al. Biliopancreatic diversion with duodenal switch. *World J Surg.* 1998;22(9):947–954.
13. Solomon H, Abarbanel J, Berginer VM, et al. Neurological deficits following gastric restriction surgery for morbid obesity. *Clin Nutr.* 1986;15[Suppl]:181–184.
14. Abarbanel JM, Berginer VM, Osimani A, et al. Neurologic complications after gastric restriction surgery for morbid obesity. *Neurology.* 1987;37(2):196–200.
15. Thaisetthawatkul P, Collazo-Clavell ML, Sarr MG, et al. A controlled study of peripheral neuropathy after bariatric surgery. *Neurology.* 2004;63(8):1462–1470.
16. Boylan LM, Sugerman HJ, Driskell JA. Vitamin E, vitamin B-6, vitamin B-12, and folate status of gastric bypass surgery patients. *J Am Diet Assoc.* 1988;88(5):579–585.
17. Brolin RE, Gorman JH, Gorman RC, et al. Are vitamin B12 and folate deficiency clinically important after roux-en-Y gastric bypass? *J Gastrointest Surg.* 1998;2(5):436–442.
18. Crowley LV, Seay J, Mullin G. Late effects of gastric bypass for obesity. *Am J Gastroenterol.* 1984;79(11):850–860.
19. Halverson JD. Micronutrient deficiencies after gastric bypass for morbid obesity. *Am Surg.* 1986;52(11):594–598.
20. MacLean LD, Rhode BM, Shizgal HM. Nutrition following gastric operations for morbid obesity. *Ann Surg.* 1983;198(3):347–355.
21. Provenzale D, Reinhold RB, Golner B, et al. Evidence for diminished B12 absorption after gastric bypass: Oral supplementation does not prevent low plasma B12 levels in bypass patients. *J Am Coll Nutr.* 1992;11(1):29–35.
22. Schilling RF, Gohdes PN, Hardie GH. Vitamin B12 deficiency after gastric bypass surgery for obesity. *Ann Intern Med.* 1984;101(4):501–502.
23. Skroubis G, Sakellaropoulos G, Pouggouras K, et al. Comparison of nutritional deficiencies after Roux-en-Y gastric bypass and after biliopancreatic diversion with Roux-en-Y gastric bypass. *Obes Surg.* 2002;12(4):551–558.
24. Chaudhry V, Umapathi T, Ravich WJ. Neuromuscular diseases and disorders of the alimentary system. *Muscle Nerve.* 2002;25(6):768–784.
25. Amaral JF, Thompson WR, Caldwell MD, et al. Prospective hematologic evaluation of gastric exclusion surgery for morbid obesity. *Ann Surg.* 1985;201(2):186–193.
26. Crowley LV, Olson RW. Megaloblastic anemia after gastric bypass for obesity. *Am J Gastroenterol.* 1983;78(7):406–410.
27. Subcommittee on the Tenth Edition of the RDAs, Food and Nutrition Board, Commission on Life Sciences, National Research Council. Water-soluble vitamins. In: Havel RJ, ed. *Recommended Dietary Allowances.* Washington, DC: National Academy Press; 1989:115–173.
28. Schlosser LL, Deshpande P, Schilling RF. Biologic turnover rate of cyanocobalamin (vitamin B12) in human liver. *AMA Arch Intern Med.* 1958;101(2):306–309.
29. Das KC, Herbert V. Vitamin B12—Folate interrelations. *Clin Haematol.* 1976;5(3):697–745.
30. Roos D. Neurological complications in patients with impaired vitamin B12 absorption following partial gastrectomy. *Acta Neurol Scand Suppl.* 1978;69:1–77.
31. Walerych WS, Venkataraman S, Johnson BC. The methylation of transfer RNA by methyl cobamide. *Biochem Biophys Res Commun.* 1966;23(4):368–374.
32. Halverson JD, Zuckerman GR, Koehler RE, et al. Gastric bypass for morbid obesity: A medical-surgical assessment. *Ann Surg.* 1981;194(2):152–160.
33. Shorvon SD, Carney MW, Chanarin I, et al. The neuropsychiatry of megaloblastic anaemia. *BMJ.* 1980;281(6247):1036–1038.
34. Grant HC, Hoffbrand AV, Wells DG. Folate deficiency and neurological disease. *Lancet.* 1965;2(7416):763–767.
35. Botez MI, Botez T, Leveile J, et al. Neuropsychological correlates of folic acid deficiency: Facts and hypotheses. In: Botez MI, Reynolds EH, ed. *Folic Acid in Neurology, Psychiatry, and Internal Medicine.* New York: Raven Press; 1979:435–461.
36. Lindenbaum J, Healton EB, Savage DG, et al. Neuropsychiatric disorders caused by cobalamin deficiency in the absence of anemia or macrocytosis. *N Engl J Med.* 1988;318 (26):1720–1728.
37. Healton EB, Savage DG, Brust JC, et al. Neurologic aspects of cobalamin deficiency. *Medicine (Baltimore).* 1991;70(4):229–245.
38. Rindi G, Ventura U. Thiamine intestinal transport. *Physiol Rev.* 1972;52(4):821–827.
39. Ziporin ZZ, Nunes WT, Powell RC, et al. Thiamine requirement in the adult human as measured by urinary excretion of thiamine metabolites. *J Nutr.* 1965;85:297–304.
40. Stryer L. *Biochemistry,* 2nd ed. San Francisco: WH Freeman; 1981.
41. Dreyfus PM, Victor M. Effects of thiamine deficiency on the central nervous system. *Am J Clin Nutr.* 1961;9:414–425.
42. Murata K. Thiaminase. In: Shimazono N, Katsura E, eds. *Review of Japanese Literature on Beriberi and Thiamine.* Tokyo: Igaku Shoin; 1965:220–254.
43. Vimokesant SL, Nakornchai S, Dhanamitta S, et al. Effect of tea consumption on thiamine status in man. *Nutrition Report International.* 1974;9:371–374.
44. Koffman BM, Greenfield LJ, Ali II, et al. Neurologic complications after surgery for obesity. *Muscle Nerve.* 2006;33(2):166–176.
45. Subcommittee on the Tenth Edition of the RDAs, Food and Nutrition Board, Commission on Life Sciences, National Research Council. Fat-soluble vitamins. In: Havel RJ, ed. *Recommended Dietary Allowances.* Washington, DC: National Academy Press; 1989:78–114.
46. Pfeifer M, Begerow B, Minne HW. Vitamin D and muscle function. *Osteoporos Int.* 2002;13(3):187–194.
47. Schott GD, Wills MR. Muscle weakness in osteomalacia. *Lancet.* 1976;1(7960):626–629.
48. Yoshikawa S, Nakamura T, Tanabe H, et al. Osteomalacic myopathy. *Endocrinol Jpn.* 1979;26[Suppl]:65–72.
49. Gloth FM, III, Lindsay JM, Zelesnick LB, et al. Can vitamin D deficiency produce an unusual pain syndrome? *Arch Intern Med.* 1991;151(8):1662–1664.
50. Plotnikoff GA, Quigley JM. Prevalence of severe hypovitaminosis D in patients with persistent, nonspecific musculoskeletal pain. *Mayo Clin Proc.* 2003;78(12):1463–1470.
51. Ronin DI, Wu YC, Sahgal V, et al. Intractable muscle pain syndrome, osteomalacia, and axonopathy in long-term use of phenytoin. *Arch Phys Med Rehabil.* 1991;72 (10):755–758.
52. Banerji NK, Hurwitz LJ. Nervous system manifestations after gastric surgery. *Acta Neurol Scand* 1971;47(4):485–513.
53. Tomasi LG. Reversibility of human myopathy caused by vitamin E deficiency. *Neurology.* 1979;29(8):1182–1186.
54. Guggenheim MA, Ringel SP, Silverman A, et al. Progressive neuromuscular disease in children with chronic cholestasis and vitamin E deficiency: Clinical and muscle biopsy findings and treatment with alpha-tocopherol. *Ann N Y Acad Sci.* 1982;393:84–95.
55. Neville HE, Ringel SP, Guggenheim MA, et al. Ultrastructural and histochemical abnormalities of skeletal muscle in patients with chronic vitamin E deficiency. *Neurology.* 1983;33(4):483–488.
56. Sugerman HJ. Preface. *Surg Clin North Am.* 2001;81:xi–xv.
57. Benotti PN. Surgery in the management of severe obesity. In: Goldstein DJ, ed. *The Management of Eating Disorders and Obesity.* Totowa, NJ: Humana Press; 1999:273–284.
58. Salas-Salvado J, Garcia-Lorda P, Cuatrecasas G, et al. Wernicke's syndrome after bariatric surgery. *Clin Nutr.* 2000;19(5):371–373.
59. Bradley JE, Brown RO, Luther RW. Multiple nutritional deficiencies and metabolic complications 20 years after jejunoileal bypass surgery. *JPEN J Parenter Enteral Nutr.* 1987; 11(5):494–498.
60. Brown GC, Felton SM, Benson WE. Reversible night blindness associated with intestinal bypass surgery. *Am J Ophthalmol.* 1980;89(6):776–779.
61. Gardner TW, Rao K, Poticha S, et al. Acute visual loss after gastroplasty. *Am J Ophthalmol.* 1982;93(5):658–660.
62. Haag JR, Smith JL, Susac JO. Optic atrophy following jejunoileal bypass. *J Clin Neuroophthalmol.* 1985;5(1):9–15.
63. Partamian LG, Sidrys LA, Tripathi RC. Iatrogenic night blindness and keratoconjunctival xerosis. *N Engl J Med.* 1979;301(17):943–944.
64. Smets RM, Waeben M. Unusual combination of night blindness and optic neuropathy after biliopancreatic bypass. *Bull Soc Belge Ophtalmol.* 1999;271:93–96.
65. Thompson RE, Felton JL. Nutritional amblyopia associated with jejunoileal bypass surgery. *Ann Ophthalmol.* 1982;14(9):848–850.
66. Yarborough GW, Wilson FA, Feman S, et al. Retinopathy following jejunoileal bypass surgery: Report of a case. *Int J Obes.* 1982;6(3):253–258.
67. Kumar N, McEvoy KM, Ahlskog JE. Myelopathy due to copper deficiency following gastrointestinal surgery. *Arch Neurol.* 2003;60(12):1782–1785.
68. Schleper B, Stuerenburg HJ. Copper deficiency-associated myelopathy in a 46-year-old woman. *J Neurol.* 2001;248(8):705–706.
69. Weir DG, Gatenby PB. Subacute combined degeneration of the cord after partial gastrectomy. *BMJ.* 1963;5366:1175–1176.
70. Chang CG, Helling TS, Black WE, et al. Weakness after gastric bypass. *Obes Surg.* 2002;12(4):592–597.
71. Smith SC, Goodman GN, Edwards CB. Roux-en-Y gastric bypass: A 7-year retrospective review of 3,855 patients. *Obes Surg.* 1995;5(3):314–318.
72. Mancall EL. Nutritional disorders of the nervous system. In: Aminoff MJ, ed. *Neurology and General Medicine.* New York: Churchill Livingstone; 1989:323–339.
73. Nelson J. Neuropathological studies of chronic vitamin E deficiency in mammals including humans. In: Porter R, Whelan J, eds. *Biology of Vitamin E.* London: Pitman; 1983: 92–105.
74. Macgregor AM, Thoburn EK. Meralgia paresthetica following bariatric surgery. *Obes Surg.* 1999;9(4):364–368.

75. Grace DM. Meralgia paresthetica after gastroplasty for morbid obesity. *Can J Surg.* 1987;30(1):64–65.
76. Ghent WR. Further studies on meralgia paresthetica. *Can Med Assoc J.* 1961;85:871–875.
77. Hsia AW, Hattab EM, Katz JS. Malnutrition-induced myopathy following Roux-en-Y gastric bypass. *Muscle Nerve.* 2001;24(12):1692–1694.
78. Khurana RN, Baudendistel TE, Morgan EF, et al. Postoperative rhabdomyolysis following laparoscopic gastric bypass in the morbidly obese. *Arch Surg.* 2004;139(1):73–76.
79. Dixon JB, Dixon ME, O'Brien PE. Birth outcomes in obese women after laparoscopic adjustable gastric banding. *Obstet Gynecol.* 2005;106(5 Pt 1):965–972.
80. Grange DK, Finlay JL. Nutritional vitamin B12 deficiency in a breastfed infant following maternal gastric bypass. *Pediatr Hematol Oncol.* 1994;11(3):311–318.
81. Campbell CD, Ganesh J, Ficicioglu C. Two newborns with nutritional vitamin B12 deficiency: Challenges in newborn screening for vitamin B12 deficiency. *Haematologica.* 2005;90[12 Suppl]:ECR45.
82. Kennedy WR. Opportunities afforded by the study of unmyelinated nerves in skin and other organs. *Muscle Nerve.* 2004;29(6):756–767.
83. Brolin RE. Gastric bypass. *Surg Clin North Am.* 2001;81(5):1077–1095.
84. Byrne TK. Complications of surgery for obesity. *Surg Clin North Am.* 2001;81(5):1181–1193.

CHAPTER 40

Gastrointestinal Transplantation

Jeffrey S. Kutcher • Fred K. Askari

OBJECTIVES

- To review the common neurologic complications of pancreatic transplantation
- To explain how pancreatic transplantation effects diabetic neuropathy
- To describe the neurologic complications and disease states associated with small bowel transplantation
- To review the neuropathology of intestinal failure and small bowel transplantation

CASE VIGNETTE

A 52-year-old man presents with a chief complaint of cognitive concerns and difficulty at work. He is a purchasing agent at a large corporation and reports having increasing difficulty generating his monthly reports. His manager has started reassigning his work load to other employees and he is concerned that he will eventually lose his job. His concern is worsened by frequently missed work days over the past 3 years because of exacerbations of his long-standing Crohn disease. His wife is concerned that he has become moody and forgetful at home. His history is difficult to complete because he is inattentive, circumferential, and emotionally labile. His wife finishes most of his answers for him.

On physical examination, he is thin, appears his stated age, but is somewhat ill-kempt. He reports decreased sensation to light touch in his feet bilaterally, with normal sensation above the ankles. His vibratory sensation is diminished at the toes bilaterally, as is his position sensation. His deep tendon reflexes are barely detectable in the ankles and diffuse mild atrophy is noted of the intrinsic muscles of both feet. The remainder of his neurologic examination is unremarkable.

His gastroenterologist has recently ordered several blood tests and the patient has brought with him results showing a normal hemoglobin, hematocrit, and mean corpuscular volume (MCV). His serum cobalamin level is also normal. These results are compared with previous studies performed 8 months ago, which were also normal. Although the patient denies any current use of supplements, his wife reports that he was receiving weekly B_{12} shots "for a few months last year."

DEFINITION

This chapter focuses on the neurologic concerns of patients who have received or will receive a small bowel or pancreas transplantation. Issues central to immunosuppression, liver transplantation, and other diseases of the pancreas and gut are discussed in other chapters.

PANCREATIC TRANSPLANTATION

Pancreatic transplantation is performed in patients with severe, difficult to regulate, insulin-requiring diabetes, usually type I, who are experiencing widespread end-organ damage, including peripheral neuropathy, retinopathy, and nephropathy (1). The primary goals of pancreatic transplantation are to reduce insulin dependency and improve the secondary complications of diabetes. The procedure generally involves whole organ transplantation, with concurrent renal transplantation. Pancreatic cell transplant is being studied. Although pancreatic transplantation may improve the symptoms of a peripheral (2) or autonomic (3) diabetic neuropathy, the procedure itself can also lead directly to neurologic complications.

SMALL BOWEL TRANSPLANTATION

Small bowel transplantation is a life-saving procedure for patients with intestinal failure. Common causes of intestinal failure include volvulus, gastroschisis, and necrotizing enterocolitis in children and bowel ischemia, Crohn disease, and trauma in adults (4). Many diseases or conditions that lead to small bowel transplantation will also involve the nervous system directly as a result of a nutritional malabsorption syndrome (5). Posttransplantation neurologic complications occur as well. Although survival outcomes continue to improve for small bowel transplantation, patients continue to experience a significant burden of neurologic disease.

EPIDEMIOLOGY

PANCREATIC TRANSPLANTATION

As of December 31, 2004, the International Pancreas Transplant Registry had recorded >23,000 pancreas transplantations worldwide, with approximately 74% performed in the United States (6). An earlier report on the same registry estimated that 94% of the procedures were performed for patients with type I diabetes, with the remaining 6% having type II (7). Before pancreas transplantation, nearly all patients presented with a significant polyneuropathy as a result of their diabetes. Following pancreas transplantation, studies have shown that many patients experience an improvement in their polyneuropathy. Navarro et al. (8), followed an initial study group of 115 patients for up to 10 years following pancreas transplantation. They describe consistent improvement in motor nerve testing in 60% of the study group. Sensory nerve testing (50%), cardiorespiratory reflexes (30%), and sweat testing (45%) were also improved in the same population. A control group of patients that did not receive pancreas transplantation was also followed, with more than 50% of these patients showing significant worsening of their neurophysiologic studies (8).

Neurologic complications following transplantation have frequently been described, including peripheral nerve lesions (93%), seizures (13%), cerebrovascular events (13%) central nervous system infections (10%), and metabolic encephalopathies (7%) (9,10). Complications thought to be secondary to the transplantation procedure itself, however, are felt to be rare (10).

SMALL BOWEL TRANSPLANTATION

As of May 31, 2003, 923 patients had received small bowel transplants worldwide (4). The number of worldwide cases per year has increased from 11 in 1990 to 140 in 2003, with >75% being performed in the United States (4). Outcome data for small bowel transplantation has been consistently worse than outcome data for other solid organ transplantation. The past 8 years, however, have seen some improvement in the rate of successful small bowel engraftment. For patients receiving small bowel transplantation before 1994, 1-year survival was estimated at 71% as compared with 77% for patients who received transplantation between 1998 and 2003 (11,12). A strong expression of histocompatability antigens, the large numbers of leukocytes, and significant microorganism colonization together are felt to be responsible for the inherent difficulty seen in successful small bowel transplantation (13).

Although the neurologic effects of the conditions that lead to intestinal failure, as well as the effects of total parenteral nutrition (TPN) itself, are well described, little is known about the rates of direct neurologic complications resulting from the small bowel transplantation procedure itself.

ETIOLOGY AND PATHOGENESIS

PANCREATIC TRANSPLANTATION

As mentioned, nearly all pancreatic transplantations are performed in patients with type I diabetes. The etiology and pathogenesis of diabetic polyneuropathy is described in other chapters. No known etiology is thought to be specific to the pancreatic transplantation procedure to account for seizures, cerebrovascular events, metabolic encephalopathies, and central nervous system infections. These complications are felt to occur for reasons common to all solid organ transplantation procedures.

SMALL BOWEL TRANSPLANTATION

In adults, the most common underlying reason for small bowel transplantation is bowel ischemia (23%). Crohn disease (14%), trauma (10%), and volvulus (7%) are other common causes. Whatever the underlying diagnosis, the immediate need for transplantation is brought on by intestinal failure. Malabsorption syndromes are common, including those that often lead to neurologic dysfunction, such as deficiencies in B_{12} and the fat-soluble vitamins: Vitamins A, D, and E. Vitamin B_6 (pyridoxine) deficiency is rare, seen in cases of excessive alcohol intake with poor diet and in newborns without dietary supplementation.

Before transplantation, most patients have been using TPN for an extended period, in some cases, >3 years (5). The central nervous system effects of TPN, especially the deposition of manganese in the basal ganglia, have been well described (5). Other neuropathologic changes are felt to be common among patients waiting for small bowel transplantation, as well as for those who have had the procedure. In one small retrospective analysis, neuropathologic abnormalities were found at autopsy or brain biopsy in 12 of 13 patients (92%) who had received a small bowel transplant. In the same study, all four patients who died while awaiting the procedure were also found to have neuropathologic changes such as ischemia, atrophy, Alzheimer type II gliosis, and infection (5).

CLINICAL MANIFESTATIONS/SPECIAL SITUATIONS

SMALL BOWEL TRANSPLANTATION

The neurologic manifestations of diseases associated with small bowel transplantation are mainly secondary to the malabsorption syndromes.

- Vitamin A deficiency most commonly presents with an impairment of night vision. An associated dryness and keratinization of the cornea can then lead to total blindness.
- Vitamin B_{12} (cobalamin) deficiency most commonly affects the nervous system via a peripheral neuropathy causing symmetric distal parasthesias. Spinal cord involvement is heralded by spasticity and weakness, as well as severe proprioceptive and vibration sensation. Psychosis or a global dementia is evidence of cerebral involvement.
- Vitamin D, known mainly for its role in bone disease, can also cause a proximal myopathy.
- Vitamin E deficiency can be the cause of a rare spinocerebellar degenerative disorder in which ataxia, weakness, and proprioceptive loss can be seen.

DIAGNOSTIC APPROACH

PANCREATIC TRANSPLANTATION

The diagnosis of diabetic polyneuropathy, common to nearly all patients who have had or who are waiting for a pancreatic transplantation, is usually suggested by the history and physical examination. If necessary, the condition can be further defined by nerve conduction studies.

The complications of the transplantation procedure itself can be diagnosed using the investigation techniques typical for each diagnosis, such as diffusion magnetic-resonance images of the brain to help identify cerebral infarcts, electroencephalogram to look for evidence of a possible seizure or seizure focus, and serum metabolic profiles to determine possible causes of metabolic encephalopathy.

SMALL BOWEL TRANSPLANTATION

Careful laboratory evaluation can usually uncover the malabsorption syndromes. Vitamin B_{12} deficiency can be identified by an abnormal Schilling test, which uses radio-labeled cobalamin compounds to test absorption. The presence of the interferon (IF) antibody can also diagnose pernicious anemia but is only 50% to 60% sensitive. Plasma retinol levels can be checked to diagnose vitamin A deficiency. Vitamin D deficiency can be diagnosed by demonstrating a low level of 25 hydroxylated (OH) vitamin D in the serum. Further evidence of the malabsorption of vitamin D include a raised serum parathyroid hormone, low urine calcium secretion, and hypophosphatemia. Pyridoxine deficiency can be diagnosed directly via serum levels. Folic acid also can be measured directly in the serum and patients typically have a megaloblastic anemia.

Vitamin E deficiency can be more difficult to confirm because evidence indicates that tissue levels of vitamin E do not correlate with those found in the serum (14). Vitamin E levels in the serum, in large part, are determined by the amount of circulating lipids. If vitamin E deficiency is suspected on clinical grounds, high performance liquid chromatography can used for conformation.

TREATMENT

PANCREATIC TRANSPLANTATION

Pancreatic transplantation has been found to significantly decrease the progression of diabetic peripheral neuropathy. In some cases, progression is halted completely, whereas in others, even a small degree of symptomatic improvement has be described (8). The treatment of possible neurologic complications of the procedure itself, such as cerebral infarction or seizure, is not specific to the pancreatic transplantation population.

SMALL BOWEL TRANSPLANTATION

Deficiencies of vitamins A, D and E, can be treated directly with oral supplementation. B_{12} deficiency can be corrected with the intramuscular administration of cyanocobalamin, typically on a weekly schedule of 1,000 μg every week for 4 to 6 weeks. If maintenance is required, a lower dose of 100 μg every month is required.

CLINICAL RECOMMENDATIONS OF THE VIGNETTE

The patient is experiencing manifestations of B_{12} (cobalamin) deficiency. The deficiency is almost certainly a result of his Crohn disease, although care should be taken to ascertain his dietary patterns, looking for a deficit in consumption rather than absorption. It is important to note that patients with neurologic effects of B_{12} deficiency will have normal blood counts 25% of the time (15). Patients with Crohn disease, in general, have a significant degree of malabsorption and would be unlikely to have normal cell counts. This patient, however, was reported to have used B_{12} supplementation in the past, which could account for his normal laboratory evaluation. Reeducation regarding his primary disease, its effects on vitamin absorption, and the importance of an adequate intake of vitamins should be stressed and this patient should be restarted on weekly intramuscular injections of cobalamin.

SUMMARY

Patients who have received, or are being considered for, pancreatic transplantation likely already have had a long experience with neurologic disease in the form of peripheral neuropathy. They are also likely to have retinopathy and renal disease. For patients with substantial end-organ damage, pancreatic transplantation offers an independence from insulin and possible improvement in symptoms of diabetic polyneuropathy. These benefits typically outweigh the risks of other neurologic complications for the transplantation procedure itself.

Small bowel transplantation is performed in patients who are experiencing intestinal failure. These patients are at high risk of developing malabsorption syndromes, as well neurologic effects from the chronic use of TPN. Small bowel transplants require a high level of immunosuppression, increasing the risk of posttransplant complications. A successful procedure, however, can help minimize the deleterious effects of the underlying disease process on the nervous system. Active research to improve outcomes of small bowel and pancreatic transplantation may increase the general applicability of these procedures.

REFERENCES

1. Sutherland D, Gruessner A, Gruessner R. Pancreas transplantation: A review. *Transplant Proc.* 1998;30:1940–1943.
2. Muller-Felber W, Landgraf R, Scheuer R, et al. Diabetic neuropathy 3 years after successful pancreas and kidney transplantation. *Diabetes.* 1993;42:1482–1486.
3. Hathaway D, Abell T, Cardoso S, et al. Improvement in autonomic function following pancreas-kidney versus kidney-alone transplantation. *Transplant Proc.* 1993;25:1306–1308.
4. Grant D, Abu-Elmagd K, Reyes J, et al. 2003 report of the intestine transplant registry. *Ann Surg.* 2005;241:607–613.
5. Idoate M, Martinez A, Bueno J, et al. The neuropathology of intestinal failure and small bowel transplantation. *Acta Neuropathol.* 1999;97:502–508.
6. Gruessner A, Sutherland D. Pancreas transplantation outcomes for United State (US) and non-US cases as reported to the United Network for Organ Sharing (UNOS) and the International Pancreas Transplant Registry (IPTR) as of June 2004. *Clin Transpl.* 2005;19 (4):433–455.
7. Gruessner A, Sutherland D. Pancreas transplantation outcomes for United State (US) and non-US cases as reported to the United Network for Organ Sharing (UNOS) and the International Pancreas Transplant Registry (IPTR) as of May 2003. *Clin Transpl.* 2003;21–51.
8. Navarro X, Sutherland D, Kennedy W. Long-term effects of pancreatic transplantation on diabetic neuropathy. *Ann Neurol.* 1997;42:727–736.
9. Kiok M. Neurologic complications of pancreas transplants. *Neurol Clin.* 1988; 6:367–376.
10. Kenney W, Navarro X, Goetz F, et al. Effects of pancreatic transplantation on diabetic neuropathy. *N Engl J Med.* 1990;322:1031–1037.
11. Abu-Elmagd K, Reyes J, Bond G, et al. Clinical intestinal transplantation: A decade of experience at a single center. *Ann Surg.* 2001;234:404–416.
12. Tzakis A, Kato T, Nishida S, et al. Preliminary experience with campath 1H (C1H) in intestinal and liver transplantation. *Transplantation.* 2003;75:1227–1231.
13. Newell K. Transplantation of the intestine: Is it truly different? *Am J Transplant.* 2003;3:1–2.
14. Fong J. Alpha-tocopherol: Its inhibition on human platelet aggregation. *Experientia.* 1976;32:639–641.
15. Karnaze D, Carmel R. Neurologic and evoked potential abnormalities in subtle cobalamin deficiency states, including deficiency without anemia and with normal absorption of free cobalamin. *Arch Neurol.* 1990;47:1008–1012.

CHAPTER **41**

Commonly Used Gastrointestinal Drugs

John C. Morgan • Brian W. Mitchell • Kapil D. Sethi • Robert R. Schade

OBJECTIVES

- To identify neurologic complications associated with commonly used gastrointestinal drugs
- To describe the treatment of these drug-related complications
- To provide an understanding of these neurologic complications that are avoidable with alternative choices of pharmacotherapy

CASE VIGNETTE

A 53-year-old right-handed woman with a history of insulin-dependent diabetes mellitus and associated gastroparesis presents for evaluation of a resting tremor in her right hand and slowing of her movements. She was prescribed metoclopramide (10 mg before meals four times per day) for the gastroparesis 5 years earlier by her primary care physician. On interview, she described gradual onset of resting tremor in her right hand, first noted 1 year ago. The tremor had progressively worsened to the point where it was present most of the time. She also noted reduced arm swing, a decrease in the size of her handwriting, and some slowing of her gait where she could not keep up with her friends while walking.

On examination she had a masked face and hypophonic voice. Resting tremor was evident in her right hand during most of the interview and examination. She also had slowing of rapidly alternating movements in her right arm and leg more than the left hemibody. She had cogwheel rigidity evident in the right arm. Her handwriting revealed micrographia; her gait demonstrated reduced right arm swing and she had reduced stride length with good turns. She had normal postural reflexes on the pull test.

INTRODUCTION

Gastrointestinal (GI) disorders are very prevalent and drugs used to treat these disorders are widely prescribed throughout the world. Commonly used gastrointestinal drugs are listed in the Table 41-1. Most drugs used in the treatment of GI disorders do not cause significant neurologic side effects, with some notable exceptions, and clinicians should be aware of side effects associated with these drugs should they occur. With some gastrointestinal drugs, causality and mechanistic details are well established (parkinsonism with phenothiazine antiemetics); however, for many of these drugs, there is predominantly an association with neurologic complications in susceptible patients without firm evidence of causality.

ANTIBIOTICS AND ANTIPARASITICS

Numerous antibiotics and antiparasitics are used in the treatment of GI disease. Amoxicillin, clarithromycin, tetracycline, and metronidazole are commonly used for *Helicobacter pylori* eradication. Metronidazole and ciprofloxacin are commonly used for GI infections in patients with inflammatory bowel disease (Crohn disease and ulcerative colitis). Clarithromycin therapy was associated with visual hallucinations in a young woman (1) and in a patient with end-stage renal disease (2). Clarithromycin is associated with other neuropsychiatric disturbances as well. Metronidazole is commonly used for anaerobic infections and parasites; extended therapy with this drug can cause a predominantly sensory peripheral neuropathy (3) that usually (but not always) improves or resolves on discontinuation of the drug (4).

Prolonged therapy with metronidazole is also associated with a toxic encephalopathy and diffuse brain magnetic resonance imaging (MRI) changes (5,6) more commonly in the setting of liver disease. The authors were consulted regarding a 49-year-old man with hepatitis C and Crohn disease who was being treated with metronidazole (500 mg four times daily) for an enteric fistula and paraspinal infection with blood cultures growing *Enterococcus faecium*. He developed dysesthesias and paresthesias in his extremities within 1 month and within 3 months he developed dysarthria and ataxia and was unable to ambulate or feed himself. Brain MRI revealed diffuse hyperintensity in the basal ganglia (Fig. 41-1A), inferior olives, midbrain, and cerebral peduncles on T2-weighted images. Metronidazole was discontinued and, in parallel with remarkable clinical improvement, repeat imaging 3 months later revealed virtually complete resolution of the basal ganglia hyperintensity (Fig. 41-1B), however inferior olivary hyperintensity remained

TABLE 41-1. Commonly Used Gastrointestinal Drugs by Symptoms or Disease State

CONSTIPATION

Laxatives: bulk forming, emollient, hyperosmolar, lubricant, stimulant
Chloride channel antagonists: lubiprostone (Amitiza)
5-HT_4 partial agonists: tegaserod (Zelnorm)

DIARRHEA

Adsorbent or absorbent agents: activated attapulgite (Kaopectate), calcium polycarbophil
Anticholinergics: dicyclomine (Bentyl)
Antimotility Agents: atropine sulfate or diphenoxylate (Lomotil), loperamide (Imodium)
Antisecretory agents: bismuth subsalicylate (Pepto-Bismol)

GASTROESOPHAGEAL REFLUX DISEASE (GERD)

Antacids: aluminum, calcium and magnesium salts, sodium bicarbonate or a combination thereof
Histamine antagonists (H_2 blockers): cimetidine (Tagamet), famotidine (Pepcid), nizatidine (Axid), ranitidine (Zantac)
Proton-pump inhibitors (PPI): esomeprazole (Nexium), lansoprazole (Prevacid), omeprazole (Prilosec), pantoprazole (Protonix), rabeprazole (Aciphex)
Prokinetic agents: cisapride, erythromycin, metoclopramide (Reglan)

***HELICOBACTER PYLORI* ERADICATION**

Antibiotics: amoxicillin, clarithromycin (Biaxin), metronidazole (Flagyl), tetracycline
PPI: as above
Bismuth salts: bismuth subsalicylate (Pepto Bismol)

INFLAMMATORY BOWEL DISEASE (IBD)

Antibiotics: metronidazole (Flagyl), ciprofloxacin (Cipro)
Antiinflammatories: balsalazide, mesalamine, olsalazine, sulfasalazine
Biological therapies: infliximab (Remicade)
Corticosteroids: budesonide, hydrocortisone, methylprednisolone (Solu-Medrol), prednisone
Immunomodulators: azathioprine (Imuran), cyclosporine (Neoral, Sandimmune), 6-mercaptopurine (Purinethol), methotrexate, tacrolimus (Prograf)

IRRITABLE BOWEL SYNDROME (IBS)

Anticholinergic agents: dicyclomine (Bentyl)
Prokinetic agents: tegaserod (Zelnorm)

NAUSEA AND VOMITING

Anticholinergics: scopolamine (Transderm Scop)
Antihistamines: dimenhydrinate (Dramamine), diphenhydramine (Benadryl), meclizine (Antivert)
Dopamine antagonists: chlorpromazine (Thorazine), droperidol (Inapsine), metoclopramide (Reglan), prochlroperazine (Compazine), promethazine (Phenergan), domperidone (Motilium—not in the United States)
Serotonin (5-HT_3) antagonist: dolasetron (Anzemet), granisetron (Kytril), ondansetron (Zofran)
Others: dexamethasone, methylprednisolone (Solumedrol), trimethobenzamide (Tigan)

(not shown). Similar clinical and MRI findings have been reported in metronidazole-induced encephalopathy by other authors (5–7). The cause of metronidazole-induced encephalopathy is unknown; however, possibly it may be caused by reversible interstitial edema or mitochondrial toxicity of the drug.

Some antiparasitics are associated with neurologic side effects. Levamisole is an antihelminthic drug that is a common adjuvant to 5-fluorouracil (5-FU) in the therapy of colon cancer (8). This drug is associated with a leukoencephalopathy that resembles acute disseminated encephalomyelitis (ADEM) (8,9). It appears monophasic, with ataxia and dysarthria as common clinical manifestations (8). Neuroimaging reveals periventricular enhancing lesions and supratentorial lesions in approximately half of affected patients and a lymphocytic pleocytosis in the cerebrospinal fluid (CSF) is also common (8). If the levamisole is discontinued, patients have good recovery in most cases, but many patients are also treated with steroids, intravenous immunoglobulin, or both (8).

ANTIDIARRHEALS

Numerous drugs are used in the treatment of diarrhea and a few have been associated with neurologic side effects. Bismuth salts are widely used throughout the world for diarrhea and dyspepsia and they are occasionally associated with significant neurologic effects in patients abusing the drug. Patients who are symptomatic typically present with an encephalopathy-associated myoclonus (10). Most features of bismuth encephalopathy are reversible; however, tremor can be both an acute and chronic problem associated with bismuth neurotoxicity in many patients (10,11). Autopsies of patients with bismuth-induced encephalopathy have demonstrated higher levels of bismuth in gray matter relative to white matter, perivenular lymphocytic infiltration, and abundant intracytoplasmic lipofuscin (12).

A case-control study of drug use preceding Guillain-Barré syndrome revealed loperamide (a peripherally acting opiate agonist) was used more often in cases than in controls (13). This finding has not been replicated, and it may be an artifact of the frequent GI bacterial or viral illnesses (often associated with diarrhea) that precede the development of Guillain-Barré syndrome in many patients. Also loss of consciousness was reported in a 2-year-old child treated with loperamide who was successfully treated with naloxone (14). Numerous reports are found of neurologic toxicity in the setting of diphenoxylate-atropine sulfate (Lomotil) overdose, especially in children (15). Patients can present with aspects of either opioid intoxication or atropine toxicity. Atropine toxicity is typified by central nervous system (CNS) hyperexcitability, hypertension, fever, and skin flushing. Diphenoxylate overdose can be associated with hypoxia, respiratory depression, abnormal muscle tone, cerebral edema, and even death (15).

ANTIEMETICS

Antiemetics, which are widely used in children and adults, include antihistamines (dimenhydrinate, diphenhydramine, meclizine), phenothiazines (promethazine and prochlorperazine), and 5-hydroxytryptamine-3 (5-HT_3) antagonists (ondansetron, alosetron, cilansetron). Phenothiazines have antihistaminic, anticholinergic, and dopamine antagonist properties and these drugs can cause acute dystonic reactions (e.g., cervical dystonia, oculogyric crisis) that can be life-threatening in some cases (laryngospasm). In a large prospective study of adult patients treated for nausea and vomiting or headache in the emergency department, 4% of patients developed acute dystonia following treatment with prochlorperazine (16). Many more patients (16%) developed akathisia (16). Acute dystonic reactions and akathisia usually occur immediately or

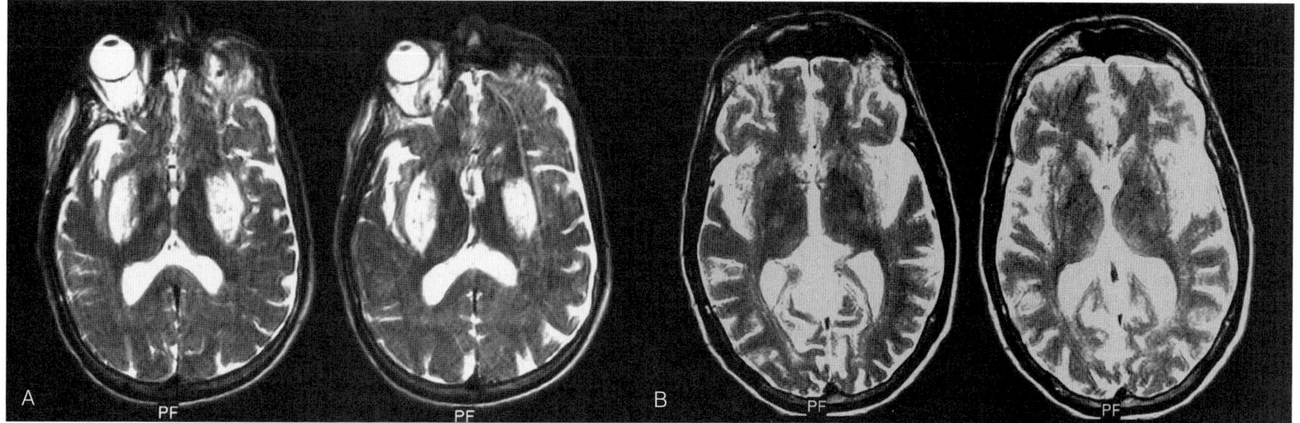

FIGURE 41-1. Metronidazole-induced encephalopathy. (A) T2-weighted magnetic resonance imaging (MRI) of the brain in a man with Crohn disease on chronic metronidazole therapy showing marked hyperintensity in the bilateral basal ganglia. **(B)** Repeat MRI of the brain 3 months after discontinuing metronidazole demonstrating nearly complete resolution of the basal ganglia lesions.

within 2 to 3 days of initiating therapy. Most patients respond to discontinuing the drug or treatment with diphenhydramine or anticholinergics.

Risk factors for acute dystonic reactions include younger age, male gender, cocaine use, and a history of such a reaction previously. In patients at higher risk, it may be prudent to use anticholinergics to prevent acute dystonic reactions. Tardive dystonia and tardive dyskinesia can also occur with these agents in chronically treated patients. Phenothiazine antiemetics can also cause drug-induced parkinsonism, given their dopamine-blocking properties, perhaps more often in the elderly (17).

Ondansetron, alosetron, and cilansetron are 5-HT_3 antagonists that are powerful and expensive antiemetics. Although neurologic side effects with these drugs are not commonly reported, ondansetron may improve cerebellar tremor (18).

ANTIINFLAMMATORY DRUGS

Antiinflammatory drugs are typically used in the setting of inflammatory bowel disease. Sulfasalazine is widely used for Crohn disease and ulcerative colitis and this drug is rarely associated with encephalopathy and focal neurologic signs in this setting (19). Infliximab, a recombinant monoclonal antibody against inflammation-promoting tumor necrosis factor-α (TNF-α), is commonly used for both Crohn disease and rheumatoid arthritis and has been associated with neurologic complications, including CNS demyelinating disease and peripheral neuropathy in numerous patients with both diseases (20–22). Infliximab has also been associated in retrobulbar optic neuritis, aseptic meningitis, and brachial plexitis (23).

HISTAMINE (H_2) ANTAGONISTS

Cimetidine, famotidine, nizatidine, and ranitidine are widely used for gastroesophageal reflux disease (GERD) and are well known to cause CNS effects in the elderly and in those with impaired hepatic or renal function. Common CNS manifestations of H_2 antagonists are typical of an encephalopathy or delirium (confusion, disorientation, lethargy, somnolence) (24–26). Some patients may experience mania (27), auditory and visual hallucinations (28), and even electroencephalographic (EEG) changes and seizures (29).

The altered mental status that can occur in these patients is frequently associated with elevated plasma concentrations, particularly in elderly patients with impaired renal function (25). In elderly patients and in patients with hepatic and renal impairment, these drugs should be used with caution and perhaps initiated at lower doses (25,26). As consulting neurologists, the authors routinely recommend discontinuing H_2 antagonists in patients with altered mental status and recommend proton-pump inhibitors for gastrointestinal prophylaxis or the treatment of GERD in the hospital setting.

In patients who are symptomatic, discontinuing the offending drug is the best practice. Most patients experience a relatively rapid recovery from the CNS effects of H_2 antagonists (days to weeks), but occasionally patients have a longer course of symptoms (27). A neurobehavioral syndrome was reported in 46 patients withdrawn from either cimetidine or ranitidine and the authors associated this withdrawal syndrome with decreased levels of prolactin (H_2 antagonists typically cause hyperprolactinemia) (30). A similar independent series of patients could not be found in the literature with a "neurobehavioral syndrome" associated with the withdrawal of H_2 antagonists and perhaps this condition is absent or mild and unrecognized in most patients.

Dystonic reactions are also reported to occur with H_2 antagonists. Cimetidine has been associated with two reports of acute dystonic reactions in women (31,32). The woman in the most recent case report had an acute dystonic reaction following prochlorperazine administration for nausea and vomiting 1 week earlier, and a similar episode of masseter spasm and oculogyric crisis followed the intravenous administration of cimetidine (32). Ranitidine was also associated with development of a subacute cranial dystonia that recurred on rechallenge (33). The authors suggested that the cholinergic effects of ranitidine could be associated with dystonic reactions with H_2 antagonists (33). Interestingly, however, H_1 antagonists such as diphenhydramine, and H_2 antagonists, such as cimetidine, have been shown to attenuate dystonic reactions in a rat model (34).

Cimetidine also exacerbated action or postural tremors in three patients, with propranolol use significantly improving the tremor in all patients (35). The authors suggested that histaminergic pathways may normally be involved in suppression of physiologic and essential tremors (35).

IMMUNOMODULATORY AGENTS

Numerous immunosuppressive agents are used for inflammatory bowel disease, including 6-mercaptopurine, azathioprine, cyclosporine, steroids, and tacrolimus. These drugs are covered in detail elsewhere in the book; however, clinicians should be aware that cyclosporine and tacrolimus can be associated significant neurologic side effects, including reversible posterior leukoencephalopathy and tremor (36). These neurologic side effects are most often reported in renal and liver transplant immunosuppression; however, they are also reported to occur in patients with gastrointestinal disease (37).

LAXATIVES

Constipation is an extremely common problem and many patients use numerous prescribed and over-the-counter medications to treat it. Few nervous system adverse events occur with use of these drugs, however, there are a few of note. Senna is an anthraquinone cathartic commonly used for constipation and concern was that this drug was associated with death of myenteric plexus neurons. This initial concern was not confirmed in further studies (38). If patients abuse laxatives (as can occur in eating disorders), then clinicians should be aware that numerous neurologic side effects can occur because of electrolyte imbalances.

PROKINETIC AGENTS

Prokinetic agents include cisapride, erythromycin, metoclopramide, and tegaserod. Cisapride was removed from the pharmaceutical market in the United States in 2000 after it was associated with life-threatening cardiac arrhythmias. Cisapride was associated with akathisia in a child in one case report (39) and was also noted to aggravate parkinsonian tremor in two patients (40). Metoclopramide use is commonly overlooked as a cause of drug-induced parkinsonism and tardive dyskinesia in clinical practice (41). In a study of diabetic and nondiabetic veterans, the relative risk for developing tardive dyskinesia was 1.67 (95% CI of 0.93 to 2.97) and for drug-induced parkinsonism 4.0 (95% CI of 1.5 to 10.5), respectively, in those treated with metoclopramide versus controls (42). Discontinuing therapy with metoclopramide is indicated in patients with tardive dyskinesias or drug-induced parkinsonism or tremors. It can take patients 6 months or more to recover from drug-induced parkinsonism after the drug is discontinued. Some patients may have underlying parkinsonism that was accentuated by the drug before the patient would have typically been symptomatic.

The authors have seen numerous patients with socially disabling tardive dyskinesia associated with metoclopramide use, and dopamine depleting agents (e.g., tetrabenazine) may be the most effective therapy for these patients.

Tegaserod is a 5-HT_4 partial agonist and is approved for the treatment of both irritable bowel syndrome and chronic idiopathic constipation. This drug may ameliorate constipation associated with Parkinson disease while not worsening parkinsonism, unlike metoclopramide (43).

PROTON-PUMP INHIBITORS

Proton-pump inhibitors (PPI), including esomeprazole, lansoprazole, omeprazole, pantoprazole, and rabeprazole, are now standard therapy for GERD, erosive esophagitis, and *H. pylori* eradication. Relatively few neurologic adverse events have been reported with use of these drugs beyond headache. Headache was commonly reported in clinical trials with these drugs as an adverse event ranging from 1.3% to 8.8%, depending on the drug studied and the study population (44). In a large, prospective community-based study in the Netherlands, lansoprazole was associated with a headache frequency of 2.5% in lansoprazole users, with an incidence density of 7.2 per 1,000 patient-months of drug use (44). Two thirds of the patients had tension headache, whereas one third had headaches typical of migraine. Women, patients with previous analgesic use, and patients reporting several adverse events were more likely to report headache with lansoprazole use (44). Of 25 patients, 20 (80%) had reduction or cessation of their headache following discontinuance of the drug. Perhaps lansoprazole and other PPI exacerbate underlying headache syndromes in susceptible patients.

One report exists of sensory axonal neuropathy temporally associated with lansoprazole (45) and two other reports of sensorimotor axonal neuropathy and sensory neuropathy associated with omeprazole (46,47). Neuropathy symptoms typically improve on discontinuation of these drugs; however, a woman treated with lansoprazole had continued paresthesias and dysesthesias 2 years later (45).

CLINICAL RECOMMENDATIONS OF THE VIGNETTE

Discontinuing the metoclopramide in this patient resulted in return of some gastroparetic symptoms that were present before treatment. She experienced improvement in her parkinsonism over time, with reduced resting tremor, and improved bradykinesia evident on examination at 3 months. By 9 months, she denied symptoms and only mild cogwheel rigidity was evident in her right arm. She was followed for another year without progression of symptoms or parkinsonian signs.

SUMMARY

Most clinicians encounter patients with GI disease and prescribe or recommend over-the-counter drugs to treat these disorders. Many of these drugs can be associated with neurologic side effects and it is important to be aware of these side effects in practice. A summary of the gastrointestinal drugs most commonly associated with neurologic side effects is presented in Table 41-2. Most of these neurologic complications are largely reversible on discontinuation of the offending drug; however, some can be a medical emergency requiring immediate treatment (acute laryngospasm associated with an antiemetic). Other patients may suffer permanent neurologic sequelae (tardive dyskinesia related to prolonged metoclopramide use). Further knowledge is needed regarding those at risk for these side effects and how to prevent them from occurring, if possible.

TABLE 41-2. Gastrointestinal Drugs Most Commonly Associated with Neurologic Complications

Drug Class	*Example(s)*	*Gastrointestinal Use(s)*	*Neurologic Complication(s)*
Antibiotics	Metronidazole	IBD, *Helicobacter pylori**	Peripheral neuropathy, encephalopathy
Anti-inflammatory	Infliximab	Crohn disease	Aseptic meningitis, brachial plexitis, central nervous system demyelination, peripheral neuropathy, retrobulbar neuritis
Bismuth salts	Bismuth subsalicylate	Dyspepsia*	Encephalopathy with myoclonus, tremor
Histamine (H_2) antagonists	Cimetidine, famotidine, ranitidine	GERD*	Acute dystonia, delirium, hallucinations, worsening of preexistent tremor
Immunomodulators	Azathioprine	IBD	Neuropathy
	Cyclosporine, tacrolimus	IBD	Reversible posterior leukoencephalopathy, tremor
	Methotrexate	IBD	Leukoencephalopathy
Phenothiazines	Prochlorperazine, promethazine	Antiemetics	Acute and tardive dystonia or dyskinesias, akathisia, parkinsonism
PPI	Omeprazole, lansoprazole	GERD*	Headaches, neuropathy
Prokinetics	Metoclopramide	Gastroparesis*	Acute and tardive dystonia or dyskinesias, akathisia, parkinsonism

*Examples.
IBD, inflammatory bowel disease; GERD, gastroesophageal reflux disease; PPI, proton-pump inhibitors.

REFERENCES

1. Jimenez-Pulido, Navarro-Ruiz A, Sendra P, et al. Hallucinations with therapeutic doses of clarithromycin. *Int J Clin Pharmacol Ther.* 2002;40:20–22.
2. Steinman MA, Steinman TI. Clarithromycin-associated visual hallucinations in a patient with chronic renal failure on continuous ambulatory peritoneal dialysis. *Am J Kidney Dis.* 1996;27:143–146.
3. Coxon A, Pallis CA. Metronidazole neuropathy. *J Neurol Neurosurg Psychiatry.* 1976;39:403–405.
4. Duffy LF, Daum F, Fisher SE, et al. Peripheral neuropathy in Crohn's disease patients treated with metronidazole. *Gastroenterology.* 1985;88:681–684.
5. Ahmed A, Loes DJ, Bressler EL. Reversible magnetic resonance imaging findings in metronidazole-induced encephalopathy. *Neurology.* 1995;45:588–589.
6. Horlen CK, Seifert CF, Malouf CS. Toxic metronidazole-induced MRI changes. *Ann Pharmacother.* 2000;34:1273–1275.
7. Seok JI, Yi H, Song YM, et al. Metronidazole-induced encephalopathy and inferior olivary hypertrophy: Lesion analysis with diffusion-weighted imaging and apparent diffusion coefficient maps. *Arch Neurol.* 2003;60:1796–1800.
8. Wu VC, Huang JW, Lien HC, et al. Levamisole-induced multifocal inflammatory leukoencephalopathy: Clinical characteristics, outcome, and impact of treatment in 31 patients. *Medicine (Baltimore).* 2006;85:203–213.
9. El Kallab K, El Khoury J, Elias E, et al. Encephalopathy induced by antihelminthic use of levamisole: Report of two patients. *J Med Liban.* 2003;51:221–227.
10. Buge A, Rancurel G, Poisson M, et al. 20 cases of acute encephalopathy with myoclonus during treatments with orally-administered bismuth salts [in French]. *Ann Med Interne (Paris).* 1974;125:877–888.
11. Gordon MF, Abrams RI, Rubin DB, et al. Bismuth subsalicylate toxicity as a cause of prolonged encephalopathy with myoclonus. *Mov Disord.* 1995;10:220–222.
12. Escourolle R, Bourdon R, Galli A, et al. Neuropathologic and toxicologic study of 12 cases of bismuth encephalopathy [in French]. *Rev Neurol.* 1977;133:153–163.
13. Stricker BH, van der Klauw MM, Ottervanger JP, et al. A case-control study of drugs and other determinants as potential causes of Guillian-Barre syndrome. *J Clin Epidemiol.* 1994;47:1203–1210.
14. Chanzy S, Moretti S, Mayhet H, et al. Loss of consciousness in a child due to loperamide [in French]. *Arch Pediatr.* 2004;11:826–827.
15. McCarron MM, Challoner KR, Thompson GA. Diphenoxylate-atropine (Lomotil) overdose in children: An update (report of eight cases and review of the literature). *Pediatrics.* 1991;87:694–700.
16. Olsen JC, Keng JA, Clark JA. Frequency of adverse reactions to prochlorperazine in the ED. *Am J Emerg Med.* 2000;18:609–611.
17. Stephen PJ, Williamson J. Drug-induced parkinsonism in the elderly. *Lancet.* 1984;2(8411):1082–1083.
18. Rice GP, Lesaux J, Vandervoort P, et al. Ondansetron, a 5-HT antagonist, improves cerebellar tremor. *J Neurol Neurosurg Psychiatry.* 1997;62:282–284.
19. Schoonjans R, Mast A, Van Den Abeele G, et al. Sulfasalazine-associated encephalopathy in a patient with Crohn's disease. *Am J Gastroenterol.* 1993;88:1416–1420.
20. Thomas CW, Jr., Weinshenker BG, Sandborn WJ. Demyelination during anti-tumor necrosis factor alpha therapy with infliximab for Crohn's disease. *Inflamm Bowel Dis.* 2004;10:28–31.
21. Dubcenco E, Ottaway CA, Chen DL, et al. Neurological symptoms suggestive of demyelination in Crohn's disease after infliximab therapy. *Eur J Gastroenterol Hepatol.* 2006;18:565–566.
22. Jarand J, Zochodne DW, Martin LO, et al. Neurological complications of infliximab. *J Rheumatol.* 2006;33:1018–1020.
23. Arias M, Arias-Rivas S, Dapena D, et al. Brachial plexitis and myelitis and herpes-zoster lumbar plexus disorder in a patient treated with infliximab [in Spanish]. *Neurologia.* 2005;20:374–376.
24. Sonnenblick M, Rosin AJ, Weisberg N. Neurological and psychiatric side effects of cimetidine—Report of 3 cases with review of the literature. *Postgrad Med J.* 1982;58:415–418.
25. Slugg PH, Haug MT, 3rd, Pippenger CE. Ranitidine pharmacokinetics and adverse central nervous system reactions. *Arch Intern Med.* 1992;152:2325–2329.
26. Odeh M, Oliven A. Central nervous system reactions associated with famotidine: Report of five cases. *J Clin Gastroenterol.* 1998;27:253–254.
27. Von Einsiedel RW, Roesch-Ely D, Diebold K, et al. H(2)-histamine antagonist (famotidine) induced adverse CNS reactions with longstanding secondary mania and epileptic seizures. *Pharmacopsychiatry.* 2002;35:152–154.
28. Price W, Coli L, Brandstetter RD, et al. Ranitidine-associated hallucinations. *Eur J Clin Pharmacol.* 1985;29:375–376.
29. Van Sweden B, Kamphuisen HA. Cimetidine neurotoxicity. EEG and behavior aspects. *Eur Neurol.* 1984;23:300–305.
30. Rampello L, Raffaele R, Nicoletti G, et al. Neurobehavioral syndrome induced by H2-receptor blocker withdrawal: Possible role of prolactin. *Clin Neuropharmacol.* 1997;20:49–54.
31. Romisher S, Felter R, Dougherty J. Tagamet-induced acute dystonia. *Ann Emerg Med.* 1987;16:1162–1164.
32. Peiris RS, Peckler BF. Cimetidine-induced dystonic reaction. *J Emerg Med.* 2001;21:27–29.
33. Davis BJ, Aul EA, Granner MA, et al. Ranitidine-induced cranial dystonia. *Clin Neuropharmacol.* 1994;17:489–491.
34. Van't Groenewout JL, Stone MR, Vo VN, et al. Evidence for the involvement of histamine in the antidystonic effects of diphenhydramine. *Exp Neurol.* 1995;134:253–260.
35. Bateman DN, Bevan P, Longley BP, et al. Cimetidine induced postural and action tremor. *J Neurol Neurosurg Psychiatry.* 1981;44:94.
36. Ponticelli C, Campise MR. Neurological complications in kidney transplant recipients. *J Nephrol.* 2005;18:521–528.
37. Sood A, Midha V, Sood N. Reversible posterior leukoencephalopathy due to oral cyclosporine in severe ulcerative colitis. *Indian J Gastroenterol.* 2003;22:233–234.
38. Kiernan JA, Heinicke EA. Sennosides do not kill myenteric neurons in the colon of the rat or mouse. *Neuroscience.* 1989;30:837–842.
39. Elzinga-Huttenga J, Hekster Y, Bijl A, et al. Movement disorders induced by gastrointestinal drugs: Two pediatric cases. *Neuropediatrics.* 2006;37:102–106.
40. Sempere AP, Duarte J, Cabezas C, et al. Aggravation of parkinsonian tremor by cisapride. *Clin Neuropharmacol.* 1995;18:76–78.
41. Sethi KD, Morgan JC. Drug induced movement disorders. In: Jankovic JJ, Tolosa E, eds. *Parkinson's Disease & Movement Disorders,* 5th ed. Philadelphia: Lippincott Williams & Wilkins; 2006:394–408.
42. Ganzini L, Casey DE, Hoffman WF, et al. The prevalence of metoclopramide-induced tardive dyskinesia and acute extrapyramidal movement disorders. *Arch Intern Med.* 1883;153:1469–1475.
43. Sullivan KL, Staffetti JF, Hauser RA, et al. Tegaserod (Zelnorm) for the treatment of constipation in Parkinson's disease. *Mov Disord.* 2006;21:115–116.
44. Claessans AA, Heerdink ER, van Eijk JT, et al. Determinants of headache in lansoprazole users in The Netherlands: Results from a nested case-control study. *Drug Saf.* 2002;25:287–295.
45. Rajabally YA, Jacob S. Neuropathy associated with lansoprazole treatment. *Muscle Nerve.* 2005;31:124–125.
46. Faucheux JM, Tournebize P, Viguier A, et al. Neuromyopathy secondary to omeprazole treatment. *Muscle Nerve.* 1998;21:261–262.
47. Sellapah S. An unusual side effect of omeprazole: Case report. *Br J Gen Pract.* 1990;40:389.

PART V Liver Diseases/Biliary System

CHAPTER 42

Neurologic Problems Seen During the Management of the Patient with Viral Hepatitis

Anne Mai • Hugo E. Vargas

OBJECTIVES

- To review the manifestations of neurologic problems associated with viral hepatitis
- To discuss the current understanding of cryoglobulinemic disorders in chronic viral liver disease
- To review the management strategies for cryoglobulinemia and polyarteritis nodosa in the setting of chronic viral hepatitis
- To review the neuropsychiatric complications of viral hepatitis treatment

INTRODUCTION

Viral hepatitis has received increasing levels of attention in the last 20 years. Improved understanding of the pathophysiology, virology, and natural history of hepatitis B virus (HBV) infection, and the cloning of the hepatitis C virus (HCV) coupled with a better understanding of its pathophysiologic potential have led to a veritable revolution in hepatology. The diagnosis, staging, and management of both viral entities have progressed immensely. Along with that progress has come a better understanding of the nonhepatic manifestations of these diseases. This chapter focuses on the principal neurologic complications of infections with these viruses to provide the internist with a guide to the diagnosis, treatment, and long-term management of these disorders.

HEPATITIS B

HBV, a DNA virus of the genus *hepadnaviridae*, is an encapsulated, partially double-stranded, circular DNA structure that takes advantage of the host's eukaryotic cellular machinery to make a number of structural and nonstructural proteins that direct its life cycle (1,2). Although exclusively pathogenic to humans, several closely related viruses have been identified in ducks and woodchucks that have been used to extrapolate on the biology of HBV. This virus infects approximately 1.25 million people in the United States and 350 million worldwide, making it one of the most important human pathogens (1,2). The virus is contagious to close contacts of the index case, likely through saliva, body fluids, and blood contact (1,2). Since the introduction of highly effective vaccines in the early 1980s (3), major improvements have occurred in the epidemiology of this disease, both in Western and Far East countries. The introduction of recombinant interferons-α (IFN-α) and subsequent antimetabolite antivirals targeted against specific HBV replicative mechanisms have revolutionized the management of this disease in the last decade (1,2).

In internal medicine practices, the patients seen with this disease can be subdivided in two large groups: Those with acute HBV who acquired the disease as adults and chronic HBV carriers. The first group will have a resolution rate of approximately 90%, without specific intervention. Less than 1% will have acute hepatic failure requiring the attention of a liver transplantation service. The remaining 10% will go on to chronic carrier state. These patients, together with those who acquired the disease perinatally (conversion to chronic carrier in this setting is >90%, and generally is caused by vertical transmission or early childhood exposure in endemic regions in sub-Saharan Africa, the Middle and Far East) constitute most patients who will be targets for anti-HBV therapy and who also are likely to experience extrahepatic complications of HBV.

HEPATITIS C

HCV is an RNA virus within its own genus *hepaciviridae* within its close relatives in the *flaviviridae* family (4). Although long suspected as the cause of what was then known as non-A–non-B hepatitis, it was not cloned until 1989 (5). This pivotal moment has led to the development of serologic tests that have helped in the diagnosis and management of the infection and have led to the much improved screening of the blood supply, making transfusion-related HCV infection a thing of the past in most industrialized countries (6–8). Despite the progress, our understanding of the natural history of this disease is limited by the slow and variable course observed. Today most new infections are caused by illicit intravenous drug use and, to a lesser degree, from sexual transmission. Many undiagnosed cases of HCV infection remain a challenge to society because a significant number will develop cirrhosis, with the accompanying plethora of complications.

HCV is hepatotrophic, but also able to replicate in the peripheral mononuclear blood cells and other tissue compartments, including possibly kidney, thymus, pancreas, and the central nervous system (CNS) (9,10). This facility to replicate may help the virus evade immunologic and pharmacologic targeting. Despite the best therapy, more than 45% of patients do not respond long term. Because as many as 4 million Americans may be infected with HCV, understanding the impact of therapy is of paramount importance for clinicians. The extensive and prolonged course of therapy required for the eradication of HVC causes the appearance of secondary effects of IFN that need to be recognized and managed. Many of these effects are neurologic and should be aggressively diagnosed and treated.

Internists should also recognize the importance of both HBV and HCV in the subpopulation of patients who harbor the human immunodeficiency virus (HIV). Despite that these patients are living longer because the HIV disease is under better control, hepatic infections are an important cause of morbidity and mortality in these patients (6,11,12). It is important to recognize that these hepatitis viruses may be in the background and that HIV can influence the course of these hepatitidies, even if they are replicating at very low levels (12).

The following sections cover important complications of viral hepatitis and outline their management. Also discussed are a number of complications of IFN treatment that need to be understood and identified for appropriate treatment.

CASE VIGNETTE 1

A 55-year-old white man presents with recent diagnosis of HCV. He has a remote history of intravenous drug use (30 years before evaluation) and no symptoms of hepatic decompensation. He has mild hypertension and no other medical problems. On examination, he has normal appearance and has no appreciable affect problems. Blood pressure is within normal limits. Abdominal examination demonstrates slightly enlarged liver span, no splenomegaly. Neurologic evaluation shows normal motor function and a slight sensory deficit in the distal lower extremities. Dermatologic survey shows an erythematous, raised macular rash involving the distal two thirds of his legs in a uniform bilateral pattern and not involving his feet. His laboratory tests demonstrate hepatitis with aspartate aminotransferase (AST) 102 IU/mL, alanine aminotransferase (ALT) 160 IU/mL, and total bilirubin of 1.2 mg/dL. International normalized ratio (INR) and albumin are in the normal range. Serum creatinine is 1.6 mg/dL.

Mixed Cryoglobulinemia (MC)

DEFINITION/EPIDEMIOLOGY

Cryoglobulins are serum immunoglobulins that reversibly precipitate at cold temperatures and they are associated with systemic vasculitis. According to their molecular composition, cryoglobulins are classified into three groups: Type I are monoclonal immunoglobulins that are associated with lymphoproliferative disorders; type II and type III are considered mixed cryoglobulineminas (MC) containing a mixture of polyclonal IgG and mono- (type II) or polyclonal (type III) IgM (rheumatoid factor activity) (13). MC can be secondary to autoimmune diseases, chronic infections, or lymphoproliferative disorder or can occur as a primary condition without any underlying systemic disease (i.e., essential mixed cryoglobulinemia) (13).

HCV is highly prevalent in MC; in fact, 80% to 90% of patients previously thought to have essential MC have demonstrable serologic markers for HCV infection (14,15). Less frequently, hepatitis B may also be associated with type II cryoglobulinemia (14,16,17). The presence of elevated levels of mixed cryoglobulins is common in patients infected with HCV with an incidence ranging from 46% to 56% (15,18–20). Most cryoglobulinemic HCV-infected patients are asymptomatic or have nonspecific symptoms. Vasculitis sequelae are relatively rare, being found in <10% of these patients. Patients who are symptomatic commonly present with skin involvement (purpura), polyarthralgias, or fatigue and may also manifest with more severe organ involvement of the kidney (glomerulonephritis) or nervous system (14,15,21). The most common neurologic involvement is peripheral neuropathy, with an incidence of 7% to 90%, depending on the series reported (15,21–23). The peripheral neuropathy in patients with HCV with cryoglobulinemia is more severe than in patients with cryoglobulinemia not associated with HCV, mainly because of increased motor involvement (15,22,23). CNS symptoms, including strokes, encephalopathy, communicating hydrocephalus, and seizures, have been reported, but are rare (24–26).

ETIOLOGY AND PATHOGENESIS

Vasculitis in the setting of HCV infection is thought to be mediated by the deposition of HCV containing immune complexes in the walls of small- and medium-sized blood vessels of target organs, activating inflammatory mediators—including the complement system—causing a systemic vasculitis. In the case of peripheral neuropathy, damage of local blood vessels from immune-complex deposition could lead to local ischemic changes and eventually to axonal degeneration in peripheral nerves. The mechanism that triggers the vasculitis in the setting of hepatitis C infection and MC is not completely understood (27). It has been hypothesized that HCV has a direct role in the production of MC via its infection of B lymphocytes. This is bolstered by the response to antiviral and antilymphocytic therapies that have been used in the management of this process (28–30). The various CNS features have been studied less extensively, but presumably result, at least in part, to a vasculopathy or vasculitis of the CNS from cryoglobulin-induced inflammation of small vessels (24–26).

CLINICAL MANIFESTATIONS

Peripheral neuropathy may be the presenting symptom of MC in approximately 15% of patients, but neurologic symptoms present almost exclusively in association with purpura of the lower extremities (which may in turn be precipitated by cold temperatures), polyarthralgias, and fatigue (22). Distal lower extremity paresthesias, burning pain, and numbness are the most common neurologic symptoms (22,26). Subsequent weakness may develop as part of a generalized sensorimotor peripheral neuropathy or mononeuritis multiplex (22,31). The degree of weakness is variable, but has been reported to be less frequent than sensory deficits. The pattern of peripheral nerve involvement can be asymmetric as in mononeuritis multiplex (31), but more commonly is distal and symmetric (22). Findings on neurologic examination may include sensory loss (in a stocking distribution with distal peripheral neuropathy), diminished deep tendon reflexes, and variable degree of weakness, usually limited to the lower extremities. The clinical course of the more common distal symmetric sensorimotor peripheral neuropathy is usually insidious, whereas mononeuritis multiplex can present acutely with more severe deficits at the onset (22). Prominent symptoms of restless leg syndrome have been reported in a group of patients with symmetric sensory neuropathy associated with mixed cryoglobulinemia (32). Restless leg syndrome has been thought to result from moderate sensory loss from the neuropathy (32).

Few case reports are found of CNS involvement. Clinically, patients have presented with diffuse encephalopathy. In addition, both ischemic and, lesser frequently, have been described hemorrhagic strokes in association with CNS vasculitis (24–26).

DIAGNOSIS

The diagnostic evaluation of patients suspected to have MC is the demonstration of a cryoprecipitate of measurable quantity from the patient's serum. This approach is fraught with laboratory errors and must be handled with care (33). Other laboratory findings can include low serum levels of total complement or C4, increased rheumatoid factor activity, increased erythrocyte sedimentation rate (ESR), increased antinuclear antibody (ANA) levels, abnormal liver function tests, and possibly increased cerebrospinal fluid (CSF) protein concentrations. HIV, as well as hepatitis B and C viral, profiles should be done. In testing for hepatitis C, confirmation of viral antibody should be done with RNA polymerase chain reaction (PCR) of the serum. HCV antibodies in the cryoprecipitate have been used in earlier studies, but should not be necessary today, given the well understood relationship between MC and HCV infection. When patients report symptoms of a peripheral neuropathy, then nerve conduction studies and electromyography (EMG) should be performed to document the extent of involvement. Follow up of these patients has helped to document progression (23,24).

Electrophysiologic studies typically confirm the neuropathy as an axonopathy, with EMG evidence of denervation and low amplitude nerve action potentials on nerve conduction studies. Cutaneous nerve biopsy may be useful to verify the presence of vasculitis and exclude other causes of neuropathy. Biopsy of the skin and muscle can increase the yield for diagnosis when evidence of systemic involvement is seen. Patients with suspected CNS involvement and severe manifestations should have magnetic resonance imaging (MRI) to evaluate for ischemic lesion(s) and possibly cerebral arteriography to help document CNS vasculitis (24).

TREATMENT

Traditionally, neurologic involvement has been equated with severe disease—one that required aggressive immunosuppressant therapy. Data from individual and small case series suggest, however, that patients with HCV associated-mixed cryoglobulinemia have had minimal improvement in neurologic symptoms when treated with corticosteroids, cyclophosphamide, or plasmapheresis.

With the establishment of HCV infection being associated with mixed cryoglobulinemia, the focus of attention has shifted from immunosuppression to antiviral therapy. The use of IFN, alone or in combination with ribavirin, has been evaluated in a small series of patients with mixed cryoglobulinemia (33). Although IFN-based therapy has demonstrated some clinical benefit in vasculitic manifestations when evidence of virological response is seen, the results in treating neurologic complications (i.e., peripheral neuropathy) have been varied and overall have been disappointing (20,23,30,34). Furthermore, in rare case reports, IFN-based therapy was thought, possibly to have exacerbated or worsened the peripheral neuropathy (30,35,36).

In a recent study evaluating pegylated IFN-α_{2b} plus ribavirin in nine patients with hepatitis C associated-mixed cryoglobulinemia, greater efficacy was demonstrated in terms of a higher sustained virologic response than had been previously reported with IFN-α and ribavirin (37). In addition, all patients had resolution of baseline vasculitic symptoms, including those related to peripheral neuropathy. Of the seven patients with peripheral neuropathy, three had objective improvement on serial electrophysiologic studies (37).

Other treatment options that have been recently investigated include rituximab, an anti-CD20 monoclonal antibody used in treatment of B-cell non-Hodgkin lymphoma and other antibody-mediated autoimmune diseases (28,29,38,39). Rituximab has been shown to be efficacious in the treatment of skin manifestations, nephrologic manifestations and subjective symptoms of peripheral neuropathy, although the evidence of resolution on electrodiagnostic studies has been mixed (28,29,38,39). Plasmapheresis has also been used in severe cases with mixed results (20,33,40,41).

As CNS manifestations of MC rarely occur, no randomized controlled studies exist. Anecdotal reports exist of successful outcomes using high-dose oral prednisone, plasmaphereses, or combination therapy with cyclophosphamide and intravenous methylprednisolone (41–48).

CLINICAL RECOMMENDATIONS OF THE VIGNETTE

The patient had very typical findings of MC. At the initial patient encounter, it is important to review dermatologic and neurologic findings with the patient because they may be remitting and not elicited on initial physical examination. Because dermatologic manifestations are common, a skin biopsy demonstrating leukocytoclastic vasculitis is very helpful. Complement levels should be obtained and, in patients such as the one in the vignette, an EMG or nerve conduction velocities (NCV) measurement may be considered, particularly in view of the reports that antiHCV treatment may exacerbate peripheral neuropathies. Nerve biopsy and CNS imaging are used only in extreme cases with very overt symptoms.

CASE VIGNETTE 2

A 21-year-old black man presented to the emergency department with complaints of fever, chills, and abdominal pain. He reported that he is homosexual, with only recent onset of sexual activity, and he has high risk behaviors for HIV. He has limited means and does not see a physician regularly. He reports numbness in the feet and legs and has noticed skin ulcers in the distal lower extremities. He became worried when he experienced fevers and chills and noticed blood in his stool.

On examination he is a gaunt, ill-appearing young man. He is cooperative and friendly with the examiner and his affect is appropriate. He has a fever (38.6°C) and has normal blood pressure. Pulse is 100 beats per minute. Lungs are clear, and his heart examination, other than his tachycardia is unremarkable. Increased bowel sounds are heard in his abdomen and it is diffuse tender without guarding or rigidity. Neurologic evaluation was remarkable for a pronounced sensory deficit in the left lower extremity, with minimal changes on the right. His anterior left lower extremity has a well-healed 2-cm ulceration that does not appear infected. Review of the laboratory and radiologic workup performed by the emergency department staff shows a white blood cell count of 12,000, predominantly lymphocytes, normal liver injury tests, sedimentation rate is high at 75 mm and HIV, HBV markers are pending. Serum creatinine is 2.4 mg/dL and urine analysis reveals hematuria. A computed tomographic (CT) scan of the abdomen is significant for a left renal infarct.

Polyarteritis Nodosa (PAN)

DEFINITION/EPIDEMIOLOGY

Polyarteritis nodosa (PAN) is a rare necrotizing vasculitis predominately affecting medium- and small-sized arteries (without glomerulonephritis or vasculitis of arterioles, capillaries or venules) (13). PAN typically presents as a systemic disease affecting the kidney (but not glomerulonephritis), gastrointestinal system, skin, heart, and nervous system or, not uncommonly, it is limited to one organ. It can be idiopathic without any identifiable etiologic agent, manifest during the course of other diseases (i.e., Sjogren syndrome or rheumatoid arthritis), or secondary to a known cause. It has a high association with HBV; one of the highest rates for PAN was reported from an area that was endemic for HBV infection (49). The frequency of hepatitis B-associated polyarteritis nodosa (HBV-PAN) in the developed world has declined from 36% in the 1970s to 7% to 10% in the 1990s. This has been attributed to widespread use hepatitis B vaccination and mandatory blood donor screening. Interestingly, case reports have also suggested that a causal link exists between PAN and hepatitis B vaccination; however, a review of reports submitted to the Vaccine Adverse Event Reporting System from 1990 through 2001 did not support this (50–53).

Cases reports of PAN have also been described in association with other infectious agents, including HCV (54).

Men are more frequently affected with PAN than women. The age at onset is from age 40 to 60 years and occurs in all ethnic groups. HBV-PAN may be seen in acute and chronic liver disease, and may precede or follow overt liver disease (55,56). No relationship exists between the severity of vasculitis and hepatic disease and often the underlying liver disease may be inactive. The clinical course of HBV-PAN is essentially no different than that of the idiopathic variant, although a higher morality for HBV-PAN has been reported (55). Furthermore, a prospective study of HVB-PAN showed that the frequency of gastrointestinal manifestations, malignant hypertension, renal infarction, and orchiepididymitis was higher in patients with HBV-PAN compared with those who did not have HBV-PAN (57).

ETIOLOGY/PATHOGENESIS

Two general mechanisms have been described in HBV-PAN: (*a*) viral replication can cause direct injury to the vessel wall; and (*b*) immune-mediated vascular damage as a result of deposition of circulating immune complexes or their in situ formation. The immune complexes are composed of viral antigens, more likely HBe antigen and specific antibodies (58–60). It is now well accepted that the pathogenesis in HBV-PAN is a phenomenon of the infection and not a triggered response (59).

CLINICAL MANIFESTATIONS

The clinical manifestation of PAN at the time of diagnosis can vary from case to case. Most patients present at onset with constitutional symptoms (e.g., malaise, fever, anorexia, weight loss). A retrospective study of patients with PAN (in which most were HBV-PAN cases) found that peripheral neuropathy and gastrointestinal symptoms were present in 75% and 53% of the cases, respectively, at the time of diagnosis (57,61). Virtually any organ system, with the exception of the lungs, can be involved in the vasculitis (55). Peripheral neuropathy develops in as many as 60% of patients (55). Vasculitic neuropathy is often asymmetric, predominately affecting the lower extremities and presents as (*a*) mononeuritis multiplex, (*b*) distal polyneuropathy, or (*c*) cutaneous neuropathy. It most commonly takes the form of mononeuritis multiplex or of a pure motor, sensory, or mixed sensorimotor polyneuropathy.

Central nervous involvement is less common. Palsies of cranial nerves have been reported in less than 2% of cases, with the oculomotor (III), trochlear (IV), abducens (VI), facial (VII), and acoustic (VIII) cranial nerves being most often affected (62–70). Cerebral arteritis can cause arterial thrombosis with cerebral ischemia, and intraparenchymal or subarachnoid hemorrhage. Transient symptoms of cerebral ischemia, the most commonly presenting symptom, usually presents late in the course of the disease. Global CNS dysfunction with encephalopathy and seizures results from metabolic derangements secondary to multiple organ failure. Acute or subacute myelopathy with paraparesis can occur at any cord level. Rare case reports have been made of spinal artery thrombosis, spinal subarachnoid hemorrhage, intradural spinal hematoma, and cord compression by an extramedullary hematoma secondary to a ruptured aneurysm.

DIAGNOSIS

The diagnosis of PAN requires integration of clinical, laboratory, angiography, and biopsy findings. Diagnostic criteria have been established to classify patients accurately (71). Inflammatory signs are found in most cases with an elevated erythrocyte sedimentation rate (>60 mm in the first hour) and increased C-reactive protein (72). Antineutrophil cytoplasmic antibodies (ANCA) are unusual in HBV-PAN, in contrast to other vasculitides (including microscopic polyartertitis nodosa, Wegener granulomatosis, and Churg-Strauss syndrome) and should be viewed with suspicion if found in HBV-PAN. The presence of HBV surface antigen should be sought, although the impact of HBV vaccination now has reduced the incidence to 7% to 10% or less (57,58). CSF findings are usually normal, although IL-6 may be elevated in patients with CNS involvement (73).

Saccular or fusiform aneurysms, ranging in size from 1 to 5 mm, are predominately seen in the mesenteric, renal, and hepatic arteries on visceral angiography. Although aneurysms are not pathognomonic of PAN, they are have been demonstrated in 60% to 90% of patients with PAN and are rarely seen in ANCA-associated vasculidities (66).

The gold standard for diagnosis of PAN is the demonstration of focal, segmental, pan-mural necrotizing inflammation of medium-sized arteries, with a predilection for branch points of muscular arteries (72). The predictive value of a biopsy is often proportionate to the degree of clinical involvement of that tissue (72). The most frequent tissues selected for biopsy are the skin, sural, superficial peroneal, or superficial radial nerve and muscle (less sensitive than nerve) (72). Renal biopsy is not advocated as the first choice because the risk of hemorrhage from rupturing aneurysms (72).

Electrodiagnostic studies in patients with PAN typical demonstrate an axonal polyneuropathy, with absent or markedly decreased muscle and sensory action potentials in the most affected nerves (74). The study may indicate the pattern of nerve involvement (asymmetric or symmetric, mononeuritis simplex or multiplex) and detect subclinical lesions. Patients suspected of having CNS involvement should have MRI to evaluate for ischemic or hemorrhagic lesion(s) and possibly cerebral arteriography to help document CNS vasculitis (66).

TREATMENT

Conventional treatment with steroids and immunosuppressive agents may control HBV-PAN, but their prolonged use can put the patient's favorable outcome at risk by allowing the causative virus to replicate and facilitate further progression to chronic hepatitis and cirrhosis (55,57,61,75–79). The current approach to HBV-PAN consists of initial use of steroids for rapid control of the most severe life-threatening manifestations of PAN (55,75). After 2 weeks, the steroids are rapidly tapered and discontinued. Subsequently, plasma exchanges and lamivudine, a nucleoside analog that potently inhibits HBV DNA replication, are simultaneously started. Plasma exchange is done to remove the immune complexes causing vessel inflammation and the antiviral agent is used to diminish viral replication (78). Plasma exchange is performed on a tapering schedule and maintained once a week until seroconversion to anti-HBe or after stable clinical recovery had been obtained and maintained for 2 to 3 months. Similarly, antiviral treatment should be maintained for 6 months or until clearance of HBV DNA and seroconversion is achieved. Keep in mind that long-term use of lamivudine (>6 months) can be followed by emergence of resistant mutant HBV strains; however, this may not be an issue in the present protocol in which lamivudine is used for only 6 months (78). Recent therapeutic trials on chronic HBV infection suggest that a combination of two major antiviral agents, lamivudine and IFN-α_2, might be more effective than either agents alone (80).

CLINICAL RECOMMENDATIONS OF THE VIGNETTE

The patient has a typical presentation of PAN that may be associated with a viral hepatitis. It is important to recognize that the severity of the liver disease in this entity is not related to the activity of PAN. Also it occurs generally in the recently infected. Diagnostic priorities would be to obtain HBV markers and serum ANCA because the absence of these antibodies helps to rule out other causes of vasculitis. Angiographic demonstration of the vasculitis may be of interest, although it should be carefully considered in view of the renal infarct. The management, given the severity of the manifestations, should include steroids coupled with antiviral treatment if HBV is confirmed. As always, the recognition of HIV coinfection is very important in this case.

Other Immune-mediated Neurologic Complications Associated with Viral Hepatitis

Infectious triggers are often implicated in the mechanisms of autoimmune diseases. The more well-known extrahepatic manifestations of the viral hepatitides, such as MC and PAN that have been discussed earlier in this chapter, are thought to be immune related. Other neurologic complications are associated with the viral hepatitides that have been less well described and which may also have an immunologic association.

Transverse myelitis (TM) is a sudden onset, demyelinating disorder involving the spinal cord. Symptoms include extremity weakness, numbness and tingling, bowel and bladder dysfunction, back pain, and radicular pain (in the distribution of a single spinal nerve). TM can be caused by viral infections, vascular insufficiency, systemic autoimmune disease (e.g., systemic lupus erythematosus [SLE]), paraneoplastic syndrome or occur in association with a demyelinating disorders (i.e., multiple sclerosis or neuromyelitis optica). Of cases, 20% to 40% of acute transverse myelitis are attributed to viral infections, including hepatitis A and hepatitis C. Grewal et al. (81) reported a case of biopsy proved recurrent myelitis that occurred in association with chronic HCV infection. Pathology of the spinal cord biopsy demonstrated demyelination without evidence of vasculitis. Antibodies to HCV were present in the CSF, although HCV RNA was not detected (81).

Encephalomyelitis has also been reported as a complication of chronic HCV infection in two case reports (82,83). One report described the patient as developing a progressive encephalomyelitis with rigidity. Postmortem examination demonstrated an inflammatory process consistent with findings of an encephalomyelitis. HCV RNA was also detected in the brain, but not the CSF (82). In a separate case report, another patient was described with acute disseminated encephalomyelitis (ADEM) that developed 50 days after acquiring HCV infection from a blood transfusion. MRI of the brain showed characteristic findings of ADEM, with multifocal areas of high-intensity signal involving gray and white matter with contrast enhancement (83). Similarly, a case was reported of a 9-year-old boy who developed ADEM 1 month following the diagnosis of hepatitis A virus infection. ADEM is an autoimmune demyelinating, usually monophasic disease that typically develops following an acute viral or bacterial infection or vaccination (84).

Guillain-Barré syndrome (GBS) or acute inflammatory demyelinating polyneuropathy (AIDP) is classically characterized by an acutely progressive symmetric ascending muscle weakness, paralysis, and hyporeflexia with or without sensory or autonomic symptoms. The typical patient with GBS presents 2 to 4 weeks after a relatively benign respiratory or gastrointestinal illness. Antecedent bacterial (e.g., *Campylobacter jejuni*) and viral (e.g., cytomegalovirus [CMV], Epstein Barr virus [EBV]) infections has been associated with GBS. Well-documented cases are seen of GBS that occurred during acute hepatitis A or B infection. GBS has been reported in several cases of chronic hepatitis C infection as well (85–88). Although the relationship of GBS to antiviral vaccination has been much publicized (89–97), the controversy is far from resolved.

The treatment in these viral hepatitis-associated neurologic complications is similar to what has been done in cases related to other etiologies. Immunosuppressant therapy is the standard treatment in the form of high-dose steroids and plasmapheresis for cases of transverse myelitis or ADEM and, in the case of GBS, intravenous immunoglobulins or plasmapheresis.

Interferon Treatment-associated Complications

Interferon therapy has been associated with neuropsychiatric side effects, most commonly depression and impaired cognitive function (98). Less frequently, patients may exhibit a manic condition characterized by mood instability, irritability, agitation, and occasional euphoria (99). An acute confusional state that develops rapidly after administration of high-dose IFN by either intracerebroventricular or intravenous has been reported. This, however, has infrequently occurred in patients receiving IFN therapy for HCV (99).

Neuropsychiatric symptoms are widely reported in association with hepatitis C and IFN treatment. Of the studies that have evaluated whether INF-α induces depression, most suggest that INF therapy is associated with the development of both depressive symptoms and major depression as defined by the fourth edition of the *Diagnostic and Statistical Manual of Mental Disorders* (DSM-VI) criteria (98,100). A depressive syndrome associated with IFN typically develops slowly over weeks to months of treatment. The actual prevalence rate for mood disturbances related to IFN treatment is not clear, although it is reported to vary between 16% and 58%. Variable prevalence rates have been owing to differences in methodologic considerations (e.g., prospective vs. retrospective design, use of depression-specific screening assessments vs. general adverse screening questionnaire) and definition of depression either as a single symptom or as a syndrome of related symptoms (that included fatigue and neurovegetative symptoms, such as sleep and appetite disturbance), which may or may not fully meet DSM-IV criteria for major depression (98–100). Earlier studies tended to define depression as a single symptom based on patient self-report during screening for adverse effects and subsequently found lower rates of depression than later studies that evaluated depression as a syndrome of related symptoms. Risk factors to developing IFN-induced depression appear to be related to dosage and duration of treatment, as well as to the patient's premorbid physical and psychiatric condition (98–100). The presence of clinical or subclinical depression or anxiety is predictive of developing psychiatric disturbances during IFN treatment. It is not clear if a history of psychiatric disturbance confers the same risk (101). Similarly, a history of alcohol or substance abuse does not seem to increase the risk of depression, provided that the patient remains abstinent during treatment. Preliminary reports suggest ribavirin, which is typically used in combination with IFN for HCV, may synergistically increase the likelihood of IFN-α inducing depression; however, a prospective study is needed to confirm this result. Management of IFN-induced depression can be approached in two ways: (*a*) preventive treatment in which patients who are at high risk for developing depression during IFN-α therapy are pretreated with antidepressants; and (*b*) treating patients once they become symptomatic. The available literature on patients with HCV provides support for both preventive and symptomatic treatment of IFN-induced depression (99,101–104). Currently, selective serotonin reuptake inhibitors (SSRI), particularly paroxetine, have been studied most frequently, although it does not necessarily mean it is superior to other antidepressants, especially newer ones (101,103,105). Drug–drug interactions may need to be considered in relation to antidepressants effects on the cytochrome P450 (CYP) enzyme system. In regards antidepressant dosing, patients with severe liver disease may require lower dosages of antidepressants secondary to decreased metabolism; however, patients with HCV without cirrhosis or liver failure can still receive standard doses of antidepressants during treatment with IFN-α or ribavirin. Patients receiving INF-α may benefit from antidepressants that combine serotonin and catecholamine activity, which have been shown to be more effective than SSRI in reducing chronic pain and treating fatigue—frequent symptoms that can occur in isolation from more depression-specific complaints in patients receiving INF-α therapy.

Although previously considered rare, IFN-α is capable of inducing mania, according to many reports in the literature. A European study found that 20% of patients receiving pegylated IFN-α and ribavirin for HCV developed manic or hypomanic symptoms at some point during the 24 weeks of treatment (98). Similar to the prevalence rate of IFN-induced depression, it is difficult to determine the true prevalence of IFN-induced mania, which is dependent on the criteria by which mania is defined. Many patients with mania demonstrate extreme irritability rather than euphoria. In patients treated with IFN, it is not known what percentage of those with irritability are experiencing dysphoric mania versus a depressive or fatigue-related condition.

Although original descriptions of seizures during IFN-treatment were in association with high doses of IFN-α, seizures have also been reported to occur with lower doses of IFN used in therapy for chronic viral hepatitis (106). The mechanism by which IFN-α induces seizures is uncertain, although it could be as a result of increasing excitability of neural cells or causing small vessel damage, hemorrhage, or infarction of the brain. This complication is likely related to dose and duration of IFN therapy and has been reported to occur in approximately 1% of patients (106).

As discussed, essential mixed-cryoglobulinemia is the major cause of peripheral neuropathy in patients with chronic HCV and less commonly HBV. Noncryoglobulinemic vasculitic peripheral neuropathies occur less frequently. Complications of vasculitis tend to improve on viral clearance. Therefore, antiviral therapy, such as IFN-α, is the treatment of choice. During IFN therapy for chronic HCV infection, however, both new onset and exacerbation of cryoglobulinemic and noncryoglobulinemic vasculitic neuropathies have been described (35,36). In some cases, the neuropathy occurred despite virologic response to IFN (35,36). The pathogenic mechanism of IFN-induced vasculitic neuropathy is not well known. Nonvasculitic neuropathy induced by IFN from direct neuropathic effects of IFN can also occur. Because clinically IFN-induced vasculitic and nonvasculitic neuropathy during treatment of chronic HCV typically do not differ, a nerve biopsy may be needed to differentiate the two.

Anecdotal cases describe a relationship between chronic demyelinating inflammatory demyelinating polyneuropathy (CIDP) and HCV. The underlying relationship may be an immune-mediated process triggered by HCV rather than direct toxicity of the virus itself. IFN has been used successfully as an alternative treatment for CIDP associated with, or without HCV, (107). Conversely, CIDP has also been reported as a neurologic complication of IFN in treatment of a patient with HCV (108).

Interferon therapy has been associated with extrapyramidal side effects such as akathisia, parkinsonism, chorea, tremor, and acute dystonia (109–111). The mechanism of IFN-induced extrapyramidal side effects is still unclear, although may be related to the antidopaminergic effects of IFN (112).

SUMMARY

Current management of chronic viral hepatitis has evolved over recent years to a more effective regimen of medications that have improved the benefit to patients significantly over the last 20 years. With better antiviral treatment have come opportunities to treat extrahepatic complications of viral hepatitis that may have neurologic involvement.

Hepatitis C is not infrequently responsible for mixed cryoglubulinemia. Clues to the presence of this entity are found in complaints of peripheral neuropathy, typical purpuric rash, and in more severe cases, renal insufficiency or failure. The clinician should confirm the diagnosis of HCV, measure cryoglobulins, and confirm the diagnosis using skin, renal, or nerve biopsies, as needed. Treatment should focus on an effort to suppress the virus with pegylated (PEG)-IFN-α and ribavirin, and if needed, the use of rituximab infusions or plasmapheresis. Cytotoxic agents should be used in this setting only as a last resort to save the kidney or address severe, confirmed CNS vasculitis.

Hepatitis B has recently become more rare in Western countries and select Eastern countries because of effective vaccination and preventive measures. When patients present with acute infections and evidence of systemic large vessel vasculitis, the entity of HBV-PAN should be considered and ruled out. This ANCA-negative PAN variant is felt to be directly caused by HBV and responds to efforts to decrease the viral replication. Its presentation can involve skin, kidney, gastrointestinal tract, CNS, and reproductive system. Management should include angiography, when appropriate, confirmation of HBV infection, and initiation of strong anti-HBV agents in effort to control the infection. Short courses of steroids should be considered to slow vasculitic effects.

Because of the toxic profile of PEG-IFN, all clinicians treating viral hepatitidies should have a strategy to address the neuronpsychiatric effects of these antiviral medications. Furthermore, recognition of the risk for coinfection with HIV is important in the management of this patient population, and may have an impact on the findings of neurologic symptoms.

REFERENCES

1. Lok AS, McMahon BJ. Chronic hepatitis B. *Hepatology.* 2001;34(6):1225–1241.
2. Lok AS, McMahon BJ. Chronic hepatitis B: Update of recommendations. *Hepatology.* 2004;39(3):857–861.
3. Viral Hepatitis and HIV/AIDS Integration: A Resource Guide for HIV/AIDS Programs NASTAD: National Alliance of State and Territorial AIDS Directors, 2004. Available at http://www.cdc.gov. Accessed November 19, 2006.
4. Penin F. Structural biology of hepatitis C virus. *Clin Liver Dis.* 2003;7(1):1–21, vii.
5. Choo QL, Kuo G, Weiner AJ, et al. Isolation of a cDNA clone derived from a blood-borne non-A, non-B viral hepatitis genome. *Science.* 1989;244(4902):359–362.
6. Strader DB, Wright T, Thomas DL, et al. Diagnosis, management, and treatment of hepatitis C. *Hepatology.* 2004;39(4):1147–1171.
7. Liang TJ, Rehermann B, Seeff LB, et al. Pathogenesis, natural history, treatment, and prevention of hepatitis C. *Ann Intern Med.* 2000;132(4):296–305.
8. Seeff LB. Natural history of chronic hepatitis C. *Hepatology.* 2002;36(5 Suppl 1):S35–S46.
9. Laskus T, Radkowski M, Wang LF, et al. Search for hepatitis C virus extrahepatic replication sites in patients with acquired immunodeficiency syndrome: Specific detection of negative-strand viral RNA in various tissues. *Hepatology.* 1998;28(5):1398–1401.
10. Vargas HE, Laskus T, Radkowski M, et al. Detection of hepatitis C virus sequences in brain tissue obtained in recurrent hepatitis C after liver transplantation. *Liver Transpl.* 2002; 8(11):1014–1019.
11. Soriano V, Puoti M, Sulkowski M, et al. Care of patients with hepatitis C and HIV co-infection. *Aids.* 2004;18(1):1–12.
12. Sulkowski MS, Thomas DL. Hepatitis C in the HIV-infected patient. *Clin Liver Dis.* 2003;7(1):179–194.
13. Stone JH. The classification and epidemiology of systemic vasculitis. In: Harris ED, Budd R, Genovese MC, et al., eds. *Kelley's Textbook of Rheumatology,* 7th ed. Philadelphia: WB Saunders; 2005.
14. Ferri C, Sebastiani M, Giuggioli D, et al. Mixed cryoglobulinemia: Demographic, clinical, and serologic features and survival in 231 patients. *Semin Arthritis Rheum.* 2004;33(6): 355–374.
15. Bryce AH, Kyle RA, Dispenzieri A, et al. Natural history and therapy of 66 patients with mixed cryoglobulinemia. *Am J Hematol.* 2006;81(7):511–518.
16. Galli M, Invernizzi F. Hepatitis B virus and cryoglobulinemia. *Ann Intern Med.* 1981;95(4):522.
17. Levo Y. Hepatitis B virus and essential mixed cryoglobulinemia. *Ann Intern Med.* 1981;94(2):282.
18. Ferri C, Greco F, Longombardo G, et al. Hepatitis C virus antibodies in mixed cryoglobulinemia. *Clin Exp Rheumatol.* 1991;9(1):95–96.
19. Pascual M, Perrin L, Giostra E, et al. Hepatitis C virus in patients with cryoglobulinemia type II. *J Infect Dis.* 1990;162(2):569–570.
20. Kayali Z, Labrecque DR, Schmidt WN. Treatment of hepatitis C cryoglobulinemia: Mission and challenges. *Current Treatment Options in Gastroenterology.* 2006;9(6):497–507.
21. Sene D, Ghillani-Dalbin P, Thibault V, et al. Longterm course of mixed cryoglobulinemia in patients infected with hepatitis C virus. *J Rheumatol..* 2004;31(11):2199–2206.
22. Gemignani F, Brindani F, Alfieri S, et al. Clinical spectrum of cryoglobulinaemic neuropathy. *J Neurol Neurosurg Psychiatry.* 2005;76(10):1410–1414.
23. Ammendola A, Sampaolo S, Ambrosone L, et al. Peripheral neuropathy in hepatitis-related mixed cryoglobulinemia: Electrophysiologic follow-up study. *Muscle Nerve.* 2005;31(3):382–385.
24. Cappellari A, Origgi L, Spina MF, et al. Central nervous system involvement in HCV-related mixed cryoglobulinemia. *Electromyogr Clin Neurophysiol.* 2006;46(3):149–158.
25. Petty GW, Duffy J, Houston J, 3rd. Cerebral ischemia in patients with hepatitis C virus infection and mixed cryoglobulinemia. *Mayo Clin Proc.* 1996;71(7):671–678.
26. Heckmann JG, Kayser C, Heuss D, et al. Neurological manifestations of chronic hepatitis C. *J Neurol.* 1999;246(6):486–491.
27. Agnello V. The etiology and pathophysiology of mixed cryoglobulinemia secondary to hepatitis C virus infection. *Springer Semin Immunopathol.* 1997;19(1):111–129.
28. Zaja F, De Vita S, Mazzaro C, et al. Efficacy and safety of rituximab in type II mixed cryoglobulinemia. *Blood.* 2003;101(10):3827–3834.
29. Sansonno D, De Re V, Lauletta G, et al. Monoclonal antibody treatment of mixed cryoglobulinemia resistant to interferon alpha with an anti-CD20. *Blood.* 2003;101(10):3818–3826.

30. Ferri C, Zignego AL, Longombardo G, et al. Effect of alpha-interferon on hepatitis C virus chronic infection in mixed cryoglobulinemia patients. *Infection.* 1993;21(2): 93–97.
31. David WS, Peine C, Schlesinger P, et al. Nonsystemic vasculitic mononeuropathy multiplex, cryoglobulinemia, and hepatitis C. *Muscle Nerve.* 1996;19(12):1596–1602.
32. Gemignani F, Marbini A, Di Giovanni G, et al. Cryoglobulinaemic neuropathy manifesting with restless legs syndrome. *J Neurol Sci.* 1997;152(2):218–223.
33. Tavoni A, Mosca M, Ferri C, et al. Guidelines for the management of essential mixed cryoglobulinemia. *Clin Exp Rheumatol.* 1995;[13 Suppl 13]:S191–S195.
34. Marcellin P, Descamps V, Martinot-Peignoux M, et al. Cryoglobulinemia with vasculitis associated with hepatitis C virus infection. *Gastroenterology.* 1993;104(1):272–277.
35. Beuthien W, Mellinghoff HU, Kempis J. Vasculitic complications of interferon-alpha treatment for chronic hepatitis C virus infection: Case report and review of the literature. *Clin Rheumatol.* 2005;24(5):507–515.
36. La Civita L, Zignego AL, Lombardini F, et al. Exacerbation of peripheral neuropathy during alpha-interferon therapy in a patient with mixed cryoglobulinemia and hepatitis B virus infection. *J Rheumatol.* 1996;23(9):1641–1643.
37. Cacoub P, Saadoun D, Limal N, et al. PEGylated interferon alfa-2b and ribavirin treatment in patients with hepatitis C virus-related systemic vasculitis. *Arthritis Rheum.* 2005;52(3):911–915.
38. Cai FZ, Ahern M, Smith M. Treatment of cryoglobulinemia associated peripheral neuropathy with rituximab. *J Rheumatol.* 2006;33(6):1197–1198.
39. Lamprecht P, Lerin-Lozano C, Merz H, et al. Rituximab induces remission in refractory HCV associated cryoglobulinaemic vasculitis. *Ann Rheum Dis.* 2003;62(12):1230–1233.
40. Stefanutti C, Di Giacomo S, Mareri M, et al. Immunoadsorption apheresis (Selesorb) in the treatment of chronic hepatitis C virus-related type 2 mixed cryoglobulinemia. *Transfus Apher Sci.* 2003;28(3):207–214.
41. Filippini D, Colombo F, Jann S, et al. Central nervous system involvement in patients with HCV-related cryoglobulinemia: Literature review and a case report [in Spanish]. *Reumatismo* 2002;54(2):150–155.
42. Cojocaru IM, Cojocaru M, Iacob SA, et al. Cerebral ischemic attack secondary to hepatitis C virus infection. *Rom J Intern Med.* 2005;43(3–4):255–260.
43. Younes S, Chebel S, Boukhris S, et al. Central nervous system involvement in patients with hepatitis C infection [in French]. *Rev Neurol (Paris).* 2002;158(12 Pt 1):1202–1204.
44. Ince PG, Duffey P, Cochrane HR, et al. Relapsing ischemic encephaloenteropathy and cryoglobulinemia. *Neurology.* 2000;55(10):1579–1581.
45. Fragoso M, Carneado J, Tuduri I, et al. Essential mixed cryoglobulinemia as a cause of ischemic cerebrovascular accident [in Spanish]. *Rev Neurol.* 2000;30(5):444–446.
46. Cacoub P, Sbai A, Hausfater P, et al. Central nervous system involvement in hepatitis C virus infection [in]. *Gastroenterol Clin Biol.* 1998;22(6–7):631–633.
47. Origgi L, Vanoli M, Carbone A, et al. Central nervous system involvement in patients with HCV-related cryoglobulinemia. *Am J Med Sci.* 1998;315(3):208–210.
48. Serena M, Biscaro R, Moretto G, et al. Peripheral and central nervous system involvement in essential mixed cryoglobulinemia: A case report. *Clin Neuropathol.* 1991;10(4):177–180.
49. McMahon BJ, Heyward WL, Templin DW, et al. Hepatitis B-associated polyarteritis nodosa in Alaskan Eskimos: Clinical and epidemiologic features and long-term follow-up. *Hepatology.* 1989;9(1):97–101.
50. Begier EM, Langford CA, Sneller MC, et al. Polyarteritis nodosa reports to the vaccine adverse event reporting system (VAERS): Implications for assessment of suspected vaccine-provoked vasculitis. *J Rheumatol.* 2004;31(11):2181–2188.
51. Bourgeais AM, Dore MX, Croue A, et al. Cutaneous polyarteritis nodosa following hepatitis B vaccination [in French]. *Ann Dermatol Venereol.* 2003;130(2 Pt 1):205–207.
52. Saadoun D, Cacoub P, Mahoux D, et al. Postvaccine vasculitis: A report of three cases [in French]. *Rev Med Interne.* 2001;22(2):172–176.
53. De Keyser F, Naeyaert JM, Hindryckx P, et al. Immune-mediated pathology following hepatitis B vaccination. Two cases of polyarteritis nodosa and one case of pityriasis rosea-like drug eruption. *Clin Exp Rheumatol.* 2000;18(1):81–85.
54. Canada R, Chaudry S, Gaber L, et al. Polyarteritis nodosa and cryoglobulinemic glomerulonephritis related to chronic hepatitis C. *Am J Med Sci.* 2006;331(6):329–333.
55. Guillevin L, Mahr A, Callard P, et al. Hepatitis B virus-associated polyarteritis nodosa: Clinical characteristics, outcome, and impact of treatment in 115 patients. *Medicine (Baltimore).* 2005;84(5):313–322.
56. Han SH. Extrahepatic manifestations of chronic hepatitis B. *Clin Liver Dis.* 2004;8(2): 403–418.
57. Guillevin L, Lhote F, Cohen P, et al. Polyarteritis nodosa related to hepatitis B virus. A prospective study with long-term observation of 41 patients. *Medicine (Baltimore).* 1995;74(5): 238–253.
58. Guilpain P, Servettaz A, Tamby MC, et al. Pathogenie des vascularites systemiques primitives (II): Vascularites ANCA-negatives. *Presse Med.* 2005;34(14):1023–1033.
59. Trepo C, Guillevin L. Polyarteritis nodosa and extrahepatic manifestations of HBV infection: The case against autoimmune intervention in pathogenesis. *J Autoimmun.* 2001; 16(3):269–274.
60. Michalak T. Immune complexes of hepatitis B surface antigen in the pathogenesis of periarteritis nodosa. A study of seven necropsy cases. *Am J Pathol.* 1978;90(3):619–632.
61. Guillevin L, Lhote F, Jarrousse B, et al. Polyarteritis nodosa related to hepatitis B virus. A retrospective study of 66 patients. *Ann Med Interne (Paris).* 1992;143[Suppl 1]:63–74.
62. Bourgarit A, Le Toumelin P, Pagnoux C, et al. Deaths occurring during the first year after treatment onset for polyarteritis nodosa, microscopic polyangiitis, and Churg-Strauss syndrome: A retrospective analysis of causes and factors predictive of mortality based on 595 patients. *Medicine (Baltimore).* 2005;84(5):323–330.
63. Paula De Carvalho Panzeri Carlotti A, Paes Leme Ferriani V, Tanuri Caldas C, et al. Polyarteritis nodosa with central nervous system involvement mimicking meningoencephalitis. *Pediatr Crit Care Med.* 2004;5(3):286–288.
64. Oran I, Memis A, Parildar M, et al. Multiple intracranial aneurysms in polyarteritis nodosa: MRI and angiography. *Neuroradiology.* 1999;41(6):436–439.
65. Semmo AN, Baumert TF, Kreisel W. Severe cerebral vasculitis as primary manifestation of hepatitis B-associated polyarteritis nodosa. *J Hepatol.* 2002;37(3):414–416.
66. Hurst RW, Grossman RI. Neuroradiology of central nervous system vasculitis. *Semin Neurol.* 1994;14(4):320–340.
67. Moore PM. Neurological manifestation of vasculitis: Update on immunopathogenic mechanisms and clinical features. *Ann Neurol.* 1995;[37 Suppl 1]:S131–S141.
68. Morfin-Maciel B, Medina A, Espinosa Rosales F, et al. Central nervous system involvement in a child with polyarteritis nodosa and severe atopic dermatitis. *Rev Alerg Mex.* 2002; 49(6):189–195.
69. Rumboldt Z, Beros V, Klanfar Z. Multiple cerebral aneurysms and a dural arteriovenous fistula in a patient with polyarteritis nodosa. Case illustration. *J Neurosurg.* 2003;98(2): 434.
70. Younger DS. Vasculitis of the nervous system. *Curr Opin Neurol.* 2004;17(3):317–336.
71. Lightfoot RW, Jr., Michel BA, Bloch DA, et al. The American College of Rheumatology 1990 criteria for the classification of polyarteritis nodosa. *Arthritis Rheum.* 1990;33(8): 1088–1093.
72. Hawke SH, Davies L, Pamphlett R, et al. Vasculitic neuropathy. A clinical and pathological study. *Brain.* 1991;114(Pt 5):2175–2190.
73. Hirohata S, Tanimoto K, Ito K. Elevation of cerebrospinal fluid interleukin-6 activity in patients with vasculitides and central nervous system involvement. *Clin Immunol Immunopathol.* 1993;66(3):225–229.
74. Bouche P, Leger JM, Travers MA, et al. Peripheral neuropathy in systemic vasculitis: Clinical and electrophysiologic study of 22 patients. *Neurology.* 1986;36(12):1598–1602.
75. Gorson KC. Therapy for vasculitic neuropathies. *Curr Treat Options Neurol.* 2006;8(2): 105–117.
76. Lau CF, Hui PK, Chan WM, et al. Hepatitis B associated fulminant polyarteritis nodosa: Successful treatment with pulse cyclophosphamide, prednisolone and lamivudine following emergency surgery. *Eur J Gastroenterol Hepatol.* 2002;14(5):563–566.
77. Guillevin L, Lhote F. Distinguishing polyarteritis nodosa from microscopic polyangiitis and implications for treatment. *Curr Opin Rheumatol.* 1995;7(1):20–24.
78. Guillevin L, Cohen P. Management of virus-induced systemic vasculitides. *Curr Rheumatol Rep.* 2002;4(1):60–66.
79. Cohen RD, Conn DL, Ilstrup DM. Clinical features, prognosis, and response to treatment in polyarteritis. *Mayo Clin Proc.* 1980;55(3):146–155.
80. Wicki J, Olivieri J, Pizzolato G, et al. Successful treatment of polyarteritis nodosa related to hepatitis B virus with a combination of lamivudine and interferon alpha. *Rheumatology (Oxford).* 1999;38(2):183–185.
81. Grewal AK, Lopes MB, Berg CL, et al. Recurrent demyelinating myelitis associated with hepatitis C viral infection. *J Neurol Sci.* 2004;224(1–2):101–106.
82. Bolay H, Soylemezoglu F, Nurlu G, et al. PCR detected hepatitis C virus genome in the brain of a case with progressive encephalomyelitis with rigidity. *Clin Neurol Neurosurg.* 1996;98(4):305–308.
83. Sacconi S, Salviati L, Merelli E. Acute disseminated encephalomyelitis associated with hepatitis C virus infection. *Arch Neurol.* 2001;58(10):1679–1681.
84. Tan H, Kilicaslan B, Onbas O, et al. Acute disseminated encephalomyelitis following hepatitis A virus infection. *Pediatr Neurol.* 2004;30(3):207–209.
85. Lacaille F, Zylberberg H, Hagege H, et al. Hepatitis C associated with Guillain-Barre syndrome. *Liver.* 1998;18(1):49–51.
86. Han HF, Wu JC, Huo TI, et al. Chronic hepatitis B exacerbated by Guillain-Barre syndrome: A report of two cases. *Zhonghua Yi Xue Za Zhi (Taipei).* 1999;62(9):652–656.
87. Gordon SC. Extrahepatic manifestations of hepatitis C. *Dig Dis.* 1996;14(3):157–168.
88. Ono S, Chida K, Takasu T. Guillain-Barre syndrome following fulminant viral hepatitis A. *Intern Med.* 1994;33(12):799–801.
89. Schattner A. Consequence or coincidence? The occurrence, pathogenesis and significance of autoimmune manifestations after viral vaccines. *Vaccine.* 2005;23(30): 3876–3886.
90. Khamaisi M, Shoenfeld Y, Orbach H. Guillain-Barre syndrome following hepatitis B vaccination. *Clin Exp Rheumatol.* 2004;22(6):767–770.
91. Rubinstein E. Vaccination and autoimmune diseases: The argument against. *Isr Med Assoc J.* 2004;6(7):433–435.
92. Vial T, Descotes J. Autoimmune diseases and vaccinations. *Eur J Dermatol.* 2004;14(2):86–90.
93. Blumenthal D, Prais D, Bron-Harlev E, et al. Possible association of Guillain-Barre syndrome and hepatitis A vaccination. *Pediatr Infect Dis J.* 2004;23(6):586–588.
94. Boz C, Ozmenoglu M, Aktoz G, et al. Guillain-Barre syndrome during treatment with interferon alpha for hepatitis B. *J Clin Neurosci.* 2004;11(5):523–525.
95. Seti NK, Reddi R, Anand I, et al. Guillain Barre syndrome following vaccination with hepatitis B vaccine. *J Assoc Physicians India.* 2002;50:989.
96. Piyasirisilp S, Hemachudha T. Neurological adverse events associated with vaccination. *Curr Opin Neurol.* 2002;15(3):333–338.
97. Sinsawaiwong S, Thampanitchawong P. Guillain-Barre syndrome following recombinant hepatitis B vaccine and literature review. *J Med Assoc Thai.* 2000;83(9):1124–1126.
98. Constant A, Castera L, Dantzer R, et al. Mood alterations during interferon-alfa therapy in patients with chronic hepatitis C: Evidence for an overlap between manic/hypomanic and depressive symptoms. *J Clin Psychiatry.* 2005;66(8):1050–1057.
99. Dieperink E, Ho SB, Thuras P, et al. A prospective study of neuropsychiatric symptoms associated with interferon-alpha-2b and ribavirin therapy for patients with chronic hepatitis C. *Psychosomatics.* 2003;44(2):104–112.
100. Capuron L, Gumnick JF, Musselman DL, et al. Neurobehavioral effects of interferon-alpha in cancer patients: Phenomenology and paroxetine responsiveness of symptom dimensions. *Neuropsychopharmacology.* 2002;26(5):643–652.

101. Horikawa N, Yamazaki T, Izumi N, et al. Incidence and clinical course of major depression in patients with chronic hepatitis type C undergoing interferon-alpha therapy: A prospective study. *Gen Hosp Psychiatry.* 2003;25(1):34–38.
102. Hauser P, Khosla J, Aurora H, et al. A prospective study of the incidence and open-label treatment of interferon-induced major depressive disorder in patients with hepatitis C. *Mol Psychiatry.* 2002;7(9):942–947.
103. Musselman DL, Lawson DH, Gumnick JF, et al. Paroxetine for the prevention of depression induced by high-dose interferon alfa. *N Engl J Med.* 2001;344(13):961–966.
104. Raison CL, Demetrashvili M, Capuron L, et al. Neuropsychiatric adverse effects of interferon-alpha: Recognition and management. *CNS Drugs.* 2005;19(2):105–123.
105. Gleason OC, Yates WR, Philipsen MA, et al. Plasma levels of citalopram in depressed patients with hepatitis C. *Psychosomatics.* 2004;45(1):29–33.
106. Shakil AO, Di Bisceglie AM, Hoofnagle JH. Seizures during alpha interferon therapy. *J Hepatol.* 1996;24(1):48–51.
107. Corcia P, Barbereau D, Guennoc AM, et al. Improvement of a CIDP associated with hepatitis C virus infection using antiviral therapy. *Neurology.* 2004;63(1):179–180.
108. Meriggioli MN, Rowin J. Chronic inflammatory demyelinating polyneuropathy after treatment with interferon-alpha. *Muscle Nerve.* 2000;23(3):433–435.
109. Atasoy N, Ustundag Y, Konuk N, et al. Acute dystonia during pegylated interferon alpha therapy in a case with chronic hepatitis B infection. *Clin Neuropharmacol.* 2004;27(3):105–107.
110. Horikawa N, Yamazaki T, Sagawa M, et al. A case of akathisia during interferon-alpha therapy for chronic hepatitis type C. *Gen Hosp Psychiatry.* 1999;21(2):134–135.
111. Tan EK, Chan LL, Lo YL. "Myorhythmia" slow facial tremor from chronic interferon alpha-2a usage. *Neurology.* 2003;61(9):1302–1303.
112. Sunami M, Nishikawa T, Yorogi A, et al. Intravenous administration of levodopa ameliorated a refractory akathisia case induced by interferon-alpha. *Clin Neuropharmacol.* 2000;23(1):59–61.

CHAPTER **43**

Management of Acute Liver Failure: Emphasis on Neurologic Complications

David J. Kramer • Benjamin H. Eidelman

OBJECTIVES

- To define acute liver failure (ALF), also known as fulminant hepatic failure (FHF)
- To distinguish acute liver failure from acute decompensation of chronic liver disease (AoCLF)
- To describe derangement of neurologic function in acute liver failure with emphasis on cerebral edema
- To delineate diagnostic techniques and therapeutic interventions that address the neuropathophysiology characteristic of acute liver failure

CASE VIGNETTE

The patient was transferred to a liver transplant center because of confusion and disorientation that had developed and progressed over a 12-hour period without prodrome. Her medical history was unremarkable. On examination in the emergency room, she was conscious but unable to cooperate in mental status testing. No focal abnormalities were observed and she moved her extremities on request. Laboratory studies revealed the presence of hypoglycemia, azotemia, anemia, and hyperammonemia. Other laboratory abnormalities included hyperbilirubinemia and elevated aminotransferases. Further evaluation included a negative computed axial tomography (CAT) scan of the head and negative hepatitis serology. A review of previous laboratory studies revealed mild abnormalities of liver function tests and a positive antinuclear antibody (ANA) test finding.

The patient was admitted to the general medical service with a diagnosis of hepatic encephalopathy caused by autoimmune hepatitis-induced acute liver failure. Lactulose therapy was initiated. Further laboratory test finding, including other autoimmune serology, proved negative. A liver biopsy was obtained and while awaiting the histologic findings, corticosteroids were introduced. The patient's level of consciousness deteriorated and she was transferred to the intensive care unit approximately 12 hours after hospital admission in grade 3 to grade 4 hepatic coma (Table 43-1).

Critical care included intubation for airway protection and mechanical ventilation with escalating levels of positive end-expiratory pressure and fraction of inspired oxygen (FIO_2) to address hypoxemia. The chest x-ray study revealed pulmonary edema. Pulmonary artery catheterization revealed a hyperdynamic state with high cardiac output, low central venous pressure (CVP) and low pulmonary occlusion pressure. Peripheral vascular resistance was low. Adult respiratory distress syndrome (ARDS) was diagnosed. The patient became oliguric. Creatinine increased by 1.5 mg/dL daily, but the blood urea nitrogen (BUN) remained low.

The coagulopathy was managed with transfusion of fresh frozen plasma, cryoprecipitate, and platelets guided by thromboelastography to allow placement of a ventriculostomy. Cerebrospinal fluid (CSF) was drained continuously to keep the intracranial pressure (ICP) at 10 cm H_2O or less. The patient was actively cooled to 35°C. The ICP dropped on initial placement from 22 mm Hg to 10 mm Hg.

DEFINITION

Acute liver failure is manifest by coagulopathy and encephalopathy, which develop over a period of 8 weeks in the absence of preexisting liver disease (1). In children and young adults, coagulopathy may be the dominant abnormality and encephalopathy difficult to detect. ALF is uncommon. Approximately 2,000 cases are recognized in the United States annually (2). The most common cause is acetaminophen intoxication (46%) of which half result from intentional overdose (suicide attempt) and the remainder is inadvertent, a therapeutic misadventure (3). Causes unrelated to acetaminophen include autoimmune hepatitis (5%), viral hepatitis (10%), medications (12%), and undetermined causes (15%) (4). For most of the world's population, however, viral hepatitis, in particular hepatitis B, is the major cause of ALF. Acetaminophen intoxication is nonexistent in developing countries. The cause of ALF is undetermined in nearly half of pediatric patients (5).

TABLE 43-1. Coma Grades

0	None
I	Subtle cognitive deficits. Sleep/wake reversal. Difficulty with calculations, spatial relations. No asterixis.
II	Awake, interactive, but confused. Asterixis present
III	Somnolent. Arousable with verbal/tactile stimulation, but confused. Asterixis present
IV	Comatose. No response to painful stimuli.

ALF is a medical and often neurologic emergency that requires specialized care to optimize survival. Transfer to a liver transplant center experienced in the management of such patients should occur when coagulopathy is recognized (international normalized ratio [INR] = 1.5) and before encephalopathy advances beyond grade 1 (Table 43-1). Both a candidate and a noncandidate for liver transplantation will benefit from transfer. General agreement is that liver transplantation is indicated when the risk of death from ALF exceeds 90% (6) despite aggressive intensive care. The King's College Criteria (Table 43-2) enable risk stratification in patients with ALF in the United States (7), although a lower threshold for liver transplantation is typical.

Etiology, age, concomitant degree of extrahepatic organ dysfunction, academia, and coagulopathy may be combined to identify a patient at high risk. Liver injury caused by acetaminophen intoxication usually resolves with intensive care and liver transplantation is required in less than one third of these patients. Patients for whom the etiology is undetermined or who have drug-induced liver injury (DILI) have a much worse prognosis—<20% survival without liver transplantation. Patients at the extremes of age (<10 or >40 years of age) have a worse prognosis. Patients with acetaminophen intoxication who are acidemic after resuscitation have a very poor prognosis, similar to patients with nonacetaminophen intoxication with severe coagulopathy who have a high mortality unless they can receive a transplant (Table 43-2).

TABLE 43-2. King's College Criteria: Indication for Liver Transplant in Acute Liver Failure

1. Acetaminophen overdose
   a. pH <7.3 or lactate >3 mmol/lL(after resuscitation)
   b. OR the combination of
      i. INR >6.5
      ii. Creatinine ≥3.5 mg/dL
      iii. Grade III or IV hepatic encephalopathy
2. Nonacetaminophen
   a. INR >6.5
   b. OR any three of the following
      i. INR >3.2
      ii. Age <10 or >40
      iii. Etiology not hepatitis A or hepatitis B
      iv. Interval >7 days between onset of jaundice and encephalopathy
      v. Total bilirubin ≥17.5 mg/dL

INR, international normalized ratio.
(Modified from O'Grady JG, Alexander GJ, Hayllar KM, et al. Early indicators of prognosis in fulminant hepatic failure. *Gastroenterology*. 1989;97(2):439–445; Bernal WDN, Wyncoll D, Wendon J. Blood lactate as an early predictor of outcome in paracetamol induced acute liver failure: A cohort study. *Lancet*. 2002;359:558–563; and Bernuau J, Goudeau A, Poynard T, et al. Multivariate analysis of prognostic factors in fulminant hepatitis B. *Hepatology*. 1986;6(4):648–651, with permission.)

ETIOLOGY AND PATHOPHYSIOLOGY OF INTRACRANIAL HYPERTENSION

Cerebral edema has been recognized as a cause of death with cerebral herniation in acute liver failure (8). Cerebral edema results from the combination of cytotoxocity, which induces astrocyte swelling, and cerebral hyperemia (9,10). The accumulation of glutamine is a consequence of excess ammonia is cytotoxic. The consequence of excess glutamate may be stimulation of the *N*-methyl-d-aspartate (NMDA) receptor that results in excess neuronal nitric oxide (nNOS). Other compounds such as mercaptans and thiols may act synergistically to induce cell damage. Curiously, serial CT imaging of the brain demonstrates that cerebral edema develops hours or days after the onset of coma. Clinical signs of intracranial hypertension and brainstem dysfunction may develop before cerebral edema is evident (11).

Cerebral blood flow is directly related to cerebral metabolism. In ALF, however, cerebral blood flow is often luxuriant. Cerebral blood flow is high for the metabolic demands. The relation between blood flow and cerebral oxygen consumption is given by the equation:

$$CMRo_2 = CBF \times AJVdo_2 \times 0.01$$

where

$CMRo_2$ is the cerebral consumption of oxygen (Normal: 6 mL/min/100 g brain)
CBF is cerebral blood flow (Normal: 50 mL/min/100 g brain)
$AJVdo_2$ is the oxygen content difference between arterial and jugular venous blood (Normal: 6 mL/mL)

In chronic liver disease, a decreased cerebral metabolic rate is matched by a decreased cerebral blood flow and the arterial jugular venous oxygen content difference is normal. Early in ALF, however, cerebral blood flow is markedly elevated and associated with a very low arterial jugular venous oxygen content difference. In contrast to traumatic and postcardiac arrest brain injury, where luxuriant perfusion is also a reported and $CMRO_2$ correlates inversely with survival, in ALF there is no relation between $CMRO_2$ and outcome.

It remains unclear how (or even if) cerebral hyperperfusion results in cerebral edema. Nonetheless, patients with cerebral hyperemia are susceptible to develop cerebral edema (12). Intracranial hypertension that results from cerebral hyperemia or increased cerebral blood volume is exquisitely sensitive to manipulation of intravascular volume and carbon dioxide. Controversy exists whether a reduction in cerebral blood volume to control cerebral hyperemia prevents or mitigates the development of cerebral edema.

PATHOGENESIS

Mechanism of liver injury can be direct or indirect. Acetaminophen is metabolized by the liver to a hepatotoxic intermediary. Although a secondary pathway for metabolism of acetaminophen, it can be induced by cytochrome P450 induction by alcohol or medication. Depletion of glutathione as occurs in starvation, deprives the liver of the substrate needed for the primary (nontoxic) metabolism. These conspire to make modest overdoses of acetaminophen lethal.

Indirect toxicity reflects enhanced autoimmunity. This can be recognized in autoimmune hepatitis, which can have a fulminant presentation with positive assays for autoantibodies. It is also evident in reactivation of hepatitis B, such as occurs with chemotherapy, and the enhanced immune response that occurs rarely in primary infection.

Histopathology allows broad distinction between frank hepatitis with inflammatory cell infiltrates and bridging necrosis and bland (acellular) zone 3 necrosis, such as results from ischemic hepatitis or acetaminophen intoxication. Some patients with ALF present with massive infiltration of the liver by fat. The most well-known process is Reye syndrome in which hepatic failure is usually associated with children acutely infected with influenza A who are treated with aspirin. In adults, a similar process may reflect an adverse medication reaction. Patients may be particularly susceptible to ALF if they have prior liver damage, even if subclinical. This has been observed in patients with subclinical hepatitis C who develop ALF and primary infection with hepatitis A.

Traditional teaching counsels against obtaining a liver biopsy. This recommendation reflects a high risk of bleeding after a percutaneous liver biopsy. Furthermore, sampling error can result in a complete misunderstanding of the severity of the disease process. Indeed normal, regenerating liver can be adjacent to massively necrotic liver (13). A transjugular approach to liver biopsy is less risky and allows for the recognition of underlying chronic liver disease. This would lower any expectation of spontaneous recovery and strengthen the argument for urgent liver transplantation. It also allows for the identification of acute viral injury that might be amenable to antiviral therapy. For example, herpes simplex virus can cause ALF and may respond to treatment with acyclovir. Entecavir or lamivudine treatment of early hepatitis B may also be considered.

CLINICAL MANIFESTATIONS

The neurologic manifestations often develop before the clinical features of altered hepatic function become apparent. Routine laboratory studies may not reveal major abnormalities in the early phase of the development of acute hepatic failure. Thus, the presentation may suggest a primary nervous system disorder for which a neurologic consultation may be sought. Patients with ALF often present with confusion and altered mental status. Patients can progress to a state of deep coma over a few hours. Hypoglycemia and cerebral edema can contribute to the altered mental status. Seizures can develop and be overt or subclinical. The latter may manifest as altered mental status. ICP rises initially as a consequence of cerebral hyperemia and, subsequently, from cerebral edema. Tonsilar herniation will result in brain death if the rise in ICP cannot be controlled.

Patients may be profoundly coagulopathic and spontaneous cerebral hemorrhage can occur, contributing to an increase in ICP. Invasive monitoring of ICP can be associated with significant intracranial hemorrhage, which can be located subarachnoid or intraparenchymal. In the former, should the patient survive, obstructive hydrocephalus may develop later.

CARDIAC

Cardiovascular manifestations are common and warrant monitoring such patients in the intensive care unit. As liver failure progresses, the patient becomes vasodilated and hyperdynamic. Although blood pressure is initially in the low normal range, with continued loss of hepatocellular function the patient become hypotensive. Patients can develop significant atrial and ventricular arrhythmias. Intervention to restore perfusion pressure is crucial. This requires restoration of circulating blood volume and maintenance of arterial tone—often with vasopressor support.

PULMONARY

Pulmonary edema is frequently recognized in patients with ALF. Typically, neither heart failure nor volume overload is present. Capillary leak is a component of multiple organ system failure and diagnosed as adult respiratory distress syndrome (ARDS) when low filling pressures (pulmonary artery occlusion) are measured. It resolves with improvement in liver function—spontaneous and following liver transplantation. It often heralds the development of cerebral edema.

The presence of both lung injury (acute lung injury [ALI], ARDS) and cerebral edema leads to competing mandates with regard to management. Management of ARDS with low airway pressures and tidal volumes is indicated to minimize further lung and extrapulmonary organ injury. This approach often leads, however, to significant hypercapnia. Hypercapnia can worsen cerebral hyperemia and increase cerebral edema. Because renal failure is usually present in such patients, fluid management is particularly problematic.

Pulmonary infection may be obscured by the pulmonary edema. A low index of suspicion should be maintained. The authors favor frequent bronchoalveolar lavage. This facilitates identification of *Aspergillus* organisms and other opportunistic infections.

RENAL

Renal failure is common in ALF and may reflect direct injury to the kidney; for example, acetaminophen-induced nephrotoxicity, or may be a functional impairment that results from deteriorating liver function. In the latter cause, the urine sediment is inactive and the fractional excretion of sodium is low and remains so despite restoration of renal perfusion. In the former, tubular damage can present with impaired concentrating ability (decreased to specific gravity), elevated fractional excretion of sodium, and an active sediment.

Azotemia, which usually attends renal failure caused by inadequate perfusion and primary renal failure is often absent in the setting of severe liver failure. Instead of an increased BUN, patients present with accelerating creatinine rises and oliguria. As a consequence, renal function is often overestimated. As with other causes of acute renal failure, a role for diuretics is solely to address fluid excess and it fails to protect the kidney, *per se*. Although low-dose dopamine can act as a diuretic, it should be avoided in this setting because it will certainly contribute to increased mesenteric flow in portal pressure and increase the risk of gastrointestinal hemorrhage.

INFECTIOUS DISEASE

Infection is problematic for patients with liver failure in which impaired opsonization has been recognized for more than 20 years. Hepatic dysfunction results in systemic circulation of bacteria, endotoxin, and cytokines. Infection is a significant and sometimes overwhelming stress for the liver. As liver function deteriorates, encephalopathy advances from early to late grades and extrahepatic organ function deteriorates.

Surveillance cultures and a high-level of suspicion are indicated. Bacterial infections are ubiquitous and nearly 40% of patients acquire fungal infections. The authors advocate early antibacterial and antifungal prophylaxis targeted at community-acquired staphylococci, streptococci, and common Gram-negative rods such as *Escherichia coli* and *Klebsiella* spp. Typically, the combination of ampicillin or sulbactam and fluconazole suffice for patients admitted from the community with broader spectrum antimicrobial coverage for those already hospitalized. Following liver transplantation, filamentous fungi, such as *Aspergillus*, are a major concern, particularly in patients with renal failure. Fluconazole is discontinued after surgery and AmBisome or voriconazole are initiated.

GASTROINTESTINAL

Gastrointestinal bleeding can result from stress ulceration, intrinsic peptic ulcer disease, and portal hypertension. Classic teaching, however, mandates that patients with varices be considered chronic. Consequently, portal hypertensive gastropathy may be identified as the source of bleeding. The use of H2 blockers results in significantly less bleeding. Currently, the authors used proton pump inhibitors to achieve the same objective. Bleeding from the lower gastrointestinal tract is unusual before transplant during which time it might be ascribed to diverticuli and superimposed coagulopathy. Bleeding following liver transplant can result from colitis, for example, caused by cytomegalovirus (CMV) or *Clostridium difficile*.

Pancreatitis has been recognized as a comorbid feature of ALF for more than 30 years. It is more typical of viral hepatitis, particularly hepatitis B, but can be seen with acetaminophen intoxication. It is possible that systemic hypotension and portal hypertension combined to compromised blood flow to the pancreas and one may speculate that the injury is ischemic. Pancreatitis presents a grave threat to successful liver transplantation. When severe, it can progress to pancreatic necrosis with spillage of enzymes into the retroperitoneum resulting in a phlegmon or abscess and destruction of adjacent tissues such as bowel. Death can result from pancreatitis.

Patients with ALF are typically nutritionally replete. A traditional approach is to withhold protein to minimize encephalopathy. Indeed, ileus often results from the portal hypertension or pancreatitis and patients may have delayed gastric emptying. They may be intolerant of enteral nutrition. Furthermore, it is difficult for them to tolerate lactulose should encephalopathy worsen. More recently, the marked catabolic nature of formalin to hepatic failure has been recognized. As delay often results from the unavailability of a transplant, marked muscle wasting is observed. Probably, operative success is compromised by nutritional insufficiency, however, this is not quantified. Consequently, some physicians attempt a low protein diet or nutrition supplement and monitor the serum ammonia level.

HEMATOLOGY

Patients with ALF are usually not anemic on presentation. They are often unable, however, to compensate for blood loss from laboratory testing or from the intestine and become anemic. Similarly, patients are not usually thrombocytopenic on presentation. Progressive thrombocytopenia, however, is routinely observed. This can compromise efforts at extracorporeal circulation to manage renal failure if such were attempted to treat hepatic failure. It may also compromise the choice of immunosuppressants postoperatively.

The optimal hemoglobin level in critically ill patients is controversial; in the absence of coronary artery disease, however, it appears to be <10 g/dL and approximately 7 to 8 g/dL (14,15). Although no evidence suggests that patients with liver failure should be maintained at a higher hematocrit, anemia can exacerbate cerebral hyperperfusion. Consequently, recommended target is a hemoglobin of 10 g/dL in patients with intracranial hypertension and documented cerebral hyperemia.

RECURRENCE OF DISEASE

There is concern that patients who have liver transplantation are at risk for recurrence of the primary disease. For viral hepatitis, this appears to be uncommon. Most patients with fulminant hepatitis B seroconvert and are no longer considered to have active disease.

From a neuropsychiatric perspective, patients with intentional acetaminophen intoxication might be considered at risk for recurrence of depression. It is striking that in the authors' review of their clinical experience this has not occurred, which reflects a significant pretransplant selection effect. Patients with intractable depression, with multiple serious suicide attempts, are not considered appropriate for transplantation. With that caveat, acetaminophen intoxication with suicidal intent is not a contraindication to liver transplantation if appropriate psychiatric care can be provided in the postoperative period.

DIAGNOSTIC APPROACH

Patients with ALF can present with jaundice, nausea, loss of appetite, and abdominal pain. They can also present, however, with confusion, seizures, or dyspnea. Intoxication, liver failure, or both should be considered in the presenting differential diagnosis for such patients. Hepatology and neurology input may be delayed. Emergency management of altered mental status will include establishing venous access, assaying urine and blood for toxins (including acetaminophen), and empiric treatment with dextrose, thiamine, naloxone, and flumazenil. Hypoglycemia may not be recognized until the initial laboratory data are analyzed. Stigmata of chronic liver disease are not present on examination. Nausea and right upper quadrant abdominal pain with a tender swollen liver are typical, however, of ALF. Discomfort can extend to the epigastrum and the back when pancreatitis is precipitated by ALF. Splenomegaly, caput medusa, palmar erythema, and spider angiomata all indicate chronicity.

Distinguishing ALF from acute deterioration of chronic liver disease (AoCLD) is crucial because of the high immediate mortality and risk of intracranial hypertension, cerebral edema, and herniation in the former. Wilson disease (hepatolenticular degeneration) is a hereditary (autosomal recessive) disorder of copper metabolism (specifically, cellular copper export). Liver function abnormalities are common, but only half of patients present with the classic low ceruloplasmin and Kayser-Fleischer rings. Occasionally, changes in liver function are subclinical. Subtle neuropsychiatric changes can develop. The patient with Wilson disease, however, may present dramatically between 10 and 40 years of age with ALF. Although fibrosis and cirrhosis may be well established, the cerebral hemodynamics are more compatible with acute liver failure. Prolonged survival after fulminant presentation requires liver transplantation.

Controversy attends whether patients with evidence for preexisting liver abnormalities without clinical disease, most commonly viral hepatitis, who develop ALF should be considered the same as other patients with ALF (16). Because cerebral edema, intracranial hypertension, and herniation can develop in these patients and is rare, although reported in cirrhosis (17), inclusion is appropriate for clinical purposes.

Acute alcoholic hepatitis can mimic ALF. Indeed, acute alcohol intoxication can result in hepatic necrosis. Perhaps the distinction is most important from the perspective of eligibility for liver transplantation, because the clinical course can be similar otherwise.

Once the diagnosis of ALF is made, treatable causes should be excluded or treatment initiated while in the process. To that end, recommendation is to initiate therapy with N-acetylcysteine for acetaminophen intoxication; entecavir or lamivudine for hepatitis B; and penicillin, cimetidine, and silymarin for *Amanita phylloides* ingestion.

Ongoing surveillance for metabolic complications, such as hypoglycemia electrolyte imbalance, abnormal cardiac rhythms, respiratory failure, and infection, is required. Recommendation is to routinely establish peripheral intravenous access and start a dextrose infusion. Then, obtain cultures of blood, sputum, and urine and maintain a low threshold for initiating antimicrobial therapy. Patients should be monitored in the intensive care unit with electrocardiographic (ECG) monitoring and pulse oximetry and frequent assessments of level of consciousness with tools, such as the Glasgow coma score.

Timely transfer to a liver transplant center should be arranged for those whose condition is most likely to deteriorate—preferably before the encephalopathy grade increases above 2 or the INR is >2. These patients, even if ineligible for liver transplantation, benefit from care in an experienced liver unit. Early transfer is associated with fewer complications and provides the transplant center more time to procure an appropriate organ.

Neurologic deterioration can be anticipated, but often is precipitous. The transition from stage II to stage III encephalopathy can be used as the point at which invasive monitoring, including arterial and pulmonary arterial catheterization and ICP monitoring, are instituted. This transition often correlates with patients' inability to protect their airway and a decision to electively intubate the airway and institute mechanical ventilation. Seizures are common and may present only as a disturbance of consciousness without convulsions (NCE). Consequently, continuous EEG monitoring can often be used. Prophylaxis with phenytoin is associated with less intracranial hypertension and risk of herniations (18). Alternative agents, such as propofol, can offer a similar benefit. Monitoring of cerebral blood flow requires specialized equipment. The arterial jugular venous content difference of oxygen (AJVDO_2) can be easily determined, however, by simultaneous measurements of oxygen content from arterial and jugular bulb cannulae. Cerebral hyperemia will be recognized by a narrow AJVD O_2. This information, combined with measurement of ICP, allows for appropriate management of intracranial hypertension.

Intracranial pressure monitoring is controversial. Two major concerns with this invasive procedure are the risk of bleeding and the risk of infection (19,20). The benefits derive from timely intervention before intracranial hypertension results in irreversible brain injury. Monitors can be placed in the epidural space, subdural space, or ventricles. Accuracy and fidelity improve with increasing invasiveness, but so does the risk of complications. Ventriculostomy adds a unique benefit to monitoring in that CSF can be evacuated. The pressure at which CSF drains can be kept constant avoiding sudden rises in ICP with attendant compromise before therapeutic intervention can take effect. Neurosurgic skill and rapt attention to correction of coagulopathy are essential to minimize complications.

TREATMENT

Treatment of intracranial hypertension can be tailored to the degree of cerebral hyperemia. Early in the course of ALF, cerebral blood flow and blood volume are high and ICP can be reduced by hyperventilation and a decrease in central venous pressures. Reduction in metabolic activity with propofol and with hyperthermia will also be effective. Later in the course of ALF, when cerebral edema is present, maintenance of cerebral perfusion pressure is paramount. This often requires vasopressors to maintain arterial tone and osmotic agents such as mannitol. A key caveat is that mannitol will increase ICP in the absence of normal renal function. With continuous renal replacement therapy for the management of ALF-induced renal failure, it is possible to increase the ultrafiltration rate to counter the increase in central venous pressure that attends the hyperoncotic effects of the mannitol. Hypothermia and propofol or barbiturate coma can have additional neuroprotective effects in this late phase. The adverse impact of these measures on systemic hemodynamics must be balanced, however, by the reduction in ICP and neuroprotective effects.

MANAGEMENT OF EXTRAHEPATIC ORGAN DYSFUNCTION

The diagnostic evaluation of renal failure requires an assessment of intravascular volume and cardiac output to assess renal perfusion, calculation of the fractional excretion of sodium, and a urinalysis. Typical prerenal factors are initially caused by hypovolemia. Once corrected, a function abnormality develops, which reflects acute hepatorenal syndrome with a fractional excretion of Na (FENa) <15%. This reflects renal arterial vasospasm, which can be sufficiently severe to result in acute kidney injury (acute tubular necrosis [ATN]). Direct kidney injury can result from the hepatotoxin c.f. CCl4 and acetaminophen. Management of renal failure with intermittent hemodialysis is associated with worsening pulmonary and cerebral edema (21,22). Early institution of continuous renal replacement therapy (CRRT) as continuous venous–venous hemofiltration or even hemodiafiltration affords tight control of fluid, electrolyte, and acid-base homeostasis even while patients are aggressively resuscitated.

Progress in the management of acute lung injury (ALI or ARDS) has developed with the recognition that stretch injury

TABLE 43-3. Clichy Criteria for Liver Transplantation in Acute Liver Failure

Hepatic encephalopathy grade III or IV
And
Factor V <20% in patients <30 years of age
Or
Factor V <30% in patients >30 years of age

(From Bernuau J, Goudeau A, Poynard T, et al. Multivariate analysis of prognostic factors in fulminant hepatitis B. *Hepatology.* 1986;6(4):648–651; and Bernuau J, Rueff B, Benhamou JP. Fulminant and subfulminant liver failure: Definitions and causes. *Semin Liver Dis.* 1986;6(2):97–106, with permission).

to the lung affects the most compliant (normal) lung and releases cytokines, which adversely affects extrapulmonary organ function. Consequently, efforts to limit airway pressure and lung stretch have focused on low tidal volumes, which can result in hypoventilation and has been shown to reduce the mortality in ARDS (23). This results in permissive hypercapnia, which is well tolerated in many critically ill patients. Patients with intracranial hypertension, however, are susceptible to hypercapnia, which increases cerebral blood flow, worsens cerebral hyperemia, and increases ICP. Minute ventilation should be tightly controlled to minimize unintended fluctuation in CO_2. End-tidal carbon dioxide does not reflect arterial $PaCO_2$ as dead space is increased in ALI or ARDS. Periodic arterial blood gas measurement is indicated and should be obtained whenever the neurologic assessment changes and, particularly, with increases in ICP.

Nutritional support was avoided by clinicians before liver transplantation. ALF, however, is an extremely catabolic state. Indeed, survival from prolonged intensive care before and after liver transplantation is directly impacted by the calorie deficit a patient accrues with limited nutritional support. Caloric needs must be met with attention to avoid hyperglycemia. Similarly, protein needs can be estimated from the nitrogen balance if renal function is adequate to collect a 24-hour urea nitrogen; however, 1.25 g/kg is often required to stem the negative nitrogen balance. Measurements of ammonia are indicated to avoid worsening hyperammonemia. Branched-chain enriched formulae may be needed. Zinc should be supplemented and nonabsorbable antibiotics (e.g., rifaximin or neomycin) administered. Lactulose and other cathartics are often poorly tolerated because of ileus induced by portal hypertension or pancreatitis. The enteral route is preferred, but may not be available for the same reasons. In such cases, recommendation is the slow introduction of total parenteral nutrition.

CLINICAL RECOMMENDATIONS OF THE VIGNETTE

The patient developed intractable coagulopathy. Intracranial pressure was controlled with CSF drainage via the ventriculostomy. Cholestasis worsened with the total bilirubin rising 2 to 3 mg/dL daily. Listing for transplantation was delayed 4 days because of hypoxemic respiratory failure. A variety of modalities could be used to maintain low peak airway pressures and low tidal volumes. A high mean airway pressure was maintained with positive end-expiratory pressure (PEEP) and inverse ratio ventilation. Oxygenation improved and over 48 hours, the FIO_2 was reduced. Elimination of CO_2 (ventilation) became problematic, however. Despite intracranial hypertension and narrow AJV O_2-content difference consistent with cerebral hyperemia, CO_2 tensions remained in >60 mm Hg. Ventilation could not be increased without compromising hemodynamics and potential lung recovery. Intracranial hypertension was managed, however, by lowering central venous pressures and inducing hypothermia. CRRT was used to remove volume, reduce CVP and ICP as well as to control electrolyte and acid-base imbalances. The patient was cooled 34.5°C.

Within 4 days, the patient was oxygenated with FIO_2 <60% and PEEP ≤12 cm H_2O. Dead space fell and to the patient could be ventilated. On the fourth day of hospitalization, the CSF drainage from the ventriculostomy decreased abruptly. The wave form lost its characteristic trace and ICP measurements were unreliable. A head CT scan demonstrated cerebral edema and dilation of the lateral horn on the side of the ventriculostomy with blood around the catheter and in the ventricle. Thrombotic occlusion of the ventriculostomy catheter was suspected. The ventriculostomy was flushed with tissue plasminogen activator (TPA) and drainage of blood-tinged CSF rapidly increased. The CVP trace and ICP normalized. Follow up CT demonstrated resolution of the focal hydrocephalus. The coagulopathy was corrected aggressively and low filling pressures maintained with CRRT. The patient was listed for liver transplant and a suitable donor was identified within 72 hours. A technically successful operation was evident in the small number of red blood cells transfused (5) and short surgical time, 180 minutes.

On return from the operating room, the patient was vasodilated and hypotensive despite a high cardiac output. Arterial tone was maintained with norepinephrine. The patient remained comatose and CSF drainage persisted as the threshold for the ventriculostomy was maintained at 10 cm H_2O.

Three days after liver transplantation with excellent graft function CSF drainage was discontinued. No worsening of intracerebral hemorrhage (ICH) or hydrocephalus was evident on repeat CT scan. The ICP remained well controlled (<10 mm Hg) and the drain was removed. Over the next 2 weeks the patient regained full consciousness and rapidly regained strength.

The patient's neurologic and respiratory deterioration were abrupt. Cerebral edema and pulmonary edema presented competing therapeutic imperatives. The patient would have been unable to survive liver transplantation early in her course. Yet, with aggressive support, she improved to the point that the procedure could be performed successfully. At all points after presentation, even in the face of improvement, survival with transplantation was a much higher probability than survival with intensive care alone. The neuropathophysiology of ALF often persists for several hours and even days after successful transplant. Therapeutic intervention such as hypothermia should be reversed slowly.

SUMMARY

The key steps to managing the patient with ALF include recognizing the process, determining the cause, making a triage decision for transfer to a liver transplant center, minimizing additional harm to the patient through oversight or therapeutic misadventure and timing liver transplant before the patient is too sick to benefit. The case presented highlights many of these issues.

REFERENCES

1. Trey C, Davidson CS. The management of fulminant hepatic failure. *Progress in Liver Diseases.* 1970;3:282–298.
2. Hoofnagle JH, Carithers RL, Jr., Shapiro C, et al. Fulminant hepatic failure: Summary of a workshop. *Hepatology.* 1995;21(1):240–252.
3. Larson AM, Polson J, Fontana RJ, et al. Acetaminophen-induced acute liver failure: Results of a United States multicenter, prospective study [Comment]. *Hepatology.* 2005;42(6):1364–1372.
4. Lee WM. Acute liver failure in the United States. *Semin Liver Dis.* 2003;23(3):217–226.
5. Squires RH, Jr., Shneider BL, Bucuvalas J, et al. Acute liver failure in children: The first 348 patients in the pediatric acute liver failure study group. *J Pediatr.* 2006;148(5):652–658.
6. O'Grady JG, Alexander GJ, Hayllar KM, et al. Early indicators of prognosis in fulminant hepatic failure. *Gastroenterology.* 1989;97(2):439–445.
7. Shakil AO, Kramer D, Mazariegos GV, et al. Acute liver failure: Clinical features, outcome analysis, and applicability of prognostic criteria. *Liver Transplant.* 2000;6(2):163–169.
8. Ware AJ, D'Agostino AN, Combes B. Cerebral edema: A major complication of massive hepatic necrosis. *Gastroenterology.* 1971;61(6):877–884.
9. Blei AT, Larsen FS. Pathophysiology of cerebral edema in fulminant hepatic failure. *J Hepatol.* 1999;31(4):771–776.
10. Larsen FS, Gottstein J, Blei AT. Cerebral hyperemia and nitric oxide synthase in rats with ammonia-induced brain edema [Comment]. *J Hepatol.* 2001;34(4):548–554.
11. Munoz SJ, Robinson M, Northrup B, et al. Elevated intracranial pressure and computed tomography of the brain in fulminant hepatocellular failure. *Hepatology.* 1991;13(2):209–212.
12. Aggarwal S, Kramer D, Yonas H, et al. Cerebral hemodynamic and metabolic changes in fulminant hepatic failure: A retrospective study. *Hepatology.* 1994;19(1):80–87.
13. Scotto J, Opolon P, Eteve J. Liver biopsy and prognosis in acute liver failure. *Gut.* 1973; 14:927–933.
14. Vincent JL, Baron JF, Reinhart K, et al. Anemia and blood transfusion in critically ill patients [Comment]. *JAMA.* 2002;288(12):1499–1507.
15. Hebert PC, Wells G, Blajchman MA, et al. A multicenter, randomized, controlled clinical trial of transfusion requirements in critical care. Transfusion Requirements in Critical Care Investigators, Canadian Critical Care Trials Group [Comment]; [erratum appears in *N Engl J Med.* 1999;340(13):1056]. *N Engl J Med.* 1999;340(6):409–417.
16. O'Grady JG. Fulminant hepatitis in patients with chronic liver disease. *J Viral Hepat.* 2000;7[Suppl]1:9–10.
17. Donovan JP, Schafer DF, Shaw BW, Jr., et al. Cerebral oedema and increased intracranial pressure in chronic liver disease. *Lancet.* 1998;351(9104):719–721.
18. Ellis AJ, Wendon JA, Williams R. Subclinical seizure activity and prophylactic phenytoin infusion in acute liver failure: A controlled clinical trial [Comment]. *Hepatology.* 2000; 32(3):536–541.
19. Blei AT, Olafsson S, Webster S, et al. Complications of intracranial pressure monitoring in fulminant hepatic failure [Comment]. *Lancet.* 1993;341(8838):157–158.
20. Vaquero J, Fontana RJ, Larson AM, et al. Complications and use of intracranial pressure monitoring in patients with acute liver failure and severe encephalopathy. *Liver Transplant.* 2005;11(12):1581–1589.
21. Davenport A, Finn R, Goldsmith HJ. Management of patients with renal failure complicated by cerebral oedema. *Blood Purif.* 1989;7(4):203–209.
22. Davenport A, Will EJ, Davison AM, et al. Changes in intracranial pressure during machine and continuous haemofiltration. *Int J Artif Organs.* 1989;12(7):439–444.
23. Anonymous. Ventilation with lower tidal volumes as compared with traditional tidal volumes for acute lung injury and the acute respiratory distress syndrome. The Acute Respiratory Distress Syndrome Network [Comment]. *N Engl J Med.* 2000;342(18):1301–1308.
24. Bernal WDN, Wyncoll D, Wendon J. Blood lactate as an early predictor of outcome in paracetamol induced acute liver failure: A cohort study. *Lancet.* 2002;359:558–563.
25. Bernuau J, Goudeau A, Poynard T, et al. Multivariate analysis of prognostic factors in fulminant hepatitis B. *Hepatology.* 1986;6(4):648–651.
26. Bernuau J, Rueff B, Benhamou JP. Fulminant and subfulminant liver failure: Definitions and causes. *Semin Liver Dis.* 1986;6(2):97–106.

CHAPTER 44

Hepatic Encephalopathy

Andres T. Blei • Karin Weissenborn

OBJECTIVES

- To provide an understanding of the anatomic underpinnings of liver failure, with varying contributions of hepatocellular dysfunction and portal-systemic shunting to the neurologic picture of hepatic encephalopathy
- To describe the nature of the cerebral disturbance responsible for the development of hepatic encephalopathy, focusing on the neuroanatomic and neurochemical changes that occur in this syndrome
- To dispel the notion that hepatic encephalopathy is simply a disturbance of a liver-brain interaction
- To discuss involvement of the small and large bowel, kidney, and muscle in the pathogenesis of this disorder, which indicates a multiorgan dimension to this serious neurologic complication of liver disease

CASE VIGNETTE

A 23-year-old woman presents with fatigue, which occurs mainly in the afternoons and evenings, when she feels very sleepy at work (office setting). She has been unable to participate in swim meets as she did during her high school years. She has difficulty falling asleep during the night. Her weight has remained stable. She takes no ethanol (ETOH) or drugs and is not on any medications. Over the course of a year, she has seen five physicians. Psychiatric evaluation finds no evidence of depression. Her body mass index is 24 and other physical examination findings are normal. Neurologic examination was unremarkable.

Her laboratory tests were as follows: complete blood count (CBC): white blood cells (WBC) 5.4, hemoglobin 14 g/dL, hematocrit 44%, platelets 312,000; blood urea nitrogen (BUN) 17 mg/dL, creatine 0.7 mg%; alanine aminotransferase (ALT) 23; aspartate aminotransferase (AST) 17; alkaline phosphatase 98; γ-glutamyltransferase (GGT 105); albumin 3.9, international normalized ratio (INR) 1.1; thyrotropin (TSH) 2.1; urinalysis within normal limits; arterial ammonia: 103μg/dL.

A subsequent test is ordered that provides the diagnosis.

DEFINITION AND CLINICAL EPIDEMIOLOGY

Hepatic encephalopathy (HE) can be broadly defined as the neurologic alterations that occur in the setting of liver failure. A wide range of neuropsychiatric signs and symptoms can be detected, with similarities and differences between acute and chronic liver failure. Although neurologic manifestations are present in several other liver conditions (Wilson disease, Zellwegger syndrome) or arise from products linked to hepatic metabolism (indirect bilirubin and kernicterus), HE is related to liver failure. The term *portal-systemic encephalopathy* has been used interchangeably with HE, although it carries a narrower pathophysiologic implication and a recent consensus statement has argued against its use (1).

The consensus statement did reach an agreement on three types of HE.

HE TYPE A ACUTE LIVER FAILURE

The etiology of acute liver failure (ALF) has a geographical variation. In the United States and selected countries of western Europe, acute liver injury from acetaminophen is the leading cause; infection with hepatitis E is the main cause in India. (For further detail, the reader is referred to Chapter 43, *Management of Acute Liver Failure.*) Regardless of cause, the development of encephalopathy in ALF is a poor prognostic sign. Deeper stages of encephalopathy (confusion, coma) are associated with the development of brain edema. Death can occur as a result of intracranial hypertension (2).

HE TYPE B PORTAL-SYSTEMIC BYPASS

Vascular malformations that directly link the portal vein to the systemic circulation are an uncommon cause of HE. They can occur within the liver parenchyma or represent the persistence of a ductus venosus. The age of presentation varies widely, ranging from 18 to 70 years in a large series from Japan (3). Portal vein thrombosis, acquired in different clinical settings, will also result in the development of portal-systemic shunts and can be associated with changes in cognitive function in the pediatric and adult population.

HE TYPE C CIRRHOSIS

HE is most often seen in patients with cirrhosis. The incidence of cirrhosis continues to increase as a result of epidemics of hepatitis C and obesity-related liver injury (4). It is not an early event in the course of liver failure. In the Child-Pugh classification, a three-stage prognostic tool, alterations of mental state correspond to stages B and C.

Three types of presentation of HE can occur (1):

1. Episodic encephalopathy is the most common form, generally related to a precipitating factor that triggers a toxin load to the brain.
2. Persistent encephalopathy, a rarer form of presentation, where patients may have severe liver failure or exhibit large portal-systemic shunts.
3. Minimal encephalopathy, an alteration of cognitive function detected by neuropsychologic or neurophysiologic tests.

In contrast to the encephalopathy of ALF, where the neurologic picture can by itself cause the patient's death, HE in cirrhosis carries a poor prognosis as an indicator of the severity of liver failure.

ANATOMIC BACKGROUND OF LIVER DISEASE

In cirrhosis, the interplay between three factors underlies the development of HE.

PORTAL-SYSTEMIC SHUNTING

Once the liver injury has progressed and a critical value of portal pressure has been reached, portal-systemic collaterals develop. In the most common clinical expression of such collaterals, gastrointestinal bleeding can arise from gastroesophageal varices. Some collaterals can be large and carry a large portion of the portal flow; for example, splenorenal collaterals can be associated with repeated bouts of encephalopathy (5). The placement of a radiologic portal-systemic shunt, transjugular intrahepatic porto-system shunt (TIPS), can improve portal hypertension but precipitate or aggravate HE (6).

DEGREE OF LIVER FAILURE

Patients with a preserved liver function are less susceptible to HE. If function is relatively well preserved, recurrent or persistent symptoms may be a clinical clue for the presence of a large spontaneous portal-systemic shunt (5). In the setting of poor liver function, persistent HE may indicate the presence of "acute-on-chronic" liver failure, where an acute injury is superimposed in cirrhosis.

PRECIPITATING FACTORS

Most patients with cirrhosis develop HE as a result of a precipitating factor, regardless of the degree of liver failure. Such factors result in an increased toxin load to the brain. Dehydration, often the result of diuretic therapy of ascites, is a common precipitating factor. Diuretics can also induce hyponatremia, hypokalemia, and elevations of BUN, factors that can also precipitate HE by themselves. Gastrointestinal bleeding, infection, high dietary protein, constipation, and the use of sedatives are other common precipitants. The search for such precipitants is a mainstay of the clinical management of these cases.

In ALF, the interplay of the three factors mentioned in cirrhosis is also operative. By definition, liver failure is maximal. Extrahepatic portal-systemic shunting is not a feature of the syndrome, but functionally, the inability of the liver to remove circulating toxins results de facto in a large intrahepatic shunt. Of all precipitating factors, infection is the most common. Recent studies have pointed to the importance of inflammation and infection in the development and progression of HE in this condition (see Chapter 43, *Management of Acute Liver Failure*).

PATHOGENESIS

Two dimensions to consider when examining the pathogenesis of HE are the periphery and the brain.

PERIPHERY

Traditional research has focused on the nature of purported toxins that escape hepatic uptake and reach the systemic circulation as a result of hepatic failure or portal-systemic shunting. In accordance with the anatomic underpinnings of HE, the substance(s) must originate in the splanchnic territory, have high levels in the portal vein, and undergo efficient first-pass extraction by the liver. Clinical observations indicate the substance is related to dietary protein (witness the classic descriptions of "meat intoxication") and is also related to the bacterial flora (witness the favorable clinical response to nonabsorbable antibiotics).

Ammonia

Ammonia meets all these requirements. It is a nitrogenous product arising from both bacterial metabolism in the colon as well as from deamidation of glutamine in the small bowel (glutamine is the main energetic source for this tissue). It has a high concentration in the portal vein, almost tenfold higher than in the systemic circulation, indicating an effective first-pass extraction by the liver. Hepatic metabolism of ammonia proceeds via two pathways: A low-affinity, high-capacity synthesis of urea, localized to perivenous hepatocytes, and a high-affinity, low-capacity synthesis of glutamine in pericentral hepatocytes. The dual system indicates the tight control of hepatic tissue on the ammonia load that exits the splanchnic territory (7).

In liver disease, the access of ammonia to the systemic circulation is enhanced as a result of extrahepatic portal-systemic shunts as well as a decreased hepatic uptake, the product of decreased functional mass and intrahepatic portal-systemic shunts (as seen in advanced cirrhosis). Once in the periphery, uptake occurs in muscle and brain, with amidation of glutamate to glutamine. Glutamine released into the circulation is used by other tissues, including small bowel and kidney, a process that generates ammonia. Thus, an ammonia-glutamine cycle is profoundly disrupted in liver disease.

Ammonia had been traditionally thought to cross membranes in its gaseous form, NH_3. More recent studies point at the ability of charged ammonia to cross membranes across specialized ion channels (8). In addition, ammonia or ammonium transporters may also be operative. Rh (Rhesus) proteins, traditionally located in the red blood cell in association with other proteins, include two nonerythroid members, RhBG and

RhCG (9). These are located in liver and kidney and appear to represent specific mammalian ammonium transporters. The relation of these channels and transporters with the process of hepatic encephalopathy has not been examined.

Synergism

For many years, the concept of synergism included the effect of other gut products arising from bacterial metabolism in combination with ammonia. This view has been replaced by the demonstration of synergistic effects of systemic inflammation or infection. Blood levels of tumor necrosis factor-α (TNF-α) are related to the degree of HE in cirrhosis (10). In another study, a glutamine challenge (essentially an ammonia load) was administered at the onset of a tissue infection (mainly of the urinary tract) to patients with cirrhosis. The challenge resulted in more conspicuous neuropsychologic changes at the onset of infection in contrast to the end-of-therapy findings (9). Proinflammatory cytokines may signal into brain via vagal afferents, bind to receptors in the cerebral vasculature (with subsequent transduction of signals into brain), or even cross into cerebral tissue via anatomic sites that lack a blood–brain barrier (11).

Other theories of the pathogenesis of HE based on different circulating factors have been scrutinized and rejected over the years (12). A role for circulating γ-aminobutyric acid (GABA) and endogenous benzodiazepines has not been confirmed. Correction of an altered aromatic or branched chain amino acid ratio was the basis for the administration of branched-chain amino acid solutions, with the goal of reducing false neurotransmitters in the brain. Both laboratory and clinical studies do not support the validity of this theory, Another amino acid is tryptophan, whose entry is favored into brain as result of an exchange with an increased intracerebral glutamine. Tryptophan is a precursor of serotonin and altered serotoninergic neurotransmission has been implicated in the pathogenesis of HE.

At another level, accumulation of manganese in basal ganglia may be important in the pathogenesis of extrapyramidal symptomatology in cirrhosis. Increased levels of manganese reflect the effects of portal-systemic shunting and decreased biliary excretion of the metal (13). Magnetic resonance imaging (MRI) of the brain may show a characteristic hyperresonant globus pallidus (Fig. 44-1). Of note, such changes, coupled with other alterations of white matter, have also been found in Wilson disease, where the accumulated metal is copper.

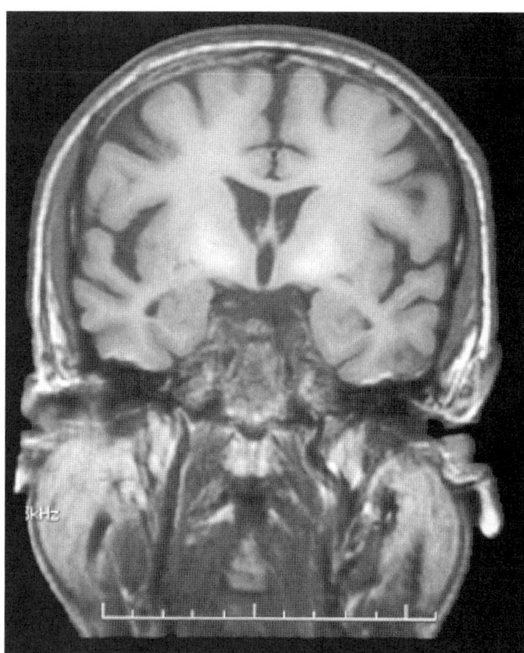

FIGURE 44-1. Bilateral pallidal intensities on (MRI), characteristic of the patient with portal-systemic shunting, which most often is a result of cirrhosis. (Courtesy of Dr. K. Weissenborn.)

BRAIN

Autopsy studies of patients who die with ALF show evidence of brain edema, mainly of the cerebral cortex. In cirrhosis, autopsy studies are striking for the lack of gross anatomic changes.

At microscopy, a consistent feature is the presence of glial changes, the so-called *Alzheimer type II astrocyte* (Fig. 44-2). Seen on immersion-fixation as an astrocyte with an enlarged, pale nucleus, such cells correspond to the swollen astrocyte seen in animal studies where brains have undergone perfusion-fixation. Involvement of astrocytes and their corresponding swelling is a key observation to understand current views on the pathogenesis of HE. The term *hepatic gliopathy* has been coined by Norenberg (14) to describe the nature of the central nervous system (CNS) disturbance.

The central role of astrocyte swelling is evident when considering the pathogenesis of brain edema in ALF. Animal and human studies point at the accumulation of glutamine in this cell as a critical initial step in the process that culminates in a net increase in brain water. Astrocytes contain glutamine synthetase and levels of glutamine in brain increase at least sixfold. The accumulation of this amino acid, effectively an organic

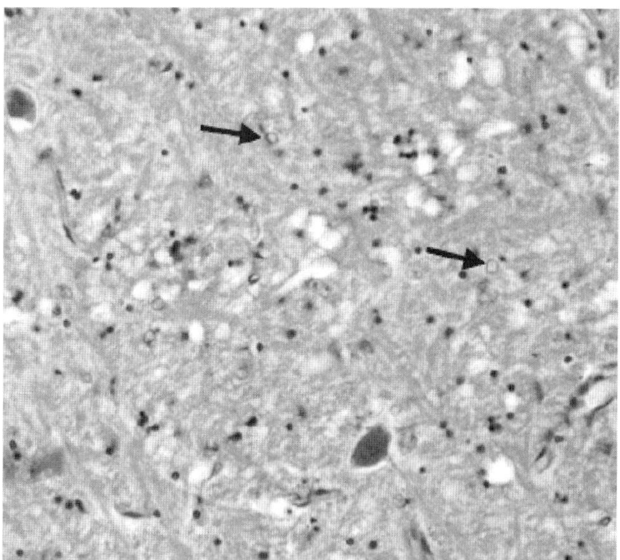

FIGURE 44-2. Large, vacuolated nucleus of astrocytes (Alzheimer type II) in a patient who died with cirrhosis and hepatic encephalopathy (HE). (Courtesy of Dr. K. Weissenborn.)

osmolyte, will result in water movement into glial cells and the compensatory reduction in the levels of other osmolytes, especially myoinositol (15). Acute release of intracellular K^+ and glutamate is seen under these conditions too.

An alternate view of the generation of astrocyte swelling points at glutamine as a "Trojan horse" (16). In glial cells, ammonia is detoxified to glutamine, but the latter is transported into mitochondria via specific transporters, where the action of phosphate-activated glutaminase results in the generation of ammonia. At this site, ammonia induces the permeability transition and the ensuing mitochondrial dysfunction results in the generation of reactive oxygen species. Such compounds would be involved in the process of astrocyte swelling, impairing the activity of membrane pumps that maintain cellular osmolarity.

Evidence of oxidative and nitrosative stress has been shown in isolated glial cells and in models of ammonia infusion (17). Whether the result of the metabolism of glutamine in mitochondria or the product of cellular swelling itself, oxidative stress in astrocytes can result in a wide range of cellular abnormalities. Impairment of the activity of the Glut-1 transporter results in increased levels of extracellular brain glutamate. Impairment of glycolysis is manifested by an increase in lactate and pyruvate levels, as assessed by MR spectroscopy (18). Generation of vasodilatory stimuli as a result of oxidative or nitrosative stress, such as nitric oxide or carbon monoxide, will result in the development of cerebral hyperemia, a common finding in animal models and humans with brain edema (19).

Low-grade brain edema has been shown in patients with cirrhosis using diffusion-weighted MR (20). Hyponatremia can contribute to the reduction in brain myoinositol, a characteristic feature on MR spectroscopy of the brain. Clinical evidence of brain swelling with evolution to intracranial hypertension is exceptionally seen in patients with cirrhosis (21). Nonetheless, the concept of low-grade brain edema has highlighted a mechanism that shares pathogenic features in the encephalopathy of both acute and chronic liver disease.

The alterations in astrocyte function are central to the abnormalities in mental state seen in HE. In this setting, normal glial-neuronal communications are disrupted, resulting in alterations of neurotransmission, including glutamatergic, GABAergic, and dopaminergic pathways. In a direct way, HE points at the importance of astrocyte integrity to the process by which consciousness is maintained.

PATHOLOGY

One exception to the inconspicuous macroscopic changes of the brain in HE is the entity already mentioned, hepatocerebral degeneration. Described by Victor et al. in 1965 (22), the entity has a clinical expression with symptoms of dysfunction of basal ganglia, such as choreoathetosis, rigidity, dystonia, and dysarthria. Neuropathologic features are similar to those seen in Wilson disease, and hence the term *acquired hepatolenticular degeneration*. These include spongiform changes and polymicrocavitation in the area of the basal ganglia, but also cortical laminar neuronal loss. Alzheimer type II astrocytes are prominently seen; manganese accumulation may be responsible for such changes (23). A myelopathic presentation may also be present. Although reversal of such changes has been reported after liver transplantation (24), the effectiveness of this approach is not fully known.

CLINICAL MANIFESTATIONS

From a neurologic perspective, several signs and symptoms can be elicited.

CHANGES IN MENTAL STATE

Patients may present with minor behavioral changes (stage I), on occasions detected by a family member. Difficulty with simple mathematical calculations can be elicited. Inversion of the sleep–wake cycle can be present, with difficulty falling asleep during the night and daytime sleepiness. Alterations of the rhythm of plasma melatonin are prominent (25). As encephalopathy progresses, lethargy is more prominent; patients are somnolent (stage II). With stage III, patients are stuporous. In stage IV, patients are in a coma, with varying degrees of response to painful stimuli. A striking feature of this sequence is the reversibility of symptoms, which in the case of a precipitant-induced coma, can fully improve within a 72-hour period.

NEUROMUSCULAR ABNORMALITIES

Asterixis

Asterixis is a classic sign of HE, although it is seen in other metabolic encephalopathies, such as uremia, CO_2 retention, and hypomagnesemia. Muscles that are tonically active undergo an involuntary very brief silent period that results in postural lapses. The pathogenesis of this condition is poorly understood, but it can be traced to alterations in basal ganglia and thalamic function. A postural tremor of varying frequency has been termed *mini-asterixis* (26); an altered thalamomotor cortical coupling underlies the genesis of this symptom.

Long-Tract Signs

Patients in deeper stages of coma can exhibit transient Babinski sign as well as clonus, which can be bilateral. Recent studies using diffusion-weighted MR note changes in the pyramidal tract consistent with edema (27).

Brain Edema

As in other neurologic or neurosurgical conditions, swelling of the brain can remain undetected until prominent elevations of the intracranial pressure occur. Monitoring for pupillary abnormalities and alterations of the oculovestibular reflex is impractical in the acute clinical setting of ALF. In cirrhosis, low-grade brain edema is not diagnosed clinically.

Extrapyramidal Symptomatology

In patients with advanced liver disease, it is common to detect hypokinesia associated with rigidity; postural tremors are less frequent. These classic parkinsonian features have an anatomic correlate, with MRI already described (Fig. 44-1) and functional studies with positron emission tomography (PET) scanning that show increased cerebral glucose utilization in basal ganglia and thalamus (28).

Hepatocerebral Degeneration

In patients with long-standing portal-systemic shunts, hepatocerebral degeneration may be diagnosed (see *Pathology* section). Extrapyramidal and cerebellar symptoms may be prominent, together with spastic paraparesis, mood alterations, and even dementia.

Respiratory Findings

Mercaptans, a product of gut bacterial metabolism of methionine, have been associated with a particular pungent breath odor, fetor hepaticus. Hyperventilation is common in patients with deep encephalopathy, the result of glutamate-induced stimulation of the respiratory center.

DIAGNOSTIC APPROACH

DIFFERENTIAL DIAGNOSIS

When a patient is not known to have liver disease, the presence of an altered mental state requires careful consideration of other causes of neurologic impairment. The search may be led by the detection of other physical signs, such as hyperreflexia, Babinski sign, and clonus. Other metabolic encephalopathies may also present with asterixis. Abnormal physical examination findings and laboratory tests suggestive of liver disease lead to the correct diagnosis.

Hyperammonemia, with varying degrees of alterations of consciousness, can be a manifestation of pathology not related to acute or chronic liver disease. Urea cycle enzyme defects can present as severe hyperammonemia in adult heterozygotes. Urine infection with *Proteus mirabilis*, a urease-containing bacterium, results in a systemic ammonia load that has been associated with encephalopathy. Hyperammonemia has been reported after chemotherapy for lymphoid tumors and after lung transplantation.

A greater challenge can be the exclusion of other causes for an abnormal mental state in patients with known liver disease. Imaging of the brain is frequently obtained in these patients to rule out structural abnormalities, especially the presence of subdural hematomas in alcoholic individuals. Patients with alcoholic cirrhosis can also develop Wernicke encephalopathy. A brain autopsy study has noted the high prevalence of unsuspected evidence for thiamine deficiency, even in patients with nonalcoholic cirrhosis (29).

DIAGNOSTIC TOOLS

Staging

The four grades of HE described above have been termed the *West Haven classification* (30). This classification combines an assessment of alterations of consciousness, behavioral changes, and neuromuscular alterations. The Glasgow coma scale can be used in patients with severe encephalopathy.

Measurements of Ammonia

An elevated ammonia level at diagnosis points to a potential hepatic origin to the change in mental function. Although serum levels correlate broadly with stages of encephalopathy, substantial overlap exists between values at different stages. Thus, repeated measurements of ammonia are not recommended for the follow up of these patients; monitoring mental state provides the important information. Arterial hyperammonemia is an important measurement in patients with ALF. Values >200 μg/dL indicate a higher risk of developing cerebral herniation (31). Arterial values are preferable in this condition, because an arteriovenous difference of ammonia can be substantial. Samples should be kept in a cold environment and promptly assayed.

Neuropsychological Testing

Patients with cirrhosis may exhibit cognitive defects in the absence of overt neurologic findings. A psychometric hepatic encephalopathy score (32) can be used to quantify this disturbance, mainly focusing on the areas of attention and psychomotor coordination. The test combines the results of the Number Connection tests A and B, the serial dotting test, the digit symbol test, and the line tracing test. It was validated against a population of normal controls as well as another cohort with chronic disease. Although originally described in a German population, it has been validated in other countries (33).

Neurophysiological Testing

In general terms, neurophysiologic tests appear to have a higher sensitivity in detecting abnormalities in asymptomatic individuals. Many of these tests, except the encephalogram (EEG) (with the classic descriptions of wave slowing), have been used for investigative purposes and have not reached the clinical arena. A recent development in the field has been the use of the critical flicker frequency (CFF) test (33,34). With this tool, the threshold frequencies at which light pulses are perceived as fused or flickering can be recorded. In two different laboratories, values between 38 and 39 Hz for the flicker frequency distinguished low-grade HE from normal subjects.

Brain Imaging (Including Functional Brain Imaging)

None of the brain imaging methods used so far provides information that can be used to make the diagnosis of HE. The pallidal hyperintensities found in about 90% of patients with cirrhosis indicate the presence of significant portal-systemic shunting, but not HE. The characteristic MR spectography (MRS) alterations, with an increase in the glutamate or glutamine signal intensity and a decrease in the myoinositol and choline signal intensity (both compared with creatine) rise with increasing grades of encephalopathy (Fig. 44-3), but can also be found in patients without clinical, neuropsychological, or neurophysiologic signs of brain dysfunction (35). Alterations of cerebral glucose utilization, as detected by ^{18}F-fluoro-desoxy-glucose-PET (Fig. 44-4), show a decrease in the utilization of the cingulated gyrus, and the dorsolateral prefrontal and the parietal cortex accompanied by a relative increase in the glucose utilization of the basal ganglia and the thalamus, which correlates with the cognitive and motor symptoms of the patients (36,37). The study of Lockwood et al. (38) on cerebral ammonia metabolism in patients with cirrhosis, indicating an increased permeability of the blood–brain barrier to ammonia in the patients was considered a

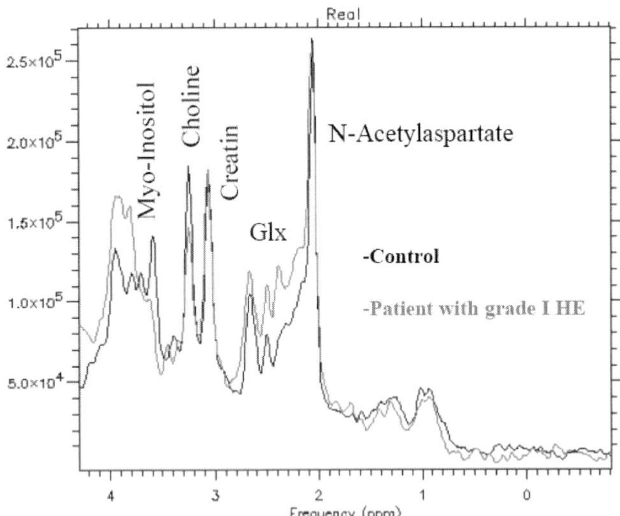

FIGURE 44-3. Magnetic resonance spectrosocopy (MRS) of a patient with cirrhosis and grade I hepatic encephalopathy (HE) as compared with a control tracing. Notice the increase in the *Glx* peak (glutamate and glutamine) and the reduced myoinositol peak, reflecting an osmotic alteration of the brain. (Courtesy of Dr. K. Weissenborn.)

milestone. It was contradicted, however, by the recent study of Keiding et al. (39) who found no alterations of the permeability surface area product for ammonia in such patients, irrespective of their grade of HE. Undoubtedly, there is a higher ammonia supply to the basal ganglia, thalamus, and cerebellum compared with cortical areas, a finding that might explain the predominance of extrapyramidal and cerebellar symptoms in these patients.

MINIMAL HEPATIC ENCEPHALOPATHY

In the 1970s, several groups reported findings of disturbed cerebral function in about 30% to 60% of patients with cirrhosis without clinically obvious signs of hepatic encephalopathy using neuropsychologic or neurophysiologic methods (40,41). These patients were considered to have *subclinical* or *latent* hepatic encephalopathy. Because this slightest grade of HE is of practical significance for the patients daily living, experts in the field discourage the use of the terms "subclinical HE" or "latent HE," because such a connotation runs the risk of considering this mildest degree of HE void of clinical significance. Instead, it was recommended to use the term *minimal HE* (1). Minimal HE interferes with the patient's ability to drive a car, their earning capability, and their quality of life (42–44).

Minimal HE is characterized by sleep disturbances and subtle behavioral changes that are more apparent to the patient's family than to the medical staff (45). The behavioral changes are predominantly caused by subtle impairment of cognitive function resulting from bilateral forebrain and parieto-occipital dysfunction (36,37). Because verbal abilities are usually preserved in this stage of HE, cerebral dysfunction is not detectable by the clinical routine examination but only by neuropsychological or neurophysiologic measures. Patients with minimal HE perform less well than healthy controls in tests of psychomotor speed, visual perception, and attention (32). Some of them also show a pathologic slowing of the EEG and prolonged latencies of exogenous and endogenous-evoked potentials, such as the visual-evoked potentials, somatosensory-evoked potentials, brainstem-evoked potentials, or the P300, for example (46). In addition, CFF has been shown to be reduced in some of these patients (33,34).

Minimal HE has prognostic significance. After a follow up of 3 years, 50% of the patients with minimal HE present with clinically overt HE compared with only 8% of patients with cirrhosis without minimal HE (34). Looking at the future, two tasks remain to be completed: (*a*) an agreement on the most appropriate method for the diagnosis of minimal HE and (*b*) proof that the classic treatment applied in the case of clinically overt HE improves the daily functioning as well as the prognosis of patients with minimal HE.

TREATMENT AND PREVENTION

Three strategies are to be followed when confronted with a patient with cirrhosis and overt HE. (See Chapter 43, *Management of Acute Liver Failure.*)

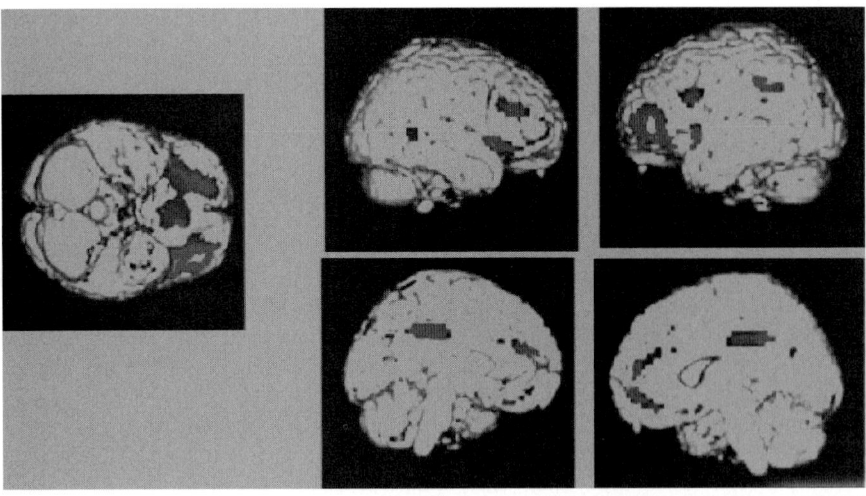

FIGURE 44-4. Cerebral regions with decreased glucose utilization in patients with cirrhosis and minimal hepatic encephalopathy (HE) as compared with controls. A decrease in the utilization of the cingulated gyrus, the dorsolateral prefrontal, and the parietal cortex accompanied by a relative increase in the glucose utilization of the basal ganglia and the thalamus is seen. (From Lockwood AH, Weissenborn K, Bokemeyer M, et al. Correlations between cerebral glucose metabolism and neuropsychological test performance in non-alcoholic cirrhotics. *Metab Brain Dis.* 2002;17(1):29–40, with permission.)

GENERAL SUPPORTIVE MEASURES

Dehydration as a result of diuretic therapy is a common complication of HE and fluid should be replaced via the intravenous route. Correction of metabolic disturbances, especially hypokalemia, is important. Hypoxemia, common in persons with cirrhosis, can also aggravate the neurologic picture. Recent studies point at deleterious effects of hyponatremia on brain function (47) and efforts should be made to normalize serum sodium levels. Patients with deeper stages of encephalopathy are at risk of aspiration and may require intubation for airway protection.

Catharsis should be assured, although most times this is provided with the use of nonabsorbable disaccharides (see later). Although protein restriction is usually instituted at the time of initial encounter with a person who is severely encephalopathic, a recent clinical trial shows no benefits from such an approach (48). Furthermore, such measures should be avoided in the long run. Patients with cirrhosis are hypercatabolic and may require up to 1.5 g/kg protein per day. Vegetable and dairy-based protein is preferred over animal protein as the dietary source. Branched-chain amino acids can be used in patients who are intolerant of dietary protein; recent studies also indicate an anabolic effect of this combination that may have a favorable impact on patient survival (49,50).

IDENTIFY AND TREAT THE PRECIPITATING FACTOR

A careful history should be obtained, including the use of hypnotics and sedatives, a common problem in these patients. General laboratory tests should be obtained, and the possibility of gastrointestinal bleeding considered, even without overt signs of hemorrhage. In patients with ascites, a diagnostic paracentesis is required to exclude spontaneous bacterial peritonitis, because such patients may present with encephalopathy as the sole clinical manifestation. Infection should be excluded in other territories, and blood and urine samples should be obtained.

PROVIDE SPECIFIC THERAPY

The armamentarium for the treatment of HE is not wide. Furthermore, therapy is not supported by large, well-designed clinical trials; a recent review of such studies point at major deficiencies in study design and limited proof of the actual efficacy of currently used therapies (51). Still, a rationale for their use and clinical experience has resulted in the wide adoption of such therapies by the practicing community.

Reduce Generation of Toxins from the Gastrointestinal Tract

Most therapies for HE target the gastrointestinal tract and attempt to reduce the generation of ammonia by the colon.

NONABSORBABLE DISACCHARIDES. Nonabsorbable disaccharides, such as lactulose and lactitol, can be administered orally or via enema, the latter useful in patients with deep HE where a quicker arousal is sought. They exert several effects on the gut, including an acidification of the lumen (via bacterial generation of lactic acid), incorporation of ammonia into bacteria, as well as a general cathartic effect. Oral administration can be started with 15 to 30 mL every 12 hours. The goal is to obtain three soft bowel movements per day. Chronic use is hampered by poor compliance, because the sweet taste is not palatable for some, whereas flatulence and abdominal cramping can be bothersome. Excessive diarrhea will result in hypernatremia, a factor that can independently alter the mental state by causing hyperosmolarity.

ANTIBIOTICS. Poorly-absorbed oral neomycin can be administered at doses from 2 to 6 g per day. An antibiotic is better suited for chronic use, although little evidence is available to support such an indication. If neomycin is provided in such a setting, renal and auditory testing should be done, because there is some absorption of this aminoglycoside. A malabsorption syndrome has also been described with chronic use. Metronidazole is another antibiotic that may be effective in treating HE. The bacterial flora affected by this antibiotic differs significantly from the one affected by neomycin, suggesting other effects, probably on the generation of ammonia by the small bowel. The dose of metronidazole in liver disease has to be lowered, because the hepatic clearance of the drug is reduced in liver failure: 250 mg twice daily should be the starting dose. Rifaximin, a nonabsorbed antibiotic, may exert positive effects in HE (52); ongoing trials should confirm these preliminary results.

Improve Hepatic Elimination of Ammonia

Zinc is a cofactor in all reactions of the urea cycle. Patients with cirrhosis and zinc deficiency will improve their ability to synthesize urea after zinc supplementation. Long-term zinc supplementation may be useful for patients with mild chronic forms of encephalopathy. The role of other approaches to improve the capacity of the liver to detoxify ammonia, such as sodium benzoate and ornithine-aspartate, is still under investigation. Ornithine-aspartate is of special interest, because it will also improve muscle elimination of ammonia via a posttranscriptional increase in the activity of glutamine synthetase (53).

Improve Abnormalities in Neurotransmission

Flumazenil, a benzodiazepine receptor antagonist, has been used to quickly reverse the sedative effects of benzodiazepine on the brain. In HE, studies using 1 mg intravenously indicate an improvement in mental function when compared with placebo (54). The effects were not striking, however, and improvement was transient. The lack of an oral formulation has precluded further research with this drug.

Bromocriptine, a dopamine agonist, may improve mental state in patients with chronic encephalopathy who exhibit extrapyramidal symptomatology. It is not commonly used and requires neurologic consultation.

CLINICAL RECOMMENDATIONS OF THE VIGNETTE

The patient had a portal vein-hepatic vein congenital communication (Fig. 44-5) that shunted all her portal blood into the systemic circulation. Her liver was intact.

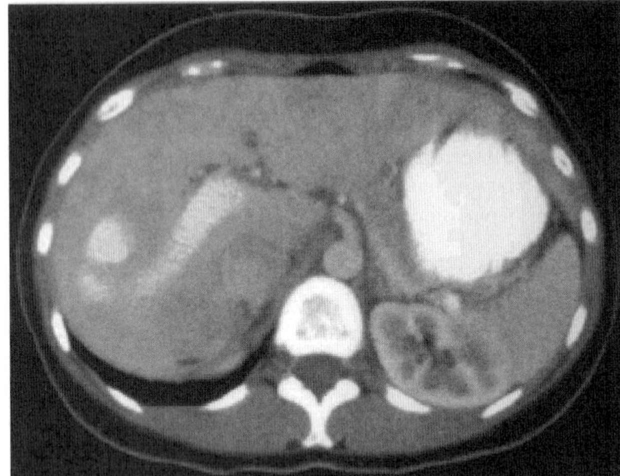

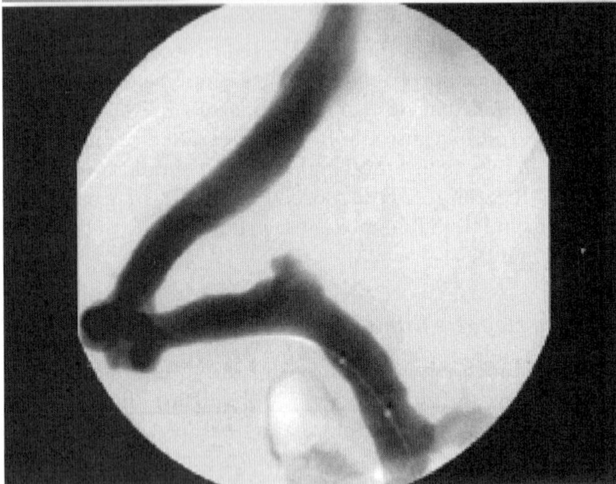

FIGURE 44-5. *(Top)* Spiral abdominal computed tomography (CT) image demonstrating a massively enlarged portal vein (PV) running toward the hepatic vein (HV). *(Bottom)* Portal venous system injection performed from the right transjugular approach. Portal venogram showing a direct connection from the portal vein (PV) and the hepatic vein (HV). (From Crespin J, Nemcek A, Rehkemper G, et al. Intrahepatic portal-hepatic venous anastomosis: A portal-systemic shunt with neurological repercussions. *Am J Gastroenterol.* 2000;95:1568–1571.

Her case has been described in detail (55). She had arterial hyperammonemia (102 μmol/L), a hyperresonant globus pallidus on MRI, MRS that showed an increase in the glutamate or glutamine peak, and a reduction in the myoinositol signal, as well as neuropsychological tests that showed deficits in the area of attention and fine motor skills. All of these abnormalities can be also seen in patients with cirrhosis and highlight the importance of portal-systemic shunting in the pathogenesis of hepatic encephalopathy. The complaint of fatigue is of special interest, as it indicates a probable central effect as a result of portal-systemic shunting.

Closure of these shunts needs to be done gradually, because the portal vein cannot accommodate a sudden occlusion. A TIPS stent was placed on the endogenous shunt, and the stent was allowed to endothelialize. The obstruction to portal flow, thus was gradual, allowing redirection of blood flow toward the liver. Once achieved (within 8 months), the patient's ammonia levels were normalized and fatigue was not a clinical feature any longer.

SUMMARY

Hepatic encephalopathy reflects the impact of acute or chronic liver failure on the brain.

Hepatocellular failure and portal-systemic shunting are the key splanchnic abnormalities that underlie the development of HE. Current views on the nature of the toxins responsible for HE highlight the roles of ammonia, manganese, and mediators of inflammation or infection.

Elimination of ammonia by muscle and kidney indicates the multiorgan nature of the abnormalities that lead to HE.

The main cellular element in the brain affected by HE is the astrocyte. Anatomic alterations (Alzheimer type II change) and functional abnormalities (development of oxidative stress) can be demonstrated. HE likely develops as a result of alterations of neuronal–astrocytic communication. Clinical manifestations in ALF include the development of brain edema and intracranial hypertension. In cirrhosis, episodic, persistent, or minimal changes can be observed.

Most of the current therapy is directed at the gut flora, using prebiotics (nonabsorbable disaccharides) and antibiotics. Therapies directed at the liver (improvement of efficiency of the urea cycle and alternatives pathways to nitrogen metabolism) may also have a role. Very few agents directed at abnormalities of neurotransmission have been tested and shown to be efficacious in HE.

REFERENCES

1. Ferenci P, Lockwood A, Mullen K, et al. Hepatic encephalopathy—Definition, nomenclature, diagnosis, and quantification: Final report of the working party at the 11th World Congresses of Gastroenterology, Vienna, 1998. *Hepatology.* 2002;35:716–721.
2. Vaquero J, Chung C, Cahill ME, et al. Pathogenesis of hepatic encephalopathy in acute liver failure. *Semin Liver Dis.* 2003;23:259–269.
3. Watanabe A. Portal-systemic encephalopathy in non-cirrhotic patients: Classification of clinical types, diagnosis and treatment. *J Gastroenterol Hepatol.* 2000;15:969–979.
4. Williams R. Global challenges in liver disease. *Hepatology.* 2006;44:521–526.
5. Riggio O, Efrati C, Catalano C, et al. High prevalence of spontaneous portal-systemic shunts in persistent hepatic encephalopathy: A case-control study. *Hepatology.* 2005;42:1158–1165.
6. Morgan MY, Amodio P. Treatment for hepatic encephalopathy: Tips from TIPS? *J Hepatol.* 2005;42:626–628.
7. Haussinger D, Lamers WH, Moorman AF. Hepatocyte heterogeneity in the metabolism of amino acids and ammonia. *Enzyme.* 1992;46:72–93.
8. Khademi S, O'Connell J, 3rd, Remis J, et al. Mechanism of ammonia transport by Amt/MEP/Rh: Structure of AmtB at 1.35 A. *Science.* 2004;305:1587–1594.
9. Peng J, Huang H. Rh proteins vs Amt proteins: An organismal and phylogenetic perspective on CO2 and NH3 gas channels. *Transfus Clin Biol.* 2006;13(1–2):85–94. Epub 2006 Mar 27.
10. Odeh M, Sabo E, Srugo I, et al. Serum levels of tumor necrosis factor-alpha correlate with severity of hepatic encephalopathy due to chronic liver failure. *Liver Int.* 2004;24:110–116.
11. Shawcross DL, Davies NA, Williams R, et al. Systemic inflammatory response exacerbates the neuropsychological effects of induced hyperammonemia in cirrhosis. *J Hepatol.* 2004; 40:247–254.
12. Butterworth RF. Pathogenesis of hepatic encephalopathy: New insights from neuroimaging and molecular studies. *J Hepatol.* 2003;39:278–285.
13. Rose C, Butterworth RF, Zayed J, et al. Manganese deposition in basal ganglia structures results from both portal-systemic shunting and liver dysfunction. *Gastroenterology.* 1999;117:640–644.
14. Norenberg MD. Astroglial dysfunction in hepatic encephalopathy. *Metab Brain Dis.* 1998;13:319–335.
15. Cordoba J, Gottstein J, Blei AT. Glutamine, myo-inositol, and organic brain osmolytes after portocaval anastomosis in the rat: Implications for ammonia-induced brain edema. *Hepatology.* 1996;24:919–923.
16. Norenberg MD, Albrecht J. Glutamine: A Trojan horse in ammonia neurotoxicity. *Hepatology.* 2006;44:788–794.
17. Schliess F, Gorg B, Haussinger D. Pathogenetic interplay between osmotic and oxidative stress: The hepatic encephalopathy paradigm. *Biol Chem.* 2006;387:1363–1370.
18. Zwingmann C, Chatauret N, Leibfritz D, et al. Selective increase of brain lactate synthesis in experimental acute liver failure: Results of a [H-C] nuclear magnetic resonance study. *Hepatology.* 2003;37:420–428.
19. Vaquero J, Chung C, Blei AT. Cerebral blood flow in acute liver failure: A finding in search of a mechanism. *Metab Brain Dis.* 2004;19:177–194.
20. Haussinger D. Low grade cerebral edema and the pathogenesis of hepatic encephalopathy in cirrhosis. *Hepatology.* 2006;43:1187–1190.

21. Donovan JP, Schafer DF, Shaw BW, Jr., et al. Cerebral oedema and increased intracranial pressure in chronic liver disease. *Lancet.* 1998;351:719–721.
22. Victor M, Adams RD, Cole M. The acquired (non-Wilsonina) type of chronic hepatocerebral degeneration. *Medicine (Baltimore).* 1965;44:345–394.
23. Burkhard PR, Delavelle J, Du Pasquier R, et al. Chronic parkinsonism associated with cirrhosis. A distinct subset of acquired hepatocerebral degeneration. *Arch Neurol.* 2003;60:521–528.
24. Weissenborn K, Tietge UJ, Bokemeyer M, et al. Liver transplantation improves hepatic myelopathy: Evidence by three cases. *Gastroenterology.* 2003;124:346–351.
25. Blei AT, Zee P. Abnormalities of circadian rhythmicity in liver disease. *J Hepatol.* 1998;29:832–835.
26. Timmermann L, Gross J, Butz M, et al. Mini-asterixis in hepatic encephalopathy induced by pathologic thalamo-motor-cortical coupling. *Neurology.* 2003;61:689–692.
27. Cordoba J, Raguer N, Flavia M, et al. T2 hyperintensity along the cortico-spinal tract in cirrhosis relates to functional abnormalities. *Hepatology.* 2003;38:1026–1033.
28. Lockwood AH, Murphy BW, Donnelly KZ, et al. Positron-emission tomographic localization of abnormalities of brain metabolism in patients with minimal hepatic encephalopathy. *Hepatology.* 1993;18:1061–1068.
29. Kril JJ, Butterworth RF. Diencephalic and cerebellar pathology in alcoholic and nonalcoholic patients with end-stage liver disease. *Hepatology.* 1997;26:837–841.
30. Atterbury CE, Maddrey W, Conn HO. Neomycin-sorbitol and lactulose in the treatment of acute portal-systemic encephalopathy. A controlled, double-blind clinical trial. *Am J Dig Dis.* 1978;23:398–406.
31. Clemmesen JO, Larsen FS, Kondrup J, et al. Cerebral herniation in patients with acute liver failure is correlated with arterial ammonia concentration. *Hepatology.* 1999;29:648–653.
32. Weissenborn K, Ennen JC, Schomerus H, et al. Neuropsychological characterization of hepatic encephalopathy. *J Hepatol.* 2001;34:768–773.
33. Romero-Gomez M, Cordoba J, Planas R, et al. A comparison of PHES and critical flicker frequency for the diagnosis of hepatic encephalopathy. *Hepatology* (in press).
34. Kircheis G, Wettstein M, Timmermann L, et al. Critical flicker frequency for quantification of low-grade hepatic encephalopathy. *Hepatology.* 2002;35:357–366.
35. Köstler H. Proton magnetic resonance spectroscopy in portal-systemic encephalopathy. *Metab Brain Dis.* 1998;13:291–301.
36. Lockwood AH, Yap EWH, Rhoades HM, et al. Altered cerebral blood flow and glucose metabolism in patients with liver disease and minimal encephalopathy. *J Cereb Blood Flow Metab.* 1991;11:331–336.
37. Lockwood AH, Weissenborn K, Bokemeyer M, et al. Correlations between cerebral glucose metabolism and neuropsychological test performance in non-alcoholic cirrhotics. *Metab Brain Dis.* 2002;17(1):29–40.
38. Lockwood AH, Yap EWH, Wong WH. Cerebral ammonia metabolism in patients with severe liver disease and minimal hepatic encephalopathy. *J Cereb Blood Flow Metab.* 1991;11:337–341.
39. Keiding S, Sorensen M, Bender D, et al. Brain metabolism of 13N-ammonia during acute hepatic encephalopathy in cirrhosis measured by positron emission tomography. *Hepatology.* 2006;43:42–50.
40. Rikkers L, Jenko P, Rudman D, et al. Subclinical hepatic encephalopathy: Detection, prevalence, and relationship to nitrogen metabolism. *Gastroenterology.* 1978;75:462–469.
41. Gilberstadt SJ, Gilberstadt H, Zieve L, et al. Psychomotor performance defects in cirrhotic patients without overt encephalopathy. *Arch Intern Med.* 1980;140:519–521.
42. Schomerus H, Hamster W, Blunck H, et al. Latent portasystemic encephalopathy: I. Nature of cerebral functional defects and their effect on fitness to drive. *Dig Dis Sci.* 1981;26:622–630.
43. Wein C, Koch H, Popp B, et al. Minimal hepatic encephalopathy impairs fitness to drive. *Hepatology.* 2004;39:739–745.
44. Groeneweg M, Quero JC, De Bruijn, et al. Subclinical hepatic encephalopathy impairs daily functioning. *Hepatology.* 1998;28:45–54.
45. Cordoba J, Cabrera J, Lataif L, et al. High prevalence of sleep disturbances in cirrhosis. *Hepatology.* 1998;27:339–345.
46. Davies MG, Rowan MJ, Feely J. EEG and event related potentials in hepatic encephalopathy. *Metab Brain Dis.* 1991;6:175–186.
47. Restuccia T, Gomez-Anson B, Guevara M, et al. Effects of dilutional hyponatremia on brain organic osmolytes and water content in patients with cirrhosis. *Hepatology.* 2004;39:1613–1622.
48. Cordoba J, Lopez-Hellin J, Planas M, et al. Normal protein diet for episodic hepatic encephalopathy: Results of a randomized study. *J Hepatol.* 2004;41:38–43.
49. Marchesini G, Bianchi G, Merli M, et al.; Italian BCAA Study Group. Nutritional supplementation with branched-chain amino acids in advanced cirrhosis: A double-blind, randomized trial. *Gastroenterology.* 2003;124:1792–1801.
50. Muto Y, Sato S, Watanabe A, et al. Effects of oral branched-chain amino acid granules on event-free survival in patients with liver cirrhosis. *Clin Gastroenterol Hepatol.* 2005;3:705–713.
51. Als-Nielsen B, Gluud LL, Gluud C. Non-absorbable disaccharides for hepatic encephalopathy: Systematic review of randomised trials. *BMJ.* 2004;328:1046. Epub 2004 Mar 30.
52. Mas A, Rodes J, Sunyer L, et al. Comparison of rifaximin and lactitol in the treatment of acute hepatic encephalopathy: Results of a randomized, double-blind, double-dummy, controlled clinical trial. *J Hepatol.* 2003;38:51–58.
53. Kircheis G, Wettstein M, Dahl S, et al. Clinical efficacy of L-ornithine-L-aspartate in the management of hepatic encephalopathy. *Metab Brain Dis.* 2002;17:453–462.
54. Als-Nielsen B, Gluud LL, Gluud C. Benzodiazepine receptor antagonists for hepatic encephalopathy. *Cochrane Database Syst Rev.* 2004;(2):CD002798.
55. Crespin J, Nemcek A, Rehkemper G, et al. Intrahepatic portal-hepatic venous anastomosis: A portal-systemic shunt with neurological repercussions. *Am J Gastroenterol.* 2000;95:1568–1571.

CHAPTER **45**

Liver Transplantation

Saša Živković • Peter K. Linden

OBJECTIVE

- To describe the pathogenesis, clinical spectrum, and diagnostic approach to neurologic complications of liver transplantation

CASE VIGNETTE

A 26-year-old man who had liver transplantation 2 months ago was found to be confused and stuporous. Primary liver failure was related to autoimmune hepatitis and alcohol cirrhosis. Postoperative course was complicated by renal failure and *Escherichia coli* sepsis, and required prolonged stay in the intensive care unit. Electromyography (EMG) was suggestive of critical illness myopathy, but a muscle biopsy had not been done. Laboratory testing showed borderline low level of tacrolimus (4.5 ng/mL; normal 5 to 20 ng/mL). On examination, he was arousable and followed commands with difficulty. Brainstem reflexes were preserved. A diffuse weakness (Medical Research Council of the U. K. [MRC] 4/5) was noted with areflexia, but no abnormal movements. Magnetic resonance imaging (MRI) of the brain showed T1 hyperintensities in basal ganglia and T2 hyperintensity in the mid pons (Fig. 45-1).

This case illustrates two important complications of liver transplantation, namely, impaired consciousness and diffuse weakness.

DEFINITION

Neurologic complications of liver transplantation can develop at any time following the procedure and are of varied etiology. A simple, but useful, classification is to divide the complications into *early*, developing within the first month, and *late*, developing at any time thereafter. Complications may be specific to transplantation, but also can include conditions common to any major surgical procedure.

EPIDEMIOLOGY

More than 6,400 liver transplantations were performed in 2005 in United States. The most common indications for liver transplantation in adults in the United States are chronic hepatitis C, alcoholic cirrhosis (or both), autoimmune hepatitis, primary biliary cirrhosis, primary sclerosing cholangitis, and, in pediatric population, primary biliary atresia and α-1 antitrypsin deficiency. Acute liver failure is most commonly caused by acetaminophen and other idiosyncratic drug toxicities. Neurologic complications affect 30% to 60% of solid organ transplant recipients, but usually do not independently affect the outcome (except for fungal central nervous system [CNS] infections) (1,2).

ETIOLOGY AND PATHOGENESIS

The etiology of most of the posttransplant neurologic disorders generally varies over the course of time following transplantation. In the early phase, postsurgical complications, metabolic disorders, anoxic encephalopathy, and toxic effects of medications are the dominant conditions contributing to neurologic disability (Table 45-1). At times more remote from the transplantation procedure, opportunistic infections become the major cause of neurologic complications. Chronic high immunosuppressive requirements increase the risk of opportunistic infections that can involve CNS after bone marrow and solid organ transplantation. The risk of infection is also determined by the intensity of prior and current epidemiologic exposure to pathogens and the type, duration, and dose of immunosuppression (3).

CLINICAL MANIFESTATIONS

EARLY POSTTRANSPLANT COMPLICATIONS

Coma or Failure to Awaken

An altered level of consciousness is the most common neurologic problem encountered in the early phase following the liver transplantation. This issue can be divided into delayed awakening after the transplantation itself or *de novo* presentation after initial recovery. Etiology includes cyclosporin or tacrolimus toxicity, metabolic encephalopathy (hepatic failure, hyperglycemia, hypoglycemia, uremia, delayed excretion or metabolism of anesthetic agents), intracerebral bleeding, hypoxic-ischemic encephalopathy, or central pontine myelinolysis (4).

Calcineurin Inhibitor Toxicity

In the early postoperative recovery period, the use of higher doses of calcineurin inhibitors increases the risk of neurotoxicity, especially with intravenous dosing, manifesting with encephalopathy, akinetic mutism, and speech apraxia (5).

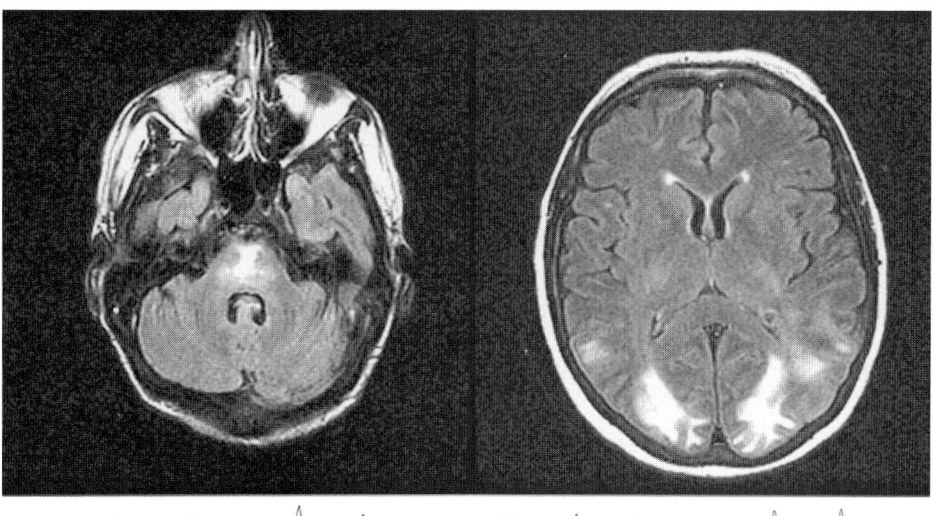

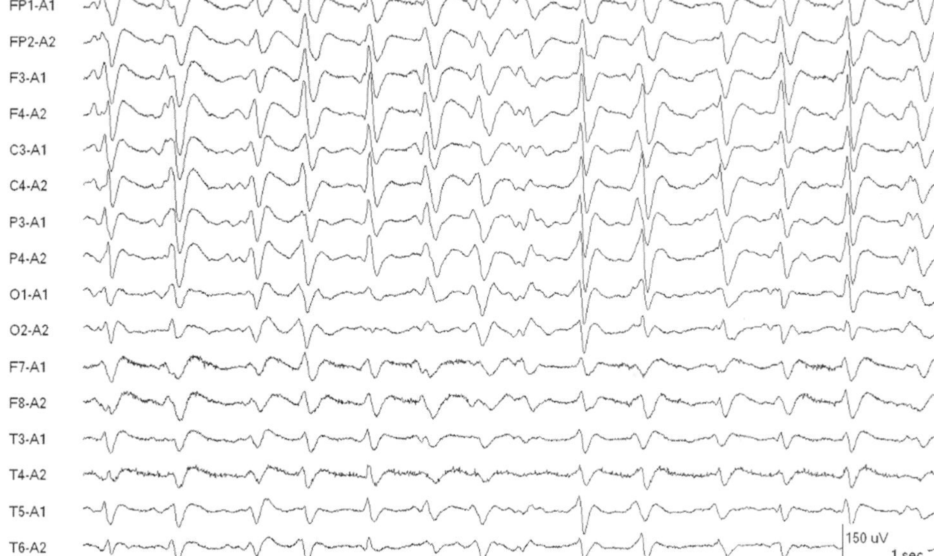

FIGURE 45-1. **Top left:** Central pontine myelinolysis: Hyperintense signal on magnetic resonance imaging (MRI) FLAIR images in mid pons. **Top right**: Posterior reversible leukoencephalopathy syndrome (PRES) related to tacrolimus neurotoxicity: Hyperintense signal on MRI FLAIR images in posterior white matter bilaterally. **Bottom:** Triphasic waves are typical electroencephalogram (EEG) finding in hepatic encephalopathy (Courtesy of Dr. R. Brenner).

Although calcineurin inhibitor neurotoxicity is more common in the acute perioperative period, it can also occur later at any other time after transplantation. Other medications can also precipitate alteration of consciousness, especially with delayed graft function and the use of sedating medications metabolized by the liver, such as benzodiazepines. Hepatic encephalopathy after liver transplantation can occur in the context of delayed graft function, severe rejection, or technical complications leading to posttransplant hepatic failure.

Other Drug Toxicity

Liver transplant recipients are at risk of drug toxicity from hepatic or renal insufficiency leading to impaired excretion or metabolism or as a result of complex drug–drug interactions. Different medications (azoles, macrolides, diltiazem) can raise the levels of calcineurin inhibitors, thus increasing the risk of neurotoxicity or unwanted enhanced immunosuppression. Serotonin syndrome is also described with concomitant use of linezolid and serotonin-uptake inhibitor antidepressants. Other commonly used drugs in the posttransplant period leading to an altered mental status include metoclopramide, haloperidol, acyclovir, foscarnet, imipenem-cilastatin, and the quinolones.

Hepatic Insufficiency

Delayed graft functioning or graft failure can manifest with hepatic encephalopathy that cannot be distinguished clinically from pretransplant hepatic failure. Associated signs of liver allograft dysfunction should be manifest, including poor bile production, hyperbilirubinemia, impaired coagulation, persistent hyperlactemia, and renal failure. Intracranial hypertension caused by cerebral edema, a common complication of acute liver failure, is usually not present in delayed graft function in the absence of intra- or postoperative cerebral hypoperfusion. Abnormal hepatic function will also affect metabolism of numerous medications metabolized by the liver.

Central Pontine Myelinolysis

Pretransplant hepatic failure is frequently associated with fluid overload and hyponatremia caused by compromised renal water

TABLE 45-1. Risk Factors for Neurologic Complications After Liver Transplantation

CENTRAL PONTINE MYELINOLYSIS
Chronic hyponatremia (with rapid correction)
CALCINEURIN INHIBITOR NEUROTOXICITY (TACROLIMUS, CYCLOSPORIN)
Intravenous use, high serum levels or sudden increases in serum levels
Hypomagnesemia
CENTRAL NERVOUS SYSTEM (CNS) INFECTIONS
Higher immunosuppression requirements
Nosocomial epidemic exposures (aspergillosis, other mycelial fungi)
Endemic exposures (e.g., coccidioidomycosis in southwestern United States)
Infectious agents from food (e.g., Listeria—raw milk, soft cheese)
INTRACRANIAL HEMORRHAGE
Coagulopathy (severe fibrinolysis, poor graft function, thrombocytopenia)
Systemic or CNS infection
CRITICAL ILLNESS MYOPATHY OR POLYNEUROPATHY
Use of corticosteroids and neuromuscular junction blockers
Multiple organ failure, sepsis

excretion and aggressive use of diuretics. Rapid correction of hyponatremia during the intraoperative or early postoperative period can increase the risk for central pontine myelinolysis (CPM) that can manifest with pseudobulbar palsy, weakness, and stupor.

Weakness

Diffuse or focal weakness can occur at any time after liver transplantation—of either central or peripheral origin. Sudden onset of focal weakness can be related to ischemic stroke or intracerebral hemorrhage. Focal lower motor neuron weakness with hyporeflexia can be related to postoperative mononeuropathies, and a few patients may develop brachial plexopathy, which may be secondary to injury from prolonged arm abduction or axillary dissection for placement of the bypass cannulae. Prolonged stay in the intensive care unit with use of corticosteroids and neuromuscular junction blocking agents can precipitate diffuse weakness caused by critical illness myopathy or neuropathy (6). Spastic paraparesis caused by spinal cord compression can be related to epidural abscess or hematoma, or hepatic myelopathy.

Neuromuscular Complications

Postoperatively, liver transplant recipients may develop mononeuropathies or brachial plexopathy. The use of neuromuscular junction blocking agents and corticosteroids can precipitate diffuse weakness caused by critical illness myopathy or neuropathy (6). Critical illness myopathy and polyneuropathy are also associated with protracted sepsis and multiple organ failure. Definite diagnosis of critical illness myopathy is established with muscle biopsy showing myosin depletion (6).

Cerebrovascular Complications

Cerebrovascular complications are relatively rare in liver transplant recipients Intracerebral hemorrhage occurs usually in the setting of severe coagulopathy or infections, whereas ischemic strokes may be associated with hypotension (*watershed infarcts*) and cardiac embolism (endocarditis, atrial fibrillation).

Seizures

New occurrence of seizures after liver transplantation is frequently related to immunosuppressant neurotoxicity and is usually not associated with CNS infection or structural lesions (7). Seizures related to calcineurin inhibitor neurotoxicity frequently originate from posterior brain regions, similarly to neuroimaging changes in posterior reversible encephalopathy syndrome.

Abnormal Movements

Involuntary movements can occur in the context of ongoing seizures related to a mass lesion, CNS infection, or, more commonly, with immunosuppressant neurotoxicity. Asterixis is seen with hepatic insufficiency, and tremor is a common side effect of calcineurin inhibitors (5). Cirrhosis can be also associated with parkinsonism that may improve following the transplantation.

LATE POSTTRANSPLANT COMPLICATIONS

Opportunistic Infections

Opportunistic CNS infections are more common 1 month or later after transplantation, but can occur at any time. The spectrum of pathogens has a temporal pattern in the posttransplant period, which may vary because of variance in epidemiologic, iatrogenic, and other host factors (3). Herpesvirus-related infections are mostly caused by cytomegalovirus (CMV), which usually occur between the first and sixth month, although CMV encephalitis is a rare occurrence. Herpes simplex virus, human herpesviruses (6,8) and Epstein-Barr virus (EBV) are less common pathogens from this family that can sporadically cause encephalitis or EBV-mediated B-cell postransplant lymphoproliferative disorder (PTLD). Progressive multifocal leukoencephalopathy caused by JC papovavirus is a very rare, demyelinating condition that is almost uniformly fatal. Aspergillosis, the most common CNS fungal pathogen, may occur early in the nosocomial setting or because of community exposure later in the posttransplant period (8). Concurrent pulmonary infection is common because this is the portal of entry for the organism. Cryptococcal meningitis occurs usually in the late posttransplant period beyond 6 months (9). Fungal CNS infections are associated with a high mortality in the range of 90%, highlighting the need for a timely and accurate diagnosis. Other causes of CNS infections after liver transplantation include *Listeria monocytogenes*, *Nocardia* spp., *Mycobacterium tuberculosis*, *Toxoplasmosis gondii*, and varicella-zoster virus. Patients with endemic exposures are also at risk of less common infections (e.g. coccidioidomycosis).

Malignancies

Transplant recipients have overall higher frequency of malignant tumors, especially skin cancers and Kaposi sarcoma. Systemic

PTLD affects 3% of liver allograft recipients and may involve the CNS in 20% of affected patients. PTLD is frequently associated with either primary or reactivated EBV infection and is more common in pediatric and adult EBV-seronegative recipients. Gliomas are also more common in transplant recipients, but the overall frequency remains low (10).

DIAGNOSTIC APPROACH

Diagnostic approach to neurologic complications after liver transplantations is based on obtaining a comprehensive history and clinical examination followed by laboratory testing, neuroimaging, and electrodiagnostic studies directed at the differential diagnosis (Table 45-2). Neuroimaging studies are important in the evaluation of focal or diffuse processes associated with neurologic complications and often direct the subsequent diagnostics. MRI of brain and spine offers superior signal resolution and is the procedure of choice in most liver transplant recipients. Cranial computed tomography (CT) may be helpful as well, particularly to rule out intracerebral hemorrhage acutely. MRI of brain is also helpful to confirm calcineurin-inhibitor toxicity typically manifesting with hyperintensities on T2-weighted images with bilateral posterior white matter involvement and sparing of the calcarine and paramedian occipital lobe regions (Fig. 45-1) (5). Additionally, imaging abnormalities may be seen in basal ganglia, cerebellum, brainstem or cortex. Contrast-enhanced MRI is superior to CT in identifying ring-enhancing abscesses or other mass lesions, and in establishing the presence of pontine or extrapontine myelinolysis. Cerebrospinal fluid analysis is needed to establish the presence and microbial etiology of suspected CNS infection, although lumbar puncture may not be necessary in patients with disseminated fungal infections (11). Serum levels of tacrolimus or cyclosporine may be helpful in determining the cause of unexplained encephalopathy or other new neurologic symptoms. Calcineurin inhibitor toxicity can occur even with *therapeutic* levels, however, particularly in the setting of hypomagnesemia or a sudden level change. An arterial ammonia level should be checked in suspected hepatic encephalopathy because of allograft insufficiency; however, the clinical correlation may be poor. Electroencephalography (EEG) might be helpful in the evaluation of altered consciousness. Hepatic encephalopathy is typically associated with triphasic waves (Fig. 45-1) and these are also found with other toxic-metabolic encephalopathies. *Triphasic-like* waves, however, can be seen in nonconvulsive status epilepticus (NCSE), and careful evaluation is needed to distinguish between NCSE and toxic-metabolic encephalopathy (12). Continuous EEG monitoring can be used in the critical care setting in patients with suspected subclinical (electrographic) status epilepticus or poorly controlled seizures. Hepatic and renal insufficiency (or failure), dialysis, and drug–drug interactions can significantly alter the levels of antiepileptic drugs (AED). It is advisable to follow free levels of AED with significant protein binding because the total serum drug level may not provide adequate information. A potential pitfall is the change of EEG pattern and disappearance of some discharges in toxic-metabolic encephalopathy after benzodiazepine use, which can be misdiagnosed as a seizure disorder and is related to a change in the state of wakefulness. Needle EMG and nerve conduction studies are helpful to document nerve entrapments and brachial plexopathy, or critical illness myopathy or polyneuropathy. Stereotactic or open brain biopsy may be needed to establish the underlying cause of mass lesions, which are most often caused by invasive fungal infection or CNS PTLD.

TABLE 45-2. Suggested Investigations in Liver Allograft Recipients

1. Review the primary liver disease and previous neurologic complications
2. Review the course of transplantation and its potential surgical and perioperative complications
3. Review possible opportunistic infection and consider lumbar puncture
   a. Consider endemic exposures
   b. Consider testing for systemic infection
4. Review potential drug side-effects (e.g., tacrolimus, cyclosporin)
5. Laboratory testing including drug levels

CENTRAL NERVOUS SYSTEM SIGNS AND SYMPTOMS

1. Cerebropinal fluid studies (other studies may also be appropriate in individual patients)
   a. Gram stain, India ink
   b. Cultures: Bacterial, fungal, viral, mycobacterial
   c. Other: Herpes simplex virus polymerase chain reaction (HSV PCR), cryptococcal antigen, toxoplasma antibody titers, PCR for mycobacteria
2. Consider electroencephalogram (EEG)
3. Consider neuroimaging studies
   a. Preferably magnetic resonance imaging (MRI) of brain or spinal cord (consider use of gadolinium)

PERIPHERAL NERVOUS SYSTEM SIGNS AND SYMPTOMS

1. Consider electromyography and nerve conduction studies
2. Consider autonomic testing
3. Consider nerve or muscle biopsy

(Modified from Pless M, Zivkovic SA. Neurologic complications of transplantation. *Neurologist.* 2002;8(2):107–120, with permission.)

TREATMENT

Treatment options for neurologic complications of liver transplantation vary from general supportive measures, immunosuppression withdrawal (calcineurin toxicity, PTLD), to specific therapies usually directed at CNS infections, which may include surgical drainage. The timely treatment of opportunistic CNS and systemic infections in transplant recipients is of paramount importance. Although specific treatment is ideal, broad empiric coverage may be necessary in the early phase as the diagnostic workup is proceeding. Thus, suspected meningitis requires coverage for *Listeria* (ampicillin), *Streptococcus pneumoniae* (ceftriaxone, vancomycin), and multiresistant gram-negatives (cefepime, meropenem) until Gram stain and culture results are available. Coverage for cryptoccal meningitis should include conventional or lipid formulations of amphotericin B plus 5-flucytosine. Patients with unexplained enhancing mass lesions are most likely to have a mycelial infection, usually *Aspergillus* spp., which requires voriconazole with or without a second antifungal (caspofungin, amphotericin B). The management of neurologic complications related to liver allograft dysfunction is supportive and coupled to the management plan for the allograft. This can include just allowing time for allograft recovery from severe preservation injury or the appropriate management of sepsis, rejection, or technical complications. Improvement in encephalopathy may sometimes only occur following liver retransplantation for refractory complications in the first allograft. Neurotoxicity of cyclosporine or tacrolimus may be lessened with switching to the alternative calcineurin inhibitor or another immunosuppressant. Reducing immunosuppression may be helpful; however, this also depends on the level host-to-graft tolerance on a case-by-case basis. Emergent inpatient treatment of seizures in transplant recipients does not differ significantly from that used in other patients. In outpatient settings, however, consider complex drug–drug interactions, potential side effects, and hepatorenal function. In most transplant patients with normal kidney function, therefore, consider using gabapentin or levetiracetam as maintenance AED. In patients with kidney insufficiency, dose of gabapentin and levetiracetam need to be adjusted and other hepatically metabolized medications, such as phenytoin, can be used. Long-term treatment with anticonvulsants is usually not needed for seizures related to cyclosporine or tacrolimus neurotoxicity. Treatment of critical illness myopathy and polyneuropathy consists of physical and occupational therapy, and the recovery may be slow.

CLINICAL RECOMMENDATIONS OF THE VIGNETTE

The patient illustrates the complexity of multiple simultaneous medical problems in liver transplant recipients. Neuroimaging findings are consistent with central pontine myelinolysis, which can occur in liver transplant recipients in the absence of rapid correction of hyponatremia. Clinical presentation usually includes quadriparesis and pseudobulbar palsy, but it can present with stupor only. The onset of CPM can be difficult to determine and critical illness myopathy or polyneuropathy might have overshadowed its symptoms. The patient did not have a history of rapid sodium correction. Sodium correction in liver allograft recipients should be performed at a slow rate (<9 mEq over first 24 hours) to decrease the risk of CPM (1). The use of corticosteroids and neuromuscular junction blockers in intensive care units should also be restricted to limit the occurrence of critical illness myopathy or polyneuropathy.

SUMMARY

Neurologic complications are a significant source of morbidity, prolonged hospitalization, and mortality in liver allograft recipients. The complex medical milieu of the liver recipient includes multiple medications, sepsis and multiorgan failure, opportunistic infection, and metabolic-toxic events that can make an early discrete diagnosis a most challenging endeavor. A careful assessment of the patient's epidemiologic risks (native disease and iatrogenic exposures) can increase the efficiency of the diagnostic process. Calcineurin inhibitor neurotoxicity is most common in the early posttransplant period and improves after decreasing the dose or after a switch to another immunosuppressant. Opportunistic CNS infections should be considered as a potential cause of unexplained neurologic complications and lumbar puncture may be needed. CPM, relatively common in liver transplant recipients, can occur in the absence of rapid correction of hyponatremia. Complicated postoperative course and prolonged recovery can lead to critical illness myopathy or polyneuropathy. Electrodiagnostic (EEG, EMG) and neuroimaging studies are helpful in determining the underlying cause of decreased responsiveness or unexplained weakness.

REFERENCES

1. Bronster DJ, Emre S, Boccagni P, et al. Central nervous system complications in liver transplant recipients—Incidence, timing, and long-term follow-up. *Clin Transplant.* 2000;14(1):1–7.
2. Pless M, Zivkovic SA. Neurologic complications of transplantation. *Neurologist.* 2002;8(2):107–120.
3. Fishman JA, Rubin RH. Infection in organ-transplant recipients. *N Engl J Med.* 1998;338(24):1741–1751.
4. Wijdicks EF. Impaired consciousness after liver transplantation. *Liver Transpl Surg.* 1995;1(5):329–334.
5. Wijdicks EF. Neurotoxicity of immunosuppressive drugs. *Liver Transpl.* 2001;7(11):937–942.
6. Campellone JV, Lacomis D, Kramer DJ, et al. Acute myopathy after liver transplantation. *Neurology.* 1998;50(1):46–53.
7. Wijdicks EF, Plevak DJ, Wiesner RH, et al. Causes and outcome of seizures in liver transplant recipients. *Neurology.* 1996;47(6):1523–1525.
8. Singh N, Avery RK, Munoz P, et al. Trends in risk profiles for and mortality associated with invasive aspergillosis among liver transplant recipients. *Clin Infect Dis.* 2003;36(1):46–52.
9. Wu G, Vilchez RA, Eidelman B, et al. Cryptococcal meningitis: An analysis among 5,521 consecutive organ transplant recipients. *Transpl Infect Dis.* 2002;4(4):183–188.
10. Schiff D, O'Neill B, Wijdicks E, et al. Gliomas arising in organ transplant recipients: An unrecognized complication of transplantation? *Neurology.* 2001;57(8):1486–1488.
11. Bonham CA, Dominguez EA, Fukui MB, et al. Central nervous system lesions in liver transplant recipients: Prospective assessment of indications for biopsy and implications for management. *Transplantation.* 1998;66(12):1596–1604.
12. Brenner RP. The interpretation of the EEG in stupor and coma. *Neurologist.* 2005;11(5):271–284.

CHAPTER **46**

Commonly Used Liver Drugs

Andrew Silverman • David R. Chabolla

OBJECTIVES

- To estimate the incidence and identify risk factors for drug-induced neurologic complications in patients with varying levels of liver disease
- To discuss how changes in drug clearance and pharmacokinetic issues related to various stages of liver disease increase the risk of neurotoxicity from medications
- To describe the clinical manifestations of drug-induced neurotoxicity at the earliest possible time, to minimize the long-term effects on patient outcomes
- To discuss the most appropriate diagnostic tests used to identify drug-induced neurotoxicity
- To describe treatment options when drug-induced neurotoxicity is identified.

CASE VIGNETTE

A 52-year-old man had received an orthotopic liver transplant (OLT) because of hepatitis C virus (HCV) cirrhosis. On the third postoperative day, he became confused late in the evening. He received tacrolimus dose number 4 at 0500 hours on the fourth postoperative day, and became aphasic later that day. Cranial computed tomography (CT) scan was normal. Cerebrospinal fluid (CSF) analysis was unremarkable. A brain magnetic resonance imaging (MRI) was not done. On day 5, his neurologic status became worse, and he was unresponsive, except to deep painful stimuli. Tacrolimus was stopped on day 4. Highest level was 14 ng/mL. Serum sodium day of transplant went from 133 to 144 in 12 hours. He was switched to cyclosporine on postoperative day 6, and showed improvement on day 7.

DEFINITION

The liver and the nervous system are closely linked from a pharmacologic perspective. Drugs used in the treatment of neurologic disorders can have an impact on liver function. Pharmacologic agents introduced to maintain liver function can become neurotoxic in the presence of liver failure, and impaired clearance of substances can have deleterious effects on both the liver and the nervous system. Few randomized, prospective clinical trials have evaluated the incidence, causes, risk factors, and causality of the relationship between drugs, liver, and brain neurotoxicity related to medications in liver disease. It is usually a diagnosis of exclusion based on symptoms, temporal relationship of the drug to the patient, and pharmacokinetic and pharmacodynamic principles. Most pharmacologic agents have the potential of inducing hepato-and neurotoxicity. From a practical perspective, it appropriate to focus on three important classes of drugs: Immunosuppressants, antibiotics, and anticonvulsants.

EPIDEMIOLOGY

IMMUNOSUPPRESSANTS

Neurotoxicity from calcineurin inhibitors (CNI) occurs in 7% to 22% for severe toxicities, such as change in mental status, dysarthria, seizures, mutism, leukoencephalopathy, central pontene myelinolysis, and coma. Less severe neurologic complications, such as tremor, peripheral neuropathies, mood changes, headache, and insomnia occur in 20% to 60% of patients (1–4). The incidence of adverse neurologic effects may be as high as 70% in patients on high-dose steroids (5,6).

ANTIBIOTICS

Ciprofloxacin and norfloxacin are commonly used for treatment and prophylaxis of spontaneous bacterial peritonitis, and levofloxacin is commonly used for treatment of posttransplant community-acquired pneumonia. More common central nervous system (CNS) side effects occur in 1% to 22% of patients. Serious CNS toxicity occurs in <1% of patients (7–9). Levofloxacin may have the lowest incidence (8). In one series, 20 of 75 (27%) courses of lactulose administration showed increases in serum sodium levels >145 mEq/L. Mortality was 41% in patients who developed hypernatremia versus 14% in patients with normal serum sodium (10).

ANTIEPILEPTIC DRUGS

Antiepileptic drugs (AED) are commonly used in the management of seizure disorders, pain syndromes, mood and behavior disorders, and headaches. In patients with liver disease, differentiation between AED-induced neurotoxicity from other sources of encephalopathy, neurotoxicity, or seizures themselves may be difficult.

ETIOLOGY AND PATHOGENESIS

GENERAL PRINCIPLES

Drug-related neurotoxicity in patients with liver failure can result from decreased total body clearance, decreased hepatic cell mass, shunting of blood away from functioning hepatocytes, decreased protein binding secondary to decreased serum albumin levels, increased volume of distribution, pharmacodynamic drug–drug interactions, and decreased function of the cytochrome P450 (CYP 450) enzyme system (11). Unlike renal function studies, no simple tests can identify appropriate clearance of drugs by the liver. Large inter- and intrapatient variability are seen in the expression of CYP 450 enzymes in patients with liver disease. It does appear that clearance decreases as liver failure worsens (11–13). Patients will have significant risk from medications that cause CNS toxicities, such as narcotics, AED, benzodiazepines, anticholinerics, and antidepressants. Understanding which drugs have impaired hepatic clearance requires understanding of phase I and phase II metabolic pathways, and for which pathways the medications are substrates (11) (Table 46-1).

TABLE 46-1. Effect of Liver Cirrhosis on Phase I and Phase II Drug Metabolism Enzymes

Enzyme	*Species*	*Effect*	*Protein/mRNA/ Activity*
CYP1A	Human	↓	mRNA, protein, activity
	Rat	↓	Protein, activity
	Rat	↔	Activity
CYP2A6	Human	↓	Activity
CYP2B	Human	↔	Activity
	Rat	↓	mRNA, protein, activity
CYP2C	Human	↓	mRNA, protein, activity
	Human	↔	Protein
	Rat	↓	Protein, activity
CYP2EI	Human	↓	mRNA, protein, activity
	Rat	↔	Protein, activity
	Rat	↓	Protein, activity
CYP3A	Human	↓	mRNA, protein, activity
	Rat	↓	Protein, activity
XO	Human	↔	Serum level/activity
	Human	↓	Serum activity
	Human	↑ virus effected ↔ nonviral	Activity
ALDH	Human	↓ Total low *km* ↔ high *km*	Activity
	Human	↔ nonalcoholic ↓ alcoholic	Activity
ADH	Human	↓ alcoholic ↔ nonalcoholic	Activity
		↓	Activity
		↔	Activity
UGT	Human	↔	mRNA, activity
	Human	↑in whole cell	Protein
	Rat	↑	mRNA, protein
SULT	Human	↓	Protein, activity
GST	Human	↔	Serum activity
	Rat	↓	Activity

mRNA, messenger RNA.
(From Elbekai RH, Hesham M, Korashy M, et al. The effects of liver cirrhosis on the regulation and expression of drug metabolizing enzymes. *Curr Drug Metab.* 2004;5:157–167, with permission.)

Inflammation is an ongoing issue in chronic active liver disease, the cirrhotic liver, and in primary nonfunction after liver transplantation. This can lead to accumulation of cytokines because of decreased clearance. Cytokines inhibit the effects of many CYP-450 enzymes related to decreased messenger RNA (mRNA) expression, decreased protein levels, their effect on nuclear factor-$\kappa\beta$, or by stimulating nitric oxide. Nitric oxide can decrease CYP-450 activity by binding directly to the protein and causing ligation, or by other mechanisms. Alcoholic liver disease can decrease CYP-450 activity by additional mechanisms, including increased free radicals and lipid peroxidation markers (11–13).

IMMUNOSUPPRESSANTS

CN-related seizures can result from inhibition of the γ-aminobutyric acid (GABA) system; delirium and tremors may be related to their depletion of presynaptic serotonin and CNI inhibition of glutaminerigic or *N*-methyl-d-aspartate (NMDA) receptors. Immunophylins, including FKBP-12, FKBP-52, and cyclophilin, and effects on calcineurin, in the CNS may play a key role in neurotoxicities. This can lead to increased concentrations of calcineurin susbstrates in neural tissues caused by inhibition of this calcium-mediated pathway. Steroids and CNI can have additive or synergistic effects via this mechanism (14–16). Risk factors for CNI neurotoxicity include hypertension, hypocholesterolemia, hypomagnesemia, history of seizure disorder, renal failure, hyponatremia before transplant, and elevated CNI trough levels (1,4,15,17,18).

The relationship between CNI levels and toxicity is not clear. Concomitant medications that increase CNI levels significantly increase the risk of neurotoxicity via CYP-450 inhibition or other mechanisms (Table 46-2). An increased risk for toxicity exists when levels are elevated, but many patients have severe neurotoxicities with therapeutic CNI trough levels (1–3,15,17). Tacrolimus and its metabolites, and cyclosporine and most of its metabolites are cleared via the biliary system, and this can be impaired in a slowly recovering liver, increasing the risk of neurotoxicity (19,20). Metabolites of cyclosporine have been bound in CSF fluid, but their role in CNI-neurotoxicity is unclear (21). Both CNI are highly bound to red blood cells, with tacrolimus approximately 70% to 90%, and cyclosporine 41% to 58%. Tacrolimus, is highly bound to albumin and α1 acid glycoprotein. Cyclosporine is approximately 90% bound to circulating lipoproteins. This binding is concentration, pH, and temperature dependent (20,21). CNI blood levels are troughs, and it is possible that C_{max}, free drug concentration, or measurements of metabolites, may be better predictors.

High-dose intravenous methylprednisolone results in competitive inhibition of CYP-450 3A4 because both CNI and methylprednisolone are CYP-450 3A4 subsubstrates (11,13). This can lead to rapid increases in CNI levels within the first few doses. Increases in the levels of methylprednisolone and prednisolone can occur, further increasing the risk of neurotoxicity (6). This may be more prominent in the liver transplant recipient because CYP-450 activity may be slow to recover at the same time that high doses of intravenous methylprednisolone are being used. This makes it difficult to predict the correct starting dose of CNI in the perioperative liver transplant recipient.

TABLE 46-2. Common Drugs Affecting CYP P450 System

Drug	*Inhibitor*	*Inducer*
Ketoconazole (KZ), Fluconazole (FZ), Itraconazole (IZ), Voriconazole (VZ), Posiconazole (PZ)	KZ (3A4/5, 2C19), FZ (2C9, 3A4/5), IZ (3A4/5), VZ (2C9, 3A4/5), PZ (3A4/5	
Erythromycin, Clarithromycin, Azithromycin[a]	3A4/5	
Omeprazole, Lansoprazole	2C19	
Metronidazole	3A4/5, 2C9	
Sertraline (ST), Fluvoxamine (FLV), Fluoxetine (FLX)	ST 3A4/5, FLV (1A2, 2C9), FLX (2C19, 2D6)	
Amiodarone	3A4/5, 2D6, 2C9	
Verapamil, Diltiazem, Nicardipine	3A4/5	
Levofloxacin (LFX), Ciprofloxacin (CPX), Norfloxacin (NFX)	CPX (1A2, 3A4/5[b]) NFX (1A2, 3A4/5[b])	
Rifampin (RIF), Rifabutin (RIB), Carbamazepine (CBZ), Phenobarbital (PB), phenytoin (PHT) Isoniazid (INH)	INH (3A4/5, 2C9)	RIF (1A2, 2B6, 2C19, 2C9, PB (2B6, 3A4/5), RIB (3A4/5), PHT (2C9, 3A4/5) CBZ (2C19, 3A4/5)
Dexamethasone		2D6, 3A4/5
Methylprednisolone	3A4/5	
Grapefruit Juice (GPF)		
St. John's Wart (SJW)	GPF (3A4/5)	SJW (3A4/5)

[a]Competitive inhibition with tacrolimus.
[b]Weak inhibitor or inducer.

ANTIBIOTICS

Fluoroquinolone-induced CNS toxicities are dose dependent. Age, decreased renal clearance, arteriosclerosis, and a damaged blood–brain barrier can increase the risk (9). Their ability to inhibit GABA receptors is thought to be the reason for the CNS effects. Previous seizure disorders, anoxia, renal dysfunction, metabolic disturbances, such as hypomagnesemia, and concomitant use with other proconvulsant agents can increase the risk of seizures (7,9). Loop diuretics have been shown to cause ototoxicity, which is related to edema of the stria vascularis in the cochlear duct. Both intravenous and oral administration can cause ototoxicity. It is usually transient but a few reports have been made of permanent ototoxicity. Higher doses and infusion rates of 15 to 25 mg/minute are more likely to cause ototoxicity, and infusion of furosemide at 4 mg/minute can reduce the incidence (22,23). When given in large doses, lactulose—a complex sugar—can cause an osmotic gradient in the gastrointestinal tract drawing water greater than sodium, this leads to contraction of the extracellular fluid volume and hypernatremia (10). Neomycin is an aminoglycoside-like antibiotic that can cause both irreversible ototoxicity and neuromuscular blockade (NMB). The risk of NMB is greatest when neomycin is used with nondepolarizing muscle relaxants (24). Large doses of metronidazole and long duration of treatment are risk factors for neuropathy, which places the patient with liver failure at high risk (25).

ANTIEPILEPTIC DRUGS

Newer AED topiramate, gabapentin, levetiracetam, and pregabalin have little to no hepatic metabolism or protein binding and do not induce or inhibit hepatic enzymes. Dose-dependent neurotoxicity, including idiosyncratic reactions related to AED administration, is common in patients with preexisting hepatic or renal dysfunction (26,27). Serum protein alterations in liver disease will increase the concentration of active free (non–protein-bound) drug, increasing the risk of neurotoxicity. Phenytoin (PHT), carbamazepine, and valproic acid (VPA) will display normal total serum drug concentrations, but have high free drug concentrations. Gabapentin, levetiracetam, and pregabalin are eliminated renally, and dosing adjustments are needed in patients with hepatorenal syndrome or other causes of renal dysfunction (26,27). Phenobarbital (PB) is not highly protein bound, but needs dosage reductions in hepatic impairment (28). Topiramate, lamotrigine, and oxcarbazepine are eliminated by both renal and non-renal methods, and careful dosing should occur (29). CYP-450 inducers carbamazepine, oxcarbazepine, PB, and PHT can cause clinically relevant drug interactions, including decreased CNI (cyclosporine, tacrolimus) and corticosteroid blood levels. There can be a delayed effect of up to 10 days, which can lead to rejection in liver transplant recipients if not recognized (19,26,–29) (Table 46-2). Valproate sodium produces a less significant reduction in CNI levels. Other CYP-450 drug interactions can occur with many drugs that are substrates for this enzyme system (29).

PATHOLOGY

IMMUNOSUPPRESSANTS

The cause of paraneoplastic limbic encephalitis (PLE) and central pontine myelinolysis (CPM) may be direct toxic effects of CNI on vascular endothelial cells in the nervous system secondary to release of endothelin, prostacyclin, and thromboxane. This leads to cerebral vasoconstriction and vasospasm, causing decreased cerebral blood flow, and then white matter edema occurs. Focal necrosis suggesting damage to the blood–brain barrier also occurs (15,17). Occipital white matter seems to be more sensitive to CNI effects, but gray–white junctions in the parietal and occipital lobes are also affected. MRI studies show cortical hyperintensity on T2 images (15,30). Neurologic effects of steroids can result from downregulation of glucocorticoid receptors on the hippocampus after exposure to high levels of endogenous or exogenous steroids (5,6).

ANTIBIOTICS

Horlen et al. (31) reported a patient with metronidazole-related MRI changes showing increased signal intensity in the inferior basal ganglia lateral to the hypothalamus, and all around the fourth ventricle.

ANTIEPILEPTIC DRUGS

Most of the neurotoxicity effects are dose dependent and reversible, although some effects are irreversible. Chronic phenytoin exposure does produce cerebellar atrophy and can lead to clinically significant unsteadiness in the elderly (32). Chronic phenytoin use can also produce a peripheral neuropathy manifested by reduced ankle reflexes and reduced sensation in the feet. Carbamazepine and oxcarbazepine can produce hyponatremia that can lead to mental status changes, dizziness, headache, and nausea, which may mimic drug-induced neurotoxicity and lead to seizures (33).

CLINICAL MANIFESTATIONS

IMMUNOSUPPRESSANTS

Calcineurin inhibitors can cause restlessness, insomnia, acute manic syndrome, fine tremors of the upper extremities, headaches, paresthesias, peripheral neuropathies, ataxia, mutism, dysarthria, an upper motor neuron type of weakness, confusion, acute psychosis, hallucinations, delirium, cortical blindness, posterior leukoencephalopathy, seizures, and coma (1–3,15–18). Signs and symptoms of OKT3 neurotoxicity include aseptic meningitis, cerebral edema, diffuse encephalopathy, seizures, and hemiparesis. Confusion, agitation, delusions, visual and auditory hallucinations, somnolence, lethargy, stupor, and coma (34). Aseptic meningitis presents within 72 hours of start of therapy (35). The most common neurologic complications of steroids include euphoria, hypomania, depression, insomnia, irritability, personality changes, anxiety, hallucinations, and psychosis (5,36). Cognitive deficits can occur, including impaired memory retention, attention, concentration, mental speed and efficiency, and occupational performance (5).

ANTIBIOTICS

Confusion, hallucinations, anxiety, restlessness, nervousness, insomnia, euphoria, nightmares, psychosis, and seizures occur in patients on fluoroquinolones (7,9). Symptoms of neomycin neurotoxicity include acute muscle flaccidity, diaphragmatic breathing, and CNS depression (24). Metronidazole can cause peripheral neuropathy, encephalopathy, and seizures (31). Symptoms of loop diuretic ototoxicity include tinnitus, bilateral hearing loss, and vestibular symptoms. Most of these are reversible within hours of stopping the drug (22,23).

ANTIEPILEPTIC DRUGS

Phenytoin can cause concentration-dependent side effects, such as sedation, lethargy, confusion, ataxia, nystagmus, coma, seizures, and difficult-to-treat cardiac arrhythmias. Peripheral neuropathy can occur, but is concentration independent. Phenobarbital can cause excessive sedation, lethargy, and coma, which are concentration dependent (28).

DIAGNOSTIC APPROACH

Optimal evaluation of suspected neurotoxicity requires a multifaceted approach and a broad differential diagnosis. Although drug-induced neurotoxicity is common, it is important to rule out nonmedication causes of neurotoxicity, including portal systemic encephalopathy, metabolic or hepatic encephalopathy, electrolytes imbalances, hypertensive crisis, hypoxic-anoxic injury, and infection. In those patients with focal neurologic findings, it is also important to consider cerebrovascular ischemic, intracranial hemorrhagic events and malignancies. Simultaneous assessment for drug-related neurotoxicity is essential (21,37–39).

Patients who are immunosuppressed pose unique diagnostic challenges when sources of neurotoxicity or encephalopathy are not quickly identified. Brain imaging with CT or MRI should be performed, even in these patients without focal neurologic findings, because of the high risk of intracranial pathology. MRI is the diagnostic test of choice to evaluate encephalopathy related to progressive leukoencephalopathy and to identify central pontine myelinolysis. In patients with a fever or leukocytosis, lumbar puncture (LP) to exclude infectious sources of encephalitis or meningitis is essential. A thorough history and physical examination are essential in the diagnosis of drug-induced neurotoxicity (21,37–39). Electroencephalography (EEG) can be considered an extension of the neurologic examination and provide clues toward the diagnosis of toxic and metabolic encephalopathies, as well as diagnose seizures and nonconvulsive status epilepticus.

Close monitoring of AED should be performed. Extreme caution should be taken if using VPA in patients with liver disease. Frequent serum determinations (total and free concentrations) and gradual dose regulation of phenytoin is necessary. In liver disease, phenytoin and phenobarbital both have a prolonged half-life, and this produces a common mistake among physicians. Excessive dosing adjustments based on nontrough and nonsteady-state measurements leads to errors in over- or under-medications. These levels should be checked every 3 to 4 days in the critically ill and neurotoxic individuals, using trough measurements for most accurate estimates of dosing. Following a dosage adjustment, additional dosage changes should only be considered after a trough steady-state assessment of concentration. Hepatic dysfunction is less of a concern with newer AED (e.g., gabapentin, levetiracetam, topiramate, and zonisamide) and routine monitoring of serum levels is not needed (26,27).

TREATMENT

First-line therapy in suspected drug-induced neurologic toxicity is discontinuation of the offending agent. If no alternative medication is available for replacement therapy, then it is prudent to restart at a reduced dose of approximately 25% to 75%

after a 24- to 48-hour hiatus (11–13). A dosing recommendation for patients with hepatic and renal dysfunction, and for elderly and pediatric patients, is available for most medications in the *Physician Desk Reference.* The assistance of a clinical pharmacist to determine appropriate dose reduction can be valuable.

The authors have begun to use levetiracetam for anticonvulsant therapy in patients with liver disease to prevent recurrent CNI-induced seizures, to alleviate drug interactions and reduce the risk of side effects from the older agents (40). In one report, a patient with recurrent seizures while on tacrolimus was successfully converted from phenytoin to levetiracetam (41). An intravenous preparation of levetiracetam has recently become available, making it potentially useful in the critically ill patient with seizures.

Magnesium replacement should also be considered to treat suspected CNI-induced seizures. It is an intracellular ion usually depleted in patients with liver cirrhosis. A recommended goal for posttransplant magnesium levels is 2 mmol/L or higher for the first 2 weeks. Keeping blood pressure normal may decrease the risk of posterior leukoencephalopathy. Careful use of concomitant medications that can increase CNI levels, with frequent monitoring of CNI levels, and may prevent some neurotoxic events. Switching CNI has been successful in treating many CNS-related adverse effects (1–4,16). Abouljoud et al. (42) showed resolution of neurotoxicity in 79% of patients switched from tacrolimus to cyclosporine-microemulsion. Always consider converting to a drug without neurotoxicity to replace current therapy. Sirolimus and mycophenolate mofetil have been used successfully in liver transplantation as CNI sparing or elimination agents (43,44). Headaches can be treated by lowering the doses of CNI, switching agents, or treating with acetaminophen with a maximal daily dose of 3 g, or oral propranolol 20 mg every 6 to 8 hours (18).

Neurologic effects from quinolones will reverse on discontinuation of the drug. Metronidazole doses should be reduced to 500 mgs twice daily intravenously, or 250 mg three times daily to four times daily orally with frequent assessments for neuropathies (11–13). Neomycin-induced neuromuscular blockade can be treated by administration of calcium gluconate (20 to 30 mg/kg); supportive care may be necessary. Physostigmine can be given for CNS manifestations because it crosses the blood–brain barrier well (24).

CLINICAL RECOMMENDATIONS OF THE VIGNETTE

The tacrolimus was discontinued, and cyclosporine was started 2 days later with marked clinical improvement. A brain MRI was obtained. Over the next few months, the patient's speech became clearer. It took more than a year for the patient to make a complete recovery. In a patient who does not improve when switching CNI, treatment with a CNI-sparing regimen should be used. One or two doses of basiliximab or daclizumab, during the switch, may help prevent acute rejection in the early posttransplant period (personal observation).

SUMMARY

Drug-induced neurotoxicity is hard to identify. It should be suspected always in patients with liver disease. Early recognition with discontinuation of the offending agent should result in complete resolution, but the effects can be permanent. Any medication used to treat liver disease should be evaluated for changes in clearance before administering to patients. Initiate new drugs at lowest dose, and titrate to effect. Use your clinical pharmacist to assist with starting doses, as well as preventing drug interactions.

REFERENCES

1. Wijdicks EFM, Wiesner RH, Krom RAF. Neurotoxicity in liver transplant recipients with cyclosporine immunosuppression. *Neurology.* 1995;45(11):1962–1964.
2. Mueller AR, Platz KP, Bechstein WO, et al. Neurotoxicity after orthotopic liver transplantation: A comparison between cyclosporine and FK506. *Transplantation.* 1994;58: 155–169.
3. Margreiter R, and the European Tacrolimus vs. Ciclosporin Microemulsion Renal Transplantation Study Group. Efficacy and safety of tacrolimus compared to ciclosporin microemulsion in renal transplantation: A randomized multicenter study. *Lancet.* 2002; 359:741–746.
4. Bonham CA, Dominguez EQ, Fukui MB, et al. Central nervous system lesions in liver transplant recipients: Prospective assessment of indications for biopsy and implications for management. *Transplantation.* 1998;66(12):1596–1604.
5. Sacks O, Shulman M. Steroid dementia: An overlooked diagnosis? *Neurology.* 2005;64:707–709.
6. Uribe M, Go VL. Corticosteroid pharmacokinetics in liver disease. *Clin Pharmacokinet.* 1979;4(3):233–240.
7. Stahlmann R, Lode H. Fluoroquinolones in the elderly. Safety considerations. *Drugs Aging.* 2003:20(4):289–302.
8. Leone R, Venegoni M, Motola D, et al. Adverse drug reactions related to the use of fluoroquinolone antimicrobials. *Drug Saf.* 2003;26(2):109–120.
9. Fish DN. Fluoroquinolone adverse effects and drug interactions. *Pharmacotherapy.* 2001;21(10 pt 2):253S–272S.
10. Nelson DC, McGrew WR, Hoyumpa AM. Hypernatremia and lactulose therapy. *JAMA.* 1983;249(10):1295–1298.
11. Elbekai JR, Korashy HM, El-Kadi AOS. The effect of liver cirrhosis on the regulation and expression of drug metabolizing enzymes. *Curr Drug Metab.* 2004;5:157–167.
12. Rodighiero V. Effects of liver disease on pharmacokinetics. *Clin Pharmacokinet.* 1999; 37(5):399–431.
13. Sonne J. Drug metabolism in liver disease: Implications for therapeutic drug monitoring. *Ther Drug Monit.* 1996;18(4):397–401.
14. Dumont FJ, Staruch MJ, Koprak SL, et al. The immunosuppressive and toxic effects of FK-506 are mechanistically related: Pharmacology of a novel antagonist of FK-506 and rapamycin. *J Exp Med.* 1992;176:751–760.
15. Bechstein WO. Neurotoxicity of calcineurin inhibitors: Impact and clinical management. *Transpl Int.* 2000;13:313–326.
16. Beresford TP. Neuropsychiatric complications of liver and other organ transplantation *Liver Transpl.* 2001;7(11)[Suppl 1]:S36–S45.
17. Gijtenbeek JMM, Ven Den Bent MJ, Vecht CJ. Cyclosporine neurotoxicity: A review. *J Neurol.* 1999;246:339–346.
18. Wijdicks EFM. Neurotoxicity of immunosuppressive drugs. *Liver Transpl.* 2001;7(11): 937–942.
19. Venkataramanan R, Swaminathan A, Prasad T, et al. Clinical pharmacokinetics of tacrolimus. *Clin Pharmacokinet.* 1995:29(6):404–430.
20. Maurer G, Lemaire M. Biotransformation and distribution in blood of cyclosporine and its metabolites. In: Kahan BD, ed. *Cyclosporine. Volume IV: Pharmacological Aspects.* Orlando, Grune & Stratton; 1987.
21. Bronster DJ, Emre S, Boccagni P, et al. Central nervous system complications in liver transplant recipients: Incidence, timing, and long-term follow-up. *Clin Transpl.* 2000;14:1–7.
22. Tuzel IH. Comparison of adverse reactions to bumetanide and furosemide. *J Clin Pharmacol.* 1981;21(11–12 pt 2):615–619.
23. Rybak LP. Ototoxicity of loop diuretics. *Otolaryngol Clin North Am.* 1993;26(5):829–845.
24. Coleman JW, Yao FY, Jalandoni SR, et al. Neomycin-induced neuromuscular blockade. *Urology.* 1981;17(3):265–267.
25. Boyce EG, Cookson ET, Bond WS. Persistent metronidazole-induced peripheral neuropathy. *DICP. The Annals of Pharmacotherapy.* 1990;24(1):19–21.
26. Hachad H, Ragueneau-Majlessi I, Levy RH. New antiepileptic drugs: Review on drug interactions. *Ther Drug Monit.* 2002;24(1):91–103.
27. Bialer M. The pharmacokinetics and interactions of new antiepileptic drugs: An overview. *Ther Drug Monit.* 2005;27:722–726.
28. Winters ME. Phenytoin. In: Koda-Kimble MA. *Basic Clinical Pharmacokinetics,* 3rd ed. Philadelphia, Lippincott Williams & Wilkins; 1994.
29. Mignat C. Clinically significant drug interactions with new immunosuppressive agents. *Drug Saf.* 1997;16(4):267–278.
30. Agildere AME, Basaran C, Cakir B, et al. Evaluation of neurologic complications by brain MRI in kidney and liver transplant recipients. *Transplant Proc.* 2006;38:611–618.
31. Horlen CK, Seifert CF, Malouf CS. Toxic metronidazole-induced MRI changes. *Ann Pharmacother.* 2000;34:1273–1275.
32. Ney G, Lantos G, Barr W, et al. Cerebellar atrophy in patients with long-term phenytoin exposure and epilepsy. *Arch Neurol.* 1994;51:767–771.
33. Van Amelsvoort T, Bakshi R, Devaux CB, et al. Hyponatremia associated with carbamazepine and oxcarbazepine therapy: A review. *Epilepsia.* 1994;35:181–188.

34. Parizel PM, Snoeck HW, Van Den Hauwe L, et al. Cerebral complications of murine monoclonal CD3 antibody (OKT3): CT and MR findings. *Am J Neuroradiol.* 1997;18:1935–1938.
35. Martin MA, Massanari RM, Nghiem DD, et al. Nosocomial aseptic meningitis associated with administration of OKT3. *JAMA.* 1988;259(13):2002–2005.
36. Sirois F. Steroid psychosis: A review. *Gen Hosp Psychiatry.* 2003;25(1):27–33.
37. Shimono T, Miki Y, Toyoda H, et al. MRI imaging with quantitative diffusion mapping of tacrolimus-induced neurotoxicity in organ transplant patients. *Eur Radiol.* 2003;13:986–993.
38. Bartynski WS, Zeigler Z, Spearman MP, et al. Etiology of cortical and white matter lesions in cyclosporin-A and FK-506 neurotoxicity. *Am J Neuroradiol.* 2001;22:1901–1914.
39. Jansen O, Krieger D, Krieger S, et al. Cortical hyperintensity on proton density-weighted images. An MR sign of cyclosporine-related encephalopathy. *Am J Neuroradiol.* 1996;17:337–344.
40. French J, Arrigo C. Rapid onset of action of levetiracetam in refractory epileptic patients. *Epilepsia.* 2005;46:324—326.
41. Chabolla DR, Harnois DM, Meschia JF. Levetiracetam monotherapy for liver transplant patients with seizures. *Transplant Proc.* 2003;35:1480–1481.
42. Abouljoud MS, Anil Kumar MS, Brayman KL, et al.; OLN-452 Study Group. Neoral rescue therapy in transplant patients with intolerance to tacrolimus. *Clin Transplant.* 2002;16:168–172.
43. Forgacs B, Merhav HJ, Lappin J, et al. Successful conversion to rapamycin for calcineurin inhibitor-related neurotoxicity following liver transplantation. *Transplant Proc.* 2005;37(4):1912–1914.
44. Smallwood GA, Steiber AC, Davis L, et al. Renal sparing effects of mycophenolate when used in long-term liver transplant recipients. *Transplant Proc.* 2002;34(5):1550.

CHAPTER 47

Red Blood Cell Disorders

Harry L. Messmore • William H. Wehrmacher

OBJECTIVES

- To describe the classification of red blood cell disorders
- To discuss the pathophysiology of representative red blood cell disorders
- To explain the diagnostic clinical and laboratory features of the most common red blood cell disorders
- To describe the usually effective therapeutic measures
- To discuss the newer diagnostic and therapeutic approaches to selected red blood cell disorders

CASE VIGNETTE

A 16-year-old girl of northern European heritage was transferred from a community hospital for evaluation of an illness characterized by fever, mental confusion, and an acute anemia with thrombocytopenia. There was no apparent infection and no evidence for a neoplastic or collagen vascular disease. Laboratory evaluation demonstrated a hemoglobin of 7.2 gm/dL, mean corpuscular volume (MCV) 80/fL, mean corpuscular hemoglobin (MCH) 30 pg per red blood cells (RBC) gm/dL RBC and a mean corpuscular hemoglobin concentration (MCHC) of 35 gm/dL RBC), hematocrit 21%, RBC count, 2.4 million/μL, leukocyte count 12,500/μL (70% segmented neutrophils 19% lymphocytes, 7% monocytes, and 4% eosinophiles), and a platelet count of 42,000 μL. Fragmented red blood cells with many helmet cells were noted on the peripheral blood smear. Reticulocyte count was 32% and no abnormal leukocytes or platelets were seen, but some platelets were large. Liver enzymes were normal, but the lactic dehydrogenase was 2,500 units (Normal = 150 to 300). Blood urea nitrogen (BUN) was elevated at 34 mg/dL, and creatine was moderately increased. The serum haptoglobin was 0. Free hemoglobin was seen in the urine, but only an occasional RBC or leukocyte, and no red or white blood cells casts were seen.

DEFINITION

Red blood cells, also known as erythrocytes, are produced in the bone marrow under the influence of erythropoietin, a hormone produced in the kidney. Anemia is a deficiency of circulating hemoglobin. Causes of anemia are numerous and include anything that interferes with RBC production or results in premature RBC destruction (hemolysis). The spleen is a unique organ having the function of monitoring circulating RBC for any defects of RBC membranes, which include those caused by the aging of RBC. So, RBC 90 to 100 days old are removed by the spleen, as are any defective RBC whose external membrane or internal hemoglobin structure renders the membrane rigid or misshapen. RBC enzyme defects that permit oxidation of hemoglobin or loss of energy also shorten RBC life.

Defects of RBC production can be entirely exclusive to the RBC, such as erythropoietin deficiency (renal disease); structural defects or replacement of bone marrow by fibrous tissue (myelofibrosis), neoplastic tissue (metastatic cancer, leukemia or multiple myeloma); or infectious processes (granulomatous). Hereditary or acquired RBC membrane defects, cytoplasmic (hemoglobin or enzyme) defects, and RBC parasites (malaria) also shorten RBC life.

Nutritional effects on RBC formation result in structural defects manifested as small (micro-), large (macro-), oval (ovalo-), or both (macro- and ovalo-) RBC or a deficiency in hemoglobin (hypochromic). Vitamin B_{12}, folic acid, and iron deficiency are common nutritional causes of anemia.

Destruction of circulatory RBC can occur because of vascular defects, autoantibodies, or the direct effects of infectious disease. Enlargement of the spleen from any cause can result in a mild anemia because of sequestering and preventing RBC from circulating.

Given that the above-described causes of anemia can be hereditary or acquired, it is essential to make an accurate clinical diagnosis before attempting treatment. Table 47-1, which outlines RBC disorders based on general causes, provides a classification help formulate a diagnostic approach to a more specific etiologic diagnosis in a particular patient. For example, this diagnostic approach helps the clinician to avoid not discriminating between the several causes of microcytosis and prevents treating a patient for an “iron deficiency” only because it is the most common cause of such a finding. It is as if the “small” RBC were the disorder when, in fact, it is what causes these small RBC that is the disorder to be treated.

Many clinical entities are associated with anemia, but in itself it is not a clinical entity, just as “heart disease” is not a clinical entity. It, however, is useful to list those entities that may be uncovered in the investigation of the cause of anemia in a particular patient. Table 47-1 lists such clinical entities that are discovered in the investigation of an anemia. Laboratory investigations are necessary to determine the cause of most chronic anemias, but acute blood loss anemia is usually self-evident. These laboratory evaluations are supplemented by certain imaging procedures.

TABLE 47-1. Disorders of Red Blood Cells (RBC)

RBC Production Deficit

PRIMARY BONE MARROW FAILURE

- Hereditary
  - Diamond-Blackfan syndrome
  - Fanconi anemia
  - Congenital dyserythropoiesis (CDA) types I, II, III

SECONDARY OR ACQUIRED BONE MARROW FAILURE

- Lack of erythropoietin
- Infectious diseases
- Drugs and chemicals
- Radiation
- Tumor infiltrates (marrow replacement); myelofibrosis
- Chronic inflammation: Anemia of chronic disorder

HEMORRHAGE

- Acute
- Chronic: Iron deficiency

NUTRITIONAL DEFECTS

- Folic acid
- Vitamin B_{12}
- Pyridoxine deficiency or inhibition
- Protein deficient diet in children (Kwashiorkor syndrome)

Excessive RBC Destruction (Hemolytic Anemia)

HEREDITARY HEMOLYTIC ANEMIA

- Hemoglobin defects (sickle cell, thalassemia syndrome)
- RBC membrane defects (spherocytosis, elliptocytosis, stomatocytosis, pyropoikilocytosis)
- RBC enzyme defects (G6PD, pyruvate kinase, glycolytic pathway, antioxidant pathway, heme synthesis pathway)

ACQUIRED HEMOLYTIC ANEMIA

- Cellular mediated (activated macrophages)
- Infectious diseases (malaria, clostridia)
- Toxic chemical (hypotonic solutions, oxidant drugs, or chemicals)
- Erythrophagocytic syndromes
- Isoimmune, alloimmune mechanisms (transfusion reactions)
- Autoimmune mechanisms
- Drug-induced mechanisms

RBC FRAGMENTATION SYNDROMES

- Mechanical disorders (prosthetic heart valve)
- Vascular disorders
- Thrombotic thrombocytopenic purpura (TTP)
- Hemolytic uremic syndrome (HUS)
- Disseminated intravascular coagulation (DIC) and associated infections
- Clostridium perfringens (gas gangrene-phosphorylase C-induced hemolysis)

ANEMIA OF ENDOCRINE ORIGIN

- Hypothyroidism
- Primary hypothyroidism
- Pan-hypopituitarism

CLINICAL MANIFESTATIONS

HISTORY

Important symptoms to consider are observed blood loss, abnormal stools, and discolored urine; painful joints and muscles; and dark urine. Cardiorespiratory distress, peripheral edema, and orthopnea can occur in the elderly or younger patients with heat disease. More subtle can be neurologic symptoms, such as peripheral neuropathy. Gastrointestinal symptoms are critically important in regard to blood loss or nutritional defects and malabsorption.

PHYSICAL EXAMINATION

Pallor, dyspnea, tachycardia, and flow murmurs are signs of very advanced anemia. Mucous membrane changes, such as smooth tongue, cheilitis, and flattening of the nails (koilonychia), are signs of chronic iron deficiency. Abnormal reflexes and impaired position sense may be a sign of vitamin B_{12} deficiency. Splenomegaly can suggest heredity or acquired hemolytic anemia and whether a lymphoma or myeloproliferative disease is present. A palpable urinary bladder or a large prostate can suggest an obstruction and subsequent renal failure that is associated with anemia. A large nodular uterus is often the common cause of chronic blood loss. Telangiectasias of the skin and mucous membranes can be causes of chronic blood loss and lead to an iron deficiency anemia. Multiple myeloma is suggested when the patient with anemia has chronic back pain with painful percussion over the vertebrae.

Epidemiology, Etiology, Pathogenesis, Diagnosis and Treatment of Specific Disorders

Primary Bone Marrow Failure

Aplastic anemia is not compatible with life before birth (panaplasia), but pure red cell aplasia on a genetic basis (*Diamond-Blackfan syndrome*) may be apparent at birth in some cases, having only partial aplasia. Another hereditary anemia of bone marrow progenitor cell origin that may be apparent at birth is *Fanconi's anemia.* Both disorders are rare and are probably under diagnosed, particularly because of unfamiliarity with the syndrome by clinicians, lack of diagnostic facilities in developing countries, and the marked heterogeneity in their clinical manifestations. Primary bone marrow failure is sometimes severe at birth, but at times not manifested until early or late adulthood. Most patients eventually die of hemopoietic or somatic cancers.

Diamond-Blackfan Syndrome

Approximately 1 to 7 per million live newborns have pure red cell aplasia on a genetic basis. No geographic or ethnically related distribution is found. Most data come from northern European and northern American sources.

The cause of Diamond-Blackfan syndrome is primarily found by genetic analysis, but not all are recessive. No distinctive features are found in the blood other than mild to severe anemia.

Failure of RBC precursor production under the normal stimulant effects of erythropoietin is owing to a genetic defect, but those genetic mutations are variable as is the severity of the anemia.

The peripheral blood RBC are normal or macrocytic. The reticulocyte count is low. The bone marrow is normal, except for a decrease in erythroid precursors. Differential diagnosis includes an acquired defect caused by virus infection or a thymic defect. Genetic studies of the patients will reveal an abnormal gene mutant called *RPS19*.

Corticosteroids are effective in 50% to 60% of patients. Severe cases require periodic transfusions. Cyclosporin-A has been useful, as has interferon and metaclopmide therapy (1).

Fanconi Anemia

Fanconi anemia (FA), an autosomal recessive pancytopenia caused by genetic defects in the stem cell population, results in chromosomal fragility and pan-hypoplasia of the bone marrow.

FA occurs equally in both sexes and has been found in northern European and in Americans originating from there. Originally, Fanconi (Switzerland) reported a family in which three boys had aplastic anemia and their parents were healthy. A similar syndrome characterized by hypoplastic bone marrow, presenting from birth to early childhood or even in adulthood, is called *dyserythropoiesis congenita (DC)*. Widespread, but subtle defects in a variety of solid organs, skin, head and neck, bone, kidney, and so on have been reported.

Genetic defects have been reported in so-called "housekeeping" genes that maintain stability and repair defects in stem cells.

Absent to severe pancytopenia may be present at birth, but eventually bone marrow hypoplasia becomes evident. The marrow may show an increase in mast cells. Physical examination may show nothing abnormal other than abnormalities of the hands and wrist bones, which are common, as are large areas of hyperpigmentation on the trunk. Short stature is common. Some patients can function well in school and even graduate from college (2).

Patients respond rapidly to small doses of androgens in terms of the anemia. Caution is advised regarding risk of hepatic neoplasms with androgens. Immunosuppressive drugs are not valuable (2).

Congenital Dyserythropoiesis

At least three phenotypes of congenital dyserythropoiesis, two are autosomally recessively inherited and one (type III) is dominantly inherited. In all three conditions, erythropoiesis is abnormal and RBC precursors are seen in the bone marrow. Nuclear abnormalities in the bone marrow (dumbbell forms, three to four small nuclei, some connected by a narrow strand of nuclear membrane) are present. Erythroid hyperplasia is also present, but reticulocytes are low. The spleen can be enlarged because of trapping of abnormal RBC.

Congenital dyserythropoiesis is rare and is neither geographically or ethnically restricted (in the United Kingdom with >60 million people, 47 cases were identified in a recent 2-year period or an incidence of 3 cases per million population per year).

A spectrum of closely related genetic defects that control nuclear membrane maturation of erythroblasts are responsible for this disease. The abnormal nuclear maturation results in failure of release of mature RBC into the circulation as rapidly as normal. In the type II variety (*hereditary erythroblastic anemia with positive acid serum test* [HEMPAS]), hemolysis can also be somewhat more brisk than in the other two varieties, the serum iron binding protein is nearly saturated and the iron stores are very high as a result (3).

Anemia appearing in children or young adults with a high MCV, variation in size and shape of peripheral RBC, splenomegaly, icterus, and normal or slightly increased reticulocyte count can signal the presence of these disorders. A bone marrow examination, which shows multinucleated RBC precursors and increased iron stores, may also point to this disorder. A positive acid serum test makes the diagnosis of HEMPAS in the type II variety that has autosomal recessive inheritance. Dominant inheritance would be typical of type III congenital dyserythropoiesis, and very large normoblasts are found. Treatment requires folic acid and vitamins, but avoidance of iron and iron-containing foods. Rare severe cases may require blood transfusions and stem cell or bone marrow transplantation. Rarely, this turns out to be the explanation for iron overload in middle aged or older persons.

Secondary or Acquired Bone Marrow Failure

A variety of factors that include drugs, chemicals, radiation, virus infections caused by immune mechanisms, (usually antibody mediated) can cause secondary or acquired bone marrow failure. Thymic tumors can cause pure red cell aplasia on an immune basis. None of these are geographically or ethnically correlated, but aplastic anemia is more prevalent in countries where chloramphenicol is widely used (Southeast Asia) (4).

Bone marrow cell precursors can be permanently damaged in drug-related cases, and stem cell or bone marrow transplant therapy is required. This is also true in certain virus infections (hepatitis C). Idiopathic autoimmune types can be responsive to immunosuppressive drugs or antithymocyte globulin. Bone marrow or stem cell transplants are less likely to be rejected if only a few blood transfusions have to be given (4).

Acute Blood Loss

No correlation is seen of acute blood loss with ethnic or geographic location.

Congenital bleeding disorders, gastrointestinal lesions, such as ulcer disease or duodenal, gastritis, and ulcer-active colitis, can each result in hemorrhagic shock—loss of 40% of the blood volume. The loss of volume results in vasoconstriction and organ ischemia as oxygenation is impaired. Reticulocytosis ensues in 6 to 12 hours with the recovery of tissue perfusion and the release of erythropoietin and iron stores are adequate (5).

Chronic Blood Loss (Iron Deficiency)

A decrease in intravascular volume may not occur in chronic blood loss. Causes include gastrointestinal lesions, therapeutic phlebotomies, meno-metrorrhagia, and chronic interstitial pulmonary hemorrhage. Chronic intravascular hemolysis can be responsible by way of urinary loss of hemoglobin. Iron chelation therapy rarely causes it. The result of chronic blood loss is iron deficiency (5).

Iron deficiency exists when all iron stores are exhausted. It is characterized by reticulocytopenia, small pale (hypochromic) RBC (low MCV, MCHC, and MCH). Serum iron is low, iron-binding capacity is elevated and the percentage of iron-binding capacity is <10%. There is low serum ferritin as a rule and elevated serum transferrin receptor levels. Treatment consists of oral ferrous sulfate until iron stores are normal, which usually takes 3 to 6 months (5,6).

Failure of iron absorption (celiac disease) can cause iron deficiency because this is a physiologic loss of approximately 1 mg daily via the stool. Normal iron stores are about 1,000 to 1,500 mg. Pregnancy also can cause iron loss in excess of absorption unless supplemental iron is given.

Nutritional Deficiencies

Folic Acid Deficiency

Folic acid deficiency is more common in women because of pregnancy and in men when alcoholism is prevalent. Poverty with low intake of fresh fruits and vegetables can cause it as well (7). Megaloblastic anemia is common throughout the world. It is rare in children.

Malabsorption syndromes are the most common cause of folic acid deficiency, other than pregnancy, hemolytic anemias, and alcoholism. The effect on the bone marrow is a failure of production of methyl donors for DNA synthesis. Tetrahydrofolate reduction releases methyl groups to vitamin B_{12}, which then methylates homocysteine to form methionine, which is necessary for nucleic acid synthesis. Defective nucleic acid synthesis results in delayed nuclear maturation in the RBC precursors (megaloblast formation). The bone marrow becomes hypercellular because of a build-up of megaloblastic RBC. Oval-shaped macrocytic RBC are released slowly into the blood. Many of these are destroyed in the spleen. Mucosal cells in the gastrointestinal tract fail to reproduce and perform an absorptive function. In pregnancy, fetal defects, especially spinal closure defects (spina bifida) occurs. Prevention is by administration of oral folic acid (1 mg daily). The bone marrow becomes normoblastic within 24 hours, and reticulocytosis occurs. Serum iron and potassium, as well as lactate dehydrogenase (LDH) levels fall rapidly and folate levels in the blood and RBC are restored (8).

Vitamin B_{12} Deficiency

Pernicious anemia is the result of a gastric disorder caused by autoantibodies to the parietal cells of the stomach, which results in atrophic gastritis and a failure to produce intrinsic factor. This, in turn, results in malabsorption of vitamin B_{12} antibodies to intrinsic factor. The problem is most common in elderly whites and middle-aged or younger blacks.

Vitamin B_{12} deficiency described above as pernicious anemia is not the most common cause of vitamin B_{12} deficiency. It occurs whenever there are no animal products in the diet (meat, milk, eggs) as in India where vegetarianism is widely practiced and in other parts of the world where it is a religious practice to avoid animal products (Seventh Day Adventists). The megaloblastic anemia described above for folic acid deficiency is identical. Hemoglobin can go as low as 4 g/dL and leukocyte and platelet counts are decreased as well. There is marked pallor and mild icterus; oral mucous membranes are atrophic. A neurologic presentation may be seen in the form of subacute combined degeneration of the spinal cord resulting in paresthesias, anesthesia, and loss of position sense, resulting in a positive Romberg test.

Blood and bone marrow findings are the same as for folic acid deficiency because of failure of the methyl groups transferal to homocysteine and to produce methionine, which is necessary for nucleic acid synthesis (9). Laboratory testing shows anemia, macroovalocytosis, hypersegmented neutrophils in the blood, giant bands in the bone marrow, and very high LDH levels in the blood. Vitamin B_{12} levels in the blood are variably low. Methylmalonic acid levels in the urine are high. When no atrophic gastritis or intrinsic factor antibodies are found, vitamin B_{12} may fail to absorb because of obstruction or inflammation of the terminal ileum, Crohn disease of the terminal ileum, or the presence of the fish tapeworm diphyllobothrium latum. A Schilling test using radioactive vitamin B_{12} with and without intrinsic factor administered orally with measurements of radioactivity in the urine may be diagnostic. Treatment is with vitamin B_{12} administration, either intramuscular or (orally in the nonpernicious anemia varieties) because of a purely dietary deficiency (10).

Hereditary Hemolytic Anemias

The hereditary hemolytic anemias consist of three major types: Hemoglobin defects, RBC membrane defects, and RBC enzyme defects.

Hemoglobin Defects

The most prevalent types of hemoglobin defects, sickle cell and thalassemia, have been discussed separately. Two smaller groups, the unstable hemoglobins and those associated with abnormal oxygen binding, are briefly discussed here.

Unstable hemoglobins are readily oxidized to methemoglobin and precipitate within the cell. Other types are so unstable that their β-chains have disintegrated, giving the appearance of a β-thalassemia major on laboratory testing. Precipitated hemoglobin appears in the RBC cytoplasm as Heinz bodies on blood smears. These unstable hemoglobins form methemoglobin, which detected by the red-brown screening test on blood and by spectrophotometry (11).

RBC Membrane Defects

The four types of hereditary RBC membrane defects are (i) hereditary spherocytosis, (ii) elliptocytosis, (iii) pyropoikilocytosis, and (iv) stomatocytosis. These names reflect the appearance of the RBC of each type on a stained blood smear. A more rare type not so distinctive on a blood smear is hereditary xerocytosis. The first four types share many common features of epidemiology, etiology, and pathogenesis as well as treatment (12).

These four types of hereditary RBC membrane defects are reflections of genetic defects not limited to any geographic area or ethnic group and found worldwide.

Genetically determined defects in synthesis of select proteins comprising the cell wall constitute the basis for the fragility of the cells. These proteins consist of α- and β-spectrin, ankyrin, pallidin (band 4.2), protein 4.1, band 3 and glycophorin C.

Hereditary Spherocytosis

Hereditary spherocytosis is the most common type of membrane defect seen worldwide. It involves ankyrin, α- and β-spectrin, band 3 and protein 4.2. Loss of membrane results in a spherocytic cell that is removed by the spleen because the rigid cell cannot traverse the systemic sinusoids (12).

The patient may be a child or even a middle-aged or older adult with mild pallor, icterus, splenomegaly, possibly gallstones, and a few or many spherocytes on the blood smear. Autoimmune hemolytic anemia must be excluded because anti-RBC antibodies also cause loss of membrane. It is usually autosomal dominant, so family studies are helpful. RBC fragility studies using hypotonic saline, glucose, and incubation are diagnostic. No treatment is necessary unless the hemoglobin is sufficiently low to be symptomatic, in which case splenectomy may be needed to relieve the symptoms. Transient *aplastic* crises caused by folic acid deficiency or an ongoing virus infection (parvovirus B_{19}) may require temporary transfusions and folic acid supplements.

Hereditary elliptocytosis is the variant of spherocytosis in terms of RBC shapes, the RBC being cigar shaped because of deficiencies in the type of cell wall proteins involved, but the fragility is similar and all the clinical and laboratory aspects are the same except that it is somewhat less severe in most cases. The proteins of the cell wall involved are glycophorin C and protein 4.1 (13).

Pyropoikilocytosis and stomatocytosis are genetic variants of elliptocytoses (ovalocytosis). A southeastern Asian form has many stomatocytes, but is mild compared with some cases of spherocytosis. Splenectomy is useful in the more advance cases of any of these four clinical entities.

Hereditary Red Blood Cell Enzyme Defects

RBC enzymes protect hemoglobin from oxidation and free radical effects. The major enzymatic pathways include glucose 6-phosphate dehydrogenase (G6PD), pyruvate kinase (PK) 5′ nucleosidase, and cytochrome B5 reductase. Many hazards, however, *await* the newly formed RBC, each of which can shorten its life span of 90 plus days when the combined total of these hazards can overcome the RBC protective mechanisms. Hemolysis begins when oxidation overcomes these enzyme systems, but anemia does not occur until RBC destruction exceeds normal by 60%, the maximum that the bone marrow can respond to with the formation of reticulocytes. The patient by this time has a low haptoglobin and physical evidence of increased bilirubin production (scleral icterus).

Optimal nutrition in terms of iron and vitamin supplements is needed to meet such challenges. Pregnancy is a state when those challenges are even more difficult to meet. G6PD is an X-linked enzyme and males manifest this deficiency, whereas females are carriers. Nature packs the reticulocytes with extra G6PD that limits the severity of this disease. When an oxidant challenge occurs, only the older RBC, (approximately one third), hemolyze (14). These challenges are much the same as those that cause precipitation of hemoglobin and Heinz body formation as described with the unstable hemoglobinopathies. The four most common RBC enzyme deficiencies are G6PD, PK, pyrimidine 5′ nucleotidase, and cytochrome B5 reductase (Cb5R), each of which is described below.

The genes for the antioxidant enzymes of the RBC are located on autosomal chromosomes, except for G6PD, which is X linked. Gene mutations for the antioxidant enzymes are extremely common in the G6PD group, but most have no clinical symptoms since as a rule, strong oxidants are needed to bring out the clinical manifestations. Because as a rule strong oxidants are needed to bring out clinical manifestations, G6PD deficiency does not cause chronic anemia, except in the extreme mutants. PK deficiency, in contrast, results in a chronic state because it is not a not and antioxidant type enzyme.

Glucose 6-phosphate Dehydrogenase (G6PD) Deficiencies

G6PD deficiencies are relatively common, distributed worldwide and in numerous mutated forms. RBC antioxidant enzyme defects are much more common in areas where severe malaria exists: The Mediterranean, African, and Southeast Asian countries. A deficiency of G6PD is thought to minimize the adverse effects of malaria and provide a survival advantage. G6PD was the first enzymopathy described; it was discovered in a University of Chicago laboratory during World War II during the study of the mechanism of hemolysis in black male volunteers given an antimalarial drug with oxidant properties. Other RBC enzyme deficiencies (e.g., PK) are found in populations from northern European and some Chinese ethnic groups. The Amish (German descent) are notably affected, possibly because of the consanguinity effect in Amish patients (15).

The inheritance is X linked and acute hemolysis of a self-limited nature can occur with exposure to oxidant drugs or infectious diseases. The enzyme serves as an antioxidant that acts in concert with other less commonly deficient antioxidant enzymes in the RBC. Its high concentration in reticulocytes protects these *younger* RBC, and hemolysis usually stops after approximately one third of the RBC are hemolyzed. This rule applies to fava bean hemolysis occurring in the Mediterranean region as well.

No specific morphologic features of the RBC exist. Anemia, transient icterus, and reticulocytosis are clues that suggest the diagnosis. Fluorescent staining for the activity of the enzyme or spectrophotometry are diagnostic, but findings may be negative immediately following a hemolytic episode. As a rule, avoidance of known precipitating triggers is the only treatment required.

Pyruvate Kinase Deficiency

The distribution of PK deficiency is worldwide with an increased prevalence in northern Europeans. Kinships of Amish (German origin) people in America have increased probability of the disease.

The genetics of PK deficiency are complex and incompletely characterized. Chronic hemolysis occurs in homozygous and double heterozygous states. Deficiency results in variable severe hemolysis as a result. The enzyme normally promotes the production of adenosine triphosphate (ATP) in the cell, providing energy for the cell.

The patient can be anemic and jaundiced at birth, causing confusion with Rh and ABO incompatibility (hemolytic disease of the newborn) problems that may quickly resolve by results of a Coombs antiglobulin test for IgG antibodies on the RBC. More commonly, it is discovered later in life. RBC morphology is nonspecific. A precise diagnosis requires biochemical assays on properly preserved RBC hemolysate. Severe cases of PK deficiency may need blood transfusions. Splenectomy is often effective, but should not be done before the age of 3 years because of the risk of overwhelming sepsis. This can be dealt with effectively by immunization with pneumococcal, *Haemophilus influenzae* and meningococcal vaccines (15).

Pyrimidine 5′ Nucleotidase Deficiency

No specific ethnic or geographical correlations are known for pyrimidine 5′ necleotidase deficiency.

Five different genes encoding for pyrimidine 5′ nucleotidase are known. The function of this enzyme is to degrade pyrimidine derived from RNA synthesis. When the enzyme is lacking, RNA residuals remain in the RBC, which has a toxic effect leading to hemolysis. Lead is a known inhibitor or pyrimidine 5′ nucleotidase, resulting in hemolysis by the same mechanism as the enzyme deficiency. Cases of lead poisoning are not immediately distinguishable from the enzyme deficiency (16).

The hemolysis is apparently mild and chronic. A diagnostic laboratory feature is basophilic stippling of the RBC on a blood smear. If lead exposure is involved, chelation therapy will reverse the process (16).

Cytochrome b5R Reductase

Cytochrome b5R reductase enzymopathy does not cause hemolysis, but it causes pathologic levels of methemoglobin to accumulate in the RBC, which results in a cyanotic appearance. Its distribution is worldwide and mostly sporadic. It is increased, however, in North American Indians (Navajo) and other tribal groups. One aboriginal tribe in Siberia is known to harbor this defect (17).

Deficiency of the cytochrome b5R reductase enzyme can be traced to a single gene. The function of the enzyme is to restore methemoglobin to hemoglobin as a natural daily housekeeping function. Absence of the enzyme results in gradual increase in the level of methemoglobin. It may permit higher levels of methemoglobin in patients with unstable hemoglobins (hemoglobin E). Diagnosis is confirmed by the presence of methemoglobin on spectrophotometry and exclusion of other causes. Erythrocytosis (rather than anemia) is a compensatory mechanism because oxygen is not carried by methemoglobin (17).

Acquired Hemolytic Anemias

No specific associations with ethnic groups or geographic distribution in acquired hemolytic anemias, a diverse category. A tendency exists for female predominance in autoimmune-mediated hemolytic anemia (Table 47-1).

As seen in Table 47-1, there are eight major categories, each with several subdivisions. Several types and causes for antibodies to RBC exist. RBC isoantibodies are type immunoglobulin M, which are natural and specific for an individual, depending on his or her blood type (ABO antigen system). Blood type A has antibodies to type B and AB. Blood type B has antibodies to types A and AB. Blood type AB has no antibodies, whereas blood type O has A, B, and AB antibodies. Transfusion of an RBC ABO antigen to which the patient has natural antiblood type antibodies will cause those RBC to be destroyed within the circulation by intravascular hemolysis, mediated by complement fixation. Renal failure, shock, and disseminated intravascular coagulation (DIC) occur (18).

Hemoglobinemia and hemoglobinuria are accompanied by fever and, eventually, oliguria. There may be spherocytes in the blood. Treatment consists of hydration and hyperosmolar fluids to attempt to protect the kidneys. Symptomatic treatment of fever is usually necessary.

Alloimmune Antibody-Mediated Hemolysis

All antibodies are generated by the immune system when RBC with antigens foreign to the recipient cause anti-RBC antibodies of the IgG type. This can cause RBC destruction, primarily extravascularly in the spleen and reticuloendothelial system after a significant titer is reached. The antigens are often minor RBC antigens (e.g., Rh, Kell, Kidd). The kidneys are not severely threatened in this type of hemolytic anemia. Diagnosis is made by the direct and indirect Coombs test that detects IgG, IgA, or complement on the RBC. The indirect Coombs test shows that the patient's serum is now reacting with the donor's RBC. Therapy consists of hydration and treatment of symptoms of fever or signs of anoxia of tissue caused by anemia. Corticosteroids may slow the rate of hemolysis, but all the incompatible cells will be destroyed. This is known as late onset (delayed) transfusion reaction. Females have this problem even without prior sensitization by a transfusion, because mismatch for minor blood groups between the fetus and the mother causes immunization of the mother that can last for years (19).

Hemolytic Disease of the Newborn

Hemolytic disease of the newborn is relatively common in populations where the Rh factor antigen is lacking in some individuals.

Variability antibodies formed by the mother is the most common cause in other minor RBC antigens, such as Kell or Kidd, which can also result in maternal immunization by a fetus carrying RBC antigens that the mother lacks. Severe anemia occurs in the fetus and the syndrome of hydrops fetalis can result in death of the fetus if it is undiagnosed. Rh negative mothers are often sensitized during their first pregnancy at the time of delivery. Administration of anti-Rh immunoglobin (RhoGAM) just before delivery is useful to prevent the fetal cells from sensitizing the mother. This is also useful in subsequent pregnancies. The autosomal dominance of the inheritance of the Rh antigen and its prevalence dictates the practice (20).

Autoimmune Hemolytic Anemia

The autoimmune hemolytic anemias (AIHA) are usually of the IgG antibody type that mediate extravascular hemolysis. They occur worldwide with no geographic or ethnic association. The idiopathic type is more common in females and can be associated with collagen disease and non-hematologic autoimmune disorders. Malignant lymphoproliferative disorders are also correlated with AIHA.

Autoimmunity is generally poorly understood. It consists of antibody formation or lymphoid cellular proliferation that is directed at autoantigens. Infections, drugs, and inflammatory and neoplastic disorders are associated with AIHA (21).

Immunoglobins G, M, and, rarely, A are the means of RBC destruction, sometimes with participation of complement. The RBC destruction can be intravascular (complement mediated) or extravascular. Splenic and reticuloendothelial cells in nonsplenic areas, including phagocytic cells in the circulation and liver, are sites of RBC destruction. Immunoglobin G is the most common autoantibody-mediated hemolysis, with IgM and IgA much less commonly found (21).

The mechanism of cell destruction in the sites is via the Fc receptor on the phagocytic cell binding to the IgG antibodies on the RBC surface. The IgGFc receptor bearing macrophage engulfs RBC membrane fragments containing IgG, releasing the RBC as a spherocyte, many of which are noted in the circulation in the classic idiopathic IgG type or in the lymphoma or collagen diseases associated types. The spherocytes then are removed by the spleen because they are now inflexible and cannot traverse the splenic sinusoids. Splenectomy may be necessary if immunosuppressant drugs are ineffective. The usual clinical and laboratory evidence of hemolysis is present. The Coombs test (direct) is usually positive (21).

Treatment with corticosteroids, antipurines, and anti–B-cell antibodies are commonly used to treat this type of AIHA. Treatment of what appears to be the underlying disease is essential but not necessarily effective. The IgG type antibodies described above are active at 37°C (warm antibodies), but some are active in the cold (below 37°C). An example is paroxysmal cold hemoglobinuria and IgG directed against that antigen. Complement is bound to the RBC causing intravascular hemolysis and hemoglobinuria. Corticosteroid therapy may be of some benefit but avoidance of cold is the only predictably effective therapy. IgM antibodies cause low-grade chronic hemolysis. They are cold reactive *agglutinating* the RBC via a monoclonal IgM kappa antibody. Splenic sequestration is only modest, with many of the RBC taken out by the liver macrophages. This antibody is sometimes induced by mycoplasma pneumoniae and is transient. Most cases are idiopathic and persist for months or years. Acrocyanosis is caused by the aggregation of RBC, which obstruct the microvasculature in cold areas, such as fingers and nose. Avoidance of cold is the most effective treatment. Immunosuppressive drugs are only modestly effective. RBC transfusions may be rapidly hemolyzed because of fresh complement being able to cause cell destruction. The complement may eventually be converted to C3b, which prevents further complement deposition, and this protects against hemolysis. Hemophagocytic syndromes are either inherited or acquired. Immune drug-induced hemolytic anemia is usually mediated by IgG.

Immune drug-induced (immune) hemolysis is not common. Antibodies generated by that mechanism are not induced by the drug alone, but rather by the mechanism by which the drug binds to a protein (either circulating or on the RBC membrane) to form an antigen (22). The drug must be bound to the RBC before the cell can be typed by complement or removed from the circulation by phagocytic cells. Antibodies can become bound to the antigen-coated RBC causing a positive Coombs test, yet hemolysis does not always occur. Thus, the drug may cause hemolysis by inducing antibodies to a drug–RBC membrane complex or to a drug-protein complex that is RBC bound. A third mechanism is the induction of IgG antibodies to RBC by some poorly understood mechanism in which anti-RBC antibodies are formed, but they do not require the presence of the drug to give rise to a positive direct antiglobulin test. Previously, this was encountered with the drug α-methyl-dopa (Aldomet) used to treat hypertension. The hemolysis was usually mild.

Red Blood Cell Fragmentation Syndromes

Intravascular hemolysis caused by physical forces results in fragmentation of RBC. Fragmentation of normal RBC occurs when blood circulates in a pathologic vascular tree. The two major subtypes are hereditary and acquired, but the latter is very rare (23).

No relationship exists to genetic or ethnic background, but certain causes are likely to be prevalent in certain societies. Mechanical heart valves cause hemolysis by physical forces, whereas DIC is caused by infection or malignancy and occurring throughout the world. March hemoglobinuria caused by foot trauma is likely to be seen among military personnel and joggers. Thrombotic thrombocytopenic purpura (TTP) and hemolytic uremic syndrome (HUS) are seen throughout the world.

The common causes of red blood cell fragmentation syndrome are mentioned above as generic mechanisms, but special mechanisms exist for TTP. TTP occurs when the enzyme that depolymerizes high molecular weight multimers of von Willebrand factor normally released from the *Weibel-Palade bodies* in endothelial cells is lacking on a hereditary or acquired basis. Lack of the gene for production of normal ADAMTS13 (the enzyme) or the presence of an antibody (acquired) to ADAMTS13 constitute known causes (24). The high molecular weight multimers cause platelets to bind to each other, embolize to arterioles, and cause partial occlusion that results in fragmentation of RBC as they pass.

HUS is similar in its final destructive mechanism as is DIC, small thrombi occluding in blood vessels. The problem in HUS, however, is caused by endothelial damage by a toxin from *Escherichia coli* 0157 originating from contaminants of food by the intestinal content of beef. This toxin attacks the kidney vasculature and results in renal failure. Some systemic vascular occlusion can occur, as it does in TTP, when arterioles throughout the body are occluded.

Hereditary Thrombotic Thrombocytopenic Purpura (Upshaw-Schulman Disease)

The gene for production of normal ADAMTS13 is absent or defective in hereditary TTP. Inheritance is autosomal recessive. ADAMTS13 is an enzyme that depolymerizes ultrahigh molecular weight multimers (UHMWM) of von Willebrand factor (25). During normal physiologic processes, HMWM are synthesized in the Weibel-Palade bodies of endothelial cells throughout the body. When the HMWM are not depolymerized, then platelets aggregate and embolize to arterioles, partially or completely occluding them. Platelets are consumed and RBC are fragmented. DIC does not occur. Hemoglobin, as well as lactic dehydrogenase (LDH), is released in large amounts, causing the haptoglobin to decrease to zero. Vascular occlusions occur in all organs, resulting in severe brain, heart, liver, and kidney dysfunction.

The patient presents at a young age in hereditary TTP, even at birth, sometimes with fever anemia, thrombocytopenia, brain dysfunction (coma, seizures), and peripheral blood smear showing RBC fragmentation (schistocytes, helmet cells). Reticulocytes in the blood are markedly increased after the first day. Erythropoietin may be slightly or modestly elevated, and ADAMTS13 levels are <1%. Emergency treatment with fresh frozen plasma (FFP) replaces the missing enzyme; hemolysis stops and platelets rise. Periodic infusions of plasma are then required. The patient may be successfully carried through pregnancy with FFP infusions.

Acquired Thrombotic Thrombocytopenic Purpura

No correlation with ethnic or geographical location exists in TTP, but correlation can be made to certain drugs (ticlopidine, clopidogrel, mitomycin) and disseminated carcinomas or human immunodeficiency virus (HIV). Etiology in most cases is not evident (idiopathic).

The pathogenesis of this idiopathic acute type is autoimmune. An IgG antibody directed to ADAMTS13 lowers its level to <10%. From this point, the pathogenesis is identical to the hereditary type.

The diagnosis based on clinical and laboratory findings is identical to the hereditary type, with the exception of the presence of a circulating antibody in this type. Treatment is supportive therapy and emergency plasma or plasma exchange transfusions, with initial exchange of 50% of the patient's plasma and subsequent daily exchanges until a stable low LDH and rising platelet counts are observed. Close follow up is required because recurrence may ensue. Other treatments directed at antibody production have been used successfully to treat refractory and recurring cases. Previously, splenectomy was successful, but plasma may have played a role in the success of that procedure. Removal of a source of antibody production may offer some explanation as well.

Hemolytic Uremic Syndrome

Hemolytic uremic syndrome is usually the acquired type related to enteric infection with toxin producing *E. coli* 0157, but a familial form has also been identified, the result of a mutation in human complement regulator protein (26). There is also 0157H type as well, which originates primarily from beef intestinal contents that contaminate ground beef, water, vegetables, fruit, and unpasteurized milk. It occurs throughout countries where beef is produced and in North America the incidence is about 8/100,000/year.

On a clinical basis, cases are described as diarrhea associated or not (D^+ or D^-), but the most common in adults is D^+ and with diarrhea followed by bloody stools, hematemesis, hematuria, and hypertension beginning 3 to 5 days after onset. The toxin adversely effects renal vascular endothelium causing fibrin-rich thrombi (27).

Stool examination for the specific *E. coli* and toxin are positive. The patient exhibits pallor, weakness, headache, seizures, and low hemoglobin and platelet counts, with no DIC. Treatment is basically supportive and no specific therapy is known to be effective. Renal dialysis becomes necessary in about 40% of cases. Long-term renal failure can occur. The rate in the acute phase is about 5%. Other RBC fragmentation syndromes include DIC, mechanical heart valves, malignant hypertension, HELLP syndrome of pregnancy (hemolysis, elevated liver enzymes, and low platelet counts), and antiphospholipid syndrome. All are associated with vasculopathy or physical factors unrelated to the RBC or from von Willebrand factor multimers.

Anemia of Endocrine Origin

Anemia of endocrine origin is caused by the lack of a demand for oxygen by the cells of the body. Pan-hypopituitarism influences the endocrine organs—thyroid and gonads, particularly the testes that promote the normal state of circulating hemoglobin.

CLINICAL RECOMMENDATIONS OF THE VIGNETTE

The clinical impression in this case is an acquired hemolytic anemia and thrombocytopenia. The differential diagnosis included disseminated vasculopathy, DIC, and TTP or HUS. Blood and urine cultures were drawn and a blood coagulation profile for DIC. A serum sample was analyzed for antibody to von Willebrand factor depolymerase (ADAMTS13). In view of the life-threatening nature of the clinical disorder, an exchange plasmapheresis was immediately started. Within 2 hours, the patient's mental status began to improve and her LDH level fell to 1,200 U/mL. A second plasma exchange brought about further improvement. She eventually recovered after plasma exchanges daily for a week. A gingival biopsy showed intraarteriolar platelet (thrombi). No apparent cause was found.

SUMMARY

Disorders of the RBC are numerous and such a disorder can be a significant factor in systemic illnesses, including neurologic diseases. This contained a discussion of how the disorders of the RBC impact a patient's general health as well as how it can, in some instances, seriously alter a patient's survival, independent of other diseases.

REFERENCES

1. Charles RJ, Sabo KM, Kidd PG, et al. The pathophysiology of pure red cell aplasia: Implications for therapy. *Blood.* 1996;87:4831–4838.
2. Kutler DI, Singh B, Satagopan J, et al. A 20-year perspective on the International Fanconi Anemia Registry (IFAR). *Blood.* 2003;101:1249–1256.
3. Wickramasinghe SN. Dyserythropoiesis and congenital dyserythropoietic anaemias. *Br J Haematol.* 1997;98:785–797.
4. Marsh JC. Management of acquired aplastic anaemia. *Blood* 2005;[Rev 19]:143–151.
5. Cook, JD, Skikne BS, Baynes RD. Serum transferrin receptor. *Annu Rev Med.* 1993;44:63–74.
6. Weiss G, Goodnough LT. Anemia of chronic disease. *N Engl J Med.* 2005;352:1011–1023.
7. Coban E, Timuragagoglu A, Meric M. Iron deficiency anemia in the elderly: Prevalence and endoscopic evaluation of the gastrointestinal tract in outpatients. *Acta Haematol.* 2003; 110:25–28.
8. Herbert V. Experimental nutritional folate deficiency in man. *Trans Assoc Am Physicians.* 1962;75:307–320.
9. Victor M, Lear A. Subacute combined degeneration of the spinal cord: Current concepts of the disease: Value of serum vitamin B_{12} determinations in clarifying some of the common clinical problems. *Am J Med.* 1956;20:896–911.
10. Hillman RS, Adamson J, Burka E. Characteristics of vitamin B_{12} correction of the abnormal erythropoiesis of pernicious anemia. *Blood.* 1968;31:419–432.
11. Rose C, Bauters F, Galacteros F. Hydroxyurea therapy in high hemoglobin carriers. *Blood.* 1996;88:2807–2808.
12. Eber S, Lux SE. Hereditary spherocytosis-defects in proteins that connect the membrane skeleton to the lipid bilayer. *Semin Hematol.* 2004;41:118–141.
13. Gallagher PG. Hereditary elliptocytosis: Spectrin and protein 4.1R. *Semin Hematol.* 2004; 41:142–164.
14. Ruwende C, Khoo S, Snow R, et al. Natural selection of hemi- and heterozygotes for G6PD deficiency in Africa by resistance to severe malaria. *Nature.* 1995;376:246–249.
15. Aizawa S, Kohderea U, Hiramoto M, et al. Ineffective erythropoieses in the spleen of a patient with pyruvate kinase deficiency. *Am J Hematol.* 2004;74:68–72.
16. Escuredo E, Marinaki AM, Duley JA, et al. The genetic basis of the interaction between pyrimidine 5′ nucleotidase I deficiency and hemoglobin E. *Nucleosides Nucleotides Nucleic Acids.* 2004;23:1261–1263.
17. Davis CA, Barber MJ. Cytochrome b5 oxidoreductase: Expression and characterization of the original familial idiopathic methemoglobinemia mutations E255- and G291D. *Arch Biochem Biophys.* 2004;425:123–132.
18. Sampathkumar P. West Nile virus: Epidemiology, clinical presentation, diagnosis, and prevention. *Mayo Clinic Proc.* 2003;78:1137–1144.
19. Bizzarro MJ, Colson E, Ehrenkranz RA. Differential diagnosis and management of anemia in the newborn. *Pediatr Clin North Am.* 2004;51:1087–1107.
20. Fibey D, Hanson U, Wesstrom G. The prevalence of red cell antibodies and pregnancy correlated to the outcome of the newborn. *Acta Obstet Gynecol Scand.* 1995;74:687–692.
21. Petz LD, Garratty G. *Immune Hemolytic Anemia*, 2nd ed. Oxford: Churchill Livingstone; 2004.
22. Salama A, Santoso S, Mueller-Eckhardt C. Antigenic determinants responsible for the reactions of drug-dependent antibodies with blood cells. *Br J Haematol.* 1991;78: 535–539.
23. Moake, JL. Thrombotic microangiopathies. *N Engl J Med.* 2002;347:589–600.
24. Zheng X, Richard KM, Goodnough LT, et al. Effect of plasma exchange on plasma ADAMTS13 metalloprotease activity, inhibitor level, and clinical outcome in patients with idiopathic and non-idiopathic thrombotic thrombocytopenic purpura. *Blood.* 2004;103: 4043–4049.
25. Furlan M, Robles R, Galbusera M, et al. von Willebrand factor-cleaving protease in thrombotic thrombocytopenic purpura and the hemolytic-uremic syndrome. *N Engl J Med.* 1998;339:1578–1584.
26. Richards A, Kemp EJ, Liszewski MK, et al. Mutations in human complement regulator, membrane cofactor protein (CD46), predispose to development of familial hemolytic uremic syndrome. *Proc Natl Acad Sci USA.* 2003;100:12966–12971.
27. Moghal NE, Ferreira MAS, Howie AJ, et al. The late histologic findings in diarrhea-associated hemolytic uremic syndrome. *J Pediatr.* 1998;133:220–223.

CHAPTER **48**

Disorders of White Blood Cells

Michael Y. Ko • Harry L. Messmore

OBJECTIVES

- To define epidemiology, etiology, and pathophysiology of different primary white blood cell disorders
- To describe the systemic manifestations of those white blood cell disorders
- To discuss the neurologic complications associated with these disorders
- To explain the diagnostic criteria and general treatment guidelines for these disorders

CASE VIGNETTE

A 32-year-old man presents with recurrent herpes zoster infections over the right truncal region, associated with burning pains on the right T10 dermatome. Treatment with acyclovir had hastened recovery in the past. His medical history is remarkable for treatment of frequent gastroenteritis. He is not taking any medications at this time. On examination, his vital signs are normal. General examination was notable for raised truncal vesicular rash. Laboratory studies demonstrated normal metabolic profile and complete blood count; suspicion of an immunodeficiency led to quantization of serum immunoglobulins. The immunoglobulin G (IgG) level was 96 mg/dL (700 to 1,600 mg/dL), immunoglobulin A (IgA) was 10 mg/dL (70 to 400 mg/dL), and immunoglobulin M (IgM) was 14 mg/dL (60 to 300 mg/dL). Subsequently, white blood cell flow cytometry demonstrated normal percentages of CD3+, CD4+, CD8+, and CD19+ T cells. The human immunodeficiency virus (HIV) enzyme-linked immunosorbent assay (ELISA) and nitroblue tetrazolium reduction test were negative. Complement levels were normal.

DEFINITION

White blood cell disorders are categorized as those caused by underproduction, overproduction, or dysfunction of a specific cell type. Underproduction of granulocytes (e.g., severe congenital neutropenia) or lymphocytes (e.g., severe combined immunodeficiency) could result in loss of the specific immunologic functions. Overproduction of certain cell types (e.g., acute myelogenous leukemia) can interfere with the function of these affected cells as well as other components of the immune system. Abnormal white blood cells that proliferate in the bone marrow or blood are characteristic of the *leukemias. Lymphomas* are characterized by aggregates of abnormal lymphocytes in lymph nodes, spleen, bone marrow, skin, and intestinal wall. If the abnormal lymphocytes are in the bone marrow or blood, the disorder is classified as a *leukemic lymphocytic lymphoma.* Dysfunction of white blood cells results in abnormal phagocytic function (e.g., *myeloperoxidase deficiency*) or depressed immunoglobulin production (e.g., *X-linked agammaglobulinemia*) that weakens resistance to particular microorganisms, or the development of a disease directly related to immunologic dysfunction. These primary immunodeficiencies include disorders causing lymphopenia, and lymphocyte and phagocytic dysfunction. Excessive proliferation of any leukocyte that circulates in the blood can cause the syndrome of leukostasis, which can be a medical or neurologic emergency.

EPIDEMIOLOGY

Primary neutropenias are rare, but the annual incidence of leukemia and lymphoma in the United States is 13 and 23 per 100,000 persons, respectively (1). The annual incidence of primary immunodeficiencies, except for *selective immunoglobulin A (IgA) deficiency,* is approximately 1 in 5,000 live births (2).

NEUTROPHILS

Neutropenia is defined as an absolute neutrophil count (ANC) <1,500 cells/mm^3. The etiology of neutropenia can reflect decreased cell production, increased cell destruction, or enhanced migration of cells into surrounding tissues. Table 48-1 lists secondary causes of neutropenia. *Severe congenital neutropenia* or *Kostmann syndrome* has an estimated incidence of 1 case per 1,000,000 persons and usually is diagnosed only in children (3).

Granulocyte dysfunction disorders are mainly phagocytic defects, and remain rare entities, representing only 9% of all primary immunodeficiencies (2). *Myeloperoxidase deficiency* is likely the most common phagocyte dysfunction, seen in approximately 1 of 2,000 persons in the United States (4). *Chediak-Higashi syndrome* (*CHS*) is a rare immunodeficiency frequently presenting before age 5, and without a gender preference (5). *Chronic granulomatous disease* (*CDS*) is diagnosed in 1 of 200 to 250,000 live births; most cases present during infancy, predominantly in males because two thirds of cases are X-linked (6).

The annual incidence of *chronic myelogenous leukemia* (*CML*) is 1–2 per 100,000 and *acute myelogenous leukemia* (*AML*) 2.7 cases

TABLE 48-1. White Blood Cell Disorders

Granulocytes	*Lymphocytes*
○ Phagocytic dysfunction	○ B-cell dysfunction
■ Chronic granulomatous disease	■ X-linked agammaglobulinemia
■ Neutrophil glucose-6-phosphate dehydrogenase deficiency	■ Selective IgA deficiency
■ Glutathione metabolism defect	■ Common variable immunodeficiency
■ Myeloperoxidase deficiency	■ Hyper IgM syndrome
■ Chediak-Higashi syndrome	■ Selective IgG subclass deficiency
■ Neutrophil specific granule deficiency	■ Antipolysaccharide antibody deficiency
○ Leukocyte adhesion dysfunction	○ T-cell dysfunction
■ Leukocyte adhesion deficiency type I and II	■ Severe combined immunodeficiency
■ Hyper-immunoglobulin E syndrome	• X-linked
○ Congenital neutropenia	• JAK3 deficiency
■ Severe congenital neutropenia (Kostmann syndrome)	• Il-7 receptor deficiency
■ Cyclic neutropenia	• Purine nucleoside phosphorylase deficiency
■ Myelokathexis	• Adenoside deaminase deficiency
■ Shwachman-Diamond-Oski syndrome	• RAG1/RAG2 deficiency
■ Reticular dysgenesis	• Omenn syndrome
■ Dyskeratosis congenita	■ Major histocompatibility complex (MHC) class I/II deficiency
○ Acquired neutropenia	■ Interferon-γ receptor deficiency
■ Postinfectious related	■ CD3 deficiency
■ Medication induced	■ IL-2 deficiency
■ Radiation induced	■ Wiskott-Aldrich syndrome
■ Chronic benign neutropenia	■ DiGeorge syndrome
■ Nonimmune chronic idiopathic neutropenia	■ DNA repair defect
■ Autoimmune neutropenia	• Ataxia-telangiectasia
■ Pure white cell aplasia	• Xeroderma pigmentosum
■ Nutritional deficiencies (folate, copper, vitamin B_{12})	• Bloom syndrome
	• Nijmegen breakage syndrome

(Modified from Ten RM. Primary immunodeficiencies. *Mayo Clin Proc.* 1998;73:865–872 and Cleary AM, Insel RA, Lewis DB. Disorders of lymphocyte function. In: Hoffman R, Benz E, Hattil S, et al.: *Hematology: Basic Principles and Practice,* 4th ed. Churchill Livingstone; 2005:831–851, with permission.)

per 100,000 people worldwide (7,8). This equates to approximately 3,400 to 4,500 new cases of CML, and 11,000 new cases of *AML* in the United States per year, but the true incidence of CML could be higher because a significant portion of patients are asymptomatic (9). Both of these leukemias are slightly more common among men than women (1.3–1.4:1) (10). CML has no particular preponderance with ethnicity, but *AML* is more common among Caucasians. Most patients with CML are in their fifth to seventh decades of life at the time of diagnosis (11). AML has a peak age of presentation that is slightly older, 65 years, and remains the most common leukemia in adults (9).

LYMPHOCYTES

Congenital immunodeficiencies typically present in children and are more common in men than women (5:1). If the immunodeficiency is milder, however, it can appear in adulthood with almost equal predilection between the sexes (1:1.4 male-to-female ratio). Congenital lymphopenias (cellular immunodeficiencies), such as severe combined immunodeficiency (SCID), account for 20% of all primary immunodeficiencies (2). Patients with SCID are evenly divided between *X-linked (X-SCID)* symptomatic male and female carriers and *autosomal recessive (AR-SCID)* etiologies and, consequently, men are three times as affected as women (12). The incidence of *X-SCID* is 1 case in 100,000 to 500,000 live births (13). Most patients with SCID present by the third month of life (12), but it can be as early as 1 month of age for X-SCID (2). *Adenosine deaminase deficiency* causes 15% of all SCID cases, and is an autosomal recessive disorder (2).

Congenital lymphocytic dysfunction, which is more commonly found in B cells, represents 70% of all primary immunodeficiencies (2). *X-linked agammaglobulinemia,* or *Bruton disease,* presents in male infants by 1 year of age and usually at a time when their maternally transmitted antibodies have degraded (12). The initial presentation, however, can be as late as 3 to 5 years of age (13). *Common variable immunodeficiency* (*CVID*) is usually diagnosed by the second or third decade of life with an equal prevalence between genders (12). Its incidence is estimated to be 1 case per 10,000 to 50,000 persons (13) and, although it may be the most frequently diagnosed primary immunodeficiency (12), *selective IgA deficiency* may be more common, with an estimated incidence of 1 case per 700 persons (12). The discrepancy between the most common and most commonly diagnosed immunodeficiency is secondary to the mild or asymptomatic nature of *selective IgA deficiency* (13) and may be as much a three times more prevalent in men (14).

Several disorders can present with variable immunodeficiencies. One of these is *DiGeorge syndrome* with a reduced T-cell count, but with variable immunocompetency dependent on the amount of coexisting thymic hypoplasia (2). The characteristic heterozygous genetic mutation seen in this syndrome has an incidence of 1 per 4,000 to 5,000 live births (15) and clinical evidence of the immunodeficiency usually presents by 6 months of age (13). The actual male-to-female ratio is not known. *Ataxia-telangiectasia* (*AT*) has an incidence of 1 case per 100,000 live births, but the AT gene is estimated to exist in approximately 2% of the population. No racial preference is found for the disease and an equal incidence is seen in both genders (16).

ETIOLOGY AND PATHOPHYSIOLOGY

NEUTROPENIA

As for the congenital neutropenias, *severe congenital neutropenia* (*SCN*), or *Kostmann syndrome*, is a disorder without a single specific genetic etiology. Mutations in the zinc-finger transcriptional repressor gene (GF1) or neutrophil elastase gene (ELA-2) have been proposed as the underlying cause, but the exact mechanism remains unknown (3).

NEUTROPHIL DYSFUNCTION

Myeloperoxidase deficiency is an autosomal recessive disorder with a mutation at 17q22–23, which leads to a reduced production of chloramines (reactive oxygen species containing chloride ions). These molecules are involved in fighting fungal infections such as Candidiasis, but other oxygen species can assist in the destruction of those same organisms. CHS is an autosomal recessive disorder, caused by an abnormal protein, and is generated from a genetic mutation at 1q42–43 (6). This transport protein is involved in the delivery or generation of granules for secretion and storage, such as melanosomes in melanocytes and lysosomes for granulocytes. The defective lysosomes or enlarged granules in the granulocytes are unable to kill the phagocytized microorganisms. Improper microtubule assembly or functioning may be a second pathophysiologic process that can also lead to an associated neutropenia.

CGD is a deficiency in reactive oxygen molecules used to kill phagocytized microorganisms (6). Mutations in the genes for the four enzymatic subunits involved in this nicotinamide adenine dinucleotide phosphate (NADPH) fueled oxygen species production can lead to *CGD* (6). A mutation of the X chromosome gene CYBB is identified in almost two thirds of *CGD* cases, whereas a NCF1 mutation, located on chromosome 7 and classified as autosomal recessive, is the second most common etiology (17).

MYELOGENOUS LEUKEMIAS

The etiology of CML is believed to be an acquired translocation between chromosomes 9 and 22 that leads to a shortened chromosome 22, or Philadelphia chromosome, and insertion of genes onto chromosome 9. Cytogenetic studies have found the Philadelphia chromosome in 90% to 95% of patients with CML (18). The *abl* oncogene from chromosome 9 combines with the *bcr* gene on chromosome 22 to encode a tyrosine kinase protein that leads to increased number of immature granulocytes. This abnormal protein can lead to uncontrolled proliferation and resistance to apoptosis (18).

AML does not have a single genetic cause and different genetic abnormalities appear to lead to the same phenotype: A decrease of mature hematopoetic cells and overproduction of immature hematopoetic cells that fail to undergo apoptosis. Exposure to ionizing radiation and benzene has been shown to increase the risk of developing AML two- to tenfold (19) and also the risk of CML. Disorders of chromosomal repair, such as AT, or aneuploidy, such as Down syndrome, also increase the risk of AML than in the general population (9). Mutations in the myeloid transcription factor, C/EBPα, can also lead to decreased functioning, but increased risk of AML in some patients (20). Myelodysplasias, such as CML, can also transform into AML (9).

LYMPHOPENIA

SCID can have multiple causes and affect the development of B and T cells. The most common form, *X-SCID*, has a genetic defect mapped to Xq13 that generates a mutated gamma chain in receptors for multiple interleukins (2, 5, 7, 11, and 15) and the loss of signaling by this mutated receptor leads to defective development of T cells and late maturation of B cells (12). The remaining cases are autosomal recessive with the most common cause being *adenosine deaminase (ADA) deficiency* (2). Lymphocytes deficient in this enzyme have an accumulation of deoxyadenosine triphosphate that blocks DNA synthesis and 2′-deoxyadenosine that eventually blocks DNA methylation.

DiGeorge syndrome usually presents with low CD3+ T-cell counts because of poor maturation in an anaplastic or hypoplastic thymus. The deletion of a gene in the long arm of chromosome 22 leads to a defect in the development of the third and fourth pharyngeal pouches, which include the thymus, parathyroid glands, and cardiac-related structures. The degree of immunoglobulin deficiency is dependent on the functionality of the T and B cells. Patients with SCID have little or no immunglobulins, whereas those with *DiGeorge syndrome* can have highly variable levels of immunoglobulins (21).

IMMUNOGLOBULIN DEFICIENCY

CVID has multiple causes, but the common endpoint is diminished immunoglobulin production by immature B cells (2). Although multiple inheritance patterns exist, a sporadic genetic mutation is likely the most common cause. With the proper stimulation, these B cells could produce their deficient immunoglobulins, but defective stimulation by T cells to B cells can result in low levels of immunoglobulins (2). *Selective IgA deficiency* is associated with normal serum IgG and IgM concentrations with usually normal immune function. Its cause is unknown, but defects in the major histocompatibility complex (MHC) may play a role in its pathogenesis (12). *X-linked agammaglobulinemia* is caused by a mutation in the *btk* gene at Xq21.2–22, which codes for a tyrosine kinase and plays an unknown role in B-cell maturation. The minimal number of mature B cells leads to diminished or absent serum IgG, IgM, and IgA concentrations (2). AT is an autosomal recessive disorder where the ATM gene at 11q22.3 is mutated (22). The affected protein is a protein kinase that participates in DNA replication, repairing of DNA damage, and cell cycle regulation (22). The immune system defect in AT is hypothesized to be from poor T-cell developmental that leads to reduced activation by antigens (23), but the thymus can also be hypoplastic and poorly organized (22).

CLINICAL MANIFESTATIONS

The main clinical manifestations of white blood cell disorders include infections by various organisms and are determined by the severity and type of dysfunction within the immune system.

NEUTROPENIA

The common site of infection among patients who are neutropenic are the mucous membranes, such as the oral cavity and sinuses, whereas the skin is the second most common infected tissue with manifestations such as ulcers, abscesses, or delayed wound healing (24). Because of a poor inflammatory response, the infected areas may not become erythematous or induce a fever. Gram-negative bacteria such as *Escherichia coli* and pseudomonas are the most common organisms, but gram-positive bacteria, such as staphylococci are reported. The chance of developing an infection is almost certain when the ANC is <100 cells/mm^3. Superinfections with fungi-like candida or aspergillus are also a common side effect associated with broad-spectrum antibiotic use. The risk of infections by parasites and viruses is not increased among patients who are neutropenic (24).

SCN also presents with similar infections of the mucous membranes, respiratory tract, gastrointestinal tract, and urinary tract, and causes ANC of <200 cells/mm^3. Of these patients, 12% will develop a myelodysplasia or even acute myeloid leukemia, but the mechanism for this transformation is unknown (3).

NEUTROPHIL DYSFUNCTION

Patients with *myeloperoxidase deficiency* are usually asymptomatic, and <5% of these patients develop a fungal infection, usually with candida (25). *CHS* and *CGD* present with recurrent infections involving skin, upper respiratory, and gastrointestinal tracts (26,27). Most common bacterial pathogens include staphylococcus, streptococcus, pneumococcus, pseudomonas, and klebsiella, and they lead to granuloma formation and poor wound healing. Patients with CHS also have hypopigmented skin, hair, and eyes from defective melanocytes, and bleeding disorders from improperly formed platelets. Older such patients develop symptoms of organ dysfunction from an infiltrative lymphoproliferative disorder (6) and this lymphoma-like disorder is not malignant and likely is triggered by a virus, such as the Epstein-Barr (28). Patients with CGD are also susceptible to fungi-like candida and aspergillus, which are destroyed by reactive oxygen species (26,27). They will present with the typical signs of an infection: Fever and elevated white blood cell counts. Microorganisms can cause abscesses in atypical places such as the liver or spleen. A chronic granulomatous inflammatory process can develop in the gastrointestinal tract, kidneys, stomach, and brain (26).

MYELOGENOUS LEUKEMIAS

Clinical manifestations of CML include typical "B symptoms" One component used in the staging of a lymphoma is indicating whether systemic symptoms are absent, "A" or present "B". These B symptoms are weight loss, intermittent temperature elevation, and night sweats, frequent infections, splenomegaly, and a leukocytosis >30,000 cells/mm^3 (29). Although up to 40% of patients are diagnosed by laboratory studies, most are asymptomatic and diagnosed while in their stable or chronic phase where <15% of peripheral cells are blasts. Within 3 to 5 years, the CML will progress to an accelerated phase where the percentage of immature lymphocytes is >15% (10). After 3 to 18 months in the accelerated phase, the CML will progress to a blast phase where the peripheral blood has >30% of leukemia-type cells and a presentation similar to acute myelogenous or lymphocytic leukemia, depending on the transformed cell type. The treatment approach is similar to AML or ALL (29). Detection of the BCR-ABL gene or its messenger RNA (mRNA) via fluorescence in situ hybridization (FISH) or polymerase chain reaction (PCR) could predict those patients with an increased risk of relapses (18). In most patients, their CML will eventually reach a blast phase.

Similar to those with CML, patients with AML typically present with bruising, fatigue, fevers, and infections. Bone marrow biopsy shows that at least 30% of cells are myeloblasts. These cells can also infiltrate other organs such as the skin and meninges (9). Approximately 10% of these patients will have white blood cell counts >100,000 cells/mm^3, that account for leukostasis or a tumor lysis syndrome. Leukostasis can lead to chest pain, shortness of breath, headaches, changes in mental status, and cranial neuropathies. Most of the *tumor lysis syndrome* manifestations are metabolic and consist of hyperuricemia, hypocalcemia, renal failure, and acidosis (9).

LYMPHOPENIA

Clinical manifestations of congenital lymphopenias and immunodeficiencies include both recurrent infections and also associated neoplasms, autoimmune disorders, and allergic conditions (2). Patients with SCID usually present early in infancy with chronic thrush, a diffuse diaper rash, or pneumocystis-related protracted cough. Untreated, these patients may die from overwhelming viral infection from varicella, herpes, cytomegalovirus (CMV), or adenoviruses (12), and remain susceptible to opportunistic infections such as pneumocystis or candida (13). Medical evaluation can show an anaplastic thymus, lymphocyte counts <1,000 cells/mm^3, and low serum immunoglobulin concentrations (12). The subset of SCID, *ADA* or *purine nucleoside phosphorlyase (PNP) deficiency*, presents with a variable immunocompetency (2). Patients who are *ADA-deficient* can have an associated chondro-osseous dysplasia (2). DiGeorge syndrome presents with recurrent fungal, viral, or opportunistic infections, such as pneumocystis, mycobacteria, and fungi (13). These patients may also have associated sequela of malformations in structures arising from the third and fourth pharyngeal pouches: Hypocalcemia from abnormal parathyroid glands and tetrology of Fallot from abnormal cardiac structures (13).

IMMUNOGLOBULIN DEFICIENCIES

CVID is also a B-cell deficiency with associated decreased immunoglobulin production and recurrent bacterial infections of the sinuses and lungs. Repeated reactivation of herpes simplex or enteric infections, such as giardia, are common. These patients are also at an increased risk of developing autoimmune diseases and malignancies, such as lymphoma or gastric carcinoma. Enterovirus infections in *CVID* can lead to a chronic meningoencephalitis or dermatomyositis (12). *Selective IgA deficiency* is uncommonly diagnosed, but may be the most common immunoglobulin production deficiency. Most patients are usually asymptomatic, but an increased risk exists of bacterial respiratory tract and sinus infections (13). This deficiency also increases the risk for autoimmune diseases and malignancies, especially hematologic neoplasms (27,30).

X-linked agammaglobulinemia also induces a reduced humoral immunity that increases the risk for bacterial sinusitis, pneumonia, and otitis. Commonly responsible bacteria for these infections are streptococcus, staphylococcus, and haemophilus, and although easily treated with antibiotics, recurrent infections can lead to chronic scarring especially of the lungs (12). Because the cellular immunity remains functioning, only rarely is an increased risk seen of viral or fungal infections, except from enteroviruses that can progress to a meningoencephalitis or dermatomyositis (27,31). The live poliovirus vaccine can induce a prolonged viremia and subsequent paralytic poliomyelitis in these patients. Serum concentrations of immunoglobulins are typically <100 mg/dL of IgG and absent IgA and IgM. Circulating T cells are in normal concentrations, whereas B cells are typically absent (12). Parasitic infection, such as giardia, is more commonly seen in all the B-cell deficiencies (27,31).

Patients with *AT* have variable cellular and humoral immunodeficiencies. Testing of their immune function can show low levels of IgG and IgA, and poorly responding lymphocytes to antigens. Approximately 50% to 80% of patients with AT have a selective IgA deficiency. Such dysfunctions typically increase the risk of bacterial infections, especially of the upper respiratory tract (22). Ataxia and telangiectasias, however, are the hallmarks of the disease. Telangiectasia is the second most common sign, usually appearing by mid childhood. Common areas for telangiectasias are the conjunctiva, eyelids, and cubital and popliteal fossas. These telangiectatic lesions rarely bleed. Other skin changes include hypopigmented and hyperpigmented spots, and graying of hair. Associated endocrine and hepatic abnormalities have been documented (22). Because of the higher susceptibility to chromosomal damage, an almost 100 times increase is seen in the incidence of cancer. In juvenile cases, this is usually acute lymphocytic leukemia. Solid tumors from areas such as the gastrointestinal tract, breasts, thyroid, liver, and skin are the major type of cancer seen in adult patients with AT.

Neurologic Complications

Disorders of white blood cell types typically lack unique neurologic complications, but put the patient at increased risk for specific infections that could involve the nervous system. The ensuing encephalitis, meningitis, or abscess cause corresponding neurologic deficits based on the involved area of the nervous system. Some white blood cell disorders, however, also have associated neurologic symptoms or findings.

NEUTROPHILS

CHS in older patients can cause a peripheral neuropathy from abnormal microtubule-related axonal transport (27). Electrodiagnostic testing demonstrates both a demyelinating and axonal pathologic process. Patients who live into adulthood may also develop dementia, parkinsonism, and spinocerebellar degeneration. Patients with CGD may rarely have a chronic inflammation involving the brain, leading to nonspecific white matter lesions (32).

AML rarely infiltrates the CNS. The meninges, however, would be the most common site for such a process. As mentioned, the leukocytosis in *AML* can cause cranial and peripheral neuropathies (9). Similarly, the elevated white blood cell counts in *CML* have been associated with retinal hemorrhages, ischemic strokes, and mental status changes (31). Peripheral neuropathies in patients with AML treated with cytosine arabinoside and patients with CML treated with chronic interferon-α (IFN-α) have been reported (33,34).

LYMPHOCYTES

The SCID subgroup of patients with *ADA* or *PNP deficient* are at higher risk of being developmentally delayed, and *PNP deficiency* can lead to mental retardation and spasticity (35). Patients with *X-linked agammaglobulinemia* have trouble clearing the live poliovirus vaccine and may develop paralytic poliomyelitis. Exposure to enteroviruses can also lead to a chronic meningoencephalitis.

Patients with CVID have an increased risk of recurrent herpes simplex exacerbations with about one fifth developing herpes zoster. Similar to X-linked agammaglobulinemia, *CVID* can predispose to a severe meningoencephalitis from enteroviruses. Associated peripheral neuropathy and subacute combined degeneration in patients with *CVID* are reported (36,37). Anaphylaxis is a known complication of intravenous immunoglobulin (IVIg) administration in some patients who are *CVID* or *selective IgA deficient* and the mechanism may be related to an anti-IgA antibody. A National Institutes of Health (NIH) consensus statement suggested that routine prescreening of IgA levels, before IVIg administration was recommended, and a low IgA IVIg formulation does exist for at risk patients (38).

Ataxia is the most common symptom of *AT*. It usually appears between 1 to 2 years of age and remains progressive throughout life and in young children, a diagnosis of Friedreich ataxia can incorrectly be made. Most children are wheelchair bound by their early teen years and other associated neurologic symptoms include dysarthria and poor coordinated eye movements (39,40).

DIAGNOSTIC APPROACH

White blood cell disorders are diagnosed based on the white blood cell count and their function. Signs of a potential immunodeficiency are listed in Table 48-2. "B symptoms" could lead to an evaluation for malignancies and, at times, elevated white

TABLE 48-2. Warning Signs of Primary Immunodeficiency Disorders

Medical History	*Physical Findings*
• Eight or more ear infections in 1 year	• Poor growth
• Two or more serious sinus infections in 1 year	• Failure to thrive
• Two or more infections in unusual areas	• Absent lymph nodes or tonsils
• Recurrent deep skin or organ abscesses	• Skin lesions, such as dermatomyositis, lupuslike rash, petechiae, telangiectasias
• Received intravenous antibiotics	• Ataxia
• Infection by an unusual or opportunistic organism	• Oral thrush or ulcers
• Family history of a primary immunodeficiency	

(Modified from Cooper MA, Pommering TL, Koranyi K. Primary immunodeficiencies. *Am Fam Physician.* 2003;68:2001–2011, with permission.)

blood cell levels are found incidentally during routine complete blood counts. Family history can also provide clues of a potential white blood cell disorder.

NEUTROPENIA

A suggestion of neutropenia comes from clinical symptoms or illnesses, such as frequent infections. Complete blood counts usually demonstrate a deficiency in neutrophils. As genetic causes for neutropenia are rare, other possible causes need to be excluded, and these are listed in Table 48-1. Antinuclear antibodies for autoimmune diseases, ELISA screen for HIV, and serum vitamin B_{12} and folate for pancytopenias are other laboratory studies that can identify the cause of a secondary neutropenia. A bone marrow aspirate can provide further information about the cause of neutropenia, and in patients with SCN shows hematopoetic cells up to the promyelocyte or myelocyte stage of development. Quantifying immunoglobulin levels identifies primary immunodeficiencies with associated neutropenias.

NEUTROPHIL DYSFUNCTION

When evaluating for a possible neutrophil dysfunction disorder, the clinical history may indicate other symptoms that are associated with particular disorders, such as the lack of pigmentation in CHS. A family history may indicate a suggestive inheritance pattern. The nature of repeated infections, such as gram-negative enteric bacteria or streptococcus, may suggest a particular type of immunodeficiency (27). The nitroblue tetrazolium test provides a quick test for NADPH oxidase activity and the dihydrorhodamine-123 fluorescence test can quantify the activity of NADPH oxidase (41). Further genetic testing can also identify a number of known mutations in the NADPH oxidase gene.

MYELOGENOUS LEUKEMIAS

Diagnostic approaches for leukemias include grading and staging of the disease process. Symptoms suggestive of a neoplastic process can lead to further evaluation and initially often begins with a complete blood count followed by bone marrow examination. Diagnostic criteria for CML include marked leukocytosis, reduced leukocyte alkaline phosphatase activity, hypercellular bone marrow with a larger proportion of myelocytes and promyelocytes, and cytogenetic evidence of a BCR-ABL gene fusion, which typically demonstrates the Philadelphia chromosome (42). The leukocytosis can be as high as 1,000,000 cells/mm^3 with associated basophilia or eosinophilia.

AML is diagnosed when abnormally elevated numbers of myeloblasts are found in bone marrow or peripheral blood. Recent World Health Organization (WHO) diagnostic criteria of AML have reduced the minimal percentage of myeloblasts in the bone marrow to 20%. Cytogenetic studies can also identify the associated genetic mutations in AML, regardless of the percentage of myeloblasts in the bone marrow (9).

LYMPHOPENIA

Similar to neutropenias, a complete blood count typically demonstrates lymphopenia, and flow cytometry further qualifies it. Analyzing the number of cells binding to certain cell surface markers helps in distinguishing particular immunodeficiencies and lymphomas. Cell typing will indicate secondary causes of lymphopenia, or whether immunoglobulin deficiencies need to be further evaluated. Routine quantification of immunoglobulins can be done, but may not be helpful in specifically identifying immunodeficiencies.

Diagnosis of SCID requires that <20% of the lymphocytes be T cells, an absolute lymphocyte count <3,000 cells/mm^3, and a mitogenic response <10% of control (43). Further genetic testing can help differentiate specific forms of SCID. DNA analysis could identify X-SCID. Mutations in other genes, such as JAK3, RAG1, RAG2, or IL-7Rα, can be used in the diagnosis of other forms of SCID. ADA deficiency is diagnosed by identifying an ADA activity of <2% of control (43). Patients with DiGeorge syndrome have CD3+ T cell counts of <500 cells/mm^3; conotruncal cardiac defects, such as tetralogy of Fallot; hypocalcemia from abnormal parathyroid glands; and a chromosomal deletion at 22q11.2.

IMMUNOGLOBULIN DEFICIENCY

Selective IgA deficiency is diagnosed by documenting IgA levels two standard deviations below normal, with otherwise normal levels of IgG and IgM. Other acceptable criteria are an IgA level <7 mg/dL, and normal amounts of IgG and IgM (43). CVID can be difficult to diagnose because it is a heterogeneous disorder, but IgG levels will be less than two standard deviations from normal values. Also, response to vaccinations should be documented, because patients with CVID have an impaired response (44). On flow cytometry, patients with X-linked agammaglobulinemia have absent B cells, but normal T-cell levels. Serum IgG levels will either be low or absent. A reduction in the amount of Bruton tyrosine kinase (BTK) protein can also help confirm the diagnosis. Diagnostic criteria for AT include a progressive cerebellar ataxia with evidence of mutations in both ATM genes. Cultured cells also show increased chromosome fragility to radiation (43).

TREATMENT

Treatment of white blood cell disorders will obviously be specific to the underlying cause or syndrome. Minimizing the risks of acquiring infections is a common treatment strategy for any immunodeficient patient. Common measures, such as frequent handwashing and good oral hygiene when immunodeficient, are also easy precautions to take.

NEUTROPENIA

For congenital or idiopathic neutropenic disorders, administration of *granulocyte colony stimulating factor (G-CSF or filgrastim)* can improve the immune systems response to future infections when given on a prophylaxis basis. SCN is now routinely treated with recombinant G-CSF. G-CSF increases the number of neutrophils and decreases the incidence of infections. Up to 90% of patients with SCN respond to G-CSF, and this treatment is recommended for life (3). Initial broad-spectrum antibiotic coverage is needed among patients who are neutropenic presenting with fever, but treatment can be reduced to a more specific antibiotic once the causative agent is found. Finally, bone marrow transplantation (BMT) has been investigated and may be beneficial, but the risks associated with the procedure remain high (45).

NEUTROPHIL DYSFUNCTION

Patients with *myeloperoxidase deficiency* usually do not require prophylactic antibiotic treatments, because most are asymptomatic. They can develop various fungal infections, however, and require aggressive management with systemic antifungal agents. CHS has been treated by BMT in the early childhood period (2). Although marrow transplantation corrects the immunologic complications and potential lymphoproliferative disorders, the pigmentation and neurologic features remain. In patients with rapidly progressive CHS, antiviral prophylaxis with acyclovir, and administration of immunoglobulins may be beneficial. Microtubule-directed medications, such as vincristine, might also offer some benefit.

Chronic granulomatous disease can initially be managed with IFN-γ (46). Antibacterial prophylaxis with trimethoprim-sulfamethoxazole (TMP-SMZ) can minimize the recurrence of bacterial infections. Prophylaxis for fungal infections has not proved to be beneficial. Finally, early and aggressive treatment with proper parenteral antibiotics is required when definite infections are discovered. The only curative therapy remains BMT, but finding an HLA antigen-matched sibling is difficult (2,26). Nonmyeloablative allogenic bone marrow transplantation is being actively studied, but it appears to be associated with a significant risk of graft-versus-host disease (47).

MYELOGENOUS LEUKEMIA

Hydroxyurea was the previous standard of care for myelogenous leukemia because of its improvement in survival rates with stabilization of lymphocyte counts (7,18). Administration of recombinant IFN-α with hydroxyurea has shown better survival outcomes (48–50). Of note, a few reports are found of patients with CML developing multiple sclerosis following administration of IFN-α (8). Patients with CML in the chronic phase who have received allogenic hematopoietic stem cell transplantation from a matched-related donor have an overall survival of 60% after 10 years and approximately 50% after 15 years. Autologous hematopoetic stem cell transplantation did not show any benefits greater than those seen with the administration of IFN-α (7). Imatinib, a selective inhibitor of the BCR-ABL tyrosine kinase, has been compared with IFN-α and cytarabine. Of patients receiving imatinib, 76% had undetectable cells with the Philadelphia chromosome (complete cytogenetic response) versus 15% among patients receiving IFN-α and cytarabine (51). Treatment for the blast crisis usually includes vincristine and prednisone. Median survival among patients with primarily lymphoid blast crisis is 12 months compared with 4.7 months among those patients with a myeloid blast crisis (18).

Standard therapy for AML is doxorubicin, daily for 3 days, and cytarabine, daily for 7 days (52). Complete remission with this regimen is seen in 65% to 75% of patients <60 years of age, and in 50% in those >60 years of age after 1 year (19). Less than 20% of patients will have a complete remission for 5 years (9). G-CSF has also been used to treat the complications of neutropenia seen in AML. No evidence indicates that G-CSF stimulates further production of leukemic cells (19). Hematopoietic stem cell transplantation, autologous and allogenic, has not shown to increase survival in patients with AML (52). Research is ongoing with other molecules, such as antiangiogenesis medications, or therapies targeted by specific surface markers (9).

LYMPHOPENIA

Treatment of primary lymphopenia and immunoglobulin deficiencies are limited to replacement of the defective lymphocyte precursors or supplementation of immunoglobulins. BMT is used in lymphopenia associated with immunodeficiency conditions, such as SCID and DiGeorge syndrome. In SCID, BMT is first line treatment, and is usually done early in the disease course because SCID is always fatal, whereas successful BMT can lead to a normal life (2,12). In cases of *adenosine deaminase deficiency* of SCID, administration of the deficient enzyme, an expensive conjugated adenosine deaminase to polyethylene glycol, has resulted in improved immune function (12). Gene therapy has also been tried, but remains experimental. BMT from an HLA antigen-identical donor is also first line treatment for severe cases of DiGeorge syndrome (2).

IMMUNOGLOBULIN DEFICIENCIES

In primary immunoglobulin deficiencies, such as X-linked agammaglobulinemia, the benefit of BMT is unclear (53). Immunoglobulin supplementation is now part of the medical therapy for all immunodeficiencies with resultant low levels of gammaglobulins regardless of the lymphocyte counts, including SCID. In X-linked agammaglobulinemia and CVID, current standard of care consists of prophylactic monthly administration of IVIg (12). The use of IVIg remains controversial in selective IgA deficiency, because of the usual mild immunodeficiency and possible anaphylactic reaction to IgA-containing IVIg with anti-IgA antibodies. No specific treatments are currently available for AT.

CLINICAL RECOMMENDATIONS OF THE VIGNETTE

The patient with recurrent viral and enteric infections, normal leukocyte counts, and moderate to severely diminished immunoglobulin levels most likely has a common variable immunodeficiency. Genetic testing in CVID would not be beneficial because multiple possible genetic mutations can present as CVID. Treatment for his condition would be monthly administration of IVIg. He will also need to be monitored for the rare complication of a chronic meningoencephalitis from enteroviruses.

SUMMARY

Disorders of white blood cells encompass many different diseases and syndromes. Common clinical presentation of these disorders is characterized by recurrent infections. Myelogenous leukemias present with "B symptoms" commonly seen in other neoplasms and evidence of bone marrow dysfunction. Treatments are specific to these individual disorders and range from BMT, to monthly administration of immunoglobulin supplementation. CML and AML may respond to chemotherapy and BMT. Unless a cure is found, life-long surveillance against microorganisms will be the main goal of management for these disorders.

REFERENCES

1. National Program of Cancer Registries—2002 Cancer (all ages). From the Center for Disease Control.
2. Ten RM. Primary immunodeficiencies. *Mayo Clin Proc.* 1998;73:865–872.
3. Ancliff PJ. Congenital neutropenia. *Blood Rev.* 2003;17:209–216.
4. Parry MF, Root RK, Metcalf JA, et al. Myeloperoxidase deficiency: Prevalence and clinical significance. *Ann Intern Med.* 1981;95:293–301.
5. Lakshman R, Finn A. Neutrophil disorders and their management. *J Clin Pathol.* 2001;54:7–19.
6. Heyworth PG, Cross AR, Curnuttle JT. Chronic granulomatous disease. *Curr Opin Immunol.* 2003;15:578–584.
7. Baccarani M, Saglio G, Goldman J, et al. Evolving concepts in the management of chronic myeloid leukemia: Recommendations from an expert panel on behalf of the European Leukemia Net. *Blood.* 2006;108:1809–1820.
8. Kataoka I, Shinagawa K, Shiro Y, et al. Multiple sclerosis associated with interferon-alpha therapy for chronic myelogenous leukemia. *Am J Hematol.* 2002;70:149–153.
9. Jabbour EJ, Estey E, Kantarjian HM. Adult acute myeloid lymphoma. *Mayo Clin Proc.* 2006;81:247–260.
10. Redaelli A, Bell C, Casagrande J, et al. Clinical and epidemiologic burden of chronic myelogenous leukemia. *Expert Rev Anticancer Ther.* 2004;4:85–96
11. Goldman J. ABC of clinical haematology: Chronic myeloid leukaemia. *BMJ.* 1997;314:657–660.
12. Rosen FS, Cooper MD, Wedgwood RJ. The Primary immunodeficiencies. *N Engl J Med.* 1995;333:431–438.
13. Cooper MA, Pommering TL, Koranyi K. Primary immunodeficiencies. *Am Fam Physician.* 2003;68:2001–2011.
14. Weber-Mzell D, Kotanko P, Hauer AC, et al. Gender, age and seasonal effects on IgA deficiency: A study of 7293 Caucasians. *Eur J Clin Invest.* 2004;34:224–228.
15. Yamagishi H. The 22q11.2 deletion syndrome. *Keio J Med.* 2002;51:77–88.
16. Swift M, Morrell D, Cromartie E, et al. The incidence and gene frequency of ataxia-telangiectasia in the United States. *Am J Hum Genet.* 1986;39:573–583.
17. Curnutte JT. Chronic granulomatous disease: The solving of a clinical riddle at the molecular level. *Clin Immunol Immunopathol.* 1993;67:S2–S15.
18. Osarogiagbon UR, McGlave PB. Chronic myelogenous leukemia. *Curr Opin Hematol.* 1999;64:241–246.
19. Rathnasabapathy R, Lancet JE. Management of acute myelogenous leukemia in the elderly. *Cancer Control.* 2003;10:469–477.
20. Mueller BU, Pabst T. C/EBPα and the pathophysiology of acute myeloid leukemia. *Curr Opin Hematol.* 2006;13:7–14.
21. Jawad AF, McDonald-Mcginn DM, Zackai E, et al. Immunologic features of chromosome 22q11.2 deletion syndrome (DiGeorge syndrome/velocardiofacial syndrome). *J Pediatr.* 2001;139:715–723.
22. Buckley RH. Primary immunodeficiency diseases due to defects in lymphocytes. *N Engl J Med.* 2000;343:1313–1322.
23. Giovannetti A, Mazzetta F, Caprini E, et al. Skewed T-cell receptor repertoire, decreased thymic output, and predominance of terminally differentiated T cells in ataxia telangiectasia. *Blood.* 2002;100:4082–4089.
24. Watts RG. Neutropenia. In: Lee GR, Foerster J, Lukens J, et al., eds. *Wintrobe's Clinical Hematology.* Vol. 1. 10th ed. Baltimore, MD: Williams & Wilkins; 1999:1862–1888.
25. Lanza F. Clinical manifestations of myeloperoxidase deficiency. *J Mol Med.* 1998;76:676–681.
26. Dinauer M, Coates T. Disorders of phagocyte function and number. In: Hoffman R, Benz E, Hattil S, et al. *Hematology: Basic Principles and Practice,* 4th ed. Philadelphia: Churchill Livingstone; 2005:787–802.
27. Lekstrom-Hines JA, Gallin JI. Immunodeficiency diseases caused by defects in phagocytes. *N Engl J Med.* 2000;343:1703–1714.
28. Kinugawa N. Epstein-Barr virus infection in Chediak-Higashi syndrome mimicking acute lymphocytic leukemia. *Am J Pediatr Hematol Oncol.* 1990;12:182–186.
29. Lydyard P, Gross C. Cells involved in the immune response. *Immunology.* 1988;65:14–I41.
30. Baehner R. Normal phagocyte structure and function. Hoffman: *Hematology: Basic Principles and Practice,* 4th ed. Churchill Livingstone; 2005:737–762.
31. Tosi M. Innate immune responses to infection. *J Allergy Clin Immunol.* 2005;1162:241–249.
32. Hadfield MG, Ghatak NR, Laine FJ, et al. Brain lesions in chronic granulomatous disease. *Acta Neuropathol.* 1991;81:467–470.
33. Saito T, Asai O, Dobashi N, et al. Peripheral neuropathy caused by high-dose cytosine arabinoside treatment in a patient with acute myeloid leukemia. *J Infect Chemother.* 2006; 12:148–151.
34. Niederle N, Kloke O, Osieka R, et al. Interferon alfa-2b in acute- and chronic-phase chronic myelogenous leukemia: Initial response and long-term results in 54 patients. *Eur J Cancer* 1991;27:[Suppl 4]:S7–S14.
35. Buckley RH. Primary cellular immunodeficiencies. *J Allergy Clin Immunol.* 2002;109:747–757.
36. Larner AJ, Webster AD, Thomas DJ. Peripheral neuropathy associated with common variable immunodeficiency. *Eur J Neurol.* 2000;7:573.
37. Yousry TA, Strupp M, Bruning R. Common variable immunodeficiency leading to spinal subacute combined degeneration monitored by MRI. *J Neurol Neurosurg Psychiatry.* 1998;64:663–666.
38. Intravenous Immunoglobulin: Prevention and Treatment of Disease. National Institutes of Health. Consensus Development Conference Statement. 1990
39. Taylor AMR, Byrd PJ. Molecular pathology of ataxia telangiectasia. *J Clin Pathol.* 2005; 58:1009–1015.
40. Crawford TO, Mandir AS, Lefton-Greif MA, et al. Quantitative neurologic assessment of ataxia-telangiectasia. *Neurology.* 2000;54:1505–1509.
41. Jirapongsananuruk O, Malech HL, Kuhns DB, et al. Diagnostic paradigm for evaluation of male patients with chronic granulomatous disease, based upon the dihydrorhodamine 123 assay. *J Allergy Clin Immunol.* 2003;111:374–379.
42. Quintas-Cardama A, Cortes JE. Chronic myeloid leukemia: Diagnosis and treatment. *Mayo Clin Proc.* 2006;81:973–988.
43. Conley ME, Notarangelo LD, Etzioni A. Diagnostic criteria for primary immunodeficiencies. Representing PAGID (Pan-American Group for Immunodeficiencies) and ESID (European Society for Immunodeficiencies). *Clin Immunol.* 1999;93:190–197.
44. Kondratenko I, Amlot PL, Webster AD, et al. Lack of specific antibody response in common variable immunodeficiency (CVID) associated with failure in production of antigen-specific memory T cells. *Clin Exp Immunol.* 1997;108:9–13.
45. Ferry C, Ouachee M, Leblanc T, et al. Hematopoietic stem cell transplantation in severe congenital neutropenia: Experience of the French SCN register. *Bone Marrow Transplant.* 2005;35:45–50.
46. Woodman RC, Erickson RW, Rae J, et al. Prolonged recombinant interferon-gamma therapy in chronic granulomatous disease: Evidence against enhanced neutrophil oxidase activity. *Blood.* 1992;79:1558–1562.
47. Horwitz ME, Barrett AJ, Brown MR, et al. Treatment of chronic granulomatous disease with nonmyeloablative conditioning and a T-cell-depleted hematopoietic allograft. *N Engl J Med.* 2001;344:881–888.
48. Hehlmann R, Berger U, Pfirrmann M, et al. Randomized comparison of interferon alpha and hydroxyurea monotherapy in chronic myeloid leukemia (CML-study II): Prolongation of survival by the combination of interferon alpha and hydroxyurea. *Leukemia.* 2003;17:1529–1537.
49. Baccarani M, Russo D, Rosti G, et al. Interferon-alfa for chronic myeloid leukemia. *Semin Hematol.* 2003;40:22–33.
50. Guilhot F, Chastang C, Michallet M, et al. Interferon alfa-2b combined with cytarabine versus interferon alone in chronic myelogenous leukemia. *N Engl J Med.* 1997;337:223–229.
51. O'Brien SG, Meinhardt P, Bond E, et al. Imatinib compared with interferon and low-dose cytarabine for newly diagnosed chronic-phase chronic myeloid leukemia. *N Engl J Med.* 2003;348:994–1004.
52. Estey EH. Therapeutic options for acute myelogenous leukemia. *Cancer.* 2001;92:1059–1073.
53. Howard V, Myers LA, Williams DA, et al. Stem cell transplants for patients with X-linked agammaglobulinemia. *Clin Immunol.* 2003;107:98–102.
54. Cleary AM, Insel RA, Lewis DB. Disorders of lymphocyte function. Hoffman: *Hematology: Basic Principles and Practice,* 4th ed. Churchill Livingstone; 2005:831–851.

CHAPTER 49

Disorders of Platelets

Joseph F. Stilwill • Mauna B. Pandya • Sucha Nand • Laura C. Michaelis

OBJECTIVES

- To define thrombocytosis and thrombocytopenia
- To describe the symptoms of quantitative platelet disorders and platelet dysfunction
- To discuss the diagnostic evaluation of platelet disorders
- To explain the neurologic complications of the myeloproliferative disorders and thrombotic thrombocytopenic purpura

CASE VIGNETTE

A 68-year-old right-handed man with a history of elevated cholesterol, presents to the emergency room with acute onset of left-sided weakness that began 5 hours before to presentation. Review of systems is positive for a burning sensation on his feet for the past 2 months. Vital signs are normal. His neurologic examination is remarkable for decreased muscle strength in his left arm and leg. Strength is normal on his right extremities. He is hypereflexic on the right side and has a right Babinski sign. Sensory examination and cranial nerve function are intact. Laboratory findings demonstrate a leukocyte count of 8.3 K/μL, hemoglobin of 14.2 g/dL, hematocrit of 42.5%, and platelet count of 1,180,000/μL. Unenhanced computed tomographic (CT) scan is normal. Magnetic resonance imaging (MRI) of the brain demonstrates an area of restrictive diffusion of the right internal capular region consistent with a recent ischemic stroke.

Platelets

DEFINITION

Platelets, which are anucleate cell fragments that circulate in the blood, are critical to the hematologic mechanisms of primary and secondary hemostasis. They are derived from megakaryocytes—multinucleated cells of the bone marrow that form long processes called *proplatelets* as they mature. From these processes, fragments of megakaryocytic cytoplasm, or platelets, are released into the peripheral circulation (1). Although these fragments were long considered inert, recent understanding illustrates that platelets are capable of elegant and choreographed activity utilizing the multiple organelles included in the cytoplasm. Circulating platelets are recruited to sites of endothelial injury by local and systemically released cytokines. Interplay of expressed receptors on the subendothelium and platelet surface activates the platelets, leading to changes in the platelet cytoskeleton and release of locally activating factors. These factors, including fibrinogen, grow factors, adenosine diphosphate (ADP), ionized calcium, and serotonin, lead to conformational changes in glycoprotein IIb/IIIa receptors, vasoactivity within the vessel, and the recruitment and aggregation of additional platelets. This initial formation of the platelet plug is the catalyst for the coagulation cascade and hemostatic regulatory elements.

Platelets typically circulate in the blood for 7 to 10 days (their average life span) before they are cleared by the reticuloendothelial system, particularly the spleen. Low levels of circulating platelets, or dysfunction of any number of their hemostatic mechanisms, can predispose an individual to bleeding, whereas high levels, although usually asymptomatic, can increase the risk of thrombosis as well as hemorrhage. As such, disorders of platelets can be characterized as either quantitative disorders or qualitative disorders. Quantitative platelet disorders include thrombocytosis (elevated number of platelets) and thrombocytopenia (reduced number of platelets); qualitative disorders include platelet dysfunction.

Thrombocytosis

DEFINITION

Thrombocytosis is defined as a platelet count >500,000/μL. It is important to exclude pseudothrombocytosis by ensuring fragmented erythrocytes or leukocytes have not been misidentified as platelets by an automated cell counter and that circulating protein abnormalities, such as mixed cryoglobulinemia, have not interfered with the smear technique. Once measurement inaccuracies have been excluded, disorders of thrombocytosis can be classified as either primary or secondary. The primary processes can be the result of inherited or acquired megakaryocytic disorders.

ETIOLOGY AND PATHOGENESIS

Reactive thrombocytosis is much more prevalent than primary thrombocytosis. In a retrospective study of 732 patients with a platelet count >500,000/μL, 87.7% were found to have reactive thrombocytosis (2). Another study found that infection was the most common cause of reactive thrombocytosis (50.1%) (3). Reactive thrombocytosis is not associated with an increased risk of thrombosis or hemorrhage above the risk of other patients with the same underlying condition, regardless of the platelet count.

In reactive thrombocytosis, inflammation causes increased levels of thrombopoietin and interleukin-6 (4). Thrombopoietin, which is produced by the liver, binds preferentially to receptors on circulating platelets. The remaining free hormone then binds to megakaryocytes in the bone marrow and stimulates production of more cells. In inflammatory conditions, the liver produces increased levels of IL-6 and, in turn, thrombopoietin, accounting for the increase in platelet count (5). Reactive thrombocytosis can also occur when the bone marrow is being stimulated to increase other cell lines, such as in acute blood loss, iron-deficiency anemia, or tissue damage, which lead to physiologic increases in erythropoietin or granulocyte growth factors. Elimination of clearance mechanisms, for example splenectomy, often leads to thrombocytosis. Additionally, secondary thrombocytosis can be seen in malignancy, rheumatologic conditions, allergic reactions, exercise, renal disease, and with use of certain medications, including vincristine, epinephrine, IL-1B, and all-trans retinoic acid. Interestingly, a familial variant of thrombocytosis also is seen in which thrombopoietin is over produced. These patients do face an increased risk of thrombosis (4).

Clonal bone marrow disorders that result in thrombocytosis are most often myeloproliferative disorders or one of the myelodysplastic syndromes. The myeloproliferative disorders are a group of related disorders of bone marrow hematopoetic stem cells. These include chronic myelogenous leukemia (CML), essential thrombocythemia (ET), polycythemia vera (PV), and myelofibrosis with myeloid metaplasia. For the most part, these are clonal disorders, which can lead to an increase in mature cells in the peripheral circulation (6). Thrombocytosis is seen in any of these disorders, but most prominently in ET and PV. The thrombocytosis seen in these disorders is not secondary to increased levels of thrombopoietin (although increased levels may be seen) but rather to dysregulation of megakaryocyte production and maturation signaling. Myelodysplastic syndromes (MDS) are characterized by abnormal cellular maturation, dysplasia, and either hyperplasia or hypoplasia of the bone marrow. Thrombocytopenia complicates MDS in 30% to 45% of cases (7).

Essential thrombocytosis is characterized by a persistent thrombocytosis (>600,000 μL) that is not reactive in nature (8). The incidence is approximately 2.5 in 100,000, and typically presents between the ages 50 and 60 years. Although patients with this disorder can be asymptomatic, clinical features include erythromelalgia (burning sensation of the hands and feet), digital ischemia, and thromboses. Both arterial and venous thromboses may be seen, and these have been reported at diagnosis in 20% to 50% of patients with ET and PV (9). Neurologic complications can be seen in up to 25% of patients. These include headache, dizziness, and focal neurologic findings thought to be secondary to cerebral ischemia (4). Fetal growth retardation and recurrent spontaneous abortions commonly occur in pregnant women with ET. Risk factors for thrombosis include a history of thrombosis, hyperlipidemia, tobacco use, and advanced age.

Polycythemia vera is characterized by inappropriate proliferation of the erythroid cell line; it can often involve an overabundance of the granulocytic and megakaryocytic cell lines as well (8). Thrombotic complications in PV are often caused by increased blood viscosity as well as thrombocytosis.

DIAGNOSTIC APPROACH

Initial evaluation of thrombocytosis should begin with complete blood count with differential, erythrocyte sedimentation rate (ESR), C-reactive protein (CRP), serum ferritin, and examination of the peripheral smear. Microcytosis and low serum ferritin strongly suggest iron deficiency anemia as the cause. Howell-Jolly bodies may be seen on examination of the peripheral smear in patients who are asplenic. Patients with chronic inflammation may show a neutrophilic leukocytosis or *left shift.* Inflammatory markers, such as CRP and ESR, can suggest a secondary thrombocytosis if elevated. If the above studies do not suggest a secondary thrombocytosis, then a bone marrow aspirate and biopsy should be performed to evaluate for a myeloproliferative disorder or myelodysplastic syndrome. In addition, mutation of the JAK2 gene may be seen in the myeloproliferative disorders, particularly PV (10). Detection of this mutation strongly suggests that one of these disorders is causing a patient's thrombocytosis.

TREATMENT

As stated, reactive or secondary thrombocytosis rarely leads to complications. Therefore, no specific treatment is necessary, other than treatment of the underlying condition. In the myeloproliferative disorders, the risk of complications does not necessarily correspond to the measured platelet level; however, therapy to reduce platelets can decrease the risk of complications. In cases of thrombosis, platelet apheresis is recommended for counts >800,000/μL. Hydroxyurea is an oral antimetabolite chemotherapy that is considered the first-line cytoreductive therapy in patients at high risk (age >60, platelet count >1,500,000/μL, history of prior thrombosis). It is given in conjunction with low-dose aspirin. Patients who are at intermediate and low risk (those without high risk features and age 40 to 60 and age <40 years, respectively) can be treated with low-dose aspirin alone. All patients with ET should have reversible cardiovascular risk factors stringently controlled (11). Alternative cytoreductive agents, including anagrelide and interferon-α (IFN-α), are available, although these are considered second-line therapies and are less commonly used.

Thrombocytopenia

DEFINITION

Thrombocytopenia is defined as a platelet count <150,000/μL. In general, significant spontaneous bleeding is not encountered until the platelet count reaches a level <20,000/μL. As the platelet count drops further, the incidence of bleeding increases (12). Critically ill patients and patients treated with chemotherapy are the most likely to develop thrombocytopenia.

ETIOLOGY AND PATHOGENESIS

Thrombocytopenia can be classified into three categories: (i) decreased platelet production in the bone marrow, (ii) increased destruction or consumption of platelets, or (iii) increased sequestration of platelets in the periphery (13).

Decreased production occurs when there is a lack of adequate megakaryocytes in the bone marrow. This can be secondary to infiltration of malignant cells, such as in leukemia, lymphoma, or other disseminated cancers. It can also be secondary to fibrosis or marrow aplasia or toxic marrow suppression from drugs, alcohol or infection. This can be easily identified on bone marrow biopsy. Certain medications (particularly chemotherapeutic agents), radiation therapy, and nutritional deficiencies (e.g., B_{12} and folate deficiency) can also result in decreased megakaryocyte production.

Splenic sequestration of platelets occurs when the spleen enlarges. In the healthy individual, approximately 30% of the body's circulating platelets are within the splenic circulation at any one time. When splenomegaly develops, larger percentages are out of circulation and the peripheral count is lower. Splenomegaly can be seen in cases of portal hypertension secondary to cirrhosis or congestive heart failure or in certain hematologic conditions, such as hereditary spherocytosis or thalassemia. It can also be secondary to a malignant infiltration such as occurs in leukemia and lymphoma or in the myeloproliferative disorders. The annual incidence of these disorders per million per year is as follows: ITP 33 and TTP-HUS. DIC has been described in up to 1% of all hospitalized patients.

Increased platelet destruction is a broad category that includes immune-mediated processes, such as immune thrombocytopenic purpura (ITP), drug-induced antiplatelet antibody formation, such as heparin-induced thrombocytopenia (HIT), postinfectious thrombocytopenia, and certain rheumatologic disorders, including systemic lupus erythematosus (SLE). Increased platelet consumption includes disseminated intravascular coagulation (DIC) and thrombotic thrombocytopenia purpura and hemolytic-uremic syndrome (TTP-HUS). In the peripartum pregnant patient, HELLP syndrome (hemolytic anemia, elevated liver enzymes, and low platelet count) is a leading cause of thrombocytopenia.

ITP is an autoimmune syndrome in which autoantibodies are directed against platelet surface protein complexes, such as glycoprotein IIb/IIIa. The antibodies target the platelet for clearance by the spleen (14). The incidence has been reported as 32 in 1 million persons (13). Patients can present with severe thrombocytopenia (<20,000) and subsequent mucocutaneous bleeding and petechiae, or they can present with an asymptomatic, mild thrombocytopenia that is incidentally detected. A complete blood count typically shows an isolated thrombocytopenia. Platelet transfusion does not often result in an increased platelet count because of the circulating antibodies, and transfusion is generally not required except in cases of severe bleeding. In general, ITP is a chronic condition that can fluctuate over time. If the platelet count is severely depressed, the patient is often first treated with corticosteroids, with or without intravenous gamma globulins (IVIG). Occasionally, further treatment with splenectomy, rituximab, or cytoreductive chemotherapy is undertaken.

HIT is also an antibody-mediated process that can occur in approximately 3% of patients treated with heparin products (~120,000 patients per year in the United States). HIT should be suspected in a patient who receives heparin and develops a 50% reduction in platelet count from baseline. The immune-mediated form of HIT (type 2) can be life-threatening. Antibodies directed against a complex of heparin and platelet factor 4 are formed; these antibodies bind to heparin/PF4 complexes and platelet receptors. This results in both platelet activation and increased platelet clearance, resulting in a paradoxical increased risk of thrombosis despite the profound thrombocytopenia. Treatment with either unfractionated or low-molecular-weight heparin can lead to HIT, although a higher percentage of those treated with unfractionated heparin develop the disorder. Treatment involves immediate discontinuation of all heparin products and treatment with alternative anticoagulation with a direct thrombin inhibitor to prevent thromboses. A nonimmune HIT, also called HAT (heparin associated thrombocytopenia), is also seen. HAT is of little clinical significance, and it is characterized by a modest thrombocytopenia that occurs 2 to 3 days after initiation of heparin and is self-limited: It is not necessary to discontinue heparin in this situation.

A number of other medications can also lead to thrombocytopenia, including thiazide diuretics, penicillins, sulfa derivatives, phenytoin, cimetidine, and quinine. Alcoholism is commonly associated with thrombocytopenia, whether because of B_{12} or folate deficiencies, increased portal hypertension, or a directly toxic effect of alcohol on the bone marrow.

Infection can reduce platelet numbers through several mechanisms. Patients with sepsis can develop thrombocytopenia because of excessive consumption of platelets, bone marrow suppression, or disseminated intravascular coagulation. The viral hepatidities, Epstein-Barr virus, cytomegalovirus, and human immunodeficiency virus (HIV) can lead to thrombocytopenia through an immune-mediated phenomenon in which antibodies to viral antigens cross-react with platelets.

DIC leads to consumption of platelets and clotting factors. The true incidence of DIC is not known, but it has been estimated to be as high as 1 per 1,000 persons. In addition to hemolytic anemia and thrombocytopenia, laboratory values often include abnormal activated partial thromboplastin time (aPTT) and prothrombin time (PT) or international normalized ratio (INR), elevated fibrin split products, elevated D-dimer, and decreased fibrinogen. DIC can be caused by infection, obstetric complications, or malignancy, such as acute leukemia or adenocarcinoma. In addition to thrombocytopenia, patients develop a consumptive coagulopathy. The disease manifests itself through both bleeding and thrombosis. Treatment is directed at the underlying cause.

TTP-HUS is potentially fatal disease with an annual incidence of 3 to 4 cases per 100,000 persons. TTP-HUS is characterized by a pentad of signs that include thrombocytopenia, microangiopathic hemolytic anemia, fever, renal insufficiency, and mental status changes. Not all of the signs will necessarily be present, but thrombocytopenia and microangiopathic hemolytic anemia are crucial for the diagnosis of TTP. Neurologic symptoms can include seizures and focal deficits, often caused by platelet-rich thrombi in the arterial and capillary microvasculature (13). Endothelial injury is thought to lead to the accumulation of unusually large von Willebrand factor in endothelial tissue. This protein is a procoagulant and, when it is not broken down by a metalloproteinase, TTP can develop. The lack of metalloproteinase can result from an inhibitor or a genetic defect (15). This can be set in motion by an infection (*Escherichia coli* 017:H7, *Shigella* spp.), medications, or malignancy. In some cases, TTP can be idiopathic. Treatment consists of exchange transfusion or plasmapheresis and infusion of fresh frozen plasma to remove the procoagulants from the circulation. The diagnosis of TTP-HUS is a clinical one, and it is important to recognize the disease early and initiate treatment immediately.

HELLP syndrome is one of the hypertensive disorders of pregnancy that may be related to preeclampsia. It is estimated to occur in 0.1% of all pregnancies. As with TTP and DIC, it is characterized by a microangiopathic, hemolytic anemia thought to be secondary to dysfunction of the uteroplacental unit (16). The liver injury seen in HELLP is caused by hepatic infarction from microthrombi. Complications include DIC, hepatic rupture, acute renal failure, pulmonary edema, and adult respiratory distress syndrome. The disease can be fatal for both the mother and fetus. Management consists of prompt delivery, blood pressure management, and supportive care.

DIAGNOSIS

In evaluating thrombocytopenia, it is important to first rule out pseudothrombocytopenia. This is a laboratory artifact in which clumping of platelets is seen in EDTA tubes. *In vitro,* a conformational change leads to exposure of antigens on platelets that are not exposed *in vivo.* Antibodies in the patient's blood react with these antigens, which leads to clumping of platelets and a low laboratory value. Testing of citrated blood will reveal the true platelet count. Pseudothrombocytopenia has no clinical significance, and no increase is seen in thrombosis or hemorrhage.

Evaluation of a patient with thrombocytopenia should always start with a careful history and physical examination. Special attention should be paid to medication and bleeding history and to the presence of splenomegaly. Evaluation of the peripheral blood smear is critical, as peripheral blood findings can guide further work up. A proposed algorithm for the diagnosis of thrombocytopenia is included in Figure 49-1.

TREATMENT

The treatment of thrombocytopenia depends on the underlying cause. In all cases, uncontrolled bleeding should prompt rapid platelet transfusion. It has been well demonstrated that spontaneous bleeding, including hemorrhagic stroke, epistaxis, or gastric bleeding, is uncommon when platelets are >20,000/μL. Transfusion parameters, however, should be appropriate to the patient and the clinical situation. Most invasive procedures can be safely performed with a platelet count between 50,000 and 75,000/μL. In some cases of thrombocytopenia, notably ITP, bleeding is uncommon, despite the low platelet counts, and transfusion should be avoided whenever possible. Among the dangers of overexposure to platelets is the development of antibodies to various HLA antigen subtypes, which can increase the risk of adverse immune reactions to future transfusions. In the prothrombotic disorders, such as HIT and TTP-HUS, unnecessary platelet transfusions can actually propagate the formation of microthrombi and worsen the clinical condition; outside of severe life-threatening bleeding, platelet transfusions are generally contraindicated in these disorders.

Platelet Dysfunction

ETIOLOGY AND PATHOGENESIS

Platelet dysfunction can be seen in a variety of acquired circumstances and in some rare, genetic conditions. Common causes of platelet dysfunction are drugs, foods, and spices, more than 100 of which have been implicated (17). The most common of these are the nonsteroidal anti-inflammatory drugs (NSAIDs). Aspirin irreversibly acetylates cyclooxygenase and inhibits the platelet aggregation and vasoconstriction. Other NSAID act in a similar manner, but their action is reversible. Clopidogrel, dipyridamole, ticlopidine, abciximab, and eptifibatide are all medications that are specifically designed to inhibit platelet aggregation, although they work through different mechanisms.

A number of other causes are found for acquired platelet dysfunction. These include profound renal and hepatic dysfunction, plasma cell dyscrasias, cardiopulmonary bypass, and the aforementioned myeloproliferative disorders. Uremia leads to defects in adhesion, aggregation, secretion, and procoagulant activity (17). The mechanism for this dysfunction is not completely understood, but the uremic toxins and anemia are both thought to play a role because bleeding improves with

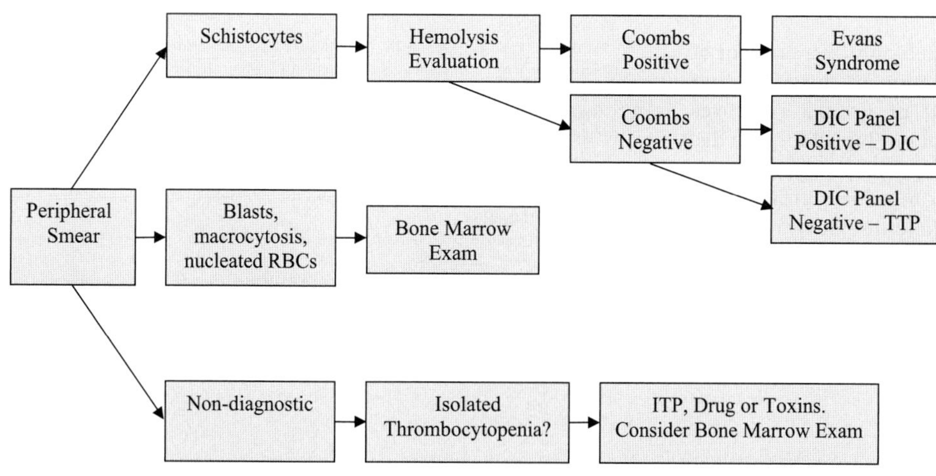

FIGURE 49-1. Diagnostic algorithm for thrombocytopenia. (Adapted from Sekhon SS, Roy V. Thrombocytopenia in adults: A practical approach to evaluation and management. *South Med J.* 2006;99(5):491–498, with permission).

dialysis and correction of anemia with exogenous erythropoietin or blood transfusion (18,19). In liver disease, there may be a defect in platelet aggregation and an increased risk of bleeding that is not related to thrombocytopenia or decreased levels of coagulation factors. The abnormal levels of protein seen in the plasma cell dyscrasias lead to defects in platelet function. Patients on cardiopulmonary bypass have dysfunction because of a variety of mechanisms, including interaction with nonphysiologic surfaces of the machine and hypothermia (20). Impairment of aggregation is thought to be the mechanism of dysfunction in the myeloproliferative disorders.

The inherited disorders of platelet function are rare. They can be secondary to abnormalities of membrane proteins, granule constituents, or metabolic reactions. These include the diagnoses of Glanzmann thrombasthenia, Bernard-Soulier syndrome, Wiskott-Aldrich syndrome, Chediak-Higashi syndrome, and Hermansky-Pudlak syndrome (21). Von Willebrand disease, a much more common disorder characterized by a deficiency of von Willebrand factor, can lead to platelet dysfunction by limiting platelet adherence to subendothelial surfaces and to other platelets. This disease is discussed in greater detail in Chapter 51.

The symptoms of platelet dysfunction are similar to those of thrombocytopenia. Mucocutaneous bleeding (epistaxis, gingival bleeding, easy bruising, hematuria) is most frequently seen. The need to evaluate for platelet dysfunction is most often encountered perioperatively or when a patient is actively bleeding.

DIAGNOSIS

Again, the first step in diagnosis is obtaining a complete blood count and review of the peripheral smear. Particular attention should be paid to the leukocyte count and differential to look for evidence of the myeloproliferative disorders. Liver and kidney function tests should be drawn to evaluate dysfunction in these organ systems. An elevation in total protein may also point toward a plasma cell dyscrasia. The bleeding time has been traditionally used to screen for platelet dysfunction. This test, however, is invasive, operator-dependent, and relatively insensitive (22). Newer diagnostic tools allow more sensitive and specific *in vitro* testing of platelet function and platelet aggregation.

TREATMENT

Acquired platelet dysfunction is corrected only by treatment of the underlying disease or discontinuation of the offending medication. As described, treatment of uremia improves platelet dysfunction. The same is true of myeloproliferative disorders and plasma cell dyscrasia. In the acute setting, desmopressin (DDAVP) has been shown to be of use in acquired platelet dysfunction and in von Willebrand disease by releasing factor VIII from endothelial cells (23). Antifibrinolytic agents, such as aminocaproic acid, can be helpful for patients with significant mucocutaneous, uterine or gastrointestinal tract bleeding; however aminocaproic acid is contraindicated for thrombotic disorders with fibrinolysis, such as DIC. Platelet transfusion may be required to control bleeding in both acquired and inherited platelet dysfunction.

CLINICAL RECOMMENDATIONS OF THE VIGNETTE

The patient likely has essential thrombocythemia complicated by an acute subcortical ischemic stroke. The patient should be treated acutely with platelet apheresis and cytoreductive therapy. Diagnostic evaluation should include a bone marrow examination with cytogenetics to evaluate other possible causes for the patient's thrombocytosis. Eventually, aspirin may be started to treat the patient's erythromelalgia.

SUMMARY

Disorders of platelets account for a wide variety of disease. They can be characterized by thrombocytosis, thrombocytopenia, and dysfunctional platelets. These disorders can lead to thromboses, bleeding, or both.

REFERENCES

1. Italiano JE, Hartwig JH. *Hematology: Basic Principles and Practice*, 4th ed. In: Hoffman R, ed. *Megakaryocyte and Platelet Structure*. Philadelphia: Churchill Livingstone; 2005.
2. Griesshammer M, Bangerter M, Sauer T, et al. Aetiology and clinical significance of thrombocytosis: Analysis of 732 patients with an elevated platelet count. *J Intern Med.* 1999;245:295–300.
3. Aydogan T, et al. Incidence and etiology of thrombocytosis in an adult Turkish population. *Platelets*, 2006;17(5):328–331.
4. Schafer AI. Thrombocytosis. *N Engl J Med.* 2004;350:1211–1219.
5. Wolber E, Fandrey J, Frackowski U, et al. Hepatic thrombopoietin mRNA is increased in acute inflammation. *Thromb Haemost.* 2001;86(6):1421–1424.
6. Schafer AI. Thrombocytosis and thrombocythemia. *Blood Rev.* 2001;15(4):159–166.
7. Steensma DP, Bennett JM. The myelodysplastic syndromes: diagnosis and treatment. *Mayo Clinic Proceedings.* 2006;81:104–130.
8. Robyn J, Sloand E. The myeloproliferative disorders. In: Rodgers G, Young N, eds. *Bethesda Handbook of Clinical Hematology.* Philadelphia: Lippincott Williams & Wilkins; 2005.
9. Pearson T. The risk of thrombosis in essential thrombocythemia and polycythemia vera. *Semin Oncol.* 2002;29[3 Suppl 10]:16–21.
10. James C, Ugo V, Le Covedic JP, et al. A unique clonal JAK2 mutation leading to constitutive signalling causes polycythaemia vera. *Nature.* 2005;434(7037):1144–1148.
11. Cambell P, Green A. *Management of Polycythemia Vera and Essential Thrombocythemia in Hematology 2005.* Atlanta: American Society of Hematology; 2005.
12. Sekhon SS, Roy V. Thrombocytopenia in adults: A practical approach to evaluation and management. *South Med J.* 2006;99(5):491–498.
13. Fogarty PF, Dunbar CE. Thrombocytopenia. In: Rodgers G, Young N, eds. *Bethesda Handbook of Clinical Hematology.* Philadelphia: Lippincott Williams & Wilkins; 2005.
14. van Leeuwen E, van der Ven J, Enelfriet C. Specificity of autoantibodies in autoimmune thrombocytopenia. *Blood.* 1982;59:23–26.
15. Moake JL. Thrombotic microangiopathies. *N Engl J Med.* 2002;347:589–600.
16. Stone JH.,HELLP syndrome: Hemolysis, elevated liver enzymes, and low platelets. *JAMA* 1998;280:559–562.
17. Crowther M, Abshire T, George JN. In: Williams ME, ed. *Hemostasis and Thrombosis*, 2nd ed. American Society of Hematology Self-assessment Program. Michael E. Williams and Marc J. Kahn, editors. Blackwell Publishing; 2005.
18. Cases A, et al. Recombinant human erythropoietin treatment improves platelet function in uremic patients. *Kidney Int.* 1992;42(3):668–672.
19. Stewart J, Castaldi P. Uraemic bleeding: A reversible platelet defect corrected by dialysis. *Q J Med.* 1967;36:409.
20. Weerasinghe A, Taylor K. The platelet in cardiopulmonary bypass. *Ann Thorac Surg.* 1998;66(6):2145–2152.
21. Nurden AT. Qualitative disorders of platelets and megakaryocytes. *Journal of Thrombosis and Haemostasis.* 2005;3:1773–1782.
22. Harrison P, Robinson M, Liesner R, et al. The PFA-100: A potential rapid screening tool for the assessment of platelet dysfunction. *Clin Lab Haematol.* 2002;24:225–232.
23. Zeigler ZR, Megaludis A, Fraley DS. Desmopressin (d-DAVP) effects on platelet rheology and von Willebrand factor activities in uremia. *Am J Hematol.* 1992;39(2):90–95.

CHAPTER **50**

Sickle Cell Anemia and Other Hemoglobinopathies

Harry L. Messmore • William H. Wehrmacher

OBJECTIVES

- To define hemoglobinopathy
- To describe the basis for the clinical features of sickle cell anemia and the common variants
- To explain the pathophysiology of sickle cell anemia in terms of blood cell and blood vessel interactions
- To discuss the thalassemia syndromes in terms of definitions and pathophysiology
- To describe current treatment options for the more common hemoglobinopathies, sickle cell anemia and thalassemia major

CASE VIGNETTE

A 27-year-old black man was examined in the emergency room for a complaint of headache and right-sided weakness. He had a lifelong history of sickle cell anemia characterized by numerous hospitalizations for pain in various parts of his body, leg ulcerations, chest pain with dyspnea, fever, and cough.

A computed tomographic (CT) scan of his brain was performed for suspected stroke. The CT showed a large hemorrhage in the left frontal parietal area. Exchange transfusions with compatible normal red blood cells were given over the next 24 hours, but the patient died in a comatose state.

DEFINITION

Hemoglobin is a tetramer of globin polypeptide chains that is present in normal red blood cells in three forms: HbA ($\alpha\alpha$-$\beta\beta$), HbA_2 ($\alpha\alpha$-$\delta\delta$), and HbF ($\alpha\alpha$-$\gamma\gamma$). HbF is fetal hemoglobin, which does not sickle, thus it is protective against sickle cell disease whenever it is the predominant hemoglobin present. Amino acid substitution can occur on a genetic basis as can complete or partial chain deletion and those defects may involve one or both chains of a pair and mixed substitutions and chain deletions can occur in the same person.

Defects in the chemical structure of the hemoglobin molecule that result in deranged function or altered physical or chemical properties resulting in injury to tissue or organ are termed *hemoglobinopathy*. The defects are genetically determined, and consist of amino acid substitution or deletions in one or more of the polypeptide chains of the molecule. Mutations that impair production or translation of a globin messenger RNA (mRNA), leading to deficient globin chain biosynthesis and partial or complete deletion of one or more of the chains are not a hemoglobinopathy, but are termed *thalassemia*.

Sickle cell anemia is an autosomal recessive disease and the clinical syndrome is commonly referred to as *sickle cell disease* (*SCD*) in which the homozygous state results from an amino acid substitution of valine for glycine in the sixth position of both of the β-globin chains of hemoglobin A. The *sickle trait* or *HbAS*, involves only one chain and the hemoglobins (HbS) concentration is usually $<50\%$; the disease involves both chains. The variants of this abnormal molecule (*hemoglobin S*) are commonly caused by an amino acid substitution in the other beta chain of HbA; for instance, the combination of an abnormal beta chain known as *hemoglobin C* results in *HbSC disease*. In combination with thalassemia (a family of various chain deletions caused by decreased synthesis of the second beta chain) that results in an absent beta chain (*beta thalassemia 0*), one beta chain is the sickle variant or hemoglobin S and the other chain is absent (beta) the patient has HbSB or *S-thalassemia* which is clinically indistinguishable from SCD. Hemoglobin F ($\alpha\alpha$-$\gamma\gamma$) hemoglobin is increased in some patients and protecting against red blood cell (RBC) sickling (1–3).

EPIDEMIOLOGY

Sickle cell anemia is the most prevalent hemoglobinopathy known; it is identified in most human races, but is most prevalent in African, Middle Eastern, and Mediterranean populations. The presence of the sickle cell gene confers a degree of protection from falciparum malaria in the heterozygote state and may explain its increased prevalence in these populations living in endemic areas. The prevalence of the genetic defect is the same in both sexes. The heterozygote (sickle cell trait $\alpha\alpha$-$\beta\beta_s$) is a benign disorder, except under unusually low oxygen tension (see pathogenesis below). Hemoglobin C, another hemoglobin beta chain defect, is prevalent in certain black populations of Africa, although less common than hemoglobin S. Intermarriage as well as spontaneous mutation may account for the finding of *HbSC*, a sickling disorder not as severe as SCD sickle cell (SS) hemoglobin in which both beta chains carry the S defect, whereas the patient with sickle cell has an S defect in one chain and a C defect in the other beta chain). *Hemoglobin CC* (*HbCC*) is relatively benign and not accompanied by RBC sickling.

One or more of the polypeptide chains of the hemoglobin molecule may have a complete or partial deletion of its alpha or beta chain. This is termed *thalassemia,* which can be the alpha or beta variety, depending on which chains are involved. This has broad distribution in south east Asia and Africa. Deletion of both alpha chains results in death in utero (4,5).

ETIOLOGY AND PATHOGENESIS

As stated, the hemoglobinopathies are genetically determined abnormalities in the hemoglobin molecule. The hemoglobin A molecule represents >95% of the hemoglobin in the red cell; hemoglobin A^2 and F are present in variable, but small amounts normally after the age of 1 year.

Hemoglobin F is a four chain molecule consisting of two alpha chains and two gamma chains ($\alpha\alpha$-$\delta\delta$). This hemoglobin is synthesized in the fetus and continues to be the major hemoglobin molecule synthesized during the first few months of postnatal life. The gamma chains and alpha chains do not have defects that cause sickling (see below). Thus, the neonate and early postnatal period do not manifest SCD. During the latter half of the first year of life, synthesis of beta chains begin to replace the gamma chains. At this time, sickle-shaped RBC begin to appear in the blood. This characteristically curvilinear shape is the result of two abnormal beta chains linked to two normal alpha chains, resulting in decreased solubility in the deoxygenated state. As a result, the hemoglobin molecules form long insoluble fibers that polymerize and force the cell to assume the *sickle* shape. These cells are inflexible and tend, partially or completely, to occlude blood vessels of the microcirculation. The abnormal cells interact with the endothelial cells to which they may become adherent through the appearance of a scavenger receptor (CD36) in the sickle cell membrane that binds to the thrombospondin molecule that, in turn, binds to the CD36 receptor site on the endothelium. The CD36 is most prominent on reticulocytes (6,7). The production of nitric oxide (NO), a natural vasodilator, is simultaneously reduced, in consequence of free hemoglobin in the blood (9).

Complete or partial vasoocclusion in various tissues and organs accounts for the lesions of SCD, which give rise to symptoms of pain, organ dysfunction, and the consequences of RBC destruction (hemolytic anemia). In early childhood, the spleen becomes congested with masses of sickled cells resulting in a *splenic crisis* (splenic enlargement and infarction). Complete loss of splenic function leads to increased susceptibility to sepsis and death from encapsulated organisms, such as the pneumococcus, as well as sepsis from other organisms because of loss of opsonic–phagocytic activity of the spleen. Infarction of bone leads to pain, and aseptic necrosis of the head of the femur and humerus. Ischemic ulcers of the skin, especially in the pretibial and malleolar areas, are occasionally encountered. The most devastating lesions, which occur in the lungs, kidneys, and brain, are caused by infarction plus inflammation. Infections are common in bone. Hematuria, papillary necrosis, and nephrotic syndrome are the result of renal involvement and the naturally low oxygen tension in the renal medulla is an important factor. Patients with sickle cell trait can have hematuria and hyposthenuria, but no other adverse clinical complications.

In addition to infarctions, inflammatory infiltrates with or without identifiable infection can lead to a severe respiratory distress syndrome and death (8). Cytokine release by leukocytes and other cells may be responsible for a major portion of the lung injury (9) and reduced oxygenation of the RBC adds to the problem. Pulmonary hypertension is a serious problem as well and its pathogenesis is probably multifactoral. It is common in β-thalassemia as well as in SCD. Because heart failure is a mechanism of death in both disorders, left-sided heart failure caused by iron overload may be one common risk factor. Pulmonary disease and low NO can be major factors in SS disease, whereas immunologic factors related to transfused blood would be a factor in β-thalassemia (9).

Strokes are a frequent problem, especially in children. These can be purely ischemic or combined with a hemorrhagic component. The veins of the retina are characteristically engorged and tortuous with pin-point occlusions of retinal arterioles frequently observed. This could reflect circulatory problems in the brain where vascular narrowing around the circle of Willis is demonstrable.

The bone marrow becomes expanded and hyperplastic, distorting the vertebral shape (*fish bone vertebrae* on x-ray study) and marked thickening of the skull bones with characteristic "*hair on end*" appearance radiographically.

CLINICAL MANIFESTATIONS

The adolescent and adult patients with sickle cell have somewhat different clinical findings on physical examination than the child. The most evident physical finding in the child is *dactylitis* (swollen tender fingers). Abdominal distention and a painful enlarged spleen and pallor are present as well.

The adolescent and adult with sickle cell may have a somewhat eunuchoid habitus, low grade tachycardia, flow murmurs, variable pulmonary rales, and skin ulcers over the tibial and malleolar areas. Frontal bossing may be seen because of thickening of the frontal portion of the calvarium. The veins of the retina are tortuous and many of the arterioles end abruptly.

SCD does not become apparent until the latter part of the first year of life. Anemia, dactylitis, frequent infections, and splenomegaly with episodes of abdominal pain caused by splenic congestion and infarction may then begin to occur. As splenic function diminishes and opsonim clearance of bacteria fails, infection of the bone and lung become frequent, with pneumococcal, salmonella, and staphylococcal infections appearing. In the first 5 to 6 years of life, infection is the leading cause of death. Vaccination with pneumococcal vaccine, *Haemophilus influenzae,* and others, along with prophylactic penicillin, has greatly reduced this risk.

Infections remain a threat throughout life; however, during adolescence and adulthood, other problems related to circulatory defects appear. Bilirubin gallstones are a cause of cholecystitis and bilary obstruction in some patients. Impaired endocrine function, especially that of the gonads, is characteristic and leads to a eunuchoid appearance because of delayed epiphysial closure. Delayed menarche sometimes occurs. Extramedullary hematopoiesis in lymph nodes and

TABLE 50-1. Management of Acute Chest Syndrome (Early Vigorous Treatment Essential)

- Antibiotics: For community acquired organisms, followed by therapy for culture-proved infections
- Oxygen
- Fluid management with attention to cardiopulmonary status, daily intake and output analysis, and daily weight
- Pain control, avoiding over sedation
- Bronchial dilators, if indicated, for obstructive airway disease
- Incentive spirometry while awake
- Red blood cell (RBC) transfusions with deteriorating respiratory function
- Corticosteroids may be helpful in the face of severe respiratory failure, especially in children

Laboratory Tests
- Complete blood count
- Chest x-ray study
- Sputum and blood cultures
- Oximetry
- Daily blood chemistries (electrolytes, liver function, renal function)
- Monitoring of blood gases
- Monitoring hemoglobin S concentration after transfusion

(Adapted from Adams RJ, Brambilla D. Discontinuing prophylactic transfusions used to prevent stroke sickle cell disease. *N Engl J Med.* 2005;353:2769–2778, with permission.)

paravertebral tissues sometimes causes nerve and spinal cord compression.

Painful crises bring the patient to medical attention frequently. Problems such as anemia, renal, pulmonary and hepatobiliary injuries, bone defects and skin lesions are also periodically occurring. Impaired growth and development are universally present, but are not so apparent until adolescence. Skeletal abnormalities consist of bone infarcts in the ribs, vertebrae, and long bones (especially femoral and humeral heads) can be very painful and crippling. The vertebrae deform into a "fish mouth" or letter H shape caused by multiple infarcts. Visceral effects include acute infarctions of the spleen, bowel, kidney, and lung.

Renal involvement is primarily medullar, with papillary necrosis, proteinuria, and hematuria. Renal vein thrombosis can occur in conjunction with nephrosis. Hepatobiliary problems include hepatitis, cholestatic jaundice, and bilirubin stones resulting from chronic hemolysis.

The blood and bone marrow findings are moderate to severe anemia; hematocrit 18% to 25% with normal or increased neutrophils and platelets; and RBC morphology consists of occasional sickled shape and target cells with Howell-Jolly bodies and nucleated RBC. In the variants of SS disease, SC (S-trait combined with C-trait) and S-Thal B 0 (S-trait combined with S-thalassemia 0), there are variant RBC shapes such as "*oat*" shapes and, in thalassemia, traits may target and hypochromic RBC.

Pulmonary disease may be chronic and not fully appreciated by the clinician. Impaired pulmonary function is attributed, in part, to multiple ischemic episodes and infection. Pulmonary emboli can be a factor as well, but venous thrombolism is not as commonly encountered as might be expected in view of the presence of inflammatory processes and vascular endothelial damage. Pulmonary hypertension can be demonstrated in many patients utilizing cardiac catheterization and measuring pressures or by demonstrating a jet through the tricuspid valve as measured by echocardiography (8,10). Leftward bowing of the interventricular septum may be present as well. The pathogenesis of the pulmonary hypertension is not entirely clear, but the endothelial defect, consisting of impaired (NO) synthesis, can be a factor. Activated platelets are present in some patients with SS disease, which can predispose to thrombosis. Thromboxane A_2 production with resultant vasoconstriction could be a factor as well. Chronic and repeated pulmonary insults are probably the most important cause.

The *acute chest syndrome (ACS)* is a common cause of death in adults with SS disease, less commonly in younger patients. This syndrome can occur as an acute exacerbation of chronic pulmonary disease where long-standing hypoxemia and pulmonary hypertension have resulted in pulmonary vascular damage and right-sided heart failure. The ACS commonly occurs in conjunction with fever, multiple organ dysfunctions, bone marrow emboli (fat emboli), and central nervous system (CNS) abnormalities. The ultimate result in many is the acute respiratory distress syndrome. Although pulmonary infection is often the inciting cause, multiple factors are likely to be responsible for this syndrome. The risk varies greatly based on prior attacks, age, cardiac status, and aggressiveness of the therapeutic approach (11).

Sudden worsening of the anemia can occur in patients who have an acute viral infection of the bone marrow RBC precursors (aplastic-crisis). The reticulocyte count falls to near zero and the marrow is devoid of RBC precursors. Viral cultures and DNA analysis of bone marrow may reveal the parvovirus B19 (12). Folic acid deficiency can also result in severe exacerbation of anemia. Glucose-6 phosphate dehydrogenase enzyme deficiency (G6PD) of the RBC occurs in approximately 8% to 10% of black males on a genetic basis. Certain oxidant drugs can also cause increased hemolysis (13).

Stroke occurs in 6% to 12% (14) of patients with SS disease and can develop in 8% of children by the age of 14, with a median age of 8 years (15) and mortality as high as 20% if untreated (16); recurrent stroke occurs in two thirds of untreated patients within 3 years of the initial event (17–19). Although manifesting as ischemic strokes in children and intracerebral and subarachnoid hemorrhage in adults, both types can be present in a single episode. Although pathological evidence indicates microvascular occlusion and sludging caused by sickling, clinical and neurodiagnostic findings are consistent with cerebral infarction and usually caused by an occlusive arteriopathy (intimal hyperplasia with superimposed thrombus). This process typically involves the distal intracranial segments of the internal carotid artery (ICA) and proximal anterior and middle cerebral arteries, but SCD can commonly cause a moyamoya-like angiographic pattern as well.

Evaluating the patient with SS disease who has had a stroke is individualized, but requires a RBC count, blood smear, hemoglobin electrophoresis, and sickling tests. MRI and angiography, and transcranial Doppler (TCD) ultrasonography studies are both valuable investigative tools and guide management because TCD can detect elevated flow velocities from intracranial arterial vasculopathy and patients at highest risk of stroke (18). Cerebral angiography can also be safely performed, but after partial exchange transfusion and using low osmolar contrast agents. By using TCD, the *Stroke Prevention Trial in Sickle Cell Anemia* (*STOP*) identified children with a high risk of stroke and demonstrated that maintenance of their hemoglobin S concentration <30% reduced their risk of cerebral infarction (20). Other risk factors, such as iron overload, upper airway obstruction, and blood pressure elevation secondary to renal disease or other causes, can contribute to stroke risk and necessitate their separate management (21).

Usually, increased iron stores are found because of increased absorption of food iron and RBC transfusions (simple transfusions). Iron overload becomes a serious problem (hemosiderosis) with cardiomyopathy, heart failure, and ischemic heart disease.

Priapism is often seen with recurrence resulting in a chronically indurated and painful organ. Hyphema is a complication of ocular involvement.

TREATMENT OF COMPLICATIONS

Sickle cell disease affects each of the tissues and organs of the body, primarily through impairment of the circulation. The mechanisms are only partially understood as discussed above. Treatments are both preventive and therapeutic. Evidence-based therapeutic guidelines are available for management of children, but randomized controlled trials (RCT) have not been done in adults. Observational data and expert opinion are the only guides to treatment in adults and for many aspects of pediatric age SCD-related problems (10).

PREVENTION OF COMPLICATIONS

Preventive measures found to be useful in children are derived from observational and RCT (17,18). Infection, stroke, and ACS commonly occur in children with SCD. Effective methods for infection prevention have been standardized and published as guidelines (10,18); a study was also published of the prevention of stroke in children at high risk (STOP trial and STOP-2 trial) (19,21). Children who had evidence of abnormal flow velocities in the anterior cerebral circulation as measured by TCD clearly had fewer strokes when given exchange transfusions of compatible RBC to lower the hemoglobin S level to 30% and maintained over a period of 30 months or more as compared with a control group of comparable size and risk who agreed to be monitored without transfusion therapy. The STOP 2 study was carried out in the same group of patients in which the incidence of stroke or recurrence of abnormal TCD was found to revert to the same risk as controls (18,19) and long-term exchange transfusion was beneficial in terms of stroke prevention, but red cell sensitization with transfusion reactions were increased over those who had simple transfusions to maintain a hemoglobin 10 g/dL. The latter group was considered to be at high risk for iron overload. These problems have not been resolved.

The incidence of ACS was decreased in the group receiving transfusion as well as in groups using other means of preventing complications. The use of orally administered hydroxyurea to promote the production of fetal hemoglobin in high concentrations, a protection against sickling, was effective in preventing stroke. Trials have been published of stroke prevention in patients 6 years of age (18,19).

Because hydroxyurea is an antineoplastic drug that impairs blood cell production that decreases leukocyte counts, it could promote infection in this infection-susceptible population. It is not routinely used, therefore, but its use is reserved for those with complicated and recurrent clinical problems, such as multiple recurrences of painful crises, priapism, ACS, or stroke (10).

Pain is the most common problem encountered in SCD. Basic therapy includes hydration with intravenous fluid, oxygen if desaturation is present, and the judicious use of narcotics (avoiding meperidine). Excessive doses of acetaminophen can cause liver toxicity and it should be used with caution. Management in dedicated sickle cell centers and daycare facilities (doctor's clinics) is ideal. Treatment of painful crises in and out of the hospital is an art gained by experience with each patient and the physician needs training and experience to give optimal care (10).

Acute Chest Syndrome

ACS has been defined as a new pulmonary infiltrate involving at least one complete segment associated with acute respiratory symptoms.

Treatment

Suggested clinical guidelines for the management of this very serious complication include antibiotic therapy to cover community-acquired organisms as well as identified non–community-acquired infections. *Mycoplasma pneumoniae*, virus, and bacterial infections should be suspected. Oxygen, respiratory therapy, pain control, and hydration are routinely recommended. RBC transfusions, simple or exchange, are sometimes used, depending on whether increased risk factors exist, such as history of recurrent episodes, heart disease, multiple infiltrates in the lungs, or acute clinical deterioration and need for ventilator support. Bronchial dilators and dexamethasone (Table 50-1) can be considered when bronchospasm is suggested or a history of asthma is present. Mortality rates of 10% have been reported in those 20 years of age and 9% in those who are older, especially in those with recurrences. Even first time cases can proceed rapidly to death, prompting the practice of vigorous early treatment (10,11).

Stroke

Acute stroke in children is treated with exchange transfusion, oxygen, and hydration. Adults are treated in the same manner (18,19). Anticoagulant and antiplatelet drugs, as well as thrombolytic agents used for strokes in nonsickling disorders, have not been evaluated in clinical trials of stroke in SCD. Blood pressure may be elevated and require control in hemorrhagic strokes. Surgical treatment of hemorrhagic stroke has not been studied, but may have some role in conjunction with exchange transfusions (18,19).

Renal Complications

For renal complications, the same potential exists for benefit from hydroxyurea as it does for patients with other complications. Hydroxyurea use to prevent renal complications has not been specifically studied in RCT. Up to 30% of adult patients develop chronic renal failure requiring long-term hemodialysis or renal transplant. Success rates for the short term are reasonably good, but because the SCD remains, long-term survival of the graft is not as probable as it is for patients with other types

TABLE 50-2. Management of Priapism

1. Priapism is best treated within 4 hours of inset; patients, as well as parents of boys, should be advised to seek prompt medical attention.
2. Urologic consultation as soon as the patient arrives at the medical facility is strongly advised.
3. Various nonsurgical measures may abort some cases. These include hydration, frequent urination, and aspiration.
4. Preventive measures in recurrent cases can include antiandrogen therapy, hydroxyurea, and or exchange transfusions, depending on the frequency and severity of recurrences.

(Adapted from Beutler E. Disorders of hemoglobin structure: Sickle cell anemia and related abnormalities. In: Lechtman M, Beutler E, Kipps T, et al. eds. *Williams Hematology*. New York: McGraw-Hill; 2006:667–700, with permission.)

of renal disease (21). Management of priapism is outlined in Table 50-2 (10).

Treatment of Thalassemia

Although the thalassemia syndromes are not discussed in detail in this chapter, it is worth noting that the homozygous state (B β-thalassemia major) is not compatible with life beyond puberty because of the ravages of severe anemia, massive hepatosplenomegally, and extramedullary hematopoiesis. Iron overload, even without transfusions, occurs. Current treatment consists of splenectomy at about 3 to 4 years of age, following immunization against pneumococcae and *Haemophilus influenzae*. Life-long transfusions of RBC are necessary. Iron overload results in cardiomyopathy, as well as multiple endocrine defects, unless chelation therapy for iron is given daily. Hemoglobinemia occurs as it does in SCD and other hemolytic diseases. Diminished NO caused by the free hemoglobin effects permits vascular spasm and ultimately some permanent vascular endothelial changes, but ischemic infarcts, renal insufficiency, and stroke are less common than in SCD. Iron chelation is the critical therapeutic measure that can prolong life up into the third and fourth decade. Stem cell transplantation is practical and has been used successfully in many patients. Genetic counseling is widely practiced as a preventive measure, utilizing blood tests to screen young adults (5,22).

Pregnancy

Prophylactic transfusions to prevent fetal loss has not been proved to be successful on a routine basis, but patients with severe painful crises or those with recurrent severe complications may benefit from transfusion therapy (Table 50-3) (24).

Pulmonary Hypertension

Approximately 30% of adult patients with SCD have systolic pulmonary artery pressure of at least 30 mm Hg (10). This is true of those who have thalassemia major as well. The pathophysiology is unclear and treatments are experimental. This is a recently recognized problem of major consequence in SCD (11,25).

TABLE 50-3. General Guidelines for Management of Patients with Sickle Cell Disease (SCD) during Pregnancy

1. Pain management is the same as that for a nonpregnant patient with SCD, provided the drug has no adverse effects on the fetus.
2. Routine folic acid supplementation, as for any pregnancy, is particularly important in patients with SCD whose folate requirements are high.
3. Prophylactic red blood cell (RBC) transfusions are not recommended for uncomplicated pregnancies in woman with SCD. They may be considered in the patient who has frequent pain crises, acute chest syndrome, severe anemia, or stroke.
4. Preeclampsia and low-birthweight newborns are the most common complication of pregnancy in patients with SCD. The patient should be followed closely for both complications by conventional methods. Management requires careful avoidance of measures that cause dehydration (medications).
5. The patient with SCD should be under the combined care of a hematologist and an obstetrician who specializes in high-risk cases, when possible.
6. Contraceptive measures considered safe are medroxyprogesterone acetate injections (repository), barrier methods, or both. History of thromboembolism or hypercoagulable state has been tested as contraindications to the use of medroxyprogesterone acetate in the product guidelines in the *Physician's Desk Reference* (PDR). SCD is a risk factor for vascular occlusion, which makes the use of this drug potentially hazardous in these patients.

(Adapted from Beutler E. Disorders of hemoglobin structure: Sickle cell anemia and related abnormalities. In: Lechtman M, Beutler E, Kipps T, et al. eds. *Williams Hematology*. New York: McGraw-Hill; 2006:667–700, and Vinchinsky EP, Haberkern CM, Neumayr L, et al. A comparison of conservative and aggressive regiments in preoperative management of sickle cell disease. The Preoperative Transfusion in Sickle Cell Disease Study Group. *N Engl J Med.* 1995;333:206–213, with permission.)

Surgery for Patients with Sickle Cell Disease

Major surgical procedures, in which shock, acidosis, or hypoxemia can occur, should be preceded (when possible) by simple or exchange transfusion of RBC to lower the hemoglobin S concentrate to 30% or less. Exchange transfusions are preferred because of the problem of fluid overload (26).

CLINICAL RECOMMENDATIONS OF THE VIGNETTE

Whether the risk of stroke was sufficiently high to justify chronic exchange transfusions prophylactically, or to treat the patient chronically with hydroxyurea to prevent stroke is not known from clinical studies. His treatment was appropriate because of data from studies in children who do benefit from such therapy. Older patients with advanced disease or multiple organ dysfunctions may not be able to tolerate the procedure sufficiently well to justify the risk (23).

Stem cell transplants (allogeneic) have proved to be successful in curing some patients and are a clinical option in patients who are having complications not well controlled by other means of therapy. Older patients with advanced disease or multiple organ dysfunctions may not be able to tolerate the procedure sufficiently well to justify the risk (18).

SUMMARY

Treatment of SCD is primarily directed at specific complications. The use of drugs, such as hydroxyurea, to induce fetal hemoglobin synthesis as well as stem cell transplantation is effective but has serious risks. A search for alternatives is clearly a high priority for safer management of such cases.

REFERENCES

1. Conley CL. Blood, pure and eloquent. In: Wintrobe MM, ed. *Sickle Cell Anemia—The First Molecular Disease.* New York: McGraw-Hill; 1979;319–371.
2. Weatherall D. Disorders of globinsyntheses: The thalassemias. In: Lechtman M, Beutler E, Kipps T, et al., eds. *Williams Hematology.* New York: McGraw-Hill; 2006:633–666.
3. Beutler E. Disorders of hemoglobin structure: Sickle cell anemia and related abnormalities. In: Lechtman M, Beutler E, Kipps T, et al., eds. *Williams Hematology.* New York: McGraw-Hill; 2006:667–700.
4. Pagnier J, Mears JG, Dunda-Belkhodja O, et al. Evidence for the multicentric origin of the sickle cell hemoglobin gene in Africa. *Proc Natl Acad Sci USA.* 1984;81:1771.
5. Lukens JN. The thalassemias and related disorders: Quantitative disorders of hemoglobin synthesis. In: Lee JR, Foerster J, Lukens J, et al., eds. *Wintrobe's Clinical Hematology,* 10th ed. Baltimore: Lippincott Williams & Wilkins; 1999:1405–1448.
6. Browne PV, Hebbel RP. CD 36-Positive reticulocytes in sickle cell anemia. *J Lab Clin Med.* 1996;27:340–347.
7. Lukens JN. The abnormal hemoglobins—General Principles. In: Lee JR, Foerster J, Lukens J, et al., eds. In: *Wintrobe's Clinical Hematology,* 11th ed. Baltimore: Lippincott, Williams & Wilkins; 2004:1247–1262.
8. Wang W. Sickle Cell Anemia and Other Sickling Syndromes. In: *Wintrobe's Clinical Hematology,* 11th ed. Baltimore: Lippincott, Williams & Wilkins; 2004:1263–1311.
9. Reiter CD, Wang X, Tanus-Santos JE, et al. Cell-free hemoglobin limits nitric oxide bioavailability in sickle cell disease. *Nat Med.* 2002;8:1338–1389.
10. Mehta SR, Appenzi-Annan A, Byrnes P, et al. Opportunities to improve outcomes in sickle cell disease. *Am Fam Phys.* 2006;74:303–310, 313–314.
11. Vinchinsky EP, Neumayr LD, Earles AN, et al. Causes and outcomes of the acute chest syndrome in sickle cell disease. National Acute Chest Syndrome Study Group. *N Engl J Med.* 2000;342:1855–1865.
12. Anderson MJ, Davis LR, Hodgson J, et al. Occurrence of infection with a parvo-virus-like agent in children with sickle cell anemia during a two year period. *J Clin Pathol.* 1982;35:744–749.
13. Buetler E. The study of glucose 6-phosphate dehydrogenase: History and molecular biology. *Am J Hematol.* 1993;42:53–58.
14. Pavlakis SG, Prohovnik I, Piomelli S, et al. Neurologic complications of sickle cell disease. *Adv Pediatr.* 1989;36:247–276.
15. Balkaran B, Char G, Morris JS, et al. Stroke in a cohort of patients with homozygous sickle cell disease. *J Pediatr.* 1992;120:360–366.
16. Powars D, Wilson B, Imbus C, et al. The natural history of stroke in sickle cell disease. *Am J Med.* 1978;65:461–471.
17. Switzer JA, Hess DC, Nichols FT, et al. Pathophysiology and treatment of stroke in sickle cell disease. Past, present and future. *Lancet Neurology.* 2006;5:501–512.
18. Kwialkowski JL, Granger S, Brombella DJ, et al. Elevated blood flow velocity in the anterior cerebral artery and stroke risk in sickle cell disease: Extended Analysis From The STOP Trial. *Br J Haematol.* 2006;134:333–339.
19. Adams RJ, Brambilla D. Discontinuing prophylactic transfusions used to prevent stroke sickle cell disease. *N Engl J Med.* 2005;353:2769–2778.
20. Pegelow CH, Adams RJ, McKie V, et al. Risk of recurrent stroke in patients with sickle cell disease treated with erythrocyte transfusions. *J Pediatr.* 1995;126:896–899.
21. Guasch A, Navarrete J, Nass K, et al. Glomerular involvement in adults with sickle cell hemoglobinopathies: Prevalence and clinical correlations of progressive renal failure. *J Am Soc Nephrol.* 2006;17:2228–2235.
22. Walters MC, Patience M, Leisenring W, et al. Stable mixed hematopoietic chimerism after bone marrow transportation for sickle cell anemia. *Biol Blood Marrow Transplant.* 2001:7:665–673.
23. Iammone R, Casella SF, Fuchs EJ, et al. Results of minimally toxic non-myoablative transplantation in patients with sickle cell anemia and beta thalassemia. *Biol Blood Marrow Transplant.* 2003:9:519–528.
24. Smith JA, Espelanet M, Bellevue R, et al. Pregnancy in sickle cell disease: Experience of the Cooperative Study of Sickle Cell Disease. *Obstet Gynecol.* 1996:87:199–204.
25. Singer S, Kuypers F, Styles L, et al. Pulmonary hypertension in thalassemia: Association with platelet activation and hypercoagulable state. *Am J Hematol.* 2006;81:670–675.
26. Vinchinsky EP, Haberkern CM, Neumayr L, et al. A comparison of conservative and aggressive regiments in preoperative management of sickle cell disease. The Preoperative Transfusion in Sickle Cell Disease Study Group. *N Engl J Med.* 1995;333:206–213.

CHAPTER 51

Bleeding Diatheses and Hemophilias

Nirmala Bhoopalam • Chris Braden • Sowjanya Reganti

OBJECTIVES

- To define the various bleeding diatheses
- To describe the clinical characteristics and laboratory abnormalities associated with selected bleeding diatheses
- To explain the principal treatments for individual bleeding diatheses
- To review how bleeding diatheses can cause or contribute to neurologic illnesses

CASE VIGNETTE

A 30-year-old man with history of epileptic seizures presented to the emergency room with swelling and pain on his right knee after a fall resulting from a generalized tonic-clonic seizure. He had a large bruise on the left thigh, and took ibuprofen for pain and swelling. Medical history was noteworthy for severe bleeding following an appendectomy 13 years ago requiring transfusion of multiple units of blood. Before that episode, he had not had any bleeding problems. After the appendectomy, he was advised to get regular infusions of "a plasma product." He received the plasma infusions for awhile, but stopped and did not have regular medical check-ups or plasma infusions for many years. Family history was remarkable for a maternal uncle who had died of an intracranial hemorrhage at the age of 10 years. Examination demonstrated right knee hemarthrosis with limited range of motion, and a large resolving hematoma on his left thigh with no other abnormalities. Neurologic examination was normal. Laboratory studies demonstrated a normocytic normochromic anemia with hemoglobin 11.8 g/dL, normal white blood cell (WBC) and platelet count. Urinalysis showed microscopic hematuria. A computed tomographic (CT) scan of the head, with and without contrast, was normal. A serum metabolic profile was remarkable for total bilirubin of 1.5 mg/dL and normal liver function studies. Hepatitis C and human immunodeficiency virus (HIV) testing were negative. Prothrombin time (PT) was normal. Activated partial thromboplastin time (aPTT) was elevated to 120 seconds. Hematology consult was requested. Mixing studies demonstrated a factor VIII inhibitor (Bethesda units 5). The factor VIII level was 1% and factor IX level was normal. Thrombin time, fibrinogen, and fibrin split products (FSP) were normal. The patient was treated with high doses of factor VIII concentrate and high dose methylprednisolone. He did not experience any more bleeding episodes and an orthopedic consult was obtained.

DEFINITION

Bleeding diathesis is abnormal excessive bleeding, either spontaneous or as a result of tissue injury. The normal hemostatic pathway involves complex interactions of vasculature, platelets, coagulation factors, and fibrinolysis. Bleeding disorders can occur because of abnormal vascular function, platelet disorders, decreased levels or abnormal function of coagulation factors, abnormal clot stabilization, fibrinolysis, or combination of these factors.

Evaluation of bleeding diathesis begins with a complete history that includes a description of bleeding events, personal and family history of bleeding, comorbidity, medications, and physical examination and laboratory findings to help establish the diagnosis (Fig. 51-1). Appropriate management depends on identifying the specific defects that have caused the bleeding disorder.

Hemophilia A

Hemophilia A is an X linked hereditary disorder caused by defective synthesis or by synthesis of dysfunctional factor VIII molecules (1,2). The estimated incidence of hemophilia A is 1 of 5,000 to 10,000 live male births. Approximately 60% have severe disease, with factor VIII activity <1% of normal. It is nearly six times more common than hemophilia B. The disease exhibits no racial predilection.

Genetics

Hemophilia A can result from multiple alterations in the factor VIII gene, including gene rearrangements; missense mutations, in which a single base substitution leads to an amino acid change in the molecule; nonsense mutations, resulting in

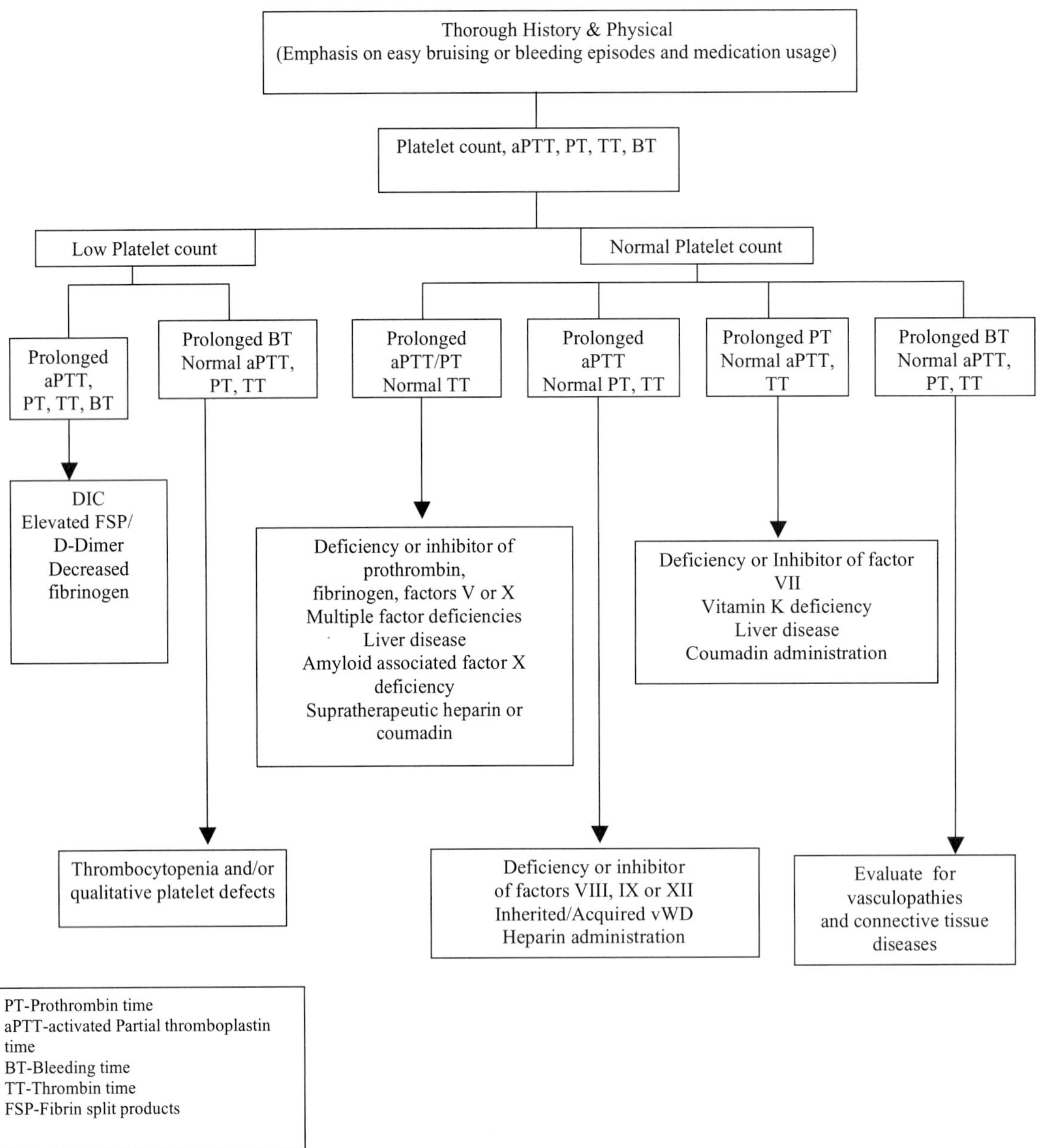

FIGURE 51-1. Approach to patients with a bleeding diathesis.

a stop codon; abnormal splicing of the gene; deletions of all or portions of the gene; or insertions of genetic elements. The factor VIII gene, one of the largest genes, is divided into 26 exons that span 186,000 base pairs. One of the most common mutations, accounting for 40% to 50% of patients, is a unique combined gene inversion and a crossing over that disrupts the factor VIII gene. Another uncommon cause of factor VIII deficiency is a mutation in the LMAN1 gene, which causes a rare autosomal recessive disease with combined deficiency of factor VIII and factor V. Hemophilia A is an X-linked recessive disorder that occurs almost exclusively in males, although women are usually carriers. It is an extremely rare disorder in women, although affected offspring from a hemophilic father and carrier mother have been reported. It can occur in females with X chromosome abnormalities, such as Turner syndrome, X chromosome mosacism, and other X chromosome defects (2).

CLINICAL MANIFESTATIONS

Hemophilia A is characterized by excessive bleeding into various organs of the body. It can result in soft tissue hematomas, hemarthroses, hematuria, and life-threatening neurologic complications that can result in intracranial bleeding and death. The disease has been broadly classified as mild (6% to 30% of normal), moderate (1% to 5% of normal) and severe (<1% of normal). Hemophilic bleeding occurs hours or days after injury; it can involve any organ and, if untreated, can continue for days or weeks. This can result in large collections of partially clotted blood exerting pressure on adjacent normal tissues causing necrosis of muscle (compartment syndromes), venous congestion (pseudophlebitis), or ischemic nerve damage. Patients with hemophilia often develop a femoral neuropathy caused by compression from an unsuspected retroperitoneal hematoma. They can also develop large calcified masses of blood and inflammatory tissue that are mistaken for neoplasms (pseudotumor syndrome) (3–5).

MILD TYPE

With mild type (6% to 30% factor VIII), patients have infrequent bleeding episodes. The disease can remain undiagnosed in the absence of an informative family history and can be discovered only because of excessive hemorrhage developing postoperatively or following trauma. In one report of ten patients with mild disease, median age at diagnosis was 14 to 62 years (6).

MODERATE TYPE

Those with moderate type (1% to 5% factor VIII) have occasional hematomas and hemarthrosis that is not always related to trauma. The hemarthropathy is less debilitating. Mean age at diagnosis was 22 months (7).

SEVERE TYPE

Most patients have the severe type of disease (<1% factor VIII). Patients with severe hemophilia are usually diagnosed shortly after birth because of an extensive cephalhematoma or profuse bleeding after circumcision. More often, children with severe hemophilia A become symptomatic after the newborn period, but within the first 2 years of life. Median age at diagnosis is 9 months (8). These patients bleed spontaneously. The frequent and recurrent nature of joint bleeding can lead to the development of a chronic hemophilic arthropathy and orthopedic disability by the time patients with hemophilia are in their 20s or 30s. Some patients with severe disease exhibit mild symptoms because of coinheritance of factor V Leiden mutation (R506) with hemophilic gene (9).

CARRIERS

Most carriers have approximately 50% factor VIII activity and experience no abnormal bleeding. Some symptomatic carriers have levels below 50%, usually because of an extremely imbalanced X chromosome. Studies in small Amish kindreds in Pennsylvania have found that postpartum bleeding and dental bleeding are the most common symptoms (1).

DIAGNOSTIC APPROACH

Careful review of family history, however, shows that approximately one third of patients with hemophilia have a negative family history. This could be because of the development of new mutations that can be seen in 25% to 30% of cases.

SCREENING TESTS

Among the screening tests are platelet count, PT, and aPTT. A normal platelet count, normal PT, and a prolonged aPTT are characteristic findings of hemophilia A. An abnormal test occurs in individuals who have less than approximately 30% of the mean normal concentration of factor VIII. Another useful test to perform with a prolonged aPTT is a mixing study. This is normally done by performing an aPTT on a 1:1 mix of patient and normal plasma and incubated at 37°C for 2 hours. That should be corrected by normal plasma in cases of factor VIII deficiency. If the aPTT is not corrected, then an inhibitor is present.

A specific clotting assay for factor VIII activity should be done, by either a one-stage or a two-stage method. Factor VIII activity is expressed as percent of normal or as units per milliliter of plasma. Chromogenic assays for factor VIII activity are also widely used, but do not always agree with the one stage-method (9). Factor VIII antigen levels are measured by immunologic assays which detect normal and most abnormal factor VIII molecules (2).

TREATMENT

General principles of therapy for hemophilia A are avoidance of aspirin, anti-inflammatory drugs, and other agents that interfere with platelet aggregation (1). Patients should be advised to exercise great caution when using over-the-counter medications. The treatment goal is to raise the patient's factor activity level following an acute bleed or, optimally, to prevent further bleeding.

FACTOR VIII REPLACEMENT THERAPY

Hemorrhagic episodes can be managed by replacing factor VIII and several plasma products, such as fresh frozen plasma (FFP) and cryoprecipitate. Affinity purified factor VIII concentrates that have undergone viral inactivation by either pasteurization or solvent-detergent treatment are favored. For most patients, recombinant factor preparations are the agents of choice in North America. The target factor level depends on the clinical setting. For major bleeding or surgery, a minimal factor activity level >50% is desirable, whereas peak levels of 30% to 40% may be sufficient for treating minor hemorrhages or for prophylaxis (4). Complications of factor replacement therapy include infection, antibody formation, transfusion-related acute lung injury, and thrombosis.

DESMOPRESSIN

Desmopressin (DDAVP; 1-deamino-8-D-arginine vasopressin) is the drug of choice for the treatment of mild or moderate hemophilia A. DDAVP is administered intravenously (0.3 μg/kg) or intranasally (150 μg in each nostril). Side effects include tachycardia, headache, and flushing, caused by the vasodilatory effects of DDAVP. Hyponatremia and volume overload, which are also seen, are caused by the antidiuretic effects of DDAVP. With repeated dosing, tachyphylaxis can occur as von Willebrand factors (vWF) stores are depleted.

ANTIFIBRINOLYTIC AGENTS

Antifibrinolytic agents, such as epsilon-aminocaproic acid (EACA) and tranexamic acid, have been used to enhance hemostasis in patients with hemophilia with oropharyngeal bleeding (13,14). The usual oral dose of tranexamic acid for adults is 1 g four times a day. EACA can be given as a loading dose of 4 to 5 g followed by 1 g/h in adults. Another regimen is 4 g every 4 to 6 hours orally for 2 to 8 days, depending on the severity of bleeding (2). Antifibrinolytic therapy is contraindicated in the presence of hematuria. Pediatric dosing is smaller, and is dependent on factor levels.

Hemophilia B

Hemophilia B is clinically indistinguishable from hemophilia A (2). It is also an X-linked recessive disorder, but it is caused by a deficiency of factor IX, also called *Christmas factor*, or *dysfunction of factor IX molecules*. The estimated incidence of hemophilia B is 1 of every 25,000 to 30,000 male births. As with hemophilia A, this disease is also found in all ethnic groups.

Genetics

The factor IX gene is located on the long arm of chromosome X. It is approximately 33 kb long, which is much smaller than the gene for factor VIII (14,15). More than 2,000 mutations in the factor IX gene are described for hemophilia B. Most are low risk missense mutations and some are gene deletions, rearrangements, and frameshifts. The Leyden phenotype of hemophilia B is characterized by severe hemophilia in childhood that becomes mild after puberty. The mutation in the Leyden phenotype occurs at nucleotide-20 in the promoter region and disrupts the hepatocyte nuclear factor 4 (HNF-4) binding site, but does not affect the overlapping site for an androgen response element, which may explain the recovery at puberty. These patients also may have less disruption of the HNF-4 binding site (15).

CLINICAL MANIFESTATION

Bleeding episodes in patients with hemophilia B are clinically identical to those in patients with hemophilia A. Classification of hemophilia B is based on clinical severity and roughly correlates with levels of factor IX coagulant activity similar to hemophilia A (severe disease <1% normal, moderate disease 1% to 5% normal, mild disease 5% to 40% normal). Hematuria, bleeding from mucous membranes, and hemarthroses resulting in chronic crippling hemarthropathy can occur as in cases of hemophilia A.

DIAGNOSTIC APPROACH

Screening tests used in the diagnosis of hemophilia B are similar to those used in hemophilia A. The only method for differentiating hemophilia B from hemophilia A is by performing a specific assay for factor IX coagulant activity.

TREATMENT

The basic treatment of hemophilia B is replacement of factor IX (2). Other therapies used are desmopressin and antifibrinolytics. To summarize, the therapeutic goal for hemophilia A and B does not have to be restoration of normal factor levels; conversion from a severe (<1%) to a mild (>5%) phenotype is sufficient to produce dramatic improvements. Issues of sustained levels of factor delivery, neutralizing antibody response, safety, and cost, however, remain to be resolved for all of these approaches (11,12). Gene therapy trials are currently ongoing for patients with both hemophilia A and B (10,11).

Hemophila C

Hemophilia C is an autosomal hereditary factor XI deficiency occurring predominantly in individuals of Ashkenazi Jewish descent. Bleeding in patients with factor XI deficiency varies from no bleeding to severe bleeding and may be detected only at the time of surgery, particularly involving the urinary tract or oral cavity. The basis for this clinical heterogeneity remains unknown. Patients who have a history of bleeding complications with surgery are at increased risk of bleeding with subsequent surgery and these patients should receive prophylactic FFP before the procedure. Purified factor XI concentrate, which is available only in Europe, is associated with thrombotic complications. Fibrinolytic inhibitors have also been used for prophylaxis in dental procedures (4).

Hemophilia in Pregnancy

A thorough personal and family history is crucial for all pregnant patients. All daughters of hemophilic fathers are potential carriers, and if a known carrier has a daughter, they too have a 50% chance of being a carrier. When a daughter of a known carrier or a female offspring of a hemophiliac patient wishes to become pregnant, it is important to initiate or discuss carrier testing for both hemophilia A and B with the patient. Carrier testing for both hemophilia A and B is done by measuring factor VIII or IX levels. Other tests includes DNA samples (chorionic sampling and blood samples from affected family members or known carriers), and analysis of restriction fragment length polymorphisms (RFLP) and complementary DNA (cDNA) probes (3,4).

Von Willebrand Disease

Von Willebrand factor is a large, multimeric protein synthesized from the vWF gene located on chromosome 12. The protein is synthesized in vascular endothelial cells and megakaryocytes and then stored in Weibel-Palade bodies. Normal vWF serves two functions: binding of factor VIII in plasma to protect it from inactivation and formation of the platelet plug by binding to exposed collagen and its receptor on platelets, known as platelet glycoprotein Ib (GPIb) (1–4,16–19).

Von Willebrand disease (vWD), in fact, is not a single entity, but a group of bleeding disorders. Collectively, this group constitutes the most common inherited bleeding diathesis in both men and women, with a prevalence of approximately 1%. Various mutations in the vWF gene give rise to quantitative or qualitative defects in the vWF protein, which interfere with the normal functions of vWF, causing both a factor VIII deficiency and development of defective platelet plugs. Three separate disease phenotypes exist: types 1, 2, and 3. The degree of clinical manifestations varies, depending on the phenotype (1,16,17,20).

CLINICAL MANIFESTATIONS

The principal clinical manifestations of vWD are easy bruising, epistaxis, mucosal bleeding, menorrhagia, and excessive, prolonged bleeding after surgical procedures. The severity of bleeding can vary, depending on the type or subtype of vWD.

TYPE 1 vWD

Patients with type vDW typically have mild to moderate bleeding, with some remaining asymptomatic. Type 1 vWD is the most common phenotype, accounting for 60% to 80% of cases. This phenotype is characterized by mild to moderate quantitative deficiencies of vWF and factor VIII (21).

TYPE 2 vWD

Type 2 vDD is divided into four subtypes: 2A, 2B, 2M and 2N. All four subtypes are characterized by qualitative abnormalities of vWF. Bleeding in patients included in these subtypes is usually more severe and usually occurs earlier in life than with patients with type 1 vWD.

SUBTYPE 2A

Patients with vWD 2A have mutations in vWD that either lead to increased destruction of the vWF protein or cause a defect in intracellular transport. Patients typically have mild to moderate bleeding and subtype 2A accounts for approximately 10% to 15% of all vWD (22,23).

SUBTYPE 2B

Patients with vWD 2B have mutations that result in increased binding of the vWF to the GPIb platelet-binding site. These vWF–platelet complexes are subsequently removed from the circulation, causing thrombocytopenia. Recent evidence also suggests impaired megakaryocytopoiesis may significantly contribute the thrombocytopenia associated with this subtype (24). Patients typically have mild to moderate bleeding and subtype 2B accounts for approximately 5% of all vWD cases.

SUBTYPE 2M

Patients with vWD 2M have mutations that lead to decreased binding of vWF to platelets. Subtype 2M is rare and patients typically have significant bleeding.

SUBTYPE 2N

Patients with vWD 2N have mutations that affect the binding site for factor VIII. These mutations cause decreased binding to factor VIII and low plasma factor VIII levels. Subtype 2N is extremely uncommon and patients may present with joint and soft tissue bleeding similar to patients with factor VIII deficiency (25).

TYPE 3 vWD

Characterized by mutations that result in a significant decrease or absence of vWF type 3 is the least common phenotype of vWD. Patients may have severe bleeding from mucosal surfaces as well as skin, soft tissues, and joints because of a decrease or absence of vWF. Symptoms usually manifest in childhood.

DIAGNOSTIC APPROACH

The diagnostic approach is based on a detailed history and physical examination, with findings of easy bruising or frequent, excessive bleeding, along with confirmatory laboratory testing. If vWD is strongly suggested, then, initial laboratory testing should include an aPTT, PT, enzyme-linked immunosorbent assay (ELISA) based vWF antigen test, vWF activity by ristocetin cofactor assay, factor VIII activity level, and a vWF multimer assay (22,25).

TREATMENT

An accurate diagnosis is essential before initiating treatment. The vWD phenotype dictates specific and appropriate intervention. Therapeutic intervention should focus on the termination of bleeding by replacing the defective or deficient proteins. Patients should also be advised to avoid aspirin and other nonsteroidal anti-inflammatory drugs that may interfere with platelet function. Currently five classes of medications are used to treat vWD, Desmopressin (DDAVP), vWF and factor VIII replacement concentrates, antifibrinolytic agents, fibrin sealant or topical thrombin, and estrogen in select cases involving female patients.

DDAVP, a synthetic analog of antidiuretic hormone, is known to induce the release of vWF and factor VIII from storage sites causing a transient increase in plasma levels of both factors. It can be administered intravenously, subcutaneously, or by intranasal spray. A significant variability is seen in the response to desmopressin, depending on the vWD phenotype. Desmopressin is effective in most patients with type 1 vWD, but has variable effectiveness in type 2 vWD because of the qualitative nature of the vWF defects. In fact, desmopressin can induce thrombocytopenia in patients with subtype 2B vWD. A test dose should be given before initiating therapy in all patients with type 2 vWD to assess for factor VIII and vWF responsiveness as well as desmopressin-induced thrombocytopenia. Desmopressin is not effective in treating type 3 vWD because these patients lack vWF in the storage sites.

Factor replacement therapy is indicated in a variety of clinical situations involving vWD. Several commercially available replacement concentrates exist and these concentrates may contain both vWF and factor VIII or vWF alone. Patients with type 1 vWD having major surgical procedures or those with severe bleeding are candidates for factor replacement with vWF-factor VIII concentrate. Factor replacement is indicated in patients with type 2 who have had a poor response with desmopressin, uncontrolled bleeding with desmopressin, or tachyphylaxis after desmopressin. Some authors advocate factor replacement as the initial therapeutic intervention in type 2 vWD. Factor replacement is the treatment of choice for type 3 vWD, but some patients may develop alloantibodies against vWF after receiving multiple transfusions. Patients developing these antibodies should be treated with recombinant factor VIII, which is devoid of vWF.

Antifibrinolytic agents are typically used as adjunct therapy. These agents help stabilize newly formed blood clots and prevent their dissolution. Currently available agents include EACA and tranexamic acid. Caution should be exercised when using these drugs because prolonged usage can result in thrombosis and usage with hematuria can cause ureteral obstruction.

Fibrin sealant and thrombin spray are used as adjunct therapy. These substances (e.g., Gelfoam, Surgicel) are typically used in patients with oral or nasal bleeding and can be applied by soaking either product with the substance and applying it directly to the site of bleeding. Estrogen therapy has been used in patients with vWD experiencing menorrhagia. The therapeutic effectiveness of estrogen appears to result, at least in part, from an increase in the synthesis of vWF (20,22,25,26).

PREGNANCY AND vWD

Most patients with vWD will not require treatment during pregnancy. Levels of vWF have been shown to increase two- to threefold during the second and third trimester. DDAVP may be used effectively in patients going into early labor with severe vWD. Patients with bleeding unresponsive to DDAVP in the peripartum period should receive factor replacement therapy (27,28).

Other Congenital Factor Deficiencies (Factors II, V, VII, IX, X, XI and XIII)

Hemophilia A, hemophilia B, and vWD account for most congenital bleeding diatheses. Congenital factor deficiencies of the remaining coagulation factors are exceedingly uncommon. Clinical manifestations include easy bruising and excessive bleeding that may be seen when patients are having a surgical procedure. Therapeutic intervention is focused on factor replacement with FFP or isolated factor concentrates, when available. It is important to remember that factor XII is prothrombotic and not associated with bleeding diatheses (4,29,30). Other rare disorders causing bleeding, with normal screening coagulation tests, are factor XIII deficiencies and abnormalities of α_2 plasmin inhibitor or plasminogen activator inhibitor-1 deficiency (4).

Acquired Bleeding Diathesis

Acquired von Willebrand Syndrome

Acquired von Willebrand syndrome (AvWS) is a rare bleeding disorder with clinical features and laboratory findings similar to those of inherited vWD (31,32). The underlying pathophysiology of the disorder is not well understood. The syndrome typically occurs in association with a variety of clinical conditions, including lymphoproliferative and myeloproliferative disorders, nonhematologic malignancies, autoimmune diseases, hypothyroidism, aortic stenosis, mitral valve prolapse, and uremia (33). In addition, several drugs have also been associated with the condition, including valproic acid, griseofulvin, and ciprofloxacin and hydroxyethyl starch (32). The most successful therapy is treatment of the underlying cause or withdrawal of the offending agent. DDAVP should be used if treatment of the underlying cause is ineffective or not possible (33,34).

Liver Disease

In chronic liver disease, increased bleeding diathesis can be associated with thrombocytopenia caused by hypersplenism. The liver plays an integral role in normal hemostasis by producing most of the coagulation factors, anticoagulants, and inhibitors of plasminogen activators. Causes of bleeding diathesis associated with fulminant hepatic failure or end-stage liver disease is multifactorial and is the end result of decreased production of coagulation factors, fibrinolysis, dysfibrinogenemia, thrombocytopenia, and occasionally disseminated intravascular coagulation (DIC). Patients with decreased clotting factors secondary to liver disease or DIC have elevated PT, aPTT, and thrombin time and abnormal bleeding time. Patients with recent liver surgery or liver transplant can have excessive bleeding because of increased activation of the fibrinolytic system. Appropriate treatment of patients with excessive bleeding caused by liver disease is determined when the underlying cause of bleeding is discovered. Typically, factor replacement with FFP or cryoprecipitate is needed. Additional therapy with platelet transfusions may also be indicated (4,29).

Vitamin K Deficiency

Vitamin K is a cofactor required for the formation of gamma-carboxyglutamic acid (Gla) residues in various coagulation factors. The Gla residues help facilitate membrane binding during the coagulation process. Vitamin K-dependent proteins include factors VII, IX, X, as well as prothrombin and proteins C and S. Abnormalities in these coagulation factors can lead to prolongation of both the PT and the aPTT. Vitamin K deficiency can result in easy bruising and mucosal bleeding and is corrected by administration of vitamin K via oral, subcutaneous, or intravenous routes (29,30).

Acquired Inhibitors to Clotting Factors

Acquired inhibitors are typically auto-antibodies directed toward specific clotting factors. Auto-antibodies can be seen in patients with rheumatologic diseases (e.g., systemic lupus erythematosis, rheumatoid arthritis), neoplasms; those who are pregnant or in the postpartum period; and patients on certain medications. Factor VIII inhibitors, which are most frequently seen, are usually antibodies that interfere with factor VIII activity. Other mechanisms of inhibition also exist; for example, patients with amyloidosis can develop bleeding symptoms secondary to amyloid interactions with factor X. Inhibitors directed against factors V, VII, IX, X, XI, and XIII are exceedingly rare. Treatment focuses on immunosuppression to decrease concentrations of the offending antibody. Treatment can also include factor replacement, steroids, and cyclophosphamide, intravenous gamma globulin (IVIG) or rituximab. Patients with acquired factor inhibitors have the potential for severe bleeding and a hematology consult is recommended when any of these disorders are suspected (4,35,36,37).

Hyperfibrinolytic States

Hyperfibrinolytic states are rare, and can be difficult to distinguish from other bleeding diatheses. Hyperfibrinolysis, which occurs when fibrinolytic activity outweighs fibrin formation, is associated with a variety of clinical conditions. Associated conditions include severe liver disease, trauma, cardiac bypass surgery; and DIC secondary to malignancy, such as metastatic prostate cancer, α_2 plasmin inhibitor deficiency, and plasminogen activator inhibitor 1. A hyperfibrinolytic state should be suspected in a bleeding patient with one of the above associated clinical conditions when the platelet count, PT, and aPTT are all normal. Treatment should focus on correcting the underlying associated state. Aminocaproic acid and tranexamic acid can used to stabilize the fibrin clot, but these compounds are contraindicated in patients with hematuria or DIC. Patients with hyperfibrinolysis have the potential for severe bleeding, and the recommendation is for a hematology consult when any of these disorders are suspected (30,37).

Hemorrhagic Vascular Disorders

Hemorrhagic vascular disorders are a group of heterogeneous disorders present with petechiae and ecchymoses. Screening coagulation tests are normal, except for prolonged bleeding time. These are the diagnoses of exclusion without a confirmatory laboratory abnormality. Physical examination findings are more important. These include vasculopathies (hereditary hemorrhagic telangiectasias), hereditary connective tissue disorders (Ehlers-Danlos disease, osteogenesis imperfecta), and acquired connective tissue disorders such as scurvy, amyloidoses, Cushing disease, and arteriovenous malformations.

In some patients with bleeding diathesis, the cause may never be established. In such cases, abuse or self-inflicted injuries may have to be considered (37).

CLINICAL RECOMMENDATIONS OF THE VIGNETTE

The patient had a typical family history, and his clinical picture indicates mild hemophilia. His hemophilia A phenotype, however, evolved to moderate and severe bleeding types with the development of an inhibitor. Development of inhibitors is more common in severe hemophiliacs, but can also occur in the mild to moderate phenotypes. To limit future bleeding episodes into the joint, he needs immune tolerance treatments with high-dose factor VIII replacement. Alternatively, porcine factor VIII or recombinant factor VIIa can be used (4). Corticosteroids, cytoxic drugs, IVIG, or rituximab are used to inhibit antibody production. He also needs orthopedic intervention and physical therapy to restore joint function.

SUMMARY

Diagnosis and management of bleeding diathesis requires a basic understanding of both hemostasis and the clinical presentation. Evaluation always begins with a description of bleeding events from present to past episodes and a family history of bleeding disorders should include at least two generations of both maternal and paternal families. Personal history should include comorbidity, medications, and life style. A complete physical examination and initial laboratory screening provide algorithmic approach to bleeding diathesis. Identification of a specific defective hemostatic abnormality guides care and management of the bleeding diathesis.

REFERENCES

1. Ragni MV. The hemophilias: Factors VIII and factor IX deficiencies. In: Young NS, Gerson SL, High KA, eds. *Clinical Hematology*. Philadelphia: Mosby Elsevier; 2006:814–841.
2. Roberts HR, Escobar M, Gilbert CW II. Hemophilia A and hemophilia B. In: Lichtman MA, Beutler E, Kipps TJ, et al., eds. *Williams Hematology*. New York: McGraw-Hill Medical; 2006:1867–1886.
3. Handin RI. Disorders of coagulation and thrombosis. Kasper DL, Braunwald E, Fauci AS, et al., eds. *Harrison's Principles of Internal Medicine*. New York: McGraw-Hill Medical: 2005:680–693.
4. Crowther M, Abshire T, George JN. Hemostasis and thrombosis. In: Williams ME, Kahn MJ, eds. *American Society of Hematology Self-assessment Program*. Washington, DC: Blackwell; 2005: 297–341.
5. Kitchens, CS. Occult hemophilia. *Johns Hopkins Med J*. 1980;146:255–259.
6. Ljung, R, Petrini, P, Nilsson, IM. Diagnostic symptoms of severe and moderate hemophilia A and B. A survey of 140 cases. *Acta Pediatr Scand*. 1990;79:196–200.
7. Escuriola EC, Halimeh, S, Kurnik, K, et al. Symptomatic onset of severe hemophilia A in childhood is dependant on the presence of prothrombotic risk factors. *Thromb Haemost*. 2001;85:218–220.
8. Lee, DH, Walker, IR, Teijel J, et al. Effect of the factor V Leiden mutation on the clinical expression of severe hemophilia A. *Thromb Haemost*. 2000;83:387–391.
9. Cinotti S, Longo G, Messori A, et al. Reproducibility of one stage, two stage and chromogenic assays of factor VIII activity: A multi center study. *Thromb Res*. 1991;61:385–393.
10. Chuah, MK, Schiedner, G, Thorrez, L, et al. Therapeutic factor VIII levels and negligible toxicity in mouse and dog models of hemophilia A following gene therapy with high-capacity adenoviral vectors. *Blood*. 2003;101:1734–1743.
11. Mingozzi, F, Liu, YL, Dobrzynski, E, et al. Induction of immune tolerance to coagulation factor IX antigen by in vivo hepatic gene transfer. *J Clin Invest*. 2003;111:1347–1356.
12. Porte RJ, Leebeek FW. Pharmacological strategies to decrease transfusion requirements in patients undergoing surgery. *Drugs*. 2002;62:2193–2211.
13. Ghosh K, Shetty S, Jijina F, et al. Role of epsilon amino caproic acid in the management of hemophilic patients with inhibitors. *Haemophilia*. 2004;10:58–62.
14. Kurachi K, Davie EW. Isolation and characterization of a cDNA coding for factor IX. *Proc Natl Acad Sci USA*. 1982;79:6461–6464
15. Reijen MJ, Peerlinck K, Maasdam D, et al. Hemophilia B Leyden: Substitution of thymine for guanine at position 21 results in disruption of a hepatocyte nuclear factor 4 binding site in the factor IX promoter. *Blood*. 1993;82:151–158.
16. Armstrong E, Konkle BA. von Willebrand disease. In: Young NS, Gerson SL, High KA, eds. *Clinical Hematology*. Philadelphia: Mosby Elsevier; 2006:830–841.
17. Johnsen J, Ginsburg D. von Willebrand disease. Hemophilia A and Hemophilia B. In: Lichtman MA, Beutler E, Kipps TJ, et al., eds. *Williams Hematology*. New York: McGraw-Hill Medical; 2006:1929–1945.
18. Triplett DA. Coagulation and bleeding disorders: Review and update. *Clin Chem*. 2000;46:1260–1269.
19. Sadler JE. New concepts in von Willebrand disease. *Ann Rev Med* 2005;56:173–191.
20. Michiels JJ, Gadisseur A, Budde U, et al. Characterization, classification and treatment of von Willebrand diseases: A critical appraisal of the literature and personal experiences. *Semin Throm Hemost*. 2005;31:577–601.
21. Sadler JE. Von Willebrand disease type 1: A diagnosis in search of a disease. *Blood*. 2003;101:2089–2093.
22. Favaroloro EJ, Lillicrap D, Lazzari MA, et al. Von Willebrand disease: Laboratory aspects of diagnosis and treatment. *Hemophilia*. 2004;10:164–168.
23. Michiels JJ, Berneman Z, Gadisseur A, et al. Classification and characterization of hereditary types 2A, 2B, 2C, 2D, 2E, 2M, 2N, and 2U (unclassifiable) von Willebrand disease. *Clin Appl Thromb Hemost*. 2006;12:397–420.
24. Nurden P, Debili N, Vainchenker W, et al. Impaired megakaryocytopoiesis in type 2B von Willebrand disease with severe thrombocytopenia. *Blood*. 2006;108:2587–2595.
25. Federici AB, Castaman G, Mannucci PM. Guidelines for the diagnosis and management of von Willebrand disease in Italy. *Haemophilia*. 2002;8:607–621.
26. Mannucci PM. Treatment of von Willebrand's disease. *N Engl J Med*. 2004;351:683–694.
27. Franchini M. Haemostasis and pregnancy. *Thromb Haemost*. 2006;95:401–413.
28. Kujovich JL. Von Willebrand disease and pregnancy. *J Thromb Haemost*. 2005;3:246–253.
29. Thompson A. Congenital bleeding disorders from other coagulation protein deficiencies. In: Young NS, Gerson SL, High KA, eds. *Clinical Hematology*. Philadelphia: Mosby Elsevier; 2006:855–866.
30. Seligsohn U, Zivelin A, Inbal A. Inherited deficiencies of coagulation factors II, V, VII, X, XI and XIII and combined deficiencies of factors V and VII and of the vitamin K dependent factors. In: Lichtman MA, Beutler E, Kipps TJ, et al., eds. *Williams Hematology*. New York: McGraw-Hill Medical; 2006:1887–1907.
31. Mohri H. Acquired von Willebrand syndrome: Features and management. *Am J Hematol*. 2006;81:616–623.
32. Vincentelli A, Susen S, Le Tourneau T. Acquired von Willebrand in aortic stenosis. *N Engl J Med*. 2003;349:343–349.
33. Franchini M, Veneri D, Lippi G, et al. The efficacy of rituximab in the treatment of inhibitor-associated hemostatic disorders. *Thromb Haemost*. 2006;96:119–125.
34. Sallah S, Saint-Remy JM. Acquired inhibitors to clotting factors. In: Young NS, Gerson SL, Higk KA, eds. *Clinical Hematology*. Philadelphia: Mosby Elsevier; 2006:842–854.
35. Vermylen J, Arnout J. Antibody-mediated coagulation factor deficiencies. In: Lichtman MA, Beutler E, Kipps TJ, et al., eds. *Williams Hematology*. New York: McGraw-Hill Medical; 2006:1947–1951.
36. Bell WR. The fibrinolytic system in neoplasia. *Semin Thromb Hemost*. 1996;22:459–469.
37. LoRusso KL, Macik BG. Chronic bruising and bleeding diathesis. In: Young NS, Gerson SL, High KA, eds. *Clinical Hematology*. Philadelphia: Mosby Elsevier; 2006:1079–1088.

CHAPTER 52

Thrombotic Disorders

William R. Broderick • Sucha Nand • Laura C. Michaelis

OBJECTIVES

- To define the acquired and inherited syndromes of abnormal thrombosis
- To recognize clinical scenarios that should prompt a hypercoagulable workup
- To delineate the testing necessary to diagnose a hypercoagulable state
- To review options and recommendations for treatment of hypercoagulable states

CASE VIGNETTE

A 24-year-old woman admitted to the hospital complained of an unrelenting, right-sided headache that she had had for 4 days. The headache was associated with nausea, vomiting, and photophobia. She characterized it as the "worst headache of her life." The patient's only medications were oral contraceptive pills and an antihistamine. Physical examination demonstrated normal fundoscopy and normal cranial nerve function. Muscle strength, coordination, reflexes, and sensory examination were unremarkable. She had a right Babinski sign. She was afebrile. Computed tomographic (CT) scan demonstrated a subtle area of increased density in the superior sagittal sinus extending to the right transverse sinus. Magnetic resonance venography (MRV) demonstrated a partial right proximal transverse sinus thrombosis.

DEFINITIONS

Thrombotic disorders stem from the disruption of the balance between hemostasis and the fluidity of blood, and the resulting disinhibition of thrombus formation. The character of the thrombi differs based on the flow conditions in the microenvironment where they form. The high-pressure, high-shear environment of the arterial system results in thrombi composed primarily of platelets. The low-pressure, low-shear environment of the venous system results in thrombi composed primarily of fibrin and trapped erythrocytes. A number of acquired and inherited conditions can disrupt the hemostatic balance (1) and vary in whether they result in arterial or venous clot.

In this chapter is discussed the thrombotic disorder most frequently encountered in clinical practice, including heparin-induced thrombocytopenia (HIT), the antiphospholipid antibody syndrome, hyperhomocysteinemia, factor V Leiden, protein C deficiency, protein S deficiency, antithrombin III (ATIII) deficiency, and prothrombin gene mutation. This list is by no means exhaustive and concentrates on the inherited predispositions to clotting disorders. Other conditions that can contribute to arterial and venous thrombotic disease, including atherosclerosis, medications, pregnancy, cancer, surgery, and liver disease, are beyond the scope of this discussion.

HEPARIN-INDUCED THROMBOCYTOPENIA

Although the pathophysiology of HIT leads to thrombocytopenia, paradoxically the clinical consequences are typically clotting, rather than bleeding. Two subtypes of this condition exist. One is a reversible fall in platelet count that occurs soon after heparin therapy is initiated. This form is typically asymptomatic and is attributed to nonimmune-mediated, drug-induced platelet agglutination. The second form is an immune-mediated disorder characterized by the formation of antibodies against the heparin-platelet factor 4 (PF4) complex. The antigen-antibody complex on the platelet surface leads to activation and further release of PF4, resulting in a positive feedback loop. The activated platelets aggregate and leave the circulation, causing thrombocytopenia and frequently thrombosis (2). Both forms of HIT should be considered when the platelet count is reduced to at least 50% or a decrease to less than 150×10^9 cells per liter after exposure to heparin. Although the milder, nonimmune-mediated form can occur shortly after therapy, the immune-mediated form typically occurs >4 days after drug initiation. Whenever possible, immune-mediated HIT should be confirmed by testing for the presence of heparin-related antibodies or a functional platelet-based assay, because nonimmune HIT is not uncommon and is not associated with thrombotic complications. In immune-mediated HIT, venous thrombosis is five times more common than is arterial thrombosis (2).

ANTIPHOSPHOLIPID ANTIBODY SYNDROME

The antiphospholipid antibody syndrome is an acute, multiorgan thrombotic microangiopathy. Clinical consequences are secondary to a heterogeneous group of autoantibodies directed again phospholipids. It is defined by the presence of vascular thrombosis, pregnancy complications, or both, and the presence of either anticardiolipin antibodies (IgG or IgM) or lupus anticoagulant antibodies (3). Venous thrombosis occurs more frequently in patients with lupus anticoagulant antibodies, whereas arterial thromboses are more common in patients with anticardiolipin antibodies.

HYPERHOMOCYSTEINEMIA

Homocysteine is an intermediary amino acid formed during the conversion of methionine to cysteine. Errors in homocysteine metabolism are caused by cofactor deficiencies (vitamin B_{12}, folate, vitamin B_6), or genetic abnormalities in enzymes, such as cystathione-B-synthase and methylene tetrahydrofolate reductase, which result in a backup in the biochemical pathways and inappropriately high levels of homocysteine in the blood, which has been shown to be both atherogenic and prothrombotic. Severe hyperhomocysteinemia, also called *homocystinuria,* is caused by severe enzyme deficiency. It is rare and results in mental retardation, peripheral neuropathy, and thrombosis early in life. Less-severe hyperhomocysteinemia is more common and increases patients' risk for both arterial and venous clots (4).

ACTIVATED PROTEIN C RESISTANCE/ FACTOR V LEIDEN MUTATION

Factor V Leiden is the most common cause of hereditary thrombophilia. There are a number of described mutations in the factor V gene. The most common is a substitution of glutamine for arginine at position 506 in the factor V molecule (factor V Leiden) causing resistance to activated protein C. Less-avid binding to activated protein C results in a longer duration of activated factor V (Va) within the prothrombinase complex, increasing coagulation via the generation of thrombin. The result is an increased risk of venous thromboembolism over the general population (5).

PROTEIN C DEFICIENCY

Protein C is a vitamin K-dependent protein synthesized in the liver. It exerts its anticoagulant function after activation to the serine protease, activated protein C (aPC). The primary effect of aPC is to inactivate coagulation factors Va and activated factor VIII (VIIIa), which are necessary for efficient thrombin generation and factor X activation (6). Protein C deficiency predominantly results in increased thrombin production and a tendency toward venous thrombosis. The deficiency is discovered in 2% to 5% of patients having a workup for new venous thromboembolism (VTE).

PROTEIN S DEFICIENCY

Protein S is a vitamin K-dependent protein that acts as a cofactor for the inhibition of factors Va and VIIIa by aPC. In type I deficiency, both total and free protein S levels are decreased. In type II deficiency, both levels are normal, but the protein S activity is reduced. In type III deficiency, the total protein S level is normal, but the free protein S level is reduced. The free form is the active form of protein S. Again, decreased levels of protein S result in increased activity of factor Va and VIIIa and a tendency toward venous thrombosis (7).

ANTITHROMBIN III DEFICIENCY

Antithrombin complexes with activated coagulation factors Xa, IXa, XIa, and XIIa and thrombin limit their activity. Values that are only slightly below normal increase the risk of venous thrombosis (8). Deficiency can arise from reduced synthesis of biologically normal protease inhibitor molecules secondary to gene mutation or deletion.

PROTHROMBIN GENE MUTATION

Prothrombin is the precursor for thrombin. A mutation in the 20210 position of the gene coding for prothrombin is associated with a 25% increase in thrombin (1). The increase in thrombin leads to increased risk of thrombosis.

EPIDEMIOLOGY

Arterial thrombosis is most often a complication of atherosclerotic vascular disease rather than an acquired or congenital thrombotic disorder. Although coronary artery thrombosis results in approximately 1.2 million myocardial infarctions yearly, only a small percentage are caused by acquired or congenital thrombotic disorders predisposing a patient to arterial "clot." VTE affects 1 of 1,000 people annually and is much more likely to be secondary to an identifiable acquired or congenital predisposition. Pulmonary embolism (PE) is a potentially fatal complication of VTE. It has been estimated that the incidence of PE is close to 500,000 cases per year, with mortality of approximately 10%. Evidence of PE is found in 25% to 30% of routine autopsies, however, suggesting the condition is much more common. PE is also a common cause of postoperative and postpartum deaths, accounting for approximately 5,000 deaths annually (1).

HIT occurs in approximately 3% of patients exposed to unfractionated heparin. The incidence is lower with low molecular weight heparins, but some risk persists. In the immune-mediated form, thrombosis occurs in approximately 25% of patients. Although VTE is five times more common than arterial thrombosis, once arterial thrombosis develops mortality may be as high as 50% (3).

Antiphospholipid antibodies were first described in patients with systemic lupus erythematosus (SLE), in whom they can be detected in 30% to 50% of cases. They have also been detected in patients with other autoimmune disorders, patients taking certain medications, patients recovering from acute viral infections, patients with human immunodeficiency virus (HIV) infection, and women with multiple fetal losses. Thrombosis occurs in 30% to 40% of patients with SLE and anticardiolipin antibodies or lupus anticoagulant, and in 15% to 30% of patients with antiphospholipid antibodies, but without SLE (1).

Estimates are that 10% of the risk of coronary heart disease is attributable to hyperhomocysteinemia. Also, homocysteine levels in patients with venous or arterial thrombotic events are 30% higher than in healthy patients. In patients with severe congenital hyperhomocysteinemia, 50% will have a thrombotic event by age 30, with a 20% mortality rate. Homocysteine levels above the 95th percentile for normal controls have been associated with a 2.5 times increased risk of deep venous thrombosis (DVT).

Approximately 5% of the caucasian North American population is heterozygous for the factor V Leiden gene mutation. The prevalence is highest in Greece, Sweden, and Lebanon where it approximates 15% in some areas. In contrast, it is essentially nonexistent in African black, Chinese, or Japanese populations. The presence of this mutation may account for 10% to 25% of patients with DVT or PE. Heterozygosity for this mutation doubles a patient's risk for thrombotic event. Homozygous patients are at a 20-fold increased risk. In addition, heterozygous women who take oral contraceptives or are pregnant increase their risk 14-fold (8).

Protein C deficiency is inherited as an autosomal dominant disorder. It can be inherited as a functional abnormality or decrease in production. Heterozygous individuals with 50% decrease in protein C activity are at risk for thrombosis. Thrombotic events typically occur after the second decade, although it is not clear what biochemical events are playing a protective role. DVT of the legs are the most common manifestation, but protein C deficiency has been documented as a cause of thrombotic stroke in the young patient (9). Protein C deficiency has a prevalence of approximately 1 in 200, but penetrance varies. The estimated increased lifetime risk of thrombotic event has been reported as high as 31-fold. Homozygous protein C deficiency or homozygous deficiency with protein C concentration <1% has been documented, but is typically fatal in newborns secondary to purpura fulminans. Acquired protein C deficiency can occur in liver disease (1).

Hereditary deficiency of protein S predisposes to thrombotic events and occurs in a prevalence of 1 in 20,000. The total protein S concentration in heterozygous individuals is typically 50% of normal and it results in (10) an 8.5 times increase in the lifetime relative risk of thrombosis (11). Little thrombotic risk is found before age 15. Approximately 50% of affected patients will have had thrombotic events by the age of 30.

Although ATIII deficiency can occur as frequently as 1 of 600 people in the general population, symptomatic disease is rarer, and is estimated to occur in between 1 of 2,000 and 1 of 5,000 people. It is also inherited as an autosomal dominant disorder. Most patients are heterozygous and demonstrate ATIII levels 40% to 70% of normal. Those who are homozygotic are extremely rare (12). In patients with ATIII deficiency, a 40-fold increased lifetime risk exists of venous thrombosis. Typically, events occur by the age of 50. An absolute annual risk of >27% has been documented in women who are ATIII deficient who use oral contraception, and some studies have demonstrated a 70% risk of pregnancy-related venous thrombosis (10).

The prothrombin G20210A mutation is the second most common inherited predisposition to thrombosis. It is an autosomal dominant gene mutation that appears to follow a geographic and ethnic distribution. The highest prevalence appears in caucasian populations from southern Europe (3%). Northern European population studies revealed a prevalence of 1.7%. The mutation infrequently occurs in Middle Eastern and Indian populations and is virtually absent in Asian and African populations. Heterozygous individuals have a two- to sixfold increased lifetime risk of VTE. That risk is increased to 15-fold in pregnancy and 16-fold when combined with oral contraceptive use. Homozygosity occurs in 0.014% of the caucasian population and confers an increased risk of venous thromboembolism before age 40. A fourfold increased risk of myocardial infarction (MI) has been demonstrated in young women with the prothrombin gene mutation, but no increased risk of stroke or MI was noted in men (10).

ETIOLOGY AND PATHOGENESIS

Two subtypes of heparin-induced thrombocytopenia exist. The first is an innocuous, transient, modest decrease in platelet count caused by heparin-induced platelet aggregation. This form of HIT is not prothrombotic. The more serious form of HIT is an antibody-mediated disorder that should be suspected when the platelet count falls to <150,000/mm^3 or <50% of baseline up to 3 weeks after heparin exposure. It occurs in approximately 1% of patients receiving unfractionated heparin and a much smaller proportion of patients receiving low molecular weight heparin. HIT is triggered by antibodies (usually IgG) directed against heparin in complex with platelet factor 4. These antibodies bind to, and activate, platelets, increase procoagulant activity, and lead to endothelial damage. These antibodies tend to disappear over a period of 3 months. The platelet count returns to normal within days of heparin cessation (3).

Antiphospholipid antibodies are a heterogeneous group of antibodies that may be found in association with autoimmune diseases or HIV infection. The two classes of antiphospholipid antibodies are (*a*) anticardiolipin antibodies and (*b*) lupus anticoagulants. Anticardiolipin antibodies can be IgG or IgM and are directed against B_2-glycoprotein 1. High titer IgG anticardiolipin antibodies are most strongly associated with clinical manifestations. Lupus anticoagulants produce a prolongation in phospholipid-dependent clotting assays such as the aPTT using a sensitive reagent, the dilute Russell viper venom time, or kaolin clotting time. The method by which antiphospholipid antibodies cause thrombosis is unclear. It has been suggested that their prothrombotic properties may be very diverse, including attenuation of activated protein C, downregulation of antithrombin III, inhibition of the anticoagulant activity of B_2-glycoprotein 1, endothelial cell activation, enhanced binding of prothrombin to biologic surfaces, enhanced adhesion molecule expression, platelet activation and aggregation, and impaired fibrinolysis (3). Others have implied that they may simply be markers of a hypercoagulable state (1).

An increased level of the non–protein-forming amino acid homocysteine, a product of methionine metabolism, is a risk factor for both premature atherosclerosis and DVT. The homocysteine levels in cells and plasma are controlled by two biochemical reactions: Remethylation of homocysteine to methionine (involving the enzyme methylenetetrahydrofolate reductase) and transulfuration, in which homocysteine condenses with serine to form cystathione (involving the Vitamin B_6-dependent enzyme cystathione-B-synthase). The thrombogenic properties of homocysteine are also not well known. In animal models, it has been shown to increase platelet adherence, activate factors V, X, and XII, inhibit protein C activation, and inhibit cell surface thrombomodulin (13). These mechanisms have not been confirmed in human studies.

The diagnosis of activated protein C (APC) resistance is made when an insufficient increase is seen in the aPTT after the addition of APC to patient serum. In >90% of cases, this resistance is caused by a point mutation in the gene that codes for factor V. The factor V Leiden mutation causes the clinical condition of activated protein C resistance and the subsequent prothrombotic state. In contrast to protein C and S deficiency and ATIII deficiency, there are sufficient levels of inactivating factors, but a factor Va that is resistant to inactivation. In addition to factor V Leiden mutation, an acquired form of APC resistance of uncertain significance also can develop during pregnancy or in patients with antiphospholipid antibodies.

When protein C is activated by the thrombin–thrombomodulin complex to APC, one of its functions is to inactivate factors Va and VIIIa and, thus, damper coagulation. In addition, APC possesses fibrinolytic activity. Patients with type I deficiency demonstrate a quantitative decrease in protein C, as well as a decrease in activity. This type of protein C deficiency is the result of point mutations that cause improper protein folding and impaired excretion from hepatocytes. Type II protein C deficiency is characterized by normal levels of protein C, but reduced activity. Patients with protein C deficiency are susceptible to both superficial vein thrombosis and DVT. Frequently, these disorders are treated with warfarin. Warfarin decreases the production of vitamin K-dependent clotting factors in the liver, including protein C, by competing for binding sites that allow vitamin K absorption into the liver. In patients with protein C deficiency, the further decrease in protein C levels can cause a loss of the function of the protein C regulatory pathway before the anticoagulant effect of warfarin is fully established. Without the anticoagulant effect of protein C, thrombosis can develop and is termed *Coumadin necrosis* if it involves the skin. This disorder begins a few days after starting warfarin and presents as painful erythematous lesions that can rapidly progress to necrosis. This effect is attenuated by coadministering heparin therapy until warfarin is therapeutic. Acquired protein C deficiency can also develop in patients with liver disease (7).

Free protein S acts as a cofactor in the inhibition of factor Va and VIIIa by APC. Hereditary protein S deficiency is classified into three subtypes. In type I deficiency, total and free protein S levels are reduced. In type II, total and free protein S levels are normal, but the protein S activity is reduced. In type III, total protein S levels are normal, but free protein S levels are reduced. Protein S levels are lower in women when pregnant or using oral contraceptives. Levels are also decreased in liver disease, inflammatory bowel disease, and nephrotic syndrome. As with protein C deficiency, skin necrosis can occur if warfarin therapy is initiated without heparin coadministration.

Antithrombin (AT) is a serine protease inhibitor that regulates coagulation by inactivating thrombin and factors IXa, Xa, XIa, and XIIa. Patients with ATIII deficiency may have either a decrease in AT synthesis with concordant decrease in activity (type I) or normal levels of AT with decreased activity (types II and III). Type I deficiency is caused by gene deletions and rearrangements that decrease synthesis of AT, resulting in parallel decreases in both the functional and immunologic levels. Type II deficiency is caused by mutations in thrombin-binding sites. Type III deficiency is caused by mutations in the heparin-binding sites. Acquired ATIII deficiency has been linked with DIC, liver disease, nephrotic syndrome, and preeclampsia, and is seen in patients taking oral contraceptives or who are pregnant (10).

Prothrombin is a precursor for thrombin. The prothrombin 20210 gene mutation results in elevated concentrations of prothrombin. The rise in prothrombin is likely caused by increased efficiency of prothrombin messenger RNA (mRNA) processing or decreased degradation of prothrombin mRNA (10). An increase in prothrombin results in an increase in thrombin and increased thrombosis.

CLINICAL MANIFESTATIONS AND DIAGNOSIS

Although people with hypercoagulable states are at great risk of thrombotic events, not all will develop overt thrombosis, and not all patients with a thrombotic event will have an identifiable hypercoagulable state. Testing is likely to identify an abnormality in 60% of patients presenting with a spontaneous venous thrombosis. Although 40% of patients with spontaneous thromboses will have normal tests, some of these people, however, will have an acquired hypercoaguable state, such as malignancy, or an inherited condition that has not yet been discovered or recognized (10).

Thrombotic disorders can be characterized by those that favor arterial thrombosis, such as HIT, antiphospholipid antibody syndrome, and hyperhomocysteinemia, or those that favor venous thrombosis, such as APC resistance, protein C and S deficiency, ATIII deficiency, and prothrombin gene mutation. Arterial hypercoagulability can lead to cerebrovascular disease and contribute to coronary disease. Venous hypercoagulability most frequently manifests itself as DVT or PE. The clinical scenarios involved in acute thrombotic stroke, DVT of the extremities, and PE are well known. Multiple risk factors contribute to these pathologic states, including arterial hypertension, hyperlipidemia, age, and cigarette smoking, for cardiovascular disease and stroke; and prolonged immobility, trauma, surgery, and malignancy for VTE.

Patients who develop venous thromboembolism without a predisposing factor, have a strong family history, present under the age of 30, or have more than one episode of VTE, should have studies for antithrombin III deficiency, protein C and S deficiency, factor V Leiden, and prothrombin gene mutation. Because an association between elevated homocysteine levels and both arterial and venous thrombotic events is recognized, homocysteine levels should be checked in this population as well.

With the possible exception of rupture of a coronary atherosclerotic plaque or acute stroke in a patient with multiple risk factors, arterial thrombosis is never a "normal" phenomenon. Patients who present with arterial thrombosis should be evaluated for antiphospholipid antibody syndrome, hyperhomocysteinemia, and, if exposed to heparin products, HIT (14).

Patients who present with stroke before the age of 45 or with minimal risk factors should also be considered for a hypercoagulable workup. This clinical scenario is frequently complicated by a patent foramen ovale (PFO), which may allow thrombosis from a venous source to cause an acute embolic stroke. In addition to the standard stroke workup, including evaluation of both the cerebral vasculature and the cardiac valves for embolic source, these patients should have transesophageal echocardiography or transthoracic echocardiograpy with bubble study to rule out PFO. The hypercoagulable workup in these patients should address both arterial and venous thrombi. Thus, screening for antiphospholipid antibodies, antithrombin III deficiency, protein C and S deficiencies, prothrombin gene mutation, factor V Leiden mutation, and homocysteine levels is appropriate.

As mentioned, pregnancy frequently exacerbates prothrombotic states. Pregnancy or the use of oral contraceptives is often the trigger that precipitates a thrombotic event in a woman with an underlying prothrombotic state. Pregnant patients who have had a thrombotic event should be tested for all of the abovementioned prothrombotic states.

Recurrent fetal loss is a significant problem in prothrombotic states. A growing body of evidence has associated protein C, protein S, and antithrombin deficiencies with fetal losses. The risk of thrombosis with ATIII deficiency is particularly high during pregnancy and in the postpartum period. The association of factor V Leiden with recurrent fetal loss was endorsed by the College of American Pathologists Consensus Conference on Thrombophilia (15).

TREATMENT

Patients with an inherited or acquired prothrombotic state present a difficult therapeutic challenge. As stated, not every patient with a prothrombotic disorder will have a thrombotic event. To date, no way exists to differentiate those that will clot from those that will not. All patients with VTE should have immediate anticoagulation therapy with unfractionated or low molecular weight heparin, or an appropriate substitute if there is a history of HIT, followed by 3 to 6 months of oral anticoagulation with warfarin. This regimen allows for recovery of the endothelium of the vessel and prevents recurrence in the damaged vascular bed. Patients with antiphospholipid antibody syndrome, ATIII deficiency, or homozygous mutations for factor V Leiden have a high risk of recurrence and should remain on lifelong oral anticoagulation. Patients with protein C and S deficiency or those who are heterozygous for factor V Leiden mutation are at a lower risk of recurrence and, therefore, may avoid lifelong anticoagulation unless they have secondary risk factors such as oral contraception use or experience a second event. Warfarin is contraindicated during pregnancy; thus, heparin products should be continued through pregnancy and warfarin started postpartum (8).

For pregnant patients known to have ATIII deficiency, but no history of thrombosis, heparin prophylaxis is recommended throughout the pregnancy. The precise regimen is controversial. Postpartum, warfarin therapy with a goal international normalized ratio (INR) of 2.0 to 3.0 is recommended for 6 weeks (12).

Treatment of patients with prothrombin gene mutation should parallel treatment of individuals who are heterozygous for the factor V Leiden mutation (10).

HIT is an extremely hypercoagulable state and, therefore, requires immediate action on suspicion of the disorder. First, all heparin-containing treatments must be discontinued, including flushes and low molecular weight heparin. Second, immediate anticoagulation should be initiated with a direct thrombin inhibitor, such as lepirudin or argatroban. Confirmatory testing with heparin-induced platelet aggregation assay is 90% specific, but is not adequately sensitive. Serotonin release assay is 100% sensitive and 97% specific, but is expensive and is must be sent out for laboratory in many institutions. Once the platelet count recovers, the patient can be transitioned to oral warfarin. Anticoagulation should be continued for 2 to 3 months (2).

Although elevated levels of homocysteine have been associated with both arterial and venous thrombosis, a reduction in recurrent thrombosis has not been demonstrated with therapeutic reduction of homocysteine. In the immediate case, thrombosis in a patient with hyperhomocysteinemia should be anticoagulated as with any of the prothrombotic states. In addition to anticoagulation, daily oral doses of folate (1 mg), vitamin B_6 (10 mg), and vitamin B_{12} (0.4 mg) effectively lower homocysteine levels. Oral anticoagulation should be continued for 3 to 6 months after a first episode of thrombosis. Life-long anticoagulation should be considered after a second or life-threatening event.

CLINICAL RECOMMENDATIONS OF THE VIGNETTE

In the patient presented, a hypercoagulable workup was initiated and the patient was started on heparin in the hospital. Once a therapeutic level was achieved, she was transitioned to warfarin and the heparin was discontinued only after her INR was recorded between 2.0 and 3.0. Her oral contraception was discontinued. Appropriate warnings were provided regarding the teratogenicity of warfarin. Hypercoagulable workup demonstrated factor V Leiden deficiency. She was discharged on warfarin and remained on anticoagulation for 2 years after the embolic event at which time it was discontinued until she became pregnant; then, low molecular weight heparin was initiated. She has had no additional hypercoagulable events.

SUMMARY

Disruption of the normal homeostatic balance between hemostasis and fluidity of blood commonly results in intravascular thrombosis. The thrombotic disorders most frequently seen in clinical practice are HIT, antiphospholipid antibody syndrome, hyperhomocysteinemia, APC resistance, protein C and S deficiencies, ATIII deficiency, and the prothrombin gene mutation. Of these, HIT, antiphospholipid antibody syndrome, and hyperhomocysteinemia contribute to arterial thrombosis, whereas the remainder predispose patients to venous thrombosis. All patients with VTE should receive anticoagulation therapy with heparin products and transitioned to oral anticoagulation with warfarin for 3 to 6 months. In certain circumstances, anticoagulation should be life-long. Patients who develop HIT should be treated as hypercoagulable and receive anticoagulation therapy immediately with a direct thrombin inhibitor. They can also be transitioned to warfarin therapy for 3 months. Patients with hyperhomocysteinemia should also have anticoagulation therapy for acute thrombosis and be treated with life-time folic acid, vitamin B_6, and vitamin B_{12}. A second thrombotic event or a life-threatening event typically prompts life-long anticoagulation.

REFERENCES

1. Humes HD, Dupont HL, eds. *Kelley's Textbook of Internal Medicine*, 4th ed. Philadelphia: Lippincott Williams & Wilkins; 2000:1734–1739.
2. Steven Coutre M. *Heparin-induced Thrombocytopenia*. UpToDate On Line 2006. Available from: www.utdol.com.
3. Andreotti F, Becker RC. Atherothrombotic disorders. *Circulation*. 2005;111:1855–1863.
4. Robert S, Rosenson M, David M, et al. *Overview of Homocysteine*. UpToDate On Line 2006. Available from: www.utdol.com.
5. Bauer KA. *Activated protein C resistance and factor V Leiden*. UpToDate On Line 2006. Available from: www.utdol.com. [cited]
6. Bauer KA. *Protein C Deficiency*. UpToDate On Line 2006. Available from: www.utdol.com. [cited; 14.3:]
7. Williams ME, Kahn MJ, eds. *American Society of Hematology Self-Assessment Program*, 2nd ed. Washington, DC: Blackwell Publishing; 2005.
8. Fauci AS, et al., eds. *Harrison's Textbook of Medicine*, 14 ed. New York: McGraw-Hill; 1998:742–743.
9. Camerlingo M, Finazzi G, Casto L, et al. Inherited protein C deficiency and nonhemorrhagic arterial stroke in young adults. *Neurology*. 1991;41:1371–1373.
10. Greer JP, Foerster J, Lukens JN, et al. *Wintrobe's Clinical Hematology*, 11th ed. Philadelphia: Lippincott Williams & Wilkins; 2004;1718–1729.
11. Martinelli I, Mannucci PM, De Stefano V, et al. Different risks of thrombosis in four coagulation defects associated with inherited thrombophilia: A study of 150 families. *Blood*. 1998;92(7):2353–2358.
12. De Stefano V, Finazzi G, Mannucci PM. Inherited thrombophilia: Pathogenesis, clinical syndromes, and management. *Blood*. 1996;87(9):3531–3544.
13. Eikelboom JW, Lonn E, Genest J, Jr., et al. Homocyst(e)ine and cardiovascular disease: A critical review of the epidemiologic evidence. *Ann Intern Med*. 1999;131(5):363–375.
14. Kahn MJ. Hypercoagulability as a cause of stroke in adults. *South Med J*. 2003;96(4):350–354.
15. Brenner B. Clinical management of thrombophilia-related placental vascular complications. *Blood*. 2004;103(11):4003–4009.

CHAPTER **53**

Lymphoproliferative Disorders

Michael Y. Ko • Harry L. Messmore

OBJECTIVES

- To define the epidemiology, etiology, and pathophysiology of several lymphoproliferative disorders
- To describe the systemic manifestations and neurologic complications of those disorders
- To discuss diagnostic criteria used to diagnose lymphoproliferative disorders
- To explain the treatments and complications of those disorders

CASE VIGNETTE

A 67-year-old woman presents with persistent fatigue and a 20-pound weight loss over the past year. On further review of systems, the patient complained of a vague and intermittent numbness in both feet and toes for about 1 year. She has a history of long-standing type 2 diabetes, but no significant surgical history. She is taking an angiotensin-converting enzyme (ACE) inhibitor for hypertension and an oral hyperglycemic agent for her diabetes. On examination, her vital signs are normal. General examination is unremarkable. No enlarged lymph nodes were found. Laboratory studies demonstrated normal metabolic profile, but the complete blood count (CBC) showed a total white blood cell count of 62,000 cells/μL. The absolute lymphocyte count is 21,000 cells/μL. Flow cytometry indicated many of the lymphocytes had the B-cell marker, CD 19. At that point, the patient refused a bone marrow biopsy.

DEFINITION

Lymphoproliferative disorders involve an abnormal accumulation of lymphocytes where each disorder has different levels of maturations and types of lymphocytes. If these cells are primarily found in the blood and bone marrow, which can disrupt the production of other hematologic cells, the disease is considered a *leukemia.* If the abnormal accumulations occur mainly in lymph nodes, the disease is called a *lymphoma.* Hodgkin lymphomas are composed of Reed-Sternberg cells, whereas non-Hodgkin lymphomas are derived from neoplastic B cells or T/natural killer (NK) cells that are not derived from a Reed-Sternberg cell (1). The World Health Organization (WHO) designated the classification of non-Hodgkin's lymphoma (NHL) by the Revised European-American Classification of Lymphoid Neoplasms, or REAL, which uses the morphology, immunology, and genetic characteristics of the abnormal lymphocyte (1). The most common of these lymphoproliferative disorders is the diffuse large B-cell lymphoma (2). Other less-common lymphomas are listed in Table 53-1. Of the lymphocytic leukemias, the chronic, or small cell, lymphocytic leukemia is the most common in adults. Although less common, primary central nervous system (CNS) lymphoma, which is a B-cell lymphoma, is also discussed because of its main involvement of the nervous system (3–5).

EPIDEMIOLOGY

NHL remains one of the more common hematopoietic-related neoplasms. In the United States alone, >50,000 new cases will be diagnosed each year (6). Along with Hodgkin lymphoma, both types comprise about 4% of all annual cancer cases (7), but NHL encompasses 80% of all lymphomas (1). Over the last 30 years, the incidence of lymphoma has doubled for unknown reasons (7). A higher incidence of human immunodeficiency virus (HIV) infections, more organ transplantation with immunosuppresion, and better diagnostic techniques and criteria can only partially account for this recent increase in lymphoma prevalence (1). It seen in all ethnic groups, however, but is slightly more common in white than black populations. Overall, the male-to-female ratio in all NHL is 1.5:1 (8). The incidence of NHL increases with age, with the highest rates found in adults >50 years of age (9). Immunodeficiencies, such as from HIV, or congenital conditions are the most common risk factor for developing NHL and will increase the risk of these disorders 10 to 100 times (10). Autoimmune diseases, such as Sjögren syndrome, and certain chronic viral infections, such as human T-lymphotrophic virus (HTLV)-1 or Epstein-Barr virus (EBV), also increase the risk of developing NHL (6). Diffuse large B-cell and follicular lymphomas are the two most common NHL and account for 31% and 22% of all lymphoma cases, respectively (6).

Chronic lymphocytic leukemia (CLL), or small lymphocytic lymphoma, is less common at 7% of all NHL cases (6), but it account for 24% of all leukemia cases (1), which translates into 7,000 new cases in the United States per year (11). Its prevalence is approximately 3 cases per 100,000 persons in the United States, and 80% will be diagnosed after 60 years of age (1).

Primary CNS lymphoma (PCL) accounts for <5% of NHL cases and a similar percentage of primary CNS malignancies (12). As with other NHL, the risk of developing PCL increases with worsening immunocompetency. Only 4% of patients

TABLE 53-1. Prevalence of World Health Organization (WHO)-classified Non-Hodgkin Lymphoma/ Lymphoproliferative Disorders

Prevalence (%)	*Lymphoproliferative Disorder*
30–33	Diffuse B-cell lymphoma
20–21	Follicular B-cell lymphoma
5–10	Mucosa associated lymphoid tissue (MALT) Lymphoma
	Peripheral T-cell lymphoma
	Small lymphocytic lymphoma
	Mantle cell lymphoma
1–2	Mediastinal B-cell lymphoma
	Anaplastic large T-cell lymphoma
	Lymphoblastic lymphoma
<1	Burkitt lymphoma
	Adult T-cell lymphoma

congenitally immunocompromised, 4% to 6% of patients with acquired immunodeficiency syndrome (AIDS), and 7% of organ transplant recipients will develop PCL (13). AIDS increases the risk of developing PCL by 3,600 times (14) and may have accounted for some of the lowering of the peak age of incidence. The median age at diagnosis of 53 to 57 years and the male-to-female ratio is 1.2 to 1.7:1 are similar those of NHL (15).

ETIOLOGY AND PATHOPHYSIOLOGY

NHL encompasses a large group of different subtypes that have different pathophysiologies. Lymphomas in western countries are typically of B-cell origin, whereas eastern countries have a higher percentage of T-cell lymphomas (7). Although acquired and congenital immunodeficient states, autoimmune diseases, and certain viral infections appear to increase the risk of developing lymphoma, the exact mechanisms for this increased incidence is unknown (9). Exposure to radiation or organophosphates has been implicated in causing NHL in some patients (1). Of the suspected infectious organisms linked with specific NHL disorders, EBV is associated with Burkitt lymphoma, HTLV-1 with adult T-cell leukemia, and human herpesvirus 8 in primary effusion lymphoma (1). Genetic abnormalities have also been implicated as possible causes for lymphoma.

Diffuse large B-cell lymphoma is most commonly caused by a gene translocation between chromosomes 18 and 14. This mutation places the *bcl-2* gene near the encoding for the immunoglobulin heavy chains and results in a lymphocyte that resists apoptosis (1). It is found only in 28% of all diffuse large B-cell lymphoma cases. Some of the remaining cases have been found to be mutations with the *bcl-6* or *c-myc* gene (6).

The cause of CLL is not known, but it is typically of B-cell origin with characteristic surface markers and morphology. No correlation has been found between exposure to viruses, chemicals, medications, or radiation (11). A genetic cause is suspected, because epidemiologic studies indicate that relatives of patients with CLL have a higher incidence of cancer in general and siblings of parents with CLL are more likely to be diagnosed earlier (6). The most common genetic abnormality yet discovered is a deletion at 13q14 of a supposed tumor suppressor gene (16). Serum studies in 2% to 3% of all CLL cases will find evidence of monoclonal expansion of B cells (6).

EBV has been implicated as the origin of PCL because its DNA has been found in the genome of malignant B cells in immunocompromised patients (10). Most cases of PCL in immunocompetent patients contain malignant B cells without the EBV genome, but are a monoclonal expansion without a single common genetic mutation or chromosomal abnormality (13). Abnormalities on chromosomes 6q, 12q, 18q, and 22q have been reported (17). Of PCL, 90% have histologic characteristics similar to a diffuse large B-cell lymphoma. The remaining 10% are composed of other cell types, such as T cells, which account for <4% of all cases (18). T cells found imbedded in histologic specimens of PCL are likely normal reactive T cells in the tumor and not a sign of a mixed B- and T-cell lymphoma. Two theories exist to where the malignant lymphocytes originate: A malignant transformation of an already resident lymphocyte in the CNS or proliferation to the CNS by an extracranial malignant lymphocyte (15).

CLINICAL MANIFESTATIONS

NON-HODGKIN LYMPHOMA

The typical initial presentation of NHL is painless lymphadenopathy, whereas systemic symptoms, such as fever, night sweats, or weight loss, are mainly seen in more aggressive forms of NHL (6). The enlarged lymph nodes are commonly found in the cervical, axillary, or inguinal regions. Occasionally, the enlarged lymph nodes will compress surrounding structures, especially if the nodes are retroperitoneal or mediastinal. Compression of these surrounding structures could cause pain in the back, pain, and abdomen, or spinal cord compression. The spleen is involved in 30% to 40% of all cases (6). Although extranodal involvement is rare initially, NHL most commonly disseminates to the brain, gastrointestinal tract, lungs, or bone marrow (6). Spread to the skull base, orbits, or testes; elevated serum lactate dehydrogenase; or higher grade malignancy correlate to an increase risk CNS metastases (13). Associated symptoms, such as anemia and thrombocytopenia from bone marrow involvement, and even peripheral neuropathy can be the initial presenting symptoms in NHL. Intravascular lymphoma (neoplastic angioendotheliomatosis) is a rare variant of NHL wherein small vessels of the skin, CNS, and endocrine glands become occluded by the neoplastic cells. These patients present with small vessel stroke syndromes, peripheral neuropathies, or skin lesions, but do not have the common risk factors for ischemic disease (13).

CHRONIC LYMPHATIC LEUKEMIA

Almost half of all patients with CLL are asymptomatic and diagnosed by an incidentally found leukocytosis on serum studies. Lymphadenopathy is the most common clinical symptom of CLL. Involvement of the spleen and liver are less common, but can be found during the initial evaluation (11). Other organs of the body, such as the skin, lungs, bones, gastrointestinal mucosal, and meninges, are less likely to be involved. Of patients with CLL, 10% to 15% will have the typical "B" symptoms of fever, fatigue, night sweats, or unexplained weight loss (19). The remaining will have symptoms related to the large number of monoclonal and poorly functioning lymphocytes and an impaired production of other hematologic cells:

Increased infections, anemia, thrombocytopenia, autoimmune-type symptoms, or hypersensitivity (20).

PRIMARY CENTRAL NERVOUS SYSTEM LYMPHOMA

Lesions of PCL are typically located in the subcortical white matter and can be multifocal. Initial symptoms can include cognitive difficulties, behavior changes, hemiparesis, language deficits, or visual problems. Focal neurologic symptoms are seen when lesions have mass effect and are less infiltrative. Approximately 70% will present with focal neurologic symptoms, whereas 43% will have behavioral symptoms. One third may have evidence of increased intracranial pressure. Seizures (14%) are a less-common initial presentation (15). This lymphoma can also be found infiltrating the eye in approximately 20% of newly diagnosed cases (14). Such patients can be initially diagnosed with sarcoidosis, rheumatoid arthritis (13), or uveitis (21). Leptomeningeal extension is seen in approximately 40% of patients, but does not usually induce the expected meningismus, headaches, or cranial neuropathies (15). Other parts of the CNS that can be involved include the choroids plexus and subarachnoid space. The spinal cord is rarely involved and such involvement would mimic a transverse myelopathy. Metastatic spread to the rest of the body, such as bones and soft tissue, is seen in <5% of patients with PCL at the time of diagnosis (13). This lack of systemic malignant lymphocytes has been theorized to be from a destruction of those lymphocytes by a competent immune system while the sequestered immune system in the CNS is unable to eliminate malignant lymphocytes (3). "B" symptoms, such as fever, weight loss, and night sweats, are usually a sign of systemic spread of the lymphoma (13).

Neurologic Complications

NON-HODGKIN LYMPHOMA

Metastatic spread of systemic lymphomas into the nervous system is a rare occurrence (22). Even with phenotypic transformation, this systemic lymphoma will rarely metastasize to the CNS (23). When lymphomas do metastasize, the CNS parenchyma is less likely to be involved than is the leptomeninges, epidural space, or peripheral nervous system (23,24). If the lymphoma does involve the brain parenchyma, the observed symptoms (e.g., headaches, confusion, nausea, or focal neurologic symptoms) are similar to those of other mass lesions. Symptoms of leptomeningeal involvement are dependent on the affected CNS region and include ataxia, headaches, cranial neuropathies, back pain, radiculopathies, visual changes, drowsiness, or confusion (22). Metastases can extend into the epidural space and compression of the spinal cord or nerve roots. Symptoms could include back pain, weakness, numbness, or bladder and bowel dysfunction (25). A radiculopathy or myelopathy can even be the initial presentation of lymphoma (26). Direct spinal cord involvement remains a very rare occurrence (27). Intravascular lymphomatosis, which mainly involves the lumen of blood vessels, presents with symptoms ranging from cranial or peripheral neuropathies to strokelike episodes and subacute encephalopathies. Examination of bone marrow and cerebrospinal fluid (CSF) does not demonstrate any abnormalities (28). Gadolinium enhanced magnetic resonance imaging (MRI) studies, however, will demonstrate enhancement along intracranial vessels (29).

Although clinical symptoms of peripheral nervous system (PNS) involvement remain rare, more cases of asymptomatic involvement via autopsy or electrodiagnostic studies are discovered (22). Approximately 5% of lymphoma cases had spinal cord or nerve root involvement (24). B-cell NHL are much more likely to have PNS involvement than other lymphomas (24). Direct infiltration or compression of nerve roots, dorsal root ganglia, plexus, and nerves would be the most obvious method of neurologic involvement (22). Hypertrophy of the cauda equina nerve roots has been reported (30). Blood vessels in the nerves and brain could also be occluded or compressed and lead to a vasculitis-type mononeuropathy multiplex or strokelike presentation (22). Inflammatory neuropathies similar to Guillain-Barré syndrome (GBS), chronic inflammatory demyelinating polyradiculopathy (CIDP), multifocal motor neuropathy, and anti–Hu-mediated neuropathy have been documented and can mimic a polyradiculopathy secondary to chemotherapy or metastatic involvement (24,31). A rare complication is pandysautonomia secondary to infiltration of autonomic nerves (22).

Paraneoplastic or antibody-mediating neuropathies mimic that seen in vasculitis, cryoglobulinemia, and amyloidosis. The paraneoplastic syndrome can also present as cerebellar degeneration, dysautonomia, or Lambert-Eaton myasthenic syndrome (LEMS) (32). Because of the immune dysregulation seen in lymphomas, herpes zoster virus or other viruses could also directly affect the peripheral nerves (22). The neuropathies from chemotherapy, metabolic derangements, or other cryptic causes are typically a mild sensory and axonal variant (22,24).

Chemotherapies have been documented to cause a toxic polyneuropathy, but other presentations exist. Stage IV NHL can present with a GBS of flaccid quadriparesis and facial diplegia. This syndrome appears partially to respond to intravenous immunoglobulins and plasmapheresis (31).

CHRONIC LYMPHATIC LEUKEMIA

The neurologic manifestations are rare in B-cell CLL. Bower et al. (33) found a complication rate of 1:1000 in stage 0 to 2 cases. The most common complication was a herpes zoster infection (7%). Fewer patients had other opportunistic infections (2%). Treatment-related complications were found in 1.5% of CLL cases. Less than 1% had direct spread of CLL into the nervous system (33). Involvement of the CNS can be meningeal with cranial neuropathies, cerebellar dysfunction, or encephalopathy (34). CSF studies can show monoclonal B cells, but are of unknown significance. This finding may signal an infiltration of the brain parenchyma found in late stage CLL (34). Sensory and motor polyneuropathy, myopathy, or even radiculopathy, especially of the cervical roots and lumbar plexus, from CLL have been reported (22).

PRIMARY CENTRAL NERVOUS SYSTEM LYMPHOMA

Neurologic complications for PCL are described in the clinical manifestations section.

DIAGNOSTIC APPROACH

Diagnosis of NHL is mainly based on biopsy of the enlarged lymph node. Biopsy of other lymph nodes or bone marrow may be needed to stage the lymphoma (6). A CBC and serum chemistries may rule out other causes for lymphadenopathy not related to lymphoma. Imaging of particular parts of the body can help differentiate the subtypes of NHL. Lymphoblastic lymphoma can present with a mediastinal mass. Burkitt lymphoma can form large abdominal masses, whereas the African Burkitt lymphoma has a tendency to present with a mass in the neck or angle of the jaw (6). Computerized tomography (CT) of the chest and abdomen may find evidence of lymphadenopathy in other regions, as well as direct involvement of other organs. Positron-emission tomography (PET) can globally scan for diffuse lymphadenopathy, as seen in diffuse B-cell lymphoma, and assist in staging (6). Chromosomal analysis has been helpful in confirming many of the more common NHL. Serum lactate dehydrogenase has been used as a marker for lymphocyte proliferation. β_2-microglobulin has been slow to predict treatment response and time to treatment failure (6). CSF evaluation can be restricted to patients with lymphoma with aggressive disease or metastatic spread to the bone marrow, testes, sinuses, eye, meninges, or epidural spaces (6). CSF studies can be as sensitive as 80% in finding neoplastic lymphocytes in patients with leptomeningeal disease (32). Patients with a suggestion of leptomeningeal or epidural disease should also have MRI of the brain and spine. Suspected nerve root or peripheral nerve involvement can be evaluated by electromyography and nerve conduction studies (32). Staging of NHL is currently done with the Ann Arbor Staging Classification (Table 53-2).

CHRONIC LYMPHATIC LEUKEMIA

Diagnostic criteria have recently been updated by the International Workshop on Chronic Lymphocytic Leukemia in 2006. The CBC usually shows an absolute lymphocyte count of >5,000 cells/μL (35). The abnormal cells are small, mature lymphocytes that have monoclonal expression of kappa or gamma light chains. Flow cytometry demonstrates at least one B-cell surface marker, such as CD 19, 20, and 23 (35). Atypical or immature cells cannot comprise >55% of the total white cell count (11). Bone marrow evaluation and prolonged lymphocytosis have been used for diagnosis, but are not required in the update criteria (11). Prognosis is dependent on the stage of the lymphoma and ranges from 2 years for patients with stage 3 or 4 to 10 years for those with stage 0 or 1 (11). More aggressive disease is seen in patients with a lymphocyte doubling time of <6 months, elevated serum thymidine kinase levels, elevated serum β_2-microglobulin levels, or other genetic mutations besides the 13q14 deletion, such as a *p53* gene mutation (11,16). Staging for CLL is done with the Rai or Binet staging systems (Tables 53-3 and 53-4) and not the Ann Arbor Staging Classification.

TABLE 53-2. Ann Arbor Staging Classification for Non-Hodgkin Lymphoma (NHL)

Stage	*Area of Involvement*
I	One lymph node region
IE	Involvement of one extranodal site
II	Two or more lymph node regions on the same side of the diaphragm
IIE	NHL in extralymphatic site with involved lymph node region on the same side of the diaphragm
III	Two or more lymph node groups on both sides of the diaphragm
IIIE	Two or more lymph node groups on both sides of the diaphragm, with an extranodal site
IV	One or more lymph node region with diffuse involvement of one or more extranodal sites

TABLE 53-3. Rai Staging System for Chronic Lymphatic Leukemia (CLL)

Rai Stage	*Definition*
0	Lymphocytosis only
I	Lymphocytosis and lymphadenopathy
II	Lymphocytosis, lymphadenopathy with hepatomegaly or splenomegaly
III	Lymphocytosis and anemia
IV	Lymphocytosis and thrombocytopenia

PRIMARY CENTRAL NERVOUS SYSTEM LYMPHOMA

The diagnostic workup for PCL should include a gadolinium-enhanced MRI and lumbar puncture with flow cytometry and cytologic evaluation of the CSF to identify the type and grade of the PCL. MRI will usually show a single lesion in about 60% to 80% of cases, with more involvement of the hemispheres and deep gray matter (75%) than the brainstem. The lesions usually enhance with gadolinium (13). CSF analysis is suggestive of a neoplastic process initially in only one sixth to one third of cases. Serial CSF studies are eventually positive in two thirds of patients who initially had negative finding on CSF studies (15). CSF PCR can also be used to find evidence of monoclonalality in the lymphocytes (36). Evidence of extracranial spread can be done with a CT scan of the chest, abdomen, and pelvis; bone marrow biopsy; and ophthalmologic evaluation of the vitreous (15). In men, testicular examination, including ultrasound studies, may also be needed. Because HIV infection is a risk factor for developing PCL, serum studies should include HIV testing, CBC, metabolic panel, and serum lactate dehydrogenase (LDH), which can

TABLE 53-4. Binet Staging System for Chronic Lymphatic Leukemia

Binet Stage	*Definition*
A	Lymphocytosis with fewer than three areas of lymph node involvement
B	Lymphocytosis with more than three areas of lymph node involvement
C	Lymphocytosis with anemia, thrombocytopenia, or both

indicate the amount of global cell turnover and be elevated in more aggressive forms of NHL (13,15).

TREATMENT

NON-HODGKIN LYMPHOMA

Preferred treatment modalities for NHL will depend on the lymphoma type and stage. Because of its systemic nature, most NHL are not treated solely with surgery or radiation therapy. In select situations, such as orchiectomy for testicular lymphoma, such treatments are appropriate. Diffuse large B-cell lymphoma is now commonly treated with cyclophosphamide, doxorubicin, vincristine, methylprednisolone, (CHOP), and rituximab, which is a monoclonal CD-20 antibody that targets B cells (6,37). This chemotherapy has resulted in a 50% curative rate (6). Overall survival after 6 years in more aggressive diffuse large B-cell lymphomas was approximately 60% in the patients receiving CHOP with rituximab versus approximately 45% in the patients who only received CHOP (38). Focal radiation of 30 to 35 Gy to involved lymph nodes can be used along with an anthracycline-based chemotherapy if the diffuse B-cell lymphoma is confined to a limited area (6). Other regimens include CHOP with etoposide or ACVBP (adriamycin [doxorubicin], cyclophosphamide, vindesine, bleomycin, and prednisone) (6). Neurologic complications of chemotherapy are varied. Possible symptoms include an encephalopathy, seizures, headaches, cerebellar signs, and peripheral neuropathies (39). Metastases to the brain and leptomeninges and involvement of peripheral nerves may respond to radiation along with the appropriate chemotherapy. Leptomeningeal lymphoma has been treated with intrathecal methotrexate or cytarabine (32). Compression or involvement of the spinal cord is a neurologic emergency and typical requires high-dose corticosteroids and radiation therapy (32).

CHRONIC LYMPHATIC LYMPHOMA

Asymptomatic CLL is not usually treated (16). Chlorambucil had been the standard of care in the past for CLL, but it did not improve overall survival (16). Other alkylating combinations, such as CHOP, showed no improvement in overall survival versus chlorambucil (11). Recent trials have explored the use of purine analogues, such as cladribine and fludarabine, and monoclonal antibodies (11). Multiple trials with fludarabine alone or in combination continued to show better response rates than those with more conventional chemotherapy survival, such as chlorambucil or CAP (cyclophosphamide, doxorubicin, prednisone) (11,40). Chlorambucil, fludarabine, and cladribine rarely cause neurologic complications (39). The use of these purine analogues is not without risk. Increased incidences of acute myelocytic leukemia, autoimmune hemolytic anemia, and myelodysplastic syndrome have been reported in exposed CLL cases (6,16). Only several studies have discussed the use of bone marrow transplantation in CLL. Because of the difficulty removing all CLL cells, autologous stem cell transplantation may not completely rid the body of CLL. Some hypothesize that by inducing a graft-versus-leukemia response with an allogenic stem cells transplantation maybe beneficial (41). Monoclonal antibodies have increased progression-free survival in most patients. Rituximab is an anti-CD20 monoclonal antibody has had 80% to 90% response rates when combined with purine nucleoside analogues (20).

PRIMARY CENTRAL NERVOUS SYSTEM LYMPHOMA

PCL is highly sensitive to corticosteroids, but the response usually does not exceed several months. Similarly, this lymphoma responds well to whole brain radiation. Focal radiation is usually not used because the lymphoma is typically diffuse in the CNS (42). Because of the invasiveness and multifocal nature of the disease, surgical resection is usually not a viable treatment option. Standard NHL chemotherapy agents do not penetrate the blood–brain barrier very well. High-dose methotrexate (MTX) is the chemotherapy of choice because of its high permeability through the blood–brain barrier and response rates of up to 80%. Median survival with MTX is up to 60 months, with 25% surviving up to 5 years. MTX in combination with other chemotherapies, such as cyclophosphamide, cytarabine, and vincristine, has been studied with variable improvement seen in survival (13). Those signal changes on MRI are seen in patients receiving chemotherapy, with their neurocognitive function remaining stable or even improving (15). Whole brain radiation therapy has been used, but it provided a median survival of only 12 to 18 months. Severe neurocognitive dysfunction, ataxia, and urinary incontinence from radiation therapy are usually seen if the patient survives sufficiently long. MRI studies of such patients show diffuse global atrophy and signal changes in the periventricular white matter (15). Ischemia from radiation-caused vascular injury has been proposed as another cause of whole brain radiation toxicity (15). The combination of radiation therapy with MTX therapy can induce an incurable severe leukoencephalopathy. Symptoms range from memory loss to a severe dementia (39). High-dose chemotherapy, including cytarabine, is being explored to avoid using whole brain radiation. Finally, autologous bone marrow transplantation has shown benefit against relapsing PCL but not in newly diagnosed PCL (13).

CLINICAL RECOMMENDATIONS OF THE VIGNETTE

The patient has systemic symptoms suggestive of a neoplastic process. The history, markedly elevated white blood cells with a predominate lymphocytosis, and lack of lymphadenopathy would be consistent with a chronic lymphocytic leukemia. Electromyographic studies in the lower extremities found an axonal sensory and motor polyneuropathy, which is likely consistent with her history of diabetes. The serum thymidine kinase levels, β_2-microglobulin levels, and lymphocyte double times were not elevated. The treatment was held. Close monitoring was initiated. In the near future, fludarabine and rituximab will be considered.

SUMMARY

Lymphoproliferative disorders encompass varied presentations and treatments. Manifestations differ among the diseases. Lymphomas typically have lymphadenopathy, whereas leukemias involve the bone marrow. Primary CNS lymphoma is its own unique entity that mainly causes multiple enhancing lesions in the brain. Non-Hodgkin lymphoma, which is more common than Hodgkin lymphoma, and chronic lymphocytic leukemia, which is the most common adult leukemia, do not frequently involve the nervous system. When the nervous system is affected, presentation ranges from focal signs from metastatic parenchymal lesions, cranial neuropathies, and altered consciousness from meningeal involvement, to peripheral neuropathies from multiple causes, such as paraneoplastic effects, or secondary to chemotherapy. Treatment is specific to the individual disorder and includes observation to radiation therapy and chemotherapy with CHOP to bone marrow transplantation. Recently discovered treatments appeared to have improved survival in these patients. Neurologic complications, however, can be a significant morbidity for these disorders.

REFERENCES

1. Bociek RG, Armitage JO. Hodgkin's disease and non-Hodgkin's lymphoma. *Curr Opin Hematol.* 1999;6:205–215.
2. Armitage JO, Weisenburger DD. New approach to classifying non-Hodgkin's lymphomas: Clinical features of the major histologic subtypes. Non-Hodgkin's Lymphoma Classification Project. *J Clin Oncol.* 1998;16:2780–2795.
3. Fine HA, Mayer RJ. Primary central nervous system lymphoma. *Ann Intern Med.* 1993;119:1093–1104.
4. Krogh-Jensen M, D'Amore F, Jensen MK, et al. Clinicopathological features, survival and prognostic factors of primary central nervous system lymphomas: Trends in incidence of primary central nervous system lymphomas and primary malignant brain tumors in a well-defined geographical area. Population-based data from the Danish Lymphoma Registry, LYFO, and the Danish Cancer Registry. *Leuk Lymphoma.* 1995;19:223–233.
5. Miller DC, Hochberg FH, Harris NL, et al. Pathology with clinical correlations of primary central nervous system non-Hodgkin's lymphoma. The Massachusetts General Hospital experience 1958–1989. *Cancer.*1994;74:1383–1397.
6. Ansell SM, Armitage J. Non-Hodgkin lymphoma: Diagnosis and treatment. *Mayo Clin Proc.* 2005;80:1087–1097.
7. Bhatia S, Robison LL. Epidemiology of leukemia and lymphoma. *Curr Opin Hematol.* 1999;6:201–214.
8. Chiu BC, Weisenburger DD. An update in the epidemiology of non-Hodgkin's lymphoma. *Clin Lymphoma.* 2003;4:161–168.
9. Clarke CA, Glaser SL. Changing incidence of non-Hodgkin lymphomas in the United States. *Cancer.* 2002;94:2015–2023.
10. Grulich AE, Vajdic CM. The epidemiology of non-Hodgkin lymphoma. *Pathology.* 2005;37:409–419.
11. Yee KW, O'Brien SM. Chronic lymphocytic leukemia: Diagnosis and treatment. *Mayo Clin Proc.* 2006;81:1105–1129.
12. Central Brain Tumor Registry of the United States. http://www.cbtrus.org. 1998–2002.
13. Baehring JM, Hochberg FH. Primary lymphoma of the nervous system. *Cancer J.* 2006;12:1–13.
14. Cote TR, Manns A, Hardy CR, et al. AIDS/Cancer Study Group: Epidemiology of brain lymphoma among people with or without acquired immunodeficiency syndrome. *J Natl Cancer Inst.* 1996;88:675–679.
15. Batchelor J, Loeffler JS. Primary CNS lymphoma. *J Clin Oncol.* 2006;24:1281–1288.
16. Wierda WG, Kipps TJ. Chronic lymphocytic leukemia. *Curr Opin Hematol.* 1999;6:253–261.
17. Weber T, Weber RG, Kaulich K, et al. Characteristic chromosomal imbalances in primary central nervous system lymphoma of the diffuse large B-cell type. *Brain Pathol.* 2000;10:73–84.
18. Fisher SG, Fisher RI. The epidemiology of non-Hodgkin's lymphoma. *Oncogene.* 2004; 23:6524–6534.
19. Pangalis GA, Vassilakopoulous TP, Dimopoulou MN, et al. B-chronic lymphocytic leukemia: Practical aspects. *Hematol Oncol.* 2002;20:103–146.
20. Shanafelt TD, Call TG. Current approach to diagnosis and management of chronic lymphocytic leukemia. *Mayo Clin Proc.* 2004;79:388–398.
21. Park S, Abad S, Tulliez M, et al. Pseudouveitis: A clue to the diagnosis of primary central nervous system lymphoma in immunocompetent patients. *Medicine.* 2004;83:223–232.
22. Kelly JJ, Karcher DS. Lymphoma and peripheral neuropathy: A clinical review. *Muscle Nerve.* 2005;31:301–313.
23. Grupka NL, Seinfeld J, Ryder J, et al. Secondary central nervous system involvement by follicular lymphoma: Case report and review of the literature. *Surg Neurol.* 2006;65: 590–594.
24. Correale J, Monteverde DA, Bueri JA, et al. Peripheral nervous system and spinal cord involvement in lymphoma. *Acta Neurol Scand.* 1991;83:45–51.
25. Grier J, Batchelor T. Metastatic neurologic complications of non-Hodgkin's lymphoma. *Curr Oncol Rep.* 2005;7;55–60.
26. Schiff D, O'Neill BP, Suman VJ. Spinal epidural metastasis as the initial manifestation of malignancy: Clinical features and diagnostic approach. *Neurology.* 1997;49:452–456.
27. Pels H, Vogt I, Klockgether T, et al. Primary non-Hodgkin's lymphoma of the spinal cord. *Spine.* 2000;25:2262–2264.
28. Glass J, Hochberg FH, Miller DC. Intravascular lymphomatosis. A systemic disease with neurologic manifestations. *Cancer.* 1993;71:3156–3164.
29. Liow K, Asmar P, Liow M, et al. Intravascular lymphomatosis: Contribution of cerebral MRI findings to diagnosis. *J Neuroimaging.* 2000;10:116–118.
30. Kumar N, Dyck PJ. Hypertrophy of the nerve roots of the cauda equina as a paraneoplastic manifestation of lymphoma. *Arch Neurol.* 2005;62:1776–1777.
31. Re D, Schwenk A, Hegener P, et al. Guillain-Barre syndrome in a patient with non-Hodgkin's lymphoma. *Ann Oncol.* 2000;11:217–220.
32. Giglio P, Gilbert MR. Neurologic complications of non-Hodgkin's lymphoma. In: Batchelor T, ed. *Lymphoma of the Nervous System.* Boston: Butterworth-Heinemann; 2004: 107–122.
33. Bower JH, Hammack JE, McDonnell SK, et al. The neurologic complications of B cell chronic lymphocytic leukemia. *Neurology.* 1997;48:407–412.
34. Cramer SC, Glaspy JA, Efird JT, et al. Chronic lymphocytic leukemia and the central nervous system: A clinical and pathological study. *Neurology.* 1996;46:19–25.
35. Binet JL, Caligaris-Cappio F, Catovsky D, et al. International Workshop on Chronic Lymphocytic Leukemia (IWCLL). Perspectives on the use of new diagnostic tools in the treatment of chronic lymphocytic leukemia. *Blood.* 2006 Feb 1;107:859–861.
36. Rhodes CH, Glantz MJ, Glantz L, et al. A comparison of polymerase chain reaction examination of cerebrospinal fluid and conventional cytology in the diagnosis of lymphomatous meningitis. *Cancer.* 1996;77:543–548.
37. Coiffier B. Current strategies for the treatment of diffuse large B cell lymphoma. *Curr Opin Hematol.* 2005;12:259–265.
38. Feugier P, Van Hoof A, Sebban C, et al. Long term results of the R-CHOP study in the treatment of elderly patients with diffuse large B cell lymphoma: A study by the Groupe d' Etudes des Lymphomes de l'Adulte. *J Clin Oncol.* 2005;23:4117–4126.
39. Wen PY, Ramkrishna N, Fisher DC. Neurological complications of lymphoma therapy. In: Batchelor T, ed. *Lymphoma of the Nervous System.* Philadelphia: Butterworth-Heinemann; 2004:149–180.
40. Keating MJ, O'Brien S, Lerner S, et al. Long-term follow-up of patients with chronic lymphocytic leukemia receiving fludarabine regiments as initial therapy. *Blood.* 1998;92: 1165–1172.
41. Rizouli V, Gribben JG. Role of autologous stem cell transplantation in chronic lymphocytic leukemia. *Curr Opin Hematol.* 2003;10:306–311.
42. Hormigo A, DeAngelis LM. Treatment of primary central nervous system lymphoma in immunocompetent patients. In: Batchelor T, ed. *Lymphoma of the Nervous System.* Philadelphia: Butterworth-Heinemann; 2004:83–95.

CHAPTER **54**

Plasma Cell Dyscrasias

Gregory Gruener • Harry L. Messmore

OBJECTIVES

- To describe the characteristics and define the plasma cell dyscrasias
- To discuss the direct and secondary metabolic or organ system manifestations of the disorders
- To explain the components of polyneuropathy, organomegaly, endoerinopathy, monoclonal gammopathy and skin changes (POEMS) syndrome as well as the significance of monoclonal gammopathy of undetermined significance (MGUS)
- To discuss the direct and indirect neurologic manifestations of plasma cell dyscrasias

CASE VIGNETTE

A 67-year-old man, with a medical history that was noteworthy for arterial hypertension and hypercholesterolemia, but controlled with a hydrochlorothiazide and diet, presents with a 3-month history of progressive fatigue and nonradicular low back pain. On examination, his vital signs are normal and his general physical examination is without clear abnormalities and, specifically, organomegaly or lymphadenopathy. His back range of motion is normal, but there is tenderness to light percussion directly over the upper lumbar spine. Laboratory studies demonstrate a normocytic normochromic anemia with a hemoglobin of 11.5 g/dL (13.5 to 17.5 g/dL), but a normal leukocyte and platelet count. A serum metabolic profile shows normal electrolytes, elevated calcium of 12.3 mg/dL (8.9 to 10.1 mg/dL), but normal phosphorus and later a normal magnesium level as well. The serum urea nitrogen is elevated to 38 mg/dL (6 to 21 mg/dL) as is the creatinine at 4.4 mg/dL (0.8 to 1.2 mg/dL). Urine analysis shows trace protein, but no white blood cells (WBC) or red blood cells (RBC) on high powered field (HPF) examination. Chest X-ray study is normal, but the lumbar spine series shows osteopenia and a lytic lesion of the T12 vertebral body.

DEFINITION

Plasma cell dyscrasias are characterized by the accumulation of malignant plasma cells in bone marrow, bone, or soft tissues. These disorders include *multiple myeloma* (MM) (accumulation of plasma cells in the bone marrow), *extramedullary plasmacytoma* (solid tumors of plasma cells in soft tissues), and *systemic amyloidosis* (deposition of amyloid fibrils in various tissues). The two most common forms of systemic amyloidosis are *amyloid A* or *AA*, secondary to a chronic inflammatory condition or *primary amyloidosis, amyloid light chain-related* (AL), in the setting of a B-cell malignancy.

EPIDEMIOLOGY

MM is uncommon in those younger than 40 years of age (2% of cases), but increases rapidly after the age of 50, with a median age of onset of 66 years and older than 70 (38%) (1). No gender preference or relationship to socioeconomic status is found. It affects blacks more commonly (male ratio of 1.9 and female of 2.4, compared with Western countries) and the incidence may be lower in Chinese and other Asians. The number of new cases in the United States in 2005 was estimated to approach 15,980 with a projected 11,300 deaths (2). The incidence of AL is one fifth that of MM, approximately 1 case per 100,000 person-years in Western countries (3).

ETIOLOGY AND PATHOGENESIS

The cause of MM is unclear, although exposure to ionizing radiation, paints, solvents, and pesticides have all been implicated. Yet MM myeloma does evolve from a premalignant condition known as *monoclonal gammopathy of undetermined significance* (MGUS), but the precise mechanism is unclear. MM is characterized by accumulation of plasma cells that represents an altered malignant cell of an earlier B-cell stage of development. Primary translocations involving the immunoglobulin heavy chain locus on chromosome 14q32 and chromosome 13 deletions (13q14 is a deletion hot spot) are frequently identified in MM, but not yet *routinely* used in staging (4–6). These chromosomal abnormalities allow expression of distinct adhesion molecules on these plasma cells and their adherence to nonmalignant bone marrow stromal cells that secrete cytokines that stimulate their growth while preventing apoptosis. MM overproduces monoclonal immunoglobulins (or an *M-protein*) that is identified by protein electrophoresis or immunofixation of serum and urine (primarily IgG in 60% to 70%, IgA 20%, only light chains in 15%, and no detectable M protein in 3%) while depressing normal immunoglobulin secretion.

Amyloidosis AL is one example of a group of disorders that manifest themselves by the accumulation of insoluble, misfolded, extracellular proteins whose altered structure allows their intermolecular bonding and aggregation that leads to a β-pleated sheet conformation. Under normal physiologic circumstances, their deposition in tissue is felt to be responsible for the toxic or pathologic manifestations (3); however, amyloid fibril accumulation may not entirely explain the observed pathologic effects. The soluble oligomeric intermediaries of amyloid may better explain the observed toxic effects; through changes in membrane permeability, they cause an altered cell function and affect survival (7).

CLINICAL MANIFESTATIONS

The clinical manifestations of MM are a confluence of their direct immunologic manifestations, associated metabolic abnormalities, and the location of their abnormal cellular or protein deposition. The most common presenting symptoms are fatigue (32%), bone pain (58%), and recurrent infections (1).

BONE DISEASE

Symptoms, which are present in 79% at diagnosis, are a diagnostic feature of MM. Although lytic lesions are the most typical, osteopenia is more common, but osteosclerotic lesions are reported as well (1). Radiation therapy for painful lesions should be deferred if possible, because the effectiveness of later chemotherapy may be impaired. Exceptions include spinal cord compression, which may necessitate steroid administration or, uncommonly, surgical decompression; weight-bearing bones when surgical fixation of fracture is impending or vertebroplasty with vertebral body compression; and when palliative treatment has failed (8).

ANEMIA

Anemia (hemoglobin <12 g/dL) was evident in 73% of patients at the time of diagnosis of MM. Usually a consequence of bone marrow replacement, renal failure, chronic disease, and an inappropriate erythropoietin response to the degree of anemia are all contributors to the anemia. Even in individuals with a mild anemia (11 to 12 g/dL), their quality of life has benefited from recombinant human erythropoietin replacement (1,9).

CRYOGLOBULINEMIA

Cryoglobulinemia is characterized by the presence of proteins, usually immunoglobulins, which precipitate at temperatures <37°C and redissolve on warming; classification is based on the type of monoclonal proteins present and a wide spectrum of clinical manifestations exist. Symptoms are caused either by a vasculitis (IgM-IgG complex deposition on a vessel wall leading to complement activation) or complexes directly causing vessel occlusion. Such vasculitic skin lesions are commonly found on the anterior aspect of the lower extremities. Although 5% to 10% of patients with MM harbor cryoglobulins, more than half have no symptoms attributed to their presence (10).

HYPERCALCEMIA

A presenting sign of hypercalcemia (calcium level ≥11 mg/dL) in 13% of patients with MM (1) requires that a free (ionized) calcium level be obtained in the asymptomatic patient to identify those patients at risk and to guide treatment. High calcium levels can result in lethargy, confusion, or constipation.

RENAL INSUFFICIENCY

Present in 19% (serum creatinine ≥2 mg/dL) of patients with MM, renal failure has multiple causes that include direct infiltration of the kidney by plasma cells or amyloid, obstruction of kidney tubules secondary to myeloma proteins (cast nephropathy) or a hyperviscosity state, predisposition to infections from an altered immune system, and hypercalcemia and elevated uric acid that lead to kidney injury or the development of a nephrotic syndrome (1). Predisposition to renal dysfunction in MM necessitates adequate hydration and careful use of intravenous contrast dye or even nonsteroidal anti-inflammatory drugs (NSAID) (11). Plasmapheresis, dialysis, and renal transplantation have all been used to treat individual cases of renal failure (12).

HYPERVISCOSITY

Hyperviscosity syndromes occur more commonly with an IgA MM (greater polymerization of the paraprotein) and manifest as shortness of breath (SOB), confusion, and chest pain. Treatment is directed at the MM; plasmapheresis is an appropriate treatment for symptomatic patients and should be continued until serum viscosity is normalized (9,13).

INFECTIOUS DISEASE

The type and intensity of antineoplastic therapy affects the bone marrow microenvironment and influences immune reconstitution. The resulting immunosuppression and end-organ toxicity directly influence later approaches to managing infections (9,14).

An increased risk of bacterial infections is related to impaired synthesis of normal immunoglobulins, defective complement activation, and impaired B- and T-cell function. Encapsulated organisms are the more frequent cause of such infections early in the course of the disease; however, with the use of chemotherapy, gram-negative infections become more frequent.

Stem cell transplantation places the patient at an increased risk of endogenous yeast and exogenous mold infections. The risk of invasive fungal infections remains high because of immunodeficiencies that render the patients susceptible and unable to successfully resolve fungal disease (15). Yeast prophylaxis with fluconazole before engraftment has since become part of the standard regimen. If fungal prophylaxis is needed during the conditioning regimen of hematopoietic stem cell transplantation, itraconazole and voriconazole should not be used (interactions with cyclophosphamide) and fluconazole or an echinocandin are the agents of choice (16). Later, following transplant, if mold coverage is desired during prolonged immunosuppression, itraconazole can be used if gastrointestinal side effects are tolerated. Transplant recipients are also predisposed to emerging infections that include viral infections, such as severe acute respiratory syndrome (SARS) and West Nile virus (17).

Administration of intravenous immunoglobulins has not been found to be either cost effective or uniformly protective and patients with MM also exhibit a poor antibody response to pneumococcal and influenza vaccines, which has an impact on prophylaxis (9).

NEUROLOGIC SYMPTOMS AND SYNDROMES

Complications in MM include direct compression (spinal cord compression, radiculopathy, or base of the skull tumors),

TABLE 54-1. Neurological Manifestations of Plasma Cell Dyscrasias

	Multiple Myeloma	*Extramedullary Plasmacytoma*	*MGUS*	*POEMS*	*Amyloidosis*	*Cryoglobulinemia*
COMPRESSIVE						
Radiculopathy	✓	✓				
Spinal cord compression	✓	✓				
Base-of-skull tumor	✓	✓				
Carpal tunnel syndrome					✓	
INFILTRATIVE						
Peripheral neuropathy					✓	
Autonomic neuropathy					✓	
Numb chin syndrome	✓					
METABOLIC						
Hypercalcemia	✓					
Uremia	✓			✓	✓	✓
Hyperviscosity	✓					✓
AUTOIMMUNE: CYTOKINE MEDIATED						
Peripheral neuropathy[a]	✓	✓	✓	✓		✓
AUTOIMMUNE: VASCULITIC						
Peripheral neuropathy						✓

(Modified from Dispenzieri A, Kyle RA. *Bailliere's Best Practice in Clinical Haematology*. 2005;18:673–688, with permission.)
[a]Although not a direct consequence of these disorders, involvement of the peripheral nervous system is a complication of treatment (chemotherapy as well as after bone marrow transplantation) and, in the setting of disease, can result in peripheral neuropathies, chronic and acute demyelinative neuropathies, plexopathies, and myasthenia gravis and polymyositis (19–24).

infiltrative (amyloid, peripheral neuropathies, and numb chin syndrome), and metabolic (hyperviscosity syndrome, hypercalcemia and uremia) (Table 54-1) (18–23). Although meningeal and cerebral involvement is reported to occur in MM, it is an unusual complication (24). Spinal cord compression can also occur in cases of epidural plasmacytoma as well as with MM involvement of bone.

The syndrome known as *POEMS* involves polyneuropathy, organomegaly, endocrinopathy, monoclonal gammopathy, skin changes (*Crow-Fukase syndrome, **p**lasma cell dyscsrasia, **e**ndocrinopathy, **p**olyneuropathy [PEP] syndrome, Takatsuki syndrome, osteosclerotic myeloma*), which may represent a remote effect of a plasmacytoma and the overproduction of *vascular endothelial growth factor* (VEGF) responsible for many of the clinical manifestations (25). Although specific major and minor criteria for diagnosis exist, the acronym POEMS represents the major (but not all) clinical manifestations of a polyneuropathy (sensorimotor), M-protein (almost always a monoclonal λ light chain), organomegaly (hepatomegaly), endocrinopathy (diabetes, amenorrhea, and gynecomastia), and skin changes (hyperpigmentation). The median survival of patients is 165 months and, whereas additional features of the syndrome can develop with time, complications seen in MM rarely develop (26). The administration of high-dose melphalan and autologous blood stem cell transplantation improved some of the symptoms in a group of such patient and was accompanied by a drop in VEGF levels, representing a treatment option (27).

DIAGNOSTIC APPROACH

MM is usually diagnosed when an increased serum protein concentration is detected in the evaluation of an anemia, renal dysfunction, or asymptomatic hypercalcemia. The initial evaluation begins with a complete blood count, metabolic profile, serum electrophoresis, and quantitative immunoglobulin determination. A bone marrow aspiration with biopsy is also performed. Radiographic surveys are used to identify sites of involvement as well as areas at increased risk for fracture. The diagnosis requires the fulfillment of at least one major (plasmacytoma is identified, bone marrow plasma cells >30%, an M-protein that is quantified as an IgG >3.5 g/dL, IgA >2.0 g/dL, or urinary light chain >1 g/24 hour urine collection) and at least one minor criterion (bone marrow plasmacytosis >10%, M-protein identified at a lower level, lytic bone lesion, reduced residual immunoglobulins). An international staging system for multiple myeloma has been developed (Table 54-2) and correlated with tumor mass as well as prognosis (28). In addition to this staging system, an independent poor prognostic risk factor—deletion of chromosome 13—has been identified in those patients who have stem cell transplantation. When this chromosomal deletion is present with a high β_2-micorglobulin level, median survival is 25 months; when either is present, it is 47 months; and when both are absent, the mean survival time had not been reached at 111 months of follow-up (5).

A plasmacytoma will present as a solid tumor in either soft tissue or bone. Although they may be cured with local radiation

TABLE 54-2. New International Staging System for Multiple Myeloma

Stage	*Criteria*	*% of Patients*	*Median survival (months)*
I	Serum β2-microglobulin <3.5 mg/L Serum albumin ≥3.5 g/dL	28.9	62
II	Not stage I or II*	37.5	44
III	Serum β2-microglobulin ≥5.5 mg/L	33.6	29

(From Merlini G, Bellotti V. Molecular mechanisms of amyloidosis. *N Engl J Med.* 2003;349:583–596, with permission.)
*Serum β2-microglobulin <3.5 mg/L and serum albumin <3.5 g/dL or serum β2-microglobulin 3.5 to 5.5 mg/L, and irrespective of serum albumin level.

therapy, those identified in bone will also initially respond, but 50% will progress to a MM, and two third of those within 3 years after diagnosis.

MGUS is identified as an M-protein on electrophoresis, usually an IgG, present at a level of 3.0 g/dL or less. It is identified in 3.2% of persons 50 years of age or older and 5.3% of persons 70 years of age or older (29). None of the other major or minor criteria of MM are present. With prolonged follow-up, 50% of patients will die of another illness, 20% will continue to demonstrate an M protein, 10% an increase in immunoglobulin that does not require treatment, and in 25%, a lymphoproliferative disorder develops (two third are MM). No reliable indicators of prognosis exist at the time of initial discovery and the risk of progression to a malignancy is indefinite, which is the rationale for continued patient monitoring (30).

AL usually presents in the sixth or seventh decade and with weight loss and fatigue. The expected median survival is 13.2 months (31). Peripheral neuropathy may be the presenting feature in 20% of patients and autonomic involvement (cardiovascular, gastrointestinal or urogenital) is frequently found. Systemic features of the disease include hepatomegaly, macroglossia, cardiomyopathy, and proteinuria within a nephrotic range. Immunofixation electrophoresis of urine or serum detects immunoglobulins or light chains in 90% of patients, but unlike MM, this monoclonal protein does not increase over time and the number of patients with <10% monoclonal plasma cells on bone marrow examination is 60% (32). In the remaining cases, diagnosis is aided by the use of free-light chain assays, which allows monitoring for their disappearance following treatment (31) and biopsy of involved tissue to identify amyloid deposition by its birefringence when viewed under polarized light, or immunohistochemistry that allows identification of the specific type of amyloid present (33).

TREATMENT

The treatment of MM has evolved from melphalan and prednisone (melphalan-prednisone regimen) (34) to the administration of non-myeloablative doses of melphalan followed by peripheral-blood stem cell (PBSC) transplant (6,35,36). Presently, two sequential courses of myeloablative therapy, each followed by PBSC transplant have resulted in 7-year event-free rates of 20% and overall survival rates of 40%, twice the rates obtained with single transplantations (37,38). When thalidomide is incorporated into high-dose therapy for myeloma, the frequency of complete responses increased and event-free survival extended, but at the expense of adverse effects and without improving overall survival (37). The addition of thalidomide to melphalan and prednisone in elderly patients (60 to 85 years) increased their 2-year event-free survival (27% to 54%) and 3-year survival rates (80% versus 64%), but whether overall survival advantage was improved is unclear. Again, this was accompanied by increased toxicity manifested as infections, thromboembolism, and neurologic effects (39).

The two treatment strategies being explored in MM include (*a*) tumor eradication with the use of a combination of all, or most of, the available agents and high-dose therapy with stem cell transplantation or (*b*) reserving new agents for sequential treatment of relapse and as a means of controlling the growth or regrowth of tumor, thereby converting MM into an indolent disease (38). The primary treatment modalities of newer therapies are directed at overcoming drug resistance (thalidomide, Lenalidomide and bortezomib) and targeting the bone marrow microenvironment.

The role of genomic profiling of cancers (4) to identify molecular phenotypes that predict sensitivity to targeted therapy and models as to how resistance develops (on the basis of turnover rate, mutation rate, and effective tumor size and mutation fitness) suggests that treatment resistance may exist before, and not necessarily acquired during, treatment (40). Such knowledge may assist with the sequencing and extent of therapy, "predicting" those susceptible to complications or specific manifestations and allowing better prognostication (9).

The current recommendation is to administer bisphosphonates to all patients with MM with evidence of one or more lytic lesions on skeletal radiography (8,41). Their administration can significantly reduce the number of skeletal events. When hypercalcemia is associated with minimal or no symptoms, then treatment with systemic chemotherapy is appropriate. In those with high calcium levels, hydration with isotonic saline and corticosteroids is usually effective. The administration of bisphosphonates (pamidronate [2] or zoledronic acid) is also helpful in lowering and normalizing calcium levels quickly (8). (Reports of osteonecrosis of the mandible in patients receiving intravenous therapy with these drugs prompt caution in their use.) In patients with MM with anemia and low erythropoietin levels, its administration may reduce the need for RBC transfusions (8,9).

Treatment of primary (AL) amyloidosis has consisted of both high-dose melphalan and autologous stem cell transplantation and attempts to stratify risk of treatment based on age and extent of organ involvement (31,43). Unlike MM, the multisystem involvement in AL necessitates careful pretransplantation planning to address and minimize side effects and toxicities related to chemotherapeutic regimens. Gastrointestinal (hemorrhage), cardiac (including arrhythmias), and renal involvement, as well as associated autonomic dysfunction, predisposes to such complications. Involvement of two major organ systems or cardiac involvement places candidates at high risk for dying during the peritransplantation period and also at risk for stem cell transplant using high-dose regiments (31). Attempts to develop a risk-adapted approach to planning treatment could allow selective interventions with a different chemotherapeutic regimen (e.g., dexamethasone-melphalan or dexamethasone-thalidomide) where the potential toxicity of stem cell transplantation makes them ineligible candidates (44–46).

CLINICAL RECOMMENDATIONS OF THE VIGNETTE

The association of anemia, hypercalcemia, renal failure, and an osteopenia or lytic bone lesion in this clinical setting is consistent with the presentation of multiple myeloma. The next steps are qualitative and quantitative characterization of the abnormal protein with serum protein electrophoresis (SPEP) and immunofixation studies of serum and urine. For staging, β2-microglobulin level and bone marrow aspiration and biopsy are performed. Further characterization of the extent of bone disease with a skeletal survey and whether local treatment with radiation therapy (RT) of the thoracic spine lesion is indicated depends on the extent of involvement and risk of spinal cord compression as well as any delay in a definitive treatment of the MM. It would be appropriate to assess the immediate need for further treatment of the hypercalcemia or observe the response to treatment of the MM and the use of bisphosphonates.

SUMMARY

The clinical presentation of plasma cell dyscrasias can be nonspecific early in the illness, but the later pattern of associated laboratory and diagnostic tests allows diagnosis of a spectrum of disorders from the premalignant MGUS to multiple myeloma. The manifestations of plasma cell dyscrasias reflect an altered immunologic state as well as the effects of their abnormal proteins on other organ system and tissue functions. Interventions attempt to balance reconstitution of the immune state with side effects of treatment and to manage and prevent associated metabolic and organ system dysfunction. Clarification of the underlying pathophysiology, as well as advancements in cancer treatment biology, will lead to focused interventions and result in an extension of disease-free survival while limiting side effects.

REFERENCES

1. Kyle RA, Gertz MA, Witzig TE, et al. Review of 1027 patients with newly diagnosed multiple myeloma. *Mayo Clin Proc.* 2003;78:21–33.
2. www.cancer.org/downloads/stt/Estimated_New_Cancer_Cases_and_Deaths_by_Sex_forAll_Sites,_US,_2005.pdf.
3. Merlini G, Bellotti V. Molecular mechanisms of amyloidosis. *N Engl J Med.* 2003;349: 583–596.
4. Shaughnessy J. Primer on Medical genomics Part IX: Scientific and clinical applications of DNA microarrays—Multiple myeloma as a disease model. *Mayo Clin Proc.* 2003;78: 1098–1109.
5. Facon T, Avet-Loiseau H, Guillerm G, et al. Chromosome 13 abnormalities identified by FISH analysis and serum beta2-microglobulin produce a powerful myeloma staging system for patients receiving high-dose therapy. *Blood.* 2002;118:1041–1047.
6. Rajkumar SV, Kyle RA. Multiple myeloma: Diagnosis and treatment. *Mayo Clin Proc.* 2005;80:1371–1382.
7. Glabe CG, Kayed R. Common structure and toxic function of amyloid oligomers implies a common mechanism of pathogenesis. *Neurology.* 2006;66[Suppl 1]:874–878.
8. Barosi G, Boccadoro M, Cavo M, et al. Management of multiple myeloma and related disorders: Guidelines form the Italian Society of Hematology (SIE), Italian Society of Experimental Hematology (SIES) and Italian Group for Bone Marrow Transplantation (GITMO). *Haematolgica.* 2004;89:717–741.
9. Barlogie B, Shaughnessy J, Tricot G, et al. Treatment of multiple myeloma. *Blood.* 2004;103:20–32.
10. Mohammed K, Rehman HU. Cryoglobulinemia. *Acta Medica Austriaca.* 2003;3:65–68.
11. Yussim E, Schwartz E, Sidi Y, et al. Acute renal failure precipitated by non-steroidal anti-inflammatory drugs (NSAIDs) in multiple myeloma. *Am J Hematol.* 1998;58:142–144.
12. Johnson WJ, Kyle RA, Pineda AA, et al. Treatment of renal failure associated with multiple myeloma: Plasmapheresis, hemodialysis and chemotherapy. *Arch Intern Med.* 1990;150: 863–869.
13. Gertz MA, Kyle RA. Hyperviscosity syndrome. *J Intensive Care Med.* 1995;10:128–141.
14. Brown JMT. The influence of the conditions of hematopoietic cell transplantation on infectious complications. *Curr Opin Infect Dis.* 2005;18:346–351.
15. Brown JMY. Fungal infections in bone marrow transplant patients. *Curr Opin Infect Dis.* 2004;17:347–352.
16. van Burik JH. Role of new antifungal agents in prophylaxis of mycoses in high risk patients. *Curr Opin Infect Dis.* 2005;18:479–483.
17. Kumar D, Humar A. Emerging viral infections in transplant patients. *Curr Opin Infect Dis.* 2005;18:337–341.
18. Dispenzieri A, Kyle RA. Neurological aspects of multiple myeloma and related disorders. *Bailliere's Best Practice in Clinical Haematology.* 2005;18:673–688.
19. Rabinstein AA, Dispenzieri A, Micallef IN, et al. Acute neuropathies after peripheral blood stem cell and bone marrow transplantation. *Muscle Nerve.* 2003;28:733–736.
20. Adams C, August CS, Maguire H, et al. Neuromuscular complications of bone marrow transplantation. *Pediatr Neurol.* 1995;12:58–61.
21. Rodriguea V, Kuehnle I, Heslop HE, et al. Guillain-Barré syndrome after allogenic hematopoietic stem cell transplantation. *Bone Marrow Transplant.* 1998;22:873–881.
22. Tse S, Saunders EF, Silverman E, et al. Myasthenia gravis and polymyositis as manifestations of chronic graft-versus-host disease. *Bone Marrow Transplant.* 1999;23:397–399.
23. Wen PY, Alyea EP, Simon D, et al. Guillain-Barré syndrome following allogenic bone marrow transplantation. *Neurology* 1997;49:1171–1714.
24. Patriaraca F, Zaja F, Silvestri F, et al. Meningeal and cerebral involvement in multiple myeloma patients. *Ann Hematol.* 2001;80:758–762.
25. Scarlato M, Previtali SC, Carpo M, et al. Polyneuropathy in POEMS syndrome: Role of angiogenic factors in the pathogenesis. *Brain.* 2005;128:1911–1920.
26. Dispenzieri A, Kyle RA, Lacy MQ, et al. POEMS syndrome: Definitions and long-term outcome. *Blood.* 2003;101:2496–2506.
27. Kuwabara S, Misawa S, Kanai K, et al. Autologous peripheral blood stem cell transplantation for POEMS syndrome. *Neurology.* 2006;66:105–107.
28. Greipp PR, Sam Miguel J, Durie BG, et al. International staging for multiple myeloma. *J Clin Oncol.* 2005;23:3412–3420.
29. Kyle RA, Therneau TM, Rajkumar SV, et al. Prevalence of monoclonal gammopathy of undetermined significance. *N Engl J Med.* 2006;354:1362–1369.
30. Kyle RA, Therneau TM, Rajkumar SV, et al. Long-term follow-up of 241 patients with monoclonal gammopathy of undetermined significance: The original Mayo Clinic Service 25 years later. *Mayo Clin Proc.* 2004;79:859–866.
31. Comenzo R, Gertz MA. Autologous stem cell transplantation for primary systemic amyloidosis. *Blood.* 2002;99:4276–4282.
32. Kyle Ra, Gertz MA. Primary systemic amyloidosis: Clinical and laboratory features in 474 cases. *Semin Hematol.* 1995;32:45–59.
33. Gertz MA. Diagnosing primary amyloidosis. *Mayo Clin Proc.* 2002;77:1278–1279.
34. Alexanian R, Haut A, Khan AU, et al. Treatment for multiple myeloma. Combination of chemotherapy with different melphalan dose regimens. *JAMA.* 1969;208:1680–1685.
35. Barlogie B, Alexanian R, Dicke KA, et al. High-dose chemotherapy and autologous bone marrow transplantation for resistant multiple myeloma. *Blood.* 1987;70:869–872.
36. Vesole DH, Barlogie B, Jagannath S, et al. High dose therapy for refractory multiple myeloma: Improved prognosis with better supportive care and double transplant. *Blood.* 1994;84:950–956.
37. Barlogie B, Tricot G, Anaissie E, et al. Thalidomide and hematopoietic-cell transplantation for multiple myeloma. *N Engl J Med.* 2006;354:1021–1030.
38. Cavo M, Baccarani M. The changing landscape of myeloma therapy. *N Engl J Med.* 2006;354:1076–1078.
39. Palumbo A, Bringhen S, Caravita T, et al. Oral melphalan and prednisone chemotherapy plus thalidomide compared with melphalan and prednisone alone in elderly patients with multiple myeloma: Randomized controlled trial. *Lancet.* 2006;367:825–831.
40. Sawyers CL. Calculated resistance in cancer. *Nat Med.* 2005;11:824–825.
41. Berenson JR, Hillner BE, Kyle RA, et al. American Society of Clinical Oncology clinical practice guidelines: The role of bisphosphonates in multiple myeloma. *J Clin Oncol.* 2002;20:3719–3736.
42. Gucalp R, Theriault R, Gill I, et al. Treatment of cancer associated hypercalcemia: Double-blind comparison of rapid and slow intravenous infusion regimens of pamidronate disodium and saline alone. *Arch Intern Med.* 1994;154:1935–1944.
43. Dispenzieri A, Kyle RA, Lacy MQ, et al. Superior survival in primary systemic amyloidosis patients undergoing peripheral blood stem cell transplantation: A case-control study. *Blood.* 2004;103:3960–3963.
44. Jaccard A, Moreau P, Leblond V, et al. Best therapy for primary amyloidosis, a not-yet-solved question. *Blood.* 2004;104:2990–2991.
45. Goodman HJB, Hawkins PN. The role of PBSCT in treatment of Al amyloidosis is far from settled. *Blood.* 2004;104:2991.
46. Palladini G, Perfetti V, Perlini S, et al. The combination of thalidomide and intermediate-dose dexamethasone is an effective but toxic treatment for patients with primary amyloidosis (AL). *Blood.* 2005;105:2949–2951.

CHAPTER **55**

Bone Marrow Transplantation

Gregory Gruener • Harry L. Messmore

OBJECTIVES

- To describe the dichotomous role played by the histocompatibility complex compatibility in necessitating specific interventions (and potential complications) that complicate transplantation, while the same issues are responsible for its success when performed as a treatment of malignancies
- To provide background information on the process of hematopoietic stem cell transplantation
- To explain the pathophysiology, clinical manifestations, and treatment options for graft-versus-host disease as well as acute and chronic toxicity

CASE VIGNETTE

A 22-year-old man had hematopoietic stem cell transplantation from a related family donor for T-cell leukemia. Although mild thrombocytopenia persisted 2 months later, he had no immediate difficulties during the immediate preparatory regimen or for the ensuing 2 months after transplant, but required low doses of prednisone, because of recurrent skin rash (assumed graft-versus-host). He subsequently developed an upper respiratory infection (URI), not accompanied by any other systemic symptoms that resolved after 1 week. However, two weeks later he began to notice distal lower extremity paresthesias and then, during the next week, the gradual development of lower extremity weakness, unaccompanied by bladder dysfunction, but significantly impairing his ambulation.

Examination showed normal vital signs and general physical examination. His cranial nerves and upper extremity strength were normal, but had weakness (4-/5) in the lower extremities, which was worse distally. He had generalized muscle stretch areflexia. Sensory examination was normal as was sacral sensation and rectal tone. Gait was impaired because of weakness. Complete blood count (CBC) and complete metabolic profile (CMP) were normal. A chest X-ray study (CXR) was normal. Cerebrospinal fluid (CSF) was acellular. A borderline increase was noted in protein content, but normal glucose level. Electromyelographic (EMG) study demonstrated increased distal latencies in the peroneal and tibial nerves and absent F-waves in all extremities. Sensory responses were normal.

DEFINITION

HEMATOPOIETIC STEM CELL TRANSPLANTATION

Because bone marrow transplantation is less frequently performed and to reflect the multiple sites or origin of such stem cells, hematopoietics stem cell transplantation (HSCT) (now the preferred and more inclusive term) is primarily used for hematologic and lymphoid cancers, but increasingly for other disorders, both neoplastic as well as autoimmune. The transplantation source can either be *syngenic* (between identical twins), *autologous* (recipients serve as their own donor), or *allogenic* (a nonidentical genetic donor). In adults, peripheral blood has become the primary source of stem cells for transplantation and it is increasingly used as the source in children. The goal of transplantation is cure of the disease and through the newly transplanted immune system to detect and eliminate neoplastic cells.

EPIDEMIOLOGY

It 2003, approximately 9,600 autologous transplantations (>80% for multiple myeloma and lymphoma) and 7,300 allogenic transplantations (almost 70% for acute leukemia and myelodysplasia) were performed in North America (1). Yet, despite their potential benefit, transplantation continues to be clinically underused (2).

ETIOLOGY AND PATHOGENESIS

ROLE OF THE HISTOCOMPATABILITY COMPLEX

The *major histocompatibility complex* (MHC) or antigens are a set of molecules displayed on cell surfaces and responsible for lymphocyte recognition and "antigen presentation" that ultimately results in the immune system's ability to recognize *self* and *nonself*. The MHC is responsible for both favorable and detrimental immune reactions related to the different histocompatibilities of allogenic grafts, but absent if the donor is genetically identical to the recipient.

The MHC is encoded by several genes in the human leukocyte region (HLA) within chromosome 6; *class I molecules* are encoded by HLA-A, HLA-B, and HLA-C genes; *class II molecules* are encoded by HLA-DR, HLA-DQ, and HLA-DP genes; the region between them encodes *class III* molecules, which includes complement components. At this time, hundreds of different known alleles (each encoding a unique HLA protein or antigen) exist for each of those HLA genes.

Although class I and II molecules are structurally similar and serve to present antigen to T cells, their functions differ significantly. Class I molecules present *endogenous* antigens or those generated by the metabolic activity of that cell (and in some cases fragments of viral or tumor proteins that may exist within them) to cytotoxic T cells (CTL) and they are found on virtually every cell. The presentation of these antigens serves as an indicator of internal cellular activity and any alterations and dysfunction, thus, this antigen–MHC complex normally identifies a *self-antigen*. CTL identify cells presenting abnormal antigens and initiate their destruction, thereby serving as a *self-monitor*. Class II molecules present *exogenous* antigens (e.g., bacterial cell or viral fragments that are engulfed and processed within the cell) to helper T cells (TH-cells) and are only found on B cells, macrophages, and other antigen-presenting cells (APC). These activated TH-cells can activate B cells to then produce antibody, which would lead to the destruction of the pathogen from which that antigen was derived (3).

Minor histocompatibility antigens are represented by a small fraction of HLA molecules; they initiate weaker responses than the MHC and are encoded by genes on the Y chromosome. They account for a higher incidence of graft-versus-host disease (GvHD) and a lower relapse rate of underlying disease among male recipients of marrow transplants from female donors than among male recipients of transplants from male donors.

Just as the recipient's T cells recognize foreign antigens from the HSCT donor, which leads to graft rejection, donor T cells also recognize recipient antigens that lead to both the detrimental GvHD and the beneficial graft-versus-tumor (GvT) effects. This, in part, explains the dilemma where donor T cells are responsible for the GvT effects and the lower rate of relapse in allogenic transplantation compared with transplantation from an identical twin, but accompanied by a higher incidence of GvHD in allogenic transplants. Recently, a group of regulatory T cells (natural killer and CD4+CD25+ T cells) were identified that modulate the effector T cells responsible for GvHD, allow the GvT response to occur as well as immune system reconstitution within the donor, and offer a potentially new avenue of immune *manipulation* that may favor GvT effects, yet limit GvHD (4,5).

HEMATOPOIETIC AND TUMOR STEM CELLS

Hematopoietic stem cells have the capacity to produce daughter cells that retain stem cell properties and do not become specialized, but remain self-renewing as well as pluripotent. These stem cells are otherwise quiescent and demonstrate several unique qualities, including the ability to repair DNA efficiently, resist apoptosis, and excrete toxic drugs by means of adenosine triphosphate (ATP)-binding cassette (ABC) transporters (6).

Tumors are also believed to arise from normal stem cells and retain their mechanism for self-renewal (7,8). Although malignant cells have a limited capacity to reproduce, they are constantly replenished from these malignant stem cells. As with normal stem cells, they are also quiescent and, therefore, insensitive to chemotherapy; they repair their DNA efficiently, resist apoptosis, and also remove toxic foreign molecules from the cell (chemotherapeutic drug pumps) by means of the same ATP-binding transporters (6). These characteristics may explain why malignant stem cells can then survive radiation and chemotherapy given in preparation for hematopoietic stem cell transplantation. They can still be eliminated, however, by immunologically active donor T cells and this is the present rationale and foundation for current understanding of the effectiveness of stem cell transplantation in the treatment of malignancies (9).

SOURCES OF HEMATOPOIETIC STEM CELLS: PERIPHERAL BLOOD STEM CELLS

Peripheral blood has increasingly replaced bone marrow collection as the source of stem cells for both autologous and most allogenic HSCT. Hematopoietic stem cells are normally known to be continuously released from the bone marrow into the peripheral blood circulation, but eventually return again to the marrow. Identified by the presence of a cell surface molecule, CD34, their release into the peripheral blood can be increased by the use of granulocyte colony stimulating factor (G-CSF), which also results in T-cell differentiation (10), and by further inhibiting stem cell return (as with the use of AMD3100) has improved the yield of stem cells that are then collected during leukapheresis (11). Although autologous transplantation does not induce GvHD and is better tolerated in older or high-risk recipients, the associated lack of a GvT effect limits its effectiveness because tumor cell contamination of the autologous transplant increases the chance of a relapse.

SOURCES OF HEMATOPOIETIC STEM CELLS: UMBILICAL CORD BLOOD

Collected immediately after birth, umbilical cord blood (UCB) is rich in hematopoietic stem cells. In addition, HLA antigen typing mismatches appear to be better tolerated (possibly a reflection of the immaturity of these cord blood lymphocytes) and less likely to cause GvHD while maintaining a GvT effect. These less stringent HLA antigen requirements could permit this donor pool to address the needs of all potential recipients; however, now it is usually considered a second choice and after an unrelated BMT has been ruled out (12). As availability and technical or transplantation limitations of this source of stem cells continues to be developed, it may eventually address those cases were an HLA antigen match is not available or autologous transplantation is not possible (13). (Prospective studies of UCB versus unrelated PBSC or bone marrow transplant [BMT] have yet to be performed.) The role or applicability of human embryonic stem cells as a source of hematopoietic stem cells has not yet been defined (14).

PREPARATORY REGIMENS BEFORE TRANSPLANTATION

The original role for myeloablative treatment preparations was to eliminate malignant cells before HSCT and allow the immunosuppression that permits a bone marrow engraftment to occur. The indirect effects of such treatments (potentiating the antitumor response of donor and host T-cells through the release of tumor antigens to antigen-presenting cells), however, has led to a proliferation of T cells. This proliferation of T cells would then attack the surviving tumor cells (15) that would be identified as playing the more important role of eradicating residual tumor cells (GvT, response).

The new preparatory treatment regimens have continued to combine tumor-specific or effective regimens and minimize acute and chronic toxicity while enhancing engraftment, minimizing GvHD, and augmenting GvT activity (16). These newer low-intensity nonmyeloablative therapies, which are based on the fact that the GvT effect is more important than the intensity of the preparatory regimen, allow engraftment while lessening epithelial injury and reducing the incidence of acute GvHD (17).

The specific preparatory regimens are chosen on the basis of the tumor type, health and age of the recipient, and HSCT source. They combine radiation (either total body radiation or selective radiation that makes use of tagged antibodies against related antigens) (18), tumor-specific chemotherapeutic (and immunotherapy) (15) regimens, infusion of donor T cells (to potentate graft antitumor effects), and at times serial HSCT. These modifications have allowed a greater range of tumor types and individuals typically at higher risk for toxicity (those older than 65) to now have transplantation (4,19,20).

TRANSPLANTATION AND ENGRAFTMENT

Peripheral blood stem cell infusions tend to be well tolerated, but the rate of engraftment depends on the source of stem cells, choice of prophylaxis against GvHD, and whether hematopoietic growth factors were used. Although complete and sustained engraftment is the general rule after transplantation, marrow function does not return in some cases. Treatment in those cases usually involves removal of all potentially myelosuppressive agents, short course of myeloid growth factors, and in some cases, a second transplant (21).

CLINICAL MANIFESTATIONS

Pretransplant regimens are associated with a substantial array of toxicity. After transplantation, in addition to acute GvHD, the major noninfectious transplant-related complications include veno-occlusive disease, idiopathic pneumonia syndrome, and multiorgan dysfunction syndrome, reflecting the primary target organs of injury that include the skin, gastrointestinal system, and liver. After allogenic transplantation, the major causes of death include GvHD, infection, and organ toxicity damage (these rates increase if the underlying neoplastic disease is active; frequencies of these complications are similar in autologous transplants, but lower). After autologous transplantation the major cause of death is relapse from the underlying malignancy.

EARLY COMPLICATIONS

Oral *mucositis* is one of the most common complications of these myeloablative preparative regimens or when methotrexate is used to prevent GvHD. In addition to basic oral hygiene treatment regimens, nonpharmacologic approaches (oral cryotherapy as well as low-level laser) and pharmacologic (chlorhexidine, amifostine, recombinant human keratinocyte growth factor, pentoxifylline, glutamine) have all been used, but with variable response rates and often still necessitating palliative care. Oral mucositis remains a serious complication following transplantation (22).

Hepatic veno-occlusive disease (*sinusoidal obstruction syndrome*) is a syndrome characterized by painful hepatomegaly, jaundice, ascites, and fluid retention. Damage to sinusoidal endothelium obstructs the hepatic circulation, causing central lobular hepatocyte injury; no effective treatment is currently for this syndrome (23). This remains a serious complication of high-dose chemotherapy and approximately 30% of patients may die.

Although most cases of pneumonia that occur are caused by microbial agents, *transplantation-related lung injury* (idiopathic interstitial pneumonia) occurs in 11% to 17% of patients, with a mortality rate that can exceed 60% (24). The identified pathologic processes implicate donor lymphocytes as primarily responsible for injuring the lung (25).

While mimicking acute GVHD in some respects, systemic inflammatory syndromes can occur following hematopoietic cell transplantations. These syndromes include *disseminated intravascular coagulation (DIC), capillary leak syndrome, engraftment syndrome, hemophagocytic lymphohistiocytic disorders,* and *macrophage activation syndrome* (26,27). Although they appear to have distinct clinical, laboratory, and unique pathogenesis, overlapping features exist and diagnostic criteria continue to be established. Exclusion of infection and the rapid establishment of their diagnosis allow appropriate treatment (immunosuppressive) that may eventually improve outcome.

Transplantation-related infections result from the associated immunodeficiency; injuries to the mouth, gut, and skin; and predisposition from indwelling catheters. During the first few weeks after transplantation, the greatest risk is of disseminated bacterial infections and broad spectrum antibiotics, and prophylaxis for *Candida albicans* as well as *Pneumocystis carinii* that are often provided. Although viral infections, such as cytomegalovirus (CMV) are more aggressively handled, herpes simplex as well adenoviral infections also continue to contribute to posttransplant morbidity (28).

Acute GvHD is an immune response accentuated and possibly stimulated by injury resulting from the preparative regimen used before transplantation, but with the principal risk factor being HLA antigen mismatch between donor and recipient. The injury is primarily confined to the gastrointestinal tract, where Peyer patches have a central role in attracting donors T cells to the site of injury, and this process contributes to the development of GvHD (29). Attempts to remove T cells from the transplantation population helps prevent acute GvHD, but is also associated with an increased evidence of graft rejection and tumor relapse. (Cytokines are critical to GvHD and their genetic variants influence its development. Inactivation of the chemokines that attract donor T cells to Peyer patches eliminates most deaths from GvHD in mice transplant models.)

The clinical presentation is a manifestation of the primary sites of injury in acute GvHD: Skin (rash), gastrointestinal tract (diarrhea), and liver. Clinical staging is based on the extent of their involvement. Attempts to decrease the incidence of GvHD by prophylaxis have included immunosuppressive medication, early posttreatment radiation, antithymocyte antibody, or monoclonal antibodies against T cells or their receptors (4). Complications of treating acute GvHD can lead to an immunodeficiency state that predisposes to fatal infections.

Pretreatment minor neurologic signs and mild cognitive impairment were felt to be secondary to treatment (chemotherapy as well as radiation therapy [RT]) or the underlying disease. The accompanying neuroradiologic evaluations identified mild white matter changes, but not extensive. New neurologic abnormalities after BMT are frequent (57%), but symptoms, such as tremor or headache, predominated. Acute GvHD is the main risk factor for these symptoms, but assigning GvHD, the associated effects of renal and liver dysfunction, or drug or treatment toxicity as the etiology is somewhat problematic. Polyneuropathy, muscle weakness, tremor, or confusional states may, therefore, have multiple causes (30).

Guillain-Barré syndrome (GBS) has been reported, but it is usually associated with a viral infection. Similar clinical syndromes precipitated by the conditioning regimen (role of cytosine arabinoside as a possible neurotoxic effect) (31) and additional cases lacking the associated EMG and CSF findings of GBS (32) suggest that the pathogenesis, prognosis, and clinical interventions or treatments for this syndrome are not equivalent.

DELAYED EFFECTS

Late effects of transplantation have included musculoskeletal stiffness, cramps, weakness and joint swelling, sexual dysfunction, memory and attention concerns, urinary frequency, or incontinence. Infertility, sexual problems, developmental problems with children, depression, and anxiety, as well as an increased risk of secondary cancers, are also encountered as delayed effects of transplantation (33). These symptoms are based on the unique clinical predisposition to specific organ system dysfunction and complicated by the unique social circumstances that affect quality of life and induce psychosocial issues (34). These clinical circumstances and the increasing number of transplant survivors, necessitates their indefinite clinical and laboratory follow-up.

Chronic GvHD occurs in 20% to 70% of individuals after allogenic hematopoietic stem cell transplantation, which originally was defined as occurring 100 days after transplantation, recent definitions hinge on its different clinical manifestations (35). It is not simply a continuation of acute GvHD, and innovations that have improved acute GvHD have not affected chronic GvHD. Although acute GvHD is highly associated with chronic GvHD, 25% to 35% of cases derive de novo and 20% to 30% of those with acute GvHD do not develop chronic GvHD (36).

Chronic GvHD clinically resembles an autoimmune disease, such as scleroderma or Sjögren's syndrome (37). Clinically, it can be associated with bronchiolitis, keratoconjunctivitis sicca, esophageal stricture, malabsorption, cholestasis, hematocytopenia, and generalized immunosuppression (38). Treatment usually includes prednisone or cyclosporine. When it eventually resolves, immunosuppressive therapy can be withdrawn, but can necessitate immunosuppressive treatments for a median of 1 to 3 years. When immunosuppressive therapy is administered, susceptibility to bacterial infections may necessitate prophylactic antibiotic usage (39).

Chronic GvHD affecting the CNS or peripheral nervous system (PNS) is uncommon. Painful neuropathy can occur as a sequelae of treatment related neurotoxicity as well as associated systemic dysfunction. Myopathies related to steroids (40) as well as polymyositis, demonstrating clinical and laboratory presentations similar to the idiopathic form, have been seen and at times not associated with GvHD. Treatment of polymyositis with steroids, cyclosporin as well as tacrolimus, can result in remission, but recurrence can also occur when steroids are tapered (41). Myasthenia gravis has also been reported in the setting of GvHD. Cases have been reported of individuals who presented either acutely or subacutely with focal neurologic signs (42), encephalopathy, or neurocognitive impairment; multifocal CNS white matter changes were shown on MRI and some had brain biopsy for suspicion of a cerebral vasculitis. Evidence of cerebral (granulomatous) angiitis or vasculitis was identified on biopsy, demonstrating morphologic similarity between those CNS infiltrates and ones described in other involved organs in chronic GvHD, and suggesting a similar pathologic process (43,44).

Within the first year after transplantation 18% of patients developed neurologic complications, with CNS infections being most common (11%), and subdural hematoma the most common cerebrovascular complication (3%). Neurologic complications led to the death of 9% of subjects and fungal or bacterial infections of the CNS and cerebrovascular events were the most common causes (30). Although similar causes are responsible for the early neurologic complications observed in children having HSCT, treatment-related toxicities (cyclosporine A neurotoxicity, irradiation, and chemotherapy) are perhaps more frequent (45).

DIAGNOSTIC APPROACH AND TREATMENT

General guidelines for ancillary and supportive care of acute and chronic GvHD, as well as recommendations concerning monitoring, have been developed (46). These guidelines summarize current recommendations and address those organ systems most often affected: Skin, mouth, and oral cavity; eyes; vulva and vagina; gastrointestinal tract; liver; lungs; hematopoietic, neurologic, immunologic, and infectious diseases; and the musculoskeletal system. The specific recommendations are not included in this chapter, but generally include treatment of symptoms, recommendations for patient education, preventive measures, prevention and management of infections, and follow-up guidelines.

Posttransplant immunodeficiencies also increase the risk for serious infection from varicella zoster virus, CMV, and *Streptococcus pneumoniae.* The role and types of vaccine-mediated immunization continues to be developed (38).

CLINICAL RECOMMENDATIONS OF THE VIGNETTE

The patient demonstrates the acute development of an ascending syndrome of symmetric weakness associated with areflexia and intact sensory function; at this time, autonomic function is normal as well. The clinical characteristics and CSF and EMG findings support the initial clinical diagnosis of GBS. The initial impression would suggest that it may have been caused by the antecedent infection (assumed viral). In patients who have had HSCT, it is important to search for other potential viral infections that require evaluation, as well as the possibility of the patient developing GvHD. Support and monitoring (respiratory) need to be undertaken and interventions (either plasma exchange [PE] or intravenous gamma globulin [IVIG]) may be necessary if the weakness progresses. As in all acute medical developments in patients after HSCT, the effects of the underlying illness and preexisting or earlier treatments have to be included within the *standard* differential diagnosis.

SUMMARY

HSCT has continued to evolve and is now used in an increasing number of both neoplastic and non-neoplastic disorders. Associated morbidity and mortality are significant and occur both in regard to the preparative treatments, immunosuppression, and finally are immune mediated through both the host and transplanted stem cells. When used in patients with neoplasms, it is no longer believed that the role of preparative treatment is to eradicate all of the patient's tumor cells, but to allow the introduction of a new donor immune system in the recipient. This transplanted immune system will then exert a graft-versus-disease effect which can be further amplified by the infusion of donor lymphocytes (47).

REFERENCES

1. Pasquini M. Report on state of the art in blood and marrow transplantation. Center for International Blood and Bone Marrow Transplant; May 2006 Newsletter.
2. Paivanas T. New center provides resources for large transplant-related studies. Oncology *News International* 2005;14:51–52, 73.
3. Milford EL, Carpenter CB. Adaptive Immunity: Histocompatibility antigens and immune response genes. Section 6, Chapter 5 in ACP Medicine 2004. Available at: www.acpmedicine.org.
4. Lowsky R, Takahashi T, Liu YP, et al. Protective conditioning for acute graft-versus-host disease. *N Engl J Med.* 2005;353:1321–1331.
5. Gregori S, Bacchetta R, Hauben R, et al. Regulatory T cells: Prospective for clinical application in hematopoietic stem cell transplantation. *Curr Opin Hematol.* 2005:12;451–456.
6. Dean M, Fojo T, Bates S. Tumor stem cells and drug resistance. *Nature Rev Cancer.* 2005;5:275–284.
7. Krivtsov AV, Twomey D, Feng Z, et al. Transformation form committed progenitor to leukemia stem cell initiated by MLL-AF9. *Nature.* 2006;442:818–822.
8. Jordan CT, Guzman ML, Noble M. Cancer stem cells. *N Engl J Med.* 2006;355:1253–1261.
9. Bleakley M, Riddell SR. Molecules and mechanisms of the graft-versus-leukaemia effect. *Nature Rev Cancer.* 2004;4:371–380.
10. Morris ES, MacDonald KPA, Hill GR. Stem cell mobilization with G-CSF analogs: A rational approach to separate GVHD and GVL? *Blood.* 2006;107:3430–3435.
11. Flomenberg N, Devine SM, DiPersio JF, et al. The use of AMD3100 plus G-CSF for autologous hematopoietic progenitor cell mobilization is superior to G-CSF alone. *Blood.* 2005;106:1867–1874.
12. Schoemnas H, Theunissen K, Maertens J, et al. Adult umbilical cord blood transplantation: A comprehensive review. *Bone Marrow Transplant.* 2006;38:83–93.
13. Bone Marrow Donors Worldwide. Available at: www.bmdw.org.
14. Priddle H, Jones DRE, Burridge PW, et al. Hematopoieses from human embryonic stem cells: Overcoming the immune barrier in stem cell therapies. *Stem Cells.* 2006;24:815–824.
15. Lake RA, Robinson BW. Immunotherapy and chemotherapy—A practical partnership. *Nature Rev Cancer.* 2005;5:397–405.
16. Burroughs L, Storb R. Low-intensity allogenic hematopoietic stem cell transplantation for myeloid malignancies: Separating graft-versus-leukemia effects from graft-versus-host disease. *Curr Opin Hematol.* 2004:12;45–54.
17. Socié G. Graft-versus-host disease β: From the bench to the bedside? *N Engl J Med.* 2005;353:1396–1397.
18. Gopal AK, Pagel JM, Rajendran JG, et al. Improving the efficacy of reduced intensity allogenic transplantation for lymphoma using radioimmunotherapy. *Biol Blood Marrow Transplant.* 2006:12;697–702.
19. Satwani P, Harrison L, Morris E, et al. Reduced-intensity allogenic stem cell transplantation in adults and children with malignant and nonmalignant diseases: End of the beginning and future challenges. *Biol Blood Marrow Transplant.* 2005:11;403–422.
20. Baron F, Sandmaier BM. Current status of hematopoietic stem cell transplantation after nonmyeloablative conditioning. *Curr Opin Hematol.* 2005:12;435–443.
21. Nemunaitis J, Singer JW, Becker CD, et al. Use of recombinant human granulocyte macrophage colony stimulating factor in graft failure after bone marrow transplantation. *Blood.* 1990;76:245.
22. Saadeh CE. Chemotherapy- and radiotherapy-induced oral mucositis: Review of preventive strategies and treatment. *Pharmacotherapy.* 2005;25:540–554.
23. Hogan WJ, Maris M, Storer B, et al. Hepatic injury after nonmyeloablative conditioning followed by allogenic hematopoietic cell transplantation: A study of 193 patients. *Blood.* 2004;103:78–84.
24. Kantrow SP, Hackman RC, Boeckh M, et al. Idiopathic pneumonia syndrome: Changing spectrum of lung injury after marrow transplantation. *Transplantation.* 1997; 63:1079–1086.
25. Cooke KR, Yanik G. Acute lung injury after allogenic stem cell transplantation: Is the lung a target of graft-versus-host disease? *Bone Marrow Transplant.* 2004;34:753–765.
26. Sreedharan A, Bowyer S, Wallace CA, et al. Macrophage activation syndrome and other systemic inflammatory conditions following BMT. *Bone Marrow Transplant.* 2006;37:629–634.
27. Maiolino A, Biasoli I, Lima J, et al. Engraftment syndrome following autologous hematopoietic stem cell transplantation: Definition of diagnostic criteria. *Bone Marrow Transplant.* 2003;31:393–397.
28. Lee Am, Bollard CM, Myers GD, et al. Adenoviral infections in hematopoietic stem cell transplantation. *Biol Blood Marrow Transplant.* 2006;12:243–251.
29. Hill GR, Ferrara JL. The primacy of the gastrointestinal tract as a target organ in acute graft-versus-host disease: Rationale for the use of cytokine shields in allogenic bone marrow transplantation. *Blood.* 2000;95:2754–2759.
30. Sostak P, Padovan CS, Yousry TA, et al. Prospective evaluation of neurological complications after allogenic bone marrow transplantation. *Neurology.* 2003;60:842–848.
31. Rodriguez V, Kuehnle I, Heslop HE, et al. Guillain-Barré syndrome after allogenic hematopoietic stem cell transplantation. *Bone Marrow Transplant.* 2002;29:515–517.
32. Fujisaki G, Kami M, Murashige N, et al. Guillain-Barré syndrome associated with rapid immune reconstitution following allogenic hematopoietic stem cell transplantation. *Bone Marrow Transplant.* 2006;37:617–619.
33. Syrjala KL, Langer SL, Abrams JR, et al. Late effects of hematopoietic cell transplantation among 10 year adult survivors compared with case matched controls. *J Clin Oncol.* 2005;23:6596–6606.
34. Rizzo JD, Wingard JR, Tichelli A, et al. Recommended screening and preventive practices for long-term survivors after hematopoietic cell transplantation: Joint recommendations of the European Group for Blood and Marrow transplantation, Center for International Blood and Marrow transplant Research, and the American Society for Blood and Marrow Transplantation (EBMT/CIBMTR/ASBMT). *Bone Marrow Transplant.* 2006;37:249–261.
35. Lee SJ. New approaches for preventing and treating chronic graft-versus-host disease. *Blood.* 2005;105;4200–4206.
36. Tivol E, Komorowski R, Drobyski WR. Emergent autoimmunity in graft-versus-host disease. *Blood.* 2005;105:4885–4891.
37. Rapoport AP. Immunity for tumors and microbes after transplantation: If you build it, they will (not) come. *Bone Marrow Transplant.* 2006;37:239–247.
38. Tiwol E, Komorowski R, Drobyski WR. Emergent autoimmunity in graft-versus-host disease. *Blood.* 2005;105:4885–4891.
39. Koi S, Leisening W, Flowers ME, et al. Therapy for chronic graft-versus-host disease: A randomized trail comparing cyclosporine plus prednisone versus prednisone alone. *Blood.* 2002;100:48–51.
40. Lee HJ, Oran B, Saliba RM, et al. Steroid myopathy in patients with acute graft-versus-host disease treated with high-dose steroids. *Bone Marrow Transplant.* 2006;38:299–303.
41. Couriel DR, Beguelin GZ, Giralt S, et al. Chronic graft-versus-host disease manifesting as polymyositis: An uncommon manifestation. *Bone Marrow Transplant.* 2002;30:543–546.
42. Solaro C, Murialdo A, Giunti D, et al. Central and peripheral nervous system complications following allogenic bone marrow transplantation. *Eur J Neurol.* 2001;8:77–80.
43. Padovan CS, Bise K, Hahn J, et al. Angiitis of the central nervous system after allogenic bone marrow transplantation. *Stroke.* 1999;30:1651–1656.
44. Ma M, Barnes G, Pulliam J, et al. CNS angiitis in graft vs. host disease. *Neurology.* 2002;59:1994–1997.
45. Faraci M, Lanino E, Dini G, et al. Severe neurologic complications after hematopoietic stem cell transplantation in children. *Neurology.* 2002;59:1895–1904.
46. Couriel D, Carpenter PA, Cutler C, et al. Ancillary therapy and supportive care of chronic graft-versus-host disease: National Institutes of Health consensus development project on criteria for clinical trials in chronic graft-versus-host disease: V. Ancillary therapy and supportive care working group document. *Biol Blood Marrow Transplant.* 2006;12:375–396.
47. Schattenberg AVMB, Dolstra H. Cellular adoptive immunotherapy after allogenic stem cell transplantation. *Curr Opin Oncol.* 2005;17:617–621.

CHAPTER 56

Commonly Used Hematologic Drugs

Athena Kostidis • Harry L. Messmore

OBJECTIVES

- To describe the common neurologic toxicities of cancer chemotherapy
- To describe the common neurologic toxicities of biological agents used in the treatment of neoplastic disease
- To discuss some of neurotoxic syndromes that be a result of multidrug regimens

CASE VIGNETTE

A 61-year-old woman with history of breast cancer had painful dysesthesias and tingling in both feet that began shortly after her first dose of paclitaxel. Symptoms were initially mild, but escalated in severity with each subsequent dose, abated after the third administration. Her pain was so severe that it interfered with sleep, and the dysesthesias progressed to mid-shin level. Also noted were a sense of imbalance since these symptoms began and a numbness and tingling in the fingertips bilaterally, but no weakness.

Examination showed a decrease in light touch, pin-prick, and vibration in the feet, bilaterally to the level of the ankle was found. Proprioception was intact. Muscle stretch reflexes were hypoactive in the upper extremities and patella bilaterally, and absent at the ankles. Gait showed a sensory ataxia. Laboratory studies demonstrated normal values of hemoglobin A1C, folate, vitamin B_{12}, thyroid-stimulating hormone (TSH), free T4, and vitamin E. Complete blood count, comprehensive metabolic panel, and serum protein electrophoresis were unremarkable.

DEFINITION

Neurotoxicity is a common phenomenon from cancer chemotherapies (Table 56-1). Toxicity can be related to the dose of the medication as well as to the route of administration. It can be mild and transient; severely affect the patient's quality of life; and persist after treatment is discontinued; or it can progress for sometime after therapy is completed ("coasting"). Finally, many of these neurotoxicity syndromes are seen when certain chemotherapeutic agents are combined. It is important to recognize these toxicities in patients with cancer who develop neurologic dysfunction, and to differentiate them from progression of disease, opportunistic infection, and metabolic abnormalities.

ANTIMETABOLITES

Cytosine Arabinoside

Cytosine arabinoside (Cytarabine, Ara-C) is a pyrimidine analog used to treat leukemias, lymphomas, and leptomeningeal metastases. Neurotoxicity is dependent on the dose and route of administration. At conventional doses, there is no significant toxicity. With high-dose regimens, several neurologic complications are known to occur, including seizures, encephalopathy, and rarely peripheral neuropathy. Cerebellar dysfunction occurs with increased frequency in the older population, and typically presents with dysarthria, nystagmus, and ataxia (1). In addition, high-dose regimens can be toxic to the cornea, producing conjunctival injection and corneal opacities. Intrathecal administration can produce fever, acute encephalopathy, aseptic meningitis, and an ascending myelopathy (2).

Fludarabine

Fludarabine (Fludara) is a purine analog used in the treatment of chronic lymphocytic leukemia. Patients receiving conventional doses may experience reversible neurologic toxicity, including hemiparesis, paresthesias, gait disorder, encephalopathy, and blurred vision (3). At higher doses, a delayed progressive encephalopathy (and even coma) can occur (1). Numerous cases have been reported of patients who developed progressive multifocal leukoencephalopathy with a negative JC virus polymerase chain reaction (PCR) after treatment with standard-dose fludarabine (4).

5-Fluorouracil

5-Fluorouracil (5-FU) is a pyrimidine analog used in the treatment of breast cancer, as well as gastrointestinal and head and neck tumors. Adverse neurologic effects include encephalopathy (5), cerebellar ataxia, optic neuropathy, and extrapyramidal syndromes. Ocular motility disorders, such as disturbance

TABLE 56-1. Neurologic Complications of Cancer Therapies (1,3)

ACUTE ENCEPHALOPATHY		
Asparaginase	Fludarabine	Mitomycin C
BCNU	5-Fluorouracil	Paclitaxel
Carboplatin	GM-CSF	Procarbazine (HD)
Cisplatin	Ifosfamide	Suramin
Cyclophosphamide	Interferons	Tamoxifen
Cytosine arabinoside (HD)	Interleukins	Thalidomide
Denileukin	Levamisole	Thiotepa (HD)
Doxorubicin (IT)	Mechloramine	Vinca alkaloids
Etoposide (IT or IA)	Methotrexate	
ASEPTIC MENINGITIS		
Cytosine arabinoside (IT)	Doxorubicin (IT)	Methotrexate (IT)
CEREBELLAR SYNDROME		
Cytosine arabinoside (HD)	Interleukin-2	Thalidomide
5-Fluorouracil	Mitotane	Vinca alkaloids
Ifosfamide	Procarbazine	
CORTICAL BLINDNESS		
Carboplatin	Fludarabine	Methotrexate (HD)
Cisplatin	GM-CSF	Vinca alkaloids
Erythropoietin	Interleukin-2	
DEMENTIA		
BCNU (IA and HD)	Interferon-α	Procarbazine
Cytosine arabinoside	Interleukin-2	Fludarabine
Methotrexate		
DIZZINESS		
Cyclophosphamide	Mitotane	Rituximab
Hydroxyurea Rituximab	Octreotide	Trastuzumab
EXTRAPYRAMIDAL SYNDROME		
5-Fluorouracil	Interferon-α	Ifosfamide
Vincristine		
HEADACHE		
Asparaginase	Gemtuzumab	Octreotide
Cisplatin	Hydroxyurea	Rituximab
Corticosteroids	Interferons	Temozolomide
Danazol	Interleukins	Thalidomide
Denileukin	Mechlorethamine	Trastuzumab
Etoposide (IA)	Methotrexate (IT)	TNF
HEARING LOSS		
Cisplatin	Mitotane	Oxaliplatin
Interferons (IT)	Mechlorethamine	Suramin
MOOD DISORDERS		
Asparaginase	Interferons	Procarbazine
Cladribine	Interleukin-2	Pyrazoloacridine
Corticosteroids	Mechlorethamine	Suramin
Danazol	Pentostatin	Thalidomide
MYELOPATHY		
BCNU (HD)	Doxorubicin (IT)	Mitoxantrone (IT)
Cisplatin	Goserelin	Thiotepa (IT)
Corticosteroids	Interferon-alpha	Vincristine (IT)
Cytosine arabinoside (IT)	Leuprolide	
Docetaxel	Methotrexate (IT)	
PERIPHERAL NEUROPATHY		
Carboplatin	Oprelvekin	Teniposide
Cisplatin	Oxaliplatin	Thalidomide
Cladribine	Paclitaxel	TNF
Docetaxel	Procarbazine	Vinca alkaloids
Etoposide	Suramin	

(*continued*)

TABLE 56-1. ***(Continued)***

SEIZURES		
Asparaginase	Dacarbazine	Ifosfamide
Busulfan (HD)	Etoposide (IA)	Interferon (IT)
BCNU	Erythropoietin	Levamisole
Carboplatin (IA)	5-Fluorouracil	Mechlorethamine
Chlorambucil (HD)	Fludarabine	Methotrexate
Cytosine arabinoside (IT or HD)	GM-CSF	Thalidomide
		Vinca alkaloids
VASCULOPATHY AND STROKE		
Asparaginase	Doxorubicin	Imatinib
Bleomycin	Erythropoietin	Methotrexate
Carboplatin (IA)	Estramustine	Tamoxifen
Cisplatin	Gemtuzumab	Toremifene
VISUAL DISTURBANCE		
BCNU (IA)	Cytosine arabinoside	Pamidronate
Carboplatin	Etoposide	Suramin
Chlorambucil	5-Fluorouracil	Tamoxifen
Cisplatin (IA)	Fludarabine	Toremifene
Corticosteroids	Interleukin-2	Vincristine
Cyclophosphamide	Paclitaxel	Zoledronic acid

BCNU, carmustine; GM-CSF, granulocyte macrophage colony-factor; TNF, tumor necrosis factor; HD, high-dose; IT, intrathecal; IA, intraarterial.

of convergence, can also occur (6). If used in combination with levamisole, multifocal inflammatory leukoencephalopathy can occur. In patients with a deficiency of dihydropyrimidine dehydrogenase, toxicity may be more severe, manifesting as encephalopathy and coma (7). A case series has described focal dystonia after treatment with 5-fluorouracil; four patients developed oromandibular dystonia and blepharospasm. Two of those patients were treated with 5-FU, one received doxorubicin alone, and one was treated with both (8).

Hydroxyurea

Hydroxyurea is used in the treatment of myeloproliferative disorders and may produce mild drowsiness, headache and dizziness (3).

Methotrexate

Methotrexate is the most widely used antimetabolite, used primarily against leukemias, lymphomas, breast cancer, and head and neck cancer. Intrathecal administration is used for leptomeningeal carcinomatosis (7). Methotrexate can cause significant neurologic toxicity in the acute, subacute, and chronic stages of treatment. Acutely, it can cause an aseptic meningitis marked by headache, nuchal rigidity, somnolence, confusion, dizziness, nausea, vomiting, and seizures (9). An acute encephalomyelopathy can also occur with intrathecal methotrexate and one case reported a patient who developed fatal acute encephalomyelitis within 24 hours of a single dose of intrathecal methotrexate during his third cycle of chemotherapy. This patient was also on cyclophosphamide, vincristine, doxorubicin, and dexamethasone (10). Subacute toxicity from methotrexate can cause strokelike episodes, but these episodes are usually self-limited. Some evidence suggests restricted diffusion on magnetic resonance imaging (MRI) in those patients who experienced subacute methotrexate toxicity. Notably, both clinical symptoms and diffusion abnormalities resolved within 1 to 4 days (9). Chronically, intrathecal or intravenous methotrexate can cause a leukoencephalopathy characterized by cognitive dysfunction, behavioral abnormalities, spasticity, gait ataxia, and urinary incontinence (3).

ANTIMICROTUBULE AGENTS

Vincristine

Vincristine, the most neurotoxic of the Vinca alkaloids, arrests cell division by inhibiting microtubule formation. Vincristine is often used in combination with other agents in the treatment of acute lymphocytic leukemia, non-Hodgkin lymphoma, neuroblastoma, and Wilm tumor (11). The primary neurologic toxicity is a peripheral neuropathy. This typically presents as paresthesias in the distal extremities, with loss of reflexes, followed by motor weakness. Pain in the limbs can also occur. Mononeuropathies, cranial nerve palsies, and sensorineural hearing loss have also been described (7). Vincristine can also cause an autonomic neuropathy characterized by constipation and, rarely, more severe symptoms, such as ileus, orthostatic hypotension, and impotence. Central nervous system (CNS) toxicity mainly presents as an encephalopathy or seizures. Self-resolving episodes of cortical blindness, ataxia, and extrapyramidal syndromes have also been described (6). Finally, myeloencephalopathy can occur with intrathecal administration (7).

Paclitaxel

Paclitaxel (Taxol) blocks the cell cycle phase by polymerization and stabilization of microtubules. It is used in the treatment of ovarian, breast, and lung carcinoma (7). The principal toxicity of paclitaxel is a peripheral neuropathy, which is primarily sensory and mostly spares motor function; a combined sensorimotor polyneuropathy is less frequently seen, but has also been reported (12). The peripheral neuropathy can be dose limiting and presents as paresthesias, numbness, and burning pain in the limbs, with impaired vibration and proprioception and loss of reflexes (13). At high doses, paclitaxel can also cause an acute encephalopathy (7).

PLATINUM ANALOGUES

Cisplatin

The primary adverse neurologic effect of cisplatin is a sensory neuropathy or neuronopathy. This manifests as paresthesias, dysesthesias, sensory ataxia, and impairment of vibration and proprioception. Pain and temperature modalities are only minimally affected, and motor function is typically spared (7). The symptoms can persist or even worsen after discontinuation of the drug in up to 60% of patients. Ototoxicity, manifesting as hearing loss and tinnitus, has been reported with cisplatin use. Retinal toxicity can also occur with symptoms of blurred vision and abnormal color perception (14). CNS toxicity can also occur and particularly with intraarterial administration of cisplatin. Headache, encephalopathy, and seizures have been reported (7), as well as a small risk of cerebrovascular thrombosis with ischemic infarction and cortical blindness (15).

Carboplatin

Carboplatin, rarely, produces a sensory neuropathy in about 4% of patients. Ototoxicity can occur in up to 1% of patients (11).

ALKYLATING AGENTS

Nitrosureas

CARMUSTINE (BCNU). BCNU is used in the treatment of primary CNS neoplasms as well as melanoma and lymphoma. At high doses, ocular toxicity, myelopathy, and encephalopathy can develop (3). With intravenous or intraarterial infusion, blindness can result from an optic neuropathy. Intracarotid infusion can cause retinal ischemia and white matter changes, which resemble radiation necrosis within the vascular territory of the infusion (1,2).

ESTRAMUSTINE. Estramustine is used in the treatment of advanced prostate cancer, and has rarely been associated with stroke (6).

Mustards

IFOSFAMIDE. Ifosfamide is the most neurotoxic of the mustard class of alkylating agents. It is used in the treatment of many solid tumors, such as ovarian, testicular, sarcomas, lymphomas, and head and neck cancers. Associated neurotoxicities include encephalopathy, ataxia, extrapyramidal dysfunction, hallucinations, seizures, and coma (1,16). Several reports are found of nonconvulsive status epilepticus in patients receiving intravenous ifosfamide (16,17).

CYCLOPHOSPHAMIDE. Cyclophosphamide has little neurologic toxicity, but at high doses, encephalopathy, dizziness, and blurred vision can occur (7).

Other Alkylating Agents

BUSULFAN. Busulfan is used in the treatment of chronic myelocytic leukemia and in combination therapy for allogeneic bone marrow transplantation. Its use has been associated with dose-dependent focal and generalized seizures, especially in the bone marrow transplant population (3,18). One case was reported of a patient developing myasthenia gravis after busulfan therapy (19).

THIOTEPA. Thiotepa is used in breast, ovarian, and bladder cancers, as well as lymphoma. Intrathecal administration is sometimes used for leptomeningeal metastases. Intrathecal injection can result in a myelopathy (11). High intravenous doses can also result in confusion, behavioral changes, and somnolence (6).

PROCARBAZINE. Procarbazine is a monoamine oxidase inhibitor used in advanced Hodgkin disease and CNS neoplasms. It is associated with encephalopathy and, occasionally, ataxia (11). Peripheral neuropathy presenting as paresthesias and loss of muscle stretch reflexes occurs in about 17% of patients (7).

ANTINEOPLASTIC ANTIBIOTICS

Doxorubicin

Doxorubicin (Adriamycin) is an anthracycline antibiotic, effective against lymphomas, leukemias, sarcomas, and many other solid tumors. Perhaps the most important dose-limiting toxicity is acute and chronic cardiac toxicity, characterized by arrhythmias, pericarditis, or cardiomyopathy (11). Cardiac thrombi may thus form and lead to embolic strokes. Furthermore, intracarotid injections may be associated with hemorrhagic cerebral infarctions. Intrathecal administration can cause a severe myelopathy or an aseptic meningitis (1,20).

Mitoxantrone

Mitoxantrone, an analog of doxorubicin, is largely free of neurotoxicity when given intravenously. Intrathecal administration, however, is associated with nerve root damage and myelopathy; therefore, this route of therapy is no longer used (6).

Bleomycin

Bleomycin is an antibiotic complex that results in DNA fragmentation. It is used in combination therapy against testicular cancer and also in the management of lymphomas and head and neck cancers (11). Vascular toxicity associated with cerebral infarction has been described with bleomycin use, but only when it had been combined with cisplatin with or without vinblastine and etoposide in a multidrug regimen (21,22).

TOPOISOMERASE INHIBITORS

Etoposide

Etoposide (VP-16) is used in the treatment of lung cancer, leukemias, and testicular cancer. In standard doses, it is largely free of neurotoxicity. In high doses, encephalopathy, seizures (23), headache (7), and peripheral neuropathy can occur (2).

MISCELLANEOUS CHEMOTHERAPY

L-Asparaginase

L-asparaginase acts by deaminating the amino acid L-asparagine, ultimately resulting in apoptosis (11). It is typically used in combination therapy for acute lymphocytic leukemia. In high doses, encephalopathy, seizures, and even coma can occur. L-asparaginase also causes a reduction in plasminogen, fibrinogen, antithrombin, and protein-C levels, leading to cerebrovascular complications in 1% to 2% of patients (15). Cerebrovascular complications, such as sinovenous or arterial thromboses, are usually characterized by sudden focal neurologic deficits or seizures in patients receiving L-asparaginase (6).

Thalidomide

Thalidomide is a glutamic acid derivative used in the treatment of multiple cancers, including multiple myeloma, acute myeloid leukemia, breast cancer, and in renal, prostate, and colon tumors. Its dose-limiting toxicity is peripheral neuropathy. Symptoms are distal sensory loss and paresthesias, largely sparing motor function. Evidence suggests that the risk of neuropathy is very low if the dose is <20 g (24). The neuropathy can persist, even when treatment is discontinued. Somnolence is also a fairly common side effect of thalidomide (2).

HORMONAL THERAPY

Tamoxifen

Tamoxifen is a nonsteroidal antiestrogen used in the treatment of estrogen-receptor positive breast cancer. Although neurologic toxicity is fairly uncommon, difficulties with central vision, retinal changes in the macula, dizziness and ataxia may be seen in patients on high dose therapy (2). Tamoxifen has also been associated with thromboembolic complications in 1% to 2% of patients (1).

BIOLOGICAL THERAPIES

Interferon-α

Interferon-α (IFN-α) is a naturally occurring cytokine used in the treatment of hematologic malignancies as well as Kaposi sarcoma, melanoma, and renal cell carcinoma. At low doses, flulike symptoms, such as headache, fever, and myalgias, can occur (3). In higher dosages, an encephalopathy marked by somnolence, memory dysfunction, and seizures has been described (25). Patients taking IFN-α are also at risk of developing depression with frontal-subcortical dysfunction (26). Pretreatment with paroxetine may lessen those symptoms (27). Other possible toxicities include parkinsonism with intention tremor and, rarely, brachial plexopathy, oculomotor palsy, and myasthenia gravis (2).

Interleukins

Interleukin-2 (IL-2) is used in the treatment of renal cell carcinoma, melanoma, and lymphoma (11). IL-2 produces toxicity by increasing vascular permeability, and causes hallucinations, agitation, seizures, coma, and transient focal neurologic deficits. Carpal tunnel syndrome has also been reported, possibly related to edema surrounding the median nerve (2). When combined with granulocyte macrophage colony-stimulating factor (GM-CSF), acute multifocal cerebral venous thrombosis, acute subdural hemorrhage, and subarachnoid hemorrhage have occurred (28).

Rituximab

Rituximab (Rituxan) is a monoclonal antibody used in the treatment of B-cell lymphomas. Neurologic toxicity is not prominent, but mild to moderate dizziness, headache, paresthesias, and lethargy have been reported (29).

Growth Factors

COLONY-STIMULATING FACTORS: GRANULOCYTE COLONY-STIMULATING FACTOR (G-CSF) AND GM-CSF. These agents are often used in patients with nonmyeloid tumors who are receiving chemotherapy. A syndrome of acute disorientation, agitation, cortical blindness, and seizures can occur in patients taking GM-CSF (30). A similar syndrome has also been reported with G-CSF. In one case, however, the patient was also taking vincristine, ifosfamide, and etoposide and this syndrome may have been the result of a multidrug regimen (31).

Erythropoietin

Erythropoietin is used in the treatment of chronic anemia and end-stage renal failure. Its use is associated with hypertension and hypertensive posterior leukoencephalopathy. The most common symptoms include headache, lethargy, seizures, nausea, and visual disturbance (e.g., cortical blindness, hemianopia, or visual neglect). Posterior white matter signal abnormalities are often seen on MRI of these patients (32). Thrombotic events, such as transient ischemic attacks and cerebral venous thrombosis, can also occur with its use (33).

CLINICAL RECOMMENDATIONS OF THE VIGNETTE

The quality and timing of this patient's symptoms, as well as the physical examination findings, support a diagnosis of chemotherapy-induced peripheral neuropathy. Electrophysiologic studies demonstrated a predominantly moderate sensory neuropathy affecting both lower limbs. The patient had tried gabapentin in adequate doses, and it did not relieve her symptoms. A trial of duloxetine, starting at 30 mg daily and titrating to 60 mg daily, did provide significant relief of the paresthesias and dysesthesias. This was combined with a course of physical therapy, which significantly improved the stability of her gait.

SUMMARY

Cancer chemotherapies can cause many adverse neurologic effects, involving both the peripheral and central nervous systems. It is important to be aware of the potential adverse effects because many of them are dose limiting. Furthermore, many clinically relevant multidrug interactions can have a negative impact on the nervous system. Further research is needed in the area of neuroprotection against these harmful side effects. By being aware of these issues, chemotherapy regimens can be altered appropriately to optimize the quality of life for patients.

REFERENCES

1. Posner JB. *Neurologic Complications of Cancer.* Contemporary Neurology Series, 1995;45: 282–310.
2. New PZ. Neurologic Complications of Chemotherapeutic and Biological Agents. *Continuum.* 2005;11(5):116–152.
3. Plotkin SR, Wen PY. Neurologic complications of cancer therapy. *Neurol Clin N Am.* 2003;20:279–318.
4. Verstappen CCP, Heimans J, Hoekman K, et al. Progressive multifocal leukoencephalopathy after fludarabine therapy for low grade lymphoproliferative disease. *Am J Hematol.* 2002;70(1):51–54.
5. Kim YA, Chung HC, Choi HJ, et al. Intermediate dose 5-fluorouracil-induced encephalopathy. *Jpn J Clin Oncol.* 2006;36(1):55–59.
6. Biller J. Complications of chemotherapy, In: Biller J, ed. *Iatrogenic Neurology,* 1st ed. Woburn, MA: Butterworth-Heinemann; 1998:439–459.
7. Verstappen CCP, Heimans J, Hoekman K, et al. Neurotoxic complications of chemotherapy in patients with cancer. *Drugs.* 2003;63(15):1549–1563.
8. Brashear A, Siemers E. Focal dystonia after chemotherapy: A case series. *J Neurooncol.* 1997;34:163–167.
9. Haykin ME, Gorman M, van Hoff J, et al. Diffusion-weighted MRI correlates of subacute methotrexate-related toxicity. *J Neurooncol.* 2006;76:153–157.
10. Brock S, Jennings HR. Fatal acute encephalomyelitis after a single dose of intrathecal methotrexate. *Pharmacotherapy.* 2004;24(5):673–676.
11. Haskell CM. Antineoplastic agents. In: CM Haskel, ed. *Cancer Treatment,* 5th ed. Philadelphia: WB Saunders; 2001:111–213.
12. Mielke S, Sparreboom A, Mross K. Peripheral neuropathy: A persisting challenge in paclitaxel-based regimens. *Eur J Cancer.* 2006;42:24–30.
13. Hausheer FH, Schilsky RL, Bain S, et al. Diagnosis, management, and evaluation of chemotherapy-induced peripheral neuropathy. *Semin Oncol.* 2006;33:15–49.
14. Visovsky C. Chemotherapy-induced peripheral neuropathy. *Cancer Invest.* 2003;21(3): 439–451.
15. Rogers L. Cerebrovascular complications in cancer patients. *Neurology Clinics of North America.* 2003;21:167–192.
16. Primavera A, Audenino D, Cocito L. Ifosfamide encephalopathy and nonconvulsive status epilepticus. *Can J Neurol Sci.* 2002;29(2):180–183.
17. Kilickap S, Cakar M, Onal IK, et al. Nonconvulsive status epilepticus due to ifosfamide. *Ann Pharmacother.* 2006;40(2):332–335.
18. La Morgia C, Mondini S, Guarino M, et al. Busulfan neurotoxicity and EEG abnormalities: A case report. *Neurol Sci.* 2004;25(2):95–97.
19. Djaldetti M, Pinkhas J, de Vries A, et al. Myasthenia gravis in a patient with chronic myeloid leukemia treated by busulfan. *Blood.* 1968;32:336.
20. Jordan B, Pasquier Y, Schnider A. Neurological improvement and rehabilitation potential following toxic myelopathy due to intrathecal injection of doxorubicin. *Spinal Cord.* 2004;42(6):371–373.
21. Samuels BL, Vogelzang NJ, Kennedy BJ. Vascular toxicity following vinblastine, bleomycin and cisplatin therapy for germ cell tumors. *Int J Androl.* 1987;10(1):363–369.
22. Brouha ME, Bleomendal HJ, Kappelle LJ, et al. Cerebral infarction and myocardial infarction due to cisplatin-containing chemotherapy. *Ned Tijdschr Geneeskund.* 2003;147(10):457–460.
23. Keime-Guibert F, Napolitano M, Delattre J. Neurological complications of radiotherapy and chemotherapy. *J Neurol.* 1998;245:695–708.
24. Cavaletti G, Beronio A, Reni L, et al. Thalidomide sensory neurotoxicity. *Neurology.* 2004; 62:2291–2293.
25. Ulbricht D, Metz RJ, Ries F, et al. Alpha-interferon encephalopathy. *Neurology.* 2003;61(9): 1301.
26. Meyers CA, Scheibel RS, Forman AD. Persistent neurotoxicity of systemically administered interferon-alpha. *Neurology.* 1991;41(5):672–676.
27. Capuron L, Gumnick JF, Musselman DL, et al. Neurobehavioral effects of interferon-alpha in cancer patients: Phenomenology and paroxetine responsiveness of symptom dimensions. *Neuropsychopharmacology* 2002;26(5):643–652.
28. Hotton KM, Khorsand M, Hank JA, et al. A phase Ib/II trial of granulocyte-macrophage-colony stimulating factor and interleukin 2 for renal cell carcinoma patients with pulmonary metastases. *Cancer.* 2000;88(8):1892–1901.
29. Foran JM, Rohatiner AZ, Cunningham D, et al. European Phase II study of rituximab (chimeric anti-CD20 monoclonal antibody) for patients with newly diagnosed mantle-cell lymphoma and previously treated mantle-cell lymphoma, immunocytoma, and small B-cell lymphocytic lymphoma. *J Clin Oncol.* 2000;18(2):317–324.
30. Kastrup O, Diener HC. Granulocyte-stimulating factor filgrastim and molgrastim induced recurring encephalopathy and focal status. *J Neurol.* 1997;244:274–275.
31. Leniger T, Kastrup O, Diener HC. Reversible posterior leukencephalopathy syndrome induced by granulocyte stimulating factor filgrastim. *J Neurol Neurosurg Psychiatry.* 2000;69:280–281.
32. Delanty N, Vaughan C, Frucht S, et al. Erythropoietin-associated hypertensive posterior leukoencephalopathy. *Neurology.* 1997;49(3):686–689.
33. Finelli PF, Matthew CD. Cerebral venous thrombosis associated with epoetin alfa therapy. *Arch Neurol.* 2000;57(2):260–262.

PART VII Oncologic Diseases

CHAPTER 57

Paraneoplastic Disorders of the Central Nervous System

Edward J. Dropcho

OBJECTIVES

- To survey the variety of clinical manifestations of paraneoplastic disorders affecting the central nervous system (CNS)
- To discuss the diagnostic approach to patients with suspected CNS paraneoplastic disorders, including the appropriate use of antineuronal antibodies as diagnostic markers
- To describe the management approaches for patients with CNS syndromes

CASE VIGNETTE

A 67-year-old woman with a long history of cigarette smoking awoke with vertigo, nausea, and blurred vision. Over the next 2 weeks, she developed slurred speech, vomiting, clumsiness, and "staggering." Examination revealed opsoclonus, moderate dysarthria, limb dysmetria, and severe gait ataxia. Brain magnetic resonance imaging (MRI) scan was normal. Cerebrospinal fluid (CSF) showed a white blood count (WBC) of 5, protein 78, and no oligoclonal bands. Chest X-ray study was normal. Anti-Yo antibodies were detected in her serum.

DEFINITION

Neurologic paraneoplastic disorders are nonmetastatic syndromes not attributable to toxicity of cancer therapy, cerebrovascular disease, coagulopathy, infection, or toxic or metabolic causes.

EPIDEMIOLOGY

Almost any type of tumor has been associated with paraneoplastic disorders, but for most paraneoplastic neurologic syndromes there is an overrepresentation of one or a few particular neoplasms. Small cell lung carcinoma is the tumor most often associated with CNS paraneoplastic phenomena in adults. Approximately 1% to 3% of patients with small cell lung carcinoma develop Lambert-Eaton myasthenic syndrome or another paraneoplastic syndrome. Other tumors over represented among patients with paraneoplastic syndromes include breast carcinoma, ovarian carcinoma, Hodgkin lymphoma, thymoma, and testicular germ cell tumors (1,2).

ETIOLOGY AND PATHOGENESIS

Most neurologic paraneoplastic disorders are believed to be autoimmune diseases, although with some exceptions, the exact immunopathogenetic mechanisms remain unclear. The central theory of autoimmunity for paraneoplastic disorders postulates that tumor cells express *onconeural* antigen(s) identical or antigenically related to molecules normally expressed by neurons and, in rare instances, an autoimmune response initially arising against the tumor subsequently attacks neurons expressing the same or related antigen(s).

Since the mid-1980s, a steadily growing list of antineuronal antibodies have been identified in the sera of patients with paraneoplastic disorders (Table 57-1). The neuronal molecular targets of many of these autoantibodies have been cloned and characterized (3,4). Some paraneoplastic antibodies have selective neuronal reactivity and are highly restricted to patients with a particular clinical syndrome, such as antirecoverin antibodies in patients with retinal degeneration, and anti-Yo or anti-Tr antibodies in patients with cerebellar degeneration. Most paraneoplastic autoantibodies show a more widespread or pan-neuronal reactivity and are associated with a variety of clinical neurologic syndromes, or with multifocal encephalomyelitis. Overall, the most prevalent such antibodies are anti-Hu and anti-CV2. It is not rare for patients with small cell lung carcinoma to have more than one type of autoantibody (5). Except for antibodies against cell-surface receptors or membrane ion channels, nearly all paraneoplastic antibodies associated with CNS syndromes react with intracytoplasmic or intranuclear neuronal proteins. Protein antigens reacting with antineuronal antibodies are known to be expressed by tumors from affected patients, supporting the general theory of an autoimmune response arising against shared onconeural antigens.

For some CNS paraneoplastic syndromes antineuronal autoantibodies are directly involved in causing clinical disease:

- Antibodies against voltage-gated potassium channels can cause neuronal injury or dysfunction in some patients with limbic encephalitis (6).
- Antibodies against voltage-gated calcium channels (7) or glutamate receptors (8) can directly mediate Purkinje cell injury in some patients with paraneoplastic cerebellar degeneration.

TABLE 57-1. CNS Paraneoplastic Disorders and Autoantibodies

Clinical Syndrome	*Associated Tumor(s)*	*Autoantibodies*
Multifocal encephalomyelitis	SCLC	Anti-Hu (ANNA-1), anti-CV2 (CRMP-5), anti-amphiphysin, anti-Ri, ANNA-3
	Various carcinomas	Anti-Ma1, anti-Hu, anti-CV2
Limbic encephalitis	SCLC	Anti-Hu, anti-CV2, PCA-2, ANNA-3 anti-amphiphysin, anti-VGKC, anti-VGCC, anti-Zic4
	Testicular, breast	Anti-Ma2
	thymoma,	Anti-VGKC, anti-CV2
	ovarian teratoma,	Anti-neuropil
	ovarian, others	Anti-Yo, anti-Ma1, anti-Ri
Cerebellar degeneration	SCLC, others	Anti-Hu, anti-CV2, PCA-2, ANNA-3, anti-amphiphysin, anti-VGCC, anti-Ri, anti-Zic4
	Hodgkin lymphoma,	Anti-Tr, anti-mGluR1
	breast, ovarian	Anti-Ri, anti-Yo, anti-amphiphysin
Opsoclonus-myoclonus	SCLC	Anti-Hu, anti-Ri, anti-CV2, anti-amphiphysin
	Neuroblastoma,	Anti-Hu, others
	testicular, others	Anti-Ma2
Extrapyramidal syndrome	SCLC, thymoma	Anti-CV2, anti-Hu
Brainstem encephalitis	SCLC, breast, others	Anti-Hu, anti-Ri
	Testicular	Anti-Ma2
Optic neuritis	SCLC	Anti-CV2
Retinal degeneration	SCLC, others	Anti-recoverin
	Melanoma	Anti-bipolar cell
Myelopathy	SCLC, thymoma	Anti-CV2, anti-amphiphysin
Stiff-person syndrome	Breast, SCLC, others	Anti-amphiphysin, anti-Ri, anti-GAD
Motor neuron disease	SCLC, others	Anti-Hu

SCLC, small cell lung carcinoma.

- Antiamphiphysin antibodies can directly contribute to causing paraneoplastic stiff-person syndrome (9).
- Autoantibodies probably exert a direct cytotoxic effect in patients with paraneoplastic retinal degeneration, perhaps in concert with cellular immune effectors (10).

For most of the CNS syndromes associated with antineuronal antibodies, the antibodies are probably an epiphenomenon or *footprint* for autoimmunity and not directly involved in causing neuronal injury. Recent studies of anti-Yo, antibody-associated paraneoplastic cerebellar degeneration (11), anti-Hu, antibody-associated encephalomyelitis or sensory neuronopathy (12), and anti-Ma2, antibody-associated limbic encephalitis (13) implicate cell-mediated immune effectors in causing neuronal injury. For these disorders, it is postulated that onconeural antigens released by apoptotic tumor cells are presented to T lymphocytes in draining peripheral lymph nodes, initiating a Th1 helper response that eventually gains access to the CNS and attacks neurons expressing the antigens (14). Many unanswered questions remain regarding how this exactly happens. To date, no fully successful animal models have reproduced cell-mediated paraneoplastic disorders in the CNS.

PATHOLOGY

The pathologic hallmarks of CNS paraneoplastic disorders are neuronal loss and infiltration of inflammatory mononuclear cells. In patients with multifocal encephalomyelitis (especially those with small cell lung cancer), these changes are patchy and can involve any or all areas of the cerebral hemispheres, limbic system, basal ganglia, cerebellum, brainstem, spinal cord, dorsal root ganglia, and autonomic ganglia. Patients with a predominantly cerebellar syndrome show severe, diffuse loss of Purkinje cells throughout the cerebellar cortex, and a lesser degree of neuronal loss in the granular cell layer and deep cerebellar nuclei. Patients with predominant limbic encephalopathy show extensive neuronal loss, gliosis, and microglial nodules in the hippocampus and amygdala (13,15). Similar, but less severe, changes are often present in the parahippocampal gyrus, cingulate gyrus, insular cortex, orbital frontal cortex, basal ganglia, and diencephalon. Some adults and children with paraneoplastic opsoclonus-myoclonus have no definable neuropathologic lesions at autopsy. In these patients, immune-mediated neuronal injury or dysfunction in the brainstem or cerebellum may have occurred without causing actual neuronal death.

In CNS paraneoplastic disorders, the inflammatory changes accompanying neuronal loss include parenchymal and perivascular infiltration of T and B lymphocytes and plasma cells. The degree of inflammation does not correlate very well with the degree of neuronal loss. By the time of autopsy, some patients have minimal inflammatory changes; in these cases, the autoimmune or inflammatory process may have *burned out.*

CLINICAL MANIFESTATIONS

Paraneoplastic disorders can affect any part(s) of the CNS. For most patients, the neurologic syndrome is the presenting feature of a previously undiagnosed neoplasm. Many patients can be grouped into a recognizable clinical neurologic syndrome predominantly affecting one anatomic location or system, such as cerebellar degeneration or limbic encephalitis (Table 57-1) (4). Other patients do not neatly fit into this scheme, because they have signs and symptoms of more than one syndrome. In most patients with small cell lung cancer and many patients with other neoplasms, paraneoplastic disorders are subsets of a diffuse and multifocal "paraneoplastic encephalomyelitis" in which individual patients may show predominant involvement of particular parts of the nervous system.

Several CNS syndromes should always raise the possibility of a paraneoplastic etiology, including subacute cerebellar degeneration, limbic encephalopathy, opsoclonus-myoclonus in children or adults, and unexplained multifocal encephalomyelitis (16,17). It is important to keep in mind, however, that no neurologic syndrome is absolutely pathognomonic for a paraneoplastic etiology; all of the syndromes listed in Table 57-1 have their "nonparaneoplastic" counterparts.

MULTIFOCAL ENCEPHALOMYELITIS

Small cell lung carcinoma is by far the tumor most commonly associated with paraneoplastic encephalomyelitis, with a scattering of patients with a variety of other neoplasms (18–21). The most common clinical manifestation of encephalomyelitis is subacute sensory neuronopathy reflecting involvement of the dorsal root ganglia (see Chapter 58). Other patients have a predominant clinical syndrome of focal cortical encephalitis, limbic encephalitis, extrapyramidal movement disorder, subacute cerebellar degeneration, brainstem encephalitis, or motor neuron disease. Regardless of an individual patient's predominant clinical manifestations, nearly all display signs and symptoms of multifocal involvement of the CNS and dorsal root ganglia. Patients may additionally show involvement of the peripheral nervous system, including sensorimotor polyneuropathy, mononeuritis multiplex, autonomic system failure, or Lambert-Eaton syndrome (see Chapter 58, *Paraneoplastic Disorders of the Peripheral Nervous System*).

The most common clinical course of paraneoplastic encephalomyelitis is deterioration over a period of weeks to months, and then stabilization at a level of severe neurologic disability, regardless of treatment (see below). Subsequent stepwise or gradual neurologic deterioration is less common and tends to occur in patients with less than complete response of the associated small cell lung cancer to treatment (20).

LIMBIC ENCEPHALITIS

Approximately 50% to 60% of reported patients with paraneoplastic limbic encephalitis have small cell lung carcinoma (15,22,23). Other associated neoplasms include testicular germ cell tumors (13), thymoma (24), Hodgkin lymphoma (25), ovarian teratoma (26), and a number of carcinomas.

Paraneoplastic limbic encephalitis generally has a subacute onset evolving over days to weeks. Patients typically present either with an amnestic syndrome or psychiatric disorder; most patients eventually develop features of both (15,22,23). The memory loss includes short-term anterograde amnesia and a variable period of retrograde amnesia. Denial of the deficit and confabulation are common. The affective disorder usually includes some combination of depression, anxiety, emotional lability, and personality change. Hallucinations and paranoid delusions can occur. Generalized or partial complex seizures occur in most patients; they may be the initial neurologic feature and can be medically intractable. Less common manifestations of limbic or diencephalic dysfunction include abnormal sleep–wake cycles, disturbed temperature regulation, labile blood pressure, inappropriate secretion of antidiuretic hormone, and elements of the Klüver-Bucy syndrome, such as hyperphagia and hypersexuality (13).

Most patients with paraneoplastic limbic encephalitis have antineuronal autoantibodies, depending on the associated tumor (Table 57-1). Of particular note are the recent associations of antivoltage-gated potassium channel (anti-VGKC) antibodies with thymoma (2), of anti-Ma2 antibodies in young men with testicular germ cell tumors (13), and of "novel neuropil antibodies" in young women with ovarian teratoma (24,26). Some patients with anti-Ma2 antibodies have a clinically *pure* limbic encephalitis, whereas most present with a combined syndrome reflecting involvement of the limbic system, diencephalon (e.g., sleep disorder or autonomic dysfunction), and brainstem (especially ocular motor disturbance) (13). Some patients with anti-VGKC antibodies have *Morvan's fibrillary chorea* featuring neuromyotonia, dysautonomia, insomnia, and encephalopathy (27). Patients with "novel neuropil antibodies" can have a *typical* limbic encephalopathy, whereas others have a more acute and severe clinical course with psychosis, seizures, lethargy, and central hypoventilation requiring extended ventilatory support (24,26).

The course of paraneoplastic limbic encephalitis is variable and unpredictable. A few patients with clinically pure limbic encephalitis show spontaneous remission of the neurologic condition before any treatment (28). A significant proportion of patients will have neurologic improvement with tumor treatment, immunotherapy, or both (see below).

CEREBELLAR DEGENERATION

Of patients with paraneoplastic cerebellar degeneration, 90% have small cell lung carcinoma, Hodgkin lymphoma, or carcinomas of the breast, ovary, or female genital tract (1,29–31). The clinical features are similar regardless of the associated tumor type. Typically, the onset is fairly abrupt. Signs and symptoms reflect diffuse dysfunction of the cerebellum, including dysarthria and severe appendicular and gait ataxia. Abnormalities of oculomotor function are common and include nystagmus, particularly downbeat nystagmus, disruption of smooth pursuit movements, ocular dysmetria, and opsoclonus. Superimposed on the cerebellar deficits, symptoms or signs of multifocal encephalomyelitis develop in many patients. Paraneoplastic cerebellar degeneration can also occur in conjunction with paraneoplastic peripheral neuropathy or Lambert-Eaton myasthenic syndrome, usually in patients with small cell lung carcinoma (32).

Virtually all *paraneoplastic antibodies* react with antigens in the cerebellum and can be associated with clinical cerebellar dysfunction (Table 57-1). Anti-Yo, anti-Tr, and anti-mGlu1 glutamate receptor antibodies are associated with a pure cerebellar syndrome (31,33), whereas the other paraneoplastic antibodies occur in patients with a variety of clinical presentations, including cerebellar dysfunction or multifocal encephalomyelitis.

The neurologic deficits in paraneoplastic cerebellar degeneration generally worsen over a period of several weeks to months and then stabilize at a level of severe disability. Only about one third of patients can walk independently, and many patients cannot sit up or feed themselves. Significant neurologic improvement, either spontaneously or after successful treatment of the associated tumor, is distinctly unusual (see below).

OPSOCLONUS-MYOCLONUS

Opsoclonus is defined as continuous, multidirectional rapid eye movements (saccadic oscillations) without an intersaccadic interval. Paraneoplastic opsoclonus most commonly occurs in children with neuroblastoma (4). Opsoclonus as a remote effect of cancer is less common in adults, with small cell lung carcinoma and breast carcinoma together accounting for approximately 70% of reported cases (34–36). The neurologic symptoms and signs that accompany paraneoplastic opsoclonus in adults are heterogeneous. Nearly all patients have one or more of the following: (*a*) spontaneous and stimulus-sensitive limb myoclonus, sometimes also involving the palate, face, larynx, or respiratory muscles; (*b*) pancerebellar dysfunction, including limb, truncal, and gait ataxia, which varies in severity from mild to incapacitating; and (*c*) signs and symptoms of brainstem dysfunction, including vertigo, vomiting, dysphagia, gaze palsy, jaw opening dystonia, and laryngospasm. Patients may have additional signs and symptoms that reflect multifocal encephalomyelitis. Antineuronal antibody associations are listed in Table 57-1.

As a group, adults with paraneoplastic opsoclonus have a better neurologic outcome than patients with paraneoplastic cerebellar degeneration or encephalomyelitis. In some patients, the opsoclonus and other neurologic features spontaneously improve before any therapy. Patients may show significant neurologic improvement with successful treatment of the associated tumor or immunotherapy (35,36) (see below).

EXTRAPYRAMIDAL SYNDROMES

Chorea, athetosis, dystonia, or parkinsonism are rare manifestations of paraneoplastic encephalitis, occurring most often in association with small cell lung carcinoma (37,38) and also with lymphoma, thymoma, or other tumors (13). The extrapyramidal features can occur with or without other signs of multifocal encephalomyelitis.

BRAINSTEM ENCEPHALITIS

Paraneoplastic *brainstem encephalitis* manifests as a variety of gaze palsies or other ocular motor disturbance, possibly together with dysarthria, dysphagia, facial weakness, vertigo, central respiratory failure, or other signs and symptoms referable to the brainstem. This most commonly occurs in the setting of multifocal encephalomyelitis associated with small cell lung carcinoma (39) or in patients with testicular germ cell tumor who generally have additional limbic or hypothalamic involvement (13).

OPTIC NEURITIS

Optic neuritis is a rare complication of breast carcinoma, small cell lung carcinoma, or other tumors. Nothing is clinically distinctive about the optic neuritis in these patients, who have decreased visual acuity, afferent pupillary defects, cecocentral scotomas, and disc edema. Visual symptoms can occur with or without other signs and symptoms of multifocal encephalomyelitis (40). A few reported patients had combined optic neuritis and myelopathy resembling Devic disease (41).

MYELOPATHY

Patients with paraneoplastic encephalomyelitis associated with small cell lung cancer, breast carcinoma, thymoma, or other tumor may present with a predominant myelopathy syndrome. Some of these patients have myelopathy with rigidity, myeloradiculopathy, or Devic's disease (41–43). Paraneoplastic necrotizing myelopathy is a rare syndrome which is probably distinct from the multifocal patchy involvement of the spinal cord in cases of encephaloymelitis (44). This syndrome has occurred in association with a variety of carcinomas and lymphoid tumors, without a clear preponderance of any specific tumor type. Most patients suffer rapid deterioration of function and a progressively ascending level of flaccid paralysis and numbness, often leading to death from respiratory failure or medical complications.

STIFF-PERSON SYNDROME

A syndrome of muscle rigidity and spasms, which clinically resembles the *stiff-person syndrome,* is associated with a variety of neoplasms, including small cell lung carcinoma, thymoma, Hodgkin lymphoma, and carcinoma of the breast or colon (45,46). The rigidity is probably caused by multifocal encephalomyelitis affecting the spinal cord or brainstem. Patients develop progressive aching and rigidity of the axial and proximal limb musculature, usually asymmetric at onset. Superimposed are painful and sometimes violent spasms, either occurring spontaneously or triggered by voluntary movement, passive movement, or sensory stimuli. The most severely affected patients may develop opisthotonos and respiratory difficulty.

MOTOR NEURON DISEASE

Motor neuron dysfunction as a paraneoplastic phenomenon occurs in a variety of different settings. Lower motor neuron signs and symptoms reflecting anterior horn cell involvement are among the presenting or predominant manifestations in up to 25% of patients with multifocal encephalomyelitis associated with anti-Hu or other antibodies (18,21). A more problematic issue is how often, if ever, isolated motor neuron disease or amyotrophic lateral sclerosis (ALS) is a paraneoplastic syndrome (47). No convincing epidemiologic evidence indicates that nonhematologic neoplasms occur in patients with ALS any more frequently than would be expected in an age-matched control population. Despite the absence of a clear epidemiologic link between motor neuron disease and neoplasia, the relationship in small subsets of patients is probably more than coincidental. There are several well-described patients with a lower motor neuron syndrome or combined upper and lower motor neuron syndrome who had significant neurologic improvement after resection of lung or renal carcinomas (48).

An association exists between ALS or *progressive spinal muscular atrophy* and lymphoproliferative disease, including Hodgkin lymphoma, non-Hodgkin lymphoma, and chronic lymphocytic leukemia (49). In approximately half of reported patients, the neurologic symptoms preceded diagnosis of the lymphoproliferative disease. Most patients with an ALS-like syndrome have progressive weakness leading to a fatal outcome despite treatment of the associated lymphoproliferative disease.

DIAGNOSTIC APPROACH

The clinical management of cases of patients with known or suspected paraneoplastic syndromes includes four components: (*a*) verification that the disorder is in fact paraneoplastic; (*b*) identification of the associated tumor; (*c*) treatment of the tumor; and (*d*) suppression of the autoimmune effectors causing neuronal injury.

Differential diagnosis of patients with a suspected paraneoplastic disorder varies with whether there is a known cancer diagnosis. Among patients with neurologic dysfunction and a known cancer diagnosis, the level of suspicion for a paraneoplastic disorders depends on the neurologic syndrome, tumor histology, and presence of antineuronal antibodies. Tumor metastases and neurotoxicity of cancer treatments are far more common than paraneoplastic disorders and should always be considered, as should metabolic derangements and CNS infection. For patients without a previous cancer diagnosis, the level of suspicion for a paraneoplastic disorder depends on patient age, gender, risk factors (especially cigarette smoking), the neurologic syndrome, and the presence of antineuronal antibodies (17).

Neuroimaging and CSF evaluation are often abnormal in CNS paraneoplastic disorders, but do not in themselves prove a paraneoplastic etiology. Brain MR scans in patients with paraneoplastic encephalomyelitis may (or may not) show focal lesions in the cerebral cortex, limbic system, basal ganglia, brainstem, or spinal cord in patients with corresponding clinical involvement. Brain MR scans in patients with paraneoplastic cerebellar degeneration or opsoclonus-myoclonus are usually normal early in the course of the illness, and later show nonspecific diffuse cerebellar atrophy. Brain MR scans in at least two thirds of patients with paraneoplastic limbic encephalitis show areas of abnormal T2-weighted or fluid-attenuated inversion recovery (FLAIR) signal in the mesial temporal lobe and amygdala bilaterally, and less commonly in the hypothalamus and basal frontal cortex (13,15,22,23). Some patients additionally have lesions in the extratemporal cerebral hemispheres, diencephalon, or brainstem.

Most patients with CNS paraneoplastic syndromes have abnormal CSF, including some combination of mildly elevated protein, mild mononuclear pleocytosis, elevated IgG index, or oligoclonal bands. Normal CSF does not exclude a paraneoplastic diagnosis.

Good, but not perfect, correlations exist among particular paraneoplastic syndromes, antineuronal antibody specificities, and associated tumor types (Table 57-1). The practical clinical value of antineuronal antibodies is that when present, they greatly increase the index of suspicion for a paraneoplastic condition, and the type of antibody can help guide the search for the associated tumor (5,16,17). Antineuronal antibody assays do, however, have important practical clinical limitations:

- A given clinical syndrome can be associated with one of several autoantibodies.
- Conversely, a given autoantibody can be associated with a variety of clinical presentations.
- For most, if not all, CNS syndromes, some patients have antineuronal autoantibodies and yet never develop a demonstrable tumor. The prime example is nonparaneoplastic limbic encephalitis associated with anti-voltage-gated potassium channel antibodies (50,51). The presence of antibodies, therefore, does not absolutely indicate an underlying neoplasm.
- Some autoantibodies are present at low titers in patients with tumor without any accompanying clinical neurologic manifestations.
- Patients with a suspected paraneoplastic syndrome may not have demonstrable antineuronal antibodies, or may have *atypical* or incompletely characterized antibodies not detected in commercially available assays. Some patients initially determined to be *negative* for the more common antibodies eventually are found to have newly recognized antibodies as the list of paraneoplastic antibodies grows. A negative antibody assay, therefore, does not rule out the possibility of a paraneoplastic disorder and the presence of an underlying neoplasm.

The tumor workup for adults should include CT or MR scans of the chest and abdomen, as well as mammography and pelvic examination or imaging in women. Chest CT or MR scanning is more sensitive than plain chest X-ray studies in detecting a lung neoplasm. Testicular ultrasound may detect a small germ cell tumor in young men. Total-body [^{18}F]fluorodeoxyglucose positron emission tomography (FDG-PET) scanning may demonstrate a neoplasm in patients with suspected paraneoplastic disorders, with or without autoantibodies, in whom other imaging studies are negative or equivocal (52,53). For patients with any of the syndromes, it is not uncommon for the tumor to be found only after repeated searches.

TREATMENT

For at least some patients with CNS paraneoplastic disorders, successful tumor treatment is associated with better neurologic outcome. Patients with some syndromes, most notably limbic encephalitis (13,15,24) and opsoclonus-myoclonus (35,36), often show neurologic improvement solely with successful tumor therapy. Some patients with cerebellar degeneration and Hodgkin lymphoma, and exceptional patients with carcinoma, improve neurologically after successful tumor treatment (1,31,33).

If paraneoplastic disorders are truly autoimmune diseases, theoretically they should respond to immunosuppressive or immunomodulatory treatment. Several factors make it difficult to interpret the published literature regarding immunotherapy for CNS paraneoplastic disorders:

- These syndromes are relatively rare. For some of the syndromes, only a few well-characterized cases have been published.
- Most reports are anecdotal and nearly all published series are retrospective. Prospective studies of plasma exchange plus cyclophosphamide (54) or of immunoadsorption therapy (55) for CNS syndromes included patients with a variety of clinical syndromes and associated antineuronal antibodies.

- A reporting bias is noted, in that patients who respond to treatment are more likely to be published than those who do not respond.
- Paraneoplastic cerebellar degeneration, encephalomyelitis or sensory neuronopathy, and other syndromes often stabilize spontaneously (although at a level of severe disability), so that it is difficult to interpret reports of "disease stabilization" with immunotherapy.
- Perhaps the greatest difficulty in evaluating immunotherapy for paraneoplastic disorders is the confounding effect of tumor treatment. When patients receive concomitant tumor treatment and immunotherapy, it is difficult to discern the impact of each therapy on the neurologic outcome. For many, if not most, patients, immunotherapy is more likely to be effective when the tumor is also treated successfully (13,16,21).

The two most prevalent paraneoplastic CNS syndromes in adults (i.e., multifocal encephalomyelitis or sensory neuronopathy and cerebellar degeneration), however, usually have a poor prognosis despite aggressive tumor treatment and a variety of immunosuppressive therapies (21,31,56). Patients with other CNS syndromes, including opsoclonus-myoclonus (55,57), limbic encephalitis (13,15,24), or stiff-person syndrome (45) have a somewhat higher likelihood of neurologic improvement with immunotherapy, suggesting that the immune-mediated neuronal dysfunction or injury is less severe or of a sort more likely to be reversible.

Even for the *unfavorable* syndromes, such as encephalomyelitis and cerebellar degeneration, a few patients do show a meaningful neurologic response to immunotherapy (1,54,58). For these few responders, the only factors that sometimes correlate with neurologic improvement are successful tumor treatment, and the duration and severity of neurologic deficits before diagnosis and initiation of therapy. For patients who are already stabilized at a plateau of severe neurologic disability for more than several weeks, subsequent improvement with any intervention is not impossible but extremely unlikely. The decision whether to try immunosuppressive therapies, therefore, must be based on the particular syndrome and on the individual patient's circumstances.

Corticosteroids and intravenous gamma globulin (IVIG) are the most commonly used immunotherapies for paraneoplastic disorders. Patients generally receive an initially high dose of intravenous or oral steroid (predinisone, methylprednisolone, dexamethasone) followed by a slow or rapid taper. No clear evidence indicates the optimal drug, dose, route of administration, or schedule of corticosteroids. IVIG can be tried alone or in combination with corticosteroids. Plasma exchange could arguably be reserved for syndromes that are definitely antibody mediated, but reports exist of improvement in patients with other syndromes as well (54). Chronic oral or pulsed intravenous cyclophosphamide have also been used for a variety of paraneoplastic disorders (54), with anecdotal responses and no definite evidence supporting a particular schedule or dose. One small study of immunoadsorption with a staphylococcus protein A column showed neurologic improvement in some patients with varied paraneoplastic disorders (55). There are anecdotal responses to rituximab in patients with cerebellar degeneration, encephalomyelitis, or limbic encephalitis (59).

Several potential explanations are found for the disappointingly poor response to immunotherapy in many patients. As noted above, the continuing presence of even a small tumor burden seems to provide an *antigenic drive* for further neuronal injury. Also likely, current immunotherapies do not adequately gain access to the CNS, and do not effectively abrogate an ongoing autoimmune response that is "sequestered" in the CNS. For many if not most CNS syndromes, however, it is likely that patients have already undergone neuronal death or irreversible injury by the time the diagnosis of a paraneoplastic disorder is made.

Theoretic concern is that if paraneoplastic disorders arise from an immune response directed against the tumor, attempts to treat the neurologic disorder with immunosuppression may adversely affect the evolution of the tumor. At this time, no definite evidence suggests that patients given immunosuppressive treatment have a worse tumor outcome (20,60).

CLINICAL RECOMMENDATIONS OF THE VIGNETTE

The presence of anti-Yo antibodies is a strong indicator of an underlying carcinoma of the breast, ovary, or adnexa, so the tumor search should be directed at these organs. Immunotherapy with prednisone and IVIG could be offered before or after tumor treatment; the patient should be informed that the likelihood of significant neurologic improvement with anti-Yo-associated paraneoplastic cerebellar degeneration is low, despite aggressive tumor treatment and immunotherapy.

SUMMARY

Paraneoplastic disorders can affect the CNS in a wide variety of syndromes. These disorders are uncommon relative to other neurologic complications of systemic cancer, but affected patients frequently have severe and permanent neurologic morbidity. Paraneoplastic disorders are believed to be autoimmune diseases, but the details of their immunopathogenesis remain largely unknown. Early recognition of these syndromes, at least for some patients, will maximize the likelihood of a good neurologic outcome.

REFERENCES

1. Rojas-Marcos I, Rousseau A, Keime-Guibert F, et al. Spectrum of paraneoplastic neurologic disorders in women with breast and gynecologic cancer. *Medicine.* 2003;82:216–223.
2. Vernino S, Lennon VA. Autoantibody profiles and neurological correlations of thymoma. *Clin Cancer Res.* 2004;10:7270–7275.
3. Musunuru K, Darnell RB. Paraneoplastic neurologic disease antigens: RNA-binding proteins and signaling proteins in neuronal degeneration. *Annu Rev Neurosci.* 2001;24: 239–262.
4. Dropcho EJ. Remote neurologic manifestations of cancer. *Neurol Clin.* 2002;20(1):85–122.
5. Pittock SJ, Kryzer TJ, Lennon VA. Paraneoplastic antibodies coexist and predict cancer, not neurological syndrome. *Ann Neurol.* 2004;56:715–719.
6. Kleopa KA, Elman LB, Lang B, et al. Neuromyotonia and limbic encephalitis sera target mature Shaker-type K+ channels: Subunit specificity correlates with clinical manifestations. *Brain.* 2006;129:1570–1584.
7. Fukuda T, Motomura M, Nakao YK, et al. Reduction of P/Q-type calcium channels in the postmortem cerebellum of paraneoplastic cerebellar degeneration with Lambert-Eaton myasthenic syndrome. *Ann Neurol.* 2003;53:21–28.
8. Coesmans M, Sillevis Smitt PA, Linden DJ, et al. Mechanisms underlying cerebellar motor deficits due to mGluR1-autoantibodies. *Ann Neurol.* 2003;53:325–336.
9. Sommer C, Weishaupt A, Brinkhoff J, et al. Paraneoplastic stiff-person syndrome: Passive transfer to rats by means of IgG antibodies to amphiphysin. *Lancet.* 2005;365:1406–1411.
10. Ohguro H, Yokoi Y, Ohguro I, et al. Clinical and immunologic aspects of cancer-associated retinopathy. *Am J Ophthalmol.* 2004;137:1117–1119.

11. Albert ML, Austin LM, Darnell RB. Detection and treatment of activated T cells in the cerebrospinal fluid of patients with paraneoplastic cerebellar degeneration. *Ann Neurol.* 2000;47:9–17.
12. Rousseau A, Benyahia B, Dalmau J, et al. T-cell response to Hu-D peptides in patients with anti-Hu syndrome. *J Neurooncol.* 2005;71:231–236.
13. Dalmau J, Graus F, Villarejo A, et al. Clinical analysis of anti-Ma2-associated encephalitis. *Brain.* 2004;127:1831–1844.
14. Roberts WK, Darnell RB. Neuroimmunology of the paraneoplastic neurological degenerations. *Curr Opin Immunol.* 2004;16:616–622.
15. Gultekin SH, Rosenfeld MR, Voltz R, et al. Paraneoplastic limbic encephalitis: Neurological symptoms, immunological findings and tumour association in 50 patients. *Brain.* 2000;123: 1481–1494.
16. Candler PM, Hart PE, Barnett M, et al. A follow up study of patients with paraneoplastic neurological disease in the United Kingdom. *J Neuro Neurosurg Psychiatry.* 2004;75:1411–1415.
17. Graus F, Delattre JY, Antoine JC, et al. Recommended diagnostic criteria for paraneoplastic neurological syndromes. *J Neuro Neurosurg Psychiatry.* 2004;75:1135–1140.
18. Dalmau J, Graus F, Rosenblum MK, et al. Anti-Hu-associated paraneoplastic encephalomyelitis/sensory neuronopathy: A clinical study of 71 patients. *Medicine.* 1992;71:59–72.
19. Lucchinetti CF, Kimmel DW, Lennon VA. Paraneoplastic and oncologic profiles of patients seropositive for type I antineuronal nuclear autoantibodies. *Neurology.* 1998;50:652–657.
20. Keime-Guibert F, Graus F, Broet P, et al. Clinical outcome of patients with anti-Hu-associated encephalomyelitis after treatment of the tumor. *Neurology.* 1999;53:1719–1723.
21. Graus F, Keime-Guibert F, Rene R, et al. Anti-Hu-associated paraneoplastic encephalomyelitis: Analysis of 200 patients. *Brain.* 2001;124:1138–1148.
22. Alamowitch S, Graus F, Uchuya M, et al. Limbic encephalitis and small cell lung cancer: Clinical and immunological features. *Brain.* 1997;120:923–928.
23. Lawn ND, Westmoreland BF, Kiely MJ, et al. Clinical, magnetic resonance imaging, and electroencephalographic findings in paraneoplastic limbic encephalitis. *Mayo Clin Proc.* 2003;78:1363–1368.
24. Ances BM, Vitaliani R, Taylor RA, et al. Treatment-responsive limbic encephalitis identified by neuropil antibodies: MRI and PET correlates. *Brain.* 2005;128:1764–1777.
25. Deodhare S, O'Connor P, Ghazarian D, et al. Paraneoplastic limbic encephalitis in Hodgkin disease. *Can J Neurol Sci.* 1996;23:138–140.
26. Vitaliani R, Mason W, Ances B, et al. Paraneoplastic encephalitis, psychiatric symptoms, and hypoventilation in ovarian teratoma. *Ann Neurol.* 2005;58:594–604.
27. Liguori R, Vincent A, Clover L, et al. Morvan's syndrome: Peripheral and central nervous system and cardiac involvement with antibodies to voltage-gated potassium channels. *Brain.* 2001;124:2417–2426.
28. Sillevis Smitt P, Grefkens J, de Leeuw B, et al. Survival and outcome in 73 anti-Hu positive patients with paraneoplastic encephalomyelitis/sensory neuronopathy. *J Neurol.* 2002;249: 745–753.
29. Hammack JE, Kotanides H, Rosenblum MK, et al. Paraneoplastic cerebellar degeneration: Clinical and immunologic findings in 21 patients with Hodgkin's disease. *Neurology.* 1992;42:1938–1943.
30. Peterson K, Rosenblum MK, Kotanides H, et al. Paraneoplastic cerebellar degeneration: A clinical analysis of 55 anti-Yo antibody-positive patients. *Neurology.* 1992;42:1931–1937.
31. Shams'ili S, Grefkens J, de Leeuw B, et al. Paraneoplastic cerebellar degeneration associated with antineuronal antibodies: Analysis of 50 patients. *Brain.* 2003;126:1409–1418.
32. Mason WP, Graus F, Lang B, et al. Small-cell lung cancer, paraneoplastic cerebellar degeneration and the Lambert-Eaton myasthenic syndrome. *Brain.* 1997;120:1279–1300.
33. Bernal F, Shams'ili S, Rojas I, et al. Anti-Tr antibodies as markers of paraneoplastic cerebellar degeneration and Hodgkin's disease. *Neurology.* 2003;60:230–234.
34. Ridley A, Kennard C, Scholtz CL, et al. Omnipause neurons in two cases of opsoclonus associated with oat cell carcinoma of the lung. *Brain.* 1987;110:1699–1709.
35. Anderson NE, Budde-Steffen C, Rosenblum MK, et al. Opsoclonus, myoclonus, ataxia, and encephalopathy in adults with cancer: A distinct paraneoplastic syndrome. *Medicine.* 1988;67:100–109.
36. Bataller L, Graus F, Saiz A, et al. Clinical outcome in adult onset idiopathic or paraneoplastic opsoclonus-myoclonus. *Brain.* 2001;124:437–443.
37. Vernino S, Tuite P, Adler CH, et al. Paraneoplastic chorea associated with CRMP-5 neuronal antibody and lung carcinoma. *Ann Neurol.* 2002;51:625–630.
38. Kinirons P, Fulton A, Keoghan M, et al. Paraneoplastic limbic encephalitis and chorea associated with CRMP-5 neuronal antibody. *Neurology.* 2003;61:1623–1624.
39. Chong DJ, Strong MJ, Shkrum MJ, et al. A 58-year-old woman with progressive vertigo, deafness and weakness. *Can J Neurol Sci.* 2005;32:103–108.
40. Guy J, Aptsiauri N. Treatment of paraneoplastic visual loss with intravenous immunoglobulin. *Arch Ophthalmol.* 1999;117:471–477.
41. Cross SA, Salomao DR, Parisi JE, et al. Paraneoplastic autoimmune optic neuritis with retinitis defined by CRMP-5-IgG. *Ann Neurol.* 2003;54:38–50.
42. Antoine JC, Camdessanche JP, Absi L, et al. Devic disease and thymoma with anti-central nervous system and antithymus antibodies. *Neurology.* 2004;62:978–980.
43. Pittock SJ, Lucchinetti CF, Parisi JE, et al. Amphiphysin autoimmunity: Paraneoplastic accompaniments. *Ann Neurol.* 2005;58:96–107.
44. Ojeda VJ. Necrotizing myelopathy associated with malignancy: A clinicopathologic study of two cases and literature review. *Cancer.* 1984;53:1115–1123.
45. Dropcho EJ. Antiamphiphysin antibodies with small cell lung carcinoma and paraneoplastic encephalomyelitis. *Ann Neurol.* 1996;39:659–667.
46. Wessig C, Klein R, Schneider MF, et al. Neuropathology and binding studies in anti-amphiphysin-associated stiff-person syndrome. *Neurology.* 2003;61:195–198.
47. Rosenfeld MR, Posner JB. Paraneoplastic motor neuron disease. *Adv Neurol.* 1991;56: 445–459.
48. Forman D, Rae-Grant AD, Matchett SC, et al. A reversible cause of hypercapnic respiratory failure: Lower motor neuronopathy associated with renal cell carcinoma. *Chest.* 1999;115: 899–901.
49. Gordon PH, Rowland LP, Younger DS, et al. Lymphoproliferative disorders and motor neuron disease: An update. *Neurology.* 1997;48:1671–1678.
50. Thieben MJ, Lennon VA, Boeve BF, et al. Potentially reversible autoimmune limbic encephalitis with neuronal potassium channel antibody. *Neurology.* 2004;62:1177–1182.
51. Vincent A, Buckley C, Schott J, et al. Potassium channel antibody-associated encephalopathy: A potentially immunotherapy-responsive form of limbic encephalitis. *Brain.* 2004;127:701–712.
52. Linke R, Schroeder M, Helmberger T, et al. Antibody-positive paraneoplastic neurologic syndromes: Value of CT and PET for tumor diagnosis. *Neurology.* 2004;63:282–286.
53. Younes-Mhenni S, Janier MF, Cinotti L, et al. FDG-PET improves tumour detection in patients with paraneoplastic neurological syndromes. *Brain.* 2004;127:2331–2338.
54. Vernino S, O'Neill BP, Marks RS, et al. Immunomodulatory treatment trial for paraneoplastic neurological disorders. *NeuroOncology.* 2003;6:55–62.
55. Batchelor TT, Platten M, Hochberg FH. Immunoadsorption therapy for paraneoplastic syndromes. *J Neurooncol.* 1998;40:131–136.
56. Keime-Guibert F, Graus F, Fleury A, et al. Treatment of paraneoplastic neurological syndromes with antineuronal antibodies (anti-Hu, anti-Yo) with a combination of immunoglobulins, cyclophosphamide, and methylprednisolone. *J Neurol Neurosurg Psychiatry.* 2000;68:479–482.
57. Pittock SJ, Lucchinetti CF, Lennon VA. Anti-Neuronal nuclear autoantibody type 2: Paraneoplastic accompaniments. *Ann Neurol.* 2003;53:580–587.
58. Uchuya M, Graus F, Vega F, et al. Intravenous immunoglobulin treatment in paraneoplastic neurological syndromes with antineuronal antibodies. *J Neurol Neurosurg Psychiatry.* 1996;60:388–392.
59. Shams'ili S, de Beukelaar J, Gratama H, et al. An uncontrolled trial of rituximab for antibody associated paraneoplastic neurological syndromes. *J Neurol.* 2006;253:16–20.
60. Rojas I, Graus F, Keime-Guibert F, et al. Long-term clinical outcome of paraneoplastic cerebellar degeneration and anti-Yo antibodies. *Neurology.* 2000;55:713–715.

CHAPTER **58**

Paraneoplastic Disorders of the Peripheral Nervous System

Edward J. Dropcho

OBJECTIVES

- To survey the variety of clinical manifestations of paraneoplastic disorders affecting the peripheral nervous system
- To describe the diagnostic approach to patients with suspected paraneoplastic disorders, including the appropriate use of antineuronal antibodies as diagnostic markers
- To discuss the management approaches for patients with peripheral nervous system syndromes

CASE VIGNETTE

A 61-year-old man with a long history of cigarette smoking presents with a 4-month history of generalized fatigue and difficulty climbing stairs. Examination is unremarkable except for proximal weakness, worse in the legs than arms, and absent or diminished muscle stretch reflexes. On questioning, the patient reports dry mouth and erectile dysfunction. Needle electromyelographic (EMG) studies show diminished motor unit amplitudes, with an incremental response after exercise. A chest X-ray study shows a 2-cm hilar mass.

DEFINITION

Neurologic paraneoplastic disorders are nonmetastatic syndromes that are not attributable to toxicity of cancer therapy, cerebrovascular disease, coagulopathy, infection, or other toxic or metabolic causes.

EPIDEMIOLOGY

Myasthenia gravis associated with thymoma is the oldest known and most common neurologic paraneoplastic disorder, with the first descriptions dating back more than 100 years. Up to 20% of patients with myasthenia gravis have thymoma, and at least 10% of patients with thymoma have myasthenia. Small cell lung carcinoma is the solid tumor most often associated with paraneoplastic disorders: Approximately 1% to 3% of patients develop Lambert-Eaton myasthenic syndrome or another paraneoplastic syndrome. The incidence of neuropathy associated with plasma cell dyscrasias, overall, is low, but varies among disease subtypes; the most striking association is among patients with osteosclerotic myeloma, one half of whom develop polyneuropathy.

ETIOLOGY AND PATHOGENESIS

Most, if not all, peripheral nervous system paraneoplastic disorders are believed to be autoimmune diseases. Some syndromes are associated with serum autoantibodies against neuronal or peripheral nerve antigens (Table 58-1). The proven or postulated immunopathogenetic mechanisms for these disorders fall into four main categories:

1. Autoantibodies against shared tumor-neuronal (*onconeural*) antigens are the direct cause of neurologic disease:
   - Lambert-Eaton myasthenic syndrome is caused by antibodies that bind to, and downregulate, voltage-gated calcium channels (VGCC) at the presynaptic neuromuscular junction, leading to reduction in the quantal release of acetylcholine by a nerve impulse (1).
   - Antibodies against voltage-gated potassium channels in patients with neuromyotonia are believed to cause prolonged motor neuron depolarization, leading to abnormal spontaneous muscle activity (2).
2. A cellular immune reaction against onconeural antigens causes neuronal or nerve injury, analogous to several central nervous system (CNS) paraneoplastic disorders (3) (see Chapter 57). Patients can also develop antineuronal antibodies, but the antibodies are an epiphenomenon or are not the primary effectors of neurologic disease:
   - Paraneoplastic sensory neuronopathy is believed to be caused by a cell-mediated immune attack against sensory neurons in the dorsal root ganglia (4,5).
   - Gastrointestinal dysmotility associated with small cell lung cancer can result from a combined cellular–humoral immune reaction against myenteric plexus neurons (6).
3. Neoplastic plasma cells produce monoclonal paraproteins (immunoglobulins) that react with peripheral nerve antigens and cause neuropathy:
   - Passive antibody transfer studies in animals strongly implicate anti-myelin–associated glycoprotein (anti-MAG) IgM as the direct mediator of complement-dependent nerve injury (7).

TABLE 58-1. Peripheral Nervous System Paraneoplastic Disorders and Autoantibodies

Clinical Syndrome	*Associated Tumor(s)*	*Autoantibodies*
Sensory neuronopathy	SCLC, others Plasma cell dyscrasias	Anti-Hu, anti-CV2, ANNA-3, anti-Ma1, anti-amphiphysin Anti-disialosyl ganglioside
Neuromyotonia	Thymoma, SCLC, Hodgkin lymphoma	Anti-VGCC
Acute demyelinating polyneuropathy	Hodgkin lymphoma, various solid tumors (rare)	
Chronic demyelinating Polyneuropathy	Plasma cell dyscrasias Osteosclerotic myeloma, various solid tumors	Anti-MAG
Sensorimotor axonal polyneuropathy	SCLC, thymoma, others Plasma cell dyscrasias	Anti-Hu, anti-CV2, ANNA-3
Vasculitic neuropathy	SCLC, other solid tumors	Anti-Hu
Autonomic insufficiency	SCLC	Anti-Hu, anti-ganglionic AChR
LEMS	SCLC	Anti-VGCC
Myasthenia gravis	Thymoma	Anti-AChR, anti-striated muscle
Polymyositis	Various tumors	

LEMS, Lambert-Eaton Myasthenic Syndrome; SCLC, small cell lung carcinoma; ANNA-3, Anti-Neuronal Nuclear Antibody; VGCC, voltage-gated calcium channel; anti-MAG, anti-myelin–associated glycoprotein.

- Immunization of rabbits with GD1b ganglioside induces an ataxic neuropathy, supporting a direct immunopathogenetic role for anti-GD1b antibodies in patients with sensory neuropathy (8).

4. Disorders that arise from other or poorly understood immune mechanisms:
   - The pathogenesis of neuropathy in patients with osteosclerotic myeloma or POEMS (polyneuropathy, organomegaly, endocrinopathy, monoclonal gammopathy, skin changes) syndrome may be related to elevated serum levels of *proinflammatory* cytokines rather than to any direct effect of the paraprotein (9).
   - The pathogenesis of myasthenia gravis associated with thymoma is complex and depends on intratumoral production of autoreactive T lymphocytes (10,11).

PATHOLOGY

The neuropathologic hallmark of paraneoplastic sensory neuronopathy is severe dropout of primary sensory neurons in the dorsal root ganglia and gasserian ganglia. There is a highly variable degree of infiltration by T and B lymphocytes, plasma cells, and macrophages, often in a perivascular distribution. Most patients with sensory neuronopathy have multifocal encephalomyeloneuritis (see Chapter 57).

Biopsied nerves from patients with chronic demyelinating paraneoplastic polyneuropathy typically show loss of myelinated fibers and segmental demyelination. This is seen in patients with anti-MAG antibodies, osteosclerotic myeloma, and anti-GD1 ganglioside antibodies. Anti-MAG–associated neuropathy additionally shows deposition of anti-MAG IgM and complement on myelin sheaths, and a characteristic widening of the myelin lamellae at the minor dense lines (12).

The pathology of Lambert-Eaton syndrome is ultrastructural: Electron microscopy shows marked depletion of presynaptic active zones (the sites of synaptic vesicle exocytosis), paucity and disorganization of active zone intramembrane particles, and aggregation of the active zone particles into clusters (13). Active zone particles contain P/Q-type VGCC that mediate the quantal release of acetylcholine in response to nerve impulses and which are the targets of anti-VGCC antibodies.

The pathology of several peripheral nervous system syndromes does not differ from that of their nonparaneoplastic counterparts and will not be discussed further here. These include sensorimotor axonal polyneuropathy, Guillain-Barré syndrome, vasculitic neuropathy, polymyositis, and myasthenia gravis.

CLINICAL MANIFESTATIONS

Paraneoplastic disorders can affect any part(s) of the peripheral nervous system. In most patients, the neurologic syndrome is the presenting feature of a previously undiagnosed neoplasm. Many patients can be grouped into a recognizable clinical syndrome (Table 58-1). Some clinical syndromes (e.g., chronic demyelinating polyneuropathy) are associated with varied tumor types and are caused by one of a number of different immune mechanisms. It is not rare for patients with a peripheral nervous system paraneoplastic disorder to have concomitant CNS involvement, especially when associated with small cell lung carcinoma (see Chapter 57).

Several syndromes should always raise the possibility of a paraneoplastic cause, including Lambert-Eaton myasthenic syndrome and severe sensory neuronopathy (14,15). As with CNS syndromes, no peripheral neurologic syndrome is absolutely pathognomonic for a paraneoplastic etiology.

SENSORY NEURONOPATHY

The most common clinical manifestation of paraneoplastic encephalomyelitis is subacute sensory neuronopathy reflecting involvement of the dorsal root ganglia (16–19). More than 90%

of reported patients have small cell lung carcinoma. Early symptoms are patchy or asymmetric numbness and paresthesias, often involving face, trunk, or proximal limbs. The symptoms eventually spread to involve all limbs. Burning dysesthesias and severe aching or lancinating pain are common. Examination reveals severe sensory ataxia, predominant impairment of vibration sense and proprioception, frequent pseudoathetosis, and hypoactive or absent muscle stretch reflexes. Most patients have additional signs and symptoms that reflect a multifocal encephalomyelitis (see Chapter 57). Some patients develop concomitant Lambert-Eaton myasthenic syndrome, a component of motor neuropathy, or peripheral nerve microvasculitis presenting as mononeuritis multiplex (18,20). The antibodies and tumors associated with paraneoplastic sensory neuronopathy are essentially the same as with paraneoplastic encephalomyelitis (Table 58-1).

The clinical course of paraneoplastic sensory neuronopathy in patients with small cell lung carcinoma is fairly stereotyped. By far the most common pattern is deterioration over a period of weeks to months, and then stabilization at a level of severe neurologic disability, regardless of treatment. Subsequent stepwise or gradual neurologic deterioration is less common. In a few patients with minimal CNS manifestations, a sensory neuronopathy takes a relatively indolent course independent of any treatment (21).

NEUROMYOTONIA

Patients with small cell lung carcinoma, thymoma, Hodgkin lymphoma, or plasmacytoma may develop peripheral nerve hyperexcitability, which manifests as *the cramp-fasciculation syndrome* or as a syndrome of diffuse muscle stiffness, cramps, and myokymia similar to *neuromyotonia* or *continuous muscle fiber activity* (Isaacs' syndrome) (22,23). Patients with thymoma may concurrently have myasthenia gravis, and some patients have limbic encephalitis or *Morvan fibrillary chorea* (see Chapter 57).

DEMYELINATING NEUROPATHIES AND CARCINOMA OR LYMPHOMA

Several reports describe an acute, predominantly motor polyradiculoneuropathy occurring in the setting of a number of primary neoplasms, particularly lymphomas. The clinical features, electrophysiologic findings, CSF, and peripheral nerve pathology in these patients are indistinguishable from Guillain-Barré syndrome (24). Several well-documented cases describe patients with lymphoma, carcinoma, or melanoma who develop a sensorimotor polyneuropathy that fulfills the clinical and electrophysiologic diagnostic criteria for chronic demyelinating polyneuropathy (CIDP) (25,26). In some patients with acute or chronic demyelinating polyneuropathy, the tumor association may be fortuitous.

DEMYELINATING NEUROPATHY AND ANTI-MAG ANTIBODIES

Many patients presenting with an *idiopathic* polyneuropathy are discovered to have a monoclonal gammopathy. Most of these patients have monoclonal gammopathy of undetermined significance or nonmalignant monoclonal gammopathy. A few have or will eventually develop multiple myeloma, plasmacytoma, Waldenstroms macroglobulinemia, non-Hodgkin lymphoma, chronic lymphocytic leukemia, or Castleman syndrome (27). In some patients with neuropathy, the IgM paraprotein reacts with MAG and several cross-reacting glycolipids (28,29). A male predominance is seen with onset usually after age 60 years. Patients with anti-MAG antibodies generally develop a slowly progressive, predominantly sensory, neuropathy, which can be present for several years before the diagnosis is established. Proprioception and vibratory sense are selectively affected. Intention tremor and ataxia are each present in up to one-half of patients at initial presentation. Muscle stretch reflexes are diminished or absent. Romberg test may be positive. Cranial nerves and autonomic functions are usually unaffected. Approximately 20% of patients have a predominantly motor neuropathy. Although the progression is slow, the neuropathy is frequently debilitating.

DEMYELINATING NEUROPATHY AND OSTEOSCLEROTIC MYELOMA/POEMS SYNDROME

Patients with osteosclerotic myeloma frequently develop a predominantly motor polyneuropathy, presenting with distal weakness and, to a lesser extent, sensory symptoms, which progress proximally. Examination shows weakness and disproportionate loss of vibration sense and proprioception. Muscle stretch reflexes are diminished or absent. Pain or autonomic involvement are rare. The neuropathy is usually slowly progressive, but can be severely disabling. Some patients with neuropathy and osteosclerotic myeloma have the multisystem POEMS syndrome (30,31).

SENSORY NEUROPATHY AND ANTIDISIALOSYL GANGLIOSIDE ANTIBODIES

A syndrome of sensory neuropathy and antidisalosyl ganglioside antibodies is rare relative to other neuropathies associated with plasma cell dyscrasias. Patients usually have an IgM paraprotein in the setting of nonmalignant monoclonal gammopathy. The paraprotein binds to GD1b and to several other gangliosides which bear disialosyl groups. Patients present with numbness, paresthesias, and gait ataxia (32,33). The clinical course can be steadily progressive, acute relapsing and remitting, or chronic worsening with acute relapses. Examination shows severe loss of proprioception and vibratory sense, with relative sparing of pain and temperature sensations. Patients are frequently unable to walk because of severe sensory ataxia. Weakness, if any, is mild. Some patients have ophthalmoparesis or other cranial nerve or bulbar involvement. Muscle stretch reflexes are usually absent. This syndrome resembles subacute sensory neuronopathy associated with small cell lung cancer.

VASCULITIC NEUROPATHY

Peripheral nerve microvasculitis can occur in association with lymphomas or with carcinoma of the lung, prostate, uterus, kidney, or stomach (20,34,35). The clinical presentation is either that of mononeuritis multiplex, or of an asymmetric distal sensorimotor neuropathy. Pain is common. Patients usually have an elevated sedimentation rate, but rarely have cutaneous vasculitis or other systemic symptoms.

OTHER NEUROPATHIES

Rather than the more common sensory neuronopathy, a few patients with small cell lung cancer and anti-Hu antibodies have a mixed sensorimotor polyneuropathy with a mixed axonal-demyelinating electrophysiologic pattern (36). A few patients with anti-Hu antibodies have what appears to be a primary demyelinating polyneuropathy superimposed on sensory neuronopathy (37), or a mononeuritis multiplex with nerve vasculitis. Patients with anti-CV2 antibodies, most of whom have small cell lung carcinoma, may develop a sensorimotor polyneuropathy with mixed axonal-demyelinating electrophysiologic features (38). Some of these patients have both anti-Hu and anti-CV2 antibodies.

Distal, slowly progressive axonal sensorimotor polyneuropathy occurs in patients with a wide variety of carcinomas and hematologic neoplasms. Most affected patients have had significant weight loss and are in an advanced or preterminal phase of their illness. The neuropathy itself is generally not a major source of disability. The exact cause of the polyneuropathy in these patients is usually unclear and is probably multifactorial.

AUTONOMIC INSUFFICIENCY

Paraneoplastic autonomic dysfunction most commonly occurs as a part of encephalomyelitis in patients with small cell lung carcinoma or, rarely, in patients with lymphoma, thymoma, or other carcinomas. In some patients, the autonomic symptoms overshadow other manifestations of encephalomyelitis. These patients may develop severe and progressive gastrointestinal dysmotility, including gastroparesis, chronic intestinal pseudoobstruction, and severe constipation (39,40). Patients may also have other features of sympathetic or parasympathetic dysfunction. Associated antineuronal antibodies include anti-Hu antibodies, which react with neurons in the sympathetic ganglia and myenteric plexus (39,40), and antibodies against neuronal ganglionic acetylcholine receptors (41).

LAMBERT-EATON MYASTHENIC SYNDROME

Approximately one half of patients with Lambert-Eaton syndrome have an associated neoplasm, which is small cell lung carcinoma in >90% of well-documented cases (42,43). The clinical features of Lambert-Eaton syndrome are indistinguishable between paraneoplastic and nonparaneoplastic cases (1,42,44). Most patients have a gradual onset of weakness and fatigue. Symmetric weakness predominantly affects proximal leg muscles and, to a lesser extent, shoulder girdle muscles. Muscle aches or distal paresthesias are not uncommon. Muscle stretch reflexes are characteristically diminished or absent. Approximately 75% of patients have symptoms of sympathetic or parasympathetic autonomic dysfunction, including dry mouth, impotence, blurred vision, constipation, difficulty with micturition, and reduced sweating (45). About one third of patients have mild dysphagia, ptosis, or diplopia, and rare patients have respiratory failure.

One clinical feature that distinguishes paraneoplastic from nonparaneoplastic Lambert-Eaton syndrome is that some patients with a neoplasm have concomitant cerebellar degeneration, encephalomyelitis, sensorimotor polyneuropathy, or other *overlap* syndromes (46,47) (see Chapter 57). In these patients, either weakness or CNS symptoms can dominate the clinical presentation.

MYASTHENIA GRAVIS

Median age at presentation for patients with myasthenia gravis and thymoma is 40 to 50 years, which is older than for those with nonthymoma myasthenia. Patients with myasthenia or thymoma may have other systemic or neurologic autoimmune disorders, including neuromyotonia (see above) (48). The thymoma in patients with myasthenia is almost never symptomatic of itself and is usually discovered radiographically shortly after the diagnosis of myasthenia. A few patients have the clinical onset of myasthenia up to several years after thymoma resection, in the absence of tumor recurrence. Nothing is distinctive about the clinical neurologic features of myasthenia among thymoma versus nonthymoma cases.

Nearly all patients with myasthenia or thymoma have anti-acetylcholine receptor antibodies; those with thymoma cannot be distinguished based on the titer or antigenic binding characteristics of the acetylcholine receptor antibodies. Autoantibodies against striated muscle are present in 80% to 90% of patients with myasthenia or thymoma, and include antibodies against titin and the ryanodine receptor (49,50). These antibodies are also found with a much lower prevalence among patients with myasthenia without thymoma.

MYOPATHIES

Most published evidence indicates a significantly higher than expected incidence of cancer among patients with dermatomyositis and, to a lesser degree, with polymyositis (51,52). Except perhaps for ovarian carcinoma, no clear-cut overrepresentation exists of any particular tumor type compared with an age-matched control population. Nothing is distinctive about the neurologic symptoms, EMG findings, muscle pathology, clinical course, or response to immunotherapy in patients with paraneoplastic myositis. A possible exception may be a higher incidence of cutaneous necrosis in patients with paraneoplastic dermatomyositis compared with those with nonparaneoplastic syndrome (53).

Severe necrotizing myopathy is a rare complication of lung carcinoma or other neoplasms (54). Patients develop severe, rapidly progressive weakness, with marked elevation of serum creatine kinase. Muscle biopsy or autopsy show diffuse, extensive muscle fiber degeneration and necrosis, with minimal or no inflammatory reaction. A few patients improved after tumor resection and corticosteroids, whereas others were severely disabled or died of bulbar and respiratory weakness.

DIAGNOSTIC APPROACH

As with CNS syndromes, the clincal management of patients with known or suspected peripheral nervous system paraneoplastic syndromes includes four components: (*a*) verification that the disorder, in fact, is paraneoplastic; (*b*) identification of the associated tumor; (*c*) treatment of the tumor; and (*d*) suppression of the autoimmune effectors causing neuronal injury.

Among patients with neurologic dysfunction and a known cancer diagnosis, the level of suspicion for a paraneoplastic disorder depends on the neurologic syndrome, tumor type, and presence of antineuronal antibodies. In the differential diagnosis it is important to keep in mind that peripheral neuropathy is a common and often dose-limiting toxicity of several chemotherapy agents (55).

For patients without a previous cancer diagnosis, the level of suspicion for a paraneoplastic disorder depends on patient age, gender, risk factors (especially cigarette smoking), the neurologic syndrome, and the presence of antineuronal antibodies (15). As described, most peripheral nervous system paraneoplastic disorders are clinically indistinguishable from their nonparaneoplastic counterparts and, in most patients, the neurologic syndrome is the presenting feature of the tumor. A paraneoplastic cause, therefore, should be considered in all patients who present with neuromyotonia, Lambert-Eaton syndrome, myasthenia gravis, and dermatomyositis. The overall incidence of a neoplasm in patients presenting with peripheral neuropathy is low, but is higher in certain clinical subtypes. For example, severe rapidly progressive sensory neuronopathy is much more likely to be paraneoplastic than a mild, distal, slowly progressive axonal polyneuropathy (26,56,57).

Electrophysiology is of value in characterizing the clinical syndrome in patients with suspected paraneoplastic disorders, but cannot itself differentiate a paraneoplastic versus nonparaneoplastic etiology.

The characteristic electrophysiologic profile of paraneoplastic sensory neuronopathy includes severely reduced amplitude or complete absence of sensory nerve potentials, with normal or only slightly reduced sensory nerve conduction velocities if a response can be elicited (17,26). Most patients do show at least some abnormalities in motor nerve conduction studies, with or without symptoms of a mixed sensorimotor polyneuropathy (36,58); motor conduction studies are almost always less affected than sensory nerve studies. Needle EMG may show denervation in patients with a component of motor neuropathy or encephalomyelitis and anterior horn cell involvement.

Electrophysiologic studies in patients with anti-GD1b paraprotein usually resemble those of carcinoma-associated sensory neuronopathy. Patients have low amplitude or absent sensory nerve potentials (33). Motor nerve conduction study findings are usually normal or slightly abnormal, although some patients have temporal dispersion and conduction block.

The electrophysiology of neuropathy-associated with anti-MAG antibodies or osteosclerotic myeloma or POEMS syndrome shows features of primary demyelination, similar to the findings in patients with idiopathic chronic demyelinating polyneuropathy (59). Disproportionate prolongation of distal motor latencies may distinguish anti-MAG neuropathy from other chronic demyelinating neuropathies (60).

Needle EMG in cases of neuromyotonia shows repetitive bursts of rapidly firing motor unit discharges (myokymic potentials) or very high frequency trains of discharges (22). Fibrillations and fasciculations may also be present.

The characteristic electrophysiologic profile of Lambert-Eaton myasthenic syndrome includes: (*a*) reduced amplitude of muscle action potentials evoked by a supramaximal stimulus; (*b*) a marked increase in compound muscle action potential amplitude after several seconds of maximal voluntary contraction (postexercise facilitation); (*c*) a decremental response to 2 to 5 Hz repetitive nerve stimulation; and (*d*) an incremental response to 20 to 50 Hz stimulation (61). Many laboratories test for facilitation after maximal voluntary contraction rather than performing 20 to 50 Hz stimulation (62,63).

Nothing is distinctive about the electrophysiologic features of myasthenia gravis or polymyositis among paraneoplastic versus nonparaneoplastic cases.

For the peripheral nervous system syndromes associated with autoantibodies, the presence of antibodies confirms the clinical diagnosis and may indicate the likely associated tumor (Table 58-1). For example, 90% of patients with Lambert-Eaton syndrome have serum antibodies against P/Q-type VGCC (64), and approximately 50% of patients with neuromyotonia have anti–voltage-gated potassium channel antibodies (22). It is important to remember that the presence of autoantibodies is not absolute proof of a paraneoplastic cause, except for plasma cell dyscrasias in which tumor cells make the autoantibody. Conversely, absence of antibodies does not rule out a paraneoplastic condition.

The tumor workup for an adult with a suspected peripheral nervous system paraneoplastic disorder should include computed tomographic (CT) or magentic resonance (MR) scans of the chest and abdomen, as well as mammography and pelvic examination or imaging in women. The strong link between these neurologic syndromes and small cell lung carcinoma or thymoma places particular importance on high-quality chest scanning. Total-body fluorodeoxyglucose positron emission tomography (FDG-PET) scanning may demonstrate a neoplasm in patients with suspected paraneoplastic disorders (with or without autoantibodies) in whom other imaging study findings are negative or equivocal (65,66). It is not uncommon for the tumor to be found only after repeated searches. Reports have been made of patients with Lambert-Eaton syndrome and cigarette smoking in whom "blind" bronchoscopy in the absence of a definite radiographic pulmonary lesion diagnosed an otherwise occult small cell lung carcinoma (1).

Patients with suspected paraprotein-associated neuropathy should have serum immunofixation, because a low level of paraprotein can be missed in a routine serum protein electrophoresis. Radiographic skeletal survey should be done in patients with a suspected osteosclerotic myeloma.

TREATMENT

Some patients with peripheral nervous system paraneoplastic disorders show neurologic improvement with successful tumor treatment. This includes Lambert-Eaton syndrome (1,67), neuromyotonia, and probably vasculitic neuropathy and polymyositis as well. Patients with myasthenia gravis and thymoma generally improve after thymoma resection. Data are conflicting to whether patients with myasthenia and thymoma have a worse or equivalent long-term neurologic outcome after thymectomy compared to patients with myasthenia but without thymoma (68,69). Patients with myasthenia and thymoma usually require chronic immunosuppression therapy after thymectomy (48).

Patients with anti–MAG-associated neuropathy may show neurologic improvement with agents directly cytotoxic for neoplastic plasma cells, including chlorambucil, cyclophosphamide, or fludarabine. Improvement or stabilization of the neuropathy does not always correlate with a reduction in paraprotein levels (70,71). Plasmapheresis or intravenous gamma globulin (IVIg) is also sometimes effective, whether alone or in combination with chemotherapy (72,73). Recent studies show neurologic improvement after treatment with the monoclonal antibody rituximab, which rapidly depletes circulating B lymphocytes (74).

Some of the few published reports describe patients with anti-GD1b ganglioside sensory neuropathy who responded to treatment with corticosteroids, cyclophosphamide, IVIg, or plasmapheresis (33).

Treatment of patients with osteosclerotic myeloma or POEMS syndrome includes some combination of surgical resection of the myeloma, if possible, localized radiation, prednisone, or chemotherapy (31,75). Plasmapheresis or IVIg does not appear to be beneficial. Anecdotal responses to tamoxifen, retinoic acid, or thalidomide have been resported. Selected patients may benefit from myeloablative chemotherapy with autologous stem cell transplantation (76).

Many patients with Lambert-Eaton syndrome benefit from drugs that facilitate neuromuscular transmission. 3,4-Diaminopyridine (an orphan drug) is the most effective (1,67). Pyridostigmine or guanidine may also be useful. For patients with paraneoplastic Lambert-Eaton syndrome who still have severe weakness despite tumor treatment and pharmacologic treatment, several therapeutic options exist for removal of autoantibodies or suppression of autoantibody production (1,67). Prednisone or azathioprine are generally effective, but improvement may not be apparent for several weeks or longer. Cyclosporine has been occasionally used for treatment of patients who do not respond to, or tolerate, corticosteroids or azathioprine. Plasma exchange or IVIg produces significant but temporary improvement in most patients.

Paraneoplastic syndromes affecting the peripheral nervous system are generally more likely to improve with tumor treatment or immunosuppressive treatment than are CNS syndromes. Syndromes caused by autoantibodies reacting with neuronal cell surface receptors or ion channels are more likely to respond to immunotherapy, probably because the antibodies do not usually cause axonal degeneration or neuronal cell death.

Sensory neuronopathy and autonomic insufficiency associated with small cell lung cancer also involve the peripheral nervous system, but patients rarely show significant neurologic improvement, despite tumor treatment or a variety of immunosuppressive therapies (18,19,77). A few patients do show a meaningful neurologic response to immunotherapy (78). For most patients, however, it is likely that neurons in the dorsal root ganglia and autonomic ganglia have already been irreversibly injured or killed by the autoimmune response before any treatment is initiated.

CLINICAL RECOMMENDATIONS OF THE VIGNETTE

The neurologic examination, EMG findings, and chest X-ray study are highly suggestive for Lambert-Eaton myasthenic syndrome associated with small cell lung carcinoma. Serum anti–VGCC antibodies would virtually clinch the diagnosis of Lambert-Eaton syndrome. If it is proved that the patient has small cell lung cancer, the usual approach would be to treat the tumor and use pyridostigmine, 3,4-diaminopyridine, or both as initial therapy, and to defer immunotherapy, depending on the patient's neurologic response.

SUMMARY

Paraneoplastic disorders can affect the peripheral nerves, neuromuscular junction, or muscle, most commonly in association with small cell lung carcinoma, thymoma, or plasma cell dyscrasias. Early recognition of these syndromes will maximize the likelihood of a good oncologic and neurologic outcome.

REFERENCES

1. Sanders DB. Lambert-Eaton myasthenic syndrome: Diagnosis and treatment. *Ann NY Acad Sci.* 2003;998:500–508.
2. Tomimitsu H, Arimura K, Nagado T, et al. Mechanism of action of voltage-gated K+ channel antibodies in acquired neuromyotonia. *Ann Neurol.* 2004;56:440–444.
3. Roberts WK, Darnell RB. Neuroimmunology of the paraneoplastic neurological degenerations. *Curr Op Immunol.* 2004;16:616–622.
4. Bernal F, Graus F, Pifarre A, et al. Immunohistochemical analysis of anti-Hu-associated paraneoplastic encephalomyelitis. *Acta Neuropathol.* 2002;103:509–515.
5. Plonquet A, Gherardi RK, Creange A, et al. Oligoclonal T-cells in blood and target tissues of patients with anti-Hu syndrome. *J Neuroimmunol.* 2002;122:100–105.
6. De Giorgio R, Bovara M, Barbara G, et al. Anti-HuD-induced neuronal apoptosis underlying paraneoplastic gut dysmotility. *Gastroenterology.* 2003;125:70–79.
7. Monaco S, Ferrari S, Bonetti B, et al. Experimental induction of myelin changes by anti-MAG antibodies and terminal complement complex. *J Neuropathol Exp Neurol.* 1995;54:96–104.
8. Kusunoki S, Hitoshi S, Kaida K, et al. Monospecific anti-GD1b IgG is required to induce rabbit ataxic neuropathy. *Ann Neurol.* 1999;45:400–403.
9. Scarlato M, Previtali SC, Carpo M, et al. Polyneuropathy in POEMS syndrome: Role of angiogenic factors in the pathogenesis. *Brain.* 2005;128:1911–1920.
10. Marx A, Muller-Hermelink HK, Strobel P. The role of thymomas in the development of myasthenia gravis. *Ann NY Acad Sci.* 2003;998:223–236.
11. Chuang WY, Strobel P, Gold R, et al. A CTLA4(high) genotype is associated with myasthenia gravis in thymoma patients. *Ann Neurol.* 2005;58:644–648.
12. Lopate G, Kornberg AJ, Yue J, et al. Anti-MAG antibodies: Variability in patterns of IgM binding to peripheral nerve. *J Neurol Sci.* 2001;188:67–72.
13. Fukunaga H, Engel AG, Osame M, et al. Paucity and disorganization of presynaptic membrane active zones in the Lambert-Eaton myasthenic syndrome. *Muscle Nerve.* 1982;5:686–697.
14. Candler PM, Hart PE, Barnett M, et al. A follow up study of patients with paraneoplastic neurological disease in the United Kingdom. *J Neurol Neurosurg Psychiatry.* 2004;75:1411–1415.
15. Graus F, Delattre JY, Antoine JC, et al. Recommended diagnostic criteria for paraneoplastic neurological syndromes. *J Neurol Neurosurg Psychiatry.* 2004;75:1135–1140.
16. Dalmau J, Graus F, Rosenblum MK, et al. Anti-Hu-associated paraneoplastic encephalomyelitis/sensory neuronopathy: A clinical study of 71 patients. *Medicine.* 1992;71:59–72.
17. Chalk CH, Windebank AJ, Kimmel DW, et al. The distinctive clinical features of paraneoplastic sensory neuronopathy. *Can J Neurol Sci.* 1992;19:346–351.
18. Graus F, Keime-Guibert F, Rene R, et al. Anti-Hu-associated paraneoplastic encephalomyelitis: Analysis of 200 patients. *Brain.* 2001;124:1138–1148.
19. Sillevis Smitt P, Grefkens J, de Leeuw B, et al. Survival and outcome in 73 anti-Hu positive patients with paraneoplastic encephalomyelitis/sensory neuronopathy. *J Neurol.* 2002;249:745–753.
20. Eggers C, Hagel C, Pfeiffer G. Anti-Hu-associated paraneoplastic sensory neuropathy with peripheral nerve demyelination and microvasculitis. *J Neurol Sci.* 1998;155:178–181.
21. Graus F, Bonaventura I, Uchuya M, et al. Indolent anti–Hu-associated paraneoplastic sensory neuropathy. *Neurology.* 1994;44:2258–2261.
22. Hart IK, Maddison P, Newsom-Davis J, et al. Phenotypic variants of autoimmune peripheral nerve hyperexcitability. *Brain.* 2002;125:1887–1895.
23. Vernino S, Lennon VA. Ion channel and striational antibodies define a continuum of autoimmmune neuromuscular hyperexcitability. *Muscle Nerve.* 2002;26:702–707.
24. Vital C, Vital A, Julien J, et al. Peripheral neuropathies and lymphoma without monoclonal gammopathy: A new classification. *J Neurol.* 1990;237:177–185.
25. Antoine JC, Mosnier JF, Lapras J, et al. Chronic inflammatory demyelinating polyneuropathy associated with carcinoma. *J Neurol Neurosurg Psychiatry.* 1996;60:188–190.
26. Antoine JC, Mosnier JF, Absi L, et al. Carcinoma associated paraneoplastic peripheral neuropathies in patients with and without anti-onconeural antibodies. *J Neurol Neurosurg Psychiatry.* 1999;67:7–14.
27. Kyle RA, Therneau RM, Rajkumar SV, et al. A long-term study of prognosis in monoclonal gammopathy of undetermined significance. *N Engl J Med.* 2002;346:564–569.
28. Ponsford S, Willison H, Veitch J, et al. Long-term clinical and neurophysiological follow-up of patients with peripheral neuropathy associated with benign monoclonal gammopathy. *Muscle Nerve.* 2000;23:164–174.
29. Eurelings M, Moons KG, Notermans NC, et al. Neuropathy and IgM M-proteins: Prognostic value of antibodies to MAG, SGPG, and sulfatide. *Neurology.* 2001;56:228–233.
30. Soubrier MJ, Dubost JJ, Sauvezie BJ. POEMS syndrome: A study of 25 cases and a review of the literature. *Am J Med.* 1994;97:543–553.
31. Dispenzieri A, Kyle RA, Lacy MQ, et al. POEMS syndrome: Definitions and long-term outcome. *Blood.* 2003;101:2496–2506.
32. Eurelings M, Ang CW, Notermans NC, et al. Antiganglioside antibodies in polyneuropathy associated with monoclonal gammopathy. *Neurology.* 2001;57:1909–1912.

33. Willison HJ, O'Leary CP, Veitch J, et al. The clinical and laboratory features of chronic sensory ataxic neuropathy with anti-disialosyl IgM antibodies. *Brain.* 2001;124:1968–1977.
34. Younger DS, Dalmau J, Inghirami G, et al. Anti–Hu-associated peripheral nerve and muscle microvasculitis. *Neurology.* 1994;44:181–183.
35. Oh SJ. Paraneoplastic vasculitis of the peripheral nervous system. *Neurol Clin.* 1997; 15(4):849–863.
36. Oh SJ, Gurtekin Y, Dropcho EJ, et al. Anti-Hu antibody neuropathy: A clinical, electrophysiological, and pathological study. *Clin Neurophysiol.* 2005;116:28–34.
37. Antoine JC, Mosiner JF, Honnorat J, et al. Paraneoplastic demyelinating neuropathy, subacute sensory neuropathy, and anti-Hu antibodies: Clinicopathological study of an autopsy case. *Muscle Nerve.* 1998;21:850–857.
38. Antoine JC, Honnorat J, Camdessanche JP, et al. Paraneoplastic anti-CV2 antibodies react with peripheral nerve and are associated with a mixed axonal and demyelinating peripheral neuropathy. *Ann Neurol.* 2001;49:214–221.
39. Condom E, Vidal A, Rota R, et al. Paraneoplastic intestinal pseudo-obstruction associated with high titres of Hu autoantibodies. *Virchows Arch.* 1993;423:507–511.
40. Lee HR, Lennon VA, Camilleri M, et al. Paraneoplastic gastrointestinal motor dysfunction: Clinical and laboratory characteristics. *Am J Gastroenterol.* 2001;96:373–379.
41. Vernino S, Lennon VA. Neuronal ganglionic acetylcholine receptor autoimmunity. *Ann NY Acad Sci.* 2003;998:211–214.
42. O'Neill JH, Murray NM, Newsom-Davis J. The Lambert-Eaton myasthenic syndrome: A review of 50 cases. *Brain.* 1988;111:577–596.
43. Wirtz PW, van Dijk JG, van Doorn PA, et al. The epidemiology of the Lambert-Eaton myasthenic syndrome in the Netherlands. *Neurology.* 2004;63:397–398.
44. Chalk CH, Murray NM, Newsom-Davis J, et al. Response of the Lambert-Eaton myasthenic syndrome to treatment of associated small cell lung carcinoma. *Neurology.* 1990;40:1552–1556.
45. O'Suilleabhain P, Low PA, Lennon VA. Autonomic dysfuncton in the Lambert-Eaton myasthenic syndrome: Serologic and clinical correlates. *Neurology.* 1998;50:88–93.
46. Mason WP, Graus F, Lang B, et al. Small-cell lung cancer, paraneoplastic cerebellar degeneration and the Lambert-Eaton myasthenic syndrome. *Brain.* 1997;120:1279–1300.
47. Graus F, Lang B, Pozo-Rosich P, et al. P/Q-type calcium-channel antibodies in paraneoplastic cerebellar degeneration with lung cancer. *Neurology.* 2002;59:764–766.
48. Lovelace RE, Younger DS. Myasthenia gravis with thymoma. *Neurology.* 1997;48[Suppl 5]: S76–S81.
49. Baggi F, Andreetta F, Antozzi C, et al. Anti-titin and antiryanodine receptor antibodies in myasthenia gravis patients with thymoma. *Ann NY Acad Sci.* 1998;841:538–541.
50. Buckley C, Newsom-Davis J, Willcox N, et al. Do titin and cytokine antibodies in MG patients predict thymoma or thymoma recurrence? *Neurology.* 2001;57:1579–1582.
51. Buchbinder R, Forbes A, Hall S, et al. Incidence of malignant disease in biopsy-proven inflammatory myopathy: A population-based cohort study. *Ann Intern Med.* 2001;134:1087–1095.
52. Hill CL, Zhang Y, Sigurgeirsson B, et al. Frequency of specific cancer types in dermatomyositis and polymyositis: A population-based study. *Lancet.* 2001;357:96–100.
53. Basset-Seguin N, Roujeau JC, Gherardi R, et al. Prognostic factors and predictive signs of malignancy in adult dermatomyositis. *Arch Dermatol.* 1990;126:633–637.
54. Levin MI, Mozaffar T, Al-Lozi MT, et al. Paraneoplastic necrotizing myopathy: Clinical and pathologic features. *Neurology.* 1998;50:764–767.
55. Dropcho EJ. Neurotoxicity of cancer chemotherapy. *Semin Neurol.* 2004;24(4):419–426.
56. Camerlingo M, Nemni R, Ferraro B, et al. Malignancy and sensory neuropathy of unexplained cause: A prospective study of 51 patients. *Arch Neurol.* 1998;55:981–984.
57. Molinuevo JL, Graus F, Serrano C, et al. Utility of anti-Hu antibodies in the diagnosis of paraneoplastic sensory neuropathy. *Ann Neurol.* 1998;44:976–980.
58. Camdessanche JP, Antoine JC, Honnorat J, et al. Paraneoplastic peripheral neuropathy associated with anti-Hu antibodies: A clinical and electrophysiological study of 20 patients. *Brain.* 2002;125:166–175.
59. Min JH, Hong YH, Lee KW. Electrophysiological features of patients with POEMS syndrome. *Clin Neurophysiol.* 2005;116:965–968.
60. Isoardo G, Migliaretti G, Ciaramitaro P, et al. Differential diagnosis of chronic dysimmune demyelinating polyneuropathies with and without anti-MAG antibodies. *Muscle Nerve.* 2005;31:52–58.
61. Tim RW, Massey JM, Sanders DB. Lambert-Eaton myasthenic syndrome: Electrodiagnostic findings and response to treatment. *Neurology.* 2000;54:2176–2178.
62. Maddison P, Newsom-Davis J, Mills KR. Distribution of electrophysiological abnormality in Lambert-Eaton myasthenic syndrome. *J Neurol Neurosurg Psychiatry.* 1998;65: 213–217.
63. Oh SJ, Kurokawa K, Claussen GC, et al. Electrophysiological diagnostic criteria of Lambert-Eaton myasthenic syndrome. *Muscle Nerve.* 2005;32:515–520.
64. Motomura M, Lang B, Johnston I, et al. Incidence of serum anti-P/Q-type and anti-N-type calcium channel autoantibodies in the Lambert-Eaton myasthenic syndrome. *J Neurol Sci.* 1997;147:35–42.
65. Linke R, Schroeder M, Helmberger T, et al. Antibody-positive paraneoplastic neurologic syndromes: Value of CT and PET for tumor diagnosis. *Neurology.* 2004;63:282–286.
66. Younes-Mhenni S, Janier MF, Cinotti L, et al. FDG-PET improves tumour detection in patients with paraneoplastic neurological syndromes. *Brain.* 2004;127:2331–2338.
67. Newsom-Davis J. Therapy in myasthenia gravis and Lambert-Eaton myasthenic syndrome. *Semin Neurol.* 2003;23(2):191–198.
68. Durelli L, Maggi G, Casadio C, et al. Actuarial analysis of the occurrence of remissions following thymectomy for myasthenia gravis in 400 patients. *J Neurol Neurosurg Psychiatry.* 1991;54:406–411.
69. de Perrot M, Liu J, Bril V, et al. Prognostic significance of thymomas in patients with myasthenia gravis. *Ann Thorac Surg.* 2002;74:1658–1662.
70. Nobile-Orazio E, Meucci N, Baldini L, et al. Long-term prognosis of neuropathy associated with anti-MAG IgM M-proteins and its relationship to immune therapies. *Brain.* 2000;123: 710–717.
71. Gorson KC, Ropper AH, Weinberg DH, et al. Treatment experience in patients with anti-myelin-associated glycoprotein neuropathy. *Muscle Nerve.* 2001;24:778–786.
72. Oksenhendler E, Chevret S, Leger JM, et al. Plasma exchange and chlorambucil in polyneuropathy associated with monoclonal IgM gammopathy. *J Neurol Neurosurg Psychiatry.* 1995;59:243–247.
73. Comi G, Roveri L, Swan A, et al. A randomised controlled trial of intravenous immunoglobulin in IgM paraprotein associated demyelinating neuropathy. *J Neurol.* 2002;249:1370–1377.
74. Renaud S, Fuhr P, Gregor M, et al. High-dose rituximab and anti-MAG-associated polyneuropathy. *Neurology.* 2006;66:742–744.
75. Kuwabara S, Hattori T, Shimoe Y, et al. Long term melphalan-prednisolone chemotherapy for POEMS syndrome. *J Neurol Neurosurg Psychiatry.* 1997;63:385–387.
76. Dispenzieri A, Moreno A, Suarez GA, et al. Peripheral blood stem cell transplantation in 16 patients with POEMS syndrome. *Blood.* 2004;104:3400–3407.
77. Keime-Guibert F, Graus F, Broet P, et al. Clinical outcome of patients with anti-Hu-associated encephalomyelitis after treatment of the tumor. *Neurology.* 1999;53:1719–1723.
78. Oh SJ, Dropcho EJ, Claussen GC. Anti-Hu-associated paraneoplastic sensory neuronopathy responding to early aggressive immunotherapy: Report of two cases and review of the literature. *Muscle Nerve.* 1997;20:1576–1582.

CHAPTER **59**

Radiation Therapy in Neurologic Disease

Edward Melian

OBJECTIVES

- To describe what radiation therapy is and how it is used in the modern era
- To explain the role of radiation in the treatment of benign and malignant diseases that originate in, or affect, the central and peripheral nervous systems
- To discuss the acute and late effects of radiotherapy on the central and peripheral nervous systems

CASE VIGNETTE

A 48-year-old woman was diagnosed with a right frontal lobe glioblastoma multiforme after presenting with left-sided focal seizure activity (Fig. 59-1A). She had subtotal resection followed by 60 Gy in 30 fractions external beam radiotherapy using intensity modulation with concurrent temozolamide chemotherapy follow by monthly temozolamide. She remained steroid dependent since surgery. Nine months later, she developed increased seizure activity. Magnetic resonance imaging (MRI) showed an enhancing lesion, with poorly defined margins just slightly greater than the original tumor volume (Fig. 59-1B). Neurologic examination showed 4/5 strength on the left and normal on the right. She had a left pronator drift. On Mini-Mental Status Examination (MMSE) she scored 30 of 30, and was appropriate in conversation. She had marked cushingoid features, had difficulty rising from a chair, and tired easily.

DEFINITION: RADIATION THERAPY

Ionizing radiation was first described by Conrad Roentgen in Germany in 1895 (1). He showed how it could be used for imaging and, within 3 months, the first patient was treated with radiation therapy in Chicago, by Emil Grubbe, who was still in medical school at the time (2). Early radiation devices used either Crooks tubes to accelerate electron into target to create X-rays used for imaging and treatment, or pieces of radioactive substances such as radium or radon.

The linear accelerator or LINAC is currently the predominant machine used for radiotherapy. It uses microwaves to create electromagnetic waves that accelerate electrons to very high energies and then slam them into a metal target to create high-energy photons. For reasons of radiation safety, faster dose rates, and ability to achieve higher energy photons, the linear accelerator has replaced older machines that relied on radioactive substances, such as radium, cesium, and cobalt. The linear accelerator can also withdraw the metal target and treat with the high-energy electrons alone. Because of their mass, these electrons travel a limited distance in tissue proportional to their energy and are used to treat superficial lesions only. Contemporary LINAC are designed to rotate the beam isocentrically about the patient. By placing the treated lesion at the isocenter of the machine, treatment can be delivered from multiple angles by rotating the gantry and table without the need to move the patient. This allows for rapid multiple-field treatment with greater precision because the patient needs to be positioned only once for most daily treatments. Until recently, other particles, such as protons and helium nuclei, could be accelerated only by very large costly machines, which are available in just a few locations worldwide.

Brachytherapy is the placement of radioactive sources close to, or into, the targeted lesion. It has a long history in radiation therapy, perhaps originating when Pierre Curie failed to remove a piece of radioactive pitchblend from his pocket and inadvertently gave himself a radiation burn of the skin. Brachytherapy has been used for the treatment of intracranial lesions, but to some extent now been replaced by highly focused external beam techniques. It is still used, however, in the treatment of many lesions, including gynecologic tumors, prostatic carcinomas, breast cancers, and soft tissue sarcomas, including peripheral nerve sheath tumors. Brachytherapy tends to create a very high-dose region around the sources and a sharp fall-off in dose as it moves away from the sources. Commonly used isotopes are iodine–125, cesium-137, iridium-192, and palladium-103. They increase the dose given to the area treated while giving a lesser dose to surrounding structures; however, the intense dose in the high-dose region can be associated with increase risk for tissues intimately associated with the irradiated region.

RADIOBIOLOGY

The beneficial and deleterious effects of radiotherapy on tumors and normal tissues are caused by the ability to induce cell death. Most of the cell death is believed to be caused by DNA damage,

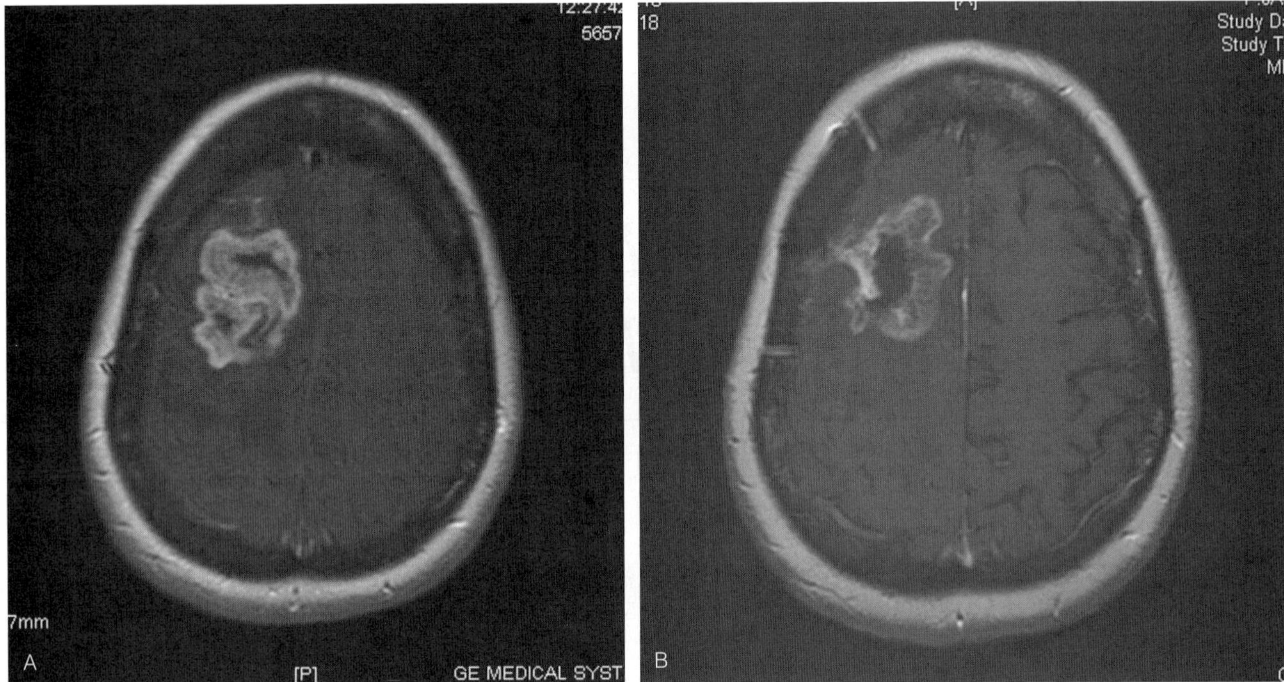

FIGURE 59-1. Glioblastoma multiforme at diagnosis **(A)**, and same brain lesion 9 months after 60 Gy irradiation **(B)**. Note softer borders zone. Differential diagnosis includes recurrent or persistent tumor versus radiation injury.

mostly double-strand breaks, which clinically manifests itself when the cell attempts to undergo mitosis and the process fails, leading to cell death. Apoptosis or cell-mediated death can occur between mitotic cycles, especially at higher single radiation doses such as those given in radiosurgery. Unlike drug therapy, radiation does not rely on the circulatory system to get to its target. The photon interactions with matter are enhanced by the presence of oxygen, which is theorized to fixate radiation injury done to the DNA. Although the exact mechanism is not agreed on, it has been shown that greater doses of radiation are needed to induce cell death in hypoxic regions. Mitotic and G2 phase of the cell cycle are the most sensitive to ionizing radiation, whereas S phase and late G1 are the most resistant. Giving fractionated radiotherapy allows the surviving fraction of cells to reoxygenate and redistribute through the cell cycle, thereby making them more sensitive to the next fraction of radiation. Although most radiotherapy is given in fractionated treatment because of the aforementioned biology, a technique known as stereotactic radiosurgery exists where a single high dose or a few high doses of radiation are given to a small volume in an attempt to obliterate the target and take advantage of a sharp fall-off in dose at the edge of the target to spare normal tissues. This technique was initially used in the brain and delivered by devices such as the Gamma Knife (Elekta AB, Stockholm, Sweden), Cyberknife (Accuray, Sunnyvale, CA), and Novalis (Brain Lab, Feldkirchen, Germany) (Fig. 59-2A). It is now being used elsewhere in the body as well. Most of these devices use multiple cross-firing beams to create the sharp fall-off in doses at the treatment volume edge. The exception to this is proton beam radiosurgery where the physics of the proton particle stopping at a specified depth is used (3).

HOW IS TREATMENT PLANNED AND DELIVERED

Most modern day radiation therapy is image based, especially when the targets are intracranial. This involves strict immobilization of the patient, either in a mask system or when submillimeter precision is needed, with invasive stereotactic headframes (Fig. 59-3A and B). The patient is then scanned using computed tomography (CT) and or MRI with localizing fiducials, either on the patient or attached to the frame. The data from the scans are transferred to a treatment-planning computer where targets and normal tissues can be delineated. Using computer simulation, custom-shaped beams that match the lesions geometry are either placed by the treatment planner or assigned by a computer optimization process to best target the lesion and decrease dose to normal tissue. A three-dimensional dose display shows the planners the result of their efforts. An interactive process then ensues to choose the best beam energy, beam angle, and beam shaping to achieve the goal of encompassing the target with the desired dose and minimizing dose to normal brain and other critical structures (Fig. 59-3B). The process of creating a treatment plan from volumetric imaging such as CT and MRI, and performing full volume dose calculation is referred to as *three-dimensional conformal radiotherapy.* The full volume calculation has been critical in allowing for more uniform treatments and limiting *hot spots* within the target volume that may have gone unnoticed previously. A newer development has been the ability to break each beam down into smaller segments or beamlets and adjust the dose given to each segment of each beam. This is known as *intensity modulation.* This technology has now been combined with sophisticated computer processing to allow for inverse treatment planning. The computer program is given a desired dose for the lesion and limitations to what dose each normal tissue can be given. These sophisticated computer programs will then modify each beamlet to help spare critical normal tissues within the beamlets' pathway and make up for the decreased dose by that beamlet by increasing the dose in a beamlet from a different beam that may not transverse the critical tissue.

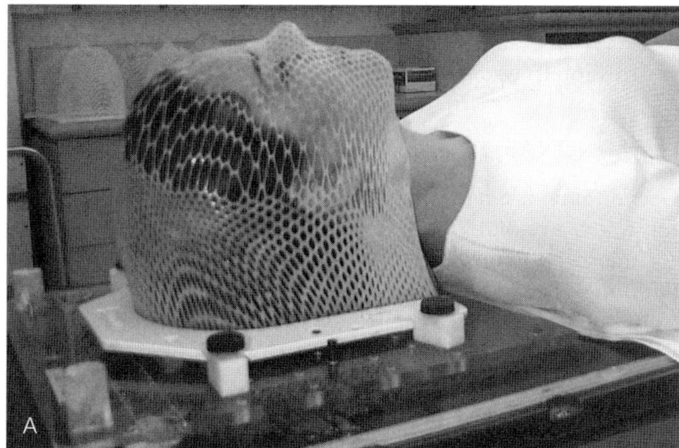

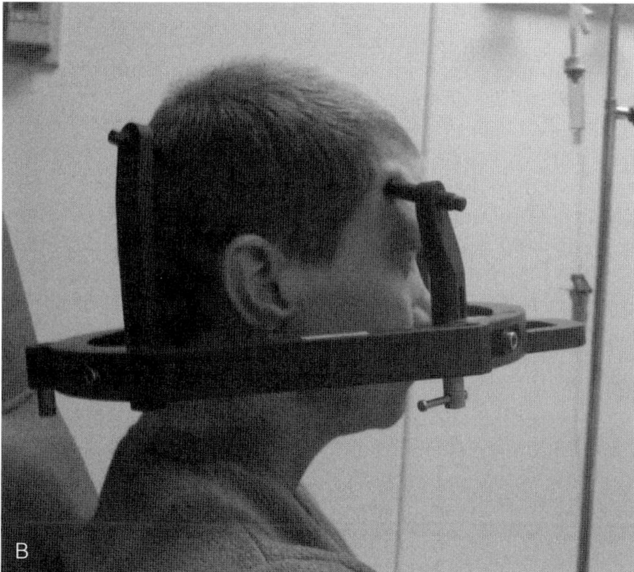

FIGURE 59-2. Immobilization devices for radiation therapy of the brain. Mask system **(A)** have between 3–5 mm reproducibility. Fixed frame systems **(B)** have 1 mm or less reproducibility.

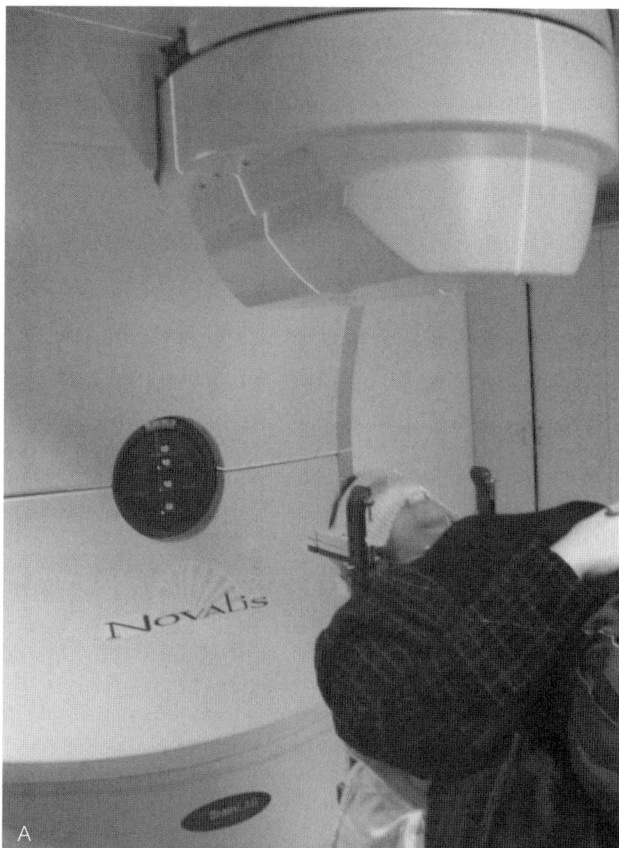

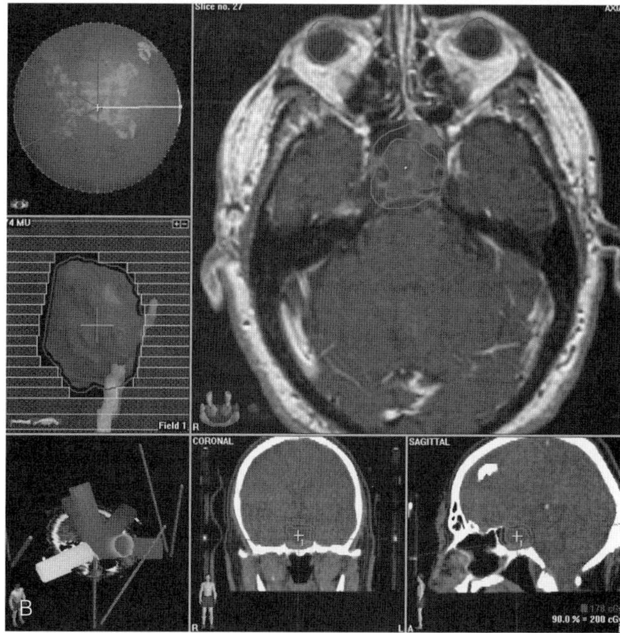

FIGURE 59-3. Modern linear accelerator (LINAC) with patient for stereotactic fractionated radiosurgery. **(A)** Treatment planning station for radiotherapy. **(B)** This is where beams are arranged and dose displayed.

Thousands of reiterations are performed to find the *best fit* to the desired doses. This process is known as *intensity modulated radiotherapy*. This technique is especially useful for irregular targets adjacent to critical normal tissues, such as is found in tumors and other lesions at the skull base. Care must be taken in its use because some of the computer optimization planning programs will give excellent conformality of the prescription dose at the targets edge, but pay a price in creating hotter regions within the target. This is good for solid tumor lesions, such as meningiomas and metastases, but less ideal for infiltrative lesions, such as gliomas, where tumors cells and functioning brain tissue are often intermixed.

TREATMENT: USE OF RADIOTHERAPY IN MALIGNANT AND BENIGN DISORDERS

HIGH GRADE GLIOMAS

Grade III and IV glial tumors, also known as anaplastic astrocytomas and glioblastomas, are the most common malignant brain tumors. The value of radiotherapy in these tumors has been well established since the 1970s when well-done trials in the United States and Europe showed that doses of 60 Gy would double the median survival for these patients from 4 to 5 months to 8 to 11 months (4–6). An improvement in the number of months patients spend in good performance status has been shown. To date, attempts at increasing the dose further with traditional techniques have not been shown to further improve survival (7). Brachytherapy boosts and radiosurgical boosts have also failed to increase survival (8,9). Both of these techniques do appear to aid some patients in the salvage setting, although level-one evidence is lacking (10,11). Although tumor cells have been found at autopsy to be present far from the primary site (12), the clinical pattern of failure remains within 2 cm of the enhancing lesion and this is the volume targeted by most radiation oncologists (13,14). A recent trial has established daily temozolamide chemotherapy during the radiation as the standard of care (15).

LOW GRADE GLIOMAS

Doses of 45 to 54 Gy have been shown to improve disease-free survival and decrease symptoms in those patients who have symptoms (15,16). Two-dose escalation studies have failed to find additional value in doses beyond 45 to 50 Gy (17–19). A European Organisation for Research and Treatment of Cancer (EORTC) randomized study comparing observation with radiotherapy confirmed an improvement in disease-free survival, but did not show an improvement in overall survival (15). This trial really compared radiotherapy at diagnosis against radiotherapy at progression as most patents who did not receive radiotherapy received treatment at progression. The presence of symptoms and prognostic factors (e.g., patient age, tumor size, extent of resection, and crossing of the corpus callosum) have been used to try to determine which patients to treat after diagnosis and which to observe until progression before using radiation (20).

OLIGODENDROGLIOMA

Similar to other gliomas, radiotherapy improves symptoms and disease-free survival for low and high grade oligodendrogliomas (21,22). Two randomized trials failed to show additional benefit to adding procarbazine, lomustine, and vincristine (PCV) chemotherapy, either before or after radiation for grade 3 oligodendrogliomas, but did show a modest benefit in progression-free survival (23,24). Whether PCV can replace radiotherapy as initial treatment and save the radiation for salvage is not known. More recently, temozolamide is being used in the treatment of grade 3 oligodendrogliomas, although how best to combine it with radiotherapy is not known (25,26). Grade-for-grade, patients with these tumors have longer survival and better response to radiotherapy (as well as chemotherapy) than the astrocytic lineage gliomas with median survivals approaching 10 years. Response to radiotherapy and survival for the mixed oligoastrocytic tumors tend to fall in between the pure oligocytic and pure astrocytic tumors (27). Doses used are the same as low and high grade astrocytic gliomas.

EPENDYMOMAS

The value of radiation in these tumors appears to mirror that of the astrocytic low grade gliomas with similar disease-free and overall survivals. In the rare noninvasive ependymoma, surgery alone is adequate; for the more common infiltrating tumor, postoperative radiotherapy is given. Although older literature shows treatment of the craniospinal axis, this is no longer done. If proper CSF sampling and MR imaging of the craniospinal axis is done, these tumors can be treated with local fields only and not craniospinal radiation because the pattern of failure remains local even in grade 3 lesions (28). Doses of 50 to 54 Gy yield 45% progression free survival, and 55% overall survival at 5 years.

GERMINONAS

Germinomas are perhaps the most radiocurable of intracranial tumors. Doses of 45 to 50 Gy for gross disease and 25 to 30 Gy for microscopic disease give long-lasting, complete response and long-term survival for >90% of patients (29–31). Historically, craniospinal treatment fields were advocated because of the finding that about 10% of these tumors would disseminate through the CSF (31,32). Improved imaging of the craniospinal axis also improves the ability to find those patients with disseminated disease. The current tendency is to treat an initial field, covering either the whole brain, or the whole ventricular system, and then boost the gross tumor (30,32,33). Although these tumors are very sensitive to chemotherapy as well, attempts to use chemotherapy alone have had unacceptable results, and one major trial was stopped early (35–37). Protocols using systemic chemotherapy, combined with local field radiation, have had only mixed results (37). This may still be a preferred option for younger patients. Because of the excellent response and control rates with chemotherapy and radiotherapy, the role of surgery should be to confirm the diagnosis and excessive risks need not be taken.

NONGERMINOMA GERM CELL TUMORS

Nongerminomatous germ cell tumors are approached in a similar fashion to germinomas, with the exception that their response rate to radiation and their radiocurability is not nearly as good, with 5-year survival rates with radiotherapy alone hovering at 30% to 40%. Usually, chemotherapy is added to the radiation because some small single trials and retrospective reviews show an increase in 5-year survivals to 50% to 60% (38,39). Because of the small number of these patients, it is not likely that a randomized trial will be done successfully.

PITUITARY ADENOMA

Doses of 50 Gy given with fractionated stereotactic techniques are used for nonfunctional Adenomas, with local control rates of 95% at 5 years and >90% at 10 years (40–43). Most prolactinomas can now be treated medically, but radiation is still useful for those that fail medical and surgical management, as well as other functional adenomas not controlled surgically (43,44). Single dose radiosurgery has been advocated by some and the success rate is similar, but not better than fractionated treatment. Both techniques allow a significant decrease in volume irradiated to the treatment dose. We prefer to avoid the risk of high single doses of radiation close to the optic nerves and chiasm.

MENINGIOMAS

Meningioma, the most common benign intracranial tumor, is well treated by radiotherapy (45-49). For many years, it was not clear how useful radiation was against these tumors because the lesions did not typically shrink or resolve after treatment. With the advent of improved intracranial imaging (CT and

MRI scanners), which allow for better follow up for these patients, it is now clear that radiation prevents progression of most of these lesions, yielding 5- and 10-year progression-free survival of 95% and 90%, respectively (45–49). The current trends are to decrease the irradiated volume in treating meningiomas by using stereotactic fractionated and stereotactic single dose (radiosurgery) techniques. Both of these achieve excellent control rates while treating less normal tissue (49,50). The success of radiotherapy has allowed a less morbid surgical approach, which is aimed at decreasing mass effect and pressure on normal brain and cranial nerves and not fixated on total tumor removal if the risks to normal tissues are high.

ACOUSTIC AND OTHER NEUROMAS

Although base of skull surgery has been the predominant treatment approach for acoustic and other neuromas, the role of radiation has become better defined (50–53). Lesions with significant mass effect need to be approached surgically and are not candidates for radiotherapy or radiosurgery. Most of these lesions, however, are small lesions for which stereotactic radiotherapy or radiosurgery is a reasonable option and no need exists for an extensive base of skull operation. Local control rates are 80% to 90% and complication rates are 30% to 50% for hearing loss and 15% to 30% for facial or trigeminal nerve injury, rates that compare favorably with base of skull surgery. Recent decrease in the radiosurgical dose given and the use of fractionated stereotactic techniques have now pushed these complication rates down to <30% and <10%, respectively (52,53).

CRANIOPHARYNGIOMAS

Although craniopharyngiomas are benign lesions and gross total resection is curative, because of their location and at times intricate association with the optic chiasm and or hypothalamus gross total resection can be perilous to the patient's neurologic function. Subtotal resection, combined with postoperative radiotherapy, has been shown to produce equal survival rates and should be a favored option when total resection is deemed excessively risky (54,55). Doses of 54 Gy in 27 to 30 fractions are typically given. Because of the proximity of the optic chiasm, optic nerves, hypothalamus, and temporal lobes as well as the younger age group that is afflicted with these tumors, the conformal stereotactic techniques of radiotherapy are typically used and, in young children, are associated with better long-term cognitive function (56).

ARTERIOVENOUS MALFORMATIONS

The role of single dose radiation is firmly established as a treatment option for small arteriovenous malformations (AVM) (57–60). Doses of 15 to 25 Gy are used, with larger volumes getting lower doses because of safety concerns. AVM <2 cm have >80% obliteration rates at 3 years. For lesions >3 cm, this rate drops to 50%. Because it takes 6 months for the risk of bleeding to begin to decrease and usually 2 to 3 years for complete obliteration during which a risk of hemorrhage still exists, embolization, surgery, or both are preferred options when the AVM is safely approachable by these modalities (60).

MEDULLOBLASTOMA

The incorporation of radiotherapy and specifically craniospinal radiotherapy into the treatment of medulloblastoma is one of the great success stories of 20th century medicine. A few scattered case reports of long-term survival after surgery alone became a 20% survival rate after adding cranial radiotherapy. The shift to full craniospinal radiation in the 1960s and 1970s increased survival to >50% (61–63). Coupling a platinum-based chemotherapy regimen with radiotherapy has improved survival in patients with a poor prognosis (64) and has allowed a decrease in craniospinal dose from 36 Gy to 24 Gy in those with a standard prognosis (65–67). Posterior fossa boosts to the primary site are being replaced by boosts to the tumor bed alone. Boost doses take the total dose to 54 to 55.8 Gy to the tumor bed. Attempts at withholding or delaying the radiation has led to unacceptable failure rates and is now done only for the youngest age groups where the long-term toxicity at the radiation is more severe (68). Current studies continue to look at how to decrease the craniospinal dose without compromising survival.

PRIMARY CENTRAL NERVOUS SYSTEM LYMPHOMAS

Primary central nervous system (CNS) lymphomas appear histologically similarly to their diffuse large B-cell extracranial counterparts, but their response to treatments, including radiotherapy, has not been nearly as successful. Through most of the 20th century, treatment consisted of whole brain radiotherapy. Although benefit improved with increasing dose up to 50 Gy, no further benefit was seen in pushing past 50 Gy (69). Good initial responses, but frequent relapses, and median survivals of close to a year were seen in most series. The findings in initial trials of similar chemotherapy to that used in systemic lymphomas were negative (70,71). The addition of high-dose systemic and intrathecal methotrexate to 45 Gy whole brain radiation created a quantum leap forward, with median survivals extending to near 3 years and more (72,73). This came at a significant cost of 20% to 30% late neurologic injury, mostly in the form of global dementia (72–75). This was seen more often in patients older than 60 years (75), where most long-term survivors received injury. Trials withholding the radiation and treating using chemotherapy alone or decreased dose radiotherapy have shown more early relapses than the combined modality treatment (75–77). While a current national trial is still combining chemotherapy with the radiation, many institutions, including our own, prefer to treat with up-front chemotherapy and hold the radiation in case of relapse to decrease the risk of dementia (78), thereby accepting a decreased risk of survival for a decreased risk of dementia. High dementia rates in survivors have been reported by this approach as well (79,80).

ACUTE AND LATE EFFECTS OF RADIOTHERAPY

The benefits of radiotherapy, as with other medical therapeutics, come at the risk of side effects and complications for normal tissues. Complications from radiotherapy are dose and volume dependent. These effects and complications can be grouped into three time-phased categories: Early, delayed, and late. For an effect to be ascribed to radiation treatment, the end organ should be within the irradiated volume (e.g., a patient cannot have a radiation-induced brachial plexopathy if the only radiation was to the pelvis for a localized prostate cancer). Reported incidence rates vary widely, perhaps owing to the combination of early deaths, which prevent many patients from having the chance to develop late complications; multiple confounding factors, such as the underlying disease process itself; or other treatments, such as chemotherapy or surgery. The unclear denominator in many studies because of patients lost to follow up, or death likewise can make the interpretation of the absolute risk difficult. Age at date of radiotherapy is also important, with both children, especially those <3 years (when brain myelination is completed), and the elderly being at greater risk for radiation-induced injury.

EARLY EFFECTS

Early effects occur during the course of radiotherapy and tend to resolve once the treatment has concluded. Hair loss, skin and soft tissue erythema and edema, acute nausea, and emesis are all examples of acute effects. For the most part, they are managed with symptomatic treatments, such as skin moisturizers and antiemetics. When the brain is irradiated, the most serious acute complication is an increase in perilesional edema. This edema is usually proportional to volume irradiated, total dose, and dose given per fraction. Typically, the effect is a worsening of previously present symptoms and can be confused with tumor progression. Single or oligofractionated whole brain regimens have been associated with a greater likelihood of significant acute edema and have even been known to precipitate acute death (81–83). These regimens are no longer used for whole brain irradiation. Another common, and probably under reported, acute effect is a serous otitis, which can develop during the later stages of a course of radiotherapy. It is usually self-limiting, but can be treated with tympanostomy tubes. These should not be done prophylactically as risk of infection and nonhealing increases (84–86).

DELAYED EFFECTS

The delayed effects in brain and spinal cord irradiation are thought to be secondary to transient demyelination, with or without radiation-induced edema. Seen more commonly in children, it manifests as an increased lethargy called "somnolence syndrome." Demyelination also can be associated with a transient worsening of neurologic function. It responds to, and can be prevented, by increased corticosteroid doses (87,88). In children with acute leukemia and primary CNS lymphoma patients, demyelination can be magnified by the use of high-dose methotrexate-based systemic and intrathecal chemotherapy. In the spinal cord, this demyelination can cause a phenomenon known as *Lhermitte syndrome.* This is an electric shocklike sensation down the spine and radiating to the legs after neck flexion. Incidence varies with dose per fraction and total dose >50 Gy, but does not exceed 10% and is self-resolving after a few months (89–91). These delayed effects have not been shown to increase the risk of late radiation injury. They often may mimic tumor progression.

LATE EFFECTS

Late effects from radiotherapy are seen from 6 months after radiation therapy onward, continuing potentially to manifest any time during the patient's life. Most are secondary to radiation therapy's effects on the vasculature, either with direct effect on the vessels serving the normal tissues or indirect effect of progressive fibrosis or neovascularization in response to loss of the original vessels. Certain patients appear to be significantly more radiosensitive and more likely to experience late effects from treatment. Other than rare genetic disorders, such as xeroderma pigmentosum—a defective DNA repair mechanism—the full genetics behind these differences in radiosensitivity has not been elucidated. If this were possible, doses may be pushed higher for the remainder of the general population. Some clinical disorders increase the incidence of late effects (e.g., diabetes mellitus, hypertension, and a subpopulation of the patients with connective tissue disorders, such as active rheumatoid arthritis). All of these appear to have in common an increased risk of vascular injury.

BRAIN NECROSIS

The risk of late radionecrosis of the brain has a threshold of 50 to 54 Gy in standard fractionation of 1.8 to 2 Gy per day (92–94). Larger dose per fraction increases the risk and forces the total dose given to be decreased. Likewise, if the volume of irradiated brain is small, as in radiosurgery, standard tolerance doses can often be exceeded without certainty of injury. Brain necrosis is seen most commonly at 12 to 15 months after radiotherapy and should correlate to the high-dose volume of the radiation therapy. Although once thought to be inexorably progressive, it is now known that brain necrosis caused by radiotherapy can decrease and, at times, resolve with corticosteroid treatment; a role for hyperbaric oxygen may exist as well (95).

GLOBAL BRAIN INJURY

Diffuse white matter injury can be seen following wide field or whole brain radiotherapy. These findings correlate with a global dementia clinical picture, often times with gait abnormalities, cognitive changes, and fatigue. MRI T2 findings are the most sensitive to these changes, with abnormalities seen in patients, both symptomatic and asymptomatic, and can be seen in doses as low as 20 Gy (96). The incidence of clinically significant dementia varies, depending on whether looking at all patients treated or only at long-term survivors, with incidences of 1% to 5% and 11% being reported in nearly simultaneous articles (97,98). Whole brain radiotherapy has been the most commonly reported association with this injury and dose per fraction the greatest risk factor. It is also difficult to truly ascertain the cause of the global dysfunction (97–100). In a potentially underpowered study of approximately 20 patients in each of three groups, Taphoorn et al. (101) showed no differences in neuropsychological testing, performance status, or neurologic examination, in patients with low grade glioma treated with or without radiotherapy. In contrast, the control group of age-matched patients treated for hematologic malignancies without radiation outperformed both groups of patients with low grade glioma in neuropsychological testing. This implies an affect from the tumor more than from the treatment as the cause for the neuropsychological dysfunction. Normal pressure hydrocephalus should always be in the differential diagnosis because it is a potentially treatable condition.

Diffuse leukoencephalopathy in children is a syndrome seen in those who have received a combination of high-dose systemic methotrexate, intrathecal methotrexate, and cranial radiation, usually for the treatment of acute lymphocytic leukemia (ALL). It is also seen in patients with primary CNS lymphoma who also receive a similar combination of methotrexate and whole brain radiotherapy. In these patients, significant global brain injury is seen in 30% of those <60 years of age and up to 50% to 80% in patients >60 years of age who are long-term survivors. Vascular and white matter injury are seen, at times, leading to dementia and death (80,102,103).

OPTIC NERVE INJURY

Compounded data from irradiation of pituitary adenomas (a large patient population, with long-term follow-up, and similar size target volume) show an incidence of optic nerve or chiasm injury of 1.5% at doses of 45 to 50 Gy in 1.8 to 2 Gy fractions (104). University of Florida data showed no optic nerve injury in 106 optic nerves treated to a dose of 59 Gy or less, whereas in >59 Gy, the risk was 11% for patients treated at <1.9 Gy per fraction, but 47% for patients treated at or above 1.9 Gy per fraction (105,106). In contrast, the optic nerves and chiasm are intolerant to single doses of radiosurgery with maximal tolerated dose being 8 to 10 Gy (107).

OTHER CRANIAL NERVE INJURY

The tolerance of the cranial nerves varies widely. The optic nerve and chiasm are the most sensitive, with injury threshold at 50 Gy in fractionated doses and 8 Gy in single doses, as noted above. The eighth cranial nerve is also fairly sensitive to radiation, with injury thresholds at 12 to 14 Gy for a single dose and 60 Gy in fractionated treatment. The facial nerve has been reported to have dysfunction after single doses of 14 to16 Gy, with at least 50% of these patients regaining facial function. In contrast, the remaining cranial nerves are fairly radioresistant to either large doses of fractionated radiotherapy or single doses of radiosurgery. Sixty to 70 Gy of fractionated doses and 20 to 24 Gy single dose radiosurgery are given to these nerves with relative impunity (104,108).

HYPOTHALAMIC-PITUITARY DYSFUNCTION

Late hypothalamic-pituitary dysfunction has become a more recognized late effect from radiotherapy, dating to reporting of 58% dysfunction in survivors of medulloblastoma in 1969 (61). With proper modern treatment planning, the pituitary gland can be completely avoided or given limited dose for most lesions, which are not within a few centimeters of the gland. When the pituitary receives doses of >45 Gy, eventual dysfunction is seen in at least 50% of patients (109–111). Incidence is higher in patient with primary pituitary adenomas and those who received chemotherapy and surgery (112). Dysfunction can affect quality of life and eventually survival. Therefore, patients require interval pituitary hormone monitoring, typically yearly, and replacement as needed can prevent them from ever becoming symptomatic.

SECOND MALIGNANCY

Risk of second malignancy after ionizing radiation to the head is real and increases steadily over time. The overall risk for any one patient remains low. Patients treated with doses >45 Gy for pituitary adenoma (a patient population with long follow up after radiotherapy), showed an absolute second malignancy rate of 0% to 2% even at 10 to 20 years (112–115). This risk must be weighed against the potential benefits of the treatment for the current lesion. Meningiomas, gliomas, and sarcomas are the most frequently reported tumors after cranial radiation with a review article listing 312 total cases of radiation-induced meningiomas in the world literature (113). The relative risk for gliomas and meningiomas in a population of children irradiated for tinea capitis was 2.6 and 9.5, respectively, with 25 year follow up (116). The relative risk for the same gliomas and meningiomas in a population of childhood cancer survivors was 6.8 and 9.9, respectively (117). The difference perhaps caused by the greater total dose and dose per fraction given the childhood cancer survivors or a greater genetic susceptibility to malignancy once an initial malignancy has been diagnosed.

LATE SPINAL CORD INJURY

Late spinal cord injury from radiation therapy manifests itself as a progressive upper motor neuron neuropathy. Increase in T2 signal within the cord itself can, but does not have to, be seen. A single institution review of 1,000 patients treated with spinal cord doses of >40 Gy found only two cases of spinal cord injury (118). Most clinicians cap the dose at near 50 Gy, although risk of injury may be still <5% at 60 Gy (111). In the emerging field of spinal radiosurgery, early data appears to show that 10 Gy to 10% of the volume of the cord adjacent to the lesion is safe (119).

CEREBROVASCULAR EFFECTS

The frequency of cerebrovascular (CVA) events is increased by radiotherapy. The best evidence may come from patients treated for pituitary adenomas. Although a study in the United States failed to show a statistically significant difference, it did show a difference, a relative risk (RR) of 2.0 between patients irradiated and the general population (120). A study in Great Britain confirmed the increase in comparison to the general population, RR 4.1 with an actuarial risk of 10% at 10 years (121). Both studies have been criticized because of the lack of a truly appropriate control group and a Swedish study with 342 pituitary cases using matched pituitary cases as controls failed to find a correlation between risk of a CVA effect and radiation dose (122). The fact remains, however, that ionizing radiation can increase intimal hyperplasia as seen in a study of carotid artery comparison irradiated and nonirradiated neck in the same patients (123). A recent sibling matched pair analysis of leukemia and brain tumor survivors show a RR of CVA of 6.4 for doses of 30 Gy and 29.0 for doses of 50 Gy (124). This is evidence for a nonlinear relationship between dose and risk, with greater risk per unit dose at the high end. Small vessels as well can be affected and the effects of closing these small vessels can lead to neovascularization, late fibrosis, and global tissue injury. An extreme example of this is the moyamoya disease, where abnormal collateral vessels develop in a response to previous radiation (125). It has been predominately described in children <5 years of age receiving radiation, but can also be seen in adults. An association also exists between radiation and CNS cavernous malformations and other occult CNS vascular malformations (126,127).

BRACHIAL PLEXOPATHY AND LUMBAR PLEXOPATHY

The pathophysiology of brachial plexopathy, lumbar plexopathy, and other peripheral nerve injuries is believed to be entrapment of the nerves by progressive perineural fibrosis and not a direct effect of the radiation on the nerves. This hypothesis is supported by data showing that most patients treated with repeat localized brachytherapy for sarcomas, where the dose given can be extremely high (90 plus Gy), do not suffer injury (128). The best described injury is brachial plexopathy after irradiation for breast cancer. The neurologic injury usually begins a few years after treatment, but can develop at any time. Sensory change and weakness dominate the presentation, with significant pain being seen only in a few cases. Indeed, if much pain is present, the patient needs to be carefully evaluated for a diffuse recurrence, which can infiltrate the nerves and mimic a radiation-induced plexopathy (129). Dose per fraction is very important, as noted in a randomized trial of 45 Gy in 15 fractions versus 54 Gy in 30 fractions (130). The former group had a brachial plexopathy rate of 6%, whereas the latter despite the higher total dose, had a rate of 1%.

CLINICAL RECOMMENDATIONS OF THE VIGNETTE

The patient was taken for craniotomy for diagnostic and therapeutic purpose. A near total resection was obtained, with the pathology showing a mixture of radiation necrosis and recurrent or persistent tumor. Her seizures were controlled following the resection and her dependence on steroids decreased, but was not resolved. This is a typical presentation of the dilemma between recurrent tumor and radiation injury and this outcome; the presence of both is often seen in patients with glioblastoma multiforme. Although the tumor did not resolve, it also did not progress after the initial radiotherapy. The second resection improved her quality of life. She remains at very high risk for further progression.

SUMMARY

Radiation has a wide range of uses and tremendous benefit for patients with neurologic diseases. The use of ionizing radiation also carries substantial risks to normal tissues, and should not be used when equal less-injurious modalities are available. Developments in technology help to limit the volumes irradiated to high doses and decrease some of these risks. The volume irradiated to low doses by these technologies is sometimes increased, however, and how this will affect risks of second malignancies and other late effects is not entirely clear. It is hypothesized that the overall effect will be at substantial net gain for patients because even second malignancies increase exponentially with does given. Because of the late development of many of the radiation-induced injuries, it is critical that patients be followed and monitored throughout their lives. As more patients are long-term survivors of their diseases, they will be seen more often in the internist's clinic and knowledge of previous radiotherapy will be critical to maximizing their health care benefit.

REFERENCES

1. Roentgen WC. On a new kind of rays. Translation of a paper read before the Physikalische-medicinischen Gesellschaft of Wurzburg on December 28, 1895. *Br J Radiol.* 1931;432.
2. Hodges PC. *The Life and Times of Emil H. Grubbe.* Chicago: University Chicago Press; 1964.
3. Hall EJ. *Radiobiology for the Radiologist,* 6th ed. Philadelphia: Lippincott Williams & Wilkins; 2006.
4. Walker MD, Alexander E, Jr., Hunt WE, et al. Evaluation of BCNU and/or radiotherapy in the treatment of anaplastic gliomas. A cooperative clinical trial. *J Neurosurg.* 1978;49(3):333–343.
5. Walker MD, Green SB, Byar DP, et al. Randomized comparisons of radiotherapy and nitrosoureas for the treatment of malignant glioma after surgery. *New Engl J Med.* 1980;303(23):1323–1329.
6. Kristiansen K, Hagen S, Kollevold T, et al. Combined modality therapy of operated astrocytomas grade III and IV. Confirmation of the value of postoperative irradiation and lack of potentiation of bleomycin on survival time: A prospective multicenter trial of the Scandinavian Glioblastoma Study Group. *Cancer.* 1981;47(4):649–652.
7. Chang CH, Horton J, Schoenfeld D, et al. Comparison of postoperative radiotherapy and combined postoperative radiotherapy and chemotherapy in the multidisciplinary management of malignant gliomas. A joint Radiation Therapy Oncology Group and Eastern Cooperative Oncology Group study. *Cancer.* 1983;52(6):997–1007.
8. Laperriere NJ, Leung PM, McKenzie S, et al. Randomized study of brachytherapy in the initial management of patients with malignant astrocytoma. *Int J Radiat Oncol Biol Phys.* 1998;41(5):1005–1011.
9. Souhami L, Seiferheld W, Brachman D, et al. Randomized comparison of stereotactic radiosurgery followed by conventional radiotherapy with carmustine to conventional radiotherapy with carmustine for patients with glioblastoma multiforme: Report of Radiation Therapy Oncology Group 93-05 protocol. *Int J Radiat Oncol Biol Phys.* 2004;60(3): 853–860.
10. Sneed PK, Larson DA, Gutin PH. Brachytherapy and hyperthermia for malignant astrocytomas. *Semin Oncol.* 1994;21(2):186–197.
11. Shaw E, Scott C, Souhami L, et al. Single dose radiosurgical treatment of recurrent previously irradiated primary brain tumors and brain metastases: Final report of RTOG protocol 90-05. *Int J Radiat Oncol Biol Phys.* 2000;47(2):291–298.
12. Concannon JP, Kramer S, Berry R. The extent of intracranial gliomata at autopsy and its relationship to techniques used in radiation therapy of brain tumors. *Am J Roentgenol Radium Ther Nucl Med.* 1960;84:99–107.
13. Hochberg FH, Pruitt A. Assumptions in the radiotherapy of glioblastoma. *Neurology.* 1980;30(9):907–911.
14. Wallner KE, Galicich JH, Krol G, et al. Patterns of failure following treatment for glioblastoma multiforme and anaplastic astrocytoma. *Int J Radiat Oncol Biol Phys.* 1989;16 (6):1405–1409.
15. van den Bent MJ, Afra D, de Witte O, et al; EORTC Radiotherapy and Brain Tumor Groups and the UK Medical Research Council. Long-term efficacy of early versus delayed radiotherapy for low-grade astrocytoma and oligodendroglioma in adults: The EORTC 22845 randomised trial. *Lancet.* 2005;366(9490):985–990. Erratum in *Lancet.* 2006; 367(9525):1818.
16. Rogers LR, Morris HH, Lupica K. Effect of cranial irradiation on seizure frequency in adults with low-grade astrocytoma and medically intractable epilepsy. *Neurology.* 1993;43(8):1599–1601.
17. Karim AB, Maat B, Hatlevoll R, et al. A randomized trial on dose-response in radiation therapy of low-grade cerebral glioma: European Organization for Research and Treatment of Cancer (EORTC) Study 22844. *Int J Radiat Oncol Biol Phys.* 1996;36(3):549–556.
18. Kiebert GM, Curran D, Aaronson NK, et al. Quality of life after radiation therapy of cerebral low-grade gliomas of the adult: Results of a randomised phase III trial on dose response (EORTC trial 22844). EORTC Radiotherapy Co-operative Group. *Eur J Cancer.* 1998;34(12):1902–1909.
19. Shaw E, Arusell R, Scheithauer B, et al. Prospective randomized trial of low- versus high-dose radiation therapy in adults with supratentorial low-grade glioma: Initial report of a North Central Cancer Treatment Group/Radiation Therapy Oncology Group/Eastern Cooperative Oncology Group study. *J Clin Oncol.* 2002;20(9):2267–2276.
20. Pignatti F, van den Bent M, Curran D, et al; European Organization for Research and Treatment of Cancer Brain Tumor Cooperative Group; European Organization for Research and Treatment of Cancer Radiotherapy Cooperative Group. Prognostic factors for survival in adult patients with cerebral low-grade glioma. *J Clin Oncol.* 2002;20(8): 2076–2084.
21. Lindegaard KF, Mork SJ, Eide GE, et al. Statistical analysis of clinicopathological features, radiotherapy, and survival in 170 cases of oligodendroglioma. *J Neurosurg.* 1987;67(2): 224–230.
22. Macdonald DR. Low-grade gliomas, mixed gliomas, and oligodendrogliomas. *Semin Oncol.* 1994;21(2):236–248.
23. van den Bent MJ, Carpentier AF, Brandes AA, et al. Adjuvant procarbazine, lomustine, and vincristine improve progression-free survival but not overall survival in newly diagnosed anaplastic oligodendrogliomas and oligoastrocytomas: A randomized European Organisation for Research and Treatment of Cancer phase III trial. *J Clin Oncol.* 2006;24(18):2715–2722.
24. Cairncross G, Berkey B, Shaw E, et al. Phase III trial of chemotherapy plus radiotherapy compared with radiotherapy alone for pure and mixed anaplastic oligodendroglioma: Intergroup Radiation Therapy Oncology Group Trial 9402. *J Clin Oncol.* 2006;24(18): 2707–2714.
25. van den Bent MJ, Taphoorn MJ, Brandes AA, et al; European Organization for Research and Treatment of Cancer Brain Tumor Group. Phase II study of first-line chemotherapy with temozolomide in recurrent oligodendroglial tumors: The European Organization

for Research and Treatment of Cancer Brain Tumor Group Study 26971. *J Clin Oncol.* 2003;21(13):2525–2528.
26. Taliansky-Aronov A, Bokstein F, Lavon I, et al. Temozolomide treatment for newly diagnosed anaplastic oligodendrogliomas: A clinical efficacy trial. *J Neurooncol.* 2006;79(2):153–157.
27. Shaw EG, Scheithauer BW, O'Fallon JR. Supratentorial gliomas: A comparative study by grade and histologic type. *J Neurooncol.* 1997;31(3):273–278.
28. Wallner KE, Wara WM, Sheline GE, et al. Intracranial ependymomas: Results of treatment with partial or whole brain irradiation without spinal irradiation. *Int J Radiat Oncol Biol Phys.* 1986;12(11):1937–1941.
29. Bamberg M, Kortmann RD, Calaminus G, et al. Radiation therapy for intracranial germinoma: Results of the German cooperative prospective trials MAKEI 83/86/89. *J Clin Oncol.* 1999;17(8):2585–2592.
30. Haas-Kogan DA, Missett BT, Wara WM, et al. Radiation therapy for intracranial germ cell tumors. *Int J Radiat Oncol Biol Phys.* 2003;56(2):511–518. Erratum in: *Int J Radiat Oncol Biol Phys.* 2003;57(1):306.
31. Schoenfeld GO, Amdur RJ, Schmalfuss IM, et al. Low-dose prophylactic craniospinal radiotherapy for intracranial germinoma. *Int J Radiat Oncol Biol Phys.* 2006;65(2):481–485. Epub 2006.
32. Dearnaley DP, A'Hern RP, Whittaker S, et al. Pineal and CNS germ cell tumors: Royal Marsden Hospital experience 1962–1987. *Int J Radiat Oncol Biol Phys.* 1990;18(4):773–781.
33. Rogers SJ, Mosleh-Shirazi MA, Saran FH. Radiotherapy of localised intracranial germinoma: Time to sever historical ties? *Lancet Oncol.* 2005;6(7):509–519.
34. Bouffet E, Baranzelli MC, Patte C, et al. Combined treatment modality for intracranial germinomas: Results of a multicentre SFOP experience. Societe Francaise d'Oncologie Pediatrique. *Br J Cancer.* 1999;79(7–8):1199–1204.
35. Kellie SJ, Boyce H, Dunkel IJ, et al. Intensive cisplatin and cyclophosphamide-based chemotherapy without radiotherapy for intracranial germinomas: Failure of a primary chemotherapy approach. *Pediatric Blood Cancer.* 2004;43(2):126–133.
36. Farng KT, Chang KP, Wong TT, et al. Pediatric intracranial germinoma treated with chemotherapy alone. *Zhonghua Yi Xue Za Zhi (Taipei).* 1999;62(12):859–866.
37. Haddock MG, Schild SE, Scheithauer BW, et al. Radiation therapy for histologically confirmed primary central nervous system germinoma. *Int J Radiat Oncol Biol Phys.* 1997;38(5):915–923.
38. Robertson PL, DaRosso RC, Allen JC. Improved prognosis of intracranial non-germinoma germ cell tumors with multimodality therapy. *J Neurooncol.* 1997;32(1):71–80.
39. Buckner JC, Peethambaram PP, Smithson WA, et al. Phase II trial of primary chemotherapy followed by reduced-dose radiation for CNS germ cell tumors. *J Clin Oncol.* 1999;17(3):933–940.
40. Park P, Chandler WF, Barkan AL, et al. The role of radiation therapy after surgical resection of nonfunctional pituitary macroadenomas. *Neurosurgery.* 2004;55(1):100–106; discussion 106–107.
41. McCollough WM, Marcus RB, Jr., Rhoton AL, Jr., et al. Long-term follow-up of radiotherapy for pituitary adenoma: The absence of late recurrence after greater than or equal to 4500 cGy. *Int J Radiat Oncol Biol Phys.* 1991;21(3):607–614.
42. Grigsby PW, Simpson JR, Emami BN, et al. Prognostic factors and results of surgery and postoperative irradiation in the management of pituitary adenomas. *Int J Radiat Oncol Biol Phys.* 1989;16(6):1411–1417.
43. Tsang RW, Brierley JD, Panzarella T, et al. Role of radiation therapy in clinical hormonally-active pituitary adenomas. *Radiother Oncol.* 1996;41(1):45–53.
44. Olafsdottir A, Schlechte J. Management of resistant prolactinomas. *Nature Clinical Practice Endocrinology & Metabolism.* 2006;2(10):552–561.
45. Goldsmith BJ, Wara WM, Wilson CB, et al. Postoperative irradiation for subtotally resected meningiomas. A retrospective analysis of 140 patients treated from 1967 to 1990. *J Neurosurg.* 1994;80(2):195–201. Review. Erratum in: *J Neurosurg* 1994;80(4):777. PMID: 8283256.
46. Barbaro NM, Gutin PH, Wilson CB, et al. Radiation therapy in the treatment of partially resected meningiomas. *Neurosurgery.* 1987;20(4):525–528.
47. Taylor BW, Jr., Marcus RB, Jr., Friedman WA, et al. The meningioma controversy: Postoperative radiation therapy. *Int J Radiat Oncol Biol Phys.* 1988;15(2):299–304.
48. Kondziolka D, Levy EI, Niranjan A, et al. Long-term outcomes after meningioma radiosurgery: Physician and patient perspectives. *J Neurosurg.* 1999;91(1):44–45.
49. Milker-Zabel S, Zabel-du Bois A, Huber P, et al. Fractionated stereotactic radiation therapy in the management of benign cavernous sinus meningiomas : Long-term experience and review of the literature. *Strahlenther Onkol.* 2006;182(11):635–640.
50. Noren G, Greitz D, Hirsch A, et al. Gamma knife surgery in acoustic tumors. *Acta Neurochir Suppl (Wien).* 1993;58:104–107.
51. Kondziolka D, Lunsford LD, McLaughlin MR, et al. Long-term outcomes after radiosurgery for acoustic neuromas. *N Engl J Med.* 1998;339(20):1426–1433.
52. Friedman WA, Bradshaw P, Myers A, et al. Linear accelerator radiosurgery for vestibular schwannomas. *J Neurosurg.* 2006;105(5):657–661.
53. Combs SE, Thilmann C, Debus J, et al. Long-term outcome of stereotactic radiosurgery (SRS) in patients with acoustic neuromas. *Int J Radiat Oncol Biol Phys.* 2006;64(5):1341–1347.
54. Suh JH, Gupta N. Role of radiation therapy and radiosurgery in the management of craniopharyngiomas. *Neurosurg Clin N Am.* 2006;17(2):143–148, vi–vii.
55. Stripp DC, Maity A, Janss AJ, et al. Surgery with or without radiation therapy in the management of craniopharyngiomas in children and young adults. *Int J Radiat Oncol Biol Phys.* 2004;58(3):714–720.
56. Merchant TE, Kiehna EN, Kun LE, et al. Phase II trial of conformal radiation therapy for pediatric patients with craniopharyngioma and correlation of surgical factors and radiation dosimetry with change in cognitive function. *J Neurosurg.* 2006;104[2 Suppl]:94–102.
57. Colombo F, Pozza F, Chierego G, et al. Linear accelerator radiosurgery of cerebral arteriovenous malformations: An update. *Neurosurgery.* 1994;34(1):14–20; discussion 20–21.
58. Pollock BE, Lunsford LD, Kondziolka D, et al. Patient outcomes after stereotactic radiosurgery for "operable" arteriovenous malformations. *Neurosurgery.* 1994;35(1):1–7; discussion 7–8.
59. Maruyama K, Kondziolka D, Niranjan A, et al. Stereotactic radiosurgery for brainstem arteriovenous malformations: Factors affecting outcome. *J Neurosurg.* 2004;100(3):407–413.
60. Soderman M, Andersson T, Karlsson B, et al. Management of patients with brain arteriovenous malformations. *Eur J Radiol.* 2003;46(3):195–205.
61. Bloom HJ, Wallace EN, Henk JM. The treatment and prognosis of medulloblastoma in children. A study of 82 verified cases. *Am J Roentgenol Radium Ther Nucl Med.* 1969;105(1):43–62.
62. Landberg TG, Lindgren ML, Cavallin-Stahl EK, et al. Improvements in the radiotherapy of medulloblastoma, 1946–1975. *Cancer.* 1980;45(4):670–678.
63. Castro-Vita H, Salazar OM, Scarantino C, et al. Medulloblastomas. *Reirsta interamericana de radiología.* 1980;5(3):77–82.
64. Packer RJ, Siegel KR, Sutton LN, et al. Efficacy of adjuvant chemotherapy for patients with poor-risk medulloblastoma: A preliminary report. *Ann Neurol.* 1988;24(4):503–508.
65. Packer RJ, Goldwein J, Nicholson HS, et al. Treatment of children with medulloblastomas with reduced-dose craniospinal radiation therapy and adjuvant chemotherapy: A Children's Cancer Group Study. *J Clin Oncol.* 1999;17(7):2127–2136.
66. Packer RJ, Gajjar A, Vezina G, et al. Phase III study of craniospinal radiation therapy followed by adjuvant chemotherapy for newly diagnosed average-risk medulloblastoma. *J Clin Oncol.* 2006 1;24(25):4202–4208.
67. Gottardo NG, Gajjar A. Current therapy for medulloblastoma. *Current Treatment Options in Neurology.* 2006;8(4):319–334.
68. Kortmann RD, Kuhl J, Timmermann B, et al. Postoperative neoadjuvant chemotherapy before radiotherapy as compared to immediate radiotherapy followed by maintenance chemotherapy in the treatment of medulloblastoma in childhood: Results of the German prospective randomized trial HIT '91. *Int J Radiat Oncol Biol Phys.* 2000;46(2):269–279.
69. Nelson DF, Martz KL, Bonner H, et al. Non-Hodgkin's lymphoma of the brain: Can high dose, large volume radiation therapy improve survival? Report on a prospective trial by the Radiation Therapy Oncology Group (RTOG): RTOG 8315.*Int J Radiat Oncol Biol Phys.* 1992;23(1):9–17.
70. Schultz C, Scott C, Sherman W, et al. Preirradiation chemotherapy with cyclophosphamide, doxorubicin, vincristine, and dexamethasone for primary CNS lymphomas: Initial report of radiation therapy oncology group protocol 88–106. *J Clin Oncol.* 1996;14(2):556–564.
71. Mead GM, Bleehen NM, Gregor A, et al. A medical research council randomized trial in patients with primary cerebral non-Hodgkin lymphoma: Cerebral radiotherapy with and without cyclophosphamide, doxorubicin, vincristine, and prednisone chemotherapy. *Cancer.* 2000;89(6):1359–1370.
72. DeAngelis LM, Yahalom J, Thaler HT, et al. Combined modality therapy for primary CNS lymphoma. *J Clin Oncol.* 1992;10(4):635–643.
73. DeAngelis LM, Seiferheld W, Schold SC, et al, for the Radiation Therapy Oncology Group Study 93-10. Combination chemotherapy and radiotherapy for primary central nervous system lymphoma: Radiation Therapy Oncology Group Study 93-10. *J Clin Oncol.* 2002;20(24): 4615–4617.
74. Poortmans PM, Kluin-Nelemans HC, Haaxma-Reiche H, et al. Organization for Research and Treatment of Cancer Lymphoma Group. High-dose methotrexate-based chemotherapy followed by consolidating radiotherapy in non-AIDS-related primary central nervous system lymphoma: European Organization for Research and Treatment of Cancer Lymphoma Group Phase II Trial 20962. *J Clin Oncol.* 2003;21(24):4483–4488. Epub 2003.
75. Gavrilovic IT, Hormigo A, Yahalom J, et al. Long-term follow-up of high-dose methotrexate-based therapy with and without whole brain irradiation for newly diagnosed primary CNS lymphoma. *J Clin Oncol.* 2006;24(28):4570–4574.
76. Batchelor T, Carson K, O'Neill A, et al. Treatment of primary CNS lymphoma with methotrexate and deferred radiotherapy: A report of NABTT 96-07. *J Clin Oncol.* 2003;21(6):1044–1049.
77. Hochberg FH, Tabatabai G. Therapy of PCNSL at the Massachusetts General Hospital with high dose methotrexate and deferred radiotherapy. *Ann Hematol.* 2001;80[Suppl 3]:B111–B112.
78. Omuro AM, Ben-Porat LS, Panageas KS, et al. Delayed neurotoxicity in primary central nervous system lymphoma. *Arch Neurol.* 2005;62(10):1595–1600.
79. Lai R, Abrey LE, Rosenblum MK, et al. Treatment-induced leukoencephalopathy in primary CNS lymphoma: A clinical and autopsy study. *Neurology.* 2004;62(3):451–456.
80. Herrlinger U, Kuker W, Uhl M, et al; Neuro-Oncology Working Group of the German Society. NOA-03 trial of high-dose methotrexate in primary central nervous system lymphoma: Final report. *Ann Neurol.* 2005;57(6):843–847.
81. Hindo WA, DeTrana FA 3rd, Lee MS, et al. Large dose increment irradiation in treatment of cerebral metastases. *Cancer.* 1970;26(1):138–141.
82. Young DF, Posner JB, Chu F, et al. Rapid-course radiation therapy of cerebral metastases: Results and complications. *Cancer.* 1974;34(4):1069–1076.
83. Borgelt B, Gelber R, Larson M, et al. Ultra-rapid high dose irradiation schedules for the palliation of brain metastases: Final results of the first two studies by the Radiation Therapy Oncology Group. *Int J Radiat Oncol Biol Phys.* 1981;7(12):1633–1638.
84. Chowdhury CR, Ho JH, Wright A, et al. Prospective study of the effects of ventilation tubes on hearing after radiotherapy for carcinoma of nasopharynx. *Ann Otol Rhinol Laryngol.* 1988;97(2 Pt 1):142–145.
85. Morton RP, Woollons AC, McIvor NP. Nasopharyngeal carcinoma and middle ear effusion: Natural history and the effect of ventilation tubes. *Clin Otolaryngol Allied Sci.* 1994;19(6):529–531.
86. Ho WK, Wei WI, Kwong DL, et al. Randomized evaluation of the audiologic outcome of ventilation tube insertion for middle ear effusion in patients with nasopharyngeal carcinoma. *J Otolaryngol.* 2002;31(5):287–293.

87. Faithfull S, Brada M. Somnolence syndrome in adults following cranial irradiation for primary brain tumours. *Clin Oncol (R Coll Radiol)*. 1998;10(4):250–254.
88. Mandell LR, Walker RW, Steinherz P, et al. Reduced incidence of the somnolence syndrome in leukemic children with steroid coverage during prophylactic cranial radiation therapy. Results of a pilot study. *Cancer*. 1989;63(10):1975–1978.
89. Jones A. Transient radiation myelopathy (with reference to Lhermitte's sign of electrical paraesthesia). *Br J Radiol*. 1964;37:727–744.
90. Fein DA, Marcus RB, Jr., Parsons JT, et al. Lhermitte's sign: Incidence and treatment variables influencing risk after irradiation of the cervical spinal cord. *Int J Radiat Oncol Biol Phys*. 1993;27(5):1029–1033.
91. Word JA, Kalokhe UP, Aron BS, et al. Transient radiation myelopathy (Lhermitte's sign) in patients with Hodgkin's disease treated by mantle irradiation. *Int J Radiat Oncol Biol Phys*. 1980;6(12):1731–1733.
92. Marks JE, Baglan RJ, Prassad SC, et al. Cerebral radionecrosis: Incidence and risk in relation to dose, time, fractionation and volume. *Int J Radiat Oncol Biol Phys*. 1981;7:243–249.
93. Sheline GE, Wara WM, Smith V. Therapeutic irradiation and brain injury. *Int J Radiat Oncol Biol Phys*. 1980;6(9):1215–1228.
94. Ruben JD, Dally M, Bailey M, et al. Cerebral radiation necrosis: Incidence, outcomes, and risk factors with emphasis on radiation parameters and chemotherapy. *Int J Radiat Oncol Biol Phys*. 2006;65(2):499–508.
95. Ohguri T, Imada H, Kohshi K, et al. Effect of prophylactic hyperbaric oxygen treatment for radiation-induced brain injury after stereotactic radiosurgery of brain metastases. *Int J Radiat Oncol Biol Phys*. 2007;67(1):248–255.
96. Reddick WE, Russell JM, Glass JO, et al. Subtle white matter volume differences in children treated for medulloblastoma with conventional or reduced dose craniospinal irradiation. *Magnes Reson Imaging*. 2000;18(7):787–793.
97. DeAngelis LM, Delattre JY, Posner JB. Radiation-induced dementia in patients cured of brain metastases. *Neurology*. 1989;39(6):789–796.
98. DeAngelis LM, Mandell LR, Thaler HT, et al. The role of postoperative radiotherapy after resection of single brain metastases. *Neurosurgery*. 1989;24(6):798–805.
99. Crossen JR, Garwood D, Glatstein E, et al. Neurobehavioral sequelae of cranial irradiation in adults: A review of radiation-induced encephalopathy. *JCO*, 1994;12(3):627–642.
100. Taylor BV, Buckner JC, Cascino TL, et al. Effects of radiation and chemotherapy on cognitive function in patients with high-grade glioma. *JCO*. 1998;2195–2201.
101. Taphoorn MJ, Schiphorst AK, Snoek FJ, et al. Cognitive functions and quality of life in patients with low-grade gliomas: The impact of radiotherapy. *Ann Neurol*. 1994;36(1):48–54.
102. Abrey LE, Yahalom J, DeAngelis LM. Treatment for primary CNS lymphoma: The next step. *J Clin Oncol*. 2000;18(17):3144–3150.
103. Thiessen B, DeAngelis LM. Hydrocephalus in radiation leukoencephalopathy: Results of ventriculoperitoneal shunting. *Arch Neurol*. 1998;55(5):705–710.
104. Stelzer KJ. Acute and long-term complications of therapeutic radiation for skull base tumors. *Neurosurg Clin N Am*. 2000;11:4:597–604.
105. Parsons JT, Bova FJ, Fitzgerald CR, et al. Radiation optic neuropathy after megavoltage external beam irradiation: Analysis of time dose factors. *Int J Radiat Oncol Biol Phys*. 1994;30:755–763.
106. Parsons JT, Fitzgerald CR, Hood CI, et al. The effects of irradiation on the eye and optic nerve. *Int J Radiat Oncol Biol Phys*. 1983;9(5):609–622.
107. Leber KA, Bergloff J, Pendl G. Dose response tolerance of the visual pathways and the cranial nerves of the cavernous sinus to stereotactic radiosurgery. *J Neurosurg*. 1998;88:43–50.
108. Schultheiss T, Kun L, Ang K, Stephens L. Radiation responses of the central nervous system. *Int J Radiat Oncol Biol Phys*. 1995;31(5):1093–1113.
109. Brada M, Rajan B, Traish D, et al. The long-term efficacy of conservative surgery and radiotherapy in the control of pituitary adenomas. *Clin Endocrinol*. 1993;38:571–578.
110. Agha A, Sherlock M, Brennan S, et al. Hypothalamic-pituitary dysfunction after irradiation of nonpituitary brain tumors in adults. *J Clin Endocrinol Metab*. 2005;90(12): 6355–6360.
111. Darzy KH, Shalet SM. Hypopituitarism after cranial irradiation. *J Endocrinol Invest*. 2005;28[5 Suppl]:78–87.
112. Cohen LE. Endocrine late effects of cancer treatment. *Curr Opin Pediatr*. 2003; 15(1):3–9.
113. Breen P, Flickinger JC, Kondziolka D, et al. Radiotherapy for nonfunctional pituitary adenoma: Analysis of long-term tumor control. *J Neurosurg*. 1998;89:933–938.
114. McCord M, Buatti JM, Fennell EM, et al. Radiotherapy for pituitary adenoma: Long-term outcome and sequelae. *Int J Radiat Oncol Biol Phys*. 1997;39(2):437–444.
115. Minniti G, Traish D, Ashley S, et al. Risk of second brain tumor after conservative surgery and radiotherapy for pituitary adenoma: Update after an additional 10 years. *J Clin Endocrinol Metab*. 2005;90(2):800–804. Epub 2004
116. Ron E, Modan B, Boice JD, Jr., et al. Tumors of the brain and nervous system after radiotherapy in childhood. *N Engl J Med*. 1988;319(16):1033–1039.
117. Neglia JP, Robison LL, Stovall M, et al. New primary neoplasms of the central nervous system in survivors of childhood cancer: A report from the Childhood Cancer Survivor Study. *J Natl Cancer Inst*. 2006;98(21):1528–3157.
118. Marcus RB, Jr., Million RR. The incidence of myelitis after irradiation of the cervical spinal cord. *Int J Radiat Oncol Biol Phys*. 1990;19(1):3–8.
119. Ryu S, Jin JY, Jin R, et al. Partial volume tolerance of the spinal cord and complications of single-dose radiosurgery. *Cancer*. 2007;109(3):628–636.
120. Flickinger JC, Nelson PB, Taylor FH, et al. Incidence of cerebral infarction after radiotherapy for pituitary adenoma. *Cancer*. 1989;63(12):2404–2408.
121. Brada M, Burchell L, Ashley S, et al. The incidence of cerebrovascular accidents in patients with pituitary adenoma. *Int J Radiat Oncol Biol Phys*. 1999;45(3):693–698.
122. Erfurth EM, Bulow B, Svahn-Tapper G, et al. Risk factors for cerebrovascular deaths in patients operated and irradiated for pituitary tumors. *J Clin Endocrinol Metab*. 2002; 87(11):4892–4899.
123. Dorresteijn LD, Kappelle AC, Scholz NM, et al. Increased carotid wall thickening after radiotherapy on the neck. *Eur J Cancer*. 2005;41(7):1026–1030.
124. Bowers DC, Liu Y, Leisenring W, et al. Late-occurring stroke among long-term survivors of childhood leukemia and brain tumors: A report from the Childhood Cancer Survivor Study. *J Clin Oncol*. 2006;24(33):5277–5282.
125. Desai SS, Paulino AC, Mai WY, et al. Radiation-induced moyamoya syndrome. *Int J Radiat Oncol Biol Phys*. 2006;65(4):1222–1227.
126. Amirjamshidi A, Abbassioun K. Radiation-induced tumors of the central nervous system occurring in childhood and adolescence. Four unusual lesions in three patients and a review of the literature. *Child's nervous system*. 2000;16(7):390–397.
127. Novelli PM, Reigel DH, Langham Gleason P, et al. Multiple cavernous angiomas after high-dose whole-brain radiation therapy. *Pediatr Neurosurg*. 1997;26(6):322–325.
128. Nori D, Schupak K, Shiu MH, et al. Role of brachytherapy in recurrent extremity sarcoma in patients treated with prior surgery and irradiation. *Int J Radiat Oncol Biol Phys*. 1991;20(6):1229–1233.
129. Stoll BA, Andrews JT. Radiation-induced peripheral neuropathy. *BMJ*. 1966;1: 834–837.
130. Posniak HV, Olson MC, Dudiak CM, et al. MR imaging of the brachial plexus. *AJR Am J Roentgenol*. 1993;161:373–379.

CHAPTER 60

Chemotherapy

Scott E. Smith

OBJECTIVES

- To identify expected or frequently seen neurologic toxicities associated with cancer chemotherapeutics
- To describe the etiology of these toxicities
- To discuss common treatments for these toxicities
- To review long-term neurologic sequelae of chemotherapy

CASE VIGNETTE

The patient is a 42-year-old woman who has been diagnosed with stage 3 invasive ductal carcinoma of the right breast and has had a right breast lumpectomy with right axillary lymph node dissection. She has been rendered surgically NED (no evidence of disease) and proceeds to undergo adjuvant chemotherapy with doxorubicin (Adriamycin) and cyclophosphamide every 2 weeks for four cycles (dose-dense fashion), followed by paclitaxel every 2 weeks for four cycles. She develops mild to moderate nausea and fatigue with the Adriamycin and cyclophosphamide component of the chemotherapy regimen and as well as a somewhat disabling peripheral neuropathy of the digits and both hands and feet, described as severe "numbness and tingling with burning," which occasionally awakens her from sleep. This peripheral neuropathy developed after her third cycle of paclitaxel and was somewhat relieved with a 50% dose reduction in the paclitaxel with the fourth cycle of this chemotherapy. Supportive care with amitriptyline and gabapentin relieved most of the neuropathic pain and the patient finished her chemotherapy with no further complaints.

Fourteen months after completion of chemotherapy, she presented to her oncologist for routine follow up and also complained of fever, severe fatigue, and epistaxis. A complete blood count revealed her leukocyte count to be 1,000/uL, her hemoglobin was 7.2 g/dL, and her platelet count was 14,000/uL. The patient was admitted to the hospital for neutropenic fever and workup for her pancytopenia ensued, which ultimately involved a bone marrow aspiration and biopsy. The bone marrow revealed a hypercellular marrow (95%) with 80% myeloblasts, consistent with acute myeloid leukemia (AML). Cytogenetic analysis revealed a complex karyotype, including monosomy 7, trisomy 8, and 11q11.2 deletion in all cells tested. The diagnosis of secondary AML was made and the patient was begun on empiric antibiotics for her fever, as well as transfusions of eryrthrocytes and platelets. Also begun was high-dose cytarabine to treat her AML. After the second dose of chemotherapy, the patient developed dysarthria and cerebellar ataxia. Further cytarabine was held and the patient was switched to mitoxantrone and etoposide for further anti-AML chemotherapy and all anticholinergic agents were held (including, prochlorperazine and diphenhydramine). The ataxia resolved slowly over the subsequent 2 weeks and the patient achieved a complete remission and went on for high-dose chemotherapy and allogeneic stem cell transplant without further neurologic problems.

DEFINITION

Neurologic toxicity is a common problem seen in patients having chemotherapy for various malignancies. Defined, it is any untoward change in the central, peripheral, or autonomic nervous system, whether it is permanent or transient, associated with chemotherapeutic agents. Indeed, for some chemotherapeutic agents, neurologic toxicities are the dose-limiting toxicities of the drugs. With the aging patient population and increased successes in treating patients with these malignancies, neurologic sequelae are seen more frequently in the internist's office and are having a larger, long-term impact on a patient's performance status and quality of life.

When trying to understand the neurologic problems encountered with cancer treatment, it is very important to understand the type and location of the malignancy, other modalities of treatment involved with the patient's care (surgery and radiation therapy can also impart neurologic symptoms), and, finally, the specific chemotherapeutic agent used and its associated mechanism of action. The vignette used above is an example of the neurologic toxicity associated almost purely with the specific chemotherapeutics; however, if an example of a patient with a glioblastoma multiforme was given, in which the patient had received surgical, radiation therapy, local chemotherapy (Carmustine [BCNU] wafer), and finally systemic chemotherapy, with multiple central nervous system (CNS) toxicities, it is a much more difficult task to assign toxicities to the respective treatment modality.

Nevertheless, in dealing with chemotherapy-related neurologic toxicity, it helps to understand the location of the defect. Peripheral neuropathies are a frequent toxicity seen with agents used to disrupt microtubule formation, including taxanes and vinca alkaloids. It is understood that these agents also disrupt microtubule function within the axon and, especially for the taxanes, this is seen in a dose-dependent fashion. Other agents traditionally exhibit their toxicities in the CNS, such as high-dose cytarabine which can cause apoptosis of cholinergic neurons within the CNS.

It is also important to understand that the toxicities of these agents can be somewhat predictable, but also can have a dramatic interperson variance to the point where it is virtually impossible to predict the long-term effect of these agents on quality of life and potential for permanent disability.

EPIDEMIOLOGY

With hundreds of thousands of patients being treated with chemotherapeutics each year in the United States alone and a slowly increasing survivorship, the number of patients with neurologic problems associated with cancer treatment is increasing. It is also obvious that the incidence of these toxicities will be a function of the individual agents used and that use of these agents depends on cancer type, stage, location, and other factors.

ETIOLOGY AND PATHOGENESIS

To properly identify the etiology and pathogenesis of the neurologic manifestations of the associated chemotherapeutic agents, it is important to evaluate each drug or class of drug for its inherent toxicities and the likelihood for neurotoxicity and whether it is likely to be transient or permanent. Table 60-1 lists chemotherapeutic drugs and their potential for neurotoxicity.

TABLE 60-1. Chemotherapeutic Drugs and Their Potential for Neurotoxicity

HIGH RISK
L-Asparaginase
Bortezomib
Carboplatin
Cisplatin
Cytarabine
Docetaxel
Fludarabine
5-Fluoruracil
Ifosfamide
Interleukin-2
Interferons
Methotrexate
Oxaliplatin
Paclitaxel
Pentostatin
Procarbazine
Thalidomide
Vinblastine
Vincristine
Vinorelbine
POTENTIAL FOR TRANSIENT NEUROTOXICITY
Busulfan (high-dose)
Chlorambucil
Dacarbazine
Etoposide (high-dose)
Gemcitabine
Interferons (low-dose)
Interleukin-2
Teniposide
POTENTIAL FOR PERMANENT NEUROTOXICITY
Bortezomib
Cisplatin
Cytarabine
Docetaxel
5-Fluorouracil
Ifosfamide
Paclitaxel
Thalidomide

PATHOLOGY

Certain drugs or classes of drugs with relatively well understood mechanisms of action bear special attention.

5-Fluorouracil (5-FU) was one of the earliest chemotherapeutics to become available for the treatment of various malignancies, most notably of the aerodigestive tracts. Its neurologic toxicity is rarely seen, with an incidence of only 5% to 7%. It, however, has of rapid onset and is generally not considered to be dose related. The toxicities include cerebellar findings, including gait abnormalities, dysarthria, ataxia, nystagmus, and dysmetria (1). Also seen are generalized somnolence, confusion, seizures, and, occasionally, coma. Although the cause of these toxicities is not fully understood, they are thought to be from either the drug itself or its metabolites, because patients who lack the catabolizing enzyme for 5-FU (dihydropyrimadine dehydrogenase-DPD) tend to have higher frequencies of 5-FU–induced neurotoxicity, including peripheral neuropathies (2).

The platinum-based agents, which are also associated with significant neurologic toxicities, include cisplatin, carboplatin, and oxaliplatin. These drugs function by intercalating into the DNA and altering the normal DNA structure and its replicative potential before cell division. It is believed that platinum itself in the inorganic form accumulates in the neurons and can be seen in high accumulations in the dorsal root ganglia on autopsy findings of patients with prior platinum-induced neuropathy (3). Whereas nephrotoxicity is the dose-limiting toxicity for cisplatin, neurotoxicity is the major dose-limiting factor for oxaliplatin (4) and this tends to represent itself as a peripheral neuropathy that tends to be cumulative. The platinum-induced peripheral neuropathies tend to be first noticed in the feet rather than the hands, such as seen with vinca alkaloid use. In fact, loss of ankle reflexes may be the first sign of neurotoxicity in these patients.

Vinca alkaloids (including vincristine, vinblastine, and vinorelbine) are widely known for their neurologic toxicities. The neurologic toxicity of vincristine is its only dose-limiting toxicity. Vincristine neurotoxicity can occur in the central, autonomic, and peripheral nervous systems (5). Any nerve can affected, although the initial manifestations typically seen are suppression of the muscle stretch reflexes and paresthesias of the digits of both hands and feet. With continued use, these paresthesias migrate proximally and can engulf the entire hand or foot. Proprioception, nociception, and vibratory sensation are usually spared with Vinca-induced neuropathy. Patients may also exhibit cranial nerve paralysis, as well as severe autonomic dysfunction leading to constipation or ileus. Vincristine binds to subunit B of tubulin, which causes interruption of the microtubule function in neuronal axons. Concurrent or sequential use of two antimicrotubule agents, such as vinblastine and paclitaxel, causes enhanced neurotoxicity, whereas combinations with agents, such as cisplatin, do not typically enhance the neurotoxicity (6).

Cytarabine is one of the few chemotherapeutic agents (along with methotrexate) administered both intravenously (IV) and intrathecally. Both routes of administration can lead to significant neurotoxicity, most of which is evidenced as CNS abnormalities, such as cerebellar dysfunction, encephalopathy, seizures, necrotizing leukoencephalopathy, and basal ganglia necrosis. Peripheral neuropathies may also be evident. In lower doses (<1,000 mg/m^2), neurologic findings are less common; however, if high doses of cytarabine (>1,000 mg/m^2) are used, the incidence of these toxicities are upward of 30% to 35% (7). Many of the cerebellar toxicities are transient and will diminish over a short period of time (8). Occasionally, the cerebellar ataxia can be of sufficient seriousness to warrant endotracheal intubation for airway protection.

Methotrexate-like cytarabine is commonly used by intrathecal (IT) or parenteral administration. In addition, it can be given orally and is frequently used to treat nonmalignant states, such as autoimmune disorders. In low dose forms, nephrotoxicity is the only major concern. It perturbs folate metabolism via inhibition of dihydrofolate reductase and many of its toxicities can be bypassed or *rescued* with the use of folinic acid. When high doses are used, folinic acid is regularly used to counteract many of the gastrointestinal toxicities, such as severe mucositis. It is readily eliminated via the urine at a pH >5.7. If the urine pH is <5.7, methotrexate and its major metabolite, 7-hydroxymethotrexate, may precipitate in the renal tubules, leading to renal dysfunction and delayed drug clearance and increased toxicity. When given intrathecally, methotrexate can cause direct meningeal irritation and result in headache, nausea, vomiting, and nuchal rigidity initially, or have delayed symptoms, such as seizures, hemiparesis, paraparesis, somnolence, or cranial nerve dysfunction. The risk for these symptoms is increased for regimens in which both IT and high-dose IV infusion are used. Long-term side effects of repeated IT infusion can include acute death (very rarely, secondary to necrotizing leukoencephalopathy) (9); severe dementia, ataxia, seizures, and dysphasia. Many of the acute abnormalities and possibly some of the long-term toxicities can be secondary to impairment in neurotransmitter production directly by the methotrexate or accumulation of homocysteine, adenosine, or other amino acids. Aminophylline sometimes has been used to antagonize the adenosine receptor and reduce the neurotoxicity of methotrexate (10,11).

Taxanes are represented by paclitaxel and docetaxel. As with vinca alkaloids, the mechanism of action is believed to be inhibition of axonal microtubular function. A cumulative dose relationship appears to exist with both docetaxel and paclitaxel. Single doses of paclitaxel >175 mg/m^2 given every 3 weeks produces greater neurotoxicity than lower doses. Cumulative doses of docetaxel also are shown to produce higher rates of peripheral neuropathies than lower cumulative doses. These toxicities are similar to those seen with platinum agents and may show stocking-glove paresthesia, burning pain, perioral paresthesias, loss of vibratory sensation, decreased muscle stretch reflexes, and orthostatic hypotension (12), which may be dose-limiting toxicities. In addition, proximal muscle weakness, optic neuropathy, and encephalopathy have also been noted; however, it is unclear whether these represent taxane-related toxicity or whether these are from the high-dose corticosteroids given before treatment to ameliorate any hypersensitivity reaction that may occur because of the polyethoxylated castor oil (Cremophor) used to emulsify the taxane. The effects of these toxicities tend to wane over time, assuming dose reduction or cessation of therapy once the toxicities are noted (13).

Procarbazine is frequently used in chemotherapy regimens that also contain vinca alkaloids; therefore, its true incidence of neurotoxicity is not truly known, but is thought to be approximately 20%. Although both peripheral and central toxicities have been noted, most frequently seen are lethargy, confusion, depression, hallucinations, and psychosis. When present, the peripheral neurotoxicities include loss of muscle stretch reflexes and peripheral neuropathies similar to those seen with vinca alkaloid use. Cessation of therapy may not result in resolution of peripheral manifestations for many weeks to months; however, central symptoms tend to respond quickly (14,15).

Purine analogs, such as cladribine, pentostatin, and especially fludarabine, have long been known to produce severe neurotoxicities. In early studies, fludarabine given in doses >80 to 90 mg/m^2/day given for >5 days resulted in altered mental status, dementia, quadriparesis, and coma, which did not necessarily resolve on drug cessation, and many patients went on to die from their progressive neurologic toxicities. The recommended dose of 25 mg/m^2/day for 5 days every 28 days results in mild instances of neurotoxicity, with an incidence of 10% to 20%, although severe toxicity may still ensue and may present after cessation of therapy (16). Administration of cladribine and pentostatin (17) can be lethal from a neurologic standpoint when given in myeloablative doses, with symptoms similar to those seen with higher doses of fludarabine.

Ifosfamide is structurally similar to cyclophosphamide, but it causes neurotoxicity where cyclophosphamide does not. The difference in toxicity appears to be mediated via toxic metabolites that accumulate in large doses with ifosfamide and, to a much lesser extent, with cyclophosphamide. These toxicities can be extreme, with nightmares, auditory and visual hallucinations, incontinence, confusion, agitation, perseveration, and cerebellar and cranial nerve dysfunction. Peripheral neuropathies have also been seen with ifosfamide use; other manifestations can include myoclonus and spasticity (18). These symptoms may not ensue until 5 to 7 days into therapy and are not necessarily dose dependent. Methylene blue and benzodiazepines have been used to counteract many of these symptoms (19).

Interleukin-2 is a unique drug on this list because it is a naturally occurring drug; when given in either low or high doses, however, it has an unusual list of neurotoxicities, many of which may be related to the capillary leak syndrome. Many patients also exhibit hallucinations, agitation, combativeness, seizures, and coma, which tend to resolve on cessation of the drug (20). The capillary leak syndrome may also be responsible for carpal tunnel syndrome caused by median nerve compression secondary to the increased edema (21).

CLINICAL MANIFESTATIONS AND SPECIAL SITUATIONS

The neurologic toxicities associated with chemotherapy administration can be complex and subtle. Adding to the difficulty of toxicity assessment is that many of the common regimens used in cancer treatment involve multiagent chemotherapy as well as multimodality treatment, including combinations of chemotherapy along with radiation therapy and surgical intervention. If toxicity is believed to be secondary to drug administration, it is important to be cognizant of the myriad of supportive drugs used to ameliorate the toxic chemotherapy effects. These supportive drugs themselves can be sources of other neurologic effects, such as the anticholinergic effects of diphenhydramine or prochlorperazine, which can lead to constipation or other autonomic side effects. Also, benzodiazepines and other agents, such as ondansetron, can alter mental status or cause headaches, respectively.

DIAGNOSTIC APPROACH

Neurologic toxicities from chemotherapy are approached much the same way as other neurologic symptoms. A thorough history, neurologic examination, and understanding of the frequent drug toxicities are useful for most cases. In complex cases (e.g., those dealing with nervous system tumors or metastases), it may be difficult to differentiate between the natural progression of CNS disease from the toxicities of its treatment. In these cases, neurologic examination may need to be aided with other diagnostic modalities, including magnetic resonance imaging (MRI), computed tomographic (CT) scan, lumbar puncture with flow cytometry of the cerebrospinal fluid (CSF), or even CNS biopsy. For peripheral lesions, electromyelography and nerve conduction velocities (EMG/NCV) are sometimes helpful in delineating the cause of some neuropathies.

TREATMENT

Treatment of neurologic toxicities related to chemotherapy is mainly expectant, except where specific modalities have been noted. The most common toxicity seen in long-term, cancer survivors is peripheral neuropathy. This neuropathy can be debilitating and painful and can have a dramatic impact on performance status and quality of life. Although many of the neuropathies will lessen in severity or resolve completely over time with cessation of the offending agent, many drugs and therapies have been used to help reduce the symptoms. From a pharmacologic standpoint, tricyclic antidepressants and γ-aminobutyric acid (GABA) analogs, such as gabapentin, have been used with some success and newer agents (e.g., pregabalin) as well as serotonin and norepinephrine reuptake inhibitors are also showing some promise at reducing these symptoms. In extreme cases, surgical intervention has been attempted.

Prevention has also been examined because many of the neurotoxicities are predictable. Amifostine has shown some promise in reducing the severity of paclitaxel- and platinum-based neurotoxicities. Calcium and magnesium infusions during oxaliplatin therapy may help abate the cold-related dyesthesias frequently seen with its administration.

Other toxicities, such as severe dementia (*chemo-brain*) can be seen and are difficult to manage. Treatment approaches similar to organic causes of dementia have been used with limited success. Acetylcholinesterase inhibitors have been used and have had modest results.

CLINICAL RECOMMENDATIONS OF THE VIGNETTE

The patient had multiple neurologic toxicities associated with her chemotherapy regimens. Nausea, vomiting, and fatigue frequently ensue after initiation of therapy and can respond to good supportive care. The moderate to severe neuropathy associated with her paclitaxel use also responded to supportive care and to a change in drug dose. The secondary leukemia is really an unfortunate, nonneurologic consequence of her prior therapy, which actually led to other treatment modalities that, in fact, did cause neurologic sequelae. Her cerebellar dysfunction promptly resolved with cessation of cytarabine and changing therapy to mitoxantrone and etoposide, which did not lead to further impairment. The patient is alive and without severe neurologic impairment because of prompt evaluation and management of the potentially life-threatening toxicities.

SUMMARY

Neurologic toxicities secondary to chemotherapy are but a few of the side effects commonly encountered in the treatment of patients with cancer. Cytotoxic drugs, by definition, are drugs intended to kill human cells and it is stunning that patients do not have more frequent toxicities than those already described. In addition to this, many of the chemotherapy agents have extremely narrow and unpredictable therapeutic windows. Nevertheless, it is possible for the astute clinician to recognize and anticipate certain toxicities. This can only be done effectively with a team approach. Oncology pharmacists are highly trained and invaluable in setting up and following clinical algorithms for the chemotherapy preparation and administration. Infusion nurses are on the front line of drug administration and frequently are the first to notice toxicities and immediately report these toxicities to the oncologists who then make appropriate decisions for clinical management. The patient necessarily bears the brunt of the toxicities and works with the rest of the team to get relief. Despite this, neurotoxicities take a toll on patients with cancer.

REFERENCES

1. Lucato LT, McKinney AM, Short J, et al. Reversible findings of restricted diffusion in 5-fluorouracil neurotoxicity. *Australas Radiol.* 2006;50(4):364–368.
2. Milano G, Etienne MC, Pierrefite V, et al. Dihydropyrimidine dehydrogenase deficiency and fluorouracil-related toxicity. *Br J Cancer.* 1999;79:627–630.
3. Gregg RW, Molepo JM, Monpetit VJA, et al. Cisplatin neurotoxicity: The relationship between dosage, time and platinum concentration in neurologic tissues, and morphologic evidence of toxicity. *J Clin Oncol.* 1992;10:795–803.
4. Kiernan MC, Krishnan AV. The pathophysiology of oxaliplatin-induced neurotoxicity. *Curr Med Chem.* 2006;13(24):2901–2907.
5. Weiden PL, Wright SE. Vincristine neurotoxicity. *N Engl J Med.* 1972;286:1369–1370.
6. Parimoo D, Jeffers S, Muggia FM. Severe neurotoxicity from vinorelbine-paclitaxel combinations. *J Natl Cancer Inst.* 1996;88:1079–1080.
7. Baker WJ, Royer GI, Weiss RB. Cytarabine and neurologic toxicity. *J Clin Oncol.* 1991;9:679–693.
8. Omuro AM, Abrey LE. Chemotherapy for primary central nervous system lymphoma. *Neurosurg Focus.* 2006;21(5):E12.
9. Shore T, Barnett MJ, Phillips GL. Sudden neurologic death after intrathecal methotrexate. *Med Pediatr Oncol.* 1990;18:159–161.
10. Bernini JC, Fort DW, Griener KC. Aminophylline for methotrexate-induced neurotoxicity. *Lancet.* 1995;345:544–547.
11. Jahnke K, Doolittle ND, Muldoon LL, et al. Implications of the blood–brain barrier in primary central nervous system lymphoma. *Neurosurg Focus.* 2006;21(5):E11
12. Chaudhry V, Rowinsky EK, Sartorius SE, et al. Peripheral neuropathy from taxol and cisplatin combination chemotherapy: Clinical and electrophysiological studies. *Ann Neurol.* 1994;35(3):304–311.
13. Kouroussis Ch, Androulakis N, Vamvakas L, et al. Phase I study of weekly docetaxel and liposomal doxorubicin in patients with advanced solid tumors. *Oncology.* 2005;69(3):202–207.
14. Brunner KW, Young CW. A methylhydrazine derivative in Hodgkin's disease and other malignant neoplasms: Therapeutic and toxic effects studied in 51 patients. *Ann Intern Med.* 1965;63:69–86.

15. Yamanaka R, Morii K, Shinbo Y, et al. Modified ProMACE-MOPP hybrid regimen with moderate-dose methotrexate for patients with primary CNS lymphoma. *Ann Hematol.* 2005;84(7):447–455.
16. Zabernigg A, Maier H, Thaler J, et al. Late-onset fatal neurologic toxicity of fludarabine. *Lancet.* 1994;344:1780.
17. Jehn U, Bartl R, Dietzfelbinger H, et al. Long-term outcome of hairy cell leukemia treated with 2-chlorodeoxyadenosine. *Ann Hematol.* 1999;78(3):139–144.
18. Leyvraz S, Herrmann R, Guillou L, et al. Treatment of advanced soft-tissue sarcomas using a combined strategy of high-dose ifosfamide, high-dose doxorubicin and salvage therapies. *Br J Cancer.* 2006;95(10):1342–1347.
19. Kupfer A, Aeschlimann C, Wermuth B, et al. Prophylaxis and reversal of ifosfamide encephalopathy with methylene-blue. *Lancet.* 1994;343:763–764.
20. Yang JC, Rosenberg SA. An ongoing prospective randomized comparison of interleukin-2 regimens for the treatment of metastatic renal cell cancer. *Cancer J Sci Am.* 1997;[3 Suppl 1]:S79–S84.
21. Puduvalli VK, Sella S, Austin SF, et al. Carpal tunnel syndrome associated with interleukin-2 therapy. *Cancer.* 1996;77:1189–1192.

CHAPTER 61

Disorders of Carbohydrate Metabolism

Rosario Maria S. Riel-Romero

OBJECTIVES

- To describe the wide range of clinical features associated with disorders of carbohydrate metabolism.
- To illustrate the underlying biochemical defect in McArdle disease or glycogen storage disease type V.
- To review the diagnostic approach to disorders of carbohydrate metabolism
- To explain glycogen storage disease can present as exercise intolerance

CASE VIGNETTE

An 18-year-old boy presented with decreased exercise tolerance. He complains of easy fatigability and muscle cramping during track competitions. During a recent meet where he ran the 200-meter dash, he noticed that his muscles became painful and swollen. In addition, when he went to the restroom and voided, he was surprised to note that his urine was burgundy colored. He feels somewhat weaker lately and seems less able to compete effectively during sports events. To alleviate fatigue, he has learned to rest for awhile before resuming exercise. On laboratory investigation, creatine kinase (CK) was elevated at 39,000, and both aspartate aminotransferase (AST) and alanine aminotransferase (ALT) were high at 970 and 290 U/L, respectively. Urine myoglobin was positive. He also developed acute renal failure during his hospitalization with blood urea nitrogen (BUN) at 92 mg/dL and a creatinine of 9.3 mg/dL. Two weeks later, CK levels fell to 900 and liver transaminases normalized. Urine myoglobin became undetectable.

DEFINITION

The metabolic pathways involving the synthesis and degradation of carbohydrates generate most of the energy necessary to sustain life. Glucose, galactose, fructose, and glycogen are the most important substrates in these biochemical pathways. Glucose obtained from dietary sources and generated through gluconeogenesis and glycogen degradation in the liver enables humans to maintain homeostasis and euglycemia. The processes of glycolysis (the conversion of glucose to glycogen to pyruvate) and mitochondrial oxidative phosphorylation (whereby pyruvate is converted to carbon dioxide and water) generates ATP, the cell's currency of energy (1).

Glycogen is the primary storage form of glucose in most animals and is most abundant in the liver and the muscle. Breakdown of liver glycogen provides a glucose supply when blood glucose begins to fall. Glycogen stored in the muscle provides a fuel source during short-term, high-energy situations, such as exercise. Defects in glycogen metabolism usually results in an abnormal accumulation of glycogen in body tissues.

Glycogen storage diseases are heritable disorders affecting glycogen metabolism. These are generally characterized by genetically determined enzymatic blocks in the synthesis and degradation of glycogen, resulting in an abnormal quality and quantity of glycogen (2). Glycogen storage diseases can involve the liver and muscle (cardiac and skeletal) or combinations thereof. Hence, they are also classified as *liver glycogenosis* or *muscle glycogenosis*. The numeric classification of these diseases is still widely accepted and currently more than 12 forms of glycogen storage diseases (GSD) exist (Table 61-1).

Glucose is initially phosphorylated to glucose-6-phosphate in a reaction catalyzed by hexokinase. The enzyme phosphoglucose isomerase then converts glucose-6-phosphate to glucose-1-phosphate which, in association with uridine triphosphate (UTP) and as mediated by UDPG-phosphorylase (uridine diphosphoglucose), is transformed to UDP-glucose. UDP-glucose then provides the glucose unit needed by glycogen synthase. When the active form of glycogen synthase (UDP-glucose-glycogen-glucosyl transferase) has generated a glucosyl chain that is 6 to 12 units long, a branching enzyme (amylo1,4-1,6 transglucosidase) then transfers this section and links it to an alpha 1,6 position on the same or a neighboring glycogen primer.

During glycogen degradation, phosphorylase cleaves the sequential glucosyl units from alpha-1, 4-glucosyl-linked glycogen primers, generating glucose-1-phosphate. The three phosphorylase isoenzymes are differentially activated by cyclic adenosine monophosphate (AMP) and by phosphorylase kinase. Phosphorylase kinase is then activated by protein kinase, of which there are different isoenzymes as well.

TABLE 61-1. Features of the Disorders of Carbohydrate Metabolism

Disorders	*Basic Defects*	*Clinical Presentation*	*Comments*
Liver Glycogeneses			
Type/Common Name			
Ia/Von Gierke	Glucose-6-phosphatase	Growth retardation, hepatomegaly, hypoglycemia; elevated blood lactate, cholesterol, triglyceride, and uric acid levels	Common, severe hypoglycemia
Ib	Glucose-6-phosphate translocase	Same as type Ia, with additional findings of neutropenia and impaired neutrophil function	10% of type Ia
II/Pompe Infantile	Acid maltase (acid α-glucosidase)	Cardiomegaly, hypotonia, hepatomegaly, onset: birth–6 mo	Common, cardiorespiratory failure leading to death by age 2 yr
Juvenile Adult	Acid maltase (acid α-glucosidase)	Myopathy, variable cardiomyopathy; onset: childhood	Residual enzyme activity
IIIa/Cori or Forbes	Acid maltase (acid α-glucosidase)	Myopathy, respiratory insufficiency; onset: adulthood	Residual enzyme activity
	Liver and muscle debrancher deficiency (amylo, 1,6 glucosidase)	Childhood; hepatomegaly, growth ratardation, muscle weakness, hypoglycemia, hyperlipidemia, elevated transaminase levels; liver symptoms improve with age	Common, intermediate severity of hypoglycemia
IIIb	Liver debrancher deficiency; normal muscle enzyme activity	Liver symptoms same as in type IIIa; no muscle symptoms	15% of type III
IV/Andersen	Branching enzyme	Failure to thrive, hypotonia, hepatomegaly, splenomegaly, progressive cirrhosis (death usually before 5th yr), elevated transaminase levels	Rare neuromuscular variants exist
VI/Hers	Liver phosphorylase	Hepatomegaly, mild hypoglycemia, hyperlipidemia, and ketosis	Rare, benign glycogenosis
Phosphorylase kinase deficiency	Phosphorylase kinase	Hepatomegaly, mild hypoglycemia, hyperlipidemia, and ketosis	Common, benign glycogenosis
Glycogen synthetase deficiency	Glycogen synthetase	Early morning drowsiness and fatigue, fasting hypoglycemia, and ketosis	Decreased liver glycogen store
Fanconi-Bickel syndrome	Glucose transporter-2(GLUT-2)	Failure to thrive, rickets, hepatorenomegaly, proximal renal tubular dysfunction, impaired glucose and galactose utilization	GLUT-2 expressed in liver, kidney, pancreas, and intestine

Muscle Glycogeneses			
Type/Common Name			
V/McArdle	Myophosphorylase	Exercise intolerance, muscle cramps, increased fatigability	Common, male predominance
VII/Tarui	Phosphofructokinase	Exercise intolerance, muscle cramps, hemolytic anemia, myoglobinuria	Prevalent in Japanese and Ashkenazi Jews
Phosphoglycerate kinase deficiency	Phosphoglycerate kinase	As with type V	Rare, X-linked
Phosphoglycerate mutase deficiency	M subunit of phosphoglycerate mutase	As with type V	Rare, majority of patients are African-American
Lactate dehydrogenase deficiency	M subunit of lactate dehydrogenase	As with type V	Rare
Galactose Disorders			
Galactosemia with transferase deficiency	Galactose-1-phosphate uridyltransferase	Vomiting, hepatomegaly, cataracts, aminoaciduria, failure to thrive	African-American patients tend to have milder symptoms
Galactokinase deficiency	Galactokinase	Cataracts	Benign
Generalized uridine diphosphate galactose-4-epimerase deficiency	Uridine diphosphate galactose 4-epimerase	Similar to transferase deficiency with additional findings of hypotonia and nerve deafness	A benign variant exists
Fructose Disorders			
Essential fructosuria	Fructokinase	Urine reducing substance	Benign
Hereditary fructose intolerance	Fructose-1-phosphatase aldolase	Acute: vomiting, sweating, lethargy Chronic: failure to thrive, hepatic failure	Prognosis good with fructose restriction
Disorders of Gluconeogenesis			
Fructose-1,6-diphosphatase deficiency	Fructose-1,6-disphosphatase	Episodic hypoglycemia, apnea, acidosis	Good prognosis, avoid fasting
Phosphoenolpyruvate carboxykinase deficiency	Phosphoenolpyruvate carboxykinase	Hypoglycemia, hepatomegaly, hypotonia, failure to thrive	Rare
Disorders of Pyruvate Metabolism			
Pyruvate dehydrogenase complex defect	Pyruvate dehydrogenase	Severe fatal neonatal to mild late onset, lactic acidosis, psychomotor retardation, and failure to thrive	Most commonly due to E1 α-subunit defect X-linked
Pyruvate carboxylase deficiency	Pyruvate carboxylase	Same as above	Rare, autosomal recessive
Respiratory chain defects(oxidative phosphorylation disease)	Complex I to V, many mitochondrial DNA mutations	Heterogeneous with multisystem involvement	Mitochondrial inheritance
Other Carbohydrate Disorders			
Pentosuria	L-Xyluose reductase	Urine reducing substance	Benign

(From Yaun-Tsong Chen. Defects in metabolism of carbohydrates. In: Behrman RE, Kligman R, Jenson HB, et al, eds. *Nelson Textbook of Pediatrics,* 17th ed. Philadelphia: WB Saunders; 2004:470, with permission.)

Phosphorylase degrades the glycogen chains until only four glucosyl units are left before a branch point or an 1,6 linkage. Debranching enzyme transfers a block of three glucose residues from one branch to the end of another branch using oligo→1, 4→1, 4 glucan transferase. Debranching enzyme hydrolyzes the 1, 6 linkage using amylo-1, 6-glucosidase. Glucose-1-phosphate that is liberated is converted to glucose-6-phosphate by phosphoglucomutase. Glucose-6-phosphate is converted to fructose-6-phosphate by phosphoisomerase. Fructose-6-phosphate, in a reaction mediated by phosphofructokinase, the rate-limiting enzyme in glycolysis, is changed to fructose-1, 6-diphosphate, which is ultimately converted to pyruvate.

LIVER GLYCOGENOSIS

The glycogen storage disorders mainly affecting the liver are as follows:

1. GSD I (or Von Gierke disease or *glucose-6-phosphatase deficiency*). The three subtypes are (a) type 1a, which is characterized by deficiency of the enzyme; (*b*) type 1b, which is characterized by a defect in the microsomal membrane transport system of glucose-6-phosphate; and (*c*) type 1c, which is caused by a defect in the microsomal phosphate or pyrophosphate transport.
2. GSD III (or Cori/Forbes or *debranching enzyme* or *amylo-1, 6-glucosidase deficiency*)
3. GSD IV (or Andersen disease or *branching enzyme deficiency*)
4. GSD VI (or Hers disease or *liver phosphorylase deficiency*)
5. Phosphorylase kinase deficiency
6. Glycogen synthetase deficiency and glucose transporter defect 2 (GLUT-2) or Fanconi-Bickel syndrome, hepatic glycogenosis with renal Fanconi syndrome) (2).

MUSCLE GLYCOGENOSIS

The GSD principally affecting muscle are divided into two groups:

1. Diseases characterized by cardiomyopathy, muscle weakness, or muscle atrophy, exemplified by acid α-glucosidase (GSD II or Pompe disease)
2. Diseases characterized by fatigue, exercise intolerance, rhabdomyolysis, and myoglobinuria. The latter includes GSD V or McArdle disease, which is a deficiency of *myophosphorylase* and deficiencies of phosphofructokinase (GSD VII or Tarui disease), phosphoglycerate kinase, phosphoglycerate mutase, or lactate dehydrogenase (2).

EPIDEMIOLOGY

The frequency of all forms of GSD is approximately 1 in 20,000 (3). the most commonly presenting GSD in early childhood are glucose-6-phosphatase deficiency (GSD I), lysosomal acid α-glucosidase deficiency (GSD II), debrancher enzyme (GSD III), and liver phosphorylase kinase deficiency. Myophosphorylase deficiency usually presents in early adulthood. Haller (4) estimated the prevalence of McArdle disease in the Dallas, Fort Worth area as 1 in 100,000 (4). Fukuda et al. (5) performed a nation-wide survey in Japan in 2001 to clarify the frequency of muscle GSD and found 80% are GSD II, V, and III.

ETIOLOGY AND PATHOGENESIS

Skeletal muscle utilizes different fuel sources during different situations to produce ATP. For instance, the main energy sources of skeletal muscle in a fed state are blood fatty acids, which are oxidized to produce acetyl coenzyme A (acetyl CoA), which then proceeds to the Krebs cycle and the mitochondrial respiratory chain to produce ATP. For short bursts of high-intensity activity, glucose, fatty acids, glycogen stores, and preformed phosphate compounds are generally used.

Impaired ability to metabolize muscle glycogen as in *Debrancher enzyme, myophosphorylase,* and muscle *phosphorylase kinase* will result in failure to sustain intense, high-energy activity. Similarly, enzymatic deficiencies along the glycolytic (Embden-Meyerhof) pathway, such as deficiencies of *phosphofructokinase, phosphoglycerate kinase, phosphoglycerate mutase,* and *lactate dehydrogenase,* will result in a similar clinical picture. After muscle glycogen stores are depleted, however, fatty acids become more essential as fuel sources. Hence, defects in the β-oxidation of fatty acids and defects in the carnitine cycle can also result in the inability to perform sustained exercise and in impaired exercise tolerance (5).

Other factors thought to contribute to exercise intolerance in McArdle disease is the lack of increase in muscle perfusion during exercise (6) and a reduced level of skeletal muscle tissue sodium-potassium adenosine triphosphatase (ATPase) pump (7).

PATHOLOGY

Muscle biopsy generally shows excessive subsarcolemmal deposition of normal glycogen with deficient levels of myophosphorylase (8–10). DiMauro and Hartlage (11), in 1978, reported the pathologic findings in a girl who presented with a downhill clinical course of muscle weakness and respiratory failure with death at 13 weeks of age. Muscle histochemistry demonstrated increased glycogen and immunodiffusion studies revealed a complete lack of phosphorylase activity. Roubertie et al. (12) also reported a 6-year-old girl who had extensive muscle necrosis after a near-drowning episode secondary to cramps induced by myophosphorylase deficiency. This was confirmed by ultrastructural studies of muscle in McArdle disease that demonstrated excessive glycogen in the subsarcolemmal and intermyofibrillar spaces, with disruption of the myofibrillar structure at the level of the I band (13).

CLINICAL MANIFESTATIONS

As with the patient in the vignette, the symptoms of McArdle disease usually begin early in adulthood and late in middle age. Clinical heterogeneity is common, however, and a few scattered reports show it presenting at earlier ages. DiMauro and Hartlage (11) described an infant with weakness and progressive respiratory insufficiency. Horneff et al. (14) reported a 13-year-old girl who presented with muscle pain and weakness, with increased levels of serum CK, positive rheumatoid factor, increased erythrocyte sedimentation rate (ESR), circulating complexes, and complement consumption, suggesting an inflammatory myopathy, and whose muscle biopsy showed an absence of myophosphorylase activity (14). Ito et al. (15) reported a 14-month-old girl with mild hypotonia and hypercreatine kinase-emia during febrile episodes only and whose muscle biopsy was compatible with McArdle disease. Milstein et al. (16) described a premature female infant with joint contracture and signs and symptoms of perinatal asphyxia whose muscle biopsy was also consistent with McArdle disease. On the other extreme, Hewlett and Gardner-Thorpe (17) described a 74-year-old man with McArdle disease whose symptoms began at the seventh decade of life, with proximal weakness, muscle wasting of the shoulder girdle, and calf hypertrophy. Still other clinical manifestations are late onset and diagnosed incidentally after the discovery of high CK values (18).

Muscle cramping and fatigue often occur after strenuous exercise, but generally resolve after a period of rest, after which exercise can be resumed with ease, the so-called "second wind phenomena." This is explained by a switch in the metabolic pathways from endogenous glycolysis during short bursts of high-intensity exercise to the oxidation of fatty acids as a fuel source. Haller (7) also postulated that the lack of increase in muscle perfusion during exercise and a reduced level of muscle sodium-potassium ATPase pump contribute to exercise intolerance.

A number of reports describe acute renal failure as a presenting sign of McArdle disease. One of these described a 36-year-old man who had seizures after binge drinking, followed by massive rhabdomyolysis, and his acute renal failure was diagnosed by histochemical studies of muscle to be McArdle disease (19). Another report describes a 45-year-old man who developed rhabdomyolysis and acute renal failure after skiing and gardening (20). Walker et al. (21) presented the case of a 33-year-old nurse who was diagnosed with McArdle disease only after presenting with rhabdomyolysis and recurrent cryptogenic renal failure secondary of occult seizures. Tsushima et al. (22) also reported a 64-year-old man with McArdle disease who had acute renal failure requiring hemodialysis after an asthmatic attack. Another atypical presentation of McArdle disease is statin-induced myositis (23).

DIAGNOSIS

The diagnosis of GSD V is reached through a combination of typical clinical features, increased serum basal serum CK, and a flat response to lactate during the ischemic forearm test. Confirmatory tests would include a quantitative assay for myophosphorylase activity in the muscle and molecular genetic testing.

Ischemic lactate forearm test has been used to evaluate the response of plasma lactate levels to exercise in patients with McArdle disease. The drawbacks to this test include pain and a potential for muscle damage, lack of specificity for McArdle disease because patients with both Cori/Forbes disease and Tarui disease and those who are deconditioned and unmotivated can generate a flat lactate response to the test (24). Meinck et al. (25) reported massive rhabdomyolysis and myoglobinuria following ischemic lactate forearm test. More recently, the nonischemic forearm exercise test for McArdle disease proposed by Kazemi-Esfarjani et al. (26) has gained more favor as a diagnostic tool.

During the nonischemic forearm lactate test, values for lactate, ammonia, pH, and P_{CO_2} are obtained at rest, during exercise, and recovery. Exercise consists of 2 minutes of rhythmic handgrip at 50% maximal voluntary contraction without blocked blood circulation. In controls, lactate values increase five- to sixfold above the baseline values. In McArdle disease, plasma lactate values do not increase after exercise and postexercise lactate-to-ammonia peak ratios are clearly decreased (*flat lactate curve*).

Electromyographic findings in early McArdle disease have been described as high-amplitude motor unit potentials caused by the subsarcolemmal vacuoles of glycogen deposition (27).

MOLECULAR GENETICS

McArdle disease is inherited through an autosomal recessive mode of inheritance. The gene, PGYM, which encodes for myophosphorylase, has been identified and is on chromosome 11 (28). Remarkable genetic heterogeneity is seen in patients with this disease. Thus far, more than 30 mutations, including nonsense, missense, and splice junction mutations, in the PGYM gene have been described. Targeted mutation analysis of the most common mutations, R49X and G204S, can be done. R49X, a nonsense mutation at codon 49 in exon 1, wherein thymidine is substituted for cytosine, changing arginine to a stop codon, is commonly seen in patients of European and United States descent (29). The G204S mutation consists of the substitution of adenine for guanine at codon 204 in exon 5, changing glycine to serine. A third mutation, W797R, is commonly seen in affected individuals of Spanish ancestry, and consists of the substitution of cytosine for adenine at codon 542 in exon 1 changing lysine to threonine. Among individuals of central European lineage, the Y84X is prevalent (30,31).

TREATMENT

In a single blind, randomized, placebo-controlled crossover study where 12 patients with McArdle disease were given sucrose or placebo, Vissing and Haller (32) showed that supplemental glucose or sucrose markedly improves exercise intolerance in affected individuals.

Vorgerd et al. (33) showed that creatinine supplementation of an initial load of 150 mg/kg/day and 60 mg/kg/day for 5 weeks both significantly lowered phosphocreatine on 31P-MRS during exercise and increased workload tolerance. This was not confirmed by the same group in 2002 who demonstrated that high-dose creatine worsened exercise-induced myalgia (34). O'Reilly et al. (35) did not observe any benefit to creatine supplementation. In general, avoidance of strenuous isometric and aerobic exercise appears to improve exercise intolerance. Exercise intolerance can also be improved with fructose or glucose ingestion (36).

High-protein diet has not been shown to be clearly beneficial (37). Because vitamin B_6 stores are depleted in McArdle disease, vitamin B supplementation may be helpful (38). Finally, longevity, in general, is not affected in McArdle disease.

CLINICAL RECOMMENDATIONS OF THE VIGNETTE

The patient most likely has McArdle disease based on clinical symptoms of exercise intolerance, rhabomyolysis, and myoglinuria with prolonged and intense exercise. Confirmatory diagnosis using nonischemic forearm exercise test and testing for any mutation in the PGYM gene should be done. Management consists of the avoidance of strenuous aerobic exercise and warming up before exercise. Supplementation with creatine and pyridoxine may be beneficial.

SUMMARY

Glycogen storage disease, in particular McArdle disease, should be considered in the differential diagnosis of exercise intolerance with associated with muscle cramps, Fatigue, and rhabdomyolysis. McArdle disease is a deficiency of myophosphorylase, a key enzyme in muscle glycogen breakdown. Molecular genetic analysis of the PGYM gene is a useful confirmatory test.

The mainstays of management include avoidance of strenuous exercise and creatine and vitamin B_6 supplementation. Longevity is unaffected.

REFERENCES

1. Yuan-Tsong Chen. Glycogen storage diseases. In: Scriver CR, Beaudet AL, Sly WS, et al., eds. *The Metabolic and Molecular Basis of Inherited Disease*, 8th ed. New York: McGraw-Hill; 2001:1521–1551.
2. Yaun-Tsong Chen. Defects in metabolism of carbohydrates. In: Behrman RE, Kligman R, Jenson HB, et al., eds. *Nelson Textbook of Pediatrics*, 17th ed. Philadelphia: WB Saunders; 2004:469–475.
3. Hoffman GF, Nyhan WL, Zschoche J, et al. Inherited metabolic diseases. In: *Core Handbooks in Pediatrics*, 1st ed. Philadelphia: Lippincott Williams & Wilkins; 2002:238–263.
4. Haller RG. Treatment of McArdle disease. *Arch Neurol.* 2000;57:923–924.
5. Fukuda T, Sygie H, Ito M, et al. Nation-wide survey on muscle glycogen storage disease (MGSDs) and comparison with our experiences in diagnosis of MGSDs. *Rinsho Shinkeigaku.* 2003:43(5):243–248.
6. Jehenson P, Leroy-Willig A, de Keriulier E, et al. Impairment of muscle-induced increase in muscle perfusion in McArdle's disease. *Eur J Nucl Med.* 1995;22:1256.
7. Haller RS, Clausen T, Vissing J. Reduced levels of skeletal muscle Na+K+ATPase in McArdle disease. *Neurology.* 1998;50(1):37–40.
8. Martinuzzi A, Schievano G, Nascimbeni A, et al. McArdle disease: The unsolved mystery of the reappearing enzyme. *Am J Pathol.* 1999:154:1893–1897.
9. Getachew E, Prayson R. Pathology quiz: A man with exertion-induced cramps and myoglobinuria. *Arch Pathol Lab Med.* 2003;127:1227–1228.
10. Chiado-Piat L, Mongini T, Doriguzzi C, et al. Clinical spectrum of McArdle disease: three cases with unusual expression. *Eur Neurol.* 1993:33(3):208–211.
11. DiMauro S, Hartlage PL. Fatal infantile form of muscle phosphorylase deficiency. *Neurology.* 1978;28(11):1124–1129.
12. Roubertie A, Patte K, Rivier F, et al. McArdle disease in childhood: Report of a new case. *Eur J Paediatr Neurol.* 1998;2:269–273.
13. Schotland D, Spiro D, Rowland L, et al. Ultrastructural studies of muscle in McArdle disease. *J Neuropathol Exp Neurol.* 1965;24(4):629–644.
14. Horneff G, Paetzke I, Neuen-Jacob E. Glycogenosis type V (McArdle's disease) mimicking atypical myositis. *Clin Rheumatol.* 2001;20(1):57–60.
15. Ito Y, Saito K, Shishikura K, et al. 1-year-old infant with McArdle disease associated with hyper-creatine kinase-emia during febrile episodes. *Brain Dev.* 2003;25(6):438–441.
16. Milstein JM, Herron TM, Haas JE. Fatal infantile muscle phosphorylase deficiency. *J Child Neurol.* 1989;4(3):186–188.
17. Hewlett RH, Gardner-Thorpe C. McArdle's disease—What limit to the age of onset? *S Afr Med J.* 1978;53(2):60–63.
18. Gospe SM, El-Schahawi S, Shanske C, et al. Asymptomatic McArdle's disease associated with hyper-creatine kinase-emia and absence of myophosphorylase. *Neurology.* 1998;51(4): 1228–1229.
19. Haslinger B, Kuchle C, Sitter T, et al. Acute renal failure due to rhabdomyolysis in McArdle's disease following binge drinking with seizures. *Dtsch Med Wochenschr.* 2001;126(45):1265–1268.
20. Kranck S, Wacker P, Milliet N, et al. One rare case report of acute renal insufficiency in rhabdomyolysis. *Rev Med Suisse Romande.* 2002;122(11):539–541.
21. Walker AR, Walker BA, Tschetter K, et al. McArdle's disease presenting as recurrent cryptogenic renal failure due to occult seizures. *Muscle Nerve.* 2003;28:640–643.
22. Tsushima K, Koyama S, Ueno M, et al. Rhabdomyolysis triggered by an asthmatic attack in a patient with McArdle disease. *Intern Med.* 2001;40(2):131–134.
23. Livingstone C, Al Riyami S, Wilkins P, et al. McArdle's disease diagnosed following statin-induced myositis. *Ann Clin Biochem.* 2004;41(Pt 4):338–340.
24. Lindner A, Reichert N, Eichhorn M, et al. Acute compartment syndrome after ischemic work test in a patient with McArdle's disease. *Neurology.* 2001;56(12):1779–1780.
25. Meinck HM, Goebel HH, Rumpf KW, et al. The forearm ischemic work test-hazardous to McArdle patients? *J Neurol Neurosurg Psychiatry.* 1982;4:1144–1146.
26. Kazemi-Esfarjani P, Skomorowska E, Jensen TD, et al. Non-ischemic forearm exercise test for McArdle disease. *Ann Neurol.* 2002;52:153–159.
27. Suzuki S, Sato H, Nogawa S, et al. Early electromyographic findings in asymptomatic siblings with McArdle's disease. *Eur Neurol.* 2002;47:245–246.
28. DiMauro S, Andreu AL, Bruno C, et al. Myophosphorylase deficiency (glycogenosis type V: McArdle disease. *Curr Mol Med.* 2002;2(2):189–196.
29. Bartrum C, Edwards RH, Clague J, et al. McArdle's disease: A nonsense mutation in exon 1 of the muscle glycogen phosphorylase gene explains some but not all cases. *Hum Mol Genet.* 1993;2:1241–1243.
30. Martin MA, Rubio JC, Buchbinder J, et al. Molecular heterogeneity of myophosphorylase deficiency (McArdle's disease): A genotype-phenotype correlation study. *Ann Neurol.* 2001;50:574–581.
31. Martin MA, Rubio JC, Wevers RA, et al. Molecular analysis of myophosphorylase deficiency in Dutch patients with McArdle's disease. *Ann Hum Genet.* 2003;68;17–22.
32. Vissing J, Haller RG. The effect of oral sucrose on exercise intolerance in patients with McArdle's disease. *N Engl J Med.* 2003:349:2503–2509.
33. Vorgerd M, Grehl T, Jager M, et al. Creatine therapy in myophosphorylase deficiency (McArdle's disease): A placebo-controlled crossover trial. *Arch Neurol.* 2000;57(7): 956–963.
34. Vorgerd M, Zange J, Kley R, et al. Effect of high-dose creatine therapy on exercise intolerance in McArdle's disease: Double-blind, placebo-controlled crossover study. *Arch Neurol.* 2002;57(70):956–963.
35. O'Reilly DS, Carter R, Bell E, et al. Exercise to exhaustion in the second-wind phase of exercise in case of McArdle disease with and without creatine supplementation. *Scott Med J.* 2003;48(2):46–48.
36. Haller RG, Vissing J. Spontaneous "second wind" and glucose-induced "second-wind" in McArdle disease. *Arch Neurol.* 2002;59(9):1395–1402.
37. Jensen KE, Jacobson J, Thomsen C, et al. Improved energy kinetics following high protein diet in McArdle's syndrome. A 31P magnetic resonance spectroscopy study. *Acta Neurol Scand.* 1990;81(6):499–503.
38. Phoenix J, Hopkins P, Bartram C, et al. Effect of vitamin B6 supplementation in McArdle's disease: A strategic case study. *Neuromuscul Disord.* 1998;8(3–4):210–212.

CHAPTER **62**

Disorders of Lipoprotein Metabolism

Rosario Maria S. Riel-Romero

OBJECTIVES

- To present the neurologic and nonneurological clinical manifestations of the disorders of lipoprotein metabolism, with emphasis on abetalipoproteinemia or Bassen-Kornzweig disease
- To describe the underlying biochemical processes in lipoprotein metabolism, in general, and in abetalipoproteinemia in particular.
- To present the genetics of selected disorders of lipoprotein metabolism
- To discuss the present management of selected disorders of lipoprotein metabolism

CASE VIGNETTE

A 29-year-old white man, a product of a consanguineous relationship, was referred for dysarthria and involuntary body movements. His medical history was remarkable for repeated hospitalizations during infancy for failure to thrive, vomiting, and diarrhea. During early childhood, he began to have problems walking and running and would often fall. On examination, the patient was wheelchair-bound. He had difficulty articulating words. He had pes cavus, kyphoscoliosis with generalized muscle weakness. Funduscopic examination showed a pigmentary retinopathy. Vibratory and proprioception senses were severely impaired. Muscle stretch reflexes were absent. Peripheral blood smear examination was positive for spiculated erythrocytes.

DEFINITION

Disorders of lipoprotein metabolism can either cause decreases or increases in specific types of lipoproteins. These disorders can cause symptoms secondary to lipid deposition in tissues or premature atherosclerosis. Other disorders manifest as neurologic diseases characterize by abnormal movements or peripheral neuropathy and other lipoprotein disorders lead to gastrointestinal symptoms, such as pancreatitis and steatorrhea. Lipoprotein electrophoresis is a valuable diagnostic tool in these disorders (1).

The disorders associated with hypercholesterolemia and normal triglycerides (serum <100 mg/dL) generally indicate an elevation of low-density lipoprotein (LDL), suggesting involvement of the LDL pathway, either in the LDL receptor (familial hypercholesterolemia [FH]) and in the receptor-binding region of apo B. Among these diseases are FH, familial defective apoprotein B-100, sitosterolemia, and polygenic hypercholesterolemia. Sitosterolemia is a rare autosomal recessive disorder associated with increased intestinal absorption of plant-derived sterols, such as cholesterol and sitosterol (2).

Diseases characterized by hypercholesterolemia and moderately elevated triglycerides (100 to 1,000 mg/dL) are familial combined hyperlipidemia (FCHL), familial dysbetalipoproteinemia (type III hyperlipidemia), and familial hypertriglyceridemia. The diseases associated with hypercholesterolemia and severely elevated triglycerides (>1,000 mg/dL) are familial chylomicronemia syndrome (lipoprotein lipase deficiency and apolipoprotein C-11 deficiency) and type V hyperlipoproteinemia (HLP). Disorders of high-density lipoprotein (HDL) metabolism include familial APOA-1 deficiency and structural APOA-1 mutation, Tangier disease, familial lecithin-cholesterol acyltransferase deficiency, and primary alpha-lipoproteinemia (2).

On the other hand, conditions associated with low cholesterol levels include abetalipoproteinemia, familial hypobetalipoproteinemia, chylomicron retention disease (Andersen disease), and Smith-Lemli-Opitz syndrome. Additional disorders of cholesterol metabolism are mevalonate kinase deficiency, Conradi-Hunnermann syndrome, CHILD syndrome (congenital hemidyspolasia with ichthyosiform erthroderma and limb defects), cerebral xanthomatosis, cholesterol ester storage or Wolman disease, and Niemman-Pick C (1).

Abetalipoproteinemia is a rare, autosomal recessive disorder of lipoprotein metabolism that was first described by Bassen and Kornzweig in an 18-year-old girl with pigmentary retinopathy and acanthocytosis (3). These acanthocytes are abnormal red blood cells and account for most of circulating erythrocytes and form rouleaux poorly.

After ingestion of fats, lipids are hydrolyzed by intestinal and pancreatic lipases. The resulting free-fatty acids and cholesterol are re-esterified in the intestinal epithelium to triglycerides and cholesterol esters. They are then packaged with phospholipids, cholesterol, Apo A-I, Apo A-IV and Apo B-48 to form chylomicrons. Chylomicrons are secreted into lymph and pass through the thoracic duct and then to the circulation where they are then repackaged with apo E and apo C apolipoproteins. Within the chylomicrons, triglycerides are hydrolyzed by *lipoprotein lipase*, an enzyme requiring Apo C-II as a cofactor. Free-fatty acids are then stored in adipose tissue as triglycerides or transferred to muscle for β-oxidation. The resultant triglyceride-poor molecules are then called *cholesterol remnants* (2,4).

Lipoproteins are macromolecular complexes that transport lipids in the circulation. The protein complexes of these complexes are called *apolipoproteins*. Apolipoproteins function in a variety of ways, including serving as cofactors for enzymes, ligands for cell-surface receptors, and as structural proteins.

The major lipids transported by lipoproteins are cholesterol, triglycerides, phospholipids, and fat-soluble vitamins, especially vitamin E.

The major types of lipoprotein particles are as follows:

1. Chylomicrons (dietary lipoproteins)
2. Very low-density lipoproteins (VLDL)
3. HDL
4. LDL
5. Cholesterol and triglyceride remnants

Chylomicrons, dietary lipoproteins formed in the small intestine, contain Apo A-I, Apo A-IV and Apo B-48. VLDL, which are secreted by the liver, contain esterified and unesterified cholesterol, triglycerides, phospholipids, and apo B-100, apo C-II, and apo E. HDL are secreted by the liver's nascent and mature particles composed of phospholipids and apo A-I and A-II. The metabolism of HDL involves several transfer proteins, such as ATP-binding cassette protein A1 (*ABCA-1*), cholesterol ester transfer protein (*CETP*), and other enzymes, such as lecithin cholesterol acyltransferase (*LCAT*), which enlarge the HDL particle and form cholesterol esters (2,4).

EPIDEMIOLOGY

Familial hypercholesterolemia is among the most common inborn errors of metabolism. Heterozygotes number about 1 of 500 people worldwide and homozygotes number about 1 of 1,000,000 persons. FCHL occurs in about 1 of 200 adults. Familial dysbetalipoproteinemia occurs in 1 of 700 people. Smith-Lemli–Opitz has an estimated incidence of 1 of 40,000 births (2,5).

Approximately 100 isolated cases of abetalipoproteinemia have been reported, about a third of these caused by consanguineous marriages. All pedigrees described are compatible with an autosomal recessive mode of inheritance. Of note, males outnumber females 3 to 2 (2).

ETIOLOGY AND PATHOGENESIS

In FH, the defect lies in a mutation in the gene coding for the LDL receptor, which is located in the cell surface. These receptors form an endocytic vesicle that binds LDL from the plasma (6). Familial dysbetalipoproteinemia is caused by a mutation in the gene for apolipoprotein E (apo E), impairing its ability to bind to liver receptors and clear chylomicrons and LDL remnants from the plasma (5). The molecular basis of familial hypertriglyceridemia is not clear, but is likely to be related to impaired hydrolysis of triglyceride-rich lipoproteins, VLDL, chylomicron, or apo C-III overload (2).

Familial chylomicronemia results from mutations in the genes coding for lipoprotein lipase on the apo C-II (2). Tangier disease is caused by mutations in ABCA1, a cellular protein facilitating efflux of cholesterol to lipid-poor apoA-1 (7). Familial lecithin-cholesterol acyltransferase deficiency is caused by functional impairment of LCAT, a plasma enzyme that esterifies free cholesterol in circulating plasma lipoproteins (8).

Among the conditions characterized by low cholesterol, Smith-Lemli-Opitz results from a defect in the gene encoding for 7-dehydrocholesterol δ-7 reductase, which converts 7-dehydrocholesterol to cholesterol. Chylomicron retention disease or Anderson disease is characterized by absent chylomicrons, low HDL, and low LDL levels (2). The molecular basis of this disorder lies in either in a faulty glycosylation process impairing secretion and formation of chylomicrons or in defective apo B-48s secretion (9,10). In abetalipoproteinemia, LDL, chylomicrons, and lipoproteins of the VLDL that contain B lipoproteins are absent. Cholesterol and triglycerides are reduced because these lipoproteins are responsible for their plasma transport. Lipoprotein lipase (LPL) activity is also reduced as is LCAT activity (2). Wetterau et al. advanced the premise that the absence of a microsomal triglyceride transfer protein, which mediated the transfer of lipid molecules from their sites of synthesis to nascent lipoprotein particles in the endoplasmic reticulum caused abetalipoproteinemia (11). Subsequently, genetic mutations involving the MTP gene (GeneBank X59657) were found in association with abetalipoproteinemia (12).

CLINICAL MANIFESTATIONS

Familial or polygenic hypercholesterolemia is manifested by lipid deposition in tissues such as tendon xanthomas, arcus corneal, premature atherosclerosis, coronary artery disease, and lipema retinalis) (6). The pathognomonic sign of Tangier disease are enlarged and orange tonsils coupled with peripheral neuropathy (7). Classic LCAT deficiency is characterized by anemia, progressive proteinuria, renal failure, corneal opacities, and atherosclerosis (8). LPL and apo C-I deficiency are characterized by recurrent abdominal pain, lipema retinalis, hepatoslenomegaly, and tuberoeruptive xanthomas. Blood can also appear lipemic (13). Distinctive features of familial dysbetalipoproteinemia are palmar xanthomas and tuberoeruptive xanthomas on the elbows, knees, and buttocks, which can coalesce to grapelike structures (5).

Smith-Lemli-Opitz is an autosomal recessive disorder characterized by dysmorphisms, including epicanthal folds, blepharoptosis, syndactyly, micrognathia, microcephaly, and mental retardation (2). Central nervous system abnormalities have included agenesis of the corpus callosum, cerebellar hypoplasia, holoprosencephaly, enlarged ventricles, and frontal lobe hypoplasia (14).

The features of abetalipoproteinemia affect multiple organs, but its most serious and prominent manifestations are neurologic in nature. In the neonatal and early childhood period, affected infants develop celiac syndrome with diarrhea with foul-smelling bulky stools, fat malabsorption, osteomalacia, and failure to thrive (15). The absorption of vitamin K and A is impaired in abetalipoproteinemia, but the administration of even modest supplemental amounts can restore levels to normal. In contrast, the transport of tocopherol is severely impaired in abetalipoproteinemia. Because most plasma tocopherol is transported via LDL to the peripheral tissues, a defect in the formation of chylomicrons but also in the function of LDL apparently underlies the tendency of affected individuals to be vitamin E deficient despite large oral or intramuscular administration of vitamin E. This deficiency causes fat malabsorption and ataxia. Liver cirrhosis has been reported in abetalipoproteinemia (16).

Among the hematology manifestations of abetalipoproteinemia, the markedly unusual red blood cell morphology, now called *acanthocytosis*, has attracted much attention. The malformed red blood cells form rouleaux poorly, leading to extremely low sedimentation rates. The erythrocytes acanthocytic form affects the abnormal composition and distribution of lipids in the red blood cell envelope (17).

The neurologic symptoms of abetalipoproteinemia are the most prominent and disabling. These appear between the ages of 2 and 17 years. One third of patients become symptomatic before the age of 10. The first sign of nervous system involvement is the loss of deep tendon reflexes, which can lead to the consideration of Friedrich's ataxia. Vibratory and position sense in the distal extremities are often impaired, causing ataxia and a positive Romberg sign. By the third and fourth decade, most untreated patients are severely ataxic, dysmetric, and dysarthric. Kyphoscoliosis, lordosis, pes cavus, and pes equinovarus deformities are common. Death usually occurs in the fifth decade of life or earlier (18).

Affected individuals usually develop a pigmentary retinopathy not dissimilar to other forms of retinitis pigmentosa. In the first decade, the initial signs are diminished night and color vision. During adulthood, patients may experience gradually enlarging annular scotoma, with macular sparing that diminishes visual acuity and would ultimately lead to blindness by the fourth decade of life. Ophthalmoplegia, possibly caused by the aberrant regeneration of the oculomotor nerve, has been reported have ptosis and anisocoria (18–20).

Mental retardation has been described but it is difficult to ascribe solely to the disease because specific anomalies of the cerebral cortex pathology are lacking. Rather, causative factors for cognitive deficiency may be specific nutritional deficiencies and because many cases are products of consanguineous relationships, the role of other genetic factors may also be partly responsible.

PATHOLOGY

Most pathologic studies of affected patients with hypercholesterolemia show a diffuse and severe atherosclerosis of the aorta and coronary arteries, with lipid deposition in the aortic and mitral valves (21). Corneal studies in LCAT deficiency showed extracellular vacuoles, with acid mucopolysccharide and amyloid deposits in the stroma (22). Renal changes in a patient with LCAT showed extensive lipid deposition in the glomerular basement membrane and the mesangium (23). Cabin et al. (24) described the histopathologic findings in five patients with familial dysbetalipoproteinemia. All patients demonstrated severe and diffuse atherosclerosis with prominent involvement of the left main coronary artery (24). On the other hand, colonoscopic studies of patients with Tangier disease show a *cobblestone* appearance, with irregular yellow-orange discoloration and polyps. Foamy histiocytes had been seen in the mucosa and submucosa of the colon, rectum, and gallbladder (25).

The characteristic neuropathologic finding in abetalipoproteinemia is the widespread demyelination of the axons of large sensory neurons of the spinal ganglia, fasciculus cuneatus, fasciculus gracilis, posterior columns, and cerebellar molecular layer. Lazaro et al. (26) described the quadriceps femoris muscle pathology of a 29-year-old man with abetalipoproteinemia, including type II fiber predominance, increase in central nuclei, dense lipid inclusions ceroid, and lipofuscin. Kott et al. (27) had similar findings of ceroid accumulation in the muscle of a 26-year-old man with abetalipoproteinemia, a phenomenon believed to be related to vitamin E deficiency.

The major pathologic features in the visual system include loss of photoreceptors, loss or attenuation of the pigment epithelium, preservation of the submacular pigment epithelium, and excessive lipofuscin accumulation, particularly of the posterior funiculus (28). Wong and Heon (29) described helicoid peripapillary chorioretinal degeneration in abetalipoproteinemia.

Avigan et al. (30) reported the morphologic features of liver tissue of a patient with abetalipoproteinemia. Lobular architecture was intact with no fibrosis, and electron microscopic studies of the rough endoplasmi reticulum, smooth endoplasmic reticulum, and Golgi apparatus were normal. Acanthocytes were also present in the sinusoids. Lipid droplets were not bound to the membranes and were not found either in the endoplasmic reticulum or the Golgi apparatus, suggesting impaired lipoprotein assembly and secretion, causing lipid accumulation in the hepatocytes (30). Muscle fibers show punctuate deposits of acid phosphatase activity and giant lyzosomes, and concentric laminated bodies, which are now referred to as *Mallory bodies*, a marker for hepatocyte injury (31). Intestinal biopsy has shown fat vacuoles in apical villous cytoplasm and normal villi (32).

Wickman et al. (33) demonstrated that sural nerves on abetalipoproteinemia may have decreased number of large fibers, small fibers, and clusters of regenerating fibers. Paranodal degeneration was also seen in some teased fibers (32).

DIAGNOSIS

Lipoprotein electrophoresis is the traditional laboratory approach to the diagnosis of disorders of lipoprotein metabolism and transport. FCHL is characterized by elevations in both cholesterol and triglycerides, with moderately reduced HDL. In familial dysbetalipoproteinemia, both cholesterol and triglycerides are often elevated to the same degree, but the most reliable biochemical marker for this disease is the apo E phenotype. Homozygous E2 allele (E2/E2 genotype) is the commonly seen in this disease (5,8).

Familial hypertriglyceridemia is characterized by moderately elevated triglycerides, without concomitant significant elevation in cholesterol. Lipoprotein lipase and apo C-III deficiency usually show severe elevations of triglycerides, >1,000 mg/dL, as well as cholesterol levels. Low HDL levels are characteristic of LCAT deficiency, Tangier disease, and familial APOA-1 deficiency and structural APOA-1 mutations. Low cholesterol levels are seen in abeta- and hypolipoproteinemia as well as Smith-Lemli-Opitz syndrome (2).

Characteristically, affected patients with abetalipoproteinemia show evidence of fat malabsorption and laboratory findings of low cholesterol levels, typically 20 to 50 mg/dL, low serum triglycerides (2 to 13 mg/dL), low total serum lipids (80 to 285 mg/dL), and low levels of fat-soluble vitamins, particularly vitamin E (<1.3 μg/dL, with normal values of 5 to 15 μg/dL). In addition, as the disease name implies, there is a complete lack of serum β-lipoprotein and all apolipoprotein β-containing lipoproteins, such as chylomicrons, VLDL, and LDL (18).

Acanthocytosis on peripheral blood smear is not exclusively found in abetalipoproteinemia. Acanthocytes are mature erythrocytes with numerous spiny projections. Whole blood may not reveal acanthocytosis. The best procedure to detect red blood cell acanthocytosis uses dilution of whole blood samples 1:1 with heparinized saline followed by incubation for 60 minutes at room temperature. Wet cell monolayers are then analyzed by phase contrast microscopy (34).

TREATMENT

Therapy of FH is multifactorial and includes diet, exercise, and the use of statins or bile-binding resins (colestipol and cholestyramine). Homozygotes for FH, however, are usually resistant to therapy (6). The most effective treatment for this subset of patients is LDL apheresis, a method of directly removing LDL from the plasma by use of a continuous-flow blood cell separator. In combination with nicotinic acid, this treatment promotes regression of the tendon xanthomas and retards the progression of atherosclerosis (35).

Familial chylomicronemia syndrome is best treated with restriction of dietary fats. Medium-chained triglycerides can be used for supplementation because they are not absorbed directly into the portal vein and do not form chylomicrons (6).

Familial dysbetalipoproteinemia is managed with dietary fat restriction and the use of statins, nicotinic acid, and fibric acid derivatives. Gemfribozil, a molecule structurally similar to clofibrate, appears to be the drug of choice for this disorder (36).

Restriction of triglycerides containing long chained fatty acids to approximately 15 g/day appears to mitigate the gastrointestinal manifestations of abetalipoproteinemia. Vitamin E supplementation at 100 mg/kg/day has also been shown to inhibit the progression of the neurologic disorder and retinal lesions (37). Additionally, vitamin A at 200 to 400 IU/kg/day and vitamin K at 5 mg/day can be beneficial as well. Azizi et al. (38) reported neuralgic and visual improvement in an 11-year-old girl treated with parenteral vitamin A and vitamin E for 2 1/2 years. Similarly, Bishara et al. (39) reported arrest of retinal degeneration in eight patients with abetalipoproteinemia treated with a combination of vitamin A and E as measured by electroretinogram (39). This was corroborated by case reports of Hegele et al. (40, 41). Chowers et al. (42) showed that combined oral vitamin A and E supplementation that is initiated before 2 years of age can markedly attenuate the severe retinal degeneration that is associated with untreated abetalipoproteinemia. Serial assessments of neurophysiologic functions can be done using somatosensory potentials (43).

CLINICAL RECOMMENDATIONS OF THE VIGNETTE

The patient has the symptoms of abetalipoproteinemia. Diagnostic evaluation should include a lipoprotein profile and a peripheral blood smear. The latter should be done by using dilutions of whole blood samples with heparinized saline followed by incubation for 60 minutes at room temperature and phase-contrast microscopy analysis for the presence for acanthocytes.

Treatment is mainly supportive, with fat-soluble vitamin A and E supplementation at 100 mg/kg/day and 200 to 400 IU/kg/day respectively. Vitamin K at 5 mg/kg/day should also be given. Objective methods of monitoring disease progression would include periodic electroretinograms and somatosensory evoked potentials.

SUMMARY

Abetalipoproteinemia is a rare disorder of lipoprotein metabolism that can present with neurologic symptoms. The neurologic manifestations of abetalipoproteinemia include areflexia, loss of vibratory and position sense, ataxia, dysarthria, and, possibly, cognitive decline. The ophthalmologic complications of abetalipoproteinemia can be very debilitating as are the neurologic symptoms, and they are characterized by a pigmentary retinopathy, in most cases, and opthalmoplegia, ptosis, and anisocoria in some cases.

Therapy is supportive, consisting mainly of high-dose vitamin E supplementation.

REFERENCES

1. Rader DJ. Genetic dyslipoproteinemias. In: Blau N, Duran M, Blaskovics ME, et al., eds. *Physician's Guide to the Laboratory Diagnosis of Metabolic Disease*, 2nd ed. Berlin: Heidelberg; New York: Springer; 2005.
2. Tershakovec AM, Rader DJ. Disorders of lipoprotein metabolism and transport. In: Behrman RE, Kligman R, Jenson HB, et al., eds. *Nelson Textbook of Pediatrics*, 17th ed. Philadelphia: WB Saunders; 2004.
3. Bassen FA, Kornzweig AL. Malformation of the erythrocyte in a case of atypical retinitis pigmentosa. *Blood.* 1950;5:381–387.
4. Havel RJ, Kane JP. Introduction: Structure and metabolism of plasma lipoproteins. In: Scriver CR, Beaudet AL, Sly WS, et al., eds. *The Metabolic and Molecular Bases of Inherited Disease*, 8th ed. New York: McGraw-Hill; 2001:2701–2716.
5. Mahley RW, Rall Sc. Type iii hyperlipoproteinemia (dysbetalipoproteinemia): The role of apolipoprotein E in normal and abnormal lipoprotein metabolism. In: Scriver CR, Beaudet AL, Sly WS, et al., eds. *The Metabolic and Molecular Bases of Inherited Disease*, 8th ed. New York: McGraw-Hill; 2001:2835–2862.
6. Goldstein JL, Hobbs HH, Brown MS. Familial hypercholesterolemia. In: Scriver CR, Beaudet AL, Sly WS, et al., eds. *The Metabolic and Molecular Bases of Inherited Disease*, 8th ed. New York: McGraw-Hill; 2001:2863–2914.
7. Assman G, von Eckardstein A, Brewer HB, Jr. Familial alphalipoproteinenmia: Tangier disease. In: Scriver CR, Beaudet AL, Sly WS, et al., eds. *The Metabolic and Molecular Bases of Inherited Disease*, 8th ed. New York: McGraw-Hill; 2001:2937–2980.
8. Santamaria-Fojo S, Hoeg JM, Assman G, et al. Lecithin cholesterol acyltransferase deficiency and fish-eye disease. In: Scriver CR, Beaudet AL, Sly WS, et al., eds. *The Metabolic and Molecular Bases of Inherited Disease*, 8th ed. New York: McGraw-Hill; 2001:2817–2837.
9. Levy E, Marcel Y, Deckelbaum RJ, et al. Intestinal apo B synthesis, lipids and lipoproteins in chylomicron retention disease. *J Lipid Res.* 1987;87:1263–1274.
10. Lacaille F, Bratos M, Bouma ME, et al. Andersen disease: Clinical and morphologic study of 7 cases. *Archives Françaises de pediatric* [abstract]. 1987;46:491–498.
11. Wetterau JR. Aggerbeck LP, Bouma ME, et al. Absence of microsomal triglyceride transfer protein in individuals with abetalipoproteinemia. *Science.* 1992;258(5084):999–1001.
12. Narcisi TM, Shoulders CC, Chester SA, et al. Mutation of the microsomal triglyceride transfer protein gene in abetalipoproteinemia. *Am J Hum Genet.* 1995;57(6):1298–1310.
13. Baunzell JD, Deeb SS. Familial lipoprotein lipase deficiency, apo C-II deficiency and hepatic lipase deficiency. In: Scriver CR, Beaudet AL, Sly WS, et al., eds. *The Metabolic and Molecular Bases of Inherited Disease*, 8th ed. New York: McGraw-Hill; 2001:2789–2816.
14. Haas D, Kelley RI, Hoffman GF. Inherited disorders of cholesterol biosynthesis. *Neuropediatrics.* 2001;32:113–122.

15. Menkes JH, Wilcox WR. Inherited metabolic diseases of the nervous system. In: Menkes JH, Sarnat HB, Maria BL, eds. *Textbook of Child Neurology*, 7th ed. Philadelphia: Lippincott Williams & Wilkins; 2006.
16. Partin JS, Partin JC, Schubert WK, et al. Liver ultrastructure in abetaliproteinemia: Evolution of micronodular cirrhosis. *Gastroenterology*. 1974;67(1):107–118.
17. Lange Y, Ateck TL. Mechanism of red blood cell acanthocytosis and echinocytosis in vivo. *J Membr Biol.* 1984;77:153.
18. Kane JP, Havel RJ. Disorders of the biogenesis and secretion of lipoprotein containing the B lipoproteins. In: Scriver CR, Beaudet AL, Sly WS, et al., eds. *The Metabolic and Molecular Bases of Inherited Disease*, 8th ed. New York: McGraw-Hill; 2001:717–2752.
19. Cohen DA, Bosley TM, Savino PJ, et al. Primary regeneration of the oculomotor nerve: Occurrence in a patient with abetalipoproteinemia. *Arch Neurol.* 1985;42(8):821–823.
20. Matsuo M, Nomura S, Hara T, et al. A variant form of hypobetalipoproteinaemia with ataxia, hearing loss and retinitis pigmentosa. *Dev Med Child Neurol.* 1994;36(11):1015–1020.
21. Aliev G, Castellani RJ, Petersen RB, et al. Pathobiology of familial hypercholesterolemic atherosclerosis. *J Submicrosc Cytol Pathol.* 2004;36:225–240.
22. Viestenz A, Schlotzer-Schrebardt U, Hoffmann-Rummelt C, et al. Histopathology of corneal changes in LCAT deficiency. *Cornea.* 2002;21(8):834–837.
23. Ohta Y, Yamamoto S, Tsuchida H, et al. Nephropathy of familial lecithin-cholesterol acyltransferase deficiency: Report of a case. *Am J Kidney Dis.* 1986;7(1):41–46.
24. Cabin HS, Schwartz DE, Virmani R, et al. Type III Hyperlipoproteinemia: Quantification, distribution, and nature of atherosclerotic arterial narrowing in five necropsy patients. *Am Heart J.* 1981;102:830–835.
25. Frosini G, Marini M, Galgani P, et al. Tangier disease: An unusual diagnosis for an endoscopist. *Endoscopy.* 1994;26:373.
26. Lazaro RP, Dentinger MP, Rodichock LD, et al. Muscle pathology in Bassen-Kornzweig syndrome and vitamin E deficiency. *Am J Clin Pathol.* 1986;86(3):378–387.
27. Kott E, Delpre G, Kadish U, et al. Abetalipoproteinemia (Bassen-Kornzweig syndrome). Muscle involvement. *Acta Neuropathol (Berl).* 1977;37(3):255–258.
28. Cogan DG, Rodriguez M, Chu FC, et al. Ocular abnormalities in abetalipoproteinemia. A clinicopathologic correlation. *Ophthalmology.* 1984;8:991–998.
29. Wong AM, Heon E. Helicoid peripapillary chorioretinal degeneration in abetalipoproteinemia. *Arch Ophthalmol.* 1998;116(2):250–251.
30. Avigan MI, Ishak KG, Gregg RE, et al. Morphologic features of the liver in abetalipoproteinemia. *Hepatology.* 1984;4(6):1223–1226.
31. Higuchi I, Yamano T, Kurijama M, et al. Histochemical and ultrastructural pathology of skeletal muscle in an 8 year-old patient with abetalipoproteinemia. *Acta Neuropathologica.* 1993;86(5):29–31.
32. http://www.pathologyoutlines.com/smallbowel.html. Delpre G, Kadish U, Glantz Avidor I. endoscopic assessment in abetalipoproteinemia (Bassen-Kornzweig syndrome). *Endoscopy.* 1978;10(1):59–62.
33. Wickman A, Buchanan F, Pezeshkpour GM, et al. Peripheral neuropathy in abetalipoproteinemia. *Neurology.* 1985;35(9):1279–1289.
34. Jung HH, Darek A, Dobson-Stone C, et al. McLeod Neuroacanthocytosis Syndrome. http://www.genetests.org accessed October, 2006.
35. Stein EA, Adolph R, Rice V, et al. Non-progression of coronary atherosclerosis in homozygous familial hypercholesterolemia after 31 months of repetitive plasma exchange. *Clin Cardiol.* 1986;9:115–119.
36. Larsen ML, Illingworth DR, O'Malley JP. Comparative effects of gemfribozil and clofibrate in type III hyperlipoproteinemia. *Atherosclerosis.* 1994;106:235–240.
37. Muller DPR, Lloyd JK. Effect of large oral doses of vitamin E on the neurologic sequelae of patients with abetalipoproteinemia. *Ann N Y Acad Sci.* 1982;393:133–144.
38. Azizi E, Zaidman JL, Eshar J, et al. Abetalipoproteinemia treated with parenteral and oral vitamin A and E and medium chained triglycerides. *Acta Paediatr Scand.* 1978;67916): 796–801.
39. Bishara S, Merin S, Cooper M, et al. Combined vitamin A and E therapy prevents retinal electrophysiological deterioration in abetalipoproteinemia. *Br J Ophthalmol.* 1982;66(12): 767–770.
40. Hegele RA, Angel A. Arrest of neuropathy and myopathy in abetalipoproteinemia with high dose vitamin E therapy. *Can Med Assoc J.* 1985;132(1)41–44.
41. Runge P, Muller DP, McAllister J, et al. Oral vitamin E supplements can prevent the retinopathy of abetalipoproteinemia. *Br J Ophthalmol.* 1986;70(3):166–173.
42. Chowers I, Banin E, Merin S, et al. Long-term assessment of combined vitamin A and E treatment for the prevention of retinal degeneration in abetalipoproteinemia and hypobetalipoproteinemia patients. *Eye.* 2001;15(Pt 4):525–530.
43. Fagan ER, Taylor MJ. Longitudinal multimodal evoked potential studies in abetalipoproteinemia. *Can J Neurol Sci.* 1987;14(4):617–621.

CHAPTER **63**

Disorders of Amino Acid Metabolism

Rosario Maria S. Riel-Romero

OBJECTIVES

- To explain how homocystinuria can be a cause of stroke in a young adult
- To present the major clinical manifestations of selected amino acid disorders with, emphasis on homocystinuria
- To review the underlying biochemical defects in amino acid disorders
- To outline the diagnostic approaches and current therapy for amino acid disorders

CASE VIGNETTE

A previously well 20-year-old man had cataract surgery. Postoperatively, he developed a left hemiparesis. He was somewhat mentally delayed compared with peers and he had needed special help in school. He had no history of antecedent infection, head or neck trauma, seizures, or previous surgeries. On physical examination, he was a tall and slender young man with sparse and brittle blond hair, long tapering fingers, mild scoliosis, and prominent livedo reticularis. He had aphakia on the right and glaucoma on the left eye. On neurologic examination, he had some degree of psychomotor retardation, but was alert and cooperative. He was weaker in the left arm and leg compared with the right with 3/5 strength on his left upper and lower extremities. Muscle stretch reflexes were brisker on the left and a left extensor toe sign was elicited.

Laboratory investigation was as follows: Magnetic resonance imaging (MRI) of the brain showed a recent wedge-shaped infarct on the right hemisphere. Urinary excretion of homocysteine and plasma levels of homocysteine and methionine were elevated. Urinary cyanide and nitroprusside metabolic screens were positive. Skin biopsy was done and cultured fibroblasts revealed a deficiency of cystathionine β-synthetase.

DEFINITION

Amino acid disorders result from abnormalities in the breakdown of amino acids in the cytosol. In contrast to the clinical organic acidurias, aminoacidopathies do not involve coenzyme A (CoA)-activated metabolites (1). These abnormalities are often secondary to a deficiency of a key enzyme in the metabolic pathway, resulting from the accumulation of toxic intermediates that cause the clinical symptoms of the disease. This is the case in the accumulation of phenylalanine, phenylpyruvic acid, and phenylacetic acids in phenylketonuria as it is in the case of homocysteine overload in homocystinuria.

Disorders in the intestinal or renal transport of amino acids can cause clinical symptoms as well. This is exemplified by Hartnup disease, where an essential amino acid, tryptophan, is not effectively absorbed, and can cause renal calculi. Among the more common amino acid disorders are phenylketonuria, maple syrup urine disease, homocystinuria, and tyrosinemia and nonketotic hyperglycinemia (1). These are generally diagnosed through quantitative analysis of plasma for amino acids and urine for organic acids.

The classic organic acidurias are characterized by deficiencies of enzymes in the mitochondrial catabolism of CoA-activated carboxylic acids. These are generally diagnosed through analysis of organic acids in the urine or acylcarnitines in the blood. Examples of organic acidurias are proprionic academia, methylmalonic aciduria, isovaleric aciduria, the glutaric acidurias I and II, and the multiple carboxylase deficiency syndrome (1).

EPIDEMIOLOGY

The most common treatable aminoacidopathy, phenylketonuria (PKU), has an estimated prevalence in the United States of 1 of 14,000 to 1 of 20,000 live births (2). Nonketotic hyperglycinemia (NKH), a rare condition caused by a defect in the glycine cleavage enzyme, is common in northern Finland where the prevalence is 1 of 12,000 (3). Maple syrup urine disease (MSUD), a disease caused by the defects in branched chain α-ketoacid dehydrogenase, has an estimated prevalence of 1 of 185,000 (4). Tyrosinemia type I, caused by a deficiency of the enzyme fumarylacetoacetate, has a worldwide prevalence of 1 of 100,000 to 1 of 120,000 (5).

Mudd et al. (6) estimated the prevalence of homocystinuria to be 1 of 200,000 to 1 of 335,000. In Ireland, Naughten et al. (7) estimated the prevalence to be 1 of 65,000. Linnebank et al. (8) screened 200 unrelated German control subjects and found a frequency of heterozygosity of 1.5% for 1278T, corresponding to a calculated frequency of homozygosity of 1 of 17,800 and, in Norway, Refsum et al. (9) estimated the prevalence rate at 1 of 64,000 using genotyping in 1,133 random samples. Using DNA sequencing to diagnose pyridoxine-responsive CBS 833T→C mutation, Gaustades et al. (10) put the Danish prevalence of homocystinuria at 1 of 20,000. The Qatari population has been shown to have the highest worldwide prevalence at 1 of 3,000 (11).

ETIOLOGY AND PATHOGENESIS

The amino acid disorders are caused by genetic mutations that encode for specific proteins, often enzymes, resulting in a functional and structural change in these proteins. Many mutations are benign polymorphisms that simply reflect individual variations and they are clinically insignificant. Some genetic mutations, however, result in disease states that are often severe, if not lethal, if diagnosis and treatment are delayed. For instance, the deficiency of the phenylalanine hydroxylase (PAH) in phenylketonuria causes high levels of phenylalanine, phenylpyruvic acid, and phenylacetate. Without early treatment, affected patients experience severe and irreversible central nervous system (CNS) damage. Similarly, untreated maternal PKU can result in a toxic embryopathy or fetopathy characterized by mental retardation, microcephaly, low birthweight, congenital heart disease, and dysgenesis of the corpus callosum. (12). The lack of branched chain α-ketodehydrogenase activity in all forms of MSUD results in the accumulation of branched chain ketoacids valine, leucine, and isoleucine. Experiments with microenviroments similar to MSUD have revealed that excess branched chain amino acids may alter synthesis of catecholamines and serotonin and interfere with the glutamine or glutamate cycle in the brain (13).

In NKH, a primary defect in the 4-protein glycine cleavage enzyme complex causes an accumulation of glycine in all body tissues and fluids. Excessive glycine, an excitatory cortical neurotransmitter at the *N*-methyl-d-aspartate (NMDA) receptor level, hypothetically, can result in intractable seizures and inexorable brain damage commonly seen in affected patients (5).

In hereditary tyrosinemia (tyrosinemia type I), a deficiency of fumarylacetaoacetate hydrolase (FAH), causes a wide spectrum of symptoms involving the hepatic, renal, and central nervous systems. The exact mechanism by which these symptoms occur is unknown. One hypothesis suggests that tyrosine metabolites affect free sulfhydryl groups and glutathione metabolism, both of which have protective effects on the body (14,15).

Homocystinuria can result from any of the following: (*a*) cystathione β-synthetase deficiency (classic homocystinuria); (*b*) methylcobalamin formation defects; or (*c*) methyltetrahydrofolate reductase deficiency, among others.

Homocysteine, a nonprotein-forming, sulfur amino, is metabolized through remethylation and transulfuration. During remethylation, homocysteine acquires a methyl group from *N-5 methyltetrahydrofolate* (MTHF) or from betaine to form methionine. The reaction involving MTHF is vitamin B_{12}-dependent and occurs in all tissues. It is catalyzed by *methylenetetrahydrofolate reductase* and *methionine synthetase.* The reaction with betaine is confined to the liver and is vitamin B_{12}-independent. Adenosine triphosphate (ATP) then activates methionine to form *S-adenosylmethionine* (SAM). SAM, through a reaction catalyzed by *methionine adenosyltransferase,* donates a methyl group to various acceptor molecules and regenerates *S-adenosylhomocysteine* (SAH) and adenosine, which then become available for another cycle of methyl group transfer (6,16).

During transulfuration, homocysteine condenses with serine in a reaction catalyzed by a pyridoxal-5′-phosphate (PLP)-containing enzyme, *cystathione β-synthetase* (CBS) to form cystathione. Cystathione is hydrolyzed to form cysteine and α-ketoglutarate by another PLP-containing enzyme, *γ-cystathionase.* Excess cysteine is oxidized to taurine and S-sulfocysteine which are excreted in the urine. Hence, during transulfuration, excess homocysteine, not otherwise required for remethylation, is catabolized to deliver inorganic sulfates needed for the synthesis of heparin sulfate, heparin, dermatan sulfate, and chondroitin sulfate. Sulfite, a byproduct of cysteine oxidation, is oxidized by *sulfite oxidase* to sulfate (Fig. 63-1).

The relationship between elevated homocysteine levels and arterial disease was first suggested by McCully (17) who described autopsy evidence of premature arterial thrombosis in a patient with hypercysteinemia. Since then, strong evidence in the literature suggesting the role of hyperhomocysteinemia in the development of premature and recurrent venous thromboembolic disease have emerged (18–20). In the den Heijer et al. (21) study, fasting homocysteine levels in 269 subjects 70

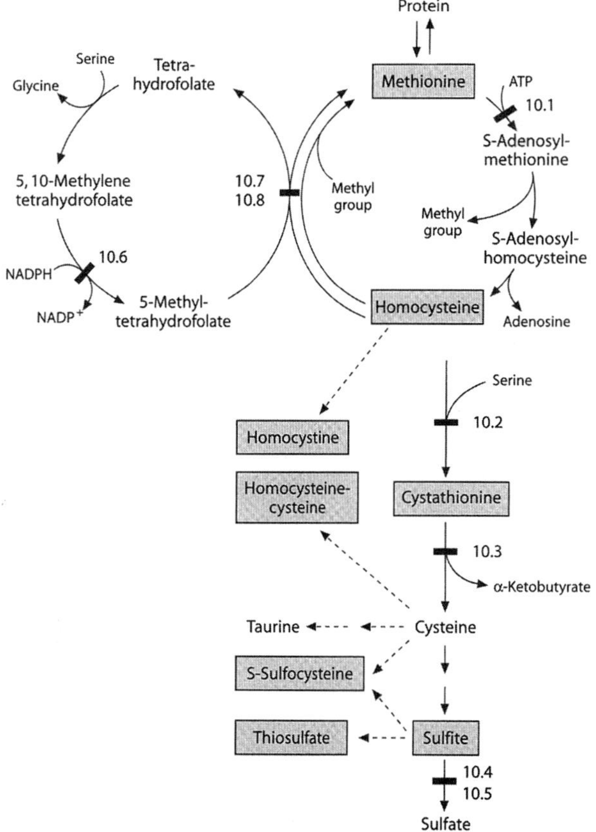

FIGURE 63-1. Pathway of homocysteine metabolism. (From Skovby F. Disorders of sulfur amino acids. In: Blau N, Duran M, Blaskovics ME, et al., eds. *Physician's Guide to the Laboratory Diagnosis of Metabolic Diseases,* 2nd ed. Berlin, Heidelberg, New York: Springer Verlag; 2003:246, with permission.)

years of age and younger with a first episode of deep vein thrombosis and in matched controls were measured. Homocysteine levels >95% were found in 105 patients. The effects of hyperhomocystenemia appeared to be independent of other risk factors for thrombosis, such as protein C, protein S, antithrombin deficiencies, and activated protein C resistance (21). High concentrations of homocysteine have been shown to inhibit prostacyclin synthesis and activation of factor V and plasminogen (18,22,23). Lentz et al. (24) showed that mild hyperhomocysteinemia in a monkey model impaired the response of resistance vessels to vasodilators and decreased thrombomodulin anticoagulant activity (24). Graeber et al. (25) found that homocysteine alters the arachidonic acid metabolism of normal platelets *in vitro* and increases two cyclooxygenase products, namely thromboxane A2 and 12-hydroxy-5,8,10-heptadecatrienoic acid (25). Other authors postulate that homocysteine cause endothelial cell injury by decreasing the levels of glutathione peroxidase, thus promoting direct cell injury by peroxides and impairing peroxide inactivation (26,27).

PATHOLOGY

In PKU, phenylalanine itself is thought to be the primary neurotoxic agent. In patients with untreated phenylketonuria, brain architecture and development are altered, with changes in myelination, number, and arborization of dendritic processes, and in neuronal density (28). Histopathologic studies of MSUD confirm neuroimaging data suggesting that MSUD is primarily a white matter disease with spongy degeneration of the cerebral hemispheres, pyramidal tracts of the spinal cord, and corpus callosum (29). Ferriere et al. (30) also described muscle fiber destruction in MSUD.

Similarly, autopsy studies of children with NKH have demonstrated diffuse vacuolation of the myelin, thinning of the corpus callosum, and hydrocephalus (31–33). The neuropathologic findings in tyrosinemia range from axonal degeneration and dysmyelination of the peripheral nerves to various degrees of spongiosis in the optic tracts, subcortical and cerebellar white matter, corpus callosum, and spinal cord (34).

The primary pathologic abnormalities in homocystinuria are structural changes in the blood vessels, including arteries, veins, and dural sinuses (35). The tunica intima is usually thickened and fibrosed, compromising vessel lumen. Tunica media has increased collagen content and the elastic fibers are described as frayed and split. Arterial and venous thrombosis are described in many organs, including the brain where infarcts are often seen. Saggital and transverse sinus thrombosis in children (36,37) have been reported as bilateral carotid dissection causing strokes in a 35-year-old woman with homocystinuria (38).

Other organ systems, such as the eyes and skeletal system, show characteristic changes. Ectopia lentis in the inferonasal direction is common and is hypothesized to be secondary to homocysteine-induced breakage of disulfide bridges in fibrillin, a glycoprotein localized in the ocular zonule (39). This hypothesis is supported by the work of Hubmacher et al. (40), which showed structural and functional alteration in fibrillin-1 in recombinant proteins incubated with homocysteine (40) and by Hutchison et al. (41) who showed that homocysteine alters intramolecular cbEGF (epidermal growth factor) domain disulfide bonds causing domain misfolding and, possibly, altering connective tissue function (41). Bilateral corneal fibrosis, characterized as membrane-bound inclusions containing fibrogranular material in the corneal epithelium and keratocytes, has been reported in a 21-year-old woman with homocystinuria (42).

CLINICAL MANIFESTATIONS

The aminoacidopathies can present suddenly in early infancy and childhood, with acute catastrophic deterioration into seizures and coma or by a chronic course characterized by episodic exacerbations and remissions. Affected newborns may appear normal until seizures, strokes, and developmental delay become apparent between 5 and 9 months of age (35). An older child with homocystinuria may have sparse blond hair, fragile skin, and hip muscle weakness. In classic homocystinuria, the diagnosis can be made in early childhood secondary to multiorgan disease or only in adulthood after a thromboembolic event.

Affected individuals with phenylketonuria appear normal at birth. Untreated, they develop moderate to profound mental retardation, seizures, and adventitious body movements. Some may manifest a transient seborrheic or eczematoid rash. These children have a characteristic unpleasant odor of phenylacetic acid, which has been variously described as *musty* or *mousy* (5).

The clinical presentation of tyrosinemia I can start in the early neonatal period, which portends a graver prognosis characterized by severe liver failure and coagulopathy. After 6 months, infants may have a milder picture of liver dysfunction, failure to thrive, rickets, and renal disease. Acute episodes of peripheral neuropathy, indistinguishable from porphyric crisis, characterize the neurologic picture of tyrosinemia. Renal disease in tyrosinemia is characterized by renal tubular acidosis, aminoaciduria, and hypophoshaturia (5).

Infants with MSUD are often normal at birth, but quickly develop poor feeding, vomiting, seizures, lethargy, and coma within the first few days of life. In the intermittent form of MSUD, seemingly normal children develop acute behavior changes, lethargy, and even coma during periods of intercurrent illness or catabolic states (5).

Most patients with NKH have the classic or neonatal form of MSUD, which presents with hypotonia, poor feeding, lethargy, and myoclonic seizures in the first few days of life. Rapid deterioration to coma and death commonly follows. Surviving patients often have intractable epilepsy and profound cognitive deficiency (5).

Classic homocystinuria is characterized by involvement of the eye, and skeletal, vascular, and central nervous systems. One or several systems can be involved in a given individual. Expressivity of clinical manifestations is also variable, and can include myopia, ectopia lentis, cataracts, corneal opacities, glaucoma, and iridodonesis (43). A *Marfanoid* habitus, with long limbs and excessive height, characterize affected individuals. Skeletal abnormalities can include pes cavus, genu valgum, scoliosis, pectus excavatum, and pectus carinatum, and biconcave or *fish* vertebrae.

Thromboembolism is a major complication and cerebrovascular accidents have been described in both infants and young adults. Other neurologic problems include seizures, mental retardation, and dystonia. Two siblings have been described with dystonia and parkinsonism appearing in the first and second decades of life (44). Psychiatric problems are likewise common and include psychosis (45), obsessive-compulsive disorder, depression, anxiety, and personality disorders (46). The vitamin B_6-responsive forms have a mean intelligent quotient (IQ) of 79 versus 56 in the vitamin B_6-unresponsive variants (46).

Two clinical conditions can mimic homocystinuria. Marfan syndrome is also characterized by an asthenic habitus, ectopia lentis, and arachnodactyly as well. Sulfite oxidase deficiency can present with ectopia lentis, although more superotemporal rather then inferonasal as in classic homocystinuria (6).

Among the atypical presentations of homocystinuria would be as *shaken baby syndrome*, with retinal hemorrhages and intracranial bleeding (47) as well as megaloblastic anemia corrected by folate and vitamin B_{12} administration (48).

DIAGNOSIS

Specific diagnosis is often crucial in disorders of amino acid metabolism because specific treatment must to be initiated as soon as possible to ensure the best possible outcome. Diagnosis often requires the measurements of serum amino acids, urine organic acids, pH, glucose, ammonia, bicarbonate, and liver enzymes.

Ideally, mass screening of newborn infants for the aminoacidopathies should be carried out, but this is technologically difficult and may be economically impossible for some countries. In the United States, babies are screened for PKU routinely at birth, using either the bacterial inhibition assay of Guthrie or by tandem mass spectrometry. Hyperphenylalaninemia is defined as a quantitative plasma phenylalanine value of >2 mg/dL or 120 μM (49). In MSUD, branched chain amino acids (BCAA) are generally elevated in the blood, urine, and cerebrospinal fluid. The presence of *alloisoleucine* in conjunction with low levels of plasma alanine, glutamine, and lysine is virtually pathognomonic of the disease (50). Hepatorenal tryosinemia is characterized by increased plasma tyrosine and tyrosinuria, coupled with increased succinylacetone levels in both plasma and urine. Enzymatic assays of fumarylacetoacetate activity in liver biopsy specimens, erythrocytes, and lymphocytes can be carried out as well. The diagnosis of Hartnup disease is based on the presence of aminoaciduria restricted only to the neutral amino acids (5).

The major biochemical features of classic homocystinuria are increased plasma concentrations of homocystine (a symmetric disulfide), homocysteine (the thiol compound in the methionine metabolic pathway), and methionine; increased excretion of urinary homocysteine; and reduced cystathione β-synthase (CBS) enzyme activity in cultured fibroblasts. Cystathione β-synthase activity can also be assayed in cultured amniocytes and, therefore, prenatal diagnosis is possible. Classic homocystinuria can be detected using Guthrie blood spot cards to screen for elevated methionine levels by tandem mass spectroscopy or bacterial inhibition assay. Most screening, however, is for methionine and not for homocysteine or homocystine. Hence, other causes of hyperhomocysteinemia, such as methylenetetrahydrofolate reductase deficiency and cobalamin cofactor (cbl) defects, which can result in normal or low levels of methionine, may not be detected. Another criticism of current newborn screening methods is the low detection for milder forms of homocystinuria (1). Among nearly 1 million newborns in a 20-year period in Taiwan, only 17 cases of hypermethionemia and 1 case of homocystinuria were detected using dried blood spots (51).

In all suspected individuals, quantitative serum and plasma amino acids tests should be done. It is crucial to know that the thiol compounds in blood are unstable. Homocysteine can bind with sulfhydryl-containing compounds, including protein cystine; without deproteinizing the plasma or serum sample, homocystine and homocysteine-cysteine mixed disulfide can become undetectable after only 1 day in storage at −20°C. The measurement of total plasma homocysteine can be a more accurate diagnosis of homocystinuria because it can be measured with deproteination. Additionally, false–negative results for homocystinuria can occur in the setting of vitamin B_6 supplementation as some vitamin B_6-responsive forms can have dramatic responses to even low doses of pyridoxine (52).

Direct assay of enzyme activity in cultured fibroblasts, liver biopsy specimens, and lymphocytes can be done to confirm CBS deficiency.

MOLECULAR GENETIC DIAGNOSIS OF HOMOCYSTINURIA

Classic homocystinuria secondary to deficiency of cystathione β-synthase is an autosomal recessive disease. Heterozygotes for CBS deficiency may be difficult to distinguish from controls because biochemical tests may be nonspecific. Guttormsen et al. (53) showed that methionine loading test may not be a reliable tool to differentiate pyridoxine-responsive homocystinuria from nonpyridoxine responsive homocystinuria (53). To distinguish between the two entities, a pyridoxine challenge test can be done. While on a normal diet, baseline plasma amino acids are obtained. Pyridoxine (100 mg) is orally given to the subjects. Vitamin B_6 responsiveness is suggested by a reduction of 30% or more of plasma homocystine or methionine.

The gene for homocystinuria had been cloned and is mapped to chromosome 21q22.3 (54). The gene for CBS maps to the subtelomeric region on human chromosome 21q and to proximal mouse chromosome 17. It has 23 exons, is >2,500 base pairs, and encodes for a polypeptide of 551 amino acids. More than 130 mutations have been described. The two most common mutations, I278T and G307S, are found in exon 8. The G307S mutation is the primary cause of the disease in Ireland and is frequently seen in individuals with Irish, Scottish, English, French, and Portuguese ancestry. Mutation p.I278T, which is very prevalent, has been found in all European countries wherein it has been searched, with the exception of the Iberian peninsula, and is known to respond to vitamin B_6. On the other hand, mutation p.T191M is prevalent in Spain, Portugal, and parts of South America and is not pyridoxine responsive (55).

Direct sequence analysis of the entire coding region of the gene can also be performed with a yield of 95% for mutation detection.

TREATMENT

Although symptomatic management is necessary, the therapy of the aminoacidopathies is often directed at decreasing the levels of toxic metabolites that accumulate in the tissues as a result of an enzymatic block. Hence, in PKU, it is vital to lower the phenylalanine levels as soon as possible. In hepatorenal tyrosinemia, treatment with NTBC (2-[2-Nitro-4-trifluromethylbenzoyl]-1, 3-cyclohexanedione) has been effective and markedly improves long-term hepatic and neurologic outcome. Liver transplantation in hepatorenal tyrosinemia has shown promising results as well (56).

Similarly, the treatment of homocystinuria is directed at controlling elevated levels of plasma homocysteine to prevent or minimize the metabolic sequelae, particularly thromboembolism.

Vitamin B_6 therapy at doses of 100 to 200 mg/day in both B_6 responsive and nonresponsive forms is recommended. A protein-restricted diet is required to reduce methionine intake. To prevent malnutrition, a methionine-free amino acid formula can be used. Betaine treatment at doses of 6 to 9 g/day provides an alternative remethylation pathway to convert excess homocysteine to methionine (57). Cerebral edema has been reported in extreme hypermethionemia (58,59).

Folate and vitamin B_{12} supplementation, cofactors of methionine synthase, facilitate the conversion of homocysteine to methionine. Periodic monitoring of plasma levels of methionine, homcystine, and homocysteine guide and optimize metabolic control (60).

Women of childbearing age with homocystinuria are at increased risk for postpartum thromboembolism. Injection with low molecular-weight heparin during the last 2 weeks of pregnancy and the first 6 weeks postpartum, coupled with aspirin throughout pregnancy, is recommended. Similarly, affected patients are at increased risk for thromboembolism during and after surgery. To minimize this risk, one and one half maintenance fluids should be given before, during, and after surgery until oral fluids can be taken (60).

CLINICAL RECOMMENDATIONS OF THE VIGNETTE

The patient appears to have the clinical features of homocystinuria, as well as laboratory evidence of cystathione β-synthetase deficiency. He can likewise have molecular genetic testing for any of the known genetic mutations. Vitamins B_6 and B_{12}, folate, and betaine should be started, along with a low-protein diet. Periodic evaluations of plasma homocysteine, homocysteine, and methionine levels should be performed. If at all possible, future surgeries should be avoided.

SUMMARY

Classic homocystinuria is a common cause of cerebrovascular events in the young adult. It is caused by deficiency of cystathione β-synthase (CBS). Classic homocystinuria affects multiple organ systems, including the eyes, and skeletal, vascular, and the central nervous systems.

Diagnosis rests on the presence of increased elevations of homocysteine and other metabolites of homocysteine metabolism in the plasma and on demonstration of low or undetectable enzyme activity in cultured fibroblasts, liver samples, or lymphocytes, coupled with detection of genetic mutations in the CBS gene. Management consists of low methionine, cystine-supplemented diet and supplementation with vitamins B_6 and B_{12}, folate, and betaine. Avoidance of surgery is advised as the risk of thromboembolism after surgery is high.

REFERENCES

1. Hoffman GF, Nyhan WL, Zschoche J, et al. *Inherited Metabolic Diseases. Core Handbooks in Pediatrics*, 1st ed. Philadelphia: Lippincott Williams & Williams; 2002.
2. Paul DB. The history of newborn phenylketonuria screening in the United States. Available at: http://www.genome.gov/10002397. Accessed October, 2006.
3. Applegarth DA, Tome JR. Nonketotic hyperglycinemia (glycine encephalopathy): Laboratory diagnosis. *Mol Genet Metab.* 2001;74:139–146.
4. Naylor EW. Newborn screening for maple syrup urine disease (branched chain aciduria). In: Bickel H, Guthrie R, Hammersen G, eds. *Neonatal Screening for Inborn Errors of Metabolism.* Berlin: Springer Verlag; 1980;19.
5. Rezvani I. Defects in metabolism of amino acids. In: Behrman RE, Kligman R, Jenson HB, et al., eds. *Nelson Textbook of Pediatrics*, 17th ed. Philadelphia: WB Saunders; 2004:399–433.
6. Mudd SH, Levy ML, Kraus JP. Disorders of transulfuration In: Scriver CL, Beaudet AL, Sly WS, eds. *The Metabolic and Molecular Basis of Inherited Diseases*, 7th ed. New York: McGraw-Hill; 2001:1279.
7. Naughten ER, Yap S, Mayne PD. Newborn screening for homocystinuria: An enzymatic defect. *Science.* 1964;43:1443–1445.
8. Linnebank M, Homberger A, Junker R, et al. High prevalence of the 1278T mutation of the human cystathione beta-synthase detected by a novel screening application. *Thromb Haemost.* 2001;85(6):986–988.
9. Refsum H, Fredriksen A, Meyer K, et al. Birth prevalence of homocystinuria. *J Pediatr.* 2004;144:830–832.
10. Gaustadnes M, Ingerslev J, Rutiger N. Prevalence of congenital homocystinuria in Denmark. *N Engl J Med.* 1999;340:1513.
11. El-Said MF, Badin R, Bassist MS, et al. A common mutation in the *CBS* gene explains a high incidence of homocystinuria in the Qatari population. *Hum Mutat.* 2006;27(7):719.
12. Levy ML, Lobbrgt D, Sansaricq C, et al. Comparison of phenylketonuric and non-phenylketonuric sibs from untreated pregnancies in a mother with phenylketonuria. *Am J Med Genet.* 1992;44:439–442.
13. Huang Y, Zeilke RH, Tildon JT. Elevation of amino acids in the interstitial space of the rat brain following infusion of large neutral and keto acids by microdialysis: Leucine infusion. *Dev Neurosci.* 1996;18:415.
14. Stoner E, Starkman H, Wellner D, et al. Biochemical studies of a patient with hereditary hepatorenal tyrosinemia: Evidence of glutathione deficiency. *Pediatr Res.* 1984;18(12):1332–1336.
15. Jorquera R, Tanguay RM. The Mutagenicity of the tyrosine metabolite fumarlyacetoacetate is enhanced by glutathione depletion. *Pediatr Res.* 1984;18(12):1332–1336.
16. Skovby F. Disorders of sulfur amino acids. In: Blau N, Duran M, Blaskovics ME, et al., eds. *Physician's Guide to the Laboratory Diagnosis of Metabolic Diseases*, 2nd ed. Berlin, Heidelberg, New York: Springer Verlag; 2003:243–260.
17. McCully KS. Vascular pathology of hypercysteinemia: Implications of the pathogenesis of arteriosclerosis. *Am J Pathol.* 1969:56;111–128.
18. Wang J, Dudman NP, Wilcken DE. Effects of homocysteine and related compounds on prostacyclin production by cultured human endothelial cells. *Thromb Haemost.* 1993;70(6):1047–1052.
19. Israelson B, Brattstrom LE, Hultberg BL. Homocystinuria and myocardial infarction. *Atherosclerosis.* 1988;72:227–233.
20. Coull BM, Malinow MR, Beamer N, et al. Elevated plasma homocysteine in acute stroke and transient ischemic attack: A possible independent risk factor for stroke. *Stroke.* 1990;21(4):572–576.
21. den Heijer M, Koster T, Blom HJ, et al. Hyperhomocysteinemia as a risk factor for deep vein thrombosis. *N Engl J Med.* 1996;334(12):759–762.
22. Rodgers GM, Kane WH. Activation of endogenous factor V by a homocysteine-induced vascular endothelial cell activator. *J Clin Invest.* 1986;77:1909–1916.
23. Hajjar KA. Homocysteine-induced modulation of tissue plasminogen activator binding to its endothelial cell membrane receptor. *J Clin Invest.* 1993;91:2873–2879.
24. Lentz RS, Sobey CG, Piferu DJ, et al. Vascular dysfunction in monkeys with diet-induced hyperhomocysteinemia. *J Clin Invest.* 1996;98(1):24–29.
25. Graeber JE, Slott JH, Ulane RE, et al. Effect of homocysteine and homocystine on platelet and vascular arachidonic acid metabolism. *Pediatr Res.* 1982;16(6):490–493.
26. Stamler JS, Osborne JA, Jaraki M, et al. Adverse vascular effects of homocysteine are modulated by endothelial-derived relaxing factor and related oxides of nitrogen. *J Clin Invest.* 1993;91:308–318.
27. Upchurch GR, Jr., Welch GN, Freedman JE, et al. Homocysteine attenuates endothelial glutathione peroxidase and thereby potentiates peroxide-mediated injury. *Circulation.* 1993;92:1–228.
28. Huttenlocher PR. The neuropathology of phenylketonuria: Human and animal studies. *Eur J Pediatr.* 2000;159[Suppl 2]:S107–S108.
29. Kamei A, Takashima S, Chan F, et al. Abnormal dendritic development in maple syrup urine disease. *Pediatr Neurol.* 1992;8(2):145–147.
30. Ferriere G, de Castro M, Rodriguez J. Abnormalities of muscle fibers in maple syrup urine disease. *Acta Neuropathol.* 1984;63(3):249–254.
31. Dobyns WB. Agenesis of the corpus callosum and gyral malformations are frequent manifestations of nonketotic hypergylcinemia. *Neurology.* 1989;39:817.
32. Sener RN. Nonketotic hyperglycinemia: Diffusion magnetic resonance imaging findings. *J Compt Assist Tomogr.* 2003;27(4):538–540.

33. Van Hove JL, Kishnani PS, Demaerel P, et al. Acute hydrocephalus in nonketotic hyperglycinemia. *Neurology.* 2000;54(3):754–756.
34. Mitchell GA, Larochelle J, Lambert M, et al. Neurologic crisis in hereditary tyrosinemia. *N Engl J Med.* 1990;322:432–437.
35. Menkes JH, Wilcox WR. Inherited metabolic diseases of the nervous system. In: Menkes JH, Sarnat HB, Maria BL, eds. *Child Neurology,* 7th ed. Philadelphia: Lippincott Williams & Wilkins, 2006:29–141.
36. Vorstmann E, Keeling D, Leonard J, et al. Sagittal sinus thrombosis in a teenager: Homocystinuria associated with reversible antithrombin deficiency. *Dev Med Child Neurol.* 2002;44 (7):498.
37. Buoni S, Molinelli M, Mariottini A, et al. Homocystinuria with transverse sinus thrombosis. *J Child Neurol.* 2001;16(9):688–690.
38. Weiss N, Demeret S, Sonneville R, et al. Bilateral internal carotid artery dissection in cystathionine β-synthase deficiency. *Eur Neurol.* 2006;55(3):177–178.
39. Sakai LY. Disulfide bonds crosslink molecules of fibrillin in connective tissue space. In: Tamburro A, Davidson J, eds. *Elastin: Chemical and Biologic Aspects.* Galatinia, Italy: Congedo; 1990:2.
40. Hubmacher D, Tiedemann K, Bartels R, et al. Modification of the structure and function of fibrillin-1 by homocysteine suggests a potential pathogenetic mechanism in homocystinuria. *J Biol Chem.* 2005;280(41):34946–34955.
41. Hutchinson S, Aplin RT, Webb H, et al. Molecular effects of homocystine on cbEGF domain structure: insights into the pathogenesis of homocystinuria. *Mol Biol.* 2005; 346(3):833–844.
42. Rao SK, Krishnakumar S, Sudhir RR, et al. Bilateral corneal fibrosis in homocystinuria: Case report and transmission electron microscopic findings. *Cornea.* 2002;21(7): 730–732.
43. Sudarshan A, Kopietz L. Corneal changes in homocystinuria. *Ann Ophthalmol.* 1986;18(2):60.
44. Ekinci B, Apaydin H, Vural M, et al. Two siblings with homocystinuria presenting with dystonia and Parkinsonism. *Mov Disord.* 2004;19(8):962–964.
45. Ryan MM, Sidhu RK, Alexander JM. Homocystinuria presenting as psychosis in an adolescent. *J Child Neurol.* 2002;17:859–860.
46. Abbott MH, Folstein SE, Abbey H, et al. Psychiatric manifestations of homocystinuria due to cystathione beta-synthase deficiency: Prevalence, natural history, and relationship to neurologic impairment and vitamin B_6-responsiveness. *Am J Med Genet.* 1987;26(4): 959–969.
47. Francis PJ, Calver DM, Barnfield P, et al. An infant with methylmalonic aciduria and homocystinuria (cblC) presenting with retinal haemorrhages and subdural haematoma mimicking non-accidental injury. *Eur J Pediatr.* 2004;163(7):420–421.
48. Ishida S, Isotani H, Furukawa K, et al. Homocystinuria due to cystathionine β-synthetase deficiency associated with megaloblastic anemia. *J Intern Med.* 2001;250:453–456.
49. Scriver CR, Kaufmann JC. Hyperphenylalaninemia: Phenylalanine hydroxylase deficiency. In: Scriver CL, Beaudet AL, Sly WS, eds. *The Metabolic and Molecular Basis of Inherited Diseases,* 7th ed. New York: McGraw-Hill; 2001:1667–1724.
50. Chuang DT, Shih VE. Maple syrup urine disease (branched chain ketoaciduria). In: Scriver CL, Beaudet AL, Sly WS, eds. *The Metabolic and Molecular Basis of Inherited Diseases,* 7th ed. New York: McGraw-Hill; 2001:1971–2006.
51. Chien YH, Chiang SC, Huang A, et al. Spectrum of hypermethioninemia in neonatal screening. *Ear Hum Dev.* 2005 Jun: 81(6);529–533.
52. Smith KL, Bradley L, Levy HL, et al. Inadequate laboratory technique for amino acid analysis resulting in missed diagnosis of homocystinuria. *Clin Chem.* 1998;44(4):897–898.
53. Guttormsen AB, Veland PM, Krugle WD, et al. Disposition of homocysteine in subjects heterozygous for homocystinuria due to cystathionine β-synthase deficiency: Relationship between genotype and phenotype. *Am J Med Genet.* 2001;100(3):204–213.
54. Munke M, Kraus JP, Ohura T, et al. The gene for cystathione beta-synthase (CBS) maps to the subtelomeric region on human chromosome 21q and to proximal mouse chromosome 17. *Am J Hum Genet.* 1988;42(4):550–559.
55. Urreizti R, Asteggiano C, Bermudez M, et al. The p.T191M mutation of the *CBS* gene is highly prevalent among homocystinuric patients from Spain, Portugal, and South America. *J Hum Genet.* 2006;51(4):305–313.
56. Grompe M. The pathophysiology and treatment of hereditary tyrosinemia type I. *Semin Liver Dis.* 2001;21(4):563–567.
57. Lawson-Yuen A, Levy HL. The use of betaine in the treatment of elevated homocysteine. *Mol Genet Metab.* 2006;88(3):201–207.
58. Yaghmai R, Kashani AH, Geragthty MT, et al. Progressive cerebral edema associated with high methionine levels and betaine therapy in a patient with cystathionine β-synthase (CBS) deficiency. *Am J Med Genet.* 2002;108(1):57–63.
59. Devlin AM, Hajipour L, Gholkar A, et al. Cerebral edema associated with betaine treatment in classical homocystinuria. *J Pediatr.* 2004:144(4):545–548.
60. Picker JD and Levy HL. Homocystinuria caused by Cystathione Beta-Synthase Deficiency. http://www.genetests.org. Accessed September, 2006.

CHAPTER **64**

Disorders of the Metabolism of Purines and Pyrimidines

Rosario Maria S. Riel-Romero

OBJECTIVES

- To describe adenosine deaminase deficiency, a disorder of purine metabolism, which can present as immunodeficiency
- To discuss the other signs and symptoms of selected disorders of purine and pyrimidine metabolism, with emphasis on adenosine deaminase deficiency
- To explain the biochemical basis of adenosine deaminase deficiency
- To review the diagnostic tests used to ascertain these disorders
- To present the existing therapy for these diseases

CASE VIGNETTE

A 35-year-old woman was seen because of a 2-week history of shortness of breath and fever. Chest X-ray film demonstrated acute pneumonia superimposed on long-standing signs of bronchiectasis. Her medical history was noteworthy for recurrent pneumonia and chronic sinusitis. Family history was positive for a brother who had died at 2 years of age of *Pseudomonas* sepsis and *Pneumocystis carinii* pneumonia. The patient was successfully treated with broad-spectrum antibiotics. Three years later, she presented with dementia. Neurologic evaluation demonstrated progressive multifocal encephalopathy secondary to the JC virus and she was subsequently found to have acquired immunodeficiency syndrome (AIDS).

DEFINITION

The inherited disorders of purine and pyrimidine metabolism encompass a wide variety of diseases with broad spectrums of clinical features. Heritable errors in purine nucleotide synthesis include *phosphoribosylpyrophosphosphate synthetase superactivity* and *adenylsuccinase deficiency*. Inborn errors in purine catabolism include *adenosine deaminase deficiency, xanthine oxidoreductase deficiency*, and *purine nucleoside phosphorylase deficiency*. Disorders of the purine salvage pathway are exemplified by *hypoxanthine-guanine phosphoribosyltransferase (HPRT) deficiency* (Lesch-Nyhan syndrome) and *adenine phosphoribosyltransferase (APRT) deficiency*. Some disorders of pyrimidine metabolism include *hereditary orotic aciduria (uridine monophosphate synthase deficiency), dihydropyrimidine dehydrogenase deficiency, and dihydropyriminidase deficiency*.

Purines and pyrimidines are the building blocks of nucleic acids and other intermediate metabolites in carbohydrate and lipid metabolism. In the body, purine compounds are derived by either dietary ingestion of purine compounds or purine synthesis *de novo*. The pathway of purine synthesis *de novo* consists of eleven enzymatic reactions on a ribose-5-phosphate backbone, culminating in the synthesis of inosine monophosphate (IMP) and the generation of adenosine monophosphate (AMP) or guanosine monophosphate (GMP), which, in turn, are crucial in RNA and DNA synthesis. Uric acid is the end product of purine catabolism (1).

Purine metabolism is characterized by interconversions. Hence, IMP yields AMP through a reaction catalyzed by *adenylosuccinate synthetase* and guanosine triphosphate (GTP). GMP is derived from IMP through a reaction using adenosine triphosphate (ATP) to transfer an amido group from glutamine to xanthine monophosphate (XMP).

In general, purine catabolism involves the dephosphorylation of AMP, IMP, and XMP to their corresponding ribonucleosides as catalyzed by *purine 5′ nucleotidases* and *phosphatases*. Nucleosides inosine, guanosine, and xanthosine are cleaved by *purine nucleoside phosphorylase* to their respective purine bases, hypoxanthine, guanine, and xanthine. Adenosine nucleotide and nucleoside catabolism is through the deamination of AMP to IMP by *AMP deaminase*. Adenosine or deoxyadenosine is converted to inosine or deoxyinosine by *adenosine deaminase*. Guanine is changed to xanthine by *guanine deaminase*. Hypoxanthine is converted to xanthine and xanthine is converted to uric acid by *xanthine oxidase*, an iron and molybdenum cofactor containing flavoprotein. During the formation of uric acid, superoxide anion and hydrogen peroxide, thence, hydroxyl radicals are generated (2).

Pyrimidines are formed by the condensation of carbamylphosphate and aspartate to yield orotic acid and the key substrate, uridine monophosphate. Other nucleotides, such as cytidine and thymidine monophosphate, are also found in this pathway. Carbamylphosphate is generated from glutamine and carbon dioxide as well as ATP by *carbamylphosphate synthetase II (CPS II)* and condenses with aspartate in a reaction catalyzed by *aspartate transcarbamylase (AST)*. Carbamyl aspartate is converted to dehydro-orotic acid by *dehydro-orotase (DHO)*. All these three enzymes are coded for by one gene. Dehydro-otic acid is converted to orotic acid by *dehydro-orotate dehydrogenase (DHODH)*. Orotate is then changed to orotidine-monophosphate (OMP) by *orotate phosphoribosyl transferase (OPRT)*. OMP is then converted to uridylic acid or uridine monophosphate (UMP) by *orotidine 5′ monophosphate decarboxylase (ODC)*. DHODH, OPRT, and ODC are coded for by a second gene. UMP is converted to uridine by *uridine monophosphate hydrolase* (1,2).

Pyrimidine nucleotides are converted to their respective nucleosides. *Cytidine deaminase* deaminates cytidine to uridine. Uridine is reduced to uracil by *uridine phosphorylase*. Uracil is converted to dihydrouracil by *dihydropyrimidine dehydrogenase* (DHPDH). Dihydrouracil is then changed to uredoproprionic acid by *dihydropyriminidase* (DHP), which is then changed to β-alanine (1,2).

Uridine diphosphate is converted to deoxyuridine diphosphate and deoxyuridine monophosphate and deoxythymidine monophosphate and ultimately to thymidine. Thymidine, as with uracil, is converted to DHPDH. Dihydrothymidine is then converted to uredobutyric acid by dihydropyriminidase or amidohydrolase. Uredobutyric acid is then changed to β-aminobutyric acid and, thus, to R-methylmalonic acid semialdehyde (1,2).

Adenosine deaminase (ADA) and purine nucleoside phosphorylase (PNP) catalyze steps in purine nucleoside metabolism. In 1972, Giblett et al. reported the association of immunodeficiency and the lack of adenosine deaminase activity. Three years later, the first case of PNP deficiency was described (3).

EPIDEMIOLOGY

Gout, a disease characterized by hyperuricemia, uric acid nephrolithiasis, and recurrent attacks of inflammatory arthritis, secondary to urate crystal deposition, affects >1% of adults in the United States. Adenosine deaminase deficiency is responsible for 15% to 17% of patients with severe combined immunodeficiency (SCID) and 30% to 40% of patients with autosomal recessive SCID. Among 225 patients treated over a combined period of 53 years, 32 (14%) were adenosine deaminase deficient (2).

Since its original description in two brothers with hyperuricemia and self-injurious behavior in 1964, Lesch-Nyhan syndrome (LNS) has become a well-described clinical entity, with a prevalence of 1 of 100,000 to 1 of 300,000 live births in the United States (4). APRT deficiency type I, associated with a complete absence of APRT enzyme activity in erythrocyte lysates, has been described in 140 patients, 45 of whom are Japanese. Patients with APRT have 5% to 25% residual enzyme activity and accounts for 75% of Japanese patients with APRT deficiency (5). Myoadenylate deficiency has been reported in >200 patients (6).

ETIOLOGY AND PATHOGENESIS

GOUT

The gouty state is predicated on a state of hyperuricemia. Hyperuricemia, in turn, depends on multiple factors, including the size of the purine nucleotide pool, increased turnover of preformed purines, the catabolism of nucleic acids, the rate of uric acid excretion, and the presence of other diseases characterized by the increased production of uric acid (e.g., malignancy, sickle cell disease, obesity, hyperlipidemia, and glycogen storage disease) (7). Uric acid is poorly soluble; most is mainly excreted by the kidneys and the rest through intestinal bacterial uricolysis. Any alteration in the processes can tax the homeostatic mechanisms by which normal serum uric acids are maintained. Primary gout, however, is a heterogenous condition and the exact biochemical defect has not been identified (Scriver). A defect in the renal fractional clearance of gout is one of the possible mechanisms. The preponderance of gout among families has long been recognized. Familial juvenile gouty nephropathy is an autosomal dominant disorder characterized by severely impaired renal clearance of uric acid that results in nephropathy and death (8).

LESCH-NYHAN SYNDROME

Neychev and Miltev (9) proposed a hypothesis explaining the relationship between uric acid overproduction and the neurobehavioral symptoms in Lesch-Nyhan syndrome. They theorized that accelerated purine and histidine synthesis in LNS results in histamine and AICAR (5-aminoimidazole-4-carboxamidenibotide) accumulation. These two compounds can potentially cause an imbalance in the excitatory and inhibitory pathways in the basal ganglia (9). On the other hand, Deustch et al. (10) suggested that the deficiency of guanine-based purines in LNS can impair the transduction of signals dependent on GTP-protein–coupled second messenger systems and interfere with the modulation of glutaminergic neurotransmission. The ensuing glial reuptake of L-glutamate can account, in part, for the neurologic complications of spasticity, choreoathetosis, mental retardation, and compulsive self-mutilation seen in LNS (10).

The gene for hypoxanthine guanine phosphoribosyltransferase has been localized to the long arm of the X chromosome; it has no exons and is about 44 kb long (11). Thus far, about 302 mutations in the gene encoding for hypoxanthine-guanine phosphoribosyltransferase have been identified. These genotypes are associated with widely heterogeneous phenotypic expressions (12).

HEREDITARY OROTIC ACIDURIA

Hereditary orotic aciduria or *uridine monophosphate synthase deficiency*, a disorder of pyrimidine *de novo* synthesis, is associated with a deficient activity of orotate phosphoribosyltransferase and orotidine-5′-monophosphate decarboxylase. Affected individuals have megaloblastic anemia, orotic acid crystalluria, and a propensity for infection. The depletion of pyrimidine metabolites then leads to defective DNA and RNA synthesis, slowing of cell division, and megaloblastosis. Additionally, Girot et al. (13) postulated that the excessive amounts of adenosine inhibit PP-ribose-P synthetase, causing even more orotic acid accumulation and pyrimidine nucleotide depletion as well as immunocyte toxicity.

ADENOSINE DEAMINASE DEFICIENCY

Patients affected by adenosine deaminase deficiency exhibit severe lymphopenia and immunodeficiencies that can be life-threatening. Blackburn and Kellems (14) postulated that the metabolic basis of the immunodeficiency is related to the sensitivity of lymphocytes to the accumulation of deoxy ATP (dATP), inducing apoptosis and leading to cellular demise (14). Herschfield (15) proposed that adenosine interferes with nuclear factor kappa-beta (NF-k-β) activation in antigen-receptor–mediated immunosuppression is partially responsible for immunosuppression associated with adenosine deaminase deficiency (15). In adenosine deaminase deficiency, the increased dATP levels inhibit ribonucleotide reductase, blocking DNA replication, dividing cells and inducing DNA strand breaks in nondividing lymphocytes. In addition, the accumulation of dATP activates caspase 9, a protease involved in apoptosis and can lead to depletion of cellular ATP. Aberrant signal transduction mediated by adenosine acting through G-protein–associated receptors or caused by erroneous or impaired functioning of T-cell–associated adenosine deaminase complexing protein CD26 or dipeptidyl peptidase IV, also impairs lymphocyte function (3,16).

Adenosine deaminase deficiency is an autosomal recessive disorder. The gene for the disorder is located on chromosome 20 q13.1; it has 32,040 base pairs, 12 exons, and 11 introns. Human adenosine deaminase has a 40,762-d peptide composed of 363 amino acids. The gene has been sequenced and, to date, >67 mutations have been identified. A good correlation appears to exist between quantitative adenosine deaminase activity and clinical phenotype. Of these mutations, 41 are missense mutations (3).

CLINICAL MANIFESTATIONS

As illustrated above, the clinical manifestations of the inborn errors of purine and pyrimidine metabolism are widely disparate, ranging from hyperuricemia, gouty arthritis, and acute renal failure (as in gout) to prominent and disabling neurologic symptoms, such mental retardation, choreoathetosis, dystonia, compulsive self-injury (as in LNS) to anemia (as in hereditary orotic aciduria and LNS) and immunodeficiency (as in adenosine deaminase deficiency).

Adenosine deaminase deficiency typically presents by 1 month of age, with life-threatening infections (17). IgM may be detected early, but IgG deficiency manifests at about 3 months of age when maternal supply has be exhausted. Pneumonia, and skin and gastrointestinal infections secondary to variety of pathogens, including bacterial, viral, fungal, and protozoan, have been reported. Diarrhea, malnutrition, and failure to thrive ensue. Hypoplasia or absence of lymphoid tissue may provide an early clue to the diagnosis. Cupping and flaring of the costochondral junctions are seen (18). Neurologic symptoms include sensorineural hearing loss (19), nystagmus, abnormal movements, head lag, and spasticity. The exact mechanism for the occurrence of neurologic dysfunction is uncertain. Left untreated, SCID caused by adenosine deaminase deficiency can be fatal by 1 to 2 years of age because of complications of infection (3).

Delayed-onset adenosine deaminase deficiency has been described in patients presenting with a less severe form SCID after 1 year of life, but within the first decade. These individuals are often given initial diagnoses of asthma, recurrent otitis media, chronic allergy, and so on. By 2 to 3 years of age, affected patients present with serious infections requiring hospitalization.

As in the vignette, patients with SCID caused by adenosine deaminase deficiency presenting after the first decade, have been reported in the literature (20). These reports suggest that, in some cases, the degree of immunodeficiency may be compatible with longer survival times. This fact is important to note because patients with adenosine deaminase deficiency must be diagnosed as early as possible, preventing subsequent neurologic deterioration.

Abnormal humoral immunity can also manifest as autoimmune thyroid disease (21), autoimmune hemolytic anemia, or insulin-dependent diabetes mellitus (22).

Other clinical features of adenosine deaminase deficiency unrelated directly to immune function include hepatobiliary disease (23), transient renal tubular acidosis, urinary tract malformations, pelvic dysplasia, and shortening of vertebral transverse processes (24,25).

PATHOLOGY

The neuropathologic studies for LNS have included focal softening, gliosis, cerebellar cell loss, demyelinating lesions, and cerebral edema (26). Sural nerves in LNS have been mainly normal, except for a report describing loss of large myelinated fibers and lipidlike inclusions in the Schwann cells (27). Harris et al. (28) performed magnetic resonance imaging (MRI) studies of the brains of a series of patients with LNS. Volumetric measurements confirmed a 34% decrease in caudate volume, 17% decrease in total cerebral volume, and a 12% decrease in putamen volume (28). Wong et al. (29) showed a reduction of dopamine transporter binding in the caudate and putamen of patients with LNS on positron emission tomography (PET) studies (29).

In most autopsy cases of adenosine deaminase deficiency, thymic hypoplasia, with loss of corticomedullary demarcations and absent lymphocytes and Hassal bodies, have been described (3). Monforte-Munoz et al. (30) described an 8-year-old girl with adenosine deaminase deficiency in which Epstein-Barre virus (EBV) was detectable in leiomyomas involving the gallbladder, liver, spleen, pancreas, lung, and intestinal tract. Mice with adenosine deaminase deficiency have also been reported to have smaller spleens, with poorly formed germinal centers, impaired B-cell development, and increased B-cell receptor-mediated apoptosis (31).

DIAGNOSIS

Uric acid elevation is the only biochemical alteration specific to a disorder of purine metabolism. This is not true for disorders of pyrimidine metabolism. Because some patients, particularly children, have a high clearance rate of uric acid, 24-hour urinary concentrations of uric acid are more reliable than a single sample. The specimen should be collected early in the morning; it should be frozen and sent on dry ice to prevent bacterial growth, which can spuriously lower the levels of purines and pyrimidines in the sample. Before collection of the sample, patients are asked to stop the intake of methylxanthines, such as coffee, tea, chocolate, and so on. A urinary tract infection must also be excluded before the test.

Most defects of the metabolism of purines and pyrimidines can be detected by high-performance liquid chromatography (HPLC) with ultraviolet light detection. Certain marker metabolites are increased in different diseases. For instance, xanthine is elevated in *xanthine oxidoreductase* deficiency and *molybdenum cofactor* or *sulfite oxidase* deficiency or uracil and thymine in *dihydropyrimidine dehydrogenase* and *dihydropyrimidase* deficiency. Adenosine and 2-deoxyadenosine are increased in *adenosine deaminase* deficiency, whereas succinlyamideimidazole carboxide ribonucleoside (SAICAR) is the marker metabolite of *adenylsuccinate lyase* (ASL) deficiency (3,32). The diagnosis of myoadenylate deficiency partly rests on the lack of increase of ammonia levels during the forearm ischemic test (6).

The diagnosis of adenosine deaminase deficiency is based on low or nonexistent adenosine deaminase levels in hemolysates using either spectrophotometric assays or radiochemical methods, such as HPLC or paper chromatography separation techniques. Prenatal diagnosis is performed by direct enzyme assay of chorionic villi or second trimester assay of adenosine deaminase activity in cultured amniotic cells (33). Cultured cells are preferable to noncultured cells (34).

In 2002, Frycak et al. (35) suggested that atmospheric pressure ionization mass spectrometry of purine and pyrimidine markers of inherited metabolic disease can be used in the diagnosis of adenosine deaminase deficiency. Subsequently, Carlucci et al. (36) have developed a capillary electrophoresis method for measuring deoxyadenosine metabolites, and activity of adenosine deaminase, S-adenosyl-L-homocysteine hydrolase, and purine nucleoside phosphorylase.

In general, obligate heterozygotes are difficult to diagnose using erythrocytes, cultured skin fibroblasts, cultured amniocytes, and chorionic villus fibroblasts because of an overlap between about 10% of normal individuals and some obligate heterozygotes. In previously studied families with a known genotype, DNA analysis had been used to confirm heterozygosity and prenatal diagnosis of adenosine deaminase deficiency (37).

TREATMENT

Hyperuricemia is treated with allopurinol, a xanthine oxidase inhibitor blocking conversion of hypoxanthine to less soluble xanthine, and a low-purine diet. Myoadenylate deficiency has been treated with oral ribose and xylitol (38,39). Hereditary orotic aciduria is effectively treated in most cases with uridine (40). In adenosine deaminase deficiency, while supportive care is provided in terms of treatment of specific infections, avoidance of live viral vaccines and irradiated blood products, and prophylaxis for *Pneumocystis carinii*, herpes virus, and fungal organisms are useful. The mainstays of therapy are (*a*) histocompatible HLA antigen-identical bone marrow transplantation; (*b*) pegylated adenosine deaminase (PEG-ADA) enzyme replacement therapy; and (*c*) somatic gene cell therapy. Treatment choice should be individualized because each of the three has its own limitations.

Marrow from HLA antigen-identical siblings is considered the best choice, but successful transplants have been reported using marrow from HLA antigen-haploidentical parents, and HLA antigen-matched unrelated donors. Nonetheless, haploidentical transplants have higher failure rates in adenosine deaminase deficiency than in other types of SCID. On the other hand, 102 of 131 patients with SCID who have had bone marrow transplantation at Duke University Medical Center survived after the transplant, some up to 12 years. Of HLA antigen-identical bone marrow transplants, 100% (15 of 15) survived and 75% of HLA antigen-haploidentical bone marrow also survived. Survival appeared unrelated to the underlying genotype (41).

Many reacquired T-cell functions, but only 30% to 40% of cases of SCID treated in children achieved reconstitution of B-cell functions.

Withholding myeloablative or immunosuppressive therapy or graft-versus-host prophylaxis, in some cases, may result in reconstitution of B- and T-cell functions and full hematopoeitic engraftment with reduced toxicity (42,43).

Enzyme replacement therapy with PEG-ADA is another treatment choice for adenosine deaminase deficiency. Patients are given biweekly or weekly intramuscular transfusions of long-circulating adenosine deaminase, normalizing dATP in blood cells. Within weeks, lymphocyte counts and immune functions return. PEG-ADA appears to be effective in many patients and failures are related to the severity of genotype associated with the disruption of the enzyme's active site (44).

PEG-ADA is a purified bovine ADA, modified by covalent attachment of the inert polymer monomethoxypolyethylene glycol. B-cells increase during the first month and T-cells follow suit in the next 6 to 12 weeks. While effective, continued treatment with PEG-ADA is needed to maintain immune function and therapy can be expensive. On the other hand, toxicity is less compared with bone marrow transplantation.

The morbidity and mortality of bone marrow transplantation and the cost of PEG-ADA treatment have led to the clinical trials using retroviral-mediated gene transfer of the normal ADA gene into autologous peripheral blood lymphocytes or human stem cells (45,46).

Auti (47) has designed a protocol of stem cell gene therapy, coupled with low-intensity myeloablation in the absence of PEG-ADA, to confer selective pressure to gene-corrected cells. He proved that, in the absence of systemic detoxification with PEG-ADA, gene-corrected lymphocytes gained selective advantage over untransduced cells. Additionally, both the immune and metabolic defects of adenosine deaminase deficiency appear to be corrected.

CLINICAL RECOMMENDATIONS OF THE VIGNETTE

The patient presented with a history of failure to thrive in early childhood and chronic infections and now has a serious life-threatening infection, AIDS. If other predisposing factors, such as intravenous drugs use, transfusion of tainted blood, and unprotected sex, could be excluded, workup should consider other factors, such as a congenital immunodeficiency syndrome, among which is SCID secondary to adenosine deaminase deficiency. ADA deficiency SCID is suggested by severe T-cell deficiency, poor mitogenic and antigenic responses, and by low or absent adenosine deaminase activity on hemolysates using spectrophotometric analysis. Supportive management should include treatment of intercurrent infections and prophylaxis against *P. carinii* and the avoidance of live vaccines and nonirradiated blood products. Given the fact that the patient has already developed significant neurologic and metabolic sequelae, the definitive management by either allogeneic bone marrow transplantation or PEG-ADA enzyme replacement has to be carefully considered.

SUMMARY

Adenosine deaminase deficiency should be considered in the differential diagnosis of immunodeficiency in both adults and children. The diagnosis is established by spectrophotometric or radiochemical assay of enzyme activity in hemolysates. Early diagnosis is crucial to prevent the onset of life-threatening infections and to obviate the neurologic and metabolic sequelae of the disease. Prenatal diagnosis can be made by enzyme assays of cultured fibroblasts or chorionic villus sampling.

The definitive treatment of choice is bone marrow or stem cell transplantation from an HLA antigen-identical sibling donor. If this is not possible, an unrelated HLA antigen-identical or a haploidentical donor may be used instead. Alternatively, PEG-ADA enzyme replacement therapy can be considered. Somatic gene therapy can also be a useful alternative in the future.

REFERENCES

1. Purines and pyrimidines: Approach to diseases of nucleotide metabolism. In: Hoffman GF, Nyhan WL, Zschocke J, et al., eds. *Selected Groups of Metabolic Diseases. Core Handbooks in Pediatrics: Inherited Metabolic Diseases.* Philadelphia: Lippincott Williams & Wilkins; 2002:334–343.
2. Becker MA. Hyperuricemia and gout. In: Scriver CR, Beaudet AL, Sly WS, et al., eds. *The Metabolic and Molecular Bases of Inherited Disease,* 8th ed. New York: McGraw-Hill; 2001:2513–2536.
3. Giblett ER, Anderson JE, Cohen F, et al. Adenosine deaminase deficiency in two patients with severely impaired cellular immunity. *Lancet.* 1972:18;2(7786);1067–1069.
4. Giblett ER, Amman AJ, Wara DW, et al. Nucleoside-phosphorylase deficiency in a child with severely defective T-cell immunity and normal B-cell immunity. *Lancet.* 1:1010,1975.
5. Sahota AS, Tischfield JA, Kamatani N, et al. Adenine phosphoribosyltransferase deficiency and 2,8-dihydroxyadenine lithiasis. In: Scriver CR, Beaudet AL, Sly WS, et al., eds. *The Metabolic and Molecular Bases of Inherited Disease,* 8th ed. New York: McGraw-Hill; 2001:2571–2584.
6. Sabina RL, Holmes EW. Myoadenylate deaminase deficiency. In: Scriver CR, Beaudet AL, Sly WS, et al., eds. *The Metabolic and Molecular Bases of Inherited Disease,* 8th ed. New York: McGraw-Hill; 2001:2627–2638.
7. Alepa FP, Howell RR, Klinsberg JR, et al. Relationship between glycogen storage disease and tophaceous gout. *Am J Med.* 1967;42:58–66.
8. Calabrese G, Simmonds HA, Cameron JS, et al. Precocious familial gout with reduced fractional urate clearance and normal purine enzymes. *QJ Med.* 1990;75:441–450.
9. Neychev VK, Mitev VI. The biochemical basis of the neurobehavioral abnormalities in the Lesch-Nyhan syndrome: A hypothesis. *Med Hypothesis* 2004;63:131–134.
10. Deustsch SL, Long KD, Rosse RB, et al. Hypothesized deficiency of guanine-based purines may contribute to the abnormalities of neurodevelopment, neuromodulation, and neurotransmission in Lesch-Nyhan syndrome. *Clin Neuropharmacol.* 2005;28:28–37.
11. Jinnah HA, Harris JC, Nyhan WL, et al. The spectrum of mutations causing hypoxanthine guanine phosphoribosyl transferase deficiency: An update. *Nucleosides Nucleotides Nucleic Acids.* 2004;23:1153–1154.
12. Shows TB, Brown JA. Localization of genes coding for PGK, HPRT, and G6PD on the long arm of the X chromosome in somatic cell hybrids. *Birth Defects.* 1975;11(3):256–259.
13. Girot R, Hanel M, Perignon JL, et al. Cellular immune deficiency in two siblings with hereditary orotic aciduria. *N Engl J Med.* 1983;308:700–704.
14. Blackburn MR, Kellems RE. Adenosine deaminase deficiency: Metabolic basis of immune deficiency and pulmonary inflammation. *Immunology.* 2005;86:1–41.
15. Herschfield MS. New insights into adenosine-receptor mediated immunosuppression and the role of adenosine in causing the immunodeficiency associated with adenosine deaminase. *Eur J Immunol.* 2005;35(10):31–41.
16. Aldrich MB, Blackburn MR, Datta SK, et al. Adenosine-deaminase deficient mice: Models for the study of lymphocyte development and adenosine signaling. *Adv Exp Med Biol.* 2000;486–493.
17. Ozdemir O. Severe combined immune deficiency in an adenosine deaminase-deficient patient. *Allergy Asthma Proc.* 2006;27(2):172–174.
18. Wolfson JJ, Cross VF. The radiographic findings in 49 patients with combined immunodeficiency. In: Pollara B, Pickering RJ, Meuwissen HJ, et al., eds. *Combined Immnunodeficiency Disease and Adenosine Deaminase Deficiency: A Molecular Defect.* New York: Academic; 1975:225.
19. Tanaka C, Hara T, Suzuki I, et al. Sensorineural deafness in siblings with adenosine deaminase deficiency. *Brain Dev.*1996;18:304.
20. Ozsabin H, Arredondo-Vega FX, Santisteban I, et al. Adenosine deaminase deficiency in adults. *Blood.* 1997:15;89(8):2849–2855.
21. Geffner ME, Steihm E, Stephure D, et al. Probable autoimmune thyroid disease and combined immunodeficiency disease. *Am J Dis Child.* 1986;140:1194.
22. Notarangelo L, Stoppoloni G, Toraldo R, et al. Insulin-dependent diabetes mellitus and severe atopic dermatitis in a child with adenosine deaminase deficiency. *Eur J Pediatr.* 1992;151(11):811–814.
23. Bollinger ME, Arredondo-Vega FX, Santisteban I, et al. Brief report: Hepatic dysfunction as a complication of adenosine deaminase deficiency. *N Engl J Med.* 1996;334;1367–1371.
24. Hirschhorn R. Clinical delineation of adenosine deaminase deficiency. In: Elliott K, Whelan J, eds. *Enzyme Defects and Immune Dysfunction.* Ciba Foundation symposium 68. New York: Excerpta Medica; 1978:35–54.
25. Buckley RH, Schiff RI, Schiff SE, et al. Human severe combined immunodeficiency: Genetic, phenotypic, and functional diversity in one hundred eight infants. *J Pediatr.* 1997;130:378.
26. Jinnah HA, Friedman T. Lesch-Nyhan disease and its variants. In: Scriver CR, Beaudet AL, Sly WS, et al., eds. *The Metabolic and Molecular Bases of Inherited Disease,* 8th ed. New York: McGraw-Hill; 2001:2537–2570.
27. Origuchi Y, Miyoshino S, Mishima K, et al. Quantitative histologic study of the sural nerve in Lesch-Nyhan syndrome. *Pediatr Neurol.* 1990; 6(5):353–355.
28. Harris JC, Lee RR, Jinnah HA, et al. Craniocerebral magnetic resonance imaging measurement and findings in Lesch-Nyhan syndrome. *Arch Neurol.* 1998;55(4):547–553.
29. Wong DF, Harris JC, Naidu S, et al. Dopamine transported are markedly reduced in Lesch-Nyhan syndrome in vivo. *Proc Natl Acad Sci U S A.* 1996;93(11):5539–5543.
30. Monforte-Munoz H, Kapoor N, Saavedra JA. Epstein-Barr virus-associated with severe combined immunodeficiency: Case report and review of the literature. *Pediatr Dev Pathol.* 2003;6(5):449–457.
31. Aldrich MB, Chen W, Blackburn MR, et al. Impaired germinal center maturation in adenosine deaminase deficiency. *J Immunol.* 2003;171(10):5562–5570.
32. Van den Berghe G, Jaeken J. Adenylsuccinate lyase deficiency. In: Scriver CR, Beaudet AL, Sly WS, et al., eds. *The Metabolic and Molecular Bases of Inherited Disease,* 8th ed. New York: McGraw-Hill; 2001:2653–2662.
33. Linch DC, Levinsky RJ, Rodeck CH, et al. Prenatal diagnosis of three cases of severe combined immunodeficiency: Severe T cell deficiency during the first half of gestation in fetuses with adenosine deaminase deficiency. *Clin Exp Immunol.* 1984;56(2):223–232.
34. Dooley T, Fairbanks LD, Simmonds HA, et al. First trimester diagnosis of adenosine deaminase deficiency. *Prenat Diagn.* 1987;7:561.
35. Frycak P, Huskova R, Adam T, et al. Atmospheric pressure ionization mass spectrometry of purine and pyrimidine markers of inherited metabolic disorders. *J Mass Spectrom.* 2002;37(12):1242–1248.
36. Carlucci F, Tabucchi A, Auiti A, et al. Capillary electrophoresis in diagnosis and monitoring of adenosine deaminase deficiency. *Clin Chem.* 2003;49(11):1830–1838.
37. Hirshhorn R. Adenosine deaminase deficiency. *Immunodeficiency Reviews.* 1990;2(3);175–198.
38. Patten BM. Beneficial effect of D-ribose in a patient with myoadenylate deficiency. *Lancet.* 1982;1;1071.
39. Brevyland M, Ebinger G. Beneficial treatment with xylitol in a patient with myoadenylate deaminase. *Clin Neuropharmacol.* 1994;17:492–493.
40. Alvarado CS, Livingstone LR, Jones ME, et al. Uridine-responsive hypogammaglobulinemia and congenital heart disease in patient with hereditary orotic aciduria. *J Pediatr.* 1988;113(5):867–871.
41. Buckley RH, Schiff RI, Schiff SE, et al. Human severe combined immunodeficiency: Genetic, phenotypic, and functional diversity in one hundred eight infants. *J Pediatr.* 1997;130:378.
42. Rubocki RJ, Parsa JR, Herschfield MS, et al. Full hematopoietic engraftment after allogeneic bone marrow transplantation without cytoreduction in a child with severe combined immunodeficiency. *Blood.* 2001;97(3):809–811.
43. Amrolia P, Gaspar HB, Hassan A, et al. Nonmyeloablative stem cell transplantation for congenital immunodeficiencies. *Blood.* 2000;96(4):1239–1246.
44. Herschfield MS. PEG-ADA replacement therapy for adenosine deaminase deficiency: An update after 8.5 years. *Clin Immunol Immunopathol.* 1995;76(3 Pt 2):S228–S232.
45. Muul LM, Ushong LM, Soenen SL, et al. Persistence and expression of the adenosine deaminase gene for 12 years and immune reaction to gene transfer components: Long-term results of the first clinical gene therapy trial. *Blood.* 2003;101(7);2563–2569.
46. Blaese RM. Development of gene therapy for immunodeficiency: Adenosine deaminase deficiency. *Pediatr Res.* 1993;[1 Suppl]:S49–S53; discussion S53–S55.
47. Auti A. Gene therapy for adenosine deaminase deficiency severe combined immunodeficiency. Best practice and research. *Clin Hematol.* 2004;17(3):505–516.

CHAPTER **65**

Disorders of Porphyrins

Arun A. Kalra • Roger E. Kelley

OBJECTIVES

- To define the porphyrias and become aware of their biosynthetic pathway
- To describe how to diagnose and treat diseases caused by abnormal porphyrin metabolism
- To discuss the newer therapeutic directions that involve porphyrins

CASE VIGNETTE

A 20-year-old young man is brought to the emergency room (ER) after he was found unconscious in his apartment. He has been complaining of abdominal pain during the last week. He denies a history of illicit ingestion, drinking alcohol, headaches, seizurelike activity, lightheadedness, or syncope. Family history is remarkable for a psychiatric disorder affecting several members of his father's family. In the ER, he appears to have postictal automatisms, with lip-smacking and other facial movements. During the examination, he has a generalized tonic seizure. After drawing blood for glucose, electrolytes, drug screen, and alcohol level, he received lorazepam. He then is given glucose, thiamine, and fosphenytoin intravenously. Examination shows stable vital signs, with no fever, normal funduscopic examination, no neck stiffness, postictal somnolence, but no focal neurologic deficit. On becoming more aware of his surroundings, he becomes agitated with threatening gestures, experiences apparent visual and auditory hallucinations, and proceeds to pull out his indwelling urinary catheter causing a bladder tear.

DEFINITION

Porphyrins, which are intermediate products in the heme biosynthetic pathway, are cyclic tetrapyrroles such as heme. Heme is the ferrous iron complex of protoporphyrin IX. It serves as a component of many of the so-called *hemoproteins,* which include hemoglobin and mitochondrial cytochromes. All of the intermediates in this pathway, except protoporphyrin IX, the last product, are called *porphyrinogens.* On contact with air, they are rapidly oxidized to porphyrins. The presence of carboxylic acid side chains determines the extent of their water solubility (1,2). This pathway is shown in Figure 65-1. The kidneys excrete uroporphyrin, reflective of its solubility, whereas protoporphyrin, the least soluble, is excreted via stool. All porphyrins emit an intense red fluorescence when exposed to light around 400 nm wavelength, whereas porphyrinogens do not fluoresce. This provides a sensitive way to detect porphyrins. Defects in the heme pathway lead to diseases called *porphyrias* and, depending on the nature and extent of the defect, they have variability in terms of manifestations.

EPIDEMIOLOGY

Porphyrias are present worldwide, although less prevalent in the United States overall. In psychiatric populations, reflective of potential psychotropic effects, the prevalence tends to be higher. They are seen more often in women than in men, and are very rare in children (1). The worldwide prevalence of all porphyrias varies between 0.5 and 10 per 100,000 persons, depending on locale (3).

There are seven porphyrias, with either a dominant or recessive inheritance pattern, and each of the acute disorders has many potential mutations. They are classified as *hepatic* or *erythropoietic,* based on the site of production of the major porphyrins (1–5). Five belong in the hepatic group: Acute intermittent porphyria (AIP), variegate porphyria (VP), hereditary coproporphyria (HC), and delta-aminolevulinate dehydratase deficiency (ALAD), also known as doss porphyria, and porphyria cutanea tarda. The erythropoietic group has two types: Congenital erythropoietic porphyria and erythropoietic protoporphyria, both of which have a nonacute onset (Fig. 65-2).

ETIOLOGY AND PATHOGENESIS

The precursors glycine and succinyl coenzyme A are converted by the enzyme aminolevulinic acid (ALA) synthetase into ALA. This is the rate-limiting step of heme synthesis. The end-product, heme, promotes feedback regulation via this conversion reaction. Two moles of ALA combine to form porphobilinogen (PBG). The hallmark of all these conditions is an increase in the production of the porphyrin precursors ALA and PBG, generally in the liver, secondary to induction of heme biosynthesis. The other porphyrins, such as uroporphyrin and coproporphyrin, are readily excreted because these serve no physiologic function. They do, however, produce the fluorescence of excreted byproducts of the heme biosynthetic pathway. The excessive

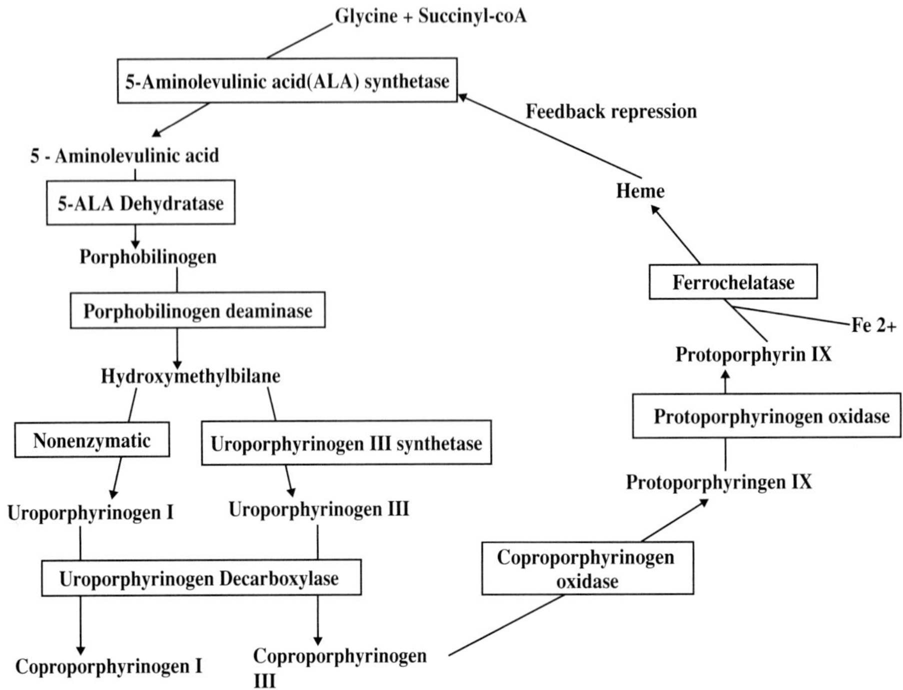

FIGURE 65-1. Pathways of heme biosynthesis.

circulating porphyrins are neurotoxic. The central nervous system (CNS) is somewhat protected, because of the blood–brain barrier, whereas the peripheral and autonomic nervous systems are vulnerable because they lack similar protection (3). The hypothalamus and limbic system tend to be the most susceptible areas of the brain. Vascular injury leads to increased permeability, which can present as reversible cerebral edema. The most common presenting symptom of most porphyrins is abdominal pain and this is thought to be caused by autonomic neuropathy (2). The exact mechanism by which these increased porphyrins are neurotoxic is still not clarified, although overproduction of circulating porphyrins appears to be the primary culprit. Potential mechanisms of this pathogenic process include the following:

1. Direct toxicity of the accumulation of ALA or PBG is believed to be an integral aspect of the neurotoxicity. The following hypothesis has been put forth (2,6):

   Interacting with γ-aminobutyric acid (GABA) receptors at high concentrations can inhibit uptake of GABA and glutamate in rat cortex, and at low concentrations, it shows agonistic activity at presynaptic GABA receptors, by inhibiting the release of GABA from nerve endings. Such accumulation has been postulated to generate free radicals, which can be involved in lipid peroxidation, resulting in tissue damage.

   Other factors that could come into play: Affect on motor nerve conduction, alteration of acetylcholine release or Na^+/K^+ adenosine triphosphatase (ATPase) activity, or interference with other aspects of neuronal function. ALA, however, is excreted in high levels in patients even when they are asymptomatic.
2. Interaction through altered heme levels via tryptophan: Decreased heme also causes reduction in important heme-related enzymes, such as tryptophan deoxygenase in the liver; this raises the tryptophan levels which, in the brain, leads to potential excess production of the neurotransmitter serotonin, which can give rise to psychiatric manifestations and peripheral nerve dysfunction (2,6).

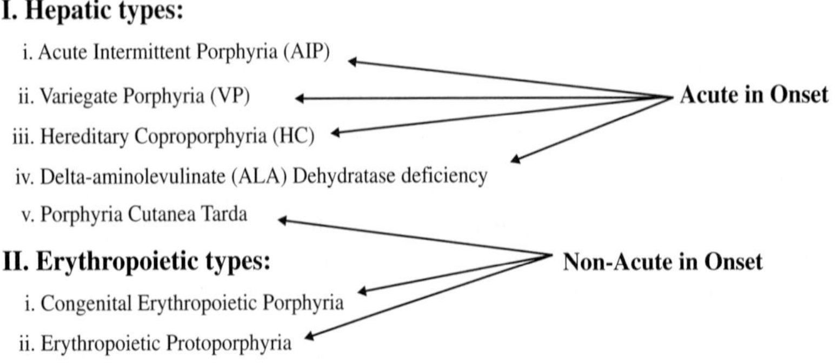

FIGURE 65-2. Porphyrias.

TABLE 65-1. Deficient Enzymes and Their Inheritance

Disease	*Deficient Enzyme*	*Inheritance*
ALA dehydratase deficiency porphyria	ALA dehydratase	AR
Acute intermittent porphyria	Porphobilinogen (PBG) deaminase	AD
Congenital erythropoietic porphyria	Uroporphyrinogen III cosynthetase	AR
Porphyria cutánea tarda	Uroporphyrinogen decarboxylase	AD or acquired
Hereditary coproporphyria	Coproporphyrinogen oxidase	AD
Variegate porphyria	Protoporphyrinogen oxidase	AD
Erythropoietic protoporphyria	Ferrochetalase	AD

AD, autosomal dominant; AR, autosomal recessive.

Also, via the cytochrome P-450 system: Involvement of this system can lead mitochondrial cytochrome levels to be reduced, because of heme deficiency and impaired adenosine triphosphate (ATP) production, resulting in neuronal impairment (7).

3. In the cutaneous forms, porphyrins are activated by long wave ultraviolet light and can generate oxygen radicals, which leads to tissue damage.
4. Various drugs can be triggers for porphyrias. It has been also postulated that some do so by causing oxidative stress, with the CNS very sensitive to free radical production because of its low antioxidant capacity. Rodriguez et al. (8) have demonstrated induction of heme oxygenase in a mouse model in support of this possible mechanism. Some drugs increase synthesis of hepatic cytochrome P-450 utilizing large amounts of heme, which causes disinhibition of ALA synthetase-1, although the exact site of action of heme remains speculative (7). Some chemicals directly induce ALA synthetase and cytochrome P-450 (1,2,7).

Although, the porphyries are caused by inherited enzymatic defects, their phenotypic expression is reflective of the environmental milieu. Certain factors, such as drugs, hormones, changes in nutrition, and so on can precipitate the clinical condition by affecting heme metabolism. The drugs precipitate their effect by causing marked decrease in the heme in cytochrome P-450 system. This causes reduction of heme in the regulatory pool, of the liver, which stimulates ALA synthetase-1. Other chemicals, however, can induce ALA synthetase and the cytochrome P-450 without such a depletion of the heme pool. Handschin et al. (9) recently showed that the transcription of ALAS-1 is downregulated by heme and upregulated by the peroxisome proliferator-activated receptor gamma coactivator 1α (PGC-1α). Its transcription, in turn, is controlled by glucose availability, with hypoglycemia leading to increase of PGC-1α. Fasting and starvation increase the synthetase activity of ALA, probably via PGC-1α (8). Increasing the carbohydrate intake causes downregulation of ALA synthetase activity, but its exact mechanism is unknown.

In AIP, HC, and VP, the enzyme activity is usually at 50% of normal function, whereas in patients with ALAD it is only at 5% of normal. Close to 80% of the patients remain symptom-free until the instigating factor comes into play. Many have only one attack in their lifetime; very few have recurrent episodes. In patients with acute porphyrias, during the acute attack and while asymptomatic, the porphyrin precursors (ALA and PBG) show a high level, which is marked in an acute attack. Abnormal porphyrin metabolism was restored to normal in a patient with acute porphyria after liver transplant, indicating that liver has a major role in the disease (3).

The deficient enzymes and their inheritance are shown in Table 65-1 (2–5).

CLINICAL MANIFESTATIONS

All of the acute porphyrias have gastrointestinal and neurologic symptoms only, except for patients with VP and HC, who can have blistering lesions on the sun-exposed skin (1–5). AIP is the most common of the acute porphyries, but they all can be associated with dark urine. Common symptoms and signs are discussed next.

GASTROINTESTINAL

Abdominal pain, of neurologic origin, is the most common symptom. Usually it is characterized as constant pain, which can be colicky, lasting for hours. It can be differentiated from a surgical abdomen by the absence of guarding and rebound tenderness. Rarely, fever and leukocytosis may accompany it. Other gastrointestinal symptoms, such as nausea, vomiting, ileus, constipation, and diarrhea, occur less often. On rare occasions, abdominal pain and tachycardia are absent.

NEUROLOGIC

In descending order of frequency, neurologic symptoms include autonomic or peripheral motor more than sensory neuropathy, neuropsychiatric symptoms, cranial neuropathy, and seizures. Other cerebral, cerebellar, or basal ganglionic symptoms have been seen, but with less frequency. Pain, a common symptom, can involve the head, chest, back, abdomen, or extremities. The latter is indicative of sensory nerve entrapment, whereas approximately one third of patients complain of numbness. Motor weakness can be seen at the start or later in the evolution of the acute attack. Most often, it begins in the arms, in a proximal distribution, rather than distally or in the legs. Peripheral motor neuropathy tends to be asymmetric. Rarely, this can progress to paralysis of respiratory muscles. Cases have been reported of patients who resemble those with Guillain-Barré syndrome (10,11) and AIP is in the differential diagnosis of such a presentation. A clinical picture resembling the Miller-Fisher variant of Guillain-Barré syndrome may be seen or there can be more of an encephalopathy (12). Of note, the presentation may be further confounded with the presence of albumino-cytologic dissociation in cerebrospinal fluid (CSF). In the presence of electrophysiologic studies revealing axonal polyradiculopathy, predilection for proximal muscles with asymmetric weakness, abdominal pain, and psychiatry manifestations, the diagnosis tends to become more apparent. Seizures can be caused by hyponatremia, from syndrome of inappropriate secretion of anti-diuretic hormone (SIADH), direct CNS involvement or both and has an incidence of 10% to 20%.

PSYCHIATRIC

The incidence of psychiatric symptoms is approximately 50%, ranging from mild dysthymic state to severe psychosis, with agitation, confusion, and hallucinations.

CARDIOVASCULAR

The most common cardiovascular presentations are tachycardia and hypertension, with the latter seen less often. These are presumably caused by overproduction of catecholamines and autonomic neuropathy. Although generally mild, they can become severe.

HYPONATREMIA

Hyponatremia can result from hypothalamic involvement, related to SIADH, or to excess loss of sodium via the kidneys or gastrointestinal tract.

DERMATOLOGIC

Congenital erythropoietic porphyria is very rare and is associated with severe photosensitivity, bullous skin lesions on light-exposed skin, and a hemolytic anemia. Cutaneous photosensitivity is the primary manifestation of protoporphyria, which is related to a partial deficiency of ferrochelatase—the final enzyme in the heme biosynthetic pathway that converts protoporphyrin to heme.

EXACERBATING OR PRECIPITATING FACTORS

Other exacerbating or precipitating factors can include infections, ethanol, pregnancy, steroids—gonadal (exogenous or endogenous), fasting or low-calorie diet, intercurrent illness, cigarette smoking, surgery (including dental extraction), as well as a variety of drugs and the menstrual cycle.

Formulations

1. Anticonvulsants: These can be barbiturates, carbamazepine, phenytoin, ethosuximide, clonazepam (at large doses), primidone, valproic acid, diazepam (at large doses), felbamate, lamotrigine, tiagabine, oxcarbamazepine, and topiramate.
2. Antibiotics: Among those associated with porphyria are sulfonamides, rifampin, griseofulvin, chloramphenicol, erythromycin, doxycycline, chloroquine, and metronidazole.
3. Hormones: These primarily consist of oral contraceptives, progesterone, synthetic progestins, and estrogens.
4. Other medications: Furosemide, diclofenac, and other nonsteroidal anti-inflammatory drugs (NSAID), pyrazinamide, ergot compounds, cimetidine, nifedipine, imipramine, metoclopramide, methyldopa, oxycodone, captopril, or any other ACE inhibitor.

SAFE DRUGS IN PORPHYRIAS

Some drugs are listed as safe to use in patients with acute porphyrias, but caution is recommended. Any drug could be a trigger, even if it had not been so previously (2–5). As more is learned about the porphyrias and their mutations, some subtypes may not be found to tolerate some of the drugs previously felt to be safe. The safe drugs include aspirin, atropine, beta-blockers, codeine, corticosteroids, digitalis, gabapentin, gentamicin, insulin, indomethacin, morphine, penicillin, prochlorperazine, warfarin, and thyroxine. For a detailed list of safe and unsafe drugs, check the web site of the porphyrin foundations at: http://www.porphyria-europe.com or http://www.uct.ac.za/depts/porphyria (2–5).

DIAGNOSTIC APPROACH

Porphyrias are often considered as a diagnostic option late into the clinical presentation. The three primary clues for AIP are unexplained severe abdominal pain, which may have resulted in unsuccessful abdominal surgery in the past, an axonal motor neuropathy, and psychiatric manifestations. This, in association with a potential precipitating factor, should help in the identification of porphyria as a possible explanation. Because most carriers of abnormal enzymes may remain asymptomatic, a negative family history may not be useful. Conversely, a "positive" history of porphyria in the patient might not be accurate because of a relatively high percentage of false–positive findings. Therefore, the physician should try to confirm prior test results, if at all possible, unless clear clinical and laboratory findings support the diagnosis. If these are unavailable, or there is any doubt, the tests should be rerun. Generally, treatment should not be delayed for a clinical presentation compatible with porphyria.

Once porphyria is suspected, based on the above symptoms or positive family history, then PBG and ALA, which are markedly increased in urine in all acute porphyrias except ALAD (in which only ALA is increased), should be measured. An effort should be made toward confirmation because one dose of hemin therapy will lower the PBG level drastically. A number of commercial tests are now available. The test by Mauzerall-Granick and other closely related tests are the most reliable, specific, and quantitative analyses, and they test both ALA and PBG levels. Many other tests are qualitative, lack specificity, have a high rate of false–positive findings, and test for only PBG. There is a rapid semiquantitative test (Trace PBG Kit, made by Thermo Trace in Texas), which detects levels of PBG >6 mg/L and has a color chart (normal levels, 0 to 4 mg; in acute porphyries, 20 to 200 mg). Because such testing is now available, collecting 24-hour urine specimens is no longer necessary (5).

The American Porphyria Foundation recommends that all hospitals should carry the Trace PBG kits for quick check (5). Their further recommendation is to refrigerate or freeze (without additives), a single-void specimen of urine, which should be shielded from light, for later quantification of ALA, PBG, and total porphyrins. In patients with marked renal dysfunction, the serum levels, of the above, should be measured instead. If the test shows a markedly increased level of ALA only, then the likely diagnosis is ALAD. In this case, before initiating treatment, other causes of increased ALA should be ruled out, such as lead or styrene poisoning, and tyrosinemia type 1. All these products inhibit ALA dehydratase, and lead does this by displacing the cofactor zinc. If testing reveals both ALA and PBG to be increased, then further differentiation of AIP, HC, and VP is performed by testing porphyrin levels in urine, feces, and plasma. Urinary porphyrins will be increased in all three. In AIP, however, it will be mostly uroporphyrin; the increase is primarily for coproporphyrins for the other two. Fecal porphyrins will be normal to slightly increased in AIP, markedly increased in the other two, whereas protoporphyrin is increased only in VC. In addition, plasma porphyrins will be normal to slightly increased in AIP and HC, but markedly increased in VC (1–5). This differentiation is not urgent and is not important before treatment. Once the above testing is finished, proceed next to DNA and enzymatic testing, trying to find the defective gene and mutations, if any. Mutation analysis is currently performed at Mount Sinai Hospital in New York. Genetic counseling should be provided to patients and their families once the disorder is established.

In a case report of an 18-year-old patient with diffuse encephalopathy, brain magnetic resonance imaging (MRI) showed multiple contrast-enhancing subcortical white matter lesions, diffusion weighted MR was normal, and MR spectroscopy excluded tissue necrosis and demyelination (12). This is differentiated from posterior reversible encephalopathy by its intense contrast enhancement (13).

TREATMENT

Treatment for an acute attack of porphyrias is much the same for all types. Once the diagnosis is made, the very first thing that must be done is to look for possible instigating factors and attempt to eliminate them. This can be difficult because often more than one precipitating factor for the attack is identified. Generally speaking, in view of the potential consequences, physicians should err on the side of being overly cautious and eliminate any and all factors that have a reasonable possibility of being the culprit. The treatment is then divided into specific and symptomatic.

Specific treatment consists of heme, approved by the US Food and Drug Administration (FDA) 20 years ago, and which works by suppressing the hepatic enzyme ALA synthetase. This results in a decrease in both ALA and PBG through the regulatory feedback loop. One double blind, placebo-controlled study has been done on 12 patients, which found a trend toward clinical improvement in conjunction with dramatic decrease in urinary PBG. In addition to the relatively small number of patients in this trial, another drawback was the failure to mention removal of possible precipitating factors for the attack. This raises the possibility of at least some of the attacks being self-limited because of removal of the offending agent. A few open-label studies have demonstrated dramatic response, along with decreased hospital stay (2). The true efficacy, however, is subject to question because of study design (2).

Heme as heme arginate, is more stable in solution, and needs no reconstitution. It is not presently available in the United States, however. Another preparation that is available in the United States, is hemin. It is reconstituted with sterile water just prior to infusion, but is unstable because it forms degradation products very quickly in this solution. These products tend to be sticky and adhere to platelets, endothelial cells, and clotting factors, causing transient coagulation effects, anaphylactic reactions, and phlebitis or thrombophlebitis at the injection site, which can be severe. Daily infusions in this situation could be hazardous. Therefore, the Foundation suggests using albumin to reconstitute, because it increases the stability and, thus, decreases the chance of side effects. It is not uncommon to see fever and malaise associated with treatment. Two isolated reports describe circulatory collapse and acute renal failure, but both patients recovered fully. It is the experience of the expert panel, chosen by the American Porphyria Foundation, that hemin is safe during pregnancy (2–5). Biochemical effects last only for 1 week and this is generally sufficiently long to ameliorate the clinical problems. Repeated treatments with hemin can induce heme oxygenase, which reduces its effectiveness. With the addition of an inhibitor of heme oxygenase, such as tin or zinc mesoprotoporphyrin, at the time of treatment, it is possible to prolong the effective duration of heme. However, this is not yet approved (2). It is given at a dose of 3 to 4 mg/kg/day intravenously, for 3 to 5 consecutive days, in conjunction with 10% intravenous glucose. Heme has greater effectiveness than glucose, although glucose alone can be used to treat patients with very mild pain without paresis. Heme cannot be used orally because it is broken down by heme oxygenase in the gut.

Symptomatic treatment depends on the symptoms and their severity. The following treatment approaches are suggested for various symptoms: Beta-blockers for tachycardia, hypertension, and arrhythmia; chlorpromazine for nausea, vomiting, and hallucinations; diazepam or lorazepam for anxiety, insomnia, and seizures (either prolonged or status epilepticus); opiates for severe pain in the abdomen, extremities, or back; antibiotics, except sulfonamides, for infections; gabapentin for seizure control, if prolonged treatment is necessary (for seizures also correct hyponatremia, if present); intravenous fluids for vomiting or diarrhea with secondary dehydration; mechanical ventilation for respiratory muscle compromise; lactulose for constipation; aspirin or acetaminophen for mild pain or fever; fluid restriction for mild SIADH and 3% saline infusion for more severe SIADH, and 300 g of carbohydrates daily. In addition, physical therapy, occupational therapy, and speech therapy may be part of the rehabilitative process, depending on neurologic sequelae. An indwelling catheter or nasogastric tube, mobilization, and antiembolus measures may be necessary as part of supportive care. Women with cyclic symptoms, during the luteal phase of menstrual cycle, should receive oral contraceptives. In case of contraindications to the use of oral contraceptives, then leutinizing hormone or leuprolide can be beneficial. For seizure control, vigabatrin has also been shown to be safe, but is not FDA approved and is unavailable in the United States. On occasion, intravenous magnesium can be used for seizures during the acute attacks (2–5). Patients with ALAD who do not respond to treatment tend to have a poor prognosis. Only seven such cases have been reported in the literature, however (1).

PORPHYRINS IN TREATMENT

Metalloporphyrins are porphyrins with a metal attached equally to the nitrogen atom on all four pyrrole rings. They can be found in nature (e.g., chlorophyll), and can also be artificially created. The addition of the metal changes the biochemical characteristics. These agents are used in many different areas, such as contrast agents for MRI, MR spectroscopy, and so on. *In vitro* and animal model studies have demonstrated that they possess antioxidant properties, similar to superoxide dismutase and catalase, with the ability to inhibit lipid peroxidation as well as broad-spectrum scavenging capability for reactive oxygen and nitrogen-free radicals such as peroxynitrite. These properties may translate into benefit for humans with various disease processes that may benefit from free radical scavengers. Crow et al. (14) published a study in the mice model of amyotrophic lateral sclerosis (ALS) using catalytic antioxidant, manganese porphyrin (MnP). In contrast to previous such studies in ALS, they used it at symptom onset, showing increase in survival time by threefold. Motor architecture was better preserved with less gliosis than in placebo, as per immunohistochemical studies of the spinal cord. They postulate that this might be a promising agent in treatment of ALS (14).

In a rat model of spinal cord injury, MnP was demonstrated to be beneficial with the intrathecal route being superior to intravenous (15). In another rat model, iron porphyrin, administered 6 hours after middle cerebral artery ligation, showed neuroprotection and a decrease in injury induced by DNA fragmentation (16). In a rat model of Huntington disease (17), excitotoxic brain damage involves *N*-methyl-d-aspartate (NMDA) receptors and glutamate. The use of iron porphyrin, in a dose escalation study, ameliorated mitochondrial dysfunction and lipid peroxidation in a dose-dependant fashion. The DNA fragmentation was observed to be reduced within 24 hours, whereas circling behavior showed improvement within 6 days of treatment. Recent evidence in a study of newborn pigs suggests that activation of heme oxygenase (HO), at seizure onset, helps increase cerebral blood flow during ictus and maintain normal function in cerebral vessels postictus. It is theorized that seizures promote prolonged dysfunction of cerebral vessels associated with HO downregulation. In this study, newborn pigs treated 48 hours after induced seizures had tin protophyrin-HO downregulated and cobalt protophyrin (CoP)-HO upregulated compared with placebo. Decreased vascular reactivity was seen in the placebo group. The authors theorized that CoP prevented the cerebral vascular dysfunction by upregulating HO and that this finding may have implications in certain neurologic diseases (18). In addition, specially designed metalloporphyrin agents are being tested in humans for potential use in oncology. The goal is for the agents to go selectively to cancer cells to enhance their destruction in conjunction with chemo- or radiotherapy. Furthermore, such agents have photosensitizing properties because of their porphyrin nature. When retained in tumor cells and activated by light, termed *photopdynamic therapy*, singlet oxygen is produced, which can induce cancer cell death.

CLINICAL RECOMMENDATIONS OF THE VIGNETTE

The patient's history of unexplained abdominal pain, along with the history of an apparent familial psychiatric disorder might well have raised suspicion of acute intermittent porphyria. Such a presentation warrants careful evaluation of what might be predisposing this patient to seize on a metabolic basis, assuming that his brain imaging reveals no structural lesion and his cerebrospinal fluid examination demonstrates no evidence of an infectious process. The possibility of alcohol-related seizure exists as well as the possibility of illicit drug ingestion or of a prescribed medication that has the potential to lower the seizure threshold. He might also be predisposed by sleep deprivation and must be evaluated for possible recent head trauma as an inciting factor. In retrospect, the agitated state associated with the administration of the anticonvulsant phenytoin is suggestive of AIP. If this is the case, the phenytoin needs to be stopped and replaced with an agent that does not have the potential to aggravate or promote the metabolic disorder. In the interim, a single-void urine specimen should be obtained for the Trace PBG test and, if positive, treatment with hemin started.

SUMMARY

Porphyrins are widely distributed in the body. Elevated accumulation, through metabolic inborn errors in the heme synthesis, can lead to an array of clinical manifestations, including severe neurologic impairment. AIP should be considered in the differential diagnosis of a patient presenting with a motor neuropathy, unexplained severe abdominal pain, a psychiatric disorder that is not readily classified, especially with a familial predisposition, and the potential identification of a characteristic precipitating factor for such an attack. Initiation of treatment, along with removal of the offending agent, can make a substantial difference in outcome. Metalloporphyrins are porphyrins with a central metal attachment. They have antioxidant properties and experimental evidence suggests they hold promise for use in a variety of CNS disorders, as well as in oncology.

REFERENCES

1. Anderson K, Sassa S, Bishop D, et al. *The Metabolic and Molecular Bases of Inherited Disease.* New York: McGraw-Hill; 2001.
2. Chemmanur AT, Bonkovsky HL. Hepatic porphyrias: Diagnosis and treatment. *Clin Liver Dis.* 2004;8:807–838.
3. Kauppinen R. Porphyrias. *Lancet.* 2005;365:241–252.
4. Dombeck TA, Satonik RC. The porphyrias. *Emerg Med Clin N Am.* 2005;23:885–899.
5. Anderson K, Bloomer J, Bonkovky H, et al. Recommendations for the diagnosis and treatment of the acute porphyrias. *Ann Intern Med.* 2005;142:439–450.
6. Winkler AS, Peters TJ, Elwes RDC. Neuropsychiatric porphyria in patients with refractory epilepsy: Report of three cases. *J Neural Neurosurg Psychiatry.* 2005;76:380–383.
7. Herrick AL, McColl KEL. Acute intermittent porphyria. *Best Pract Res Clin Gastroenterol.* 2005;19(2):235–249.
8. Rodríguez JA, Martinez MC, Gerez EB, et al. Heme oxygenase, aminolevulinate acid synthetase and the antioxidant system in the brain of mice treated with porphyrinogenic drugs. *Cell Mol Biol (Noisy-le-grand).* 2005;51(5):487–494.
9. Handschin C, Lin J, Rhee J, et al. Nutritional regulation of hepatic heme biosynthesis and porphyria through PGC-1alpha. *Cell.* 2005;122:505–515.
10. Phillips JD, Kushner JP. Fast track to the porphyrias. *Nat Med.* 2005;11(10):1049–1050.
11. Keung Y, Chuahirun T. Acute intermittent porphyria with seizure and paralysis in the puerperium. *J Am Board Fam Pract.* 2000;13(1):76–79.
12. Periasamy V, Shubaili A, Girsh Y. Diagnostic dilemmas in acute intermittent porphyria. A case report. *Medical Principles and Practice.* 2002;11(2):108–111.
13. Maramattom B, Zaldivar R, Glynn S, et al. Acute intermittent porphyria presenting as a diffuse encephalopathy. *Ann Neurol.* 2005;57(4):581–584.

14. Crow JP, Caligasan NY, Chen J, et al. Manganese porphyrin given at symptom onset markedly extends survival if ALS mice. *Ann Neurol.* 2005;58(2):258–265.
15. Sheng H, Spasojevic I, Warner DS, et al. Mouse spinal cord compression injury is ameliorated by intrathecal cationic manganese (III) porphyrin catalytic antioxidant therapy. *Neurosci Lett.* 2004;366(2):220–225.
16. Thiyagarajan M, Kaul CL, Sharma SS. Neuroprotective efficacy and therapeutic time window of peroxynitrite decomposition catalysts in focal cerebral ischemia. *Br J Pharmacol.* 2004;142(5):899–911.
17. Pérez-De La Cruz V, González-Cortés C, Galván-Arzate, et al. Excitotoxic brain damage involves early peroxynitrite formation in a model of Huntington's disease in rats: Protective role of iron porphyrinate 5,10,15,20-tetrakis (4-sulfonatophenyl)porphyrinate iron (III). *Neuroscience.* 2005;135(2):463–474.
18. Parfenova H, Carratu P, Tcheranova D, et al. Epileptic seizures cause extended postictal cerebral vascular dysfunction that is prevented by HO-1 overexpression. *Am J Physiol Heart Circ Physiol.* 2005;288(6):H2843–H2850.

CHAPTER 66

Disorders of Heavy Metals

Roger E. Kelley • Jonathan Glass

OBJECTIVES

- To explain the importance of heavy metals on central and peripheral nervous system metabolic function
- To describe the array of various neurodegenerative processes associated with heavy metals
- To provide insight into potential assessments of heavy metal-mediated disturbance in neurologic disease
- To explain how the pathophysiology of heavy metal-mediation of neurologic disease can lead to more effective therapeutic approaches to heavy metal poisoning

CASE VIGNETTE

A 68-year-old reclusive man has lived alone near a contaminated pond for a number of years. He is seen only on occasion, but is observed to fish in the pond. He has avoided people for years, but literally crawls to his neighbor because he is increasingly unable to ambulate well. For several months, he has had progressive gastrointestinal pain and symptoms of stomatitis. His neighbor notes that he is dysarthric with tremulousness. In addition, he is quite weak and unsteady on his feet. He is brought to the local hospital where he is admitted onto the neurology service. The admitting neurology resident notes muscle atrophy, fasciculations along with hyperreflexia and bilateral Babinski signs, and prepares to present him to neurology grand rounds as a newly diagnosed case of amyotrophic lateral sclerosis (ALS). The neurology program director notes the patient's anxiety and psychotic features, along with a fine tremor of the hands and head. He recommends 24-hour urine for heavy metal screening and the pathology department calls immediately when testing reveals a markedly elevated excretion of mercury in the urine.

DEFINITION

Heavy metals include mercury, lead, zinc, arsenic, bismuth, thallium, and manganese. Toxic exposure can result in various disruptions of central or peripheral nervous system function. The degree of neurologic effect is generally reflective of the level and duration of exposure. It is important to recognize that metals are vital for biochemical function in the body (1). For example, the alkali metal ions K^+ and Na^+ are crucial in the depolarization and repolarization process associated with neural transmission. Calcium ion fluxes are part of signal transduction within cells, including those of the nervous system. Zinc (Zn) appears to play a role in central nervous system (CNS) function, perhaps serving as an inhibitory neuromodulator of glutamate release. Redox metal ions include copper (Cu), iron (Fe), and manganese (Mn). These metals are components of metalloenzymes, which are key components of metabolic pathways within nervous system tissue. Although not usually included as a heavy metal, Fe deposition has been implicated in the pathogenesis of both Alzheimer and Parkinson diseases (2). The Fe enzyme tyrosine hydroxylase mediates the formation of dopamine from tyrosine. The copper enzyme dopamine β-hydroxylase transforms dopamine to norepinephrine. Involved in neuroprotection is the Cu/Zn superoxide dismutase located within the cytosol. Also involved in neuroprotection is Mn superoxide dismutase located within the mitochondria. Mn is an important component of this mitochondrial enzyme.

EPIDEMIOLOGY

The frequency of heavy metal intoxication reflects societal patterns and industrialization (2). Careful attention to limiting exposure and effective removal of pesticides and industrial wastes protects against mercury exposure. Potential occupational hazards still exist, however, including exposure during the manufacture of thermometers, vacuum pumps, incandescent lamps, mirrors, and x-ray machines, as well as the potential for exposure to toxic fumes in the manufacturing process of pulp and paper and also electrochemicals. Firefighters who have chronic exposure to mercury-containing vapors as part of the fire extinguishing process have been reported to be susceptible to polyneuropathy. From a historical perspective, hatmakers who were exposed to mercury in the processing of felt for men's hats, in the 19th and early 20th centuries, had the potential to develop psychosis. Such exposure was the basis of the "Mad Hatter" in Lewis Carroll's classic novel *Alice in Wonderland.*

Increasing concerns exist about the mercury content in certain fish and this can lead to epidemics of mercury poisoning in susceptible regions. The best recognized was so-called *Minamata disease,* which was an affliction of Japanese villagers in the 1950s. This was attributed to ingestion of fish with high concentrations of methyl mercury. Concern continues about chronic mercury exposure in dental amalgam, which is quite ubiquitous. In addition, there has been conjecture about thimerosal-containing immunoglobulin shots, used as vaccines, having the potential to produce neurotoxicity in susceptible children because of genetic polymorphism.

Lead poisoning has been a major issue for children who ingest lead-based paints. This can lead to severe manifestations and is preventable by the removal of lead-based paints in living quarters and other areas where children or mentally challenged individuals might be exposed to such paint products. It has been estimated that up to 3 to 4 million children in the United States, up through the 1980s, had potentially toxic levels of lead using a serum threshold of 10 to 15 $\mu g/dL$. Toxic levels in adults can be seen with industrial manufacturing exposure such as that associated with dusts from inorganic lead salts as well as toxic fumes from lead smelting, storage battery manufacture, pottery glazing, painting, mining, printing, and work in certain foundries. Bismuth salts are part of formulations to treat gastrointestinal disorders. Excessive intake of such formulations can lead to bismuth intoxications.

Arsenic exposure, historically, has been a surreptitious means of murder. Forms of arsenic were part of the treatment for syphilis in the preantibiotic era. This led to inadvertent poisoning in years past. In addition, arsenic is found in various pesticides, herbicides, and rodenticides. It is also used in various manufacturing processes, exposure to which has the potential to promote signs and symptoms. Accidental ingestion can result in toxic manifestations.

Manganese toxicity, traditionally, has been described in manganese miners who do not have proper ventilation within the mines. This can lead to a neurologic disorder resembling Parkinson disease. Recently some concern has been raised about the potential for welders to be exposed to manganese-containing vapors to a degree that can result in involvement of the CNS (3). The initial report of this possible association has generated considerable controversy, however, and most epidemiologic data, to date, has not supported welding as a significant occupational risk for manganese-induced parkinsonism.

Thallium poisoning is now sporadic and can be seen with accidental ingestion of thallium-containing poisons used to kill rodents. It is also possible to see toxicity from excessive exposure to depilatory agents. Before the antibiotic era, thallium was a component of various formulations used to treat venereal disease, tuberculosis, and ringworm. Excessive ingestion, with secondary toxicity, was not uncommon. Thallium toxicity is now considered rare, however.

PATHOGENESIS

Excessive lead (Pb) exposure can interfere with neurotransmitter release (1). For example, synaptotagmins are a family of Ca^{2+}-binding proteins located on the membranes of synaptic vesicles. Synaptotagmins are involved in neurotransmitter release. One possible mechanism of Pb toxicity is the greater affinity of Pb^{2+} for the synaptotagmin than for Ca^{2+}. Lead has an adverse effect on multiple proteins, primarily by binding to the Ca^{2+} binding structures, including the "EF-hand" motif and C2 domains, both of which have a high affinity for lead. The binding results in decreased function of a diverse group of proteins in the nervous system and elsewhere as protein kinase C, calmodium, and N-methyl-d-aspartate (NMDA) receptor subtype of the glutaminergic receptors.

The degree of lead exposure is reported to dictate the neurologic sequelae (2). Excessive lead exposure can lead to neuronal death as well as to alteration of cellular architecture. There can be associated formation of neurofibrillary tangles, and a predilection for hippocampal involvement has been observed in an animal model looking at the effect of lead dosing. Lead toxicity is associated with both smaller brain volume and white matter lesions that are seen long term, by magnetic resonance imaging (MRI) brain scan, in approximately one third of subjects with excessive occupational lead exposure. The cumulative lead load was determined by X-ray fluorescence of the tibial bone and expressed as microgram per gram of bone mineral. This was observed for both organic lead (tetraethyl and tetramethyl) as well as for inorganic lead exposure. Clinically, cumulative lead exposure dosage correlates with cognitive decline.

Lead, as a divalent metallic cation, competes with calcium and zinc ions for a variety of protein-binding sites, including polycysteine coordination arrays found, for example, in aminolevulinic acid (ALA) dehydrogenase. Accumulation of 5-aminolevulinate is associated with both lead poisoning and acute intermittent porphyria (AIP). This accumulation can result in damage to γ-aminobutyric acid (GABA) receptors in both conditions (4). Transcription factors, with zinc finger motifs, also have a greater affinity for lead than for zinc and this can have pathogenic implications in lead toxicity (5). Lead is typically absorbed either by ingestion or inhalation. In the gastrointestinal tract, lead shares the iron uptake pathway in the distal duodenum and completes with iron for absorption. Nutritional status is a significant factor in biological susceptibility lead absorption. Iron deficiency decreases absorption and retention of ingested Pb^{2+}. Age at onset of exposure is also considered a significant risk factor because children absorb significantly more Pb^{2+} than adults. Hence, in individuals who have low dietary iron, lead absorption is enhanced. This has implications, from a socioeconomic standpoint, because disadvantaged children will tend to have a higher incidence of dietary-induced iron deficiency and have a greater potential for living in housing with lead-contaminated paint and have greater exposure to lead from gasoline combustion associated with certain urban areas.

Mercury toxicity can occur through inhalation of mercury vapors, oral ingestion, or through the skin. The three potential forms of mercury exposure include elemental mercury, also known as quicksilver; inorganic mercury salts; and organic mercury compounds. Mercury intoxication can lead to neuronal death and gliosis of the cortex, especially the calcarine cortex. Selective involvement of motor neurons results in a neurologic picture that can simulate ALS (6). Also in mercury poisoning is often seen severe involvement of the granular layer of the cerebellum with Purkinje cells relatively spared. An axonal form of neuropathy can also be seen. Both mercury and mercury-containing thimerosal can inhibit methionine synthetase, an enzyme important in neural development. Inhibition of methionine synthetase leads to reduction in glutathione, which is an important antioxidant and detoxifying agent.

Manganese can be neurotoxic at higher concentrations, with a predilection for the globus pallidus and striatum. This is in contradistinction to idiopathic Parkinson disease, in which there is predilection for involvement of the substantia nigra pars compacta. This is seen in association with loss of striatal dopamine and intracytoplasmic inclusions termed *Lewy bodies.* It has been reported that the potential for neurotoxicity with excessive manganese exposure can be accentuated by excessive Fe ingestion (1). This might be related to a synergistic transport effect through the blood–brain barrier. Both Zn and Mn can influence neurotransmitter release at the synaptic cleft and this might well have an impact on neurologic manifestations. Although Zn might serve as an inhibitory neuromodulator of glutamate release, Mn may serve to promote excitatory neurotoxicity. It has also been proposed that Mn may interact with α-synuclein in triggering cell death in dopaminergic cells. It is also possible that Mn can induce production of nitric oxide (NO), a neurotoxin, within microglial cells. This could have a deleterious effect on contiguous neurons. Thus, a number of potential mechanisms can lead to selective toxicity of Mn on the extrapyramidal system (1).

Arsenic poisoning results in multiple punctuate hemorrhages within the cerebral white matter. There are pericapillary zones of degeneration, associated with accumulation of erythrocytes, on microscopic examination.

CLINICAL MANIFESTATIONS

LEAD INTOXICATION

Excessive lead exposure is associated with cerebral edema and encephalopthy. The cerebral involvement is characterized by headache, vomiting, confusion that can progress to delirium, stupor, and even coma. Papilledema is seen as reflective of increased intracranial pressure and this can be seen in association with abducens palsy. There can be a seizure predisposition. Long term, accelerated cognitive decline associated with reduced brain volume and white matter lesions can be seen by MRI brain scan (7). Generally, dementia associated with excessive lead exposure requires blood levels exceeding a threshold of 80 μg/dL. There can also be an effect on the peripheral nervous system with motor (axonal-type) neuropathy (8). The neuropathy has a predilection for the extensor innervated muscles. Reflective of this is the not uncommon finding of a radial nerve palsy associated with a wrist drop. This can occur in an isolated fashion and be misdiagnosed as pressure palsy from malposition of the arm. A common peroneal palsy related to lead intoxication can also be seen. Nonneurologic manifestations can include the gingival lead line, as well as gastrointestinal symptoms related to colic from lead-induced porphyria. Also seen is hypochromic anemia resulting from Pb^{2+} -induced inhibition of ALA dehydrogenase and ferrochelatase, two enzymes in the heme synthestic pathway. Additionally, stippling of the red blood cells can occur because lead interferes with RNA degradation by inhibition of pryimidine-5′-nucleotidase.

MERCURY INTOXICATION

Systemic manifestations of mercury toxicity can include gingivitis, stomatitis, abdominal pain, excessive salivation, and anorexia (2). Neurologic symptoms can include fine tremor, initially starting in the hands and spreading to the tongue and perioral region. Over time, there can be involvement of both the arms and the legs. Paresthesias are not uncommon with mercury poisoning and can involve the perioral region as well as the extremities. Bulbar findings can include dysarthria and dysphagia. There can be lower motor neuron findings of weakness, atrophy, and fasciculations. When long tract signs, such as hyperreflexia and extensor plantar response occur, the clinical picture can simulate ALS. In addition, neurobehavioral manifestations can be seen, such as agitation, irritability, as well as psychosis is severe cases.

BISMUTH INTOXICATION

Bismuth toxicity can present as psychomotor slowing, with impairment of attention and concentration. This can progress to agitation, delirium, and even coma. Muscle twitching can be seen, which can progress to myoclonus; headache and sleep disturbance, including insomnia, can occur. In severe cases, along with significant encephalopathy, there can be ataxia with gait instability.

MANGANESE INTOXICATION

It is well recognized that chronic exposure to high levels of manganese, such as occurs as an occupational hazard of manganese mining, can cause parkinsonism. Unlike typical Parkinson disease, there is less in terms of resting tremor and more in terms of bradykinesia, dystonia, and gait impairment, especially when walking backwards (9). In addition, postural tremor, hypophonia, and micrographia can be seen. Prominent neurobehavioral manifestations can occur, such as aggressive behavior. Furthermore, there is limited, if any, response to levodopa administration in manganese-induced parkinsonism.

THALLIUM INTOXICATION

Acute thallium exposure can cause an encephalopathy. Ongoing exposure can be associated with a subacute myelopathy or optic neuropathy. Over time, there can be evolution of an axonal-type of polyneuropathy (10). Thallium poisoning is also typically accompanied by pronounced hair loss.

ARSENIC INTOXICATION

As with acute intoxication with most heavy metals, arsenic can cause an encephalopathy similar to that seen with other toxins. Generally, 1 to 2 weeks after ingestion, a peripheral neuropathy develops, which is associated with distal weakness, sensory loss, and painful dysesthesias (10). The neuropathic involvement tends to peak at roughly 1 month, assuming that the ingestion is not ongoing. Electrophysiologic monitoring can reveal progression of nerve conduction delay for up to several months. A pronounced myalgia may be noted and a subacute myelopathy has also been described. Nonneurologic manifestations can include skin pigment changes, hair loss, and gastrointestinal symptoms, including diarrhea; as well as white striations of the fingernails termed *Mees lines*. The more characteristic neurologic manifestations are summarized in Table 66-1.

DIAGNOSTIC ASSESSMENT

Lead toxicity should be suspected from the clinical scenario of peripheral and CNS signs, the presence of a gingival lead line, gastrointestinal symptoms, and a hypochromic anemia with basophilic stippling of the erythrocytes. It is important to be aware of the social and workplace factors that can result in lead levels >10 μg/dL, which is a serum lead level considered an action point. Recent data suggest, however, that in children irreversible neurologic changes can occur at levels below this limit,

TABLE 66-1. Characteristic Neurologic Manifestation of Heavy Metal Intoxication

	Heavy Metal					
	Mercury	*Lead*	*Manganese*	*Arsenic*	*Thallium*	*Bismuth*
Encephalopathy	+	+	+	+	−	+
Increased intracranial pressure	−	+	−	−	−	−
Motor neuron dysfunction	+	−	−	−	−	−
Parkinsonism	+	−	+	−	−	−
Dementia	+	+	+	−	−	−
Seizures	+	−	−	−	−	+
Tremor	+	−	+	−	−	−
Ataxia	+	+	+	−	−	+
Myoclonic jerks	−	−	−	−	−	+
Mononeuropathy	−	+	−	−	−	−
Axonal polyneuropathy	+	+	−	+	+	−
Optic atrophy	−	−	−	−	+	−
Ophthalmoplegia	−	−	−	−	+	−

strongly suggesting that no threshold exists for lead toxicity. In addition, because lead interferes with heme synthesis, the heme precursor delta-amino-levulinic acid is elevated >20 mg/dL while urinary coproporphyrin excretion is elevated at >150 mg/24 hour. The half-life of lead in the blood is about 35 days, reflecting both the half-life of the erythrocytes to which it is bound and the gradual elution of lead from those binding sites. As a consequence, with intermittent exposure to lead, blood level measurements may be misleadingly low and this necessitates analysis of other tissue. Lead deposition within bone, such as the tibia, can be detected with X-ray fluorescence study or by examination of deciduous teeth or nail or hair clippings.

Mercury intoxication can be detected in the serum as well by 24-hour urine collection of mercury. The level of mercury in whole blood, in the normal state, is <10 μg/L. Toxic levels are those >50 μg/L. Computed tomographic (CT) brain scan, in chronic mercury brain involvement, can demonstrate hypoattenuation within the calcarine cortex and cerebellum.

Manganese toxicity typically reveals bilateral globus pallidus and corpus striatum signal intensity increase on T1-weighted MRI brain scan. Unlike idiopathic Parkinson disease, which is associated with reduced fluorodopa uptake within the striatum, by positron emission tomographic (PET) scan, the PET scan is normal in manganese-induced parkinsonsism (9).

Excessive ingestion of bismuth can be detected by radiographs of the intestine. In addition, bismuth can be detected within either serum, urine, or cerebrospinal fluid of the affected patient.

Arsenic poisoning is best detected by increased levels of arsenic in the hair and urine. Arsenic deposition can be detected in hair within 2 weeks of exposure and can persist for years. A hair concentration of >0.1 mg arsenic per 100 mg hair is considered abnormal. Urinary excretion of arsenic of >0.1 mg arsenic per liter of urine is abnormal with levels >1 mg/L of urine not uncommon in the acute period. There is chronic elevated excretion within the urine and feces reflective of the deposition of arsenic within the long bones.

Thallium toxicity is typically seen in the context of excessive exposure along with the neuropathy, often characterized by severe sensory loss, often painful, with a much milder motor component as well as pronounced diffuse hair loss. This metal can be detected on 24-hour urine collection.

TREATMENT

The best therapeutic approach is obviously prevention or removal of the offending toxin as quickly as possible. Continuing risk exists, however, for exposure to heavy metals and ready recognition of the culprit can make all the difference in terms of reversible versus irreversible nervous system damage. Lead intoxication is treated with chelation therapy. The response to chelation therapy can be dramatic, with resolution of extensive brain lesions, based on serial MRI scans, observed (11). This can include intravenous administration of either dimercaprol (BAL), ethylene diamine tetra-acetic acid (EDTA), or penicillamine with EDTA, the most commonly used chelator. More recently, however, dimercaptosuccinate acid (DMSA), also known as *succimer*, which can be given orally, and with fewer side effects, has become the chelator of choice. This agent is especially attractive for use in children. The drug is rapidly absorbed through the gastrointestinal system. The drug reaches peak levels at 1 to 2 hours and peak mercury excretion, in the urine, takes place within 2 to 4 hours. The gastrointestinal absorption can vary among patients, however, and this can have a significant impact on the potential of this water-soluble chelating agent to be effective.

Chronic mercury poisoning is usually treated with penicillamine, which promotes urinary excretion of this heavy metal. On the other hand, BAL has the potential to promote increased mercury deposition within the brain and should be avoided. Succimer, useful for lead poisoning, also has the ability to promote urinary excretion of mercury.

Dimercaprol (BAL) is generally the chelating agent of choice for bismuth intoxication. The parkinsonism of manganese toxicity is best managed with discontinuation of exposure. Some patients have subjective response to levodopa, but this has been difficult to demonstrate objectively.

Thallium toxicity is best addressed by removal of the exposure and oral potassium chloride may accelerate thallium excretion in the urine.

CLINICAL RECOMMENDATIONS OF THE VIGNETTE

The patient needs to be properly diagnosed and protected from further mercury poisoning. In the acute stage, penicillamine would probably be the agent of choice for the promotion of the removal of the mercury via urinary excretion. Succimer would be a reasonable alternative, but the response to this chelating agent, because of variable oral absorption, would probably make it a less attractive choice.

SUMMARY

The potential continues to exist for central and peripheral nervous system dysfunction related to excessive exposure to heavy metals. The exposure is often subtle, but cumulative over time, which can obscure the explanation. Prevention is paramount and removal of lead-based paints has been a great stride in terms of the prevention of plumbism in children. Industrial exposure is still a potential concern for heavy metal exposure, especially if there is not proper oversight of the work environment with special attention to identification of the exposure levels along with protective clothing and adequate ventilation. Many of the reports of heavy metal poisoning are now generated in Third World countries where the work environment is not as well monitored as in modern industrialized nations and where a greater potential may exist for exposure to unregulated remedies that are promoted to a more naïve patient population. Early recognition and removal of exposure is paramount in the therapeutic approach. Chelating agents remain the mainstays of interventional therapy.

REFERENCES

1. Crichton RR, Ward RJ. *Metal-based Neurodegeneration.* Hoboken, NJ: John Wiley & Sons; 2006.
2. Ibrahim D, Froberg B, Wolf A, et al. Heavy metal poisoning: Clinical presentations and pathophysiology. *Clin Lab Med.* 2006;26:67–97.
3. Racette BA, McGee-Minnich L, Moerlein SM, et al. Welding-related parkinsonism: Clinical features, treatment, and pathophysiology. *Neurology.* 2001;56:8–13.
4. Adhikari A, Penatti CA, Resende RR, et al. 5-aminolevulinate and 4,5-dioxovalerate ions decrease GABA(A) receptor density in neuronal cells, synaptosomes, and rat brain. *Brain Res.* 2006;1093:95–104.
5. Garza A, Vega R, Soto E. Cellular mechanisms of lead neurotoxicity. *Med Sci Monit.* 2006;12:RA57–RA65.
6. Tamm C, Duckworth J, Hermanson O, et al. High susceptibility of neural cells to methylmercury toxicity: Effects on cell survival and neuronal differentiation. *J Neurochem.* 2006;97:69–78.
7. Stewart WF, Schwartz BS, Davatzikos C, et al. Past adult lead exposure is linked to neurodegeneration measured by brain MRI. *Neurology.* 2006;66:1476–1484.
8. Thomson RM, Parry GJ. Neuropathies associated with excessive lead exposure. *Muscle Nerve.* 2006;33:732–741.
9. Olanow CW. Manganese-induced parkinsonism and Parkinson's disease. *Ann NY Acad Sci.* 2004:1012:209–223.
10. Rusyniak DE, Furbee RB, Kirk MA. Thallium and arsenic poisoning in a small midwestern town. *Ann Emerg Med.* 2002;39:307–311.
11. Atre AL, Shinde PR, Shinde SN, et al. Pre- and post-treatment MR imaging findings in lead encephalopathy. *AJNR Am J Neuroradiol.* 2006;27:902–903.

CHAPTER **67**

Disorders of Bone and Bone Mineral Metabolism

Arun A. Kalra • Roger E. Kelley

OBJECTIVES

- To review the nature and type of disorders of bone and its minerals
- To discuss how to diagnose and treat the diseases caused by abnormal bone metabolism
- To describe potential therapeutic approaches for disorders of bone and bone mineral metabolism

CASE VIGNETTE

A 60-year-old man with a history of arterial hypertension, chronic renal insufficiency, and gout was admitted to the hospital with new onset of slurred speech and right-sided weakness. On examination, he was alert with stable vital signs. Neurologic examination showed dysarthria, right central facial paresis, and right hemiplegia. Computed tomographic (CT) brain scan demonstrated an early left middle cerebral artery (MCA) infarction. Urinalysis revealed trace protein. Routine blood work was normal. He was treated with aspirin. On the tenth hospital day, he had a depressed level of alertness with evolution of the left MCA infarct on CT. Cerebrospinal fluid (CSF) was unremarkable. Renal ultrasound showed small kidneys. Further testing revealed a serum calcium of 13 mg/dL, increased urinary calcium excretion, and low levels of intact parathyroid hormone (PTH). Whole body imaging failed to demonstrate a neoplastic process. Chest X-ray was unremarkable with no radiologic evidence to suggest sarcoidosis. He received intravenous fluids, His level of alertness slowly began to improve. On the 24th day of admission, however, the hypercalcemia returned, his renal function deteriorated, and he once again became less responsive.

DEFINITION

Bone is a dynamic organ with constant modeling and remodeling (1). The disorders that affect the bone and its mineralization are collectively called *metabolic bone disorders.* The list of diseases considered in this group is diverse; it can include genetic diseases, infiltrative bone disease, hyperparathyroid bone disease (i.e., osteitis fibrosa cystica, as well as Paget disease of bone), renal osteodystrophy, osteoporosis, osteomalacia, and rickets. An intimate relationship exists between various metabolic disorders and bone disease because bone serves as a reservoir for essential ions, including calcium, sodium, magnesium, and phosphorus. The most common primary bone disorders are osteoporosis, osteomalacia, and rickets. These bone disorders are usually associated with low bone mass with abnormal bone mass defined by the following equation: Bone mineral density (BMD)/bone mineral content (BMC) either one standard deviation greater or 2.5 standard deviations lower than the young adult mean value (2). It is important to understand that the low bone density as measured on dual-energy X-ray absorptiometry (DEXA) scan is not synonymous with osteoporosis, although it can reflect low bone mass.

Bone mass loss is a naturally occurring age-related phenomenon. It typically starts by age 35 to 45 years with a rate of loss of 0.5% to 1.0%. However, in women this loss pattern increases tenfold at the time of menopause. Pathologic conditions associated with bone loss also include osteomalacia and rickets. Osteoporosis is defined as a metabolic bone disease characterized by congruent loss of bone mineral and bone matrix, with an end result of weaker thinner bones with retention of normal composition. This condition tends to be aggravated by hormonal factors, exogenous steroid, thyroxine administration, and the older antiepileptic drugs (AED), such as phenytoin, carbamazepine, and valproic acid, which can also accelerate this process (3). On the other hand, osteomalacia and rickets are both associated with abnormality of calcification. In osteomalacia, there is abnormal calcification of the normally occurring organic matrix of bone called *osteoid.* Rickets is typically a childhood disorder in which there is impairment of provisional calcification of endochondral bone growth at the open epiphyses.

Bone is termed *osteopenic* when the mineral content is decreased with reduced bone mass. This term is often used synonymously with *osteoporosis* and appears to imply the evolution of the process to the point of pathologic state of osteoporosis associated with enhanced tendency for fractures and the common occurrence of curvature of the spine. Clinically, the risk of bone fracture has been incorporated into the concept of "bone quality" (1,2). This accounts for the contribution of bone architecture, bone turnover, reparative processes, and mineralization. Osteoporosis is often subclassified into primary, related to age, and hormonal factors, as well as secondary related to exogenous agents, conditions such as Cushing disease, and immobilization.

EPIDEMIOLOGY

Osteoporosis has become a well-recognized epidemic, with at least 20 to 30 million people affected in the United States and the most susceptible population is composed of postmenopausal women. Also increasingly recognized is the potential for AED to promote this process (3). It is estimated that 30% of all postmenopausal white women will develop fractures related to osteoporosis. This is a dynamic process in recognition of the enhanced screening for osteoporosis and the increasing armamentarium to combat it. Up to 1.3 million fractures per year have been reported in the United States related to osteoporosis, affecting up to 40% of women and 13% of men over the age of 50. Paget disease, the second most common primary bone disorder, discussed in a different chapter, affects approximately 3% of adults over age 40 in the United States. The incidence, however, appears to be falling as it probably also is for osteoporosis, which is reflective of more aggressive prevention, at least in countries with more accessible health care.

Rickets is primarily seen in children with poor nutritional intake, particularly of vitamin D. This was prominent during the 19th century and a contributing factor was inadequate sun exposure. This is much less of a factor in countries where consumption of vitamin D-fortified milk is encouraged, along with reasonable sun exposure. Rickets, however, is now once again recognized as a global health issue. This is reflective of not only vitamin D deficiency in a number of developing countries, but also calcium deficiency, acquired and inherited disorders of vitamin D, and calcium and phosphorus metabolism can also promote rickets (4). Osteomalacia is also reflective of susceptible populations. It can be related to poor nutrition, malabsorption, alcohol abuse, limited sun exposure, vitamin D deficiency, chronic phosphate depletion, systemic acidosis, certain drugs (e.g., AED, isoniazid, and rifampin), nephrotic syndrome and other renal disorders, chronic low calcium levels, and inhibitors of mineralization, such as aluminum and sodium fluoride.

ETIOLOGY

As mentioned, osteoporosis is viewed as part of the aging process, but it is accelerated by primary and secondary factors. Various metabolic processes involving calcium, vitamin D, magnesium, phosphorus, and PTH function can have an impact on the susceptibility to osteomalacia and rickets. These can be related to dietary and absorption aberrations; related to various systemic processes, especially those associated with abnormal renal function; to degree of sun exposure; to malignancies as well as drugs that can interfere with bone metabolites.

Hypercalcemia is one of the more common bone metabolic disorders encountered in the clinical realm. The differential diagnosis for clinically significant elevation of the serum calcium includes the following:

1. Primary hyperparathyroidism
2. Malignancies: Can be associated with osteolytic bone lesions, humoral factors, or production of 1,25-$(OH)_2$ with lymphoma
3. Granulomatous disease, such as sarcoid and tuberculosis
4. Milk-alkali syndrome
5. Drug-induced: Thiazide diuretics, lithium, tamoxifen, vitamin A or D intoxication
6. Immobilization associated with high bone turnover
7. Renal failure—either acute or chronic
8. Adrenal insufficiency
9. Pheochromocytoma
10. Familial hypocalciuric hypercalcemia

Hyperparathyroidism is typically related to a PTH-secreting tumor. The triad of hyperparathyroidism includes: Ostitis fibrosa cystica, renal stones (consisting of either calcium oxalate or phosphate), and duodenal ulcer.

Hypocalcemia can have myriad manifestations and there are a number of potential explanations. The differential diagnosis for clinically significant hypocalcemia includes:

1. Hypoparathyroidism
2. Parathormone resistance
3. Vitamin D deficiency
4. Vitamin D resistance
5. Hyperphosphatemia
6. Osteoblastic bone lesions (e.g., prostate carcinoma)
7. "Hungry bones" syndrome
8. Chronic renal failure
9. Acute pancreatits
10. Multiple citrated blood transfusions
11. Gram-negative sepsis

Hypoparathyroidism can be either hereditary or acquired, resulting in either deficiency of PTH or resistance to the effect of the hormone on the receptor cells (termed either *pseudohypoparathyroidism* or *pseuo-pseudohypoparathyroidism*). These conditions are typically associated with low calcium, magnesium, and phosphorus levels.

Vitamin D deficiency can be dietary or related to decreased formation of vitamin D or its metabolites. Vitamin D_2 or D_3, from the diet, is biologically inert. It is metabolized in the liver to 25-hydroxyvitamin D [25(OH)D], which is the major circulating form of vitamin D, and it is the form measured to determine vitamin D availability. 25(OH)D is activated in the kidneys to 1,25-dihydroxyvitamin D [1,25$(OH)_2$D]. This form serves to regulate calcium, phosphorus, and bone metabolism (5). Hypervitaminosis D can be seen with excessive consumption or related to abnormal conversion of 25(OH)D to 1,25$(OH)_2$D. This abnormal conversion can be seen in granulomatous disease, such as tuberculosis or sarcoidosis, or with certain T-cell lymphomas.

Phosphorus is a vital component of the structural integrity of bone in the form of hydroxyapatite crystals. Plasma phosphorus levels tend to fluctuate, unlike serum calcium and magnesium levels which are closely regulated, with variations of 30% to 50% during the day. Physiologic factors include age (higher levels in children and postmenopausal women), diet (decreased levels after large carbohydrate consumption), acidosis or alkalosis, and various hormones, such as PTH, as well as insulin and 1,25-$(OH)_2$D. The causes of hyperphosphatemia include renal failure (acute or chronic), hypoparathyroidism, parathyroid suppression, acromegaly, acidosis, catabolic conditions, the agent etidronate, tumoral calcinosis, infections, vitamin D intoxication, hyperthermia, hemolytic anemia, acute tumor lysis, excessive phosphate ingestion, and rhabdomyolysis. Causes of hypophosphatemia include hyperparathyroidism, malignancy-related humoral factors, X-linked vitamin D-resistant rickets, alcohol abuse, drugs (e.g., diuretics, steroids, calcitonin, and bicarbonate), decreased intestinal absorption, antacid overuse, vitamin D deficiency, acute gout, acute alkalosis, gram-negative bacteremia, salicylate poisoning, and excessive carbohydrate administration.

Magnesium, the second most abundant intracellular cation, after potassium, serves as a cofactor for many important enzymatic pathways. It also has an important structural role in bone crystals.

Hypermagnesemia is usually of little clinical concern because excess magnesium is usually readily excreted by the kidneys. It can be seen, however, in the setting of renal insufficiency. Hypomagnesemia can be seen in dietary deficiency states, hypoparathyroidism, malabsorption, acute or chronic diarrhea, recurrent vomiting, biliary or intestinal fistulas, excessive renal loss related to osmotic diuresis, metabolic acidosis, drugs (including diuretics, aminoglycosides, cisplatin, amphotericin B), alcoholism, and aldosteronism, acute pancreatitis and *hungry bone* syndrome.

PATHOGENESIS

Bone mineral homeostasis is maintained via regulation of intra- and extracellular calcium, phosphorus, and magnesium, along with the help of PTH, calcitriol, 1,25 dihydoxyvitamin D, as well as various cytokines and calcitonin. These interactions occur mainly in bone, the intestine, and the kidneys (6). Calcium has two important physiologic roles in the body. It is an intracellular second messenger for many hormones and neurotransmitters. 1,25-dihydroxyvitamin D serves to regulate calcium, phosphorus, and bone metabolism (5). Studies suggest that, in addition to regulating calcium homeostasis, vitamin D also has a direct effect on muscle strength because low vitamin D levels are associated with reversible weakness in osteomalacia. Calcium receptors have been identified in skeletal muscle and it has been observed that muscle pain can respond to vitamin D supplementation (7).

The human skeletal system is made up of cortical (80%) and trabecular (20%) bone, which consists of protein matrix, containing mostly osteoid, a collagen, and the minerals deposited into this matrix. Radiologic studies have demonstrated rapid deterioration of trabecular architecture annually in transmenopausal as opposed to postmenopausal women. The density of trabecular connectivity is lost much faster in postmenopausal women with osteoporosis, however, and is probably the primary cause of increased fractures (8). Various factors can contribute to this process. For example, intake of colas, including diet and noncaffeinated, were found to significantly lower the bone mass in teenage girls (9). High intake of fruits and vegetables helps to promote healthy skeletal formation in children (10). Older men with high vitamin A intake appear to have better bone mass (11), but this is not necessarily the case in women (12).

Other factors may also be important for normal bone development. For example, increased bony fragility was observed in an animal model when hydroxyproline was reduced; blood homocysteine levels may also be important (13).

In patients with spinal cord injury, BMD below the lesion is decreased and correlates well with the duration of immobilization following the injury, although the biomechanical stress does not affect the BMC (14). Similarly, it has been shown that stroke patients have decreased BMD and hemiparetic individuals develop hemiosteoporosis. This is felt to be secondary to hypercalcemia, induced by immobilization, inhibiting PTH secretion and promoting vitamin D deficiency, leading to a decrease in BMD (15). In recent years, AED have become the focus of bone health. Decreased BMD has been shown in patients on enzyme-inducing AED, such as phenytoin, carbamazepine, phenobarbital, and valproic acid, an enzyme-inhibiting AED (3). Low vitamin D level was shown to be a primary factor in some of the earlier studies, but recently low BMD was found even without low vitamin D (16). Therefore, involvement of more than one metabolic factor is postulated. This is compounded by polypharmacy and with long term use of AED (17). AED given to patients with a marginal vitamin D level can lead to osteomalacia (6). The effect of the newer AED on bone and bone mineral metabolism has not yet been determined however.

Calcium is primarily stored in bone (99% of the body's total store) and this is mostly as complex phosphate crystals called *hydroxyapatites.* These calcium salts make up half the bone mass. Bone also houses 85% of the body's phosphorous and 50% of body's magnesium. Bone cells include osteoblasts, which form osteoid, and also stimulate the differentiation of precursors to osteoclasts. Osteoclasts, bone resorbing cells, help in remodeling, and are the cells of the bone marrow. The principal stimulator of osteoclast generation is derived from the family of tumor necrosis factor protein and is termed *receptor activator of nuclear factor KB ligand* (RANKL). Osteoprotegrin, an inhibitor of osteoclast generation, and RANKL are opposing regulators of osteoclast formation. They are in an interactive relationship with PTH, vitamin D levels, prostaglandins, and other mediators of bone metabolism. Vitamin D produces its effect as a potent stimulator of osteoclast formation, whereas PTH stimulates bone resorption by a direct effect and also stimulates RANKL production by osteoblasts. PTH, when given intermittently, can stimulate bone formation (6,18).

Other hormones and local factors, such cytokines and prostaglandins, participate in this process. Calcium homeostasis is mostly maintained by the intestinal tract and that of phosphorous by the kidneys, with the help of PTH. Calcitonin, resulting from thyroid hormone response to rapid rise of plasma calcium, inhibits the resorption of calcium in kidneys and its mobilization from bones, thus reducing the serum calcium level (6). It also inhibits osteoclastic bone resorption. In adults, calcium salts are deposited in newly formed or remodeled bone; in children, however, they are deposited at the growing ends of the bones in cartilage cells.

Rickets and osteomalacia are caused by vitamin D deficiency, which can be secondary to poor sun exposure, use of too much sunscreen, inadequate vitamin D intake, and poor absorption. They can also be caused by disturbed mineral availability, secondary to transportation or supply problems, as well as to factors related to the gut, kidneys, or the bone cells. A disturbance may also occur with renal or hepatic activation of vitamin D or interference with its receptor (6). In addition, a familial resistance to vitamin D may exist, which can be associated with a

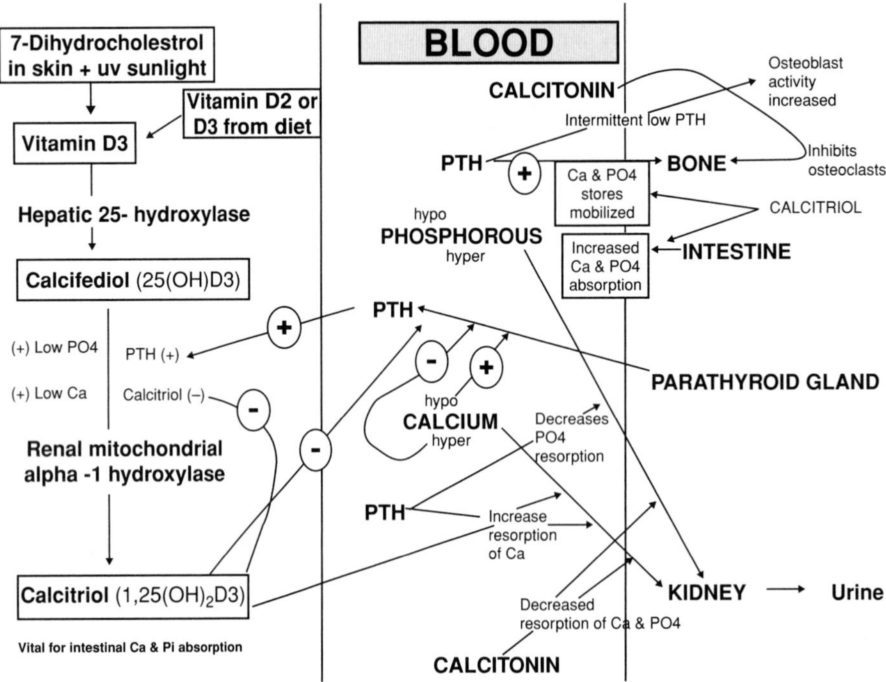

FIGURE 67-1. Bone and mineral homeostasis.

familial X-linked phosphate transport defect. High fluoride content of water and treatment with high doses of fluoride can produce osteomalacia as well (1). In rickets enlarged cartilage is seen at the growth plates, leading to *rachitic rosary* and widened cartilaginous ends of long bones. In patients with cancer with bone metastases, bone pain seems to correlate with enhanced bone resorption and hypercalcemia (19).

Calcium plays an important role in normal functioning of the body. In addition to maintenance of bony structural integrity, it serves multiple functions in biochemical processes, including cofactor in coagulation, regulation of permeation of sodium ions, neuronal activation, hormonal secretion, and excitation and contraction of muscles. In reference to muscle excitation and contraction, it is crucial that the balance between intracellular and plasma calcium be maintained with ionized calcium serving as the most important component. Outside of bone, phosphorous is present in both inorganic and organic forms, with the organic form being the key factor in various biochemical functions. Of particular importance are high-energy bonds, such as adenosine triphosphate (ATP). As with phosphorous, intracellular magnesium is essential for many cell functions (6). Magnesium is involved in bone metabolism, is integral in neuromuscular function and acts as a cofactor for various enzymatic activities. Increased magnesium intake was shown to be significantly related to higher BMD in whites, but not in blacks (20). The mechanisms involved in bone metabolism are varied and complex. Figure 67-1 illustrates some of the intricacies of these potential mechanisms (6). Determination of the specific aberration in particular disorders of bone and bone mineral metabolism can be particularly challenging because of the complexities of the interactions.

CLINICAL MANIFESTATIONS

MINERAL DISORDERS

The manifestations of mineral disorders can be diverse, depending on the array of minerals involved. Some manifestations can be common to all because they can coexist in certain maladies. Their presentation can be divided into acute, subacute, and chronic, with manifestations reflective of the change in concentration of the metabolite, over time, as well as the magnitude of the metabolic disturbance. Acute presentations are most commonly seen in the hospital setting in patients with underlying severe medical or surgical problems. Neurologic symptoms can include confusion, disorientation, hallucinations, dysarthria, dysphagia, oculomotor palsies, anisocoria, cerebellar tremor, muscle weakness, distal sensory deficits, an ascending paralysis resembling Guillain-Barré syndrome, seizures, coma, and, when untreated, can lead to death. Seizures can be seen with low calcium, phosphorous, or magnesium as well as with hyperphosphatemia. Fasciculations, tetany, manifested by carpopedal spasm, Chvostek's sign (ipsilateral facial spasm elicited by tapping on the exit of the facial nerve anterior to the ear) or Trousseau's sign (cramping of the distal muscles of the upper extremity associated with proximal compression), and laryngospasm can be seen with both hypocalcemia and hypomagnesemia. Hypercalcemia can give rise to polyuria, polydipsia, nausea and vomiting, marked dehydration, and constipation.

Hypo- and hypermagnesemia, as well as hypophosphatemia, can result in parasthesias and muscle weakness. There can also be respiratory failure, prolonged QT or PR intervals, congestive heart failure, and conduction heart block. It is not uncommon to see coexistent mineral level abnormalities, which can confuse the situation. For example, in severe hypocalcemia accompanied by hypomagnesemia, associated with acutely diminished glomerular filtration rate and dehydration, hypophosphatemia can be masked or provoked with selective correction of the hypomagnesemia (6). A particularly low serum magnesium level can lower the seizure threshold and seizure activity should respond to correction of the magnesium deficiency in such a clinical setting. A low phosphorous level, which can be associated with inadequate supplementation of phosphorous with parenteral hyperalimentation, or in certain systemic processes, can result in a clinical picture resembling Wernicke encephalopathy. This is characterized by the triad of confusion, extraocular motility impairment, and ataxia.

In newborns, hypermagnesemia can result from the administration of magnesium to the mother for preeclampsia. Hypomagnesemia can be seen in babies of diabetic mothers and can also be seen in neonatal hypoparathyroidism. Neonatal hypocalcemia can be divided into an early and late group. Patients in the early group present within the first 36 hours, whereas the latter group develops manifestations after 5 to 6 days in babies fed with high phosphate-containing milk, such as cow's milk. This is most common in babies with either low birthweight, intrauterine growth retardation, infants of diabetic mothers, mothers with hyperparathyroidism, mothers with congenital hypoparathyroidism (e.g., DiGeorge syndrome), those with certain mitochondrial disorders, and babies delivered after prolonged and difficult labor. If administration of intravenous calcium stops the seizures, in such a situation, then hypocalcemia can be presumed to be the culprit (6,21). Alteration of mineral levels can be reflective of malignancy or abnormal PTH levels and this needs to be kept in mind during the evaluation process.

BONE DISORDERS

Osteoporosis, the most common bone disorder, with equal loss of bone volume and mineral content, commonly is symptom free. Outside of effective detection by screening, it is usually recognized by a fracture. Vertebral compression fracture, the most common, can occur with or without trauma. These compression fractures can be asymptomatic, particularly those with anterior wedging. These mostly occur in the vertebrae from the thoracic 6 level to the lumbar region. They typically present with back pain, with the thoracic area most frequently involved. The nature and extent of pain often depend on the number of vertebrae fractured, which can also lead to kyphosis and loss of lumbar lordosis. Loss of height is a good indicator of compression fractures of the vertebral spine. This, however, can also be seen with vertebral disc space narrowing. This can be associated with reduction in thoracic and abdominal cavities, leading to secondary restrictive problems. Other common fracture sites include the hip and Colles' type and are usually related to trauma which can be trivial (6).

Osteomalacia and rickets typically present with bowing of long bones caused by impaired mineralization. They can have associated myopathy, a pectus deformity called *Harrison's groove*, as well as defective teeth, with problems in both the pulp and dentin. Patients with rickets typically have short stature. The calcium-deficient variety of rickets results in defective tooth enamel. The clinical picture seen in adults can be varied. Severe vitamin D deficiency can lead to muscle weakness which, along with bone pain, can lead to markedly decreased mobility in adults. When associated with compromised chest volume, it can give rise to an increased risk of pneumonia. X-ray study may reveal pseudofractures of long bones, ribs, pubic rami, and so on. With osteomalacia in young women, pelvic involvement can give rise to difficulties with vaginal delivery (6).

Metabolic bone disorders can also contribute to degenerative arthritis of the spine and can promote compressive myelopathies and radiculopathies. This tends to be most pronounced in Paget disease of bone, discussed in another chapter. It is important to assess for potential contributions of osteoporosis, osteomalacia, or rickets as a treatable aspect of the pathogenesis of cervical, thoracic, or lumber spondylosis with the potential for spinal cord or nerve root compression.

DIAGNOSTIC APPROACH

BONE MINERAL DISORDERS

Assessment of bone mineral disorders includes a thorough history to assess for all the pertinent factors as well as physical findings, family history, and coexistent disease. Hypercalcemia from hyperparathryoidism may be an incidental finding in an asymptomatic patient. In such a circumstance, the level of serum calcium elevation is usually mild. For this type of setting, check the ionized calcium level measured without venous occlusion and in the fasting state. If the value is normal, then the elevated calcium level is caused by hemoconcentration. If the value remains elevated, then measure serum albumin, blood urea nitrogen, electrolytes, creatinine, alkaline phosphatase, phosphate, 24-hour urine for calcium-to-creatinine ratio, and PTH level. If primary hyperparathyroidism is excluded, because of rapid rise or markedly high serum calcium level, with a normal PTH level, then a search for malignancy is indicated (6). All causes of hypocalcemia are accompanied by elevation of the serum phosphorous, except with vitamin D deficiency. In addition, the PTH level is elevated, except in magnesium deficiency and hypoparathyroidism.

Hypophosphatemia associated with increased urinary excretion of phosphorous points to a renal disorder as the explanation. Low vitamin D levels are indicative of dietary deficiency, malabsorption, or interference of the metabolic pathways, perhaps by a genetic enzymatic aberration. By itself, a low magnesium level is insignificant unless to a critically low degree. Potential causative factors then need to be addressed. Measurement of urinary excretion will help to determine if inappropriate excretion by the kidneys is the explanation (6).

BONE METABOLIC DISORDERS

The most important approach to bone metabolic disorders is assessment of the bone density. DEXA scan is the most common test for this and it provides accurate measurement of both BMC and BMD. Although not inexpensive, this examination tends to be reliable, despite the variability of measurement even with small changes in disease progression. In older subjects, there can be errors due to calcification in the aorta. This can be corrected at least partially by a lateral X-ray study of the spine. Osteoarthritis, however, might also have an impact on the study. Quantitative CT scan can provide an assessment of bone quality. The major limitation, outside of considerable expense, is the radiation exposure. Peripheral densitometry has certain attractive features, such as being faster, less expensive, and portable compared with the previous two, but the drawback is that it cannot be used for BMD in either the hip or the spine.

Biochemical tests currently available have a wide normal range with marked variability, which limits their use. These include (*a*) markers for bone formation, such as total bone-specific alkaline phosphatase, and osteocalcin, which is specific for skeletal tissue, but whose production is increased by calcitonin leading to falsely low values in osteomalacia and rickets; (*b*) markers for bone resorption, such as urinary calcium excretion, which is quite variable, and fasting urinary hydoxyproline levels, which are of very limited utility; and (*c*) bone biopsy from iliac crest, which can be used for definitive diagnostic purposes, but is not useful as an indicator of bone resorption. This is generally reserved to assess rare bone lesions and in cases of renal osteodystrophy (6). Women with multiple risk factors should be routinely screened at menopause and universal screening at 65 years and beyond is viewed as cost effective (2).

TREATMENT

BONE MINERAL DISORDERS

Obviously, the cause for the mineral disorder must be treated aside from correcting the mineral problem itself. For all acute severe disturbances, supportive therapy is critical, including, when indicated, mechanical ventilation for respiratory failure, temporary pacemaker for arrhythmias, and hemodialysis for renal insufficiency. For asymptomatic hypermagnesemia, cessation of supplement is adequate. For more severe (symptomatic) hypermagnesemia, give 10 to 20 mL intravenous 10% calcium gluconate over 10 to 15 minutes to temporarily antagonize the magnesium effect. Mild deficiencies of the minerals can be taken care of by oral supplement intake. This translates into magnesium at 240 mg four times daily or twice daily and phosphorous at 0.5 to 1.0 g two or three times daily. Symptomatic hypercalcemia requires urgent management by first giving intravenous 10% calcium gluconate 20 mL over 10 minutes. Surgical removal of a parathyroid gland adenoma, when present, should be curative.

Correction of low serum calcium with parenteral therapy is followed by oral calcium supplement along with vitamin D to help increase the absorption of calcium from the intestine with a target serum calcium of 8 to 9 mg/dL. Calcium carbonate is inexpensive and can be taken as 1 to 2 g three times daily initially and later 0.5 to 1 g three times daily should be adequate. Vitamin D at 400 to 1,000 IU/day should be sufficient for vitamin D dietary deficiency. With hypocalcemia, administer either vitamin D, at 50,000 IU/day initially, with a maintenance dose of 50 to 100,000 IU/day or calcitonin, with a more rapid treatment effect, given initially at 0.25 μg/day, followed by an increase every 2 to 4 weeks for a maintenance dose of 0.5 to 2.0 μg/day. The specific cause of the hypoparathryroidism or pseudohypoparathyroidism also needs to be addressed. Because PTH is unable to limit renal calcium excretion, this can lead to renal stones. After the acute treatment, the goal for long-term management is to keep the serum calcium level slightly below normal (i.e., 8 to 9 mg/dL), which helps minimize hypercalciuria. While vitamin D dose is being titrated, the serum calcium level should be closely monitored and its urinary excretion should not exceed 250 mg/24 hours. In patients with severe hyperphosphatemia, the serum phosphorous should be kept at <6.5 mg/dL. Correction of hypomagnesemia, when severe, requires electrocardiographic monitoring to assess for possible cardiac rhythm disturbance, which can be associated with the metabolic disorder.

Brain calcifications, often associated with various central nervous system (CNS) insults, can expand with the potential to aggravate the neurologic deficit, ranging from seizures to parkinsonism. Speculating that the high serum calcium contributes to ongoing cerebral injury, Loeb et al. (22) reported improvement in intractable epilepsy and headaches, as well as reduced calcium load, on follow-up CT brain scan, in two patients, using the bisphosphonate drug disodium etidronate.

BONE METABOLIC DISORDERS

Osteoporosis

Basic measures to prevent and retard the progression of osteoporosis include a regular exercise program, along with calcium and vitamin D supplementation and avoidance of precipitating factors. If an increased risk of osteoporosis exists and if the BMD is less than two standard deviations from normal, then after evaluating for the secondary causes, start antiresorptive medications and follow the BMD every 1 to 2 years. Medications giving rise to sedation or hypotension should be avoided to prevent falls. For hip and vertebral fractures, an intense rehabilitation program may be indicated.

Bisphosphonates work by inhibiting resorption or remodeling (which prevents removal of old and damaged bone) or increasing the bone mineral content (which could increase its stiffness). These agents, theoretically, can make the bone more brittle. Longer term studies are needed to address this issue. The second-generation medications (alendronate, risedronate, ibandronate) do not impair mineralization and oral treatment is simpler with weekly or monthly dosing. Zoledronic acid is being assessed for possible yearly infusion (15). The length of treatment has not been determined yet, although continued effectiveness has been observed for up to 7 years. Because of their poor oral bioavailability, which is further compromised when administered in less than 30 minutes before eating breakfast, bisphosphonates have to be taken on empty stomach and not eat breakfast for a minimum of half an hour.

Parathyroid hormone administered in low dose results in a marked increase in trabecular bone mass, with increased bone formation. Bone resorption catches up within 6 months, however, and its benefit lessens. Promotion of longer term benefit can be accomplished by cessation of treatment for a period of time and then resumption. It can be used alone or in combination with other measures. It is given parenterally and is particularly useful in steroid-induced osteoporosis. It can give rise to hypercalcemia and hypercalciuria so these potential complications require careful monitoring.

Teriparatide (rhPTH 1-34), brand name FORTEO, is the only anabolic bone agent approved in the United States. It contains recombinant human PTH and can result in a dramatic response in the spine, although it has not been demonstrated to prevent fracture. It is contraindicated in hypercalcemia, Paget disease, and bone malignancy (23). In animal models, teriparatide was associated with an enhanced risk of osteosarcoma, which was both dose- and duration of treatment dependent.

In patients with severe pain, calcitonin may be helpful because of its analgesic effect. It can also help prevent bone resorption given as 100 to 400 U intranasally, although it is not as effective as the antiresorptive agents. Hormonal replacement therapy is now more controversial because of potential side effects such as an increased risk of breast and endometrial cancer, and its vascular effects. On occasion, surgical intervention might be necessary for people with disabling vertebral fracture. In the experimental realm, the anti-RANKL agent denosumab, used as an antiresorptive treatment for osteoporosis, mimics osteoprotegrin's function (24). It has been shown to have a rapid, potent, and reversible action. A relatively low dose might be a promising avenue of therapy with an effect similar to PTH 1-34 (25).

For both osteomalacia and rickets, once contributing factors have been eliminated, initially treat with high dose vitamin D at 50,000 to 100,000 U/day. This should address deficiency related to either poor dietary intake or malabsorption. During treatment, the serum and urinary calcium should be monitored. It is advisable to avoid overtreatment because vitamin D is stored in fat and elevated stores can result in prolonged hypercalcemia. Parenteral vitamin D may be necessary in cases of severe malabsorption of vitamin D. Deficiency of α-1-hydroxylase should be treated with calcitonin and removal of the responsible tumor, if present, along with vitamin D supplement, as necessary (6). With severe vitamin D receptor defects, bone growth is rarely normal, even with large doses of calcium and phosphorous supplement.

CLINICAL RECOMMENDATIONS OF THE VIGNETTE

The patient was diagnosed with immobilization-related hypercalcemia. He was then treated with intravenous pamidronate disodium (90 mgs), saline hydration with 2,000 mL/day, and rehabilitative therapy started on the 25th hospital day. His serum calcium level, renal function, and consciousness recovered within 1 week of treatment. During a 2-year follow-up, his renal function remained stable, with no recurrence of hypercalcemia. The patient demonstrates that, in addition to a detailed history and physical examination, testing of serum calcium and urinary calcium excretion, along with serum vitamin D and PTH levels, can be helpful in the assessment. Urinary calcium is lower in reabsorptive hypercalcemia (renal-mediated), but is higher in resorptive (bone-related) and absorptive (gut-related). Vitamin D levels are higher in absorptive processes, whereas PTH levels will help to distinguish parathyroidal from nonparathyroidal mechanisms. The patient had recurrent hypercalcemia related to exacerbation of his chronic renal failure. His presentation was not related to any particular medication that could have promoted hypercalcemia and he had no evidence of a malignant process, or sarcoidosis, as an explanation. The patient illustrates the importance of recognizing the potential contribution of bone and bone mineral metabolic disorders as an explanation for what turned out to be a very treatable, and reversible, metabolic encephalopathy.

SUMMARY

Metabolic bone and mineral disorders are widely prevalent and quite intermixed. To be able to diagnose and treat these conditions, it is important to know their interaction with each other as well as with the kidneys, intestinal tract, calcitonin, vitamin D, and PTH. Methodical testing should be undertaken to evaluate possible explanations, so that proper treatment can be instituted. The patients can present with similar yet variable clinical pattern, which can be very mild to the point of being life threatening, if not treated appropriately and promptly. It should be emphasized that these simple, but important, metabolites should neither be omitted from the diet nor be taken in abundance to ensure homeostasis. For osteoporosis, DEXA scan screening of the susceptible population should be routinely performed. Effective preventive measures include proper diet and exercise, calcium and vitamin D supplementation when indicated, adequate exposure to the sun's ultraviolet light, and avoidance of agents that can promote osteoporosis, such as prolonged steroid therapy and certain anticonvulsants.

REFERENCES

1. Seeman E, Delmas PD. Bone quality—The material and structural basis of bone strength and integrity. *N Engl J Med.* 2006;354:2250–2261.
2. NIH Consensus Development Panel on Osteoporosis Prevention, Diagnosis, and Therapy. Osteoporosis prevention, diagnosis and therapy. *JAMA.* 2001;285:785–795.
3. Andress DL, Ozuna J, Tirschwell D, et al. Antiepileptic drug-induced bone loss in young males who have seizures. *Arch Neurol.* 2002;59:781–786.
4. Nield LS, Mahajan P, Joshi A, et al. Rickets: Not a disease of the past. *Am Fam Physician.* 2006;74:619–626.
5. Holick MF. Resurrection of vitamin D deficiency and rickets. *J Clin Invest.* 2006;116:2062–2072.
6. Bringhurst FR, Demay MB, Kronenberg HM. *William's Textbook of Endocrinology.* Philadelphia: WB Saunders; 2003.
7. Reginster Jean-Yves. The high prevalence of inadequate serum vitamin D levels and implications for bone health. *Curr Med Res Opin.* 2005;21:579–585.
8. Zhao JJ, Jiang Y, Recker RR, et al. Longitudinal changes in 3D micro architecture of human iliac crest bone biopsies: Transmenopausal and postmenopausal. *J Bone Miner Res.* 2003;18[Suppl 2]:S256(abst).
9. McGarland C, Robson PJ, Murray L, et al. Carbonated soft drink consumption and bone mineral density in adolescence: The Northern Ireland Young Hearts Project. *J Bone Miner Res.* 2003;18:1563–1569.
10. McGarland C, Robson PJ, Murray L, et al. Fruit and vegetable consumption and bone mineral density: North Ireland. Young Heart Project. *Am J Clin Nutr.* 2004; 80:1019–1023.
11. Stone KL, Blackwell T, Orwoll ES, et al. High vitamin A intake is not associated with low bone mineral density in older men. *J Bone Miner Res.* 2003;18[Suppl 2]:S242(abst).
12. Llich JZ, Brownbill RA, Furr HC. Prospective, 2-year study in postmenopausal women reveals negative association of vitamin A and bone mineral density of various skeletal sites. *J Bone Miner Res.* 2003;18[Suppl2]:S242(abst).
13. McLean RR, Jacques PF, Selhub J, et al. Increased plasma homocysteine concentrations are strongly associated with increased risk of hip fracture in elderly men and women. *J Bone Miner Res.* 2003;18[Suppl 2]:S4(abst).
14. Dauty M, Perrouin Verbe B, Maugars Y, et al. Supralesional and sublesional bone mineral density in spinal cord-injured patients. *Bone.* 2000;27:305–309.
15. Sato Y, Kuno H, Asoh T, et al. Effect of immobilization on vitamin D status and bone mass in chronically hospitalized disabled stroke patients. *Age Ageing.* 1999;28:265–269.
16. Pack AM. Bone disease in epilepsy. *Curr Neurol Neurosci Rep.* 2004;4:329–334.
17. Souverein PC, Webb DJ, Weil JG, et al. Use of antiepileptic drugs and risk of fractures. *Neurology.* 2006;66:1318–1324.
18. Whyte MP. The long and the short of bone therapy. *N Engl J Med.* 2006;354:860–863.
19. Berruti A, Dogliotti L, Gorzegno G, et al. Differential patterns of bone turnover in relation to bone pain and disease extent in bone in cancer patients with skeletal metastases. *Clin Chem.* 1999;45:1240–1247.
20. Ryder KM, Shorr RI, Bush AJ, et al. Magnesium intake from food and supplement is associated with bone mineral density in healthy older white subjects. *J Am Geriatr Soc.* 2005;53:1875–1880.
21. Volpe JJ. *Neurology of the Newborn,* 4th ed. Philadelphia: WB Saunders; 2001.
22. Loeb JA, Sohrab SA, Huq M, et al. Brain calcifications induce neurologic dysfunction that can be reversed by a bone drug. *J Neurol Sci.* 2006;243:77–81.
23. Close P, Neuprez A, Reginster JY. Developments in the pharmacotherapeutic management of osteoporosis. *Expert Opin Pharmacother.* 2006;7:1603–1615.
24. Yamamoto Y, Noguchi T, Udagawa N. The molecular mechanism of osteoclastic bone resorption and inhibitory drugs for bone resorption. *Clinical Calcium.* 2005;15:11–16.
25. Hollick MF. PTH (1-34): A novel anabolic drug for treatment of osteoporosis. *South Med J.* 2005;98:1114–1117.

CHAPTER 68

Paget Disease of Bone

Roger E. Kelley • Steven N. Levine

OBJECTIVES

- To illustrate the potential effect of Paget disease of bone on the central nervous system
- To illustrate the potential effect of Paget disease of bone on the peripheral nervous system
- To provide an overview of the diagnostic assessment of Paget disease of bone
- To discuss the various therapeutic approaches presently available for Paget disease of bone

VIGNETTE

A 67-year-old woman consults for progressive gait difficulty of several years duration. She "lived with it" up until recently when she began to note an increasing tendency to fall. She has had chronic arthritic pain of her neck, shoulders, and lower back for a number of years. She goes regularly to a chiropractor with transient relief. She is found to have a spastic-ataxic gait with absent biceps reflexes, hyperactive triceps and knee reflexes, with clonus of both ankles. The Babinski response is extensor on both sides. Cervical spine films reveal pronounced bony overgrowth of the cervical canal, with diffuse osteophytic formation. Coarse thickening of the vertebrae is seen with coarsening of trabecular markings and a resultant pronounced narrowing of the cervical canal with spinal cord compression, which is most marked at the C5-6 level.

DEFINITION

Paget disease of bone is a primary bone disorder characterized by increased bone resorption and increased bone formation, resulting in bone that is deposited in a disorganized, mosaic fashion (1). The bones most commonly affected include the pelvis, skull, vertebral bodies, femur, and tibia. Characteristic bone findings are seen on plain X-ray study of the involved skeleton. Typically seen are cortical thickening; focal bone loss termed *osteoporosis circumscripta*, most commonly seen in the skull or pelvis; lytic lesions within long bones, which have been termed *blade of grass* or *flamelike* lesions. As the disease progresses, features seen are a combination of cortical thickening, coarsening of trabecular margins, and both lytic and sclerotic bone lesions, which has been termed the *mixed* phase. In later disease, a so-called *burnt out* phase, primarily sclerosis with bony overgrowth is observed. Many patients are asymptomatic, but a multitude of clinical manifestations of Paget disease exist. Patients may experience pain or deformities in areas of affected bone pain, secondary degenerative arthritis, loss of hearing, and a variety of neurologic manifestations resulting from compression of either the central or peripheral nervous system (2). Rarely, patients may develop an osteogenic sarcoma.

EPIDEMIOLOGY

The cause of Paget disease of bone is unknown. It affects approximately 3% of adults in the United States and is the second most prevalent primary bone disorder after osteoporosis. The prevalence varies with higher frequency in the United States, Germany, France, Great Britain, and Australia, with a lower prevalence in Asia, the Middle East, and Scandinavian countries. It has been estimated that up to 4% of people of Anglo-Saxon lineage are affected by the disease after age 40 years. Of affected individuals, 20% to 30% have relatives with the disease (3). Of particular interest, a gradual reduction has been seen in the incidence and prevalence of Paget disease of bone in recent decades. It has been estimated that the global prevalence is now approximately 2% compared with an estimate of 5% in the 1970s.

ETIOLOGY AND PATHOGENESIS

Although the exact etiology of Paget disease remains unknown, scientific and epidemiologic studies suggest the importance of both genetic and environmental factors. An increased frequency is seen of the human leukocyte antigen (HLA) DQW1, on chromosome 6, and several other susceptibility loci on other chromosomes in this disorder. This genetic susceptibility may be related to a pathologic response to viral stimulation. Electron microscopy studies of Paget disease of bone have revealed virus-like inclusion bodies in the nuclei and cytoplasm of pagetic osteoclasts. In immunohistochemical studies of Paget disease of bone, both measles virus and respiratory syncytial virus antigens have been identified. In addition, *in situ* hybridization techniques have identified the presence of measles and canine distemper virus sequences. No specific virus has been cultured, however, and the use of polymerase chain reaction gene amplification has not produced consistent results. Sir James Paget, who described this disorder, theorized that it was inflammatory in nature and this has yet to be disproved.

Recent genetic studies have led to identification of specific mutations in the p62-sequestosome gene. It is possible that this genetic mutation promotes increased osteoclastic activity by enhancing the sensitivity of osteoclasts to RANKL (receptor activator of nuclear factor-kappaB [NF-κB] ligand), a critical factor in the regulation of osteoclast formation and function (4).

PATHOLOGY

Normal bone remodeling is a coordinated process of bone resorption followed by bone formation. This remodeling process involves the interplay of osteoclasts and osteoblasts in localized areas of bone termed *multicellular bone forming units.* The process is initiated when multinucleated osteoclasts produce areas of bone resorption, followed by new bone formation. This latter phase of bone remodeling occurs as osteoblasts line the areas where bone has been resorbed, laying down new bone matrix, which is then mineralized. Bone resorption allows strengthening and maintenance of bone integrity, by elimination of weakened bone, and this component of remodeling is not a problem as long as restorative bone formation ensues. This implies a balance between osteoblastic activity, for bone formation, with osteoclastic activity, for bone resorption. In the process of bone remodeling, osteoclastic activity precedes osteoblastic restoration.

The initial pathologic change in Paget disease of bone is osteoclast proliferation and what has been termed *giant osteoclasts.* These osteoclasts can have up to 100 nuclei and are unique to this metabolic bone disturbance (5) The osteoclastic proliferation is associated with accelerated bone resorption. In response, enhanced osteoblastic activity occurs in a compensatory fashion. During the initial phase of increased osteoclastic activity, the bones weaken because of the structural damage. This is followed by the next phase of accelerated osteoblastic activity competing with ongoing osteoclastic bone resorption. As the disease progresses, this may evolve into a phase of sclerotic, deformed bones that are susceptible to pathologic fracture. These mixed areas of blastic and lytic lesions typically involve the medial cortex of the affected bones (6). Particularly worrisome is the potential for Paget disease to evolve into sarcomatous degeneration with secondary development of bony tumors. These tumors are rare, occurring in <1% of patients with Paget disease. They can include osteogenic sarcomas, fibrosarcomas, chondrosarcomas, and benign giant cell tumors. The latter most commonly involve the skull.

On biopsy, older lamellar bone is replaced by randomly oriented bone in an intermingled pattern. In addition, the delineation between cortical and trabecular bone is no longer distinct. The finding of this so-called *mosaic pattern of interwoven bone,* with irregular segments of lamellar bone linked by multiple cement lines in a disorganized fashion, is the end product of disrupted bone turnover (7).

The potential effect on the central and peripheral nervous system reflects the location of the bones involved. This will be discussed in detail in the *Clinical Manifestations.* Paget disease of bone has a number of potential secondary effects as the primary pathologic process is restricted to bone. For example, abnormal bone growth and deformities can lead to compressive effects related to skull involvement, which can lead to dysfunction of the auditory nerve with secondary hearing loss. Spinal column involvement can lead to a compressive myelopathy or radiculopathy (8).

DIAGNOSTIC ASSESSMENT

The diagnosis of Paget disease is usually made by reviewing bone radiographs that demonstrate typical features of this disorder (9). With osteolytic activity can be seen the characteristic *blade of grass* appearance of long bones. A pattern of so-called osteoporosis circumscripta can be seen in the skull or pelvis. When evolution to a mixed phase of osteolytic and osteoblastic activity occurs, expanded bone diameter with cortical thickening and coarsening of trabecular markings are seen. In later stages, as the disease burns out, sclerosis of bone is the radiographic hallmark.

Radionuclide bone scans are more sensitive at identifying bone involvement of Paget disease, but are less specific, than plain radiographs. There is increased nucleotide uptake in affected areas of bone. Based on the pattern of which bones demonstrate increased uptake, Paget disease can usually be suspected. In occasional patients, however, it may be difficult to distinguish the bone scan findings of Paget disease from metastatic tumor. This distinction can usually be made, however, by review of the plain radiographs and only rarely is a bone biopsy required.

Laboratory findings that can be helpful in supporting the diagnosis of Paget disease of bone are increased markers of both bone formation and bone resorption. The serum alkaline phosphatase, a marker for bone formation, is almost always elevated while the serum calcium and phosphorus levels are normal. Hypercalcemia tends to be limited to patients with polyostotic Paget disease who become immobilized or those with coexistent hyperparathyroidism. Often, the diagnosis of Paget disease is first suggested when the alkaline phosphatase is noted to be high in a normocalcemic patient with no evidence of liver disease. Measurement of a serum bone-specific alkaline phosphatase can readily distinguish whether an increased alkaline phosphatase is from bone or liver disease. It can be particularly helpful in diagnosing patients suspected of having Paget disease if the total alkaline phosphatase is normal or only slightly increased.

Patients with Paget disease also have increase markers of bone resorption that can be used to assess the activity of disease. Evaluation for an increased urinary hydroxyproline often used to be undertaken. Now more sensitive tests are available to assess osteoclastic bone resorption. These include urinary excretion of N-telopeptide of type 1 collagen, C-telopeptide, deoxypyridinoline crosslinks, and serum N-telopeptide (7).

The degree of elevation of the serum alkaline phosphatase and the tests to assess bone resorption provide a rough estimate of the activity of Paget disease. Furthermore, they are used to determine the response to therapy. In many patients, simply monitoring the serum alkaline phosphatase is the easiest and most cost efficient way to determine the success of treatment.

CLINICAL MANIFESTATIONS

It is important to be aware that most patients are asymptomatic, with Paget disease of bone found as an incidental finding. It is estimated that only 5% of patients are symptomatic. Often, the disease is diagnosed when typical findings of Paget disease are found on radiographs obtained for an unrelated medical problem or because of an isolated elevation of the serum alkaline phosphatase on a chemistry panel.

Manifestations of Paget disease of bone can include bone pain, skeletal deformities, fractures, secondary osteoarthritis, increased skin temperature over areas of affected bone, and a variety of neurologic complications. Rare complications include hypercalcemia and hypercalciuria during periods of immobilization, high output cardiac failure caused by increased vascularity of the bone, or development of osteosarcoma.

Involvement of the skull, seen in approximately 40% of patients with Paget disease of bone, can have a number of potential effects on the nervous system. The skull can become enlarged, with chronic head pain. An associated erythema and warmth over the affected bone can result in a chronic sense of discomfort. Involvement of the auditory canal or acoustic meatus, as mentioned above, can compress the auditory nerves and lead to hearing loss. Hearing loss can also result from pagetic involvement of the auditory ossicles. Theoretically, any bony canal within the skull could become involved, with bony overgrowth resulting in secondary compression of the particular cranial nerve or nerves located within the affected region. Thus, compression can be seen of the jugular foramen with involvement of the glossophayngeal and vagus nerves. Alternatively, there could be compression of the optic foramen, the facial canal, Meckel's cave with involvement of the Gasserian (semilunar) ganglion of the trigeminal nerve, or involvement of the hypoglossal canal. In addition, extradural hematomas can be seen as a complication of Paget disease affecting the skull (10).

Distortion at the base of the skull, with skull softening, can lead to basilar impression. Involvement at the craniocervical junction has been termed *platybasia.* Basilar impression, or invagination, can promote brainstem compression. Typical manifestations of brainstem compression can include lower cranial nerve palsies; brainstem dysfunction, such as nystagmus, especially downbeating nystagmus, vertigo, dysarthria, ataxia, dysphagia, as well as long tract signs, secondary to involvement of the pyramidal tracts; and sensory disturbance. It is not uncommon to see *crossed findings* with compression of the brainstem such as one side of the face and the other side of the body. In addition, obstruction can be seen of the basilar cisterns, secondary to basilar impression, resulting in diffuse ventricular enlargement. The combination of dementia, incontinence, and gait instability can mimic normal pressure hydrocephalus (11).

Involvement of the spinal bone architecture can lead to spinal stenosis, with cord compression and neuroforaminal impingement. A combination of myelopathic features and radiculopathic features can also be seen. Extensive cervical spine compressive disease can actually mimic motor neuron disease where one can see upper motor neuron findings of spasticity and hyperreflexia in combination with lower motor neuron findings of atrophic weakness with fasciculations. Thus, generally a radiographic imaging should be obtained of the cervical spine in cases that clinically look like motor neuron disease without clear bulbar involvement. Thoracic spine involvement is usually manifested by either thoracic myelopathic findings or thoracic radiculopathy. Severe involvement of the thoracolumbar region can lead to a conus medullaris or cauda equina syndrome. Lumbosacral involvement can lead to lower back pain with radiculopathic features including sacroiliitis and sciatica.

TABLE 68-1. Neurological Manifestations of Paget Disease of Bone

1. Hearing loss
2. Head pain
3. Spinal pain
4. Compressive cranial neuropathy
5. Hydrocephalus
6. Basilar impression or platybasia with brainstem impingement
7. Spinal cord compression with myelopathy
8. Radiculopathy
9. Compressive mononeuropathy
10. Extradural hematoma

It is also possible that skeletal deformities related to Paget disease of bone can promote local nerve compression. Thus, elbow involvement could be associated with an ulnar palsy, wrist involvement with carpal tunnel syndrome, knee involvement with a peroneal palsy, or foot involvement with tarsal tunnel syndrome. The potential neurologic manifestations of Paget disease of bone are summarized in Table 68-1.

TREATMENT

Patients with Paget disease are treated to improve symptoms as well as to prevent or treat specific complications. Drugs that directly inhibit osteoclastic bone resorption target the underlying pathophysiologic process of Paget disease (12). In addition, general, nonspecific measures include salicylates, nonsteroidal anti-inflammatory drugs or acetaminophen for pain control, when indicated. Significant bone pain, bone deformity, hearing loss, or other neurologic involvement, as well as high output cardiac failure, related to markedly enhanced blood flow to involved bone, warrants measures to limit bone resorption. The overall goals are to normalize the markers of bone remodeling, usually the alkaline phosphatase level, alleviate bone pain, and prevent complications. Preoperative treatment, to reduce the vascularity of affected areas of bone and limit bleeding, is another indication when surgery is anticipated.

Calcitonin inhibits osteoclastic activity, with subsequent reduction of bone turnover. Subcutaneous or intramuscular injections of salmon calcitonin can lead to significant reduction in pain at the involved area and lower markers of bone formation and resorption. Nasal calcitonin spray is not approved for this indication, but has been used in limited trials. The first-line therapy is now bisphosphonates, which are recognized for their potential to dramatically reduce complications of the disease. The bisphosphonates inhibit osteoclastic bone resorption.

Etidronate, the first bisphosphonate approved to treat Paget disease, while reducing bone resorption, can also decrease bone formation. This can lead to osteomalacia, a problem rarely observed with other biphosphonates (13). The five agents presently approved in the United States for Paget disease of bone, in descending order of potency, are risedronate, alendronate, pamidronate, tiludronate, and etidronate. Zoledronic acid, currently approved to treat hypercalcemia, is the most potent bisphosphonate, and it will likely receive US Food and Drug Administration (FDA) approval to treat Paget disease in the near future (2). The overall goals are to normalize the markers of bone remodeling, usually the alkaline phosphatase level, alleviate bone pain, and prevent complications, including both neurologic and musculoskeletal. Some general comments concerning use of bisphosphonates are provided below, but a detailed discussion is beyond the scope of this chapter. Interested readers are referred to an excellent presentation of this topic by Siris and Roodman (5).

Risedronate, alendronate, tiludronate, and etidronate are oral bisphosphonates with limited absorption from the gastrointestinal tract and the potential for gastric irritation or esophageal ulceration. They must be taken on an empty stomach with a large glass of water. No food or medications should be taken 30 to 60 minutes after administration of the medication and the patient must not lie down for at least 2 hours. A 3- to 6-month course of daily therapy can significantly improve symptoms and lower the markers of bone formation and resorption. A single course of therapy will often control the disease for months or even years and treatment can be reinstituted when the alkaline phosphatase again becomes elevated (14). It should be noted that the doses and frequency of administration of the oral bisphosphonates for treating patients with Paget disease differ when some of these medications are used to treat osteoporosis.

Many believe that use of pamidronate or zoledronic acid, intravenous preparations of bisphosphonates, is the most efficacious and convenient form of therapy for Paget disease, especially for patients susceptible to gastrointestinal complications of oral bisphosphonates. Several 30 to 90 mg infusions of pamidronate administered by infusion over 2 to 4 hours or as a single 15-minute infusion of zoledronic acid can remarkably reduce symptoms and normalize the alkaline phosphatase for more than 1 year (15). Some patients may experience flulike symptoms, a low grade fever, or hypocalcemia after intravenous bisphosphonate therapy. Recently, osteonecrosis of the jaw or other skeletal sites have been reported in patients treated with biphosphonates (2). In most of these cases, affected patients had received multiple, often monthly, doses of intravenous bisphosphonates. All patients treated with bisphosphonates, oral or intravenous, should receive adequate supplementation with calcium and vitamin D to allow for normal bone mineralization and to avoid secondary hyperparathyroidism.

CLINICAL RECOMMENDATIONS OF THE VIGNETTE

The patient has cervical spondylosis with myelopathy. She has spinal cord compression at the C5-6 level. The localization of most prominent involvement is reflected by the absence of the biceps reflexes, with hyperactivity of the triceps reflexes. Corticospinal tract involvement is reflected in the hyperactivity of the triceps reflexes, mediated by C7 and C8 nerve roots, as well as by the hyperactive reflexes in the lower extremities, with positive Babinski reflexes. This is caudal to the area of primary compression at the C5-6 level, which mediates the biceps reflex. Spinocerebellar tract involvement is seen which, in combination with corticospinal tract involvement, results in a spastic-ataxic gait. The only way to achieve decompression of the spinal cord process is for surgical intervention to alleviate the spinal canal stenosis. This would require bone grafting to promote stability of the spinal bone structure, which has been affected by the Paget disease. This patient would also require long-term therapy with a bisphosphonate.

SUMMARY

Paget disease of bone is not at all uncommon, but its incidence is declining for some unexplained reason. It can have numerous potential effects on the central and peripheral nervous systems, including head pain, deafness, other cranial neuropathies; brainstem and spinal cord compression; and compressive peripheral neuropathies. It can also be associated with certain tumors and with extradural hematoma. It can result in a hydrocephalus that mimics normal pressure hydrocephalus. It is diagnosed by characteristic radiographic features and an elevated blood alkaline phosphatase level. The neurologic manifestations can be abated, or prevented, with biphosphonate therapy.

REFERENCES

1. Seeman E, Delmas PD. Bone quality—The material and structural basis of bone strength and fragility. *N Engl J Med.* 2006;354:2250–2261.
2. Whyte MP. Paget disease of bone. *N Engl J Med.* 2006;355:593–600.
3. Altman R. Paget disease of bone. In: Coe FL, Favus MJ, eds. *Disorders of Bone and Mineral Metabolism,* 2nd ed. Philadelphia: Lippincott, Williams & Wilkins; 2002:985–1020.
4. Whyte MP. Paget disease of bone and genetic disorders of RANKL/OPGRANK/NF-kappaB signaling. *Ann NY Acad Sci.* 2006;1068:143–164.
5. Siris ES, Roodman, GD. Paget disease of bone. In: Favus MJ, ed. *Primer on the Metabolic Bone Diseases and Disorders of Mineral Metabolism,* 6th ed. Philadelphia: Lippincott, Williams & Wilkins; 2006:320–330.
6. Kanis J. *Pathophysiology and Treatment of Paget Disease of Bone,* 2nd ed. London: Martin Dunitz; 1998.
7. Roodman GD, Windle JJ. Paget disease of bone. *J Clin Invest.* 2005;115:200–208.
8. Saifuddin A, Hassan A. Paget disease of the spine: Unusual features and complications. *Clin Radiol.* 2003;58:102–111.
9. Lyles KW, Siris ES, Singer FR, et al. A clinical approach to diagnosis and management of Paget disease of bone. *J Bone Miner Res.* 2001;16:1379–1387.
10. Ramesh RVG, Deiveegan K, Soundappan V. Vertex extradural hematoma in association with Paget disease of the skull. *Neurol India.* 2005;53:115–116.
11. Rooh F, Mann D, Kula RW. Surgical management of hydrocephalic dementia in Paget disease of bone: The 6-year outcome of ventriculo-peritoneal shunting. *Clin Neurol Neurosurg.* 2005;107:325–328.
12. Rousiere M, Michou L, Cornelis F, et al. Paget disease of bone. *Best Pract Res Clin Rheumatol.* 2003;17:1019–1041.
13. Miller PD, Brown JP, Siris ES, et al. A randomized double-blind comparison of risedronate and etidronate in the treatment of Paget disease of bone. *Am J Med.* 1999;106:513–520.
14. Reid IR, Miller P, Lyles K, et al. Comparison of a single infusion of zoledronic acid with risedronate for Paget disease. *N Engl J Med.* 2005;353:898–908.
15. Gutteridge DH, Retallack RW, Ward LC, et al. Bone density changes in Paget disease 2 years after iv pamidronate: Profound, sustained increases in pagetic bone with severity-related loss in forearm nonpagetic cortical bone. *Bone.* 2003;32:56–61.

PART IX Nutritional Disorders

CHAPTER 69

Nutritional Deficiency Syndromes

Martha P. Seagrave • Hrayr P. Attarian

OBJECTIVES

- To define malnutrition
- To identify the causes of protein energy malnutrition (PEM)
- To describe the neurologic manifestations of acute PEM
- To discuss the management of PEM and neurologic manifestations for best outcomes
- To discuss preventive strategies

CASE VIGNETTE

A 28-year-old morbidly obese man had a Roux-en-Y gastrojejunostomy. He lost 80 pounds in a period of 3 months. Six months later, he developed bilateral lower extremity weakness and frequent falls, followed by severe parasthesias. He was admitted to the neurology inpatient service after 7 months of continued weight loss. On examination, he had severe weakness of both lower extremities and hands. Workup, including autoimmune screen for neuropathies, heavy metal screen, and vitamin levels, showed mildly low red blood cell transketolase. Thiamine infusions did not produce significant improvement. Electromyography and nerve conduction studies (EMG/NCS) showed changes consistent with severe axonal motor and sensory polyneuropathy. He was transferred to a rehabilitation facility, and after 3 weeks of therapy, he improved sufficiently to be discharged home with outpatient physical and occupational therapy and ambulation aids.

DEFINITION

Malnutrition for the purpose of this chapter relates to protein and energy deficiency and their related physiologic effects.

Protein energy malnutrition (PEM) is the term used to describe a set of clinical conditions that result from inadequate supply of protein and calories. These deficiencies can be primary, caused by inadequate intake of protein and calories as in starvation, or secondary, originating from malabsorption, altered nutrient utilization, excessive nutrient loss, or increased demand for calories and protein. Two forms of PEM are described: *Marasmus*, with weight loss and loss of subcutaneous fat; and *kwashiorkor*, which presents additionally with peripheral edema and abdominal protuberance.

EPIDEMIOLOGY

The incidence of PEM varies by country and is significantly affected by socioeconomic influences. In developing nations, the primary cause of malnutrition is starvation, crossing all age groups, with predominantly a devastating effect on the very young. According to the United Nations Children's Fund (UNICEF), in developing nations the rate of malnutrition in children under 5 years of age is 28% and is implicated in >50% of the mortalities in this age group. The incidence is greatest in sub-Saharan Africa and in southern Asia, despite significant decremental rates in China in the past 10 years.

In the United States and industrialized countries, primary PEM is not considered a significant health problem, although hunger and food insecurity put an estimated 5.5 million children <12 years of age at risk in the United States alone (1). In contrast, secondary PEM is predominant with a higher prevalence in adults. It has been estimated that >50% of hospitalized adults in the United States have PEM. The causes are varied and cross all socioeconomic boundaries.

ETIOLOGY AND PATHOGENESIS

The rates of primary PEM worldwide are affected by a complex interplay of economics, politics, topography, climate, access to health care, and education. Politics in a region can limit access to food by making the procurement dangerous or impossible. Economics for a nation or an individual can make available food unobtainable. The topography and weather conditions affect the kinds of foods that can be produced and the reliability of a harvest, as evidenced by catastrophic natural events such as occurred in the 2005 earthquake in Pakistan and the Asian tsunami in 2004.

Health status can affect the ability of the individual to seek food or use the food that is ingested and, finally, education on how to produce, procure, and prepare foods is essential as is an understanding about how to satisfy nutritional requirements.

In industrialized nations, primary PEM can be the result of these same socioeconomic causes, but neglect, abuse, and eating disorders are sources as well.

Secondary PEM has more varied origins. Protein energy malnutrition can be a consequence of impairment of digestion, malabsorption, decreased available absorptive tissue because of inflammation, lymphatic obstruction, increased transit time, and surgical reduction in intestinal tissue (2).

Protein deficiency during starvation has been known to cause a number of cognitive problems. Neuropathies have been reported in alcohol-induced malnutrition and in patients after gastric bypass surgery.

In 1888, a British medical officer, Henry Strachan, described a syndrome of painful peripheral neuropathy, ataxia, optic neuropathy, and stomatitis among Jamaican sugarcane workers that is known as *Strachan syndrome.* More recently, this has been reported in Cuba where it is caused by malnutrition because of the lack of food and fuel imports from the former Soviet Union (3).

Protein deficiency causes alteration in neurotransmitter levels because dietary amino acids play a precursor role in neurotransmitter synthesis (tyrosine for norepinephrine and tryptophan for serotonin) and their turnover decreases with protein deficiency. Electrocardiography (EEG) shows diminution of voltage and excessive slow-rhythm activity.

The pathophysiology of neurologic problems in combined forms of nutritional deficiencies described above has not been elucidated.

PATHOLOGY

The physiologic compensatory response to starvation begins within the first 24 hours. With the absence or decrease of exogenous sources of energy, hepatic glycogen is utilized; gradually the body shifts reliance from glucose as the primary source of energy to increases in the availability and oxidation of lipids. This shift increases the production of ketone bodies from fat as an energy source, limiting the breakdown of lean muscle mass. Initially, this shift in energy utilization results in maintenance of brain function as ketone bodies, unlike lipids, cross the blood–brain barrier and provide 70% of the brain's energy requirements. This further limits the need for glucose from protein catabolism, temporarily protecting protein stores. As starvation progresses, glucose production in the kidney increases with the conversion of glutamine from muscle and the resting metabolic rate decreases. These adaptations are limited by prolonged protein energy malnutrition. As lipid supply diminishes, protein catabolism increases and death is likely secondary to poorly understood mechanisms associated with loss of body mass, protein, and lipids, and with opportunistic infections. The rate of this degradation will vary relative to the individual's initial body mass, available exogenous nutrients, and disease status (4).

Because of the role glucose plays in producing acetyl–coenzyme A, a precursor to acetylcholine, low glucose availability to the brain is associated with cognitive decline, especially verbal learning and short-term memory (5). Acetylcholine mediates memory processing and is deficient in patients with Alzheimer disease. Hypophosphatemia, especially in cases of malnutrition resulting from anorexia nervosa, causes delirium, paralysis, peripheral sensory neuropathy, and cerebral atrophy. The underlying mechanism seems to be disturbed oxidative phosphorylation and adenosine triphosphate (ATP) depletion, which causes deranged composition of phospholipids in membranes of the nervous system (6).

Optic neuropathy has been described in the setting of combined nutritional deficiencies and toxin exposure. Oxidative phosphorylation within the mitochondria involves the process of electron transfer to oxygen at one end and the production of ATP at the other end. Certain vitamins are crucial to this process, and their deficiency would lead to reductions of ATP. Similarly, certain toxins block this electron transport (7).

Animal studies have shown that protein deficiency can lead to loss of cells in the hippocampus CA1 segment and in the mossy fiber system (8,9) as well as to altered excitatory and inhibitory interaction(10) in those neurons.

Malnutrition decreases the amount of myelin and impairs the packing order of the membranes in the sheaths (11).

Autopsy results have shown that short apical dendrites, fewer spines, and dendritic spine abnormalities in cortical neurons occur in severe infant malnutrition (12).

Sural nerve biopsies in individuals with malnutrition resulting from bariatric surgery have revealed prominent axonal degeneration and perivascular inflammation (13).

Muscle biopsies in patients with anorexia nervosa have shown myopathic changes with severe type 2 fiber atrophy, but with separation and segmental loss of myofibrils and abundant glycogen granules (14).

NEUROLOGIC MANIFESTATIONS OF MALNUTRITION

Neurological manifestations of malnutrition can be divided into three categories:

1. Developmental delay and behavior issues in children
2. Cognitive problems in the already developed brain
3. Neuropathies

Below is discussed all those issues in the setting of different malnutrition syndromes.

MALNUTRITION AND BRAIN DISORDERS

Cognitive impairment in the elderly may be caused by poor nutrition (15), and cerebral atrophy is a common occurrence in patients on long-term parenteral therapy (16). In addition, malnutrition during infancy alters intellectual development by interfering with overall health as well as the child's energy level and rates of motor development and growth (17).

Protein-calorie malnutrition (kwashiorkor) is a problem not only in poor and developing countries where kwashiorkor is common, it is also found in some hospitalized patients with a long duration of stay in developed countries.

Children with marasmus or marasmic-kwashiorkor have various degrees of psychomotor delay and mental retardation, including language deficits, lower intelligence quotient (IQ) scores and poorer performances on various tests of intersensory perception. Severe protein calorie malnutrition in the first year of life causes severe intellectual deficits. In the second year of life, it can produce mental retardation. A short, acute episode of kwashiorkor does not necessarily have lasting cognitive deficits; it depends on the degree to which it is superimposed on the chronic lack of sufficient food that is responsible for marasmus (18).

ANOREXIA NERVOSA

Adolescents with anorexia nervosa can experience structural and functional brain changes. Structural brain abnormalities (enlarged ventricles primarily) are among the most common, early, and substantial consequences. The results of functional neuroimaging studies suggest that brain metabolism may be altered and the neuropsychologic profile shows cognitive dysfunction (19). Both cognitive and neuromuscular problems occur in adults with anorexia nervosa as well (6).

Nutritional optic neuropathy presents with slowly progressive bilateral painless loss of central vision without complaints of positive visual phenomena such as photopias. Sometimes other neurologic symptoms, such as paresthesias, ataxia, or hearing impairment, are associated (20).

Nutritional neuropathy is generally a slowly progressive entity; however, situations occur in which the onset may be acute or subacute.

- *Alcoholic neuropathy* can deteriorate suddenly in a Guillain-Barré-like fashion (21). Alcoholic neuropathy is often asymptomatic. When present, symptoms begin with paresthesias and burning feet, and develop into painful calves, numbness, cramps, weakness, and sensory ataxia. On examination, patients have primarily vibration and deep sensation loss in the distal lower extremities together with weakness, areflexia, calf tenderness, and orthostatic hypotension (22). Leg ulceration and neuropathic joint degeneration can occur. These changes are not always reversible.
- *After gastric restriction procedures* for weight loss, or following weeks of intractable vomiting, such as in hyperemesis gravidarum, a severe axonal neuropathy can develop (13). Sometimes in the above setting, an encephalopathy, similar to Wernicke-Korsakoff can occur (4,23).
- *Gluten sensitivity neuropathy* is an autoimmune disorder where gluten induces an antibody reaction in susceptible individuals against Purkinje cells and other nervous system tissue, leading to a variety of neurologic disorders, including cerebellar ataxia, neuropathy, and myoclonus (24).

DIAGNOSTIC APPROACH

A detailed history, as always, is the place to start. It should include a social history, including living situation, emotional health, dietary intake and sources, medications, drug and alcohol use, travel history, weight history, and physical activity. Medical history should be elicited: chronic disease, gastrointestinal and endocrine disease, pregnancy history, if appropriate; eating disorders, and psychiatric issues. Surgical history should identify abdominal and endocrine procedures. Family history should specifically address digestive and malabsorption conditions, endocrine disorders, cancer, and eating disorders. On physical examination, height and weight should be determined.

The patient should be weighed unclothed, when possible, or in a medical gown and values should be compared with the norm for age. Head circumference should be checked in infants and children. Some clinicians use anthropomorphic measurements to estimate body fat. Because of a major clinician variation when using these instruments, it is recommended that only trained individuals rely on this measurement and that the same individual should assess this measurement on a particular patient, when feasible. Appearance should be documented, including skin and hair texture, quality, tone and color, body habitus, and conjuctiva. Calluses on the fingers and enamel erosion on the teeth may be signs of an eating disorder. Examine for peripheral edema (25).

Orthostatic blood pressure and pulse should be obtained; temperature should be measured and the heart auscultated to identify arrhythmias and bradycardia.

Perform an abdominal examination looking for decreased bowel sounds, hepatomegaly, abdominal masses, and pain. A detailed neurologic examination is necessary; look for affect and responsiveness, assess cognitive function, and look for muscle wasting. A comprehensive workup must include a complete blood count with differential; blood chemistries, including albumin levels; liver and kidney function tests; electrolytes; and thyroid function studies. A basic metabolic panel will give information on electrolyte and glucose levels. An ECG looking for a prolonged QT interval, and nonspecific ST-T segment changes and bone densitometry should be performed (26). If malnutrition is suspected, then serum levels of specific vitamins and minerals can be measured. Urinalysis, urine, stool, and blood cultures, as well as a chest X-ray study should be considered because most patients with PEM are immunocompromised and will not present with expected symptoms to infectious agents. Phosphate levels should also be checked because hypophosphatemia is a major cause of neurologic problems in patients with anorexia nervosa (6).

In neuropathies, EMG/NCV studies can be done and, if needed, a sural nerve biopsy (13).

Neuropsychologic tests are generally not specific and not likely to be of help in identifying malnutrition as an underlying cause for a central nervous system (CNS) disorder (18).

TREATMENT

The management of neurologic disorders that are secondary to malnutrition is directed toward the treatment of the underlying nutritional deficiency, and sometimes the results can be reversible.

In the case of severe PEM, when possible, the patient should be admitted for evaluation and treatment. Continuous cardiac monitoring should be started and intravenous access established. The initial goal is stabilization. Oral and enteral feeding are the preferred methods of treatment because parenteral feedings increase the risk of the most significant complication associated with the treatment of PEM—refeeding syndrome. This condition is the result of introducing carbohydrates and fluids too rapidly, which results in electrolyte imbalance, glucose intolerance, and fluid retention. Hypophosphatemia is the most likely cause of neurologic manifestations of the refeeding syndrome as a result of increased intracellular uptake of phosphate from a relative increased insulin release. To avoid this, introduce frequent small amounts of oral nutrition or continuous slow drip or infusion, with phosphorus, potassium, and magnesium supplementation. Sodium should be limited during the early phases of refeeding, making traditional rehydration supplementation contraindicated. The risk of refeeding syndrome can last up to 5 days. Close monitoring of electrolytes and glucose levels is essential.

Once a patient has been stabilized, malabsorption issues can be addressed and treated and a dietary plan should be established. Reevaluation of neurologic function should be done and rehabilitation for persistent neurologic symptoms can be instituted.

CLINICAL RECOMMENDATIONS OF THE VIGNETTE

Neurologic complications can arise from general malnutrition after gastric bypass surgery, even if specific vitamin levels are normal. General malnutrition after gastric bypass surgery can be prevented by getting a dietary consult and following the recommendations may have prevented the neurologic complications associated with it in the patient.

SUMMARY

In conclusion, malnutrition can cause a variety of significant neurologic problems. These can be prevented or treated early on if the proper diagnosis is made. Malnutrition and its neurologic complications are not only a problem of developing countries, but do occur in certain populations and certain circumstances in the developed world.

REFERENCES

1. Wheler CA, Scott RI, Anderson JJ. Community Childhood Hunger Identification Project: A survey of childhood hunger in the United States. Washington (DC): Food Research and Action Center; 1995.
2. Kumar V, Fausto N, and Abbas A, eds. *Robbins and Cotran Pathologic Basis of Disease*, 7th ed. Philadelphia: WB Saunders; 2005.
3. Roman GC. An epidemic in Cuba of optic neuropathy, sensorineural deafness, peripheral sensory neuropathy and dorsolateral myeloneuropathy. *J Neurol Sci.* 1994;127(1): 11–28.
4. Judge BS, Eisenga BH. Disorders of fuel metabolism: Medical complications associated with starvation, eating disorders, dietary fads, and supplements. *Emerg Med Clin North Am.* 2005;23(3):789–813, ix.
5. Nicolas AS, Andrieu S, Nourhashemi F, et al. Successful aging and nutrition. *Nutr Rev.* 2001;59(8 Pt 2):S88–S91; discussion S-91–S-92.
6. Haglin L. Hypophosphatemia in anorexia nervosa. *Postgrad Med J.* 2001;77(907):305–311.
7. Johns DR, Sadun AA. Cuban epidemic optic neuropathy. Mitochondrial DNA analysis. *J Neuroophthalmol.* 1994;14(3):130–134.
8. Cintra L, Aguilar A, Granados L, et al. Effects of prenatal protein malnutrition on hippocampal CA1 pyramidal cells in rats of four age groups. *Hippocampus.* 1997;7(2):192–203.
9. Cintra L, Granados L, Aguilar A, et al. Effects of prenatal protein malnutrition on mossy fibers of the hippocampal formation in rats of four age groups. *Hippocampus.* 1997;7(2):184–191.
10. Schweigert ID, de Oliveira DL, Scheibel F, et al. Gestational and postnatal malnutrition affects sensitivity of young rats to picrotoxin and quinolinic acid and uptake of GABA by cortical and hippocampal slices. *Brain Res Dev Brain Res.* 2005;154(2):177–185.
11. Vargas V, Vargas R, Marquez G, et al. Malnutrition and myelin structure: An X-ray scattering study of rat sciatic and optic nerves. *Eur Biophys J.* 2000;29(7):481–486.
12. Benitez-Bribiesca L, De la Rosa-Alvarez I, Mansilla-Olivares A. Dendritic spine pathology in infants with severe protein-calorie malnutrition. *Pediatrics.* 1999;104(2):e21.
13. Thaisetthawatkul P, Collazo-Clavell ML, Sarr MG, et al. A controlled study of peripheral neuropathy after bariatric surgery. *Neurology.* 2004;63(8):1462–1470.
14. McLoughlin DM, Spargo E, Wassif WS, et al. Structural and functional changes in skeletal muscle in anorexia nervosa. *Acta Neuropathol (Berl).* 1998;95(6):632–640.
15. Abalan F, Manciet G, Dartigues JF, et al. Nutrition and SDAT. *Biol Psychiatry.* 1992;31(1):103–105.
16. Idoate MA, Martinez AJ, Bueno J, et al. The neuropathology of intestinal failure and small bowel transplantation. *Acta Neuropathol (Berl).* 1999;97(5):502–508.
17. Brown JL, Pollitt E. Malnutrition, poverty, and intellectual development. *Sci Am.* 1996;274(2):38–43.
18. Scrimshaw NS. Malnutrition, brain development, learning, and behavior. *Nutr Res.* 1998;18(2):351–379.
19. Kerem NC, Katzman DK. Brain structure and function in adolescents with anorexia nervosa. *Adolesc Med.* 2003;14(1):109–118.
20. Sadun AA, Martone JF, Muci-Mendoza R, et al. Epidemic optic neuropathy in Cuba. Eye findings. *Arch Ophthalmol.* 1994;112(5):691–699.
21. Wohrle JC, Spengos K, Steinke W, et al. Alcohol-related acute axonal polyneuropathy: A differential diagnosis of Guillain-Barre syndrome. *Arch Neurol.* 1998;55(10):1329–1334.
22. Monforte R, Estruch R, Valls-Sole J, et al. Autonomic and peripheral neuropathies in patients with chronic alcoholism. A dose-related toxic effect of alcohol. *Arch Neurol.* 1995;52(1):45–51.
23. Kinsella L. Nutrition-related neuropathies. In: Gilman S, ed. *MedLink Neurology.* San Diego: MedLink Corporation. Available at www.medlink.com. Accessed May 2006.
24. Hadjivassiliou M, Grunewald RA, Davies-Jones GA. Gluten sensitivity as a neurological illness. *J Neurol Neurosurg Psychiatry.* 2002;72(5):560–563.
25. Halsted CH. Clinical evaluation of the malnourished patient. In: Kasper DL, Braunwald E, Fauci AS, et al., eds. *Harrison's Internal Medicine*, 16th ed. Hightstown, NJ: McGraw-Hill Companies; 2006.
26. Pritts SD, Susman J. Diagnosis of eating disorders in primary care. *Am Fam Physician.* 2003;67(2):297–304.

CHAPTER **70**

Hydrosoluble Vitamins (Except B_{12} and Folate)

Noor A. Pirzada

This chapter deals with diseases of the nervous system resulting from deficiency of the hydrosoluble vitamins, except for vitamin B_{12} and folic acid. The important members of this group are thiamine, pyridoxine, and niacin. Isolated deficiency of other hydrosoluble vitamins, such as riboflavin, biotin, and pantothenic acid is rare and no well-defined clinical syndrome attributable to deficiency of these agents is described. In the case of vitamin C, neurologic manifestations are not a prominent feature of clinical deficiency. Inherited metabolic diseases that respond to vitamin therapy are not discussed in this chapter.

OBJECTIVES

- To review the dietary sources and metabolic role of the hydrosoluble vitamins
- To describe the pathophysiology and pathology of disease states resulting from deficiency of these vitamins
- To explain the signs and symptoms resulting from deficiency of the hydrosoluble vitamins
- To review the diagnosis, treatment, and prognosis of the diseases resulting from such vitamin deficiencies

CASE VIGNETTE

A 56-year-old white woman was brought to the emergency room by the police because she was noted to be very unsteady while walking and was also confused. On examination, the patient was noted to be emaciated and disheveled, with a regular pulse of 100 beats per minute and blood pressure of 130/80 mm Hg. General physical examination showed no obvious external injuries, an odor of alcohol was noted on her. On neurologic examination she was able to comprehend only one-step commands and was disoriented to time, place, and person. She had a reduced attention span and could not retain any information. Intermittently, she appeared agitated and was experiencing visual hallucinations. Her word output was normal and speech was not slurred. Examination of the cranial nerves revealed bilateral restriction of abduction, left worse than right, and bilateral horizontal and vertical nystagmus. Her muscle strength was normal bilaterally. Sensory examination was notable for decreased pinprick sensation distally over her feet and legs. Muscle stretch reflexes were 1+ in the arms and absent in the lower extremities. Finger-nose testing was normal and a mild clumsiness was noted on the heel-to-shin testing bilaterally. She had a markedly ataxic wide-based gait, which was out of proportion to the limb ataxia. A computed tomographic (CT) scan of the brain revealed generalized cerebral atrophy.

Thiamine (Vitamin B_1)

EPIDEMIOLOGY AND ETIOLOGY

Thiamine is most abundant in cereal grains such as rice, and in legumes, yeast, and pork. The outer layers of cereal grains are especially rich in the vitamin and, hence, machine-milled rice is a poor source of thiamine. The recommended daily allowance of this vitamin is 0.5 mg per 1,000 kcal. The total body store is 30 to 100 mg and large amounts are present in skeletal muscle, heart, liver, kidneys, and brain. The half-life of thiamine is about 2 weeks and, because limited quantities are stored in the body, this supply must be constantly replenished. Thiamine requirements are increased during pregnancy, lactation, and thyrotoxicosis. Increased loss of thiamine from the body can occur with hemodialysis, peritoneal dialysis, and diuretic therapy. Patients at high risk for thiamine deficiency also include people with alcohol dependence, infants breast-fed by undernourished mothers, and populations that derive most of their carbohydrate from milled rice. Other conditions associated with thiamine deficiency include prolonged total parenteral nutrition, hyperemesis gravidatum, anorexia nervosa, gastric or jejunal bypass, and severe malabsorption.

PATHOPHYSIOLOGY AND PATHOLOGY

The metabolically active form of thiamine, which is called *thiamine pyrophosphate* (TPP), is involved in the intermediary metabolism of carbohydrates. TPP is involved with the three enzyme systems: (*a*) pyruvate dehydrogenase, which converts pyruvate to acetyl coenzyme A; (*b*) α-ketoglutarate dehydrogenase, which converts α-ketoglutarate to succinate in the krebs cycle; and (*c*) transketolase, which catalyzes the pentose monophosphate shunt. TPP deficiency leads to elevated levels of serum pyruvate and, occasionally, lactate, reduced red blood cell (RBC) transketolase activity, and decrease in oxygen uptake and transketolase activity in the brainstem. The requirement for thiamine is greatest during periods of high metabolic demand or high glucose intake and, therefore, symptoms of thiamine deficiency can be acutely precipitated during periods of intravenous administration of glucose in undernourished patients.

Thiamine deficiency causes peripheral neuropathy, congestive cardiomyopathy, and the Wernicke-Korsakoff syndrome. The primary change in the peripheral nerves is segmental demyelination associated with axonal degeneration, which is most marked in the distal portions of the peripheral nerves. The autonomic nerves can also be involved. In chronic cases, retrograde changes can be found in the spinal cord in the form of chromatolytic changes in the anterior horn cells and secondary degeneration in the posterior columns. The pathologic changes in Wernicke encephalopathy involve predominantly the brainstem and the hypothalamus. Lesions are typically found centrally, in the mammillary bodies, along the walls of the third ventricle, in the medial dorsal nucleus of the thalamus, the periaqueductal gray matter of the mesencephalon, the floor of the fourth ventricle, and in the superior cerebellar vermis. The characteristic lesion is one of subtotal tissue necrosis involving neurons, axons, and myelin to variable degrees. Within the lesions is a glial response that is chronologically appropriate to the age of the destructive lesions. Inflammatory changes are lacking. In some cases, hemorrhages are found and probably these hemorrhagic changes are secondary, rather than primary events. Occasionally, vascular proliferation is encountered. The clinical findings reflect the pathologic changes, with the ophthalmoplegias being caused by lesions in the periaqueductal gray matter and pontine tegmentum, nystagmus by lesions involving the vestibular complex at the pontomedullary junction and truncal ataxia being related to lesions in the superior cerebellum vermis. The changes in attention, cognition, and memory are probably caused by lesions in the mammillary bodies and the medial and posterior thalamus (1).

CLINICAL MANIFESTATIONS

PERIPHERAL NEUROPATHY

Thiamine deficiency is also called *beriberi*. Beriberi affecting predominantly the peripheral nervous system is known as *dry beriberi*. Thiamine deficiency can also affect the heart and, if congestive heart failure is the major manifestation, the condition is called *wet beriberi*. Early symptoms of thiamine deficiency include lethargy, fatigue, and muscle cramps. Later, burning dysesthesias as well as numbness and tingling occur, which start in the toes and the feet and then spread to the upper extremities. These sensory symptoms are followed by sensory loss. Cramps in the feet and calf muscles are common. Patients may also complain of restless legs and sharp lancinating pains similar to those seen in tabes dorsalis. A mild distal weakness then occurs in the feet and hands. Examination shows sensory loss in a glove-and-stocking distribution, with diminished deep tendon reflexes and distal weakness in the hands and feet. Sometimes encountered are signs and symptoms of autonomic dysfunction, including hypotension and pupillary abnormalities, as well as hyperhidrosis of the extremities. Cranial nerve involvement of the facial muscles, vocal cords, and tongue has been described, but is uncommon. In the alcoholic population, the presence of Wernicke-Korsakoff syndrome and cerebellar degeneration can complicate the neurologic picture. Peripheral neuropathy can also develop in alcoholic patients with no obvious nutritional deficiency, suggesting a primary toxic effect of alcohol on the peripheral nervous system.

Wernicke-Korsakoff Syndrome

Wernicke encephalopathy is an acutely or subacutely evolving condition. Patients with thiamine deficiency may become acutely symptomatic when given large doses of carbohydrate, such as the alcoholic patient receiving intravenous glucose. The frequency of Wernicke-Korsakoff syndrome from autopsy studies ranges from 0.8% to 2.8% and the disorder is probably underdiagnosed in patients while they are alive. Clinical features of Wernicke encephalopathy include ophthalmoplegia, ataxia, and mental status changes (2). Bilateral sixth nerve palsies are most common, but any pattern of decreased ocular motility can be found, including gaze palsies and internuclear ophthalmoplegia. Patients usually complain of diplopia. Nystagmus is typically encountered and occurs in both the horizontal and vertical planes. In cases of severe sixth nerve palsies, the nystagmus may be lacking in the abducting eye and becomes apparent only as the ophthalmoplegia subsides with treatment. Ataxia, a prominent feature of this condition, involves the trunk and gait, sometimes with truncal titubation. Limb ataxia as noted on the finger-nose and heel-to-knee tests may be minimal. Mental status changes include agitation, a global confusional state, perceptional distortions, and hallucinations. Rarely, coma can occur. Other findings include hypothermia and postural hypotension, which reflect involvement of the hypothalamic and brainstem autonomic pathways. Polyneuropathy is present in >80% of patients with the Wernicke-Korsakoff syndrome.

Korsakoff syndrome is the chronic stage of the Wernicke-Korsakoff syndrome and typically follows Wernicke encephalopathy, emerging as the ocular symptoms and encephalopathy subside with treatment. Some patients may not be encephalopathic and may show the Korsakoff amnestic state when first seen. The characteristic feature of this amnestic disorder is a defect in learning (anterograde amnesia) and a loss of past memories (retrograde amnesia). Attention and immediate memory, as judged by the patient's ability to repeat a series of numbers, are intact, but short-term retrograde memory is markedly affected. The anterograde amnesia is always coupled with a disturbance of past remote memory (retrograde amnesia) and covers a period that antedates the onset of the illness by several years. Social behavior and other aspects of cognitive function are relatively preserved. Confabulation is frequently encountered in Korsakoff syndrome, but is not invariable and is not pathognomonic of Korsakoff syndrome.

DIAGNOSTIC APPROACH

Diagnosis of both beriberi and Wernicke encephalopathy are based on recognizing the appropriate clinical features in a patient with history of alcoholism or nutritional deficiency. Thiamine status can be assessed by several tests, including RBC transketolase activity, thiamine pyrophosphate stimulation of RBC transketolase (the TPP effect), and the 24-hour urinary excretion of thiamine (3). Serum thiamine levels are of limited usefulness because the level does not reliably reflect tissue concentrations. RBC transketolase activity, with or without TPP challenge, is the most accurate diagnostic tool, which is difficult to find commercially. Pyruvate accumulates in the blood in thiamine deficiency and measurement of serum pyruvate levels may help in making the diagnosis. In beriberi, nerve conduction studies may show an axonal neuropathy with reduced amplitudes of motor and sensory responses, mildly reduced conduction velocity, and neurogenic changes on electromyography (EMG). In Wernicke encephalopathy, magnetic resonance imaging (MRI) may show abnormal signal in the periaqueductal gray matter and midline structures, which corresponds to the pathologic lesions (4).

TREATMENT

For polyneuropathy caused by thiamine deficiency, restoration of a well-balanced diet with supplemental thiamine and other members of the B group is the mainstay of therapy. In the early stages, parenteral vitamin preparations should be used. An intramuscular dose of 50 to 100 mg per day may be used initially for 3 to 5 days, followed by 50 to 100 mg daily by mouth, along with other supplemental vitamins. Symptomatic treatment of pain and paresthesias includes use of tricyclic antidepressants (e.g., amitriptyline), as well as anticonvulsants (e.g., neurontin and carbamazepine). Recovery can be slow and incomplete and, in advanced cases, there may be severe motor and sensory residual deficits, even in individuals who maintain a normal diet.

To avoid precipitating Wernicke disease, intravenous thiamine should be given to all alcoholic and malnourished patients before the administration of intravenous glucose. The body's dose of thiamine is exhausted in 7 to 8 weeks in the chronic alcoholic or the malnourished patient, and the administration of glucose may serve to precipitate Wernicke disease or cause an early form of the disease to progress rapidly. It has become standard practice in emergency departments to administer 50 to 100 mg of thiamine simultaneously with intravenous fluids that contain glucose. Thiamine should also be administered to patients in unexplained stupor or coma. When Wernicke encephalopathy is diagnosed, it should be treated with intravenous thiamine (100 mg) daily, which is continued throughout the acute period. Patients should then be maintained on 100 mg daily of oral thiamine and daily multivitamins. The ocular manifestations of Wernicke encephalopathy show the most dramatic improvement after thiamine is administered. Recovery often begins within hours after starting treatment and almost always within several days. Failure of the ocular palsies to respond to thiamine should raise doubts about the diagnosis and the sixth nerve palsies and gaze palsies recover completely within a week or two, but the nystagmus may persist longer. Improvement of ataxia is more delayed and about 40% of patients recover completely. The remainder shows incomplete recovery, with a residue of wide-based unsteady gait. The early symptoms of encephalopathy invariably improve, but as they do, the memory disorder of Korsakoff psychosis becomes obvious. Once established, the memory disorder shows significant recovery in only about 20% of patients and the remainder are left with varying degrees of permanent disability. Many patients require some form of supervision, either at home or in an extended care facility.

Pyridoxine (Vitamin B_6)

EPIDEMIOLOGY AND ETIOLOGY

The recommended daily allowance of pyridoxine is 2 mg. It is widely and uniformly distributed in all foods, including enriched breads, cereals and grains, chicken, orange and tomato juice, bananas, and avocados. Because of the widespread occurrence of the vitamin in food, pure pyridoxine deficiency is uncommon, except when the pyridoxine content of food is destroyed or converted to less available protein-bound forms during processing, as has happened in infant formulas. Pyridoxine deficiency can be associated with medications that act as pyridoxine antagonists. Such medications include isoniazid, hydralazine, cycloserine, and d-penicillamine. Other patients at risk for pyridoxine deficiency include those with malnutrition, alcoholics, infants of vitamin B_6-deficient mothers, as well as prisoners of war and refugees.

PATHOPHYSIOLOGY AND PATHOLOGY

The active form of pyridoxine is pyridoxal phosphate. It is a coenzyme for amino acid metabolism, particularly tryptophan and methionine. By inhibiting methionine metabolism, pyridoxine deficiency leads to accumulation of compounds that inhibit nerve lipid and myelin synthesis. Because tryptophan is required for endogenous production of niacin, pyridoxine deficiency can produce a secondary niacin deficiency indistinguishable from primary pellagra. Pyridoxine is also involved in synthesis of neurotransmitters such as γ-aminobutyric acid (GABA), dopamine, and other catecholamine and serotonin neurotransmitters. Pyridoxine is unique among the water-soluble vitamins because both a deficiency and toxicity can result in peripheral neuropathy. Mega doses of pyridoxine produce a sensory neuropathy, usually in doses of >2 g a day (5), but it has also been reported with long-standing use of doses as low as 200 mg per day (6). Sural nerve biopsies have shown axonal degeneration of both large- and small-diameter myelinated fibers. Experimental studies have shown pyridoxine-induced neuronal cell body degeneration in the dorsal root ganglion. Pyridoxine deficiency peripheral neuropathy is a predominantly sensory neuropathy affecting the arms and legs.

CLINICAL MANIFESTATIONS

Pyridoxine deficiency causes a mixed distal symmetric polyneuropathy. Patients complain of numbness and tingling in the extremities, especially involving the legs, followed later by pain and tenderness in the calf muscles. Examination reveals impairment of touch and pinprick sensation distally over the extremities with reflex loss. Distal weakness can occur in the legs, but is very uncommon in the upper extremities.

Pyridoxine excess causes a sensory neuropathy or neuronopathy (7). It begins with numbness and paresthesias in the toes. Gait instability is a common complaint and perioral numbness may occur. Neurologic examination reveals impairment of large-fiber sensory modalities, including proprioception and vibration. A positive Romberg sign and sensory ataxia are often noted and, with severe position sense loss, pseudoathestosis may be seen. Touch, temperature, and pain are less affected. Deep tendon reflexes are depressed, but muscle strength is usually normal.

DIAGNOSTIC APPROACH

Pyridoxine levels in the blood can be measured. Pyridoxine excess neuropathy shows an absence or severe reduction in the amplitude of the sensory nerve action potentials. Sensory conduction velocities are mildly reduced. Compound muscle action potential amplitudes and motor nerve conductions are normal. Needle EMG studies are normal. Sural nerve biopsy shows axonal degeneration of both large and small diameter myelinated fibers.

TREATMENT

Up to 10% of patients who are on isoniazid may develop peripheral neuropathy, but the incidence may be as high as 50% in slow acetylators of isoniazid. The intake of vitamin B_6 from 150 to 450 mg per day prevents the neuropathy and should be used by patients on this medication. Once established, the neuropathy may not resolve completely, but may improve with the replacement of vitamin B_6.

Pyridoxine-induced neuropathy is reversible on stopping the drug, although some worsening may occur for 2 to 3 weeks after it is stopped. Such worsening is attributed to a metabolite that remains stored in nonneural body tissues and is subsequently released into the systemic circulation or may result from toxic metabolites that have not been cleared from the neural tissue. Most symptoms disappear within 6 months, but residual deficits can last for many years.

Niacin (Vitamin B_3)

EPIDEMIOLOGY AND ETIOLOGY

Niacin includes both nicotinic acid and nicotinamide and the term *niacin* was introduced to prevent confusion with the tobacco-derivative nicotine. Niacin can be formed in the body from the essential amino acid tryptophan. In the human, an average of about 1 mg of niacin is formed from 60 mg of dietary tryptophan. Although it is endogenously produced, exogenous intake is required to prevent a deficiency. Niacin is found in legumes, peanuts, coffee, tea, meat, liver, and fish. Many foods, especially cereals such as maize, contain bound forms of niacin from which the vitamin is not nutritionally available. Niacin deficiency is called *pellagra* and the word is derived from the Italian pelle agra, which means rough skin. Pellagra still occurs in parts of Africa and Asia, mostly in populations dependent on maize as the principal source of carbohydrate. In the United States, pellagra was common in the south, but has largely disappeared because of enrichment of bread with niacin. It may still occur, however, in alcoholics and in patients taking isoniazid (8).

PATHOPHYSIOLOGY AND PATHOLOGY

Nicotinic acid and nicotinamide form the metabolically active nicotinamide adenine dinucleotide (NAD) and NAD phosphate (NADP), an end product of tryptophan metabolism. Many enzymes are dependent on NAD and NADP to carry out oxidation reduction reactions, and these enzymes are involved in the synthesis and breakdown of carbohydrates, fats, and amino acids. Pathologic changes in pellagra are found the cerebrum, spinal cord, and peripheral nerves and roots. Chromatolytic changes are seen involving most prominently the large Betz cells of the motor cortex and a similar neuronal change may be found throughout the central gray matter. Symmetric degenerative changes are found in the posterior and lateral columns of the spinal cord. The peripheral nerves show a patchy loss of myelin and axons.

CLINICAL MANIFESTATIONS

The symptoms of pellagra are referable to the gastrointestinal tract, the skin, and the central nervous system and, therefore, the classic triad of the three Ds: dermatitis, diarrhea, and dementia. Both central and peripheral nervous systems can be involved. Central nervous system involvement takes the form of an encephalopathy with irritability, insomnia, confusion, and cognitive impairment (9). Extrapyramidal or cerebellar deficits can develop and the optic nerves can be involved. Such a presentation is common among alcoholics. Peripheral neuropathy and myelopathy have also been reported, especially in prisoners of war. There may be associated deficiency of thiamine and pyridoxine, typically among alcoholics (10). Dementia and confusion are almost constant findings, followed by diarrhea (50%) and dermatitis (30%) (11). The skin lesions are a photosensitive dermatitis noted over the parts of the body exposed to the sun. Affected skin lesions are initially erythematous and associated with itching, followed later by blistering and vesiculation. As the dermatitis progresses, the affected skin becomes thickened and hyperpigmented. In addition to diarrhea, other gastrointestinal manifestations include nausea, vomiting, and glossitis.

DIAGNOSTIC APPROACH

The diagnosis of pellagra is mainly clinically based on appropriate signs and symptoms and the response to replacement therapy. Although nicotinic acid metabolites can be measured in the urine, this measurement is impractical and unnecessary. Diagnosis can be difficult if diarrhea and dermatologic changes are absent. Unexplained progressive encephalopathy in an alcoholic patient that is not responsive to thiamine therapy should suggest the possibility of pellagra.

TREATMENT

Pellagra can be treated initially with 25 mg of niacin given intravenously two to three times a day. Other B vitamins, especially pyridoxine, should also be given. Oral nicotinic acid can then be continued in a dose of 50 mg several times a day. Such therapy can reverse most of the signs and symptoms of niacin deficiency and the prognosis for resolution of neurologic symptoms is good.

DISEASES CAUSED BY DEFICIENCY OF MULTIPLE VITAMINS

Nutritional Amblyopia or Tobacco Alcohol Amblyopia

Nutritional amblyopia is a condition in which there is selective involvement of the optic nerves. In developed countries, it is seen most frequently in chronic and malnourished alcoholics. Previously, it was observed in prisoners of war during World War II and the Korean War who were confined for long periods under conditions of dietary deprivation. The condition is characterized by defective vision, which is insidious in onset and progressive in course. At first, there is inability to read small print or distinguish colors, which leads eventually to serious impairment of visual acuity. On examination, patients have bilateral and symmetric loss of visual acuity, with bilateral central, cecocentral, or paracentral scotomas. Funduscopic examination is often unrewarding and, even in severely affected patients, the optic disks may show only mild pallor. Pathologic changes are found in the optic tracts affecting predominately the papillomacular bundle, with loss of myelin and axis cylinders (12). Although the condition is labeled *tobacco alcohol amblyopia*, neither agent has been proved to play a significant role in its pathogenesis. The underlying cause is most likely a nutritional deficiency of multivitamins such as vitamin B_{12}, thiamine, folate, and riboflavin (13). Treatment with a combination of an adequate diet and supplemental B vitamins results in recovery, even if the patient continues to smoke and consume alcohol as before.

Syndrome of Amblyopia, Painful Neuropathy, and Orogenital Dermatitis (Strachan Syndrome)

The syndrome of amblyopia, painful neuropathy, and orogenital dermatitis is a condition that was first described by Strachan in 1897 among Jamaican sugar cane workers and was originally known as *Jamaican neuritis*. It was then described in many other parts of the world, especially in malnourished populations in tropical countries. Subsequently, many cases were described among prisoners of war during World War II, mostly in North Africa and the Far East. A relatively recent outbreak occurred in Cuba during the period of 1991–1994 and coincided with a period of food shortage (14). The clinical features consist of a sensory polyneuropathy leading to sensory ataxia, optic atrophy with loss of vision, deafness, vertigo, and a combination of stomatoglossitis, genital dermatitis, and corneal degeneration. Only a few neuropathologic studies have been conducted of this syndrome. Other than the changes in the papillomacular bundle of the optic nerve, the changes most often described have been a loss of medullated fibers in the posterior columns. The association of this condition with dietary deprivation and the response of the optic and peripheral nerve symptoms to treatment with B vitamins suggest a deficiency of multivitamins as the cause.

DISEASES PRESUMED CAUSED BY NUTRITIONAL DEFICIENCY

Alcoholic Cerebellar Degeneration

Cortical cerebellar degeneration, a complication of chronic alcoholism, is the most common of the acquired degenerations of the cerebellum. Men are affected more frequently than women and the incidence peaks in the middle decade of life. The usual presentation is with progressive unsteadiness in walking that worsens over weeks or months. On examination, the most prominent finding is truncal ataxia, which is demonstrated by a wide-based gait and difficulty with tandem walking. Limb ataxia is much milder than truncal ataxia and is more pronounced in the legs than in the arms. Nystagmus is uncommon and dysarthria, tremor, and hypotonia are rare. Pathologically, selective atrophy of the anterior and superior parts of the cerebellar vermis is found and, histologically, the cell loss involves all neuronal types in the cerebellum, although the Purkinjie cells are the most severely affected (15). The vermian atrophy can be noted on imaging studies of the brain. There may be associated polyneuropathy or Wernicke's encephalopathy. When patients become abstinent and improve their nutritional status, improvement in cerebellar symptoms can occur, but this is slow and often incomplete. Well-documented cases exist of a similar type of cerebellar degeneration, occurring in conditions of severe nutritional depletion without alcohol abuse. This has led some investigators to suggest that alcoholic cerebellar degeneration is caused by nutritional deficiency, particularly of thiamine and does not result from the toxic effects of alcohol.

Marchiafava-Bignami Disease

A rare condition, Marchiafava-Bignami disease, is encountered largely in nutritionally depleted chronic alcoholics. Originally, it was thought to appear most often in middle-aged or elderly men of Italian descent, who drank large quantities of red wine. It is now clear, however, that the disease is not restricted to Italians and consumption of red wine is not an invariable feature, but the most important underlying factor is chronic and severe nutritional depletion. The disease usually has its onset in middle or late adult life and the neurologic presentation can vary considerably. Cognitive slowing, personality and behavioral changes, seizures, tremor and rigidity, coma, and focal motor deficits can all occur to a varying extent. Primitive reflexes may be prominent. Although the disease is usually progressive, some patients may show remission. Most common pathologic changes are symmetric degeneration of the myelin sheath in the mid zone of the corpus callosum, with relatively good preservation of the axons and without significant inflammatory changes (16). Similar changes can be found in the anterior commissure, optic chiasm, and the cerebellar peduncles. These lesions may be identified readily on MRI (17). Treatment consists of nutritional support and abstinence from alcohol. Some patient's condition will improve, but it is not clear if this is related to vitamin supplementation or is a reflection of the natural history of the disease and no specific nutritional defect has been identified.

CLINICAL RECOMMENDATIONS OF THE VIGNETTE

The patient's clinical features suggest that she is a malnourished alcoholic who has presented with features of Wernicke encephalopathy. Findings supporting this diagnosis include the bilateral sixth nerve palsies, nystagmus, and gait ataxia, which is out of proportion to limb ataxia. The higher mental functions indicate an encephalopathy, which is common in patients with this condition, and, with treatment, the encephalopathy improves to reveal the classic findings of Korsakoff amnestic syndrome. The depressed deep tendon reflexes and the distal hypoesthesia in the lower extremities suggest an associated nutritional polyneuropathy, which is present in about 80% of these cases.

An imaging study of the brain is required to rule out a posterior fossa hemorrhage or infarction, as well as a condition such as subdural hematoma. Given the patient's fever, a workup would also be needed for evidence of infection and a metabolic panel should be ordered to rule out metabolic causes of confusion and encephalopathy. The diagnosis of Wernicke encephalopathy is primarily a clinical one, based on appropriate clinical findings in a malnourished and alcoholic patient while excluding other causes for a similar presentation. This patient needs immediate treatment with intravenous thiamine. It is imperative that the patient should not receive intravenous fluids containing glucose until intravenous thiamine has been given, because this can worsen the Wernicke encephalopathy. The intravenous thiamine should be continued for several days and then the patient should receive long-term oral thiamine, as well as vitamin B supplements. As part of long-term management, the most important measures are establishment of a well-balanced, nutritious diet and a decrease in the patient's alcohol intake.

SUMMARY

Neurologic diseases caused by vitamin deficiency are still a serious problem in many developing countries because of chronic dietary deprivation. Such diseases are especially likely to be seen under circumstances such as famine, extreme poverty, and incarceration of prisoners in war camps. Deficiency diseases, however, are also common in the United States and many other developed countries. In western countries, they are usually caused by dietary deficiencies secondary to chronic alcoholism or malabsorption from diseases of the gastrointestinal tract. Clinical manifestations are varied and reflect involvement of both the central and peripheral nervous systems.

REFERENCES

1. Victor M, Adams RD, Collins GH. *The Wernicke-Korsakoff Syndrome.* Philadelphia: FA Davis; 1971.
2. Rueler JB, Girard DE, Cooney TG. Wernicke's encephalopathy. *N Engl J Med.* 1985;312:1035–1039.
3. Leigh D, McBurney A, McIlwain H. Erythrocyte transketolase activity in the Wernicke-Korsakoff syndrome. *Br J Psychiatry.* 1981;139:153–156.
4. Victor M. MR in the diagnosis of Wernicke-Korsakoff syndrome. *Am J Roentgenol.* 1990;155(6):1315–1316.
5. Schaumburg H, Kaplan J, Windebank A, et al. Sensory neuropathy from pyridoxine abuse: A new megavitamin syndrome. *N Engl J Med.* 1983;309:445–448.
6. Parry GJ, Bredesen DE. Sensory neuropathy with low dose pyridoxine. *Neurology.* 1985;35:1366–1468.
7. Dalton K, Dalton MJT. Characteristics of pyridoxine overdose neuropathy syndrome. *Acta Neurol Scand.* 1987;76:8–11.
8. Ishii N, Nishihara Y. Pellagra encephalopathy among tuberculous patients: Its relation to isoniazid therapy. *J Neurol Neurosurg Psychiatry.* 1985;48:628–634.
9. Jollife N, Bowman KN, Rosenblum LA, et al. Nicotinic acid deficiency encephalopathy. *JAMA.* 1940;114:307–312.
10. Ishii N, Nishihara Y. Pellagra among chronic alcoholics: Clinical and pathological study of 20 necropsy cases. *J Neurol Neurosurg Psychiatry.* 1981;44:209–215.
11. Shah DR, Singh SV, Jain IL. Neurological manifestations in pellagra. *J Assoc Physicians India.* 1971;19:443–446.
12. Victor M, Mancall EL, Dreyfus PM. Deficiency amblyopia in the alcoholic patient: A clinicopathological study. *Arch Ophthalmol.* 1960;64:1–33.
13. Potts AM. Tobacco amblyopia. *Surv Ophthalmol.* 1973;17:313–339.
14. Roman GC. An epidemic in Cuba of optic neuropathy, sensorineural deafness, peripheral sensory neuropathy and dorsolateral myeloneuropathy. *J Neurol Sci.* 1994:127(1):11–28.
15. Victor M, Adams RD, Mancall EL. A restricted form of cerebellar degeneration occurring in alcoholic patients. *Arch Neurol.* 1959;1:579–688.
16. King LS, Meehan MC. Primary degeneration of the corpus callosum. (Marchiafava's disease). *Arch Neurol Psychiatry.* 1936;36:547–568.
17. Kawamura M, Shota J, Yagishita T, et al. Marchiafava-Bignami disease: Computed tomographic scan and magnetic resonance imaging. *Ann Neurol.* 1985;18:103–104.

CHAPTER 71

Fat Soluble Vitamins

Nancy Hammond • Yunxia Wang

Vitamins A, D, K, and E are lipid-soluble vitamins, which play important roles in physiologic functions such as bone growth, normal bone density, visual adaptation to darkness, and maintenance of normal function of the immune system and the coagulation system. Neurologic manifestations of liposoluble vitamin deficiencies, predominantly vitamin E deficiency, have long been recognized. Recently, more attention has been paid to the role of vitamins A and D as antioxidants, and their relationship to various neurologic diseases.

OBJECTIVES

- To describe the pathogenesis of fat-soluble vitamin deficiencies
- To describe the common neurologic manifestations of fat-soluble vitamin deficiencies
- To identify the causes, treatment, and prognosis of the neurologic consequences of fat-soluble vitamin deficiencies
- To discuss conditions mimicking fat-soluble deficiencies

CASE VIGNETTE

A 45-year-old right-handed woman presented with progressive 2-year history of gait imbalance, numbness and tingling in both feet, and a 6-month history of weakness in both hands and legs. She has fallen on a few occasions over the past 2 months because of gait unsteadiness. She denied headache, vertigo, or visual disturbances. She had a history of Crohn disease for the last 27 years, with bowel resection 7 years ago, and she has had chronic diarrhea and steatorrhea for the last 5 to 6 years. Her family history was not contributory. Physical examination demonstrated a "petite" woman, slightly >100 pounds, and 5 feet 3 inches in height. General examination was unremarkable except for a well-healed surgical lower abdominal scar. Neurologic examination demonstrated dysarthric speech, bilateral gaze-evoked nystagmus, and motor strength of 4/5 in hip flexors and finger extensors. Muscle strength was 4±5 otherwise. Vibratory sense was diminished distally at the toes and ankles. Muscle stretch reflexes were absent. She was markedly clumsy on finger-to-nose and heel-to-shin evaluation. Her gait was wide-based and ataxic.

Extensive workup was performed and was noncontributory, including normal serum vitamin B_{12} level, serum copper level, creatine kinase (CK), and human immunodeficiency virus (HIV) titer. Nerve conduction studies showed minimal reduced median motor conduction velocities at 42 meters per second (m/s) (normal, >48 m/s) and peroneal motor conduction velocities at 40 m/s (normal >42 m/s), with normal compound muscle action potential (CMAP) amplitude. Plasma vitamin E level was undetectable (normal, 3.5 to 15.8 mg/L). Magnetic resonance imaging (MRI) of the brain, and visual- and brainstem-evoked auditory potentials were normal. Somatosensory-evoked potentials (SSEP) were prolonged in the posterior tibial nerves, consistent with abnormal somatosensory conduction in the spinal cord.

The diagnosis of severe vitamin E deficiency was made. Once vitamin E replacement therapy began, the patient showed improved muscle tone and modest improvement in ataxia.

Vitamin E Deficiency

ETIOLOGY

Vitamin E is abundant in the diet. The main dietary sources are vegetable oils and wheat, which are stored in the body fat. Dietary vitamin E is incorporated into chylomicrons in the small intestine and then bounds to α-tocopherol transfer protein (aTTP) in the liver. In humans, α-tocopherol is the active form of vitamin E, and it is delivered to cells via low-density lipoproteins and very low-density lipoproteins.

Vitamin E deficiency is defined as a low serum fasting vitamin E level or a low vitamin E-to-lipid ratio. Most instances of vitamin E deficiencies occur in patients with fat malabsorption or transport deficiency (Table 71-1). Idiopathic vitamin E deficiency is uncommon.

PATHOGENESIS

The pathogenesis of vitamin E deficiency is poorly understood. Vitamin E is an antioxidant and a free-radical scavenger. It is postulated that the neurologic manifestations of vitamin E deficiency are primarily related to the loss of this protective function. Isolated vitamin E deficiency is an autosomal recessive disorder caused by a mutation in the aTTP gene on chromosome 8q13 (1). Autopsy studies show neuroaxonal dystrophy and accumulation of lipid pigments, with the dorsal root ganglia and the cuneate and gracillis fasciculi most commonly involved.

TABLE 71-1. Etiologies of Vitamin E Deficiency

FAT MALABSORPTION
Cystic fibrosis
Chronic cholestasis
Short bowel syndrome
Celiac disease
Intestinal lymphangiectasia
DEFICIENT TRANSPORT
Abetalipoproteinemia
Hypo-betalipoproteinemia
Isolated vitamin E deficiency (aTTP mutation)

aTTP, α-tocopherol transfer protein.

NEUROLOGIC MANIFESTATIONS

Vitamin E deficiency is responsible for a wide range of neurologic dysfunctions, including a slowly progressive syndrome of cerebellar ataxia, dysarthria, areflexia, ophthalmoplegia, impaired proprioception, absent vibratory sensation, and generalized muscle weakness (Table 71-2). Retinitis pigmentosa and cardiomyopathy can occur in patients with hereditary causes of vitamin E deficiency. Symptoms can develop within 5 to 10 years of onset of the deficiency. Findings on neurologic examination vary from dysarthria and nystagmus, to head titubation, decreased sensation, especially proprioception and vibration; hypo- or areflexia, ataxia, to proximal muscle weakness, and extensor plantar responses. Pes cavus, and scoliosis may be present. Nerve conduction velocities can be normal or mildly slow. Sensory nerve action potential amplitudes are often reduced or absent and, at times, normal. F-wave latencies can be prolonged, indicating a demyelinating process. Electromyography is often normal, although signs of mild denervation can occur. SSEP may show abnormalities consistent with posterior column involvement (2).

CONDITIONS MIMICKING VITAMIN E DEFICIENCY

Friedreich Ataxia

Friedreich ataxia is an autosomal recessive disorder with onset before the age of 25 years. It is characterized by gait and limb ataxia, dysarthria, areflexia, and impaired or absent proprioceptive and vibratory sensations, with mixed upper and lower motor neuron findings, including muscle atrophy, muscle weakness, and extensor plantar responses. Cardiomyopathy is frequently found.

TABLE 71-2. Neurologic Manifestations of Vitamin E Deficiency

Ataxia
Bulbar palsy
Cognitive impairment
Dysautonomia
Myoclonic dystonia
Myopathy
Polyneuropathy
Seizures
Spinocerebellar degeneration

Spinocerebellar Ataxia

Spinocerebellar ataxias are a heterogeneous group of disorders characterized by cerebellar, optic, and peripheral nerve symptoms. The discussion of this diffuse group of neurologic disorders is beyond the scope of this chapter.

Vitamin B_{12} (Cobalamin) Deficiency

Detailed description of neurologic manifestations of vitamin B_{12} deficiency are presented in Chapter 72.

TREATMENT

Treatment of vitamin E deficiency can reverse or halt the progression of the neurologic symptoms. Treatment begins with oral supplementation of vitamin E, 400 mg twice daily, with a gradual increase in the dose until normalization of serum vitamin E levels. Malabsorption syndromes may require treatment with water-miscible or intramuscular preparations.

Vitamin D

ETIOLOGY

The primary source of vitamin D in humans is its production in the skin from solar ultraviolet B (UVB) radiation (3). 7-dehydro-cholesterol (provitamin D_3) is hydrolyzed to previtamin D_3 in the human skin keratinocytes by UVB radiation, then converted to vitamin D_3 by a thermal reaction in the skin. Vitamin D_3 then undergoes hydroxylation in the liver to 25-hydroxy vitamin D (25[OH]D). A second hydroxylation occurs in the kidney to 1,25-dihydroxyvitamin D (1,25[OH]$_2$D), the biologically active form of vitamin D; this step is induced by parathyroid hormone (PTH) and hypophosphatemia, and is inhibited by 1,25(OH)$_2$D.

Dietary sources of vitamin D are rare. Natural dietary sources of vitamin D include oily fishes, such as salmon, mackerel, sardines; cod liver oil, egg yolks, and fermented yeast. In the United States, dietary products, such as milk, cereals, orange juice, yogurt, and margarine, are fortified with vitamin D.

PATHOGENESIS

Vitamin D acts on diverse tissues throughout the body (Table 71-3). The vitamin D receptor (VDR) triggers an increase in intestinal absorption of calcium and phosphorus. When circulating vitamin D levels are low, the intestine absorbs only 10% to 15% of dietary calcium, as compared with 30% to 40% in the presence of adequate vitamin D levels (3). The VDR triggers osteoblasts to release biochemical signals leading to mature

TABLE 71-3. Actions of Vitamin D

Kidney	Increase calcium resorption (indirectly through PTH)
Bone	Demineralization
Intestine	Increase calcium absorption
Parathyroid	Increase secretion of PTH

PTH, parathyroid hormone.

TABLE 71-4. Risk Factors for Vitamin D Deficiency

Age
Higher latitude
Pigmented skin
Sunscreen use
Clothing
Medication use
High body fat content
Fat malabsorption

osteoclasts, which act to dissolve the bone minerals, thereby releasing calcium into the blood (3). Low calcium levels then signal the release of PTH, leading to increased resorption of calcium by the kidney, increased calcium mobilization from the bone, and stimulation of $1,25(OH)_2D$ production.

Vitamin D deficiency is very common in all demographic population. Vitamin D deficiency is associated with various conditions (Table 71-4). Older age reduces the amount of cutaneous vitamin D production; for example, a 70-year-old person exposed to the same amount of sunlight makes 25% of the vitamin D compared with that of a person 20 years of age (3). Physical factors that reduce UVB exposure have been shown to impair or eliminate vitamin D_3 production in the skin. Similarly, dark pigmentation, medication use, fat malabsorption, and age reduce cutaneous vitamin D production, and higher body mass index is associated with lower circulating 25(OH)D levels (4).

CLINICAL MANIFESTATIONS

Vitamin D deficiency in children inhibits the normal mineralization of the growth plates, leading to widening of the epiphyseal plates and bulging of the costochondral junctions, resulting in rickets, kyphoscoliosis, and bowing of the long bones. In adults, vitamin D deficiency at levels <10 ng/mL is associated with osteomalacia and increased bone fragility (5).

NEUROLOGIC MANIFESTATIONS

Rickets in infants is characterized hypotonia and generalized muscle weakness (6). Older children and adults usually present with pain, proximal muscle weakness, waddling gait, and prominent hip and nonspecific bone pain (7). The incidence of myopathy in osteomalacia is between 73% and 97% (8). Vitamin D deficiency has been associated with increased risk of fall in ambulatory nursing home residents who are not exposed to sufficient sunlight (4). Calcium and vitamin D supplementation can reduce body sway and the number of falls. Electrophysiologic study findings are frequently abnormal, showing slowed nerve conduction velocities, and myopathic motor unit action potentials. Findings on muscle biopsy include type II fiber atrophy and infiltration of the interfibrillary spaces with fat, fibrosis, or glycogen (9).

TREATMENT

The 25(OH)D levels should be maintained at a level of 30 to 50 ng/mL. Oral or parenteral routes can be used. Oral doses of 50,000 international units (IU) of vitamin D once a week for 8 weeks should be given and patients should be reevaluated with follow up and 25(OH)D levels. Sunlight, either natural or artificial is another option for vitamin D replacement (4).

Unlike deficiency state, reports of vitamin D toxicity are rare. Hypervitaminosis D is often associated with hypercalcemia or hypercalciuria (10). Dehydration, polyuria, polydipsia, vomiting, fatigue, and irritability can occur.

Vitamin A

DEFINITION

Vitamin A is a generic term for a group of related compounds. Preformed vitamin A includes retinol and retinal, which are found in animal foods, fortified foods, and pharmaceutical supplements. Provitamin A is referred to as beta-carotene and other carotenoids found in plants that can be converted by the body to retinal.

Vitamin A is absorbed through the small intestine, either as retinol or carotene, and then converted to retinyl palmitate, which is stored in the liver (11).

Vitamin A deficiency is an endemic nutrition problem throughout the developing world, especially affecting the health and survival of infants, young children, and pregnant and lactating women. Isolated vitamin A deficiency is uncommon in developed countries and is largely the result of malabsorption or abnormal metabolism.

Symptoms of vitamin A deficiency are mainly ophthalmologic, including night blindness secondary to rod dysfunction, xerophthalmic, dry eyes, keratitis and kerataomalacia, phthisis bulbi, and Bitot spots. Neurologic manifestations of vitamin A deficiency are uncommon. Ataxia, incoordination, and severe bulbar weakness have been reported.

Vitamin A toxicity, which is rare, is associated with drowsiness, irritability, headache, and vomiting. Idiopathic intracranial hypertension (ITT) has been reported with vitamin A overdose following excessive ingestion of vitamin A-rich liver (12) or carrots. The diagnosis of ITT is based on the triad of headache, papilledema, and elevated intracranial pressure with a normal cerebrospinal fluid constituency, in the absence of abnormality on imaging studies. Elevated serum and cerebrospinal fluid (CSF) retinol levels have been reported in patients with ITT (13).

Vitamin K

DEFINITION

Vitamin K is abundant in green leafy vegetables, such as spinach, lettuce, broccoli, brussel sprouts, and cabbage; it is also synthesized by bacteria in the colon. Vitamin K plays a pivotal role in the production of coagulation proteins: It controls the formation of coagulation factors II, VII, IX, and X in the liver, and coagulation proteins C and S.

Bleeding is the major manifestation of vitamin K deficiency and is predominantly encountered in neonates and infants because of lack of vitamin K transportation across the placenta to the fetus, low level of vitamin K in breast milk, and low bacterial synthesis. Newborn and infants are at high risk of intracranial hemorrhage (ICH) secondary to vitamin K deficiency. Because of the risk and severity of vitamin K deficiency-related ICH, the American Academy of Pediatrics recommends vitamin K injections to be administered intramuscularly in a single dose of 0.5 to 1 mg to all newborns (14).

CLINICAL RECOMMENDATIONS OF THE VIGNETTE

Vitamin E deficiency state was thought to explain the patient's neurologic findings. Once vitamin E replacement therapy was initiated, the patient showed improvement in muscle strength and modest improvement in ataxia. She remained areflexic despite the normalization of the serum vitamin E level to 4.6 mg/L.

SUMMARY

Idiopathic fat-soluble vitamin deficiency is uncommon in developed countries because of diets rich in lipid-soluble vitamins. It often results in conditions associated with low dietary intake, such as chronic illness, malnutrition, alcoholism, multiple abdominal surgeries, long-term parenteral nutrition, malabsorption, cholestatic disease, parenchymal liver disease, cystic fibrosis, and inflammatory bowel disease. Multiple combined fat-soluble vitamin deficiencies can occur. Early recognition of fat-soluble vitamins deficiency is pivotal for improvement of neurologic function.

REFERENCES

1. Jackson CE, Amato AA, Barohn RJ. Isolated vitamin E deficiency. *Muscle Nerve.* 1996;19(9):1161–1165.
2. Puri V, Chaudry N, Tatke M, et al. Isolated vitamin E deficiency with demyelinating neuropathy. *Muscle Nerve.* 2005;32(2):230–235.
3. Holick MF. Sunlight and vitamin D for bone health and prevention of autoimmune diseases, cancers, and cardiovascular disease. *Am J Clin Nutr.* 2004;80[6 Suppl]:1678S–1688S.
4. Holick MF. High prevalence of vitamin D inadequacy and implications for health. *Mayo Clin Proc.* 2006;81(3):353–373.
5. Eriksen EF, Glerup H. Vitamin D deficiency and aging: Implications for general health and osteoporosis. *Biogerontology.* 2002;3(1–2):73–77.
6. Prineas W, Stuart-Mason A, Henson RA. Myopathy in metabolic bone disease. *BMJ.* 1965;I:1034–1036.
7. Plotnikoff GA, Quigley JM. Prevalence of severe hypovitaminosis D in patients with persistent, nonspecific musculoskeletal pain. *Mayo Clin Proc.* 2003;78(12):1463–1470.
8. Russell JA. Osteomalacic myopathy. *Muscle Nerve.* 1994;17(6):578–580.
9. Pfeifer M, Begerow B, Minne HW. Vitamin D and muscle function. *Osteoporos Int.* 2002;13(3):187–194.
10. Jacobus CH, Holick MF, Shao O, et al. Hypervitaminosis D associated with drinking milk. *N Engl J Med.* 1992;326(18):1173–1177.
11. Blomhoff R, et al. Vitamin A metabolism: New perspectives on absorption, transport, and storage. *Physiol Rev.* 1991;71(4):951–990.
12. Rodahl K, Moore T. The vitamin A content and toxicity of bear and seal liver. *Biochem J.* 1943;37(2):166–168.
13. Tabassi A, Salmasi AH, Jalali M. Serum and CSF vitamin A concentrations in idiopathic intracranial hypertension. *Neurology.* 2005;64(11):1893–1896.
14. Controversies concerning vitamin K and the newborn. American Academy of Pediatrics Committee on Fetus and Newborn. *Pediatrics.* 2003;112(1 Pt 1):191–192.

CHAPTER 72

Cobalamin (B_{12}) Deficiency

Yunxia Wang • Carla Aamodt • Richard Barohn

OBJECTIVES

- To describe the pathogenesis of B_{12} deficiency
- To describe the common neurologic manifestations of B_{12} deficiency
- To identify the causes, treatment, and prognosis of the neurologic consequences of B_{12} deficiency
- To discuss conditions mimicking B_{12} deficiency

CASE VIGNETTE

A 60-year-old man had a 6-month history of gait unsteadiness and bilateral hand numbness. He had noticed worsening of his symptoms with increasing gait imbalance, and had to use a walker for ambulation. Three months later, he developed numbness in his feet. He had no mental changes, visual disturbances, or bowel or bladder incontinence. Examination showed decreased pinprick and light touch in hands, and diminished vibration and joint proprioception in the toes. Muscle strength showed minimal weakness in foot dorsiflexors and hip flexors. Patellar jerks were brisk; ankle reflexes were absent. He had bilateral plantar extensor response.

Laboratory workup showed a white blood cell count of 5,400, hemoglobin of 15.5, hematocrit of 45.5, and a mean corpuscular volume (MCV) of 98 (reference range, 82 to 99). Serum B_{12} level was 300 pg/mL (reference range, 200 to 900 pg/mL).

ETIOLOGY, PATHOGENESIS, AND PATHOLOGY

Vitamin B_{12} (cobalamin), which is present in animal and dairy products, is synthesized in specific microorganisms. Humans depend on nutritional intake for their vitamin B_{12} supply. Vitamin B_{12} deficiency has been observed in 5% to 15% of individuals over the age of 65 years (1). Up to 90% of cases of vitamin B_{12} deficiency are caused by pernicious anemia (15% to 20%) and food-cobalamin malabsorption (0 to 70%) (2). Except for strict vegetarians, B_{12} deficiency rarely occurs in industrial countries as a result of inadequate dietary intake, but rather as a consequence of malabsorption, gastrectomy, gastric bypass surgery, ileal disease, pancreatic insufficiency, and exposure to nitrous oxide from general anesthesia or recreational use (Table 72-1).

Vitamin B_{12} is an integral component of two biochemical reactions in human; the conversion of L-methylmalonyl coenzyme A into succinyl coenzyme A and the formation of methionine by methylation of homocysteine. The transmethylation reaction is essential to DNA synthesis and to the maintenance of the myelin sheath by the methylation of myelin basic protein. Vitamin B_{12} is liberated from food and binds to R proteins (transcobalamin I and III) in the acidic environment of stomach. It is separated from the R protein in the duodenum where it binds to intrinsic factor. The vitamin B_{12}–intrinsic factor complex is then absorbed in the terminal ileum. Impaired ability to absorb vitamin B_{12} that bound in food protein and pernicious anemia are the common cause of vitamin B_{12} deficiency among the known causes; however, no specific cause is identified in a significant number of patients. Genetic disorders are well characterized, although rare, causes of B_{12} deficiency, mostly in children.

Pernicious anemia is a classic cause of cobalamin deficiency, mainly in patients more than 60 years of age. This autoimmune disorder is seen in up to 20% of vitamin B_{12} deficiency cases. It is characterized by the destruction of the gastric mucosa, and the presence of parietal cell antibodies in 85% to 90% of cases, and intrinsic factor antibody in 50% of patients. The disorder is more common in blacks and in patients with northern European background.

Chronic exposure to nitrous oxide has been associated with B_{12} myelopathy and axonal polyneuropathy. The mechanism by which nitrous oxide induces vitamin B_{12} deficiency is through inhibiting the conversion of homocysteine and methyltetrahydrofolate (MTHF) to methionine and 5-methylene-tetrahydrofolate (THF), which are required for myelin sheath protein and DNA synthesis.

Histopathologic studies have shown breakdown and vacuolization of central myelin under B_{12} deficiency states (3). Thoracic cord is often involved first. In contrast to the demyelinating features seen in the spinal cord, axonal neuropathy is seen on nerve biopsies and nerve conduction studies in vitamin B_{12} polyneuropathy.

COMMON NEUROLOGIC MANIFESTATIONS OF B_{12} DEFICIENCY

Vitamin B_{12} deficiency is associated with hematologic, neurologic, and psychiatric manifestations (Table 72-2). Neurologic manifestations of B_{12} deficiency are often the first or most prominent clinical features of the disease. These vary, depending on the location of the pathology. Subacute combined

TABLE 72-1. Causes of Vitamin B_{12} Deficiency

- Inadequate intake (vegans, chronic alcohol abuse)
- Lack of intrinsic factor or parietal cells from autoimmune disease or surgical procedure (pernicious anemia, atrophic gastritis, gastrectomy, gastric bypass surgery)
- Other gastrointestinal causes (ileal malabsorption, ileal resection)
- Disruption of gastric acidic environment (prolonged use of proton pump inhibitors, prolonged use of histamine H_2 receptor blockers, elderly)
- Defective transport (transcobalamin II deficiency)
- Exposure to nitrous oxide

degeneration, neuropsychiatric symptoms, peripheral neuropathy, and optic neuropathy are the classic neurologic consequences of B_{12} deficiency. Patients may present with neurologic symptoms regardless of a normal hematologic picture.

SUBACUTE COMBINED DEGENERATION OF THE SPINAL CORD

Subacute combined degeneration of the spinal cord is the most common neurologic consequence of vitamin B_{12} deficiency. Pathology occurs in the posterior columns and lateral cortical spinal tracts, with initial involvement of the thoracic cord and extension in either direction (4). Tingling and numbness in hands, arms, thorax, and legs, with loss of vibration sensation and joint proprioception, broad-based ataxia gait, and Lhermitte sign are the early clinical presentations resulting from dorsal column involvement. Spastic weakness, hyperreflexia, and plantar extension responses usually occur in advanced state, secondary to involvement of the lateral corticospinal tracts. Loss of ankle reflexes is often seen in these patients because polyneuropathy often occurs in the presence of myelopathy.

PERIPHERAL NEUROPATHY

Vitamin B_{12} deficiency-related peripheral neuropathy (PN) can represent up to 8% of all PN cases evaluated at tertiary centers (5). Differentiating vitamin B_{12} deficiency-related polyneuropathy from cryptogenic polyneuropathy can be difficult on clinical grounds only. Clinical features useful to identify vitamin B_{12} deficiency-related PN are the acuteness of symptoms onset and concomitant involvement of upper and lower extremities (i.e., numbness hand syndrome). In the setting of peripheral neuropathy, myelopathic findings (e.g., Hoffman signs, spastic weakness, brisk knee reflexes, and extensor plantar responses) should raise the suspicion of cobalamin deficiency.

TABLE 72-2. Neuropsychiatric Manifestations of Vitamin B_{12} Deficiency

NEUROLOGIC

- Peripheral neuropathy
- Subacute combined degeneration of the spinal cord
- Optic neuropathy
- Anosmia
- Decreased taste
- Autonomic dysfunction
- Cognitive deficits
- Dementia

PSYCHIATRIC

- Personality change
- Depression
- Psychosis
- Megaloblastic mania

PSYCHIATRIC MANIFESTATIONS

Psychiatric symptoms attributable to vitamin B_{12} deficiency have been described for decades. Isolated psychiatric symptoms in vitamin B_{12} deficiency are rare, often seen associated with neurologic symptoms. These symptoms seem to fall into several clinically separate categories, including slow mentation, confusion, memory changes, delirium (with or without hallucinations, delusions, or both), depression, acute psychotic states, and, more rarely, reversible manic (megaloblastic madness), and schizophreniform states (6). Historical data show that James D. Duke had severe depression because of vitamin B_{12} deficiency secondary to pernicious anemia; he donated $19 million to build Duke University in an attempt to relieve guilt feelings.

OPTIC NEUROPATHY

A less common neurologic complication of vitamin B_{12} deficiency is optic neuropathy. Patients may present with optic atrophy, retrobulbar neuritis, centrocecal scotoma, macular hemorrhage, or peripheral constriction of visual fields (7).

DIAGNOSTIC APPROACH

Diagnosis of B_{12} deficiency is usually made in the presence of typical neurologic symptoms, hematologic abnormalities, and serum vitamin B_{12} levels <200 pg/mL, although a significant proportion of patients with vitamin B_{12} deficiency may have serum levels that are within the normal range. Measurement of the serum metabolites methylmalonic acid (MMA) and homocysteine (Hcy) can improve the sensitivity significantly in patients with low normal range of B_{12} (300 to 400 pg/mL) when high clinical suspicion exists (8). Although elevated MMA and Hcy suggest B_{12} deficiency, it is necessary to rule out other conditions associated with such abnormal levels, such as renal insufficiency and hypovolemia. Isolated Hcy can also be seen in hypothyroidism, deficiency of folate acid and pyridoxine, cigarette smoking, and advanced age.

The Schilling test is performed to diagnose pernicious anemia. Today, it is difficult to obtain a Schilling test because of the unavailability of the radioisotope. Antiintrinsic factor and antiparietal cell antibodies can be helpful in the diagnosis of pernicious anemia with high specificity and low sensitivity for the former and high sensitivity and low specificity for the latter.

In typical cases with myelopathic symptoms, increased T2 signal intensity is seen in the posterior column on magnetic resonance imaging (MRI) studies.

CONDITIONS MIMICKING VITAMIN B_{12} DEFICIENCY

Various causes of myelopathy should be considered in the differential diagnosis of B_{12} deficiency.

Vitamin E is a major lipid-soluble essential vitamin and chain-breaking antioxidant in the body that plays an important role in protecting the integrity of membranes by scavenging free radicals. Vitamin E deficiency can lead to prominent posterior column dysfunction and sensory loss, in addition to ataxia and retinitis pigmentosa. The combination of ataxia and peripheral neuropathy resemble Friedreich ataxia and other forms of spinocerebellar ataxias.

Copper-deficiency myelopathy has been described in patients with gastric-intestinal bypass surgery, in patients consuming excessive zinc supplementation, and can occur for unknown causes (9). Copper deficiency can coexist with vitamin B_{12} deficiency because copper is absorbed in the stomach mucosa. The clinical picture of copper deficiency is similar to B_{12} deficiency. Patients present with signs and symptoms of pathology that primarily involve the posterior columns and lateral corticospinal tracts. Predominant complaints include paresthesia in the feet, ataxia, and limb weakness. Similarly to B_{12} deficiency, neurologic symptoms in copper deficiency-myelopathy are not always associated with hematologic abnormalities. Some patients may have low-normal B_{12} levels and may be diagnosed with B_{12} deficiency; despite the treatment with B_{12} supplementation and normalization of MMA and Hcy, these patients can continue to deteriorate and the neurologic symptoms may only stabilize or improve following copper supplementation.

Patients with acquired immunodeficiency syndrome (AIDS) may rarely develop myelopathic symptoms, which are usually preceded by other neuropsychiatric manifestations. The most prominent spinal cord disease in AIDS is vacuolar myelopathy, which is seen in 20% to 55% of patients with AIDS at autopsy. Clinically, patients may present with minimal signs of myelopathy, such as paresthesia and brisk reflexes. The correlation between cerebrospinal fluid (CSF) viral load and the presence or severity of myelopathy is unclear (10).

Multiple sclerosis (MS) presenting with spinal cord pathology can mimic myelopathy secondary to B_{12} deficiency. Patients with B_{12} deficiency may also have subcortical white matter lesions on MRI of the brain, which can be misdiagnosed as MS plaques. Clinically, MS is often seen in young women, whereas B_{12} deficiency myelopathy is more common in the elderly. The presence of oligoclonal band, increased IgG index, and, elevated protein in the CSF is suggestive of the diagnosis of MS, whereas B_{12} deficiency may only show mildly elevated CSF protein count.

TREATMENT

Early diagnosis is critical because patients with advanced disease may be left with major residual disability. Common treatment regimen includes administration of vitamin B_{12} (1,000 μg) intramuscularly (IM) daily for 5 to 7 days, followed by 1,000 μg IM monthly. B_{12} levels should be monitored to determine response to treatment. Initial severity and duration of symptoms, and the initial hemoglobin measurements correlate with the residual neurologic damage after cobalamin therapy. This inverse correlation between severity of anemia and neurologic damage is not understood. Neurologic response usually occurs within the first 6 months of therapy, although further improvement may occur with time. No clear evidence indicates that folic acid therapy precipitates or exacerbates B_{12} deficiency-related neuropathy, however, pharmacologic doses of folic acid can reverse the hematologic abnormalities of cobalamin deficiency, masking early recognition of symptoms, therefore, resulting in the development or progression of neurologic symptoms.

CLINICAL RECOMMENDATIONS OF THE VIGNETTE

Based on clinical presentation and borderline B_{12} level, further laboratory tests, including MMA, Hcy, and serum copper levels, were performed on the patient. Copper level was normal, whereas MMA and Hcy levels were elevated. Further testing for antiparietal cell and antiintrinsic factor antibodies were negative. The patient was treated with daily IM injections of 1,000 μg B_{12} for the first week, followed by 1,000 μg monthly injections. His balance improved, although he continued to complain of paresthesias in his feet.

SUMMARY

Myelopathy and peripheral neuropathy are the most common neurologic manifestations of cobalamin deficiency. Early diagnosis and treatment are crucial because the neurologic deficit can be permanent in advanced stages. Elevated levels of methylmalonic acid and homocysteine are a much more sensitive diagnostic clue than a low serum B_{12} level. Food-bound B_{12} malabsorption and pernicious anemia are common causes of vitamin B_{12} deficiency in the elderly. Genetic defects or uncommon conditions, such as recreational use of nitrous oxide, should be considered in younger patients presenting with vitamin B_{12} deficiency. Other conditions mimicking vitamin B_{12} deficiency, especially copper deficiency, should be ruled out.

REFERENCES

1. Pennypacker LC, Allen RH, Kelly JP, et al. High prevalence of cobalamin deficiency in elderly outpatients. *J Am Geriatr Soc.* 1992;40(12):1197–1204.
2. Andres E, Loukili NH, Noel E, et al. Vitamin B_{12} (cobalamin) deficiency in elderly patients. *CMAJ.* 2004;171(3):251–259.
3. Weir DG, Scott JM. The biochemical basis of the neuropathy in cobalamin deficiency. *Baillieres Clin Haematol.* 1995;8(3):479–497.
4. Worrall BB, Rowland LP. Nutritional disorders: malnutrition, malabsorption, and B_{12} and other vitamin deficiencies. In: Rowland LP, ed. *Merritt's Neurology*, 11th ed. Philadelphia: Lippincott, Williams & Wilkins; 2005:1091–1098.
5. Saperstein DS, Wolfe GI, Gronseth GS, et al. Challenges in the identification of cobalamin-deficiency polyneuropathy. *Arch Neurol.* 2003;60(9):1296–1301.
6. Hector M, Burton JR. What are the psychiatric manifestations of vitamin B_{12} deficiency? *J Am Geriatr Soc.* 1988;36:1105–1112.
7. Chavala SH, Kosmorsky GS, Lee MK, et al. Optic neuropathy in vitamin B_{12} deficiency. *Eur J Intern Med.* 2005;16(6):447–448.
8. Saperstein D, Barohn RJ. Neuropathy associated with nutritional and vitamin deficiencies. In: Dyck PJ and Thomas PK, eds. *Peripheral Neuropathy.* Vol. 2. Philadelphia: Elsevier Saunders; 2005:2051–2062.
9. Kumar N, McEvoy KM, Ahlskog JE. Myelopathy due to copper deficiency following gastrointestinal surgery. *Arch Neurol.* 2003;60(12):1782–1785.
10. Di Rocco A, Tagliati M. Remission of HIV myelopathy after highly active antiretroviral therapy. *Neurology.* 2000;55(3):456.

CHAPTER 73

Folic Acid Deficiency

Taruna K. Aurora • Pawan Suri

OBJECTIVES

- To review the epidemiology and population at risk for folic acid deficiency
- To discuss the pathogenesis of folic acid deficiency
- To describe the neurologic manifestations of folate deficiency
- To discuss the management of folic acid deficiency

CASE VIGNETTE

A 75-year-old man presented with depression and progressive decline in cognitive function. His medical history included arterial hypertension, treated with lisinopril, and prostatectomy for benign prostatic hypertrophy. He drinks two to four beers on the weekend. Vital signs and physical examination, including a detailed neurologic assessment are normal. Patient scores an 8 on depression scale and 20 of 30 points on the Mini Mental Status Examination (MMSE). Blood work shows macrocytic anemia and low serum and red blood cell folic acid levels.

EPIDEMIOLOGY

Folic acid deficiency is one of the most common vitamin deficiencies in the United States, largely owing to its association with excessive alcohol intake. It affects 5% of the total US population and pregnant women and the elderly are disproportionately affected. Up to 20% of pregnant women are folate deficient because of a fivefold higher than normal daily requirement for folate during pregnancy. Elderly people may be susceptible to folate deficiency because of social isolation, low intake of leafy vegetables and fruits, and comorbid medical conditions. According to the Department of Health and Social Security Survey, approximately 15% of elderly people living in the community are likely to be deficient in folate. The greatest risk appears to be among low-income populations and those who are institutionalized (1).

PATHOGENESIS

The pathogenesis of folate deficiency as a cause of neuropsychiatric illness is not entirely clear. A defect in methylation processes is one of the proposed mechanisms. Folate deficiency can specifically affect central monoamine metabolism and aggravate depressive disorders. Others suggest that the impact of folate deficiency on cognitive function is related to a vascular mechanism mediated by hyperhomocysteinemia. Both cobalamine and folic acid are required for the metabolism of homocysteine to methionine. As a result, deficiencies in these vitamins can lead to elevations in plasma homocysteine levels, which is a risk factor for development of atherosclerosis and venous thromboembolism (2–4).

ETIOLOGY

The causes of folic acid deficiency include the following:

- Inadequate ingestion of folate-containing foods
- Impaired absorption owing to villous atrophy seen in celiac disease, tropical sprue, or as a part of the aging process
- Impaired metabolism, leading to an inability to utilize absorbed folate, as seen in congenital enzyme deficiencies of folate pathway
- Increased excretion or loss of folate, seen in vitamin B_{12} deficiency. During the course of vitamin B_{12} deficiency, methylene tetrahydrofolic acid (MTHFA) accumulates in the serum, leading to the *folate trap phenomenon.* In turn, much folate filters through the glomerulus and is excreted in the urine. Another mechanism of excess excretion occurs in people with chronic alcoholism who have increased excretion of folate into the bile. Patients having hemodialysis also tend to lose folate during the filtration process.

CLINICAL MANIFESTATIONS AND SPECIAL SITUATIONS

NEURAL TUBE DEFECTS

A well-documented correlation is seen between folate status and intake and the risk of neural tube defects, such as spina bifida and anencephaly, probably because of the increased level of homocysteine. Intervention studies have shown that periconceptional folic acid intake of 400 μg or higher significantly reduces the risks of neural tube defects in the baby. The mechanism whereby folic acid supplementation protects against neural tube defects remains unknown (7–9).

INHERITED DISORDERS OF FOLATE TRANSPORT AND METABOLISM

Inherited disorders of folate transport and metabolism are rare disorders associated with variable and overlapping neurologic presentation. Some clinical manifestations include developmental delay associated with cognitive impairment, motor or gait abnormalities, behavioral or psychiatric symptoms, seizures, demyelinating myelopathy, and neuropathies. The age of onset of the symptoms ranges from the neonatal period to early adult life (10). Some of these disorders are listed below:

- Methylene tetrahydrofolate reductase deficiency
- Functional methyltetrahydrofolate: Homocysteine methyltransferase deficiency
- Glutamine formimotransferase deficiency
- Hereditary folate malabsorption
- Dihydrofolate reductase deficiency

DEPRESSION AND DEMENTIA

In adult patients presenting with megaloblastic anemia owing to folate deficiency, approximately two thirds have neuropsychiatric disorders, which overlap considerably with those associated with anemia caused by vitamin B_{12} deficiency (2). Depression, however is more common in patients with folate deficiency, and subacute combined degeneration of the spinal cord with peripheral neuropathy is more frequent in those with vitamin B_{12} deficiency. The degree of anemia is poorly correlated with the presence of neuropsychiatric disorders, but if these anemias are left untreated, nearly all patients would eventually develop neuropsychiatric complications. Over the past 35 years, numerous studies have shown a direct co-relationship between folate deficiency and depression and cognitive decline in epileptic, neurologic, psychiatric, geriatric, and psychogeriatric populations. Furthermore, recent studies in elderly people suggest a link between folic acid, homocysteine, aging, depression, and dementia, including Alzheimer's disease and vascular disease (5,6).

HYPERHOMOCYSTEINEMIA AND STROKE

An elevated homocysteine level is associated with increased risk of stroke through endothelial cell injury and upregulation of prothrombotic state. Hyperhomocysteinemia can be secondary to deficiency of enzymes responsible for the metabolism of methionine, including deficiency of cystathionine B-synthase, methylcobalamin synthesis, or abnormality in methylene tetrahydrofolate reductase (6). Hyperhomocysteinemia can also be encountered in various conditions, including cigarette smoking, use of oral contraceptives, following methotrexate therapy, and chronic renal insufficiency.

DIAGNOSTIC APPROACH

Folic acid deficiency should be suspected in any patient presenting with macrocytic anemia with symptoms of depression or dementia, especially in patients with seizures on antiepileptic drugs, and in those with history of excessive alcohol use. Ruling out cobalamine deficiency is imperative because treatment with folic acid in the face of vitamin B_{12} deficiency will worsen symptoms. The diagnosis of folate deficiency can be problematic when hematologic manifestations are absent. Some studies suggest that folate deficiency affects the nervous system only at certain not very well-defined critically low concentrations of folic acid or high concentrations of homocysteine.

Serum folate (reference range, 2.5 to 20 ng/mL) and serum cobalamine (reference range, 200 to 900 pg/mL) should be measured as the initial diagnostic tests. Additional follow-up tests include serum homocysteine (reference range, 5 to 16 mmol/L), which is elevated in vitamin B_{12} and folate deficiency, and serum methylmalonic acid (reference range, 70 to 270 mmol/L), which is elevated in B_{12} deficiency only. Red blood cell folate levels (reference range, >40 ng/mL) tend to reflect chronic folate status, whereas serum folate levels reflect acute folate status.

TREATMENT

No clear guidelines exist for the appropriate formulation, dose, or duration of folate therapy for the treatment of nervous system disorders. Folate deficiency is treated with oral folic acid (1 to 5 mg/day) for 1 to 4 months, or until complete hematologic recovery occurs. It is recognized that the response of neuropsychiatric disorders to vitamin therapy is usually much slower when compared with hematologic improvement. The blood–brain barrier limits the entry of folate into the central nervous system, which gets its folate through an active transport system involving methylfolate.

When replacing folate, small doses over the long term may be preferable to larger doses in the short or long term. It is not clear which folate formulation is preferable: Folic acid, folinic acid, or perhaps methylfolate (the transport form across the blood–brain barrier).

In the United States, the US Food and Drug Administration (FDA) has authorized fortification of grains with folic acid to prevent neural tube defects. Large-scale, community-based studies of folate supplementation are needed to explore the potential of the vitamin to prevent mood and cognitive disorders.

CLINICAL RECOMMENDATIONS OF THE VIGNETTE

The patient has megaloblastic anemia, with neurologic symptoms and normal serum vitamin B_{12} levels. Low red cell and plasma folate levels strongly point toward folic acid deficiency. The patient should be given folate replacement therapy and a short course of antidepressants.

SUMMARY

Folate is an important vitamin in the nervous system for all age groups. Folic acid deficiency is associated with a wide spectrum of neurologic and psychological disorders, including neural tube defects in the fetus, developmental delay in children, depression and dementia in adults, and cerebrovascular diseases. Signs of folate deficiency are often subtle, and the condition should be suspected in patients with cognitive impairment, even in the absence of hematologic abnormalities. Although the potential benefit of folic acid supplementation in the prevention of neural tube defects is well established, its role in the prophylaxis of mood disorders and cerebrovascular diseases secondary to hyperhomocysteinemia is yet to be determined in randomized clinical trials.

REFERENCES

1. United States Department of Health and Human Services. Food and drug administration food standards: Amendments of the standards of identify for enriched grain products to require addition of folic acid. *Federal Register.* 1996;61:8781.

2. Reynolds EH. Folic acid, ageing, depression, and dementia. *BMJ.* 2002;324:1512.
3. Bottiglieri T. Folate, vitamin B12, and neuropsychiatric disorders. *Nutr Rev.* 1996;54(12): 382–390.
4. Reynolds EH. Benefits and risks of folic acid to the nervous system. *J Neurol Neurosurg Psychiatry.* 2002;72:567.
5. Bottiglieri T, Laundy M, Crellin R, et al. Homocysteine, folate. Methylation and monamine metabolism in depression. *J Neurol Neurosurg Psychiatry.* 2000;69:228.
6. Selhub J, Jacques PF, Wilson PW, et al. Vitamin status and intake as primary determinants of homocysteinemia in an elderly population. *JAMA.* 1993;270:2693.
7. Mcpartin J, Halligon A, Scott JM, et al. Accelerated folate breakdown in pregnancy. *Lancet.* 1993;341:148.
8. Wald JN, Bower C. Folic acid, pernicious anemia and prevention of neural tube defects. *Lancet.* 1994;343:307.
9. Centers for Disease Control. Recommendations for the use of folic acid to reduce the number of cases of spina bifida and other neural tube defects. *MMWR Morb Mortal Wkly Rep.* 19992;41(RR-14):1.
10. Geller J, Kronn D, Jayabose S, et al. Hereditary folate malabsorption: Family report and review of the literature. *Medicine (Baltimore).* 2002;81:51.

CHAPTER **74**

Parenteral Nutrition and Neurologic Complications

Marielle A. Kabbouche

OBJECTIVES

- To define parenteral nutrition
- To identify the types of parenteral nutrition
- To recognize the neurologic complications associated with parenteral nutrition
- To discuss measures to minimize complications of parenteral nutrition

CASE VIGNETTE

A 56-year-old man had a total pancreatectomy and segmental duodenectomy for a benign pancreatic tumor. At 2 months postoperatively, he was found to be cachectic and was diagnosed with severe malnutrition. He was hospitalized because of nutritional depletion and was started on total parenteral nutrition (TPN). A few days following administration of TPN, he complained of generalized upper and lower extremity weakness, and difficulties breathing. Examination demonstrated generalized muscle weakness and limb hyporeflexia. Sensory examination was unremarkable. Ancillary studies were not contributory except for serum phosphorus level <0.25 mmol/L (normal, 1.12 to 1.45 mmol/L). He was diagnosed with refeeding syndrome.

DEFINITION

Parenteral nutrition (PN), also known as hyperalimentation, is defined as the intravenous administration of a solution of essential nutrients to patients unable to receive oral nutrition because of a variety of critical conditions, which is done to minimize lean body mass loss (1).

PN is generally categorized into partial parenteral nutrition (PPN) when only half of the daily needs are administered intravenously, or TPN.

Indications and benefits of TPN are multiple, including but not limited to surgery among critically ill patients, patients who have had gastrointestinal operations, chronic intestinal disorders (e.g., inflammatory bowel disease, malabsorption syndromes, gastrointestinal fistulas, intestinal occlusion), pancreatic diseases, oncologic or hematologic disorders, and especially those receiving chemotherapy or bone marrow transplant, as well as among elderly and neonates (2).

The two main components of PN are macronutrients and micronutrients (2–3):

1. Macronutrients
   a. Carbohydrates provide, on average, 3.5 to 4 kcal/1 g.
   b. Lipids provide, on average, 9 kcal/1 g.
   c. Amino acids provide, on average, 3 to 6.7 g kcal/1 g.
2. Micronutrients
   d. Electrolytes (sodium, potassium, calcium, magnesium, chloride, and phosphorus)
   e. Oligoelements, including zinc, copper, manganese, chromium, and selenium
   f. Liposoluble and hydrosoluble vitamins (reviewed independently in Chapters 71–73).

COMPLICATIONS OF PARENTERAL NUTRITION

PN can be associated with multiple complications (Table 74-1). Briefly reviewed in this chapter are selective metabolic complications associated with neurologic dysfunction. Most of these complications are preventable and, if diagnosed early and treated aggressively, patients have a better chance for total recovery.

NEUROLOGIC COMPLICATIONS

Despite major improvements in the delivery of PN, technical difficulties are still encountered. Nerve injuries, carotid artery laceration during central line placement with devastating sequelae, such as carotid artery dissection, arterial thrombosis, air embolism, and injury to the brachial plexus, or phrenic nerve injury can occur. Neurologic complications most often occur as the result of metabolic disturbances (4–6). Two main metabolic complications of PN associated with neurologic sequelae are reviewed:

1. Electrolyte imbalance
2. Deficiencies of microelements, especially vitamin deficiencies

TABLE 74-1. Complications Associated with PN

Mechanical	*Infectious*
IMMEDIATE	**INTRALUMINAL**
Arterial or venous puncture	Catheter infection
Catheter malposition	
Pneumohemothorax	**EXTRALUMINAL**
Air embolism	Sepsis
Carotid artery injury	
Horner syndrome	**METABOLIC**
Phrenic nerve paralysis	Electrolyte imbalance
Brachial plexus injury	Vitamin deficiencies
LATE	Oligoelements deficiencies
Obstruction of line	Acidosis or alkalosis
Catheter migration	Cholestasis or hepatic steatosis
Venous thrombosis or thromboembolism	Hyperosmolar nonketotic coma
	Hypo- or hyperglycemia
	Dehydration or fluid overload
	Refeeding syndrome

Electrolyte Imbalances

SODIUM. Any rapid change in serum sodium (Na^+) levels causes a dysfunction in the central nervous system (CNS) by altering the osmotic equilibrium between the brain and body fluids. The typical clinical features are mostly disturbances of cognition and difficulty in arousal. Myoclonus, asterixis, and seizures are common, and are usually refractory to therapy until sodium levels are corrected appropriately. Focality on examination raises suspicions of intracranial hemorrhage, including intraparenchymal or subdural, presumably as a result of brain shrinkage from osmotic changes and tearing of intracranial vessels. Neurologic symptoms can occur with high or low serum sodium levels. These complications are not frequent during PN and may only occur during false calculation of the electrolytic needs or because of an underlying associated pathology. Hypernatremia, a common consequence of dehydration, can occur from inadequate parenteral fluid replacements. Hyponatremia can be associated with a hypoosmolar state caused by fluid loss, impaired hydrogen excretion, and syndrome of inappropriate secretion of antidiuretic hormone (SIADH). Rapid correction of serum sodium by >12 mEq/L/day may lead to the syndrome of osmotic demyelination with central pontine myelinolysis (CPM) and extrapontine myelinolysis (EPM). CPM and EPM have also been reported with slow correction of hyponatremia, particularly following liver transplantation, in alcoholism and malnutrition, in rapid correction of hypernatremia, and with other electrolyte imbalances, including hypokalemia and magnesium administration. The classic clinical presentation of CPM includes spastic quadriplegia, pseudobulbar palsy, and pseudobulbar affect (6,7). The underlying pathogenesis of osmotic demyelination syndrome is not well understood; noninflammatory myelin disruption predominantly involves the central pons; other extrapontine sites can be involved, including the lateral geniculate bodies, cerebellar and cortical white–gray junctions; internal, external, and extreme capsule; thalami, and striatum (7). Characteristic lesions of increased signal intensity on T2 and diffusion-weighted magnetic imaging studies are present in the pons, basal ganglia, and cerebellum. Management is usually supportive.

POTASSIUM. Cardinal manifestations of potassium imbalance are cardiac, with cardiac arrhythmias occurring before any neurologic changes are noticed clinically.

Arrhythmia is the initial clinical picture of hyperkalemia, followed by a rapid, progressive flaccid paralysis, decreased muscle stretch reflexes, and encephalopathy. Unlike hyperkalemia, hypokalemia is more commonly associated with neuromuscular disturbances rather than encephalopathy, with symptoms such as fatigue, myalgia, and paroxysmal weakness (6).

CALCIUM. Hypercalcemia can trigger headaches, agitation, nausea, or encephalopathy. Hypocalcemia can result in increased neuromuscular irritability secondary to a decrease in ionized calcium. Patients usually complain of paresthesias, predominantly perioral and distal numbness. Muscle cramps are common, and may rarely progress to tetany. Both hypo- and hypercalcemia can lead to other neurologic symptoms, including irritability, personality changes, confusion, focal or generalized seizures, hallucinations, and psychosis. Laryngospasm and bronchospasm can also occur and may contribute to respiratory failure (6).

PHOSPHORUS. Changes in phosphorus balance are frequent with PN. They are mostly encountered in the refeeding syndrome, when TPN is administered to patients who are cachectic, including those with poor nutrition secondary to eating disorders such as anorexia nervosa and bulimia (6–8). The mechanism associated with hypophosphatemia is not known; it is thought that anabolism may lead to cellular uptake of phosphate. Hypophosphatemia is associated with skeletal muscle weakness, which can mimic a variety of myopathic or neuromuscular junction disorders, along with pulmonary, cardiac, and hematologic complications. Delirium, seizures, encephalopathy, hallucinations, and peripheral neuropathy may occur.

MAGNESIUM. Magnesium deficiency results in nonspecific clinical neurologic symptoms with peripheral, autonomic, and neuromuscular junction manifestations. CNS and psychiatric involvement is less commonly encountered. Neuropsychiatric symptoms associated with magnesium deficiency include headache, dizziness, acroparesthesias, myalgias, muscle cramps, and anxiety.

Microelements Deficiencies

THIAMINE DEFICIENCY. The most frequent neurologic complication of PN is Wernicke encephalopathy caused by thiamine deficiency. Other conditions associated with Wernicke encephalopathy include alcoholism, hyperemesis gravidarum, starvation, refeeding syndrome after prolonged intravenous feeding, inappropriate PN, anorexia nervosa, hunger strikes, drug treatment for obesity, gastric laceration, pyloric stenosis, gastrointestinal tract malignancies, lymphohemopoietic malignancies, thyrotoxicosis, chronic hemodialysis, and digitalis intoxication. Thiamine plays a role in multiple steps of human metabolism, including anaerobic glycogenesis, Krebs cycle, as well as being a cofactor in multiple steps of the pyruvate transformation. Thiamine deficiency can inhibit pyruvate dehydrogenase, resulting in accumulation of pyruvate, and, as a consequence, shifting the excess of pyruvate into lactate and lactic acid. Daily needs of thiamine in a healthy adult are approximately

2 mg/day. The clinical picture of Wernicke encephalopathy is characterized by a global confusional state, ophthalmoplegia (e.g., nystagmus, VI nerve palsy, conjugate gaze palsy) and a staggering, ataxic gait. Confusion usually occurs days to weeks after PN is started, whereas ophthalmoplegia, a late manifestation of thiamine deficiency, is often associated with truncal ataxia. Other symptoms of thiamine deficiency include hypothermia, hypotension, autonomic changes, acute high cardiac output heart failure, and severe lactic acidosis. MRI of the brain is very helpful in the diagnosis, demonstrating typical signal abnormalities in the periaqueductal gray, dorsomedial thalamus, and mammillary bodies (5,9).

Supplementing TPN with 0.5 to 1 mg/1,000 kcal/day of thiamine (daily adult needs) may prevent the neurologic manifestations of thiamine deficiency. If left untreated, the sequelae are irreversible, rapidly progressing to death. With early treatment, ocular signs usually reverse in a matter of hours in approximately 60% of the patients, and MRI changes disappear in 5 to 6 weeks. Lethargy resolves in few days, whereas gait disturbances are the slowest to recover. Some patients may be left with mild memory impairment.

OLIGOELEMENTS (ZINC, COPPER, MANGANESE, CHROMIUM, AND SELENIUM). Manganese neurotoxicity can be encountered in patients on chronic TPN, and it is associated with neuropsychologic profiles, including frontal and subcortical cognitive impairment, "parkinsonism," bradykinesia, tremor, motor neuropathy, and presence of T1 signal hyperintensities in the basal ganglia on brain MRI. Conversely, manganese deficiency is rarely associated with neurologic dysfunction, mainly seizures (10). Copper deficiency can lead to a chronic progressive spastic ataxic gait with proprioceptive deficits (copper deficiency myeloneuropathy) (11). Patients often have associated anemia, neutropenia, and increased serum zinc levels (12). Selenium, chromium, and zinc are essential trace minerals that are rarely associated with neurologic dysfunction, such as behavioral problems and memory impairment. Other symptoms, such as hyposmia, dysgeusia, and hypogeusia, have also been associated with zinc deficiency (13).

Refeeding Syndrome

Refeeding occurs when malnourished patients resume eating after a period of prolonged starvation. First described among Far East prisoners of war after World War II, the syndrome has been a recognized complication of TPN and feeding. It is more commonly encountered among patients with anorexia nervosa, cancer, and alcoholism, and after gastrointestinal operations (14–15). The physiologic basis of refeeding syndrome is not well understood. This potentially lethal syndrome may result as a consequence of dehydration and rapid repletion of fluid loss with expansion to the extracellular volume and fluid overload, with sudden shift from fat to carbohydrate metabolism. It is associated with electrolyte disorders, especially hypophosphatemia, hypoglycemia, hyperglycemia, and imbalance of trace mineral (8). Thiamine deficiency can also occur. Patients at risk of developing refeeding syndrome should be started at a reduced caloric rate of <50% of estimated requirements, with close follow up by dietitians and nutritionists, and frequent monitoring of serum phosphorus, magnesium, calcium, potassium, urea, and creatinine (8,14–15).

CLINICAL RECOMMENDATIONS OF THE VIGNETTE

The patient had neuromuscular complications caused by severe hypophosphatemia despite phosphorus supplements in the hypocaloric TPN formula. Moderate degrees of hypophosphatemia are commonly found among patients with the refeeding syndromes, mainly among those with malnutrition, resulting in depletion of total body phosphate. When patients received TPN, stimulation of insulin release that follows administration of PN, may contribute to an acute sudden shift of phosphate from the extracellular to the intracellular compartments, resulting in acute generalized muscle weakness. Intravenous supplementation of phosphorus may correct the problem, and should be followed by gradual increase in the rate of TPN administration.

SUMMARY

Patients receiving PN should be examined regularly and monitored closely. Weight measurements and intake and output should be evaluated daily. Regular monitoring of fluid and electrolytes, acid-base balance, and trace elements is essential. Special attention should be paid to avoiding refeeding syndrome among patients at risk.

REFERENCES

1. Dall'Osto H, Simard M, Delmont N, et al. Parenteral nutrition: Indications, modalities and complications: EMC. *Hepato-gastroenterologie.* 2005;2:223–248.
2. Rombeau JL, Caldwell MD, eds. *Clinical Nutrition: Parenteral Nutrition,* 2nd ed. Philadelphia: WB Saunders; 1990.
3. Koretz RL, Lipman TO, Klein S; American Gastroenterological Association. AGA technical review on parenteral nutrition. *Gastroenterology.* 2001;121:970–1001.
4. Wolfe BM, Ryder MA, Nishikawa RA, et al. Complications of parenteral nutrition. *Am J Surg.* 1986;152:93–99.
5. Melchior J. Complications of renutrition. *Ann Med Interne* (Paris). 2000;151:635–643.
6. Btaiche IF, Khalidi N. Metabolic complications of parenteral nutrition in adults, Part 2. *Am J Health Syst Pharm.* 2004;61:2050–2057.
7. Riggs JE. Neurologic manifestations of electrolyte disturbances. *Neurol Clin.* 2002;20: 227–239.
8. Marinella MA. Refeeding syndrome and hypophosphatemia. *Journal of Intensive Care Medicine.* 2005;20:155–159.
9. Attard O, Dietemann JL, Diemunsch P, et al. Wernicke encephalopathy: A complication of parenteral nutrition diagnosed by magnetic resonance imaging. *Anesthesiology.* 2006;105: 847–848.
10. Klos KJ, Chandler M, Kumar N, et al. Neuropsychological profiles of manganese neurotoxicity. *Eur J Neurol.* 2006;13:1139–1141.
11. Tan JC, Burns DL, Jones HR. Severe ataxia, myelopathy, and peripheral neuropathy due to acquired copper deficiency in a patient with history of gastrectomy. *JPEN.* 2006;30: 446–450.
12. Hedera P, Fink JK, Bockenstedt PL, et al. Myelopolyneuropathy and pancytopenia due to copper deficiency and high zinc levels of unknown origin: Further support for existence of a new zinc overload syndrome. *Arch Neurol.* 2003;60:1303–1306.
13. Henkin RI, Schechter PJ, Hoye R, et al. Idiopathic hypogeusia with dysgeusia, hyposmia, and dysosmia. A new syndrome. *JAMA.* 1971;217:434–440.
14. Crook MA, Hally V, Panteli JV. The importance of the refeeding syndrome. *Nutrition.* 2001;17:632–637.
15. Kraft MD, Btaiche IF, Sacks GS. Review of the refeeding syndrome. *Nutr Clin Prac.* 2005;20:625–633.

CHAPTER 75

Enteral Nutrition

Lisa A. Millsap • Gretchen Peyton • Michael J. Schneck

OBJECTIVES

- To identify possible complications of enteral feeding
- To identify uses for copper in the human body
- To describe neurologic symptoms of copper deficiency
- To discuss treatment options for copper deficiency

CASE VIGNETTE

A 62-year-old woman presents to the neurology clinic with gait disturbance, painful toes, and progressive leg weakness she experienced over a period of 4 months. She had a gastrectomy 10 years ago for severe peptic ulcer disease. Her nutritional status has been maintained by the use of enteral feedings via a jejunosotomy tube since the time of her surgery. Neurologic examination shows intact cranial nerve functions, wasting of distal hand muscles, generalized weakness, and muscle stretch hyperreflexia. Plantar reflexes were flexor. Proprioception was impaired bilaterally at the toes. She walked with a wide-based slightly ataxic gait.

Laboratory workup was remarkable for macrocytic anemia and leukopenia. Serum vitamin B_{12} and folate levels were normal. Cerebrospinal fluid (CSF) analysis and magnetic resonance imaging (MRI) studies of the spinal cord and brain were unremarkable. Serum copper level was 2 μmol/L (normal, 11 to 20 μmol/L). Serum ceruloplasmin level was 0.05 mg/L (normal, 0.2 to 0.6 mg/L). The patient was diagnosed with copper-related myeloneuropathy.

DEFINITION

In the strictest sense of the word, enteral feeding refers to any form of nutrition that is given using the digestive tract. Medically speaking, enteral feeding refers to tube feedings given through a variety of different tube types to the digestive tract. These tubes are placed into the stomach, the duodenum, or the jejunum with the preference being that the tube be past the third portion of the duodenum or beyond the ligament of Treitz to decrease the risk of aspiration (1).

EPIDEMIOLOGY

Enteral feedings are indicated in anyone who cannot or will not eat, who have a functional gastrointestinal tract, and in whom a safe form of access can be achieved. Patients with cancer, cerebrovascular disease, trauma, and many other diagnoses may all be excellent candidates for enteral feeding.

Complications of enteral feeding fall into three categories: Gastrointestinal, mechanical, and metabolic (1,2).

Gastrointestinal complications include nausea, vomiting, diarrhea, steatorrhea, inadequate gastric emptying, and malabsorption. These complications are the ones most commonly encountered in patients receiving enteral feedings (2,3). Malabsorption can be blamed for decreased levels of trace minerals (see further discussion in the *Etiology and Pathogenesis* section) (4,5). Many of these complications can be controlled by altering the formula, the timing of feedings, or both, and supplementing nutrients that may be lacking in the enteral formula (1).

Mechanical complications of enteral feeding include transnasal catheter dislocation or obstruction, lower esophageal sphincter incompetence, reflux of gastric contents leading to aspiration pneumonia, and ostomy site drainage leading to skin erosion (1,2). These complications can be minimized by proper (*a*) tube size selection, (*b*) placement, and (*c*) positioning of the patient during feeding (1,2).

Metabolic complications of enteral feeding include fluid and electrolyte imbalances and nutrient deficiencies (2). Pulmonary, hepatic, renal, cardiac, and pancreatic dysfunctions have all been shown to occur when fluid or electrolyte imbalances are present in patients receiving enteral nutrition. For example, hepatic encephalopathy can result if high nitrogen content formulas are used on the context of liver dysfunction. These patients can present with acute confusion, agitation, seizures, and asterixis. In advanced stages, patients can become comatose. Blood tests may show low serum albumin, high serum bilirubin, and elevated serum ammonia levels. Electroencephalographic studies are characterized by diffuse slowing and high-amplitude, low-frequency waves and triphasic waves.

Hypophosphatemia, a rare but potentially lethal complication of the refeeding syndrome, is rarely seen among patients on enteral nutrition. Patients with hypophosphatemia may exhibit hemolytic anemia, altered mental status, seizures, skeletal muscle weakness, and, rarely, abnormal movements, including asterixis. Both hypophosphatemia and hypomagnesemia can also lead to serious cardiac arrhythmias.

A more complete discussion of the metabolic complications of the refeeding syndrome is available in Chapter 74.

Copper is a trace mineral that is incorporated into many essential enzymes in the human body (Table 75-1). These

TABLE 75-1. Copper-dependent Enzymes in Humans

Enzyme	*Biologic Function*
Ceruloplasmin	Oxidation of ferrous iron and hemoglobin synthesis
Copper superoxide dismutase	Oxygen radical scavenger helps protect against oxidative injury
Cytochrome c oxidase	Adenosine triphosphate (ATP) synthesis in mitochondria
Dopamine-β-hydroxylase	Catalyzes conversion of dopamine to norepinephrine
Tyrosinase	Catalyzes tyrosine in the melanin synthesis pathway
Monamine oxidase	Breakdown of catecholamines
Diamine oxidase	Inactivation of histamines and polyamines
Lysyl oxidase	Used in collagen and elastin metabolism
Peptidylglycine-α-amidating monooxygenase	Used in the synthesis of bioactive peptides

enzymes include ceruloplasmin used in iron and copper metabolism; superoxide dismutase, which is an antioxidant; cyctochrome c oxidase used in oxidative phosphorylation; dopamine-β-hydroxylase used in catecholamine synthesis; and tyrosinase used in melanin synthesis (6–8). Hematopoieses and the structure and function of the nervous system are both dependent on enzymes that incorporate copper.

Because of the small daily dietary requirements (RDA 1.2 mg/day) and the almost ubiquitous nature of copper in the environment, copper deficiency is thought to be rare (7). Severe hematologic and neurologic sequelae have been well documented when deficiency does occur (4–6,8–10). Previous gastric surgery or malabsorption predisposes patients to this condition because copper is thought to be absorbed in the stomach and proximal small bowel (4,5,8,10,11). Excessive intake of zinc, iron, phosphorus, and calcium can impede optimal copper absorption. Vitamin C can reduce copper from a cupric state to a less bioavailable cuprous state (12). Individuals who may be at risk for copper deficiency include those with antacid ingestion, nephrosis, malabsorptive disorders, and those receiving long-term enteral nutrition (12–13).

Swayback, a neurologic dysfunction condition secondary to copper deficiency, is well known in ruminant animals (6). This deficiency leads to segmentation of myelin sheaths, with resultant axonal atrophy and destruction (10). Also microcavitation of the white matter is found in both the central and peripheral nervous systems.

The neurologic complications of copper deficiency include severe ataxia, myelopathy, and peripheral neuropathy. The symptomatology resembles subacute combined degeneration of the spinal cord secondary to vitamin B_{12} (cobalamin) deficiency.

Copper deficiency myeloneuropathy can be associated with various hematologic disorders, including macrocytic anemia, neutropenia, and, rarely, panytopenia, especially with overuse of zinc supplementation.

CLINICAL RECOMMENDATIONS OF THE VIGNETTE

The patient was diagnosed with copper deficiency myeloneuropathy and initially was treated with intravenous copper supplementation at a dose of 2 mg of copper sulfate daily. Subsequently, she was maintained on enteral copper supplementation. Within 3 months, she showed improvements in neurologic function.

SUMMARY

Diligent monitoring is necessary in patients receiving long-term enteral nutrition to avoid potential serious complications. Early identification and correction of electrolyte imbalance and supplementation of trace elements, when deficient, are important to avoid potentially devastating and irreversible neurologic complications. Oral intake of a balanced diet should be encouraged as much as possible.

REFERENCES

1. American Gastroenterological Association. American gastroenterological association medical position statement. Guidelines for the use of enteral nutrition. *Gastroenterology.* 1995;108:1280–1301.
2. Cataldi-Betcher EL, Seltzer, MH, Slocum BA, et al. Complications occurring during enteral nutrition support: A prospective study. *JPEN.* 1983;7:546–552.
3. Rombeau JL, Barot LR. Enteral nutritional therapy. *Surg Clin North Am.* 1981;61:605–620.
4. Kumar N, Low PA. Myeloneuropathy and anemia due to copper malabsorptiom. *J Neurol.* 2004; 251:747–749.
5. Hayton BA, Broome HE, Lilenbaum RC. Copper deficiency-induced anemia and neutropenia secondary to intestinal malabsorption. *Am J Hematol.* 1995:48:45–47.
6. Kumar N, Crum B, Petersen R, et al. Copper deficiency myelopathy. *Arch Neurol.* 2004;61:762–766.
7. Tapiero H, Townsend DM, Tew KD. Trace elements in human physiology and pathology: Copper. *Biomed Pharmacother.* 2003;57:386–398.
8. Kumar N, Gross JB, Ahlskog JE. Copper deficiency myelopathy produces a clinical picture like subacute combined degeneration. *Neurology.* 2004;63:33–39.
9. Gregg XT, Reddy V, Prchal JT. Copper deficiency masquerading as myelodyplaastic syndrome. *Blood.* 2002;100:1493–1495.
10. Tan JC, Burns DL, Jones HR. Severe ataxia, myelopathy, and peripheral neuropathy due to acquired copper deficiency in a patient with history of gastrectomy. *JPEN.* 2006;30: 446–450.
11. Everett CM, Matharu M, Gawler J. Neuropathy progressing to myeloneuropathy 20 years after partial gastrectomy. *Neurology.* 2006;66:1451.
12. Groff JL, Gropper SS. Microminerals. In: Graham L, ed. Advanced Nutrition and Human Metabolism. Boston: Wadsworth; 2000;12:430–434.
13. Gottschlich MM. Monitoring home and other alternate site nutrition support. In: Gottschlich MM, ed. *The Science and Practice of Nutrition Support: A Case-Base Core Curriculum.* Silver Spring, MD: American Society for Parenteral and Enteral Nutrition, 2001;35:736.

PART X Endocrine Diseases

CHAPTER 76

Pituitary and Hypothalamus

Jorge C. Kattah • William C. Kattah

OBJECTIVES

- To discuss the signs and symptoms of common disorders of the hypothalamus
- To discuss the signs and symptoms of pituitary gland and sellar tumors and inflammatory disorders
- To present the endocrine, visual, and oculomotor findings encountered in lesions of the hypothalamus and the pituitary
- To describe an up-to-date workup and protocol management of lesions involving the hypothalamus and pituitary

CASE VIGNETTE 1

A 5-month-old baby was referred for evaluation of poor vision; she was neither fixating nor following visual stimuli. She had acquired all expected developmental milestones to date and had normal growth. The light reflex was present in the left eye and absent in the right, without afferent pupil defect. Bilateral hypoplastic optic nerves were found on ophthalmoscopic examination.

CASE VIGNETTE 2

A 19-year-old female college student presented with painless, binocular loss of vision of 3-month duration, left more than right. In addition, she had a 1-year history of amenorrhea, and increased ring and shoe size. Moreover, she was unable to lose weight and had observed coarsening of her facial features. Her father had a prolactinoma that had been treated successfully. On examination, she had a visual acuity (VA) of 20/20 in the right eye and 20/200 in the left, a left temporal hemianopia, and a right superotemporal quadrantopia, normal ophthalmoscopic examination. She also had large hands and feet.

DEFINITION

The *hypothalamus* is located beneath the thalamus and bounded anteriorly by the lamina terminalis and the optic chiasm; posteriorly by the mamillary bodies; and laterally by the optic tracts. It weighs 4 g. The *pituitary gland* is housed within the anatomic confines of the sella turcica and measures 0.6 to 0.8 g in the adult: It is composed of the anterior adenohypophysis and the posterior neurohypophysis. The lateral adenohypophysis contains cells secreting growth hormone (GH) and prolactin and the medial adenohypophysis secretes the thyroid-stimulating hormone (TSH), the follicle-stimulating hormone (FSH), the luteinizing hormone (LH), and the adrenocorticotropic hormone (ACTH).

The *hypothalamus* contains neurons that regulate homeostasis and control blood pressure, body temperature, heart rate, blood osmolarity, water and food intake, and circadian rhythms. It exerts an influence on the endocrine systems by synthesis and release of peptides that regulate secretion of hormones from the pituitary, which in turn, control target glandular secretion; it modifies the activity of the autonomic nervous system in response to environmental changes and receives projections from the limbic system and the cerebral cortex concerned with motivation and drive. Table 76-1 summarizes the hypothalamic-pituitary function.

The anterior pituitary gland releases its peptides into the circulation via the pituitary portal system, thus reaching all target glands. Neurons of the supraoptic and paraventricular nuclei synthesize and transport both the antidiuretic hormone (ADH) and oxytocin to the neurohypophyisis.

EPIDEMIOLOGY

Clinically eloquent hypothalamic lesions, by definition, must be bilateral. The most common endocrinopathy in children involving the hypothalamus and pituitary gland include septo-optic dysplasia (1), Russell diencephalic syndrome (failure to thrive) (2), and precocious puberty (3). Common childhood neoplasms in this region include craniopharyngiomas, Rathke cleft cysts, germinomas, teratomas and gliomas of the optic nerve or chiasm, and hypothalamus. The latter represent 30% of all tumors in children under age 5 years and 70% under age 10 years.

In adults, hypothalamic dysfunction is frequently the result of compression exerted by pituitary tumors, meningiomas, craniopharyngiomas, metastatic tumors, and aneurysms; it is also a target of inflammatory, granulomatous, and infectious lesions. Additional causes can include head injury and the effect of therapeutic cranial irradiation; the most common neoplasms to be found in this location in adults include pituitary adenomas (10% to 15% of all intracranial tumors) occurring between ages 30 and 50 years. Craniopharyngiomas are frequently found in children (about half of the cases); however, not infrequently, they become first symptomatic in adults, even in late decades of life.

TABLE 76-1. Function of Hypothalamus

Function	*Description*
Food intake and feeding behavior	• Ventromedial nucleus: Satiety
Temperature regulation	• Anterior hypothalamus: Raises thermostat set point • Heat conservation: Vasoconstriction/increased heat production • Posterior hypothalamus: Generates heat–dissipation adaptation
Sleep-wake cycle	• Lesions anterior hypothalamus: Insomnia/agitation • Posterior hypothalamus lesions: Hypersomnolence
Memory/behavior	• Mammillary body and ventromedial hypothalamic lesion: Korsakoff syndrome • Ventromedial lesions cause rage reactions • Lateral hypothalamic lesions cause apathy
Thirst	• Supraoptic paraventricular nuclei control production of vasopressin but also has primary osmoreceptors
Autonomic regulation	• Anterior hypothalamus: Parasympathetic • Posterior hypothalamus: Sympathetic

ETIOLOGY AND PATHOGENESIS

Abnormalities in fetal central nervous system (CNS) development account for the variable clinical spectrum of septo-optic dysplasia. In milder forms, a diagnosis is made in adult life. The diencephalic syndrome is often the result of a low grade optic nerve-chiasm-hypothalamic glioma, which is likely related to the absence of a tumor suppressor gene in chromosome 17, not infrequently found among patients with neurofibromatosis (NF). NF1 is inherited as an autosomal dominant trait (4), occasionally among patients with NF-2 as well. Precocious puberty can be the result of an increased production of testosterone related to germ cell tumors, choriocarcinoma, or from secretion of gonadotrophin-releasing factors. Pituitary adenomas can arise from mutation of single pituitary cells or from hyperstimulation resulting from hypothalamic dysregulation; they are often isolated, but can occur as a component of the multiple endocrine neoplasm syndrome types 1 and 2. Craniopharyngiomas represent 3% of all intracranial tumors thought to originate from remnants of Rathke pouch.

PATHOLOGY

Congenital malformations of the visual pathways in septo-optic dysplasia are associated with different degrees of visual pathway and diencephalic formation as well as cerebral midline deformities (1–3). Most neoplasms under consideration in this region are not malignant. Optic gliomas represent benign, juvenile pilocytic astrocytomas that contain eosinophilic Rosenthal fibers in the absence of necrosis or mitotic figures.

Pituitary adenomas are benign epithelial neoplasms that can be classified by their size (microadenomas, <10 mm and macroadenomas >10 mm), their staining characteristics as acidophilic (GH secreting), basophilic (ACTH), and cromophobic, but they are more precisely identified by their immunostaining characteristics (5). Craniopharyngiomas are calcified cystic tumors of epithelial origin. The remaining tumors in this region will have specific characteristics that allow pathologic recognition. In adults, metastatic disease to the sella and pituitary/hypothalamic region occur with relative frequency (6).

Sarcoidosis and inflammatory lesions can also be found (7). In lymphocytic hypophysistis, lymphocytes infiltrate the pituitary gland (8). Histiocytic infiltration of the hypothalamus represents an idiopathic proliferation of histiocytes, eosinophiles, and plasma cells; depending on their uni- or multifocality, they are classified as *eosinophilic granuloma* and *Hand-Schuller-Christian disease.* The more aggressive form with multiorgan involvement is known as *Letterer-Siwe disease* (9).

CLINICAL MANIFESTATIONS

HYPOTHALAMIC LESIONS

Possible clinical manifestations of hypothalamic lesions are summarized in Table 76-1. In children, two principal clinical endocrine syndromes are seen: Failure to thrive (Russell diencephalic syndrome) and precocious puberty in combination with visual impairment (Table 76-2). Russell diencephalic syndrome, which usually begins between the newborn period and 4 years of age, consists of emaciation, hyperkinesis, and euphoria with preservation of linear growth (2). In both septo-optic dysplasia and gliomas in this region, central or bitemporal visual field defects and nystagmus can occur. Pendular seesaw nystagmus is a frequent finding in the glioma group. Precocious

TABLE 76-2. Common Hypothalamic Syndromes

Syndrome	*Symptom(s)*
Russell's diencephalic syndrome	• Emaciation • Hyperkinesis • Euphoria • Preservation of linear growth
Septo-optic dysplasia	• Visual loss • Nystagmus • Pituitary insufficiency • Seizures • Variable degrees of mental retardation
Precocious puberty	
Hyperprolactinemia	• Polyglandular insufficiency • Hypersomnolence • Obesity • Diabetes insipidus • Impaired thermoregulation

puberty is more frequent in boys who are taller and have premature sexual maturation (3). Mental retardation and gelastic seizures can be seen with tuber cinereum hamartomas (10).

Common hypothalamic endocrinopathies are summarized in Table 76-2 and include (*a*) moderate hyperprolactinemia secondary to diminished or absent prolactin inhibitory factor (dopamine) with amenorrhea, galactorrhea, and sterility in women and decreased libido and impotence in men; (*b*) polyglandular insufficiency caused by decreased or absent hypothalamic releasing factors; (*c*) altered circadian rhythms with hypersomnolence and secondary narcolepsy; (*d*) altered satiety sensation leading to obesity; (*e*) diabetes insipidus (DI); and (*f*) impaired thermoregulation. In addition, visual loss secondary to optic nerve, chiasm, and optic tract compression are frequently found.

The endocrine manifestations of *pituitary tumors* depend on their functional status. The most common hypersecreting tumor is the prolactinoma (11), followed by GH (12) secreting tumors. ACTH (13), TSH, and LH or FSH tumors are less common. Nonfunctional adenomas represent 25% to 30% of all pituitary tumors. The clinical symptoms and signs of the pituitary endocrine syndromes are summarized in Table 76-3. Pierre Marie, a neurologist from the Salpetriere Hospital in Paris and a disciple of Charcot, was the first to identify a pituitary mass in a patient with acromegaly. Years later, Harvey Cushing, a Johns Hopkins neurosurgeon, first described the syndrome that bears his name in a patient with a pituitary tumor. Hypersecreting adenomas usually announce themselves by their endocrine manifestations (Table 76-2). In contrast, nonfunctioning adenomas cause symptoms related to suprasellar or lateral sellar extension with visual or oculomotor symptoms, respectively (14). Whereas DI is a common syndrome in hypothalamic lesions, pituitary tumors before surgery are not associated with DI (15). Hypopituitarism may be the presenting syndrome in 61% of nonfunctioning or null cell adenomas.

Typical chiasmal compression by pituitary tumors results in bitemporal hemianopsia; however, other visual field defects, including unilateral temporal depression, a monocular central defect with contralateral temporal heminopsia, and, less frequently, incongruous, homonymous visual field defects caused by optic tract compression may be found. Symptoms are usually indolent; however, 2% will present in an abrupt manner, as a result of intratumor bleeding with rapid expansion (pituitary apoplexy) (16). Table 76-3 represents a serial endocrine protocol to evaluate pituitary function.

DIAGNOSTIC APPROACH

A thorough physical evaluation will uncover physical findings that are suggestive of specific endocrinopathies. Failure to thrive with normal linear growth in a child, precocious puberty, gigantism and acromegaly, Cushing's syndrome, gynecomastia, galactorrhea, and hypogonadism are all possible symptoms suggestive of hypothalamic/pituitary dysfunction. Acute hypotension and shock in pituitary apoplexy, adrenal insufficiency, and hypothyroidism may also be seen. Arterial hypertension in acromegaly, hyperthyroidism, and Cushing syndrome are commonly encountered. Cutaneous hyperpigmentation in Nelson syndrome, skin lesions in neurofibromatosis, and myxedema in hypothyroidism underscore the importance of a careful physical examination in the evaluation of this group of patients.

A detailed ophthalmologic evaluation with VA, color vision, ocular pressure, pupillary responses, visual fields, and oculomotor and fundoscopic examinations may yield specific localizing findings to the optic chiasm and tract that will direct the examiner in the sequence of imaging studies required (Table 76-4).

A comprehensive metabolic panel may show hypernatremia secondary to DI, hyponatremia without hyperkalemia and hypoglycemia in secondary adrenal insufficiency, and hyperglycemia in Cushing's syndrome. Increased lipids in hypothyroidism, an endocrine evaluation to detect hypopituitarism, pituitary hypersecretion, or both, should be implemented The initial basic tests should include a serum prolactin level, which may be significantly elevated in prolactinomas ($>250\ \mu g/L$). Pituitary stalk compression by a large pituitary adenoma and other causes of hyperprolactemia would not increase levels beyond this range. Additionally, morning serum cortisol, TSH, T4, LH, and FSH; estradiol in women, and testosterone in men, should be obtained. Low levels and even normal levels in some instances would be consistent with hypopituitarism. If a diagnosis of acromegaly is suspected, baseline GH and insulinlike growth factor (IGF-1) should be obtained and repeated after a 75-g oral glucose load, which would be expected to decrease GH <2 ng/mL. If Cushing's syndrome is suspected, an overnight dexamethasone suppression test with a morning cortisol level of $<5\ \mu g/mL$ should be present; an elevation of the serum level points to ACTH hypersecretion. A more thorough 2-day suppression test may be performed if the initial test finding is negative. Rarely, petrosal or cavernous sinus ACTH levels may be needed for tumor lateralization (13).

Evaluation of hypothalamic function includes serum levels of thyroid, cortisol, Estradiol, or testosterone. In hypothalamic dysfunction, lack of compensatory elevation of pituitary hormone levels and normal response to their exogenous administration is found. GH can be decreased with abnormal growth, but normal response to GH-releasing factor. Prolactin may be elevated given absence or diminution of hypothalamic dopamine. DI may be suspected by the presence of dehydration, serum hyperosmolarity, and low urinary osmolarity in the absence of renal disease. Other functions of the hypothalamus are difficult to test clinically. Polysomnography and multiple sleep latency testing (MSLT) may be required in hypersomnolent patients; shortened MSLT values are frequently found in hypothalamic narcolepsy and low levels of cerebrospinal fluid (CSF) hypocretin have been reported (17).

Neuroimaging testing should be obtained. The test of choice is a pre- and postcontrast-enhanced thin section sellar magnetic resonance imaging (MRI) (1 or 2 mm). Pre- and postcontrast, multiplanar computed tomographic (CT) scan may also be obtained. Specific imaging characteristics in the context of clinical, ophthalmologic, and endocrine signs allow a precise diagnosis before resection or medical management of the lesion.

TREATMENT

Congenital hypothalamic lesions are usually associated with hypopituitarism and the associated endocrinopathy responds well to treatment. Management of optic nerve-chiasm-hypothalamic gliomas is careful observation. In the absence of well-documented tumor growth, no need exists for specific

TABLE 76-3. Endocrinopathy: Algorithm for Evaluation of Patients with Endocrine Syndromes Related to Pituitary Tumor

*Hyperprolactinemia**,**		*Gigantisim**,** *Acromegally*		*Cushing's Syndrome**,**		*Hypopituitarism**,**		*Diabetes Insipidus**,**	
Male	Female	Labs	Imaging	Labs	Imaging	Labs	Imaging	Labs	Imaging
Galactorrhea*,**	Galactorrhea	Baseline GH & IGF – 1	Thin section MRI of Sella	Baseline cortisol ACTH	Thin section MRI of Sella	AM & PM cortisol	Thin section MRI of Sella	Serum osmolarity	Thin section MRI of Sella
		Post 75 g opal glucose load GH & IGF – 1		Dexamethasone suppression Test		T3 & T4		Urine osmolarity	
Decreased libido Hypogonadism	Amenorrhea Sterility	TSH*,**		Two-day suppression test if #2 is negative		Testosterone		Respense to intranasal vasopressin	
				Petrosal or cavernous sinus cortisol if #2 & 3 are negative		Estradiol			
Impotence		Prolactin** FSH/LH**				CMP			
Labs	Imaging								
Serum prolactin level	Thin section MRI of the Sella	ACTH**							

*All patients should have a neurophthalmology evaluation.
**All patients should have all pituitary hormones tested.

TABLE 76-4. Algorithm for Evaluation of Patients with Visual and Neurologic Symptoms Related to Pituitary Tumors

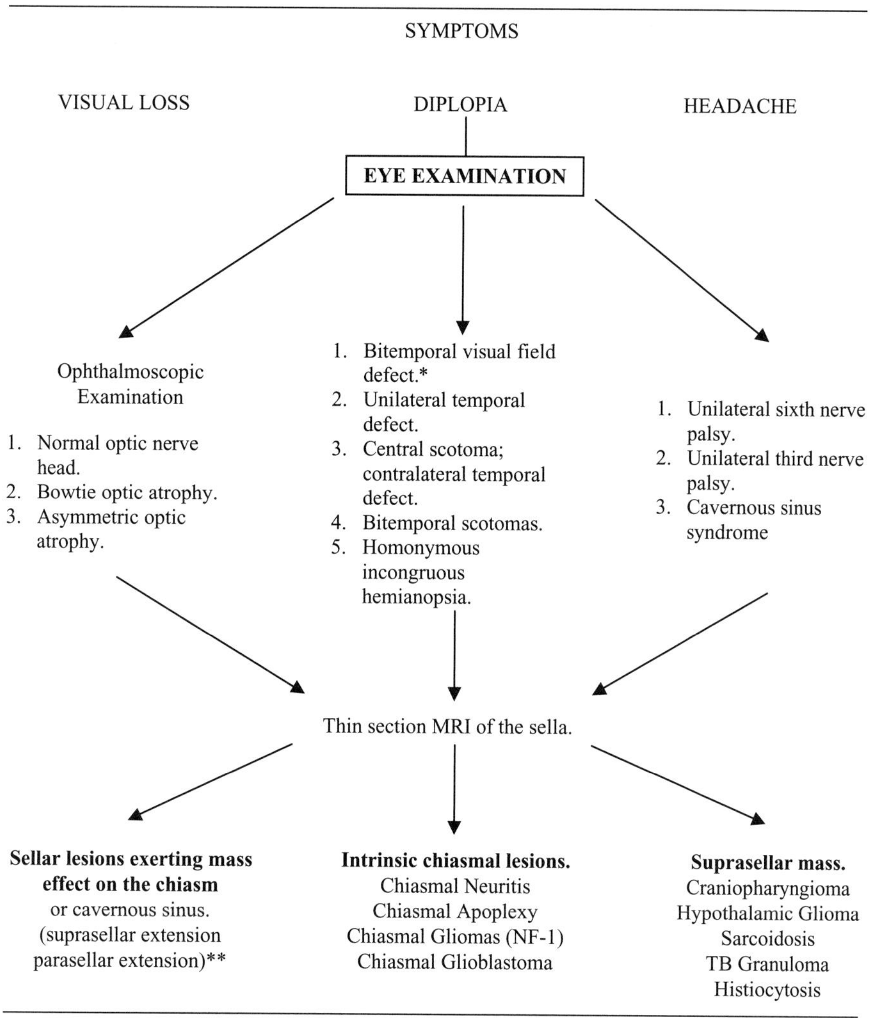

*Most common visual field defect.
**Most frequent: pituitary macroadenomas and meningiomas.

intervention. Radiotherapy can be used with good results if the tumor is growing. Symptomatic treatment of the associated endocrine and systemic abnormalities should be implemented. Tuber cinereum hamartomas associated with increased secretion of luteinizing hormone-releasing hormone (LHRH), precocious puberty, and gelastic seizures are generally managed conservatively with hormonal suppression therapy and anticonvulsants. Generally, surgery is not indicated, unless the lesion is growing with attendant complications.

Nonsecreting pituitary adenomas are usually large when first detected and associated with visual loss and eye movement abnormalities. Transphenoidal resection provides excellent results (14,18). Transnasal endoscopic resection has been used successfully as well (19). In patients with large tumors, a transcranial or staged combined transphenoidal–transcranial resection may be needed, with greater risk for complications. Residual, nonresectable pituitary tumors may require postsurgical irradiation (5,000 cGy, in fractions of <200 cGy) (20). Gamma knife radiation has overcome initial reservations about visual pathway toxicity and may become the radiotherapy modality of choice (21).

Secreting pituitary adenomas can be treated with medication; dopaminergic therapy in the case of prolactinomas is generally effective; large tumors with significant chiasmal compression and visual loss usually respond well to treatment. Bromocriptine and a long-acting dopamine agonist (cabergoline) can be used; nausea and vomiting can be a significant, dose-related complication (11,22). *GH secreting adenomas* can be treated with a combination of surgical resection, irradiation, and postsurgical somatostatin-analogs (octreotide) (12,23). A cure is considered when the levels of GH $<2\ \mu g/L$. Adenomas associated with Cushing's syndrome are generally microadenomas and should be resected. Cortisol levels are normalized within 1 to 2 years after resection. In the interim, metyrapone, aminoglutethimide, and ketacononazole can be used, because they inhibit adrenal cortisol synthesis. In unusual circumstances, dopamine agonists and octreotide could be used. Adrenalectomy does not change the size of pituitary tumor mass and involves the risk of Nelson syndrome. *TSH-secreting tumors*, which are uncommon, can be treated with a combination of transphenoidal resection and radiotherapy. Octreotide has been used successfully in this setting to improve visual field defects. *FSH-secreting tumors* are also unusual and found more frequently in middle-aged men. Transsphenoidal surgery is indicated. Octreotide has also been used with success in this setting.

Whereas large mass lesions in the pituitary region, with exception of prolactinomas, should be resected, if the lesion involves the hypothalamus and the diagnosis remains uncertain after a workup is complete, a biopsy should be obtained for treatment guidance. Pertaining to craniopharyngiomas, the size of the tumor and degree of suprasellar extension and presence of a cystic component or hydrocephalus mandate the surgical staging and extent of the resection. Generally, conservative resections followed by radiation are recommended for adult patients and complete resection for children, given the potential for radiation toxicity (24–28). Meningiomas in this region are ideally resected and a transcranial or combined transsphenoidal–transcranial approach is used. Aneurysms compressing the visual pathways or hypothalamus can be treated with clipping or endovascular occlusion. Germinomas can be resected partially with postsurgical irradiation. Sarcoid granulomas are treated with corticosteroids and steroid-sparing immunosuppressant. Lymphocytic hypophysitis respond well to steroids. Histiocytosis can be treated with a combination of surgery, irradiation, chemotherapy, and immunosuppression. Tuberculosis is treated with the usual antituberculous therapy, steroids, and, in select cases, surgical lysis of adhesions. In cysticercosis, corticosteroids and praziquantel or albendazole can be used.

CLINICAL RECOMMENDATIONS OF THE VIGNETTES

CASE VIGNETTE 1

The presence of bilateral optic nerve hypoplasia in this 5-month-old baby should raise the question of septo-optic dysplasia. Careful cerebral and orbit imaging and endocrine evaluation, should be obtained. A head MRI showed bilateral optic nerve and chiasmal hypoplasia, absent septum pellucidum, small pituitary gland with an ectopic posterior pituitary at the base of the pituitary stalk, and a narrow open lip schizencephaly in the left frontal lobe with normal corpus callosum. Endocrine evaluation showed diminished morning and afternoon cortisol levels, normal TSH and T4, and increased prolactin levels: 49.4 ng/mL (normal, 1.6 to 23.1). The patient is currently on steroids and is followed closely in anticipation of potential developmental and neurologic complications.

CASE VIGNETTE 2

The patient described symptoms and had signs suggestive of a GH-secreting macroadenoma, with suprasellar extension and compression of the optic chiasm. Besides the initial neurophthalmologic examination, endocrine evaluation and pre- and postcontrast, thin-section, multiplanar imaging of the brain is required. A head MRI, in fact, showed a pituitary tumor with suprasellar extension and compression of the chiasm. An endocrinologic evaluation showed a baseline GH level of 375.4 ng/mL (normal <7), slightly increased prolactin of 35.4 ng/mL (normal, 0.5 to 18), increased somatomedin (IGF-1) to 993 (normal, 182 to 780), increased cortisol, and normal T4. Transphenoidal resection was performed. An acidophilic adenoma stained immunologically positive against GH and had positive foci against TSH, FSH, and LH. Following surgery, she was treated with octreotide; the neurophthalmologic examination normalized and the acromegaly resolved within the ensuing year. Serial follow-up in the last 3 years demonstrated a small residual nongrowing tumor.

SUMMARY

For the clinician, familiarity with the neurologic complications of hypothalamic or pituitary disorders is critical. The translation between neurologic responses to the environment and the autonomic nervous system adjustment required takes place within these structures. This chapter provides an organized approach to the diagnosis and management of lesions or dysfunction of the hypothalamic–pituitary axis.

REFERENCES

1. Hoyt WF, Kaplan SL, Grumbach MM, et al. Septo-optic dysplasia and pituitary dwarfism. *Lancet.* 1970;1:893–894.
2. Russell A. A diencephalic syndrome of emaciation in infancy and childhood. *Arch Dis Child.* 1951;26:274.
3. Poussaint TY, Barnes PD, Nichols K, et al. Diencephalic syndrome: Clinical features and imaging findings. *AJNR.* 1997;18:1499–1505.
4. Ragge NK. Clinical and genetic patterns of neurofibromatosis 1 and 2. *Br J Ophthalmol.* 1993;77:662–672.
5. Kovacs K, Horvath E. Pathology of pituitary tumors. *Endocrinol Metab Clin North Am.* 1987;16:529–551.
6. Kattah JC, Silgals R, Manz H, et al. Presentation and management of parasellar and suprasellar metastasic mass lesions. *J Neurol Neurosurg Psychiatry.* 1985;48:44–49.
7. Winnacker JL, Becker KL, Katz S. Endocrine aspects of sarcoidosis. *N Engl J Med.* 1968;278:427–434; 483–492.
8. Honegger J, Fahlbusch R, Bornemann A, et al. Lymphocytic and granulomatous hypophysitis: Experience with nine cases. *Neurosurgery.* 1997;40:713–723.
9. Tibbs PA, Challa V, Mortara RH. Isolated histiocytosis X of the hypothalamus. Case Report. *J Neurosurg.* 1978;49:929–934.
10. Burton EM, Ball WS, Crane K. Hamartomas of the tuber cinereum: Comparison of MRI and CT findings in 4 cases. *AJNR.* 1989;10:497–502.
11. Schlechte JA. Clinical practice: Prolactinoma. *N Engl J Med.* 2003;349:2035–2041.
12. Sheppard MC. Primary medical therapy for acromegaly. *Clin Endocrinol (Oxf).* 2003;58: 387–399.
13. Orth DN. Cushing's syndrome. *N Engl J Med.* 1995;332:791–803.
14. Ebersold MJ, Quast LM, Laws ER, et al. Long-term results in transphenoidal removal of nonfunctioning pituitary adenomas. *J Neurosurg.* 1986;64:713–719.
15. Maghnie M, Cosi G, Genovese E, et al. Central diabetes insipidus in children and young adults. *N Engl J Med.* 2000;343:998–1007.
16. Bills DC, Meyer FB, Laws ER, et al. A retrospective analysis of pituitary apoplexy. *Neurosurgery.* 1993;33:602–608.
17. Culebras A. Update on idiopathic narcolepsy and the symptomatic narcolepsies. *Rev Neurol Dis.* 2005;4:203–210.
18. Trautmann JC, Laws ER. Visual status after transphenoidal surgery at the Mayo Clinic. *Am J Ophthalmol.* 1983;96:200–208.
19. Sheehan MT, Atkinson JL, Kasperbauer JL, et al. Preliminary comparison of the endoscopic transnasal vs the sublabial transseptal approach for clinically nonfunctioning pituitary macroadenomas. *Mayo Clin Proc.* 1999;74:661–670.
20. Halberg FE, Sheline GE. Radiotherapy of pituitary tumors. *Endocrinol Metab Clin North Am.* 1987;16:667–684.
21. Sheehan JP, Kondziolka D, Flickinger J, et al. Radiosurgery for residual or recurrent nonfunctioning pituitary adenoma. *J Neurosurg.* 2002;97:408–414.
22. Bevan JS, Webster J, Burke CW, et al. Dopamine agonists and pituitary tumor shrinkage. *Endocr Rev.* 1992;13:220–240.
23. Mahmoud-Ahmed AS, Suh JH, Mayberg MR. Gamma knife radiosurgery in the management of patients with acromegaly: A review. *Pituitary.* 2001;4:223–230.
24. Kennedy HB, Smith RJ. Eye signs in craniopharyngioma. *Br J Opthalmol.* 1975;59:689–695.
25. Repka MX, Miller NR, Miller M. Visual outcome after surgical removal of cranipharyngiomas. *Ophthalmology.* 1989;96:195–199.
26. Savino PJ, Paris M, Schatz NJ, et al. Optic track syndrome. A review of 21 patients. *Arch Ophthalmol.* 1978;96:656–663.
27. Fischer EG, Welch K, Shillito J, et al. Craniopharyngiomas in children. Long term effects of conservative surgical procedures combined with radiation therapy. *J Neurosurg.* 1990;73:534–540.
28. Manaka S, Teramoto A, Takakura K. The efficacy of radiotherapy for craniopharyngioma. *J Neurosurg.* 1985;62:648–656.

CHAPTER 77

Thyroid Dysfunction

Jorge C. Kattah • William C. Kattah

OBJECTIVES

- To describe the neurologic manifestations of hyperthyroidism in adults and children
- To describe the neurologic manifestations of hypothyroidism in adults and children
- To discuss the pathogenesis of these disorders, as they are relevant to their diagnosis and management

The thyroid hormones have a role in the growth and maturation of tissues, cellular respiration, and energy metabolism. The target of action in the cell is the thyroid hormone receptor complex within mitochondria, plasma membranes, and endoplasmic reticulum. There are two known cellular receptors, each encoded by a different gene and named alpha and beta. The secretion of thyroid hormone is regulated by the pituitary gland (thyroid-stimulating hormone [TSH]), which is in turn regulated by a hypothalamic peptide (thyrotropin-releasing hormone [TRH]) by a negative feedback mechanism.

Given the aforementioned role of the thyroid hormone in cellular metabolism, it is clear that disorders affecting the thyroid gland will involve every tissue in the body; those organs with a high metabolic demand will be affected to a greater extent; thus, the brain, peripheral nervous system, and muscle will be significantly symptomatic. In this chapter, are reviewed the neurologic manifestations of thyroid disorders, derived from both hyper- or hypothyroidism. Table 77-1 summarizes the most common neurologic syndromes found with thyroid gland dysfunction.

Hyperthyroidism

CASE VIGNETTE

A 36-year-old woman presents with a history of discomfort in the left eye. She has noticed a change in the appearance of her eye in the past few weeks. She does not have any other complaints in a thorough review of systems. Examination disclosed asymmetry of the palpebral fissures; the left was wider, with a decreased blinking rate and lid lag in down gaze. Exophthalmometry measured 2 mm of proptosis in the left eye and no evidence of ophthalmoplegia. The neurologic, physical, and the rest of the ophthalmologic evaluation were normal. A presumptive diagnosis of thyroid-associated ophthalmopathy (TAO) was made and workup was initiated. This case raises a question frequently found regarding the association between TAO and systemic, subclinical hyperthyroidism.

The etiologic classification of thyrotoxicosis and hyperthyroidism is listed in Table 77-1, which involves the possibilities of an abnormal thyroid stimulator (Graves disease and trophoblastic tumors), thyroid autonomy (adenoma and toxic multinodular goiter), increased hormone storage (subacute and chronic thyroiditis, including Hashimoto's), extrathyroid hormone sources, and ectopic thyroid tissue. Regardless of the source of thyrotoxicosis, most patients will present with similar overt neurologic symptoms and signs. Graves disease is discussed first. It is important to mention that goiters may be associated with hyper- and hypothyroidism as well as an euthyroid state.

DEFINITION

Graves disease has an approximate incidence of 3 cases per 100,000 in men and 16 per 100,000 in women. A bimodal age peak is seen in both sexes in the 40s and 60s. In men, the peak is about 5 years later than women. Risk factors include age, gender, and smoking. A genetic predisposition coupled with an environmentally triggered autoimmune disorder is a likely theoretical pathogenesis. Both HLA antigen (DR, B8 and DW) and genetic mapping in some patients to a location in chromosome 14, which encodes the TSH receptor, confers increased susceptibility to this disorder.

ETIOLOGY AND PATHOGENESIS

Both humoral and cell-mediated immunity are involved in the pathogenesis. The dysimmune process consists of binding antibodies against the thyroid, which increases their activity and causes hyperthyroidism. Not infrequently, thyroid disease is associated with prominent ocular signs: TAO, and it is possible that an antigenic similarity between tissues in the orbit and thyroid explain this common association (see Chapter 136). Recently, a mitochondrial protein, G2s, has been cloned, which may be the candidate cross-reactive molecule (1). It is important to mention that patients with Graves disease are frequently thyroperoxidase (formerly known as antimicrosomal) antibody positive, suggestive of coexistent Hashimoto's thyroiditis. Other causes of hyperthyroidism and their pathogenic mechanism are listed in Table 77-1.

TABLE 77-1. Hyperthyroidism and Hypothyroidism: Neurologic Complications of Thyroid Disorders

Central Nervous System (CNS)	*Peripheral and Cranial Nerves*	*Muscle*
HYPERTHYROIDISM		
Tremor	Compression of recurrent laryngeal nerve	Hypokalemic periodic paralysis
Chorea	Dysthyroid optic neuropathy	Thyroid associated ophthalmopathy[a]
Hyperreflexia		Myasthenia gravis[b]
Agitation or delirium		
Coma		
HYPOTHYROIDISM		
Cretinism (childhood)	Carpal tunnel syndrome	Myopathy
Mental retardation (juvenile)		
Encephalopathy (adults)	Facial palsy	Pseudomyotonia
Psychosis	Hearing loss	
Dementia		
Limbic encephalitis[c]		
Pseudotumor cerebri		

[a] Graves disease only.
[b] May be present in any patient with hyperthyroidism.
[c] Autoimmune related; occurs independent of normal thyroid function among patients with Hashimoto's thyroiditis.

PATHOLOGY

In *Graves disease,* the thyroid gland is diffusely enlarged, soft, and vascular. Microscopically, there is glandular hyperplasia and lymphocytic infiltration. On occasion, generalized lymphocytic hyperplasia is also noted and, in some areas, large lymphoid follicles are produced. Splenomegaly and thymus enlargement may be found as well. Muscle fiber degeneration, fatty degeneration or fibrosis of the liver, and changes and loss of adipose tissue in skin and muscle may be observed. (The changes in TAO are described in detail in Chapter 136.) All orbital contents, but particularly the eye muscles, are infiltrated by lymphocytes, mucoplysaccharides, and edema (2). In the skin, is also noted dermal infiltration with lymphocytes and mucopolysaccharides. Hyperthyroidism may also occur in association with an *isolated or multiple nodules within a goiter*, pathologically, focal hyperplasia and hypertrophy of the epithelial cells are seen, accompanied by hemorrhage, necrosis, and scarring, resulting in nodularity (known as *toxic nodular goiter*).

CLINICAL MANIFESTATIONS

In hyperthyroidism (thyrotoxicosis), the thyroid gland may be enlarged to palpation and a bruit may be heard in the thyroid owing to increased vascularity. Regardless of the cause of hyperthyroidism, the clinical manifestations are similar. TAO, however, would be unique to Graves' disease. Patients who are hyperthyroid have obvious signs of hypermetabolism, with weight loss, increased sweating, arterial hypertension, diarrhea, and agitation. Cardiac arrhythmias, spanning from tachycardia to episodic atrial fibrillation, may be seen. The neurologic manifestations are listed in Table 77-1. Patients who are asthenic and complain of muscle weakness, rarely have associated episodic hypokalemic periodic paralysis. Several movement disorders may be seen; tremor is universal and is mostly a postural-action type. Chorea is found infrequently. Hyperreflexia and pyramidal tract signs are present in many instances (3). In elderly patients, these signs may be missing and are replaced by generalized asthenia (apathetic hyperthyroidism).

Thyrotoxic crisis (thyroid storm), a fulminant increase in the clinical manifestations of thyrotoxicosis, is usually precipitated by surgery or an infection in a patient partially treated or having a condition not previously recognized. The patients are delirious or comatose with fever, tachycardia, and hypotension. It is probably secondary to a shift from protein-bound to free hormone. Common causes of hyperthyroidism are listed in Table 77-2.

DIAGNOSTIC APPROACH

Neurologic and general examination may provide diagnostic information in the clinically symptomatic patients. None of the signs observed in the central nervous system (CNS) examination are diagnostic, but the hyperthyroid syndrome can be recognized easily. Signs related to TAO, on the other hand, are very characteristic. The combination of uni- or bilateral exophthalmus, lid lag, and ophthalmoplegia are strongly suggestive of the diagnosis. Palpation and auscultation of the thyroid gland may provide useful information. Occasionally, local compression of the recurrent laryngeal nerve causes hoarseness. Once a diagnosis is suggested from the clinical findings, laboratory tests will be used for confirmation.

LABORATORY TESTS

Measurement of the concentration of free T4, T3, and TSH would be a good way to start the diagnostic workup. Normal values for T4 are 60 to 100 nmol/L (total) and 0.6 to 1.6 ng/dL; for T3, 1.2 to 3.2 nmol/L and 1.5 to 4.5 pg/L free. Normal TSH levels vary from 0.4 to 4.0 μIU/L. In primary hyperthyroidism, the TSH levels can be markedly decreased. In secondary hyperthyroidism, a rare entity, TSH levels are usually normal or increased.

TABLE 77-2. Causes of Hyperthyroidism

THYROTOXICOSIS	
1. Increased production	Secondary hyperthyroidism of pituitary origin Graves disease Trophoblastic tumors
2. Intrinsic thyroid autonomy	Hyperfunctioning adenoma Toxic multinodular goiter
3. Disorders of hormone storage	Various thyroiditis with transient thyrotoxicosis
4. Exogenous thyroid	Thyrotoxicosis factitia Hamburger toxicosis
5. Ectopic thyroid tissue	Struma ovarii Functioning follicular carcinoma

Radioactive thyroid uptake. The radioiodine active uptake (RAIU) is measured 24 hours after its administration. The RIAU varies inversely with the plasma iodine concentration and the functional state of the gland. The normal value is 10% to 30% of the administered dose. Values above normal suggest hyperthyroidism and are commonly seen in Graves disease multinodular goiter and in the early phase of Hashimoto disease (hashitoxicosis).

Antithyroglobulin antibodies are positive in patients with Graves' disease. More specifically, thyroid-stimulating antibodies (TSAb) and TSH-binding inhibitory immunoglobulin (TBII) can be found as well (4).

Imaging by *scintiscanning and ultrasound* can be useful in the evaluation of an enlarged thyroid gland.

Orbit imaging using magnetic resonance imagine (MRI) or computer tomographic CT-scan in the event of coexisting TAO will confirm the typical enlargement of the extraocular muscles with sparing of the insertion tendon. Thyroid function test results must be carefully interpreted and correlated with the clinical findings (5).

TREATMENT

The main therapeutic strategies in hyperthyroidism consist in the administration of medications that block thyroid hormone synthesis as a transient measure or by the administration of radioactive iodine leading to permanent reduction in the production of thyroid hormone and eventual hypothyroidism. The possibility of a partial surgical resection of the gland is also a consideration in selective cases, particularly in young patients. The most common antithyroid agents used include propylthiouracil (150 mg twice or three times daily) or methimazole. Some of the clinical manifestations of hyperthyroidism caused by an increased adrenergic tone can be treated with propanolol and other beta-blockers. The issue of radioactive iodine therapy in Graves' disease and its potential effect on the TAO is discussed in Chapter 136 (6).

Large doses of dexamethasone may be very effective in reducing the serum T4 levels among patients with severe thyrotoxicosis or thyroid storm. In addition, these patients may require parenteral therapy if comatose; the X-ray contrast agent, sodium ipodate, can be administered or large doses of iodine may be given.

CLINICAL RECOMMENDATIONS OF THE VIGNETTE

The patient has typical findings for TAO and yet, clinically, she does not have clinical symptoms or signs suggestive of hyperthyroidism. Testing did demonstrate a decreased TSH and positive TSAb and TBII. A thyroid releasing factor (TRF) suppression test was utilized, but the results are usually not fully conclusive.

Hypothyroidism

CASE VIGNETTE

A 79-year-old woman was seen for evaluation of an encephalopathy associated with lethargy and difficulty to thrive following an uncomplicated small bowel resection. The patient was weak and unable to sit up on her own power. She was lethargic and had prolonged myotatic reflexes in the upper extremities and absent reflexes in the lower. There were no focal signs and a TSH value of 50 μIU/L was found, thus establishing the diagnosis of hypothyroidism. For unclear reasons, however, the recommendations from the neurology consultant were not followed and the patient remained encephalopathic. A reevaluation 6 weeks later found the patient still stuporous and her TSH was now 160 μIU/L. Gradual thyroid replacement resulted in complete resolution of her encephalopathy; thus, placement in a nursing home facility was avoided for this patient.

DEFINITION

Hypothyroidism is a clinical state resulting from either an underactive thyroid gland or a failure of normal hypothalamic-pituitary stimulation. When it dates from birth, it is associated with mental retardation and other developmental abnormalities causing a syndrome known as *cretinism.* In adults, severe hypothyroidism causes mucopolysaccharide accumulation in the dermis, leading to typical facial features and a doughy induration of the skin, known as *myxedema.*

EPIDEMIOLOGY

Estimating the true incidence of hypothyroidism is difficult. Congenital hypothyroidism is present in about 1:5,000 births. Endemic goiter, caused by iodine deficient diets, can still be found in clusters throughout the world. Otherwise, most adults with hypothyroidism have Hashimoto's thyroiditis with TSH receptor and antithyroid peroxidase: Thyroid peroxidase (TPO)-blocking antibodies (formerly known as antimicrosomal antibodies) or primary thyroid atrophy. Less common causes include results of radioiodine or surgical therapy and the effect of medications thyrotoxicity (Table 77-3). Rarely, inborn

TABLE 77-3. Causes of Hypothyroidism

1. Primary with goiter	• Hashimoto's thyroiditis • Iodine deficiency • Medications blocking T4 synthesis (lithium, iodine, ethionamide and amiodarone) • Goitrogenic substances: Thiocyanates, interferon-α, interleukin Z • Glandular infiltration: Hemochromatosis, sarcoidosis, amyloidosis, cystinosis, scleroderma
2. Primary without goiter	• Autoimmune thyroid atrophy • Radioactive iodine • Surgical resection • Agenesis or hypoplasia
3. Secondary hypothyroidism Pituitary/hypothalamic	

defects in the synthesis of the hormone can lead to hypothyroidism. Regardless of the cause, an inability to synthesize adequate amounts of thyroid hormone leads to hypersecretion of TSH and, hence, goiter.

ETIOLOGY AND PATHOGENESIS

The different pathogenic mechanisms of hypothyroidism are summarized in Table 77-3. Outside the obvious postradioiodine and postsurgical cases, the most common causes include autoimmune Hashimoto's thyroiditis, toxicity of medications in adults and inborn defects of thyroid hormone synthesis or the effect of maternal iodine-therapy in newborn children. Hypothalamic or pituitary hypothyroidism is uncommon.

PATHOLOGY

In Hashimoto's thyroiditis, the gland is massively infiltrated by lymphocytes and plasma cells, which replace the normal tissue. The gland can be enlarged three or four times its normal size. In extreme cases, the normal architecture of the gland is nearly totally replaced. A less frequent cause of granulomatous, giant-cell thyroiditis, has been recognized.

In common goiter, the histologic findings vary with the stage of the goiter and consist of focal hyperplasia with colloid deposition early and late scarring and involution. Unlike Graves disease or Hashimoto thyroiditis, in uni- or multinodular goiter no lymphocytic infiltrates are found in the gland. Finally, adenomas and carcinomas of the thyroid can be found in thyroid glands that have nodular enlargement and often a diagnostic differentiation can be difficult. Needle biopsy of the lesion may be necessary.

CLINICAL MANIFESTATIONS

The most characteristic clinical neurologic findings of hypothyroidism are listed in Table 77-3. In infants and neonates, the nonneurologic findings include persistence of physiologic jaundice, constipation, somnolence, and feeding problems. A routine thyroid function profile in newborns is now mandatory. In later ages, there is delay in developmental milestones and a full-blown picture of cretinism. The systemic signs include short stature; coarse features, macroglossia, protuberant abdomen, and an umbilical hernia are the most striking characteristics. In adults, none of the clinical signs are diagnostic; however, the syndrome can be easily recognized when the thyroid hormone level is low and has been this way for some time (Table 77-1). Thyroid function must be evaluated in any patient with dementia. Palpation of the thyroid usually reveals a normal gland, except for those with goitrous hypothyroidism (7).

The association of autoimmune thyroiditis and steroid-responsive limbic encephalitis, although infrequent, is well known since the initial 1966 report from Brain et al. (8). The most recent criteria for this diagnosis include (*a*) acute encephalopathy with delirium, sensorium changes, and paranoia; (*b*) plus antimicrosomal antibodies; (*c*) euthyroid status (may be on medication); (*d*) no other cause for encephalitis; (*e*) absence of paraneoplastic, potassium voltage-gated or calcium-voltage gated antibodies; (*f*) MRI plus only for inflammatory changes in the temporal lobes; and (*g*) response to steroid therapy in most cases (9).

DIAGNOSTIC APPROACH

Following a thorough history intake and physical examination, the single most sensitive test is to measure the TSH. T4 is also decreased, but T3 may be normal. The RAIU is of limited value in hypothyroidism. The electrocardiogram (ECG) may show low voltage QRS, bradycardia and T wave inversion; in secondary hypothyroidism, low T4, T3, and TSH are found and there is a normal response to TRF stimulation. Circulating antithyroid antibodies should be ordered: Antimicrosomal, antithyroperoxidase antibodies, and antithyroglobulin. In addition, other hormone levels should be checked because autoimmune hypothyroidism can be associated with polyglandular failure, diabetes mellitus, and autoimmune-related pernicious anemia.

TREATMENT

The normal metabolic state should be restored gradually. In adults, a dose of 25 μg should be initiated and increased by 25 to 50 μg every 4 weeks until a normal state is reached. A caveat in the treatment of hypothyroidism is the possibility of coexistent hypoadrenalism and the risk of acute adrenal insufficiency with thyroid replacement, if not detected. Children require thyroid hormone doses that are disproportionably larger than those of adults.

CLINICAL RECOMMENDATIONS OF THE VIGNETTE

Thyroid function assessment is mandatory in any patient with altered mental status, metabolic encephalopathy, and dementia. It can be either the primary or a contributing cause and treatment may have rather strikingly favorable outcomes.

SUMMARY

The potential role of the thyroid in the pathogenesis of central and peripheral nervous system and muscle disorders cannot be over emphasized and must be tested in the clinical setting listed in Table 77-1.

REFERENCES

1. Gunji K, Kubota S, Swanson J, et al. Role of the eye muscles in thyroid eye disease: Identification of the principal autoantigens. *Thyroid.* 1998;6:553–556.
2. Liu GT, Volpe NJ, Galetta SJ. Neuro-ophthalmology. Diagnosis and Management. Philadelphia: WB Saunders; 2001:663.
3. Ravera JJ, Cervino JM, Fernandez G, et al. Two cases of Graves' disease with signs of a pyramidal lesion. Improvement in neurologic signs during treatment with antithyroid drugs. *J Clin Endocr.* 1960;20:876–880.
4. O'Connor G, Davies TF. Human autoimmune thyroid disease. A mechanistic update. *Trends Endocrinol Metab.* 1990;1(5):266–274.
5. Nicoloff JT, Spencer CA. The use and m*is use of the sensitive thyrotropin assays. *J Clin Endocrinol Metab.* 1990;71(3):553–558.
6. Hashizume K, Ichikawa K, Sakura A, et al. Administration of thyroxine in treated Graves' disease: Effects on the level of antibodies to thyroid-stimulating hormone receptors and on the risk of recurrence of hyperthyroidism. *N Engl J Med.* 1991;324(14):947–953.
7. O'Doherty DS, Canary JF. Neurologic aspects of endocrine disturbances. In: Baker AB, Baker LH, eds. *Clinical Neurology.* Hagerstown, MD: Harper & Row; 1974.
8. Brain L, Jellinek EH, Ball K. Hashimoto's disease and encephalopathy. *Lancet.* 1966;2:512–514.
9. Castillo P, Woodruff B, Caselli R, et al. Steroid-responsive encephalopathy associated with autoimmune thyroiditis. *Arch Neurol.* 2006;63:197–202.

CHAPTER **78**

Neurologic Complications of Parathyroid Gland Disorders: Hypoparathyroidism and Hyperparathyroidism

Michael D. Sirdofsky • Leah Kroeger

PART A: Hypoparathyroidism and Vitamin D Deficiency

OBJECTIVES

- To review possible causes of hypoparathyroidism or vitamin D deficiency
- To explain the clinical manifestations of hypocalcemia caused by either hypoparathyroidism or vitamin D deficiency
- To present the appropriate workup for hypocalcemia and explain how to differentiate between hypoparathyroidism and vitamin D deficiency
- To describe treatment for hypoparathyroidism and vitamin D deficiency

CASE VIGNETTE

An 83-year-old man presents to the neurologist with a complaint of localized pain in the shoulders and pelvis. He also states it is more difficult for him to rise from chairs and climb stairs. He occasionally has diffuse muscle cramps, but denies tetany or seizures. He admits he stays indoors for most of the day and almost never goes out in the winter months. His diet is poor as he does not cook for himself. He denies any changes in cognition and is still able to manage his finances. His examination is significant for 3 ± 5 strength in bilateral iliopsoas, otherwise strength was 5/5. Muscle stretch reflexes were brisk but symmetric. Chvostek and Trousseau signs were negative. Routine laboratory study results were as follows: Serum calcium was 6.9 mg/dL (normal, 8.8 to 10.4 mg/dL) and phosphorous level was 1.9 mg/dL (normal, 2.5 to 4.5 mg/dL).

DEFINITION

Hypoparathyroidism is defined as a deficiency of parathyroid hormone or an abnormality in the action of parathyroid hormone. Vitamin D deficiency is defined as low levels of 1,25 dihydroxyvitamin D or 25 hydroxyvitamin D in the serum. Both hypoparathyroidism and vitamin D deficiency lead to hypocalcemia. Hypocalcemia is defined as total calcium levels in the blood <8.8 mg/mL.

EPIDEMIOLOGY

Hypoparathyroidism is very rare, except in neonates and patients with renal failure. Vitamin D deficiency is becoming more recognized in children, possibly because of an increase in breastfed infants (1). Men and women are equally affected and the age of onset depends on the cause.

ETIOLOGY AND PATHOGENESIS

Normal serum calcium levels are maintained by the direct actions of the parathyroid hormone on the kidney and bone and by the indirect actions through 1,25 dihydroxyvitamin D on the intestine. Parathyroid hormone causes renal tubular cells to reabsorb calcium and stimulates renal parenchymal cells to hydroxalate 25 hydroxyvitamin D into 1,25 dihydroxyvitamin D, a more active form. Parathyroid hormone is released in response to low levels of calcium in the serum. In hypoparathyroidism, there is deficient parathyroid hormone secretion, which causes a decrease in calcium resorption and results in hypocalcemia. Most often, hypoparathyroidism is caused by a previous parathyroidectomy. The risk of hypocalcemia after surgery is increased if a subtotal or three and one-half gland parathyroidectomy has been performed. The risk of hypocalcemia is also increased if there is a history of previous neck surgery or if preoperative parathyroid hormone levels were >25 pmol/L (2).

Other causes of hypoparathyroidism include infiltrative diseases, such as iron overload caused by hemochromatosis or multiple blood transfusions or deposition of copper, as in Wilson disease, which can destroy the parathyroid glands. In some cases, parathyroid hormone is not deficient, but rather hormone resistance exists wherein not appropriate action occurs. Hypomagnesemia is an example wherein low levels of magnesium cause end-organ resistance to parathyroid hormone, and developmental defects exist in the parathyroid glands, such as in DiGeorge syndrome. This syndrome, also known as *velocardiofacial syndrome*, consists of mental retardation, congenital heart anomalies, aplasia or hypoplasia of the thymus, and hypoparathyroidism (3). In hypocalcemia caused by hypoparathyroidism, there is decreased mobilization from bone and decreased renal resorption of calcium. Phosphate levels are low, which helps distinguish hypoparathyroidism from vitamin D deficiency.

Hypocalcemia also occurs with normal or even high levels of parathyroid hormone. Often this is seen in vitamin D deficiency, which has become more common. High risk groups for vitamin D deficiency include infants being breastfed without vitamin supplementation, elderly patients who are housebound, women with strict dress codes where skin must be covered, and people taking phenytoin or phenobarbital (4). Patients with cirrhosis, renal failure, or malabsorption diseases (e.g., celiac disease) are also at risk (5). In vitamin D deficiency, parathyroid hormone levels will be high because the parathyroid gland is attempting to compensate for the low levels of calcium by increasing its absorption in the kidneys. This increase in renal calcium absorption leads to a decrease in phosphate excretion and hyperphosphatemia. Parathyroid hormone also increases bone resorption, leading to increased levels of alkaline phosphatase (6). If vitamin D is not replaced, the bone turnover continues and bone demineralization decreases lead to rickets in children and osteomalacia in adults.

CLINICAL MANIFESTATIONS

Hypocalcemia, either caused by hypoparathyroidism or vitamin D deficiency, classically presents as neuromuscular excitability, with parasthesias in the fingers, toes, and circumoral area; tetany; and muscle cramping (7). Tetany can be either overt or latent and is elicited with two maneuvers. In the first maneuver, referred to as *Chvostek sign*, percussion of the facial nerve 2 cm anterior to the tragus of the ear lobe produces twitching of the upper lip. This is fairly nonspecific, because the test can be positive in up to 25% of patients with normal levels of serum calcium (8). The second test often used to test for tetany is the *Trousseau sign*. A blood pressure cuff is inflated to the systolic blood pressure for 2 to 3 minutes, which will provoke a carpopedal spasm. The spasm is often preceded by parasthesias. Latent tetany can also be elicited in the setting of alkalosis, either with hyperventilation or administration of sodium bicarbonate. This reflects the increased binding between ionized calcium and albumin. The clinical picture is similar to opisthotonos if the spasms involve the trunk. Acute hypocalcemia can also present with mental disturbances, such as increased irritability, depression, or psychosis with agitation and insomnia (9). Evidence may be seen of increased intracranial pressure, with bilateral papilledema as is seen in pseudotumor cerebri. Hypocalcemia needs to be considered in adult onset seizures because generalized tonic–clonic seizures are not uncommon and can occur in 30% to 70% of patients with low serum calcium. Often, electroencephalogram (EEG) findings are normal between attacks. Because of an increase in smooth muscle contractions, laryngeal stridor or bronchospasms are often found. There may be prolongation of the QT interval on ECG and a decrease in myocardial contractility that can lead to congestive heart failure (10). Relatively few symptoms are seen in chronic hypocalcemia.

In hypoparathyroidism with associated hypocalcemia, retropyramidal symptoms can occur with choreathetosis, gait abnormalities, and cerebellar ataxia (11). Dysarthria and dysphagia are possible as well. Often, this correlates with intracerebral calcification in the basal ganglia, cerebellum, and cerebrum. The pathophysiology of the calcification is unknown and is often asymptomatic in patients with hypoparathyroidism. A common theory is that the symmetric calcification is secondary to microvascular degeneration caused by excessive calcium deposition in those particular, highly metabolic areas (12,13).

Hypoparathyroidism has also been linked to sensorineural deafness. It is hypothesized this is caused by low levels of calcium in the inner ear fluid for a prolonged period of time (14). This finding can be associated with steroid-resistant nephritic syndrome, which responds to renal transplantation (15). In some instances, patients have episodic stiffening of the limbs, without changes of consciousness, where they have normal EEG readings and respond to supplemental calcium (16). Not infrequently, the associated feeling of panic and coexistent parasthesias can be attributed to a psychiatric cause rather than to hypocalcemia. The clinician, therefore, must be aware of the multiple and often vague presentations of hypoparathyroidism and hypocalcemia.

Very rarely, patients present with myopathy, similar to that seen in hyperparathyroidism. Muscle biopsies reveal nonspecific myopathic features, but this damage to the muscle is believed to be secondary to tetany rather than actual myopathy (17).

Osteomalacia in adults, or rickets in children, may be increasing in incidence over the past few years because of fad, poorly balanced diets. Both are caused by vitamin D deficiency and are characterized by impairment of mineralization of bone, with an increase in bone turnover. In rickets, a child often presents with tetany, generalized tonic–clonic seizures or unexplained fractures. Patients are often underweight, shorter than expected, and have bowing of the long bones. In infants, a delay occurs in closure of the anterior fontanel and in dental eruption. X-ray studies show diffuse osteopenia, with widening or fraying of the metaphyses caused by poor calcification of newly formed bone. The bones eventually become so weak they bend or "bow." Rickets is more common in dark-skinned children, because it takes three to six times more exposure to the sun to produce similar amounts of vitamin D, compared with fairer children. Other causes, other than inadequate vitamin D intake or sunlight exposure in children, include liver disease or malabsorptive conditions (e.g., celiac disease). Antiepileptic drugs (e.g., phenytoin or phenobarbital) have been known to cause rickets because of impairment of vitamin D metabolism (1).

Osteomalacia is the term used in adults, but rickets and osteomalacia have the same pathologic process. Osteomalacia is common in the elderly, and often presents as generalized or localized bone pain. The localized pain most often involves the spine, ribs, pelvis, or shoulder girdle. Patients often complain of proximal muscle weakness, with difficulty rising from chairs or climbing stairs. On examination, a waddling gait may be noted. Reflexes may be brisk and this, with proximal weakness, may be the primary presentation of osteomalacia (18). Electromyelography (EMG) finding is often consistent with myopathy, although creatine kinase enzyme will be within normal range. Muscle biopsy may reveal interstitial fibrosis, fatty infiltration, variation in fiber size, and loss of myofibrils (19). Late in the disease process, the patient may develop kyphosis, scoliosis, or have bowing of the legs as is seen in rickets. The condition is often misdiagnosed as fibromyalgia, polymyalgia rheumatica, rheumatoid arthritis, osteoporosis, or multiple myeloma (20). It is imperative that osteomalacia be ruled out in patients with vague muscle complaints because it is easily curable with the proper management.

DIAGNOSTIC APPROACH

All patients with muscle pain or weakness, unexplained seizures, or tetany need a workup for hypocalcemia, which could relate either to hypoparathyroidism or vitamin D deficiency. It is important to distinguish between the two, because replacing the calcium alone does not benefit vitamin D deficiency. An appropriate workup includes a review of calcium and phosphorous levels in addition to the basic metabolic panel. The phosphorous level will be low in vitamin D deficiency and high in hypoparathyroidism, which will help to narrow the diagnosis. Once hypocalcemia is established with serum calcium level <8.5 mg/dL, the parathyroid hormone levels must be obtained; low levels will be diagnostic of hypoparathyroidism and normal or elevated levels will be diagnostic of vitamin D deficiency. In the latter, alkaline phosphatase will be elevated because of increased bone breakdown and 25 hydroxyvitamin D a low level, which are confirmatory. In case of doubt, an anterior iliac crest bone biopsy is the gold standard to establish osteomalacia.

The workup should also include an ECG to evaluate for QT interval prolongation and continuous monitoring may be necessary for possible arrhythmias (1). A head CT can be performed to assess for calcifications in the basal ganglia, cerebellum, or cerebrum. An EMG may be useful in patients complaining of muscle weakness or pain because myopathic units are often seen.

TREATMENT

Acute, severe hypocalcemia, which presents as seizures, tetany, or acute delirium requires emergency treatment with intravenous calcium. Calcium gluconate or calcium chloride can be used and should be given over a period of 10 to 20 minutes. In less urgent cases, a slower infusion can be used over 4 to 8 hours or oral supplementation given on an outpatient basis. With regard to vitamin D deficiency resulting in osteomalacia or rickets, 5,000 IU of vitamin D with 1 g of calcium should be given every day for 4 to 6 weeks or longer if symptoms remain. With evidence of intestinal malabsorption, larger doses of vitamin D are then required in addition to treatment of the underlying gastrointestinal disorder, if amenable to therapy.

CLINICAL RECOMMENDATIONS OF THE VIGNETTE

The patient's symptoms and low serum calcium and phosphorous levels should suggest vitamin D deficiency resulting in osteomalacia with bone pain and myopathy with proximal muscle weakness. The next step is to check both a parathyroid hormone and 25 hydroxyvitamin levels. If the parathyroid hormone level is high and the 25 hydroxyvitamin level is low, then the patient needs to be treated with vitamin D and calcium supplementation.

PART B: Hyperparathyroidism

OBJECTIVES

- To present different causes of hyperparathyroidism
- To identify the clinical manifestations of hyperparathyroidism
- To discuss the diagnosis and treatment of hyperparathyroidism

CASE VIGNETTE

A 72-year-old woman presents to the emergency room with abdominal pain. Her daughter states the patient has been feeling fatigued, not able to concentrate on crossword puzzles, and has had difficulty climbing stairs for the past few months, which preceded the onset of the abdominal pain. On examination, the patient is oriented to person, but does not know time or place. She has 4 ± 5 strength proximally in bilateral legs; otherwise, her strength is 5/5. She does not wish to complete the neurologic examination because of extreme pain.

DEFINITION

Hyperparathyroidism occurs when there is a defect in the cells of the parathyroid gland that secretes parathyroid hormone (PTH). The parathyroid glands are responsible for detecting changes in serum calcium concentration. If the serum calcium level decreases, the parathyroid glands secrete PTH, which stimulates osteoclasts to increase bone resorption. The kidneys respond to PTH by increasing calcium resorption and increasing conversion of 25 hydroxyvitamin D3 , which is synthesized in the liver, to the more potent metabolite 1,25 dihydroxyvitamin DE. This conversion is mediated by an hydroxylating enzyme found in the kidney. Vitamin D is needed for bone formation. The principal target is the intestine, where, in response to vitamin D, the intestine increases absorption of calcium and phosphate. All these organs respond to PTH in an attempt to increase calcium levels in the blood (1). With an abnormality in parathyroid tissue (e.g., an adenoma), there is inappropriate secretion of parathyroid hormone, which leads to excessive renal, bone, and intestine calcium resorption; this, in turn, leads to hypercalcemia.

EPIDEMIOLOGY

Since the early 1970s, when routine serum calcium screening was first introduced, many patients were diagnosed with hyperparathyroidism early in the course of the disease, despite being asymptomatic (2); therefore, the long-term effects of hyperparathyroidism are rarely seen today. The peak incidence for detection is in the sixth decade and is rarely found in patients <15 years of age. Women are affected two to three times more than men. In the past 10 years, the incidence of primary hyperparathyroidism has appeared to decline. Possibly, this is because of dietary changes, the use of estrogen replacement, or that ionizing radiation to the head and neck is not used as often as in the past—although the decline is poorly understood (3).

ETIOLOGY AND PATHOLOGY

Hyperparathyroidism can be either primary, secondary, or tertiary, with primary hyperparathyroidism being the most common. This diagnosis can be made by identifying an increased serum calcium level and increased PTH concentrations with an inappropriately normal or elevated 24-hour urine calcium concentration (4). Benign adenomas affecting one of the four parathyroid glands, which are the most common cause of hyperparathyroidism, can be found in approximately 85% of patients affected. Hyperplasia of all four glands is found in 15% of patients and carcinoma is found in <2% (1). In addition, the possibility exists of inherited forms of primary hyperparathyroidism. *Multiple endocrine neoplasia* type 1 (MEN-1) involves tumors of the parathyroid gland, anterior pituitary gland, and pancreatic islet cells. Of these patients, 95% will develop hyperparathyroidism, usually in the second or third decades, which resembles sporadic hyperparathyroidism. MEN type 2 consists of medullary carcinoma of the thyroid and pheochromocytoma and hyperplasia of the parathyroid gland; however, hyperparathyroidism occurs late in the disease and is more infrequent that in MEN-1 (2).

Secondary hyperparathyroidism occurs when there is a stimulus outside the normal feedback loop. The most common cause is renal failure, wherein is decreased renal conversion of 25 hydroxyvitamin D to 1,25 dihydroxyvitamin D; this results in decreased calcium absorption and hypocalcemia, leading to excessive PTH secretion. Other causes of hypocalcemia or vitamin D deficiency can also increase PTH. Inadequate vitamin D intake, for instance, needs to be considered, especially in the elderly, who may have limited exposure to sunlight combined with poor nutrition. Primary and secondary hyperparathyroidism can be differentiated by phosphate levels. Primary hyperparathyroidism causes hypophosphatemia, whereas secondary hyperparathyroidism results in hyperphosphatemia. Tertiary hyperparathyroidism occurs when secondary hyperparathyroidism is not treated. The parathyroid glands become autonomous and produce excess PTH, even if serum calcium levels are normal or elevated.

Other causes of hypercalcemia need to be ruled out when establishing the diagnosis of hyperparathyroidism; among those, hypercalcemia of malignancy, which is associated with the release of PTH-related peptides from tumor cells. The PTH-related peptide binds to the parathyroid receptor, triggering the cascade of increased bone resorption and decreased kidney excretion of calcium. Squamous cell lung, breast, prostate, and colon cancers are frequently associated with hypercalcemia and indicate a poor prognosis (5). Granulomatous diseases, such as sarcoid and tuberculosis, can cause an increase in 1,25 dihydroxyvitamin D production from macrophages within the granuloma which is typically independent from the normal negative parathyroid feedback loop causing hypercalcemia. Lastly, drug use, such antacids, lithium, and thiazide diuretics, needs to be considered when evaluating hypercalcemia, all of which can increase calcium levels. Also, vitamin D intoxication associated with use of over-the-counter supplements can lead to increased calcium resorption in the intestine (5).

CLINICAL MANIFESTATIONS

Historically, patients with kidney stones, peptic ulcer disease, bone pain, pancreatitis, and neuropsychiatric complaints may harbor either hyperparathyroidism or hypercalcemia. Now that serum calcium level is checked routinely, patients diagnosed with hyperparathyroidism are usually asymptomatic. Studies have shown, however, that more than half of the patients who appear to be asymptomatic have subtle neurobehavioral symptoms (6). These symptoms include depression, poor concentration, and irritability and sleep disturbances, which resolve with treatment (1). Patients presumed to be asymptomatic, whose muscle power and fine motor movements were objectively measured, showed slight deficits, which improved after parathyroidectomy—verifying the need for a thorough clinical examination (7). Additional pre- and postsurgical studies have shown that the same is true for respiratory muscles following surgery (8).

Patients can present with *pseudomyopathy* with proximal muscle weakness, muscle pain, and stiffness (9,10). These patients may have a waddling gait or be unable to walk. In these instances, bulbar involvement with dysphagia or hoarseness may be present (11). Rarely, the patients may have a head drop because of weakness of the neck extensors or shortness of breath because of respiratory involvement; however, the degree of weakness does not correlate with the calcium or phosphorous levels. Reflexes may be brisk, usually with down-going toes. Between 29% and 57% of patients have symptoms suggestive of an underlying neuropathy, such as decreased pain or vibratory sensation with decreased reflexes (12). EMG finding is often normal or reveals myopathic abnormalities such as small, polyphasic motor units. Rare reports are found of neurogenic changes on EMG, such as fibrillations or fasciculations with decreased recruitment and decreased nerve conduction velocities (13). Muscle biopsies usually show myopathic changes, such as type 2 fiber atrophy.

Primary hyperparathyroidism can mimic amyotrophic lateral sclerosis (ALS), with spasticity, hyperreflexia, and up-going toes, in addition to lower motor neuron findings (13,14). Some reports exist of patients who met the El Escorial criteria for ALS, but who were also found to have primary hyperparathyroidism with increased serum calcium and parathyroid hormone. Despite resection of parathyroid adenomas, the patients continued to experience progressive weakness, with death within 1 to 3 years (14,15). This led to the conclusion that primary hyperparathyroidism and ALS were unrelated diseases and the presence of hyperparathyroidism is most likely coincidental. The previous studies, which showed improvement after parathyroidectomy in patients presumed to have ALS, revealed the patients most likely did not have motor neuron disease, but rather associated myopathy; further observations are needed (13–15).

Other neurologic symptoms reported include acute paraparesis, hypotonicity of muscles with areflexia, and unsteady gait (16). Although rare, hyperparathyroidism can present as acute delirium because of changes in the levels of consciousness, global cognitive decline, and lethargy (17–19). Lower extremity radicular pain has been reported as the only manifestation of hyperparathyroidism caused by compression from a vertebral brown tumor. In these patients, weakened vertebrae can collapse, leading to cord or root compression (1,16). High bone turnover results in osteitis fibrosa cystica and bone fractures similar to that seen in vitamin D deficiency.

DIAGNOSTIC APPROACH

The first step in the workup is to check the calcium level. Calcium exists in the plasma in both a free and bound state and normal plasma concentration is between 8.5 and 10.5 mg/dL. Hypoalbuminemia affects the total serum level and, therefore, an ionized calcium level should be drawn in the setting of malnourished or critically ill patients. Once hypercalcemia is established, the second step is to measure the level of PTH in the serum; the normal reference range is 2 to 6 mol/L. If the PTH level is elevated, then the most likely diagnosis is primary hyperparathyroidism. Serum phosphorous levels should be low to low-normal. Levels of 1,25 dihydroxyvitamin D can be drawn and may be elevated because of increased conversion from 25 hydroxyvitamin D from the excess PTH. In secondary hyperparathyroidism, the PTH level will be elevated whereas the serum calcium level is low. If the phosphate level is high, then the most likely cause is renal failure. Tertiary hyperparathyroidism is difficult to distinguish from primary hyperparathyroidism, but it often occurs in the setting of chronic renal failure or renal transplantation (1).

Further studies may depend on clinical presentation. If radicular pain is present, a magnetic resonance image (MRI) of the spine is indicated to rule out a vertebral brown tumor. Other imaging studies have limited value, especially early in the disease (20). Imaging of the neck can help eliminate a parathyroid tumor as the cause, but is not routinely ordered. Parathyroid gammagraphy with sestamibi may localize the adenoma. High resolution ultrasound can be sensitive; both of these modalities are of great value in detecting the adenomatous parathyroid lesions.

Skeletal X-ray study findings are rarely abnormal today. Bone densitometry may be a more useful technique to assess bone involvement. A CT scan of the pelvis may be useful to rule out kidney stones. If familial hypocalciuric hypercalcemia is suspected, a 24-hour urine calcium excretion can be helpful. Low levels of urine calcium are diagnostic for the disease.

TREATMENT

With overt signs of hypercalcemia, such as fractures, kidney stones, or neuromuscular complaints, then surgical resection is warranted. For asymptomatic patients, surgery is more controversial, although a parathyroidectomy is often curative with rates as high as 98% in primary hyperparathyroidism (21). No large clinical trials have compared outcomes in patients with asymptomatic primary hyperparathyroidism randomly assigned to surgery versus medical management. Studies have demonstrated, however, that vague symptoms, such as fatigue or mild cognitive impairment, have markedly improved following surgery (22). Also, surgery has a relatively low perioperative mortality of 1% to 2 % with experienced surgeons, even in the elderly, which makes it a more attractive therapy for hyperparathyroidism. Guidelines for parathyroid surgery in asymptomatic hyperparathyroidism are as follows (23):

1. Serum calcium >1.0 mg/dL above the upper limit of normal
2. 24-hour urinary calcium >400 mg
3. A 30% decline in creatine clearance compared with age-matched baseline
4. Bone mineral density T-score <2.5
5. Age <50 years

Bilateral cervical exploration of all four glands was previously the standard and no preoperative localization was required. Minimally invasive parathyroidectomy is now possible, although preoperative localization of the adenoma is needed. Studies have found no significant difference in complication or cure rates (1). Complications of surgery include vocal cord paralysis (<1%) and permanent hypoparathyroidism (<4%). Most often, these complications are seen in patients who require subtotal parathyroid resection for hyperplasia or resection of carcinoma (2). In patients with advanced bone disease, parathyroidectomy may be associated with the syndrome of *osseus calcium starvation*, which can carry high morbidity and mortality rates.

Medical treatment for symptomatic hypercalcemia includes rehydration with saline followed by diuresis with furosemide. Normal saline increases the filtration and excretion of calcium, whereas furosemide inhibits calcium resorption in the distal renal tubule, thereby decreasing serum calcium levels. Bisphosphonates, such as pamidronate and zolendronic acid (Zometa), can also be used to inhibit osteoclast activity. Calcitonin use is restricted to hypercalcemic crisis; it inhibits bone resorption and augments calcium excretion, but its use is limited by vomiting and cramping as well as rebound hypercalcemia (5).

Prevention should be the main goal in secondary hyperparathyroidism, with vitamin D replacement and phosphorous reduction in patients with chronic renal failure. For treatment, vitamin D analogues (e.g., paricalcitol) are used to decrease PTH levels. Guidelines for surgery for secondary hyperparathyroidism are not well established, but surgery is used in patients who have not responded to various medical treatments and in patients who have severe hypercalcemia or severe bone disease (1).

CLINICAL RECOMMENDATIONS OF THE VIGNETTE

The patient has symptoms of kidney stones and neurobehavioral complaints and her serum calcium level should be checked. If elevated, the PTH level needs to be drawn. Calcium and PTH elevation will define hyperparathyroidism. As presented in the patient, kidney stones, proximal muscle weakness, and neurobehavioral symptoms are then an indication for parathyroidectomy. Given that she has overt symptoms of hyperparathyroidism, medical management should only be considered if contraindications to surgery exist.

SUMMARY

Routine serum calcium levels are a part of most annual patient evaluations, which has resulted in a decrease in the morbidity and mortality associated with hyperparathyroidism. Clinicians need to be aware, however, of hypercalcemia caused by hyperparathyroid in the patient presenting with vague neurologic complaints, such as muscle weakness or fatigue; or radiculopathy or neurobehavioral complaints, such as lethargy, cognitive decline, or irritability. Calcium levels need to be checked, followed by parathyroid levels to diagnose hyperparathyroidism. If both calcium and parathyroid levels are elevated, patients should be evaluated for possible parathyroidectomy given the low risk of perioperative complications and that surgery can be curative in up to 98% of patients. Secondary hyperparathyroidism, most often caused by chronic renal failure, needs to be prevented with vitamin D replacement in high risk groups.

PART A REFERENCES

1. Bloom E, Klein EJ, Shushan D, et al. Variable presentations of rickets in children in the emergency department. *Pediatr Emerg Care.* 2004;20(2):126–130.
2. Ariyan CE, Sosa JA. Assessment and management of patients with abnormal calcium. *Crit Care Med.* 2004;32(4):S146–S154.
3. Graesdal A, Suren P, Vadstrup S. DiGeorge syndrome. An underdiagnosed disease category with different clinical features. *Tidsskr Nor Laegeforen.* 2001;121(27):3177–3179.
4. Francis RM, Selby PL. Osteomalacia. *Baillieres Clin Endocrinol Metab.* 1997;11(1):145–163.
5. Lyman D. Undiagnosed vitamin D deficiency in the hospitalized patient. *Am Fam Physician.* 2005;71(2):299–304.
6. Bellazzini MA, Howes DS. Pediatric hypocalcemic seizures: A case of Rickets. *J Emerg Med.* 2003;28(2):161–164.
7. Goldman L, Ausiello D, eds. *Cecil Textbook of Medicine,* 22nd ed. Philadelphia: WB Saunders; 2004.
8. Thorton PS. Hypoparathyroidism. Emedicine.com, 2003.
9. Adorni A, Lussignoli G, Geroldi C, et al. Extensive brain calcification and dementia in postsurgical hypoparathyroidism. *Neurology.* 2005;65(9):1501.
10. Beach CB. Hypocalcemia. Emedicine.com, 2005.
11. Abe S, Tojo K, Ichida K, et al. A rare case of idiopathic hypoparathyroidism with varied neurological manifestations. *Intern Med.* 1996;35(2):129–134.
12. Nguyen HV, Gan SK. Neurological sequelae of chronic profound hypocalcemia. *Med J Aust.* 2005;182(3):123.
13. Rastogi R, Beauchamp NJ, Ladenson PW. Calcification of the basal ganglia in chronic hypoparathyroidism. *J Clin Endocrinol Metab.* 2003;88(4):1476–1477.
14. Garty BZ, Daliot D, Kauli R, et al. Hearing impairment in idiopathyic hypoparathyroidism and pseudohypoparathyroidism. *Isr J Med Sci.* 1994;30(8):587–591.
15. Hameed R, Raafat F, Ramani P, et al. Mitochondrial cytopathy presenting with focal segmental glomerulosclerosis, hypoparathyroidism, sensorineural deafness, and progressive neurologic disease. *Postgrad Med J.* 2001;77(910):523–526.
16. Stevens M, Deinum J, Willems MH. Clinical thinking and decision making in practice. A young woman with muscle cramps. *Ned Tijdschr Geneeskd.* 2001;145(17):818–821.
17. Kaminski HJ, Amato AA, Barohn RJ, et al. Myopathies associated with parathyroid disorders. Available at www.medlink.com.
18. Russell JA. Osteomalacic myopathy. *Muscle Nerve.* 1994;17(6):578–580.
19. Kaminski HJ, Ruff, RL. Hypoparathyroidism. Neurologic complications of endocrine disease. *Neurol Clin.* 1989;7:489–508.
20. Reginator AJ, Falasca GF, Pappu R, et al. Musculoskeletal manifestations of osteomalacia: Report of 26 cases and literature review. *Semin Arthritis Rheum.* 1999;28(5):287–304.

PART B REFERENCES

1. Ahmad R, Hammond JM. Primary, secondary, and tertiary hyperparathyroidism. *Otolaryngol Clin North Am.* 2004;37(4):701–713.
2. Larsen PR. *Williams Textbook of Endocrinology,* 10th ed. Philadelphia: WB Saunders; 2003.
3. Wermers RA, Khosla S, Atkinson EJ, et al. The rise and fall of primary hyperparathyroidism: A population based study in Rochester, Minnesota, 1965–1992. *Ann Intern Med.* 1997;126(6):433–440.
4. Hackett DA, Kauffman GL. Historical perspective of parathyroid disease. *Otolaryngol Clin North Am.* 2004;37(4):689–700.
5. Carroll MF, Schade DS. A practical approach to hypercalcemia. *Am Fam Physician.* 2003;67(9):1959–1966.
6. Marx SJ. Hyperparathyroid and hypoparathyroid disorders. *N Engl J Med.* 2000;343(25): 1863–1875.
7. Chou FF, Sheen-Chen SM, Leong CP. Neuromuscular recovery after parathyroidectomy in primary hyperparathyroidism. *Surgery.* 1995;117(1):18–25.
8. Kristoffersson A, Bjerle P, Stjernberg N, et al. Pre- and postoperative respiratory muscle strength in primary hyperparathyroidism. *Acta Chirurgica Scandinavia.* 1988;154(7–8): 415–418.
9. Verges B, Wechsler B, Brunet P, et al. Neuromuscular forms of hyperparathyroidism. Apropos of 2 cases. *Ann Med Interne (Paris).* 1988;139(4):254–257.
10. Aminoff, MJ. *Neurology and General Medicine,* 3rd ed. New York: Churchill-Livingstone; 2001;392.
11. Patten BM, Pages M. Severe neurological disease associated with hyperparathyroidism. *Ann Neurol.* 1984;15:453–456.
12. Kaminski H, Amato AA, Barohn RJ, et al. Myopathies associated with parathyroid disorders. www.medlink.com.
13. Kaminiski HJ, Ruff RL. Neurologic complications of endocrine diseases. *Neurol Clin.* 1989;7(3):489–508.
14. Jackson CE, Amato AA, Bryan WW, et al. Primary hyperparathyroidism and ALS: Is there a relation? *Neurology.* 1998;50(6):1795–1799.
15. Patten BM, Pages M. Severe neurological disease associated with hyperparathyroidism. *Ann Neurol.* 1984;15(5):453–456.
16. Olukoga A. Lessons to be learned: A case study approach. Primary hyperparathyroidism simulating an acute severe polyneuritis. *J R Soc Health.* 1998;118(2):103–106.
17. Pino RV, Marcos GM, et al. Acute confusional syndrome as first manifestation of primary hyperaparathyroidism. *Anales Otorhynolaringologia Ibero-Americana.* 2004;31(5):405–411.
18. Bando N. Hypercalcemic delirium associated with hyperparathyroidism and a vitamin D analog [Letter]. *General Hospital Psychiatry.* 2005;27:374–376.
19. Mustonen AO, Kiuru MJ, Stahls A, et al. Radicular lower extremity pain as the first symptom of primary hyperparathyroidism. *Skeletal Radiol.* 2004;33(8):467–472.
20. Salen P. Hyperparathyroidism. www.emedicine.com.
21. Ariyan CE, Sosa JA. Assessment and management of patients with abnormal calcium. *Crit Care Med.* 2004;32(4):5146–5154.
22. Emmelot-Vonk MH, Samson MM, Raymakers JA. Cognitive deterioration in elderly due to primary hyperparathyroidism—Resolved by parathyroidectomy. *Ned Tijdschr Geneeskd.* 2001;145(41):1961–1964.
23. Bilezikian JP, Potts JT, Jr., Fuleihan Gel-H, et al. Summary statement from a workshop on asymptomatic primary hyperparathyroidism: A perspective for the 21 century. *J Clin Endocrinol Metab.* 2002;87(12):5353–5361.

CHAPTER **79**

Disorders of the Adrenal Glands and Neuroendocrine Tumors

Tulio E. Bertorini • Angel S. Perez • Maamoon Tammaa

OBJECTIVES

- To discuss the neurologic manifestations of disorders caused by increased production of adrenal hormones such as Cushing syndrome and hyperaldosteronism, their diagnosis, and treatment
- To discuss the neurologic manifestations of disorders causing decreased production of adrenal hormones, such as in Addison disease, their diagnosis and treatment
- To discuss the neurologic manifestations of tumors of neuroendocrine origin, such as chemodectomas, pheochromocytomas, neurofibromas, and carcinoid neoplasms

CASE VIGNETTE

A 74-year-old-woman presented with a 10-year history of recurrent syncope. In the process of the workup, she was found to have bilateral lesions at the carotid artery bifurcations on carotid ultrasound. This was confirmed by magnetic resonance imaging (MRI) and magnetic resonance angiography (MRA); bilateral vascular lesions were present at the carotid bifurcations and a diagnosis of a paraganglioma was made.

Cushing Syndrome

DEFINITION

Cushing syndrome (CS) is a metabolic disorder caused by hypersecretion of cortisol, affecting carbohydrate, protein, and lipid metabolism. The syndrome consists of several features, including hypertension, obesity, and hyperglycemia. It is caused by a dysfunction affecting different areas of the hypothalamic-pituitary-adrenal axis. CS was described initially by H. W. Cushing in a study of cases of pituitary adenomas in 1932, hence Cushing disease (CD).

EPIDEMIOLOGY

Most cases of CS are caused by the exogenous administration of corticosteroids for therapeutic purposes. The actual incidence of endogenous CS is unknown. Endogenous CS can be adrenocorticotropic hormone (ACTH)-dependent or independent. ACTH-dependent CS, caused by adrenal hyperplasia, occurs in 80% to 85% of cases, including pituitary adenomas in 68%, ectopic ACTH syndrome in 12%, and ectopic corticotrophic-releasing hormone (CRH) secretion in 1%. ACTH-independent CS occurs in 15% to 20% of cases; these include adrenal adenomas in 10%, adrenal carcinoma in 8%, and micronodular hyperplasia in 1%. Exogenous use of ACTH or glucocorticoids for medical reasons (1,2) include oral steroids, intramuscular dexamethasone acetate (2), topical (Lotrisone) (2), and even inhaled glucocorticoids (nasal beclomethasone) (2). Medroxyprogesterone, a progesterone compound with some intrinsic glucocorticoid activity, may also result in clinical manifestations of CS (2).

Small cell carcinoma of the lung is an ectopic source of ACTH and, rarely, of CRH (1), and intrathoracic carcinoids, pancreatic, adrenal, or thyroid tumors might also secrete ACTH (1) and cause CS.

ETIOLOGY AND PATHOGENESIS

The adrenal glands situated in the superior pole of the kidneys have two main components, (*a*) the cortex, derived from the mesoderm, and (*b*) the medulla derived from the neuroectoderm. The medullary chromaffin cells secrete catecholamines, such as epinephrine, the secretion of which is controlled by the preganglionic sympathetic neurons. The adrenal cortex is further divided into three zones: The zona reticularis, adjacent to the medulla that secretes sex hormones; the middle zone that secretes corticosteroids; and the outer glomerular zone that secretes mineralocorticoids; the former two are under control by the hypothalamus-pituitary axis and the latter by angiotensin.

The periventricular nucleus of the hypothalamus controls the secretion of CRH (3) that is excreted in the hypophyseal portal blood to the anterior pituitary where it stimulates the synthesis and release of ACTH. ACTH, in turn, stimulates cortisol secretion by the adrenal gland. Cortisol, in turn, inhibits hypothalamic CRH synthesis and secretion of ACTH. The axis works under a circadian rhythm. ACTH peaks at 3 to 4 AM and bottoms out at 10 to 11 PM (3). Corticosteroid-binding globulin binds up to 90% of cortisol, and the rest is free plasma cortisol, that is, the biologic active form of the hormone. This is filtered into the saliva and urine, and its metabolites are detectable in the urine as 17-hydroxycorticosteroid (17-OHCS) and 17-ketosteroids (17-KS) (3). Importantly, increased levels of cortisol occur in physiologic states, such as stress, excessive exercise, and third trimester of pregnancy, and in pathologic states, such as pseudo-CS, that represents 1% to 2% of cases. Excess adrenal stimulation, caused by altered pituitary or hypothalamic regulation, may be involved in the pathogenesis of adrenal hyperplasia. Pathologically, most pituitary-independent CS cases are related to adrenal hyperplasia, and 30% of cases are caused by either adenomas or carcinomas.

CLINICAL MANIFESTATIONS

Symptoms and signs of CS involve almost all body systems, such as abnormal fat distribution, temporal wasting, central obesity, weight gain, thin skin, moon face, striae, acne, menstrual irregularities, hirsutism, and cataracts. Arterial hypertension is seen in 75% of cases, whereas CS causes increased appetite in 75% of cases. Easy bruisability and poor wound healing are seen in 40% of cases. Increased tendency to infections, hypercholesterolemia, and hypertriglyceridemia are common. Diabetes mellitus or glucose intolerance can be seen in 65% of cases. Decreased libido and impotence occurs in 50% of cases. Osteoporosis and pathologic fractures are also frequently seen.

NEUROPSYCHIATRIC MANIFESTATIONS

Symptoms of psychiatric disease can occur in more than one half of patients with CS (4,5). In some patients, these could be the presenting symptoms and include emotional lability, agitated depression, irritability, anxiety, panic attacks, and mild paranoia (4,5). Depression with weight gain and increased appetite is seen in two third of patients with CS, but anorexia and weight loss can also occur (4). Severely depressed patients can also be suicidal (4). Mania is not uncommon (4). Learning, cognition, and memory, especially short-term memory, are impaired by hypercortisolism. One study showed a selective impairment of memory functions in patients with CS (6). This appears to be related to cortical atrophy and a reduction in hippocampal volume (4,7,8). Insomnia is often an early symptom, which mostly is related to high serum cortisol concentrations during sleep caused by the absence of normal diurnal variations (4,9). Resolution of the psychiatric symptoms is variable after correction of the hypercortisolism (4,10).

Weakness and proximal muscle wasting is seen in 60% of cases, secondary to the catabolic effects of the excess glucocorticoid on skeletal muscles, in addition to physical inactivity (4,11). On the other hand, they are rare in patients with pseudo-CS (4,12). High plasma level of mineralocorticoid can cause hypokalemia, which can increase the weakness in patients with severe hypercortisolism. A high-protein diet and exercise may reverse the muscle wasting and increase strength (4). A severe myopathy could be the most prominent and distressing symptom.

Steroid myopathy manifests with proximal muscle wasting and weakness, which predominantly involves the legs, with sparing of muscles innervated by the sphincters. Patients may complain of myalgias and usually have normal serum muscle enzymes. Steroid myopathy occurs with excessive production of ACTH and glucocorticoid treatments (13). Several observations have documented that increasing amounts of steroids produce direct muscle weakness, which is reversible when steroid levels return to normal. This has been estimated to occur in about 50% to 80% of patients with CD (14).

Electromyographic (EMG) studies show normal nerve conduction velocities and, on needle examination, no denervation potentials are seen, but the motor unit action potentials could be of low amplitude. Normal motor units can also be seen.

The characteristic histologic finding of steroid myopathy is a selective atrophy of type II muscle fibers, particularly type IIB (13) (Fig. 79-1). Evidence of mitochondria aggregations and

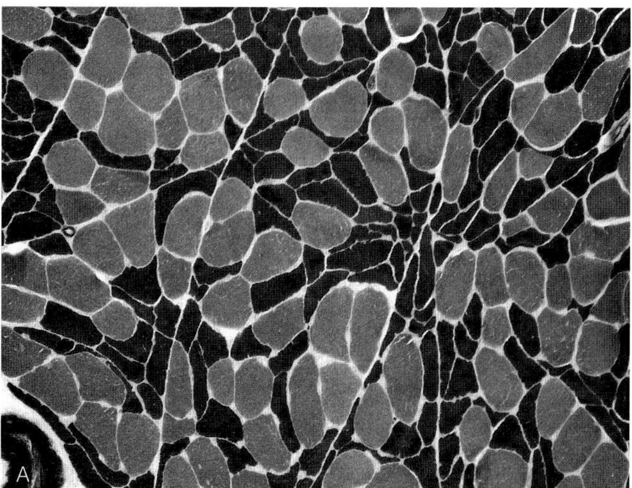

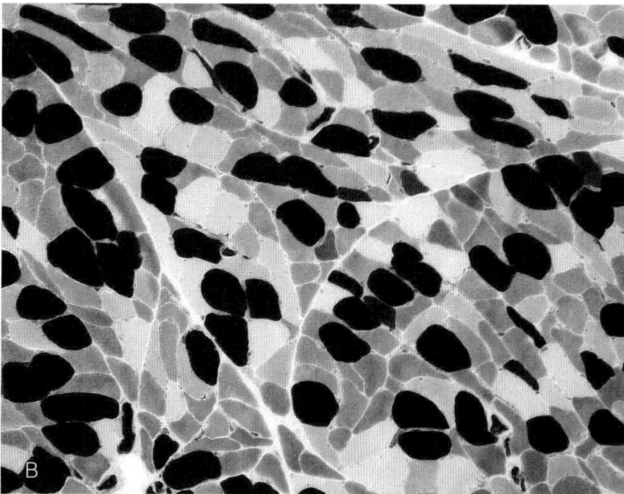

FIGURE 79-1. **(A)** Selective atrophy of type II muscle fibers. (ATPase stain, PH 9.4 ×100). **(B)** Atrophic fibers are mainly type IIB that stain intermediate with ATPasa at PH 4.6 (×100).

vacuolization may also be detected on electromicroscopy. Type II fibers have also been found to be more affected than type I fibers in steroid myopathy in experimental animals receiving corticosteroids (15).

A number of mechanisms have been proposed in the pathogenesis of steroid myopathy, and evidence indicates alteration of carbohydrate metabolism and a negative protein balance. High doses of corticosteroids stimulate protein degeneration, which is dose related. Inhibition of protein synthesis affects predominantly type II fibers. Decreased physical activity might be a contributing factor in muscle atrophy and weakness of these patients.

Treatment of steroid myopathy consists of removal of the primary cause of CS, particularly reduction of corticosteroid doses, increased mobilization, and physical therapy.

Critical illness myopathy (CIM) is a paralyzing disease predominantly observed among patients in the intensive care unit who have received high doses of steroids and neuromuscular blocking agents (16), but it has also been reported in patients not receiving steroids and in patients with myasthenia gravis receiving steroids but not paralyzing agents. The risk of developing CIM increases with the severity of the primary illness, and with renal failure and hyperglycemia.

Characteristically, patients with CIM have diffuse, but predominately proximal, muscle weakness and are usually ventilator dependent and have decreased muscle stretch reflexes. They may also have evidence of a neuropathy of the gravely ill. Serum creatine kinase (CK) could be normal or elevated.

Electrodiagnostic tests reveal low amplitude compound muscle action potentials (CMAP), with a relative preservation of sensory evoked response. The CMAP obtained by direct muscle or nerve stimulation are equally decreased in amplitude. Needle EMG shows fibrillation potentials and small polyphasic motor unit action potentials. Nerve conduction studies could also demonstrate the presence of a neuropathy (17). Muscle biopsy shows fiber muscle atrophy of both types, but mainly type II fibers. There are also atrophic angulated fibers and internalized nuclei and many features of a chronic myopathy with some evidence of muscle necrosis, basophilic stripling, moth-eaten fibers, and reduction of andenosine triphosphatase (ATPase) activity (17). Electron microscopy (EM) demonstrates a diffuse loss of thick filaments (Fig. 79-2), although this finding can sometimes occur in other conditions.

The etiology of CIM is uncertain, and several hypotheses have been proposed; particularly, a relationship may exist between CIM and the systemic inflammatory response, and thus, there is a cytokine-induced muscle injury and activation of proteases.

The treatment is nonspecific and consists of rehabilitation, physical therapy, and decreasing steroid dosages with avoidance of paralyzing blocking agents.

OTHER NEUROLOGIC MANIFESTATIONS

Of patients with CS, 20% complain of low back pain secondary to vertebral compression fractures and they can also have pathologic long bone fractures and osteoporosis, or lordotic posture from weight gain (4). Cranial nerve palsies are mostly secondary to a mechanical compression of the pituitary mass, but some cases of ocular paresis may be seen, even in the absence of mechanical compression on ocular nerves (18).

The relative severity of these symptoms varies according to several factors, including the degree and duration of hypercortisolism, the presence or absence of androgen excess, and the cause of the hypercortisolism.

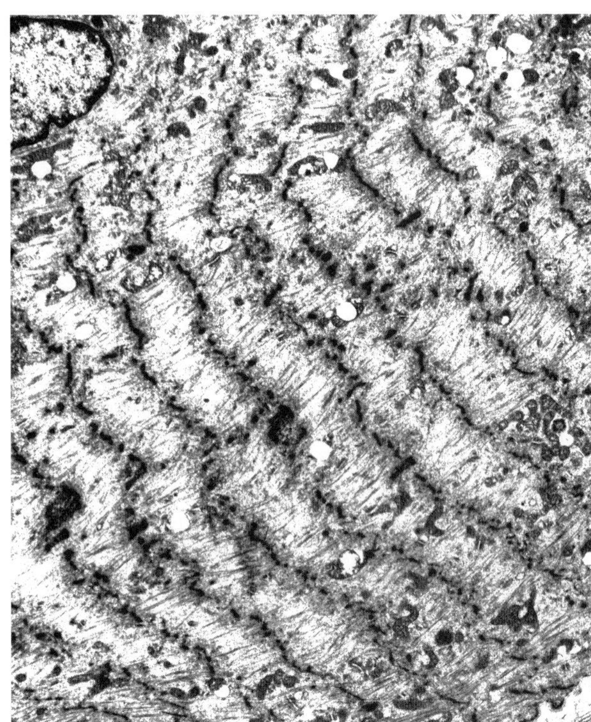

FIGURE 79-2. Electromicroscopy of a muscle biopsy in a patient with critical illness myopathy showing loss of thick filaments (×7,500).

DIAGNOSTIC APPROACH

The first step in the diagnosis of CS is demonstrating elevated urinary free cortisol (UFC), its metabolite, 17-OHCS, or the presence of inadequate suppression of cortisol secretion during the dexamethasone suppression test. The second step is to determine the cause of the hypercortisolism, whether it is ACTH-dependent (pituitary or nonpituitary ACTH-secreting tumor) or ACTH-independent (primary adrenal disease), depending on measurements of plasma ACTH using immunoradiometric assay (IRMA).

DAILY URINARY CORTISOL SECRETION

A 24-four-hour urinary cortisol excretion provides a reliable index of cortisol secretion and free serum cortisol concentration (2). Urinary cortisol can be detected by immunoassay or by structurally based techniques. CS is diagnosed if basal urinary cortisol secretion is more than three times the upper limit of normal, (2) or >50 μg/24 hours (1). Patients with CD usually have UFC levels between 100 and 500 μg/24 hours, whereas in ectopic ACTH syndrome and cortisol-secreting adrenal adenomas or carcinomas, the UFC levels are >500 μg/24 hours.

LOW-DOSE DEXAMETHASONE SUPPRESSION TESTS

The low-dose dexamethasone suppression screening test is based on the fact that dexamethasone suppresses ACTH release from the pituitary gland, leading to reductions in serum cortisol levels and in the urinary excretion of cortisol and its metabolites (2). The test is performed by administering 1 mg of dexamethasone at 11 PM to 12 AM; then, serum cortisol levels are measured at 8 AM the next morning. Normal individuals have an 8 AM serum cortisol value of <2 μg/dL (55 nmol/L) (2,20), whereas a morning plasma cortisol level >3 μg/dL suggests hypercortisolism (1). Levels of <14.3 μg/dL may be normal or may suggest CS or pseudo-CS, and the definitive diagnosis would need a confirmatory test.

LATE EVENING SERUM AND SALIVARY CORTISOL

Measurement of serum or salivary cortisol in the late evening is of great diagnostic value. Usually, patients collect samples on three consecutive evenings. The diagnosis of CS is very unlikely if the serum level is <5 μg/dL (2) or the salivary level is <1.3 ng/mL (3.6 nmol/L) when measured by radioimmunoassay (RIA), or <1.5 ng/mL (4.2 nmol/L) when measured by competitive protein-binding assay.

TEST TO IDENTIFY PATIENTS WITH PSEUDO-CUSHING SYNDROME

As the circadian rhythm is preserved in depressed patients but not in those with CS, the diagnosis of CS is unlikely if a midnight plasma cortisol level is >7.5 μg/dL. Administration of CRH and dexamethasone in sequence exploits the greater sensitivity of corticotropin secretion to dexamethasone suppression in depressed patients and the greater plasma cortisol response to exogenous CRH in patients with CS (3). Administration of naloxone stimulates releasing of CRH better in depressed patients (3). That hypercortisolism is mild and transient in depression makes plasma cortisol levels increase in response to insulin-induced hypoglycemia in depression, but not in patients with chronic CS (3).

TEST TO DETERMINE ACTH-DEPENDENT VERSUS ACTH-INDEPENDENT CS

Two to three blood specimens are collected to determine plasma cortisol and ACTH levels between 11 PM and midnight from the patients while they are collecting their urine specimens. A plasma cortisol level >15 μg/dL and an ACTH concentration <5 pg/mL is diagnostic that cortisol secretion is ACTH independent, and an ACTH concentration >15 pg/mL is diagnostic that cortisol secretion is ACTH dependent (19).

METYRAPONE STIMULATION TEST

Metyrapone blocks the conversion of 11-deoxycortisol to cortisol, leading to a low level of cortisol, which stimulates the pituitary gland to secrete more ACTH, leading to high plasma 11-deoxycortisol and urinary 17-hydroxycorticosteroid levels with low plasma cortisol levels. Patients with CD have normal or supranormal response, those with ectopic ACTH have little or no response (3).

DIAGNOSING THE SOURCE OF EXCESS ADRENOCORTICOTROPIC HORMONE SECRETION

A standard high–dose dexamethasone suppression test should be done in patients with ACTH-dependent CS. In those with adequate suppression, pituitary computed tomography (CT) or MRI should be done to rule out pituitary adenoma. In patients with inadequate suppression, an octreotide scan and chest CT or MRI should be done to rule out carcinomas. If findings are negative, pituitary CT or MRI should then be done to rule out a pituitary source of ACTH production.

TREATMENT

In most CS, primary adrenal hyperplasia responds to bilateral adrenal adrenalectomy, and unilateral adrenalectomy may be performed in those with adrenal adenoma or carcinoma (3). Adrenal enzyme inhibitors should be considered to control hypercortisolism in those patients with carcinomas.

The treatment of choice for patients with Cushing disease is transsphenoidal microadenomectomy or partial resection of the anterior pituitary (85% to 90%), which provides cure rate of about 80% among experienced neurosurgeons. Patients are considered cured if their morning plasma cortisol levels are undetectable and ACTH levels are <5 pg/mL 24 hours after the last dose of hydrocortisone 4 to 7 days after the surgery. Patients require daily glucocorticoid replacement therapy from the time of surgery until their hypothalamic-pituitary-adrenal function recovers; this takes 6 to 12 months. Adrenalectomy performed in a patient with a pituitary tumor carries the risk of Nelson syndrome, which is described in the pituitary tumor section-chapter which is described in Chapter 76.

In patients with ectopic ACTH and CRH syndromes, the treatment of choice is resection of the tumor; however, because 90% of these tumors are malignant and nonresectable, the treatment of choice is the use of adrenal enzyme inhibitors or surgical adrenalectomy.

Hyperaldosteronism

DEFINITION

Hyperaldosteronism is defined as a state of a selective increase of mineralocorticoid secretion by a primary disorder of the adrenal gland in the zona glomerulosa.

EPIDEMIOLOGY

Hyperaldosteronism is a relatively uncommon syndrome that may be related to adrenal hyperplasia or, less commonly, to an adenoma.

ETIOLOGY AND PATHOGENESIS

Hyperaldosteronism could be primary (aldosterone-secreting adenomas or carcinomas, bilateral adrenal hyperplasia), or secondary from overactivation of the renin-angiotensin system, such as in accelerated hypertension, renovascular hypertension, estrogen administration, renin-secreting tumors, and Bartter syndrome (a rare disorder with several metabolic abnormalities, including hypokalemia, metabolic alkalosis, hyperreninemia, hyperaldosteronism, and hyperplasia of the juxtaglomerular apparatus). Kearns-Sayre syndrome, a mitochondrial disease, can present with hyperaldosteronism, hypokalemic alkalosis, and symptoms similar to Bartter syndrome (21). Other causes include potassium sodium-wasting nephropathy, renal tubular acidosis, diuretic or laxative abuse, or edematous state. Hyperaldosteronism could also be caused by adrenal enzyme deficiencies (11 β-hydroxylase, 17 α-hydroxylase, and 11 β-hydroxysteroid dehydrogenase, type II) and from exogenous mineralocorticoids administrations, such as licorice, carbenoxolone, and fluorocortisone (1).

CLINICAL MANIFESTATIONS

Hyperaldosteronism manifests by hypertension in 5% of cases; hypokalemia and metabolic alkalosis may be seen as well (1). Patients with mild hypokalemia present with fatigue, muscle weakness, nocturia, and headache, whereas those with more severe hypokalemia have polyuria, polydipsia, paresthesias, and muscle weakness, such as hypokalemic periodic paralysis or a persistent myopathy (22,23). Because of these manifestations, hyperaldosteronism should be considered in patients presenting with muscle weakness associated with hypokalemia, regardless of the degree of hypertension. Patients could complain of leg pain or develop tetany secondary to metabolic alkalosis (24) with positive Trousseau or Chvostek signs. Other neurologic manifestations include static tremor, encephalopathy, and syncope. Idiopathic intracranial hypertension may be rarely seen in patients with primary hyperaldosteronism (25). Ischemic optic neuropathy has also been reported in patients with this disease. Hyperaldosteronism can also manifest with depression.

DIAGNOSIS

Hyperaldosteronism should be suspected in patients with arterial hypertension accompanied by hypokalemia, muscle weakness, or both, particularly if they are not receiving diuretics. The first step in diagnosis is to measure aldosterone and plasma renin activity (PRA) in the early morning hours. A serum aldosterone-to-PRA ratio >20 ng/dL or ng/mL/hour and a serum aldosterone level >15 ng/dL suggest the diagnosis (1).

The second step in the diagnosis is to determine whether the cause is an adrenal adenoma, or bilateral adrenal hyperplasia. The postural challenge test is useful in this differential diagnosis. The test consists of obtaining an early morning supine blood sample of aldosterone, renin, cortisol, and 18-hydrocortisone; then, tests are repeated after the patient stands for 2 hours. A plasma aldosterone level <20 ng/dL with an increase on standing suggests a bilateral hyperplasia. In adenomas, the baseline levels are >20 ng/dL, and they decrease on standing, as a result of decreased stimulation by ACTH. Also, an 18-hydrocortisone level <50 ng/dL that increases on standing suggests bilateral hyperplasia. A level >50 ng/dL that falls on standing suggests an adenoma. After these tests are performed, a CT scan of the abdomen helps to localize the tumor.

TREATMENT

The treatment of choice for unilateral adenomas is a laparoscopic adrenalectomy (26). Ablative procedure by percutaneous acetic acid injection also could be affective for unilateral adrenal adenomas (27). Both treatment types lead to a marked reduction in aldosterone secretion with orthostatic hypotension in almost all cases (28), but a lesser degree of persistent hypertension occurs in as many as 40% to 65% of patients, likely caused by nephrosclerosis after a prolonged period of uncontrolled hypertension. Mineralocorticoid receptor antagonists, such as spironolactone and eplerenone, can be used in the treatment of this disease (29) and, if patients fail to tolerate this treatment, amiloride can be used. Hydrochlorothiazide can also be added for better control of blood pressure.

Optimal treatment for idiopathic hyperaldosteronism consists of spironolactone or eplerenone, aiming to normalize blood pressure and serum potassium levels (30). In patients with bilateral hyperplasia and glucocorticoid-remediable aldosteronism (GRA), a rare autosomal dominant condition with hyperaldosteronism, can be reversed with glucocorticoid therapy (31).

Glucocorticoid Deficiency

The nervous and endocrine systems are closely interrelated, and neurologic diseases can result in endocrine dysfunction, whereas patients with endocrine diseases can develop neurologic symptoms, particularly in corticosteroid deficiency.

Primary and Secondary Hypoadrenalism

DEFINITION

Adrenal insufficiency (AI), which results from inadequate adrenocortical function, can be divided in two types: Primary AI, referring to glucocorticoid deficiency caused by diseases of the adrenal gland, and, secondary AI, which occurs as a result of pituitary or hypothalamic diseases. In both, the final result is deficiency of corticotropin (ACTH).

EPIDEMIOLOGY

It is difficult to find an epidemiologic study on the frequency of Addison disease. Patients who have been on long-standing steroid-therapy are clearly at risk on discontinuation of therapy, which should be slowly tapered. A variable prevalence of autoimmune adrenal insufficiency has been reported, from 4 to 11 per 100,000 populations.

ETIOLOGY AND PATHOGENESIS

Primary AI is always associated with mineralocorticoid deficiency, but in secondary AI the renin-angiotensin-aldosterone axis remains intact, and only ACTH is deficient.

Autoimmune disorders account for most of cases of primary AI, or Addison disease, which can be either isolated or part of the autoimmune polyglandular syndrome. Primary AI can also be caused by infections, such as tuberculosis, histoplasmosis, cryptococcosis, cytomegalovirus, and human immunodeficiency virus (HIV); less frequent causes include metastatic malignancies (mostly from lung or breast), amyloidosis, hemorrhage or infarction, hemochromatosis, surgical removal of the adrenal glands, adrenoleukodystrophies, congenital adrenal hypoplasia (CAH), and other rare hereditary disorders (32–35).

Secondary AI is more common and could be caused by glucocorticoid therapy, surgical removal of pituitary tumors, or hypopituitarism. Less common causes include tumors or infections that can affect the pituitary gland, but usually other hormonal defects are associated. Other less common causes include pituitary apoplexy, Sheehan syndrome, lymphocytic hypophysitis, radiation, idiopathic ACTH deficiency, propiomelanocortin (POMC) gene mutations, and surgical resection of parts of hypothalamus (33,34).

PRIMARY ADRENAL INSUFFICIENCY

Frequent causes of AD include autoimmune adrenalitis, infections, congenital metabolic endocrine and central nervous system (CNS) disorders, and metastatic tumors. They will be discussed as separate groups.

Isolated Autoimmune Adrenalitis

Thomas Addison described isolated autoimmune adrenalitis in 1885. This rare condition accounts for about 75% of primary adrenal insufficiency (PAI) cases. Autoimmune adrenalitis sometimes is accompanied by autoimmune thyroid disorder and other autoimmune endocrine deficiencies. The mean age at diagnosis is 40 years (range from 17 to 72 years) (33,36). Evidence of both humoral- and cell-mediated immune mechanisms directed at the adrenal cortex has been found (32,34). Addison disease (AD) is associated with significant morbidity and mortality. In this condition, the adrenal glands do not produce sufficient cortisol, and, rarely, there is also a defect of aldosterone and androgens. Clinical manifestations occur when at least 90% of the adrenal cortex has been destroyed.

Pathologically, in PAI the adrenal glands are atrophic with loss of most of the cortical cells, but the medulla is usually spared. Because epinephrine synthesis in the medulla depends on high local corticosteroid concentrations, an adrenomedullary dysfunction or destruction may be associated with PAI (37).

AD is a common component of the autoimmune polyglandular syndrome (APS). This syndrome might manifest into two separate forms: APS-1 (type 1) and APS-2 (type 2), which is described in detail in the multiple endocrine syndromes chapter (Chapter 82) (33,34). Mutations in gene autoimmune regulator at 21q 22-3 have been reported with APS-1 (34). Autoantibodies to the adrenal cortex or to 21-hidroxylase are useful markers and are predictive of the development of adrenal destruction (34,35,38).

Infections

Tuberculous adrenal insufficiency, a common cause of AD in the past, resulted from hematogenous spread of mycobacteria, with subsequent gradual destruction of the adrenal glands. Initially, the adrenal glands appear enlarged, but later, adrenal tissue becomes replaced by caseous nodules and with fibrosis becoming smaller in size. Radiographically, calcifications are present in 50% (32). Adrenal insufficiency is an increasingly common occurrence in patients with acquired immunodeficiency syndrome (AIDS), correlating with stage of progression of HIV infection (39). Cytomegalovirus is the pathogen in 50% of cases; mycobacterium avium, mycobacterium tuberculosis, toxoplasma, and pneumocystis species are pathogens causing this condition in AIDS. In addition, antiinfective medications frequently used in AIDS, such as ketoconazole (decreased adrenal steroidogenesis), rifampin, opiates (increase steroid catabolism), and trimethoprim may precipitate adrenal insufficiency (32,35). Histoplasmosis and paracoccidioidomycosis have predication for the adrenal glands and are part of the differential diagnosis in endemic areas. Prolonged antifungal treatment is indicated (40).

Adrenoleukodystrophy

Adrenoleukodystrophy (ALD) is an X-linked disorder characterized by a combination of primary adrenal insufficiency with a progressive inflammatory demyelinating process that mainly affects cerebral hemispheres, particularly the parietooccipital regions (41).

The classic form of ALD has onset in childhood and is often rapidly progressive. Deficiency of acyl Coenzyme A synthetase, results in an inability to degrade very long chain fatty acid (VLCFA) in peroxisomes, leading to accumulation and formation as cytoplasmic inclusions (41,42).

The responsible ALD gene is located in Xq28 and encodes for a peroxisomal membrane protein. All ethnic groups are affected, with a wide range of phenotypic expression, and women carriers can become symptomatic. The age of onset of cerebral ALD is 5 to 12 years. Central demyelination results in seizures, spastic tetraparesis, cortical blindness, auditory dysfunction, dementia, coma, and death (35,41,42).

Adrenomyeloneuropathy (AMN) is a variant of ALD that affects the central and peripheral nervous system, adrenal glands, and testes (42,43). AMN is a noninflammatory distal axonopathy that involves long tracts of spinal cord and lesser extension peripheral nerves (44). This is a slowly progressive disease, and the clinical presentation occurs in the third and fourth decade of age. Involvement of ascending and descending tracts of the spinal cord occurs. A mixed, motor and sensory neuropathy associated with color blindness, spastic paraparesis, and urinary and erectile dysfunction is a frequently found clinical picture (35,42,43). Up to 50% of affected males have MRI showing cerebral demyelination that is not associated with significant clinical cerebral involvement; cerebellar dysfunction is rare. AD can occur in two thirds of male patients, and gonadal dysfunction is also present (43). Some female heterozygotes have neurologic symptoms that are milder than male presentations, showing mild pyramidal involvement and urinary incontinence (34,43).

Tumors

Adrenal metastases are most commonly caused by lung and breast tumors in 40% to 60% of patients, melanoma in 30%, and stomach or colon cancer in 20%. Clinically, adrenal insufficiency in these patients is uncommon, because most of the adrenal cortex must be destroyed before clinical manifestations, and symptoms of adrenal insufficiency are mistakenly attributed to cancer (45). The benefits of glucocorticoids have been described in a few studies with bilateral adrenal metastasis (45).

Other less common causes, including adrenal hemorrhage or infarction, should be considered in patients gravely ill, affected with underlying conditions, such as infection, thromboembolic disease, coagulopathy, trauma, shock, burns, or recent surgery. In meningococcal septicemias, adrenal hemorrhage can complicate the patient's condition; pseudomona is also associated with hemorrhage (34,35). In the antiphospholipid syndrome, a lupus anticoagulant is responsible for thrombosis or hemorrhage (35).

Congenital

In adrenal dysgenesis, mutations in the dosage-sensitive sex reversal-adrenal hypoplasia gene 1 on Xp21 (DAX-1) or mutations of steroidogenic factor-1 (SF-1) have been reported. Both nuclear hormone receptors could act as coregulators and are required for normal adrenal, gonadal and hypothalamus development (46).

In congenital adrenal hypoplasia, the adrenal cortex has arrested development; an X-linked form is associated with PAI and hypogonadotrophic hypogonadism. Adrenal insufficiency is present from birth, and phenotypically, several forms do not correlate with genotype (47).

Another X-linked form of adrenal insufficiency that occurs in association with glycerol kinase deficiency has been described (48); the genetic locus was mapped to Xp21. The onset of symptoms varies from birth to childhood. Clinical presentation includes psychomotor retardation, muscular dystrophy, especial facies with hypertelorism, strabismus, drooping mouth, anorchia or cryptorchidism, short stature, and osteoporosis (48).

Familial glucocorticoid deficiency (FGD) is a rare autosomal recessive disorder in which cortisol and androgen secretions are deficient, and no adrenal response to ACTH occurs; aldosterone secretion is normal or partially deficient. Mutations of the G protein-coupled ACTH-receptor are found in 40% (type 1), but no mutations are detected in 60% (type 2). Patients with FGD type 1 are significantly taller than those with type-2. Patients are affected in early childhood. Signs include hyperpigmentation, hypoglycemia, failure to thrive, and severe infections (34,35).

In Allgrove syndrome, or triple A, is found a triad of ACTH resistance, alacrima, and achalasia. This is an autosomal recessive disorder mapping to 12q13. There is a gradual neurologic dysfunction, polyneuropathy, deafness, mental retardation, and hyperkeratosis of palms and soles; aldosterone deficiency has been seen in 15% of cases (49).

Mitochondrial diseases can present with chronic lactic acidosis, myopathy, cataracts, and nerve deafness (34). Kearns-Sayre syndrome is characterized by mitochondrial myopathy, deafness, and endocrine dysfunctions (short stature, hypogonadism, hypoparathyroidism, hypothyroidism, adrenal deficiency) (50).

In Smith-Lemli-Opitz syndrome, the primary defect is in the fetal adrenal glands. Features include a distinctive facial appearance, consisting of ptosis, inner epicanthal folds, anteverted nares and micrognathia. Other characteristics include microcephaly, mental retardation, congenital cardiac abnormalities, syndactyly, incomplete development of male genitalia in boys, and photosensitivity (34).

Congenital lipoid adrenal hyperplasia is characterized by glucocorticoid, mineralocorticoids, and sex steroid deficiencies. Mutations are found in the StAR gene that maps on 8p11; the phenotype is female (34).

Defective cholesterol metabolism because of absence of low-density lipoprotein (LDL), such as abetalipoproteinemia, or absence of LDL receptors, such as homozygous familial hypercholesteremia, have moderately impaired serum cortisol response to ACTH (32).

Finally, several drugs can inhibit cortisol biosynthesis, such as aminoglutethimide, etomidate, ketoconazole, metyrapone, and suramin. Patients with limited pituitary or adrenal reserve are most vulnerable to developing adrenal insufficiency. Other drugs that accelerate cortisol metabolism include phenytoin, barbiturates, and rifampin (32,34).

SECONDARY ADRENAL INSUFFICIENCY

Sudden cessation of chronic exogenous glucocorticoid therapy is the most common cause of adrenal insufficiency, decreased CRH or ACTH synthesis and secretion with preserved mineralocorticoid secretion is typical. This risk should be anticipated in any person who has taken more than 30 mg of hydrocortisone or equivalent glucocorticoids per day longer than 3 weeks (32). Pituitary tumors associated with low ACTH levels are described in Chapter 76. In isolated ACTH deficiency, there is no ACTH-secretory response to CRH. This is a rare disorder, possibly of an autoimmune origin (51). A defect in conversion of POMC to ACTH by prohormone convertase enzymes (PC1 and PC2) has been described. Given the ACTH, the melanocyte-stimulating hormone (MSH) is increased and results in severe obesity, skin darkening, and red hair pigmentation (52).

SYMPTOMS OF ADRENAL INSUFFICIENCY

The clinical presentation of AI depends on the rate and the degree of the hormonal deficiency. The primary type is associated with both glucocorticoid and mineralocorticoid deficiencies. The secondary type has an intact renin-angiotensin-aldosterone system. AD is often insidious in onset and is characterized by nonspecific symptoms of corticosteroid deficiency, such as chronic weakness, fatigue, general malaise, orthostatic hypotension (more marked in primary than secondary AI), dizziness, weight loss, fever, and anorexia (33,37). Some patients present with abdominal cramps, nausea, vomiting, or diarrhea alternating with constipation (32,33). Patients with AD have increased daytime fatigue, but they do not have excessive daytime sleepiness (53).

The most significant sign that differentiates both forms of AI is hyperpigmentation of the skin and mucous surfaces, present in primary AI. This is caused by high plasma corticotropin concentrations that occur as a result of decreased cortisol feedback, leading to increased MSH levels. Vitiligo may also be associated with AD. Another specific symptom of primary insufficiency is a craving for salt (32,33,36). Androgen secretion is lost in AI, and the clinical presentation is more apparent in women, who may complain of loss of axillary and pubic hair. In young patients, delayed growth and puberty would point to hypothalamic-pituitary disease. Headaches, visual disturbances, or diabetes insipidus have been seen in patients of any age (33,41). Hyponatremia, hypokalemia, acidosis, elevated creatinine, hypoglycemia, hypercalcemia, mild normocytic anemia, lymphocytosis, and mild eosinophilia have been described (33,37).

Secondary adrenal insufficiency (SAI) is associated with hypopituitarism; then, clinical presentation may be related to different hormonal deficiencies, especially luteinizing hormone (LH) or follicle-stimulating hormone (FSH), as well as thyroid-stimulating hormone (TSH) (32).

Acute adrenal crisis is a medical emergency. Patients become hypotensive and may have acute circulatory failure. Symptoms can include upper abdominal or loin pain, abdominal rigidity, severe vomiting, diarrhea, and confusion. Hyperpigmentation and vitiligo have also been described in adrenal crisis (32,33).

The neurologic manifestations of glucocorticoid deficiency are multiple and mainly related to systemic dysfunction. Mental status changes are frequent and varied. Electroencephalographic (EEG) abnormalities are seen, although seizures are unusual. Also, increased intracranial pressure, with or without cerebral edema, may occur (54). In SAI caused by hypopituitarism, symptoms are usually not as severe. Lassitude and weakness with lack of energy might resemble a myopathy and is usually caused by dehydration and hypoglycemia. In PAI, muscle or joint pain occurs in 6% to 13% of patients, but muscle biopsy is usually normal (55). Deficit of glucocorticoids, mineralocorticoids, and sometimes lack of catecholamines secretion, along with dehydration, can cause orthostatic hypotension and syncope. Loss of consciousness could also be caused by episodic hypoglycemia.

The hyponatremia that occurs in patients with AD can lead to delirium, coma, and seizures. These patients have poor response to saline infusions, but a prompt response to hydrocortisone. Acute addisonian crisis can cause weakness, fatigue, lethargy, confusion, or coma.

Hyperkalemia found in AD can cause relapses of neuromuscular symptoms, such as weakness and myalgias, mostly in legs (55). General weakness seen in AD probably results from the changes in plasma and muscle water and electrolytes.

PGA-1 can manifest with muscle cramps, myalgias, weakness, and, later, neuropsychological disturbances; one study reported muscular histologic appearance similar to hypothyroidism (55,56). The neurologic abnormalities in triple A syndrome include hyperreflexia, muscle weakness, dysarthria, ataxia, impaired intelligence, and postural hypotension (57).

Addison-Schilder syndrome is probably an X-linked disorder characterized by bronze skin, caused by PAI, and cerebral sclerosis. Abnormalities usually occur between the ages of 5 and 15 years. Patients have difficulties in learning, and ataxia or seizures. Also, blindness, deafness, hemiplegia or quadriplegia, pseudobulbar palsy, and dementia can occur (58).

Neuropsychiatric symptoms can be present in severe and long-standing AI. These include impairment of memory, confusion, delirium, stupor, depression, and psychosis. These may disappear a few days after corticosteroid therapy, but psychosis can persist for several months (59).

DIAGNOSIS

The diagnosis of AD is made by determining reduced plasma cortisol level and establishing its cause. Imaging studies of the adrenal and pituitary glands, such as CT scan or MRI, are useful. Morning plasma cortisol concentrations of <3 μg/dL indicate AI, whereas concentrations equal or more than 19 μg/dL rule out this disorder (33,60).

In PAI, corticotropin (ACTH) concentration is usually >100 pg/mL, even when cortisol level is normal. Normal ACTH level rules out PAI but might be seen in SAI. Aldosterone is low or at the lower end of normal value in PAI, whereas plasma renin activity or concentration is increased. ACTH stimulation test is the most specific test to diagnosis PAI. There is a short and a prolonged stimulation test. The short test uses 250 μg of cosyntrin (synthetic form of ACTH). Cortisol is measured at 0, 30, and 60 minutes after the injection. Normal response occurs if basal of postcosyntrin plasma cortisol level is at least 18 μg/dL or preferably >20 μg/dL (60). A normal test finding excludes PAI, but does not rule out SAI or recent onset.

The prolonged ACTH stimulation test consists of continuous infusion of cosyntrin for 24 to 48 hours. In normal subjects, plasma cortisol at 4 hours is >36 μg/dL, and beyond this time there is no further increase. A progressive increase is seen in cortisol secretion in secondary insufficiency, but little or no response in primary insufficiency (32,60). Other tests used in the evaluation of patients with suspected SAI include the insulin-induced hypoglycemia test, which produces signs of activation of the sympathetic nervous system after intravenous administration of insulin, causing hypoglycemia, which stimulates the hypothalamic-pituitary-adrenal axis (33).

In the metyrapone test, a measure of 11-deoxycortisol and cortisol after oral administration of adrenal 11-hydroxylase inhibitor (metyrapone) detects patients with mild SAI. In normal subjects, 11-deoxycortisol level is at least 7 μg/dL; patients with AI show smaller levels, and related to severity of the ACTH deficiency, simultaneously, plasma cortisol level is <8 μg/dL (60). CRH stimulates ACTH secretion. After CRH injection, plasma ACTH and cortisol should be measured. Plasma ACTH peak occurs at 15 or 30 minutes, and cortisol peaks at 30 or 45 minutes. This test can distinguish between ACTH deficiency and CRH deficiency (60).

The simultaneous presence of 21-hydroxylase and adrenal cortex antibodies permits definitive diagnosis of autoimmune AD. The presence of only one of the two autoantibodies of low titers does not necessarily exclude a non-autoimmune origin of the disease (61).

The diagnosis of ALD or AMN is established by plasma VLCFA assay as well as C24 or C22 (fatty acid with 24 and 22 carbon atoms, respectively) and C26-to-C22 ratios. Very rarely, male patients may have normal levels of C26, but all have abnormal ratios (43). No correlation exists between absolute levels of VLCFA and degree of neurologic involvement. These assays should be performed in all males with idiopathic AD and in patients with progressive paraparesis. MRI may show demyelination, and all modalities of evoked potentials may be abnormal (41,43). Prenatal diagnosis can be made by measuring VLCFA levels in cultured amniocytes and chorionic villus cells, but this should be confirmed by DNA analysis (62).

TREATMENT

Replacement of gluco- and mineralocorticoids are essential in AI; however, no clear indication is found for replacement of adrenal androgens, such as dehydroepiandrosterone (34).

Cortisol replacement is given orally with hydrocortisone or cortisone in morning and afternoon, trying to emulate the natural circadian rhythm. Usually, the initial dose is 25 mg of hydrocortisone, divided into 15 and 10 mg, or 37.5 mg of cortisone, divided in 25 and 12.5 mg. The goal is to use the smallest dose that relieves symptoms.

Mineralocorticoid replacement in PAI is accomplishment by fludrocortisone (0.05 to 2 mg daily) in a single daily dose. Hypertension, bradycardia, and suppressed renin levels are clinical signs of over treatment with mineralocorticoid (34).

Patients must be advised to double or triple the hydrocortisone daily dose temporarily with febrile illness or injury (33). In addisonian crisis, immediate high doses of intravenous hydrocortisone (100 mg every 8 hours) and isotonic saline with dextrose should be administered rapidly until hypotension is corrected. Hydrocortisone is reduced gradually as symptoms resolve and changed to oral maintenance therapy. Mineralocorticoid replacement is indicated when the dose of hydrocortisone is <100 mg/day. Management of ALD includes hormonal replacement therapy, but steroid replacement does not slow neurologic progression. A combination of 4:104 of glyceryltrioleate and glyceryltrierucate (Lorenzo's oil) normalizes VLCFA levels in X-linked ALD patients within 4 weeks (41). This should be administered before the age of 6 to reduce the probability of developing cerebral disease (63).

Patients with X-linked ALD with early evidence of inflammatory cerebral involvement might find benefit with hematopoietic stem cell transplantation. Peters et al. (64) found a 92% survival at 5 years in boys with mild involvement (intelligent quotient [IQ] >80 and limited MRI abnormality), however, this procedure has been shown to worsen neurologic conditions in patients with established severe disease (64). Family members at risk should receive genetic counseling.

Pheocromocytoma

DEFINITION

Pheochromocytomas are tumors that originate from chromaffin cells that produce, store, metabolize, and release catecholamines; they, however, can also be nonfunctional. This section also covers tumors derived from amine precursor uptake and decarboxylation (APUD) cells, which also secrete catecholamines, and include chemodectomas, pheochromocytomas, carcinoid tumors, neuroblastomas, and paragangliomas. Other APUD tumors, such as thyroid carcinoma and melanomas, will not be discussed herein.

EPIDEMIOLOGY

The incidence of pheochromocytoma is about two cases per million population (65).

ETIOLOGY AND PATHOGENESIS

Pheochromocytromas more frequently are located in the adrenal medulla, but about 10% to 27% are extra-adrenal (65), 10% are bilateral, and 10% malignant; extra-adrenal tumors are more frequently malignant (66). Receptive genes predispose individuals to develop these tumors, and it is estimated that 25% of the cases result from genetic mutations. The familial form is frequently bilateral and extra-adrenal and is usually more benign. Pheochromocytomas could also be associated with familial multiple endocrine neoplasia syndrome, familial paraglioma or carotid body tumors, Von Hippel-Lindau disease, and neurofibromatosis type 1 (67). Pathologically, they vary in size from 10 to 1,000 g, with an average of 140 g. Areas of hemorrhage may be present in the larger tumors. Microscopically, pheochromocytomas are formed by an islet of a lobulated pattern of cells that appear benign but could have malignant transformation.

CLINICAL MANIFESTATIONS

The symptoms of pheochromocytoma are variable and usually caused by an excessive release of catecholamines. The most frequent manifestation is hypertension, which could be severe and accompanied by headaches, palpitations, and diaphoresis (67). These vary with the type of catecholamines secreted; for example, tumors that primarily secrete norepinephrine usually produce sustained hypertension, whereas those that secrete primarily epinephrine produce episodic hypertensive crises and sometimes hypotension (68).

Other symptoms include sweating, tremors, weakness, and anxiety associated with the palpitations (67). The triad of episodic headaches, diaphoresis, and palpitations has a sensitivity of 89% and a specificity of 67% for pheochromocytoma (69). Hypertensive crises can be precipitated by minor surgical procedures.

Neurologic manifestations of pheochromocytoma are usually related to the changes in blood pressure. These include not only episodic headache, (70) but also cerebrovascular events (71), from dilated cardiomyopathy (72) and musculoskeletal pain caused by bone metastasis that sometimes affects vertebral bodies and causes radiculopathies (73). Rarely, patients manifest seizures (74) caused either by hypertension or cerebral infarcts. Recurrent syncopal episodes could occur from hypotension caused by vasodilatation from excessive plasma epinephrine. Symptoms that resemble *dysautonomic dysreflexia* in patients with paraplegia caused by thoracic spinal cord lesions, may also occur (75).

The differential diagnosis of pheochromocytomas is lengthy and includes, among others, hyperthyroidism, panic attacks, migraine headaches, and drug abuse; these tumors may also release other hormones, such as somatostatin and adrenal corticotropic hormone, causing symptoms and signs of Cushing syndrome. Patients with such tumors have impaired glucose tolerance. Most of these tumors, however, secrete a mixture of catecholamine without dopamine; only rarely do they secrete just dopamine or both.

DIAGNOSTIC APPROACH

The diagnosis is based on the measurement of catecholamines, particularly plasma metanephrine (76), which has a sensitivity of 99% and a specificity of 89% (77). Measurements of other plasma catecholamines, urinary metanephrine, catecholamines, and vanilmandelic acid are also useful (77). Imaging techniques used to localize the tumors include CT (78), and MRI, particularly using radioactive iodine with metaiodobenzylguanidine (MIBG) scans. The clonidine suppression test may distinguish a high secretion of catecholamine from tumors or from excessive CNS outflow (79).

TREATMENT

The therapy for pheochromocytomas consists of resection of the tumor and control of arterial hypertension with an α_1-adrenergic antagonist, such as phenoxybenzamine hydrochloride (Dibenzyline). If the hypertension is not fully controlled with an alpha-blocker, beta-blockers, such as propanolol, should be added, but their use should never precede those of an alpha-blocker, to avoid an exaggerated pressure response. Intravenous nitroprusside sodium is used in patients with severe hypertension (67). Opiates, narcotic antagonists, histamines, and sympatheticomimetic drugs should be avoided, because they might provoke a hypertensive crisis by stimulating the release of catecholamines.

Carcinoid Syndrome and Carcinoid Tumors

DEFINITION

The carcinoid syndrome (CS) consists of a variety of symptoms caused by release of polypeptides by carcinoid tumors (CTs), including episodic cutaneous flushing, associated with generalized burning sensations, and increased blood pressure and heart rate.

EPIDEMIOLOGY

CS is an uncommon syndrome; detailed epidemiologic studies are not available. The use of serotonin reuptake inhibitors (SSRI) may sometimes present with a partial serotonin syndrome.

ETIOLOGY AND PATHOLOGY

CTs have an endocrine origin and are derived from primitive stem cells that synthesize, store, and release biogenic amines, prostaglandins, and polypeptides. Tumors could manifest anywhere in the gastrointestinal tract, bronchi, and rarely other areas. Their classic cells are argentaffinic and argyrophilic.

The substances released by CTs are usually inactivated in the liver; CS develops only when the tumors have metastasized to this organ (80). The most important pathogenic mechanisms in this syndrome relates to alterations of tryptophan metabolism; under normal circumstances, only 1% of dietary tryptophan is converted to serotonin, in contrast, in CS <70% is converted to serotonin and metabolized to 5-hydroxyindoleacetic acid (5-HIAA) (81). Other CTs, particularly those of gastric and bronchial origin, lack the aromatic amino-acid decarboxylase enzyme that converts 5-hydroxytryptophan to serotonin and, thus, have elevated levels of 5-hydoxyhiptophan and histamine, but no serotonin (82). CTs originating in the colon are not associated with CS, even when they metastasize to the liver, because they do not convert tryptophan to serotonin in their metabolism (83).

The abnormalities of the tryptophan metabolism result in decreased protein synthesis, hypoalbuminemia, and a deficiency of nicotinic acid, causing pellagra with its characteristic dermatitis with erythema and scaling, diarrhea, and dementia (81). Abnormalities of Tryptophan metabolism could also cause glossitis, stomatitis, and peripheral neuropathy. The diarrhea is caused by increased intestinal motility from excessive serotonin, which also causes fibrinogenesis, resulting in peritoneal and heart valvular fibrosis (82,84). The valvular fibrosis is a potential cause of cerebral embolism.

CLINICAL MANIFESTATIONS

Patients with CS have facial venous telangiectasias similar to rosacea, which are caused by persistent vasodilatation. Other symptoms include diarrhea, bronchial spasms, peptic ulcers, and valvular heart disease. Frequent diarrhea is associated with pellagra from nicotinic acid deficiency; other vitamin deficiencies could also be present from malabsorption and abnormal protein metabolism (83). The characteristic flushing is caused by increased release of histamine, whereas increased secretion of kallikrein that is converted to bradykinin is likely the cause of the rash and of hypotension, because bradykinin is a potent vasodilator. Patients may also have bronchial spasms resembling asthma and can manifest as a *carcinoid crisis* during anesthesia characterized by severe flushing and by hypotension. This can be prevented with the use of octreotide (84,85). CTs might also secrete prostaglandins, insulin, ACTH, and other biological peptides; neurologic and clinical syndromes associated with these are rare (85).

DIAGNOSTIC APPROACH

The diagnosis of CS is based on the measurement of 5-hydroxytryptamine, 5-hydroxytryptophan, and serotonin and their metabolites in plasma, platelets, and urine (86). Imaging studies include CT and MRI, and endoscopy is also very useful (87). Additionally, positron emission tomography (PET), MIBG, and octreotide scanning can be used.

TREATMENT

The treatment consists of tumor removal (88,89) and chemotherapy with alkylating agents, doxorubicin, 5-fluorouracil, and oral somatostatin analogs (90).

Neuroblastomas

DEFINITION

Neuroblastomas are tumors that originate in primitive neural crest cells from the adrenal medulla and the paraspinal sympathetic ganglia; they correspond to the spectrum of *neuroblastic tumors* that also includes ganglioneuroblastomas and ganglioneuromas. Neuroblastomas account for 97% of all neuroblastic tumors and have a clinical heterogeneous presentation, depending on their location, histopathologic appearance, and biological characteristics (91).

EPIDEMIOLOGY

Neuroblastomas are the second most common solid tumors in childhood after brain tumors and, thus, are the most frequent extracranial tumors in this population; they are the most common malignant tumors in infancy, occurring in 1 of 1,000,000 infants, with a slight male predominance. They can be associated with Hirschsprung disease, fetal hydantoin syndrome, and Von-Recklinghausen disease (92). Neuroblastomas secrete neurogenically derived substances, such as neuron-specific enolase, ferritin, ganglioside GD2, and catecholamines, from which metabolites can be measured in urine for diagnosis and to determine a response to therapy, because they are sensitive indicators of disease status. Their elevation occurs in 75% to 90% of cases (92,93).

ETIOLOGY AND PATHOLOGY

Cytogenetic studies in neuroblastomas demonstrate chromosomal abnormalities in most cases. The most common are double-minute chromatin bodies, homogenously staining regions, and nonrandom deletions or heterozygosity of the short arm of chromosome 1 (94). A genomic amplification is found of the MYCN locus in chromosome band 2p4, which is associated with advanced tumors having a poor prognosis (94).

Pathologically, neuroblastomas consist of small round blue cells, sometimes forming rosettes (Fig. 79-3), and might present as masses in lymph nodes or the abdomen, but also as intrathoracic masses. Clinical manifestations are variable, including malaise, fever, and weight loss. They can present as painless masses in the abdomen, chest, and neck.

CLINICAL MANIFESTATIONS

Frequent neurologic manifestations in neuroblastomas include Horner syndrome, particularly in those with cervical and upper thoracic expansions (Fig. 79-4). Thoracic and abdominal tumors often invade the epidural space in a *dumbbell* fashion, compromising the spinal cord and causing symptoms of cord compression. On the other hand, bone metastasis can cause pain and limping (92). Intraorbital and intracranial invasions

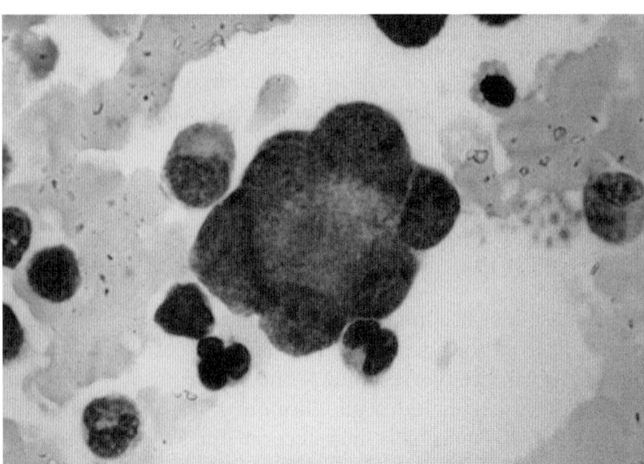

FIGURE 79-3. Metastatic neuroblastoma in bone marrow aspirate with Homer-Wright rosette. (Wright stain; ×100 magnification).

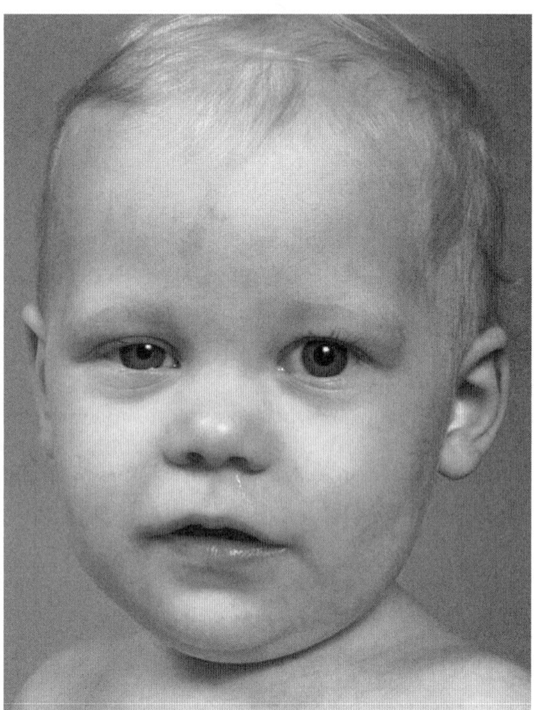

FIGURE 79-4. A child with neuroblastoma of the right upper thoracic area showing right Horner syndrome.

cause proptosis with ecchymosis, giving the child a *raccoon eye* appearance (Fig. 79-5).

Another important manifestation is the syndrome of opsoclonus, myoclonus, and truncal ataxia (OMA). Opsoclonus is a disorder of ocular motility characterized by spontaneous,

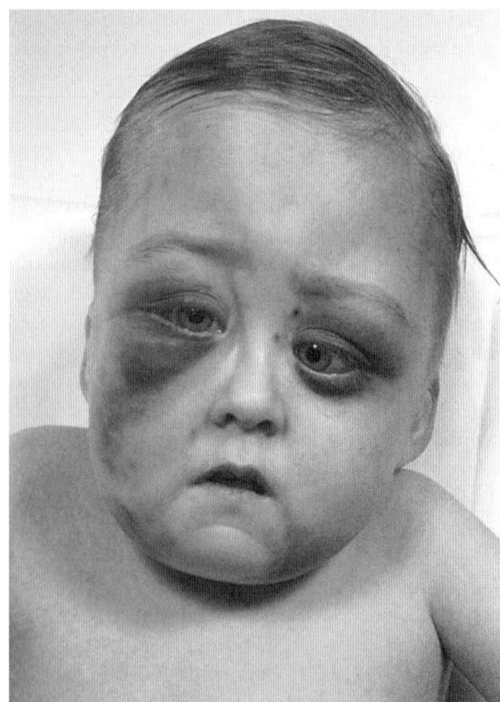

FIGURE 79-5. Intracranial neuroblastoma causing *raccoon eyes*; patient also has opthalmoplegia.

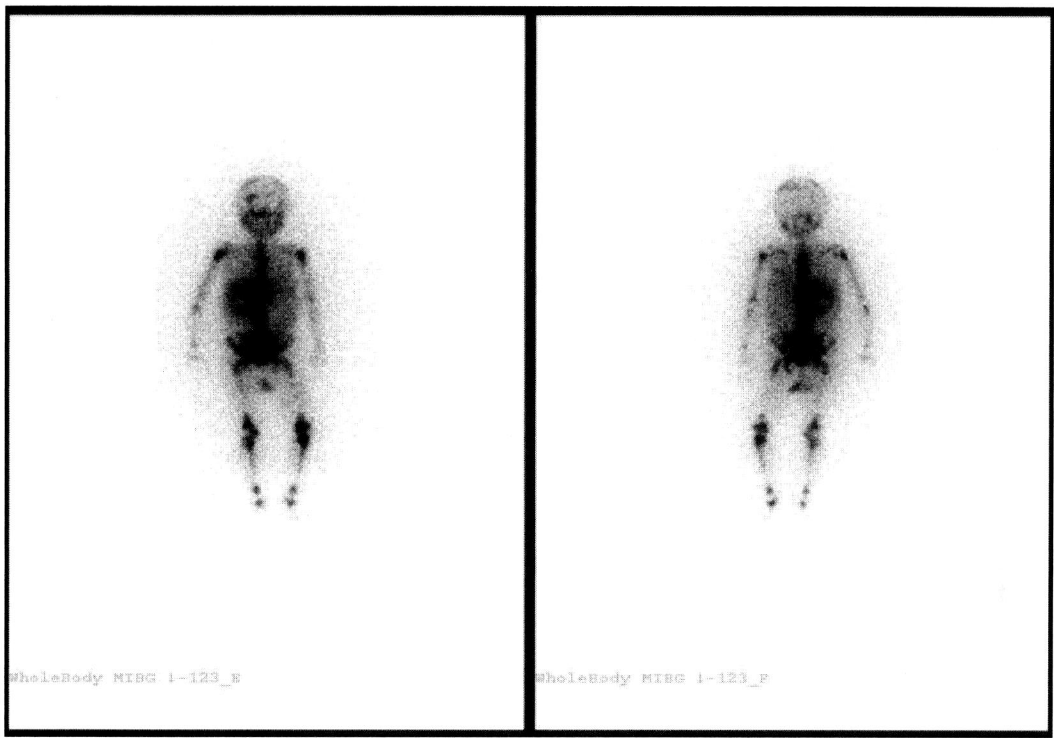

FIGURE 79-6. Methiodobenzilguidine scan in a patient with neuroblastoma showing an adrenal mass with bone metastasis.

conjugate arrhythmic saccades in all directions of gaze, without intersaccadic interval caused by dysfunction of pause cell and the result of a paraneoplastic-mediated syndrome. Opsoclonus can be accompanied by myoclonic jerks of the limbs and truncal ataxia (95).

Although opsoclonus is generally autoimmune and paraneoplastic, particularly those associated with neuroblastoma, it can be associated with various infections or metabolic disorders. Of children with OMA, 50% have a neuroblastoma and about 2% of children with neuroblastoma develop this syndrome (95). The neurologic symptoms can precede the diagnosis of the tumor in about half of the patients. Children with OMA have a mortality rate lower than those without the syndrome, but they may have a protracted course with recurrences having neurologic sequelae (96). Spinal fluid studies showed increased B- and T-cell recruitment, which correlates with relapses and progression (97). Additionally, a pathologic study demonstrated a high incidence of antibodies against CNS antigens, which are directed against Purkinje cells (98). Patients with OMA also have antibodies against the surface of cerebellar granular neurons, and these antibodies are directed against the same autoantigen in different patients (99).

DIAGNOSTIC APPROACH

The diagnosis of neuroblastoma is based on imaging, including MRI, CT, and intravenous myelogram, particularly with methiodobenzylguanidine scans (100) (Fig. 79-6), and measurement of catecholamine in blood and urine.

TREATMENT

The treatment of OMA consists in the use of corticosteroids, ACTH, and plasma exchange or IgG therapy. The type of treatment is based on a complete pathologic evaluation with assessment of genetic markers (101) and staging (Table 79-1).

Therapy of neuroblastoma usually consists of removal and radiation, chemotherapeutic agents, including cyclophosphamide, vincristine, and doxorubicin, alternating with cisplatin and etoposide and retinoid. High dose chemotherapy with bone

TABLE 79-1. International Neuroblastoma Staging System

Stage	*Description*
1	Localized tumor. Complete excision, with or without microscopic residual. Ipsilateral lymph nodes negative.
2A	Localized unilateral tumor. Incomplete gross excision. Ipsilateral lymph nodes negative.
2B	Localized unilateral tumor. Complete or incomplete excision. Ipsilateral and regional lymph nodes positive. Contralateral lymph nodes negative.
3	Unresectable unilateral tumor infiltrating across the midline, with or without lymph node involvement. Unilateral tumor with contralateral lymph node involvement. Midline tumor with bilateral infiltration or bilateral lymph node involvement.
4	Dissemination of tumor to distant lymph nodes, bone, bone marrow, liver, or other organs.
4S	Localized primary tumor in patients <1 year with limited dissemination to liver, skin, or bone marrow.

marrow transplantation might be useful in patients with poor long-term prognosis. Experimental studies include immunotherapy with antibodies targeted against GD2, neuroblastoma vaccines, and antisense oligonucleotides (101,102). Also, targeting tumor cells with drugs that induce apoptosis deposits, such as fenmetramide, or suppress angiogenesis are being investigated.

Paragangliomas or Chemodectomas

DEFINITION

Paragangliomas are part of the extra-adrenal neuroendocrine system that presents primarily in the jugular bulb (or *glomus jugulare)* (103), the middle ear (or *glomus tympanicum)* (104), or in the vagus nerve (or *glomus vagale)* (103). They are composed of chemoreceptive (or type 1) cells and sustentacular (or type 2) cells.

EPIDEMIOLOGY

These tumors represent about 0.6% of tumors of the head and neck.

ETIOLOGY AND PATHOGENESIS

Most of these tumors present as highly vascular soft tissue tumor masses.

CLINICAL MANIFESTATIONS

Mass lesions are a frequent presentation. As illustrated in the vignette, if the chemodectoma is located in the carotid body, syncope may be a possible presentation. Deafness and pulsatile tinnitus may also be present. Glomus tympanicus can also affect the seventh and oculomotor cranial nerve (105). Glomus jugularis tumors may affect cranial nerves IX, X, and XI, as they might invade the jugular foramen.

DIAGNOSIS

The diagnosis of chemodectomas is based on measurement of catecholamines in urine and with imaging, which includes CT angiogram, and MRI angiography (103,106).

TREATMENT

The treatment of choice is surgery (107). Presurgical tumor embolization may be a useful strategy to minimize surgical bleeding. Radiation is used in older patients, particularly when they are not good surgical candidates (108). Gamma knife is an excellent therapeutic choice.

CLINICAL RECOMMENDATIONS OF THE VIGNETTE

The patient had episodic syncope for at least a decade and the cause was not fully defined until bilateral chemodectomas of the carotid body were identified; they were successfully resected. Following surgery, a few months later, the patient developed episodic hypertension, which was difficult to control, and further investigation identified a unilateral pheochromocytoma, which was resected with eventual normalization of the blood pressure. The coexistence of these tumors should be kept in mind because neurologists are frequently consulted in patients with idiopathic syncope.

SUMMARY

Disorders of the adrenal glands can cause multiple neurologic complications from excessive secretion of corticosteroids (Cushing syndrome), mineralocorticoids (hyperaldosteronism), or from adrenal insufficiency. Adrenoleukodystrophy is an X-linked recessive disorder manifested by adrenal insufficiency and CNS demyelination. Neuroendocrine tumors are derived from amine precursor uptake and decarboxylation (APUD) cells in the adrenal gland or other tissues. These include chemodectomas, pheochromocytomas, carcinoid tumors, and neuroblastomas.

Acknowledgments

We would like to acknowledge the secretarial help of Cindy Culver, the editorial assistance of Mary Ann Lucas. The photographs used in Figures 79-3 through 79-6 were generously provided by Dr. Victor Santana from St. Jude Children's Research Hospital in Memphis, Tennessee.

REFERENCES

1. Andreoli TE, Carpenter C, Griggs R, et al. *Cecil Essentials of Medicine*, 6th ed. Philadelphia: WB Saunders; 2004:608–613.
2. Nieman LK. *Establishing the Diagnosis of Cushing's Syndrome.* In UpToDate, Rose, BD, (ed), UpToDate. Waltham, MA 2007. Copyright © 2007 UpToDate, Inc.
3. David N. Cushing's syndrome. *N Engl J Med.* 1995;332:791–803.
4. Nieman LK. *Clinical Manifestation of Cushing's Syndrome.* In UpToDate, Rose, BD, (ed), UpToDate. Waltham, MA 2007. Copyright © 2007 UpToDate, Inc.
5. Kelly WF. Psychiatric aspects of Cushing's syndrome. *QJM.* 1996;89:543–551.
6. Mauri M, Sinforiani E, Bono G. et al. Memory impairment in Cushing's disease. *Acta Neurol Scand.* 1993: Jn;87(1)52–55.
7. Momose KJ, Killberg RN, Kilman B. High incidence of cortical atrophy of the cerebral and cerebellar hemispheres in Cushing's disease. *Radiology.* 1971;99(2):341–348.
8. Starkman MN, Gebarski SS, Berent S, et al. Hippocampal formation volume, memory dysfunction, and cortisol levels in patients with Cushing's syndrome. *Biol Psychiatry.* 1992;32:756–765.
9. Born J, Spath-Scwalbe E. Influences of corticotropin-releasing hormone, adrenocorticotropin, and cortisol on sleep in normal man. *J Clin Endocrinol Metab.* 1989;68:904–911.
10. Dorn LD, Burgess ES, Friedman TC, et al. The longitudinal course of psychopathology in Cushing's syndrome after correction of hypercortisolism. *J Clin Endocrinol Metab.* 1997;82:912–919.
11. Ferrando AA, Stuart CA, Sheffield-Moore M, et al. Inactivity amplifies the catabolic response of skeletal muscle to cortisol. *J Clin Endocrinol Metab.* 1999;84:3515–3521.
12. Newell-Price J, Trainer P, Besser M, et al. The diagnosis and differential diagnosis of Cushing's syndrome and pseudo-Cushing's states. *Endocr Rev.* 1998;19:647–672.
13. Ubogu EE, Ruff RL, Kaminski HJ. Endocrine myopathy. In: Engel A, Franzizi-Armstrong C, eds. *Myopathy.* New York: McGraw-Hill; 1994:1713–1738.
14. Gsponer J, De Tribolet N, Deruaz JP, et al. Diagnosis, treatment, and outcome of pituitary tumors and other abnormal intrasellar masses. Retrospective analysis of 353 patients. *Medicine.* 1999;78:236–269.
15. Ferguson G, Irvin C, Cherniack R. Effect of corticosteroids on respiratory muscle histopathology. *Am Rev Respir Dis.* 1990;142:1047.
16. Bolton CF. Neuromascular complications of critical illness. *Muscle Nerve.* 2005;32: 140–163.
17. Showalter C, Engel AG. Acute quadriplegic myopathy: Analysis of myosin isoforms and evidence for calpain-mediated proteolysis. *Muscle Nerve.* 1997;20:316–322.
18. Hsu TH. Sudden onset of unilateral third nerve paresis inpatient with Cushing's syndrome. *Arch Neurol.* 1977;34(3):196–198.
19. Nieman LK. *Establishing the Cause of Cushing's Syndrome.* In UpToDate, Rose, BD, (ed), UpToDate. Waltham, MA 2007. Copyright © 2007 UpToDate, Inc.
20. Findling JW, Raff H, Aron DC. The low-dose dexamethasone suppression test: A reevaluation in patients with Cushing's syndrome. *J Clin Endocrinol Metab.* 2004;89: 1222–1226.

21. Emma F, Pizzini C, Tessa A, et al. "Bartter-like" phenotype in Kerans-Sayre syndrome. *Pediatr Nephrol.* 2006;21:355–360.
22. Bautista J, Gil-Neciga E, Gil-Peralta A. Hypokalemic periodic paralysis in primary hyperaldosteronism: Subclinical myopathy with atrophy of the type 2A muscle fibers as the most pronounced alteration. *Eur Neurol.* 1979;18(6):415–420.
23. Talib A, Mahmood K, Jairmani KL, et al. Hypokalemic quadriparesis with normotensive primary hyperaldosteronism. *Journal of the College of Physicians and Surgeons—Pakistan (JCPCP).* 2004;14:492–493.
24. Fujihara K, Miyoshi T, Yamaguchi Y, et al. Tetany as a sole manifestation in a patient with Bartter's syndrome and a successful treatment with indomethacin. *Rinsho Shinkeigaku.* 1990;30:529–532.
25. Weber KT, Singh KD, Hey JC. Idiopathic intracranial hypertension with primary aldosteronism: Report of 2 cases. *Am J Med Sci.* 2002;324:45–50.
26. Duncan JL, 3rd, Fuhrman GM, Bolton JS, et al. Laparoscopic adrenalectomy is superior to an open approach to treat primary hyperaldosteronism. *Am Surg.* 2000; 66:932.
27. Minowada S, Fujimura T, Takahashi N, et al. Computed tomography-guided percutaneous acetic acid injection therapy for functioning adrenocortical adenoma. *J Clin Endocrinol Metab.* 2003;88:5814.
28. Milsom SR, Espiner EA, Nicholls MG, et al. The blood pressure response to unilateral adrenalectomy in primary hyperaldosteronism. *QJM.* 1986;61:1141.
29. Brown JJ, Davies DL, Ferriss JB, et al. Comparison of surgery and prolonged spironolactone therapy in patients with hypertension, aldosterone excess, and low plasma renin. *BMJ.* 1972;2:729.
30. Lim PO, Young WF, MacDonald TM. A review of the medical treatment of primary aldosteronism. *J Hypertens.* 2001;19:353.
31. McMahon GT, Dluhy RG. Glucocorticoid-remediable aldosteronism. *Cardiol Rev.* 2004;12:44.
32. Larsen PR, Kronenberg HM, Melmed S, eds. *Williams Textbook of Endocrinology*, 10th ed. Philadelphia: WB Saunders; 2003.
33. Wolfgang O. Adrenal insufficiency. *N Engl J Med.* 1996;335:1206–1212.
34. Ten S, New M, MacLaren N. Addison's disease 2001. *J Clin Endocrinol Metab.* 2001;86:2909–2922.
35. Carey R. The changing clinical spectrum of adrenal insufficiency. *Ann Intern Med.* 1997;127:1103–1105.
36. May ME, Vaughan ED, Carey RM. Adrenocortical insufficiency: Clinical aspects. In: Vaughan ED, Carey RM, eds. *Adrenal Disorders.* New York: Thieme Medical; 1989: 171–189.
37. Burke C. Adrenocortical insufficiency. *J Clin Endocrinol Metab.* 1985;14:947–976.
38. Yu L. DRB1*04 and DQ alleles: Expression of 21-hydroxylase autoantibodies and risk of progression to Addison's disease. *J Clin Endocrinol Metab.* 1999;84:328–335.
39. Piedrola G, Casado JL, Lopez E, et al. Clinical features of adrenal insufficiency in patients with acquired immunodeficiency syndrome. *Clin Endocrinol (Oxf).* 1996;45:97–101.
40. Washburn RG, Bennett JE. Reversal of adrenocortical glucocorticoid dysfunction in a patient with disseminated histoplasmosis. *Ann Intern Med.* 1989;110:86–87.
41. Moser HW, Raymond GV, Dubey P. Adrenoleukodystrophy: New approaches to a neurodegenerative disease. *JAMA.* 2005;294:3131–3134.
42. Mukherjee S, Newby E, Harvey J. Adrenomyeloneuropathy in patients with Addison's disease: Genetic case analysis. *J R Soc Med.* 2006;99:245–249.
43. Spurek M, Taylor-Gjevre R, Van Uum S, et al. Adrenomyeloneuropathy as a cause of primary adrenal insufficiency and spastic paraparesis. *CMAJ.* 2004;171:1073–1077.
44. Powers JM, De Ciero DP, Moser AB, et al. Adrenomyeloneuropathy: A neuropathologic review featuring its noninflammatory myelopathy. *J Neuropathol Exp Neurol.* 2000;59: 89–102.
45. Seidenwurm DJ, Elmer EB, Kaplan LM, et al. Metastases to the adrenal glands and the development of Addison's disease. *Cancer.* 1984;54:552–557.
46. Guo W, Burris TP, McCabe ER. Expression of DAX-1, the gene responsible for X-linked adrenal hypoplasia congenital and hypogonadotropic hypogonadism, in the hypothalamic-pituitary-adrenal/gonadal axis. *Biochem Mol Med.* 1995;56:8–13.
47. Reutens AT, et al. Clinical and functional effects on mutations in the DAX-1 gene in patients with adrenal hypoplasia congenital. *J Clin Endocrinol Metab.* 1999;84: 504–511.
48. Sjarif DR, et al. Isolated and contiguous glycerol kinase gene disorders: A review. *J Inherit Metab Dis.* 2000;23:529–547.
49. Huebner A, Elias L, Clark A. ACTH resistance syndromes. *J Pediatr Endocrinol Metab.* 1999;12[Suppl 1]:277–293.
50. Artuch R, et al. Multiple endocrine involvement in two pediatric patients with Kearns-Sayre syndrome. *Horm Res.* 1998;50:99.
51. Sauter NP, Toni R, McLaughlin CD, et al. Isolated adrenocorticotropin deficiency associated with autoantibody to a corticotroph antigen that is not adrenocorticotropin or other proopiomelanocortin-derived peptides. *J Clin Endocrinol Metab.* 1990;70: 1391–1397.
52. Krude H, Biebermann H, Luck W, et al. Severe early-onset obesity, adrenal insufficiency and red hair pigmentation caused by *POMC* mutations in humans. *Nat Genet.* 1998;19:155–157.
53. Lovas K, Husebye ES, Holsten F, et al. Sleep disturbances in patients with Addison's disease. *Eur J Endocrinol.* 2003;148:449–456.
54. Schipper HM, Abrams GM. Other endocrinopathies and the nervous system. In: Aminoff MJ, ed. *Neurology and General Medicine.* New York: Churchill Livingstone; 1995:383–399.
55. Benvenga S, Rodolico C, Trimarchi F, et al. Endocrine evaluation for muscle pain. *J R Soc Med.* 2001;94:405–407.
56. Rodolico F, Toscano A, Benvenga S, et al. Myopathy as the persistently isolated symptomatology of primary autoimmune hypothyroidism. *Thyroid.* 1998;8:1033–1038.
57. Grant DB, Barnes ND, Dumic M, et al. Neurological and adrenal dysfunction in the adrenal insufficiency/alacrima/achalasia (3A) syndrome. *Arch Dis Child.* 1993;68: 779–782.
58. Charmoles ND, Hainaut H, Hariga J. Genetic contribution to the study of the Addison-Schilder syndrome. *J Neurol Sci.* 1971;14:457–462.
59. Leigh H, Kramer SI. The psychiatric manifestations of endocrine disease. *Adv Intern Med.* 1984;29:413–445.
60. Grinspoon SK, Biller BM. Laboratory assessment of adrenal insufficiency. *J Clin Endocrinol Metab.* 1994;79:923–931.
61. Falorni A, Laureti S, De Bellis A, et al. Italian Addison network study: Update of diagnostic criteria for the etiological classification of primary adrenal insufficiency. *J Clin Endocrinol Metab.* 2004;89:1598–1604.
62. Moser AB, Moser HW. The prenatal diagnosis of X-linked adrenoleukodystrophy. *Prenat Diagn.* 1999;19:46–48.
63. Moser HW, Raymond GV, Lu SE, et al. Follow-up of 89 asymptomatic patients with adrenoleukodystrophy treated with Lorenzo's oil. *Arch Neurol.* 2005;62:1073–1080.
64. Peters C, Chamas LR, Tan Y, et al. Cerebral X-linked adrenoleukodystrophy: The international hematopoietic cell transplantation experience from 1982 to 1999. *Blood.* 2004;104:881–888.
65. O'Riordain DS, Young WF, Jr., Grant CS, et al. Clinical spectrum and outcome of functional extraadrenal paraganglioma. *World J Surg.* 1996;20(7):916–921.
66. Neumann HP, Bausch B, McWhinney SR, et al. Germ-line mutations in nonsyndromic pheochromocytoma. *N Engl J Med.* 2002;346(19):1459–1466.
67. Bravo EL, Gifford RW, Jr. Current concepts. Pheochromocytoma: Diagnosis, localization and management. *N Engl J Med.* 1984;311:1298–1303.
68. Euda T, Oka N, Matsumoto A, et al. Pheochromocytoma presenting as recurrent hypotension and syncope. *Intern Med.* 2005;44(3):222–227.
69. Stein PP, Black HR. A simplified diagnostic approach to pheochromocytoma: A review of the literature and report of one institution's experience. *Medicine.* 1991;70(1): 46–66.
70. Eclavea A, Gagliardi JA, Jezior J, et al. Phaeochromocytoma with central nervous system manifestations. *Australas Radiol.* 1997;41(4):373–376.
71. Lehmann FS, Weiss P, Ritz R, et al. Reversible cerebral ischemia in patients with pheochromocytoma. *J Endocrinol Invest.* 1999;22(3):212–214.
72. Dagartzikas MI, Sprague K, Carter G, et al. Cerebrovascular event, dilated cardiomyopathy, and pheochromocytoma. *Pediatr Emerg Care.* 2002;18(1):33–35.
73. Lynn MD, Braunstein EM, Shaprio B. Pheochromocytoma presenting as musculoskeletal pain from bone metastases. *Skeletal Radiol.* 1987;16(7):552–555.
74. Leiba A, Bar-Dayan Y, Leker RR, et al. Seizures as a presenting symptom of phaeochromocytoma in a young solider. *J Hum Hypertens.* 2003;17(1):73–75.
75. Armenti-Kapros B, Nambiar PK, Lippman HR, et al. An unusual case of autonomic dysreflexia: Pheochromocytoma in an individual with tetraplegia. *J Spinal Cord Med.* 2003;26(2):172–175.
76. Eisenhofer G, Keiser H, Friberg P, et al. Plasma metanephrines are markers of pheochromocytome produced by catechol-O methyltransferase within tumors. *J Clin Endocrinol Metab.* 1998;83:2175–2185.
77. Eisenhofer G, Hunynh TT, Hiroi M, et al. Understanding catecholamine metabolism as a guide to the biochemical diagnosis of pheochromocytoma. *Rev Endocrinol Metab Dis.* 2001;2:297–311.
78. Goldstein DS, Eisenhofer G, Flynn JA, et al. Diagnosis and localization of pheochromocytoma. *Hypertension.* 2004;43:907–910.
79. Grossman E, Goldstein DS, Hoffman A, et al. Glucagon and clonidine testing in the diagnosis of pheochromocytoma. *Hypertension.* 1991;17(6 Pt 1):733–741.
80. Feldman JM. Carcinoid tumor and syndrome. *Semin Oncol.* 1987;14:237.
81. Lie JP. Carcinoid tumor, carcinoid syndrome and carcinoid heart disease. *Primary Cardiology.* 1982;8:163.
82. Maton PN. The carcinoid syndrome. *JAMA.* 1988;260:1602.
83. Modlin IM, Kidd M, Latich I, et al. Current status of gastrointestinal carcinoids. *Gastroenterology.* 2005;128:1717.
84. Wareing TH, Sawyers JL. Carcinoids and the carcinoid syndrome. *Am J Surg.* 1983; 145:769.
85. Marsh HM, Martin JK, Jr., Kvols LK, et al. Carcinoid crisis during anesthesia: Successful treatment with a somatostatin analogue. *Anesthesiology.* 1987;66:89.
86. Vinik AI, McLeod MK, Fig LM, et al. Clinical features, diagnosis and localization of carcinoid tumors and their management. *Gastroenterol Clin North Am.* 1989;18:865.
87. Kema IP, Willemse PH, De Vries EG. Carcinoid tumors. *N Engl J Med.* 1999;341(6): 453–454.
88. Kulke MH, Mayer RJ. Carcinoid tumors. *N Engl J Med.* 1999;340(11):858–868.
89. Loftus JP, van Heerden JA. Surgical management of gastrointestinal carcinoid tumors. *Adv Surg.* 1995;28:317–336.
90. Rubin J, Ajani J, Schirmer W, et al. Octreotide acetate long-acting formulation versus open-label subcutaneous octreotide acetate in malignant carcinoid syndrome. *J Clin Oncol.* 1999;17(2):600–606.
91. Goodman MT, Gurney JG, Smith MA, et al. Sympathetic nervous system tumors. In: Ries LA, Smith MA, Gurney JG, et al., eds. *Cancer Incidence and Survival among Children and Adolescents: United States SEER Program, 1975–1995.* Bethesda, MD: National Cancer Institute; 1999:35.
92. Weinstein JL, Katzenstein HM, Cohn SL. Advances in the diagnosis and treatment of neuroblastoma. *Oncologist.* 2003;8:278–292.
93. Hann HW, Levy HM, Evans AE. Serum ferritin as a guide to therapy in neuroblastoma. *Cancer Res.* 1980;40(5):1411–1413.
94. Kushner BH, Cheung NKV. Neuroblastoma—From genetic profiles to clinical challenge. *N Engl J Med.* 2005;353(21):2215–2217.

95. Rudnick E, Khakoo Y, Antunes NL, et al. Opsoclonus-myoclonus-ataxia syndrome in neuroblastoma: Clinical outcome and antineuronal antibodies—A report from the Children's Cancer Group Study. *Med Pediatr Oncol.* 2001;36:612–622.
96. Russo C, Cohn SL, Petruzzi MJ, et al. Long-term neurologic outcome in children with opsoclonus-myoclonus associated with neuroblastoma: A report from the Pediatric Oncology Group. *Med Pediatr Oncol.* 1997;28:284–288.
97. Pranzatelli MR, Travelstead AL, Tate ED, et al. B- and T-cell markers in opsoclonus-myoclonus syndrome: Immunophenotyping of CSF lymphocytes. *Neurology.* 2004;62:1526–1532.
98. Connolly AM, Pestronk A, Mehta S, et al. Serum autoantibodies in childhood opsoclonus-myoclonus syndrome: An analysis of antigenic targets in neural tissues. *J Pediatr.* 1997;130:878–884.
99. Blaes F, Fuhlhuber V, Korfei M, et al. Surface-binding auto-antibodies to cerebellar neurons in opsoclonus syndrome. *Ann Neurol.* 2005;58:313.
100. Siegel MJ, Ishwaran H, Fletcher BD, et al. Staging of neuroblastoma at imaging: Report of the radiology diagnostic oncology group. *Radiology.* 2002;223:168–175.
101. Goldsby RE, Matthay KK. Neuroblastoma: Evolving therapies for a disease with many faces. *Pediatric Drugs.* 2004;6:107–122.
102. Brignole C, Pagnan G, Marimpeitri D, et al. Targeted delivery system of antisense oligonucleotides: A novel experimental strategy for neuroblastoma treatment. *Cancer Lett.* 2003;197:231–235.
103. Glenner GG, Grimley PM. Tumors of the extra-adrenal paraganglion system (including chemoreceptors). In: *Atlas of Tumor Pathology*, Second Series. Armed Forces Institute of Pathology; 1974.
104. Cheng A, Niparko JK. Imaging quiz case 2: Glomus tympanicum tumor of the temporal bone. *Arch Otolaryngol Head Neck Surg.* 1997;123(5):549,551–552.
105. O'Leary MJ, Shelton C, Giddings NA, et al. Glomus tympanicum tumors: A clinical perspective. *Laryngoscope.* 1991;101(10):1038–1043.
106. Mafee MF, Raofi B, Kumar A, et al. Glomus faciale, glomus jugulare, glomus tympanicum, glomus vagale, carotid body tumors, and stimulating lesions: Role of MR imaging. *Radiol Clin North Am.* 2000;38(5):1059–1076.
107. van der Mey AG, Frijns JH, Cornelisse CJ, et al. Does intervention improve the natural course of glomus tumors? A series of 108 patients seen in a 32-year period. *Ann Otol Rhinol Laryngol.* 1992;101(8):635–642.
108. Pluta RM, Ram Z, Patronas NJ, et al. Long-term effects of radiation therapy for a catecholamine-producing glomus jugulare tumor: Case report. *Neurosurgery.* 1994;80(6):1091–1094.

CHAPTER **80**

Diabetes Mellitus

Gregory M. Blume

OBJECTIVES

- To present the neurologic signs and symptoms attributable to diabetes mellitus
- To describe how diabetic peripheral nerve injury can occur in a number of clinical patterns that are important to identify so that additional causes of peripheral nerve injury can be sought, when appropriate
- To illustrate how hyperglycemia, in the setting of dehydration, can present with both an altered sensorium and focal neurologic signs, including seizures
- To reinforce that the mainstay of treatment of neurologic manifestations of diabetes is still good glycemic control, but that other factors, such as immune dysfunction, can play important roles in injuring the nervous system in patients with diabetes

CASE VIGNETTE

A 48-year-old man with a 24-month history of diabetes presents with bilateral foot and leg pain described as burning and prickling. The onset of his discomfort predated the discovery of diabetes by several months and has been only partially relieved with medication. Blood glucose control has been difficult to obtain, but the patient's last hemoglobin A1c was 7.5% (upper limits of normal, 6.4%). On examination, the patient has significant loss of muscle bulk in the distal lower extremities, including the peroneal compartment and the calves, with limited movement of the toes and profound foot drop bilaterally. There is no detection of pin-prick or vibration to the wrists and knees. Muscle stretch reflexes are not obtained in the arms or legs.

DEFINITION

As one of the most common medical conditions encountered throughout the world, diabetes mellitus is usually recognized by health care professionals without difficulty. The myriad manifestations of this systemic disease can be challenging to identify and manage, however. Hyperglycemia is the core feature of the disease, although the cause of the hyperglycemia is not identical in all patients. The American Diabetes Association (ADA) classifies diabetes into four clinical classes:

- Type 1 diabetes (results from pancreatic β-cell destruction, usually leading to absolute insulin deficiency, autoimmune mechanism), usually in thin, young patients who are susceptible to ketosis and are insulin dependent
- Type 2 diabetes (results from a progressive insulin secretory defect on the background of insulin resistance), usually in older (>40 years of age), obese patients who are not susceptible to ketosis and are more likely to have a family history of diabetes
- Other specific types of diabetes (from other causes, such as genetic defects in β-cell function, genetic defects in insulin action, disease of the exocrine pancreas, and drug or chemical induced); often referred to as *secondary diabetes*
- Gestational diabetes (hyperglycemia that meets the criteria for diabetes during pregnancy, but that resolves after parturition)

The recommended test for diagnosis of diabetes in nonpregnant adults is the fasting plasma glucose (FPG) with a value of 126 mg/dL or greater being the diagnostic cut-off. Other tests that can be used include a random glucose, >200 mg/dL in the correct setting, or an abnormal oral glucose tolerance test. The details on the use of these tests in diagnosing diabetes are readily available from the ADA web site. The use of the hemoglobin A1c test for diagnosis of diabetes is not recommended at this time. *Prediabetes* is the term used for FPG values between 100 and 125 mg/dL and is considered a risk factor for future diabetes (1).

EPIDEMIOLOGY

The ADA reports that 7% of the population of the United States would meet the criteria for diabetes, but as many as one third of those individuals have not had the condition diagnosed. The importance of these numbers cannot be overstated because management of hyperglycemia can prevent or at least delay the onset of many of the complications of diabetes. Most patients who are diabetic in the United States are classified as type 2 and they account for >90% of all those who are diabetic. Gestational diabetes affects approximately 4% of all pregnant women. Concurrently, estimates are that twice as many Americans are in the prediabetic state (1).

The most common neurologic problem accompanying diabetes is peripheral neuropathy. Neuropathy is seen in 30% of patients who are diabetic overall and becomes more common the longer the disease is present (50% at 25 years). A significant difference does not appear to exist between type 1 and type 2 diabetics as far as the incidence of neuropathy. Diabetes is the most common cause of autonomic neuropathy in developed countries (2).

Lumbosacral plexopathies (diabetic amyotrophy, diabetic lumbosacral radiculoplexus neuropathy) associated with diabetes are not common and are seen in <1% of all patients who are diabetic. Mononeuropathies also occur with increased frequency in these patients and are often at common sites of entrapment (e.g., the carpal tunnel). Diabetic radiculopathies can occur at any root level. All of these focal neuropathic processes usually occur in the setting of an underlying diffuse neuropathy.

Cranial mononeuropathies occur, especially, in older adults. The most common cranial mononeuropathy involves either the third or sixth oculomotor nerves. The former is typically associated with a pupil-sparing ophthalmoplegia.

Diabetic muscle infarction is a less commonly encountered complication of chronic diabetes. This is seen more commonly in patients with type 1 diabetes with other end-organ involvement by diabetes (2).

Central nervous system (CNS) complications of diabetes include both principally metabolically mediated processes (e.g., diabetic ketoacidosis, nonketotic hyperosmolar coma, hypoglycemia) and cerebrovascular disease. The risk of cerebrovascular disease in diabetes, independent of other comorbidity (obesity, hypertension, hyperlipidemia) is unclear. The increased risk of stroke for persons with diabetes is estimated to be between a two- and fourfold increase, however, whereas mortality from stroke in patients with diabetes is also greater than the mortality from stroke in nondiabetics (3).

ETIOLOGY AND PATHOGENESIS

Peripheral nerve injury in diabetes is likely a multifactorial process, with persistent hyperglycemia as the central factor in development of neuropathy. Persistent hyperglycemia is associated with multiple mechanisms through which nerve injury can result, including accumulation of injurious compounds, increased oxidative stress, and alteration of enzymatic function and cellular membrane constituents. A direct mechanism of injury may be through increased polyol pathway activity leading to increased sorbitol and fructose. These products of the polyol pathway are thought to damage nerve cells through an as-of-yet unknown mechanism (4).

Increased oxidative stress is associated with diabetic neuropathy, although the contribution of this factor to neural injury is not completely understood (5,6). Advanced glycation endproducts (AGE) are created by both nonenzymatic glycosylation and increased aldose reductase activity. AGE are proteins that are permanently modified by glycosylation and, therefore, may have loss or alteration of function. Some of these proteins are thought to play important roles in maintaining antioxidant properties in cells (7). The activation of aldose reductase may also lead to competition for energy substrates necessary for other enzymes, including glutathione reductase. This can lead to the loss of antioxidant function of glutathione. These factors can lead to an increase in reactive oxygen species within nerve cells. Evidence has long supported nitric oxide (NO) deficiency in diabetes; however, NO production has been found to be stimulated in hyperglycemic states and can lead to damage of both the endothelium of blood vessels and the perineurium of nerves (8,9). A complete understanding of these seemingly contradictory data has not yet been achieved.

Additional effects of hyperglycemia that lead to neuron injury include depletion of myoinositol, an important membrane constituent. Coupled with oxidative injury to membrane lipids secondary to increased reactive oxygen species, the decrease in myoinositol could lead to membrane composition changes altering the function of membrane-bound proteins, such as protein kinase C, or a disturbance in ion channel function.

Microvascular insufficiency is also thought to play a role in diabetic neuropathy. This is based on histopathologic changes noted in endoneurial and epineurial blood vessel walls, as well as functional changes, such as altered blood flow or permeability of the microvasculature of the nerves in diabetic subjects.

An immunologic pathogenesis for diabetic neuropathy has also been suggested by the occurrence of various autoantibodies, including antiphospholipid antibodies, more commonly in diabetic patients with neuropathy than those without neuropathy (10). The presence of endothelial inflammatory infiltrates, noted on biopsy of the intermediate femoral cutaneous nerve in patients with the clinical syndrome of diabetic amyotrophy, may correlate with an inflammatory vasculopathy as a part of the neural injury in that syndrome (11).

Growth factor deficiency may also play a role in the pathogenesis of diabetic neuropathy. Many of the changes seen in diabetic neuropathy mimic those seen with depletion of endogenous growth factors. A decline in nerve growth factor synthesis has been linked to altered function of small nerve fibers in diabetic neuropathy (12).

The unique structure of sensory neurons may also play a significant role in the development of diabetic neuropathy. The dorsal root ganglia (DRG) lie outside the blood–brain barrier and, therefore, the cell bodies of sensory neurons lack the added protection afforded by the choroid plexus and blood–brain barrier in the maintenance of a homeostatic environment. Blood glucose shifts in the cerebrospinal fluid (CSF) tend to be less drastic than in the extracellular space occupied by the DRG. Additionally, because of the vast length of the axon, sensory neurons are metabolically very active to support basic cell maintenance and repair. Even a modest alteration in cell metabolism or a modest increase in cellular injury could unbalance the repair mechanisms in sensory neurons.

The cause of mononeuropathies or radiculopathies in patients who are diabetic is uncertain and may represent multiple processes. Possibly, an increased vulnerability of nerves to compression injury exists in the setting of diabetes and this may account for some mononeuropathies. Other mononeuropathies may be ischemic and related to endoneurial or epineurial vasculopathy or vasculitis.

The cause of cranial mononeuropathies in diabetes is not entirely understood. The oculomotor nerve is the most frequent cranial nerve injured in diabetes and this is commonly an acute injury suggesting an ischemic process. The sparing of the pupillary fibers, on the basis of anatomic knowledge of the third cranial nerve, also suggests an ischemic neural injury.

Diabetic muscle infarction is a rare complication of diabetes that is likely secondary to a diffuse microangiopathic process. Muscle biopsy shows necrotic and regenerating muscle fibers with hyalinization of arterioles and vascular occlusion (13).

Hyperglycemia can cause CNS symptoms in patients with diabetic ketoacidosis, nonketotic hyperosmolar coma, and nonketotic hyperglycemic chorea. The clinical features of diabetic ketoacidosis and nonketotic hyperosmolar coma do overlap considerably and some common features of their pathogenesis may exist. Diabetic ketoacidosis is caused by a relative or absolute deficiency of insulin. This is commonly caused by missed insulin doses, either intentionally because of fear of hypoglycemia, or unintentionally because of illness, but it can be seen in undiagnosed diabetes and in those with diabetes who have been consistent with their insulin regimen (14). The insulin deficiency leads to decreased glucose uptake by tissues and subsequent hyperglycemia. Glucagon, growth hormone, and catecholamines are released by tissues starving for glucose and these hormones lead to a breakdown of triglycerides into free fatty acids and stimulate gluconeogenesis, which further exacerbates hyperglycemia. Beta-oxidation of the free fatty acids leads to ketone body formation and metabolism takes on the guise of a fasting state. A subsequent metabolic acidosis develops as the body's buffers are depleted, whereas an osmotic diuresis occurs because of the hyperglycemia and this leads to electrolyte derangements and a shift of fluid to the intravascular compartment with intracellular dehydration. In nonketotic hyperosmolar coma, many of the same processes that occur in diabetic ketoacidosis also occur; however, ketones do not develop. In these patients, ketone formation may be inhibited because of sufficient insulin, the degree of hyperosmolarity, hepatic resistance to glucagon's actions, and, possibly, less free fatty acids released through beta-oxidation.

Diabetes is a well-recognized risk factor for cerebrovascular disease. Mechanisms are proposed by which hyperglycemia predisposes to both vascular damage and to increased thrombogenesis (15). NO, an endothelium-derived factor with both vasodilatory and antiatherosclerotic properties is decreased in diabetes. Because of the creation of reactive oxidative species, NO synthesis is significantly reduced in the presence of hyperglycemia (although, as noted previously, NO production has been found in animal models to be elevated in hyperglycemia). In addition, the formation of advanced-glycation endproducts alters the structure of vessel walls. Thrombogenesis may be increased by both platelet activation and impairment of clot breakdown. Thromboxane, a platelet activator, has been found to be raised in patients with peripheral vascular disease. Diabetes (along with hypertension and hypercholesterolemia) may increase thromboxane synthesis. Hyperinsulinemia and glucose intolerance is associated with impaired fibrinolysis.

PATHOLOGY

Most pathognomonic changes in diabetes occur within the pancreas with type 1 diabetes associated with insulitis, atrophy and fibrosis, and depletion of beta-cells. Type 2 diabetes is not associated with insulitis and shows only mild loss of beta-cells (16). Within peripheral nerves, none of the findings in diabetic neuropathy are specific for diabetes. Axonal loss, thickening and hyalinization of capillaries, and distal axonal swellings may all be seen. Focal lymphocytic infiltrates may be seen in diabetic amyotrophy, usually located perivascularly in the epineurium.

CLINICAL MANIFESTATIONS

Diabetes is the classic cause for the *stocking-glove* distribution, sensory neuropathy. The most common presentation of diabetic neuropathy is a chronic, symmetric, sensory predominate neuropathy that involves all sensory modalities. Involvement of small fiber sensory modalities leads to painful paresthesias and recurrent injury because an awareness of skin irritants is lacking. Involvement of large fiber sensory modalities contributes to the loss of deep tendon reflexes, poor balance, and neuropathic osteoarthropathy. Motor involvement is typically limited and is most commonly seen as decreased toe wiggle early in the course of neuropathy. Later on, foot drop may occur. Early, significant weakness with diabetic neuropathy should trigger a search for other superimposed causes of weakness (2).

Autonomic nerve fibers are also frequently involved, but this involvement tends to occur late in the course of neuropathy and usually is only clinically symptomatic in <5% of patients with diabetes. Autonomic neuropathy accompanies the classic symmetric, sensory neuropathy. Brittle diabetics are more likely to experience symptoms of autonomic neuropathy. Erectile dysfunction and dysfunction of bladder emptying (eventual progression to urinary retention) are frequent autonomic symptoms. Postural hypotension may be seen and can present as lightheadedness or even cognitive impairment. Both sympathetic and parasympathetic denervation contribute to cardiac impairment. The overall impact on the heart is impairment of myocardial blood flow, a fixed tachycardia, and inability to increase the heart rate to meet physiologic demands. These changes contribute to silent myocardial ischemia and increased mortality after myocardial infarction. Gastrointestinal autonomic neuropathy may present with symptoms of gastroparesis, including early satiety, nausea, epigastric pain, and postprandial bloating. The degree of gastroparesis documented with gastric motility studies, however, does not always correlate well with the degree of symptoms experienced by the patient. Constipation, nocturnal diarrhea, and fecal incontinence can also be seen with gastrointestinal autonomic neuropathy. Sudomotor involvement can lead to hypohidrosis or hyperhidrosis. The former can be problematic in maintenance of thermoregulation and as a contributing factor to diabetic skin ulceration (2).

Rapid onset of usually painful neuropathies can occur at the time of diagnosis of diabetes or when patients with poorly controlled diabetes are brought under tight control with the institution of insulin therapy. In both instances, the clinical symptoms tend to improve after maintenance of good blood sugar control over time, although electrodiagnostic evidence of neuropathy will usually persist.

Asymmetric diabetic neuropathies are much less common than the classic symmetric diabetic neuropathy. A general rule to follow is any asymmetric neuropathy in a patient with diabetes mandates a thorough evaluation for alternate or superimposed causes of neural injury. Diabetic lumbosacral plexopathies encompass several closely related syndromes, including diabetic amyotrophy (diabetic lumbosacral radiculoplexus neuropathy), proximal diabetic neuropathy, and multifocal diabetic neuropathy. These unusual neuropathies are uncommon, occurring in <0.1% of diabetic cases, and are more likely to occur in type 2 diabetes. Onset is typically subacute. These neuropathies are accompanied by pain that is often localized to the hips, thighs, and buttocks and heralds the onset of neuropathy. The pain can be intense and requires aggressive management. The common clinical feature to these neuropathies is proximal leg weakness that is asymmetric and often involves the quadriceps, psoas, and thigh adductor muscles.

Atrophy of individual muscles can be striking; some degree of distal weakness can occur. The term *multifocal diabetic neuropathy* is usually reserved for syndromes that have some degree of upper extremity involvement or thoracic radiculopathy as well. Often found is a history of recent poor diabetic control and weight loss near the time of onset of diabetic lumbosacral plexopathies (2).

Diabetic mononeuropathies involving limb or trunk nerves or roots can be either acute and accompanied by pain (presumably, ischemic in origin) or chronic. The latter can be caused by concurrent entrapment at common compression sites. Acute mononeuropathies can spontaneously recover over months to several years. The clinical symptoms seen are determined by the nerve involved. Diabetic thoracic radiculopathies can cause abdominal wall muscle weakness in addition to pain (2).

Diabetic cranial mononeuropathies have been described involving most cranial nerves. Palsies of the oculomotor, trochlear, and abducens nerves have been most commonly described and all present with binocular diplopia. Ptosis can accompany diabetic oculomotor nerve palsy. The onset is usually abrupt and often accompanied by retroorbital pain. Pupillary sparing is considered a classic finding in diabetic third nerve palsies, but does not rule out other possible causes. Facial nerve palsies are likely more common in patients with diabetes and may have worse recovery than Bell's palsies in the general population. Trigeminal nerve involvement has been described in diabetes, and symptomatically mimics trigeminal neuralgia. The facial dysesthesias and pain often resolve with better glycemic control. Reports have appeared of simultaneous, bilateral trigeminal nerve involvement with diabetes. Diabetes is considered a risk factor for anterior optic ischemic neuropathy, which presents with acute, monocular visual loss, often experienced nocturnally (2).

Diabetic muscle infarction presents with an acute, swollen, painful, and weak muscle. The pain is present at rest and intensifies with activity. This is most commonly seen in the muscles of the thigh and usually in an isolated muscle, although involvement of multiple muscles simultaneously may occur. Patients with poorly controlled, type 1 diabetes are more susceptible to this complication and generally have renal, retinal, and peripheral nerve end-organ injury. Recovery is spontaneous over several months (2).

Hyperglycemia can cause a number of symptoms related to dysfunction of the CNS, whether associated with ketones, hyperosmolarity, or neither. An alteration in mental status, ranging from mild confusion to comatose, is the most common clinical symptom associated with marked hyperglycemia. When accompanying diabetic ketoacidosis, confusion is usually seen in a patient who appears systemically ill with malaise, generalized weakness, polydipsia, polyuria, and anorexia. There are often accompanying physical signs of infection and dehydration. A sweet, fruity odor to the breath has been referred to as *ketotic breath*. Patients who experience diabetic ketoacidosis are predominantly younger, with type 1 diabetes. In the setting of nonketotic hyperosmolar coma, the term coma is misleading because many patients who fit the diagnostic criteria for this entity are not in a comatose state. The altered mental status can be associated with seizures and focal neurologic signs, including hemiparesis or cranial mononeuropathies (17). Physical signs of dehydration are usually present and signs of concurrent infection may also be seen. These patients tend to be older and with type 2 diabetes and factors may be present that have led to fluid restriction, such as immobility caused by stroke, orthopedic injury, or dementia (14). Chorea has been described in several patients with nonketotic hyperglycemia with normal serum osmolarity. These patients usually have a history of diabetes and present with subacute onset of chorea that can be unilateral or bilateral. These cases come primarily from Asian literature, suggesting a possible genetic susceptibility. The chorea usually resolves shortly after attaining an euglycemic state (18).

DIAGNOSTIC APPROACH

In most instances of neurologic symptoms associated with diabetes, the diagnosis has already been established. When a patient presents with virtually any form of neuropathy (with the exception of classic entrapment neuropathies), it is customary to obtain a FPG. This is important from both the standpoint of diabetes as an independent cause for neuropathy and as a cofactor with other causes of neuropathy. If the fasting blood sugar falls between 100 and 125 mg/dL, the patient can be classified in the fasting hyperglycemia spectrum. Levels >140 mg/dL and <199 mg/dL represent carbohydrate intolerance. A glucose tolerance test is indicated in these cases and treatment should be initiated because these patients are at risk of neuropathy, particularly if they are obese, have a positive family history of diabetes, a history of gestational diabetes, or belong to ethnic groups at high risk. Nerve conduction studies and electromyography, as well as screening tests for vitamin B_{12}, thyroid-stimulating hormone, and a serum immunofixation are warranted to rule out superimposed causes of neuropathy. In the correct setting, additional testing, including a sedimentation rate, vitamin E and copper levels, antinuclear antibodies, rheumatoid factor, genetic testing for hereditary neuropathies, and even lumbar puncture, may be warranted. Nerve biopsy rarely adds additional information in the setting of diabetic neuropathy unless marked asymmetry is present and a superimposed process is suspected.

Serum glucose measurement is standard in any setting in which normal wakefulness is impaired, with additional testing determined by the clinical setting and degree of hyperglycemia. As presented earlier, hemoglobin A1c testing is not considered a diagnostic tool in diabetes.

In the setting of any cranial mononeuropathy in a patient with diabetes, magnetic resonance imaging (MRI) of the brain with and without gadolinium is mandatory. Lumbar puncture or angiography may be warranted, depending on the MRI findings.

TREATMENT

Treatment specifics of diabetes are outside the realm of this chapter, but maintaining an euglycemic state is the most appropriate treatment for all neurologic diabetic complications. Aldose reductase inhibitors, by virtue of limiting AGE accumulation, have been evaluated for diabetic neuropathy in numerous trials with mixed results (19). Other agents, including nerve growth factor, α-lipoic acid, γ-linolenic acid, and protein kinase C inhibitors, have been investigated with some promise of limiting or reversing diabetic nerve injury. The use of intravenous gamma globulin and short-term intravenous corticosteroids has been recommended in the setting of diabetic amyotrophy (20).

Treating the hyperglycemia in states with ketoacidosis or hyperosmolarity is complex and requires vigilant monitoring of electrolytes in addition to management of hyperglycemia. The various neurologic symptoms will usually resolve with resolution of the euglycemic state.

Most treatment options available for nonacute diabetic complications, beyond glucose regulation, remains symptomatic. A wide variety of anticonvulsants, tricylic antidepressants, and antiarrhythmic agents have been tried for symptomatic relief of diabetic neuropathic pain. Topical agents, such as capsaicin cream, and therapeutic interventions, including infrared light therapy, have also become routinely used to help alleviate suffering. Treatment of the autonomic component of neuropathy is also largely symptomatic (11).

CLINICAL RECOMMENDATIONS OF THE VIGNETTE

This patient had a very rapid onset of significant sensory and motor neuropathy in the setting of uncontrolled diabetes mellitus. The degree of muscle atrophy and weakness is unusual this early in diabetes. The loss of all deep tendon reflexes and the early involvement of the upper extremities are also unusual so soon after diagnosis of diabetes. This should prompt consideration of additional causes for the patient's neuropathy or neuropathic changes, including another neuropathy, spinal stenosis, motor neuron disease, or possibly a distal myopathy. Little information could be gleaned from nerve conduction studies in the lower extremities because of the severity of the patient's neuropathy. Nerve conduction studies in the upper extremities, however, revealed marked slowing of motor conduction velocities that were nearly identical in all nerves tested. This is a characteristic finding in the demyelinating form of hereditary motor sensory neuropathy (HMSN type 1 or Charcot-Marie-Tooth disease type 1). Genetic testing confirmed the presence of HMSN type 1 that had likely been subclinical until the cooccurrence of diabetes.

The sheer numbers of patients with diabetic neuropathy make it likely that other causes for neuropathy will coexist with diabetes. Recognition of the common presentations of diabetic neuropathies will allow the clinician to pursue alternatives in appropriate cases.

SUMMARY

Diabetes is a common disease without racial or geographic boundaries. The neurologic complications are frequent and range from irritating to life-threatening in severity. Diabetic neurologic complications fit distinct clinical patterns, and recognition of those patterns allows the clinician to order appropriate testing and leads to improved treatment for the patient. Although elevated blood glucose levels are clearly correlated with diabetic complications, multiple pathways exist through which hyperglycemia can exert its long-term effects. Even as our understanding of these different pathways improves and may provide alternative treatment options, the maintenance of an euglycemic state will continue to be the mainstay of treatment for the foreseeable future.

REFERENCES

1. ADA position statement: Standards of Medical Care in Diabetes, Sections I and II. Available at: http://care.diabetesjournals.org/cgi/content/full/28/suppl_1/s4.
2. Washington University Neuromuscular Division webpage. Available at: www.neuro.wustl.edu/neuromuscular/nother/diabetes.htm.
3. Capes SE, Hunt D, Malmberg K, et al. Stress hyperglycemia and prognosis of stroke in nondiabetic and diabetic patients: A systematic overview. *Stroke.* 2001;32(10):2426–2432.
4. Diabetes Control and Complications Trial Research Group. Effect of intensive diabetes treatment on nerve conduction in the Diabetes Control and Complications Trial. *Ann Neurol.* 1995;38:869.
5. Cameron NE, Cotter MA. Metabolic and vascular factors in the pathogenesis of diabetic neuropathy. *Diabetes.* 1997;46[Suppl]:31–37.
6. Baynes JW. Role of oxidative stress in development of complications in diabetes. *Diabetes.* 1991;40:405–412.
7. Coppey LJ, Gellett JS, Davidson EP, et al. Effect of antioxidant treatment of streptozocin-induced diabetic rats on endoneurial blood flow, motor nerve conduction velocity, and vascular reactivity of epineurial arterioles of the sciatic nerve. *Diabetes.* 2001;50(80):1927–1937.
8. Pitre DA, Seifert JL, Bauer JA. Perineurium inflammation and altered connexin isoform expression in a rat model of diabetes related peripheral neuropathy. *Neurosci Lett.* 2001;303(1):67–71.
9. Wada R, Yagihashi S. Role of advanced glycation end products and their receptors in development of diabetic neuropathy. *Ann NY Acad Sci.* 2005;1043:598–604.
10. Vinik AI, Pittenger GL, Stansberry KB, et al. Phospholipid and glutamic acid decarboxylase autoantibodies in diabetic neuropathy. *Diabetes Care.* 1995;18:1225–1232.
11. Llewelyn JG, Thomas PK, King RH. Epineurial microvasculitis in proximal diabetic neuropathy. *J Neurol.* 1998; 245(11):748.
12. Vinik AI, Newlon PG, Lauterio TJ, et al. Nerve survival and regeneration in diabetes. *Diabetes Metab Res Rev.* 1995;3:139–157.
13. Trujillo-Santos AJ. Diabetic muscle infarction: An underdiagnosed complication of long-standing diabetes. *Diabetes Care.* 2003;26(1):211–215.
14. Chiasson JL, Aris-Jilwan N, Belanger R, et al. Diagnosis and treatment of diabetic ketoacidosis and the hyperglycemic hyperosmolar state. *CMAJ.* 2003;168(7):859–866.
15. Renard C, Van Obberghen E. Role of diabetes in atherosclerotic pathogenesis. What have we learned from animal models? *Diabetes Metab.* 2006;32(1):15–29.
16. Kumar V, Cotran R, Robbins S. *Robbins Basic Pathology*, 7th ed. Philadelphia, PA: Saunders; 2003.
17. Manford M, Fuller GN, Wade JP. "Silent diabetes": Non-ketotic hyperglycaemia presenting as aphasic status epilepticus. *J Neurol Neurosurg Psychiatry.* 1995;59(1):99–100.
18. Branca D, Gervasio O, Le Piane E, et al. Chorea induced by non-ketotic hyperglycaemia: A case report. *Neurol Sci.* 2005;26(4):275–277.
19. Pfeifer MA, Schumer MP, Gelber DA. Aldose reductase inhibitors: The end of an era or the need for different trial designs? *Diabetes.* 1997;6[Suppl 2]:S82–S89.
20. Dyck PJ, Windebank AJ. Diabetic and nondiabetic lumbosacral radiculoplexus neuropathies: New insights into pathophysiology and treatment. *Muscle Nerve.* 2002;25(4):77–91.

CHAPTER 81

Testis and Ovaries

Camilo E. Fadul

OBJECTIVES

- To introduce ovary and testis disease-associated nervous system syndromes
- To discuss that ovary and testis disease associated nervous system syndromes are usually related to cancer arising from these organs
- To describe neurologic disorders associated with nonmalignant ovary and testis diseases
- To present general concepts on the frequency and pathogenesis of the neurologic complications associated with ovary or testis diseases
- To describe the most frequent clinical neurologic syndromes and relate their relationship to ovary or testis disease
- To review therapeutic modalities and their outcome

Ovaries

CASE VIGNETTE

Over a 2-week period, a 56-year-old woman developed difficulty walking, bilateral arm tremor, incoordination, difficulty writing, and joint pain. On review of systems, she complained of pelvic pain. On examination, she had dysarthria, severe truncal and limb ataxia, and bilateral hypotonia. She was unable to feed herself because of the incoordination and could not walk because of the ataxia.

Testis

CASE VIGNETTE

A 26-year-old man was diagnosed with a stage III testicular embryonal carcinoma after he presented with shortness of breath, multiple pulmonary nodules on imaging, and human chorionic gonadotrophin (HCG) of 3,616 μIU/mL (normal <4 μIU/mL). Staging studies, including brain magnetic resonance imaging (MRI) (Fig. 81-1a), were otherwise negative. Patient had orchiectomy and chemotherapy with resolution of his symptoms. Three months later, while still on chemotherapy, the patient developed progressive headache, nausea, and vomiting. On examination, the only abnormality found was bilateral papilledema.

DEFINITION

Neurologic complications associated with ovary or testis pathology are rare and mostly restricted to neoplastic diseases. The cancer can affect the nervous system by direct infiltration (lumbosacral plexopathy) or by secondary seeding (brain metastases, leptomeningeal metastases) of nervous system structures. In addition, neurologic complications can be caused by indirect effects of the cancer (paraneoplastic neurologic syndromes) or by toxicity secondary to the cancer therapy (chemotherapy-induced neuropathy) (Table 81-1).

In few instances, a neurologic disorder or its treatment is associated with nonmalignant ovary or testis disease. For example, epilepsy has been reported in association to polycystic ovary syndrome, although controversy exists about a causal relationship (1). The fragile X syndrome, which is characterized by mental retardation and macroorchidism, among other clinical characteristics, is caused by a mutation in an RNA-binding protein. Impaired responsiveness to follicle-stimulating hormone with hypogonadism is one of the clinical features associated with myotonic dystrophy. Although these entities merit mention, they are not described in this chapter.

EPIDEMIOLOGY

OVARIES

Epithelial ovarian carcinoma rarely compromises the nervous system, but the incidence of neurologic complications may be increasing as a result of more effective therapeutic regimens for systemic disease. About 4% of all patients with ovarian cancer seen at a tertiary cancer center had a neurologic consultation (2). The incidence of brain metastases has been estimated in about 1% of all patients with ovarian cancer (3). Leptomeningeal disease is even less frequent and tends to occur only in patients who have parenchymal disease (2). When the neurologic complication is metastatic, most patients have advanced cancer at the time of diagnosis. Rare paraneoplastic neurologic syndromes, such as cerebellar degeneration, can be the first manifestation of an early ovarian cancer. More frequent neurologic symptoms are directly related to the cancer treatment using chemotherapy agents. Cisplatin and taxane-based chemotherapy regimens have

TABLE 81-1. Spectrum of Neurologic Complications Associated with Ovary or Testis Cancer

Type of Complication	*Ovary*	*Testis*
Tumor infiltration or metastases	Brain Lumbosacral plexus Leptomeningeal	Brain Lumbosacral plexus
Paraneoplastic syndromes	Subacute cerebellar Dermatomyositis	Limbic encephalitis Brainstem encephalitis
Chemotherapy toxicity	Cisplatin Paclitaxel	Cisplatin

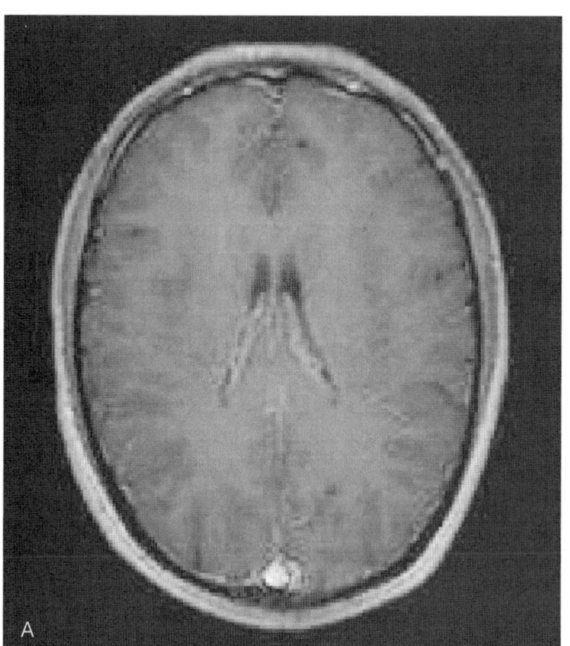

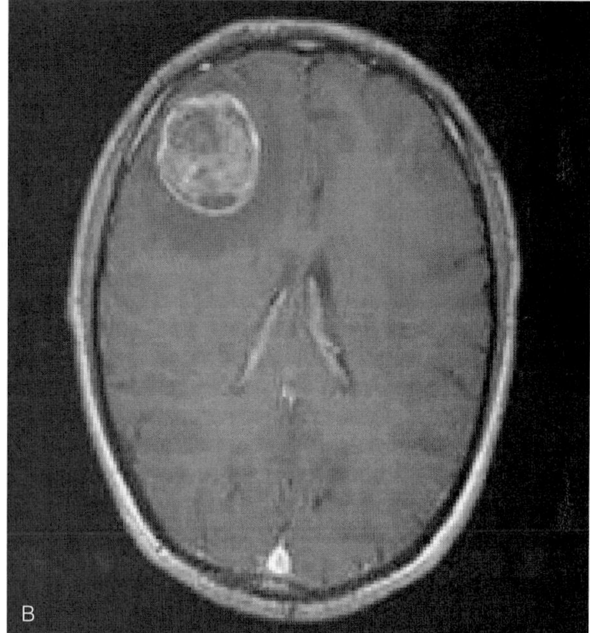

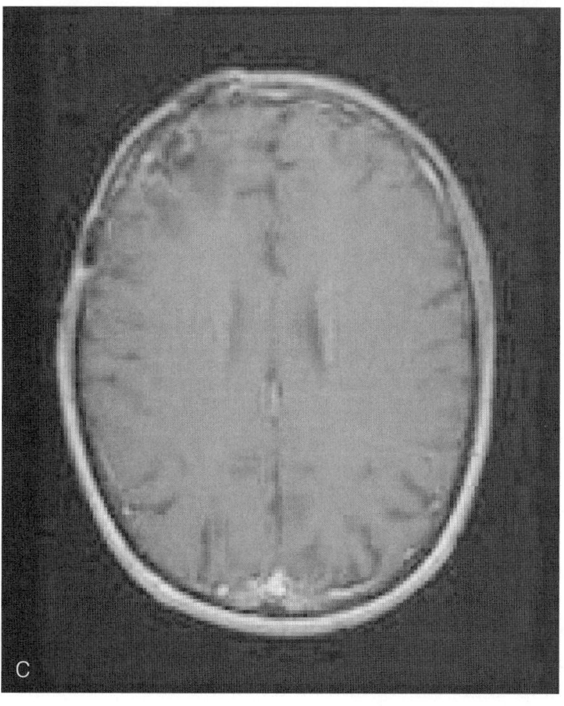

FIGURE 81-1. Case vignette. Testis. Axial postcontrast T1-weighted images of the brain (**A**) at diagnosis of testis cancer, (**B**) at diagnosis of brain metastasis, and (**C**) 3 years after initial diagnosis.

resulted in a high incidence of peripheral neuropathy that affects the quality of life of long-term survivors.

TESTIS

Testicular germ cell tumors can have a seminoma, a nonseminomatous or a mixed histology. The incidence of clinically symptomatic brain metastases in patients with disseminated germ cell tumors, usually nonseminomatous, of the testis varies between 12% and 15% (4). Cerebral involvement is a late occurrence in the course of disease, frequently associated with pulmonary metastases. A previously unrecognized distinct paraneoplastic syndrome of limbic or brainstem encephalitis associated with auto antibodies to Ma2 (brain-testis cancer related-gene family) occurs most frequently in patients with testicular cancer, although it can be seen in association with other primary tumors. Cisplatin-based chemotherapy results in a cure for many patients with testicular cancer, but neurotoxicity is an important dose-limiting side effect. Clinically relevant neuropathy symptoms can persist in approximately 20% to 25% of the long-term survivors (5), affecting their quality of life.

ETIOLOGY AND PATHOGENESIS

Metastatic deposits result from a hematogenous spread of cancer in the context of cancer cell adherence to, and invasion of, endothelium followed by proliferation and new blood vessels formation in the metastatic site (6). This is not a random process and requires specific interaction between the cancer and the organ involved. For unclear pathophysiologic reasons, it is unusual for tumors of the ovaries and testis to seed the brain without first affecting other organs such as the lung. In ovarian cancer, direct infiltration of the lumbosacral plexus and tracking along the nerve trunks is a rare complication. On the other hand, testis cancer metastasizes to pelvic lymph nodes, which can cause compression of nerve roots, trunks, and plexus. Early on the course of this microscopic invasion, severe disabling symptoms might occur that do not match puzzling unrevealing diagnostic studies.

The cause of neurologic paraneoplastic syndromes is thought to be autoimmune, although the exact pathogenesis has not been elucidated. The detection of serum and cerebrospinal fluid (CSF) antibodies that recognize antigens expressed by the normal nervous system, and in some cases the normal testis, were the first clue for the autoimmune model. Antigens identical to those found in the nervous system are expressed by cancer cells (onconeural antigens) and, once seen by the immune system, are considered "nonself," mounting an immune attack (7). The response involves both antibodies and cytotoxic T cells that react against the nervous system cell expressing that shared antigen. For example, in the case of subacute cerebellar degeneration, antibodies against the ovarian cancer target Purkinje cells and their loss is responsible for the neurologic manifestations. Nevertheless, the role of the antibodies and the cytotoxic T cells on the pathogenesis of neurologic paraneoplastic syndromes is unknown.

Chemotherapy regimens that are effective for ovarian cancer frequently combine cisplatin (platin derivative) and paclitaxel (taxanes), and for testicular germ cell tumors are usually based on cisplatin. One of the dose-limiting side effects for both platin derivatives and taxanes is the development of neuropathy. Cisplatin classically affects large sensory fibers, manifested as a purely sensory neuropathy or neuronopathy. The mechanism of neurotoxicity is unknown, but it is thought that cisplatin directly damages dorsal root ganglion neurons (8). Paclitaxel also causes a predominantly sensory neuropathy; in this case, however, both large and small fibers are affected. Its mechanism of antineoplastic action, by promoting the formation of microtubule polymers in the cell, is probably also responsible for the peripheral nervous system toxicity.

PATHOLOGY

The pathology of brain metastases reflects the same features of the primary tumor. Serous cystadenocarcinoma is the most common histologic subtype of ovarian cancer, and also the most frequently associated with central nervous system (CNS) involvement. Infrequently, an adenocarcinoma from another origin (e.g., breast) may metastasize to the ovary and the brain, giving the erroneous impression of a primary ovarian cancer spreading to the brain. Choriocarcinoma and endodermal sinus tumors are the most common histologic types of testis cancer metastasizing to the brain. Metastatic deposits, from apparently pure seminomas, can have nonseminomatous histologic features.

Pathologic changes of paraneoplastic neurologic syndromes are variable. In paraneoplastic cerebellar degeneration, a total loss of the Purkinje cells occurs without inflammatory infiltrates or pathologic changes elsewhere in the nervous system (7). In the encephalitis with Ma2 antibodies, frequently associated with testicular cancer, pathologic studies have revealed florid inflammation, with perivascular lymphocytic cuffing, variable gliosis, and neuronal degeneration. The location of these findings can be restricted to the brainstem, the hypothalamus, or the limbic system, although in most cases, multifocal involvement is present (9).

Chemotherapy-induced neuropathy causes nonspecific changes on pathologic study. The peripheral nerves after treatment with cisplatin or paclitaxel reveal axonal injury and loss, with variable secondary demyelination. In addition, cisplatin therapy will result in dorsal root ganglia neuronal loss. Lhermitte phenomenon, associated with cisplatin, is thought to be caused by localized demyelination of the posterior columns.

CLINICAL MANIFESTATIONS AND SPECIAL SITUATIONS

The clinical manifestations of brain metastases from ovary or testis cancer do not differ from those caused by seeding of other types of cancer. The neurologic symptoms are divided into nonfocal (e.g., increased intracranial pressure or personality changes), focal (e.g., weakness), or sensory symptoms, and seizures. When the clinical manifestations are nonfocal and the patient has no history of cancer, the diagnosis may be difficult, but usually a complete medical history and the examination will provide clues to suggest the diagnosis. As described, in most cases, patients have advanced disease and brain metastases are rarely the first manifestation of the ovary or testis cancer. The median interval between diagnosis of ovarian cancer and of cerebral metastases is 14.5 months and is a function of the clinical stage at diagnosis. Characteristically, patients with brain metastases are younger, have a longer survival after diagnosis of the primary cancer, and have extraperitoneal metastases, when compared with other patients with ovarian cancer (10). A few cases of leptomeningeal metastases, as a complication of epithelial ovarian cancer, have been reported and usually occur in patients who have had a prior diagnosis of parenchymal brain metastases (11). Patients with disseminated germ cell tumors of the testis might have nervous system metastases at the time of diagnosis of the cancer. In some cases, the patient might present with an acute neurologic event secondary to an intratumoral bleed, especially with choriocarcinoma (12).

Patients with neoplastic lumbosacral plexopathy experience an insidious onset of pelvic or radicular leg pain, followed weeks to months later by sensory symptoms and weakness. Plexopathy, in the absence of pain, would suggest a nonneoplastic cause for the symptoms.

Paraneoplastic subacute cerebellar degeneration is a rare entity, which most frequently relates to patients with undiagnosed epithelial ovarian cancer. The clinical profile, such as the one described in the vignette, consists in a middle-aged woman with a rapidly progressing and symmetric cerebellar syndrome. In most patients, the neurologic manifestations precede or coincide with the diagnosis of ovarian cancer, and in those with known cancer, the neurologic syndrome may be the first indication of recurrence or progression of the neoplastic disease (13). Surprisingly, although they have poor prognostic criteria, patients with ovarian cancer and paraneoplastic cerebellar degeneration have a lower metastatic volume and typically lack peritoneal implants when compared with patients without the neurologic disease. The association between dermatomyositis and occult malignancy has been controversial, as has been the impression that a disproportionately high number of the malignant tumors, among patients with dermatomyositis, are ovarian cancer. The clinical profile of the neurologic manifestations associated with ovarian primary neoplasm, consists in more acute symptoms, the development of both diseases within 1 year of each other, and the poor response to steroid therapy. Cricopharyngeal achalasia, an otherwise rare finding with dermatomyositis, is common in patients with ovarian cancer and this paraneoplastic syndrome (14). Patients with paraneoplastic encephalitis with Ma2 antibodies will have symptoms referable according to the area of involvement that could be limbic–hypothalamic, brainstem encephalitis, or both. Patients with hypothalamic dysfunction may present with somnolence, hyperthermia, abnormal weight gain, cataplexy, and gelastic seizures (9).

Cisplatin-induced neuropathy is characterized by numbness and tingling of the extremities, which are occasionally painful. Patients may lose position sense with ataxia, sometimes to the point where they cannot walk. The deep tendon reflexes disappear, although no significant weakness is found, and pinprick and temperature sensations are relatively spared. Cisplatin can also cause ototoxicity with cochlear hair cell loss and result in tinnitus and permanent hearing loss. A less frequent manifestation of cisplatin neurotoxicity is the development of Lhermitte phenomenon, a manifestation of posterior column spinal cord injury (15). Paclitaxel-induced neuropathy affects preferentially pinprick and tactile sensation, with patients complaining of paresthesias involving the hands and feet.

DIAGNOSTIC APPROACH

Once brain metastases is clinically suggested, the diagnosis is established by head MRI after the administration of contrast. This study is more sensitive than computer tomographic (CT) scan because it can identify other lesions when the impression by CT scan is of a solitary lesion and when the metastases are located in the posterior fossa. With the possibility of leptomeningeal metastases, the diagnosis is confirmed with a positive CSF cytology, unless lumbar puncture is contraindicated because of the risk of cerebral herniation. Lumbosacral plexopathy is diagnosed by CT scan or MRI, but the clinician must be aware that in initial stages of the disease these study findings may be normal.

Between 25% and 44% of brain metastases from ovarian cancer are single lesions (3,11); some may be calcified or have a cystic appearance. Extraperitoneal spread to the lung is frequently detected at diagnosis of brain metastases, although in some patients the chest X-ray study may appear normal. In patients without evidence of active ovarian carcinoma and suspicion of CNS involvement, elevated serum concentration of a tumor marker, carcinoma antigen (CA) 125, may be a useful to support the need of an MRI when the patient has no neurologic symptoms. The value of posterior determinations may correlate with response of the lesions to treatment (16). Although CSF measurement of CA 125 may be helpful for diagnosis and follow-up, the sensitivity and specificity of this marker is unknown.

Cerebral MRI is done routinely in patients who have advanced nonseminomatous germ cell testicular cancer at diagnosis and in those with limited disease but who have very high tumor markers to diagnose asymptomatic brain metastases. α-fetoprotein (AFP) and hCG are elevated in 60% of the patients with advanced germ cell tumors, and may be valuable markers for diagnosis and follow-up of nervous system involvement. Some patients also develop brain metastases after induction chemotherapy as the only site of recurrence. Thus, patients with rising serum tumor markers after their primary chemotherapy should have a brain MRI, even if they are asymptomatic from the neurologic standpoint (17).

Several autoantibodies have been identified in patients with paraneoplastic cerebellar degeneration, but the most typical is the anti-Purkinje cell antibody, also called *anti-Yo,* having a unique value as marker of underlying cancer, either ovarian, breast, or lung primary. CSF examination might reveal lymphocytic pleocytosis and oligoclonal bands. The presence of anti-Yo antibody in the CSF is more specific for paraneoplastic syndrome than when detected in the serum. MRI of the brain is initially normal, but eventually will reveal cerebellar atrophy in many cases (18). In about 60% of the patients with positive antibody, the cerebellar syndrome is the first manifestation of cancer. Because ovarian malignancies are frequently responsible, the evaluation should include a gynecological examination, tumor markers, and CT scan of chest, abdomen, and pelvis (19). If no tumor is diagnosed, a whole-body positron-emission tomography (PET) using [18F]-2-fluoro-2-deoxy-D-glucose (FDG) will help in establishing the diagnosis with a sensitivity of about 86% (20).

In a young man who presents with a diencephalic-limbic-brainstem syndrome and a positive Ma2 antibody, cancer of the testis is a high concern. The tumor is usually of the nonseminomatous type, although some cases are associated with seminoma. CSF analysis will also reveal lymphocytic pleocytosis, increased protein, and oligoclonal bands. The initial MRI will frequently reveal abnormalities in T2-weighted and fluid-attenuated inversion recovery (FLAIR) sequences involving diencephalic, brainstem, and limbic structures. Sometimes, there are areas of enhancement in the T1-weighted images with enhancement. Males with a positive antibody should have testicular ultrasound and, if abnormal, proceed with orchiectomy. If the ultrasound study is negative, recommendation is to use FDG-PET to try to identify the primary cancer (9).

TREATMENT

In the case of ovarian cancer, surgical resection of single brain metastasis, followed by radiation therapy, seems to improve survival, especially with no evidence of metastatic spread elsewhere. The role of stereotactic radiosurgery, instead of surgery, is still to be defined. Whole brain radiation therapy is the initial treatment when multiple cerebral metastases are present or in cases of widespread metastatic disease. Some response has been achieved in the treatment of cerebral metastases, with systemic administration of chemotherapeutic agents that are active against ovarian cancer and which may cross the blood–brain barrier. Only supportive care would be indicated in patients with advanced systemic disease and poor functional status. Clinical stage at diagnosis of primary ovarian cancer, number of cerebral metastases (single versus multiple), and the presence of extraperitoneal disease are the most important factors affecting outcome (10).

The treatment of brain metastases from testicular germ cell tumors depends on whether the brain metastases are present at presentation or if they have developed after induction chemotherapy. Systemic cisplatin-based chemotherapy is the foundation of treatment when brain metastases are present at the time of the initial diagnosis. Surgery and tumor resection may be required in some cases. For patients who develop the metastasis after induction chemotherapy and the response to chemotherapy is poor, the recommendation is surgery for a solitary lesion followed by whole brain radiation therapy. The 5-year cause-specific survival rate is 12% (95% CI, 8% to 16%), with a 39% survival rate in patients with an isolated brain recurrence.

Because paraneoplastic syndromes are considered to be immune mediated, two treatment approaches have been used: Removal of the source of the antigen by treating the underlying tumor, and suppression of the immune response (7). Patients diagnosed with subacute cerebellar degeneration and ovarian cancer, for the most part, have a limited stage cancer that responds to treatment, but the neurologic impairment is usually disabling and does not improve with treatment. Despite aggressive treatment of the primary neoplasm combined with plasmapheresis and corticosteroid therapy, the neurologic damage is usually irreversible. In contrast to other paraneoplastic syndromes, patients with encephalitis associated to Ma2 antibody and testis cancer are likely to show improvement or remission of neurologic symptoms (9).

CLINICAL RECOMMENDATIONS OF THE VIGNETTE

Ovaries

Pelvic pain prompted the CT scan revealing a left ovary mass. The head MRI was normal, CA 125 was elevated at 125 U/mL (normal, <35 U/mL), and anti-Yo antibodies were positive. Lumbar puncture revealed lymphocytic pleocytosis. Ovarian tumor was removed and the pathology revealed a tubulopapillary carcinoma growing on the serosa. The diagnosis was of a stage IIIc ovarian cancer with paraneoplastic subacute cerebellar degeneration. The patient received chemotherapy with cisplatin and paclitaxel with normalization of the CA 125, but she was very disabled with incomprehensible dysarthria, unable to feed herself because of limb incoordination, and restricted to a wheelchair. Despite plasmapheresis, steroids, and several courses of intravenous immunoglobulin, her functional status failed to improve. A follow-up MRI, done 1 year after onset, revealed cerebellar atrophy.

Testis

A brain MRI revealed a right frontal mass (Fig. 81-1b), which was resected, and pathology showed embryonal carcinoma. The patient had whole brain radiation therapy, and is now 3 years after diagnosis with an undetectable hCG. He continues to work, but has experienced short-term memory difficulties. A follow-up MRI (Fig. 81-1c) 3 years after diagnosis showed no evidence of metastatic disease.

SUMMARY

Diseases affecting the ovary and testis are rarely associated with neurologic complications; when they occur, however, they are usually secondary to neoplastic disease. The spectrum of neurologic involvement ranges from direct infiltration of neural structures to neurotoxicity associated with oncologic treatment. The appearance of brain metastases in the patient with ovarian cancer is a poor prognostic indicator, although treatment might alleviate symptoms and prolong survival, but eventually the patient will die from the disease. In contrast, many patients with brain metastases from testicular cancer will be cured with treatment. The possibility of an occult ovarian cancer is raised in any woman presenting with a subacute cerebellar syndrome and normal imaging studies. Likewise, the development of a subacute limbic or brainstem encephalitis in a young man is concerning for the possibility of a cancer of the testis. Because these complications are rare, the clinician must include them in the differential diagnosis when one of the neurologic syndromes previously discussed appears, because early diagnoses and treatment might prolong survival and improve quality of life.

REFERENCES

1. Harden CL. Polycystic ovaries and polycystic ovary syndrome in epilepsy: Evidence for neurogonadal disease. *Epilepsy Curr.* 2005;5(4):142–146.
2. Abrey LE, Dalmau JO. Neurologic complications of ovarian carcinoma. *Cancer.* 1999;85(1):127–133.
3. Pectasides D, Pectasides M, Economopoulos T. Brain metastases from epithelial ovarian cancer: A review of the literature. *Oncologist.* 2006;11(3):252–260.
4. Logothetis CJ, Samuels ML, Trindade A. The management of brain metastases in germ cell tumors. *Cancer.* 1982;49(1):12–18.
5. Fossa SD, de Wit R, Roberts JT, et al. Quality of life in good prognosis patients with metastatic germ cell cancer: A prospective study of the European Organization for Research and Treatment of Cancer Genitourinary Group/Medical Research Council Testicular Cancer Study Group (30941/TE20). *J Clin Oncol.* 2003;21(6):1107–1118.
6. Tosoni A, Ermani M, Brandes AA. The pathogenesis and treatment of brain metastases: A comprehensive review. *Crit Rev Oncol Hematol.* 2004;52(3):199–215.

7. Darnell RB, Posner JB. Paraneoplastic syndromes involving the nervous system. *N Engl J Med.* 2003;349(16):1543–1554.
8. Meijer C, de Vries EG, Marmiroli P, et al. Cisplatin-induced DNA-platination in experimental dorsal root ganglia neuronopathy. *Neurotoxicology.* 1999;20(6):883–887.
9. Dalmau J, Graus F, Villarejo A, et al. Clinical analysis of anti-Ma2-associated encephalitis. *Brain.* 2004;127(Pt 8):1831–1844.
10. LeRoux PD, Berger MS, Elliott JP, et al. Cerebral metastases from ovarian carcinoma. *Cancer.* 1991;67(8):2194–2199.
11. Cohen ZR, Suki D, Weinberg JS, et al. Brain metastases in patients with ovarian carcinoma: Prognostic factors and outcome. *J Neurooncol.* 2004;66(3):313–325.
12. Salvati M, Piccirilli M, Raco A, et al. Brain metastasis from non-seminomatous germ cell tumors of the testis: Indications for aggressive treatment. *Neurosurg Rev.* 2006;29(2): 130–137.
13. Hetzel DJ, Stanhope CR, O'Neill BP, et al. Gynecologic cancer in patients with subacute cerebellar degeneration predicted by anti-Purkinje cell antibodies and limited in metastatic volume. *Mayo Clin Proc.* 1990;65(12):1558–1563.
14. Peters WA, 3rd, Andersen WA, Thornton WN, Jr. Dermatomyositis and coexistent ovarian cancer: A review of the compounding clinical problems. *Gynecol Oncol.* 1983;15(3): 440–446.
15. Eeles R, Tait DM, Peckham MJ. Lhermitte's sign as a complication of cisplatin-containing chemotherapy for testicular cancer. *Cancer Treat Rep.* 1986;70(7):905–907.
16. Plaxe SC, Dottino PR, Lipsztein R, et al. Clinical features and treatment outcome of patients with epithelial carcinoma of the ovary metastatic to the central nervous system. *Obstet Gynecol.* 1990;75(2):278–281.
17. Fossa SD, Bokemeyer C, Gerl A, et al. Treatment outcome of patients with brain metastases from malignant germ cell tumors. *Cancer.* 1999;85(4):988–997.
18. Peterson K, Rosenblum MK, Kotanides H, et al. Paraneoplastic cerebellar degeneration. I. A clinical analysis of 55 anti-Yo antibody-positive patients. *Neurology.* 1992;42(10):1931–1937.
19. Frings M, Antoch G, Knorn P, et al. Strategies in detection of the primary tumour in anti-Yo associated paraneoplastic cerebellar degeneration. *J Neurol.* 2005;252(2):197–201.
20. Younes-Mhenni S, Janier MF, Cinotti L, et al. FDG-PET improves tumour detection in patients with paraneoplastic neurological syndromes. *Brain.* 2004;127(Pt 10):2331–2338.

CHAPTER 82

Multiple Endocrine Syndromes

William C. Kattah • Jorge C. Kattah

OBJECTIVES

- To describe the neurologic manifestations of multiple endocrine adenomatosis
- To describe the neurologic manifestations of the syndrome of multiple autoimmune endocrinopathy
- To provide an awareness of multiple coexistents endocrine syndromes with varied symptoms that encompass a wide spectrum of endocrine and neurologic symptoms and signs and often represent a diagnostic challenge

From the beginning of the 20th century, the occurrence of multiple endocrine neoplasms (MEN) was recognized among several members of a family. Two main syndromes, type 1 (or Wermer syndrome) and type 2 (Sipple syndrome) are predominant within MEN; other less common syndromes have been recognized as well.

Multiple autoimmune endocrinopathies (MAE) are uncommon syndromes in which polyglandular insufficiency occurs as a result of autoantibody production. The most common MAE syndromes include (*a*) multiple autoimmune endocrinopathy type 1, (*b*) multiple autoimmune endocrinopathy type 2, (*c*) POEMS (polyneuropathy, organomegaly, endocrinopathy, monoclonal gammopathy, skin changes) syndrome, (*d*) anti-insulin receptor antibody syndrome, and (*e*) endocrinopathies associated with thymomas.

CASE VIGNETTE 1

A 34-year-old man with a 5-year history of peptic ulcers and upper gastrointestinal (GI) bleeding on two different occasions had a gastrectomy (Bilroth type II) 1 year earlier. In the last months, he observed a change in his facial features, enlargement of the fingers, tingling in the hands, and weakness in his grip. On examination, he was found to have symptoms typical for carpal tunnel entrapment and acromegaly. Endocrine workup showed pertinent findings for his age, an increased human growth hormone (HGH): 16 ng/dL (normal <5 ng/dL) and somatomedin C 1,016 ng/dL (normal, 130 to 600 ng/dL). Unexpectedly, he also had hypercalcemia and elevation of the parathyroid hormone (PTH).

CASE VIGNETTE 2

A 34-year-old woman with a previous history of hypothyroidism (Hashimoto thyroiditis), primary ovarian failure, and adrenal insufficiency was admitted with progressive mental status deterioration. A brain magnetic resonance imaging (MRI) showed increased signal intensity in both medial temporal lobes fluid-attenuated inversion recovery (FLAIR) images with discrete contrast enhancement. Cerebrospinal fluid (CSF) was normal. Antipotassium channel antibodies were negative. She had a positive extractable nuclear antigens (ENA).

DEFINITION

Type 1 MEN is characterized by the presence of either parathyroid hyperplasia or adenomas, gastrinomas causing the Zollinger-Ellison syndrome, pituitary adenomas, and insulinomas (Table 82-1). MEN type 2A is characterized by the development of medullary carcinoma of the thyroid, pheochromocytomas, and hyperparathyroidism (Table 82-2). In type 2B, besides the type 2A characteristics, mucosal neuromas and a marphanoid appearance are common.

ETIOLOGY AND PATHOGENESIS

MEN type 1 (MEN-1) is an autosomal dominant disorder that results from a mutation in the MEN type 1 tumor-suppressor gene located in chromosome 11. This gene is located in the nucleus of germline cells and becomes clinically significant with inactivation of the wild-type allele (1–3). Tumors of the pancreas tend to become malignant. MEN type 2 (MEN-2) is caused by a mutation of a protooncogene present (RET) found in neural crest-derived cells, calcitonin-producing cells (C-cells) of the thyroid gland, and chromaffin cells of the adrenal glands. This syndrome can be as frequent as 0.2 per 1,000 patients. The abnormal gene is located in chromosome 10 (4).

PATHOLOGY

The pathologic manifestations of MEN-1 and MEN-2 are the common manifestations of the different neoplasms as reviewed in other section chapters. No specific abnormalities are particular to MEN-1; pheochromocytomas, when present, are frequently bilateral. Medullary carcinoma of the thyroid is universally present in children.

TABLE 82-1. Multiple Endocrine Adenomatosis (MEN) Type 1

- Hyperparathyroidism: 80% to 90%
- Pancreatic tumors: Insulinoma, glucagonoma
- Parathyroid hyperplasia: 80% to 90%
- Gastrinoma: Benign 20%; malignant 30%
- Pituitary tumors
  - Growth hormone: (GH 15%
  - Corticotropin: 5%
  - Mixed GH or prolactinomas: 15%
- Cortical adrenal tumors: 10%
- Carcinoid syndrome: 5%
- Thyroid adenomas: 5%
- Lipoma or liposarcoma: <5%

CLINICAL MANIFESTATIONS

The diagnosis of MEN must be a consideration among patients with a positive family history of endocrine tumors or the occurrence of multiple endocrine tumors in the same individual. Critical aspects in the history include previous upper GI bleeding, in addition to clinical manifestations of hyperparathyroidism and pituitary tumors, which are reviewed in other section chapters. The possibility of an insulinoma with episodic hypoglycemia, neuropsychiatric changes, seizures, coma, and focal neurologic deficits may also be found (5).

In MEN-2, the main characteristic found is the universal occurrence of medullary carcinoma of the thyroid. The clinical picture may be dominated by the presence of bilateral pheochromocytomas with hypertensive or hypotensive crisis, depending on the release of norepinephrine or epinephrine, respectively. In addition, headache, palpitations, anxiety, and paniclike reaction may be reported and recurrent syncope may occur.

In MEN-2B, multiple cutaneous and mucosal neuromas can occur, even in young children, and may be an indication for prophylactic thyroidectomy to prevent the development of medullary carcinoma of the thyroid gland. It is important to note that most pheochromocytomas and medullary carcinoma of the thyroid are sporadic and not associated with MEN.

DIAGNOSTIC APPROACH

In patients with suspected MEN-1, evaluation of parathyroid, pituitary, and pancreatic function would be indicated. Upper GI bleeding, caused by the Zollinger-Ellison syndrome, must be recognized in this clinical context. Insulinomas can present with episodic loss of consciousness and seizures. If a family member is identified with MEN, the relatives should be tested for abnormalities.

TABLE 82-2. Multiple Endocrine Adenomatosis (MEN) Type 2

MEN Type 2A	*MEN Type 2B*
Medullary carcinoma of the thyroid: 100%	Medullary carcinoma of the thyroid: 100%
Pheochromocytoma: 50%	Pheochromocytoma: 50%
Hyperparathyroidism: 10% to 60%	Marfan appearance

In MEN-2, a search for a possible medullary carcinoma of the thyroid would be critical. Pentagastrin testing can be used to investigate this possibility. Serial levels of calcitonin can also be obtained. If calcitonin levels are abnormal, early thyroidectomy may be life-saving. In addition, genetic testing is reliable. Details of the diagnosis of pheochromocytoma are described in detail in the adrenal gland function section.

TREATMENT

Management of MEN (types 1 and 2) demand a high-recognition threshold and interactive, multispecialty work. It is conceivable that patients with MEN-1 or 2 begin their search for a diagnosis at a neurologist's office with a variety of complaints, which are reviewed in the other chapters in this section. Most of the adenomas should be removed surgically. In MEN-2, a search for a silent medullary cancer of the thyroid is critical, given the likelihood of metastases and potential death.

CLINICAL RECOMMENDATIONS FOR VIGNETTE 1

The patient had peptic ulcer disease caused by increased levels of gastrin (Zollinger-Ellison syndrome). He then developed signs of acromegaly and was found to have subclinical, hyperparathyroidism. The adenomas were identified and resected.

Less common endocrine syndromes can be seen in the Von Hipple Lindau syndrome and in neurofibromatosis 1 (NF-1). In the former, tumors of the pancreas are more prevalent and, in the latter, pheochromocytomas.

Multiple Autoimmune Endocrinopathy

DEFINITION

Several types of multiple endocrine insufficiency syndromes have been recognized; most of them are inherited and are associated with the production of autoantibodies. Types 1, 2, and 3 present with the most consistent clinical syndromes (Table 82-3).

ETIOLOGY AND PATHOGENESIS

Type 1 MAE is inherited as an autosomal recessive trait; types 2 and 3 are recessive. Awareness of this coexistent endocrinopathies is necessary to recognize these syndromes.

PATHOLOGY

The findings are probably not well known, outside perhaps those in the thyroid gland, which are described in the thyroid section chapter.

CLINICAL MANIFESTATIONS

The findings in MAE 1, 2, and 3 relate to the specific endocrine failure. Any time multiple hormonal deficiencies are detected,

TABLE 82-3. Autoimmune Endocrinopathy

Type	*Classic Components*	*Less Common Components*
TYPE 1	Hypoparathyroidism Mucocutaneous-candidiasis Addison disease	Primary ovarian failure Hypothyroidism Pernicious anemia
TYPE 2 (Schmidt syndrome)	Hashimoto thyroiditis Primary adrenal failure Primary ovarian failure Diabetes mellitus	Vitiligo or pernicious anemia Myasthenia gravis Celiac disease
TYPE 3	Diabetes mellitus Hashimoto thyroiditis	Adrenal insufficiency

the possibility of MAE must be investigated and all hormonal axis function should be performed (6,7). Neurologic manifestations can be interesting because they will be the result of multiple hormonal deficiencies and, possibly, present with a very confusing differential diagnosis.

DIAGNOSTIC APPROACH

When suspecting MAE 1, 2, and 3, the initial workup can begin with a blood sugar, comprehensive metabolic panel (CMP), thyroid-stimulating hormone (TSH), luteinizing hormone (LH), and follicle-stimulating hormone (FSH), calcium, and phosphorus. Among members of the family, screening for subclinical hormonal changes should be performed every 1 to 2 years throughout the third and fourth decades.

Other less common endocrinopathy syndromes include the combination of a monoclonal gammapathy caused by a plasma cell dyscrasia known with the acronym *POEMS*, which emphasizes the presence of a polyneuropathy, organomegaly, endocrinopathy, monoclonal gammapathy, and skin changes. Hyperprolactinemia and diabetes mellitus are the most frequent hormonal abnormalities. Elevation in the spinal fluid protein can cause increased intracranial pressure and papilledema.

TREATMENT

The treatment goal in MAE would be to provide hormonal replacement as needed. If nonendocrine manifestations coexist, there could be a need for immune suppression.

CLINICAL RECOMMENDATIONS FOR VIGNETTE 2

The patient has MAE, possibly more consistent with MAE-2 or 3 in the absence of a family history. She had successful hormonal replacement; however, recurrent episodes of limbic encephalitis have required on-going immune suppression with weekly methotrexate and low-dose daily corticosteroids.

SUMMARY

Multiple endocrine syndromes involve unusual, intriguing diagnostic challenges. Awareness of the complicated array of different combinations of signs and symptoms may allow an astute clinician to provide a timely diagnosis and management. This chapter focused on their most practical characteristics.

REFERENCES

1. Friedman E, Sakaguchi K, Bale AE, et al. Clonality of parathyroid tumors in familial multiple endocrine neoplasia type 1. *N Eng J Med.* 1989:321(4):213–218.
2. Larsson C, Skogseid B, Oberg K, et al. Multiple endocrine neoplasia type 1 gene maps to chromosome 11 and is lost in insulinoma. *Nature.* 1988;322(6159):85–87.
3. Rizzoli R, Green J 3rd, Marx SJ. Primary hyperparathyroidism in familial multiple endocrine neoplasia type I. Long-term follow-up of serum calcium levels after parathyroidectomy. *Am J Med.* 1985;78(3):467–474.
4. Simpson NE. The exploration of the locus or loci for the syndromes associated with the medullary thyroid cancer (MTC) on chromosome 10. In: Brandi ML, White R, eds. *Hereditary Tumors.* New York: Raven Press; 1991:55–67.
5. Skogseid B, Eriksson B, Lundqvist G, et al. Multiple endocrine neoplasia type I: A 10-year prospective screening study in four kindreds. *J Clin Endocrinol Metab.* 1991;73(2):281–287.
6. Neufled M, Maclaren NK, Blizzard RM. Two types of autoimmune Addison's with different polyglandular autoimmune (PGA) syndromes. *Medicine.* 1981;60(5):355–362.
7. Ahonen P, Myllarniemi S, Sipula J, et al. Clinical variation of autoimmune polyendocrinopathy–candidiasis-ectodermal dystrophy (APECED) in a series of 68 patients. *N Eng J Med.* 1990;322(26):1829–1836.

CHAPTER **83**

Commonly Used Endocrine Drugs

Daniel E. Jacome • Alfredo F. Jacome

OBJECTIVES

- To present some of the neurologic adverse reactions precipitated by endocrine drugs
- To provide information on the pathogenesis of these reactions
- To illustrate the frequency of these complications to discuss the best approach in establishing the diagnosis of these disorders
- To explain how to treat or prevent the neurologic complications of endocrine drugs

CASE VIGNETTE

A 22-year-old woman with a history of systemic lupus erythematosus (SLE) was admitted to the hospital because of poor concentration, headache, diplopia, tinnitus, insomnia, and restlessness. She had been treated with 5 mg of prednisone a day, increased 3 weeks earlier to 60 mg a day, because of muscle pains and worsening facial rash. On examination, she was loquacious, did not know the day of the week, and had a short attention span. Funduscopic examination was normal. Her limb muscles were tender to palpation.

Steroid-Induced Psychiatric Syndrome

DEFINITION

Steroid-induced psychiatric syndrome (SIPS) is characterized by the acute or subacute development of abnormal behavior in patients receiving corticosteroids in whom no other origin for their symptoms is identifiable (1,2).

EPIDEMIOLOGY

The reported incidence of *steroid psychosis* has ranged from 0 to 62%, with a weighted average of 27%. *Steroid withdrawal syndrome* is classified as a different entity (3).

ETIOLOGY AND PATHOGENESIS

The etiology of SIPS is unknown, but hypercortisolemia is a primary suspect (4).

PATHOLOGY

The cognitive deficit is accompanied by a reversible diminution in the hippocampus volume (5).

CLINICAL MANIFESTATIONS AND SPECIAL SITUATIONS

Outlined below are clinical manifestations and some special situations related to steroid-induced psychiatric syndrome.

A. Affective profile: Depression, dysphoria, irritability, mood instability, suicidal ideation, mania, or hypomania.
B. Psychotic symptoms: Delirium, disorganized thought process, poor assessment of reality, depersonalization, delusions, and hallucinations (1,2).
C. Cognitive disorder: The chronic (and rarely acute) administration of corticosteroids can produce specific derangement of declarative memory caused by atrophy or dysfunction of the hippocampus (6).
D. Steroid withdrawal syndrome: Occurs with cessation of corticosteroid therapy. Dixon and Christy (3) distinguishes three variants of withdrawal:
    1. Type I: Associated with hypothalamic pituitary axis (HPA) dysfunction
    2. Type II: Caused by recrudescence of primary disease
    3. Type III: Caused by drug dependence or *steroid abstinence syndrome* (3)

DIAGNOSTIC APPROACH

It is difficult to ascertain if the patient's symptoms are caused only by SIPS or if they are also based on progression of the primary disease; central nervous system (CNS) symptoms of SLE mimics SIPS.

TREATMENT

Steroids may need to be tapered off or stopped. The patient with a history of affective illness is a probable candidate for prophylactic treatment with a mood stabilizer. Anxiolytics, neuroleptics, or antidepressants may be required.

Steroid Myopathy

DEFINITION

Steroid myopathy (SM) is an insidious illness of the striated muscles caused by endogenous or exogenous corticosteroids that results in weakness of proximal limb muscles.

EPIDEMIOLOGY

SM affects women two times more often than men, and primarily affects those with sedentary lifestyles; its incidence ranges from 7% to 60% (7). SM is more prevalent and appears earlier in patients with cancer requiring the administration of steroids (8). Acute SM is a complication of acutely ill patients receiving multiple medications and is often undiagnosed.

ETIOLOGY AND PATHOGENESIS

Pathogenic mechanisms implicated in the appearance of SM are mitochondrial dysfunction, increased protein degradation, hypokalemia, increased glutamine synthase activity, decreased protein synthesis, and abnormal carbohydrate metabolism.

PATHOLOGY

In chronic SM, the muscle biopsy will show atrophy of fast twitch, glycolitic type IIB fibers. No significant necrosis, vacuolar degeneration, or inflammation will be present. In acute SM is found either focal or diffuse myotubular necrosis of all fiber types, loss of myosin tick filaments, disorganization of myofibrils, and expression of ubiquitin in immunohistochemical stains (7).

CLINICAL MANIFESTATIONS AND SPECIAL SITUATIONS

CHRONIC STEROID MYOPATHY (CSM)

CSM is characterized by insidious onset of progressive weakness of proximal limb muscles, normally beginning in the legs, and of symmetric distribution. Muscle stretch reflexes and sensory examinations are normal. Myalgias are not common or severe. There is involvement of neck muscles, with sparing of facial and oropharyngeal muscles. Selective compromise of respiratory muscles can occur.

ACUTE STEROID MYOPATHY

Acute SM is typically of abrupt onset with tetraplegia. There is preservation of muscle stretch reflexes and sensory examination is normal. Acute SM usually follows the intravenous administration of corticosteroids to a critically ill, intubated patient in the intensive care unit (ICU), who is receiving simultaneously nondepolarizing neuromuscular blocking agents (9).

DIAGNOSTIC APPROACH

In acute SM, creatine kinase (CK) is elevated and myoglobinuria is present. In chronic SM, there is increased urinary excretion of creatine and methyl histidine or the creatine:creatinine ratio is elevated (10). CK and aldolase values are normal. Motor and sensory nerve conduction study findings are normal, but abnormalities may be found because of an underlying or concomitant illness. The electromyogram (EMG) will show occasional sharp waves, small motor units, and an early (*myopathic*) recruitment pattern.

TREATMENT

Stopping steroids or reducing the dose is the most effective step. A maintenance dose of prednisone below 30 mg a day has lesser chances of causing SM. Fluorinated steroids, such as dexamethasone, should be replaced with a nonfluorinated steroid, such as prednisone.

Endocrine Drugs and Idiopathic Intracranial Hypertension

DEFINITION

Idiopathic intracranial hypertension (IIH) has been reported after initiation of treatment with glucocorticoids, hormonal contraceptives, human growth hormone (hGH), insulin growth factor (IGF), and levothyroxine (11–16). IIH can develop after steroid withdrawal or after resection of a pituitary adenoma, if replacement therapy is not instituted (17).

EPIDEMIOLOGY

The annual incidence of IIH at the Mayo Clinic between the years of 1976 to 1990 was as follows: 0.9% per 100,000 in the general population; 1.6% per 100,000 women; 3.3% per 100,000 in people between the ages of 15 to 44 years; and 7.9% for obese women aged 15 to 44 years (18).

ETIOLOGY AND PATHOGENESIS

The exact pathogenesis of IIH in patients receiving endocrine drugs is unknown. In the example of patients with IIH following treatment with hGH, increased cerebrospinal fluid (CSF) production by the choroids plexus mediated by IGF-1 has been proposed (16).

PATHOLOGY

IIH associated to endocrine drugs has no mortality and is by definition reversible.

CLINICAL MANIFESTATIONS AND SPECIAL SITUATIONS

Typical symptoms include headaches, transient visual obscurations, intracranial noises, photopsias, diplopia, visual loss, eye pain with eye movements. Among the atypical symptoms are anosmia, weakness, numbness, ataxia, arm pain, monocular visual obscurations, seizures.

A typical sign is papilledema. Atypical signs include no papilledema, pseudopapilledema (drusen), asymmetric papilledema, cranial paresis (III, IV, VII), and cognitive disturbance. IIH after hGH replacement tends to affect children preferentially and can develop years after the initiation of treatment (19–23).

DIAGNOSTIC APPROACH

The classic triad of IIH consists of papilledema, negative neuroimaging studies (other than possible slitlike ventricles and stenosis of the intracranial venous sinuses), and a normal CSF composition under elevated pressure. Because IIH and intracranial venous thrombosis have similar symptoms, magnetic resonance venography (MRV) is indicated in all cases of IIH to rule out thrombosis. Visual field testing will document the degree of visual loss or recovery of vision over time.

TREATMENT

Treatment consists of discontinuation of the offending drug; repeated lumbar punctures (LP), diuretics, and optic nerve fenestration or ventriculoperitoneal CSF shunting, procedures reserved for cases of progressive visual loss.

Hormonal Therapy and Stroke

Hormonal Replacement Therapy (HRT) and Stroke

DEFINITION

Several studies substantiate the beneficial effects of estrogen in reducing the extent of experimental strokes in animals, and in humans the improvement of the lipid profile and blood flow. In contrast, the Women's Health Initiative (WHI) study, demonstrated in low risk, healthy postmenopausal women prescribed hormone replacement therapy (HRT) with conjugated equine estrogens alone, or in combination with hydroxyl-progesterone acetate, a 40% increased risk of stroke and a 30% increased risk of first coronary artery disease events (24–26). The women estrogen stroke trial (WEST) included women with previous strokes or transient ischemic attacks treated with 17 β-estradiol in a randomized, placebo-controlled study (27). The estrogen-treated group had almost three times the rate of fatal strokes in comparison with the placebo group. In addition, those with nonfatal strokes had worse outcomes (27). Although in the WHI study the risk of stroke was higher in the treated arm, the absolute risk of stroke resulted only in eight strokes per 10,000 women for each year of HRT.

Oral Contraceptives and Stroke

DEFINITION

Most case-controlled studies indicate an exaggerated risk of stroke in women receiving oral contraceptives, even with those of low estrogen content (24). Nevertheless, in analyzing this topic the following points should be kept in mind:

- Meta-analysis of some of the studies incriminating oral contraceptives as drugs increasing stroke risk tend to show higher estimates of stroke when the studies did not control for smoking, or in those employing case-control designs rather than a cohort design.
- New generation of oral contraceptives with an improved formulation are associated with lower risks of stroke.
- The absolute risk of stroke is low, with only four additional ischemic strokes per 100,000, in nonsmoking, normotensive women receiving low estrogen contraceptives.
- The greater the number of associated risks, the greater the chances of stroke (24).

EPIDEMIOLOGY

Stroke in women constitutes a major source of disability and the third leading cause of death. In the year 2000, 66% of stroke deaths were women (28).

ETIOLOGY AND PATHOGENESIS

Estrogens may have beneficial and deleterious effects. Among the beneficial effects are neuroprotection and endothelial function enhancement, and estrogens are antiinflammatory. Their deleterious effects include activation of coagulation, in which the effects of estrogens on coagulation are dose dependent and modified by the concomitant use of progesterone. HRT also augments the risks of thromboembolism in patients with thrombophilia. Furthermore, estrogens can enhance platelet aggregation acting through the glycoprotein II b/III, a receptor that mediates the conformational changes allowing fibrinogen binding.

PATHOLOGY

Strokes precipitated by estrogens have no specific brain pathology.

CLINICAL MANIFESTATIONS AND SPECIAL SITUATIONS

Signs and symptoms of stroke vary according to their size and location, previous strokes, metabolic and cardiac comorbidity, and age of the patient.

DIAGNOSTIC APPROACH

Neurologic examination, and neurologic and cardiovascular imaging procedures are required. Paradoxical CNS embolic strokes in patients taking oral contraceptives suggest the presence of occult deep venous thrombosis of the legs, or of the pelvis venous plexus. Testing for thrombophilia, in particular for the factor V Leiden mutation, is advisable because its presence may have facilitated the thromboembolic episode.

TREATMENT

Treatment involves discontining HRT or oral contraceptives; treat stroke according to current standards of care, including use of tissue plasminogen activator (TPA); rule out patent foramen ovale (PFO); and treat hypertension and initiate strategies for cigarette smoking cessation.

Tamoxifen and Stroke

DEFINITION

Tamoxifen is a nonsteroidal triphenyl ethylene estrogen receptor modulator that was approved in the United States for the treatment of advanced breast cancer in 1978. Over time, it became apparent that tamoxifen also reduces the chances of contralateral breast cancer among treated women. It has, however, potential serious adverse effects, including venous thromboembolism and endometrial cancer. A more recent concern has been the possibility of tamoxifen causing stroke. Geiger et al. (29) conducted a case study of first stroke after breast cancer in a cohort of Los Angeles county residents enrolled in a health maintenance organization. These authors concluded that tamoxifen is not associated to an increased risk of stroke. Bushnell and Goldstein (30) performed a meta-analysis of nine randomized control trials of tamoxifen prescribed for breast cancer. Treated women had an 82% increased risk of ischemic stroke and a 29% risk of any stroke. The absolute risk of stroke was actually very small, with an annual stroke risk of 0.053% in treated patients, versus 0.035% in controls.

EPIDEMIOLOGY

The incidence of breast cancer in the United States has been calculated at 4.28 per 1,000 person year (31).

ETIOLOGY AND PATHOGENESIS

Tamoxifen can exert its potential thrombogenic properties by decreasing the levels of protein C and antithrombin and by increasing the levels of von Willebrand factor (32).

PATHOLOGY

There is no specific neuropathology.

CLINICAL MANIFESTATIONS AND SPECIAL SITUATIONS

Stroke in patients taking tamoxifen will present with focal, multifocal, disseminated, or neuropsychiatric signs and symptoms. Older women will be overrepresented.

DIAGNOSTIC APPROACH

Alternative and more frequent causes of stroke should be ruled out in patients treated with tamoxifen. In particular, CNS metastasis from breast cancer with superimposed hemorrhage must be ruled out.

TREATMENT

History of transient ischemic attacks (TIA) or stroke is not a contraindication to treatment with tamoxifen in a patient with breast cancer, unless the stroke was of venous thromboembolic origin.

Hormonal Therapy and Migraine

DEFINITION

Migraine is a frequent primary headache disorder three times more common in women in whom estrogens play an established pathogenic role (33). Headache is a common adverse effect reported by women taking oral contraceptives (34). Women receiving HRT may also experience a worsening of their headaches, but this happens with less consistency than among women on oral contraceptives (34,35).

EPIDEMIOLOGY

Migraine with aura is a risk factor for ischemic stroke with a relative risk of 3, augmented by the use of oral contraceptives and cigarette smoking (35). Male-to-female transsexuals given antiandrogen drugs to suppress their male sex characteristics, have increased prevalence of migraine (up to 26%), in comparison to heterosexual males (36).

ETIOLOGY AND PATHOGENESIS

The amelioration of migraine during pregnancy and menopause and its worsening during menses suggest a strong pathogenic role for estrogen withdrawal (33).

PATHOLOGY

No mortality is associated with uncomplicated menstrual migraine.

CLINICAL MANIFESTATIONS AND SPECIAL SITUATIONS

Menstrual migraine is typically characterized by migraine without aura. Patients with migraine with aura can also experience accentuation of their headache, following the administration of oral contraceptives or HRT (34).

DIAGNOSTIC APPROACH

Migraine is a clinical diagnosis based on history offered by the patient.

TREATMENT

Women with a history of migraine without aura can be prescribed oral contraceptives unless they smoke or have a history of thrombophilia or thromboembolic disease. If migraine worsens with oral contraceptive use, it may represent a temporary setback.

Hormonal Therapy and Epilepsy

DEFINITION

The field of epilepsy and neuroendocrinology is complex and poorly understood; the inherent cyclical variability of plasma hormone concentrations, especially in women, has been found in multiple animal models of epilepsy and on the interplay that exists between endogenous and exogenously prescribed hormones (37).

EPIDEMIOLOGY

No large prospective study has been conducted on the effects of oral contraceptives or HRT on seizure frequency. Several early studies on the consequences of oral contraceptives in epilepsy had opposite conclusions (37). Improvement in seizure control was reported in a postmenopausal woman given HRT (38).

ETIOLOGY AND PATHOGENESIS

Clinicians agree in general terms that estrogen is proconvulsant and progesterone is anticonvulsant (39).

PATHOLOGY

No specific neuropathology is ascribed to hormone-sensitive epilepsy.

CLINICAL MANIFESTATIONS AND SPECIAL SITUATIONS

Epilepsy could be primary (genetic) or secondary to congenital or acquired lesions. Seizure frequency will vary during the different phases of the menstrual cycle.

DIAGNOSTIC APPROACH

In clinical practice, there is no indication to monitor hormone levels throughout the menstrual cycle. The patient should keep a seizure diary for at least several cycles.

TREATMENT

Oral contraceptives, HRT, or androgen replacement therapy can be safely prescribed to individuals with epilepsy. Antiepileptic drug (AED) levels, however, should be monitored on a regular basis.

Desmopressin Hyponatremic Hypervolemia

DEFINITION

Desmopressin is a synthetic analog of the endogenous pituitary hormone arginine-vasopressin (AVP) used in the treatment of primary nocturnal enuresis (PNE), central diabetes insipidus, von Willebrand disease, postsurgical bleeding, and nocturia (40,41). Desmopressin causes dilutional hyponatremia because of the hypervolemia arising from AVP-induced excessive water retention.

EPIDEMIOLOGY

Of girls, 3% and of boys, 7% have PNE by age 7. Of all children, 15% experience spontaneous remission every year. More than 37 million Europeans have nocturia (42).

ETIOLOGY AND PATHOGENESIS

Children with PNE have a blunted nocturnal release of AVP. Desmopressin administration, if accompanied by excessive water intake by the patient, can precipitate hyponatremic hypervolemia, encephalopathy, and seizures. Thumfart et al. (40) have identified three risk factors for the appearance of this complication: (*a*) Age: The younger the patient, the greater the risk of water intoxication. (*b*) Gender: Of men, 63% are affected, in contrast to 35% of women. (*c*) Time of treatment: Most cases develop during the first 3 weeks of therapy. Rapid correction of chronic hyponatremia causes central pontine myelinolysis (CPM) (43).

PATHOLOGY

No specific neuropathologic findings are diagnostic of hypervolemic hyponatremia.

CLINICAL MANIFESTATIONS AND SPECIAL SITUATIONS

Symptoms from desmopressin-induced hyponatremic hypervolemia are headache, vertigo, weakness or fatigue, nausea and vomiting, confusion, paresthesia, seizures, ataxia, and limb stiffness. Most patients present with seizures, in reality a *fortunate misfortune* because it calls for early urgent intervention before irreversible brain damage takes place.

DIAGNOSTIC APPROACH

Blood and urine electrolytes, blood urea nitrogen, serum, and urine osmolarity will establish the existence of hyponatremia and hypervolemic hemodilution. The nature of the CNS lesion will condition the selection of diagnostic testing in a patient with desmopressin-induced hypervolemic hyponatremia who exhibits changes in neurologic status after receiving desmopressin for central diabetes insipidus.

TREATMENT

Preventive treatment in the first 4 weeks of desmopressin use is indicated with fluid restriction. Special precautions should be adopted in children with attention deficit disorder and impulsive-compulsive disorder because they may have psychogenic polydipsia. Seizures should be treated according to standard protocol, but treatment beyond a few weeks is usually not necessary. Avoid using carbamazepine and oxcarbazepine. If the underlying metabolic derangement is not treated, antiepileptic drugs will be ineffective (43,44).

Complications of Dopamine Agonist Therapy of Prolactinomas

DEFINITION

CSF rhinorrhea and otorrhea are rare complications of the medical treatment of prolactinomas with bromocriptine and other dopamine agonist (DA) drugs. Bromocriptine reduces prolactin levels and diminishes the size of the pituitary tumor. Involution of the tumor, brought on by bromocriptine, can result in the herniation of the optic chiasm into the sella turcica, and delayed deterioration of vision (45, 46). Valvular heart disease, specifically valvular regurgitation, has been reported in patients with Parkinson's disease treated with pergolide, prompting discontinuation of this drug (47).

EPIDEMIOLOGY

CSF rhinorrhea following treatment of pituitary tumors with DA drugs is uncommon. Based on short case series, the incidence of visual loss in patients with prolactinoma treated with DA drugs fluctuates between 5% and 10% (46).

ETIOLOGY AND PATHOGENESIS

CSF rhinorrhea, in cases of prolactinomas treated with DA drugs, results from tumor involution and subsequent resolution of intrasellar hypertension. Visual loss in patients with prolactinoma treated with DA drugs, but not showing signs of chiasmal herniation, is perhaps a sign of vasospastic *involutional ischemia* brought on by reduction in tumor size.

PATHOLOGY

Inflammatory meningeal purulent exudates will be found in patients dying from bacterial meningitis secondary to iatrogenic or tumor-related CSF fistulas, if not treated early.

CLINICAL MANIFESTATIONS AND SPECIAL SITUATIONS

Visual loss from use of DA drugs is usually delayed even for months, but it is reversible after discontinuation of the offending drug. In contrast, CSF rhinorrhea develops within days of initiating treatment with bromocriptine.

DIAGNOSTIC APPROACH

Prolactin levels >200 mu/mL in someone with a macroadenoma >10 mm in size are diagnostic of prolactinoma. Additional diagnostic tests are MRI of the brain and of the sella turcica with multiplanar thin sections, neuroophthalmological examination, and visual fields. Contrast-enhanced MRI is employed in localizing CSF fistulas.

TREATMENT

CSF fistulas must be treated by surgical means to avoid bacterial meningitis.

Pituitary Apoplexy after Pituitary Function Tests

DEFINITION

Pituitary apoplexy (PA) is characterized by a sudden onset neurologic event of vascular origin. A preexistent pituitary adenoma is usually found.

The following drugs used in endocrine function tests can cause PA: Thyrotropin-releasing hormone (TRH), gonadotropin-releasing hormone (GnRH), insulin, glucagon, bromocriptine, dexamethasone, and clomiphene (48–50).

EPIDEMIOLOGY

Matsuura et al. (51) collected from the literature 14 cases of PA secondary to the intravenous administration of drugs used in endocrine testing. Tumor hemorrhage was evident in 92.9% of the cases (51).

ETIOLOGY AND PATHOGENESIS

PA is often the consequence of a hemorrhage or infarction of a pituitary tumor that results in its sudden expansion within the confines of the sella (52). The exact mechanisms of PA after pituitary function tests are unknown. The clinical, pathologic, imaging, and treatment features of this syndrome are reviewed in Chapter 76 on hypothalamic and pituitary lesions.

Iatrogenic Hypoglycemia

DEFINITION

Insulin and oral antidiabetic drugs can cause iatrogenic and, rarely, factitious hypoglycemia with neurologic consequences, either acute or recurrent (53). Hypoglycemia unawareness refers to the absence of warning symptoms that normally allow patients to recognize that their blood sugar level is low before they reach unconsciousness. Hypoglycemia unawareness is a major contributor of severe hypoglycemia episodes (54).

EPIDEMIOLOGY

Hypoglycemia is common in insulin-dependant diabetes mellitus (IDDM), albeit often subclinical and under recognized. Verrotti et al. (55) reported that 11.3% of 246 children and adolescents with IDDM experienced at least one episode of severe hypoglycemia over a 4-year span. Because the physiologic counterregulation response to hypoglycemia is still in place, hypoglycemia occurs less frequently in non-insulin dependant diabetes mellitus (NIDDM). According to the United Kingdom Prospective Diabetes Study, 2.4% of patients taking metformin and 3.3% of those prescribed sulfonylurea compounds, experience major episodes of hypoglycemia that require help from another person. In contrast, 11.2% of those taking insulin had hypoglycemic events (56, 57).

ETIOLOGY AND PATHOGENESIS

In established IDDM and, to a lesser extent, in NIDDM, plasma glucagon levels do not rise and plasma insulin do not fall, at lower glycemia levels (57). Because diabetics lose their first line of defense against hypoglycemia because of impaired glucagon release, they rely on the sympathetic chromaffin-epinefrine response to level off their blood sugars. With recurrent episodes of hypoglycemia, this compensatory line of defense also fails; a phenomenon labeled as *autonomic failure.*

The problem is then compounded: The patient loses awareness of hypoglycemia on one hand, and on the other, the patient is unable to compensate for hypoglycemia.

PATHOLOGY

Postmortem studies on individuals dying from hypoglycemia demonstrate cortical laminar necrosis and necrosis of the dentate gyrus of the hippocampus (58).

CLINICAL MANIFESTATIONS AND SPECIAL SITUATIONS

Neuroglycopenic and neurogenic symptoms are recognized. The former arise from brain glucose deprivation and include headache, cognitive disturbance, weakness, vertigo, confusion, lethargy, convulsions, and coma. The latter are cholinergic in nature (sweating, nausea, perioral tingling) or adrenergic (tremor, pallor, tachycardia, anxiety). Stroke can be a complication of hypoglycemia (59). Conversely, hypoglycemia mimics acute stroke and transient ischemic attacks.

DIAGNOSTIC APPROACH

Neuroglycopenic and neurogenic symptoms of hypoglycemia become evident with glycemia levels between 50 and 55 mg/dL (2.8 to 3.0 mmol/L). A glycemia of 40 mg/dL will always generate symptoms, and levels of 20 mg/dL or less will cause seizures and coma.

TREATMENT

Self-treatment is appropriate for asymptomatic and symptomatic hypoglycemic episodes with no alteration of consciousness. This is achieved by self-administering juice, milk, crackers, soft drinks, or fast-acting carbohydrate tablets. Symptoms will dissipate within 20 minutes. The unconscious or uncooperative patient will require a subcutaneous or intramuscular injection of glucagon or an immediate D50% glucose infusion (53,54). Patients with hypoglycemia secondary to sulfonylurea compounds will experience recurrent delayed hypoglycemia after initial recovery, because of the long half-life duration of these drugs.

CLINICAL RECOMMENDATIONS OF THE VIGNETTE

Repeat antinuclear antibody (ANA) titer, sedimentation rate, fibrinogen levels, and C-reactive protein to assess for possible relapse of SLE. High CK values will favor steroid myopathy over fibromyalgia. MRI of the brain will be needed to rule out unrelated lesions, CNS vasculitis, and stroke. Electroencephalogram (EEG) changes may be seen in the context of encephalopathy. If no brain lesions are encountered on MRI, a lumbar puncture is needed to rule out meningitis or meningoencephalitis (i.e., Lyme disease). CSF pressure should be measured for possible idiopathic intracranial hypertension without papilledema. If CSF pressure is elevated, an MRV must be obtained to discard intracranial venous sinus thrombosis. The differential diagnosis must also include lupus neuropsychiatric syndrome and SIPS.

SUMMARY

Behavioral disturbance and myopathy following the administration of corticosteroids frequently complicate treatment of many clinical disorders of autoimmune origin and cancer. Steroid-induced IIH can be misdiagnosed in patients with chronic headache exhibiting no papilledema. Grand mal seizures in a boy with history of enuresis is the classic presentation of desmopressin-induced hypervolemic hyponatremia. Although HRT and oral contraceptives statistically increase the chances of stroke in women, the absolute risk of stroke is low in the absence of risk factors. Oral contraceptives can aggravate or cause migraine in susceptible women. Tamoxifen increases the risk of thromboembolic disease. Patients with epilepsy can be safely prescribed HRT, oral contraceptives, and androgens, but antiepileptic drug blood levels must be monitored. Dopamine agonist drugs can induce CSF rhinorrhea, and endocrine testing with releasing hormones may cause pituitary apoplexy in patients with macroadenomas. Hypoglycemia is a major hurdle in gaining strict blood sugar control in patients with type 1 diabetes afflicted with hypoglycemia unawareness and autonomic failure.

REFERENCES

1. Brown ES, Khan DA, Nejtek VA. The psychiatric side effects of corticosteroids. *Ann Allergy Asthma Immunol.* 1999;83:495–504.
2. Sirois F. Steroid psychosis: A review. *Gen Hosp Psychiatry.* 2003;25(1):27–33.
3. Dixon R, Christy N. On the various forms of corticosteroid withdrawal syndrome. *Am J Med.* 1980;68(2):224–230.
4. Hudson JI, Hudson MS, Griffing GT, et al. Phenomenology and family history of affective disorder in Cushing's disease. *Am J Psychiatry.* 1987;144(7):951–953.
5. Starkman MN, Gebarski SS, Berent S, et al. Hippocampal formation volume, memory dysfunction, and cortisol levels in patients with Cushing's syndrome. *Biol Psychiatry.* 1992; 32(9):756–765.
6. Lupien SJ, McEwen BS. The acute effects of corticosteroids on cognition: Integration of animal and human model studies. *Brain Res Rev.* 1997;24(1):1–27.
7. Kanda F, Okuda S, Matsushita T, et al. Steroid myopathy: Pathogenesis and effects of growth hormone and insulin-like growth factor-I administration. *Horm Res.* 2001;56[(Suppl 1]: 24–28.
8. Batchelor TT, Taylor LP, Thaler HT, et al. Steroid myopathy in cancer patients. *Neurology.* 1997;48(5):1234–1238.
9. Hirano M, Ott BR, Raps EC, et al. Acute quadriplegic myopathy: A complication of treatment with steroids, nondepolarizing blocking agents, or both. *Neurology.* 1992;42(11): 2082–2087.
10. Shoji S. Myofibrillar protein catabolism in rat steroid myopathy measured by 3-methylhistidine excretion in the urine. *J Neurol Sci.* 1989;93(2):333–340.
11. Cohn GA. Pseudotumor cerebri in children secondary to administration of adrenal steroids. *J Neurosurg.* 1963;20:784–786.
12. Alder JB, Fraunfelder FT, Edwards R. Levonorgestrel implants and intracranial hypertension. *N Engl J Med.* 1995;332(25):1720–1721.
13. Ivancic R, Pfadenhauer K. Pseudotumor cerebri after hormonal emergency contraception. *Eur Neurol.* 2004;52(2):120.
14. Huseman CA, Torkelson RD. Pseudotumor cerebri following treatment of hypothalamic and primary hypothyroidism. *Am J Dis Child.* 1984;138(10):927–931.
15. Raghavan S, DiMartino-Nardi J, Saenger P, et al. Pseudotumor cerebri in an infant after L-thyroxine therapy for transient neonatal hypothyroidism. *J Pediatr.* 1997;130(3):478–480.
16. Malozowski S, Tanner LA, Wysowski D, et al. Growth hormone, insulin-like growth factor I, and benign intracranial hypertension. *N Engl J Med.* 1993;329(9):665–666.
17. Rickels MR, Nichols CW. Pseudotumor cerebri in patients with Cushing's disease. *Endocr Pract.* 2004;10(6):492–496.
18. Radhakrishnan K, Ahlskog JE, Cross SA, et al. Idiopathic intracranial hypertension (pseudotumor cerebri). Descriptive epidemiology in Rochester, Minn, 1976 to 1990. *Arch Neurol.* 1993;50(1):78–80.
19. Mathew NT, Ravishankar K, Sanin LC. Coexistence of migraine and idiopathic intracranial hypertension without papilledema. *Neurology.* 1996;46(15):1226–1230.
20. Giuseffi V, Wall M, Siegel PZ, et al. Symptoms and disease associations in idiopathic intracranial hypertension (pseudotumor cerebri): A case-control study. *Neurology.* 1991;41(2):239–244.
21. Wang SJ, Silberstein SD, Patterson S, et al. Idiopathic intracranial hypertension without papilledema. A case-control study in a headache center. *Neurology.* 1998;51(1):245–249.
22. Jacome DE. Headaches, idiopathic intracranial hypertension, and pseudopapilledema. *Am J Med Sci.* 1998;316(6):408–410.

23. Vischi A, Guerriero S, Giancipoli G, et al. Delayed onset of pseudotumor cerebri syndrome 7 years after starting human recombinant growth hormone treatment. *Eur J Ophthalmol.* 2006;16(1):178–180.
24. Bushnell CD. Oestrogen and stroke in women: Assessment of risk. *Lancet Neurol.* 2005; 4(11):743–751.
25. Writing group for the Women's Health Initiative Investigators. Risks and benefits of estrogen plus progestin in healthy post-menopausal women: Principal results from the Women's Health Initiative randomized controlled trial. *JAMA.* 2002;288:321–333.
26. The Women's Health Initiative Steering Committee. Effects of conjugated equine estrogen in postmenopausal women with hysterectomy. *JAMA.* 2004;291:1701–1712.
27. Viscoli CM, Brass LM, Kernan WN, et al. A clinical trial of estrogen-replacement therapy after ischemic stroke. *N Engl J Med.* 2001;345(17):1243–1249.
28. Bushnell CD. Hormone replacement therapy and stroke: The current state of knowledge and directions for future research. *Semin Neurol.* 2006;26(1):123–130.
29. Geiger AM, Fischberg GM, Chen W, et al. Stroke risk and tamoxifen therapy for breast cancer. *J Natl Cancer Inst.* 2004;96(20):1528–1536.
30. Bushnell CD, Goldstein LB. Risk of ischemic stroke with tamoxifen treatment for breast cancer. A meta-analysis. *Neurology.* 2004;63(7):1230–1233.
31. Cauley JA, McTiernan A, Rodabough RJ, et al. Statin use and breast cancer: Prospective results from the Women's Health Initiative. *J Natl Cancer Inst.* 2006;98(10):700–707.
32. Mannucci PM, Bettega D, Chantarangkul V, et al. Effect of tamoxifen on measurements of hemostasis in healthy women. *Arch Intern Med.* 1996;156(16):1806–1810.
33. Brandes JL. The influence of estrogen on migraine. A systematic review. *JAMA.* 2006; 295(15):1824–1830.
34. Loder EW, Buse DC, Golub JR. Headache and combination estrogen-progestin oral contraceptives: Integrating evidence, guidelines and clinical practice. *Headache.* 2005;45(3):224–231.
35. Bousser MG. Estrogens, migraine, and stroke. *Stroke.* 2004;35[Suppl 1]:2652–2656.
36. Pringsheim T, Gooren L. Migraine prevalence in male to female transsexuals on hormone therapy. *Neurology.* 2004;63(3):593–594.
37. Foldvary-Schaffer N, Harden C, Herzog A, et al. Hormones and seizures. *Cleve Clin J Med.* 2004;71[Suppl 2]:S11–S18.
38. Peebles CT, McAuley JW, Moore JL, et al. Hormone replacement therapy in a postmenopausal woman with epilepsy. *Ann Pharmacother.* 2000;34(9):1028–1031.
39. Herzog AG, Klein P, Ransil BJ. Three patterns of catamenial epilepsy. *Epilepsia.* 1997;38(10): 1082–1088.
40. Thumfart J, Roehr CC, Kapelari K, et al. Desmopressin associated symptomatic hyponatremic hypervolemia in children. Are there predictive factors? *J Urol.* 2005;174(1):294–298.
41. Lose G, Mattiasson A, Walter S, et al. Clinical experiences with desmopressin for long-term treatment of nocturia. *J Urol.* 2004;172(3):1021–1025.
42. Blanker MH, Bohnen AM, Groeneveld FP, et al. Normal voiding patterns and determinants of increased diurnal and nocturnal voiding frequency in elderly men. *J Urol.* 2000; 164(4):1201–1205.
43. Zarinetchi F, Berl T. Evaluation and management of severe hyponatremia. *Adv Intern Med.* 1996;41:251–283.
44. Rizzo V, Albanese A, Stanhope R. Morbidity and mortality associated with vasopressin replacement therapy in children. *J Pediatr Endocrinol Metab.* 2001;14(7):861–867.
45. Jones SE, James RA, Hall K, et al. Optic chiasmal herniation—An under recognized complication of dopamine agonist therapy for macroprolactinoma. *Clin Endocrinol (Oxf).* 2000;53(4):529–534.
46. Chuman H, Cornblath WT, Trobe JD, et al. Delayed visual loss following pergolide treatment of prolactinoma. *J Neuroophthalmol.* 2002;22(2):102–106.
47. Waller EA, Kaplan J, Heckman MG. Valvular heart disease in patients taking pergolide. *Mayo Clin Pisco* 2005;80(8):1016–1020.
48. Masago A, Ueda Y, Kanai H, et al. Pituitary apoplexy after pituitary function test: A report of two cases and review of the literature. *Surg Neurol.* 1995;43(2):158–165.
49. Foppiani L, Piredda S, Guido R, et al. Gonadotropin-releasing hormone-induced partial empty sella clinically mimicking pituitary apoplexy in a woman with a suspected non-secreting macroadenoma. *J Endocrinol Invest.* 2000;23(12):118–121.
50. Nagulesparan M, Roper J. Haemorrhage into the anterior pituitary during pregnancy after induction of ovulation with clomiphene. A case report. *British Journal of Obstetrics and Gynaecology.* 1978;85(2):153–155.
51. Matsuura I, Saeki N, Kubota M, et al. Infarction followed by hemorrhage in pituitary adenoma due to endocrine stimulation test. *Endocr J.* 2001;48(4):493–498.
52. Chuang CC, Chang CN, Wei KC, et al. Surgical treatment for severe visual compromised patients after pituitary apoplexy. *J Neurooncol.* 2006; Apr 28. Epub ahead of print.
53. Chiarelli F, Verrotti A, Catino M, et al. Hypoglycemia in children with type 1 diabetes mellitus. *Acta Paediatr Suppl.* 1999;88(427):31–34.
54. Cryer PE, Davis SN, Shamoon H. Hypoglycemia in diabetes. *Diabetes Care.* 2003;26(16): 1902–1012.
55. Verrotti A, Chiarelli F, Blasetti A, et al. Severe hypoglycemia in insulin-dependent diabetic children treated by multiple injection insulin regimen. *Acta Diabetol.* 1996;33(1):53–57.
56. U.K. Prospective diabetes study research group: U.K. Prospective diabetes study 16: Overview of 6 years' therapy of type II diabetes: A progressive disease. *Diabetes.* 1995;44:1249–1258.
57. Segel SA, Paramore DS, Cryer PE. Hypoglycemia-associated autonomic failure in advanced type 2 diabetes. *Diabetes.* 2002;51(3):724–733.
58. Auer RN. Hypoglycemic brain damage. *Metab Brain Dis.* 2004;19(3–4):169–175.
59. Gold AE, Marshall SM. Cortical blindness and cerebral infarction associated with severe hypoglycemia. *Diabetes Care.* 1996;19(9):1001–1003.

PART XI Musculoskeletal and Connective Tissue Diseases

CHAPTER 84

Rheumatoid Arthritis, Spondyloarthropathies, and Relapsing Polychondritis

Mihaela Mihailescu • Steven U. Brint • William I. Swedler

OBJECTIVES

- To explain how rheumatoid arthritis, ankylosing spondylitis, and relapsing polychondritis affect the central and peripheral nervous system
- To describe the subtle symptoms and signs of subluxation at the atlantoaxial joint in rheumatoid arthritis or ankylosing spondylitis
- To describe the presentation of spinal cord or root compression in ankylosing spondylitis
- To list the ways in which relapsing polychondritis can effect the nervous system

INTRODUCTION

Rheumatoid arthritis (RA), ankylosing spondylitis (AS), and relapsing polychondritis (RP) are systemic inflammatory diseases that cause arthritis. In most patients, neurologic involvement may not exist or it may be minor; in a few patients, however, the damage can be devastating or herald severe systemic illness. Each condition is driven by an immunological attack on a different tissue: Synovium (RA), enthesis (AS), or cartilage (RP). This chapter addresses the more serious neurologic complication of each disease.

CASE VIGNETTE 1

A 75-year-old man with >15 years of RA complains of slowly progressive weakness making him wheelchair bound. He has difficulty with activities of daily living, such as eating, dressing, and bathing. He has pain in the neck radiating to the occiput, but no pain in other joints. Examination demonstrates a thin man sitting upright in a wheelchair and able to arise only with assistance.

Neck range of motion is limited in all directions of movement. All muscles show atrophy. Active and passive range of motion is reduced in shoulders, elbows, wrists, hips, and knees. Flexion contractures are found in the elbows, hips, and knees. His hands have bilateral ulnar deviation of the fingers, with swan-neck deformities of the interphalangeal joints. The thumb joints are subluxed and unstable. The toes are cocked-up with hallux valgus bilaterally. No swelling or tenderness of the joints is noted. Skin examination shows subcutaneous nodules at the elbows. Neurologic examination shows weakness in many major muscle groups crossing joints that are damaged by the arthritis. No spontaneous fasciculations are noted in the muscles. Cranial nerve examination finding is normal. Muscle stretch reflexes show hyperreflexia at the biceps brachii, brachioradialis, and ankles bilaterally. Nonsustained clonus is noted in both ankles. Triceps and patellar reflexes cannot be elicited. Attempts to elicit the plantar reflexes are unsuccessful. Pinprick sensation is reduced in both feet and hands in a stocking and glove pattern.

ETIOLOGY AND PATHOGENESIS

RA is primarily a disease of synovial inflammation. Although much is known about the pathogenesis, the initiating factors are unknown. In RA, an immune attack in the synovium occurs with participation of macrophages, T cells, and B cells. A wide array of cytokines and chemokines participate, but the effectiveness of drugs that block the action of tumor necrosis factor (TNF) and interleukin-1 (IL-1) suggest that these proteins are the essential central players driving the inflammation. Synovial inflammation results in pannus, a proliferation of synovial fibroblasts with locally invasive destruction of bone, cartilage, and supporting tissues.

The most serious and life-threatening complication of RA involves the neck, either from atlantoaxial subluxation or subluxation below the axis. The pathophysiology of rheumatoid cervical spine disease results from the same synovitis that affects the peripheral joints.

The odontoid process of C2 articulates with the body of C1 and is constrained by ligaments so there is no lateral, vertical, or anterior-posterior movement of the odontoid relative to C1. To lubricate the rotational motion of the odontoid, bursal sacs are located around the dens. The synovial tissue lining these bursae develops synovitis and local expansion and proliferation of pannus can loosen or destroy the ligaments as well as erode the atlas or axis. With loss of the ligamentous constraint or bone integrity, the odontoid process can move posterior from the body of the atlas, move side to side, or protrude up through the foramen magnum. The spinal cord or the medulla oblongata can be compressed by the bony dens. In addition, a mass of synovial pannus may be causing local pressure (1,2).

Below the level of C2, synovial membrane is found in the facet joint posterior to the spinal canal. Small joints called the *uncovertebral joints* (the joints of Luschka) are anterior to the spinal cord in close proximity to the intervertebral discs. Synovitis with local damage can cause subluxation of the subaxial cervical spine, leading to cervical cord compression. Malalignment of the cervical vertebrae can cause blood flow problems in the vertebral arteries as they course cephalad in the foramen of the cervical vertebral bodies. Signs and symptoms of vertebrobasilar ischemia appear instead of local pressure (2). Although in no way can it be predicted who will develop cervical spine disease with neurologic symptoms, older age with rapid onset of early aggressive joint disease appears to correlate best.

EPIDEMIOLOGY

The worldwide prevalence of RA is approximately 1%. The frequency of cervical spine involvement from RA varies widely in reported series, the spine is commonly involved. Having cervical spine damage from RA does not necessarily mean neurologic symptoms will develop and those with neurologic disease do not necessarily die from spinal cord compression. Nonetheless, cervical spine disease caused by neurologic involvement from RA does carry a grave prognosis with a high mortality. The reason patients with RA cervical spine disease are more likely to die probably reflects the more aggressive rheumatoid disease process and a higher burden of joint damage and concomitant disability. Although hospitalizations for serious complications of RA (e.g., vasculitis and Felty syndrome) have been declining, hospitalizations for cervical spine surgery have not declined, implying that this process is still a frequent problem.

CLINICAL MANIFESTATIONS

The patient in the case vignette, illustrates the difficulties the physician faces with a patient with chronic joint deformities. Many patients with cervical spine disease have extensive damage in the peripheral joints, with concomitant lost range of motion, muscle atrophy, and weakness. These chronic rheumatoid changes can obscure the neurologic complaints and physical findings that point the clinician toward spinal cord impingement. Nonetheless, symmetric hyperreflexia and ankle clonus strongly suggest central nervous system (CNS) involvement.

Initially, patients with cervical subluxation may be asymptomatic; however, neurologic symptoms can develop insidiously. The most common complaint is pain at the base of the skull. Sometimes, the greater occipital nerve is involved. Quadriparesis may slowly progress, with long tract signs. Complaints of numbness of hands and feet may occur. Invagination of the odontoid through the foramen magnum can cause a variety of brainstem defects, including facial numbness (trigeminal involvement), dizziness, and cruciate paralysis.

In the peripheral nervous system, entrapment neuropathies are the most common problems (1). Synovial swelling from joints and tendon sheaths, as well as structural damage to joints, can compress nerves. The most common neuropathy is carpal tunnel syndrome, which results from pressure on the median nerve as it passes under the flexor retinaculum of the wrist. Less commonly, ulnar neuropathy can occur from pannus or distorted bone anatomy at the elbow or in Guyon's canal. Radial nerve injury can occur as the nerve passes anterior to the lateral epicondyle to result in loss of finger and wrist extension. Anterior tibial nerve palsy, with foot drop, can occur from popliteal space or fibular head compression. Posterior tibial nerve compression can occur in the tarsal tunnel distal to the medial malleolus to cause burning on the bottom of the foot. Treatment of compressive neuropathies entails systemic treatment of the RA, as well as possible local injection of depot corticosteroids, or surgical decompression, or both.

Polyneuropathy can also develop from RA. Usually, this manifests with dysesthesias and loss of sensation in a stocking distribution. Mononeuritis multiplex can occur when patients with RA develop a systemic necrotizing vasculitis. Necrotizing vasculitis, a rare complication, can also present with bowel infarction or digital gangrene. Muscle weakness, which is common in RA, can be multifactorial. Active myositis is not common, but can occur (1). Muscle biopsies may show type II muscle atrophy related to poor nutrition, disuse, or chronic steroid use (steroid myopathy).

DIAGNOSTIC APPROACH

Diagnosis of RA is based on finding prolonged morning stiffness, symmetric polyarthritis (at least involving the hands), skin nodules, X-ray study changes, and presence of a rheumatoid factor. In approximately 20% of patients, the rheumatoid factor is negative. Recently, it has been found that antibodies against citrullinated cyclic peptide (anti-CCP antibodies) have a very high specificity for RA (3). The inflammation can last decades and cause varying degrees of physical incapacity. Untreated, patients may be ill with inflammation beyond the joints, such as in the pleura, pericardium, lung, eye, and the nervous system.

Imaging of the cervical spine is essential when evaluating patients with RA for suspected neurologic disease. Plain x-ray study should include lateral films, with the neck taken in flexion and extension. The open mouth view will show if bone erosions have fractured the odontoid process and if movement of lateral masses of C1 relative to C2 has occurred. The lateral view should show the distance between the anterior arch of C1 and the anterior border of the odontoid process with no more than 3 mm of separation in an adult, and 5 mm in a child. Even large distances of separation (9 to 10 mm) may have no clinical consequences. More critical are measurements of the space occupied by the spinal cord. The posterior atlantodental distance (between the posterior border of the dens and the roof or posterior arch of C1) should not be <14 mm. In the neutral position, minor or no subluxation may be seen of C1 or C2, but movement may be by flexion and extension views. Below the level of C2, <14 mm indicates critical stenosis that can result in spinal cord compression (2).

The odontoid should not protrude into the foramen magnum. On plain radiography, the lines of McGregor and McRae are useful tools. McGregor's line is drawn from the posterior tip of the hard palate to the most caudal extent of the occiput. The odontoid tip should not extend >4.5 mm above this line. McRae's line is drawn from the clivus to the posterior inlet of the foramen magnum and the odontoid tip should not extend above this line. Other methods have been described as well, but all the methods using plain radiographs are limited by difficulty in clearly defining the margins of bone, especially the tip or base of C2 if erosions are present.

Magnetic resonance imaging (MRI) is now recognized as the most sensitive and specific method to diagnose cervical subluxation as well as to define the extent of compression of the neuraxis. MRI will show bone anatomy such as fracture and migration of the dens or other elements of the cervical spine. The imaging of the soft tissues will show proliferating masses of pannus that can impinge on the cord in the absence of bone damage. To improve the sensitivity of MRI for cord or brainstem compression, the study can be done with the cervical spine in flexion and extension.

MRI has surpassed other modalities of imaging, but cannot be used in all cases (e.g., contraindicated if a pacemaker is present or metal in the eye.) As a substitute, contrast myelography, preferably with computed tomographic (CT) scanning will demonstrate important details about bone damage, spinal cord impingement, and soft tissue masses.

TREATMENT

At least one study has shown that patients treated with more aggressive disease-modifying drug regimens had less progression of cervical spine disease than those treated less intensively (4). This suggests that cervical cord compression might be prevented with early aggressive systemic treatment.

Clearly, patients with cervical subluxation and signs of spinal cord compression should be referred for cervical spine stabilization or fusion. Studies that prospectively followed such patients without surgery show a high mortality rate. In one study, all patients not having surgery were dead within 8 years. Surgery to stabilize the spine leads to improved survival and better neurologic function.

Patients with RA who have radiographic evidence of subluxation and no neurologic signs may not need surgery. Some studies suggest that most of these patients will not experience disease progression, but other studies suggest that progressive neurologic deterioration can occur if not surgically fixed. The discrepancy may arise from patient sampling—rheumatologists reporting cross-sectional studies from stable RA populations versus surgeons reporting patients referred to them. In the absence of symptoms but with significant subluxation on imaging, patients should be given a hard collar to stabilize the spine.

As summarized by Kim and Hilibrand (5), cervical spine surgery should be considered if patients have (*a*) a progressive neurologic deficit, (*b*) chronic neck pain unresponsive to conservative measures with evidence of instability, (*c*) any degree of cord stenosis, (*d*) a posterior atalantoaxial distance <14 mm or subaxial cervical canal diameter <14 mm, (*e*) superior migration of the dens >5 mm above McGregor's line, or (*f*) a cervicomedullary angle <135 degrees (5).

CLINICAL RECOMMENDATIONS OF THE VIGNETTE

The patient is chronically debilitated from his RA causing damage in multiple joints of the upper and lower extremities. The findings of upper motor neuron involvement with hyperreflexia and clonus raise the suspicion for cervical cord compression. He needs urgent imaging of the cervical spine, preferably with MRI, to best delineate the thecal sac, spinal cord, and surrounding soft tissues. If significant narrowing of the spinal canal or compression of the spinal cord is found, then he will need referral to a neurosurgeon or orthopedic spine surgeon.

CASE VIGNETTE 2

A 45-year-old man with ankylosing spondylitis (AS) since the age of 25 fell in the bathtub striking his mid back. He had severe back pain and could not stand. In the emergency room, he lies quietly on the cart with an exaggerated dorsal kyphosis. His neck will not move in any direction. The thoracic spine is tender at T8. The lower extremities are plegic. Muscle stretch reflexes are normal in the arms and absent in the legs. He has bilateral Babinski signs. He has no sensation below the umbilicus and the anal sphincter is flaccid.

ETIOLOGY AND PATHOGENESIS

AS is the prototype of the family of diseases known as *seronegative spondyloarthropathies.* As the name implies, serologic tests for rheumatoid factor and antinuclear antibodies are usually negative, while the spine and peripheral joints are involved with varying degrees of inflammation. The enthesis is the tissue attacked by this group of diseases. An enthesis is the site of attachment for ligaments, tendons, and joint capsules to bone. Typically, the tough connective tissue anchoring of the intervertebral discs and sacroiliac joints, tendons such as the Achilles, and the plantar fascia are involved. A strong propensity exists for these areas of inflammation to ossify, resulting in bony joint fusion. The final endpoint of this disease is complete fusion of the spine, which becomes rigid and kyphotic.

Although a strong association exists of AS with the gene HLA-B27, testing for this is not very useful in establishing a diagnosis. Instead, diagnosis rests on finding chronic low back pain, limited chest wall expansion, limited spinal mobility, and radiographic evidence of sacroiliitis. Other diseases classified as seronegative spondyloarthropathies are psoriatic arthritis, reactive arthritis (also known as Reiter syndrome), and the arthritis of inflammatory bowel disease (specifically, ulcerative colitis and Crohn disease). Drugs that block TNF are very effective in the treatment of this group of diseases.

Cauda Equina Syndrome

EPIDEMIOLOGY AND PATHOGENESIS

Cauda equina syndrome is a rare neurologic complication of AS. First described in 1961, fewer than 100 reports are found in the literature. The pathogenesis of cauda equina syndrome in AS is not known. Theories include chronic adhesive arachnoiditis with subsequent dural ectasias and nerve root compression, demyelination from prior radiotherapy, or vascular insufficiency (6,7).

CLINICAL MANIFESTATIONS

In AS, the clinical presentation of cauda equina syndrome is characterized by an insidious onset and very slow progression. Usually, this develops in patients with long-standing disease who have marked ankylosis of the spine, often when the primary spondylitis is inactive.

Neurologic signs and symptoms are often symmetric and include diminished sensation in the lower lumbar and sacral dermatomes, wasting and weakness of the muscle innervated by these nerve roots, and decreased ankle reflexes. Frequently, urinary and rectal sphincter disturbances develop. Unlike cauda equina syndrome caused by lumbar disk herniation, only 22% of these patients complain of radicular symptoms, and only 10% will complain of worsening back pain.

DIAGNOSTIC APPROACH

Spine X-rays usually demonstrate the characteristic changes of the AS and only rarely show erosions of the pedicles, laminae, or spinous processes, with widening of the neural canal that is typical of patients with complicated cauda equina syndrome.

Myelographic images may show an enlarged caudal sac and dorsal arachnoid diverticula. CT scan of the lumbosacral spine may show the pathognomonic dorsal arachnoid diverticula filling the erosions of the pedicles, laminae, and spinous processes.

MRI is useful in showing that the enlarged caudal sac and dorsal arachnoid diverticula contain cerebrospinal fluid (CSF).

TREATMENT

No specific treatment exists for cauda equina syndrome caused by AS. Without any intervention, this condition worsens slowly over long periods of time. Neurologic deficits usually remain confined to the distribution of the sacral and lower lumbar roots. Nonsteroidal anti-inflammatory drugs (NSAID), acetazolamide, and corticosteroids have been used with contradictory results. Lumboperitoneal shunting or laminectomy of the involved levels has also been tried, although in the past, experts believed that surgery should be avoided. In a 2001 meta-analysis that reviewed 86 patients with this condition, the authors concluded that surgery has the best chance of improving neurologic dysfunction and halting the progression of the neurologic deficit, but the improvement was mild and was observed in only 40% of the patients.

Spinal Cord Compression Secondary to Vertebral Fractures

EPIDEMIOLOGY AND PATHOGENESIS

Spinal fractures are four times more frequent in AS than in the normal population. In a 12-year study of 893 patients with traumatic spinal cord injury, 15 had AS (8). Because of their rigid spine coupled with the presence of osteoporosis, patients with AS are susceptible to vertebral fractures even after minimal trauma. The most common segment involved is the lower cervical spine from C5 to C7. These fractures occur through the intervertebral disk most of the times and are very unstable. Neck hyperextension is the most common mechanism of spinal cord injury (9).

CLINICAL MANIFESTATIONS

Fractures of the AS spine are associated with a high rate of spinal cord deficits, including mild sensory loss, central cord syndrome, Brown-Sequard syndrome, or quadriplegia.

DIAGNOSTIC APPROACH

Routine X-ray study may not always identify the fracture, because the local anatomy is distorted secondary to bony proliferation and ossification of the spinal ligaments. Osteoporosis can also complicate fracture visualization. CT or MRI are better at demonstrating fractures and these should be obtained in all the patients with long-standing AS with new onset of neck or back pain in which the X-ray study fails to demonstrate a fracture line. MRI is better in delineating the epidural hematoma, which is a characteristic complication in these patients.

TREATMENT

No randomized trials have compared conservative with surgical management of vertebral fractures in patients with AS. Most authors prefer conservative treatment. Because of the high rate of complications, surgical management is indicated for patients with progressive neurologic deterioration and for those in whom the conservative treatment failed to reduce the fracture. Other neurologic complications in ankylosing spondylitis include the following:

Spinal cord compression can also occur because of either ossification of the posterior longitudinal ligament in the absence of fracture or atlantoaxial subluxation.

Similar to patients with RA, those with AS can develop atlantoaxial subluxation and vertical subluxation of the axis with a mechanism identical in RA (dens instability caused by transverse ligament erosion). This is a rare complication and usually occurs late in the course of the disease. Most patients that develop this complication have both axial and peripheral joint involvement. The initial manifestation is usually occipital pain. Cervical myelopathy, lower cranial nerve palsies, or even sudden death can occur if this is not recognized and the spine stabilized.

Vertebrobasilar ischemia (VBI) can result secondary to external compression of the vertebral arteries from bone overgrowth and ossified ligaments. Symptoms of VBI can occur with head movements. Catheter vertebral angiography is not indicated because of potential worsening of the symptoms. CT angiography or the magnetic resonance angiography (MRA) might be indicated in such cases.

Although multiple sclerosis has been suggested to be a rare complication associated with AS, this needs further epidemiologic confirmation (10).

Sensorineural hearing loss predominantly affecting high frequencies, tinnitus, ear fullness, and dizziness have been reported with some patients. Possible mechanism includes autoantibodies against inner ear antigenic epitopes, vascular inflammation of vasa vasorum, immune complex-mediated vasculitis of the inner ear, or ototoxicity from NSAID or sulfasalazine. Positive response to corticosteroids has been reported (10).

CLINICAL RECOMMENDATIONS OF THE VIGNETTE

The patient with a rigid spine from AS experienced a minor trauma to the spine followed by drastic neurologic deterioration. Plain X-ray study of the spine failed to show any fracture. His extreme kyphotic posture made it impossible for him to fit into a standard MRI scanner. CT scanning of the spine showed a fracture through the T7-T8 intervertebral disc space with encroachment on the thecal sac. Recommendation is emergent referral to a neurosurgeon or orthopedic spine surgeon for decompression of the spinal cord and fixation of the unstable fracture site.

CASE VIGNETTE 3

A 26-year-old woman with history of relapsing polychondritis (RP) complains of decreased hearing on her left ear. Her RP has been complicated by laryngeal obstruction necessitating placement of a permanent tracheostomy. Examination shows a nonverbal, but alert and cooperative woman who answers questions well by writing. Neurologic examination finding is normal, except for decreased auditory acuity in the left ear and a left peripheral facial nerve palsy.

DEFINITION

RP is a rare condition, which in most patients has manifestations limited to cartilaginous structures such as the pinna, the nose, joints, larynx, and tracheobronchial tree. In rare cases, systemic vasculitis or a necrotizing glomerulonephritis is seen. The nervous system can also be involved, with a wide array of presentations.

ETIOLOGY AND PATHOGENESIS

RP is characterized by bouts of inflammation attacking cartilaginous structures. Hyaline cartilage in the pinna, the nose, the joints, and airway (larynx, trachea, and bronchi) are most often affected. Although usually a distinct entity, polychondritis can also be seen in the course of RA and systemic lupus erythematosus (SLE). Immunologic studies have shown antibody production directed against type II collagen, the main collagen found in hyaline cartilage. T cells with reactivity against type II collagen are also found. The spectrum of disease in RP ranges from mild ear inflammation to life-threatening blockage and collapse of the airway. Interestingly, tissues other than cartilage can be involved, causing glomerulonephritis, eye inflammation, and systemic vasculitis.

CLINICAL FEATURES

Cranial neuropathies are among some of the most common neurologic complications of RP. Optic neuritis can occur alone, but is often part of a broader spectrum of neurologic involvement. Extraocular muscle palsies have been reported, some spontaneously improving without steroid therapy, whereas others improved after steroid therapy. Peripheral cranial nerve palsies have also been reported with RP (12).

More diffuse cerebral disease has also been described, including aseptic meningitis, diffuse encephalitis, limbic system encephalitis, intracranial aneurysms, stroke, intracranial granulomas, and delirium (13,14). Limited pathologic reports from patients with encephalitis have demonstrated small vessel vasculitis (9). Currently, no controlled trials can guide treatment, but high-dose corticosteroids are often successful in treating the neurologic complications.

CLINICAL RECOMMENDATIONS OF THE VIGNETTE

The patient with long-established RP was found to have dysfunction of cranial nerves VII and VIII on the left. MRI showed increased T2-weighted signal in the left internal auditory canal. Three days after administration of intravenous pulse methylprednisolone, her hearing deficit and facial palsy improved. One month later, repeat MRI showed no residual abnormalities. No further neurologic problems arose over the next 3 years of observation.

SUMMARY

Rheumatoid arthritis and ankylosing spondylitis are diseases with immunologic attack directed primarily at articular structures. Neurologic symptoms usually arise when bone and joint damage impinges on nearby nerves. Cervical spine subluxation leading to cord compression or catastrophic trauma compressing the spinal canal are the most serious sequelae of these joint diseases. A serious clinical challenge exists when evaluating a patient who already has skeletal deformities and muscle weakness arising from the arthritis. Imaging the spinal column with MRI or CT myelography is essential. Timely surgical intervention often prevents paralysis or death. Relapsing polychondritis is a rare disease and may have a rare complication of neurologic involvement. The neurologic deficits in this immunologically mediated disease often respond to systemic corticosteroids or other immunosuppressive.

REFERENCES

1. Chang DJ, Paget SA. Neurologic complications of rheumatoid arthritis. *Rheum Dis Clin North Am.* 1993;19:955–973.
2. Gurley JP, Bell GR. The surgical management of patients with rheumatoid cervical spine disease. *Rheum Dis Clin North Am.* 1997;23:317–332.
3. Van Gaalen FA, Linn-Rasker SP, van Venrooij WJ, et al. Autoantibodies to cyclic citrullinated peptides predict progression to rheumatoid arthritis in patients with undifferentiated arthritis: a prospective cohort study. *Arthritis Rheum.* 2004;50:709–715.
4. Neva MH, Kauppi MJ, Kautiainen H, et al. Combination drug therapy retards the development of rheumatoid atlantoaxial subluxations. *Arthritis Rheum.* 2001;43:2397–2401.
5. Kim DH, Hilibrand AS. Rheumatoid arthritis in the cervical spine. *J Am Acad Orthop Surg.* 2005:13:463–474.
6. Ahn NU, Ahn UM, Nallamshetty L, et al. Cauda equina syndrome in ankylosing spondylitis (The CES-AS syndrome): Meta-analysis of outcomes after medical and surgical treatments. *Journal of Spinal Disorders.* 2001;14:427–433.
7. Sparling MJ, Bartleson JD, Mcleod RA, et al. MRI of arachnoid diverticula associated with cauda equina syndrome in AS. *J Rheumatol.* 1989;16:1335–1337.
8. Young JS, Cheshire DJE, Pierce JA, et al. Cervical ankylosis with acute spinal cord injury. *Paraplegia.* 1997;15:133–139.
9. Tico N, Ramon S, Garcia-Ortun F, et al. Traumatic spinal cord injury complicating ankylosing spondylitis. *Spinal Cord.* 1998;36:349–352.
10. Thomas DJ, Kendall MJ, Whitefield AG. Nervous system involvement in ankylosing spondylitis. *BMJ.* 1974;1:148–150.
11. Atalas N, Yazgan P, Ozturk A, et al. Audiological findings in patients with ankylosing spondyltis. *The Journal of Laryngology & Otology.* 2005;119:534–539.
12. Sundaram MBM, Rajput MB. Nervous system complications of relapsing polychondritis. *Neurology.* 1983;33:513–515.
13. Stewart SS, Ashizawa T, Dudley AW, et al. Cerebral vasculitis in relapsing polychondritis. *Neurology.* 1988;38:150–152.
14. Fujiki F, Tsuboi Y, Hashimoto K, et al. Non-herpetic limbic encephalitis associated with relapsing polychondritis. *J Neurol Neurosurg Psychiatry.* 2004;75:1646–1647.

CHAPTER **85**

Systemic Lupus Erythematosus, Sjögren's Syndrome, and Scleroderma

John A. Robinson

OBJECTIVES

- To illustrate the neurologic syndromes encountered in systemic lupus erythematosus, Sjögren's syndrome, and scleroderma
- To emphasize that often a direct causal relationship does not exist between neurologic symptoms and these autoimmune diseases
- To describe the immunopathologic mechanisms of specific neurologic findings found in these autoimmune diseases
- To discuss the diagnostic and treatment strategies for neurologic syndromes associated with systemic lupus erythematosus, Sjögren's syndrome, and scleroderma

CASE VIGNETTE

A 26-year-old woman with systemic lupus erythematosus (SLE) developed fever, fatigue, and weakness. Physical examination was not remarkable, other than pallor and a maculopapular rash seen over the trunk and face. Her hemoglobin had fallen to 6.8 g/dL and serum creatinine, previously 1.7 mg/dL, had risen to 4.2 mg/dL. A marked increase was seen in the DNA antibody titer. Urinalysis revealed red blood cell casts and marked proteinuria. Her prednisone (Pred) dose of 10 mg daily was increased to 100 mg daily. Intravenous cyclophosphamide (CTX) was given, followed by two rituximab infusions 1 week apart. The Pred was reduced to 80 mg daily. Four weeks later, she was brought to the emergency department after being found hallucinating at home. Her rash had disappeared, she was afebrile, intermittently oriented to time and place, had several visual and olfactory hallucinations, and no neurologic deficits. The serum creatinine was 1.8 mg/dL.

Systemic Lupus Erythematosus and Neuropsychiatric SLE (NP-SLE)

DEFINITION

SLE is an autoimmune disease with protean clinical manifestations that vary from rash and polyarthralgias to renal failure and neuropsychiatric syndromes. The signature immunologic feature of SLE is the presence of antinuclear antibodies (ANA).

EPIDEMIOLOGY

SLE is overwhelmingly more common in postpubertal females, with a peak incidence in the third to fourth decades. The female-to-male ratio is approximately 10:1 in the years from age 15 to 40. A strong genetic component is present. Identical twins have a high concordance of SLE. Differences in prevalence are also based on socioeconomic status and race. SLE is usually more severe in Asians, Hispanics, and blacks.

ETIOLOGY AND PATHOGENESIS

Tissue deposition of immune complexes is known to be the final arbiter of organ damage in SLE, but it is not clear why patients make antibodies to nucleic acid antigens and cannot dispose of them without inciting inflammation. Many possibilities have been promoted; none are convincing. Environmental factors undoubtedly play a role in causation, but they remain largely unknown. Current fashion indicts dysfunctional T-regulator cells, abnormal DNA antigen presentation to B cells by dendritic cells, and polymorphism of Toll-like receptors as potential etiologic culprits, but very little is understood about the precise immunologic defects that cause this enigmatic disease.

The pathogenesis of neuropsychiatric SLE (NP-SLE) remains obscure but is most likely multifactorial. Although immune complexes can bind to C3b and Fc receptors in the neurovasculature and be transported across the blood–brain barrier, no evidence indicates that this occurs in patients with NP-SLE. The fruitless search for immune-mediated vasculitis in the brains of patients with NP-SLE has prompted speculation that antineuronal and antiphospholipid antibodies, common in SLE, are perturbing central nervous system (CNS) endothelium and causing neurologic symptoms. Several reports associate ribosomal P antibodies, endothelial antibodies, or antibodies directed against *N*-methyl-d-aspartate (NMDA) receptors with NP-SLE (1–3). Oligoclonal

B-cell and clonotypic lymphocyte responses are not reflected in the cerebrospinal fluid (CSF), which suggests that in situ CNS immune responses are not the cause of NP-SLE.

The most common peripheral neurologic abnormality is a mononeuritis multiplex characterized by immune complex-mediated leukocytoclastic vasculitis. Recently, a small-diameter nerve fiber neuropathy not associated with typical inflammatory pathology has been described (4).

PATHOLOGY

The histopathology of immune complex-mediated inflammation in SLE is straightforward. Complexes of nuclear antigens and IgG activate the direct complement pathway and bind C3b to the IgG heavy chain that, in turn, facilitates immune complex fixation to tissue Fc and C3 receptors. These complexes serve as a locus for perpetuating complement activation that attracts and activates neutrophils. The final result is a neutrophil-mediated leucocytoclastic vasculitis. Perineural vasculitis is the cause of mononeuritis multiplex in SLE, but the small-diameter nerve fiber neuropathy is characterized by reduction in the mean density of the fibers and not immune complex inflammation.

In CNS NP-SLE, no characteristic pathologic finding confirms the diagnosis. Indeed, it is the lack of any pathologic abnormality that often characterizes NP-SLE.

CLINICAL MANIFESTATIONS

The clinical expression of SLE depends on where the immune complexes bind to endothelial C3b and Fcγ receptors. For example, if glomeruli are the site, renal disease will be present; if the skin is the targeted site, a rash ensues.

A common misconception is that kidney disease is the most frequent source of organ-specific symptoms in SLE. It is not. Several studies have shown that NP-SLE damage is the most common cause of morbidity in SLE (5–7). Neurologic manifestations of SLE range from cognitive dysfunction to demyelinating disease, from psychosis to transverse myelitis, and from strokes to seizures and epilepsy. Although both peripheral and CNS syndromes occur in SLE, the latter are much more frequent. NP-SLE damage tends to accumulate over time, whereas a significant cause of morbidity is not associated with increased disease specific mortality. The extreme polymorphic character of the disease also makes it virtually impossible to link specific clinical findings or ANA profiles to specific neurologic syndromes. Demographic variables such as age, gender, and race are also not very helpful in predicting NP-SLE. Older age at time of SLE onset may be a weak predictor. General agreement is that a high level of overall SLE disease activity is an important predictor of NP-SLE.

Peripheral neurologic syndromes are limited to either mononeuritis multiplex, usually in patients with high SLE disease activity, or a pure small diameter nerve fiber neuropathy that appears not to be associated with high disease activity.

Two types of NP-SLE events appear to be linked to a specific autoantibody profile. Strokes and seizures are often associated with the presence of anti-phospholipid antibodies (5).

DIAGNOSTIC APPROACH

Although specific clinical and immunologic diagnostic criteria promulgated by the American College of Rheumatology are useful for research purposes, the diagnosis of SLE rests mainly on clinical suspicion and documentation of specific ANA responses.

It is of paramount importance that the diagnosis of SLE is correct. This would seem obvious, but often is the case when the diagnosis of SLE is not correct. Close to 100% certainty that SLE is not the diagnosis is when an ANA is negative, but the presence of a positive ANA is not helpful because an ANA is a highly sensitive screening test with very low specificity. Age and gender, family history, recent viral infection, and drug induction can be associated with irrelevant ANA findings. If the clinical picture is supported by acute and chronic markers of inflammation and coupled with either the presence of the Sm ANA or double-stranded DNA antibodies, the diagnosis is usually correct. Assessment of complement activation, either in the peripheral blood or CSF, is usually not helpful; it can be misleading and is not recommended.

Once the diagnosis of SLE is made, the clinician must then decide on the cause of the NP-SLE findings. In view of the vast panoply of neurologic findings that can occur in NP-SLE and the lack of strong predictors for individual neurologic symptoms, it is important to develop an intuitive strategy to decide on one of four fundamental causes of the neurologic symptoms in a patient with SLE. The symptoms can be directly related to SLE, to the presence of antiphospholipid antibodies, to accelerated atherosclerosis, or to drug toxicity.

The precise identification of the cause is vital.

Following are stylized clinical scenarios illustrating the decision paths required to treat NP-SLE.

If the patient has high overall SLE disease activity, is relatively young, has no antiphospholipid antibodies, and is not taking high doses of Pred, it is highly likely that the neurologic findings are directly related to lupus.

If the patient has either active or inactive SLE, and highly active antiphospholipid antibodies (varying combinations of high titers of IgG anti-phospholipid syndrome (APL), Russell viper venom positivity, and β_2 platelet glycoprotein I [GPI] specificity), the neurologic symptoms are likely to be thrombotic or embolic.

Because SLE is an independent risk factor for premature and accelerated atherosclerosis (8), any patient with SLE, especially a young one, may have symptomatic atherosclerotic cerebral disease.

Finally, many patients with NP-SLE are treated with very high doses of Pred and their mania, overt psychosis, and impaired cognition can be directly related to the therapy and not NP-SLE.

Multiple abnormalities have been described with single photon emission computed tomography (SPECT) and magnetic resonance imaging (MRI) (9,10). Other than a correlation of MRI with cerebral atrophy and cognitive dysfunction, neuroimaging is not helpful in NP-SLE. Cerebral angiography should not be done if the primary reason is to document a suspected SLE vasculitis because the latter is rarely, if ever, the cause of NP-SLE.

TREATMENT

The heterogeneous disease expression of SLE, with its broad spectrum of patients, makes it almost impossible to conduct meaningful clinical trials. Furthermore, the disease seems to chart a course of its own in many patients, no matter how aggressive the therapy. Corticosteroids (CS) are the time-honored treatment of SLE and clinical data suggest that CS are beneficial in mild forms of SLE only. No convincing evidence suggests that they alter its ultimate course. CS alone are not sufficient for treatment of severe forms of disease, such as advanced grades of renal disease, and no evidence indicates that CS are efficacious in NP-SLE. The serious morbidity of long-term CS use in SLE has forced the use of steroid sparing strategies. Until recently, azathioprine (AZA) was the most common drug used to keep Pred doses below 15 mg daily. Mycophenolate mofetil (MM) is rapidly replacing AZA and some evidence suggests that MM may have significant therapeutic effects in SLE (11).

In severe SLE, the treatment gold standard is intravenous CTX. This alkylating agent poses a risk of infertility, hemorrhagic cystitis, and bone marrow suppression. The recent availability of a recombinant monoclonal antibody that binds to the CD20 marker on B cells and rapidly depletes them with minimal toxicity has stimulated great interest in its use in SLE. Preliminary results suggest that this biomodulator may be effective in some patients with lupus renal disease (12).

In patients with NP-SLE, treatment is dependent on the cause of the symptoms. It cannot be assumed that the neurologic findings are secondary to lupus and to do so is dangerous. When the clinical picture does suggest that a serious neurologic finding (e.g., coma, seizures, epilepsy, stroke) is directly related to SLE, then aggressive treatment of SLE is the logical path to take. At least 1 mg/kg of Pred or equivalent should be started immediately and combined with intravenous CTX, usually at a dose of 500 to 750 mg/m^2. Infusions should be continued on a monthly basis for at least half a year and further therapy designed in concert with a rheumatologist. Some practitioners recommend, on an anecdotal basis, very high doses of methylprednisolone (1 g daily for 3 days). The lack of an immediate therapeutic effect of either CTX or rituximab poses a risk for patients with severe NP-SLE. Anecdotal reports exist of striking reversal of coma and suppression of intractable seizures with plasmapheresis used as a bridging therapy.

In patients with SLE and the APL syndrome, NP-SLE symptoms, especially seizures and thrombotic or embolic syndromes, are likely caused by the latter and not SLE. Urgent anticoagulation is mandatory. The hazards of lifetime anticoagulation and the ability of many patients with APL syndrome to break through therapeutic anticoagulation makes the use of rituximab very attractive. The use of this B-cell depleting agent, in theory, solves two problems simultaneously by eliminating B cells that produce ANA and B cells that produce phospholipid antibodies.

In patients with symptoms of cerebrovascular ischemia but relatively inactive SLE and no significant APL antibodies, it should not be assumed the symptoms are directly related to lupus. The underlying cause may actually be premature atherosclerosis, common in patients of all ages with SLE. Treatment of NP-SLE with intensified immunosuppression will not be effective.

It is common for neurologists to be asked whether sudden change in behavior, onset of hallucinations, depression, or manic behavior in a patient with SLE could be a manifestation of NP-SLE and, if so, should Pred therapy be intensified. It is imperative to consider that Pred may be the cause and that reducing, not increasing, the Pred dose is the appropriate therapy.

Sjögren Syndrome

DEFINITION

Sjögren syndrome (SjS) is an autoimmune lymphoproliferative exocrinopathy characterized by lymphocytic destruction of exocrine glands. The salivary and lacrimal glands are preferentially targeted, and their loss of function leads to the typical sicca features of keratoconjunctivitis and loss of salivary flow. Although the cardinal features of dry mouth and eyes are found in most patients with SjS, the proliferation of exocrine gland-destructive T and B lymphocytes can lead to a wide spectrum of other clinical manifestations that include renal tubular acidosis, hypergammaglobulinemic purpura, interstitial pulmonary disease, and B-cell lymphomas. Neurologic symptoms are common in SjS.

EPIDEMIOLOGY

Sjögren syndrome is very common and can affect 2% to 3% of the adult population (13). The true prevalence of CNS disease in SjS is unknown because of vagaries in classification of the disease itself and the lack of agreement on which neurologic or psychiatric symptoms are causally linked. The peak time of diagnosis is in the fifth and sixth decades of life. SjS most often occurs as a primary disorder and, similar to most other autoimmune diseases, a marked preponderance is found in women as is a coincidence with other autoimmune diseases, especially rheumatoid arthritis and SLE. Revised combinations of oral and ocular symptoms, objective ocular signs, histopathology, and the presence of SS-A and B antibodies for the diagnosis and classification of SjS have been recently proposed (14).

ETIOLOGY AND PATHOGENESIS

The etiology is completely obscure, but appears to be multifactorial and has a genetic predisposition.

PATHOLOGY

Infiltration of the salivary and lacrimal glands by CD3+ T- and CD20+ B-lymphocytes is characteristic of SjS and focal lymphocytic sialoadenitis is the histopathologic gold standard for exocrine tissue diagnosis. A high level of expertise is required to interpret oral mucosal biopsies in SjS. Other exocrine glands can be involved as can the liver, kidneys, and lungs. Up to 5% of patients will develop B-cell lymphomas originating in mucosal lymphoid tissue. At least three different mechanisms appear to cause SjS peripheral neuropathy. Sural nerve biopsy may confirm the association of a mononeuropathy or a sensory ataxic neuropathy with small vessel vasculitis. Variable degrees of large and small axon fiber loss and dorsal root, posterior column involvement, and sympathetic neuron drop-out, but no vasculitis may be present in the sural nerves of SjS. A small fiber sensory neuropathy is also frequent in SjS, which is characterized by reduced epidermal nerve density and abnormal morphology in skin biopsies (15).

CLINICAL MANIFESTATIONS

A recent review of SjS neuropathy divided patients into seven subgroups (16). Most had either sensory ataxic neuropathy, painful sensory neuropathy without sensory ataxia, or trigeminal neuropathy. Slightly less common were multiple mononeuropathies, multiple cranial neuropathies, autonomic neuropathy, and radiculopathies. Orthostatic hypotension and abnormal pupillary function were frequent. Highly relevant was the observation that many times the neurologic symptoms preceded the diagnosis of SjS.

DIAGNOSIS

The diagnosis of SjS can usually be made on a clinical basis. In the rare circumstance when the clinical picture is not entirely convincing, SS-A (Ro) and SS-B (La) antibodies will be present in almost 90% of patients with SS. A biopsy is almost never required to make the diagnosis. No strong associations exist between the presence of either SS-A or SS-B antibodies and specific neurologic abnormalities, no characteristic findings in the CSF and, although SPECT scanning, MRI, and cerebral angiography findings are frequently abnormal in SjS, they offer no diagnostic specificity (17). Sural nerve and skin biopsies can distinguish between the painful small nerve sensory neuropathy and the neuropathies associated with small vessel vasculitis.

TREATMENT

The treatment of SjS has been symptomatic. Artificial tears and salivary flow enhancers offer some relief. Biopsy documentation of neuropathic manifestations caused by small vessel vasculitis is justification for short-term Pred and long-term B-cell suppression. In patients with debilitating trigeminal and other cranial neuropathies of SjS, B-cell depletion by rituximab may offer a relatively safe therapy that can reduce or even eliminate their symptoms.

Scleroderma (Systemic Sclerosis)

DEFINITION

Scleroderma (SSc) is a multisystem autoimmune disease characterized by structural and vasoreactive abnormalities of the microvascular endothelium and deposition of collagen that culminates in dense fibrosis of the skin, gastrointestinal tract, heart, lungs, and kidneys.

EPIDEMIOLOGY

SSc is relatively rare. It has an incidence of about 19 cases per year per 1 million people and a female-to-male ratio of about 8:1 in the United States. It has a peak incidence in the fifth decade. An almost fivefold increased risk of death exists when compared with the general population (18).

ETIOLOGY AND PATHOGENESIS

Little is known about the cause(s) of SSc. Microvascular dysfunction evidenced by heightened vasospasm to multiple triggers (cold, emotional stress) and architectural changes in small arteries, arterioles, and capillaries occur early in the disease. Perturbation of vasoactive mediators (e.g., endothelin and nitric oxide) have been documented, but not causally linked to SSc. Abnormalities in a gene complex that controls tumor growth factor-β (TGF-β), a fibrogenic cytokine, in mice with a sclerodermalike disease and agonistic autoantibodies reactive with the platelet-derived growth factor (PDGF) receptor on SSc fibroblasts have recently been reported (19,20).

PATHOLOGY

There is exuberant deposition of collagen and other matrix proteins in the skin and other affected organs. The vasculopathy includes basement membrane thickening, in situ thrombosis, and distorted and irregular capillary loops that can be detected by nailfold capilloscopy.

NEUROPATHIC FINDINGS ASSOCIATED WITH SCLERODERMA

No CNS neuropathies and very few peripheral neuropathic symptoms are associated with SSC. None are uniquely related to SSC. Increased collagen deposition in the carpal tunnel can cause carpal tunnel syndrome and, rarely, trigeminal neuropathy has been reported with the disease.

DIAGNOSIS

The diagnosis of SSc is almost always a clinical one. Although most patients with SSc will have ANA, only the antitopoisomerase is relatively specific for diffuse SSc and the centromere antibody for the limited variant of SSc.

TREATMENT

No specific treatment for SSc exists and symptom subsets are treated symptomatically.

A wide spectrum of isolated peripheral neuropathies, especially carpal tunnel syndrome, caused by fibrotic entrapment or calcinosis, can occur. These should be treated as mechanical complications of SSc.

CLINICAL RECOMMENDATIONS OF THE VIGNETTE

The fatigue, weakness, pallor, elevated serum creatinine, proteinuria, and red cell casts—coupled with a change in anti-DNA titer—are strong evidence for active SLE. The patient was appropriately treated with high Pred doses and other immunosuppressive drugs. When evaluated in the emergency department, objective evidence indicated that she had gone into remission. This makes it highly unlikely that her new neuropsychiatric symptoms are caused by continuing lupus activity. At this point, the neurologist should recommend rapid reduction in Pred and the addition of a steroid-sparing drug because the odds are high that the new symptoms were Pred related.

The patient continued in remission after the addition of MM to her daily Pred maintenance. Over the next 3 years, she experienced severe sicca symptoms and progressive periodontal disease. She had almost complete loss of salivary flow and very high titers of antibodies to SS-A (Ro) and SS-B (La) antigens. She suddenly developed dysesthesia of the tongue and then numbness over the distribution of the right trigeminal nerve. She was referred to a neurologist.

A very debilitating trigeminal neuropathy can occur in SjS. All forms of treatment, including neurosurgical, however, have not been very effective. Prednisone is usually tried and, more often than not, is ineffective. Although the patient received both rituximab and cyclophosphamide (Cytoxan) 3 years ago, both agents should be reconsidered if she has no response to Pred.

SUMMARY

SLE and SjS are common autoimmune diseases that have a wide variety of neurologic complications. In SLE, it is important to decide whether (*a*) the neurologic findings are secondary to SLE, (*b*) an associated antiphospholipid antibody syndrome is present, or (*c*) premature atherosclerosis or the drugs being used to treat SLE itself are contributory. This is often difficult because there are no clinical features of SLE, other than high overall disease activity, that are strong predictors of specific neurologic syndromes and imaging studies and autoantibody analysis are usually not helpful. In SjS, peripheral neuropathies can be very debilitating, but often are secondary to B-cell hyperactivity and can be treated with prednisone or B-cell depletion. No neuropathic findings are unique to scleroderma.

REFERENCES

1. Eber T, Chapman J, Shoenfeld Y. Anti-ribosomal P protein and its role in psychiatric manifestations of systemic lupus erythematosus: Myth or reality? *Lupus* 2005;14:571–575.
2. Tin S, Xu Q, Thumboo J, et al. Novel brain reactive autoantibodies: Prevalence in systemic lupus erythematosus and association with psychoses and seizures. *J Neuroimmunol.* 2005; 169:153–160.
3. Omdal R, Brokstad K, Waterloo K, et al. Neuropsychiatric disturbances in SLE are associated with antibodies against NMDA receptors. *Eur J Neurol.* 2005;12:392–398.
4. Goransson L, Tjensvoll A, Heristad A, et al. Small-diameter nerve fiber neuropathy in systemic lupus erythematosus. *Arch Neurol.* 2006;63:401–404.
5. Mikdashi J, Handweger B. Predictors of neuropsychiatric damage in systemic lupus erythematosus: Data from the Maryland lupus cohort. *Rheumatology.* 2004;43:1555–1560.
6. Shimojima Y, Matsuda M, Gono T, et al. Relationship between clinical factors and neuropsychiatric manifestations in systemic lupus erythematosus. *Clin Rheumatol.* 2005;24:469–475.
7. Hanly J, McCurdy G, Fougere L, et al. Neuropsychiatric events in systemic lupus erythematosus: Attribution and clinical significance. *J Rheumatol.* 2004;31:2156–2162.
8. Nikpour M, Urowitz M, Gladman D. Premature atherosclerosis in systemic lupus erythematosus. *Rheum Dis Clin North Am.* 2005;31:329–354.
9. Abreu M, Jakosky A, Folgerine M, et al. Neuropsychiatric systemic lupus erythematosus: Correlation of brain MR imaging, CT and SPECT. *Clin Imaging.* 2005;29:215–221.
10. Ainiala H, Dastidar P, Loukkola J, et al. Cerebral MRI abnormalities and their association with neuropsychiatric manifestations in SLE: A population based study. *Scand J Rheumatol.* 2005;34:376–382.
11. Chan T, Li F, Tang C, et al. Efficacy if mycophenolate mofetil in patients with diffuse proliferative lupus nephritis. *N Engl J Med.* 2000;34:1156–1162.
12. Thatayatikom A, White A. Rituximab: A promising therapy in systemic lupus erythematosus. *Autoimmunity Reviews.* 2006;5:18–24.
13. Soliotis F, Mavragani C, Moutsopoulos H. Central nervous system involvement in Sjogren's syndrome. *Ann Rheum Dis.* 2004;63:616–620.
14. Vitali C, Bombardieeri S, Jonsson R, et al. Classification criteria for Sjogren's syndrome: A revised version of the European criteria proposed by the American-European consensus group. *Ann Rheum Dis.* 2002;59:554–558.
15. Chai J, Hermann D, Stanton M, et al. Painful small fiber neuropathy in Sjogren's syndrome. *Neurology.* 2005;65:925–927.
16. Mori, K, Iijima M, Koike H, et al. The wide spectrum of clinical manifestations in Sjogren's syndrome-associated neuropathy. *Brain.* 2005;128:2518–2534.
17. Morgen K, McFarland H, Pillemar S. Central nervous system disease in primary Sjogren's syndrome: The role of magnetic resonance imaging. *Semin Arthritis Rheum.* 2004;34:623–630.
18. Haustein U. Systemic sclerosis–scleroderma. *Dermatology Online Journal.* 2005. Available at: http://dermatology.cdlib.org/DOJ.html
19. Denton C, Abraham D. Transgenic analysis of scleroderma: Understanding key pathogenic events in vivo. *Autoimmunity Reviews.* 2004;3:285–293.
20. Baroni S, Santillo M, Bevilacqua F, et al. Stimulatory autoantibodies to the PDGF receptor in systemic sclerosis. *N Engl J Med.* 2006;354:2667–2676.

CHAPTER 86

Primary Vasculitides and the Nervous System

Yair Molad • Jonathan Y. Streifler

OBJECTIVES

- To describe the central nervous system (CNS) and peripheral nervous system (PNS) manifestations of vasculitis (angiitis)
- To review the diagnosis and treatment of CNS and PNS vasculitis (angiitis)
- To describe the clinical features and diagnosis of systemic vasculitic disorders that affect the nervous system

CASE VIGNETTE

A 52-year-old woman was admitted to the hospital because of headache and double vision. On physical examination, a saddle nose was noted and right abducens nerve palsy was present. Blood tests showed a sedimentation rate of 96 mm/hour. Renal and liver function tests were normal. Cranial computed tomography (CT) showed bilateral small temporal lobe lesions suspected to be caused by metastases. Cerebrospinal fluid (CSF) analysis was unremarkable with no evidence of infection or malignant cells. Brain magnetic resonance imaging (MRI) disclosed occlusion of the right internal carotid artery, extraaxial high-intensity lesion in the right middle fossa, and bilateral diffuse infiltration of the temporal lobes with bone destruction—lesions enhanced by gadolinium. A chest CT scan showed a lung infiltrate in the lingual lobe and a round lesion in the left upper lobe.

DEFINITION

Vasculitis is an organ-specific or multisystem inflammatory disorder wherein the primary pathologic insult involves blood vessel wall. Vasculitis can be either a primary disorder or secondary to other diseases, such as infections (e.g., human immunodeficiency virus [HIV], hepatitis C), autoimmune-inflammatory (e.g., rheumatoid arthritis, Sjögren syndrome, systemic lupus erythematosus, inflammatory bowel disease), hypersensitivity (e.g., drug-reaction), or neoplastic disease (e.g., paraneoplastic syndromes) (1). Current accepted classification of the vasculitides is the Chapel-Hill Consensus Conference nomenclature that is based on the size of blood vessels predominantly involved (2). The predominately large-vessel vasculitides include Takayasu arteritis (TA), giant-cell (temporal) arteritis (GCA), Cogan syndrome, and Behçet's disease (BD). The predominately medium-vessel vasculitides includes polyarteritis nodosa (PAN), cutaneous PAN, Buerger disease, Kawasaki disease, and primary angiitis of CNS (PACNS). The predominately small-vessel vasculitides include the immune-complex–mediated diseases: Goodpasture disease, leukocytoclastic vasculitis, Henoch-Schönlein purpura (HSP), hypocomplementemic urticarial vasculitis, essential mixed cryoglobulinemia (MC), and erythema elevatum diutinum; and the pauci-immune or antineutrophil cytoplasmatic antibody (ANCA)-associated vasculitis (e.g., Wegener granulomatosis [WG], Churg-Strauss syndrome [CSS], microscopic polyangiitis [MPA], and renal-limited vasculitis) (1,2).

EPIDEMIOLOGY

The primary vasculitic syndromes are characterized by an age- and organ-predilection. Generally, the annual incidence is approximately 10 to 20 per 1 million; the peak age of onset is 65 to 74 years; and these conditions are very rare in childhood, except for specific conditions: Kawasaki disease and HSP affect children yet the others, especially the ANCA-associated small-vessel vasculitides and giant-cell arteritis, affect adults above 50 years of age (2,3).

ETIOLOGY AND PATHOGENESIS

The vasculitides, which are conditions of unknown etiology, are characterized by organ tropism. For example, WG classically involves the upper and lower respiratory tract and kidneys; TA involves the aorta and its main branches, whereas the small-vessel vasculitides primarily involve the skin, peripheral nerves, and kidneys. Some of the primary vasculitides, such as WG, CSS, and GCA, are characterized by granulomatous inflammation that resembles chronic infections. The small- and medium-vessel vasculitides are divided into either immune-complex–induced or pauci-immune vasculitis. Examples of the former are mixed-cryoglobulinemia (commonly induced by hepatitis C virus), Goodpasture disease (antiglomerular basement membrane) and HSP, and the latter are the ANCA-associated vasculitides.

PATHOLOGY

The pathologic hallmark of vasculitis is an inflammation of the blood vessel wall with fibrinoid necrosis and secondary occlusion of the vessel lumen. Several vasculitides, such as WG, CSS, and GCA, are characterized by granulomatous inflammation. The histopathology of PACNS includes a granulomatous angiitis as well as a PAN-like necrotizing vasculitis, with infarct and hemorrhagic damage to the surrounding brain with myelin and axonal degeneration (4,5). PNS involvement can presents with a variety of micropathologies: Panarteritis nodosa or microscopic polyangiitis (with fibrinoid necrosis or sclerosis) or microvasculitis (without necrosis) (6).

CLINICAL MANIFESTATIONS

The CNS may be involved in 20% to 40% of patients with systemic vasculitis, frequently causing either focal or diffuse neurologic manifestations (3). Diverse neurologic manifestations have been described in patients with either primary or secondary CNS vasculitis of which headache and encephalopathy are the most common presentations (3–5,7–9). Persistent headache can be the sole feature of a vasculitic disorder, such as in GCA or PACNS, which therefore should alert the physician to search for this diagnosis (9). Neurocognitive decline as well as cranial neuropathies, spinal cord disease, and seizures are also common manifestations (4,5). Strokelike presentation is less likely to be caused by CNS vasculitis; however, atypical intracerebral and subarachnoid hemorrhages have been described.

PNS manifestations of vasculitides typically present as neuropathies of different types. The most important type is mononeuritis multiplex (MNM), which results from involvement of the vasa nervorum of different nerves at different stages of the disease, hence MNM. Yet other forms of peripheral neuropathies (PN) have been described, including symmetric sensory-motor polyneuropathy or even pure sensory neuropathy (10). The PNS is affected mainly during the course of small-vessel vasculitides.

Because PACNS is a prototype of CNS involvement, it will be thoroughly discussed first to highlight clinical manifestations and pitfalls in diagnosis also relevant to some systemic vasculitides.

PRIMARY ANGIITIS OF THE CENTRAL NERVOUS SYSTEM

PACNS, called also granulomatous angiitis of the CNS or isolated angiitis of the CNS, is the most common primary vasculitis of the CNS. A rare and often fatal disorder, PACNS is primarily an angiitis of the leptomeningeal and cortical small- and medium-size arteries, and less frequently, veins and venules (4). It affects primarily men, and presents most commonly with persistent headache accompanied by diffuse neurologic manifestations, such as cognitive decline and decrease or fluctuations of consciousness, along with focal deficits (strokelike—ischemic or hemorrhagic) and seizures. Although most patients will develop a variety of focal neurologic deficits, they usually occur in the presence of diffuse neurologic dysfunction that develops over a prolonged period of time, and rarely as an acute onset (4). Usually, no systemic clinical manifestations exist and laboratory tests, such as erythrocyte sedimentation rate (ESR), C-reactive protein (CRP), and blood count, are normal and serum autoantibodies are negative. Lumbar puncture may reveal high pressure and the CSF content will be abnormal in 80% to 90% of pathologically proved cases of PACNS (4), which is compatible with aseptic meningitis and showing modest pleocytosis, protein elevation >100 mg/dL. Evidence of intrathecal synthesis of immunoglobulin and oligoclonal bands can be also found (4,8).

Because the positive predictive value of an abnormal CSF was only 37% in a group of patients evaluated for the possibility of PACNS, a normal CSF cannot be a reliable tool for excluding the possible diagnosis of PACNS (11). CT and MRI also lack specificity (of only 36%), demonstrating multiple bilateral, supratentorial infarcts in the cortex, deep white matter, and leptomeninges (11). Indeed, a retrospective study has shown a cortical and leptomeningeal biopsy-proved pathologic evidence of angiitis in only 6 of 14 patients who presented with typical angiographic findings of brain vasculitis (60% specificity), suggesting that a definite diagnosis of PACNS should not be based solely on angiography (12) because normal angiography is noted in about 40% of patients (4,13). Hence, a histopathologic confirmation of vasculitis is essential for accurate diagnosis of CNS vasculitis. The clinical outcome has been analyzed of patients with PACNS who were diagnosed on the ground of either angiography or histopathology and has identified two different groups (4,11,12): The term *benign angiopathy of the CNS* (BACNS) is deserved for an angiographically based diagnosis of CNS vasculitis without a histopathologic evidence of vasculitis (4,15,16). Angiographically defined CNS vasculitis is usually seen in females with an abrupt onset of symptoms (most commonly, headache), usually with normal CSF findings, and eventually with a better outcome than that observed in patients with biopsy-proved PACNS (15,16). The angiographic findings of patients with BACNS are often bilateral multiple areas of smooth, symmetric narrowing, often with poststenotic dilatation of smaller, rather larger, vessels at the base of the brain (16).

Biopsy of brain and leptomeninges is still the gold standard for the diagnosis of CNS vasculitis. The biopsy site is selected according to abnormal MRI findings and, in the absence of focal lesion, the biopsy is taken from the anterior tip of the nondominant temporal lobe (4,5). The biopsy-related morbidity in patients with suspected vasculitis is 3.3%, a significantly lower rate than is related to the adverse effects of the immunosuppressive therapy (17). Moreover, because about half of patients referred for brain biopsy with a working diagnosis of CNS vasculitis are diagnosed with other disorders, a brain biopsy is necessary to make a definite diagnosis (5,17). Nevertheless, CNS vasculitis is a patchy disease, which explains why as much as 25% of biopsies are yielding a false–negative result (18). Chu et al. (17) have found a 16% false–negative rate of biopsy in a series of 30 consecutive biopsies of suspected CNS vasculitis, with a sensitivity of 84%, yielding a positive predictive value of 90% to 100%, significantly higher than for angiography (37% to 50%) and for MRI (43% to 72%) (14,18).

Treatment of PACNS is empirically based on a high dose of corticosteroids and cyclophosphamide (19,20). Such an aggressive therapy should be reserved for biopsy-proved granulomatous angiitis of CNS and be continued for 6 to 12 months after clinical remission is achieved (4). BACNS follows a more benign course for which a shorter course of high-dose corticosteroids will be sufficient for most of the patients with or without the supplement of calcium-channel blockers (4,16,21). A clinical resolution of symptoms and signs, along with improvement of the angiographic abnormalities, is expected to be the outcome in BACNS. Failure of corticosteroid therapy is suggestive of a false diagnosis and should prompt a search for other nonvasculitic diagnoses, such as infection, cerebrovascular atherosclerosis, emboli, hypercoagulable state, or malignancy (e.g., cerebral lymphoma or intravascular neoplasm) (16).

PRIMARY SYSTEMIC VASCULITIDES

CNS and PNS involvement occurs in nearly all types of systemic vasculitides, but is most commonly reported in the ANCA-associated small-vessel vasculitis, polyarteritis nodosa, Behçet disease, mixed cryoglobulinemia, TA, and GCA. The discussion in this chapter is limited to the neurologic involvement of these systemic vasculitides and to the appropriate diagnostic and therapeutic approach to them.

ANCA-Associated Small-Vessel Disease (AASVV)

WG, MPA, and CSS can cause CNS disease at any time in the course of the systemic disease; however, the involvement of the PNS is more common, presenting mainly as MNM. WG is a multisystem disease characterized by a granulomatous necrotizing vasculitis of small- to medium-size blood vessels of the lower and upper respiratory tracts and kidneys, as well as skin, eyes, heart, joints, and the nervous system. MPA is a nongranulomatous necrotizing vasculitis of small vessels affecting primarily the kidneys, lungs, skin, and PNS. CSS is also a small- to medium-size granulomatous vasculitis characterized by a history of asthma and allergic conditions, marked eosinophilia, and involvement of the lungs, skin, kidneys, gastrointestinal tract, and the heart. Together with renal-limited vasculitis, these disorders are serologically defined by serum antibodies to neutrophil cytoplasmatic enzymes of either cytoplasmatic or perinuclear immunofluorescent patterns, reacting proteinase-3 and myeloperoxidase, respectively.

Neurologic involvement has been reported in up to half of the patients with WG mainly of the PNS, whereas the CNS is involved in <10% of the patients (5). The spectrum of CNS presentation in WG includes headache, cranial neuropathies (most frequently the second, sixth and seventh nerves), seizures, aseptic meningitis, diabetes insipidus, hydrocephalus, external ophthalmoparesis, cerebrovascular events, and myelopathy (22,23). Although PN can be an early and even the sole manifestation of AASVV, CNS involvement occurs usually late in the course of the disease, frequently accompanying other disease features, and poses a high risk for mortality during the first year after diagnosis (24).

MRI is a sensitive diagnostic method for the evaluation of patients with WG who present with CNS complaints. Treatment of WG includes high-dose corticosteroids and oral cyclophosphamide for the induction of clinical remission, followed by a maintenance therapy with less-toxic immunosuppressive drugs, such as azathioprine (25). New therapies with biologic agents have been reported to be beneficial; however, well-controlled studies have not been published yet.

Mild cognitive impairment can be found in about 30% of patients with AASVV, which is related to the extent of brain MRI lesions (26).

CNS involvement of MPA is rare, whereas the CNS is affected in 25% of patients with CSS, mostly as cranial neuropathies, and to a lesser degree encephalopathy and strokelike events during the course of the disease (5). Up to 78% of patients with CSS, however, show signs of PNS involvement (mainly, MNM, including cranial), and positive ANCA, at presentation (27,28). Treatment of neurologic involvement in CSS is as in WG (25).

Polyarteritis Nodosa

PAN affects medium- and small-size arteries and typically involves the vasa nervorum of peripheral nerves. PNS, thus, is affected more frequently: MNM (including, cranial neuropathies) or PN can be early signs and a special form of PAN is limited to nerves and muscles. CNS involvement is seen in up to 40% of patients with PAN, the most common manifestations being strokes and diffuse encephalopathy with cognitive deterioration and seizures (29). Cerebral angiography can demonstrate beading in distal branches of one of the major blood vessels, representing areas of stenosis secondary to inflammation with poststenotic dilatation.

Behçet Disease

BD, a vasculitic multisystem disease, presents with oral and genital ulcers, uveitis, erythema nodosum, as well as pulmonary, cardiovascular, and gastrointestinal involvement. Neuro-Behçet is one of the most serious manifestations of BD, presenting in up to 10% of the patients as either brain small-vessel disease or cerebral venous sinus thrombosis (30–32). Parenchymal vasculitis-mediated manifestations of neuro-BD, which are more common among male patients, usually present as an attack of focal symptoms, with headache, gradual behavioral changes, or sphincteric disturbances (30). Less common features of parenchymal involvement include ophthalmoplegia and bulbar signs. MRI will demonstrate widespread lesions involving the brainstem as well (31). The other type of neuro-BD is related to venous sinus thrombosis that usually presents with headache and signs of increased intracranial pressure (30–32).

Acute attacks of neuro-BD are treated with high-dose corticosteroids with immunosuppressive drugs, such as azathioprine, cyclosporine A, cyclophosphamide, and chlorambucil. Other immunomodulators, such as interferon-α (IFN-α) and thalidomide, have also been shown to be effective in the treatment of systemic disease in BD (5). Venous sinus thrombosis is treated with anticoagulation along with corticosteroids (5).

Takayasu Arteritis

TA is a granulomatous arteritis of the aorta and its main branches. CNS involvement is related to carotid or vertebral arteries stenoses, occlusion, and even dissection, which lead to acute, intermittent, or chronic decrease in cerebral blood flow (5). The neurologic manifestations include headache, stroke, transient ischemic attack (TIA), or subclavian steal syndrome with dizziness or visual disturbances. TA usually affects young females and stroke can be the presenting feature in approximately 10% of the cases (33). Treatment consists of corticosteroids with immunosuppressive agents, together with low-dose aspirin. Endovascular stent insertion and bypass surgery have been tried with minimal success because stenosis reoccurs frequently (33)

Giant-Cell Arteritis (Temporal Arteritis)

GCA is a granulomatous giant-cell inflammation of large- to medium-size arteries that affects patients aged 50 years or older. Headache is one of the most common manifestations of the disease, frequently occurring in the temporal areas, although it can be occipital or diffuse, and is frequently accompanied by jaw claudication and visual disturbances. The latter (amaurosis fugax or acute monocular blindness) is caused by inflammation of the ophthalmic or posterior ciliary arteries (causing anterior ischemic optic neuropathy [AION]—a common ophthalmologic feature of GCA, or posterior ischemic optic neuropathy [PION]) (34). Symptoms of polymyalgia rheumatica (shoulder and pelvic girdles pain and stiffness), constitutional symptoms, such as fever and weight loss, and a markedly elevated erythrocyte sedimentation rate (ESR) are common and suggestive of the diagnosis (35), which is confirmed by a temporal artery biopsy that should be done in every case of new-onset of or change of type of headache in an elderly patient with either ophthalmic abnormality or elevated ESR. Other diagnostic techniques include ultrasonography of the artery and positron emission tomography. Although headache is the most common neurologic feature of GCA, its absence does not exclude this diagnosis.

Other less common CNS manifestations of GCA include stroke and TIA, yet stroke occurs in approximately 25% of the patients (34) and low-dose aspirin should be prescribed to all patients. Neuropsychiatric manifestations, such as dementia, mood disorders, and psychosis, were reported uncommonly in patients with GCA. In such cases, one should rule-out a possible adverse effect of steroids. Hearing loss and vertigo as well as lingual nerve involvement are rare neurologic manifestations.

The treatment of choice of GCA consists of corticosteroids (initially, prednisone 40 to 60 mg/day followed by gradual tapering) together with low-dose aspirin.

Mixed Cryoglobulinemia

Cryoglobulins are cold-precipitated proteins consisting of two or more immunoglobulin isotypes, whereas MC is a systemic vasculitis characterized by the proliferation of a B-cell clone producing pathogenic IgM with rheumatoid factor activity. Infection with hepatitis C virus (HCV) is frequently associated with MC. The clinical features of MC consist of palpable purpura (caused by leukocytoclastic vasculitis), glomerulonephritis, and neurologic involvement. PN of subacute distal axonal sensory-motor type is the most common neurologic feature of MC, but mononeuritis and mononeuritis multiplex have also been reported. A demyelinating type of PN is rare in HCV-associated MC (36). Clinical signs of PN can be found in 10.6% of patients with untreated HCV infection; electrophysiologic PN is found in 15.3% (37). It is suggested the PN in patients with HCV infection could be a direct effect of the virus rather than an MC-mediated immune effect. HCV-associated CNS vasculitis is rare and presents as strokelike episodes or progressive encephalopathy (5).

TABLE 86-1. Neurologic Features of the Major Primary Vasculitides

Disease Type	*Prevalence of CNS Involvement*	*CNS Features*	*Prevalence of PNS Involvement*	*PNS Features*
LARGE VESSEL VASCULITIDES				
Takayasu arteritis	++	HA, Str, TIA, SSS	−	
Giant cell arteritis	+++	HA, VL	+	MNM
	++	TIA, Str, CN, Sz, Enceph		MN, PN
Behçet's disease	++	Enc, Str, CD, CST, AM	+	MN
MEDIUM VESSEL VASCULITIDES				
Polyarteritis nodosa (PAN)	++	Enc, Str, Sz, CN	+++	MNM, PN
Primary angiitis of CNS (PACNS)	100%	Enc, Str, Sz, CD	−	
SMALL VESSEL VASCULITIDES				
1. Immune complex-mediated				
Goodpasture Syndrome	+	Enc, Sz, Str,	−	
Henoch-Schonlein purpura	++	HA, CD, Sz, Str	+	MNM, PN
Mixed cryoglobulinemia	+	VL, CST, Enc	+++	PN, MN, MNM
2. ANCA associated				
Wegener granulomatosis	+	Late: HA, CN, Sz, AM, SC	++	Early: MNM, PN
Churg-Strauss syndrome	++	CN, Enc, VL, Str, Sz	+++	

Key: − absent, + not common, +++ most common.
ANCA, antineutrophil cytoplasmic antibodies; HA, headache; Str, stroke; TIA, transient ischemic attack; Sz, seizure; Enc, encephalopathy; CD, cognitive decline; CN, cranial neuropathy; CST, cerebral sinus thrombosis; SC, spinal cord involvement; VL, visual loss; SSS, subclavian steal syndrome; AM, aseptic meningitis; MNM, mononeuritis multiplex; MN, mononeuropathy; PN, polyneuropathy.

Treatment of HCV-associated MC-induced vasculitis consists of antiviral therapy with IFN-α and ribavirin; remission of the vasculitic manifestations can be achieved with eradication of the HCV (38). In severe vasculitic manifestations, such as glomerulonephritis or severe neuropathy, corticosteroids, immunosuppressive drugs, and plasmapheresis are used with variable clinical response. Treatment-resistant MC-related PN can be managed with rituximab, an anti-CD20 monoclonal B-cell depleting antibody (39).

CLINICAL RECOMMENDATIONS OF THE VIGNETTE

Examination of the patient was inconclusive: Both malignancy and systemic vasculitis were reasonable options. Thus, further investigations were needed: Laboratory workup revealed a high level of serum antibody to proteinase-3 (PR3) (38 EU; normal value <15) and a leptomeningeal and cortical biopsy (right temporal) demonstrated a granulomatous inflammation and small- and medium-size vessels with no evidence of malignancy. The diagnosis was Wegener granulomatosis, which was treated with high-dose corticosteroids and oral cyclophosphamide (2 mg/kg body weight) with resolution of both headache and double vision and disappearance of the lung infiltrates and serum anti-PR3 antibody. The cyclophosphamide was switched to oral weekly methotrexate; corticosteroids were tapered off. Four years later, the patient experienced several episodes of generalized seizures that responded well to treatment with valproate.

SUMMARY

Vasculitis involving CNS or PNS vessels can present with various diffuse or focal neurologic manifestations that should alert the physician to consider such a diagnosis in the clinical evaluation of headache, encephalopathies, and focal neurologic abnormalities, including MNM or even symmetric polyneuropathy. Primary angiitis of CNS as well as CNS or PNS involvement by systemic vasculitic syndromes can cause significant, and sometimes irreversible, neurologic deficit, either focal or diffuse (Table 86-1), hence prompt early diagnosis followed by appropriate therapy is of utmost importance.

REFERENCES

1. Saleh A, Stone JH. Classification and diagnostic criteria in systemic vasculitis. *Best Pract Res Clin Rheumatol.* 2005;19:209–221.
2. Jennette JC, Falk RJ, Andrassy K, et al. Nomenclature of systemic vasculitides. Proposal of an international consensus conference. *Arthritis Rheum.* 1994;37:187–192.
3. Chin RL, Latov N. Central nervous system manifestations of rheumatologic diseases. *Curr Opin Rheumatol.* 2004;17:91–99.
4. Calabrese LH, Duna GF, Lie JT. Vasculitis of the central nervous system. *Arthritis Rheum.* 1997;40:1189–1201.
5. Siva A. Vasculitis of the nervous system. *J Neurol.* 2001;248:451–468.
6. Vital C, Vital A, Canron MH, et al. Combined nerve and muscle biopsy in the diagnosis of vasculitic neuropathy. A 16-year retrospective study of 202 cases. *J Peripher Nerv Syst.* 2006;11:20–29.
7. Sigal LH. The neurologic presentation of vasculitic and rheumatologic syndromes. *Medicine.* 1987;66:157–180.
8. Younger DS. Vasculitis of the nervous system. *Curr Opin Neurol.* 2004;17:317–336.
9. Younger DS. Headaches and vasculitis. *Neurol Clin North Am.* 2004;22:207–228.
10. Seo JH, Ryan HF, Claussen GC, et al. Sensory neuropathy in vasculitis. *Neurology* 2004;63:874–878.
11. Duna GF, Calabrese LH. Limitations of invasive modalities in the diagnosis of primary angiitis of the central nervous system. *J Rheumatol.* 1995;22:662–667.
12. Kadkhodayan Y, Moran CJ, Cross III, DT, et al. Primary angiitis of the central nervous system at conventional angiography. *Radiology.* 2004;233:878–882.
13. Rhodes RH, Madelaire C, Petrelli M, et al. Primary angiitis of the central nervous system and their relationship to giant cell arteritis. *Arch Pathol Lab Med.* 1995;119:334–349.
14. Calabrese LH. Diagnostic strategies in vasculitis affecting the central nervous system. *Cleve Clin J Med.* 2002;69[Suppl 2]:SII105–SII108.
15. Calabrese LH, Gragg LA, Furlan AJ. Benign angiopathy: A distinct subset of angiographically defined primary angiitis of the central nervous system. *J Rheumatol.* 1993;20: 2046–2050.
16. Hajj-Ali RA, Furlan A, Abou-Chebel A, et al. Benign angiopathy of the central nervous system: Cohort of 16 patients with clinical course and long-term followup. *Arthritis Rheum (Arthritis Care Res).* 2002;47:662–669.
17. Chu TC, Gray L, Goldstein B, et al. Diagnosis of intracranial vasculitis: A multidisciplinary approach. *J Neuropathol Exp Neurol.* 1998;57:30–38.
18. Calabrese LH, Furlan AJ, Gragg LA, et al. Primary angiitis of the central nervous system: Diagnostic criteria and clinical approach. *Cleve Clin J Med.* 1992;59:293–306.
19. Cupps TR, Moore PM, Fauci AS. Isolated angiitis of the central nervous system. *Am J Med.* 1983;74:97–105.
20. Younger DS, Calabrese LH, Hays AP. Granulomatous angiitis of the nervous system. *Neurol Clin.* 1997;15:821–834.
21. MacLaren K, Gillespie J, Shrestha S, et al. Primary angiitis of the central nervous system: Emerging variants. *QJ Med.* 2005;98:643–654.
22. Nishino H, Rubino FA, DeRemee RA, et al. Neurological involvement in Wegener's granulomatosis: An analysis of 324 consecutive patients at the Mayo Clinic. *Ann Neurol.* 1993;33:4–9.
23. Seror R, Mahr A, Ramanoelina J, et al. Central nervous system involvement in Wegener granulomatosis. *Medicine.* 2006;85:54–65.
24. Bourgarit A, Le Toumelin P, Pagnoux C, et al; French Vasculitis Study Group. *Medicine.* 2005;84:323–330.
25. Jayne D, Rasmussen N, Andrassy K, et al; European Vasculitis Study Group. A randomized trial of maintenance therapy for vasculitis associated with antineutrophil cytoplasmic autoantibodies. *N Engl J Med.* 2003;349:36–44.
26. Mattioli F, Capra R, Rovaris M, et al. Frequency and patterns of subclinical cognitive impairment in patients with ANCA-associated small vessel vasculitides. *J Neurol Sci.* 2002;195:161–166.
27. Sable-Fourtassou R, Cohen P, Mahr A, et al; French vasculitis study group. Antineutrophil cytoplasmic antibodies and the Churg-Strauss syndrome. *Ann Intern Med.* 2005;143: 632–638.
28. Guillevin L, Cohen P, Gayraud M, et al. Churg-Strauss syndrome. Clinical study and long-term follow-up of 96 patients. *Medicine (Baltimore).* 1999;78:26–37.
29. Moore PM, Richardson B. Neurology of the vasculitides and connective tissue diseases. *J Neurol Neurosurg Psychiatry.* 1998;65:10–22.
30. Akman-Demir G, Serdaroglu P, Taşçi B. Clinical patterns of neurological involvement in Behçet's disease: Evaluation of 2000 patients. The Neuro-Behçet Study Group. *Brain.* 1999;122:2171–2181.
31. Siva A, Kantarci OH, Saip S, et al. Behçet's disease: Diagnostic and prognostic aspects of neurological involvement. *J Neurol.* 2001;248:95–103.
32. Al-Araji A, Sharquie K, Al-Rawi Z. Prevalence and patterns of neurological involvement in Behçet's disease: A prospective study from Iraq. *J Neurol Neurosurg Psychiatry.* 2003;74: 608–613.
33. Kerr GS, Hallahan CW, Giordano J, et al. Takayasu arteritis. *Ann Intern Med* 1994;120: 919–929.
34. Nesher G. Neurologic manifestations of giant cell arteritis. *Clin Exp Rheumatol.* 2000;18[4 Suppl 20]:S24–S26.
35. Weyand CM, Goronzy JJ. Giant-cell arteritis and polymyalgia rheumatica. *Ann Intern Med.* 2003;139:505–515.
36. Boukhris S, Magy L, Senga-Mokono U, et al. Polyneuropathy with demyelinating features in mixed cryoglobulinemia with hepatitis C infection. *Eur J Neurol.* 2006;13:937–941.
37. Santoro L, Monganelli F, Briani C, et al.; HCV Peripheral Nerve Study Group. *J Neurol Neurosurg Psychiatry.* 2006;77:626–629.
38. Cacoub P, Saadoun D, Limal N, et al. PEGylated interferon alfa-2b and ribavirin treatment in patients with hepatitis C virus-related systemic vasculitis. *Arthritis Rheum.* 2005;52: 911–915.
39. Zheng F, Cai J, Ahern M, Smith M. Treatment of cryoglobulinemia associated peripheral neuropathy with rituximab. *J Rheumatol.* 2006;33:1197–1198.

CHAPTER **87**

Inflammatory Myopathies

Elizabeth G. Araujo

OBJECTIVES

- To describe the three major groups of inflammatory myopathies: Dermatomyositis, polymyositis, and inclusion-body myositis
- To discuss the different basic pathologic processes in dermatomyositis compared with polymyositis and inclusion-body myositis
- To discuss the coexistence of these diseases with other autoimmune disorders and their association with malignancies
- To describe the antisynthetase syndrome
- To explore the common treatment modalities for these conditions

CASE VIGNETTE

A 70-year-old man complains of leg weakness and inability to close his left hand. He has been experiencing lower extremity weakness for the past 3 years. Initially, he had some difficulty getting up from the floor while playing with his grandchildren, but this has progressed slowly to the point that he can no longer climb stairs. Over the last year, he has sustained four falls because his legs gave out on him. Lately, he has had problems using his left hand, and is unable to make a fist. He had no myalgias. His lipid-lowering medication was discontinued 4 months previously because of laboratory abnormalities, but he had no improvement since then.

On examination, he had quadriceps atrophy bilaterally and hip flexors were weak. A marked weakness was noted in his left third, fourth, and fifth finger flexors, and he was unable to grip with his left hand. Muscle stretch reflexes were symmetric in both upper extremities, but both patellar reflexes were absent. Sensory examination was intact. Cranial nerves were unremarkable.

Laboratory studies showed normocytic or normochromic anemia, mildly elevated creatine kinase (CK) of 430 U/L; normal aldolase, aspartate aminotransferase (AST), and alanine aminotransferase (ALT); and mildly elevated lactate dehydrogenase (LDH) of 199 U/L. Electromyelography (EMG) study showed abnormal spontaneous activity in the left tibialis anterior, rectus femoris, and biceps muscles, consistent with a myopathic process.

DEFINITION

The inflammatory myopathies, commonly referred to as idiopathic inflammatory myopathies (IIM), are a group of autoimmune disorders that affect skeletal muscle causing muscle inflammation and muscle weakness (1,2). Based on their clinical presentation and histologic findings, they can be divided into three major and distinct groups: Dermatomyositis (DM), polymyositis (PM), and inclusion-body myositis (IBM) (1,2). IIM can present as an isolated entity or in association with other autoimmune disorders, connective tissue diseases, and malignancies (3).

EPIDEMIOLOGY

IIM are rare disorders and estimates based on the old Bohan and Peter (4,5) diagnostic criteria report a prevalence of 0.6 to 1.0 per 100,000 in the general population (2,4,5). One of the problems with previous epidemiologic studies is that they failed to distinguish IBM as a separate diagnostic group. Another issue is that diagnosis was not uniformly based on muscle biopsy (6).

DM is seen in children and adults and, as with other connective tissue diseases, is more common in women than men. PM usually occurs after the second decade of life and is also more common in women. Rarely, it can affect the pediatric population (7). Both DM and PM are more common in the black population compared with the white (3). Previously considered uncommon, IBM is now recognized as the most common inflammatory myopathy in patients over the age of 50 (2). In contrast to the previous two entities, IBM is more common in men than in women and affects more whites than blacks.

ETIOLOGY AND PATHOGENESIS

Despite the many advances in understanding the IIM, the etiology of these diseases remains unknown. An autoimmune origin is suggested by the presence of autoantibodies and histocompatibility antigens, the evidence of complement activation, the identification of autoaggressive T cell, and their response to immunotherapies (8). As with other autoimmune disorders, a combination of environmental factors and genetic susceptibility act together triggering the disease.

The IIM show strong association with human leukocyte antigens (HLA). In the case of PM and DM, an increased association appears to exist with HLA DR3 phenotype. As for IBM, there is a threefold increased incidence of the DR1 phenotype, and a slight increase in the DR3 phenotype (9). Regarding possible environmental culprits, different viruses have been implicated in cases of chronic myositis (1,2,9,10).

In DM, the inflammatory infiltrates observed in the perimysial and perivascular areas consist mainly of B cells and CD4+ T cells (discussed below), which is compatible with a humorally mediated process. The earliest and most specific lesion in DM is the deposition of complement C5b-9 membranolytic attack complex (MAC) on capillaries that precedes the presence of the typical inflammatory infiltrate (11). Following the deposition of MAC, there is destruction of capillaries with focal capillary depletion, resulting in ischemia, hypoperfusion, muscle fiber destruction, and inflammation (12). This is reflected by the characteristic perifascicular atrophy seen in DM (13).

In PM and IBM, current evidence supports an antigen-directed major histocompatibility complex (MHC) class I restricted cytotoxicity process rather than a humorally mediated one (2,14,15). The inflammatory infiltrates are mainly constituted by CD8+ T cells, followed by macrophages and sparse CD4+ T cells. In normal muscle fibers, MHC class I (MHC-I) antigen is not expressed. In contrast, in PM and IBM, the muscle fibers strongly express MHC-I antigen, which are then invaded by CD8+ T cells. Because the MHC-I–CD8 complex is so specific to these two entities, its identification was recently incorporated as part of the diagnostic criteria, even in the absence of an inflammatory infiltrate (2,8,13).

Interestingly, in IBM, the cytotoxic T cells do not invade the vacuolated fibers, but only the nonvacuolated ones. This suggests that two independent processes are involved in the pathogenesis of this disease: One immunologic, similar to what is seen in polymyositis, and another degenerative (8). This could explain why patients with IBM are refractory to immunotherapies (see below).

PATHOLOGY

Muscle biopsy is the definitive test required to confirm the diagnosis and to exclude other neuromuscular diseases. The histopathologic hallmark is the presence of inflammatory infiltrates, but location and characteristics of these differ among the three entities.

In DM, cellular infiltrates are predominantly perifascicular and perivascular. B cells and CD4+ T cells are the predominant cells, but macrophages and CD8+ T cells are also found. A typical finding in biopsies of patients with DM is the presence of perifascicular atrophy.

The presence of inflammatory infiltrates within the fascicle is essential for the diagnosis of PM. T cells with a predominance of CD8+ cells invade healthy muscle fibers that express MHC class I antigen. There is evidence of necrotic fibers scattered throughout the fascicles and perifascicular atrophy is not seen (2,8,13).

The typical findings in IBM are inflammatory infiltrates within the fascicles, vacuolated muscle fibers, and detection of amyloid deposits inside the fibers (2,13,16). Like in PM, the cellular infiltrates are mostly constituted of CD8+ T cells and the muscle fibers also express MHC-I antigen.

CLINICAL MANIFESTATIONS AND SPECIAL SITUATIONS

Muscle weakness is the most common presenting symptom in all three groups of IIM (1,2,9). Muscle involvement is usually symmetric and proximal. It develops insidiously, over weeks to months, although in rare cases it can be more acute. In IBM, symptoms will progress over years until the diagnosis is confirmed (17). Patients will have difficulty in performing tasks of daily living, such as climbing stairs, getting up from a seated position, or combing the hair. Neck extensors may be involved, causing head drop (1,2,9). On examination, muscle weakness is objectively confirmed in affected muscle groups. Facial muscles are usually spared, and ocular muscles are never affected. If their involvement is suggested by physical examination, the diagnosis of IIM should be reconsidered (1). Sensory examination is intact, as well as muscle stretch reflexes, unless the degree of muscle atrophy is severe. Weakness of the oropharyngeal musculature as well as the upper third of the esophagus can cause dysphagia (1,2,9). Early recognition is important to avoid complications, such as aspiration pneumonia. In dramatic cases, respiratory muscles can be affected and patients require mechanical ventilation. Myalgias are reported in 30% of cases, but they seldom cause significant disability (2).

Constitutional symptoms, such as fever and weight loss, may be present as well as nonerosive inflammatory polyarthritis (2). Patients may report Raynaud's phenomenon, especially when they have an associated connective tissue disease, such as scleroderma. Interstitial lung disease can complicate the course of IIM and those patients are classified under a subgroup called the *antisynthetase syndrome*. Cardiac involvement was reported in 30% of patients with PM in an autopsy study, even in the absence of overt clinical manifestations (i.e., congestive heart failure) (18).

DERMATOMYOSITIS

DM is easily recognized by the presence of a skin rash that can precede or occur concomitantly with the muscle weakness. The two classic skin lesions in DM are the heliotrope sign (violaceous discoloration of both upper eye lids) and the Gottron's sign (erythematous rash, occasionally scaly, over the knuckles, but sparing the phalanges) (2,9). Patients may also have an erythematous flat rash in areas of sun exposure, such as in the face, neck, and anterior chest (usually V shaped) or in the back and shoulders (shawl sign) (1). Other cutaneous manifestations include periungual erythema and abnormalities of nailbed capillaries. In the juvenile form of this disease, patients may have calcinosis (subcutaneous calcifications), which seems to correlate with disease severity and delay in treatment. At times, DM can occur without muscle involvement, a condition referred to as *dermatomyositis sine myositis* or *amyopathic dermatomyositis* (19).

POLYMYOSITIS

PM as an isolated entity is considered a rare disorder (20). Because symptoms can mimic other myopathies, PM remains a diagnosis of exclusion, and diagnosis should be secured by muscle biopsy showing the typical changes described earlier. PM should be considered in patients who present with symmetric muscle weakness who do not have a rash, involvement of eye and facial muscles, family history of neuromuscular disease, history of exposure to drugs or toxins, endocrine disorders, dystrophy, or biochemical muscle disease. The most common myopathy misdiagnosed as PM is IBM (1,2).

INCLUSION-BODY MYOSITIS

Certain clinical findings should alert the physician for the possibility of IBM. Early involvement of the quadriceps with atrophy seems to be a characteristic feature. Patients report frequent falls from knee buckling (16,17). Distal and asymmetric muscle involvement are seen in 30% of the cases. A typical sign of IBM is involvement of finger flexors, with an inability to make a fist and to hold or manipulate objects (16,17). Mild facial muscle weakness is common in patients with IBM (2).

ASSOCIATION WITH OTHER CONNECTIVE TISSUE DISORDERS

The inflammatory myopathies can be associated with other connective tissue disorders, such as scleroderma, systemic lupus erythematous, rheumatoid arthritis, Sjögren syndrome, and mixed connective tissue disease (2). The most common association is with scleroderma (21).

ASSOCIATION WITH MALIGNANCIES

The relationship of inflammatory myopathies with malignancies has been the subject of controversy. It is generally accepted that a higher risk of malignancy exists among patients with myositis, especially in older patients with dermatomyositis. The association is much stronger in the first 5 years after diagnosis. Most experts would agree that an age- and risk-specific screening for occult malignancy is sufficient in those patients (2).

ANTISYNTHETASE SYNDROME

Antisynthetase syndrome is characterized by the association of inflammatory myopathy, fever, Raynaud phenomenon, nonerosive inflammatory arthritis, and severe interstitial lung disease. Patients also have a typical appearance of their hands (called *mechanic's hands*, with fissuring of the palms and lateral aspects of the fingers resembling the hands of a mechanic). The hallmark of this syndrome is the presence of antihistidyl-transfer RNA (tRNA) synthetase antibodies, which in 80% of affected individuals is the anti-Jo1 antibody. This syndrome is more common among women (2). Because of lung involvement, patients have a poor prognosis.

DIAGNOSTIC APPROACH

The diagnosis of inflammatory myopathies is suggested on clinical grounds, supported by the presence of elevated muscle enzymes and evidence of a myopathic process on electromyography, and confirmed by muscle biopsy. The most sensitive muscle enzyme is CK, which can be elevated up to 50 times, although in IBM this is more modest (usually up to 10 times). Aldolase, AST, ALT, and LDH may be elevated as well. Serum electrolytes, calcium, magnesium, phosphorus, and thyroid-stimulating hormone (TSH) should always be checked to exclude other causes of muscle weakness and elevated CK.

Electromyography shows increased insertional activity, with spontaneous fibrillations and bizarre high-frequency discharges, as well as short-duration and low-amplitude polyphasic units on voluntary activation. Those findings are useful to confirm a myopathic process but are not disease specific (2). About 30% of patients with IBM show signs of axonal neuropathy in the electromyography (1).

Muscle biopsy is the definitive test for the diagnosis of inflammatory myopathies (1,2,13). Skin biopsy may confirm the diagnosis in cases of DM, and avoid the need for a more invasive procedure. The following general recommendations in relationship to muscle biopsy are advisable: (*a*) open biopsy is preferred over needle guided; (*b*) muscles to be sampled should be affected clinically, but should not have significant atrophy; (*c*) in cases where muscle weakness cannot be detected by physical examination, muscle MRI may be obtained to guide biopsy site; (*d*) muscles that have been examined by EMG should not be biopsied earlier than 30 days after EMG needle examination; (*e*) the biopsy sample should be processed for frozen sections and with enzyme and immunohistochemistry staining (paraffin preparations can dissolve the granular material present in IBM making vacuoles easy to miss); and (*f*) if a biopsy fails to confirm the diagnosis despite clinical evidence of inflammatory myopathy, consider taking another sample from a different muscle, because inflammation is often spotty (13).

MAGNETIC RESONANCE IMAGING AND MYOSITIS-SPECIFIC ANTIBODIES

MRI, although not as specific as muscle biopsy, has been shown to be beneficial in assessing the presence and extent of muscle inflammation (22). In active myositis, MRI shows increased signal intensities on T2-weighted fat or non–fat-saturated images, indicating edema. In chronic myositis, high signal intensities are seen in both T1- and T2-weighted sequences, suggesting fatty tissue infiltration (22,23). MRI is particularly useful as a noninvasive tool to localize muscle inflammation for biopsy site selection in cases of absence of objective proximal muscle weakness (24). It can also be used to determine if a patient has active myositis or *burnt out* disease.

Antinuclear antibodies are detected in up to 80% of patients with DM and PM; however, they are not specific for these disorders. Antibodies against cytoplasmic antigens, such as ribonucleoproteins involved in protein synthesis (antisynthetase) or translational transport (anti–signal-recognition particle), as well as certain nuclear antigens are found in about 20% of patients (2). They have been called *myositis-specific antibodies* but their pathogenic role remains uncertain. They seem to be useful in identifying discrete subgroups of patients with characteristic clinical manifestations and prognosis (i.e., antisynthetase syndrome) (24,25).

TREATMENT

Because of the rare and heterogeneous nature of these disorders, few controlled prospective clinical trials have addressed specific treatment modalities. Another setback in the treatment of IIM is the lack of reliable outcome measures (26). Therapeutic response should be assessed by an improvement, or at least stabilization, in muscle strength rather than normalization of muscle enzyme level (chemical response) (2). In DM, improvement or resolution of the skin rash is also expected.

Despite lack of controlled studies, corticosteroids are considered the agents of choice for the initial treatment of PM and DM (1,2,26). Usually, prednisone is started in a dose of 1 mg/kg, either as a single daily dose or divided throughout the day. The latter regimen is more immunosuppressive, but carries higher toxicity potential. Another possibility, particularly in severe cases or in cases associated with interstitial lung disease, is to use intravenous pulse methylprednisolone (i.e., 1 g daily for 3 days) for rapid disease control. High doses of prednisone are kept for approximately 2 months and then reduced by 20% to 25% every month until a small dose of 5 or 10 mg/day is achieved (2,26). Patients are evaluated monthly and response should be measured as a combination of CK level, muscle strength, and functional status. The role of steroids in IBM remains controversial; in most cases, corticosteroids do not seem to be beneficial (2,16,27). Some experts feel that its use may be justified because of an improvement in endurance reported by a few patients (16).

Immunosuppressive drugs are used in different circumstances: In patients who respond to steroids but develop significant side effects (need for steroid sparing agent); in patients who relapse every time a steroid taper is attempted; in patients who failed to respond, despite a course of high-dose prednisone; and in patients with progressive weakness and lung involvement (2,26). Among the drugs used, azathioprine and methotrexate, either alone or in combination, are the most popular choices. Methotrexate is started at 7.5 mg orally weekly and can be titrated up to 25 mg. Complete blood count, liver function tests, and creatinine should be monitored every 8 weeks. Azathioprine is given orally at doses of 1.5 to 3.0 mg/ kg daily, and it has been shown to benefit some patients with polymyositis (28). Other drugs used with various rates of success are cyclosporine, cyclophosphamide, fludarabine, mycophenolate mofetil, and tacrolimus. The choice of the immunosuppressive medications largely depends on personal experience rather than on well-designed controlled trials.

Intravenous immune globulin (IVIg) is effective in the treatment of DM, but its effects are short lived and repeated infusions are required (29). IVIg has not been beneficial in cases of IBM (30).

Other aspects of management include the use of sun-blocking agents in patients with DM, speech pathology evaluation to assess for possible dysphagia and prevent aspiration, and physical and occupational therapy to help maintain functional status. Adaptive devices and the use of orthotic devices may prolong the ability to ambulate and delay the need for a wheelchair.

CLINICAL RECOMMENDATIONS OF THE VIGNETTE

The patient has classic signs of IBM: Muscle weakness progressing over years, quadriceps involvement, and finger flexor weakness. Diagnosis should be confirmed by muscle biopsy of one of the affected muscles. As mentioned, IBM is often refractory to available treatment modalities but most physicians would attempt a treatment trial with corticosteroids and, possibly, immunosuppressive medication. If the patient does not show any meaningful response after 3 to 6 months of therapy, medications should be tapered off. Supportive care should not be overlooked and the patient should be evaluated by speech pathology to assess the presence of dysphagia and address techniques that could help prevent aspiration. Physical and occupational therapy should be provided to help maintain functional capacity.

SUMMARY

The IIM are a heterogeneous group of autoimmune acquired disorders that include DM, PM, and IBM. They can occur isolated or in association with other connective tissue disorders or malignancies. They all have in common inflammation of skeletal muscle and progressive muscle weakness. The specific target antigen triggering these diseases has not yet been identified. Current understanding supports the idea that DM is a humorally mediated disease, and PM and IBM are mediated by cytotoxic T cells. In IBM, a degenerative process seems to be responsible in part for its pathogenesis and may explain why this entity is refractory to immunosuppressive therapy. The identification of myositis-specific antibodies characterizes distinct subgroups, of which the best known is anti-Jo1, in antisynthetase syndrome. Most accepted therapies have not been tested in a controlled prospective fashion, but corticosteroids and other immunosuppressive agents are the most commonly used agents.

REFERENCES

1. Dalakas MC. Polymyositis, dermatomyositis, and inclusion-body myositis. *N Engl J Med.* 1991;325:1487–1498.
2. Dalakas MC, Hohlfeld R. Polymyositis and dermatomyositis. *Lancet.* 2003;362:971–982.
3. Mastaglia FL, Phillips BA. Idiopathic inflammatory myopathies: Epidemiology, classification, and diagnostic criteria. *Rheum Dis Clin North Am.* 2002;28:723–741.
4. Bohan A, Peter JB. Polymyositis and dermatomyositis. Part 1. *N Engl J Med.* 1975;292:344–347.
5. Bohan A, Peter JB. Polymyositis and dermatomyositis. Part 2. *N Engl J Med.* 1975;292:403–407.
6. Bohan A, Peter JB, Bowman RL, et al. A computer-assisted analysis of 153 patients with polymyositis and dermatomyositis. *Medicine.* 1977;56:255–286.
7. Ramanan AV, Feldman BM. Clinical features and outcomes of juvenile dermatomyositis and other childhood onset myositis syndromes. *Rheum Dis Clin North Am.* 2002;28:833–857.
8. Dalakas MC. Inflammatory disorders of muscle: Progress in polymyositis, dermatomyositis and inclusion body myositis. *Curr Opin Neurol.* 2004;17:561–567.
9. Plotz PH, Dalakas M, Leff RL, et al. Current concepts in the idiopathic inflammatory myopathies: Polymyositis, dermatomyositis, and related disorders. *Ann Intern Med.* 1989;111: 143–157.
10. Nagaraju K, Plotz PH. Animal models of myositis. *Rheum Dis Clin North Am.* 2002;28: 917–933.
11. Emslie-Smith AM, Engel AG. Microvascular changes in early and advanced dermatomyositis: A quantitative study. *Ann Neurol.* 1990;27:343–356.
12. Dalakas MC. Immunopathogenesis of inflammatory myopathies. *Ann Neurol.* 1995;37(S1): S74–S86.
13. Dalakas MC. Muscle biopsy findings in inflammatory myopathies. *Rheum Dis Clin North Am.* 2002;28:779–798.
14. Hohlfeld R, Engel AG. Coculture with autologous myotubes of cytotoxic T cells isolated from muscle in inflammatory myopathies. *Ann Neurol.* 1991;29:498–507.
15. Hofbauer M, Weissner S, Babbe H, et al. Clonal tracking of autoaggressive T cells in polymyositis by combining laser microdissection, single-cell PCR, and CD3-spectratype analysis. *Proc Natl Acad Sci U S A.* 2003;100:4090–4095.
16. Engel WK, Askanas V. Inclusion-body myositis: Clinical, diagnostic, and pathologic aspects. *Neurology.* 2006;66(S1):S20–S29.
17. Sekul EA, Dalakas MC. Inclusion body myositis: New concepts. *Semin Neurol.* 1993;13: 256–263.
18. Denbow CE, Lie JT, Tancredi RG, et al. Cardiac involvement in polymyositis: A clinicopathologic study of 20 autopsied patients. *Arthritis Rheum.* 1979;22:1088–1092.
19. Stonecipher MR, Jorizzo JL, White WL, et al. Cutaneous changes of dermatomyositis in patients with normal muscle enzymes: Dermatomyositis sine myositis? *J Am Acad Dermatol.* 1993;28:951–956.
20. van der Meulen MF, Bronner IM, Hoogendijk JE, et al. Polymyositis: An overdiagnosed entity. *Neurology.* 2003;61: 316–321.
21. Troyanov Y, Targoff IN, Tremblay JL, et al. Novel classification of idiopathic inflammatory myopathies based on overlap syndrome features and autoantibodies: Analysis of 100 French Canadian patients. *Medicine.* 2005;84:231–249.
22. Reimers CD, Finkenstaedt M. Muscle imaging in inflammatory myopathies. *Curr Opin Rheum.* 1997;4:475–485.
23. Dion E, Cherin P, Payan C, et al. Magnetic resonance imaging criteria for distinguishing between inclusion body myositis and polymyositis. *J Rheumatol.* 2002;29:1897–1906.
24. Targoff IN, Miller FW, Medsger TA, et al. Classification criteria for the idiopathic inflammatory myopathies. *Curr Opin Rheum.* 1997;9:527–535.
25. Love LA, Leff RL, Fraser DD, et al. A new approach to the classification of idiopathic inflammatory myopathy: Myositis-specific autoantibodies define useful homogeneous patient groups. *Medicine.* 1991;70:360–374.
26. Oddis CV. Idiopathic inflammatory myopathy: Management and prognosis. *Rheum Dis Clin North Am.* 2002;28:979–1001.
27. Griggs RC. The current status of treatment for inclusion-body myositis. *Neurology.* 2006;66:S30–S32.
28. Bunch TW. Prednisone and azathioprine for polymyositis: Long-term follow up. *Arthritis Rheum.* 1981;24:45–48.
29. Dalakas MC, Illa I, Dambrosia JM, et al. A controlled trial of high-dose intravenous immune globulin infusions as treatment for dermatomyositis. *N Engl J Med.* 1993;329:1993–2000.
30. Dalakas MC, Koffman B, Fujii M, et al. A controlled study of intravenous immunoglobulin combined with prednisone in the treatment of IBM. *Neurology.* 2001;56:323–327.

CHAPTER 88

Heritable Connective Tissue Diseases

Silvina B. Tonarelli • Oscar Benavente

The term "heritable connective tissue disorder" applies to a well-characterized, but unknown group of connective tissue diseases caused by mutations in genes encoding extracellular matrix constituents as collagens. The phenotype of each disorder is determined by the organ distribution of the affected extracellular matrix. The cell–matrix interactions critically determine biological functions in all tissues, and consequently matrix gene mutations can underlie functional failures of internal organs, the nervous system, and blood vessels (1).

Four inherited connective tissue disorders are described in this chapter that can present neurologic manifestations: Vascular Ehlers-Danlos syndrome (type IV), Marfan syndrome, osteogenesis imperfecta, and pseudoxanthoma elasticum. Also briefly depicted are neurofibromatosis and autosomal dominant polycystic kidney disease, because of the high prevalence of neurologic manifestations.

OBJECTIVES

- To describe the most common manifestations of selective heritable connective tissue disorders
- To discuss the important neurologic findings of these diseases
- To provide information about the main molecular defects and the type of inheritance in each of these conditions
- To explain the implications for screening in asymptomatic patients
- To explore the different treatments and recommendations in special situations

CASE VIGNETTE 1

A 25-year-old woman presents with headaches and transient left hemiparesis after a minor trauma while skiing. On examination, she has several bruises and hyperextensibility of the skin, findings that are common in other family members.

Vascular Ehlers-Danlos Syndrome

DEFINITION

Ehlers-Danlos syndrome (EDS) encompasses at least 10 clinically and genetically heterogeneous connective tissue disorders characterized by fragility of tissues, joint hypermobility, and skin hyperextensibility (2,3) (Table 88-1). Some patients with EDS develop peripheral neuropathy caused by lax ligaments. Clubfoot and congenital dislocation of the hip have been reported (4). Vascular or ecchymotic EDS (type IV) has special importance to neurologists and neurosurgeons because of the high frequency of neurovascular complications.

EPIDEMIOLOGY

The incidence of EDS type IV is estimated at 4% of the total cases of EDS. It affects males and females with nearly equal frequency. Approximately 5% of patients with EDS type IV have their first vascular event by age 20 years, and 80% by age 40 years (4). The median survival time of EDS type IV is approximately 50 years. The main cause of death is spontaneous rupture of large arteries and hollow organs, specially the uterus and colon. Risk of uterine and vessel rupture is especially high during pregnancy (5).

ETIOLOGY AND PATHOGENESIS

The underlying defect of EDS type IV is an abnormality of collagen type III, a main component of distensible tissues, such as skin, blood vessels, and hollow viscera (6).

The inheritance is autosomal dominant, resulting from heterozygous mutations in the COA3A1 on chromosome 2, ensuing in structural defects of procollagen type III.

PATHOLOGY

Pathologic examination of the arteries may show fragmented elastic fibers, absent elastin, decreased collagen content, and distorted collagen fibril architecture (7).

CLINICAL MANIFESTATIONS

Clinical diagnosis of EDS type IV is based on at least two of the following diagnostic criteria: Easy bruising; translucent skin with visible veins; typical facial features of thinness, sunken cheeks, protruding eyes, thin nose and lips, and lobeless ears; and arterial, intestinal, or uterine rupture. Compared with others types of EDS, the hyperextensibility of skin and joint hypermobility is mild and often limited to the digits (8–10).

TABLE 88-1. Classification of Ehlers-Danlos Syndrome

	Type	*Skin*	*Joint*	*Other Features*	*Inheritance*	*Primary Defect*
Classic type	I	+++	+++	Normal wound healing	AD	Collagen V defect
	II	++	++	Vascular and intestinal		Tenascin-X
	II/III			complications	AR	deficiency
Hypermobile type	III	+	+++	Arthritis	AD	?
Vascular type	IV	+++	+	Rupture of arteries, intestine, uterus. Pneumothorax, acrogeria	AD	Collagen type III
	V	++	+		X linked	?
Kyphoscoliotic type	VI	+++	+++	Rupture of arteries and the eye globe; hypotonia, kyphoscoliosis	AR	Deficiency in lysyl hydroxylase
Arthrochalasic	VIIA/B	++	+++	Fractures and hip luxations	AD	Collagen type I
Dermatosparatic	VII C	++++	+	Skin doughy and lax	AR	Procollagen 1
	VIII	++	++	Periodontal disease	AD	?
	IX	+	+	Exostoses, occipital horns, mental retardation	X linked	Copper transporting
	X	+	++	Platelet dysfunction	?	Defect in fibronectin?

AD, autosomal dominant; AR, autosomal recessive.

Cardiovascular manifestations include ventricular and atrial septal defects, aortic insufficiency, bicuspid aortic valve, mitral valve prolapse, and papillary muscle dysfunction. EDS type IV is a rare cause of stroke in the young, but should be suspected in patients with otherwise unexplained cervicocephalic arterial dissections, intracranial aneurysms, or carotid cavernous sinus fistula (11–17). Intracranial aneurysms can be the initial manifestation, most commonly involving the internal carotid artery, typically in the cavernous sinus. Rupture of intracranial aneurysms in this location can result in spontaneous carotid-cavernous sinus fistula (17,18). Some patients develop carotid-cavernous fistulae spontaneously or following minor trauma. Clinical presentation of carotid-cavernous fistulae can include diplopia, pulsatile exophthalmus, thrill, and tinnitus. Endovascular treatment is preferred over surgery, although with a high mortality rate (50%) (12). Cervical arterial dissections of extracranial and intracranial segments of the vertebral or carotid arteries are known complications of vascular EDS (15,19).

DIAGNOSTIC APPROACH

Diagnosis of vascular EDS is made with fibroblast culture and biochemical studies of collagen metabolism that confirm the presence of the abnormal type III procollagen molecules. Also, identification of mutations in the type III procollagen gene (COL3A1) on chromosome 2 corroborates the diagnosis (4,10,20). Noninvasive diagnostic methods, such as computerized tomography angiography (CTA) or magnetic resonance angiography (MRA), are recommended for the diagnosis of neurovascular complications (cervical dissections or intracranial aneurysms). Routinely screening for asymptomatic intracranial aneurysms is generally not advisable given the high risk of complications with digital catheter angiogram and uncertainty about best treatment (16,21).

TREATMENT

Although no available specific therapies currently exist, awareness of the diagnosis of EDS type IV has major practical implications. Women should be advised about pregnancy and followed at specialized centers (4). Management of skin and joint problems should be conservative and preventive. Surgical or endovascular treatment of asymptomatic intracranial aneurysms is indicated in selected cases (19,22). Treatment of cervicocephalic arterial dissection associated with EDS should be conservative.

CASE VIGNETTE 2

A 50-year-old woman had lower back pain confined to the sacral area and urinary incontinence. Remarkable findings on examination were pectum excavatum, joint laxity, and ectopia lentis.

Marfan Syndrome

DEFINITION

Marfan syndrome (MS) is an autosomal dominant connective tissue disorder that involves many organs, but its more notorious manifestations are in the skeletal, ocular, and cardiovascular systems.

EPIDEMIOLOGY

The prevalence of MS is estimated at 2 to 3 cases per 10,000 individuals, but it is a condition that tends to be under diagnosed because of its variability and age dependence. No ethnic or demographic preference appears to exist (23).

ETIOLOGY AND PATHOGENESIS

MS is characterized by variable clinical expression explained by the large number of mutations in the gene encoding fibrillin-1 (FBN1) on chromosome 15q21.1, with a second locus at 3p24.2-p25 (24–27). About 30% of cases are sporadic (28). FBN1 is one of the major components of the microfibrils. The microfibrils are important constituents of the extracellular matrix distributed throughout the body in elastic tissues, such as the aorta and skin, and in nonelastic tissues, such as the ciliary zonules of the ocular lens (29). The distribution of these microfibrils explains the variety of findings of MS.

PATHOLOGY

Although many reports of autopsies, histopathology, and ultrastructure are available, no changes are entirely characteristics of MS.

CLINICAL MANIFESTATIONS

Patients with MS (Table 88-2) have a disproportionate stature, with long arms and legs. The ribs also overgrow and push the sternum either in (pectus excavatum) or out (pectus carinatum). Joint laxity and hypermobility are common. Skeletal muscle development is poor, causing an asthenic habitus (28). Main cutaneous and integument manifestations are striae athropicae, occurring in areas of flexural stress; and recurrent hernia. Dural ectasia or dilatation of the dural sac usually occurs at the L5-S1 level (30). Mild cases are often asymptomatic, but moderate to severe lumbosacral dural ectasia can lead to low back pain or radicular pain caused by nerve root compression in the lumbosacral canal. Neurosurgical repair of these dural ectasias can provide symptomatic relief (31,32). Ectopia lentis, myopia, strabismus, astigmatism, glaucoma, and cataracts are the most frequent ocular problems. Mitral valve prolapse, coarctation of the aorta, mitral annulus calcification, dilation of the main pulmonary artery, and dilation or dissections of the descending thoracic or abdominal aorta are frequently found cardiovascular manifestations (33,34). Aneurysmal dilation and dissection of the ascending aorta may account for brain ischemia or paraparesis because of involvement of spinal cord arteries (35). Pregnant women have an increased risk of aortic dissection (28,36). Intracranial aneurysms (saccular or fusiform) and intracranial dissecting aneurysms have also been described. Evidence for this association is based, however, on small case series and the true prevalence is unknown (37–43). Cardiovascular manifestations remain the main cause of death. Childhood mortality is often related to aortic and mitral valve insufficiency. Mortality in adults is often associated with spontaneous aortic rupture or aortic dissection (44).

DIAGNOSTIC APPROACH

Diagnosis is based on thorough clinical examination, including measurements of body proportions, ophthalmologic evaluation, radiographs, and echocardiography of the aorta. A family history is an essential part of the diagnosis, in conjunction with genetic family tests or mutation identification.

TREATMENT

The cornerstones of management are timely diagnosis, prospective appraisal, prophylactic intervention, and genetic counseling.

TABLE 88-2. Marfan Syndrome: Phenotypic Manifestations

SKELETAL SYSTEM

Major criterion: Pectus carinatum or severe pectus excavatum; positive wrist and thumb signs. Reduced upper to lower segment ratio or arm span to height ratio >1.05; scoliosis of >20° or spondylolithesis; reduced extension of the elbows (<170°); medial displacement of the medial malleolus associated with pes planus; protrusio acetabulae of any degree (ascertained on X-ray, computed tomography [CT], magnetic resonance imaging [MRI])

Minor criteria: Pectus excavatum of moderate severity, joint hypermobility, highly arched palate with dental crowding, facial appearance (dolicocephaly, malar hypoplasia, enophthalmos, retrognathia, downslanting, palpebral fissures)

OCULAR SYSTEM

Major criterion: Ectopia lentis

Minor criteria: Flat cornea, increased axial length of globe (>23.5 mm), hypoplastic iris or hypoplastic ciliary muscle causing miosis

CARDIOVASCULAR SYSTEM

Major criteria: Dilatation or dissection of the ascending aorta, with or without aortic regurgitation, and involving at least the sinuses of Valsalva

Minor criteria: Mitral valve prolapse, with or without mitral valve regurgitation; dilatation of main pulmonary artery, in absence of valvular or peripheral pulmonic stenosis, under the age of 40 years; calcification of the mitral annulus under the age of 40 years; or dilatation or dissection of the descending thoracic or abdominal aorta under the age of 50 years

PULMONARY SYSTEM

Minor criteria: Spontaneous pneumothorax, or apical blebs (radiographic evidence)

SKIN AND INTEGUMENT

Minor criteria: Either striae atrophicae not associated with marked weight changes, pregnancy, or repetitive stress, or recurrent or incisional herniae

DURA

Major criterion: Lumbosacral dural ectasia

FAMILY HISTORY

Major criteria: Having a first-degree relative who meets diagnostic criteria listed below independently. Presence of a mutation in FBN1* known to cause Marfan syndrome

Presence of a haplotype around FBN1*, inherited by descent, known to be associated with unequivocally diagnosed Marfan syndrome in the family

REQUIREMENTS FOR DIAGNOSIS OF MARFAN SYNDROME

For the index case:

Major criterion in at least two different organ systems and a third must be involved

For a family member:

Major criterion in the family history and one major criterion in an organ system and involvement of a second organ system

FBN1*, fibrillin 1.

Pseudoxanthoma Elasticum

DEFINITION

Pseudoxanthoma elasticum (PXE) is an inherited connective tissue disease characterized by progressive calcification and fragmentation of elastic fibers in the skin, eyes, and cardiovascular system (45).

EPIDEMIOLOGY

PXE has a high heterogeneity regarding age of onset, extent, and severity of organ involvement. The prevalence of PXE is estimated at 1 of 100,000 individuals. The mean age of clinical onset is 13 years, although delayed onset in the fifth or sixth decade of life has been reported.

ETIOLOGY AND PATHOGENESIS

Mutations that cause PXE are in the adenosine triphosphate-binding cassette subtype C number 6 (ABCC6) genes, which encode an adenosine triphosphate-dependent transmembrane transporter. Autosomal recessive and autosomal dominant forms have being described. The locus has been mapped to chromosome 16p13.1, but the mechanism still remains unknown (46).

PATHOLOGY

Skin biopsy shows fragmentation of elastic fibers, with calcification and secondary proliferation of the intima (47). An increased content of glycosaminoglycans in affected elastic tissue has been demonstrated.

CLINICAL MANIFESTATIONS

The clinical spectrum of the disease ranges from mild manifestations to severe or fatal cardiovascular complications. The typical skin changes consist of yellowish grouped papules beginning on the lateral aspect of the neck giving rise to a *plucked chicken* appearance. Other sites of predilection include the axillae, periumbilical area, groin, perineum, and thighs. Similar lesions can occur in the soft palate, inner aspect of the lips, and vagina. Laxity and thickening are prominent in the axilla, groin, neck, and antecubital and popliteal spaces (48). Absence of skin or mucosal membrane lesions does not exclude PXE (49). Opthalmoscopic examination may show a mottled appearance of the retina, as well as angiod streaks caused by the breakdown of the elastic lamina of Bruch's membrane. Visual loss is generally caused by development of a choroidal neovascular membrane or infarction of the anterior visual pathways, most commonly involving the orbital segment of the optic nerve. Macular degeneration and retinal hemorrhages may be present (50–54). Cardiovascular complications are common because calcification of the internal elastic lamina of mostly medium-sized arteries causes arterial stenosis, occlusion, or aneurysmatic disease (55). Increased risk of ischemic infarction is common in the fifth or sixth decades. Cerebral ischemia can be caused by large artery, or less frequently, by small vessel disease. Multiple cerebral infarctions are not unusual (56–58). Early onset of arteriosclerosis and arterial hypertension are common. Many patients have vascular claudication of the lower extremities and abdominal ischemia. A network of abnormal vessels between the external carotid and internal carotid arteries (rete mirabile), associated with carotid artery hypoplasia, may be present (59–61). Mitral valve prolapse is the most common valvular dysfunction (62–64). Intracranial aneurysms, spontaneous dissections of cervical arteries, arteriovenous malformations, and cervical spinal cord ischemia associated with PXE have been described (57,65–67). Gastrointestinal bleeding occurs primarily in adults.

DIAGNOSTIC APPROACH

Serial echocardiographic assessments and routine opthalmoscopic examinations are valuable in patients with PXE and skin biopsy confirms the diagnosis.

TREATMENT

Careful control of vascular risk factors (arterial hypertension, hyperlipidemia, diabetes) helps to minimize the arterial complications. Precaution with antiplatelet treatment for secondary stroke prevention is critical because of increased risk of gastrointestinal hemorrhage.

Osteogenesis Imperfecta

DEFINITION

Osteogenesis imperfecta (OI), also known as *brittle bone disease*, consists of a heterogeneous group of inheritable, mostly autosomal dominant, connective tissue disorders.

EPIDEMIOLOGY

OI affects about 1 of 10,000 individuals. Phenotypic presentation is varied, ranging from death in the perinatal period to a normal lifespan with only minimal increase in fractures (68,69).

ETIOLOGY AND PATHOGENESIS

The molecular defect results from mutations in the genes encoding the chains of type I collagen, the major protein of the extracellular matrix of bone, tendons, and skin (70). Mild forms of the disease are caused by a decrease of the synthesis of type I procollagen. More severe phenotype presentations are secondary to mutations leading to structural defects of type I procollagen. Type I procollagen molecules contain two pro α_1 chains, and a single pro α_2 chain. The COL1A1 gene encoding the pro α_1 chain is located on the long arm of chromosome 17, whereas the COL1A2 gene is located on the long arm of chromosome 7 (71).

CLINICAL MANIFESTATIONS

OI is mainly characterized by extreme fragility of bone, blue sclerae, hearing loss, defective dentition, and growth retardation. OI type I is the mildest form. Affected individuals have nearly normal stature, with little or no bone deformity. Fractures are frequent during childhood, and decrease in frequency after puberty. Blue sclerae and hearing loss are common. In the perinatal lethal or type II form, most infants die from respiratory failure within 24 hours of birth. OI type III is characterized by progressive bony deformity, fractures at birth, and growth failure. Restrictive lung disease, dentinogenesis imperfecta, and hearing loss are common. Basilar impression compressing the brainstem may account for sleep apnea, headaches, and upper motor neuron signs. One of the most common forms of OI is type IV, characterized by normal sclerae hue, dentinogenesis imperfecta, mild deformity, tendency to fractures, and moderately short stature. OI is also associated with a variety of cerebrovascular complications, including cerebral aneurysms, vertebral artery dissections, spontaneous carotid-cavernous fistulas, and Moya-Moya. OI has been associated with macrocephaly, hydrocephalus, basilar impression resulting from platysbasia, trigeminal neuralgia, and cerebral atrophy (72). Adults with mild OI may also present with manifestations of complex regional pain syndromes. Tendon ruptures are not rare.

DIAGNOSTIC APPROACH

Confirmation of the diagnosis of OI by analysis of collagens produced by cultured dermal fibroblasts or by direct gene analysis is readily available.

TREATMENT

Physiotherapy, rehabilitation, and orthopedic surgery are the mainstay of treatment for patients with OI. Recent studies suggest that therapies, such as biophosphonate and bone marrow transplantation, may hold promise.

Neurofibromatosis

DEFINITION

Neurofibromatosis is an inherited disease that includes at least two different autosomal dominant disorders caused by a different gene: Neurofibromatosis type 1 (NF1), also known as von Recklinghausen disease, and neurofibromatosis type 2 (NF2) (73–75).

EPIDEMIOLOGY

NF1 is one of the most common autosomal disorders, with a prevalence of 1 of 4,000 persons and a complete penetrance in adulthood. NF2, is much less frequent, occurring in about 1 of 50,000 people.

ETIOLOGY AND PATHOGENESIS

NF1 is caused by mutations in the gene (NF1) encoding neurofibromin, a protein with a centrally located domain homologous to the guanosine triphosphatase (GTPase)-activating protein, and located on chromosome 17q11.2 (76–78). NF2 is caused by a mutation of the NF2 gene on chromosome 22, resulting in a protein product schwannomin.

PATHOLOGY

Neurofibromatosis type 1 involves tissue of mesodermal and ectodermal origin. Vascular pathology in NF1 includes a concentric growth of the intima, disruption of the elastica, and molecular aggregates of proliferating smooth muscle cells.

CLINICAL MANIFESTATIONS

Clinical features of NF1 include subcutaneous and plexiform neurofibromas, café-au-lait spots, axillary and inguinal freckling, Lisch nodules (pigmented hamartomas) of the iris, visual pathway gliomas (Fig. 88-1), pheochromocytoma, skeletal deformities (thinning of the cortex of long bones, pseudoarthrosis, and scoliosis), and dural ectasia (79). Vascular occlusive disease is not uncommon in childhood or adolescence, mainly involving the supraclinoid internal carotid artery segment and often associated with a Moya-Moya-like pattern of collateral vessels (80,81). Intracranial aneurysms and fistula formation have also been reported (82–85). Renal artery stenosis with ectasia or aneurysm formation is common, but renovascular hypertension is rare (86). NF2 is primarily limited to the nervous system, and is characterized by bilateral vestibular schwannomas (acoustic neuromas) and various other tumors of the central nervous system (CNS). NF2 is not known to be associated with vascular and skin manifestations (79).

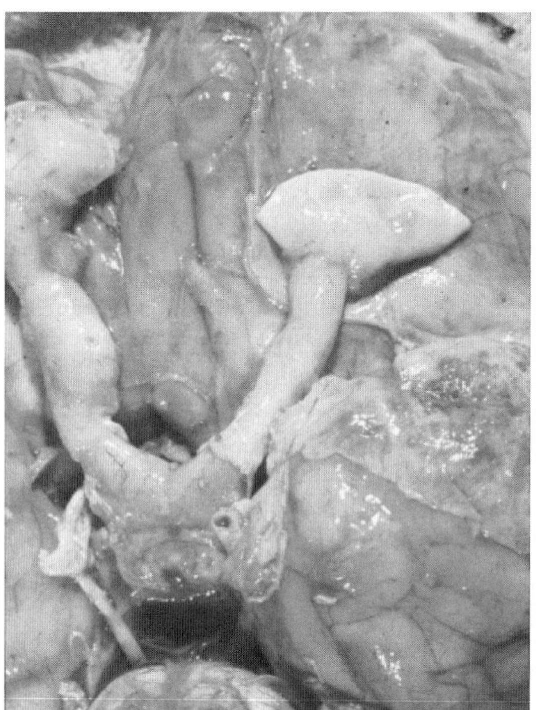

FIGURE 88-1. Optic visual pathway gliomas in neurofibromatosis type 1 (NF1).

DIAGNOSTIC APPROACH

The diagnosis of NF1 is made by the characteristics lesions of the skin and peripheral nerves. The NF2 can be diagnosed from the family history and the findings of neurofibromas at surgery.

TREATMENT

The skin tumors should not be removed unless they are cosmetically objectionable or show an increase in size that suggests malignant change. Cranial and spinal neurofibromas are amenable to excision. Surgical repair of intracranial aneurysms can be complicated by excessive vascular fragility.

Autosomal Dominant Polycystic Kidney Disease

DEFINITION

Autosomal dominant polycystic kidney disease (ADPKD) is a systemic heritable disorder characterized by cyst formation in the kidney and liver, and by gastrointestinal and cardiovascular abnormalities (87).

EPIDEMIOLOGY

ADPKD is the most common monogenetic disorder, affecting 1 of 400 to 1,000 persons in all racial groups worldwide. ADPKD is usually recognized in adults between the third and fourth decades of life.

ETIOLOGY AND PATHOGENESIS

ADPKD is a genetically heterogeneous disease, with mutations identified on genes on chromosome 16p13.3 (PKD1) and on chromosome 4q21-23 (PKD2) (88). Patients with mutations in the PKD1 gene are more severely affected, but intracranial aneurysms are a manifestation of both types. Polycystin-1 and polycystin 2 are the proteins encoded by the PKD1 and PKD2 genes, respectively. Both are integral membrane proteins, with large extracellular domains that probably play a major role in maintaining the structural integrity of the connective tissue extracellular matrix (89).

CLINICAL MANIFESTATIONS

ADPKD is clinically characterized by the presence of cysts in the kidneys, liver, pancreas, spleen, ovaries, and seminal vesicles. Other frequently encountered findings include mitral valve prolapse, intracranial aneurysms, intracranial dolichoectasia, cervicocephalic dissections, arachnoid cysts, and spinal meningeal diverticula. Patients also have an increased risk for developing gastrointestinal diverticula and inguinal hernias. ADPKD can cause secondary arterial hypertension in young adults (90). ADPKD accounts for 2% to 7 % of all patients with intracranial aneurysms (87) (Fig. 88-2). Rupture of intracranial aneurysms is the best known and most feared extrarenal complication and a frequent cause of death among these patients. Screening patients for asymptomatic intracranial aneurysms is often done with MRA; in approximately 10% of cases, one aneurysm is found. In these asymptomatic patients, the size of the aneurysms is usually <6 mm. Subarachnoid hemorrhage (SAH) in patients with ADPKD occurs at an early age, but mortality rates are similar to patients without ADPKD (91). The presence of concomitant polycystic liver disease plus a family history of intracranial aneurysms in patients with ADPKD increase the risk of harboring an intracranial aneurysm.

DIAGNOSTIC APPROACH

In patient with a family history of ADPKD, a diagnosis can be made if one of the radiologic tests (ultrasound, CT, or MRI) shows diffuse cysts in both kidneys and cysts in the liver, pancreas, or brain. Gene linkage studies can be done with a high grade of certainty (87).

TREATMENT

No specific treatment is available to preserve renal function in ADPKD. Arterial hypertension should be treated to keep the blood pressure within the normal range (90). A family history of cerebral aneurysms is an indication for angio-MRI (91). All patients with ADPKD and new onset of headache or neurologic symptoms should be evaluated to rule out intracranial aneurysms.

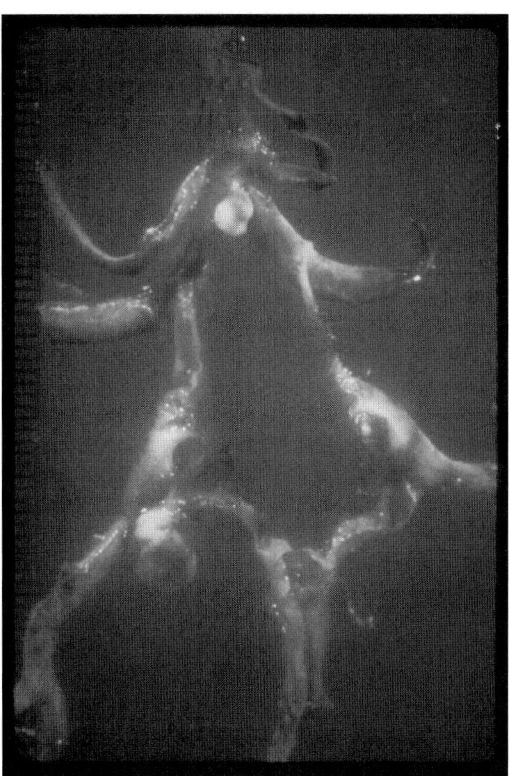

FIGURE 88-2. Circle of Willis in a patient with autosomal dominant polycystic kidney disease (ADPKD) shows multiple intracranial aneurysms.

CLINICAL RECOMMENDATIONS OF THE VIGNETTES

Case 1: EDS type IV should always be considered in young patients with vascular complications, such as arterial cervical dissection as seen in this patient. The diagnosis of EDS is more likely when patients have a positive family history and other systemic findings compromising the skin and joints. Confirmation of the diagnosis of EDS type IV is important and the diagnosis of cervical dissection should be done with noninvasive methods, such as MRA on CTA. Choice of treatment of cervicocephalic arterial dissections in these patients is extremely difficult because antithrombotic treatment can cause excessive bleeding, and stents or surgical treatments carry a high risk of complications.

Case 2: In this patient, the MRI of the lumbar and sacral spinal showed extensive dural ectasia at the L5-S1 level. The patient exemplifies the importance of recognizing dural ectasia, a rare condition in the general population, but one of the most common major criteria of MS.

SUMMARY

The inherited connective tissue diseases represent an uncommon, but well-characterized group of conditions with a defect in the extracellular matrix. Despite their low prevalence, these are important disorders because of the high frequency of complications, mainly neurovascular. The phenotype of each of these diseases is determined by the involved system. Critical is an early diagnosis, with selection of the appropriate tests and adequate management, including genetic counseling. In this chapter were described the most relevant manifestations of these disorders, with particular emphasis on treatment and screening of the asymptomatic carriers.

REFERENCES

1. Bruckner-Tuderman L, Bruckner P. Genetic diseases of the extracellular matrix: More than just connective tissue disorders. *J Mol Med.* 1998;76(3–4):226–237.
2. Burrows NP. The molecular genetics of the Ehlers-Danlos syndrome. *Clin Exp Dermatol.* 1999;24(2):99–106.
3. Royce PM and Steinmann B. *Connective Tissue and Its Heritable Disorders. Molecular, Genetic, and Medical Aspects.* Second Edition. Wiley-Liss. New York, New York. 2000.
4. Pepin M, Schwarze U, Superti-Furga A, et al. Clinical and genetic features of Ehlers-Danlos syndrome type IV, the vascular type. *N Engl J Med.* 2000;342(10):673–680.
5. Rudd NL, Nimrod C, Holbrook KA, et al. Pregnancy complications in type IV Ehlers-Danlos syndrome. *Lancet.* 1983;1(8314-5):50–53.
6. Pyeritz RE. Ehlers-Danlos syndrome. *N Engl J Med.* 2000;342(10):730–732.
7. Lauwers G, Nevelsteen A, Daenen G, et al. Ehlers-Danlos syndrome type IV: A heterogeneous disease. *Ann Vasc Surg.* 1997;11(2):178–182.
8. Dany F, Fraysse A, Priollet P, et al. [Dysmorphic syndrome and vascular dysplasia: An atypical form of type IV Ehlers-Danlos syndrome]. *J Mal Vasc.* 1986;11(3):263–269.
9. Germain DP. Clinical and genetic features of vascular Ehlers-Danlos syndrome. *Ann Vasc Surg.* 2002;16(3):391–397.
10. Germain DP, Herrera-Guzman Y. Vascular Ehlers-Danlos syndrome. *Ann Genet.* 2004; 47(1):1–9.
11. Debrun GM, Aletich VA, Miller NR, et al. Three cases of spontaneous direct carotid cavernous fistulas associated with Ehlers-Danlos syndrome type IV. *Surg Neurol.* 1996;46(3):247–252.
12. Fox R, Pope FM, Narcisi P, et al. Spontaneous carotid cavernous fistula in Ehlers Danlos syndrome. *J Neurol Neurosurg Psychiatry.* 1988;51(7):984–986.
13. Koh JH, Kim JS, Hong SC, et al. Skin manifestations, multiple aneurysms, and carotid-cavernous fistula in Ehlers-Danlos syndrome type IV. *Circulation.* 1999;100(13):e57–e58.
14. Lach B, Nair SG, Russell NA, et al. Spontaneous carotid-cavernous fistula and multiple arterial dissections in type IV Ehlers-Danlos syndrome. Case report. *J Neurosurg.* 1987;66(3):462–467.
15. North KN, Whiteman DA, Pepin MG, et al. Cerebrovascular complications in Ehlers-Danlos syndrome type IV. *Ann Neurol.* 1995;38(6):960–964.
16. Schievink WI, Link MJ, Piepgras DG, et al. Intracranial aneurysm surgery in Ehlers-Danlos syndrome type IV. *Neurosurgery.* 2002;51(3):607–611; discussion 611–613.
17. Schievink WI, Piepgras DG, Earnest FT, et al. Spontaneous carotid-cavernous fistulae in Ehlers-Danlos syndrome type IV. Case report. *J Neurosurg.* 1991;74(6):991–998.
18. Ruby ST, Kramer J, Cassidy SB, et al. Internal carotid artery aneurysm: A vascular manifestation of type IV Ehlers-Danlos syndrome. *Conn Med.* 1989;53(3):142–144.
19. Kurata A, Oka H, Ohmomo T, et al. Successful stent placement for cervical artery dissection associated with the Ehlers-Danlos syndrome. Case report and review of the literature. *J Neurosurg* 2003;99(6):1077–1081.
20. Lee B, D'Alessio M, Vissing H, et al. Characterization of a large deletion associated with a polymorphic block of repeated dinucleotides in the type III procollagen gene (COL3A1) of a patient with Ehlers-Danlos syndrome type IV. *Am J Hum Genet.* 1991;48(3):511–517.
21. Cikrit DF, Miles JH, Silver D. Spontaneous arterial perforation: The Ehlers-Danlos specter. *J Vasc Surg.* 1987;5(2):248–255.
22. Schievink WI. Cerebrovascular Involvement in Ehlers-Danlos syndrome. *Current Treatment Options in Cardiovascular Medicine.* 2004;6(3):231–236.
23. Fuchs J, Rosenberg T. Congenital ectopia lentis. A Danish national survey. *Acta Ophthalmol Scand.* 1998;76(1):20–26.
24. Collod G, Babron MC, Jondeau G, et al. A second locus for Marfan syndrome maps to chromosome 3p24.2-p25. *Nat Genet.* 1994;8(3):264–268.
25. Dietz HC, Pyeritz RE, Hall BD, et al. The Marfan syndrome locus: Confirmation of assignment to chromosome 15 and identification of tightly linked markers at 15q15-q21.3. *Genomics.* 1991;9(2):355–361.
26. Kainulainen K, Pulkkinen L, Savolainen A, et al. Location on chromosome 15 of the gene defect causing Marfan syndrome. *N Engl J Med.* 1990;323(14):935–939.
27. Magenis RE, Maslen CL, Smith L, et al. Localization of the fibrillin (FBN) gene to chromosome 15, band q21.1. *Genomics.* 1991;11(2):346–351.
28. Pyeritz RE. The Marfan syndrome. *Annu Rev Med.* 2000;51:481–510.
29. Sakai LY, Keene DR, Engvall E. Fibrillin, a new 350-kD glycoprotein, is a component of extracellular microfibrils. *J Cell Biol.* 1986;103(6 Pt 1):2499–2509.
30. Knirsch W, Kurtz C, Haffner N, et al. Dural ectasia in children with Marfan syndrome: A prospective, multicenter, patient-control study. *Am J Med Genet.* 2006;140(7):775–781.
31. Ho NC, Hadley DW, Jain PK, et al. Case 47: Dural ectasia associated with Marfan syndrome. *Radiology.* 2002;223(3):767–771.
32. Foran JR, Pyeritz RE, Dietz HC, et al. Characterization of the symptoms associated with dural ectasia in the Marfan patient. *Am J Med Genet.* 2005;134(1):58–65.
33. Ho NC, Tran JR, Bektas A. Marfan's syndrome. *Lancet.* 2005;366(9501):1978–1981.
34. Lazarevic AM, Nakatani S, Okita Y, et al. Determinants of rapid progression of aortic root dilatation and complications in Marfan syndrome. *Int J Cardiol.* 2006;106(2):177–182.
35. Spittell PC, Spittell JA, Jr., Joyce JW, et al. Clinical features and differential diagnosis of aortic dissection: Experience with 236 cases (1980 through 1990). *Mayo Clin Proc.* 1993;68(7): 642–651.
36. Abecassis P, Lecinq A, Roger-Christoph S, et al. [Management of delivery in patients with Marfan's syndrome presenting aortic dilatation]. *J Gynecol Obstet Biol Reprod (Paris).* 2004; 33(5):416–420.
37. Hainsworth PJ, Mendelow AD. Giant intracranial aneurysm associated with Marfan's syndrome: A case report. *J Neurol Neurosurg Psychiatry.* 1991;54(5):471–472.
38. Higashida RT, Halbach VV, Hieshima GB, et al. Cavernous carotid artery aneurysm associated with Marfan's syndrome: Treatment by balloon embolization therapy. *Neurosurgery.* 1988;22(2):297–300.
39. Matsuda M, Matsuda I, Handa H, et al. Intracavernous giant aneurysm associated with Marfan's syndrome. *Surg Neurol.* 1979;12(2):119–121.
40. Ohtsuki H, Sugiura M, Iwaki K, et al. [A case of Marfan's syndrome with a ruptured distal middle cerebral aneurysm]. *No Shinkei Geka.* 1984;12(8):983–985.
41. Resende LA, Asseis EA, Costa LS, et al. [Marfan syndrome and giant intracranial aneurysms: Report of a case]. *Arq Neuropsiquiatr.* 1984;42(3):294–297.
42. Schievink WI, Parisi JE, Piepgras DG, et al. Intracranial aneurysms in Marfan's syndrome: An autopsy study. *Neurosurgery.* 1997;41(4):866–870; discussion 871.
43. van den Berg JS, Limburg M, Hennekam RC. Is Marfan syndrome associated with symptomatic intracranial aneurysms? *Stroke.* 1996;27(1):10–12.
44. Januzzi JL, Marayati F, Mehta RH, et al. Comparison of aortic dissection in patients with and without Marfan's syndrome (results from the International Registry of Aortic Dissection). *Am J Cardiol.* 2004;94(3):400–402.
45. Pope FM. Historical evidence for the genetic heterogeneity of pseudoxanthoma elasticum. *Br J Dermatol.* 1975;92(5):493–509.
46. van Soest S, Swart J, Tijmes N, et al. A locus for autosomal recessive pseudoxanthoma elasticum, with penetrance of vascular symptoms in carriers, maps to chromosome 16p13.1. *Genome Res.* 1997;7(8):830–834.
47. Lebwohl M, Schwartz E, Lemlich G, et al. Abnormalities of connective tissue components in lesional and non-lesional tissue of patients with pseudoxanthoma elasticum. *Arch Dermatol Res.* 1993;285(3):121–126.
48. Inamadar AC, Palit A. Pseudoxanthoma elasticum. *Postgrad Med J.* 2004;80(943):297.
49. Lebwohl M, Phelps RG, Yannuzzi L, et al. Diagnosis of pseudoxanthoma elasticum by scar biopsy in patients without characteristic skin lesions. *N Engl J Med.* 1987;317(6): 347–350.
50. Coleman K, Ross MH, Mc Cabe M, et al. Disk drusen and angioid streaks in pseudoxanthoma elasticum. *Am J Ophthalmol.* 1991;112(2):166–170.
51. Yap EY, Gleaton MS, Buettner H. Visual loss associated with pseudoxanthoma elasticum. *Retina.* 1992;12(4):315–319.
52. Clarkson JG, Altman RD. Angioid streaks. *Surv Ophthalmol.* 1982;26(5):235–246.
53. Takeshita T, Ozaki M. Central retinal artery occlusion in a patient with pseudoxanthoma elasticum. *Hiroshima J Med Sci.* 2003;52(2):33–34.
54. Murthy S, Prasad S. Pseudoxanthoma elasticum and nonarteritic anterior ischaemic optic neuropathy. *Eye.* 2004;18(2):201–202; discussion 202.
55. Kevorkian JP, Masquet C, Kural-Menasche S, et al. New report of severe coronary artery disease in an eighteen-year-old girl with pseudoxanthoma elasticum. Case report and review of the literature. *Angiology.* 1997;48(8):735–741.
56. Pavlovic AM, Zidverc-Trajkovic J, Milovic MM, et al. Cerebral small vessel disease in pseudoxanthoma elasticum: Three cases. *Can J Neurol Sci.* 2005;32(1):115–118.
57. van den Berg JS, Hennekam RC, Cruysberg JR, et al. Prevalence of symptomatic intracranial aneurysm and ischaemic stroke in pseudoxanthoma elasticum. *Cerebrovasc Dis.* 2000;10(4):315–319.
58. Wako K, Nakayama S, Taniguchi A, et al. [A case of pseudoxanthoma elasticum associated with asymptomatic multiple cerebral infarction, hypothyroidism, glucose tolerance abnormality and multiple congenital anomalies]. *Rinsho Shinkeigaku.* 1993;33(7):759–764.
59. Araki Y, Imai S, Saitoh A, et al. [A case of carotid rete mirabile associated with pseudoxanthoma elasticum: A case report]. *No To Shinkei.* 1986;38(5):495–500.
60. Koo AH, Newton TH. Pseudoxanthoma elasticum associated with carotid rete mirabile. Case report. *Am J Roentgenol Radium Ther Nucl Med.* 1972;116(1):16–22.
61. Yasuhara T, Sugiu K, Kakishita M, et al. Pseudoxanthoma elasticum with carotid rete mirabile. *Clinical Neurology and Neurosurgery.* 2004;106(2):114–117.
62. Lebwohl MG, Distefano D, Prioleau PG, et al. Pseudoxanthoma elasticum and mitral-valve prolapse. *N Engl J Med.* 1982;307(4):228–231.
63. Challenor VF, Conway N, Monro JL. The surgical treatment of restrictive cardiomyopathy in pseudoxanthoma elasticum. *Br Heart J.* 1988;59(2):266–269.
64. Fukuda K, Uno K, Fujii T, et al. Mitral stenosis in pseudoxanthoma elasticum. *Chest.* 1992;101(6):1706–1707.
65. Munyer TP, Margulis AR. Pseudoxanthoma elasticum with internal carotid artery aneurysm. *AJR Am J Roentgenol.* 1981;136(5):1023–1024.
66. Chalk JB, Patterson MC, Pender MP. An intracranial arteriovenous malformation and palatal myoclonus related to pseudoxanthoma elasticum. *Aust N Z J Med.* 1989;19(2):141–143.
67. Kito K, Kobayashi N, Mori N, et al. Ruptured aneurysm of the anterior spinal artery associated with pseudoxanthoma elasticum. Case report. *J Neurosurg.* 1983;58(1):126–128.
68. Sillence DO, Rimoin DL, Danks DM. Clinical variability in osteogenesis imperfecta-variable expressivity or genetic heterogeneity. *Birth Defects Original Article Series.* 1979;15(5B):113–129.
69. Tsipouras P, Borresen AL, Dickson LA, et al. Molecular heterogeneity in the mild autosomal dominant forms of osteogenesis imperfecta. *Am J Hum Genet.* 1984;36(6):1172–1179.
70. Wenstrup RJ, Willing MC, Starman BJ, et al. Distinct biochemical phenotypes predict clinical severity in nonlethal variants of osteogenesis imperfecta. *Am J Hum Genet.* 1990;46(5): 975–982.
71. Wallis GA, Sykes B, Byers PH, et al. Osteogenesis imperfecta type III: Mutations in the type I collagen structural genes, COL1A1 and COL1A2, are not necessarily responsible. *J Med Genet.* 1993;30(6):492–496.
72. Charnas LR, Marini JC. Communicating hydrocephalus, basilar invagination, and other neurologic features in osteogenesis imperfecta. *Neurology.* 1993;43(12):2603–2608.

73. Neurofibromatosis. Conference statement. National Institutes of Health Consensus Development Conference. *Arch Neurol.* 1988;45(5):575–578.
74. Gutmann DH, Aylsworth A, Carey JC, et al. The diagnostic evaluation and multidisciplinary management of neurofibromatosis 1 and neurofibromatosis 2. *JAMA.* 1997;278(1):51–57.
75. Mulvihill JJ, Parry DM, Sherman JL, et al. NIH conference. Neurofibromatosis 1 (Recklinghausen disease) and neurofibromatosis 2 (bilateral acoustic neurofibromatosis). An update. *Ann Intern Med.* 1990;113(1):39–52.
76. Andersen LB, Ballester R, Marchuk DA, et al. A conserved alternative splice in the von Recklinghausen neurofibromatosis (NF1) gene produces two neurofibromin isoforms, both of which have GTPase-activating protein activity. *Mol Cell Biol.* 1993;13(1):487–495.
77. Fain PR, Barker DF, Goldgar DE, et al. Genetic analysis of NF1: Identification of close flanking markers on chromosome 17. *Genomics.* 1987;1(4):340–345.
78. Barker D, Wright E, Nguyen K, et al. Gene for von Recklinghausen neurofibromatosis is in the pericentromeric region of chromosome 17. *Science.* 1987;236(4805):1100–1102.
79. Yohay K. Neurofibromatosis types 1 and 2. *Neurologist.* 2006;12(2):86–93.
80. Fujimura T, Terui T, Kusaka Y, et al. Neurofibromatosis 1 associated with an intracranial artery abnormality, moyamoya disease and bilateral congenital large hairy pigmented macules. *British Journal of Dermatology.* 2004;150(3):611–613.
81. Sobata E, Ohkuma H, Suzuki S. Cerebrovascular disorders associated with von Recklinghausen's neurofibromatosis: A case report. *Neurosurgery.* 1988;22(3):544–549.
82. Benatar MG. Intracranial fusiform aneurysms in von Recklinghausen's disease: Case report and literature review. *J Neurol Neurosurg Psychiatry.* 1994;57(10):1279–1280.
83. Hoffmann KT, Hosten N, Liebig T, et al. Giant aneurysm of the vertebral artery in neurofibromatosis type 1: Report of a case and review of the literature. *Neuroradiology.* 1998;40(4): 245–248.
84. Kamiyama K, Endo S, Horie Y, et al. [Neurofibromatosis associated with intra- and extracranial aneurysms and extracranial vertebral arteriovenous fistula]. *No Shinkei Geka.* 1985; 13(8):875–880.
85. Kubota T, Nakai H, Tanaka T, et al. A case of intracranial arteriovenous fistula in an infant with neurofibromatosis type 1. *Child's Nervous System.* 2002;18(3–4):166–170.
86. Greene JF, Jr., Fitzwater JE, Burgess J. Arterial lesions associated with neurofibromatosis. *Am J Clin Pathol.* 1974;62(4):481–487.
87. Gabow PA. Autosomal dominant polycystic kidney disease. *N Engl J Med.* 1993;329(5):332–342.
88. Kimberling WJ, Kumar S, Gabow PA, et al. Autosomal dominant polycystic kidney disease: Localization of the second gene to chromosome 4q13-q23. *Genomics.* 1993;18(3): 467–472.
89. Dobin A, Kimberling WJ, Pettinger W, et al. Segregation analysis of autosomal dominant polycystic kidney disease. *Genet Epidemiol.* 1993;10(3):189–200.
90. Kelleher CL, McFann KK, Johnson AM, et al. Characteristics of hypertension in young adults with autosomal dominant polycystic kidney disease compared with the general U.S. population. *Am J Hypertens.* 2004;17(11 Pt 1):1029–1034.
91. Levey AS, Pauker SG, Kassirer JP. Occult intracranial aneurysms in polycystic kidney disease. When is cerebral arteriography indicated? *N Engl J Med.* 1983;308(17): 986–994.

CHAPTER **89**

Spinal Stenosis

Elaine M. Adams • Alexander J. Nemeth • Vijaya K. Patil

OBJECTIVES

- To discuss the clinical manifestations of spinal stenosis
- To describe the anatomy and pathogenesis of spinal stenosis
- To explain the role of diagnostic testing in the evaluation of spinal stenosis
- To discuss the therapeutic options for patients with spinal stenosis

CASE VIGNETTE

The patient is a healthy 70-year-old man who had slowly progressive back and leg pain over several years. The pain involved the buttocks and thighs; it occurred primarily with walking, and was relieved with sitting. He felt weak and unsteady when the pain was at its maximum. At first, the pain occurred after walking long distances, but now occurs after walking only three to four blocks. He had no sensory complaints, and bowel and bladder functions were normal. The patient's medical history includes hypertension and hyperlipidemia.

Examination showed no tenderness over the spine. Straight leg raise was normal. Lumbar motion was decreased in all directions. Hip and knee examination was normal. Neurologic examination was unremarkable, except for hypoactive lower extremity reflexes. Femoral, popliteal, and pedal pulses were symmetrically present and strong.

DEFINITION

Spinal stenosis is anatomically defined as a diminished cross-sectional area of the spinal canal resulting in impingement of the spinal cord or exiting nerve roots (1). The clinical syndromes associated with spinal stenosis include myelopathy with cervical canal stenosis and neurogenic claudication with lumbar stenosis. Radicular and polyradicular symptoms can occur as well. Radiographic findings of spinal stenosis can be found in asymptomatic patients. Despite the high frequency of these widely recognized clinical scenarios, specific diagnostic criteria are lacking.

EPIDEMIOLOGY

Spinal stenosis is a common clinical syndrome. It is one of the most frequent causes of cervical myelopathy and the leading diagnosis associated with spine surgery among patients >65 years of age in the United States (2). The exact prevalence of the disease is unknown. Symptoms typically begin in the fifth to eighth decade, with increasing incidence with advancing age, correlating with progression of degenerative processes in the spine. The disease can present at a younger age, however, with 21% of those with cervical stenosis and 9.8% of patients with lumbar stenosis presenting <51 years of age in a large series (3,4). Congenital spinal stenosis can present with symptoms in childhood. A slight female predominance is seen in the lumbar spine and a 3:2 male-to-female ratio is seen in the cervical spine (5).

ETIOLOGY AND PATHOGENESIS

Narrowing of the spinal canal occurs most commonly as a result of degenerative disease of the intervertebral disc, facet joints, and surrounding structures, although other acquired diseases and congenital abnormalities can also occur (Table 89-1). Three normal variants of the spinal canal are seen: Round, ovoid, and trefoil. The trefoil (triangular) predisposes to lateral stenosis. The common anatomic factors that contribute to stenosis include protrusion of the disc, osteophytes from facet joints or uncovertebral joints, and hypertrophy of the ligamentum flavum (6). Central stenosis is most commonly associated with neurogenic claudication, whereas lateral stenosis predisposes to radicular complaints. Extension of the lumbar spine reduces the cross section of the spinal canal, increasing the mechanical impingement of its contents. This provides an anatomic correlate for the clinical findings in lumbar spinal stenosis of increased pain with walking and reduced pain with forward flexion. In addition to direct mechanical pressure on spinal contents, ischemic neuritis has been postulated to contribute to pain from spinal stenosis. Venous engorgement with elevated epidural and intrathecal pressures and relative arterial insufficiency has been demonstrated in spinal stenosis (7). Focal inflammation has also been considered a cofactor in the symptoms of spinal stenosis, but little evidence is available to confirm its role (8).

PATHOLOGY

The pathology of spinal stenosis most commonly is degeneration of the spine. The ligamentum flavum undergoes fibrotic and chondrometaplastic changes with progressive thickening.

TABLE 89-1. Causes of Spinal Stenosis

CONGENITAL–DEVELOPMENTAL
- Idiopathic
- Achondroplasia

ACQUIRED
- Degenerative disease
- Disc, ligament, facet joints
- Spondylolisthesis
- Postsurgical
- Posttraumatic
- Paget disease
- Diffuse idiopathic skeletal hyperostosis
- Fluorosis
- Uric acid or calcium pyrophosphate dihydrate deposition disease (CPPD) tophi

Disc degeneration and rupture of the annulus fibrosus occur. Osteoarthritic changes of the intervertebral joints produce bony hypertrophy and spurs. At the nerve root, endoneural edema is an early finding. As injury becomes more severe, demyelination and axonal injury may follow (7).

CLINICAL MANIFESTATIONS

LUMBAR STENOSIS

Patients with lumbar spinal stenosis commonly present with neurogenic claudication. This consists of back and leg pain that occurs with walking and is relieved by rest. Pain is usually bilateral and can be associated with poor balance, numbness, paresthesas, and weakness. Bowel or bladder symptoms are unusual. Because lumbar extension narrows the spinal canal, a flexed posture, such as leaning on a shopping cart, reduces symptoms. For the same reason, patients may have more difficulty walking downhill than uphill. Increasing age, severe lower extremity pain, and absence of pain when seated were the historical findings most strongly associated with a diagnosis of spinal stenosis (9). Symptoms of acute radiculopathy or chronic facet arthritis may be combined with the findings of spinal stenosis.

Physical examination finding is often normal, except for decreased spinal motion, a common finding in the elderly. Neurologic examination may demonstrate weakness (18% to 52%), or sensory loss (32% to 58%) in a mono- or polyradicular distribution (1). Wide-based gait and decreased vibratory sensation can also occur. Muscle stretch reflexes may be decreased or absent. The most common levels affected, in descending order, are L4-5, L5-S1 and L3-4, L2-3, with frequent multilevel disease. Reproduction of leg pain with lumbar extension for >30 seconds has also been associated with lumbar spinal stenosis (10).

CERVICAL STENOSIS

Spinal stenosis in the cervical spine produces a radiculomyelopathy, most commonly in C5-6, C6-7, or C4-5. Patients present with neck and shoulder pain combined with numbness, paresthesias, or weakness in the arms and hands. Compression of the dorsal columns produces leg weakness and unsteady gait. Urinary irritability is frequent, although rectal or urinary incontinence is uncommon. Lhermitte's phenomenon can occur with neck flexion or extension.

Physical examination demonstrates sensory loss and or weakness in the distribution of the involved roots. Muscle stretch reflexes in the upper extremity can be decreased or increased, depending on the level of compression. Lower extremity spasticity and weakness can be present, with associated impaired vibratory and position sense in the feet. Lower extremity hyperreflexia is usually present along with a Babinski sign. Rarely, asymmetric involvement may present as a partial Brown-Sequard syndrome. Transient spinal cord injury, with temporary weakness and numbness, has been described during athletic competition in young athletes with previously unrecognized cervical spinal stenosis (11).

DIAGNOSTIC APPROACH

The differential diagnosis of back and leg pain is broad. In addition to lumbar spinal stenosis, other degenerative processes in the spine (e.g., facet arthritis, herniated discs, and spondylolistheis) can occur in isolation or as a component of the stenotic process. Osteoarthritis of the hip and trochanteric bursitis can produce activity-related leg pain. Vascular claudication may be the most difficult condition to distinguish from spinal stenosis. Increased pain with uphill walking, impotence, and absence of neurologic symptoms or signs, coupled with diminished pedal pulses, favor a vascular cause of pain. In patients with recent onset of symptoms, infection and tumor need to be considered. Red flag symptoms of fever, weight loss, severe rest pain, and history of cancer or progressive neurologic defects should prompt immediate evaluation.

The findings in cervical spinal stenosis can be similar to other causes of cervical cord compression, including tumor, herniated disc, syringomyelia, and arteriovenous malformation. Rheumatoid arthritis and ankylosing spondylitis can also cause subluxation and myelopathy. In addition, multiple sclerosis, amyotrophic lateral sclerosis, subacute combined degeneration (vitamin B_{12} deficiency), neurosyphilis, adrenoleukodystrophy, human T-lymphotrophic virus-1 (HTLV-1) or human immunodeficiency virus (HIV) infection, and parasagitital brain lesions can present with clinical features that mimic cervical spinal stenosis. The diagnostic approach, therefore, begins with a thorough history and physical examination to search for clues of systemic diseases and neurologic abnormalities. Diagnosis of spinal stenosis is confirmed with radiographic studies.

IMAGING

When spinal stenosis is suspected clinically, cross-sectional imaging yields the greatest information regarding the various causes and the potential effect of stenosis on the central canal. Plain films remain a screening measure for alignment, fracture, and degenerative changes, but offer little information regarding the status of true central canal. Magnetic resonance imaging (MRI) is the preferred imaging modality because it can be used to assess the etiologic factors and the potential effect of the underlying canal stenosis on the spinal cord better than either nonenhanced computed tomography (CT) or CT myelogram. The causative factors of spinal stenosis most frequently are related to degenerative changes, among many other causes. The specific contributing degenerative changes

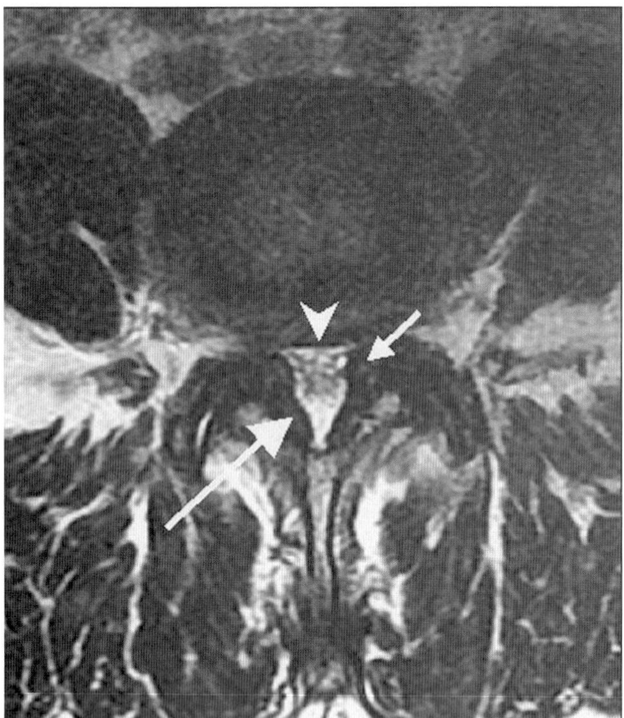

FIGURE 89-1. Axial T2-weighted magnetic resonance imaging (MRI) demonstrates moderate central canal stenosis at the lumbar intervertebral disc level L3-L4 as a result of a combination of diffuse disc bulge (*arrowhead*), ligamentum flavum thickening (*large arrow*), and facet arthrosis (*small arrow*). The cauda equina nerve roots in the central canal are crowded on the basis of the moderate central canal stenosis.

seen on MRI include intervertebral disc disease, ligamentum flavum thickening, and uncovertebral and facet arthrosis (Fig. 89-1). Nonenhanced CT assesses bony abnormalities very well, but is limited for disc disease, ligamentum flavum thickening, and spinal cord parenchyma, and the degree of spinal stenosis may be underestimated. CT myelogram offers a better evaluation of the disc and ligamentum flavum and, therefore, accurately gauges spinal stenosis, but also does not assess the spinal cord parenchyma. An additional advantage of MRI is in assessment of signal changes related to cord edema or myelomalacic changes. These findings demonstrate the degree to which spinal stenosis results in spinal cord injury. When factors, such as a pacemaker or others, preclude MRI use, the next best test is CT myelogram if the patient can tolerate lying prone for approximately 20 minutes; nonenhanced CT can be used if the patient cannot tolerate this study. Finally, imaging findings may be seen in asymptomatic patients. Matsumoto et al. (12) studied 497 asymptomatic patients using MRI and found evidence of disc degeneration in 12%, to 17% of those in their 20s, and from 86% to 89% of those >60 years of age (12).Therefore, allowance for false–positive findings should be assumed when correlating MRI results with a patient's symptoms.

ELECTRODIAGNOSTIC STUDIES

Elecrodiagnostic testing is useful in the diagnosis of spinal stenosis. Physiologic abnormalities associated with the stenosis can be defined and other disorders that may mimic spinal stenosis, such as polyneuropathy or focal neuropathy, can be detected. Because spinal stenosis progresses, electrophysiologic changes occur, including conduction block, axonal loss, and demyelination. Studies of sensory nerve action potential are typically normal. Motor nerve conduction studies are abnormal with axonal loss. H-reflexes and F waves can provide additional information, especially in lumbar canal stenosis. Abnormal spontaneous activity (fibrillations and positive sharp waves) and neurogenic motor unit potentials may be found in needle electromyography in two or more muscles innervated by the same nerve root, but different peripheral nerves. In the Nardin et al. (13) study, the finding that MRI and electromyelography (EMG) may concur in only 60% of patients suggests that the two tests provide complementary diagnostic information (13).

TREATMENT

Despite the high prevalence of spinal stenosis, a paucity of controlled trials exist to support clinical practice. Recent reviews of surgical and nonsurgical therapy state that no conclusions are possible regarding the relative effectiveness of current treatment options (14,15). Recommendations are based on observational studies and expert opinion. The goal of treatment is to reduce pain and improve function. Several long-term prognostic studies suggest that most patients will have stable or improved symptoms with conservative therapy (16–18). Treatment options include medications, exercise and physical therapy, spinal injections, and surgery.

Nonsteroidal anti-inflammatory drugs and acetaminophen are reasonable first steps in relieving pain (19).Opiods can be used for more severe pain. Muscle relaxants are often prescribed, but have not been shown to be more effective than simple analgesics. Antidepressants, gabapentin, and pregabalin have been useful in diabetic and postherpetic neuropathy, but their role in spinal stenosis is untested. Advanced age and frequent comorbid diseases mandate periodic reassessment of benefit and potential toxicity from any regimen chosen.

Aerobic and strengthening exercises are standard therapy for low back pain, although the effectiveness in spinal stenosis is less clear (20). Flexion-based lumbar stabilization exercises, core muscle strengthening, and flexibility regimens for the hips are commonly prescribed and may increase the neuroforaminal opening (21). Bracing may be useful, particularly when vertebral instability contributes to the stenosis. No evidence supports the use of acupuncture or spinal manipulation (22,23). Randomized trials of epidural steroid injections have shown mixed results, both negative and positive (24,25). Patients with disc herniation may have a more favorable response.

Decompression or laminectomy, with or without fusion, is the standard surgical therapy for refractory spinal stenosis. No large randomized trials, however, have compared the relative benefit of surgical and nonsurgical treatments (15). In the cervical spine, moderate to severe neurologic deficits are generally agreed to indicate surgical consideration. In the lumbar spine, intractable pain is more often the motivation to consider surgery; radicular symptoms are more responsive to surgery than is back pain. Two large meta-analyses of retrospective surgical series suggested that, on average, 64% to 90% of patients would obtain a satisfactory outcome short term after surgery (26,27). A single, small randomized trial reported better outcome with surgery, but methodologic flaws preclude firm conclusions (28). Most observational studies report a high frequency of recurrent symptoms after several years postoperative (14). The results of current randomized trials may provide data to better guide surgical decisions for patients with spinal stenosis (29).

CLINICAL RECOMMENDATIONS OF THE VIGNETTE

The patient presented with findings suggestive of lumbar spinal stenosis. Vascular claudication produces similar symptoms, but is unlikely with normal pedal pulses. An MRI of his lumbar spine should be performed. If spinal stenosis is confirmed, treatment options should be discussed with the patient. Conservative therapy with analgesics and physical therapy is reasonable, given his normal neurologic examination findings. If his condition does not improve, epidural steroids or surgical decompression can be considered. The patient should be aware that, although surgery may result in greater improvement in the first few years, reoccurrence of symptoms is common.

SUMMARY

Spinal stenosis is a common condition that occurs in the cervical or lumbar spine. It is most often caused by degenerative conditions involving the discs, intervertebral joints, and ligaments that impinge on the spinal cord, cauda equina, or exiting nerve roots. Clinical findings include myeloradiculopathy in the cervical spine, and neurogenic claudication in the lumbar area. MRI best confirms diagnosis, although radiographic abnormalities can be found in asymptomatic individuals. EMG can be useful to assess correlation of symptoms and anatomic findings. Treatment options include analgesics, physical therapy, epidural injections, and surgical decompression. In long-term outcome studies, approximately one half of patients have stable symptoms, one quarter improved, and one quarter worsened.

REFERENCES

1. Katz JN, Dalgas M, Stucki G, et al. Diagnosis of lumbar spinal stenosis. *Rheum Dis Clin North Am.* 1994;20(2):471–483.
2. Deyo RA, Ciol MA, Cherkin DC, et al. Lumbar spinal fusion. A cohort study of complications, reoperation and resource use in the Medicare population. *Spine.* 1993;18:1463–1470.
3. LeBan MM, Green ML. Young cervical spinal stenotic. A review of 118 patients younger than 51 years of age. *Am J Phys Med Rehabil.* 2004;83(2):162–165.
4. LeBan MM, Imas A. Young lumbar spinal stenotic. Review of 268 patients younger than 51 years. *Am J Phys Med Rehabil.* 2003;82(1):69–71.
5. Bartleson JD, O Duffy JD. Spinal stenosis. In: Koopmon WJ, ed. *Arthritis and Allied Conditions,* 14th ed. Philadelphia: Lippincott Williams & Wilkins; 2001:2042–2053.
6. Botwin KP, Gruber RD. Lumbar spinal stenosis: Anatomy and pathogenesis. *Phys Med Rehabil Clin N Am.* 2003;14:1–15.
7. Akuthota V, Lento P, Sowa G. Pathogensis of lumbar spinal stenosis pain: Why does an asymptomatic stenotic patient flare? *Phys Med Rehabil Clin N Am.* 2003;14:17–28.
8. Cavanaugh JM, Ozaktay AC, Yamashita T, et al. Mechanisms of low back pain: A neurophysiologic and neuroanatomic study. *Clin Orthop Rel Res.* 1997;335:166–180.
9. Katz JN, Dalgas M, Stucki G, et al. Degenerative lumbar spinal stenosis. Diagnostic value of the history and physical exam. *Arthritis Rheum.* 1995;38(q):1236–1241.
10. Thomas SA. Spinal stenosis: History and physical exam. *Phys Med Rehabil Clin N Am.* 2003;14:29–39.
11. Bailes JE. Experience with cervical stenosis and temporary paralysis in athletes. *J Neurosurg Spine.* 2005;2:11–16.
12. Matsumoto M, Fujmura Y, Suzuki N, et al. MRI of cervical intervertebral discs in asymptomatic subjects. *J Bone Joint Surg B.* 1998;80(1):19–24.
13. Nardin R, Patel M, Gudas T, et al. Electromyography and magnetic resonance imaging in the evaluation of radiculopathy. *Muscle Nerve.* 1999;22:151–155.
14. Atlas SJ, Delitto A. Spinal stenosis: Surgical versus nonsurgical treatment. *Clin Orthop Related Res.* 2006;443:198–207.
15. Gibson JN, Wadell G. Surgery for degenerative lumbar spondylosis: Updated Cochrane Review. *Spine.* 2005;30(20):2312–2320.
16. Tadokoro K, Miyamotoh H, Sumi M, et al. The Prognosis of conservative treatment for lumbar spinal stenosis. Analysis of patients over 70 years of age. *Spine.* 2005;30(21):2458–2463.
17. Atlas SJ, Keller RB, Wu YA, et al. Long-term outcomes of surgical and non-surgical management of lumbar spinal stenosis; 8 to 10 year results from the Maine Lumbar Spine Study. *Spine.* 2005;30(8):936–943.
18. Amundsin T, Weber H, Nordal HJ, et al. Lumbar spinal stenosis: Conservative or surgical management? A prospective 10-year study. *Spine.* 2000;25:1424–1436.
19. Van Tulder MW, Scholten RJ, Koes BW, et al. Nonsterodidal anti-inflammatory drugs for low back pain: A systematic review within the framework of the Cochrane Collaboration Back Pain Review Group. *Spine.* 2000;25:2501–2513.
20. Fritz JM, Delitto A, Welch WC, Erhard RE. Lumbar spinal stenosis: A review of current concepts in evaluation, management and outcome measurements. *Arch Phys Med Rehabil.* 1998; 79:700–708.
21. Vo AN, Kamen LB, Shih VC, et al. Rehabilitation of orthopedic and rheumatologic disorders. Lumbar spinal stenosis. *Arch Phys Med Rehabil.* 2005;86(1):569–576.
22. Assendelft WJ, Morton SC, Yu EI, et al. Spinal manipulative therapy for low back pain. A meta-analysis of effectiveness relative to other therapies. *Ann Intern Med.* 2003;138:871–881.
23. Furlan AD, VanTulder MW, Cherkin DC, et al. Acupuncture and dry needling for low back pain: An updated systematic review within the framework for the Cochrane Collaboration. *Spine.* 2005:30:944–963.
24. Ng L, Chaudhary N, Sell P. The efficacy of cortico steroids in periradicular infiltration for chronic radicular pain: A randomized double-blind controlled trial. *Spine.* 2005;30:857–862.
25. Riew KD, Yin Y, Gilula L, et al. The effect of nerve-root injection on the need for operative treatment of lumbar radicular pain. A prospective randomized, controlled, double-blind study. *J Bone Joint Surg.* 2000; 82A:1589–1593.
26. Turner JA, Ersek M, Herron, L et al. Surgery for lumbar spinal stenosis: Attempted meta-analysis of literature. *Spine.* 1992;17:1–8.
27. Mardjetko SM, Connolly PJ, Shott S. Degenerative lumbar spondylosis: A meta-analysis of the literature 1970–93. *Spine.* 1994;19:2256S–2265S.
28. Amundsen T, Weber H, Nordal HJ, et al. Lumbar spinal stenosis: Conservative or surgical management? A Prospective 10-year study. *Spine.* 2000;25:1424–1435.
29. Birkmeyer NJ, Weinstein JN, Tosteson AN, et al. Design of the Spine Patient Outcomes Research Trial (sport). *Spine.* 2002;27:1361–1372.

CHAPTER 90

Bone Tumors

Timothy B. Rapp

OBJECTIVES

- To discuss the prevalence of bone tumors
- To explain the pathophysiology of metastatic bone disease
- To define a logical workup algorithm for bony tumors
- To describe the general treatment guidelines for metastatic bone disease

CASE VIGNETTE

A healthy 49-year-old man had a 6-week history of pain radiating from the lower back into both buttocks, thighs, calves, and the plantar aspect of his left foot, and no history of trauma. The pain had begun insidiously after taking a shower, and had progressed to the point the patient can no longer find a comfortable position for rest or sleep. He describes the pain as searing, and is now requiring narcotics to control it. Over the past 24 hours, he has noticed diffuse lower extremity weakness making ambulation difficult. He also reports difficulty beginning his urinary flow over the past day. He has no history of previous back problems or spine surgery. The patient has only recently seen a primary care physician, and reports he is otherwise healthy. There is no family history of neurologic, orthopaedic, or oncologic problems. He works as a stock trader. He has smoked one pack of cigarettes per day for 30 years. Examination is remarkable for significant tenderness to palpation over the midline in the lower back. Range of motion of the lower back is difficult to assess secondary to patient compliance because of the severe pain. Diffuse muscle weakness is noted in both hip flexors, quadriceps, plantar and dorsiflexors, and great toe extensors. He also has loss of two point discrimination and pin-prick sensation up to level of the inguinal crease, including the perianal region. Symmetric lower extremity hyporeflexia is noted and plantar responses are flexor bilaterally. Rectal tone is normal, and he has intact bulbocavernosus reflex. Radiographic evaluation demonstrates compression fractures of T12 and L2, with an epidural mass at T12 (Figs. 90-1–90-3).

DEFINITION

The patient described above exemplifies a condition diagnosed as cauda equina syndrome secondary to a pathologic T12 burst fracture from metastatic lung carcinoma. Cauda equina syndrome is generally defined as a diffuse, symmetric lower extremity flaccid paralysis, saddle anesthesia, in association with urinary retention. The diagnosis of a cauda equina syndrome is a medical and surgical emergency because of the potential for irreversible neurologic injury. Direct compression of the conus medullaris secondary to the mass effect from the retro pulsed bone fragments and direct epidural tumor expansion cause the clinic presentation.

EPIDEMIOLOGY

Metastatic bone disease is the most common type of bone cancer. The thoracolumbar spine is the most common site within the skeleton afflicted with metastatic bone disease. The true incidence of metastatic bone disease is unknown (1), but autopsy studies have shown that up to 70% of patients with cancer have subclinical microscopic metastatic bone disease at death (1,2). Cauda equina syndrome is an uncommon but potentially devastating neurologic manifestation of metastatic cancer to the spine.

ETIOLOGY AND PATHOGENESIS

The development of metastatic bone disease is a multifactorial process that is currently an area of intense laboratory research. Paget's soil hypothesis (3) and Ewing's circulation theory (4) form the groundwork from which much of the current research focuses.

The physiologic milieu of the bone, including nutritional value, oxygen tension, and hormonal environment, are likely important host factors that create the proper microenvironment for metastatic cells. Specific cell-surface receptors, prostaglandins, and vascular- and endothelial-like growth factors are tumor-specific mediators that can affect the development of metastatic disease in the skeleton (6). Once the tumor begins to grow within the medullary cavity of the bone, osteoclast-activating factors likely play a large role in the development of unchecked bone resorption and destruction that leads to clinical symptoms and pathologic fracture and allows local extension of the tumor mass (5,6). Development of metastatic bone disease is most common in the anterior spine. This observation can be partially explained secondary to the vertebral vein system originally described by Batson (7). This retrograde low-pressure venous drainage system provides secondary outflow of blood from the thoracic and abdominal cavities. Convergence of these veins into a plexus surrounding the anterior vertebral

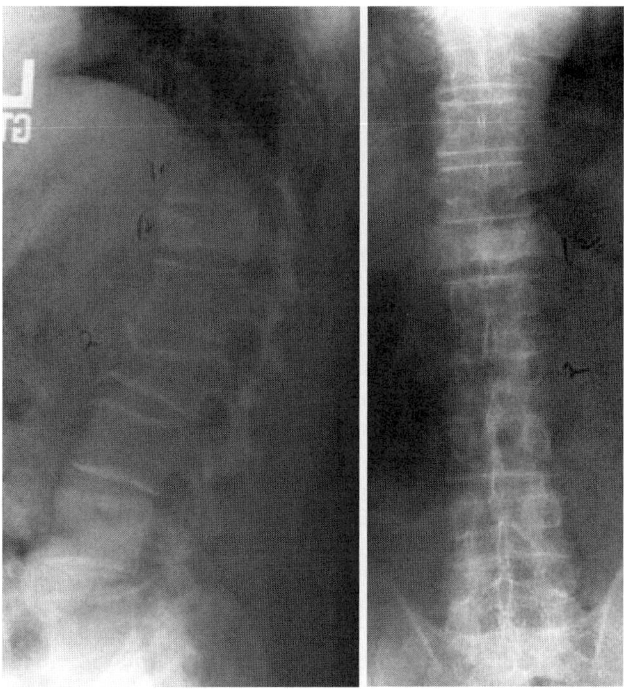

FIGURE 90-1. Posterior-Anterior and lateral radiographs of the lumbar spine showing compression fractures of the T12 and L2 vertebral bodies.

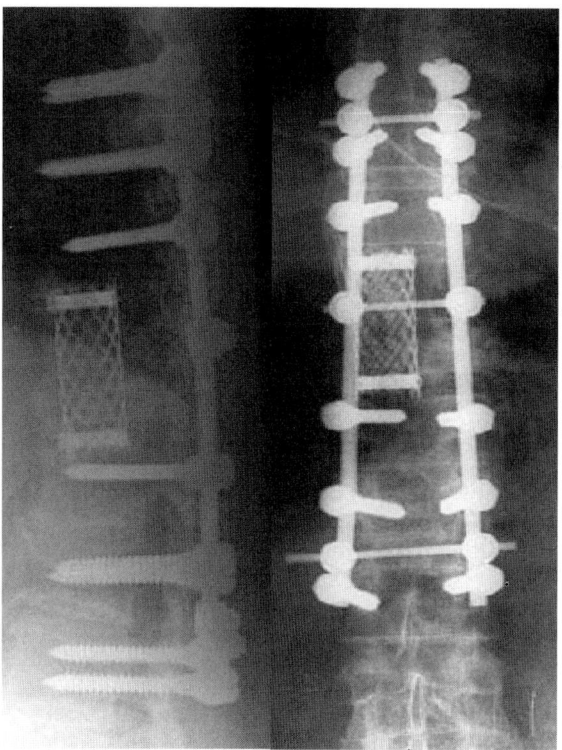

FIGURE 90-3. The patient had surgical decompression via an anterior vertebrectomy followed by posterior segmental spinal instrumentation to stabilize the spinal column.

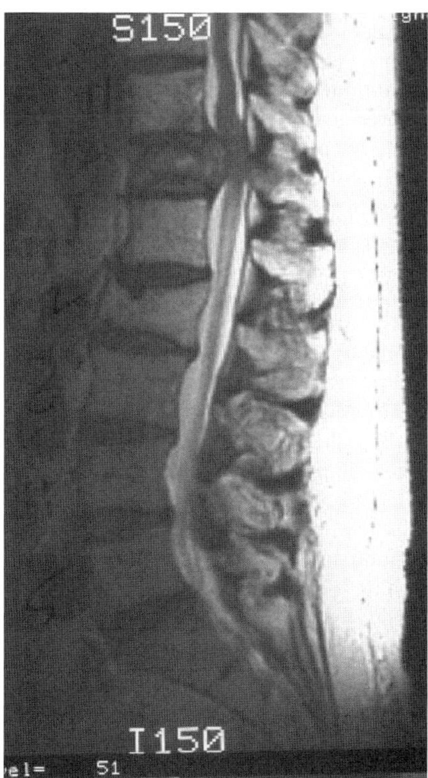

FIGURE 90-2. Saggital magnetic resonance image (MRI) of the lumbar spine showing pathologic fractures of T12 with epidural extension of the tumor mass and fracture contents causing direct compression of the spinal cord. Also noted is a pathologic compression fracture and focal kyphosis at L2.

bodies allows direct access of hematogenous tumor cells to the spinal column (7).

Physiologically, the metastatic cells disrupt the skeletal system's three primary functions: Hematopoiesis, mineral metabolism, and structural support. Because of the replacement of bone marrow by tumor cells and other side effects of systemic treatment, such as chemotherapy and radiation therapy, the patients often exhibit anemia and thrombocytopenia. Unless directly related to the use of chemotherapy, leukopenia is a late finding. Patients can also present with hypercalcemia of malignancy secondary to disrupted mineral metabolism and high levels of bone turnover. The symptoms of hypercalcemia are often nonspecific (e.g., fatigue, anorexia, nausea). A high level of clinical suspicion should be maintained for this possibility because life-threatening cardiac arrhythmias can develop in patients with undiagnosed and untreated hypercalcemia. The most obvious clinical ramification of metastatic bone disease is compromise of the structural support the skeleton provides to the body. The most morbid and orthopaedically severe manifestation of this involvement is the development of a pathologic fracture. Pathologic fracture and associated local tumor growth can have significant neurologic consequences when having an affect on the vertebral column.

PATHOLOGY

The development of metastatic bone disease is generally thought to be a late manifestation of the underlying malignancy. Up to 10% of metastatic bone disease, however, presents without a known primary tumor (8). The invasion of bony elements by malignant cells is often subclinical and diagnosed by routine bone scintigraphy during the staging of patients with carcinoma. Untreated or unresponsive to nonsurgical management, tumors can eventually decrease the structural integrity of the cancellous bone to the point that spinal fractures can occur. The retropulsion of bone fragments that can occur with such fractures, coupled with the local growth of the tumor mass, can cause spinal canal compromise and potential impingement of the spinal cord, cauda equina, or individual nerve roots. Rapid neurologic deterioration (progressive deficits over a 24-hour period) is a poor prognostic sign for functional nerve recovery. Conversely, most patients with a slower clinical decline, can expect to regain ambulatory function after treatment (9).

CLINICAL MANIFESTATIONS AND SPECIAL SITUATIONS

Formal treatment of patients with neurologic compromise secondary to metastatic bone disease is discussed below. An emerging technique, kyphoplasty, deserves special consideration in patients with these conditions. This minimally invasive technique involves inserting a small catheter into the diseased bone, inflating a small balloon to expand the collapsed elements, and injecting bone cement into the resulting void. Although successful in relieving pain for most patients, this technique is relatively contraindicated for patients with epidural expansion of the tumor because of the risk of cement extravasation during the procedure resulting in permanent paralysis (10,11). Multimodality treatment of metastatic disease and improvement in the technical aspects of this procedure may allow expansion of its indications in the future.

DIAGNOSTIC APPROACH

For patients with a known history of metastatic carcinoma, a presumptive diagnosis of metastatic bone disease can be made by plain radiography. Permeativelike radiolucent lesions, with or without concomitant pathologic fractures, are the hallmark of metastatic bone disease. Metastatic disease is the most common cause of a destructive bone lesion in patients >40 years of age. In patients with a less *classic* radiographic appearance, a remote history of cancer, or a history of metastatic cancer without known bone involvement, computed tomography (CT)-guided biopsy can be used to verify the pathologic process before proceeding with definitive treatment of metastatic disease.

As presented in the case vignette, patients can present with metastatic bone disease and associated neurologic signs and symptoms, without a known history of malignancy. Therefore, an expeditious and cost-effective treatment algorithm should remain in the armamentariums of treating physicians. For any patient presenting with a concerning pathologic lesion of bone, a thorough history and physical examination are mandatory. In some series, up to 8% of primary carcinomas presenting with metastatic bony disease could be palpated after a thorough screening medical examination (12). For other patients, laboratory tests consisting of a complete blood count (CBC), erythrocyte sedimentation rate (ESR), C-reactive protein (CRP) to workup the possibility of osteomyelitis, a serum protein electrophoresis (SPEP) to identify the protein spike associated with myeloma (the second most common cause of a destructive bone lesion in patients >40 years of age), and a prostate-specific antigen (PSA) are recommended. Plain radiographs of the chest followed by CT scanning of the chest, abdomen, and pelvis identify approximately 70% of primary lesions in this patient population (12). If this workup fails to identify a likely primary source, a whole body bone scan is recommended before CT-guided or open biopsy to identify other potential concerning areas within the skeletal system, perhaps identifying a more anatomic desirable sight for biopsy. Despite this diagnostic algorithm, 10% of patients presenting with biopsy proved metastatic disease will not be rendered a primary diagnosis. The primary tumor is rarely identified at autopsy (12,13). Biopsy is recommended for all patients with no known history of metastatic bone disease before proceeding with definitive management.

TREATMENT

Treatment of metastatic bone disease can be complex, requiring a multidisciplinary approach. Treatment modalities can include, either alone or in combination, medical management with chemotherapy, corticosteroids and bisphosphonates, external beam radiation treatment, and surgery.

CHEMOTHERAPY

The use of systemic chemotherapy for patients with widespread metastatic disease has some limited use in attempts at palliation and slowing disease progression. Hormonal modulating chemotherapy, such as the use of estrogen receptor antagonists in metastatic breast cancer and testosterone receptor antagonists in metastatic prostate cancer, has been shown to offer patients improved length of survival (14). More toxic systemic treatments have been offered; most show little to very modest improvement in patient survival and they are associated with the significant side effects.

BISPHOSPHONATES

The use of bisphosphonates in patients with known metastatic bone carcinoma is increasing. Their mechanism of action involves forming strong bonds with the hydroxyapatite crystals of bone. These bonds can withstand the hydrolytic enzymes produced by osteoclasts and some tumor cells, preventing further bone destruction. These drugs are generally well tolerated by patients. Bisphosphonates have been shown to significantly decrease both the development of pathologic fractures and the intensity of pain associated with metastatic bone disease (15). These drugs have also shown promise as prophylactic agents against the development of metastatic bone disease (16).

CORTICOSTEROIDS

The use of intravenous corticosteroids for patients presenting with neurologic symptoms secondary to metastatic disease is widely practiced. Stabilization and possible improvement in neurologic symptoms after their administration are often observed. Despite their widespread clinical use in these types of situations, a clear understanding of the mechanism and strong clinical criteria for patients that benefit from such intervention are lacking.

EXTERNAL BEAM RADIATION

Most primary carcinomas (breast, prostate, and lung) are responsive to external beam radiation. Because of the relative lack of side effects, ease of administration, and effectiveness, most patients presenting with neurologic symptoms secondary to bony metastatic disease can be effectively treated with radiation. Doses in the range of 25 to 30 Gy fractionated over 2 to 4 weeks are common protocols. Up to 80% of patients can expect complete or partial relief of their pain symptoms and up to 30% may experience abatement of their neurologic symptoms (17). Postoperative radiation therapy is recommended in nearly all cases to help minimize the risk of local recurrence and the progressive destruction, neurologic compromise, and surgical implant failure associated therein (18).

SURGERY

Surgical management may be indicated for patients with acute onset of rapid neurologic deterioration secondary to metastatic disease or for patients with slowly progressive neurologic deficits that are refractory to appropriate nonsurgical modalities. General principles of spinal surgery for neurologic compromise include complete decompression of neurologic elements and spinal stabilization to prevent further vertebral collapse. These are large surgical interventions associated with significant operative time, blood loss, and the associated perioperative physiological stress. Patients offered this degree of surgical intervention should be in an otherwise reasonable degree of cardiopulmonary health to withstand the physiologic stress induced by such surgery and have reasonable life expectancies to experience the benefits the surgery may provide. Predicting life expectancy in patients with metastatic disease is difficult, with little scientific data to help guide this determination. Improvement in neurologic symptoms and prevention of further instability can be expected in up to 80% of appropriate surgical candidates treated with surgery and postoperative radiation therapy (19).

CLINICAL RECOMMENDATIONS OF THE VIGNETTE

A high index of suspicion should exist for patients presenting with a history of protracted axial or extremity pain and associated neurologic symptoms. Certain *red flags*, such as a history of cancer, weight loss, fatigue, fevers, night pain waking patients from sleep, and progressive neurologic deficits, may alert the clinician to the possibility of metastatic bone disease. Medical management involving the use of bisphosphonates, external beam radiation, and systemic chemotherapy (when indicated) should remain the front line of treatment for patients with metastatic bone cancer and stable or slowly progressive neurologic signs. For patients who present with the acute onset of cauda equina syndrome, or less significant but rapidly progressive neurologic deficits, and are reasonable surgical candidates, surgical decompression and spinal stabilization is the most definitive approach. The patient in this vignette presented with the rapid development of a cauda equina syndrome secondary to tumor extension and direct bony compression from a pathologic fracture of T12. Because of the patient's rapid neurologic deterioration and the long-term consequences of further decline, the logistical delay in starting radiation treatment and receiving the clinical benefits from such treatment, the patient was treated with an urgent T12 vertebrectomy, cord decompression, and instrumented spinal stabilization. Postoperative external beam radiation therapy was used in this case and is generally recommended to help diminish the risk of rapid local recurrence of metastatic disease.

SUMMARY

Metastatic bone disease is the most common bone tumor. Many patients with cancer will be diagnosed with bone metastasis annually. Further, a significant subgroup of patients will sustain pathologic fractures. These fractures notably compromise the patient's function and potentially affect treatment of underlying malignancies. Neurologic manifestations of metastatic bone carcinoma are uncommon, but have devastating consequences if not diagnosed. Cauda equina syndrome, presented in this case vignette, is a medical and surgical emergency. Early recognition and treatment of these clinical scenarios can spare patients the significant morbidity associated with the deterioration of their skeletal system and the functional loss associated with irreversible nerve or spinal cord injury. For patients with the gradual onset of neurologic signs and symptoms secondary to a metastatic bone carcinoma, the initial management consists of medical treatment with bisphosphonates and the use of external beam radiation. Most patients can be successfully treated in this manner.

Patients presenting with a more rapid clinical course, or who have progressive neurologic decline despite appropriate medical management, may be candidates for surgical decompression and stabilization. Surgical determinations must take into account the overall health of the patient. Such spinal stabilizations are associated with large intraoperative blood loss and the associated physiologic stresses, and should be considered only for patients with reasonable baseline cardiopulmonary function and life expectancies. The results of surgical intervention, with return or preservation of patient's ambulatory function as the benchmark, are good in properly selected individuals.

REFERENCES

1. American Cancer Society Statistics. Online. Available at www.cancer.org/. Accessed July 29, 2006.
2. Mundy GR. Metastasis to bone: Causes, consequences and therapeutic opportunities. *Nature Rev Cancer.* 2002;2:584–593.
3. Ewing J. *Neoplastic Diseases: A Textbook on Tumors*, 3rd ed. Philadelphia: WB Saunders; 1928.
4. Paget S. The distribution of secondary growths in cancer of the breast. *Lancet.* 1889;1:571.
5. Pederson L, Winding B, Foged NT, et al. Identification of breast cancer cell line-derived paracrine factors that stimulate osteoclast activity. *Cancer Res.* 1999;59(22):5849–5855.
6. Guise TA. Molecular mechanisms of osteolytic bone metastases. *Cancer.* 2000;88[12 Suppl]:2892–2898.
7. Batson OV. The function of the vertebral vein system in metastatic processes. *Ann Intern Med.* 1942:16:38.
8. Rougraff BT. *Surgery for Bone and Soft-tissue Tumors.* Philadelphia: Lippincott-Raven; 1998.
9. Bednar DA, Brox WT, Vivani GR. Surgical palliation of spinal oncologic disease: A review and analysis of current approaches. *Can J Surg.* 1991;34:129–131.
10. Fourney DR, Schomer DF, Nader R, et al. Percutaneous vertebroplasty and kyphoplasty for painful vertebral body fractures in cancer patients. *J Neurosurg.* 2003;98[1 Suppl]:21–30.
11. Spivak JM, Johnson MG. Percutaneous treatment of vertebral body pathology. *J Am Acad Orthop Surg.* 2005;13(1):6–17.
12. Rougraff BT, Kneisl JS, Simon MA. Skeletal metastases of unknown origin: A prospective study of a diagnostic strategy. *J Bone Joint Surg [Am].* 1993;75:1276–1282.
13. Katagiri H, Takahashi M, Inagaki J, et al. Determining the site of the primary cancer in patients with skeletal metastasis of unknown origin: A retrospective study. *Cancer.* 1999;86(3):533–537.

14. Schally AV, Nagy A. Chemotherapy targeted to cancers through tumoral hormone receptors. *Trends Endocrinol Metab.* 2004;15(7):300–310.
15. Hortobagyi GN, Theriault RL, Porter L, et al. Efficacy of pamidronate in reducing skeletal complications in patients with breast cancer and lytic bone metastases. Protocol 19 Aredia Breast Cancer Study Group. *N Engl J Med.* 1996;335(24):1785–1791.
16. Diel IJ, Solomayer EF, Costa SD, et al. Reduction in new metastases in breast cancer with adjuvant clodronate treatment. *N Engl J Med.* 1998;339(6):357–363.
17. Tong D, Gillick L, Hendrickson FR. The palliation of symptomatic osseous metastases: Final results of the Study by the Radiation Therapy Oncology Group. *Cancer.* 1982;50(5):893–899.
18. Townsend PW, Rosenthal HG, Smalley SR, et al. Impact of postoperative radiation therapy and other perioperative factors on outcome after orthopedic stabilization of impending or pathologic fractures due to metastatic disease. *J Clin Oncol.* 1994;12(11):2345–2350.
19. Klimo P Jr, Schmidt MH. Surgical management of spinal metastases. *Oncologist.* 2004;9(2):188–196.

CHAPTER **91**

Commonly Used Drugs (COX-2 Inhibitors, NSAID, Corticosteroids)

Rodney Tehrani • Baltazar R. Espiritu

OBJECTIVES

- To discuss the pharmacology of nonsteroidal anti-inflammatory drugs and corticosteroids
- To describe the mechanisms of action of nonsteroidal anti-inflammatory drugs and corticosteroids
- To identify the adverse events related to the use of nonsteroidal anti-inflammatory drugs and corticosteroids
- To describe the proper techniques of corticosteroid withdrawal

CASE VIGNETTE

A 65-year-old man began a treatment of ibuprofen for osteoarthritis of the knee. After 3 months of nonspecific flulike symptoms and muscle pain, he presented with an acute onset of headache, fever, meningism, and dizziness. Cerebrospinal fluid (CSF) analysis disclosed an increased cell count (145 cells/mm^3, predominantly polymorphonuclear cells and macrophages), increased protein (1,230 mg/L), but a normal glucose level. Blood and CSF cultures, viral serologies, and antinuclear factor were all negative. Symptoms improved after ibuprofen was stopped. Subsequently the patient occasionally took aspirin and mefenamic acid without any adverse effect. A follow-up CSF analysis was normal.

Nonsteroidal Anti-inflammatory Drugs

DEFINITION

Nonsteroidal anti-inflammatory drugs (NSAID) are a family of medications used for their anti-inflammatory, antipyretic, and analgesic properties.

EPIDEMIOLOGY

Estimate is that >60 million prescriptions for NSAID are written yearly in the United States, with 17 million Americans being regular daily users. Approximately 50% of the 17 million regular users are over the age of 60 years. Currently, at least 20 different NSAID preparations are available for use in the United States. Table 91-1 lists commonly used NSAID (1).

PHARMACOLOGY

NSAID are completely absorbed after oral administration. Once absorbed, they are tightly bound to albumin and have minimal first-pass hepatic metabolism.

Serum levels of NSAID can be affected by a variety of factors. Patients with hypoalbuminemia or those on highly protein-bound medications may have higher levels of free serum NSAID concentrations. Patients with altered gastrointestinal blood flow have different absorption rates. Enteric coating preparations of NSAID can affect absorption through the gastrointestinal (GI) mucosa.

NSAID are primarily metabolized in the liver and excreted by the kidneys. Hepatic and renal function must be considered when prescribing a NSAID. Most NSAID are metabolized through the P450 CYP2C9 isoenzyme.

The various NSAID have significant differences in their plasma half-lives. This fact is important in explaining the variable responses patients experience with the use of different NSAID. Table 91-2 lists the half-lives of various NSAID.

MECHANISM OF ACTION

NSAID inhibit cyclooxygenase (COX), resulting in a decrease prostaglandin production. COX is required for the conversion of arachidonic acid to prostaglandins (Fig. 91-1).

The two isoforms of COX are as follows: COX-1, located on chromosome 9, and expressed on most tissues, is important for modulating renal blood flow, maintaining the GI mucosa, and platelet aggregation. COX-1 is inhibited by all NSAID to some degree. COX-2, located on chromosome 1, is thought to be an inducible enzyme expressed at times of inflammation. It is also found in the kidneys and brain. COX-2 has an effect of

TABLE 91-1. Commonly Used Nonsteroidal Anti-Inflammatory Drugs (NSAID)

Generic Name	*Trade Name*	*Family*
Naproxen	Aleve, Naprosyn, Anaprox	Propionic acid
Ibuprofen	Motrin, Advil	Propionic acid
Diclofenac	Voltaren	Acetic acid derivatives
Indomethacin	Indocin	Acetic acid derivatives
Etodolac	Lodine	Acetic acid derivatives
Aspirin	Many names	Carboxylic acid
Salsalate	Disalcid, Salflex	Carboxylic acid
Meloxicam	Mobic	Enolic acid
Nabumetone	Relafen	Naphthylkanones
Celecoxib	Celebrex	COX-2 inhibitors

glomerular blood flow and renal electrolyte balance. As with COX-1, COX-2 is inhibited by all NSAID to some degree (2,3).

Until recently, adverse effects of NSAID were attributed to COX-1 inhibition. Anti-inflammatory and analgesic effects were attributed to COX-2 inhibition. These beliefs led to the development of specific COX-2 inhibitors, hoping for fewer or no side effects. Questions and concerns about the safety of specific COX-2 inhibitors in regards to cardiovascular and cerebrovascular events have arisen with their use, however. The exact mechanisms are unknown, but may possibly be secondary to the effects of COX-2 inhibitors on prostaglandin I2 levels, which are antithrombotic. Presently, celecoxib (Celebrex) is the only specific COX-2 inhibitor available in the United States market.

ADVERSE EVENTS

Adverse effects of NSAID are numerous. NSAID can potentially affect any organ system, ranging from the GI tract to the central nervous system(CNS) to hypersensitivity reactions.

Gastrointestinal side effects of NSAID include nausea, vomiting, diarrhea, or constipation. They also include gastric irritation that can progress to peptic ulcer disease and potentially life-threatening GI bleeding. The gastric mucosal irritation is the result of the inhibition of prostaglandin synthesis. NSAID can also cause hepatotoxicity, with elevated liver enzymes to fulminate hepatic failure (3,4).

As with the GI tract, the renal system can be affected by NSAID in multiple ways. They can cause sodium retention and interstitial nephritis, in addition to alterations in renal plasma flow. NSAID inhibition of prostaglandins can also decrease renin release, with resultant hyperkalemia.

Patients with allergic rhinitis, nasal polyposis, and asthma have an increased risk of anaphylaxis with NSAID use. The exact mechanism is unknown. Several theories exist, however, ranging from decreased prostaglandin synthesis to alterations in the arachidonate metabolism pathways.

NSAID can also inhibit platelet aggregation by reversibly inhibiting platelet COX-1. It is important to note that only aspirin has been studied as prevention of cardiovascular events

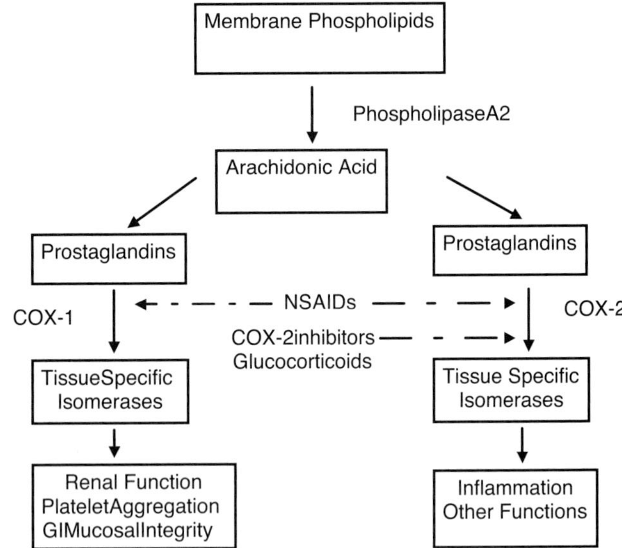

FIGURE 91-1. Action of nonsteroidal anti-inflammatory drugs (NSAID) on prostaglandins biosynthesis. (*Dotted lines* indicate mean inhibitory effects.)

secondary to its irreversible inhibition of COX-1. COX-2 is not expressed by platelets, but a concern of an increase rate of cardiovascular events with specific COX-2 inhibitors has resulted with their withdrawal from the market except for celecoxib (Celebrex).

Other adverse events with NSAID use include skin rash and photosensitivity to CNS manifestations, including headaches, meningitis, hallucinations, tinnitus, vertigo, and depression (5).

Corticosteroids

PHARMACOLOGY

Corticosteroids are life-sustaining cholesterol derivatives produced in the adrenal cortex under the influence of both the hypothalamus and pituitary gland, (hypothalamic-pituitary-adrenal axis [HPA]). The hypothalamus produces corticotropin-releasing hormone, which stimulates the pituitary gland to synthesize the adrenocorticotropic hormone to signal production of cortisol, the main endogenous corticosteroid. Synthetic derivatives of corticosteroids are available for therapy, with dexamethasone being the most potent (Table 91-3).

Corticosteroids are potent suppressors of inflammation, and their use in a variety of inflammatory and autoimmune diseases makes them among the most frequently prescribed classes of drugs. Because corticosteroids exert their effects on almost every organ system, the clinical use of, and withdrawal from,

TABLE 91-2. Half-Lives of Various Nonsteroidal Anti-Inflammatory Drugs (NSAID)

NSAID	*Aspirin*	*Diclofenac*	*Motrin*	*Indomethacin*	*Nabumetone*	*Meloxicam*	*Celebrex*
Half-life	0.25 h	1.1 h	2.1 h	4.7 h	26 h	17 h	11 h

TABLE 91-3. Relative Pharmacologic Potencies, Equivalent Dosage, and Biologic and Plasma Half-life (t 1/2) of Corticosteroid Preparations

Drug	*Equivalent Pharmacologic Dose (mg)*	*Anti-inflammatory Potency*[a]	*Mineralocorticoid Potency*[b]	*Plasma t 1/2 (h)*	*Biologic t 1/2 (h)*	*HPA Axis Suppression (mg)*[c]
Hydrocortisone	20	1	2	1.5	8–12	20–30
Cortisone	25	0.8	2	1.5	8–12	20–35
Prednisone	5	2.7	1	2.7	12–36	7.5
Prednisolone	5	4	1	2.75	12–26	7.5
Methylprednisolone	4	5	0	3	12–26	7.5
Triamcinolone	4	5	0	4.2	24–48	5–7.5
Dexamethasone	0.75	30	0	5	36–54	1–1.5

[a]Compared with hydrocortisone, which is assigned a value of 1.
[b]Range, 0 to 4.
[c]Daily dose that usually leads to hypothalamic-pituitary-adrenal (HPA) suppression.

corticosteroid use are complicated by a number of serious side effects, some of which are life threatening. Therefore, the decision to use corticosteroids always requires careful consideration of the relative risks and benefits in each patient. The effects of corticosteroids include alterations in carbohydrate, protein, and lipid metabolism; maintenance of fluid and electrolyte balance; and preservation of normal function of the cardiovascular system, the immune system, the kidney, skeletal muscle, the endocrine system, and the nervous system (Table 91-4). Corticosteroids enhance catecholamine production and modulate β-adrenergic receptor synthesis, regulation, coupling, and responsiveness. Additionally, corticosteroids bestow the individual with the capacity to resist such stressful circumstances as noxious stimuli and environmental changes. The anti-inflammatory and immunosuppressive actions of corticosteroids also provide a protective mechanism in the physiologic setting. Several immune mediators associated with the inflammatory response can decrease vascular tone, which then could lead to cardiovascular collapse if unopposed by the adrenal corticosteroids. In fact, in the setting of severe stress, the daily production rate of cortisol can rise at least tenfold (6).

MECHANISMS OF ACTION

Corticosteroids actions are mediated through several mechanisms that include induction of gene transcription, activation of transcription of inhibitory proteins, inhibition of gene transcription, and alteration of messenger RNA (mRNA) stability. Corticosteroids bind to specific receptors and interact with transcriptional coactivators to regulate the expression of corticosteroid-responsive genes. Corticosteroids have been shown to increase the expression of proteins responsible for the metabolic effects of corticosteroids and to decrease the expression of other genes, such as genes for COX-2, inducible nitric oxide synthase (iNOS-2), and inflammatory cytokines and enzymes. The negative regulation of these genes is responsible for the anti-inflammatory and immunosuppressive effects of corticosteroids. As a consequence of the time required to modulate gene expression and protein synthesis, most effects of corticosteroids become apparent after several hours. In addition to these genomic effects, some immediate actions of corticosteroids may be mediated by membrane-bound receptors (7).

SIDE EFFECTS OF CORTICOSTEROID THERAPY

The development of side effects depends on the type of corticosteroid, dose, duration of exposure, and a multitude of host, tissue, and cell variables. Some important side effects include osteoporosis, infection, adrenal insufficiency, and corticosteroid withdrawal syndromes.

TABLE 91-4. Systemic Effects of Corticosteroids

Cells	"Stabilization" of liposomal membranes
	Inhibition of macrophage response to migration inhibition factor
	Lymphocyte sensitization blocked
	Cellular response to inflammatory mediators blocked
	Inhibition of fibroblast proliferation
Central Nervous System	Benign intracranial hypertension or pseudotumor cerebri
	Alteration in mood, depression, insomnia, euphoria; appetite increase
	Lower seizure threshold
	Psychoses
Cardiovascular System	Positive inotropic effect
	Increased blood pressure (increased blood volume)
Gastrointestinal Tract	Decreased calcium and iron absorption
	Facilitation of fat absorption
	Increased acid, pepsin, and trypsin
	Structural alteration of mucin
Skeletal Muscle	Weakness (excess and deficiency)
	Muscle atrophy (chronic excess)
Skin	Atrophy and thinning (chronic excess)
	Calcinosis cutis
Hematopoietic System	Decrease in peripheral lymphocytes, monocytes, eosinophils
	Increase in peripheral neutrophils, platelets, red blood cells
	Decreased clotting time
	Decreased phagocyte competence
Kidneys	Increased reabsorption of water, sodium, chloride
	Increased excretion of potassium, calcium
	Increased extracellular fluid
Bone	Inhibition of collagen synthesis by fibroblasts
	Acceleration of bone resorption
	Antagonism of vitamin D

OSTEOPOROSIS

Corticosteroids inhibit bone formation, resulting in osteoporosis. The extent of osteoporosis depends on the maximal dose and cumulative duration of corticosteroid therapy. Men and postmenopausal women are most susceptible to developing osteoporosis; those in whom the disease process itself causes bone loss have the highest risk. Osteoporosis is caused by the inhibition of ovarian and testicular sex hormones and adrenal androgens. Secondary hyperparathyroidism caused by the inhibition of calcium absorption by corticosteroids causes osteoclast activation and osteoblast inhibition. Therapeutic and preventive measures, therefore, should include adequate intake of calcium (1,500 mg/day) and vitamin D (400 to 800 IU/day). Sex hormone replacement for men and postmenopausal women and bisphosphonate therapy for high-risk patients should be considered (8).

ADRENAL INSUFFICIENCY

Administration of corticosteroids suppresses endogenous HPA axis function, resulting in secondary adrenal insufficiency. Any patient receiving more that 20 mg of prednisone per day for 1 month may develop HPA suppression. The risk of adrenal insufficiency occurs during periods of corticosteroid tapering. Patients may require supplemental corticosteroid therapy, especially during general anesthesia, surgery, trauma, or an acute infectious disease. An adrenocorticotropic hormone (ACTH) stimulation test can be used to determine the existence of adrenal insufficiency.

INFECTIONS

Excess corticosteroid use increases the incidence and severity of infections by impairing inflammatory and immune responses. Dosages of prednisone in the range of 20 to 60 mg/day after 14 days of treatment and cumulative doses >700 mg suppress host defense mechanisms and increase the risk of infection after 14 days of treatment. Patients are at risk for infections with facultative intracellular microbes, such as mycobacterium, *Pneumocystis carinii,* and fungi and severe pyogenic infections. Most viral infections should not be a concern for patients on corticosteroids, with the exception of herpes virus infections. Infections can be masked by high-dose corticosteroids and, therefore, increased vigilance is required to detect these life-threatening conditions.

CORTICOSTEROIDS WITHDRAWAL SYNDROMES

Administration of corticosteroids can result in HPA suppression, resulting in adrenal atrophy. The specific corticosteroid dose, duration, frequency, time, and route of administration determine the extent of adrenal suppression. Pituitary-adrenal suppression will usually not occur with a dose of corticosteroids <40 mg of prednisone or equivalent that is given in the morning for <5 to 7 days or with alternate day therapy of <40 mg of prednisone (9). Pituitary-adrenal suppression can occur with short courses of larger doses or long courses of lower dose corticosteroids. In such cases, sudden withdrawal of steroid therapy can be hazardous and possibly fatal because of the adrenal insufficiency. Symptoms resulting from the adrenal insufficiency caused by steroid withdrawal include fatigue, weakness, arthralgia, dyspnea, anorexia, nausea, desquamation of the skin, orthostatic dizziness and hypotension, fainting, and hypoglycemia.

Recovery of HPA function can take up to 9 months. When a patient has received supraphysiologic doses of corticosteroid for a prolonged period of time, it is necessary to decrease the dose gradually. A typical reduction protocol involves decreasing the steroid dose by 2.5 to 5 mg every 3 to 7 days if prednisone is used. For disease flare-ups during the reduction phase, the dose can be increased, and subsequent reduction can be accomplished with a more gradual reduction, switching to alternate dosing, or adding another type of immunosuppressive agent.

CLINICAL RECOMMENDATIONS OF THE VIGNETTE

The patient provides an example case of nonsteroidal-induced meningitis. Two months after the events presented in this case, a single dose of 600 mg ibuprofen was administered, and within 90 minutes, the patient presented with fever, chills, headache, and nuchal rigidity. CSF analysis revealed 200 cells/mm^3 with 69% neutrophils, and elevated protein (1,160 mg/L). The recurrence of symptoms on re-exposure confirmed the suggested diagnosis of ibuprofen-induced aseptic meningitis. This patient should no longer be exposed to NSAID.

SUMMARY

NSAID and corticosteroids are the most widely used anti-inflammatory drugs for the treatment of various conditions. The analgesic effect of NSAID contributes to the widespread use of this class of drugs. Corticosteroids are used in a variety of inflammatory and autoimmune diseases for their anti-inflammatory action. NSAID and corticosteroid require that clinicians know the pharmacology as well as the side effects.

REFERENCES

1. Baum C, Kennedy DL, Forbes MB. Utilization of nonsteroidal anti-inflammatory drugs. *Arthritis Rheum.* 1985;28:686–692.
2. Abramson SB, Weissmann G. The mechanisms of action of nonsteroidal anti-inflammatory drugs. *Arthritis Rheum.* 1989;32:1–9.
3. Wolfe MM, Lichtenstein DR, Singh G. Gastrointestinal toxicity of nonsteroidal anti-inflammatory drugs. *N Engl J Med.* 1999;340:1888–1899.
4. Garcia Rodriguez LA, William R, Derby LE, et al. Acute liver injury associated with nonsteroidal anti-inflammatory drugs and the role of risk factors. *Arch Intern Med.* 1994;154: 311–316.
5. Hoppmann RA, Peden JG, Ober SK. Central nervous system side effects of nonsteroidal anti-inflammatory drugs. Aseptic meningitis, psychosis and cognitive dysfunction. *Arch Intern Med.* 1991;151:1309–1313.
6. Lamberts SWJ, Bruining HA, DeJong FH. Corticosteroid therapy in severe illness. *N Engl J Med.* 1997;337:1285–1292.
7. Norman AW, Mizwicki MT, Norman DP. Steroid-hormone rapid actions, membrane receptors, and a conformational ensemble model. *Nature Reviews Drug Discovery.* 2004;3:27–41.
8. Saag KG. Glucocorticoid-induced osteoporosis. *Endocrinol Metab Clin North Am.* 2003;32: 135–157.
9. Coursin DB, Wood KE. Corticosteroid supplementation for adrenal insufficiency. *JAMA.* 2002;287:236–240.

CHAPTER 92

Bacterial Meningitis

Edwin Swiatlo • Ethel S. Rose

OBJECTIVES

- To describe the epidemiology and explain the risk factors for bacterial meningitis and common pathogens associated with different demographic groups
- To explore the clinical manifestations of bacterial meningitis and the sensitivity and specificity of physical findings
- To describe a diagnostic algorithm for bacterial meningitis and the utility of various imaging and laboratory tests
- To discuss the complications of bacterial meningitis, such as septic thrombophlebitis, brain abscess, and paraspinous infections
- To discuss the antibiotics that are effective in treating meningitis and its complications
- To provide an awareness of the indications for adjunctive therapy such as steroids, and invasive procedures such as surgery and cerebrospinal fluid shunts.

CASE VIGNETTE

A 19-year-old male college student is brought to the school clinic by classmates because of fever and progressive lethargy that had developed over the past 24 hours. The patient has difficulty providing any history because of the severe lethargy, but his classmates report that the patient complained of a sore throat and coldlike symptoms 3 days before presentation. He has no known chronic medical conditions or significant history of health problems. On examination, the patient has a temperature of 38.8°C and a petechial rash is noted on the trunk. Aside from the lethargy and poor ability to concentrate, the only other pertinent physical finding is conjunctival suffusion. The patient is transferred to a local hospital and antibiotics are started in the emergency department. Computed tomography (CT) of the head was obtained without contrast and no abnormalities were noted. A lumbar puncture was performed and cerebrospinal fluid (CSF) analysis showed 770 cells/mm^3, of which 80% were polymorphonuclear leukocytes (PMN). Gram stain of CSF showed pairs and short chains of somewhat elliptical gram-negative cocci. After 48 hours, the patient's temperature returned to normal and his mental status improved to his normal baseline. The patient was discharged from the hospital after 8 days with no residual effects and in his normal state of good health.

DEFINITION

CSF, which is secreted by capillary networks in the choroid plexus of the lateral ventricles, flows through the third and fourth ventricles and then into the subarachnoid space via the foramina of Magendie and Luschka. Within the subarachnoid space, CSF flows down the spinal canal and upward over the convexity of the brain. Bacterial meningitis is characterized by the presence of bacterial cells and inflammation in the subarachnoid space of the central nervous system (CNS). The hallmark of this inflammatory response is the presence of white blood cells in the CSF and, in the case of pyogenic bacterial meningitis, elevated levels of serum proteins which are normally absent or present in very low concentration.

EPIDEMIOLOGY

Bacterial meningitis in adults (persons >16 years of age) has an annual incidence of approximately 4 to 6 cases per 100,000 population. The incidence and demographic distribution of meningitis in the United States was profoundly affected by the widespread implementation of the *Haemophilus influenzae* type b (Hib) vaccine. Before this vaccine was available, bacterial meningitis was primarily a disease of children <2 years of age. Further shifts in the epidemiology of meningitis are sure to be noted following the recent introduction of a conjugate vaccine for *Streptococcus pneumoniae* (pneumococcus) and a conjugate vaccine for *Neisseria meningitidis* (meningococcus). Currently, meningitis is most common in young adults. Passive reporting systems used to collect data render temporal and geographic comparisons unreliable, however. Blacks and Native Americans have a higher incidence of meningitis than whites. These differences are generally attributed to socioeconomic conditions, which are known to predispose to invasive bacterial infections, such as overcrowded living conditions, limited access to health care, and low educational level. When corrected for socioeconomic status, the difference in meningitis incidence between blacks and whites in the United States is not significant (1).

ETIOLOGY AND PATHOGENESIS

At least 80% of all cases of bacterial meningitis in adults are caused by *S. pneumoniae* and *N. meningitidis*. Less common causes of community-acquired meningitis are non-typeable

Haemophilus influenzae, group B and *Viridans streptococci*, and *Listeria monocytogenes*. The latter is especially associated with persons with hematologic malignancies or defects in cell-mediated immunity, including those receiving chronic steroid therapy. Alcoholism is also considered a risk factor for *Listeria* meningitis. Enteric gram-negative organisms, pseudomonas, and staphylococci are rare causes of community-acquired infection and are associated primarily with iatrogenic complications of invasive CNS procedures (2).

The development of bacterial meningitis progresses through well-defined phases. The most common pathogens of meningitis are commensal organisms that colonize the upper respiratory tract and cause no disease in most colonized individuals. The integrity of the mucosal epithelium and humoral immune mediators, such as IgA, and components of the innate immune system, such as lysozyme and lactoferrin, provide an effective barrier to invasion by colonizing bacteria. How and why bacteria breach the respiratory epithelial barrier are not completely understood, but antecedent viral respiratory infections are thought to be an important predisposing factor in many cases. Viral infections are known to cause paralysis and death of ciliated respiratory epithelial cells important for bacterial clearance. Mucosal epithelial cells have been shown to take up bacteria by endocytosis and transport them to the basolateral cell surface (3). Here, bacteria have access to subepithelial lymphatics and blood vessels, which allows dissemination.

Once in the bloodstream, bacteria encounter an array of host defense mechanisms. The major meningeal pathogens all express a polysaccharide capsule that inhibits the interaction of bacteria with phagocytic cells in the absence of specific antibody. Preexisting antibodies to capsular polysaccharide are highly protective against invasive disease and underlie the rationale for currently available pneumococcal, meningococcal, and Hib vaccines. In the absence of specific antibodies, nonspecific activation of the alternative complement pathway by the bacterial cell wall and outer membrane components is the primary means of host defense. This results in either activation of the terminal components of the common complement pathway and cell lysis or deposition of C3b and opsonophagocytosis. Bacterial pathogens, however, express a number of cell-surface proteins that inhibit complement activation and may confer sufficient survival advantage to allow replication in the bloodstream (3).

Blood-borne bacteria must cross the blood–brain barrier (BBB) to gain access to the subarachnoid space. At the anatomic level, the BBB consists of vascular endothelial cells, basement membrane, and microglial and astrocyte processes. The exact location of bacterial transmigration into the CNS is not fully defined, but the choroid plexus is thought to be a major site of invasion because of its high blood flow. CNS pathogens express a number of receptors that are specific for choroid plexus and cerebral capillaries. Attachment and movement across endothelial barriers occur by either transcellular or paracellular routes in a manner generally analogous to that seen with invasion of the blood from respiratory epithelial surfaces (3). In the CSF, host defense mechanisms are severely limited. Cells and most proteins are effectively excluded from the CSF by the BBB and bacteria can replicate, at least initially, with relatively little host interference. Bacterial products from the peptidoglycan cell wall and outer membrane (for gram-negative organisms) induce intense inflammatory responses, which are responsible for most of the pathology and adverse sequelae of bacterial meningitis. A vast array of cytokines, chemokines, reactive oxygen species, and nitric oxide have been implicated in the pathology of meningitis (3,4).

PATHOLOGY

Bacterial invasion of the subarachnoid space results in direct damage to the brain parenchyma, the most serious consequence of meningitis. An intense exudative response covers the base and convexities of the brain. Early in the course of bacterial meningitis, this exudate consists primarily of neutrophils, but evolves to a mixture of neutrophils with macrophages and lymphocytes as the infectious process progresses. An ominous result of such an exuberant inflammatory response is elevation of intracranial pressure from edema and potential herniation of the brainstem.

Cerebral vasculature is susceptible to the local inflammatory response and vessel walls can be infiltrated by inflammatory cells. Activation of the coagulation cascade can produce septic thrombosis of vessels of any size, with subsequent ischemia and neuronal death. Host inflammatory mediators, as well as bacterial toxins and products, can damage hair cells of the inner ears and lead to the hearing impairment that is noted in a minority of cases of meningitis. The causes of neuronal injury and death are numerous and potentially synergistic, and identifying all components that have an impact on the pathway from bacterial invasion of the CNS to cell death is a complex undertaking. Nevertheless, additional information on the pathogenesis of bacterial meningitis is identifying more targets for intervention to reduce the morbidity and mortality associated with this infection (4).

CLINICAL MANIFESTATIONS

The clinical presentation of bacterial meningitis is variable, but at least 90% of patients present with headache and fever. Alteration of mental status, as defined by a Glasgow Outcome Scale score below 14, occurs in nearly 75% of patients (5). Focal neurologic deficits are generally seen in about 10% to 20% of patients with meningitis, but one large study found focal deficits in 50% of patients (5). Seizures occur in 10% to 15% of patients and respiratory failure requiring mechanical ventilation occurs in about 25%. Rash can be present in up to 25% of patients, depending on the patient population and pathogen. When rash occurs, it is usually petechial and associated with meningococcal meningitis in children and adults younger than 30 years of age.

A number of noninfectious diseases can mimic bacterial meningitis and present with many of the same signs and symptoms as infection. Hypersensitivity reactions, chemical meningitis, vasculitis, autoimmune disorders, and invasion of the CNS by malignancies are some of the more commonly seen diseases that can be confused with bacterial meningitis (6). Examination of the CSF can be helpful in ruling out these disorders and guiding specific therapy, which differs significantly from that for bacterial infection.

DIAGNOSTIC APPROACH

Because of the high morbidity and mortality associated with bacterial meningitis, and its rapidly fulminant course if left untreated, any suspicion of meningitis should initiate a diagnostic evaluation. The crucial starting point begins with a complete history and physical examination. In many cases, the patient's mental status may preclude acquiring a history directly from the patient. In such cases, family members or persons who may have had a chance to observe the patient in the days before presentation are invaluable. Important data include any underlying medical conditions the patient may have, as well as prescription and nonprescription drugs being taken. A history of antecedent upper respiratory infections can be helpful, as well as any recent history of invasive procedures, particularly intrathecal injections or sinus surgery. The patient's social situation is helpful in identifying risk factors for meningitis. Injection drug users are at high risk for gram-negative and staphylococcal bacteremia, although this rarely progresses to meningitis. Crowded living conditions, most notably college dormitories or military barracks, facilitate person-to-person spread of respiratory bacteria, such as meningococci.

The common physical manifestations of meningitis are described above, however, the sensitivity of the history and physical examination in the diagnosis of bacterial meningitis is low. Less than one half of patients with meningitis present with the classic triad of fever, neck stiffness, and altered mental status. Lumbar puncture (LP) is absolutely essential for anyone suspected of having bacterial meningitis. The conundrum facing clinicians is whether to perform an LP before imaging the brain to rule out elevated intracranial pressure as thoroughly as possible. Removal of CSF from the lumbar spine reduces the counterpressure against intracranial fluid and, when intracranial pressure is elevated, can result in cerebral herniation. Clinical trials and retrospective studies have helped define which patients are likely to have abnormal brain imaging and be at high risk for herniation (7,8). Patients with new-onset seizures, significant impairment of consciousness, papilledema, focal neurologic deficits, and immunosuppressive comorbidity should have neuroimaging before LP.

Examination of CSF is mandatory in the diagnostic evaluation of bacterial meningitis. Blood cultures should also be performed at the time of presentation, because nearly all cases of meningitis in adults result from bacteremia. These cultures will help make a microbiologic diagnosis and guide therapy in those patients in whom imaging is indicated and therapy is started before a LP can be done. The opening pressure of CSF is elevated in most patients with meningitis, but the degree of elevation has no prognostic significance. The most common findings in the CSF of patients with meningitis are pleocytosis, elevated protein, and depressed glucose level. The pleocytosis is usually a neutrophil predominance with 500 to >10,000 cells/mm^3. Over time, mononuclear cells may increase, which may suggest a diagnosis of viral or *Mycobacterium tuberculosis* meningitis. Protein levels are elevated, often markedly so, to as much as 100 mg/dL or greater. CSF glucose is usually depressed to levels below 40% of simultaneously measured serum glucose.

Identification of the pathogen in CSF is helpful, not only in diagnosis but also in guiding therapy. Gram stain of CSF has a sensitivity of 60% to 90% and almost 100% specificity (9). The success of both Gram stain and culture of CSF is influenced by any antibiotics that are administered before LP. Even one dose of an antibiotic active against the pathogen can drastically reduce the sensitivity of Gram stain and culture. Bacterial antigen tests may be helpful in these situations, although their sensitivity is only about 75%. This underscores the importance of obtaining blood cultures immediately on presentation of any patient suspected of having bacterial meningitis and collecting CSF as rapidly as possible.

TREATMENT

Bacterial meningitis is associated with high morbidity and mortality, and the single best predictor of a poor outcome is delay of antibiotic administration (10). The most common reason for delay in antibiotic administration is neuroimaging. If imaging is to be performed before an LP is done, antibiotics should be given before the study. If no imaging is required, an LP should be performed promptly and therapy should be started immediately following the procedure. The choice of initial antibiotic therapy is based on the most likely pathogens according to the patient's age and concurrent medical conditions (Table 92-1). Therapy can be adjusted following culture of blood and CSF and susceptibility testing. Antibiotics that achieve significant levels in the CSF are required so as to quickly sterilize the CSF and prevent relapse (11,12). With the prevalence of pneumococci resistant to β-lactam antibiotics combination therapy with a third-generation cephalosporin and vancomycin has become

TABLE 92-1. Empiric Antibiotic Therapy for Adults with Community-Acquired Bacterial Meningitis

Age (years)	*Common Pathogens*	*Antimicrobial Therapy*
16–50	*Neisseria meningitidis* *Streptococcus pneumoniae*	Vancomycin + 3rd generation cephalosporin[a]
>50	*S. pneumoniae* *N. meningitidis* *Listeria monocytogenes* *Haemophilus* Enteric gram-negative bacilli	Vancomycin + 3rd generation cephalosporin + ampicillin
Risk factors present[b]	*S. pneumoniae* *N. meningitidis* *Haemophilus* *L. monocytogenes*	Vancomycin + 3rd generation cephalosporin + ampicillin

[a]Recommended agents are ceftriaxone or cefotaxime.
[b]Risk factors include alcoholism, immunosuppression, and hematologic malignancies.

the standard empiric therapy of meningitis (13). Some authorities would recommend adding rifampin to this regimen, although clinical studies on the efficacy of this agent in meningitis are not available. Patients who are at risk for meningococcal infection should be placed in respiratory isolation for 48 hours or until a microbiologic diagnosis can be made. Although the length of therapy for bacterial meningitis has not been completely established, most would recommend 10 to 14 days of therapy. Infections with gram-negative enteric organisms should be treated for 21 days because of the high rate of relapse associated with shorter courses of therapy. Meningitis caused by *Listeria* spp. should also be treated for 21 days because these infections frequently occur in persons with impaired immune responses and sterilization of the CSF is frequently delayed in these cases.

It is becoming increasingly evident that adjunctive steroids can reduce mortality and neurologic sequelae in bacterial meningitis. Bacteria seen on Gram stain of CSF, a leukocyte count of >1,000 cells/mm^3 in the CSF, and a CSF opening pressure >200 mm H_2O are widely regarded as indications for steroid therapy (14,15). Dexamethasone is the steroid of choice and should be started before, or with, the first dose of antibiotics. The recommended dose is 10 mg every 6 hours for 4 days. Patients who have evidence of adrenal insufficiency will require longer therapy with physiologic doses of steroids. In certain cases, steroids can be detrimental, specifically in those patients who develop septic shock. Glycerol appears to have some utility in preventing neurologic sequelae in children with bacterial meningitis, but this agent has not been studied in adults (16). The inflammatory response in the CSF is a logical target for therapeutic intervention. Research on host immune responses in the CNS has provided tremendous insight for potential immunomodulatory therapeutic targets and inflammation-modulating agents may be developed in the future as adjunctive therapy for meningitis (4).

In addition to antibiotic therapy and steroids (when indicated), supportive care is critical in the therapy of bacterial meningitis. Patients with septic shock should be monitored in an intensive care setting to provide optimal cardiovascular support. Patients with bacterial meningitis are at risk for hyponatremia, although the mechanism by which this occurs has not been clearly identified (7). Careful fluid resuscitation should be instituted, with the caveat that overly vigorous fluid replacement can worsen intracranial pressure.

Although seizures are not common in meningitis, their occurrence is an indication for anticonvulsant therapy. In rare cases, status epilepticus can cause progressive decline in mental status or a waxing and waning level of consciousness. When status epilepticus is suspected, an electroencephalogram is indicated. Although most cases of bacterial meningitis present with elevated intracranial pressure, this generally resolves relatively quickly with antibiotic therapy and steroids, in certain situations. When clinical response is slow or alterations in mental status persist, an LP should be performed to measure intracranial pressure. Persistently elevated CSF pressure may require a temporary lumbar drain or ventriculostomy. Repeated LP is also suggested for patients with infections caused by organisms with high minimal inhibitory concentrations to cephalosporins to demonstrate sterilization of the CSF. CSF cultures should be sterile by 24 hours following institution of effective antibacterial therapy.

In addition to hearing loss, other complications of bacterial meningitis can occur, although they are much less frequent. Because of the intense inflammatory response that sometime involves the cerebral vasculature, septic emboli or thrombi can result in cerebral infarction, with subsequent focal neurologic deficits. Treatment of this complication is dependent on effective antibiotic therapy and rapid resolution of the infection. Subdural empyema can cause a rapid clinical deterioration and is more commonly seen in persons with a history of sinusitis or recent sinus surgery. Imaging is required to make this diagnosis and surgical drainage is necessary, in most cases. In addition to cerebral complications, bacterial meningitis can result in pyogenic complications of the spinal cord. Paraspinous or epidural abscesses of the spine are rare complications of meningitis, but are suggested by persistent fever, focal neurologic deficits, or back pain. Accurate delineation by CT or magnetic resonance imaging (MRI) of these infections is indicated, because they frequently require surgical drainage.

Despite the availability of potent antibacterial drugs and steroids, bacterial meningitis is still associated with significant morbidity and mortality. Preventive measures are the most effective strategy for minimizing the impact of this infection. Since the use of Hib vaccine was initiated in 1986, this pathogen has been virtually eliminated as a cause of invasive disease in the United States. Protein-polysaccharide conjugate vaccines are now available for seven capsule types of the pneumococcus and four capsule types of meningococcus. These vaccines should greatly reduce the incidence of bacterial meningitis in children and young adults as they become widely deployed in these high-risk populations.

CLINICAL RECOMMENDATIONS OF THE VIGNETTE

The patient illustrates a common manifestation of bacterial meningitis. The age and living situation of the patient put him at risk for meningococcal meningitis. The appearance of a petechial rash is also consistent with this syndrome. Because the patient's mental status was considered to be significantly altered, a decision was made to image the brain before performing an LP. The decision to image, however, should not delay the administration of appropriate empiric antibiotics in suspected meningitis. Blood and CSF cultures from this patient grew meningococcus that was susceptible to ceftriaxone. Three months after this acute episode, the patient received the tetravalent meningococcal conjugate vaccine. Invasive meningococcal infections are reportable diseases and the state health department should be notified. Health department workers can also follow up with close contacts of the index patient to help assess the need for prophylactic antibiotics.

SUMMARY

Bacterial meningitis is an acute infection of the CNS that requires a high index of suspicion and prompt diagnostic and therapeutic intervention to prevent death and permanent neurologic impairments. Combination antimicrobial therapy should be directed at the most common pathogens until a microbiological diagnosis can be made and susceptibility testing completed. In certain cases, steroids should be used to reduce inflammation and lower intracranial pressure.

Immunization against the most common causes of bacterial meningitis is now available and should be widely implemented in high-risk groups to reduce the morbidity and mortality of this potentially devastating infection.

REFERENCES

1. Short WR, Tunkel AR. Changing epidemiology of bacterial meningitis in the United States. *Curr Infect Dis Rep.* 2000;2:327–331.
2. Morris A, Low DE. Nosocomial bacterial meningitis, including central nervous system shunt infections. *Infect Dis Clin N Am.* 1999;13:735–750.
3. Leib SL, Tauber MG. Pathogenesis of bacterial meningitis. *Infect Dis Clin N Am.* 1999;13:527–548.
4. van der Flier M, Geelen SPM, Kimpen JLL, et al. Reprogramming the host response in bacterial meningitis: How best to improve outcome? *Clin Microbiol Rev.* 2003;16:415–429.
5. van de Beek D, de Gans J, Spanjaard L, et al. Clinical features and prognostic factors in adults with bacterial meningitis. *N Engl J Med.* 2004;351:1849–1859.
6. De Marcaida JA, Reik L. Disorders that mimic central nervous system infections. *Neurol Clin.* 1999;17:901–941.
7. van de Beek D, de Gans J, Tunkel AR, et al. Community-acquired bacterial meningitis in adults. *N Engl J Med.* 2006;354:44–53.
8. Hasbun R, Abrahams J, Jekel J, et al. Computed tomography of the head before lumbar puncture in adults with suspected meningitis. *N Engl J Med.* 2001;345:1727–1733.
9. Zunt JR, Marra CM. Cerebrospinal fluid testing for the diagnosis of central nervous system infections. *Neurol Clin.* 1999;17:675–689.
10. Aronin SI, Peduzzi P, Quagliarello VJ. Community-acquired bacterial meningitis: Risk stratification for adverse outcome and effect of antibiotic timing. *Ann Intern Med.* 1998;129:862–869.
11. Andes DR, Craig WA. Pharmacokinetics and pharmacodynamics of antibiotics in meningitis. *Infect Dis Clin N Am.* 1999;13:595–618.
12. Sinner SW, Tunkel AR. Antimicrobial agents in the treatment of bacterial meningitis. *Infect Dis Clin N Am.* 2004;18:581–602.
13. Ahmed A. A critical evaluation of vancomycin for treatment of bacterial meningitis. *Pediatr Infect Dis J.* 1997;16:895–903.
14. de Gans J, van de Beck D. European dexamethasone in adulthood bacterial meningitis study investigations. *N Engl J Med.* 2002;347:1549–1556.
15. Aronin SI. Bacterial meningitis: Principles and practical aspects of therapy. *Curr Infect Dis Rep.* 2000;2:337–344.
16. Kilpi T, Peltola H, Jauhiainen T, et al. Oral glycerol and intravenous dexamethasone in preventing neurologic and audiologic sequelae of childhood bacterial meningitis. *Pediatr Infect Dis J.* 1995;14:270–278.

CHAPTER **93**

Stroke Complicating Systemic and Central Nervous System Infections

Augusto A. Miravalle • José Biller • James J. Corbett

OBJECTIVES

- To review the cerebrovascular complications of common systemic and central nervous system infections
- To review the mechanisms for vascular injury during these infections
- To describe the pathology and clinical manifestations of various cerebrovascular syndromes associated with these infections

CASE VIGNETTE

A 42-year-old right-handed man had a sudden onset of slurred speech and right arm weakness. He has a 2-month history of generalized malaise, intermittent episodes of occipital headaches, and confusion. He was born and lives in Anatolia, Turkey, and admits drinking raw goat milk. Examination showed mild hepatomegaly, dysarthria, right homonymous hemianopsia, and right faciobrachial paresis. Ancillary investigations demonstrated elevated C-reactive protein (CRP), and positive serum agglutination test for Brucella. Transthoracic and transesophageal echocardiography showed no evidence of valvular vegetation or intracardiac thrombi. Magnetic resonance imaging (MRI) of the brain demonstrated small foci of restricted diffusion in the left insula, medial posterior left temporal lobe, posterior limb of internal capsule, and both occipital lobes. Cerebrospinal fluid (CSF) analysis showed slight lymphocytic pleocytosis, elevated protein content, and decreased glucose levels. Brucella agglutination titers in CSF were strongly positive. He was started on tetracycline, rifampin, and gentamicin, with significant improvement of his condition.

DEFINITION

Arterial and venous strokes are a common complication of systemic or central nervous system (CNS) infections. The most common systemic infections resulting in stroke are infective endocarditis (IE), systemic bacterial infections, parasitic diseases, and acquired immunodeficiency syndrome (AIDS). CNS infections, including acute bacterial meningitis, acute encephalitides, subacute or chronic meningoencephalitides, and space-occupying lesions, can also produce stroke syndromes. Tables 93-1 and 93-2 summarize the most important characteristics for each group.

EPIDEMIOLOGY

SYSTEMIC INFECTIONS

Cerebrovascular involvement is a common complication in IE (Fig. 93-1). Reported in 30% of cases, it has remained stable over time, despite the development of many effective antimicrobial therapies (1–3). Ischemic strokes are more frequent than hemorrhages. Ischemic stroke accounts for 70% to 90% of vascular events complicating IE, whereas intracerebral hemorrhage (ICH) and venous sinus thrombosis are reported in <25% of cases. Infective (mycotic) aneurysms are recognized in 1% to 5% of IE cases (3). No statistical differences have been reported in the rate of stroke among patients with native valve and prosthetic valve endocarditis, but neurologic complications are more common with mechanical prosthetic heart valves compared with bioprosthetic heart valves. This is thought to be influenced by anticoagulation therapy, time interval between prosthetic heart valve placement, and development of IE (3,4). Regardless the cause or type of valve, mitral valve endocarditis is associated with an increased rate of stroke compared with IE involving other heart valves. The most commonly implicated organisms are *Streptococcus viridans* and *Staphylococcus aureus* accounting for >50% of cases (5).

During sepsis, ICH and brain infarcts are recognized in 7% to 10% of patients. *S. aureus, S. pneumoniae, Escherichia coli, Listeria monocytogenes*, and anaerobes are the most common etiologic agents (6,7). Neurologic involvement can be seen in 10% of cases of brucellosis, and acute, or subacute meningoencephalitides, and CNS vasculitis are frequent presentations. Cerebrovascular complications develop in 20% of patients with trichinosis and Chagas disease (8,9). Hemorrhagic brain

TABLE 93-1. Cerebrovascular Complications in Selective Systemic Infections

Systemic Infections	Stroke							
SYNDROME	**FREQUENCY**	**ONSET**	**I**	**H**	**V**	**L/M**	**SM**	**MECHANISM**
Infective endocarditis	++	Days to weeks	+++	+	+	++	+	Septic embolization Mycotic aneurysm rupture Immune complex damage
Sepsis	+	1 Week	++	++	+	+−	++	Septic embolization DIC Endotoxin damage
Parasitic Diseases	++	Variable	+	++	++	++	+	Septic embolization Direct parasite obstruction Vasculitis
AIDS or other immune disorders	++	Variable	++	+−	+−	++	+	Direct viral damage Immune complex damage Primary HIV angiitis

AIDS, acquired immunodeficiency syndromes; I, ischemia; H, intracerebral hemorrhage; V, venous thrombosis; L/M, large and medium sized vessels; Sm, small vessel stroke; DIC, disseminated intravascular coagulation; HIV, human immunodeficiency virus; +++, very frequent complication; ++, frequent complication; +, common complication; +−, occasionally observed; −, not reported.

infarcts caused by venous intracranial sinus thrombosis are not uncommon in patients with trichinosis. Although stroke syndromes are barely recognized during *Plasmodium falciparum* infection, diffuse petechial hemorrhages involving the subcortical white matter, are seen in almost 80% of autopsies (Fig. 93-2) (10–14). CNS vascular involvement in AIDS, which is reported in one fourth of autopsies, may result from primary human immunodeficiency virus (HIV) infection or opportunistic infections (15). Aspergillosis, cryptococcosis, disseminated candidiasis, toxoplasmosis, nocardia infections, histoplasmosis, free-living amebas, tuberculosis, and syphilis are among some of the opportunistic infections associated with CNS vasculopathy in patients with AIDS (Figs. 93-3 and 93-4). Ischemic lesions occur more frequently than hemorrhages (16–19).

CENTRAL NERVOUS SYSTEM INFECTIONS

Stroke can complicate acute and subacute meningoencephalitides with an estimated incidence of 30% to 40% of cases (20). Herpes zoster virus (HZV), herpes simplex virus (HSV), enteroviruses, cytomegalovirus, human T-lymphotrophic virus-1 (HTLV-1), dengue, mumps, eastern equine, California, Japanese, St. Louis, West Nile, stealth, junin, puumala, and Nipah viruses have been occasionally associated with CNS vasculopathy (21–31). In general, ischemia is the most frequent mechanism during bacterial infections, whereas hemorrhagic lesions are more common in cases of viral encephalitides. Punctate cerebral hemorrhages may be seen in the course of rickettsial infections. In addition, intracranial venous sinus thrombosis has been reported in 2% to 24% of cases of pyogenic brain abscesses and subdural empyema (20).

ETIOLOGY AND PATHOGENESIS

SYSTEMIC INFECTIONS

Embolization to large and small arteries is the most common mechanism responsible for ischemia in IE, whereas rupture of

TABLE 93-2. Cerebrovascular Complications in Central Nervous System (CNS) Infections

CNS Infections	Stroke							
SYNDROME	**FREQUENCY**	**ONSET**	**I**	**H**	**V**	**L/M**	**SM**	**MECHANISM**
Acute meningitis	++	1 week	+++	+−	+	++	+	Vasospasm/vasculitis Aneurysmal rupture Septic thrombosis
Acute encephalitides	+−	Week to months	++	++	+−	+	++	Direct viral damage Vasculitis
Subacute meningoencephalitides	++	Months to years	+++	+	+−	++	++	Aneurysmal rupture Hydrocephalus Panarteritis
Space-occupying lesions	+	Variable	++	+−	++	+	+−	Vasculitis, vasospasm Abscess rupture Venous thrombosis

I, Ischemia; H, intracerebral hemorrhage; V, venous thrombosis; L/M, large and medium size vessels; Sm, small vessel stroke; +++, very frequent complication; ++, frequent complication; +, common complication; +−, occasionally observed; -, not reported.

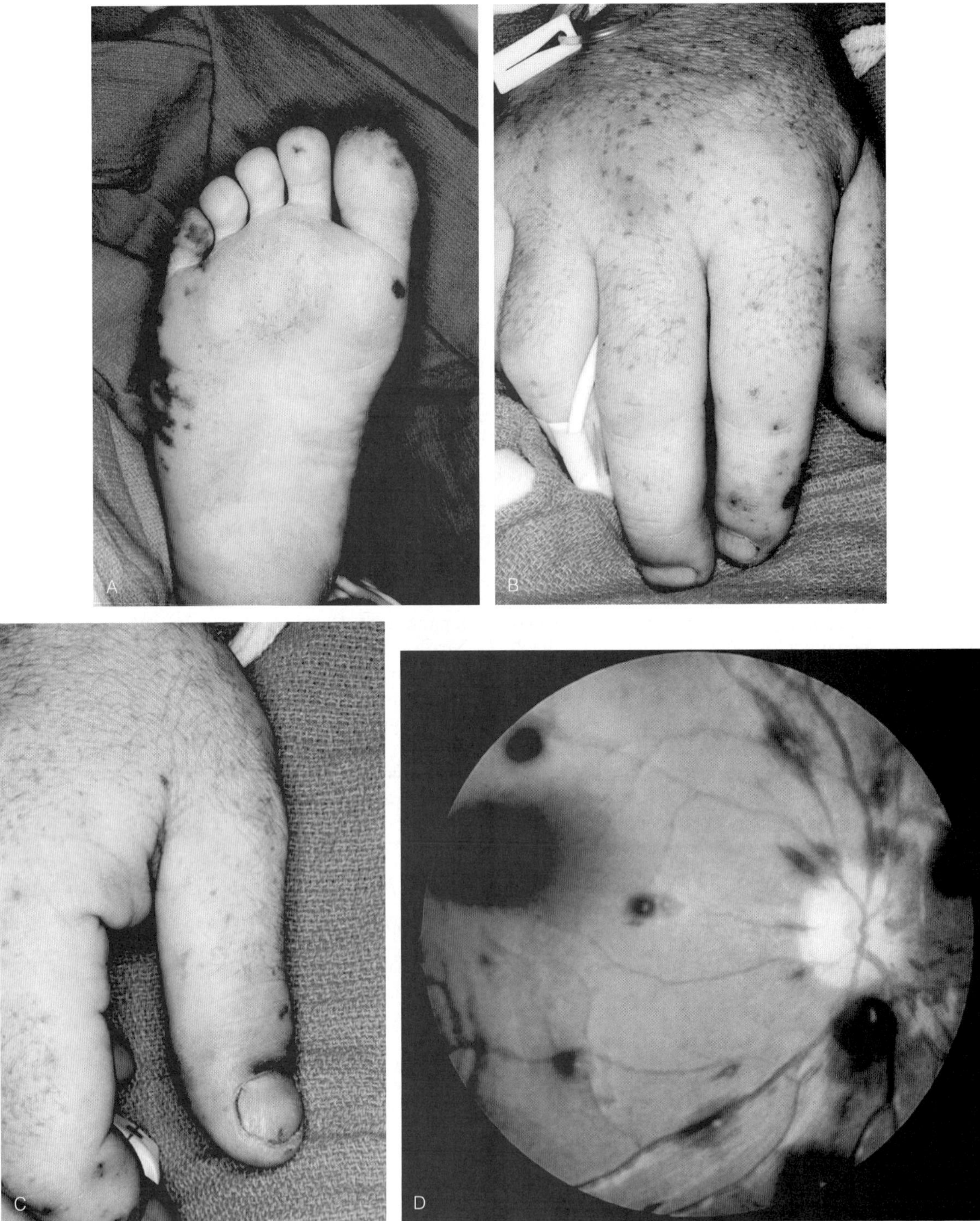

FIGURE 93-1. (**A–C**) Petechiae, splinter hemorrhages (nonblanching), Janeway lesions (macular, blanching, erythematous lesions on palms and soles), and Osler's nodes (painful violaceous nodules) are common systemic findings in subacute infective endocarditis IE. (**D**) Roth spots are white centered, hemorrhagic lesions of the retina, also seen in the setting of IE.

a mycotic aneurysm, septic arteritis, hemorrhagic transformation of bland infarctions, and immune complex vasculopathy commonly cause ICH. The pathogenesis of mycotic aneurysms is related to segmental occlusion of vasa vasorum, with subsequent invasion and weakening of the muscularis and aneurysmal formation (32). The bacteriology of mycotic aneurysms is quite heterogeneous, with *S. aureus, S. viridans,* and *Salmonella* species, as the most commonly implicated organisms. During sepsis, levels of antithrombin and proteins C and S are decreased, platelet aggregation increased, and antiphospholipid antibodies are formed, all of which increase the risk of thromboembolic complications (6). Increased concentration of endotoxins, interleukin-1, and tumor necrosis factor are also important causes of coagulation disturbances. In addition, ICH

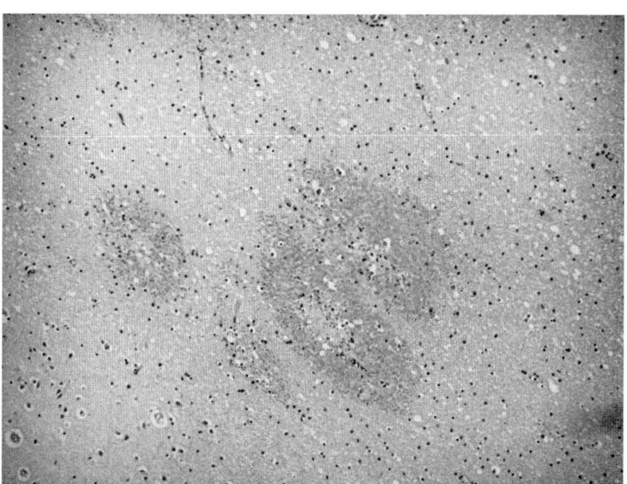

FIGURE 93-2. Low power photomicrograph of cerebral malaria. Perivascular intraparenchymal hemorrhage is seen around necrotic arterioles and venules (H&E stain). Courtesy of Henry Brown, MD, PhD, Department of Pathology, Section of Neuropathology, Loyola University Chicago.

can occur as a complication of disseminated intravascular coagulation (DIC). Intracranial sinus venous thrombosis can be associated with septic embolism and abscess formation, especially following anaerobic sepsis. Cerebrovascular involvement during neurobrucellosis can occur as cardioembolic phenomena from Brucella endocarditis, rupture of a mycotic aneurysm, or inflammatory vasculitis in the context of brucella meningoencephalitides. Direct parasite obstruction of brain blood vessels, toxic vasculitis, and hypereosinophilia-related endothelial damage are some of the proposed pathogenetic mechanisms in cerebrovascular involvement with *Trichinella* infection (8). In patients with cerebral malaria, cerebrovascular disease can be either secondary to occlusion of cerebral vessels by parasitized red blood cells, or cytokine-related endothelial damage with subsequent activation of the coagulation cascade. Primary HIV angiitis of the CNS is thought to result from direct infection of endothelial cells by HIV, immune complex deposition, or impaired regulation of cytokines. Among opportunistic infections associated with AIDS, vasculitis caused by *Aspergillus* is by direct invasion of hyphae into blood vessels, coagulative necrosis of vessel walls and subsequent thrombosis, hemorrhages, or aneurysm formation (33). Disseminated candidiasis is also associated with aneurysm formation, thrombotic brain infarction, ICH, and subarachnoid hemorrhages (34).

CENTRAL NERVOUS SYSTEM INFECTIONS

Radiologic and pathologic findings suggest different phases of the development of cerebral arteriopathy in the setting of acute bacterial meningitis (Fig. 93-5) (35). An active vascular response to the surrounding inflammatory subarachnoid exudate occurs early in the course of the disease, causing cerebral vasospasm. Vessel encroachment by purulent exudates and infiltration of the arterial walls by inflammatory cells, can lead to dilatation, intimal thickening, myonecrosis, and subendothelial edema. Hemorrhages can result from inflammatory destruction of vessel walls and from aneurysmal formation (36). Septic thrombosis of the superior sagittal sinus can be caused by spread of the meningeal infectious process to the intracranial veins via the diploic veins. Direct spread of HZV along intracranial branches of the trigeminal nerve has been proposed as a plausible pathogenetic mechanism for stroke. Several mechanisms have been implicated in the development of cerebral vasculitis during CNS tuberculosis, including strangulation of vessels by dense exudates at the base of the brain; spreading of inflammatory infiltrates through the adventitia to the intima of the vessel walls that results in necrotizing panarteritis; and stretching of vessels by dilated ventricles. Immune-mediated vasculitis has been postulated as the mechanism of cerebrovascular involvement in cases of neuroborreliosis (NB) (37). In neurocysticercosis, an intense inflammatory reaction in the subarachnoid space, triggered by adjacent cysticerci, results in vascular endothelial damage, atheromalike deposits, and further vascular occlusion (38). Rhinocerebral mucormycosis can be complicated with cavernous sinus thrombosis by direct extension from the paranasal sinuses (39).

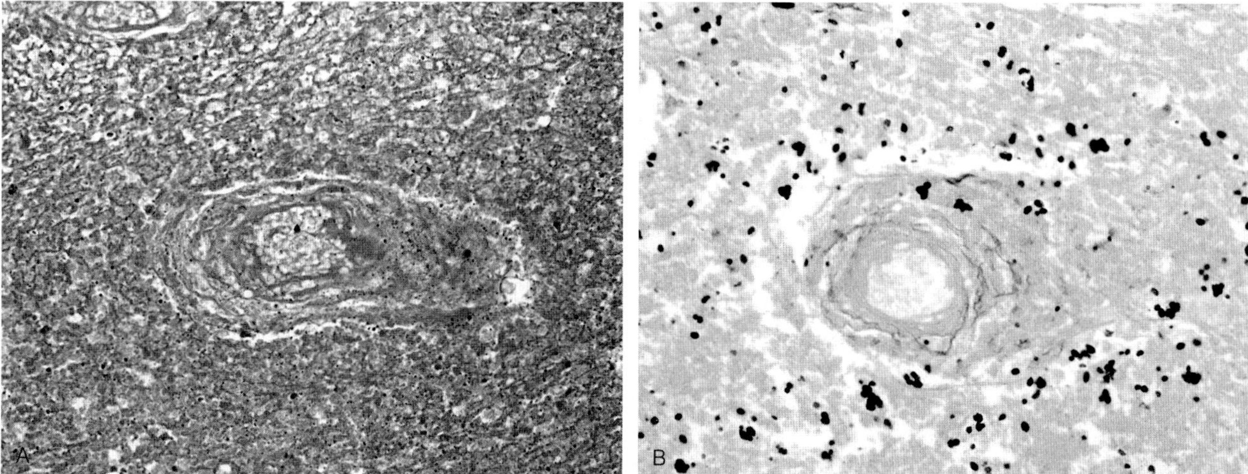

FIGURE 93-3. **(A)** Medium power photomicrograph of histoplasmosis reveals inflammation extending into the wall of an arteriole, causing vascular necrosis and thrombosis (H&E stain). **(B)** Methionine silver stain showing intravascular and intraparenchymal yeast forms, ranging from 2 to 5 μmol in size. Courtesy of Henry Brown, MD, PhD, Department of Pathology, Section of Neuropathology, Loyola University Chicago.

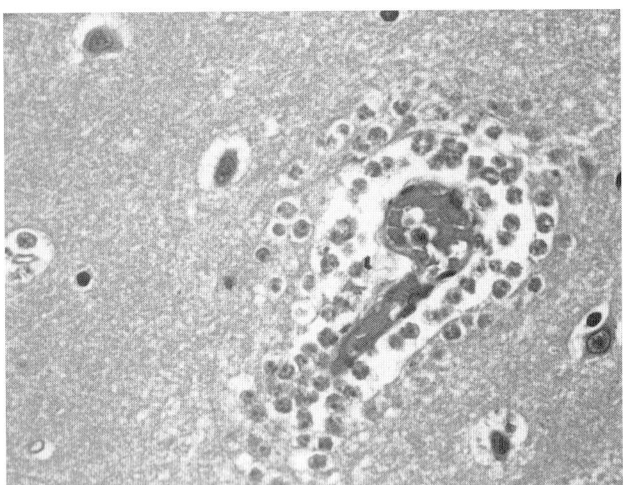

FIGURE 93-4. High power photomicrograph of infection with the amebae *Naegleria fowlerii*. Only a scant inflammatory response occurred with organisms present in the Virchow-Robin space around cerebral vessels (H&E stain). Courtesy of Henry Brown, MD, PhD, Department of Pathology, Section of Neuropathology, Loyola University Chicago.

PATHOLOGY

Cerebrovascular complications during infections can involve large, medium-size, or small vessels, as well as major intracranial venous sinuses or cortical veins. Specific differences have been recognized between the different organisms.

SYSTEMIC INFECTIONS

Large and medium-sized vessel involvement is common in the setting of IE, trypanosomiasis, and fungal infections. Small vessel vasculitis has been seen associated with bacterial sepsis, malaria, and neurobrucellosis. Sinus venous thrombosis is recognized after *Trichinella* and anaerobic infections.

CENTRAL NERVOUS SYSTEM INFECTIONS

Bacterial meningoencephalitis in adults usually involves large and medium-sized cerebral arteries, particularly the supraclinoid portion of the internal carotid artery (ICA), the middle cerebral artery (MCA) and the anterior cerebral artery (ACA). Small and medium-sized vessel inflammation is most common among children, especially with gram-negative bacilli and group B streptococci meningoencephalitides. HZV usually cause thrombosis of large and medium-sized vessels (40), whereas small vessel vasculitis is commonly described in HSV and rickettsial encephalitides. Stroke during treponemal infection results from two pathologic processes: Heubner and Nissl arteritis. Heubner arteritis is characterized by inflammatory occlusion of large and medium-sized arteries, whereas Nissl arteritis characteristically affects small perforating vessels (41). Small and medium-sized vessels are also seen in cases of cerebral infarction secondary to tuberculosis (TB) meningitis and neuroborreliosis (NB) (42).

CLINICAL MANIFESTATIONS

SYSTEMIC INFECTIONS

Patients with cardioembolic stroke secondary to IE may present with single cortical, small, or large disseminated vascular lesions. During the course of *S. aureus, Enterococcus* or *E. coli* endocarditis, embolization tends to occur early and is often multiple, with larger emboli and poor prognosis (5). Recurrent ischemic strokes are rare, occurring at a rate of 0.3% per day, usually before antimicrobial treatment is begun. In bacterial sepsis, strokes usually occur within the first week of the first positive culture.

CENTRAL NERVOUS SYSTEM INFECTIONS

In acute bacterial meningitis, focal neurologic deficits usually present during the first 5 days after infection. Hemiparesis, altered mental status, coma, and cranial nerve palsies are the most commonly observed clinical findings. During varicella infections, stroke usually develops 2 months after onset of skin rash, and approximately 4 to 15 weeks after onset of herpes zoster ophthalmicus (43). In rickettsial infections, focal neurologic signs are typically seen a few days after onset of skin rash (44).

Meningovascular syphilis often develops 7 years after infection (45). Some weeks before stroke onset, patients usually experience prodromal symptoms. Cognitive impairment is a frequent complaint. Cerebral vasculitis as a complication of tuberculosis, NB, and fungal infections usually has an insidious onset, with headaches, seizures, or focal deficits months after initial symptoms.

DIAGNOSIS

Diagnosis of vascular involvement in the context of infections should be suggested, based on the presence of focal neurologic deficits accompanying or complicating the course of the disease. Cranial CT or MRI must be performed in all patients developing focal neurologic signs. Magnetic resonance angiography (MRA), CT angiography (CTA), or catheter cerebral angiography may be invaluable in further delineating the morphology of the vessels involved. Blood serology and CSF analysis are often critical in reaching a definitive diagnosis. In the setting of CNS infection, CSF usually shows higher pleocytosis, protein content, lactate concentration, and higher opening pressure in patients with vascular complications than among those without stroke (46,47).

TREATMENT

Therapeutic regimens should aim to eradicate the infectious pathogens and treat the neurologic complications. Antimicrobial therapy should be started as soon as possible when infection is suspected. Appropriate regimens should be implemented according to each pathogen.

Prompt use of antimicrobials significantly reduces the incidence of emboli in patients with IE. In cases of native valve IE complicated by nonhemorrhagic strokes, anticoagulation is not indicated to prevent recurrences (48). If a cardioembolic stroke develops in an anticoagulated patient with mechanical valve IE, anticoagulation is often withheld for at least 48 hours. Before reinstituting anticoagulation, it is recommended that serial brain imaging be performed to rule out hemorrhagic transformation. Aspirin does not appear to reduce the risk of embolic events in patients with IE, and may be associated with an increased risk of bleeding (49). The

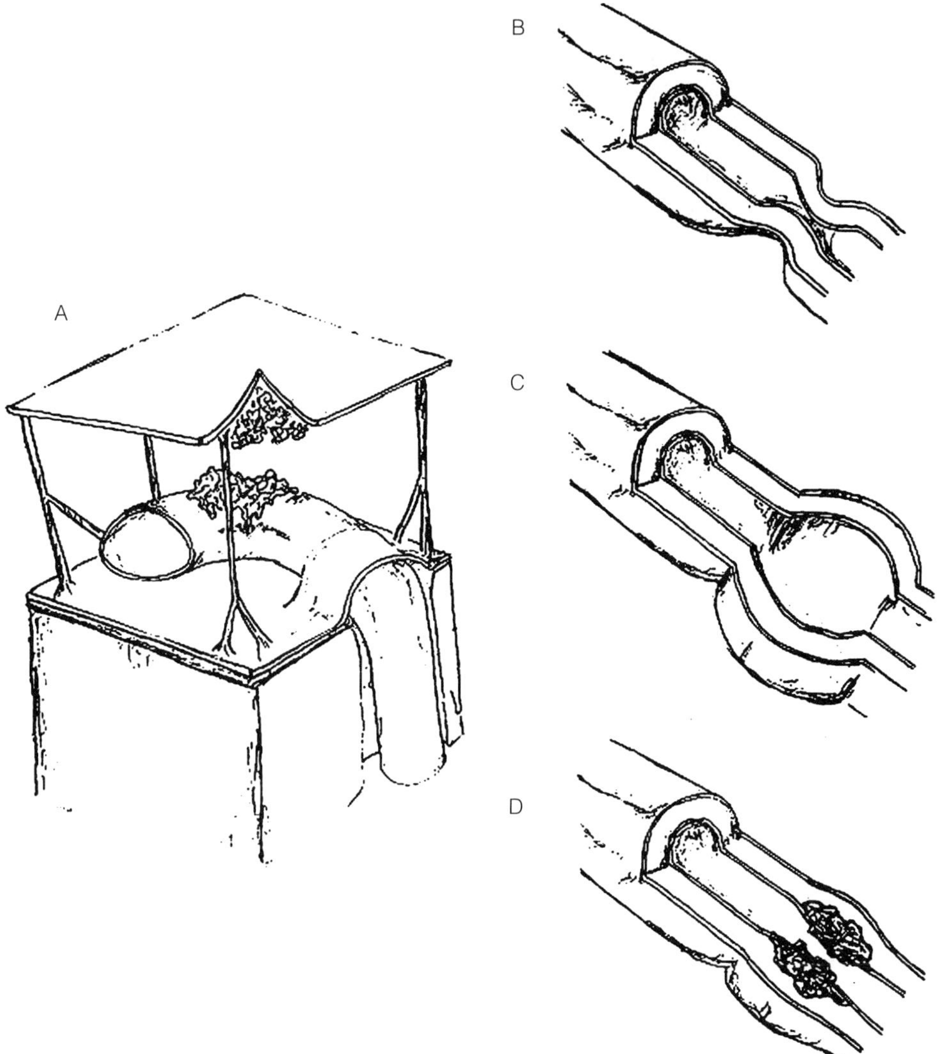

FIGURE 93-5. Pathogenesis of arteritis secondary to acute pyogenic meningitis. **(A)** During acute pyogenic meningitis, purulent exudates surround the arteries in the subarachnoid space. **(B)** Spasm of the vessel wall secondary to direct irritation by the inflammatory infiltrate. **(C)** Vasodilatation and aneurysm formation as a result of the prolonged smooth muscle cells contraction. **(D)** Subendothelial edema and myonecrosis develop, possibly associated with impaired diffusion of nutrients and metabolites to the endothelial cells.

evolution of mycotic aneurysms is unpredictable, and even with proper antimicrobial therapy, these aneurysms can regress, develop *de novo*, or rupture, with an estimated mortality rate of 80%. Occlusion of the aneurysm has been recommended early in the course of the disease process. Endovascular approaches have been recognized as a more effective and less invasive option compared with open craniotomy and aneurysmal clipping (50).

Anticoagulant use in cases of septic sinus venous thrombosis remains controversial. In a retrospective analysis of cavernous septic sinus thrombosis, anticoagulation did not affect mortality, but apparently decreased morbidity, including ophthalmoplegia, blindness, stroke, hypopituitarism, and seizures. In cases of septic cortical vein thrombosis, as well as in cases of lateral or superior sagittal sinus thrombosis, anticoagulation is generally not recommended, because it can be associated with an increased risk of hemorrhagic transformation (51).

CLINICAL RECOMMENDATIONS OF THE VIGNETTE

The patient presented with clinical and radiologic evidence of cerebral ischemia involving multiple vascular territories. On the basis of clinical history, serologic data, and imaging studies, inflammatory vasculitis secondary to neurobrucellosis was considered as a possible mechanism of cerebrovascular damage.

Brucella remains an important pathogen in endemic areas, including Saudi Arabia and Mediterranean countries. Consumption of contaminated foods and occupational contact remain the major sources of infection. Hematologic, gastrointestinal, cardiorespiratory, and musculoskeletal manifestations are common. Neurobrucellosis affects 5% to 10% of patients with systemic brucellosis. Common CNS manifestations are meningitis (the most common), encephalitis, ischemic and hemorrhagic strokes, myelitis, and brain and epidural abscesses.

Common peripheral nervous system manifestations include radiculitis, polyradiculopathy, and polyneuropathy. Prevention of human brucellosis depends on the control of the disease in animals (52,53). The treatment recommended for acute brucellosis in adults is rifampicin (600 to 900 mg) and doxycycline (200 mg) daily for a minimum of 6 weeks. Infections with complications, such as meningoencephalitis or endocarditis, require combination therapy with rifampicin, a tetracycline, and an aminoglycoside.

SUMMARY

Cerebrovascular involvement is a common complication in systemic and CNS infections. Ischemia, the most frequent mechanism, can involve large, medium, or small arteries; major intracranial venous sinuses; or other intracranial venous structures. Diagnosis should be suspected clinically, but confirmatory imaging, serology, and CSF analysis are frequently needed. Treatment should target infectious pathogens and, in selective cases, anticoagulation may be indicated.

REFERENCES

1. Pruitt AA. Neurological complications of infective endocarditis. In: Vlessis AA, Bolling SF, eds. *Endocarditis. A Multidisciplinary Approach to Modern Treatment.* Boston: Blackwell; 1999:177–179.
2. Cabell CH, Pond KK, Peterson GE, et al. The risk of stroke and death in patients with aortic and mitral valve endocarditis. *Am Heart J.* 2001;142(1):75–80.
3. Salgado AV. Central nervous system complications of infective endocarditis. *Stroke.* 1991;22(11):1461–1463.
4. Salgado AV, Furlan AJ, Keys TF, et al. Neurologic complications of endocarditis: A 12-year experience. *Neurology.* 1989;39(2 Pt 1):173–178.
5. Hart RG, Foster JW, Luther MF, et al. Stroke in infective endocarditis. *Stroke.* 1990; 21(5):695–700.
6. Valtonen V, Kuikka A, Syrjanen J. Thrombo-embolic complications in bacteraemic infections. *Eur Heart J.* 1993;14[Suppl K]:20–23.
7. Bitsch A, Nau R, Hilgers RA, et al. Focal neurologic deficits in infective endocarditis and other septic diseases. *Acta Neurol Scand.* 1996;94(4):279–286.
8. Nikolic S, Vujosevic M, Sasic M. Neurologic manifestations in trichinosis. *Srp Arh Celok Lek.* 1998;126(5–6): 209–213.
9. Carod-Artal FJ, Vargas AP, Melo M, et al. American trypanosomiasis (Chagas' disease): An unrecognized cause of stroke. *J Neurol Neurosurg Psychiatry.* 2003;74(4):516–518.
10. Brewster DR, Kwiatkowski D, White NJ. Neurological sequelae of cerebral malaria in children. *Lancet.* 1990;336(8722):1039–1043.
11. Leopoldino JF, Fukujima MM, Gabbai AA. Malaria and stroke. Case report. *Arq Neuropsiquiatr.* 1999;57(4):1024–1026.
12. Saraswat DK. Case of cerebral malaria presenting as subarachnoid haemorrhage. *J Assoc Physicians India.* 1994;42(9):756.
13. Obama MT, Dongmo L, Nkemayim C, et al. Stroke in children in Yaounde, Cameroon. *Indian Pediatr.* 1994;31(7):791–795.
14. Pham-Hung G, Truffert A, Delvallee G, et al. Cerebral infarction in pernicious malaria. Diagnostic value of computed tomography. *Ann Fr Anesth Reanim.* 1990;9(2):185–187.
15. Nogueras C, Sala M, Sasal M, et al. Recurrent stroke as a manifestation of primary angiitis of the central nervous system in a patient infected with human immunodeficiency virus. *Arch Neurol.* 2002;59(3):468–473.
16. Correa-Nazco VJ, Miguelez M, Laynez P, et al. Multiple hemorrhagic cerebral toxoplasmosis and AIDS. *Enferm Infecc Microbiol Clin.* 1999;17(10):531–532.
17. Mamidi A, DeSimone JA, Pomerantz RJ. Central nervous system infections in individuals with HIV-1 infection. *J Neurovirol.* 2002;8(3):158–167.
18. Mochan A, Modi M, Modi G. Stroke in black South African HIV-positive patients: A prospective analysis. *Stroke.* 2003;34(1):10–15.
19. Pinto AN. AIDS and cerebrovascular disease. *Stroke.* 1996;27(3):538–543.
20. Pfister HW, Borasio GD, Dirnagl U, et al. Cerebrovascular complications of bacterial meningitis in adults. *Neurology.* 1992;42(8):1497–1504.
21. Ribai P, Liesnard C, Rodesch G, et al. Transient cerebral arteriopathy in infancy associated with enteroviral infection. *Eur J Paediatr Neurol.* 2003;7(2):73–75.
22. Rabaud CH, Ghiringelli CB, Dauendorffer JN, et al. Echovirus 30 meningitis: A new cause for cerebral venous thrombosis? *J Infect.* 2002;44(1):53.
23. Ise K. A case of multiple cerebral infarctions associated with mumps, showing right hemiparesis, hemichorea and aphasia. *No To Hattatsu.* 1993;25(3):291–293.
24. Koeppen AH, Lansing LS, Peng SK, et al. Central nervous system vasculitis in cytomegalovirus infection. *J Neurol Sci.* 1981;51(3):395–410.
25. Leber SM, Brunberg JA, Pavkovic IM. Infarction of basal ganglia associated with California encephalitis virus. *Pediatr Neurol.* 1995;12(4):346–349.
26. Saposnik G, Del Brutto OH; Iberoamerican Society of Cerebrovascular Diseases. Stroke in South America: A systematic review of incidence, prevalence, and stroke subtypes. *Stroke.* 2003;34(9):2103–2107.
27. Nimmannitya S, Thisyakorn U, Hemsrichart V. Dengue haemorrhagic fever with unusual manifestations. *Southeast Asian J Trop Med Public Health.* 1987;18(3):398–406.
28. Alexeyev OA, Morozov VG. Neurological manifestations of hemorrhagic fever with renal syndrome caused by Puumala virus: Review of 811 cases. *Clin Infect Dis.* 1995;20(2): 255–258.
29. Lam SK, Chua KB. Nipah virus encephalitis outbreak in Malaysia. *Clin Infect Dis.* 2002;34[Suppl 2]:S48–S51.
30. Martin WJ. Stealth viral encephalopathy: Report of a fatal case complicated by cerebral vasculitis. *Pathobiology.* 1996;64(2):59–63.
31. Miller JD, Ross CA. Encephalitis. A four-year survey. *Lancet.* 1968;1(7552):1121–1126.
32. Molinari GF, Smith L, Goldstein MN, et al. Pathogenesis of cerebral mycotic aneurysms. *Neurology.* 1973;23(4):325–332.
33. Sharma RR, Gurusinghe NT, Lynch PG. Cerebral infarction due to Aspergillus arteritis following glioma surgery. *Br J Neurosurg.* 1992;6(5):485–490.
34. Nagashima T, Miyanoshita A, Sakiyama Y, et al. Cerebral vasculitis in chronic mucocutaneous candidiasis: Autopsy case report. *Neuropathology.* 2000;20(4):309–314.
35. Yamashima T, Kashihara K, Ikeda K, et al. Three phases of cerebral arteriopathy in meningitis: Vasospasm and vasodilatation followed by organic stenosis. *Neurosurgery.* 1985;16(4):546–553.
36. Gironell A, Domingo P, Mancebo J, et al. Hemorrhagic stroke as a complication of bacterial meningitis in adults: Report of three cases and review. *Clin Infect Dis.* 1995;21(6): 1488–1491.
37. Wilke M, Eiffert H, Christen HJ, et al. Primarily chronic and cerebrovascular course of Lyme neuroborreliosis: Case reports and literature review. *Arch Dis Child.* 2000;83(1): 67–71.
38. Barinagarrementeria F, Cantu C. Frequency of cerebral arteritis in subarachnoid cysticercosis: An angiographic study. *Stroke.* 1998;29(1):123–125.
39. Onerci M, Gursel B, Hosal S, et al. Rhinocerebral mucormycosis with extension to the cavernous sinus. A case report. *Rhinology.* 1991;29(4):321–324.
40. Kleinschmidt-DeMasters BK, Gilden DH. Varicella-zoster virus infections of the nervous system: Clinical and pathologic correlates. *Arch Pathol Lab Med.* 2001;125(6):770–780.
41. Nakane H, Okada Y, Ibayashi S, et al. Brain infarction caused by syphilitic aortic aneurysm. A case report. *Angiology.* 1996;47(9):911–917.
42. Halperin JJ. Nervous system Lyme disease. *Vector Borne Zoonotic Dis.* 2002;2(4):241–247.
43. Moriuchi H, Rodriguez W. Role of varicella-zoster virus in stroke syndromes. *Pediatr Infect Dis J.* 2000;19(7):648–653.
44. del Brutto OH. Cerebrovascular disease in the tropics. *Rev Neurol.* 2001;33(8):750–762.
45. Conde-Sendin MA, Hernandez-Fleta JL, Cardenes-Santana MA, et al. Neurosyphilis: Forms of presentation and clinical management. *Rev Neurol.* 2002;35(4):380–386.
46. Chang CJ, Chang WN, Huang LT, et al. Cerebral infarction in perinatal and childhood bacterial meningitis. *QJM.* 2003;96(10):755–762.
47. Taft TA, Chusid MJ, Sty JR. Cerebral infarction in hemophilus influenzae type B meningitis. *Clin Pediatr (Phila).* 1986;25(4):177–180.
48. Eleftherios M, Calderwood SB. Infective endocarditis in adults. *N Engl J Med.* 2001(18) 345:1318–1330.
49. Chan KL, Dumensnil JG, Cujec B, et al. Investigators of the Multicenter Aspirin Study in Infective Endocarditis. A randomized trial of aspirin on the risk of embolic events in patients with infective endocarditis. *J Am Coll Cardiol.* 2003;42(5):775–780.
50. Chapot R, et al. Endovascular treatment of cerebral mycotic aneurysms. *Radiology.* 2002;222:389–396.
51. Levine S, Twyman RE, Gilman S. The role of anticoagulation in cavernous sinus thrombosis. *Neurology.* 1988;38:517–522.
52. Adaletli I, et al. Vasculopathic changes in the cerebral arterial system with neurobrucellosis. *AJNR Am J Neuroradiol.* 2006;27:384–386.
53. Al-Sous MA, et al. Neurobrucellosis: Clinical and neuroimaging correlation. *AJNR Am J Neuroradiol.* 2004;25:395–401.

CHAPTER 94

HIV/AIDS

Harold Henderson

OBJECTIVES

- To discuss the epidemiology of major syndromes causing neurologic dysfunction in setting of HIV/AIDS
- To describe current concepts of the neuropathogenesis of HIV infection
- To explain the clinical manifestations of major opportunistic infections and neoplasms of the nervous system in persons with HIV/AIDS
- To describe the clinical manifestations of primary HIV-associated neurologic disorders
- To explain important principles of diagnosis and treatment of neurologic disorders occurring in persons with HIV/AIDS

CASE VIGNETTE 1

A 27-year-old man is brought to an emergency room after having a generalized tonic–clonic seizure. He had been complaining of a headache, poor appetite, and fatigue for about 1 week. He has no prior history of seizures, has never been under the care of a doctor, and is taking no medications. He is bisexual. Physical examination findings include a temperature of 101.2°F, generalized muscle wasting, whitish plaques on the posterior oropharynx, and a left hemiparesis.

CASE VIGNETTE 2

A 33-year-old-woman is brought by her mother to see a physician. The daughter has been having some difficulty with memory and a slowness of thinking, which has affected her job performance as a bank teller in the past 2 to 3 weeks. The mother says that these symptoms began more than 6 months ago. The mother only recently found out that her daughter tested positive for human immunodeficiency virus 1 (HIV-1) infection several years ago, but the daughter had never sought any care. Examination findings include decreased short-term memory, poor attention span, inability to perform simple mathematics problems, and a slight lack of balance when turning while walking.

DEFINITION

Disorders of the nervous system that occur in persons living with HIV or acquired immunodeficiency syndrome (AIDS) can involve either the central nervous system (CNS) or the peripheral nervous system (PNS). CNS disorders can be classified further as nonfocal diseases, such as the AIDS dementia complex (ADC), and diseases caused by focal brain lesions, such as toxoplasmosis or primary CNS lymphoma. Neurologic disorders that occur in persons infected with HIV-1 can also be categorized in another way: Primary disorders that are directly related to HIV infection, for example ADC and peripheral neuropathy; and secondary disorders in the form of opportunistic infections and neoplasms of the CNS (1–3) (Table 94-1). In addition, many of the drugs used in the treatment of HIV/AIDS can cause neurologic syndromes because of toxicity or drug interactions. Finally, multiple neurologic disorders can coexist in an individual patient.

EPIDEMIOLOGY

Neurologic manifestations of HIV/AIDS are common. Before the widespread use of highly active antiretroviral therapy (HAART) in the mid 1990s, 50% or more of persons infected with HIV developed a neurologic complication during their lifetime. Because of the beneficial effects of HAART in the treatment of HIV/AIDS and preventing immune system deterioration, the incidence of neurologic disease has dramatically decreased over the past decade, especially opportunistic infections, such as cryptococcal meningitis and toxoplasmosis (4). Persons with HIV live much longer in the HAART era, however, so the prevalence of primary disorders (e.g., dementia and peripheral neuropathy) remains relatively high. Recent surveillance data from the HAART era indicate that about 5% of newly diagnosed cases of AIDS in the United States listed the AIDS dementia complex as the initial AIDS-defining event.

ETIOLOGY, PATHOLOGY, AND PATHOGENESIS

The major neurologic complication directly caused by HIV-1 is ADC, which has also been referred to as HIV dementia, HIV encephalopathy, and the HIV-associated cognitive motor complex. The primary pathologic feature of ADC is the formation of syncytia. Autopsy studies of persons with ADC show encephalitis with syncytia formation characterized by the presence of multinucleated giant cells caused by the fusion of infected macrophages and microglial cells. Astrocytosis and infiltration of the perivascular space with mononuclear cells are also seen. Perivascular aggregates of inflammatory cells are sometimes associated with

TABLE 94-1. Major Neurologic Manifestations of Human Immunodeficiency Virus (HIV) Disease

Diagnosis	*CD4+ Count*	*Signs and Symptoms*	*Diagnostic Studies*
HIV/AIDS dementia	Usually <200	Memory loss, behavioral change, motor dysfunction	MRI/CT head, neuropsychologic studies
CMV encephalitis	<50	Progressive confusion, weakness	MRI/CT head, CSF PCR CMV
Cryptococcal meningitis	<200	Fever, headache, neck stiffness, cranial nerve palsies	CSF and serum cryptococcal antigen, CSF India ink and fungal culture
Cerebral toxoplasmosis	<200	Headache, fever, seizures, confusion	MRI/CT head, toxoplasma serology
PML	<200	Focal weakness, ataxia, visual symptoms	MRI/CT head, CSF PCR JC virus, brain biopsy
CNS lymphoma	<100	Confusion, memory loss, hemiparesis, seizures	MRI/CT head, brain biopsy
Neurosyphilis	Any	Dementia, seizures, cranial palsies	CSF and serum VDRL, elevated CSF, WBC protein
Distal sensory polyneuropathy	<200	Numbness, paresthesias, pain	NCS
Inflammatory demyelinating polyneuropathy	Any	Progressive weakness, paresthesias	NCS, EMG
Ascending CMV polyradiculopathy	<50	Progressive leg weakness, bladder dysfunction, decreased reflexes	CSF pleocytosis, CSF CMV PCR and culture
Vacuolar myelopathy	<200	Gait dysfunction, leg weakness	MRI spinal cord

MRI, magnetic resonance imaging; CT, computed tomography; CSF, cerebrospinal fluid; PML, progressive multifocal leukoencephalopathy; PCR, polymerase chain reaction; CNS, central nervous system; VDRL, venereal disease research laboratory test; CMV, cytomegalovirus; NCS, nerve conduction study; EMG, electromyography, GBS, Guillain-Barré syndrome; IDP, inflammatory demyelinating polyneuropathy.
(Adapted from Simpson DM, Tagliati M. Neurologic manifestations of HIV infection. *Ann Intern Med.* 1994;121:769, with permission.)

microinfarcts, and it has been suggested that increased vascular permeability and an alteration of the blood–brain barrier (BBB) may be present. Quantitative neuronal cell loss and a reduction in neural cell size are frequently found.

The neuropathogenesis of HIV infection is complex and not completely understood (5). HIV penetration across the BBB into the CNS can occur during both early and late stages of HIV disease. This may be in the form of either cell-free HIV virions or via infected monocytes that cross the BBB. Once present in the CNS, monocytes differentiate into macrophages and microglial cells, both of which can support continued HIV replication and disseminate throughout the nervous system. Astrocytes and primary brain endothelial cells can also be infected by HIV. Some studies have found an association between clinical dementia and high cerebrospinal fluid (CSF) HIV-1 viral load levels, but this correlation is not complete, and a wide overlap exists between CSF viral loads in those with dementia and those who are not (2,3).

Neuronal damage caused by HIV can be related to the release of toxic viral envelope proteins, such as gp120, or the regulatory proteins Tat, Nef, and Vpr. These proteins may be directly neurotoxic or may indirectly cause toxicity via the induction of the release of inflammatory cytokines. Tat and Vpr may also induce apoptosis (programmed cell death). Alternatively, HIV neuropathogenesis can be mediated indirectly through the release of cytokines by HIV-infected macrophages and microglial cells, which may in turn cause the release of other proinflammatory or toxic agents. Elevated levels of factors such as tumor necrosis factor-α (TNF-α), IL-1, RANTES, MIP-1α, MIP-1β, platelet-activating factor, and nitric oxide, have all been found in the brain or CSF of persons infected with HIV and may ultimately lead to the development of neurocytotoxicity. A similar cytokine-mediated toxic pathway is thought to be involved in the development of HIV-related peripheral neuropathy.

Secondary neurologic complications of HIV disease, such as toxoplasmosis or primary CNS lymphoma, are related to the profound immunodeficiency that occurs in persons with AIDS. These complications usually occur when absolute CD4 counts have fallen to below 200/mm^3.

Nonfocal Brain Disorders

CLINICAL MANIFESTATIONS, DIAGNOSIS, AND TREATMENT

AIDS DEMENTIA COMPLEX

Patients with a mild, early stage of ADC usually complain of difficulty with memory and ability to concentrate, and decreased attention span. Mental tasks, such as reading or balancing a checkbook, which were once easy to perform, now require more effort and take more time to complete. Slowness of thinking is common, and frequently the person loses his or her train of thought. Apathy and withdrawal from social activities often follow. As ADC progresses, motor abnormalities, such as lack of coordination, slow or unsteady gait, and altered handwriting, occur. The ability to work and perform more demanding activities of daily living is lost. Patients with the most advanced stage of ADC have profound deficits in cognitive and motor functioning;

they are no longer able to care for themselves and may be in a nearly vegetative state. Seizures are uncommon.

ADC most commonly occurs in persons with CD4 counts $<200/mm^3$ and generally follows an insidious course with development and progression of neurologic deficits over weeks to months. It is primarily a clinical diagnosis based on recognition of the characteristic cognitive and motor abnormalities with the exclusion of alternative causes. The differential diagnosis includes depression, substance abuse, progressive multifocal leukoencephalopathy (PML), CNS lymphoma, and non-HIV viral encephalitis. The mental status examination shows short-term memory deficits, psychomotor slowing, and the inability to do simple calculations. Unsteadiness of gait and abnormal reflexes are additional common findings. CSF analysis may show a mild pleocytosis and an elevated protein, but these CSF abnormalities are not specific for dementia; CSF analysis is useful mainly to exclude such disorders as neurosyphilis or cryptococcal meningitis. The most common finding on imaging studies of the brain, either computed tomography (CT) or magnetic resonance imaging (MRI), is brain atrophy, although the presence of atrophy is not specific for the diagnosis of ADC. MRI findings of multiple hyperintense signals on T2-weighted images in the subcortical white matter are more characteristic.

The treatment of choice for ADC is HAART. Epidemiologic studies of ADC in the HAART era show clearly that effective anti-HIV drug therapy can prevent dementia. Small treatment studies and multiple anecdotal experiences from HIV caregivers indicate that HAART can also stop or reverse the progression of dementia in the presence of established ADC in a significant proportion of patients. The treatment effect of HAART is not clearly related to the ability of specific anti-HIV agents to penetrate into the CNS. Historically, the improved outcomes for persons with ADC date to the advent of the protease inhibitors in 1996–1997, despite that protease inhibitors in general have poor CNS penetration. Beneficial affects on ADC have also been seen in association with HAART regimens that do not contain a protease inhibitor. It is unknown whether specific HAART drug combinations are more effective for ADC than others, and the optimal regimen is not known at present. HIV drug susceptibility should be documented, and HAART regimens capable of suppression of plasma viral loads to undetectable levels should be used in the same way as in the treatment of systemic HIV disease.

CYTOMEGALOVIRUS ENCEPHALITIS

Cytomegalovirus (CMV) encephalitis is a disease of late-stage AIDS, occurring in patients with CD4 counts $<50/mm^3$, often in the presence of other CMV-related syndromes, such as retinitis. It is uncommon in the era of HAART. The clinical presentation of CMV encephalitis tends to be similar to ADC, but it is characterized by a more acute onset. Fever, delirium, hyponatremia, and cranial nerve abnormalities may be present and serve to distinguish CMV encephalitis from ADC. Meningeal or periventricular enhancement may be seen on MRI of the brain. The presence of CMV DNA in the CSF as detected by the polymerase chain reaction (PCR) is both sensitive and specific, and is the diagnostic test of choice.

A course of intravenous ganciclovir (5 mg/kg every 12 hours for 14 days), followed by a single 5 mg/kg daily dose indefinitely as maintenance therapy, is the standard treatment approach for CMV encephalitis. Intravenous foscarnet (90 mg/kg every 12 hours for 14 days), followed by a single 90 mg/kg daily dose as maintenance, is an alternative. Oral valganciclovir (900 mg every 12 hours) is equivalent to standard intravenous ganciclovir therapy for the treatment of CMV retinitis, but no studies have evaluated the oral agent in the treatment of CMV encephalitis. Combination therapy with ganciclovir and foscarnet has also been advocated. In the pre-HAART era, when effective drug treatment of underlying HIV disease was not available, the prognosis for persons with CMV encephalitis was poor, but it is likely better in the current era.

CRYPTOCOCCAL MENINGITIS

Cryptococcus neoformans is the most common cause of meningitis in persons with AIDS. A subacute presentation with fever, malaise, weight loss, and headache is common. Cranial nerve palsies, blindness, and seizures are sometimes present, and patients with severe cryptococcal meningitis will have decreased mental status. The diagnosis is usually made by a positive CSF cryptococcal antigen titer, visualization of cryptococcal yeasts on CSF India Ink smear, or a positive CSF fungal culture. Elevated intracranial pressure (ICP) is common and may be associated with increased morbidity and mortality, so the CSF opening pressure should be measured routinely when a lumbar puncture is performed on someone with HIV/AIDS. (See also Chapter 95.)

Initial treatment of cryptococcal meningitis should be with intravenous amphotericin B (0.7 to 1.0 mg/kg/day) and oral flucytosine (25 mg/kg every 6 hours) (6). Lipid preparations of amphotericin can be used to decrease the incidence of nephrotoxicity. Once signs and symptoms of meningitis have stabilized (usually, 1 to 2 weeks), antifungal therapy can be changed to oral fluconazole (200 mg twice daily for 8 weeks). At that time, if sufficient clinical improvement is seen, the dose of fluconazole can be decreased to 200 mg daily as maintenance therapy. Elevated ICP is associated with complications, such as blindness, and an overall poorer outcome; if present, ICP should be aggressively treated by physical drainage of CSF, either via frequent, repeated lumbar puncture (every day if necessary) or the placement of an intraventricular shunt. Standard medical therapy for increased ICP in the form of mannitol and corticosteroids is not known to be effective in the setting of cryptococcal meningitis.

Nonfocal Brain Disorders

CLINICAL MANIFESTATIONS, DIAGNOSIS, AND TREATMENT

FOCAL BRAIN DISORDERS

Toxoplasmosis

Toxoplasma encephalitis (TE) is caused by the reactivation of previously acquired infection in the presence of severe immunodeficiency. CD4 counts are nearly always $<200/mm^3$ and are usually $<100/mm^3$. The widespread usage of trimethoprim-sulfamethoxazole (TMP-SMX) prophylaxis for pneumocystis pneumonia has resulted in a marked decrease in the incidence of toxoplasmosis since daily usage of oral TMP-SMX can also prevent the occurrence of TE. HAART has also contributed to the decline in cases of toxoplasmosis. The most common presenting symptoms of TE are headache, fever, confusion, and lethargy, with seizures occurring in about 30% of patients. Focal neurologic physical examination findings are common and include hemiparesis, cranial nerve palsies, and ataxia. The clinical syndrome generally develops over a period of a few days to a few weeks.

A presumptive diagnosis of toxoplasmosis can be made on the basis of a compatible clinical presentation, positive toxoplasma serology, and typical neuroimaging studies. Approximately 95% of patients with TE have detectable IgG antibodies to *Toxoplasma gondii*. Thus, a positive test result confirms prior infection and is supportive but not diagnostic of active disease, whereas a negative toxoplasma serologic test result should cast doubt on the diagnosis of TE. CT or MRI scans of the brain typically reveal multiple, bilateral focal lesions that enhance with contrast in a ring pattern. Lesions are most commonly present in the basal ganglia, thalamus, and cortex, and they can be edematous. MRI is more sensitive than CT for the detection of multiple lesions. This radiographic appearance is not specific for toxoplasmosis, however, and single, contrast-enhancing lesions in particular may also be compatible with primary CNS lymphoma.

In patients with the characteristic clinical syndrome and radiologic findings and detectable antitoxoplasma antibodies, initiation of empiric treatment of TE is indicated. Standard treatment consists of the combination of oral pyrimethamine (initial dose, 200 mg followed by 50 to 75 mg/day) and oral sulfadiazine (6 g/day in four divided doses for 6 to 8 weeks). Folinic acid (5 to 10 mg/day) is recommended to decrease the hematologic toxicity of pyrimethamine. Clindamycin (1,800 mg/day in three to four divided doses) can be substituted for sulfadiazine in patients with sulfa allergy. Corticosteroids are commonly used to decrease marked cerebral edema. Most patients improve clinically and radiologically within 1 to 2 weeks. If improvement does not occur within this period of time, diagnostic reevaluation should be performed. Maintenance therapy is necessary to prevent relapse of TE, and this usually consists of pyrimethamine (50 mg/day) with sulfadiazine (2 to 4 g/day in four divided doses) or clindamycin (300 to 450 mg three times daily).

Primary Central Nervous System Lymphoma

Patients with CNS lymphoma generally have advanced AIDS with CD4 counts $<100/mm^3$. The usual clinical presentation is subacute, lasting weeks, and includes lethargy, confusion, and memory loss. Focal neurologic signs, such as hemiparesis, are common and seizures can occur. CT or MRI of the head usually shows single or multiple mass lesions that enhance with contrast. Deep lesions involving the white matter, subependymal enhancement, and more diffuse, weak contrast enhancement are radiologic characteristics of CNS lymphoma that may serve to help distinguish it from toxoplasmosis. Epstein-Barr virus (EBV) DNA can almost always be detected in CNS lymphoma tumor cells from persons with AIDS. CSF analysis for EBV DNA by PCR has a sensitivity of 80% to 90% and is specific for the diagnosis of primary CNS lymphoma in the setting of AIDS. If a definitive diagnosis cannot be made noninvasively, a stereotactic brain biopsy would then be necessary.

The treatment of CNS lymphoma usually consists of whole brain radiotherapy over a period of 3 to 4 weeks. Chemotherapy has a high level of toxicity and is poorly tolerated by most patients. In the pre-HAART era, prognosis was very poor and average survival with therapy was 4 to 6 months. In the HAART era, survival rates have dramatically improved.

Progressive Multifocal Leukoencephalopathy

PML is caused by infection with the JC virus. In the setting of immunodeficiency, the JC virus can cause lysis of oligodendrocytes and widespread demyelination. PML is a white matter disease, characterized by demyelination and loss of tissue, rather than a CNS mass effect. Most patients have CD4 counts of about $200/mm^3$ or less, and have symptoms of limb incoordination, difficulty with gait, hemiparesis, altered mental status, and visual and speech disturbances. Focal neurologic findings on physical examination are very common. Some aspects of PML are suggestive of the ADC.

PML generally has a characteristic appearance on MRI, and this imaging modality is thus favored over CT for diagnosis. PML typically appears as single or multiple hypodense, nonenhancing lesions of the white matter with no mass effect. The lesions are usually bilateral and asymmetric, and most often involve the white matter adjacent to the cortex, but may be anywhere. In a few patients, lesions may involve the gray matter and show faint, irregular enhancement. JC viral DNA detected in the CSF is highly specific for the diagnosis of PML, and has a sensitivity of at least 75%. Brain biopsy would be needed for diagnosis if analysis of the CSF for JC virus by PCR was negative.

No specific treatment exists for PML (7). Various chemotherapeutic agents (cidofovir, cytarabine, interferon-α) have been administered in an effort to treat patients with PML, but to date none show any definite benefit over and above that obtained with HAART alone. Before the HAART ear, median survival with PML was 2 to 4 months. Although there is considerable variability, most patients with PML in the HAART era have a significantly improved prognosis. The median survival is now in the range of 10 to 12 months, and some patients have what appears to be a complete remission associated with HAART therapy.

Peripheral Neuropathies

CLINICAL MANIFESTATIONS, DIAGNOSIS, AND TREATMENT

DISTAL SENSORY POLYNEUROPATHY

Distal sensory polyneuropathy (DSP) is an axonal neuropathy, and the most common cause of peripheral neuropathy in HIV/AIDS (2). Symptomatic neuropathy occurs in about 35% of patients, usually when CD counts are $<200/mm^3$. Common symptoms are numbness, paresthesias, and pain starting usually in the feet. The sensory symptoms often progress to the level of the ankle or further up to the knee, and the hands may be affected as well. Contact with the skin in affected areas with shoes or bedclothes may be intolerable, and patients may have difficulty walking or disrupted sleep patterns. Hyporeflexia of the lower extremities is a common examination finding.

The diagnosis is primarily a clinical one based on the presence of the typical sensory abnormalities in a person infected with HIV. The results of nerve conduction and electromyographic studies can support the diagnosis of DSP. The major differential diagnosis is with neuropathy caused by the toxicity of some anti-HIV nucleoside analogs, specifically zalcitabine, stavudine, didanosine, and, to a lesser extent, zidovudine. Symptomatic neuropathy can occur in up to 30% of patients treated with these agents, and is not clinically distinguishable from DSP. Distinction between the two depends on a history of the onset of symptoms temporally related to the initiation of one of the specific nucleosides, and improvement of the symptoms with withdrawal of the drug.

Current treatment of DSP is primarily symptomatic. The incidence of DSP seems to have declined with the availability of HAART; however, anti-HIV drug therapy seems to have minimal effect on this polyneuropathy once it is established. Drugs used most commonly in an attempt to relieve neuropathic symptoms include gabapentin, lamotrigine, and the tricyclic antidepressants. Narcotic pain relievers may be necessary for patients with severe symptoms.

INFLAMMATORY DEMYELINATING POLYNEUROPATHY

The clinical syndrome known as inflammatory demyelinating polyneuropathy (IDP) can have an acute presentation, with features similar to Guillain-Barré syndrome, or can manifest in a more chronic form. IDP can occur during any stage of HIV disease, but most commonly it is diagnosed during earlier stages when immune system function is still preserved and CD4 counts are $>200/\text{mm}^3$. Patients with IDP present with weakness beginning in the distal extremities and ascending to more proximal muscle groups, and respiratory compromise may ultimately occur. Reflexes are absent and sensory symptoms are minimal.

The diagnosis of IDP can be confirmed with nerve conduction studies that show a decrease in nerve conduction velocity. Biopsy of the sural nerve shows perivascular mononuclear cell infiltration with segmental demyelination. IDP is thought to be an autoimmune disorder, and the approach to treatment is the same as in persons who are HIV negative (2,8). Plasmapheresis, corticosteroids, and intravenous immunoglobulin have all been used with success.

ASCENDING CYTOMEGALOVIRUS POLYRADICULOPATHY

CMV can cause a rapidly progressive polyradiculopathy in some patients with advanced AIDS, with CD4 counts characteristically $<50/\text{mm}^3$. Initial clinical features are paresthesias of the lower extremities and sacral area, and back pain is common. This progresses very rapidly over a period of days to an areflexive paraparesis with loss of bladder and bowel function. The upper extremities, on occasion, may be involved, as well.

Diagnosis can be made by recognition of the typical clinical syndrome, together with CSF analysis. The CSF white blood cell count is usually high (>500) and the glucose is abnormally low. Cultures of the CSF for CMV are frequently positive, and CMV DNA can be detected via PCR. Because of the rapid progression of ascending polyradiculopathy, in the presence of a compatible clinical picture, empiric anti-CMV therapy is indicated before the diagnosis has been confirmed. Treatment is similar to the treatment of CMV encephalitis (see above) with ganciclovir or related anti-CMV agents; if it is started sufficiently early, irreversible necrosis of nerve roots can be prevented and significant clinical benefit can be achieved.

Spinal Cord Syndrome

CLINICAL MANIFESTATION, DIAGNOSIS, AND TREATMENT

VACUOLAR MYELOPATHY

Vacuolar myelopathy frequently coexists in patients with AIDS dementia, and is a disease of advanced AIDS. Patients usually complain of weakness of the legs and a spastic gait that progresses to paralysis and sphincter dysfunction. Sensory impairment is mild or absent. On histopathology, the spinal cord shows a vacuolated appearance of the white matter, primarily in the posterior and lateral columns. CSF analysis and MRI of the spinal cord are generally unremarkable and are mainly useful in eliminating other causes of spinal cord syndromes, such as varicella-zoster infection and inflammatory demyelinating polyneuropathy-1 (HTLV-1) myelopathy. Treatment is generally HAART and supportive care.

CLINICAL RECOMMENDATIONS OF VIGNETTE 1

The patient has historical and examination findings that suggest underlying AIDS and a focal neurologic disease. The presence of fever implies an opportunistic infection. The next step in the evaluation should be a CT or MRI of the brain, with and without contrast. Toxoplasma serology should be obtained; if the imaging study shows ring-enhancing focal lesions, empiric antitoxoplasma therapy should be started.

CLINICAL RECOMMENDATIONS OF VIGNETTE 2

The patient has known HIV-1 infection and has a subacute clinical syndrome of progressive cognitive deficits and some impairment of balance. An absolute CD4 count and an HIV-1 viral load should be obtained to further assess the stage of HIV disease. Brain imaging and CSF analysis is indicated to assess for the presence of such disorders as non-HIV viral encephalitis and PML. Her presentation is highly suggestive of AIDS dementia, and successful HAART therapy will be critical in improving her prognosis.

SUMMARY

The neurologic manifestations of HIV/AIDS are diverse and can manifest as focal brain disorders, nonfocal brain disorders, peripheral nervous system diseases, or spinal cord syndromes. The incidence of many of these conditions has dramatically decreased in the HAART era, and some may be directly treated by antiretroviral therapy. Neurologic disorders that result from opportunistic infections also require the correct antimicrobial therapy, in addition to HAART. Diagnosis of the various syndromes, some of which are now very uncommon, may require a high index of suspicion.

REFERENCES

1. Simpson DM, Tagliati M. Neurologic manifestations of HIV infection. *Ann Intern Med.* 1994;121:769.
2. Price RW. Neurologic disease. In: Dolin R, Masur H, Saag M, eds. *AIDS Therapy.* Philadelphia: Churchill-Livingstone; 2003:737–757.
3. Koralnick I. Neurologic diseases caused by human immunodeficiency virus-1 and opportunistic infections. In: Mandell GL, Bennett JE, Dolin R, eds. *Principles and Practice of Infectious Disease.* Philadelphia: Elsevier; 2005:1583–1600.
4. Sacktor N. The epidemiology of human immunodeficiency virus-associated neurological disease in the era of highly active antiretroviral therapy. *J Neurovirol.* 2002;8(2):115.
5. Simpson DM, Cikurel K. Pathogenesis of neurologic complications of HIV. *Clinical Care Options*; 2006. Available from http://www.clinicaloptions.com.
6. Van Der Horst CM, Saag M, Cloud G, et al. Treatment of cryptococcal meningitis associated with the acquired immunodeficiency syndrome. *N Engl J Med.* 1997;337:15.
7. Koralnick IJ. New insights into progressive multifocal leukoencephalopathy. *Curr Opin Neurol.* 2004;17:365.
8. LindenbaumY, Kissel JT, Mendell JR. Treatment approaches for Guillain-Barré syndrome and chronic inflammatory demyelinating polyradiculoneuropathy. *Neurol Clin.* 2001;19:187.

CHAPTER **95**

Fungal Infections of the Central Nervous System

Dorota Krezolek • Jaime Belmares-Avales

OBJECTIVES

- To explain the risk factors for the development of a central nervous system (CNS) infection
- To familiarize the reader with the most common human fungal CNS pathogens
- To describe the main clinical syndromes associated with fungal CNS infections
- To discuss the treatment options for the most common fungal CNS infections

CASE VIGNETTE

A 56-year-old man with history of diabetes mellitus had right periorbital pain and monocular blurred vision of the right eye for the past 2 weeks. He has been on oral hypoglycemics, but took them inconsistently. On examination, he was afebrile. Visual acuity was 20/100 OD, and 20/20 OS. He had right eye proptosis, right upper eyelid ptosis, and weakness of abduction, supraduction, and infraduction of the right eye. Blood glucose level was 704 mg/dL. Unenhanced computed tomographic (CT) scan showed a mass lesion in the right maxillary and ethmoid sinuses extending into the right orbit.

DEFINITION

The fungal agents most commonly involved in CNS infections are yeasts, filamentous fungi (moulds), and dimorphic fungi. Main clinical syndromes include meningitis, meningoencephalitis, and focal CNS lesions. Many fungal species have been implicated as agents of CNS infection (Table 95-1), but only the most common ones are discussed in this chapter. Cryptococcal neuroinfection in human immunodeficiency virus and acquired immunodeficiency syndrome (HIV/AIDS) is discussed in Chapter 94.

EPIDEMIOLOGY

For the last two decades, the number of invasive fungal infections has increased dramatically (1). Factors implicated with this observations include the HIV epidemic, and the growing number of patients receiving potentially inmmunosuppressive therapies, such as antineoplastic agents, systemic corticosteroids, or tumor necrosis factor-α (TNF-α) antagonists. Other risk factors include prolonged hospitalization, parenteral nutrition, invasive catheters, and prolonged therapy with broad spectrum antibiotics. At particularly high risk are hematopoetic stem cell and solid organ transplant recipients. Fungal CNS infections are serious disorders, difficult to recognize and treat, and often associated with a very high mortality rate (2,3).

Most of the important fungal pathogens have a natural habitat in the surrounding environment. Some (e.g., *Cryptococcus* or *Aspergillus*) are found worldwide. Others are endemic to specific geographic areas. For example, *Coccidioides* are endemic in deserts of the southwestern United States and parts of Mexico, and Central and South America, whereas *Blastomyces* and *Histoplasma* are prevalent in wooded areas of the Mississippi and Ohio River valleys. Thus, a history of travel or residence in the endemic area, or of activities leading to potential exposures, is very important when evaluating the patient with a suspected fungal infection.

ETIOLOGY AND PATHOGENESIS

Yeasts, such as *Candida* or *Cryptococcus*, exist predominately in a unicellular form and reproduce by budding. Moulds (e.g., *Aspergillus*, zygomycetes) produce filamentous forms called hyphae, and spores that are their main means of reproduction. Dimorphic fungi, such as *Histoplasma*, *Coccidioides*, or *Blastomyces*, grow as moulds in the environment, and as yeasts in the host tissues. Some of these fungi are capable of invading seemingly immunocompetent hosts (e.g., *Cryptococcus*). Others are found predominantly among hosts with impaired immune system. *Aspergillus, Histoplasma, Zygomycetes*, and *Coccidioides* are most commonly acquired through inhalation of spores into the lungs, where the primary infection develops. This primary infection is often asymptomatic and contained by the cellular immune response. In immunosuppressed patients, the infection can become disseminated and progress to organs such as the skin, bones, and CNS, among others.

Candida species are common commensals of the skin and gastrointestinal tract. *Candida* species also frequently colonize

TABLE 95-1. Types of the Central Nervous System (CNS) Infections Caused by Various Fungal Species

Meningitis	*Brain Lesions*	*Spinal Cord Lesions*
Alternaria sp.	*Alternaria sp.*	*Aspergilus sp.*
Aspergillus sp.	*Aspergilus sp.*	*Blastomyces dermatitidis*
Blastomyces dermatitidis	*Blastomyces dermatitidis*	*Candida sp.*
Bipolaris hawaiiensis	*Bipolaris spicifera*	*Coccidioides immitis*
Candida sp.	*Candida sp.*	*Cryptococcus neoformans*
Cladophialophora bantiana	*Chaetomium strumarium*	*Histoplasma capsulatum*
Coccidioides immitis	*Cladophialophora bantiana*	*Paracoccidioides brasiliensis*
Cryptococcus neoformans	*Coccidioides immitis*	
Histoplasma capsulatum	*Culvularia pallescens*	
Paracoccidioides brasiliensis	*Cryptococcus neoformans*	
Pseudallescheria boydii	*Exophiala dermatitidis*	
Sporotrichium scheneckii	*Histoplasma capsulatum*	
Scedosporium prolificans	*Ochroconis gallopava*	
Zygomycetes	*Paracoccidioides brasiliensis*	
	Penicillium sp.	
	Pseudallescheria boydii	
	Ramichloridium mackenziei	
	Sporotrichium scheneckii	
	Zygomycetes	

(Modified from Salaki JS, Louria DB, Chmel C. Fungal and yeast infections of the central nervous system, a clinical review. *Medicine.* 1984;63(2):108–132 and Sutton DA, Slifkin M, Yakulis R, et al. U.S. case report of cerebral phaeohyphomycosis caused by *Ramichloridium obovoideum (R. mackenziei)*: Criteria for identification, therapy, and review of other known dematiaceous neurotrophic taxa. *J Clin Microbiol.* 1998;36(3):708–715, with permission.)

indwelling intravenous and urinary catheters (4). More than 150 species of *Candida* exist, but only a few are regarded as frequent human pathogens: *C. albicans, C. krusei, C. parapsilosis, C. tropicalis,* and *C. glabrata. Candida* species exhibit both budding and filamentous forms called *pseudohyphae.*

C. albicans can produce true hyphae *in vivo* and *in vitro* and, as such, can be differentiated from other *Candida* species (4,5). Candidiasis can range from local mucous membrane infections to systemic processes with multiorgan failure. Invasion occurs in the setting of an imbalance in their ecologic niche and skin or mucous membrane damage, which constitute the first protective barrier against an invasion (4).

Common routes of invasion include indwelling catheters, implantation of prosthetic materials (e.g., cardiac valves), or severe burns. Associated conditions and risk factors include diabetes mellitus, malignancy, parenteral nutrition, and prolonged use of antibiotics, corticosteroids, or other immunosuppressants (2–4). Premature babies are at risk for disseminated candidiasis (6).

CNS candidiasis is a rare condition, observed more commonly among critically ill premature babies and neurosurgical patients, particularly those with CNS shunts (7,8). CNS candidiasis often presents as a subacute or chronic meningitis; multiple brain micro- or macroabscesses may be observed in cases of disseminated infection (4,6).

Aspergillus can colonize the respiratory tract and paranasal sinuses, but invasive infection is infrequent and primarily occurs among immunosuppressed hosts. The species most frequently encountered are *A. fumigatus, A. flavus, A. terreus,* and, less commonly, *A. niger.* Most important risk factors include prolonged neutropenia, bone marrow and solid organ transplantation, chronic granulomatous disease, stages of advanced AIDS, and prolonged corticosteroid use. In the setting of alveolar macrophage dysfunction, inhaled conidia germinate and form hyphae capable of invading solid tissues. Vascular invasion is a hallmark of aspergillosis. CNS invasion, which is reported in 10% to 20% of patients with disseminated disease, usually results from hematogenous dissemination (2,3). Another important route of invasion is direct extension from the paranasal sinuses, orbit, or ear (9).

Zygomycetes are the second most common filamentous fungi in human pathology (after *Aspergillus*). Species most commonly involved are *Rhizopus, Absidia, Rhizomucor,* and *Mucor.* The route of infection, risk factors, and clinical presentation of zygomycosis (also called *mucormycosis*) are similar to those described for invasive aspergillosis. Angioinvasion can result in thrombosis, tissue infarction, and necrosis, as well as remote septic emboli. Hyperglycemia, acidosis, and iron-overload states facilitate the growth of the fungus. Diabetes mellitus and ketoacidosis are the most common risk factors in cases of rhinocerebral zygomycosis (10,11). Infection is clinically indistinguishable from aspergillosis, with a faster progression and higher mortality.

Histoplasma capsulatum is a soil-based, dimorphic fungus most often associated with river valleys. Outdoor activities and exposure to soil, or to bird or bat waste, can result in inhaling of the conidia. In the lungs, the conidia transform into the yeast form. Phagocytosed by macrophages, yeasts are able to survive and migrate intracellularly into lymph nodes and distant organs, such as the liver and spleen. In immunocompetent hosts, the activated macrophages are able to contain the infection, although some organisms remain viable within granulomas and may reactivate if the host immunity becomes impaired. Immunocompromised hosts can develop primary disseminated histoplasmosis (PDH). Patients primarily at risk for PDH or reactivation of a dormant disease include those with HIV/AIDS with CD4 lymphocyte count <200, recipients of anti-TNF-α therapy, immunosuppression following solid organ transplants, and those with hematologic malignancies (12). CNS involvement can occur in isolation and can present as encephalitis, acute or chronic meningitis, encephalopathy, or, in rare cases, with a mass lesion of histoplasmoma (12).

Blastomyces dermatitidis grows as the mycelial form at room temperature, and as the yeast form at 37°C. The fungus resides in warm, moist soil of wooded areas rich in organic debris and decaying vegetation. Exposure is mainly through outdoor activities, especially involving gardening or construction. Inhaled spores transform within the lungs into the broad-budding yeasts that induce a host cell-mediated response. These processes lead to a systemic pyogranulomatous disease, ranging from an asymptomatic or mild self-limiting pulmonary disease to a chronic indolent infection or a primary progressive and disseminated disease (13). As in histoplasmosis, dormant infections can reactivate if the cellular immunity of the infected individual becomes compromised. CNS involvement is rare, except in patients with AIDS (in whom it is reported in up to 40% of blastomycosis cases) and presents as meningitis or a brain abscess (14).

Coccidioides spp. grow as a mold a few inches below the surface of the desert soil. Mycelia produce spores called *arthroconidia* that are easily detached and able to spread suspended in the air and viable for a prolonged period of time. *C. immitis* and *C. posadasii* are the two known species. Following inhalation, arthroconidia transform into multicellular bodies called *spherules.* Enlarging spherules produce internal septations and endospores that are released into the tissues after several days. Each endospore can than evolve into a new spherule. In the laboratory, the organisms show a reversion to the mycelial form on culture. *Coccididioides* is highly pathogenic, and even a single inhaled arthoconidium can produce a symptomatic infection (15).

Primary coccidioidomycosis ranges from a limited and often unrecognized disease to an acute pneumonia (valley fever). In some cases, coccidioidomycosis can progress into an extrapulmonary disease. Meningitis is the most common and most serious form of extrapulmonary coccidioidomycosis (16). Other affected organs include skin and subcutaneous tissues, bones, liver, eye, prostate, and other parts of the urogenital tract.

The main risk factor for coccidioidomycosis is residence in, or travel to, endemic areas, especially during dry seasons. Extrapulmonary disease can develop in a course of weeks to months from the primary infection, usually in immunocompromised hosts, such as solid organ transplant recipients, patients with HIV/AIDS or hematologic malignancies, or those receiving prolonged steroid therapy (15).

PATHOLOGY

The immune response induced by fungi in the host results in granulomatous inflammation. Histologic specimens show granulomas with multinucleated giant cells, neutrophils, lymphocytes, and few epithelial cells. Fibrosis may be present. Angioinvasion with neutrophil infiltrates and hyphae, and formation of mycotic aneurysms can be seen in zygomycosis and aspergillosis. Pathology of infected tissues may demonstrate infarction, necrosis, or subarachnoid hemorrhage (SAH) (9). Candidiasis produces brain micro- and macroabscesses, epidural abscesses, or meningeal inflammation. Angioinvasion with mycotic aneurysm and tissue infarction can be seen (2,3). Visualization of fungal forms, such as various forms of yeasts and hyphae, in many cases, can help establish the cause of the underlying lesions.

CLINICAL MANIFESTATIONS

Fungal meningitis is a subacute or chronic illness. Symptoms develop over a period of weeks to months, or even years. As in acute meningitis, patients may present with fever, headache, meningismus, and altered sensorium. Symptoms are usually more subtle, however, with gradual onset and with low grade or no fever (17). Fungi most commonly involved in cases of meningitis are yeasts (e.g., *Candida and Cryptococcus)* and the dimorphic fungi (Table 95-1). *Candida* meningitis, on the other hand, can present with an abrupt onset and more frequently than in other fungal etiologies, with fever (4).

As is often the case, clinical presentation can vary, depending on the patient's immune status. A typical example of this difference is cryptococcal meningitis in patients with HIV/AIDS, where patients often present with subtle to minimal symptoms, frequently limited to headaches and lethargy. By contrast, patients without AIDS tend to have a subacute disease, with headache, fever, meningismus, and mental status changes. In cryptococcisis, blastomycosis, or coccidioidomycosis, the infection can be complicated with basilar meningitis, encephalitis, epidural abscess, or vasculitis (2,3). In these cases, patients present with cerebral palsies or other focal symptoms. Clinical presentation is often unspecific and mimics other infectious and noninfectious diseases, such as collagen vascular or chronic granulomatous diseases, or metabolic encephalopathies (Table 95-2).

TABLE 95-2. Differential Diagnosis of Chronic Meningitis

BACTERIAL	Tuberculosis Lyme disease Brucellosis Syphilis
FUNGAL	Candidiasis Cryptococcosis Histoplasmosis Blastomycosis Coccidioidomycosis Aspergillosis Sporotrichosis
PARASITIC	*Acanthamoeba* *Angiostrongylus cantonensis*
NONINFECTIOUS	Systemic lupus erythematosus (SLE) Polyarteritis nodosa Sjögren syndrome Wegener granulomatosis Sarcoidosis Behçet disease Neoplastic meningitis Granulomatous angiitis

(Modified from Behlau I, Ellner JJ. Chronic meningitis. In: Mandell G, Bennett J, eds. *Principles and Practice of Infectious Diseases.* New York: Elsevier; 2005:1132–1135, with permission.)

Focal CNS lesions caused by fungal agents, including brain abscesses, subdural empyemas, or epidural abscesses, can be mistaken for primary or metastatic CNS neoplasms or bacterial abscess (2,3). Patients may develop focal brain lesions via contiguous invasion (e.g., from sinusitis), hematogenous dissemination, or trauma. Initial clinical manifestations can include headaches, nausea, vomiting, seizures, alteration in the level of alertness, and focal neurologic findings. Fever is rarely present. Additionally, patients with fungal brain abscesses caused by *Aspergillus* species or the zygomycetes can present with a strokelike syndrome because of the angiophilic propensity of these organisms (2,3,10,11).

Rhinocerebral mucormycosis presents with nasal congestion, erythema and swelling of the periorbital area, proptosis, ophathalmoplegic and blurred vision, and may progress rapidly to visual loss and serious encephalitis. *Aspergillus* and zygomycetes are the most frequently implicated etiologic agents. Although their clinical presentations are similar, an important differentiating feature in favor of rhinocerebral zygomycosis is its association with diabetic hyperglycemia and ketoacidosis.

Other fungal agents that can some times present as mass lesions include *Cryptococcus, Candida, Histoplasmosis, Coccidioides,* and *Paracoccidioides.* Certain rare molds were reported to cause CNS invasion in the setting of trauma or near drowning (Table 95-1) (18).

Focal spinal cord lesions are rare and usually associated with disseminated mycoses. Spinal infection can occur via direct invasion of fungus from adjacent anatomic structures, such as vertebrae, mediastinum, or lung, or as a result of dissemination via CSF or hematogenously. Spinal cord lesions often produce a typical sequence of back pain, radicular pain, and motor and sensory findings below the level of the lesion, progressing to irreversible paralysis if untreated, and requiring emergency surgical intervention. Fungal agents most commonly involved in brain and spinal cord lesions are listed in Table 95-1. The frequency depends on the host status and geographic location (18,19).

DIAGNOSTIC APPROACH

The symptomatology of fungal CNS infection is often similar to many other CNS disorders of infectious and noninfectious causes (17). The list of disorders presenting as chronic meningitides is particularly extensive (Table 95-2). A thorough understanding of the epidemiology of these infections is essential in developing a hierarchic differential diagnosis and a rational workup.

A previous history of pulmonary diseases, diabetes mellitus, iron overload states, of travel to areas of endemic mycoses, occupational or recreational exposure to soil or birds, and intravenous drug use are all important elements of the initial evaluation. Specific risk factors for candidiasis include use of long-term intravenous catheters or other prosthetic devices, abdominal trauma, use of parenteral nutrition, and prolonged antibiotic therapy. Poorly controlled diabetes mellitus, and diabetic ketoacidosis are associated with zygomycosis. Hematologic malignancies, HIV/AIDS, persistent neutropenia, bone marrow or solid organ transplant, and prolonged steroid therapy are frequently encountered risk factors for reactivation of dormant pathogens or for the development of an invasive fungal disease (2,3).

The diagnostic workup includes detailed neuroimaging, analysis of blood and CSF, and, in some cases, tissue for microbiologic and pathologic testing. Noncontrast brain CT is an adequate procedure to exclude the presence of a mass lesion before performing a lumbar puncture. Contrast CT or MRI, however, is often necessary for a more detailed evaluation of CNS lesions. MRI is particularly useful in detecting very small lesions, meningeal enhancement, hydrocephalus, and enhancing abscesslike lesions.

CSF analysis helps in establishing the presence of meningeal involvement, but is not pathognomonic for a fungal etiology. Opening pressure is typically elevated in cases of cryptococcal and candidal meningitis. Elevated CSF protein and variably decreased glucose levels are usually present. White blood cell counts range from approximately 100 to several hundred per cubic millimeter and, in most cases of fungal meningitis, a lymphocytic pleocytosis pattern Is seen (20). CSF eosinophilia, although not always present, is very characteristic of coccidioidomycosis (16).

Microbiologic and serologic testing, although time consuming, are crucial for establishing the diagnosis. Body fluids and tissue specimens should be sent for fungal smear, culture, and histology with the use of special staining. The appropriate testing is dictated by clinical setting and suspected etiology.

Candida spp. are usually isolated form CSF or blood specimens. The ability to produce true hyphae (germ tube test) is used in differentiating *C. albicans* from other *Candida* species (5). A positive CSF culture should not be considered to result from contamination, although in some cases, it can reflect a colonization of the CNS catheter (21). Detection of mannan, a candidal surface antigen in body fluids, appears promising in a rapid diagnosis and possibly differentiation of true infection from colonization (3,22). Identification and susceptibility testing is necessary for appropriate therapy for non-*albicans* species.

Cryptococcal meningitis can be diagnosed by visualization of encapsulated yeast in the CSF via India ink staining or by CSF culture. Detection of polysaccharide antigen in the CSF or serum, via an enzyme-linked immunosorbent assay (ELISA) can establish a diagnosis before the culture is available. The test is sensitive and specific in approximately 90% of cases (3).

The diagnosis of *aspergillosis* and *zygomycosis* can be established by isolating the organisms in the CSF culture, blood, or tissue specimen. The presence of a mass lesion in the appropriate clinical setting requires obtaining tissue for fungal smear and cultures and proper histopathology with fungal stains. In the Gomori methenamine silver (GMS) or periodic acid–Schiff (PAS) stain, *Aspergillus* usually presents with thin, septate, narrow-angle branching hyphae, in contrast to the broad, nonseptate, right-angle branching hyphae of zygomycetes (20). Microbiologic and histologic testing is time consuming and findings are often negative despite ongoing infection. Several serologic assays have been developed to increase the diagnostic yield. The galactomannan antigen, a component of the *Aspergillus* cell wall, can be detected using ELISA or enzyme immunoassay (EIA). Its detection in the serum of high-risk patients was shown to have a negative predictive value of 95% to 98%. The positive predictive value, however, was much lower (54%). Only preliminary reports of testing the CSF are available. Other techniques, such as detection of other components of fungal wall or fungal DNA using CSF PCR, are in preliminary stages (3,23).

In *Histoplasma* meningitis, CSF cultures detect the organism in 25% to 65% of cases. The diagnostic yield improves larger CSF volumes (≥20 mL) (12). The mainstay of diagnosis is

Histoplasma antigen detection in the urine and CSF (12). Serologic testing is less useful because of a 3- to 6-week delay, both in the development of a detectable antibody response following an acute infection and of a fourfold titer increase in cases of reactivation. Immunocompromised hosts, such as patients with HIV/AIDS, frequently do not develop detectable levels (12). Histologic tests with GMS or Grocott silver stains are also utilized to evaluate tissue specimens or body fluids.

Microbiologic testing is not helpful in the diagnosis of meningitis caused by *Blastomyces* and *Coccidioides,* because these organisms frequently fail to grow in the CSF. A presumptive diagnosis of blastomycosis can be made with the visualization of budding yeasts in clinical specimens, but a definitive diagnosis requires demonstration of growth of the mycelial forms and reversion into the yeast form at 37°C. Serologic tests for antibodies are neither specific nor sensitive. Tests for the presence of *Blastomyces* antigen in various body fluids, including CSF, have been developed. The urine antigen can be detected in 80% to 90% of patients with disseminated blastomycosis, and is the most useful additional test (13).

Coccididioides meningitis is usually diagnosed by the detection of serum complement fixation antibodies, because CSF cultures are negative most of the time. Although most antibody detection assays are highly specific (approximately 90%), a negative result does not rule out the infection. Repeated testing might be necessary to increase the sensitivity (15,16).

TREATMENT

In general, treatment goals for fungal CNS infections include eradication of the infection, control of symptoms, and preservation or return of the patient's neurologic function. With the exceptions to be described below, amphotericin B deoxycholate can usually be substituted by a lipid amphotericin B compound. Doses of conventional amphotericin B and of lipid-based amphotericin B typically range from 0.7 to 1 mg/kg/day, and 3 to 5 mg/kg/day, respectively.

Candida CNS infections are treated with intravenous amphotericin B dexocycholate plus oral flucytosine (25 mg/kg four times daily) (22). Flucytosine serum levels should be adjusted to achieve serum concentrations of 40 to 60 μg/mL. Therapy is continued for 4 weeks after resolution of signs and symptoms. Fluconazole is used as follow up and as a long-term suppressive treatment (22). Caspofungin has been successfully used in one case of refractory meninigitis (23).

Voriconazole is the treatment of choice for *invasive aspergillosis* (24). Initial loading dose is 400 mg twice daily for 1 day, followed by a maintenance dose of 200 mg twice daily. Side effects are rash, transient visual disturbances, and elevated liver function tests (25). Neurosurgical interventions, such as debridement or removal of fungal brain lesions, can have a significant impact on survival (26). The length of therapy has not been standardized; it depends on the patient's response and immune status.

Lipid amphotericin compounds (5 mg/kg/day) are the primary agents in the treatment of *zygomycosis,* with a reported success rate of 60% to 70% in combination with surgery (27). Numerous case series suggest that posaconazole is effective as salvage therapy, with success rates ranging from 60% to 80% (28).

The best treatment for *CNS histoplasmosis* remains unclear (29). Liposomal amphotericin B is a more effective therapy of progressive disseminated histoplasmosis in patients with AIDS (30). Wheat et al. (31) suggest that patients with meningitis or focal brain lesions in the setting of immunosuppression or progressive primary histoplasmosis receive liposomal amphotericin B at 3–5 mg/kg/day for a total of 150 mg/kg over 6 to 12 weeks. This is followed by itraconazole (200 mg two times daily) or fluconazole (600 to 800 mg for up to 1 year). In other patients, amphotericin B can be stopped after 2 to 4 weeks, and is followed by an oral azole for 6 to 12 months (31). Immunosuppressed patients should continue therapy until at least 1 year after immune reconstitution and resolution of all signs and symptoms associated with their infection (32).

Initial treatment of *Blastomycosis* is amphotericin B (0.7 to 1 mg/kg/day) with a total dose of at least 2 g, followed by itraconazole 200 mg two times daily for 6 to 12 months. Many authors recommend lifelong therapy in patients with a history of immunosuppression (14).

Coccidioidal meningitis is treated with oral fluconazole (400 mg/day). Itraconazole is an alternative. Therapy is continued for life in those patients who respond. Intrathecal amphotericin B is used in those who are unresponsive to azole (33).

CLINICAL RECOMMENDATIONS OF THE VIGNETTE

The patient had additional neuroimaging studies with gadolinium-enhanced MRI. The previously noted mass lesion was described as invading the right para nasal sinuses, orbit, and optic nerve, with evidence of meningeal enhancement in the anterior cranial fossa. Prompt evaluation by an ear nose and throat (ENT) specialist and biopsy of the mass was performed. The pathology demonstrated granulomatous inflammation. Broad, nonseptate, right-angle branching hyphae were seen in fungal staining. The patient's presentation is consistent with rhinocerebral zygomycosis (or mucormycosis) in an individual with hyperglycemia. The patient was started on lipid formulation of amphotericin B. He had an orbital exenteration, with total ethmoidectomy and partial maxillectomy, within 1 day of diagnosis. The request was made for obtaining posaconazole for compassionate use.

SUMMARY

CNS fungal infections most commonly arise as complications of other chronic diseases or invasive therapies. The incidence is increasing, often along with the growing population of immunocompromised hosts. The symptomatology is nonspecific and a thorough understanding of the epidemiology of these infections is essential in reaching an accurate diagnosis. Clinical outcomes are still unsatisfactory, despite improved diagnostic tools and the availability of potent new antifungal agents.

REFERENCES

1. Tietz HJ, Martin H, Koch S. Incidence of systemic mycoses in autopsy material. *Mycoses.* 2004;47:40–46.
2. Pagano L, Caira M, Falcucci P, et al. Fungal CNS infections in patients with hematologic malignancy. *Expert Review of Anti-infective Therapy.* 2005;3:775–785.
3. Mattiuzzi G, Giles JF. Management of intracranial fungal infections in patients with haematological malignancies. *Br J Haematol.* 2005;131:287–300.
4. Edwards JE. *Candida* species. In: Mandell G, Bennett J, eds. *Principles and Practice of Infectious Diseases.* New York: Elsevier; 2005:2938–2957.
5. Gow NA. Germ tube growth of *Candida albicans. Current Topics in Medical Mycology.* 1997;8:43–55.

6. Fernandez M, Moylett EH, Noyola DE, et al. Candidal meningitis in neonates: A 10-year review. *Clin Infect Dis.* 2002;31:458–463.
7. Nguyen MH, Yu VL. Meningitis caused by *Candida* species: An emerging problem in neurosurgical patients. *Clin Infect Dis.* 1995;21:323–327.
8. Montero A, Romero J, Vargas JA, et al. *Candida* infection of cerebrospinal fluid shunt devices: Report of two cases and review of the literature. *Acta Neurochir (Wien).* 2000;142:67–74.
9. Sundaram C, Umbala P, Laxmi V, et al. Pathology of fungal infections of the central nervous system:17 years' experience from Southern India. *Histopathology.* 2006;49:396–405.
10. Pagano L, Ricci P, Tonso A, et al. Mucormycosis in patient with haematological malignancies: A retrospective clinical study of 37 cases. *Br J Haematol.* 1997;99:331–336.
11. Sundaram C, Mahadevan A, Laxmi V, et al. Cerebral zygomycosis. *Mycoses.* 2005;48:396–407.
12. Deepe GS. *Histoplasma capsulatum.* In: Mandell G, Bennett J, eds. *Principles and Practice of Infectious Diseases.* New York: Elsevier; 2005:3012–3026.
13. Chapman SW. *Blastomyces dermatitidis.* In: Mandell G, Bennett J, eds. *Principles and Practice of Infectious Diseases.* New York: Elsevier; 2005:3026–3040.
14. Chapman SW, Bradsher RW, Campbell GD, et al. Practice guidelines for the management of patients with blastomycosis. Infectious Diseases Society of America. *Clin Infect Dis.* 2000; 30:679–683.
15. Galgani J. Coccidioides species. In: Mandell G, Bennett J, eds. *Principles and Practice of Infectious Diseases.* New York: Elsevier; 2005:3040–3051.
16. Johnson RH, Einstein HE. Coccidioidal meningitis. *Clin Infect Dis.* 2006;42:103–107.
17. Behlau I, Ellner JJ. Chronic meningitis. In: Mandell G, Bennett J, eds. *Principles and Practice of Infectious Diseases.* New York: Elsevier; 2005:1132–1135.
18. Salaki JS, Louria DB, Chmel C. Fungal and yeast infections of the central nervous system. A clinical review. *Medicine.* 1984;63:108–132.
19. Guermazi A, Benchaib N, Zagdanski AM, et al. Cerebral and spinal cord involvement resulting from invasive aspergillosis. *Eur Radiol.* 2002;12:147–150.
20. Lyons RW. Fungal infections of the CNS. *Neurol Clin.* 1986;49:159–163.
21. Geers TA, Gordon SM. Clinical significance of Candida species isolated from cerebrospinal fluid following neurosurgery. *Clin Infect Dis.* 1999;28:1139–1147.
22. Pappas PG, Rex JH, Sobel JD, et al. Guidelines for treatment of candidiasis. Infectious Diseases Society of America. *Clin Infect Dis.* 2004;38:161–189.
23. Liu KH, Wu CJ, Chou CH, et al. Refractory candidal meningitis in an immunocompromised patient cured by caspofungin. *J Clin Microbiol.* 2004;42:5950–5953.
23. Stevens DA, Kan VL, Judson MA, et al. Practice guidelines for diseases caused by Aspergillus. Infectious Diseases Society of America. *Clin Infect Dis.* 2000;30(4):696–709.
24. Herbrecht R, Denning DW, Patterson TF, et al. Voriconazole vs. amphotericin B for primary therapy of invasive aspergillosis. *N Engl J Med.* 2002;347:728–732.
25. Johnson LB, Kauffman CA. Voriconazole: A new triazole antifungal agent. *Clin Infect Dis.* 2003;36:630–637.
26. Schwartz S, Ruhnke M, Ribaud P, et al. Improved outcome in central nervous system aspergillosis, using voriconazole treatment. *Blood.* 2005;106:2641–2645.
27. Roden MM, Zaoutis TE, Buchanan WL, et al. Epidemiology and outcome of zygomycosis: A review of 929 reported cases. *Clinical Infectious Diseases.* 2005;41:634–653.
28. van Burik JA, Hare RS, Solomon HF, et al. Posaconazole is effective as salvage therapy in zygomycosis: A retrospective summary of 91 cases. *Clin Infect Dis.* 2006;42:e61–e65.
29. Wheat J, Sarosi G, McKinsey D, et al. Practice guidelines for the management of patients with histoplasmosis. Infectious Diseases Society of America. *Clin Infect Dis.* 2000;30:688–695.
30. Johnson PC, Wheat LJ, Cloud GA, et al. Safety and efficacy of liposomal amphotericin B compared with conventional amphotericin B for induction therapy of histoplasmosis in patients with AIDS. *Ann Intern Med.* 2002;137:105–109.
31. Wheat LJ, Musial CE, Jenny-Avital E. Diagnosis and management of central nervous system histoplasmosis. *Clin Infect Dis.* 2005:40;844–852.
32. Galgiani JN, Ampel NM, Blair JE, et al. Coccidioidomycosis. Guidelines from the Infectious Diseases Society of America. *Clin Infect Dis.* 2005;41:1217–1223.
33. Salaki JS, Louria DB, Chmel C. Fungal and yeast infections of the central nervous system, a clinical review. *Medicine.* 1984;63(2):108–132.
34. Sutton DA, Slifkin M, Yakulis R, et al. U.S. case report of cerebral phaeohyphomycosis caused by *Ramichloridium obovoideum (R. mackenziei)*: Criteria for identification, therapy, and review of other known dematiaceous neurotrophic taxa. *J Clin Microbiol.* 1998;36(3):708–715.

CHAPTER **96**

Rickettsia

John E. Greenlee • DeVon C. Hale

OBJECTIVES

- To demonstrate a typical case of the most common—and most dangerous rickettsial infection in North America, Rocky Mountain spotted fever
- To describe the epidemiology, pathogenesis, clinical features, and treatment of the major rickettsial and ehrlichial illnesses causing neurologic disease
- To review the pathogenesis and clinical features of infection by *Coxiella burnetii*, the agent of Q fever

CASE VIGNETTE

An 18-year-old man was brought to the emergency room on July 4 because of extreme headache, confusion, and difficulty walking. He had been in excellent health until 2 days before admission, when he developed fever, chills, myalgias, and severe headache. Seven days before admission, he had been hiking in dense brush and on the following morning had removed several ticks from his legs and back.

On admission, the patient was confused, complaining of an extreme headache. General physical examination in the emergency room was essentially unremarkable. The patient had a petechial rash on his forearms and trunk. Neurologic examination was pertinent for mild nuchal rigidity, engorgement of retinal vessels, and a mild right hemiparesis involving the leg greater than the arm, with a right Babinski sign. Hematocrit was 40%. White blood count was 7,500/mm^3, with 85% polymorphonuclear leukocytes. Platelets were 79,000 mm^3. Aspartate aminotransferase (AST) and alanine aminotransferase (ALT) were mildly elevated. Cerebrospinal fluid (CSF) showed 17 white blood cells, 60% polymorphonuclear leukocytes, per cubic millimeter glucose was 62 mg/dL with simultaneous blood glucose of 108 mg/dL, and protein of 120 mg/dL. Magnetic resonance imaging (MRI) of the brain was normal, except for prominent perivascular spaces.

The patient was treated presumptively as having Rocky Mountain spotted fever and received 100 mg of doxycycline twice daily over a 10-day course. He made a rapid recovery. Three months after his admission, however, he still complained of fatigue and difficulty concentrating. Serologic tests for Rocky Mountain spotted fever, reported back 7 days after his admission, revealed elevated titers of IgM antibody, with minimally elevated titers of IgG antibody.

DEFINITION

Bacteria of the order Rickettsiales fall into two families: Rickettsiaceae and Anaplasmataceae. These, in turn are divided into four genera: *Rickettsiae* and *Orientia* (Rickettsiaceae); and *Ehrlichia* and *Anaplasma* (Anaplasmataceae) (Fig. 96-1). The taxonomy of these organisms has recently undergone extensive (and somewhat controversial) revision, and one organism previously considered rickettsial, *C. burnetii*, is now considered to belong to the order, Legionellales (Fig. 96-1). With the exception of the etiologic agent of epidemic typhus, *Rickettsia prowazekii*, Rickettsiales are agents of arthropods and of wild or domestic animals, rather than of man. In this chapter are discussed the diseases caused by Rickettsiales. Because infections caused by *C. burnetii*, have long been grouped with rickettsial diseases, this agent is also discussed.

EPIDEMIOLOGY

Rickettsiaceae and Anaplasmataceae are worldwide in distribution and comprise a large number of organisms, only a small number of which are known to infect humans (1). The major Rickettsiales known at present to cause neurologic disease humans are discussed below.

FAMILY RICKETTSIA: SPOTTED FEVER GROUP

Rickettsia Rickettsi (Rocky Mountain Spotted Fever)

R. rickettsii is the major rickettsial agent causing human disease in the North America, and is also the one most frequently causing severe illness (2,3). Rocky Mountain spotted fever has been reported in 44 states and, despite its name, is most common in southeastern United States (Maryland, Virginia, the Carolinas, and Georgia), and in Oklahoma (Fig. 96-2). The illness also occurs in Central and South America. In the United States, the arthropod species serving as both reservoirs and vectors for the agent are the Rocky Mountain spotted tick, *Dermacentor andersonii*, and the American dog tick, *D. variabilis*. Because these tick species are active in warmer months, 90% of cases of Rocky Mountain spotted fever occur between April and September. Cases can occur outside this range, however, in states with earlier spring and later frosts. Rocky Mountain spotted fever is usually thought of as a rural disease. Ticks are ubiquitous, however, and *R. rickettsii* has also been associated with urban outbreaks.

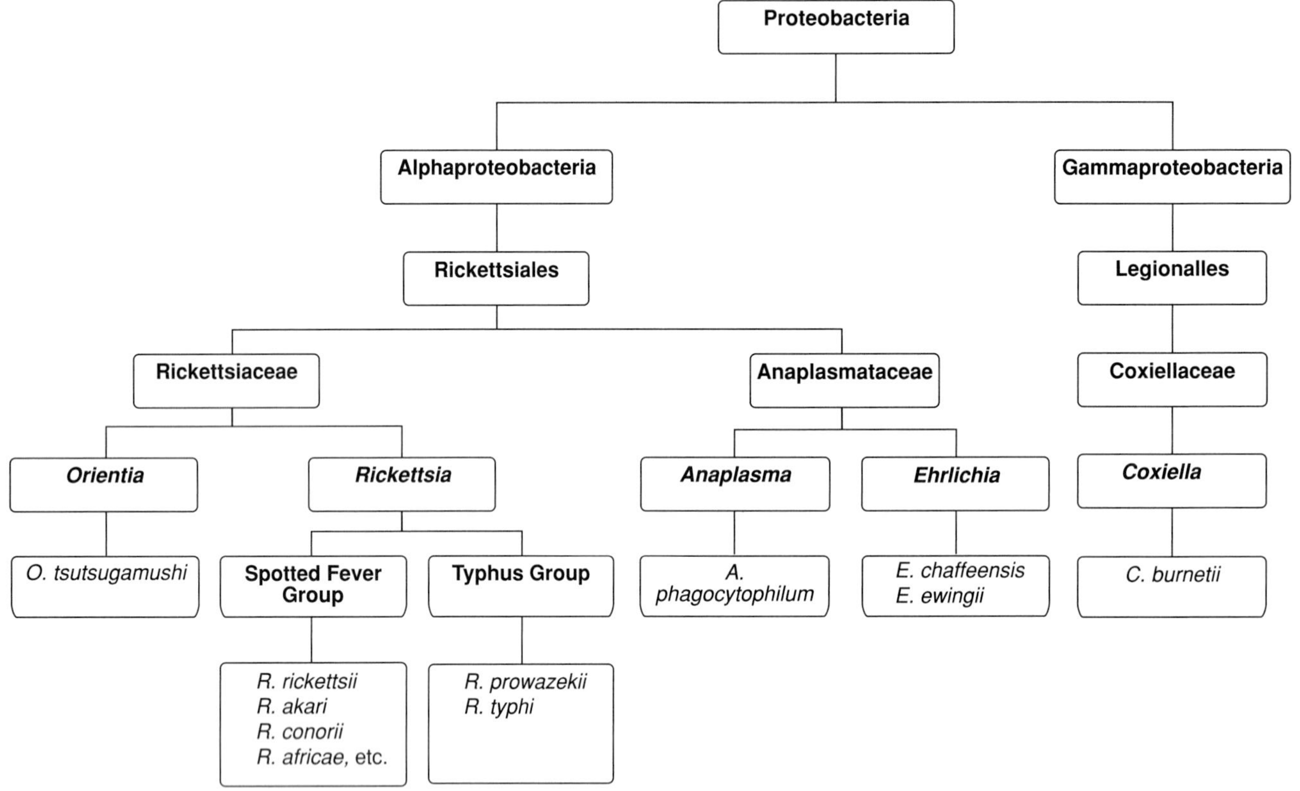

FIGURE 96-1. Taxonomy of the Rickettsiales and of *Coxiella burnetii.*

R. rickettsii is associated with 500 to 1,200 reported cases of human disease annually. Although host immunity is long-lasting, it is possible for an individual to be reinfected years after the initial event.

Rickettsia Akari (Rickettsialpox)

R. akari, an agent of mice, is present worldwide. The agent is transmitted to humans by the mouse mite, *Allodermanysus sangineus.* High prevalence of antibody to the agent has been reported in intravenous drug users (3).

FAMILY RICKETTSIA: TYPHUS GROUP

Rickettsia Prowazekii (Epidemic Typhus; Louse-borne Typhus; Brill-Zinsser Disease)

R. prowazekii is the only agent known to spread directly from human to human and is associated with two human conditions: An acute illness, epidemic typhus, and a much milder illness, Brill-Zinsser disease, which represents reactivation of latent infection. *R. prowazekii* replicates in, and is transmitted by, lice (4). Epidemic typhus is believed to occur when reactivated infection (Brill-Zinsser disease) occurs in a setting of crowding and poor hygiene, which facilitates louse-borne transmission of the organism among individuals. For this reason, epidemic typhus has been a recurring, grim companion of war, social collapse, and human destitution throughout history and throughout the world. The agent has also been detected in the American flying squirrel, *Glaucomys volans,* and human cases in the United States have been associated with contact with this animal (5). Other reservoirs for this agent may also exist (6). In 2001, an isolated case of epidemic typhus, with polymerase chain reaction (PCR) identification of *R. prowazekii,* was reported in a patient who acquired the disease after exposure to brackish water and sand flies at Padre Island, Texas (6). The source of the infection and the vector involved remain completely unknown.

Rickettsia Typhi (Endemic, or Murine Typhus)

R. typhi (formerly *R. mooserii*), an agent of rats, is transmitted between rats and to humans by the rat flea, *Xenopsylla cheopis.* The agent is worldwide in distribution (1). In North America, murine typhus has most frequently been reported in the southeastern United States and along the Gulf of Mexico. Endemic typhus has become less frequent since the 1940s. Because the illness is rarely severe, however, it is probably significantly underreported. Endemic typhus is most common in urban settings and in individuals who have close contact with rats, especially in individuals working in granaries or food storage areas.

MAJOR RICKETTSIACEAE CAUSING NEUROLOGIC DISEASE OUTSIDE NORTH AMERICA

Many other Rickettsiaceae cause human infection outside North America. Most of these are only infrequently associated with neurologic disease. Two agents, however, are important causes of human neurologic illness. The most important of these is *Orientia*

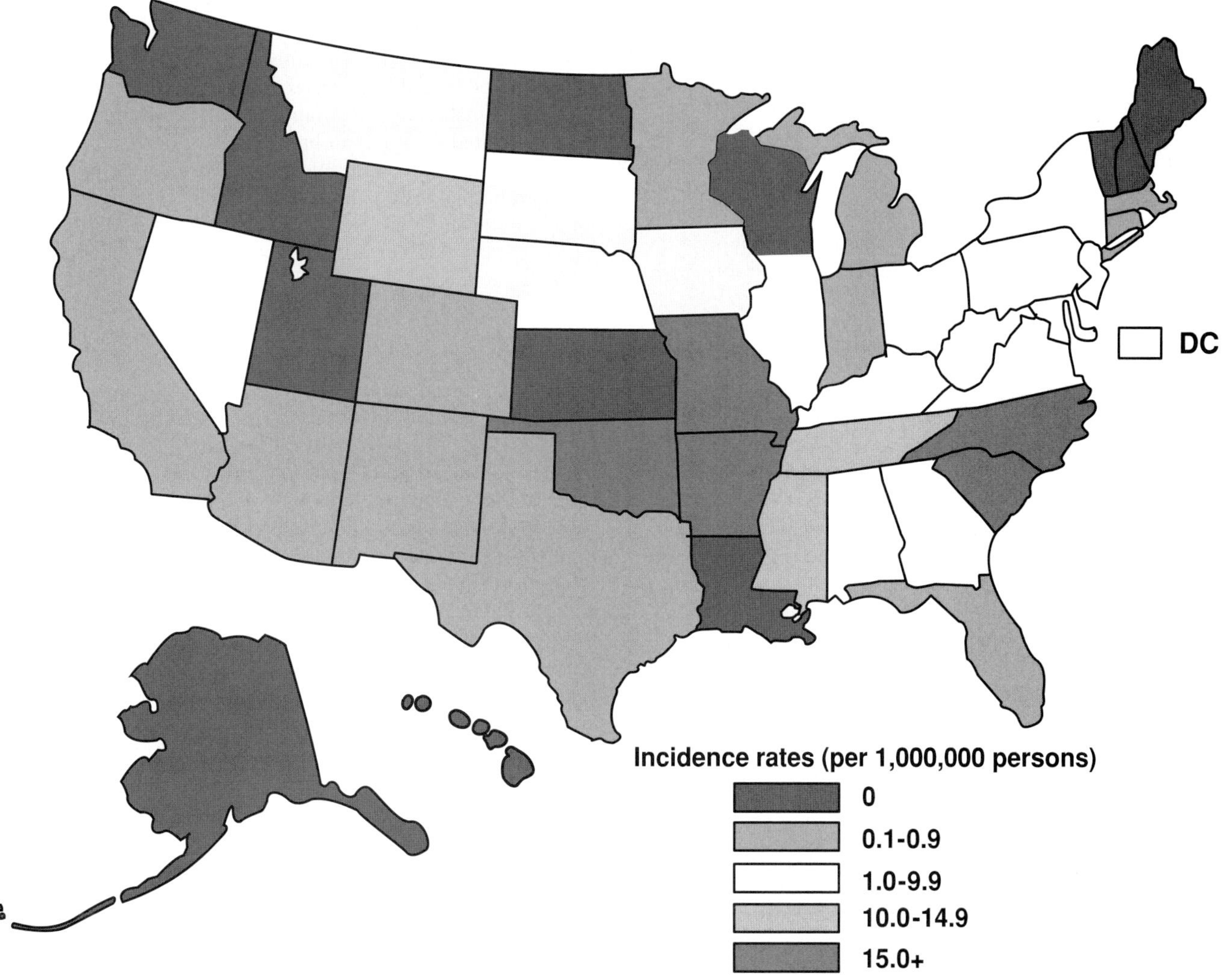

FIGURE 96-2. Distribution of Rocky Mountain spotted fever in the United States, 2002. (From the United States Department of Health and Human Services, Centers for Disease Control and Prevention, with permission.)

tsutsugamushi, the agent of scrub typhus. *O. tsutsugamushi* is found in a triangle, including northern Japan, eastern Australia, eastern Russia, China, and the Indian subcontinent, with over a billion individuals exposed to the agent (1,7). *O. tsutsugamuhsi* is transmitted by the bite of trombiculid mite larvae. Human exposure occurs during seasonal emergence of larvae; in temperate regions, this is usually in autumn and, to a lesser extent, in spring. *R. conorii* (Boutonneuse fever, Marseilles fever, Astrakan fever, Kenyan tick typhus, Indian tick typhus, Israeli spotted fever) causes an illness similar to, but less severe than, Rocky Mountain spotted feverlike illness in the Mediterranean basin, Africa, and India. A third agent, *R. africae,* is widely endemic in Africa and is a frequent cause of infections in patients recently returned from that continent. Although *R. africae* is associated with headache, it only rarely causes serious neurologic disease.

Family Anaplasmataceae

Anaplasma phagocytophilum (human granulocytic ehrlichiosis) is an agent that has been isolated in North America, Europe, and Asia (1,7). Deer are thought to be a major reservoir, and ticks (*Ixodes scapulari* in eastern North America, *I. pacificus* in western North America, *I. ricinus* in Europe, and *I. persulcatus* in Asia) are the major vectors.

E. chaffeensis (human monocytic ehrlichiosis) has been reported only in North America and has been identified in patients in middle eastern, mid-Atlantic, and southeastern United States, as well as in California (1,7). White tail deer are the major reservoir. The American (lone star) tick, *Amblyomma americanum,* is the most common vector, but the agent has also been recovered from two other tick species, *D. variabilis* and *I. pacificus.*

E. ewingii has been identified predominantly in the southeastern, mid-Atlantic, and south central United States (1,7). The agent has been detected in white tail deer, but has also been found in domestic dogs. As with *E. chaffeensis, E. ewingii* can be isolated from *A. americanum,* as well as from *D. variabilis. E. ewingii* tends to cause more severe infection in immunocompromised patients, including patients with human immunodeficiency virus (HIV).

Family Legionellales

As noted, *C. burnetii* (Q fever) is an intracellular pathogen that has long been considered "rickettsia-like." Genomic and 16sRNA sequence analysis, however, indicate that this agent more properly belongs to the order Legionellales, and that its closest relative causing human disease is *Legionella pneumophila.* Its animal reservoirs include cattle, sheep, goats, and domestic pets, and its infection, Q fever, is a worldwide condition (1,7). Unlike the agents described above, *C. burnetii* is spread to humans via the respiratory route, without need for an arthropod vector.

ETIOLOGY AND PATHOGENESIS

The classic rickettsia, such as *R. prowazekii* and *R. rickettsii,* produce human illness following transmission of these agents by arthropod vectors. The organism can be introduced into the host directly by the bite of the arthropod vector or by contamination of skin at the site of the bite when the vector defecates after a blood meal (1,4). Following inoculation, the organisms attach to, and are phagocytized by, vascular endothelial cells. Organisms then escape from the phagosome, replicate intracellularly, and are released into the circulation. The effects of rickettsial infection, including rash, interstitial loss of fluid across damaged capillaries, and organ injury, are secondary to the vasculitis caused by infection of vascular endothelia in small arteries, capillaries, and veins (8).

Rocky Mountain spotted fever exemplifies the pathogenesis of rickettsial infections leading to severe illness. Capillary infection results in increased vascular permeability, with loss of interstitial fluid, albumin, and sometimes fibrinogen or even red blood cells into the surrounding tissue. Local edema, including both pulmonary and cerebral edema, can result, as can hypovolemia, hypoalbuminemia, and consequent hypotension and shock. Hypovolemia, in turn, can lead to the syndrome of inappropriate secretion of antidiuretic hormone (SIADH) and hyponatremia. Capillary injury can also result in focal hemorrhage, as represented by the rash, or in actual capillary or small vessel occlusion. Host response to this process is usually mononuclear. Thrombocytopenia can be observed in 32% to 52% of patients, suggesting platelet consumption within foci of infection. Actual disseminated intravascular coagulation, although reported, is unusual. Brains of fatally infected patients demonstrate lymphocytic perivascular inflammatory infiltrates; nodules composed of neutrophils, histiocytes, and microglial cells; and occlusion of small blood vessels, resulting in microscopic areas of infarction. Lymphocytic infiltrates may be found in meninges and surrounding cranial nerves (3,9).

The Anaplasmataceae, unlike the Rickettsiaceae, infect white blood cells rather than vascular endothelia. *E. chaffeensis* replicates in monocytes, whereas *A. phagocytophilum* and *E. ewingii* replicate in polymorphonuclear leukocytes. As with Rickettsiaceae, these organisms are incorporated into the host cell in a phagosome. Unlike Rickettsiaceae, however, Anaplasmatacea can replicate intracellularly to form a multicompartmented entity termed a *morula.* Organisms are released following the lysis of the host cell (7).

The pathogenesis of Q fever differs from that of the Rickettsiales (10). The causative agent of Q fever, *C. burnetii,* exists both as large and small variants and also as a spore stage, which allows the organism to survive for weeks or months in wool, fresh meat in cold storage, skim milk, soil, and even formalin-fixed tissues. *C. burnetii* is believed to be maintained in nature in ticks or other arthropods, and infection of nonhuman species is thought to be spread by these vectors in much the same fashion as are Rickettsiaceae and Anaplasmacea. Major animal reservoirs associated with human infection have been cattle, sheep, goats, and cats. Infection in animals is usually asymptomatic, although both abortion and stillbirth can occur. Organisms are shed into the environment in urine, feces, milk, and, in particular, placentas. Human infection with *C. burnetii* results from inhalation of organisms rather than by introduction of the agent by an arthropod vector. The organism replicates initially in pulmonary macrophages and lung parenchyma followed by systemic spread (10).

A number of questions concerning the infections caused by Rickettsiales remain unanswered. Although most of the manifestations of infections with the spotted fever group are thought to be caused directly by replication of the causative agent, the extent to which the infection may be exacerbated by host immune response is not well understood. This question is important in deciding whether corticosteroids might play a role in restoring capillary integrity in severe infection. Q fever, as discussed below, can also cause protracted infection, and the factors that determine persisting infection rather than recovery are not well defined. The relationship between infection by *Anaplasma* and the clinical symptoms seen in affected patients are also not well understood. Finally, *R. prowazekii,* the agent of typhus, remains a significant puzzle. As mentioned, it is thought that epidemic typhus begins with one or more cases of recrudescent typhus—Brill-Zinsser disease—in conditions of overcrowding and poor hygiene and where lice can flourish. This sequence of events, however, implies that the agent is able to achieve prolonged—perhaps lifelong—infection in its human host. To date, the cells and organs in which *R. prowazekii* persists are completely unknown, as are the host factors that contain persistent infection.

CLINICAL MANIFESTATIONS

Neurologic symptoms have long been recognized as complications of rickettsial infections, and the word "typhus" itself comes from the Greek word "τγφοω," whose meaning, *hazy or smoky,* describes the mental status of affected individuals. Although neurologic symptoms of infection by Rickettsiales vary from mild to life-threatening, headache is almost invariably present and may be the presenting complaint.

ROCKY MOUNTAIN SPOTTED FEVER

Rocky Mountain spotted fever represents the major—and most severe—rickettsial infection in North America (3). Two thirds of patients are under 15 years of age, and most cases occur between the ages of 5 and 9. Adults, in particular men, may be infected as a consequence of outdoor occupational activity. The incubation period, from vector exposure to onset of symptoms, is usually 7 days, but can range between 2 and 14 days. The disease usually begins with fever, myalgias, and headache. Nausea, vomiting, and diarrhea are common. The hallmark of Rocky Mountain spotted fever is a cutaneous petechial rash, which will be present in 49% of patients within 3 days and will eventually be present in up to 91% of individuals. The rash usually begins in wrists and ankles, but may also begin more centrally. Involvement of palms and soles, considered classic for the disease, will be found in up to 82% of patients, but tends to appear later in the course of illness. In occasional patients, the characteristic rash may not be present or may be overshadowed by neurologic or other symptoms (11,12). The endothelial infection caused by the agent can result in loss of capillary integrity or in actual vascular occlusion. Skin necrosis and even gangrene of fingers or toes can occur. Retinal involvement can produce retinal edema, hemorrhages, arterial occlusion, or macular star changes (13). Major systemic organs, including lungs, heart, kidneys, gastrointestinal tract, liver, and muscles, can be involved individually or in combination. Lung involvement can manifest as pulmonary edema or pleural effusions. Renal failure, caused by tubular necrosis, is a frequent occurrence in severe cases. Death can occur within 8 to 15 days of onset if appropriate therapy is not administered. Mortality in untreated cases of Rocky Mountain spotted fever may be as high as 30%, but with treatment, it is 3% to 4%. The disease tends to be more severe in adults than in children. Severe morbidity and mortality are associated with delay in reaching diagnosis and initiating appropriate antibiotic therapy. Factors increasing risk are male sex and absence of a history of tick exposure, rash, or classic symptoms, leading the physician to ignore Rocky Mountain spotted fever as a possible diagnosis. Mortality is higher in blacks, in particular in the presence of glucose-6-phosphate dehydrogenase deficiency.

Neurologic involvement has been reported in up to 23% of cases of Rocky Mountain spotted fever and is particularly common in severe cases (3,7,9). Symptoms and signs are most commonly nonfocal and consist of headache, lethargy, and confusion; as well as meningismus and encephalopathic symptoms. Death can result from cerebral edema. Signs of focal neurologic injury may also be present. These include hemiplegia, hemianopsia, or aphasia; signs of cerebral, brainstem, or cerebellar involvement, and transverse myelitis (9). Cranial nerve palsies can also occur, and involvement of cranial nerve VIII, can cause deafness. Wei and Baumann (14) have reported a case in which serologically diagnosed Rocky Mountain spotted fever was followed by acute disseminated encephalomyelitis. Late neurologic effects of infection, which are not uncommon after severe infection, can include persistent headache, intellectual impairment, focal deficits, including tardive dyskinesias, and deafness (3,7,9).

OTHER RICKETTSIAL INFECTIONS

The clinical features of epidemic typhus are less well described in recent literature, but classic descriptions emphasize the consequences of vascular occlusion and altered capillary permeability, much as for Rocky Mountain spotted fever (4). The same is true for infections caused by *R. typhi* and *O. tsutsugamushi*, where neurologic symptoms can range from nonspecific findings of headache or irritability to focal deficits to seizures, stupor, and coma. Neurologic symptoms in infections caused by *R. akari* (rickettsialpox) are usually confined to headache and myalgias.

Acute Febrile Cerebrovasculitis

In 1986, Wenzel et al. (15) reported a series of five patients in rural Virginia who presented with the abrupt onset of fever, headache, altered mentation, multifocal neurologic signs, and CSF pleocytosis. All five had had recent exposure to forests or freshly cut firewood or contact with flea-infested dogs. Two of the patients died, one of fulminant cerebral edema within 24 hours of admission. Brain biopsy samples in two patients and autopsy findings in another showed vasculitis involving venules and capillaries, typical of rickettsial infections. Serologic studies on paired specimens in four patients showed significant cross-reacting antibody responses to rickettsial (typhus-group) antigens in the indirect hemagglutination, latex agglutination, and IgM microimmunofluorescence tests, and reactivity with typhus group antigens was suggested by subsequent immunoblot studies. A similar patient was reported by Linneman et al. in 1989 (16). In none of these cases was an agent isolated or visualized by histology or electron microscopy, and material from these cases has not been subsequently studied by PCR methods.

Anaplasma and Ehrlichia

Illnesses caused by Anaplasma and Ehrlichia characteristically have their onset approximately 10 days after exposure, with fever, chills, and myalgias. Neurologic complications, more commonly associated with *E. chaffeensis*, have included headache, aseptic meningitis, meningoencephalitis, and cranial nerve palsies (7). CSF may contain a lymphocytic pleocytosis, with normal glucose and elevated protein. In some cases, CSF leukocytes can contain *E. morulae* (7). *A. phagocytophilum* has been associated with meningismus, but not with frank meningitis, and CSF pleocytosis has not been reported. Rhabdomyolysis has been reported during infection with these agents, however, and postinfectious complications have also been described, including brachial plexopathies or demyelinating polyneuropathy (7).

Q Fever

Infection with *C. burnetii* is often asymptomatic or trivial, but can also cause life-threatening acute or chronic disease. The major acute systemic syndrome associated with the organism is an atypical pneumonia. More chronic manifestations can include endocarditis, osteomyelitis, and pulmonary fibrosis. Reported neurologic manifestations are extensive and can include meningitis, encephalitis, myelitis, cranial nerve palsies, optic neuritis, and a variety of focal findings (7).

DIAGNOSTIC APPROACH

Virtually all of the infections associated with Rickettsiaceae have protean manifestations, and cutaneous findings, such as rash, may be late in developing or may fail to appear. For this reason, the possibility of rickettsial infection, in particular Rocky Mountain spotted fever, should be kept in mind in the patient presenting with fever and neurologic signs in areas where the organism is endemic—*regardless of whether a rash is present* (17). Diagnostic suspicion should be increased with a history of being in a rural or woodland setting, exposure to ticks, myalgias, gastrointestinal complaints, or altered consciousness. Exposure to livestock, and especially to stillborn or aborted animals, should raise the possibility of Q fever. All of the conditions discussed herein, except Q fever, are most common in spring and summer months (April through September); however, patients occasionally present earlier or later in the year. The season of Rocky Mountain spotted fever, it should be noted, overlaps with that of West Nile virus infection and also Colorado tick fever, both of which can be associated with cutaneous rash.

Routine hematologic studies and blood chemistries are rarely of specific diagnostic help, although blood chemistries may provide evidence of specific organ injury or dehydration caused by internal fluid shifts. Hyponatremia caused by SIADH and thrombocytopenia are common (7). CSF studies may demonstrate a mixed pleocytosis of lymphocytes and neutrophils. Protein is usually elevated, reflecting loss of capillary integrity, but glucose level is almost always normal. Rarely, Rocky Mountain spotted fever has been associated with a CSF eosinophilia. MRI and computed tomography (CT) often fail to show abnormalities in patients with Rocky Mountain spotted fever or in other rickettsioses; abnormal findings, when present, are often subtle. MRI may show prominent perivascular spaces. In severe cases, infarctions, cerebral edema, and meningeal enhancement may also be present (18). Spinal cord and cauda equina enhancement have also been described. In a series of 44 patients studied by Bonawitz et al. (18), the presence on MRI of abnormalities suggested a higher risk of death. MRI findings in other rickettsial illnesses are less well described but are probably similar.

Detection of IgG antibody in blood is the diagnostic procedure most commonly used for Rickettsiales infection (1,7). The test most often used for Rocky Mountain spotted fever is an indirect immunofluorescence assay, although enzyme-linked immunosorbent assay (ELISA) and other methods have been used. Detection of IgG antibodies from a single sample, however, has two important limitations. First, IgG antibody may not be detectable at the time of presentation. Second, detection of IgG antibody in a single sample does not discriminate between ongoing and prior infection. For these reasons, assay of serum for specific IgM antibodies may be of great value in reaching a diagnosis early in the clinical course. Comparison of acute and convalescent antibody titers, although not of immediate value at the time of patient presentation, may allow retrospective diagnosis. An important point to keep in mind, is that, in Rocky Mountain spotted fever, both IgG and IgM antibodies may be absent, despite fatal outcome (19). Rapid diagnosis can also be achieved using PCR methods, on blood or tissue samples, and PCR products can be sequenced to allow more precise diagnosis. Immunostaining of skin biopsies can also be used for rapid diagnosis and may provide the diagnosis where serology is negative (19). The classic serologic test for Rocky Mountain spotted fever and other rickettsial infections has been the Weil-Felix test, which does not involve rickettsial antigens but rather is an agglutination assay using Proteus OX-19 and Ox-2. Although this test is still sometimes ordered, it is relatively insensitive and should not be used in place of more modern, much more accurate diagnostic assays (1,7).

Actual isolation of rickettsial organisms is offered by the Centers for Disease Control and Prevention (CDC) and should not be undertaken lightly by clinical laboratories: Rickettsial agents are highly infectious, and transmission of Rocky Mountain spotted fever by aerosol has been documented among laboratory workers. A sobering thought in this regard, and one to keep in mind, is that both Ricketts and Von Prowazek died of rickettsial illnesses.

Diagnosis of infections caused by *Anaplasma* or *Ehrlichia* is also usually made by serologic methods, as indicated by the presence of IgM antibodies, by seroconversion or by a fourfold rise in antibody titer between acute and convalescent samples (7). The antigens of *E. chaffeensis, E. ewingii,* and *A. phagocytophilum* exhibit considerable cross-reactivity. More rapid diagnosis can be made by identification of morulae in blood or CSF or by PCR analysis of blood or CSF.

TREATMENT

Although tetracycline and chloramphenicol have been used for many years for the treatment of rickettsial infections, doxycycline, given as 100 mg every 12 hours, is currently considered the drug of choice for infections caused by Rickettsia, *Anaplasma, Ehrlichia,* and *C. burnetii.* In children, the drug is administered as 4 mg/kg of body weight in divided doses given twice daily. Chloramphenicol can be given (50 to 75 mg/kg/day in four divided doses) and is sometimes used in pregnancy to avoid staining of bones or teeth in the fetus. The drug has no proved advantage over the tetracyclines, however, and limited data suggest that its use in Rocky Mountain spotted fever may carry a higher mortality (20). Antibiotics are given until the patient has been afebrile for 2 days, usually involving a course of at least 7 days (3).

The systemic complications of these infections may require additional supportive treatment. In Rocky Mountain spotted fever and other severe rickettsial infections, the combination of intravascular volume depletion and severe loss of fluid into the interstitium may require meticulous hemodynamic and fluid management to maintain both oxygenation and organ perfusion. Renal injury, if sufficiently severe, may require short-term hemodialysis. Severe cerebral edema, where present, can present the greatest challenge to prevent a fatal outcome, and monitoring of intracranial pressure should be considered in this setting. Although corticosteroids are of unproved worth in severe rickettsial infections overall, they may warrant consideration in life-threatening severe cerebral edema. Infections by Anaplasmataceae are usually less severe, but can cause severe or fatal injury, in particular in persons immunosuppressed or infected with HIV. In addition to its direct neurologic consequences, Q fever can cause an endocarditis, with embolization to the brain.

CLINICAL RECOMMENDATIONS OF THE VIGNETTE

Rickettsial or ehrlichial illness should be suspected in any febrile patient with neurologic signs presenting in an endemic area from the end of winter through the following autumn, *regardless of whether or not a rash is present.* Because patients can present without a rash, treatment should be initiated presumptively with doxycycline or, less optimally, tetracycline or chloramphenicol. Blood should be sent for serology, including both IgM and IgG antibody assays. Rapid diagnosis may require PCR analysis of blood or, in some cases, immunofluorescence staining of biopsy from cutaneous lesions.

SUMMARY

Rickettsiales, with the exception of *R. prowazekii,* are zoonotic organisms, all of which are transmitted to humans by arthropod vectors. In the case of Rocky Mountain spotted fever, transmission almost invariably occurs between April and September. These agents, including those causing Rocky Mountain spotted fever, can cause fatal systemic and neurologic illness. Clinicians should have a high index of suspicion for infection by these organisms, in particular when the patient has a history of sylvatic exposure or known exposure to ticks or other arthropod organisms. Although most of these agents produce a cutaneous rash in at least some individuals, a characteristic rash may not be present at the time of diagnosis, and treatment should be initiated presumptively while diagnostic tests are being run. Q fever should be suspected in patients presenting with a history of exposure to wool, sheep, cattle, or goats, in particular if pneumonia is present or with evidence of endocarditis. Diagnosis is usually confirmed by detection of IgM and IgG antibodies. Antibody response may not be detectable, even in the presence of fatal disease, however, and immunofluorescence of skin biopsies or PCR methods may be required for diagnosis.

REFERENCES

1. Saah AJ. Rickettsioses and ehrlichioses. In: Mandell GL, Bennett JE, Dolan R, eds. *Principles and Practice of Infectious Diseases*, 5th ed. Philadelphia: Churchill Livingstone; 2000:2033–2035.
2. Sexton DJ, Kaye KS. Rocky Mountain spotted fever. *Med Clin North Am.* 2002;86(2):351–360, vii–viii.
3. Walker DH, Raoult D. Rickettsia rickettsii and other spotted fever group rickettsiae (Rocky Mountain spotted fever and other spotted fevers). In: Mandell GL, Bennett JE, Dolan R, eds. *Principles and Practice of Infectious Diseases*, 5th ed. Philadelphia: Churchill Livingstone; 2000:2035–2042.
4. Wolbach SB, Todd JL, Polfrey FW. *The Etiology and Pathology of Typhus.* Cambridge: Harvard University Press; 1922.
5. Duma RJ, Sonenshine DE, Bozeman FM, et al. Epidemic typhus in the United States associated with flying squirrels. *JAMA.* 1981;245:2318–2323.
6. Massung RF, Davis LE, Slater K, et al. Epidemic typhus meningitis in the Southwestern United States. *Clin Infect Dis.* 2001;32:979–982.
7. Raoult D. Rickettsioses, ehrlichioses, and Q fever. In: Scheld WM, Whitley RJ, Marra CM, eds. *Infections of the Central Nervous System*, 3rd ed. Philadelphia: Lippincott Williams & Wilkins; 2004:423–439.
8. Kim JH, Durack DT. Rickettsiae. In: Scheld WM, Durack DT, Whitley RJ, eds. *Infections of the Central Nervous System*, 2nd ed. Philadelphia: Lippincott-Raven; 1997:403–416.
9. Miller JQ, Price TR. The nervous system in Rocky Mountain spotted fever. *Neurology.* 1972;22:561–566.
10. Marrie TJ. Coxiella burnetti (Q fever). In: Mandell GL, Bennett JE, Dolan R, eds. *Principles and Practice of Infectious Diseases*, 5th ed. Philadelphia: Churchill Livingstone; 2000:2043–2050.
11. Garg P, Blass DA. Rocky Mountain spotted fever manifested by cerebritis and pneumonitis. *Md Med.* 1987;36(4):343–345.
12. Westerman EL. Rocky mountain spotless fever. A dilemma for the clinician. *Arch Intern Med.* 1982;142:1106–1107.
13. Vaphiades MS. Rocky Mountain spotted fever as a cause of macular star figure. *J Neuroophthalmol.* 2003;23(4):276–278.
14. Wei TY, Baumann RJ. Acute disseminated encephalomyelitis after Rocky Mountain spotted fever. *Pediatr Neurol.* 1999;21(1):503–505.
15. Wenzel RP, Hayden FG, Groschel DH, et al. Acute febrile cerebrovasculitis: A syndrome of unknown, perhaps rickettsial, cause. *Ann Intern Med.* 1986;104(5):606–615.
16. Linnemann CC, Jr., Pretzman CI, Peterson ED. Acute febrile cerebrovasculitis. A non-spotted fever group rickettsial disease. *Arch Intern Med.* 1989;149(7):1682–1684.
17. Tenenbaum MJ, Markowitz SM. Rocky Mountain spotted fever: Diagnostic dilemma of the atypical presentation. *South Med J.* 1980;73(11):1527–1529.
18. Bonawitz C, Castillo M, Mukherji SK. Comparison of CT and MR features with clinical outcome in patients with Rocky Mountain spotted fever. *AJNR Am J Neuroradiol.* 1997;18(3):459–464.
19. Paddock CD, Greer PW, Ferebee TL, et al. Hidden mortality attributable to Rocky Mountain spotted fever: Immunohistochemical detection of fatal, serologically unconfirmed disease. *J Infect Dis.* 1999;179(6):1469–1476.
20. Holman RC, Paddock CD, Curns AT, et al. Analysis of risk factors for fatal Rocky Mountain spotted fever: Evidence for superiority of tetracyclines for therapy. *J Infect Dis.* 2001;184(11):1437–1444.

CHAPTER **97**

Protozoa and Metazoa

Ana-Claire L. Meyer • Glenn E. Mathisen

OBJECTIVES

- To describe the three most commonly diagnosed parasitic infections of the nervous system
- To review the breadth of parasitic diseases of the nervous system
- To discuss an approach to the differential diagnosis when confronted with parasitic infection of the nervous system

CASE VIGNETTE

A 41-year-old man with no medical history presents with 3 weeks of severe occipital headache and progressive visual loss. The headache waxes and wanes, involves his whole head, and is not more severe at any particular time of day. When the pain is severe, he has some associated nausea, but no vomiting. In addition, he describes gradual blurring of vision in both eyes, leading to difficulty reading and an inability to distinguish color, which caused him to stop working as a landscaper. He moved from Guatemala to Philadelphia 2 years before presentation. Review of systems is negative.

On physical examination, he is alert and able to answer questions appropriately. Visual acuity is 20/40 OD and 20/50 OS; he is unable to distinguish colors with Ishihara plates and has bilateral papilledema on dilated fundoscopic examination. He has a mild, bilateral partial sixth nerve palsy, right greater than left; finding from the remainder of the examination is otherwise normal. Computed tomography (CT) and magnetic resonance imaging (MRI) were performed (Fig. 97-1).

DEFINITION

Parasitic infections are widespread within the animal kingdom and have adapted to, and co-evolved with, *homo sapiens* for millions of years. Humans harbor more than 70 species of protozoa and 300 species of helminths, although only a few commonly cause human disease (1). Although distributed worldwide, parasites flourish in tropical latitudes. Within these areas, the burden of disease disproportionately affects people in poor or politically unstable regions, where diseases, such as malaria and trypanosomiasis, have increased in incidence over the past few decades.

Various human and environmental factors contribute to this resurgence of human parasitic disease. Perhaps chief among these, population growth in both rural and urban areas, without corresponding improvements in the public health infrastructure, leads to increased prevalence of vectors and pathogens. Another important factor is increased trade and travel, which brings people from nonendemic areas into contact with parasites, such as malaria. Furthermore, changes in land use have increased the populations of vectors, such as mosquitoes, ticks, copepods, and snails. Finally, global warming lengthens the growth season of many vectors, which may extend their area of distribution (2).

The resultant proliferation of parasites and their vectors has enormous implications for human disease. Neurologic infections, although less common than systemic ones, often result in severe morbidity and high mortality. For example, human African trypanosomiasis, cerebral malaria, and amebic encephalitides have very high mortality rates; survivors often have devastating neurologic deficits. Moreover, neurocysticercosis is the leading cause of acquired epilepsy worldwide. In this chapter, are discussed in detail three parasitic infections of the nervous system: Neurocysticercosis, toxoplasmosis, and schistosomiasis. These, however are only a small subset of the parasitic infections that can affect the nervous system (Table 97-1).

Despite the public health importance and often devastating effects of these infections, relatively little is known about their pathophysiology and molecular mechanisms. Consequently, effective treatments exist for few parasitic infections, and no vaccines are currently available. Lack of funding and political instability hamper research and fragment control efforts. Control of most parasitic diseases would require only safe drinking water, uncontaminated food, and improved housing, which remain inaccessible to most of the world, however.

Neurocysticercosis

EPIDEMIOLOGY

Neurocysticercosis is distributed worldwide, but is endemic in much of Latin America, Africa, and Asia. Immigration by carriers, however, has led to an increasing incidence in Europe and North America (3). Each year, neurocysticercosis results in more than 50,000 deaths and is the leading cause of acquired epilepsy worldwide (4).

ETIOLOGY AND PATHOGENESIS

Human infections with *Taenia solium* can result in either of two clinical syndromes: Taeniasis or cysticercosis. Taeniasis, human

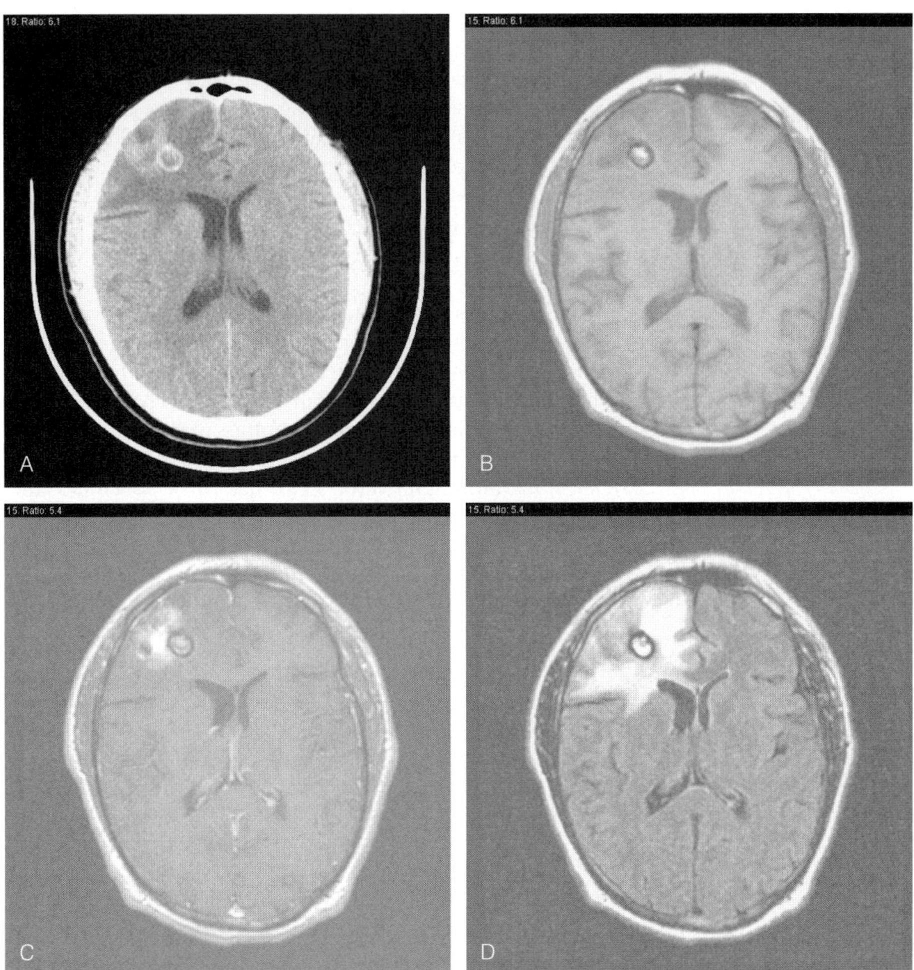

FIGURE 97-1. Images from the case vignette. Noncontrast computed tomography (CT) of the head. Hyperdense ring with a hypodense center and surrounding hypodensity in the right frontal lobe (**A**). Axial T1-weighted magnetic resonance image (MRI) of the brain. Complex mass lesion in the right frontal lobe with an eccentric bright nodule (representing scolex) (**B**). Axial T1-weighted, postgadolinium MRI of the brain. Subtle enhancement within the complex lesion, a thick enhancing calcified ring, and significant surrounding enhancement (**C**). Axial T2/fluid-attenuated inversion recovery (FLAIR) sequence on MRI of the brain. Hypointense ring of calcification, eccentric hyperintense nodule, surrounded by subtle mass effect and diffuse hyperintensity which relatively spares the gray matter (**D**).

infection with the adult tapeworm, typically results from ingestion of the tapeworm larvae, cysticerci, in uncooked or poorly cooked meat, especially pork. Cysticercosis, on the other hand, results from the ingestion of food or water containing *T. solium* eggs, owing to fecal contamination from a foodhandler or in water used for irrigation. In many cases of cysticercosis, the source of infection is unknown; however, cases may be associated with a symptom-free tapeworm carrier in the household (5).

PATHOLOGY

After the eggs are ingested, gastric acids liberate the embryos inside, which then actively cross the bowel wall and enter the bloodstream. Embryos are carried all over the body, particularly to subcutaneous tissues, muscles, heart, brain, and eyes (3,6). There, they develop into round or oval vesicles called *cysts* that vary in size from a few millimeters to 2 cm. In the brain, the most common locations are the basal ganglia or the gray–white junction of the cerebral hemispheres; however, cysts can be found throughout the brain parenchyma, subarachnoid space, ventricles, and spinal cord (3). Cysts develop at individual rates in a predictable pattern. Initially, noncystic embryos develop into thin-walled cysts, which may have a mural nodule that represents the scolex and are often surrounded by edema (6). Over the next few years, the cyst can grow in size; however, cysts eventually degenerate, an event marked by worsening edema, thickening of the cyst wall, and increased protein content within the cyst. Following this, the cyst fluid is gradually adsorbed, and finally the dead larvae calcify (3).

CLINICAL MANIFESTATIONS

The central nervous system (CNS) is involved in 60% to 90% of patients with cysticercosis. The clinical presentation is variable and depends on the location of the cysts and the overall severity of infection. Common presenting symptoms are headache, focal or generalized seizures, intracranial hypertension, or focal neurologic signs (3,5). Focal signs typically develop over a subacute time course. Children and teenagers with recent infection may present with an acute encephalitis, extensive edema, and marked intracranial hypertension (3). Intracranial hypertension and hydrocephalus can also result from giant parenchymal cysts or cysts in the cerebral ventricles and basal cisterns. Or, ventricular obstruction can be secondary to ependymal inflammation, with subsequent fibrosis. Acute intermittent hydrocephalus (Bruns syndrome) is characterized by recurrent bouts of nausea, vomiting, and headache resulting from intermittent obstruction by mobile intraventricular cysts (3,6).

TABLE 97-1. Human Parasitic Infections of the Nervous System

PROTOZOANS

1. Malaria: *Plasmodium falciparum*
2. Amoebiasis: *Acanthamoeba, Balamuthia, Naegleria fowler, Entamoeba histolytica*
3. Trypanosomes
4. Human African Trypanosomiasis: *Trypanosoma brucei gambiens, T. b. rhodesiense*
5. American trypanosomiasis: *Trypanosoma cruzi*
6. Toxoplasmosis: *Toxoplasma gondii*

HELMINTHS

Cestodes

1. Neurocysticercosis: *Taenia solium*
2. Echinococcosis: *Echinococcus granulosus*
3. Other Cestodes: *Diphyllobothrium latum, Spirometra spp., Taenia multiceps*

Nematodes

1. Angiostrongyliasis: *Angiostrongylus cantonensis*
2. Gnathostomiasis: *Gnathostoma spinigerum*
3. Toxocariasis: *Toxocara cani, T. cati*
4. Strongyloidiasis: Strongyloides stercoralis
5. Trichinosis: Trichinella spiralis
6. Other Nematodes: *Baylisascaris procyonis, Wuchereria bancrofti, Micronema deletrix, Dracunculus medinensis, Dipetalonema perstans, Onchocerca volvulus, Loa Loa*

Trematodes

1. Schistosomes: *Schistosoma mansoni, S. japonicum, S. hematobium, S. mekongi, S. intercalatum*
2. Paragonimus: *Paragonimus westermani, P. mexicanus, P. miyazakii*

ECTOPARASITES

1. Tick paralysis

Stroke is seen primarily in patients with subarachnoid neurocysticercosis; most patients present with lacunar infarcts related to basilar inflammation, which results in endarteritis of small penetrating arteries in the brainstem, internal capsule, or subcortical white matter (3). Large vessel strokes are uncommon. Spinal cord lesions are uncommon, accounting for approximately 1% of cases in some series; although intramedullary cysts are occasionally described, lesions are usually found in the subarachnoid space (3). Ocular cysticerci can result in decreased visual acuity or visual field deficits. Although asymptomatic involvement of skeletal muscle is common (e.g., calcified cysts on plain radiographs), some patients, most commonly in Asia and Africa, may develop generalized weakness, muscle enlargement, and pain, either at presentation or after initiation of cysticidal treatment (4,5).

DIAGNOSTIC APPROACH

The presence of new onset seizures or focal neurologic signs in a patient from an endemic area should suggest the possibility of neurocysticercosis. The diagnosis can be challenging, particularly in resource-limited areas; therefore, a detailed set of clinical diagnostic criteria have been proposed by Garcia and De Brutto (5). In many settings, CT or MRI is available and may provide evidence of neurocysticercosis. On CT, viable cysts appear as hypodense, rounded, cystic lesions, which often enhance with intravenous contrast. Edema may be observed in degenerating cysts. End-stage, nonviable cysts are heavily calcified and appear as punctate hyperintensities. The appearance on MRI is also variable, depending on the stage of infection. Initially, the cysts are usually hypointense on both T1- and T2-weighted images. A hyperintense eccentric nodule, representing the scolex, may be observed. As the cyst degenerates, the cyst fluid and capsule become hyperintense on T2 images, often with ring enhancement and surrounding edema (Fig. 97-1) (4,5).

Serologic assays for cysticercal antibodies in serum or CSF may be helpful in confirming infection, especially in patients with an atypical clinical or radiographic presentation. The enzyme-linked immunoelectrotransfer blot (EITB) is preferred to the enzyme-linked immunosorbent assay (ELISA), because the ELISA cross-reacts with other common cestode infections (3). Of note, although overall EITB has 100% specificity and 98% sensitivity, a positive test indicates infection, but cannot specify infection of the nervous system. Further, in patients with a single brain lesion, almost 30% have negative finding on EITB (5). In nonendemic areas or when imaging findings or serologic studies are inconclusive, biopsy of the lesion is frequently performed.

TREATMENT

Because of questions of efficacy and toxicity, the use of cysticidal medications for the treatment of neurocysticercosis has been the subject of much debate. Despite the uncertainties, several treatment principles emerge to help guide therapy in the individual patient. Patients frequently become symptomatic when a viable cyst dies; in these cases, corticosteroids alone may be used. Symptomatic patients with moderate infections and viable cysts are usually given cysticidal treatment. Concomitant corticosteroids are recommended because symptoms often worsen secondary to the inflammatory reaction to degenerating cysts. Cysticidal treatment and high-dose steroids can be given with care for subarachnoid cysts, giant cysts, or racemose cysts; however, placement of a ventriculoperitoneal shunt before initiating therapy is recommended because of the risk of an inflammatory reaction and subsequent hydrocephalus (4). High doses of steroids alone (up to 32 mg/day of dexamethasone) are used for arachnoiditis, encephalitis, or ependymitis (4). Surgical resection may be necessary for intraventricular, giant, spinal, or ocular cysts (3). Patients with massive infections of viable cysts or numerous degenerating cysts may develop a severe inflammatory reaction and endarteritis of the leptomeninges after cysticidal treatment, resulting in stroke or increased intracranial pressure. The benefit of cysticidal treatment in these patients is not known, and generally not recommended. Because low-level infections usually resolve without intervention, the necessity of treatment in a patient with one or only a few viable cysts is debated. Small, calcified lesions represent the sequelae of previous infection; cysticidal therapy is not recommended unless concurrent viable cysts are present (3,6).

Albendazole and praziquantel both destroy 60% to 85% of viable intracranial cysticerci and are the primary cysticidal drugs used for treatment of neurocysticercosis. Albendazole is administered at doses of 15 mg/kg/day up to 1 month. A small, randomized, controlled trial suggests that the duration of treatment can be shortened to 1 week without decreasing efficacy (7). Albendazole has better penetration into the CSF and is the drug of choice for subarachnoid and ventricular cysts. Dosage recommendations for praziquantel vary; typically, praziquantel is given at 50 mg/kg/day for 15 days. Seizures should be treated with antiepileptic medications. The ideal duration of treatment is not known; however, in one prospective study, up to 50% of patients had recurrent seizures after antiepileptic drugs were withdrawn (4,5).

Toxoplasmosis

EPIDEMIOLOGY

The widely distributed obligate intracellular protozoan parasite, *Toxoplasma gondii,* causes toxoplasmosis. Over one half billion of the world's population have serum antibodies to *T. gondii,* although most infected adults are asymptomatic. Once uncommon, symptomatic reactivation of latent disease in the CNS is increasing because of the greater number of patients receiving immunosuppressive therapies and the growth of the human immunodeficiency virus and acquired immunodeficiency syndrome (HIV/AIDS) pandemic. Congenital toxoplasmosis is a consequence of primary maternal infection during pregnancy and has a birth prevalence from 1 to 10 per 10,000 live births (8).

ETIOLOGY AND PATHOGENESIS

The definitive hosts of *T. gondii* are members of the cat family. Sexual replication of the parasite occurs in the cat intestine, resulting in the production of large numbers of oocysts in the feces. Human infection most commonly follows handling or ingestion of poorly cooked meat that contains viable tissue cysts. Infection can also occur after exposure to water, food, or soil contaminated with infected cat feces and viable oocysts. Recently, transmission via transplanted organs has been documented (8). Maternal-fetal transmission occurs when the mother develops primary infection during gestation, although prior maternal infection poses little or no risk to the fetus (8). After humans ingest the oocysts or tissue cysts, tachyzoites, the rapidly multiplying asexual form of the parasite, develop and invade all nucleated cells. Their replication leads to death of the host cell as well as neighboring cells and incites a strong inflammatory response. This immune response stimulates the production of cysts, which renders the tachyzoites undetectable by the immune system. Tachyzoites can be re-released from cysts, causing recrudescence of infection, or remain latent for years as bradyzoites (8).

PATHOLOGY

Cysts can form in brain, skeletal, and heart muscle. Within the brain, *T. gondii* has a predilection for the basal ganglia, but cysts can be found throughout the cerebral hemispheres and brainstem. On histologic examination of active lesions, multiple enlarging foci of necrosis and microglial nodules are observed. Necrotic areas frequently calcify. Cysts and tachyzoites are seen, but only the latter is pathognomonic of active infection. Tachyzoites are observed within, and in proximity to, necrotic areas, as well as in glial nodules, perivascular regions, and regions of unaffected brain. In infants, periaqueductal and periventricular vasculitis and necrosis develop, often leading to obstruction of the aqueduct of Sylvius or foramen of Monro, with subsequent obstructive hydrocephalus (9).

CLINICAL MANIFESTATIONS

The clinical manifestations of toxoplasmosis are varied. Although primary infection is usually asymptomatic, patients can develop a self-limited and nonspecific illness that resembles mononucleosis. These individuals present with low-grade fever, fatigue, and malaise; an isolated nonsuppurative cervical or occipital lymphadenopathy may occur, usually lasting between 4 and 6 weeks. In rare cases, immunocompetent individuals develop myocarditis, polymyositis, pneumonitis, hepatitis, or encephalitis. Although *Toxoplasma* chorioretinitis can occur as the result of acute infection, it more commonly represents a reactivation of congenital disease (8). In immunocompromised patients, the disease is almost always caused by reactivation of a latent infection. Toxoplasmosis in this setting can be life-threatening and most commonly affects the CNS. Patients with *Toxoplasma* encephalitis may initially complain of nonspecific symptoms, such as fever, headache, and malaise. These may be present for several weeks before the acute development of a confusional state, which may be accompanied by focal neurologic signs. Meningeal signs are rare. *Toxoplasma* encephalitis, rarely is associated with chorioretinitis, pneumonitis, or multiorgan involvement, leading to acute respiratory failure and hemodynamic compromise (8). In patients with HIV/AIDS, abscesses may form (Fig. 97-2).

Although late maternal infections usually result in normal-appearing newborns, maternal infection in the first or second trimester can lead to severe congenital toxoplasmosis and intrauterine death. About 85% of newborns with congenital toxoplasmosis have subclinical infection (8). In the remainder, abnormalities observed *in utero* resemble those caused by other TORCH (toxoplasmosis; other infections: Namely hepatitis B, syphilis, and herpes zoster, the virus that causes chickenpox; rubella, formerly known as German measles; cytomegalovirus [CMV]; and herpes simplex virus, the cause of genital herpes) infections, and can include intracranial calcifications, ventricular dilation, hepatic enlargement, ascites, and increased placental thickness. In the neonate, manifestations include hydrocephalus, microcephaly, chorioretinitis, strabismus, blindness, seizures, psychomotor or mental retardation, and hematologic findings, such as thrombocytopenia or anemia. The classic triad of chorioretinitis, hydrocephalus, and cerebral calcifications is rare (8).

DIAGNOSTIC APPROACH

Toxoplasmosis can be diagnosed via indirect serologic methods or directly by histology, PCR, and various isolation techniques (tissue cell culture or mouse inoculation). Among the various serologic methods, the most common screening test is the

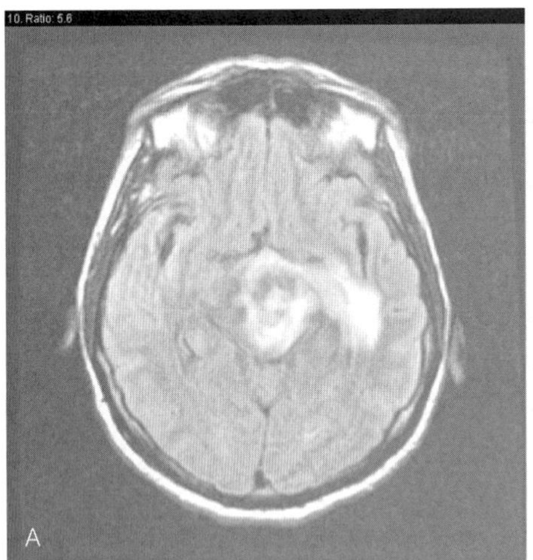

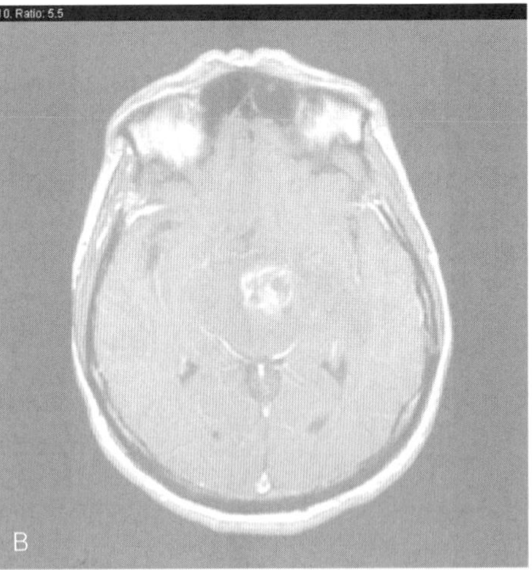

FIGURE 97-2. Toxoplasmosis. Axial T2/fluid-attenuated inversion recovery (FLAIR) sequence on magnetic resonance image (MRI) of the brain at the junction of the midbrain and basal ganglia. A complex mass lesion is seen in the left midbrain. On images not shown here, it extends into the pons and thalamus. Marked hyperintensity and mass effect surround the mass, consistent with edema (**A**). Axial T1-weighted postgadolinium MRI of the brain. An irregularly enhancing mass with a necrotic center is seen in the left midbrain (**B**).

enzyme-linked immunoassay (EIA) for IgM and IgG. IgM antibodies indicate recent infection and usually develop within 2 weeks; they can persist for more than a year despite resolution of active infection. IgG antibodies usually appear within 2 weeks of infection and peak at 6 to 8 weeks; they remain positive indefinitely and are helpful in confirming previous infection. The Sabin Feldman Dye test (SFDT) for total specific IgG is the gold standard, although it can be performed only in reference centers, and is typically used as a confirmatory test (10). Serologic testing is an important part of evaluating patients for possible congenital toxoplasmosis infection. Seronegative pregnant women are at risk of infection during pregnancy. Subsequent maternal seroconversion is suggested by the presence of IgM, IgG in rising titers, and low avidity IgG. Additional evaluation, including amniocentesis with antibody and PCR testing, is needed to confirm fetal infection. If available, immunosorbent agglutination assay test (IAAT) is useful to detect IgM or IgA in neonates where antibody titers may be low (10). In immunocompromised patients, clinical disease is usually secondary to reactivation of latent disease; therefore, serologic studies do not identify active disease but rather identify patients at risk of disease. Definitive diagnosis may require biopsy or PCR testing of CSF, blood, or urine; demonstration of organisms in cell culture or mouse inoculation studies may also prove helpful. PCR sensitivity can be decreased if testing is performed on patients who have already received treatment for toxoplasmosis (8).

Toxoplasma brain lesions on MRI are isointense or slightly hypointense with respect to brain parenchyma on T1-weighted images, and are hyperintense or isointense on T2-weighted images. After administration of contrast, thin, smooth ring enhancement is common (Fig. 97-2) (11). In an immunocompromised patient, presence of IgG antibodies and compatible radiographic imaging should prompt suspicion of *Toxoplasma* encephalitis and supports initiation of empiric antibiotics. Because toxoplasmosis has a radiographic appearance similar to other disease processes, such as tumors, especially primary CNS lymphoma, tuberculomas, and abscesses, failure to respond to therapy suggests an alternative diagnosis and the need for biopsy (8).

TREATMENT

In immunocompetent patients, *Toxoplasma* lymphadenitis typically resolves on its own without treatment. Chorioretinitis is usually treated with pyrimethamine, sulfadiazine, and folinic acid. If the chorioretinitis is minimal, treatment can be deferred because these lesions occasionally resolve on their own in immunocompetent patients. In severe cases, corticosteroids are added to the regimen. Treatment of pregnant women with evidence of acute infection during their pregnancy decreases the incidence of neonatal toxoplasmosis. Practices vary widely among centers; in general, women with acute infection early in pregnancy should be treated with spiramycin, and after 12 to18 weeks of gestation, treatment with pyrimethamine, sulfadiazine, and folinic acid may be initiated. Regardless of therapy during pregnancy, the infant should be treated throughout the first year of life (10).

Immunocompromised patients with toxoplasmosis in the CNS require intensive multidrug treatment with pyrimethamine, sulfadiazine, and folinic acid for at least 4 to 6 weeks after resolution of all symptoms. Administer pyrimethamine as a 200 mg loading dose, followed by 50 to 75 mg daily. The second drug should be either sulfadiazine (1 to 1.5 g every 6 hours) or clindamycin (600 to 1,200 mg every 6 hours), depending on the patient's allergic history. This regimen should always include folinic acid (10 to 20 mg daily) to minimize the risk of hematologic toxicity. Following primary therapy, maintenance with half doses of the induction regimen should be continued for the life of the patient as long as the patient remains in an immunocompromised state. In patients with HIV/AIDS, continue therapy until the viral load is undetectable and the CD4 count is >200 cells/mm^3. Alternative regimens for treatment of toxoplasmosis can include trimethoprim, clarithromycin, atovaquone, azithromycin, or dapsone (8).

Schistosomiasis

EPIDEMIOLOGY

In Cairo in 1851, Theodor Bilharz described the parasitic infection that is now known as *schistosomiasis* (formerly called bilharzia). More than 200 million people in 74 countries are infected; of these, 120 million people are symptomatic, and 20 million have severe disease. Despite this worldwide distribution, 85% of cases are located in sub-Saharan Africa. Moreover, travelers to endemic countries are also at risk (12). Five species of schistosomes cause human disease: *Schistosoma haematobium*, *S. mansoni*, *S. intercalatum*, *S. japonicum*, and *S. mekongi* (13,14). *S. haematobium*, *S. mansoni*, and *S. intercalatum* are found in sub-Saharan Africa. *S. mansoni* is additionally found in Brazil, Venezuela, and the Caribbean. *S. japonicum* has largely been eliminated from Japan, but is found in China, Indonesia, and the Philippines. *S. mekongi* infection can be found in Cambodia and Laos along the Mekong river (12).

ETIOLOGY AND PATHOGENESIS

Schistosomiasis is caused by a sexually dimorphic parasitic trematode. Direct contact with fresh water that harbors cercariae, the free-swimming larval form of the parasite, results in infection. Cercariae penetrate the skin, enter capillaries, are carried through the pulmonary vasculature to the systemic circulation, and finally settle into the portal or pelvic venous system. After maturation, the adult worms attach themselves in pairs to the mesenteric veins or vesicular venous plexus. Egg production begins 4 to 6 weeks after infection and continues for the life of the worm, usually about 3 to 5 years, but sometimes much longer. Eggs pass from the lumen of the blood vessel into the intestinal or bladder mucosa and then out of the body in urine or feces. The eggs hatch once they reach fresh water and the larvae seek out and infect the species specific host snails, where they undergo a complex life cycle, ultimately resulting in the release of cercariae into bodies of fresh water (12).

PATHOLOGY

Most eggs embolize from the mesenteric or vesicular veins to intraabdominal and pulmonary sites; however, eggs can reach the CNS via pulmonary arteriovenous shunts, portopulmonary anastomoses (e.g., azygos vein), or retrograde venous flow from the portal vein to the Batson epidural venous plexus. In addition, ectopic adult worms sometimes migrate to sites close to the CNS where they lay eggs, resulting in local inflammation (12,13). For unknown reasons, the eggs of *S. japonicum* cause brain lesions, whereas *S. mansoni* and *S. haematobium* typically affect the lower spinal cord. Once deposited in tissue, the eggs secrete antigenic products that generate an intense periovular granulomatous reaction. Although egg deposition is frequently clinically asymptomatic, large numbers of eggs may generate sufficient inflammation, vascular damage, and mass effect to cause clinical symptoms (13).

CLINICAL MANIFESTATIONS

Hours to days after contact with contaminated water, patients may develop an intensely pruritic, localized maculopapular eruption, which represents the penetration of cercariae through intact skin. Within 2 to 12 weeks, patients may develop Katayama fever, a form of acute schistosomiasis, which is associated with the initial systemic dissemination of the parasite. This is seen most commonly in highly endemic regions, especially in adults infected for the first time. Common symptoms of acute schistosomiasis include fever, headache, generalized myalgias, right upper quadrant pain, hematuria, and bloody diarrhea. On physical examination, patients often show signs of generalized lymphadenopathy, tender hepatomegaly, and splenomegaly. Marked peripheral eosinophilia may also be observed (12). Depending on the infective species, patients with chronic schistosomiasis frequently develop fibro-obstructive disease of the liver, intestines, or genitourinary tract. *S. mansoni*, *S. japonicum*, and *S. mekongi* cause intestinal and hepatic lesions, leading to periportal hepatic fibrosis and portal venous hypertension. *S. haematobium* causes primarily urinary tract pathology, including hematuria, dysuria, chronic cystitis, and obstructive uropathy. Recurrent *S. haematobium* infections are associated with increased risk for squamous cell carcinoma of the bladder. In children, severe infection affects growth, nutrition, activity, and school performance (12).

Symptomatic neurologic involvement can be cerebral or spinal (13). Cerebral schistosomiasis is thought to affect 2% to 4% of individuals infected with *S. japonicum*. The clinical manifestations include an acute encephalitis or encephalomyelitis concurrent with, or immediately after, the systemic manifestations of the acute phase of infection. The encephalitis is transient, lasting several days or weeks, and treatment usually

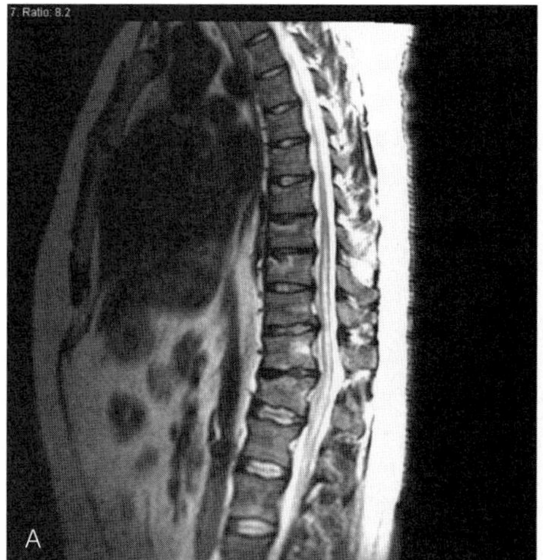

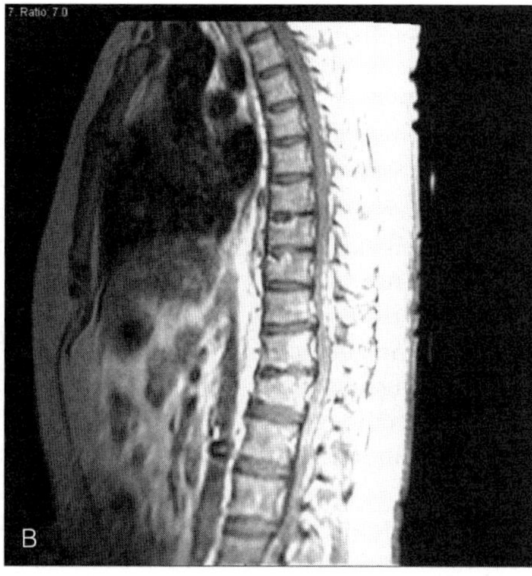

FIGURE 97-3. Spinal schistosomiasis. Sagittal T2-weighted magnetic resonance image (MRI) of the thoracic spine. Marked hyperintensity is seen in the center of the cord, extending from the midthoracic region to the conus medullaris (not shown) (**A**). Sagittal T1-weighted postgadolinium MRI of the thoracic spine. Irregular enhancement is seen within the cord from the midthoracic region to the conus medullaris (not shown), and patches of spotty nodular enhancement are seen along the posterior aspect of the cord in the midthoracic and low thoracic regions (**B**).

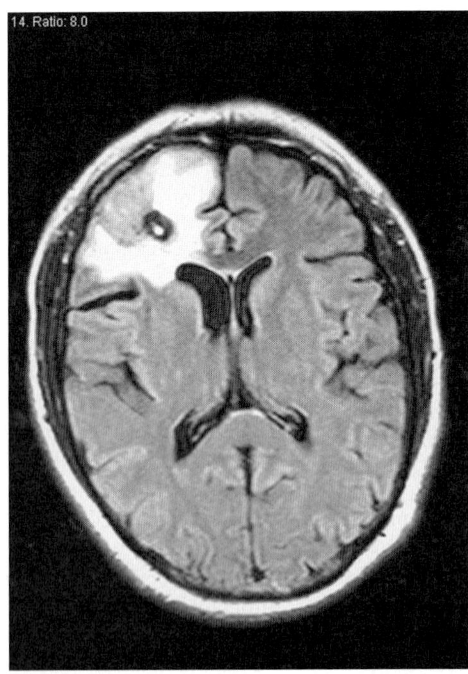

FIGURE 97-4. Case follow-up. Axial T2/fluid-attenuated inversion recovery (FLAIR) sequence magnetic resonance image (MRI) of the brain, one month after treatment. The appearance of the lesion is approximately the same, although the surrounding edema is somewhat lessened.

results in complete recovery. Rarely, cerebral schistosomiasis presents as a slowly expanding mass lesion, resulting in focal neurologic signs, increased intracranial pressure, or seizures (13). Spinal schistosomiasis is usually caused by infection by *S. mansoni* and *S. haematobium* and commonly presents as a myeloradiculopathy. Clinical symptoms usually begin with lumbar or lower extremity pains, often radicular in nature. They are followed within hours or days by leg weakness, dermatomal sensory loss, and autonomic, bladder, and erectile dysfunction. Symptoms are usually maximal within 1 to 2 weeks of onset. Hallmarks of spinal schistosomiasis include rapid progression, disease ascending through the levels, and variable severity of disease, including permanent paraplegia (13,14). A review of cases reported in the literature suggests the levels most frequently involved are low thoracic (T6-T12), followed by lumbar, then by lumbosacral, and cauda equina (15). The differential diagnosis is broad and includes transverse myelitis, cord compression, and nutritional deficiencies.

DIAGNOSTIC APPROACH

No noninvasive way exists to definitively diagnose cerebral or spinal involvement. Indirect immunologic tests, such as ELISA against *S. mansoni* adult microsomal antigen (MAMA), are available through the Centers for Disease Control and Prevention (CDC) with immunoblot testing for other *Schistosoma* species. Some studies suggest that ELISA testing using egg antigen provides greater diagnostic sensitivity and specificity for infection, although the specific utility of these tests in diagnosing neurologic infections is not known (16).

Cerebral schistosomiasis should be suspected in patients from endemic areas who present with encephalitis, especially those with schistosomal eggs in the stool or positive schistosomal serology findings. In both cerebral and spinal schistosomiasis, CSF typically shows increased protein and lymphocytosis; eosinophils may or may not be present (13,14). In patients with typical spinal lesions, although other causes of spinal cord pathology must be eliminated, a history of exposure, eggs in the stool or urine, and positive schistosomal antibodies in the CSF are strongly suggestive of schistosomiasis. Spinal CT usually shows a hyperdense, enhancing area surrounded by a hypodense halo. Spinal MRI typically demonstrates hyperintensity on T2 and fluid-attenuated inversion recovery (FLAIR) with linear and nodular contrast enhancement (Fig. 97-3). Myelography and CT myelography generate nonspecific findings,

TABLE 97-2. Clinical Manifestation of Parasitic Diseases of the Nervous System

MENINGITIS OR ENCEPHALITIS	
Eosinophilic meningitis	*Angiostrongylus cantonensis* *Gnathostoma spinigerum* *Toxocara* *Trichinella spiralis*
Acute meningitis or encephalitis	*Plasmodium falciparum* *Naegleria fowleri* *Trypanosoma cruzi* *Taenia solium* *Schistosoma* *Strongyloides stercoralis* *Baylisascaris procyonis* *Wuchereria bancrofti* *Micronema deletrix*
Chronic meningitis or encephalitis	*Acanthamoeba, Balamuthia* *Toxoplasma gondii*
ENCEPHALOPATHY	*Trypanosoma brucei* *Trichinella spiralis*
SPACE-OCCUPYING LESIONS	
Obstructive hydrocephalus	*Toxoplasmosis* *Taenia solium* *Echinococcus granulosum*
Cerebrum, cerebellum, brainstem	*Toxoplasma gondii* *Taenia solium* *Taenia multiceps* *Echinococcus granulosum* *Spirometra* *Trichinella spiralis* *Paragonimus*
Spinal cord	*Diphyllobothrium latum* *Dracunculus medinensis* *Schistosoma*
Abscess	*Entamoeba histolytica* *Toxoplasma gondii*
INTRACEREBRAL HEMORRHAGE	*Spirometra* *Gnathostoma spinigerum*
MYOSITIS	*Trichinella spiralis*
RADICULITIS	*Schistosoma* *Gnathostoma spinigerum*
ASCENDING PARALYSIS	*Ectoparasites* *Schistosoma*
BLINDNESS	*Toxoplasma gondii* *Taenia solium* *Toxocariasis* *Loa Loa* *Onchocerca volvulus*

including enlargement of the spinal cord, most frequently the conus medullaris, and thickening of the cauda equina (14).

TREATMENT

Treatment with praziquantel and corticosteroids is most efficacious when given soon after presentation. Treatment, even 2 weeks postparalysis, has led to recovery. Therefore, any patient with a nontraumatic paraparesis and a possible exposure merits presumptive treatment. Praziquantel is only active against the adult worm; however, corticosteroids diminish the granulomatous inflammation associated with egg deposition. Praziquantel (60 mg/kg/day) is administered daily in two divided doses for 3 days. A 5-day course of methylprednisolone (500 mg twice daily) is followed by prednisone (1.5 to 2.0 mg/kg/day) in three divided doses for 3 to 4 weeks and a subsequent gradual taper; the methylprednisolone can be omitted, if desired. Surgical approaches should be used only for cases with evident cord compression, diagnostic uncertainty, or those whose condition deteriorates despite treatment (13).

CLINICAL RECOMMENDATIONS OF THE VIGNETTEE

In the initial case presentation, the findings on CT and MRI suggest a heavily calcified lesion with surrounding edema, which could represent neurocysticercosis infection. Whether the cyst is viable or already degenerating is difficult to definitively state based on imaging; the calcification and edema would suggest a degenerating cyst, whereas the presence of the scolex (the eccentric nodule within the cyst) indicates viable infection. Cysticercal immunoblot assay was sent, but results were not available. Because the patient's clinical symptoms were mild, his radiographic findings were consistent with active neurocysticercosis, and he came from an endemic region, brain biopsy was deferred and empiric therapy was initiated with a 10-day course of albendazole and a longer dexamethasone taper. The patient demonstrated clinical and radiographic improvement at a follow up visit 1 month later (Fig. 97-4). Cysticercal immunoblot results, which were available at that time, were negative.

SUMMARY

Parasitic infections of the nervous system are underrecognized. Overall, they are rare in the United States, although several populations are particularly at risk: Malnourished patients, pediatric patients (especially, those with pica), travelers to endemic regions, and patients immunocompromised secondary to transplants, chronic corticosteroids, HIV/AIDS, and pregnancy. Parasitic infections of the nervous system have myriad presentations that cover the breadth of neurology (Table 97-2). Awareness of the presentation of these infections is essential because many parasitic infections respond promptly to early appropriate treatment; without treatment, they can result in lasting neurologic deficits or death.

REFERENCES

1. Cox F. History of human parasitology. *Clin Microbiol Rev.* 2002;15(4):595–612.
2. Sutherst R. Global change and human vulnerability to vector-borne disease. *Clin Microbiol Rev.* 2004;17(1):136–173.
3. Garcia H, Gonzalez A, Evans A, et al. *Taenia solium* cysticercosis. *Lancet.* 2003;361:547–556.
4. Del Brutto O. Neurocysticercosis. *Semin Neurol.* 2005;25(3):243–251.
5. Garcia H, Del Brutto O. Neurocysticercosis: Updated concepts about an old disease. *Lancet Neurol.* 2005;4:653–661.
6. Hawk M, Shahlaie K, Kim K, et al. Neurocysticercosis: A review. *Surg Neurol.* 2005;63:123–132.
7. Garcia H, Gilman R, Horton J, et al. Albendazole therapy for neurocysticercosis: A prospective double-blind trial comparing 7 versus 14 days of treatment. Cysticercosis Working Group in Peru. *Neurology.* 1997;48(5):1421–1427.
8. Montoya J, Liesenfeld O. Toxoplasmosis. *Lancet.* 2004;363:1965–1976.
9. Bhopale G. Pathogenesis of toxoplasmosis. *Comp Immunol Microbiol Infect Dis.* 2003;26:213–222.
10. Rorman E, Zamir C, Rilkis I, et al. Congenital toxoplasmosis—Prenatal aspects of *Toxoplasma gondii* infection. *Reprod Toxicol.* 2006;21:458–472.
11. Chang K, Han M. MRI of CNS parasitic disease. *J Magn Reson Imaging.* 1998;8:297–307.
12. Ross A, Bartley P, Sleigh A, et al. Schistosomiasis. *N Engl J Med.* 2002;346(16):1212–1220.
13. Ferrari T. Involvement of central nervous system in the schistosomiasis. *Mem Inst Oswaldo Cruz.* 2004;99[Suppl 1]:59–62.
14. Nascimento-Carvalho C, Moreno-Carvalho O. Neuroschistosomiasis due to *Schistosoma mansoni*: A review of pathogenesis, clinical syndromes, and diagnostic approaches. *Rev Inst Med Trop S. Paulo.* 2005;47(4):179–184.
15. Ferrari T. Spinal cord schistosomiasis. A report of 2 cases and review emphasizing clinical aspects. *Medicine (Baltimore).* 1999;78(3):176–190.
16. Doenhoff M, Chiodini P, Hamilton J. Specific and sensitive diagnosis of schistome infection: Can it be done with antibodies? *Trends Parasitol.* 2004;20(1):35–39.

CHAPTER **98**

Syphilis

Joseph R. Berger • Stephen Raffanti

OBJECTIVES

- To describe the clinical stages of syphilis
- To discuss the signs and symptoms of neurosyphilis
- To discuss the laboratory evaluation of neurosyphilis
- To describe treatment guidelines for neurosyphilis
- To explore challenges of the patient infected with both human immunodeficiency virus (HIV) and neurosyphilis

CASE VIGNETTE

A 22-year-old bisexual man presented with a generalized seizure in August 1990. His examination was normal. A computed tomographic (CT) scan of the brain demonstrated a contrast-enhancing right parietal lesion. A cranial magnetic resonance image (MRI) showed slight edema surrounding a right parietal lesion with gadolinium enhancement of the lesion and adjacent meninges. HIV serology was positive and his CD4 lymphocyte count was 227. Toxoplasmosis serology was negative. Cerebrospinal fluid analysis showed 14 white blood cells (98% lymphocytes), protein of 71 mg/dL, and glucose of 67 mg/dL. A brain biopsy showed an inflammatory infiltrate and perivascular lymphocytes and plasma cells. He was treated with phenytoin for his seizures. Although histopathologic study of the biopsy tissue revealed no evidence of toxoplasmosis tachyzoites, sulfadiazine and pyrimethamine were initiated for suspected toxoplasmosis. Zidovudine, the only antiretroviral medication then available, was also initiated for his HIV infection.

At age 18 during routine screening at the time of blood donation, he was found to be HIV seropositive. He sought no medical treatment at that time. In February 1990, he was demonstrated to have a positive VDRL test. He was treated with weekly intramuscular benzathine penicillin (2.4 million units) for 3 weeks.

After 14 days of sulfadiazine and pyrimethamine, no improvement in the mass lesion was seen. In September, he returned to the clinic because of headache, recurrent seizures, and onset of left hemisensory loss. A repeat MRI showed that the right parietal lesion was larger and exhibited a greater degree of perilesional edema. A positron emission tomographic (PET) scan revealed that the lesion was hypometabolic. A repeat biopsy showed polyclonal T cells, excluding the possibility of primary central nervous system (CNS) lymphoma. Laboratory studies revealed a serum VDRL test of 1:64 and serum fluorescent treponemal antibody (FTA-ABS) test was positive. He was then treated with 10 days of intravenous aqueous penicillin and a short course of dexamethasone. A repeat MRI obtained approximately 1 month after the completion of this regimen showed a near complete resolution of the lesion.

This patient had a syphilitic cerebral gumma that was initially misdiagnosed as CNS toxoplasmosis. At the time of his initially positive syphilis serology, cerebrospinal fluid (CSF) analysis was not performed. The demonstration of abnormalities in the CSF at that time would have suggested the possibility of asymptomatic neurosyphilis and resulted in treatment with high dose (12 to 24 million units) of aqueous penicillin daily administered in divided doses every 4 hours.

DEFINITION

Syphilis is the systemic disease caused by the spirochete *Treponema pallidum.* The clinical manifestations of syphilis are usually defined by the stage of the illness and the likelihood of infectious or long-term sequelae. Clinical and laboratory evaluation is essential for accurate diagnosis. Neurosyphilis is the result of CNS involvement with the disseminated infection. Although usually associated with late stage disease, significant evidence indicates that dissemination occurs early in the infection and CNS involvement can occur at any stage of the illness.

EPIDEMIOLOGY

In the preantibiotic era, the incidence of infectious syphilis in the United States was as high as 66 cases per 100,000 persons. The rates have since declined significantly (3.9 cases per 100,000 persons in 1956) and have fluctuated in approximately 10-year cycles. The more recent epidemics have been related to special populations and illicit drug use, principally the exchange of sex for crack cocaine. In the 1970s, a significant increase in syphilis rates was reported among men who had sex with men. In 1990, the case rate was 20 cases per 100,000 persons, which dropped to 3.2 cases per 100,000 persons in 1997, possibly reflecting increased priority and resources given to syphilis control programs (1,2). Worldwide, it is estimated that 3.5 million new cases of syphilitic infection present per year (2).

Neurosyphilis is common in association with HIV infection. Prevalence rates of CSF VDRL test-reactive neurosyphilis have been reported to be between 1.0% and 2.0% for large cohorts of persons who are HIV-seropositive (3). This prevalence rate is significantly higher if only patients with serologic evidence of syphilis are included. In some HIV-infected populations, the prevalence rate of a reactive serum fluorescent treponemal antibody absorption test approaches 50% (3).

ETIOLOGY AND PATHOGENESIS

The causative organism of syphilis is *T. pallidum* subsp. Pallidum is a spirochete ranging in size from 0.10 to 018 μm in diameter and 6 to 20 μm in length. Organisms are visible using dark field microscopy, which shows a slender, threadlike organism, moving in characteristic undulating motion with an average of 8 to 14 windings. Hours after infection, spirochetemia results in hematogenous dissemination of *T. pallidum* to virtually any organ, including the CNS. Antibodies to *T. pallidum* are detectable within 10 to 21 days of infection. This response is of little consequence in containing the infection, but can alter the course of the disease. Cellular immunity appears to be important in controlling the infections, as evidenced by immunity during rechallenge. The degree of protection is directly proportional to the extent of the response. Impairment of cellular immunity caused by immunosuppressive agents, pregnancy, or HIV infection appears to result in a more aggressive presentation, with higher rates of treatment failure with standard treatment.

Studies of CSF abnormalities occurring in association with early (primary or secondary) syphilis have detected abnormalities in 16% to 48% of cases. These results are suggestive of early invasion of the CNS by the organism. The presence of CSF abnormalities does not necessarily predict the development of neurosyphilis. In the Oslo study, for example, 9.4% of the men and 5.0% of the women ultimately developed neurosyphilis (4).

PATHOLOGY

Neurosyphilis is the consequence of the invasion of the CNS by *T. pallidum* and the associated immunologic response. In syphilitic meningitis, the earliest neurologic complication of syphilis, invasion of the meninges by the spirochete, results in an infiltration of the meninges by lymphocytes and, to a lesser degree, plasma cells. This cellular infiltration may follow blood vessels into the brainstem and spinal cord along the Virchow-Robin spaces. Necrosis of the media and proliferation of the intima of small meningeal vessels accompany *T. pallidum* invasion of the vessel walls.

Late stages of neurosyphilis can be divided into meningovascular and parenchymatous disease. The inflammation observed in the former parallels that observed with syphilitic meningitis. The classic lesion is an endarteritis obliterans of medium and large vessels. Syphilitic lesions of the brain and spinal cord occur as a secondary event. Gummas of various sizes, from microscopic to mass-producing lesions, can be observed. Pathologically, the gummas are thick, tough, rubbery lesions of fibrous trabecula, with lymphocytic and plasma cell infiltration of the outer layers. Treponemes are seldom seen in the gumma.

Parenchymatous neurosyphilis is typified by tabes dorsalis and general paresis. The pathology of tabes dorsalis predominates in the dorsal roots and posterior columns of the lumbosacral and lower thoracic levels, but is not confined to those areas. The predominant findings are believed to result from irreversible changes to the dorsal root fibers, but the exact pathogenesis of this disorder is not known. In general paresis, the meninges may be thickened and, on rare occasion, the brain may appear normal. The architecture of the cerebral cortex is disrupted, and neuronal loss accompanies astrocytic and microglial proliferation. *T. pallidum* can be demonstrated in the cerebral cortex. Ependymal granulations are commonly observed.

CLINICAL MANIFESTATIONS AND SPECIAL SITUATIONS

The clinical stages of syphilis are typically classified as (*a*) primary infection (ulcer or chancre); (*b*) secondary infection (rash, mucocutaneous lesions, lymphadenopathy); and (*c*) tertiary infection (cardiac, ophthalmologic, or auditory manifestations; neuropsychiatric abnormalities; or gummatous lesions). Patients with serologic evidence of syphilis, but no clinical features, have latent infection. Latent syphilis acquired in the preceding year is considered early latent syphilis, whereas all other cases are considered late latent or latent syphilis of unknown duration. The classification of early latent syphilis is based on the likelihood of an infectious mucocutaneous relapse in untreated patients. Approximately 90% of relapses occur in the first year (4).

Although the classification of the stages of syphilis can aid the clinician, this disease can present as unusual and oftentimes confusing clinical scenarios. The primary lesion of syphilis, the chancre, is a painless ulcerated lesion with indurated borders that develops at the site of inoculation. Painless regional adenopathy is seen frequently with genital lesions (5). In most cases, the chancre develops within 3 weeks of exposure. The principal clinical manifestation of primary syphilis is the development of the chancre, but analysis of the CSF from patients with primary and secondary syphilis have demonstrated the presence of spirochetes in 30% of subjects (6). The primary lesion usually resolves over a period of weeks, and is followed by the manifestations of secondary syphilis. Up to one third of patients still have their primary lesion when they develop secondary syphilis, but most patients with secondary syphilis do not recall a primary lesion (7).

Secondary syphilis can be a subtle disease. Almost every descriptive term has been used in reporting the dermatologic manifestations of secondary syphilis. The rash can range from macular, maculopapular, and follicular to pustular. As a rule, the rash is generalized, nonpruritic and heals without scarring. The palms and soles are often involved. Approximately 7% of patients demonstrate *moth-eaten*, patchy alopecia. Genital mucus patch lesions (condyloma lata) are extremely contagious and usually harbor high titers of spirochetes on their surface. Systemic symptoms can also occur in the setting of secondary syphilis. Mild malaise, anorexia, jaundice, fatigue, headache, and low-grade fever can occur. Asymptomatic meningitis can occur in up to 40% of patients. Other neurologic complications of secondary syphilis include ocular disease and cranial nerve palsies. Inflammatory ocular complications of secondary syphilis include episcleritis, scleritis, interstitial keratitis, iridocyclitis, vitreitis, uveitis, and optic nerve involvement. Tinnitus and deafness has been reported 20% of patients with secondary syphilis (8).

Tertiary syphilis is characterized by cardiovascular, osseous, skin, and neurologic complications. Cardiovascular involvement generally occurs 10 to 30 years after infection. Clinically apparent neurologic complications of tertiary syphilis affect fewer than 10% of untreated patients. Neurosyphilis, the occurrence of neurologic complications caused by *T. pallidum* infection, can present during early or late syphilis. The most common form of neurosyphilis currently diagnosed is asymptomatic neurosyphilis. Individuals with this form of neurosyphilis come to medical attention because of serologic evidence of syphilis in the absence of neurologic sequelae. The CSF shows evidence of neurosyphilis; these patients are at risk for developing symptomatic disease. Of the symptomatic disorders of neurosyphilis, the earliest manifestation is *syphilitic meningitis,* which typically occurs within the first 12 months of infection and may accompany features of secondary syphilis. Most patients with CSF abnormalities occurring in association with secondary syphilis are neurologically asymptomatic; 5% of all patients with secondary syphilis will have associated meningitis. Headaches, meningismus, impaired vision, cranial nerve palsies (chiefly, in descending order of frequency, VII, VIII, VI, and II), hearing loss, tinnitus, and vertigo may be observed in isolation or in combination in upward of 40% of patients with secondary syphilis. The symptoms of syphilitic meningitis include headache, photophobia, and a stiff neck. Some encephalopathic features result from vascular compromise or increased intracranial pressure. These include confusion, lethargy, seizures, aphasia, and hemiplegia. Seizures may be the initial manifestation of neurosyphilis. *Meningovascular syphilis* can affect the brain or spinal cord. It typically occurs 6 to 7 years after the initial infection, but can manifest as early as 6 months after the primary infection. Many of the stroke eponyms described at the turn of the last century were the consequence of meningovascular syphilis producing discrete lesions of the brainstem.

Syphilitic meningomyelitis (Table 98-1) is characterized by slowly progressive weakness and paresthesia of the lower extremities. Eventually, bowel and bladder incontinence and paraplegia supervene. Examination demonstrates a spastic paraparesis or paraplegia, with brisk lower extremity reflexes, loss of the superficial abdominal reflexes, and impaired sensory perception, with vibratory and position sense being disproportionately affected. *Syphilitic transverse myelitis* can also be observed, resulting in an acute onset of lower extremity paraplegia and sensory loss. An acute infarction of the anterior spinal artery results in paraplegia and loss of pain and temperature sensation below the level of the lesion, with preservation of vibratory and position sense. The characteristic spinal cord syndrome associated with parenchymatous neurosyphilis is *tabes dorsalis.* This disorder usually has a latency of 15 to 30 years following infection. The most distinctive symptom is shooting or lightninglike pains that typically affect the legs and abdomen. On occasion, these pains have been mistaken for surgical emergencies. Touch of the affected areas may trigger the pain. Pupillary abnormalities are observed in more than 90% of patients; the hallmark abnormality is Argyll Robertson pupils: Miotic, irregular pupils exhibiting light-near dissociation. The gait is ataxic, with an associated foot-stomping character caused by an associated impaired position sense. Romberg test is positive. The impaired sensory perception also leads to the development of Charcot joints, because of repeated trauma to, and ulcers of, the toes and soles of the feet. The impaired sense of deep pain may be demonstrated by its absence on squeezing the testicles (Pitre sign), the ulnar nerves (Biernacki sign), or Achilles tendons (Abadie sign). Impotence and bladder dysfunction are expected. The lower extremity reflexes are absent. Optic atrophy and cranial nerve palsies are frequently observed. Paraparesis may also be seen as a consequence of syphilitic aortic dissection (9).

TABLE 98-1. Syphilis of the Spinal Cord

Syphilitic meningomyelitis
Syphilitic spinal pachymeningitis
Spinal cord gumma
Syphilitic hypertrophic pachymeningitis
Spinal vascular syphilis
Syphilitic poliomyelitis
Tabes dorsalis
Miscellaneous
Syringomyelia
Syphilitic aortic aneurysm with dissection
Charcot vertebra with compression of the spinal cord

General paresis is a manifestation of parenchymatous neurosyphilis and, as with tabes dorsalis, usually develops after a long hiatus (15 to 30 years) from the time of infection. General paresis accounted for a substantial percentage of psychiatric illness in the preantibiotic era. In addition to a progressive dementia, these patients display a wide variety of psychiatric disturbances, including emotional lability, paranoia, illusions, and delusions of grandeur, hallucinations, and inappropriate behavior. Tremors of the tongue, postural tremors of the extremities, hyperreflexia, hypomimetic facies, dysarthria, chorioretinitis, optic neuritis, and pupillary abnormalities, including Argyll Robertson pupils, are seen. MRI of the brain of patients with general paresis has demonstrated frontal and temporal atrophy and increased ferritin in the basal ganglia (10).

Gummas of the nervous system present chiefly as space-occupying lesions. Gummas affecting the brain can result in progressive focal neurologic manifestations, seizures, or increased intracranial pressure. A dural enhancement on MRI similar to that observed with meningiomas may be found with cerebral gummas. Gummas can also affect the spinal cord as well.

Concomitant HIV infection can significantly alter the natural history of neurosyphilis (11). Syphilis appears to be not only more aggressive, but also more difficult to treat when it occurs in association with HIV infection (12). These observations suggest that the host's immune response is critical in controlling this infection. The inability of the patient who is HIV-infected to establish delayed hypersensitivity to *T. pallidum* may prevent secondary syphilis from evolving to latency, or may cause a spontaneous relapse from a latent state. This impairment of delayed hypersensitivity may account for a more rapid progression of neurosyphilis in those infected with HIV than would otherwise be expected. *T. pallidum* can be isolated from the CSF of patients who are HIV-seropositive with primary, secondary, and latent syphilis. (6). Despite the associated immunosuppression, serum nontreponemal titers at the time of presentation of neurosyphilis in those who are HIV-infected are typically high, averaging 1:128 (13). In HIV infection, acute, symptomatic, syphilitic meningitis during the course of secondary syphilis is not uncommon. A decrease in the latent period owing to the development of some neurosyphilitic manifestations has been suggested. The development of meningovascular syphilis within 4 months of primary infection, despite the administration of accepted penicillin regimens, and relapse of neurosyphilis in individuals infected with HIV after appropriate doses of benzathine penicillin (12), have been reported. Although the characteristic ophthalmologic abnormality of syphilis is the Argyll Robertson pupil, other conditions result from *T. pallidum* infection, including interstitial keratitis, chorioretinitis, and optic atrophy. Syphilitic optic atrophy is notoriously difficult to treat effectively, and progression is observed in as many as 50% of patients, despite treatment. Otitic syphilis occurs with hearing loss, either acute or gradual (14). Vertigo can also occur. Syphilitic eighth nerve dysfunction is largely a late manifestation of congenital syphilis, but it is also seen in acquired illness.

DIAGNOSTIC APPROACH

The diagnosis of neurosyphilis relies on clinical assessment and supporting serologic tests. The two categories of serological study are (*a*) nontreponemal tests, which are flocculation tests using cardiolipin, lecithin, and cholesterol as antigen; and (*b*) treponemal tests, which rely on specific treponemal cellular components as antigens. Nontreponemal tests include the VDRL, rapid plasma reagin (RPR), Wasserman, and Kolmer. The treponemal tests include the fluorescent treponemal antibody absorption test, FTA/ABS microhemagglutination assay, hemagglutination treponemal test for syphilis, and the treponemal immobilization test (TPI).

No readily applicable gold standard exists for the diagnosis of neurosyphilis. The presence of a reactive VDRL test in the CSF is specific, with rare reports of false–positive findings, but the test is not sufficiently sensitive to exclude the diagnosis of neurosyphilis on the basis of a negative study. The serum VDRL test is positive in 72% of patients with primary syphilis, nearly 100% of patients with secondary syphilis, 73% of patients with latent syphilis, and 77% of patients with tertiary syphilis. Therefore, approximately 25% of patients with neurosyphilis are anticipated to have a negative serum VDRL test finding. Its frequency of reactivity appears to vary with the clinical form of neurosyphilis and its presence in asymptomatic neurosyphilis may be substantially lower than in symptomatic disease. The CSF VDRL test is too insensitive to be relied on to exclude the diagnosis of neurosyphilis. CSF cultured in rabbit testicles had *T. pallidum* isolated from the CSF of 12 of 40 (30%) patients with primary and secondary syphilis, but the CSF VDRL test proved positive in only 4 (33%) of these 12 patients (6). Therefore, measures other than a reactive CSF VDRL test must be relied on to establish the diagnosis of neurosyphilis. The frequency with which the CSF VDRL test finding is negative in the presence of neurosyphilis is not known, but has been estimated to exceed 25%. In many respects, neurosyphilis is a diagnosis established on clinical grounds. To date, no consensus exists regarding diagnostic criteria and the physician should probably refrain from rigid adherence to narrow guidelines in making the diagnosis.

A cardinal requirement for the diagnosis of neurosyphilis is a reactive serum treponemal test. Neurosyphilis should be diagnosed in anyone with serologies reactive for a treponemal test occurring in association with a reactive CSF VDRL test finding. A diagnosis of neurosyphilis should be considered in patients with serologic evidence of syphilis and one or more of the following abnormalities in their CSF: A mononuclear pleocytosis, an elevated protein, increased immunoglobulin G, or the presence of oligoclonal bands. Undoubtedly, neurosyphilis is over diagnosed using these criteria. Newer generation tests for syphilis and neurosyphilis, in particular those using the polymerase chain reaction (PCR) (15) and monoclonal antibodies (16), are more sensitive, but require further study before widespread adoption. An alternative approach that has been proposed for patients infected with HIV who are suspected of having neurosyphilis despite negative CSF VDRL findings is to couple the CSF FTA, which is 100% sensitive, with the percentage of CSF cells that are B lymphocytes (≥9% in fresh specimens) (17).

Coinfection with HIV considerably complicates the interpretation of CSF abnormalities because a mononuclear pleocytosis, increased protein, increased immunoglobulin G, and the presence of oligoclonal bands may all be found with HIV infection in the absence of neurosyphilis (18). A schema has been proposed for the diagnosis of neurosyphilis in the presence of HIV infection (Table 98-2).

Although not diagnostic of neurosyphilis, radiologic studies may be suggestive and are certainly helpful in excluding other pathologies. Radiologic manifestations of neurosyphilis include meningeal enhancement, CSF enhancement (19), hydrocephalus, gummas, periostitis, generalized cerebral atrophy, and stroke. Gummas appear as avascular, dural-based masses with surrounding edema that on MRI are characteristically isointense with gray matter on T1-weighted image and hyperintense on T2-weighted image. Dense contrast enhancement is usually observed. Orbital periostitis typically involves the roof and supraorbital rim. These lesions may be hyperplastic, resulting in tender osteophytic nodules and exostoses (20). The periorbital inflammation can infiltrate the extraocular muscles and cranial nerves (21). MRI may also demonstrate multiple, bilateral, discrete white matter lesions involving deep periventricu-

TABLE 98-2. Diagnosing Neurosyphilis in the Presence of Human Immunodeficiency Virus (HIV) Infection

DEFINITE NEUROSYPHILIS

1. + blood treponemal serology (e.g., FTA-ABS, MHA-TP), and so on
2. + CSF VDRL

PROBABLE NEUROSYPHILIS

1. + blood treponemal serology
2. − CSF VDRL
3. CSF mononuclear pleocytosis (>20 cells/mm^3)
   Or + CSF protein (>60 mg/dL)
   Neurologic complications compatible with neurosyphilis, such as cranial nerve palsies, stroke, and so on, or evidence of ophthalmologic syphilis

POSSIBLE NEUROSYPHILIS

1. + blood treponemal serology
2. − CSF VDRL
3. CSF mononuclear pleocytosis (>20 cells/mm^3)
   Or + CSF protein (>60 mg/dL)
   No neurologic or ophthalmologic complications compatible with syphilis

FTA-ABS, fluorescent treponemal antibody; MHA-TP, microhemagglutination assay; CSF, cerebrospinal fluid.

lar and subcortical regions (20). Large vessels may exhibit segmental constriction or occlusion (20). Smaller vessels, usually Sylvian branches of the middle cerebral artery, may display focal stenoses with or without adjacent dilatation (20), which suggests that neurosyphilis must be excluded in any person suspected of having limbic encephalitis.

In a review of 35 patients with documented neurosyphilis (3 HIV-seronegative and 32 HIV-seropositive), Brightbill et al. (22) found that 31% had normal brain imaging, 23% had cerebral infarction, and 20% had nonspecific cerebral white matter lesions. Cerebral gummas and extraaxial enhancement indicating meningitis were each noted in 2 of 35 (6%) patients and arteritis was demonstrated in 2 of 4 (50%) having either magnetic resonance angiography or conventional cerebral angiography (22).

TREATMENT

The Centers for Disease Control and Prevention (CDC) has recently released updated guidelines on the treatment of sexually transmitted diseases (23). Penicillin G, administered parenterally, is still the treatment of choice for all stages of syphilis. The preparations used, dosage, and length of treatment depend on disease stage. Combinations of benzathine and procaine penicillin or forms of oral penicillin are not appropriate for the treatment of syphilis. Benzathine penicillin G (2.4 million units) given intramuscularly in a single dose, is the recommended treatment regimen in adult patients with primary, secondary, or early latent syphilis. The recommended treatment regimen for adult patients with late latent syphilis or latent syphilis of unknown duration is benzathine penicillin G (7.2 million units) total, administered intramuscularly as three doses (2.4 million units) each at 1-week intervals. Treatment recommendations are the same regardless of HIV status, although some clinicians recommend additional treatment of patients who are HIV-infected with early syphilis to include a total of 7.2 million units of benzathine penicillin G. No controlled trials, however, have demonstrated improved treatment response with this approach.

CNS involvement can occur during any stage of syphilis, and treatment of neurosyphilis is indicated for any patient with evidence of neurologic involvement. The recommended regimen for neurosyphilis is aqueous crystalline penicillin G (18 to 24 million units) a day, administered intravenously (3 to 4 million units) every 4 hours or by continuous infusion, for 10 to 14 days. An alternative regimen is procaine penicillin (2.4 million units) given intramuscularly once daily plus oral probenecid (500 mg) four times daily, for 10 to 14 days.

Patients with penicillin allergies should be offered alternative regimens, keeping in mind that fewer data exist to support efficacy. Doxycycline and tetracycline-based regimens have been used for years and limited data suggest efficacy. More recently ceftriaxone-based regimens have been used in penicillin-allergic patients with early syphilis. Azithromycin has been associated with resistance and treatment failures. Patients with neurosyphilis and penicillin allergies should be desensitized and treated with penicillin as described above.

Although treatment failure can occur with any regimen, assessing response to therapy can be difficult. Nontreponemal test titers should decline after effective treatment. In primary, secondary, and early latent syphilis, patients should be reexamined clinically and serologically 6 and 12 months following treatment. Patients who have persistent signs or symptoms or fail to have a fourfold decrease in the nontreponemal test titer at 12 months (24 months for late latent syphilis or latent syphilis of unknown duration) have probably failed treatment and should be reevaluated and retreated. Patients treated for neurosyphilis should have follow-up clinical, serologic, and CSF evaluation. If CSF pleocytosis was present initially, CSF examination should be repeated every 6 months until normal. If the cell count has not decreased after 6 months, or the CSF is not normal after 2 years, retreatment should be considered. Patients with a history of syphilis and those who are HIV-infected may have a slower serologic and CSF response. Decisions regarding retreatment in these individuals should be based on clinical and serologic findings, as well as the likelihood of reinfection.

CLINICAL RECOMMENDATIONS OF THE VIGNETTE

Although the adoption of safer sexual practices as a consequence of the acquired immunodeficiency syndrome (AIDS) pandemic has been associated with a decline in the incidence of syphilis in some populations, a high index of suspicion for the disease should be maintained. Serologic testing with nonspecific antibodies (e.g., VDRL and RPR) may fail to identify individuals with neurosyphilis and specific antibody tests should be performed, coupled with an analysis of the CSF in individuals in whom neurosyphilis is in the differential diagnosis. Neurosyphilis can present in unexpected fashions, such as CNS mass lesions (as in the Case Vignette), cranial neuropathies, or myelopathy, to name a few. These are treatable and potentially reversible disorders; therefore, it is incumbent on the physician to think of, and establish, the diagnosis.

SUMMARY

Five hundred years after it was first described, syphilis still presents significant clinical challenges. No single laboratory test can be used to diagnose neurosyphilis. The diagnosis of neurosyphilis depends on the careful review of clinical, serum, and CSF findings. The physician must have a high level of suspicion for neurosyphilis in the patient with treponemal-specific serologic evidence of infection with *T. pallidum* and neurologic or psychiatric abnormalities. Evaluation should include CSF analysis with the goal of administering high dose penicillin therapy in patients with a reasonable likelihood of neurosyphilis. Follow up should be scheduled for regular clinical, serologic and CSF evaluation. All patients with positive serology for syphilis should be screened for HIV infection.

REFERENCES

1. Nakashima AK, Rolfs RT, Flock ML, et al. Epidemiology of syphilis in the United States, 1941–1993. *Sex Transm Dis.* 1996;23:16–23.
2. WHO Office of Information. Sexually transmitted infections increasing—250 million new infections annually. WHO Feature 1990;152:1–6.
3. Berger JR. Neurosyphilis in human immunodeficiency virus type 1-seropositive individuals. A prospective study. *Arch Neurol.* 1991;48:700–702.
4. Gjestland T. The Oslo study of untreated syphilis: An epidemiologic investigation of the natural course of syphilis infection based upon a restudy of the Boeck-Bruusgaard material. *Acta Derm Venereol.* 1955;35[Suppl 34]:1–368.
5. DiCarlo RP, Martin DH. The clinical diagnosis of genital ulcer diseases in men. *Clin Infect Dis.* 1997;25:292–298.
6. Lukehart SA, Hook EW, 3d, Baker-Zander SA, et al. Invasion of the central nervous system by *Treponema pallidum:* Implications for diagnosis and treatment. *Ann Intern Med.* 1988;109: 855–862.
7. Chapel TA. The signs and symptoms of secondary syphilis. *Sex Transm Dis.* 1980;7:161–164.

8. Morrison A. On syphilis and the ear—An otologist's view. *Genitourinary Medicine.* 1992;68: 420–422.
9. Kellett MW, Young GR, Fletcher NA. Paraparesis due to syphilitic aortic dissection. *Neurology.* 1997;48:221–223.
10. Zifko U, Wimberger D, Linner K, et al. MRI in patients with general paresis. *Neuroradiology.* 1996;38:120–123.
11. Katz DA, Berger JR. Neurosyphilis in acquired immunodeficiency syndrome. *Arch Neurol.* 1989;46:895–898.
12. Berry CD, Hooten TM, Collier AC, et al. Neurologic relapse after benzathine penicillin therapy for secondary syphilis in a patient with HIV infection. *N Engl J Med.* 1987;316:1587–1589.
13. Flood JM, Weinstock HS, Guroy ME, et al. Neurosyphilis during the AIDS epidemic: San Francisco, 1985–1992. *J Infect Dis.* 1998;177:931–940.
14. Darmstadt GL, Harris JP. Luetic hearing loss: Clinical presentation, diagnosis, and treatment. *Am J Otolaryngol.* 1989;10:410–421.
15. Hay PE, Clarke JR, Taylor-Robinson D, et al. Detection of treponemal DNA in the CSF of patients with syphilis and HIV infection using the polymerase chain reaction. Genitourinary Medicine. 1990;66:428–432.
16. Whang KK, Lee MG, Lee W, et al. Production and characterization of monoclonal antibodies to Treponema pallidum. *J Dermatol Sci.* 1992;4:26–32.
17. Marra CM, Tantalo LC, Maxwell CL, et al. Alternative cerebrospinal fluid tests to diagnose neurosyphilis in HIV-infected individuals. *Neurology.* 2004;63:85–88.
18. Hollander H. Cerebrospinal fluid normalities and abnormalities in individuals infected with human immunodeficiency virus. *J Infect Dis.* 1988;158:855–858.
19. Good CD, Jager HR. Contrast enhancement of the cerebrospinal fluid on MRI in two cases of spirochaetal meningitis. *Neuroradiology.* 2000;42:448–450.
20. Harris DE, Enterline DS, Tien RD. Neurosyphilis in patients with AIDS. *Neuroimaging Clin N Am.* 1997;7(2):215–221.
21. Smith JL, Byrne SF, Cambron CR. Syphiloma/gumma of the optic nerve and human immunodeficiency virus seropositivity. *J Clin Neuroophthalmol.* 1990;10:175–184.
22. Brightbill TC, Ihmedian IH, Post MJ, et al. Neurosyphilis in HIV-positive and HIV-negative patients: Neuroimaging findings. *AJNR Am J Neuroradiol.* 1995;16:703–711.
23. Centers for Disease Control. Sexually Transmitted Diseases Treatment Guidelines, 2006. *MMWR Morb Mortal Wkly Rep.* 2006;55/RR-11:1–94.

CHAPTER **99**

Lyme Disease

A. Arturo Leis • Stanley W. Chapman

OBJECTIVES

- To describe the ecology and epidemiology of Lyme disease in the United States and Europe
- To explain the pathogenesis and clinical manifestations of Lyme disease, especially neuroborreliosis
- To review the clinical and serologic diagnosis of Lyme disease
- To describe the current treatment recommendations for the different clinical manifestations of Lyme disease

CASE VIGNETTE

A 27-year-old woman had experienced intermittent headache, low-grade fever, slight neck pain, and nausea for the past 2 weeks. She then developed difficulty in blinking of the right eye that progressed to inability to close the eye, drooling after drinking or brushing her teeth, and inability to whistle. She also noticed a loss of facial movement and "deadness" in the right side of her face although the affected part was neither numb nor tingling. Two days later, she developed similar symptoms of slightly lesser severity in the left side of her face accompanied by an alteration of taste and sensitivity to sounds (hyperacusis). One week later she noticed numbness in the perineal region and slight difficulty in urinating. In addition, she had ill-defined midback pain accompanied by increasing abdominal distention that was particularly evident in the lower abdomen on straining. She denied other symptoms, although she recalled that she had a red rash in the left axilla that she attributed to "heat rash." The rash persisted for several weeks and had only recently resolved.

Neurologic examination revealed slight nuchal rigidity, bilateral peripheral seventh nerve palsies, bilateral lower abdominal wall weakness, and slightly decreased sensation in the perineum, although anal reflexes remained normal. Examination of cerebrospinal fluid (CSF) showed lymphocytic pleocytosis and an increase in total protein. Electrophysiologic studies demonstrated denervation of the lower thoracic and upper lumbar paraspinal muscles and the internal oblique and transversus abdominis muscles.

Antibodies against *Borrelia burgdorferi* were present in both the serum and the CSF, and the patient was diagnosed with neuroborreliosis associated with early disseminated Lyme disease. Her symptoms were alleviated by administration of ceftriaxone (2 g/day) for 15 days.

DEFINITION

Lyme disease, the most common tick-borne illness in the United States and Europe, clinically presents with dermatologic, neurologic, rheumatologic, and cardiac manifestations (collectively known as borreliosis) (1,2). The clinical manifestations of Lyme disease can be generally divided into three stages: *Early localized, early disseminated,* and *late disease.* Lyme disease is caused by the spirochetes of the *Borrelia burgdorferi sensu lato complex,* which has been shown to be composed of at least 12 genospecies and genomic groups (3,4).

Evidence is slowly accumulating to suggest that Lyme disease may be a more complex condition than borreliosis alone (5,6). The same tick species that transmits *B. burgdorferi* may also be infected with, and transmit, *Anaplasma phagocytophilum* (previously referred to as *Ehrlichia phagocytophila*) and *Babesia microti.* Hence, coinfection with ehrlichiosis or babesiosis may contribute to the clinical syndrome of Lyme disease (5,6). Additionally, coinfection may also explain clinical treatment failures during the early stages of disease.

ETIOLOGY

Borrelia burgdorferi sensu lato, the spirochetes that cause human Lyme borreliosis, is a genetically and phenotypically divergent species. In the past several years, various molecular approaches have been developed and used to determine the phenotypic and genetic heterogeneity within the spirochetes and their potential association with distinct clinical syndromes (4). On the basis of these molecular studies, *B. burgdorferi sensu lato* includes at least 12 genospecies and genomic groups (3,4). Only three species are known to cause human disease (3,4). *B. burgdorferi (sensu stricto)* is the only causative organism of Lyme disease in the United States. In Europe and Asia, *B. afzelii, B. garinii,* and *B. burgdorferi* are the most common causes of Lyme disease (1,4). Genetic variability within Borrelia species is believed to have a considerable impact on the epidemiology, pathogenicity, and clinical picture of Lyme borreliosis (3).

ECOLOGY AND EPIDEMIOLOGY

Borrelia species are maintained in nature by complex zoonotic transmission cycles involving a large variety of vertebrates as hosts and hard ticks of the genus Ixodes as vectors (1,7). Occasionally, infected ticks feed on humans and transmit Lyme disease, but human infection is not relevant to the transmission cycle. More than 300 animal species have been reported as natural hosts for Ixodes and in excess of 50 vertebrate species have been identified as reservoir hosts for *B. burgdorferi* (8), including migratory birds, squirrels, rodents, other small mammals, and deer.

B. burgdorferi spirochetes persist for many months in a latent state in midguts of infected ticks. After a tick attaches to a mammalian host and ingests a blood meal, spirochetes multiply and gradually move to the salivary glands. In animal experiments, almost invariably a delay of at least 36 hours occurs between the time of tick attachment and transmission of *B. burgdorferi* in the tick saliva (9,10). The spirochete then remains in the mammalian skin for several days before dissemination via the bloodstream. Spirochetes persist in low numbers in infected mammals, yet are efficiently acquired by feeding ticks following attachment.

In the eastern United States, Lyme disease is transmitted primarily by the hard-shelled deer ticks *Ixodes dammini* or *I. scapularis* and in the western United States by *I. pacificus* (11). In Europe, *I. ricinus* is the most common tick vector (12,13). Lyme disease is most prevalent in the American Northeast (Connecticut, Maryland, Massachusetts, New Jersey, New York, Pennsylvania, and Rhode Island), where it is endemic; in the upper Midwest (Minnesota and Wisconsin); and in the Northwest (California) (9). Human cases of Lyme disease have been reported from most states in the United States, however. In Europe, *Lyme borreliosis* is most frequent in central Europe and Scandinavia (up to 155 cases per 100,000 individuals) (1). Most cases of Lyme disease occur during the summer months, from late spring to early fall. Genetic variability within and between each Borrelia species has a considerable impact on epidemiology and transmission mechanisms. Different genospecies of *B. burgdorferi sensu lato* can be maintained in nature by distinct transmission cycles involving the same vector tick species, but different vertebrate host species (10). Moreover, the distribution of distinct genospecies varies with the different geographic area and over time (3). The present knowledge of ecology and epidemiology of *B. burgdorferi sensu lato* is incomplete and further information on the distribution of different *Borrelia* species and subspecies in their natural reservoir hosts and vectors is needed. In view of the great number of potentially effective reservoirs for *B. burgdorferi sensu lato,* control of Lyme disease by reduction in numbers of reservoir hosts will be difficult to achieve.

PATHOGENESIS AND PATHOLOGY

The pathogenesis of Borrelia diseases is not fully understood. Rates of infection and the clinical manifestations and severity of disease, however, are most likely related to a complex interaction of the different species, inoculum in size at time of infection, and the immunogenetic background of the human host. *B. burgdorferi* spirochetes, as with many other pathogens, have evolved complex mechanisms for evading the immune response, including antigenic variation in which genetic or epigenetic changes result in rapid, sequential shifts in a surface-exposed antigen (14). Lyme disease Borrelia are known to possess the VIsE antigenic variation system (15), in which segmental recombination results in the establishment of a large repertoire of variants in the surface lipoproteins. The degree of variation is so high that mammals could harbor thousands of different variants at any one time, resulting in altered surface epitopes. Efforts by the immune system to keep up with the sequence variation are thus confounded (14,15). Changes in cell surface antigens may help to explain why Lyme disease can have different manifestations at different times, and why recurrences and late sequelae can appear for many years. In addition, evidence exists for differential gene expression by Borrelia in the tick vector as opposed to the mammalian host, which represent two very different environments. Stage-specific protein expression can also contribute to pathogenesis. During tick feeding, Lyme disease Borrelia proteins may be induced that are vital to the transmission of *B. burgdorferi* from tick to mammal (16).

Other than peripheral nerves, *B. burgdorferi* has been visualized in biopsy specimens of skin and other affected organs. Local tissue injury by *B. burgdorferi* results in the clinical manifestations of disease. Additionally, *B. burgdorferi* has significant modulating affects on local and systemic immunity of the host, which further affects the inflammatory changes seen in Lyme disease (17). For example, the persistence or recurrence of arthritis after appropriate therapy is thought to be immunologically mediated.

CLINICAL MANIFESTATIONS AND SPECIAL SITUATIONS

The clinical manifestations of Lyme disease are divided into three phases: Early localized, early disseminated, and late disease (Table 99-1). Early localized disease, which occurs a few days to a month after infection, is associated with the characteristic skin rash called *erythema migrans* (6). Early disseminated disease occurs weeks to months after infection. Multiple organs may be involved, including the skin with multiple erythema migrans lesions, the heart, the brain, and peripheral nerves. Late Lyme disease, which develops months to years after infection, most commonly presents with arthritis (acute or chronic), skin lesions, and neurologic symptoms. Clinical features of each of these stages may overlap and some patients may present with later stages of disease absent a history suggestive of earlier phases of Lyme disease.

TABLE 99-1. Clinical Stages of Lyme Disease

Early Localized Disease: A few days to 1 month after tick bite
- Erythema migrans
- Other signs and symptoms: Fatigue, malaise, myalgias, arthralgias, lymphadenopathy

Early Disseminated Disease: Days to 1 year after tick bite
- Neurologic disease: Meningitis, encephalitis, cranial neuropathy, peripheral neuropathy, and myelitis
- Carditis: Conduction abnormalities, cardiomyopathy, and myocarditis
- Musculoskeletal disease: Migratory polyarthritis or arthralgias
- Skin disease: Multiple erythema migrans lesions
- Less common manifestations: Lymphadenopathy, hepatic and ocular disease

Late Disease: Months to years after tick bite
- Musculoskeletal: Migratory polyarthritis and chronic monoarticular arthritis
- Neurologic disease: Chronic encephalopathy, peripheral neuropathy
- Cutaneous: Acrodermatitis chronica atrophicans

Early localized disease typically presents with skin lesions of erythema migrans, which are pathognomonic of Lyme disease.* This sign is the only one that enables a reliable clinical diagnosis in everyday medical practice (2), but the rash is present in only about 40% to 80% of patients with confirmed borreliosis (17). The rash usually appears as a solid red, expanding lesion, which can be round or oval, and flat or slightly raised. It can also appear as a central spot surrounded by clear skin that, in turn, is ringed by an expanding red rash (a *bull's-eye* or *targetlike* appearance). The erythema migrans lesion usually develops 1 to 2 weeks after tick detachment and is typically 5 cm or more in diameter. It is the primary or solitary skin lesion in most patients having Lyme disease in the United States, with the remaining patients having multiple skin lesions that arise following hematogenous dissemination from the primary site (6). The erythema migrans lesion often appears on the axilla, groin, popliteal fossa, back, or nape of the neck, where attached ticks are likely to go unrecognized. This distribution may aid in the diagnosis of Lyme disease, because these locations are unusual for community-acquired cellulitis or other solitary rashes (6). Erythema migrans is usually not painful or pruritic. In contrast to the erythema migrans lesion, there may be an initial immediate hypersensitivity reaction to tick saliva, which results in a small rash that should not be mistaken for erythema migrans. Most patients with erythema migrans have symptoms resembling an acute viral infection, including fatigue, arthralgias, headache, and neck pain, with or without fever (6).

Other skin manifestations of Lyme disease include *B. lymphocytoma* (formerly designated lymphadenosis benigna cutis) and acrodermatitis chronica atrophicans (18,19). These cutaneous manifestations, however, are rarely seen in the United States, because of a firm association with *B. Afzelii* infection, which does not occur in North America (2). Borrelial lymphocytoma is a solitary bluish-red swelling with a usual diameter of a few centimeters, consisting of a dense lymphocytic infiltration of cutis and subcutis (18,19). Acrodermatitis chronica atrophicans is a relatively frequent chronic skin manifestation of Lyme borreliosis, typically occurring years after the acute infection (18). This is in contrast to erythema migrans and borrelial lymphocytoma, which occur in early Lyme disease.

Neuroborreliosis, or nervous system involvement, is a frequent manifestation of disseminated Lyme disease that can occur at any time during the course of this disease. Signs and symptoms of neuroborreliosis sometimes develop in a characteristic sequence: Tick bite followed by erythema migrans, features of aseptic meningitis or radiculitis, and finally other focal neurologic symptoms (20,21).

The neurologic manifestations of Lyme disease can be protean, however, leading to erroneous diagnoses and diagnostic wanderings. In one series of 330 patients with neuroborreliosis, the most common symptom occurring within 6 months of illness was painful spinal meningoradiculitis alone (37%) or combined with cranial nerve involvement (29%) (21). Other signs and symptoms of this early stage of neuroborreliosis included isolated meningitis, meningoencephalitis, meningomyelitis, and erythema migrans associated mono- or polyneuropathy. In fewer than 9% of the patients, did the disease run a chronic course, with disease duration of between 6 months and 9 years, manifesting as chronic progressive encephalomyelitis or acrodermatitis chronica atrophicans associated mono- or polyneuropathy. Cerebrovascular neuroborreliosis was rare (1%), occurring during early or later stages, and was characterized by recurrent transient ischemic attacks (TIA) or strokes (21).

In another series, the most common chronic neurologic manifestation of Lyme disease was a mild encephalopathy that began 1 month to 14 years after the onset of the disease and was characterized by memory loss, mood changes, or sleep disturbance (22). The second most common chronic neurologic manifestation was axonal polyneuropathy with distal paresthesias or radicular pain (22). Rarely, leukoencephalitis with periventricular white-matter lesions occurred (22). The myelitis in chronic Lyme disease can be associated with spasticity, ataxic gait, and bladder dysfunction. Most of these patients, however, also have additional signs of encephalitis or cranial nerve palsies (20).

Other central nervous system (CNS) manifestations of neuroborreliosis include various ophthalmic and ocular manifestations (23); opsoclonus-myoclonus syndrome (24); focal or secondarily generalized seizures (25,26); hemiparesis (27), aphasia (28), cerebellitis, and cerebellar signs (29); movement disorders, including parkinsonism (30); chorea (31); dyskinesias (31); and dystonia (21). As many as 10% of European patients develop features of disseminated encephalomyelitis that can resemble those seen in multiple sclerosis (2).

Other investigators have also found that early neuroborreliosis typically manifests with involvement of cranial and peripheral nerves (2,32). In fact, the combination of lymphocytic meningitis, polyradiculoneuritis, and cranial nerve palsies is known as *Bannwarth syndrome* or *Garin-Bujadoux-Bannwarth syndrome*, in honor of Garin and Bujadoux, French physicians who in 1922 postulated a spirochetal infection invoking the typical dermatologic and neurologic manifestations (33), and Bannwarth, who in 1941 described several cases of chronic lymphocytic meningopolyneuritis and erythematous skin lesions (34). Pain is the most pronounced clinical symptom of radiculoneuritis, with or without accompanying motor or reflex changes (35). The pain can be severe; it is often in the thoracic or abdominal region and more pronounced during the night (2). In Europe, Bannwarth syndrome represents the most common manifestation of acute neuroborreliosis (20), with radicular symptoms occurring about twice as often as cranial neuropathies, whereas this ratio is reversed in the United States (35). Although this difference may reflect biologic differences between European and American Borrelia strains, it may also represent under diagnosis of this syndrome in the United States (35).

Any cranial nerve can be affected in early neuroborreliosis, but facial nerves, by far, are the most frequently involved, with bilateral peripheral facial palsies occurring in up to 50% of the cases (36). Prognosis of borrelial peripheral facial palsy is usually regarded as favorable. In one series of 124 such palsies in 101 patients seen between 1975 and 1984, the spontaneous recovery

*Beginning in the 1980s, a new illness characterized by an erythema migrans rash and flulike symptoms was reported in the southeastern United States after tick bite by the lone star tick (*Amblyomma americanum*). Serologic tests in these patients were not diagnostic of infection *B. burgdorferi*. This clinical syndrome has been given a variety of names, but is most often referred to as *Southern Tick-Associated Rash Illness* (STARI). The causative agent of STARI is thought to be *B. lonestari*. At present, many questions remain unanswered in regard to etiology, epidemiology, clinical spectrum, treatment, and prognosis of STARI. For further discussion, see Sexton, DJ. Southern Tick-Associated Rash Illness (STARI) Up-To-Date 2006. http://www.cdc.gov/ncidod/dvbid/stari/index.htm

rate was 99.2% (36). A more recent controlled, prospective study using neurophysiologic and standardized clinical tests, however, revealed signs of persistent slight-to-moderate facial motor dysfunction in about half of 24 patients examined 3 to 5 years after the facial palsy (37). Permanent facial weakness and hemifacial spasm have been reported in up to 5% of patients (20). In approximately 15 to 20% of patients with cranial neuropathies, multiple cranial nerves are involved (35).

Other peripheral manifestations of neuroborreliosis include brachial and lumbosacral plexopathies; isolated mononeuropathies, including carpal tunnel syndrome and other entrapment neuropathies; and mononeuropathy multiplex with involvement of varying numbers of peripheral nerves (35). A diffuse polyneuropathy can also occur, which occasionally mimics Guillain-Barré syndrome (35,38). In most cases, however, electrodiagnostic findings suggest an axonal loss process rather than a demyelinating neuropathy (35,39). Motor nerves can also be involved, leading to asymmetric paresis (2). Acute Lyme neuropathy can also present with abdominal protrusion or increasing abdominal girth associated with denervation of thoracic paraspinal muscles and abdominal muscles (40,41).

In children with North American Lyme disease, the most frequent neurologic symptom was headache, and the most common sign was facial palsy (42). Less common manifestations were sleep disturbance and papilledema associated with increased intracranial pressure. Signs and symptoms of peripheral nervous system involvement were infrequent (42). The most common clinical syndromes were mild encephalopathy, lymphocytic meningitis, and cranial neuropathy. In contrast to adult patients with neurologic Lyme disease, meningoradiculitis (Bannwarth syndrome) and peripheral neuropathy syndromes were rare (42). A "pseudotumor cerebrilike" syndrome appears to be unique to North American pediatric Lyme disease (42).

Articular manifestations, after neuroborreliosis, are the most frequent extracutaneous manifestations of Lyme disease (43,44). *B. burgdorferi* is the most frequently identified of the pathogenic species during Lyme arthritis (44). Brief attacks of arthritis or arthralgias may develop in the early disease stage, but typical Lyme arthritis manifests weeks to months after the infection as intermittent mono- or oligoarthritis (43). The arthritis affects predominantly the large joints, especially the knees. The diagnosis of Lyme arthritis is based mainly on clinical grounds and confirmed by laboratory tests. A small percentage of patients may develop chronic arthritides.

Cardiac manifestations of Lyme disease can occur in up to 8% of patients (45). Cardiac complications usually occur in the early phase of the disease, a median of 21 days from the onset of erythema migrans (45). Signs of borrelial heart involvement include atrioventricular block, myocarditis, pericarditis, intraventricular conduction disturbances, bundle branch block, and congestive heart failure (45). Although the clinical course of Lyme carditis is usually benign and most patients recover completely, temporary cardiac pacing may be required in as many as a third of cases (46). Cardiomyopathy has also been associated with *B. burgdorferi* in Europe, but not in the United States (47). It is highly uncommon to observe respiratory or gastrointestinal symptoms in Lyme disease.

DIAGNOSTIC APPROACH

The diagnosis of Lyme disease is based on the history of travel to, or residence in, a Lyme disease endemic region; the presence of signs and symptoms associated with Lyme disease; and the selective use of laboratory tests. The CDC has published an epidemiologic definition of Lyme disease (48). This strict definition is useful for epidemiologic and clinical research, but was not intended to be used by clinicians for the diagnosis of Lyme disease. Although the presence of these CDC criteria confirms a diagnosis of Lyme disease, reliance on these criteria alone will result in failure to identify many patients with Lyme disease.

The diagnosis of early localized Lyme disease can usually be made on clinical grounds. The characteristic erythema migrans rash, with or without systemic symptoms, is seen in up to 80% of patients during the first month after tick bite and is diagnostic for early localized Lyme disease. History of a tick bite, however, is reported in only 30% of patients diagnosed with Lyme disease. Thus, the absence of a history of tick bite should not be used to rule out this infection. Likewise, serologic tests are usually negative for Lyme-specific antibodies during the early stage of disease. Prompt antibiotic therapy can also reduce antibody response to infection. For this reason, serologic studies are not indicated for the diagnosis of patients presenting with early localized Lyme disease.

Early disseminated disease usually occurs weeks to months after infection. Some patients with disseminated disease, however, may present with no history of Lyme disease. Neurologic or cardiac manifestations are most common in patients with early disseminated Lyme disease. Multiple erythema migrans lesions may also be present. Bannwarth syndrome, a lymphocytic meningitis in association with a facial nerve palsy and other radicular neuropathies, is a classic presentation and is diagnostic of early disseminated infection. Patients with early disseminated disease are usually positive for IgM and possibly IgG Lyme-specific antibodies.

Diagnosis is most complicated in patients who present with signs and symptoms of late disease, with or without a history of Lyme disease or tick bite. Patients with late disease may present with neurologic, cardiac, arthritic, or skin disease (Table 99-1). Serologic tests may be useful in this group of patients in establishing a diagnosis of late Lyme disease. Serologic tests currently used for the diagnosis of Lyme disease include enzyme-linked immunoabsorbent assay (ELISA) and western (immuno) blot assay. The ELISA is the usual first screening test, but it is associated with a high rate of false–positive results, especially in patients with other borrelial diseases, other spirochetal diseases, viral illnesses, and autoimmune disease. It is estimated that 5% of the normal population will have a positive Lyme disease ELISA because of these cross-reacting antibodies. Owing to the high frequency of false–positive results, all positive ELISA tests should be confirmed with a western blot analysis. The CDC has proposed specific criteria for the interpretation of western blot results that correlate with clinically proved disease. (49) Great care is required, however, in the interpretation of weakly positive results. Further complicating a serologic diagnosis, significant laboratory-to-laboratory variation in test results has been reported. Additionally, many commercial laboratories are using tests for the diagnosis of Lyme disease whose accuracy and clinical correlation has not been established (e.g., urine antigen test, lymphocyte transformation test) or are evaluating western blot results by criteria that have not been clinically validated (50).

Serologic tests are frequently misused for the diagnosis of patients who present with chronic nonspecific complaints, such as fatigue, myalgias, and arthralgias. On the basis of these tests, many patients are misdiagnosed with "chronic Lyme disease." It is controversial whether chronic Lyme disease exists and many of the patients given this diagnosis actually have fibromyalgia, either as a primary disorder or as a post-Lyme disease syndrome. The diagnosis of Lyme disease should never be made in the absence of clinical findings compatible with Lyme disease or based on serology obtained in patients without evidence of exposure to *B. burgdorferi* (48–50).

TREATMENT

Antibiotics are the mainstay for treatment of active *B. burgdorferi* infection. Specific treatment recommendations relate to the stage of the disease and clinical manifestations. Antibiotic therapy is given to arrest active infection and to prevent progression to the latter stages of disease. Practice guidelines from the Infectious Diseases Society of America were published in 2000 (51). The initial clinical trials on the therapy of early localized Lyme disease used 3 weeks as treatment duration. More recent trials, however, support a shorter duration of therapy of 14 to 21 days.

EARLY LOCALIZED DISEASE

Oral therapy with doxycycline, amoxicillin, and cefuroxime axetil has proved effective in the treatment of early localized Lyme disease, irrespective of the presence or severity of associated systemic symptoms. Of note, macrolides, including azithromycin, are less effective compared with doxycycline and amoxicillin. Azithromycin, therefore, is reserved for patients who are unable to tolerate doxycycline, amoxicillin, and cefuroxime axetil. The dosage and duration of first-line drugs are noted in Table 99-2.

EARLY DISSEMINATED DISEASE

The treatment of early disseminated Lyme disease relates to the specific clinical manifestations (Table 99-3). Oral therapy with doxycycline or amoxicillin, at the same dosage and duration noted for early localized disease, is effective in the treatment of isolated facial nerve palsy, in patients with first- or second-degree atrioventricular block and in those patients presenting with predominately musculoskeletal symptoms. Intravenous therapy with ceftriaxone (2 g twice daily) or cefotaxime (2 g three times daily) is recommended for treatment of patients with neurologic disease other than isolated facial nerve palsy, and for patients with third-degree atrioventricular heart block. Intravenous ceftriaxone or longer courses of oral agents are recommended for patients with true arthritis that is persistent or relapses after an initial course of oral therapy.

LATE LYME DISEASE

Late manifestations of Lyme disease include arthritis, encephalopathy, and neuropathy. In general, the clinical response to antibiotic treatment of late Lyme disease is slow. In some patients, symptomatic improvement may take weeks or months. Intravenous therapy with ceftriaxone or cefotaxime is recommended for patients with central nervous or peripheral nervous system disease (Table 99-4). Patients with arthritis without clinical evidence of neurologic disease should receive initial therapy with oral doxycycline or amoxicillin for 28 days. Patients who have recurring arthritis should be treated with a

TABLE 99-2. Treatment Recommendations: Early Localized Lyme Disease

DOXYCYCLINE

Adults: 100 mg twice daily for 10 to 21 days
Children: 1 to 2 mg/kg twice daily (maximum,100 mg dose) for children >8 years of age for 14 to 21 days
Doxycycline is not recommended for children under 8 years of age or pregnant women.

AMOXICILLIN

Adults: 500 mg three times daily for 14 to 21 days
Children: 25 to 50 mg/kg/day divided every 8 h (maximum dose 500 mg) for 14 to 21 days

CEFUROXIME AXETIL

Adults: 500 mg twice daily for 14 to 21 days
Children: 30 mg/kg/day in divided doses (maximum dose 500 mg) for 14 to 21 days

TABLE 99-3. Treatment Recommendation: Early Disseminated Lyme Disease

NEUROLOGIC DISEASE	
Isolated cranial nerve palsy	Oral therapy with doxycycline or amoxicillin. Dose and duration as used for early localized disease
Meningitis or radiculopathy	Intravenous therapy with ceftriaxone (2 g daily) or cefotaxime (2 g three times daily) for 14 to 28 days
CARDIAC DISEASE	
First- or second-degree heart block	Oral regimen with doxycy cline or amoxicillin. Dose and duration as utilized for early localized disease
Third-degree heart block	Intravenous therapy with ceftriaxone or cefotaxime (2 g daily) for 14 to 21 days

TABLE 99-4. Treatment Recommendation: Late Lyme Disease

ARTHRITIS	
Without neurologic disease	Oral regimen with dose and duration as noted in Table 99-2
Recurrent	Repeat oral regimen or intravenous therapy in dose and duration as noted for meningitis
Persistent	Symptomatic therapy after two courses of antibiotics
CENTRAL NERVOUS SYSTEM OR PERIPHERAL NERVOUS SYSTEM DISEASE	
	Intravenous therapy with ceftriaxone or cefotaxime as noted for meningitis in Table 99-3

second course of oral antibiotics or ceftriaxone intravenously. Persistent arthritis following antibiotic therapy is most likely mediated through immune processes and should be treated with nonsteroidal anti-inflammatory drugs. Arthroscopic synovectomy may also be useful in selected patients.

CLINICAL RECOMMENDATIONS OF THE VIGNETTE

The patient presented with neurologic manifestations diagnostic of early disseminated Lyme disease. The presence of lymphocytic meningitis, facial nerve palsy, and other radiculopathies (Bannwarth syndrome) is a classic presentation and is diagnostic of early disseminated Lyme disease. Despite the lack of a history of tick bite, the presence of a red rash preceding the onset of neurologic manifestations most likely represented erythema migrans that is seen in patients with early localized disease.

Diagnosis was initially based on clinical findings and serologic studies were appropriately utilized for confirmation. Although most patients with early disseminated disease can be treated with oral antibiotics, the presence of meningitis in this case necessitated the use of parenteral therapy with ceftriaxone. Prompt recognition and the appropriate treatment of neuroborreliosis in this case resulted in an excellent clinical response.

SUMMARY

Lyme disease is the most common tick born illness in the Untied States and Europe. In the United States, most cases are caused by *Borrelia burgdorferi*. In addition to *B. burgdorferi*, *B. afzelii*, and *B. garinii* are common causes of Lyme disease in Europe and Asia. Coinfection with ehrlichiosis or babesiosis is being more commonly recognized and may explain some of the treatment failures to antibiotics reported in patients with early Lyme disease. The best method of preventing infection of *B. burgdorferi* is to avoid tick exposure. The routine use of preventive antibiotics or serologic tests following tick bite is not recommended. Rather, patients should be counseled to seek medical attention for the development of a skin rash or febrile illness within the first month after a tick bite.

The clinical manifestations of Lyme disease are protean and patients may present with signs and symptoms of skin, neurologic, rheumatologic, or cardiac disease. The manifestations of Lyme disease are divided into three stages: Early localized, early disseminated, and late disease. The diagnosis of early localized disease is based on clinical grounds by recognition of the characteristic erythema migrans rash. In patients with clinical manifestations of early disseminated disease, the presents of IgM, IgG, or both Lyme-specific antibodies may be useful in confirming a diagnosis. Serologic tests include a screening ELISA and confirmatory western blot analysis. Current serologic tests, however, must be interpreted with great caution. First, cross-reacting antibodies result in a high rate of false–positive test findings and reduce their specificity. Further, frequent laboratory-to-laboratory variations in results have been documented. Thus, serologic studies should not be performed on patients without clinical manifestations or evidence of exposure to *B. burgdorferi*.

Antibiotics are the mainstay for the treatment of active infection with *B. burgdorferi*. Specific antibiotic recommendations relate to the stage of the disease and clinical manifestations. Intravenous treatment is recommended for patients presenting with meningitis, third-degree heart block, and the neurologic manifestations (e.g., encephalopathy and neuropathy) associated with late disease. Some experts recommend intravenous therapy for the treatment of patients who have recurrent arthritis after an initial oral regimen. Oral therapy with doxycycline or amoxicillin is recommended for adults and children presenting with the other manifestations of Lyme disease. No convincing evidence indicates that a chronic Lyme disease or post-Lyme disease syndrome exists.

REFERENCES

1. Wilske B. Epidemiology and diagnosis of Lyme borreliosis. *Ann Med.* 2005;37:569–579.
2. Stanek G, Strle F. Lyme borreliosis. *Lancet.* 2003;362:1639–1647.
3. Derdakova M, Lencakova D. Association of genetic variability within the *Borrelia burgdorferi sensu lato* with the ecology, epidemiology of Lyme borreliosis in Europe. *Ann Agric Environ Med.* 2005;12:165–172.
4. Wang G, van Dam AP, Schwartz I, et al. Molecular typing of *Borrelia burgdorferi sensu lato*: Taxonomic, epidemiological, and clinical implications. *Clin Microbiol Rev.* 199912:633–653.
5. Owen DC. Is Lyme disease always poly microbial? The jigsaw hypothesis. *Med Hypotheses.* 2006;67:860–864.
6. Wormser GP. Early Lyme disease. *N Engl J Med.* 2006;354:2794–2801.
7. Gern L. The biology of the Ixodes ricinus tick. *Ther Umsch.* 2005;62:707–712.
8. Kurtenback K, Peacey M, Rijpkema SG, et al. Differential transmission of the genospecies of *Borrelia burgdorferi sensu lato* by game birds and small rodents in England. *Appl Environ Microbiol.* 1998;64:1169–1174.
9. Piesman J, Maupin GO, Campos EG, et al. Duration of adult female *Ixodes dammini* attachment and transmission of *Borrelia burgdorferi*, with description of a needle aspiration isolation method. *J Infect Dis.* 1991;163:895–897.
10. Sood SK, Salzman MB, Johnson BJ, et al. Duration of tick attachment as a predictor of the risk of Lyme disease in an area in which Lyme disease is endemic. *J Infect Dis.* 1997;175:996–999.
11. Dennis DT, Nekomoto TS, Victor JC, et al. Reported distribution of *Ixodes scapularis* and *Ixodes pacificus* (Acari: Ixodidae) in the United States. *J Med Entomol.* 1998;35:629–638.
12. Talleklint L, Jaenson TG. Transmission of *Borrelia burgdorferi s.l.* from mammal reservoirs to the primary vector of Lyme borreliosis, *Ixodes ricinus* (Acari: Ixodidae), in Sweden. *J Med Entomol.* 1994;31:880–886.
13. Hanincova K, Schafer SM, Etti S, et al. Association of Borrelia afzelii with rodents in Europe. *Parasitology.* 2003;126:11–20.
14. Norris SJ. Antigenic variation with a twist—The Borrelia story. *Mol Microbiol.* 2006;60: 1319–1343.
15. Zhang JR, Hardham JM, Barbour AG, et al. Antigenic variation in Lyme disease borreliae by promiscuous recombination of VMP-like sequence cassettes. *Cell.* 1997;89:275–285.
16. Pal U, de Silva AM, Montgomery RR, et al. Attachment of *Borrelia burgdorferi* within *Ixodes scapularis* mediated by outer surface protein A. *J Clin Invest.* 2000;106:561–569.
17. Sigal L. The immunology and potential mechanisms of immunopathogenesis of Lyme disease. *Anu Rev Immunol.* 1997;15:63.
18. Asbrink E. Cutaneous manifestations of Lyme borreliosis. Clinical definitions and differential diagnoses. *Scand J Infect Dis Suppl.* 1991;77:44–50.
19. Strle F, Pleterski-Rigler D, Stanek G, et al. Solitary borrelial lymphocytoma: Report of 36 cases. *Infection.* 1992;20:201–206.
20. Kaiser R. Neuroborreliosis. *J Neurol.* 1998;245:247–255.
21. Oschmann P, Dorndorf W, Hornig C, et al. Stages and syndromes of neuroborreliosis. *J Neurol.* 1998;245:262–272.
22. Logigian EL, Kaplan RF, Steere AC. Chronic neurologic manifestations of Lyme disease. *N Engl J Med.* 1990;323:1438–1444.
23. Lesser RL, Kornmehl EW, Pachner AR, et al. Neuro-ophthalmologic manifestations of Lyme disease. *Ophthalmology.* 1990;97:699–706.
24. Peter L, Jung J, Tilikete C, et al. Opsoclonus-myoclonus as a manifestation of Lyme disease. *J Neurol Neurosurg Psychiatry.* 2006;77:1090–1091.
25. Oksi J, Kalimo H, Marttila RJ, et al. Inflammatory brain changes in Lyme borreliosis. A report on three patients and review of literature. *Brain.* 1996;119:2143–2154.
26. Mourin S, Bonnier C, Bigaignon G, et al. Epilepsy disclosing neuroborreliosis. *Rev Neurol (Paris).* 1993;149:489–491.
27. Zhang Y, Lafontant G, Bonner FJ, Jr. Lyme neuroborreliosis mimics stroke: A case report. *Arch Phys Med Rehabil.* 2000;81:519–521.
28. Hammers-Berggren S, Grondahl A, et al. Screening for neuroborreliosis in patients with stroke. *Stroke.* 1993;24:1393–1396.
29. Arav-Boger R, Crawford T, Steere AC, et al. Cerebellar ataxia as the presenting manifestation of Lyme disease. *Pediatr Infect Dis J.* 2002;21:353–356.
30. Cassarino DS, Quezado MM, Ghatak NR, et al. Lyme-associated parkinsonism: A neuropathologic case study and review of the literature. *Arch Pathol Lab Med.* 2003;127:1204–1206.
31. Piccolo I, Thiella G, Sterzi R, et al. Chorea as a symptom of neuroborreliosis: A case study. *Ital J Neurol Sci.* 1998;19:235–239.
32. Kristoferitsch W, Spiel G, Wessely P. Meningopolyneuritis (Garin-Bujadoux, Bannwarth). Clinical aspects and laboratory findings. *Nervenarzt.* 1983;54:640–646.

33. Garin C, Bujadoux A. Paralysie par les tiques. *J Med Lyon.* 1922;71:765–767. Reprinted: *Clin Infect Dis.* 1993;16:168–169.
34. Bannwarth A. Chronische lymphocytare meningitis, entzundliche polyneuritis und "rheumatismus." *Arch Psychiatr Nervenkr.* 1941;113:284–376.
35. Halperin JJ. Lyme disease and the peripheral nervous system. *Muscle Nerve.* 2003;28:133–143.
36. Clark JR, Carlson RD, Sasaki CT, et al. Facial paralysis in Lyme disease. *Laryngoscope.* 1985;95:1341–1345.
37. Bagger-Sjoback D, Remahl S, Ericsson M. Long-term outcome of facial palsy in neuroborreliosis. *Otol Neurotol.* 2005;26:790–795.
38. Horneff G, Huppertz HI, Muller K, et al. Demonstration of *Borrelia burgdorferi* infection in a child with Guillain-Barre syndrome. *Eur J Pediatr.* 1993;152:810–812.
39. Logigian EL, Steere AC. Clinical and electrophysiologic findings in chronic neuropathy of Lyme disease. *Neurology.* 1992;42:303–311.
40. Krishnamurthy KB, Liu GT, Logigian EL. Acute Lyme neuropathy presenting with polyradicular pain, abdominal protrusion, and cranial neuropathy. *Muscle Nerve.* 1993;16: 1261–1264.
41. Daffner KR, Saver JL, Biber MP. Lyme polyradiculoneuropathy presenting as increasing abdominal girth. *Neurology.* 1990;40:373–375.
42. Belman AL, Iyer M, Coyle PK, et al. Neurological manifestations in children with North American Lyme disease. *Neurology.* 1993;43:2609–2614.
43. Krause A, Herzer P. Early diagnosis of Lyme arthritis. *Z Rheumatol.* 2005;64:531–537.
44. Sibilia J, Jaulhac B, Limbach FX. Rheumatologic manifestations of Lyme borreliosis. *Rev Med Interne.* 2002;23:378–385.
45. Nagi KS, Joshi R, Thakur RK. Cardiac manifestations of Lyme disease: A review. *Can J Cardiol.* 1996;12:503–506.
46. Pinto DS. Cardiac manifestations of Lyme disease. *Med Clin North Am.* 2002;86:285–296.
47. Haddad FA, Nadelman RB. Lyme disease of the heart. *Front Biosci.* 2003;8:s769–s782.
48. www.cdc.gov/epo/dphsi/casedef/lyme_disease_current.htm. Accessed 2006.
49. CDC. Recommendations for test performance and interpretation from the Second National Conference on Serologic Diagnosis of Lyme Disease. *MMWR Morb Mort Wkly Rep.* 1995;44:590–591.
50. CDC. Notice to readers recommendations for test performance and interpretation from the second national conference on serologic diagnosis of Lyme disease. *MMWR Morb Mort Wkly Rep.* 1995;44(31);590–591.
51. Wormser, GP, Nadelman, RB, Dattwyler, RJ, et al. Practice guidelines for the treatment of Lyme disease. *Clin Infect Dis.* 2000;31[Suppl]1:S1.

CHAPTER 100

Tuberculosis

Maria E. Santiago • Shehla P. Islam

OBJECTIVES

- To describe the typical presentation of tuberculosis (TB) of the nervous system
- To discuss the methods of diagnosing tubercular meningitis and their limitations
- To explain the importance of appropriate treatment with antituberculous drugs, and adjunctive use of steroids
- To describe the problems in management of human immunodeficiency virus (HIV) and TB coinfection

CASE VIGNETTE

A 28-year-old previously healthy black woman was brought to the emergency room by her family with a history of 2 to 3 days of lethargy and confusion. For the past several weeks, she had been complaining of a headache, which had progressively worsened. She did not use tobacco, alcohol, or any drugs. She had worked as a nursing assistant at a nursing home for the past 3 years.

On examination, she had a temperature of 103°F. She was somnolent, but responsive to voice, indicated by eye opening. Her right pupil was 3 mm and reactive to light, whereas the left was 4.5 mm and sluggish. She moved all four limbs spontaneously, but would not follow commands. Muscle stretch reflexes were 2+. Laboratory data included a normal complete blood count (CBC). A screening computed tomographic (CT) scan of the head showed no intracranial abnormalities. Magnetic resonance imaging (MRI) of the brain was also done on admission (Fig. 100-1). Cerebrospinal fluid (CSF) examination showed a white blood cell (WBC) count of 188/mm^3, 84% lymphocytes, protein 252 mg/dL, and glucose 24 mg/dL, with a serum glucose of 115 mg/d:. Gram stain was negative. Empiric treatment for viral and bacterial meningitis was initiated.

DEFINITION

Tuberculosis is an infection caused by an obligate aerobe, *Mycobacterium tuberculosis* or Koch bacillus, capable of affecting any part of the body at any age. Pulmonary tuberculosis is the most common presentation. The most typical clinical presentation of neurotuberculosis includes cranial or spinal meningitis and single or multiple tuberculomas in spine or cranium (1). Central nervous system (CNS) TB can be present as the only manifestation of the disease, or as a component of TB existing elsewhere in the body.

EPIDEMIOLOGY

Tuberculosis remains one of the most important communicable diseases worldwide and a major cause of serious illness in terms of morbidity and mortality. In developing countries, the incidence of TB is associated with poor socioeconomic status, HIV or acquired immunodeficiency syndrome (AIDS) epidemics and limited resources for public health. Additionally, genetic factors appear to play a role in certain African communities where the population is seemingly more predisposed to pulmonary involvement with tuberculosis (2).

Despite decreasing number of cases in the last few decades in the United States and other developed countries, TB remains a serious public health problem, especially in individuals infected with HIV, and inner-city and immigrant population, with drug-resistant TB becoming a major problem (3).

Traditionally, active disease had been considered to result from reactivation of a latent infection acquired earlier in life. Epidemiologic studies and DNA analysis, however, demonstrated that recently acquired infection was present in up to 40% of the new cases of TB in a study conducted in New York City in 1994 (4).

ETIOLOGY AND PATHOGENESIS

Tuberculosis results from an infection by an acid-resistant intracellular obligate aerobic organism, *Mycobacterium tuberculosis.* TB is propagated by aerosolized bacilli carried in small droplets when a person with active pulmonary TB coughs, sneezes, or speaks. If these tiny particles are inhaled by a susceptible individual, the bacilli reach the lungs where macrophages and sensitized T lymphocytes will attempt to contain the infection in the form of a granuloma. From this point, the mycobacteria can spread hematogenously to other organs, including the CNS, either during primary infection, or later, after reactivation of disease. Rupture of small tubercles (Rich's foci) in the subependymal area, followed by invasion of the subarachnoid or ventricular space by TB bacilli, leads to inflammation and disease symptoms (5).

PATHOLOGY

The hallmark of TB is the presence of epithelioid cell granulomas characterized by accumulation of mononuclear inflammatory cells and Langhan's giant cells with necrosis or caseation.

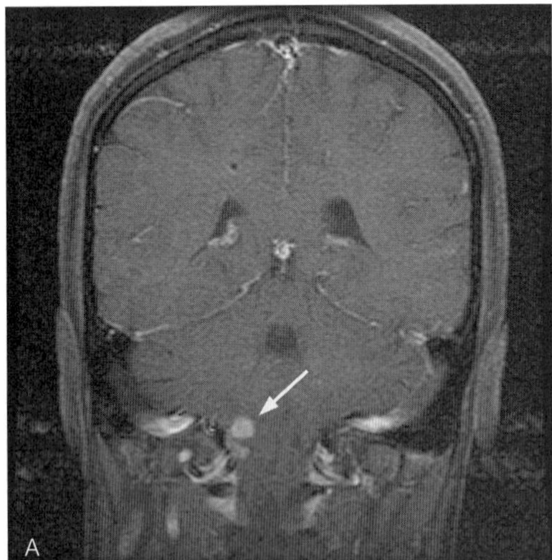

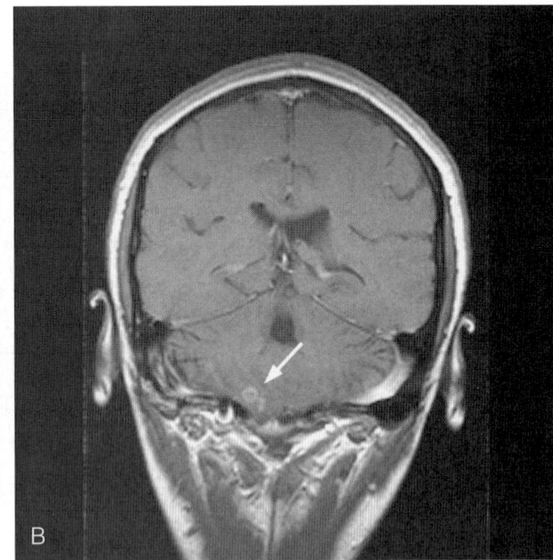

FIGURE 100-1. Magnetic resonance imaging (MRI) of the brain demonstrates a small round area of contrast enhancement (arrows), likely representing a tubercular granuloma, in this case of tuberculosis (TB) meningitis (**A**). A follow-up MRI of the brain (**B**) 6 months later shows partial resolution of the lesion. Patient had no neurologic complications.

These granulomas can house dormant bacilli that remain silent for years to later reactivate and cause bacteremia, potentially able to seed any organ. In the nervous system, these granulomas, also called *tuberculomas*, can expand and behave as a space-occupying lesion, causing mass effect secondary to surrounded inflammatory response or invade the subarachnoid space causing meningitis. Adhesive inflammatory exudates lead to obstruction and hydrocephalus. TB can involve the spinal cord with or without intracranial involvement.

CLINICAL MANIFESTATIONS

The symptoms and complications of TB can be explained by various pathologic processes: Granulomas that coalesce forming space-occupying tuberculomas; adhesive exudates that obstruct CSF and lead to hydrocephalus; and vasculitis causing infarction. TB meningitis is the most common presentation. The initial presentation is usually preceded by several days to weeks of fatigue, irritability, apathy, myalgias, and fever. The typical signs of meningeal irritation soon follow, including headache, neck rigidity, nausea and vomiting, and drowsiness or altered mental status. In up to 24% of patients, evidence is seen of cranial nerve palsies. The most commonly affected cranial nerves are VI, III, IV, VII, and VIII. TB primarily affects the base of the cranium (basal meningitis), manifested by involvement of several lower cranial nerves causing dysphagia or dysarthria. Occasionally, TB meningitis will present as an acute meningitis, resembling bacterial or viral meningitides; behavioral disturbances; rapidly dementing illness; stroke; encephalopathy; or signs of increased intracranial pressure, such as papilledema or pseudotumor cerebri. In more complicated cases (5% to 10%), the patients may present with coma, seizures, and focal neurologic deficits, such as hemiparesis (6,7). Peripheral WBC count is usually normal, but anemia may be seen. Hyponatremia is also commonly encountered in TB meningitis in both adults and children. It is thought to be caused either by secretion of the syndrome of inappropriate antidiuretic hormone (SIADH) or the secretion of plasma atrial natriuretic factor.

In children, the most common findings are alteration of consciousness and focal neurologic deficits. Seizures, fever, vomiting, and meningeal signs are also seen. Hydrocephalus was present in up to 94% of the patients evaluated in some series (8). In some instances, children may present with nonspecific symptoms, such as abdominal pain, constipation, or behavioral problems. Farinha et al. (8) reported duration of the symptoms in their series ranged from 3 days to 6 months.

Tuberculomas consist of TB granulomas that can be single or multiple; anywhere in the brain, cerebellum, and spinal cord parenchyma; and present with signs and symptoms of space-occupying lesions, such as headaches, papilledema, seizures, and focal neurologic deficits. The granulomas may be surrounded by varying degrees of edema and reactive tissue, causing mass effect, making these lesions often difficult to differentiate from primary or secondary malignant neoplasms (7).

Spinal TB presents commonly with back pain, paraparesis, kyphosis, bowel and bladder dysfunction, and sensory disturbance. Spinal TB may present as inadequately treated osteomyelitis, compression fractures, or as involvement of the vertebral space causing Pott disease (tuberculous spondylitis). Thoracic spine, especially T10 is commonly involved and can be seen in plain X-rays involving the vertebral body and intervertebral space. MRI is the best modality for evaluating this disorder (1,9,10).

The presentation of individuals with HIV infection differs little from patients not infected (11), although the likelihood of finding active TB in other sites is higher. TB meningitis can resemble other CNS infections occurring in the HIV population, including cryptococcal meningitis.

DIAGNOSIS

Early diagnosis of TB meningitis is essential in preventing morbidity and mortality, but remains difficult, owing to the nonspecific clinical features early on, and the lack of sensitive and rapid diagnostic techniques. A high index of suspicion is therefore necessary. A history of TB exposure is useful, as are findings of pulmonary TB. Skin testing with purified protein derivative (PPD) may not be of much value. In high prevalence areas, a positive test finding does not imply active disease, and up to 20% of patients with active disease have a negative skin test. A positive test in the right clinical setting and low prevalence area, however, should increase the suspicion for TB.

CSF evaluation typically demonstrates normal or elevated opening pressure, low glucose, elevated protein in the 80 to 400 mg/dL range, and pleocytosis, typically 200 to 400 WBC/μL (predominantly lymphocytes). In some cases, especially in intraparenchymal tuberculomas or miliary TB, the CSF study may be normal. In other circumstances, CSF might show marked polymorphonuclear response initially resembling acute bacterial meningitis.

The bacteriologic diagnosis depends on direct visualization of acid fast bacilli (AFB) by microscopy using acid-fast staining methods, and mycobacterial culture. Meticulous technique and culture of a large volume CSF can lead to a diagnosis in up to 80% of patients. Early diagnosis is imperative, however, and sensitivity of direct microscopy remains in the 50% to 60% range. This has led to evaluation and use of nucleic acid amplification tests. In a study comparing *M. tuberculosis* direct test (MTD) with Zeihl-Neelson staining (ZN), the sensitivity was found to be 38% and 52%, respectively, improving to 64% if the two techniques were combined (12). Both tests were highly specific. After 5 to 15 days of treatment, the sensitivity of ZN dropped dramatically to 2%, whereas that of the MTD test was 28%. Other studies also support these data. This suggests that conventional microscopy might be a more expeditious and less costly way of diagnosing TB meningitis, and the nucleic acid tests are best used in situations where treatment has been initiated.

CT and MRI are the imaging studies commonly used. Noncontrasted CT studies during the acute stage may show only a hypodense area caused by cerebritis. Tuberculomas might be iso- or hyperdense if they are immature, or even calcified if healed, on noncontrasted CT scans. In contrasted CT studies, tuberculomas typically appear as well-delineated, oval or round lesions surrounded by a ring or irregular area of enhancement. On MRI studies, tuberculomas are isointense on T1-weighted images, and have a hyperintense central region with hypointense rim on T2-weighted images and marked enhancement on contrasted studies.

TREATMENT

Treatment of neurotuberculosis involves chemotherapy to eradicate infection, management of increased intracranial pressure, and use of steroids to reduce inflammation. It is not as well defined as that of pulmonary TB, and the ideal choice of drugs and duration of treatment have not been established. The principles, however, are essentially the same. Guidelines have been published by the British Thoracic Society (BTS) (13), as well as joint guidelines from the Infectious Diseases Society of America (IDSA), the American Thoracic Society (ATS), and the Centers for Disease Control and Prevention (CDC) (14).

The mainstay of treatment is an initial phase using a combination of four first-line drugs: Isoniazid (INH); a rifamycin, usually Rifampin (RIF); pyrazinamide (PZA); and ethambutol (EMB) or streptomycin (SM), followed by a continuation phase, mainly consisting of INH and RIF (Table 100-1). EMB is favored by IDSA/ATS as the fourth drug, but the BTS recommends either SM or EMB. INH and PZA readily pass the blood–brain barrier into the CSF, achieving high concentrations. CSF levels of RIF are only 10% to 20% of the level in serum, although they may be higher in the presence of inflamed meninges. These levels are adequate for clinical efficacy. INH is bactericidal to rapidly multiplying bacilli and the key drug in the first 2 weeks of therapy. Thereafter, RIF acts to

TABLE 100-1. Treatment Recommendations for Tuberculosis (TB) Meningitis with Nonresistant *Mycobacterium tuberculosis*

Drug	*Dose*	*Frequency*[a]	*Cerebrospinal Fluid Concentration*	*Duration*
INITIAL PHASE				
Isoniazid		Daily	Excellent	2 months
Rifampin[b]		Daily	10% to 20% of serum[c]	2 months
Pyrazinamide		Daily	Excellent	2 months
Ethambutol		Daily	Fair[d]	
or				2 months
Streptomycin		5 days/week	Very low	
CONTINUATION PHASE				
Isoniazid		2 to 3 times/week		7–10 months
Rifampin		2 to 3 times/week		7–10 months

[a]Intermittent dosing recommendations are available after the initial days of treatment. Intermittent dosing recommendations in individuals infected with human immunodeficiency virus (HIV) are dependent on the CD4 cell count.
[b]Other forms of rifamycins, including rifabutin, can be used in appropriate doses.
[c]This may be higher in the presence of inflamed meninges.
[d]Cerebrospinal fluid (CSF) penetration occurs in meningitis, but efficacy in this condition is not established.

sterilize by killing slowly dividing bacteria. The other agents aid in the activity of INH and RIF. As mentioned, the exact duration of therapy is not well determined, but the usual standard of practice in case of susceptible agents is 2 months of intensive therapy, followed by 7 to 10 months of the continuation phase. The World Health Organization (WHO) recommends the standard therapy for a total of 6 months, but the BTS, and IDSA/ATS take a more conservative approach, suggesting the longer duration (15).

Drug-resistant disease is an increasing problem worldwide. The risk of drug resistance is greater in the presence of high bacillary load, as well as in an inadequate drug regimen. One of the factors influencing the latter is patient compliance, and this is maximized by the institution of directly observed therapy (DOT). In DOT, designated personnel watch the patient ingest the prescribed medication. Most Third World countries with a high incidence of TB, however, do not have the resources for this.

If resistance is present to only INH *or* RIF, the remaining first-line agents can be used for a prolonged period, and the regimen can be strengthened by the use of fluoroquinolones (FQ) (14). Evidence indicates the efficacy of FQ in TB, but their utility in neurotuberculosis is not well defined. In the presence of resistance to both INH and RIF, second-line agents and FQ must be used. These include para-amino-salicylic acid (PAS), cycloserine, amikacin, ethionamide, and others. These agents, however, are less effective and less well tolerated than the first-line drugs, and their role in TB meningitis is even less clearly defined.

The adjunctive use of steroids has been debated for more than 50 years. In theory, corticosteroids would counter the inflammation in TB, which is felt to be responsible for much of the neurologic damage. Early studies were limited, however, by small size and failed to show clear benefit in survival rates. A meta-analysis done in 2000 suggested that corticosteroids were helpful in children. A randomized, controlled trial done in Vietnamese patients using dexamethasone showed a clear benefit of survival with the use of steroids in individuals not infected with HIV, but no decrease in severe disability was noted (16). This trial also showed that treatment with dexamethasone was associated with fewer adverse events. Most groups, including the IDSA/CDC, recommend the use of steroids in TB meningitis, especially in more severe disease. The suggested dose is 12 mg/kg/day for adults and children >25 kg of body weight for 3 weeks, followed by a tapered dosage over 3 more weeks.

Treatment recommendations for TB in individuals infected with HIV, in general, is the same as those in for individuals not infected, and this remains true for TB meningitis as well. Several issues must be kept in mind. The incidence of resistance in these individuals appears to be higher, especially against rifamycins. Therapy should be monitored with vigilance, and slow response may warrant longer duration of therapy. DOT is the preferred method of treatment in this population.

Another difficulty in treating patients infected with HIV is the interaction between drugs used for highly active antiretroviral therapy (HAART) and the rifamycins. In most situations, the dose of medications must be adjusted. Of the rifamycins, rifabutin appears to have fewer interactions and is often the rifamycin of choice in patients on HAART. Intermittent TB therapy can also pose a problem in patients with HIV, because this leads to acquired rifamycin resistance. Because of the increased frequency of such resistance in patients with absolute CD4 counts of $<100/\mu L$, it is recommended that twice weekly drug administration *not* be used in these patients in the continuation phase (17). Once-weekly INH-rifapentine in the continuation phase is not recommended in any individual infected with HIV. Finally, the role of steroids in this population remains controversial.

In summary, HIV and TB coinfection is a complicated process, and is best managed by individuals trained in treatment of both diseases.

The treatment of tuberculomas can include chemotherapy or a combination of chemotherapy and surgery. Steroids may reduce the associated inflammation. In high incidence areas, such as India, tuberculomas are confirmed by biopsy and treated with antituberculous drugs (18).

Hydrocephalus is a fairly common complication. It can be treated with diuretics or serial lumbar punctures, but neurosurgical intervention may be needed, especially in more severe cases (13,19).

TB meningitis was uniformly fatal before the advent of antituberculous drugs and remains a disease with a high morbidity and mortality. Complications, such as hydrocephalus; residual neurologic deficits, including cranial nerve palsies and hemiparesis; and strokes, are a consequence of the previously described pathology, and continue to occur despite treatment.

CLINICAL RECOMMENDATIONS OF THE VIGNETTE

The patient presented with symptoms consistent with meningitis that evolved over a period of a few weeks. The initial CSF picture was very consistent with TB meningitis and, in a high incidence area, this presentation should lead to immediate initiation of antituberculous therapy along with adjunctive steroids. In this case, suspicion of aseptic meningitis was reasonable, although such low glucose is unusual. Cryptococcal meningitis would also be a consideration, especially if the patient was HIV positive. Both the HIV ELISA and CSF cryptococcal antigen test findings were negative. Treatment for TB meningitis was begun 3 to 4 days after the initial presentation. This was prompted by the patient's declining mental status, a positive PPD (previously documented as negative at her workplace), negative routine bacterial cultures, and the CSF picture. Interestingly, additional history revealed that the patient had recently cared for a nursing home resident who was diagnosed with pulmonary TB.

Culture for acid-fast bacilli (AFB) was not done on the initial sample, but a second CSF sample obtained after the initiation of antituberculous therapy was negative for AFB smear and culture. Nucleic acid amplification done on the second CSF, however, proved positive for *M. tuberculosis*. The patient also developed hydrocephalus, requiring a shunt. The patient was started on steroids and gradually improved over the next 4 weeks. She was discharged in a stable condition, with no significant neurologic deficits.

SUMMARY

Tuberculosis of the nervous system most commonly presents as meningitis. The significant inflammation it causes renders it a disease with significant morbidity and mortality. Early diagnosis is hampered by the low sensitivity of available diagnostic techniques, and a high index of suspicion is needed for prompt initiation of treatment. Complications include hydrocephalus, cranial nerve palsies, and hemiparesis. Mainstay of treatment is similar to that of pulmonary TB with four first-line drugs initially, but with a longer continuation phase. The management of HIV–TB coinfection is complicated, and best accomplished by specialists trained in the treatment of both diseases.

REFERENCES

1. Al-Deeb SM, Yaqub BA, Sharif HS, et al. Neurotuberculosis: A review. *Clin Neurol Neurosurg.* 1992;94[Suppl] S30–S33.
2. Bellamy R, Ruwende C, Corrah T, et al. Variations in the NRAMP1 gene and susceptibility to tuberculosis in West Africans. *N Engl J Med.* 1998;338:640–644.
3. Porkert MT, Sotir M, Parrott-Moore P, et al. Tuberculous meningitis at a large inner-city medical center. *Am J Med Sci.* 1997; 313(6):325–331.
4. Alland D, Kalkut GE, Moss AR et al. Transmission of tuberculosis in New York City. An analysis by DNA fingerprinting and conventional epidemiologic methods. *N Engl J Med.* 1994;330:1710–1716.
5. Solbrig MV, Healy JF, Jay CA. Infections of the nervous system. In: Bradley WG, 3rd, Daroff RB, Fenichel GM, et al., eds. *Neurology in Clinical Practice*, 3rd ed. Woburn: Butterworth-Heinemann (MA); 2000:1317–1352.
6. Sûtlas PN, Ünal A, Forta H, et al. Tuberculous meningitis in adults: Review of 61 cases. *Infection.* 2003;31:387–391.
7. Garcia-Monco JC. Tuberculosis del sistema nervioso central. In: Micheli F, Nogues MA, Asconape JJ, et al., eds. *Tratado de Neurologia Clinica.* Buenos Aires: Panamericana; 2002: 1021–1039.
8. Farinha NJ, Razali KA, Holzel H, et al. Tuberculosis of the central nervous system in children: A 20-year survey. *J Infect.* 2000;41:61–68.
9. Nussbaum ES, Rockswold GL, Bergman TA, et al. Spinal tuberculosis: A diagnostic and management challenge. *J Neurosurg.* 1995;83(2):243–247.
10. Schlesinger N, Lardizabal A, Rao J, et al. Tuberculosis of the spine: Experience in an inner city hospital. *J Clin Rheumatol.* 2005;11(1):17–20.
11. Berenguer J, Moreno S, Laguna F, et al. Tuberculous meningitis in patients infected with HIV. *N Engl J Med.* 1992;326:668–672.
12. Thwaites GE, Caws M, Chaw TT, et al. Comparison of conventional bacteriology with nucleic acid amplification (amplified mycobacterium direct test) for diagnosis of tuberculous meningitis before and after inception of antituberculous chemotherapy. *J Clin Microbiol.* 2004;42:996–1002.
13. British Thoracic Society. Chemotherapy and management of tuberculosis in the United Kingdom: Recommendations 1998. *Thorax.* 1998;53:536–548.
14. CDC. Treatment of tuberculosis. *MMWR Recomm Rep.* 2003;52:1–77.
15. Donald P, Schoeman J. Tuberculous meningitis. *N Engl J Med.* 2004;351:1719–1720.
16. Thwaites GE, Nguyen DB, Nguyen HD, et al. Dexamethasone for the treatment of tuberculous meningitis in adolescents and adults. *N Engl J Med.* 2004;351:1741–1751.
17. CDC. Acquired rifamycin resistance in persons with advanced HIV disease being treated for active tuberculosis with intermittent rifamycin-based regimens. *MMWR Morb Mort Wkly Rep.* 2002;51:214–215.
18. Mandell G, Dolin R, Bennett J. *Principles and Practice of Infectious Diseases.* Philadelphia: Elsevier; 2005.
19. Thwaites G, Hien T. Tuberculous meningitis: Many questions, too few answers. *Lancet Neurol.* 2005;4:160–170.

CHAPTER **101**

Malaria

Gretchen L. Birbeck • Terrie E. Taylor

OBJECTIVES

- To describe the relevant details to be obtained in a travel history
- To explain the other potential mechanisms for exposure to malaria
- To provide an awareness of the global burden of malaria
- To offer a working knowledge of risk factors for severe malaria
- To discuss how to recognize the clinical signs and symptoms of malaria.
- To explain how to order and interpret appropriate diagnostic studies and undertake rational patient management when treating malaria in a developed world setting
- To describe the basic pathophysiology of malaria as it relates to clinical presentation and care, particularly in terms of complicated malaria

CASE VIGNETTE

A 27-year-old woman presents to her primary care doctor with fever, chills, myalgias, and headache for the past 12 hours. She reports anorexia and malaise for 1 day. The headache is severe, bifrontal, and associated with photophobia. She tried to take acetaminophen before the office visit, but vomited the medication. On examination, her temperature is 39.2°C, blood pressure is 140/90 mm Hg, heart rate is 110 beats per minute, respirations are 14 breaths per minute. General physical examination demonstrates mild abdominal tenderness with slight guarding, and a palpable spleen tip. She had some degree of photophobia evident when a funduscopic examination was attempted, but no neck stiffness. Examination is otherwise unremarkable.

She returned 2 weeks ago from a 1-month stay in Zambia, which included time spent in both urban and rural settings. Before her trip, she received counseling from the University's Travel Clinic, including some vaccinations and mefloquine for malaria prophylaxis. She reports good adherence with the mefloquine, despite experiencing sleeplessness and disturbing dreams after each weekly dose and one episode of visual hallucinations. She is referred to the emergency department by her primary care physician for further assessment and possible lumbar puncture. She presents to the emergency room 6 hours later. She remains febrile, has become confused, and is somewhat combative when staff attempt to place an intravenous line.

DEFINITION

Malaria disease refers to the clinical manifestation caused by infection with one of four species of *Plasmodium* capable of infecting humans (1). Human malaria infections result from four distinct *Plasmodium* species: *P. falciparum, P. vivax, P. ovale, and P. malariae.* Among these, only *P. falciparum* is life-threatening and, therefore, it will be the focus of this chapter.

EPIDEMIOLOGY

Although previously much more widely distributed through warmer regions of Europe and North America, today malaria is primarily a problem of tropical regions, usually in the less-developed countries (2). An estimated 300 to 500 million malaria infections occur annually with approximately 1 million malaria-related deaths. More than 90% of malaria-related mortality occurs among children and pregnant women, primarily in sub-Saharan Africa. In highly endemic regions, repeated childhood infections result in acquired immunity developing by mid to late childhood. Therefore, the malaria-related mortality among children <5 years of age is high, but adult infections (except during pregnancy) are rarely serious. In regions with lower levels of endemicity, serious adult infections are more common.

Despite global efforts to combat malaria, the burden of the disease continues to rise. Because of the development of drug resistence, chloroquine, the mainstay of treatment before the 1990s, is now useless against *P. falciparum* in most regions. Other inexpensive and simple treatment options, such as sulfadoxine-pyrimethamine (SP), are also rapidly becoming ineffective. Alternative treatment regimens are significantly more expensive and may have a higher risk of adverse reactions.

Malaria incidence has remained relatively stable in the United States over the past 5 years, with approximately 1,300 cases annually, many of these among military personnel. More than 27 million Americans traveled overseas in 2006. The US population includes 51 million foreign residents, many of whom travel to their country of origin after being abroad sufficiently long to have their acquired immunity wane (~2 years). As military campaigns expand and more people take advantage of opportunities for international travel, malaria rates in developed countries may increase.

In addition to travel-related exposure, malaria can be transmitted accidentally, via blood transfusion; congenitally, through organ transplant; or by accidental inoculation. Years ago, malaria therapy (with *P. vivax*) was a recognized approach for the treatment of syphilis. Today, some practitioners have been known to use malaria to treat another spirochetal infection, Lyme disease. Residents of nonendemic regions residing near international airports have contracted malaria presumably from imported mosquitoes (called "airport malaria"). Even travelers who did not actually disembark in an endemic region, but simply waited in the plane while it was refueling, have been known to contract malaria ("runway malaria"). A thorough travel history, thus, is an essential part of the evaluation of a febrile or unconscious patient.

ETIOLOGY AND PATHOGENESIS

All four plasmodial species are intracellular parasites transmitted by the bite of the female *Anopheles* mosquito (3). The incubation period for *P. falciparum* is 7 to 30 days (mean, 10 days), possibly longer in the setting of prophylaxis use. Sporozoites are rapidly taken into the liver where they multiply asexually until the schizont ruptures sending merozoites into the peripheral circulation where they enter red blood cells (RBC) and begin further replication. As the *P. falciparum* parasite matures further, the infected RBC develop knoblike projections on the outer membrane; these mediate cytoadherence to endothelial cell surfaces, resulting in sequestration of the maturing parasite in various peripheral capillary beds, including brain, gut, and lung. Sequestration allows the parasite to evade splenic clearance, but the phenomenon may be at least partially responsible for the severe illness produced by *P. falciparum*. No other plasmodial species exhibits this behavior; the entire life cycle occurs in the peripheral (circulating) blood. *P. falciparum* has several other characteristics that distinguish it from the other *Plasmodium* species infecting humans and they, too, may contribute to its more clinically ominous profile.

1. *P. falciparum* has the ability to infect RBC of any age; the other species are limited to either immature or older RBC. Thus, the proportion of RBC vulnerable to infection is larger for *P. falciparum*.
2. *P. falciparum* undergoes rapid replication in both exoerythrocytic and erythrocytic stages, and so a heavier parasite burden is more likely.
3. *P. falciparum* schizonts undergo sequestration in critical tissues (brain, kidney, lung, gut). Platelets and uninfected cells can also stick to these cytoadherent cells, causing sludging and microvascular obstruction with secondary ischemia.
4. *P. falciparum* in most regions has developed multidrug resistance to previously effective, inexpensive agents. Resistance patterns have an impact on both treatment regimens and the efficacy of prophylactic medications and malaria infection rates in the region.

PATHOLOGY

Three primary mechanisms are believed to account for the pathologic effects of malaria: Mechanical, immune-mediated, and metabolic (1, 4).

Mechanical obstruction via infected RBC cytoadhering to vascular endothelium causes microthrombotic injuries evident in several organ systems, including the brain. In cerebral malaria (CM), cerebral capillaries and venules are plugged by parasite-filled erythrocytes. Retinal abnormalities evident through direct and indirect ophthalmoscopy provide premorbid evidence of parasite-induced sequestration and are predictive of outcome. These ophthalmologic findings include retinal whitening, hemorrhages, unique vessel abnormalities, papilledema, and cotton wool spots. Clinically evident large vessel strokes are recognized complications of severe malaria. Hemolysis occurs when infected RBC lyse and the lifespan of uninfected RBC is also shortened as bystander red cells are mechanically filtered by the engorged splenic system. These two mechanisms contribute to the anemia typically seen. Hemolysis can cause hemoglobinuria, acute tubular necrosis, and renal failure ("black water fever"). Severe renal involvement is more likely in adults.

Metabolic perturbations common in severe malaria include hypoglycemia, lactic acidosis, arterial hypotension, and hypoxia. Hypoxia caused by coma and comorbid pulmonary pathology can occur. Poor local central nervous system (CNS) oxygenation as a result of focal sludging in cerebral vasculature may play a role in hypoxia-induced injury, even among those with adequate oxygen saturation based on blood gas results. Hypoglycemia is especially problematic in children, pregnant women, and persons receiving quinine therapy. Parenteral doses (intravenous or intramuscular) of quinine in >10 mg/kg over 2 hours increase insulin secretion and can produce hypoglycemia. Hypoglycemia at the time of presentation, before any treatment, has been found to predict mortality and neurologic deficits. Blood glucose levels may not adequately reflect the local CNS environment with focal sludging or regions of excess metabolic stress related to focal, prolonged seizure activity. Metabolic demands are likely increased by the hyperpyrexia. Malarial fevers can remain at >40°C for the first 2 to 3 days after initiating treatment with antimalarials and antipyretics. Recurrent seizures represent another metabolic challenge associated with severe malaria. Continuous seizures, both focal and generalized status epilepticus, commonly occur during cerebral malaria.

Malaria infection is associated with a vigorous immune response resulting in what has been termed a *cytokine cascade* with high levels of circulating tumor necrosis factor-α (TNF-α), interferon-γ (IFN-γ), and phosphoglycolipids, with subsequent induction of nitric oxide. These circulating factors may play a role in bone marrow suppression with severe anemia and thrombocytopenia. Endothelial damage caused by a nonspecific immune-mediated inflammatory response with release of vasoactive substance can also result in increased metabolic demands and subsequent injury. Clinical trials have been conducted using pentoxifylline, steroids, and other immune-modulating drugs in attempts to improve outcome. To date, no one study has shown any benefit.

CLINICAL MANIFESTATIONS

Prodromal symptoms include malaise, anorexia, headache, nausea, and myalgias. Chills, alternating with spiking temperatures and then breaking sweats, follow. Headache is usually a prominent feature even in uncomplicated malaria. Diarrhea and vomiting can occur, especially in children. Classic fever patterns (tertian, quatern) only develop later in the disease progression as schizont rupture becomes synchronous and should not be relied on for diagnosis (3, 4).

TABLE 101-1. Malaria-Related Complications and Their Pathophysiology

Complication	*Pathophysiology*
Severe malaria	1. Infected RBC rupture from parasite 2. Noninfected RBC destruction as bystanders 3. Dyserythropoiesis caused by cytokine cascade
Hypoglycemia	1. Poor oral intake 2. Anaerobic glycolysis 3. Decreased gluconeogenesis 4. Marginal nutritional status at baseline 5. Increase glucose utilization by infected RBC (70 times baseline) 6. Quinine stimulation of insulin release
Renal failure (acute tubular necrosis)	1. Hemolysis 2. Shock
Acute respiratory distress syndrome[a]	1. Cytokine cascade 2. Parasite sequestration with secondary alveolar macrophage infiltration and edema
Cerebral malaria	1. Mechanical sludging and ischemia from sequestration 2. Seizures 3. Focal hypoxia not present systemically 4. Stroke(s) 5. Cytokine cascade[b]
Shock ("algid" malaria)	1. Cytokine cascade 2. Comorbid sepsis

RBC, red blood cells.
[a]Must assure patient is not volume overloaded or in failure.
[b]Given the rapid return to consciousness that commonly occurs in deeply comatose children, this almost certainly plays a role but the details remain unclear.

On examination, patients with malaria are generally miserable and can exhibit signs typically associated with meningeal irritability (photophobia, neck stiffness). Pallor may be evident at presentation or can develop within 1 to 2 days after initiating treatment. An enlarged spleen is common. In individuals with CNS symptoms, a funduscopic evaluation should be completed to look for retinal findings of cerebral malaria. Some, such as papilledema are being nonspecific, but others (whitened vessels, retinal whitening) are likely diagnostic of cerebral malaria.

Severe malaria in children is characterized by severe malarial anemia (SMA), cerebral malaria (CM), or both. Anemia occurs because of active destruction of infected RBC, bystander destruction of uninfected RBC, and bone marrow suppression. CM is clinically defined as *P. falciparum* infection with an altered level of consciousness, seizures, or both. Adults with severe malaria often experience multisystem organ failure in addition to CNS involvement. Renal failure, acute respiratory distress syndrome (ARDS), and hypotension with hemodynamic parameters consistent with sepsis can occur. See Table 101-1 for malaria-related complications and pathogenesis.

DIAGNOSTIC APPROACH

The greatest challenge to diagnosing malaria outside the tropics is to consider the possibility of malaria in the differential diagnosis (3). If malaria is not considered early in the case of a seriously ill, nonimmune person infected with *P. falciparum,* the diagnosis may well be made on postmortem examination. For the awake patient who presents with headache, fever, and a travel history in hand, malaria will be considered immediately, it is hoped. Diagnostic challenges more frequently arise when patients present in coma without a history readily available or present with malaria-related complications, such as renal failure, ARDS, or severe anemia, that rapidly become the focus of clinical attention before an adequate exposure history is obtained. Malaria prophylaxis, regardless of the regimen used and even with excellent adherence, does not guarantee someone will remain malaria free.

The gold standard test is light microscopy of both thin and thick blood smears, using any of the Romanovsky-type stains. Initially a thick blood smear should be conducted to search for evidence of parasites. Once parasites have been established, a thin film (ideally collected at the same time) should be stained and examined for speciation and quantification. Identifying the species will guide antimalarial treatment. High parasite burdens (generally >5% RBC infected in nonimmune individuals) indicates the need for close, inpatient observation. Maintaining a high level of awareness for the development of malaria complications is warranted. Although the malaria parasite should be visible on a thick blood smear examined by a sufficiently experienced microscopist, the parasite burden in the peripheral blood may not reflect the sequestered parasite load, and few laboratory staff in developed countries have much experience identifying *P. falciparum.* Furthermore, *P. falciparum* in nonimmune individuals can be life-threatening even with a relatively low level of parasitemia. If malaria is being considered and the first blood smear finding is negative, thick smears should be repeated every 4 hours for a full 24 hours, and viewed shortly after collection.

The nonimmune, seriously ill patient with a potential exposure to malaria should be treated even if the smear is negative. Delays in treatment could be fatal and increase the risk of long-term sequelae.

In addition to light microscopy, several rapid diagnostic tests (RDT) are currently available that detect malaria-specific antigens indicating a recent or active infection. Note that speciation is still necessary, and that not all RDT offer this option. Most hospital laboratories are unlikely to have malaria RDT at hand, but antigen panels will remain positive for some days after treatment initiation and may offer the opportunity for diagnosis, even when treatment has resolved the parasitemia and light microscopy has failed to confirm the clinical diagnosis.

People from malaria-endemic regions, particularly highly endemic regions, develop premunition and may have asymptomatic parasitemia. Even if the blood smear is positive for such individuals with an acute severe illness, other diagnoses should at least be considered. Asymptomatic parasitemia does not occur among nonimmune people, and any level of parasitemia should be considered pathologic in this group.

Common laboratory findings associated with malaria include anemia, thrombocytopenia, hyponatremia, and mildly elevated liver transaminases. Low-grade disseminated intravascular coagulation (DIC) can occur, especially in adults with multisystem organ failure, but full-blown DIC is uncommon. A metabolic acidosis, with or without respiratory compensation, is also likely. High lactate levels have been correlated to poor outcomes in Africa-based studies (5).

TREATMENT

Treatment will be largely determined by the antimalarial agents available, and whether the patient is sufficiently stable to take an oral agent (under close observation) or requires parenteral treatment (6). In the United States, the only approved regimen (and routinely available) for severe malaria with *P. falciparum* is intravenous quinidine gluconate, which should be given with doxycycline, tetracycline, or clindamycin. Elsewhere, intravenous quinine or a parenteral artesunate should be used. Dosing regimen are detailed in Table 101.2.

In addition to antimalarials, supportive care should include aggressive management of hypoglycemia, which can be severe and recurrent. Antipyretics are typically warranted, especially in children at risk of fever-associated seizures. Seizures should be managed initially with rapid acting benzodiazepines. If necessary, long-lasting agents (phenytoin or phenobarbitone) should be used. No data are available on the use of intravenous valproic acid for seizures caused by severe malaria. Given the somewhat compromised state of the liver and preexisting thrombocytopenia, however, this drug should probably be avoided. In a developed setting with recourse to ventilation, respiratory support may be needed to allow for adequate treatment of seizures. Nonconvulsive *status epilepticus* should be considered in anyone with malaria and coma. Appropriate electroencephalograph (EEG) monitoring is warranted until the patient regains consciousness. Hyponatremia and acidosis generally resolve with adequate hydration and blood replacement. Aggressive treatment with hypertonic solutions or bicarbonate is not generally necessary. A high parasitemia precedes a drop in hemoglobin and this should be anticipated; therefore, type and cross-match may be advisable, even if transfusion is not warranted on admission. Steroids and prophylactic anticonvulsants have not been shown to be effective. For high levels of parasitemia, exchange transfusion has been advocated by some. This will not eradicate sequestered parasites and, if used, consideration should be given to the impact of the exchange on antimalarial levels in blood and tissue.

Uncomplicated malaria caused by *P. falciparum* can be treated with chloroquine when certain that the infection was acquired in a region where chloroquine sensitivity still prevails. If in doubt or the infection was acquired in a chloroquine-resistant region, oral atovaquone-proguanil, quinine, and artesunate, or mefloquine can be used. Close observation is needed. Any vomiting or clinical deterioration requires that the patient receive parenteral therapy. The other plasmodial species remain for the most part sensitive to chloroquine, but treatment of *P. ovale* or *P. vivax* must be followed by an agent that can clear hypnozoite from the liver and prevent relapse. Primaquine is the drug of choice for hypnozoite clearance, but screening for G6PD deficiency must precede use of this drug. It is important to recognize that national drug policies for the treatment of malaria in malaria endemic regions are developed for the country's native population and treatment recommendations may not be adequate for the nonimmune adult traveler.

Even with appropriate therapy, cerebral malaria can result in CNS sequelae, including stroke-related deficits, epilepsy, cognitive dysfunction, and behavioral abnormalities. In developed country settings, long-term follow-up should be planned to assess for these outcomes and provide appropriate rehabilitation, support, and treatment.

TABLE 101-2. Treatment Regimen for Severe *P. falciparum* Malaria[a]

Medication	*Dosing*
Artesunate (only available in the United States via the CDC)	2.4 mg/kg IM or IV followed by 1.2 mg/kg at 12 hours, and 24 hours. Then daily for 6 days.
Quinine	20 mg/kg over 4 hours slow IV infusions as a loading dose. Then 10 mg/kg every 8 hours in adults, every 12 hours in children until able to take orally. Complete 5 to 7 days. In regions with reported quinine resistence, consider additional treatment with tetracycline, doxycycline, clindamycin, or azithromycin for 5 days.
Quinidine gluconate plus doxycycline, tetracycline,[b] or clindamycin	6.25 mg/kg base (10 mg/kg salt) over 1 to 2 hours. Then 0.0125 mg base/kg/min continuous infusion for 24 hours. Change to oral treatment when parasite density is <1% and the patient is taking oral medications. Doxycycline 100 mg IV every 12 hours and switch to orals when patient able. Complete treatment in 7 days. Clindamycin 10 mg/kg loading dose IV, followed by 5 mg/kg every 8 hours until patient can take orally. Complete treatment in 7 days.
Alternate choices: Rectal artesunate or artemesinin, IM artemesinin, or mefloquine per NGT.	

CDC, Centers for Disease Control and Prevention; IM, intramuscularly; IV, intravenous; NGT, nasogastric tube.
[a]Readers are encouraged to access up-to-date treatment recommendations via the internet. See References.
[b]Tetracycline and doxycycline should be avoided in children and pregnant women.

CLINICAL RECOMMENDATIONS OF THE VIGNETTE

The patient's abrupt decline warrants rapid assessment and intervention. The "ABC" assessment should include a bedside evaluation for hypoglycemia. A parenteral antimalarial drug (Table 101-2) should be given immediately. Thick and thin blood films should be taken immediately to look for malaria parasites and antimalarial treatment should be initiated, pending results (Table 101-2). If available, a RDT searching for malaria antigens should be completed. If not, repeat blood films every 4 hours should be taken until parasites are identified or another diagnosis explaining the patient's clinical condition is confirmed. A brain CT scan and lumbar puncture, as well as pancultures, should be obtained to rule out other causes of her illness or comorbid septicemia. CT findings of cerebral malaria vary widely, and may be normal. Large vessel strokes, generalized cerebral edema, venous sinus thrombosis, venous infarcts, and hydrocephalus can also be seen, however, and should be initiated while further CNS assessment. Nontyphi salmonella septicemia is a common coinfection with severe malaria in both children and adults. The differential diagnosis should include other potential tropical causes for the traveler. Details depend on the locations in which they traveled and related exposures. In this young woman, a pregnancy test should be done because pregnancy would increase her susceptibility to malaria and would also guide treatment. Additional supportive care with antipyretics and intravenous fluids, and, possibly, blood tranfusion as well.

Admission to an intensive care unit is warranted to assure close assessment, particularly for interim seizures or other organ system involvement. Cardiac monitoring is recommended for administration of quinidine. Frequent neurologic assessment should be done using the Glasgow Coma scale in adults, and the Blantyre Coma scale in children. Hemoglobin and glucose levels should be reassessed closely, and volume status, electrolytes, and liver functions should also be monitored.

SUMMARY

Severe malaria caused by *P. falciparum* can be a rapidly fatal condition among nonimmune persons if diagnosis and treatment are delayed. A high level of suspicion must be maintained in travelers as well as in individuals with other potential exposures. Treatment options likely depend on the setting and vary country to country. Given the rapidly evolving resistence patterns and treatment options, the best sources of information are up-to-date websites and public health agencies expert in the disease (World Health Organization, US Center for Disease Control and Prevention). For US health care providers needing assistance with diagnosis or management of suspected cases of malaria should call the CDC Malaria Hotline: 770-488-7788 (M-F, 8 AM to 4:30 PM, Eastern time). For emergency consultation after hours, call: 770-488-7100 and request to speak with a CDC Malaria Branch clinician.

REFERENCES

1. John D, Petri W. Malaria. *Medical Parasitology*. St. Louis: Saunders Elsevier; 2006:79–106.
2. CDC. Malaria. 2006 [cited; Available from: http://www.cdc.gov/malaria/[accessed 11 April 2007]
3. World Health Organization. *Management of Severe Malaria*. 2000 [accessed 18 September 2006]; Available from http://www.wpro.who.int/sites/rdt/using_rdts/RDT+Instructions+and+ Training.htm
4. Warrell D, Gilles H. *Essential Malariology*, 4th ed. New York: Oxford University Press; 2002.
5. Newton CR, Valim C, Krishna S, et al. and for the Severe Malaria in African Children Network. The prognostic value of measures of acid/base balance in pediatric falciparum malaria, compared with other clinical and laboratory parameters. *Clin Infect Dis*. 2005; 41:948–957. Epub 2005 Aug 23. PMID. 16142658.
6. World Health Organization. http://www.who.int/malaria/docs/hbsm_toc.htm

CHAPTER 102

Other Tropical Infections

Ana-Claire L. Meyer • Glenn E. Mathisen

OBJECTIVES

- To discuss the three common preventable neurologic diseases still prevalent worldwide
- To review the epidemiology, current prevention, and control efforts for these diseases

CASE VIGNETTE

A 22-year-old man presented to a clinic complaining of nausea, vomiting, and right flank pain. He immigrated from El Salvador to the United States 15 months before the onset of symptoms. Urinalysis showed hematuria and pyuria. He was sent home with oral antibiotics and pain medication for a urinary tract infection. On the following day, he presented to the emergency department with continued right flank pain. He also had throat tightness and difficulty swallowing, and told nurses he could not breathe when looking at water. His complaints were thought to stem from an allergic reaction. His symptoms improved with the administration of steroids and diphenhydramine. He was diagnosed with nephrolithiasis, and again sent home with additional pain medication. On the third day, he returned to the same emergency department with shortness of breath and difficulty swallowing. He left before seeing a physician.

Over the next 24 hours, the patient's family noted he became increasingly agitated and confused, claiming to be "a disciple of God." They called 911 and he was transported to another hospital when he was found to be anxious, combative, salivating profusely, and afraid to swallow his own secretions. His temperature was 101.8°F. Pulse was 141 beats per minute. Oxygen saturation was 98%. Laboratory evaluation was notable for a serum potassium level of 2.8 mmol/L and a white blood cell (WBC) count of 14,800 mm^3, with 79% neutrophils. Abdominal computed tomography (CT) was consistent with nephrolithiasis. Notes from the emergency department documented he ran out of the building during his CT scan, and had to be retrieved. He was started on intravenous fluid and antibiotics, with little improvement. Throughout the course of his admission he became increasingly violent and remained combative, confused, agitated, afraid of swallowing, and with excessive salivation. A CT of the head showed no intracranial pathology. Repeat CT scan of the abdomen showed the presence of extraluminal mediastinal air. A lumbar puncture was delayed because of the abdominal radiographic findings. An esophagogram was attempted to evaluate for a possible esophageal tear. During the procedure, the patient developed cardiopulmonary arrest. Resuscitation efforts were unsuccessful (1).

DEFINITION

A wide variety of infectious diseases that affect the nervous system are endemic in tropical latitudes, including human immunodeficiency virus (HIV) and acquired immunodeficiency syndrome (AIDS), tuberculosis, leprosy, malaria, viral encephalitides, and parasitic diseases. Developing countries are disproportionately represented in the tropical latitudes and bear the burden of these diseases because of the unequal distribution of health resources. The focus of this chapter is on preventable diseases, those that remain significant sources of morbidity and mortality in the developing world despite simple, effective preventive measures. Effective vaccines have been available for decades for poliomyelitis, rabies, and tetanus. Although these diseases have been largely eliminated from developed countries, they remain a serious problem in developing countries where access to immunization can be limited.

Poliomyelitis

EPIDEMIOLOGY

Crippling diseases resembling poliomyelitis were first described in antiquity, although the first poliomyelitis outbreaks did not occur until the 19th century (2). For the next century, each summer and fall, epidemics were reported in the northern hemisphere. In 1952, the polio epidemic reached a peak in the United States, with more than 21,000 paralytic cases of the disease (2). In 1955, the inactivated poliovirus vaccine (IPV) was developed, and was followed quickly by the development of the oral trivalent polio vaccine (OPV) in 1963. Massive immunization campaigns in the United States dramatically decreased the incidence of polio such that the last domestically acquired wild polio case was reported in 1979. Worldwide, poliomyelitis, remains a problem (2). In 1988, the World Health Organization (WHO) began working toward the global eradication of poliomyelitis. Currently, vaccine coverage is estimated at 85% of the worldwide population. This initiative has decreased the incidence of polio from 52,795 cases in 1980, to 1,259 in 2004.

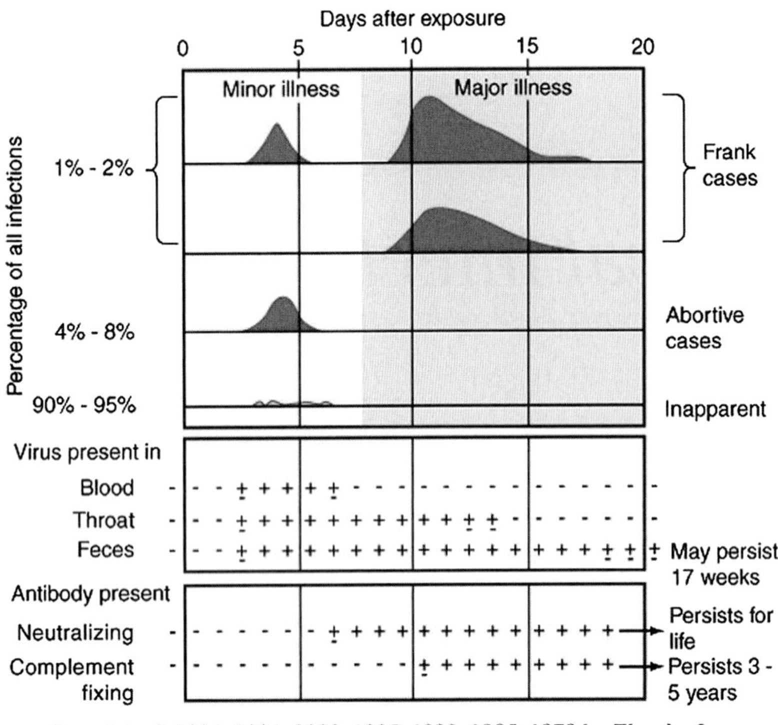

FIGURE 102-1. Poliovirus infection. (From Modlin JF. Chapter 168: Poliovirus. Principles and Practice of Infectious Diseases, ed. Mandell GL, Bennett JE, Dolin R. 6th ed. Philadelphia, Elsevier, 2005, with permission.)

Only four countries still have endemic transmission: India, Pakistan, Nigeria, and Afghanistan (3).

ETIOLOGY AND PATHOGENESIS

Poliomyelitis is caused by an infection with an RNA enterovirus of the family Picornaviridae. The poliovirus has three subtypes with minimal heterotypic immunity between the serotypes (one subtype does not confer immunity to the other subtypes). Poliovirus enters through the mouth and multiplies in the pharynx and gastrointestinal (GI) tract. The virus then invades local lymphoid tissue and enters the bloodstream. It is not known whether the poliovirus reaches the nervous system via retrograde axonal transport in peripheral nerves or by hematogenous spread. Replication of poliovirus in the spinal cord and brainstem leads to the destruction of motor neurons and thereby to the clinical manifestations of the disease (2,4,5).

PATHOLOGY

A mononuclear infiltrate into the perivascular lymphatic spaces of the meninges is noted in early acute infection. This is followed by an acute interstitial meningitis without exudate that is most marked on the anterior surface of the spinal cord, especially the anterior fissure. Histologically, neurons are observed in all stages of degeneration in the anterior horn of the spinal cord, motor nuclei of the brainstem, reticular formation, vestibular nuclei, cerebellar nuclei, hypothalamus, and thalamus. In severe cases, a striking absence of neurons is accompanied by a hyperemic perivascular infiltrate, hemorrhage, edema, and a diffuse cellular infiltrate. Early lesions are frequently found in the dorsal root ganglia (6).

CLINICAL MANIFESTATIONS

The clinical manifestations of infection with poliovirus are variable. Approximately 95% of patients are asymptomatic. Despite the lack of symptoms, these individuals continue to shed virus in the stool for several weeks and may infect others. A small percentage (4% to 8%) of patients develop *abortive poliomyelitis,* a nonspecific "viral" illness characterized by fever, sore throat, nausea and vomiting, diarrhea, and myalgias, in varying combinations. These individuals recover completely in 1 week and do not develop neurologic symptoms. Another 1% to 2% of patients develop *nonparalytic poliomyelitis,* an aseptic meningitis lasting 2 to 10 days that is followed by a complete recovery. Less than 1% of infections result in paralytic polio. Patients have an initial prodrome *(minor illness)* for 1 to 3 days that resembles abortive poliomyelitis and represents the onset of viremia. After a short period of recovery (2 to 5 days), fever recurs accompanied by malaise and signs of aseptic meningitis. These symptoms herald the onset of the *major illness,* a phase characterized by severe myalgias, frank weakness, and paralysis (Fig. 102-1) (2,4,7).

Spinal poliomyelitis is the most common presentation. Onset is sudden and swift and may occur over hours. Hyperesthesia and muscle tenderness are frequently present and are worse in the limb that might subsequently become paralyzed. Asymmetric weakness is the hallmark of poliomyelitis, with variable involvement of one or both legs, arms, trunk, and spinal and cranial nerves. The weakness can be ascending or descending. In the legs, the quadriceps, anterior tibial muscles, and the extensor hallucis longus are most frequently affected, whereas in the arm, the most commonly affected muscles are the deltoids and finger extensors. The diaphragm and lateral abdominal muscles are often involved. Sphincter involvement is rare in children, but can occur in adults (6). During the early stages, the muscle stretch reflexes are preserved, and may even be hyperreflexic. During the later stages, physical examination shows a flaccid paralysis accompanied by coarse fasciculations and absent muscle stretch reflexes.

Bulbar symptoms may accompany weakness in bulbospinal forms. Cranial nerve involvement may be subtle and signs are almost always unilateral. Involvement of cranial nerves (C.N.) IX and X is commonly observed and results in hoarseness, which may progress to aphonia and dysphagia. The facial nerve (C.N. VII) is also frequently affected; less commonly affected are the nerves to the extra-ocular muscles (C.N. III, IV, VI), while the optic nerves are spared. Nystagmus is occasionally observed, as is unilateral tongue weakness. Ataxia, especially spastic ataxia, is not uncommon. Unusual clinical presentations include Landry's paralysis, where an ascending paralysis is associated with a characteristic arrhythmia in which sinus rhythm alternates with abrupt changes in rate. On rare occasions, patients may present with encephalitis; this is most common in infants (6).

DIAGNOSTIC APPROACH

In contrast to other enteroviruses, poliovirus is rarely cultured from the cerebrospinal fluid (CSF) and diagnosis rests on serologic studies or isolation of the virus from the stools or the pharynx. It is possible to isolate the virus from the CSF, but it is rarely found. If polio is isolated from a patient with an acute flaccid paralysis, genomic sequencing or oligonucleotide mapping is necessary to determine whether the virus is wild type or vaccine type. Neutralizing antibodies appear early and may be at high levels by the time the patient is hospitalized, so a rising titer may not be observed. CSF shows a lymphocytic pleocytosis (10 to 200 cells/mm^3) and mild elevation in protein levels (40 to 50 mg/100 mL) (2). Differential diagnosis includes infections with other enteroviruses (e.g., coxsackievirus A7 and enterovirus 71), tick-borne encephalitis, and flavivirus (Japanese encephalitis and West Nile virus). Other processes, such as Guillain-Barré syndrome, acute intermittent porphyria, HIV neuropathy, diphtheria, myasthenia gravis, and botulism, can mimic some of the symptoms and signs (4).

TREATMENT

Treatment of paralytic polio is largely supportive. Pain relief, respiratory and nutritional support, and prevention of the complications of severe illness, such as pneumonia and deep vein thrombosis, are essential. Strict bed rest is important during the early stages of the disease. Soon thereafter, physical and occupational therapy should begin, initially focusing on frequent passive movements, stretching, and splinting to prevent contractures. Subsequently, intensive rehabilitation and support are essential to a functional recovery (4). With modern medical care, mortality from paralytic poliomyelitis is 2% to 5% for children and 15% to 30% for adults. With bulbar involvement, mortality increases to 25% to 75% (2).

PREVENTION

Clearly, the best treatment for poliomyelitis is to prevent the disease by immunization. Available vaccines include the IPV based on the Salk preparation, and the live oral polio vaccine developed by Sabin. IPV and OPV are roughly equivalent in efficacy, both containing all three polio subtypes, although current IPV preparations result in higher antibody titers than OPV (8). OPV provides better intestinal immunity and costs less. Fecal shedding of virus following vaccination with OPV leads to increased "herd" immunity in a community; this is a distinct advantage in countries where widespread vaccination is impossible. The rare occurrence of vaccine-associated paralytic polio (VAPP) following OPV has dampened enthusiasm for live polio vaccines in developed countries. This complication occurs most commonly in children or adults who are immune deficient; although the exact mechanism is unclear, prolonged carriage of the virus can lead to strain mutation with reversion to neurovirulence. Since 1980, there have been 152 cases of VAPP in the United States; because of this complication, in 2000, the Centers for Disease Control and Prevention (CDC) recommended that only IPV be used for vaccination in the United States. Children should be vaccinated with IPV at 2, 4, and 6 to 18 months of age, with a booster dose at 4 to 6 years of age. Adults who have never been vaccinated may receive the first dose at any time, with a second dose 1 to 2 months later, and a third dose 6 to 12 months thereafter (2).

Recently, a postpolio syndrome has been described where patients with residual impairments following paralytic poliomyelitis develop new disabilities many years later. Typical symptoms include weakness, pain, fatigue, progressive muscular atrophy, impairment of activities of daily living, or respiratory symptoms. The severity of the initial symptoms seems to predispose to later functional deterioration. The existence of postpolio syndrome as a separate clinical entity, however, remains somewhat controversial (4).

Rabies

EPIDEMIOLOGY

Rabies was first described more than 4,000 years ago in the Eshuma Code in Babylon. Until the development of the first rabies vaccine by Louis Pasteur, rabies infection was universally fatal. Each year, approximately 1 to 3 deaths are reported in the United States, although 25,000 to 40,000 people are treated for exposure at a cost of about $1,000 per person. Postexposure prophylaxis is too costly for many developing countries; therefore, worldwide, rabies encephalitis results in 30,000 to 70,000 deaths each year (9). Rabies is found in animal reservoirs of all but a few countries. Countries free of rabies are primarily islands with strict quarantine laws (10). In developed countries, domesticated animals account for 10% of exposures and wild animals, in particular skunks, foxes, raccoons, and bats, account for the other 90%. Since 1985, in the United States, 32 of 35 cases of indigenous human rabies were caused by insectivorous bat strains of the rabies virus, many of these with no clear history of a bat bite (11). In developing countries, dogs account for most exposures (10).

ETIOLOGY AND PATHOGENESIS

Rabies is caused by a bullet-shaped RNA rhabdovirus that is a member of the family Rhabdoviridae and genus Lyssavirus. Rabies, the first of seven lyssavirus genotypes to be identified, is responsible for almost all human disease; other genotypes may rarely cause a rabieslike encephalitis (10,11). Genetic sequencing can currently identify various species-specific rabies viruses (e.g., bat versus raccoon) and is helpful in determining the source of the virus in a specific case (10,11). Rabies is primarily transmitted by saliva in the bite of an infected animal. Isolated reports, however, indicate transmission via skin abrasions, aerosolized virus contaminating mucous membranes, corneal transplantation, and, most recently, transmission following solid organ donation (12). Transplacental infection has not been reported in humans (9,10).

PATHOLOGY

The bite of a rabid animal injects virus-laden saliva through skin into muscle and subcutaneous tissues. After local replication in the infected muscle, retrograde transport in sensory or motor nerves carries the virus at a rate of about 50 to 100 mm/day to the central nervous system (CNS), where there is massive replication of the virus on the endoplasmic reticulum within neurons. Although the exact mechanism is unknown, direct transmission is thought to occur across synaptic junctions. Following infection of the CNS, the virus spreads via the peripheral nervous system to many tissues, including skeletal and cardiac muscle, adrenal glands, kidney, retina, cornea, pancreas, and the nerves around hair follicles. Productive viral replication with budding from plasma membranes takes place predominantly in the salivary glands; this leads to infection of the saliva and plays a role in subsequent transmission of the virus (10).

Despite the devastating clinical effects of rabies, surprisingly few histopathologic changes are seen; the brain may appear normal at early stages, and even late disease and death can occur with only minimal changes, even on electron microscopy (10). Inflammation is most marked in the midbrain and medulla oblongata in furious rabies, and in the spinal cord in paralytic rabies. Perineural and perivascular mononuclear cell infiltration and neuronophagia may be observed. Vascular lesions, such as thrombosis or hemorrhage, have also been described. Negri bodies are pathognomonic intracytoplasmic inclusions; often few in number, they are found in up to 80% of cases on postmortem examination (Fig. 102-2). Additional findings can include ganglion cell degeneration in the brain, spinal cord, and peripheral nerves, or focal degeneration of the salivary and lacrymal glands, pancreas, and adrenal medulla (13).

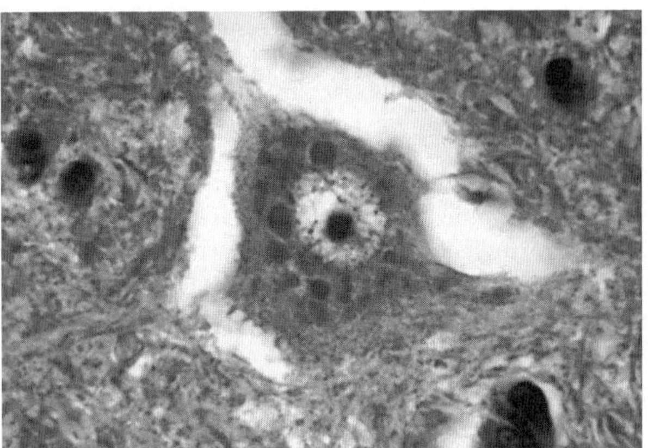

FIGURE 102-2. Negri bodies in a Purkinje cell. Hematoxylin and eosin stain. (From Perl D. Image 3377. In: Public Health Image Library, Centers for Disease Control and Prevention, www.phil.cdc.gov; 1971, with permission.)

CLINICAL PRESENTATION

Rabies typically presents with one of two major clinical syndromes: (*a*) furious rabies, a form of acute encephalitis, and (*b*) paralytic (dumb) rabies. Following exposure, the incubation period varies widely, and depends on the location of the bite; bites on the head and neck have the shortest incubation periods and those on the lower legs the longest (13). The average incubation period is 20 to 60 days, but ranges from as short as 10 days to as long as a year or more. The initial symptoms or the prodrome consists of nonspecific symptoms, such as fever, malaise, or headache; the presence of itching or paresthesia at the site of a healed bite wound is transient but can be a clue to rabies in a suspect case. The acute neurologic syndrome develops 2 to 7 days after onset of the prodrome and may include autonomic disturbances, such as excessive salivation, sweating, and labile blood pressure. An encephalitic picture develops and is characterized by irritability, anxiety, agitation and delirium, hyperreflexia, nuchal rigidity, and visual and auditory hallucinations. Patients frequently become combative and exhibit violent tendencies, sometimes spitting on, or attempting to bite, those around them. The symptoms culminate in manic behavior alternating with lethargy (10).

Hydrophobia is a pathognomonic sign in rabies; the patient develops a pathologic fear of swallowing, and attempts to drink result in painful laryngospasm combined with inspiratory muscle spasm. With progression of disease, this can be provoked by drafts—aerophobia—which may be accompanied by extension of the back and arms, and result in convulsions or cardiorespiratory arrest. Coma develops 7 to 10 days after onset of the acute neurologic syndrome and is characterized by prolonged apnea, generalized flaccid paralysis, and seizures. Although death may be delayed by life-support measures, patients typically die within 2 to 3 days after onset of paralysis because of respiratory and vascular collapse (10,13). The differential diagnosis for furious rabies includes delirium tremens, botulism, diphtheria, drug ingestion (phenothiazines and amphetamines), plant ingestion, and tetanus.

Paralytic rabies accounts for <20% of cases and usually results from vampire bat bites or occurs in individuals who received preexposure vaccination. Flaccid paralysis develops after the prodrome. It typically begins in the bitten limb and may ascend symmetrically or asymmetrically, with pain and fasciculations in the affected muscles. Mild sensory disturbances are common. Paraplegia and sphincter disturbances follow, and finally respiratory and swallowing muscles are involved. Hydrophobia is rare, but may be noted in the terminal phases. The course is somewhat slower, with most patients surviving up to 30 days without intensive care unit support (13). The differential diagnosis for paralytic rabies is Guillain-Barré syndrome, poliomyelitis, arbovirus encephalitis, and *Herpes simiae* (from monkey bites) (13).

DIAGNOSIS

Any acute neuropsychiatric presentation with a history of recent travel to a rabies endemic region, a recent bite, or bat contact should raise suspicion for rabies (11). If the animal is available, it should be monitored for symptoms and, on developing symptoms, should be immediately killed. Rabies antigen may be detected by direct immunofluorescence (DFA) or polymerase chain reaction (PCR). The best test for early diagnosis is DFA of a nuchal skin biopsy. Other tests, such as PCR of the CSF or saliva, and DFA of the serum, have high specificity but relatively low sensitivity; further, many patients die before they develop detectable antibodies (10,13).

TREATMENT

Traditionally, rabies has been a universally fatal disease in unvaccinated patients. Intensive care can prolong life, but has not changed mortality, and, therefore, for most unvaccinated patients, palliative care alone is recommended. Nevertheless, in a recent case an unvaccinated 15-year-old girl survived rabies infection after treatment with ribavirin and amantadine and coma induction with ketamine and benzodiazepines (14). A few vaccinated patients have survived, albeit with devastating neurologic sequelae (10).

PREVENTION

Again, the most effective treatment is prevention (Table 102-1). Prevention efforts focus on eliminating infection in vectors, preexposure prophylaxis in high risk individuals, and prompt postexposure prophylaxis (10,11). Postexposure treatment begins with prompt, thorough cleaning of the wound. In experimental animals, wound cleaning alone was very successful in preventing transmission (13). The local public health department should be consulted for assistance in deciding whether to administer postexposure prophylaxis. Active and passive immunization should be given to those with high risk of exposure (Table 102-1). Vaccine failures have occurred with deviation from the vaccination schedule and vaccination in the gluteal area. Of note, no evidence indicates that rabies immune globulin (RIG) or vaccines cause fetal abnormalities, so pregnancy should not be a contraindication to vaccination (10).

In the United States, human RIG (HRIG) and human diploid cell vaccines (HDCV), rabies vaccine adsorbed (RVA), or purified chick embryo cell vaccines (PCEV) have replaced older formulations. Modern rabies vaccines can cause local pain and swelling at the injection site, but they have much lower rates of immune complex reaction and Guillain-Barré-like syndromes (10). Common complications are pain and soreness around the injection site. Equine RIG, although less expensive, carries a risk of serum sickness and is not recommended if HRIG is available. The nervous tissue rabies vaccines, the Semple (sheep brain) vaccine, suckling mouse brain vaccine, and Fermi vaccine are far less efficacious and have substantially higher risks of neurologic side effects. In many parts of the world, however, these are the only treatments available (10,11).

TABLE 102-1. Rabies Prevention Strategies

Strategy	*Target Population*	*Modality*
Eliminate infection in vectors	Domestic and stray dogs	Vaccination program Fertility control
	Wildlife: Fox, coyote, raccoon	Wildlife vaccination program
	Insectivorous bats	No known methods: Avoid contact
Preexposure prophylaxis	Exposure to rabid animals (animal handlers, veterinarians)	Three doses rabies vaccine, intramuscularly (IM), into deltoid; days 0, 7, 21, or 28
	Laboratory workers	Boosters every 6 to 24 months when antibody titers wane
	Travelers to endemic countries with no access to health care	Three doses rabies vaccine IM into deltoid; days 0, 7, 21, or 28 No boosters
Strategy	*Modality*	
Postexposure prophylaxis	Clean wound: Scrub edges of wound and punctures thoroughly	Soap, iodine, 40% to 70% alcohol, quarternary ammonium compounds (cetrimide 0.1%)
	Consult local health department to determine whether vaccination necessary	Healthy, immunized domestic animal (dog, cat, ferret)→ observe for 10 days, vaccinate patient only if animal becomes sick Sick domestic animal or any wild animal→ vaccinate patient
	Active vaccination	***Previously immunized*** Two doses rabies vaccine IM into deltoid; days 0, 3 ***Not immunized*** Five doses rabies vaccine IM into deltoid; days 0, 3, 7, 14, 28
	Passive vaccination[a]	***Not immunized*** 20 IU/kg body weight given into wound if anatomically feasible, otherwise into buttocks

[a]Avoid giving larger than recommended doses of rabies immune globulin (RIG) or administering the drug more than 7 days after the first dose of the rabies vaccine, because both may decrease the response to active immunization.

(From Hankins D, Rosekrans J. Overview, prevention, and treatment of rabies. *Mayo Clin Proc.* 2004;79:671–676, with permission.)

Tetanus

EPIDEMIOLOGY

Tetanus has been described since antiquity, with clinical descriptions appearing as early as the 5th century BCE. Passive immunization for treatment and prophylaxis was first used in World War I, and tetanus toxoid was first widely used in World War II (2). Currently, tetanus is endemic in over 90 countries, but vaccine deployment is incomplete (15). The WHO estimates that 51% of pregnant women, and 80% of those <1 year of age are immunized (3). Case estimates and estimates of mortality from tetanus vary widely because case reporting is not accurate. The WHO estimates that about 250,000 neonatal deaths from tetanus occur per year, which represents 7% of total neonatal deaths worldwide and >95% of tetanus deaths worldwide. Africa alone accounts for about half of the cases (3). In contrast, 20 to 60 cases per year occur in the United States, although, of concern, a recent national survey showed that 20% of adolescents, and 69% of adults >70 years of age did not have protective levels of antibody (15).

ETIOLOGY AND PATHOGENESIS

The causative agent for tetanus is *Clostridium tetani*, an obligate anaerobic, spore-forming gram-positive bacilli (15). The spores are extremely stable; some will even survive boiling for 15 minutes (2). *C. tetani* is widely distributed in the environment, especially in soil, and is found in the intestinal flora of domestic animals, livestock, and humans (15). Tetanus most commonly develops in wounds with low tissue oxygen tension, where anaerobic growth can occur. The most common types of infections that lead to tetanus are deep penetrating wounds on the extremities, postpartum or postabortion infections of the uterus, nonsterile intramuscular injections (especially of quinine), and infection following compound fractures. Even minor trauma can lead to disease, however, and in 30% of patients no portal of entry is apparent. Neonatal tetanus occurs in infants born to mothers who were not vaccinated or who lack appropriate postvaccination titers. In these cases, lack of access to sterile delivery facilities and sterile surgical instruments for cutting the umbilical cord, and female or male circumcision places infants at high risk, as does certain other traditional practices, such as applying sheep or cow dung to umbilical cord stumps (15,16).

PATHOLOGY

C. tetani may acquire a plasmid that produces two toxins, tetanolysin and tetanospasmin. Tetanospasmin—the primary toxin responsible for clinical symptoms—is a zinc metalloprotease that cleaves synaptobrevin, a membrane protein necessary for the export of intracellular vesicles. Absence of synaptobrevin inhibits release of glycine and γ-aminobutyric acid (GABA) in inhibitory neurons. Interneurons of the spinal cord are the first affected, followed by preganglionic sympathetic neurons in the lateral horns, and finally parasympathetic centers. Motor neurons are also affected, leading to decreased acetylcholine release, but the clinical effects are minimal (17). Disinhibited efferent discharge from motor neurons in the spinal cord and brainstem lead to the classic clinical manifestations of intense muscular rigidity and spasm. Although similar in appearance to convulsions, in tetanic spasms, the reflex inhibition of antagonist muscle groups is lost; both agonist and antagonist muscle groups contract simultaneously, which can lead to tendon avulsion, tendon rupture, or fractures. Disinhibited autonomic discharge leads to disturbances in autonomic control, especially sympathetic overactivity and excessive plasma catecholamine levels. Toxin binding is thought to be irreversible, and recovery likely requires the growth of new nerve terminals (17).

CLINICAL PRESENTATION

Neonatal tetanus develops within a week of birth; infants present with high fever, inability to suck, opisthotonus, vomiting, and spasms, which are often mistaken for convulsions. Differential diagnosis should include hypocalcemia, hypoglycemia, meningitis, meningoencephalitis, and seizures. Neonatal mortality rates reach 75% to 80% (16).

In adults, the incubation period (time between inoculation and symptoms) ranges from 24 hours to several months, and is dependent on the distance the toxin must travel from the wound site to reach the CNS, and may be dependent on the amount of toxin. The most common form in adults is *generalized tetanus*. The initial symptoms can be headache, local rigidity and pain at the site of the wound, or trismus (lockjaw), the inability to fully open the mouth because of rigidity of the masseters. Generalized stiffness and rigidity leading to opisthotonus frequently develop and are punctuated by painful spasms, which are elicited by minor stimuli, such as noise, touch, or simple medical and nursing procedures (15). Spasms are excruciatingly painful and most prominent during the first 2 weeks; they can be uncontrollable, leading to respiratory arrest and death. Autonomic disturbance develops several days after the spasms and reaches a peak during the second week of disease. Autonomic storms with elevation of plasma catecholamine levels up to 10 times over normal are common. Persistent tachycardia and hypertension, vasoconstriction, and pyrexia can alternate with profound hypotension, bradycardia, or recurrent cardiac arrest. Profuse salivation, increased bronchial secretions, gastric stasis, ileus, diarrhea, and acute renal failure are also observed (15). Differential diagnosis includes tetany, strychnine poisoning, dystonic reactions, rabies, and orofacial infection (15).

Local tetanus, another form of tetanus in adults, which is characterized by muscle rigidity localized to the wound site, has low mortality. A special form of local tetanus, *cephalic tetanus*, results from injuries to the head or face, and instead of rigidity, often presents with a unilateral lower motor neuron facial nerve palsy. Although traditionally this form has higher mortality, modern case reports suggest that milder, unrecognized cases may be more common than previously thought (18).

DIAGNOSIS

Diagnosis of tetanus remains clinical. Most patients with tetanus do not have detectable antibody levels, although patients can develop tetanus despite adequate titers; therefore, positive tetanus antibodies should not be used to exclude tetanus. *C. tetani* is difficult to culture and is only cultured from about 30% of wounds, so negative cultures should also not be used to exclude tetanus (16).

TREATMENT

In individuals with clinical signs of tetanus, wound débridement, passive immunization, and antibiotics are recommended. Metronidazole is given to patients to eliminate any remaining viable bacteria. Previously, penicillin G was used, but a few studies suggest that metronidazole may be superior to penicillin, and that penicillin may act as a competitive antagonist of GABA, thereby worsening clinical symptoms (15,17). Severe tetanus requires 3 to 5 weeks of intensive care unit support, which consists of three primary components: Control of rigidity and spasms, control of autonomic dysfunction, and supportive care (Table 102-2) (2,17).

With regard to prognosis, mortality and outcomes vary dramatically, depending on available facilities. In developing countries without facilities for prolonged intensive care, unit care, and respiratory support, mortality still exceeds 50%, primarily from airway obstruction, respiratory failure, or renal failure. In the United States, mortality in adults <30 years of age approaches zero, but in those >62, approaches 52% (15,17). Recently, Thwaites et al. (20) developed a prospective scoring system, which may be superior to previous scoring systems.

PREVENTION

Tetanus is preventable with vaccination. In the United States, the tetanus antitoxoid vaccine is recommended for all persons at least 6 weeks old (Table102-3) (20). Neonatal tetanus can be prevented by vaccinating the mother before, or during, pregnancy; passive transfer of antitoxoid antibodies then occurs, and the fetus is protected during delivery and in the neonatal period. Tetanus toxoid has not been associated with fetal malformations and is deemed safe to use during pregnancy. This regimen is 90% effective; immunization failures have been reported, although they usually are caused by subpotent toxoid preparation (16). For guidelines for tetanus prophylaxis after a wound, vaccination and tetanus immune globulin are used in select circumstances (Table 102-4) (2,15,20).

TABLE 102-2. Treatment of Severe Tetanus

1. Wound débridement	Direct effects on clinical course unclear
2. Passive immunization	Shorten disease course, reduce severity
3. Antibiotics	Metronidazole 500 mg three times daily for 7 to 10 days
4. Intensive Care Unit Support	
• Control of rigidity and spasms	Benzodiazepines Phenobarbitone Chlorpromazine Propofol
• Control of autonomic dysfunction	Fluid loading Sedation with morphine and benzodiazepines Magnesium sulfate (Beta-blockers relatively contraindicated)
• Supportive care	Early enteral nutrition and gastrostomy tube Tracheostomy
• Active immunization	Once clinical condition has stabilized

(From Cook T, Protheroe R, Handel J. Tetanus: A review of the literature. *Br J Anaesth.* 2001;87(3):477–487, with permission.)

TABLE 102-3. Vaccination Guidelines for Tetanus Prevention (20)

Population	*Vaccine Formulation*	*Time Schedule*
Children	DtaP[a]	Three doses at 2, 4, 6 months of age Boosters at: 15–18 months of age, 4–6 years old
Adults	Td[b]	Boosters every 10 years
Pregnant women	Td[b]	If previously unvaccinated: Three doses 4–6 weeks apart • 2nd dose at least 4 weeks before delivery; • 3rd dose post-partum If previously vaccinated with full series: • Booster required within 10 years

[a]DtaP (diptheria, tetanus, pertussis).
[b]Td (tetanus, diptheria).
(From Nagachinta T, Cortese M, Roper M, et al. Chapter 13: Tetanus. Manual for the surveillance of Vacceni-Preventable Diseases. 3rd edition. Wharton M, Hughes H, and Reilly M. Centers for Disease Control and Prevention, eds. 2002. http://www.cdc.gov/nip/publications/surv-manual/deFault.htm; Accessed 8/25/06, with permission.)

CLINICAL RECOMMENDATIONS OF THE VIGNETTE

Postmortem examination of the patient showed histopathologic evidence of rabies encephalomyelitis with Negri bodies and perivascular cuffing on hematoxylin and eosin stain of brain tissue (Fig. 102-2). Direct fluorescent antibody staining for rabies antigen was performed by the CDC and confirmed the diagnosis. Genetic sequencing identified the virus as a canine variant from El Salvador. Additional history did not reveal any evidence of animal bites or exposures. Although rabies was suspected by an infectious disease physician who evaluated the patient, the case was not reported to the public health department until after his death; this delay in diagnosis resulted in the need for postexposure prophylaxis in more than 30 close contacts and 9 of 76 health care workers who provided care for the patient. Many states require mandatory reporting of suspected rabies cases to prevent additional exposure and injury.

SUMMARY

Despite effective, safe, and inexpensive preventative treatments, polio, tetanus, and rabies are frequently encountered in the developing world. Effective long-term control of vaccine-preventable disease requires effective public health and health infrastructure, which many developing countries still lack. Concerted efforts over several decades have led, however, to the near global eradication of poliomyelitis, which serves as a

TABLE 102-4. Tetanus Prophylaxis As Part of Wound Management

Wound Type	*Vaccination Status*	*Treatment*
Major wound[a]	Unknown vaccine status	Tetanus toxoid vaccine
	Incomplete vaccine series	Tetanus immune globulin[b]
	Complete series, last booster >5 years ago	Tetanus toxoid vaccine
	Complete series, recent booster	No treatment necessary
Minor wound	Unknown vaccine status	Tetanus toxoid vaccine
	Incomplete vaccine series	
	Complete series, last booster >10 years ago	Tetanus toxoid vaccine
	Complete series, recent booster	No treatment necessary

[a]Major wounds include wounds contaminated with dirt, feces, soil, and saliva; puncture wounds; avulsions; and wounds resulting from missiles, crushing, burns, or frostbite.
[b]If human antitetanus immune globulin not available, equine may be used.
(From Atkinson W, Hamborsky J, McIntyre L, et al. Chapter 6: Tetanus. Centers for Disease Control and Prevention. *Epidemiology and Prevention of Vaccine-Preventable Diseases.* Atkinson W, Hamborsky J, McIntyre L, et al. eds. 10th ed. Washington DC: Public Health Foundation, 2006 and Nagachinta T, Cortese M, Roper M, et al. Chapter 13: Tetanus. In: Manual for the Surveillance of Vaccine-Preventable Diseases, 3rd ed: Wharton M, Hughes H, and Reilly M. Centers for Disease Control and Prevention, eds., 2002 http://www.cdc.gov/nip/publications/surv-manual/default.htm; Accessed 8/25/2006.)

model by which other vaccine-preventable diseases may be eliminated.

REFERENCES

1. Case courtesy of Moon Kim MD. Acute Communicable Disease Service, Los Angeles County Public Health, Los Angeles County Department of Health Services, Los Angeles, California.
2. Atkinson W, Hamborsky J, McIntyre L, et al. Chapter 6: Tetanus. Centers for Disease Control and Prevention. *Epidemiology and Prevention of Vaccine-Preventable Diseases.* Atkinson W, Hamborsky J, McIntyre L, et al. eds. 10th ed. Washington DC: Public Health Foundation, 2006.
3. *WHO Vaccine-Preventable Disease Monitoring System 2005 Global Summary.* Geneva: World Health Organization; 2005.
4. Howard R. Poliomyelitis and the postpolio syndrome. *BMJ.* 2005;330:1314–1319.
5. Racaniello V. One hundred years of poliovirus pathogenesis. *Virology.* 2006;344:9–6.
6. Peabody F, Draper G, Dochez A. *A Clinical Study of Acute Poliomyelitis.* New York: Rockefeller Institute for Medical Research, 1912.
7. Modlin JF. Chapter 168: Poliovirus. Principles and Practice of Infectious Diseases, ed. Mandell GL, Bennett JE, Dolin R. 6th ed. Philadelphia, Elsevier, 2005.
8. McBean A, Thoms M, Albrecht P, et al. Serologic response to oral polio vaccine and enhanced-potency inactivated polio vaccines. *Am J Epidemiol.* 1988;128(3):615–628.
9. Rupprecht C, Gibbons R. Prophylaxis against rabies. *N Engl J Med.* 2004;351:2626–2635.
10. Hankins D, Rosekrans J. Overview, prevention, and treatment of rabies. *Mayo Clin Proc.* 2004;79:671–676.
11. Warrell M, Warrell D. Rabies and other lyssavirus disease. *Lancet.* 2004;363:959–969.
12. Srinivasan A, Burton E, Kuehnert M, et al. Transmission of rabies virus from an organ donor to four transplant recipients. *N Engl J Med.* 2005;352:1103–1111.
13. McKay N, Wallis L. Rabies: A review of UK management. *Emerg Med J.* 2005;22:316–321.
14. Willoughby R, Tieves K, Hoffman G, et al. Survival after treatment of rabies with induction of coma. *N Engl J Med.* 2005;352:2508–2514.
15. Farrar J, Yen L, Cook T, et al. Tetanus. *J Neurol Neurosurg Psychiatry.* 2000;69:292–301.
16. Sheffield J, Ramin S. Tetanus in pregnancy. *Am J Perinatol.* 2004;21(4):173–182.
17. Cook T, Protheroe R, Handel J. Tetanus: A review of the literature. *Br J Anaesth.* 2001;87(3):477–487.
18. Jagoda A, Riggio S, Burguieres T. Cephalic tetanus: A case report and a review of the literature. *Am J Emerg Med.* 1988;6(2):128–130.
19. Thwaites C, Yen L, Glover C, et al. Predicting the clinical outcome of tetanus: The tetanus severity score. *Trop Med Int Health.* 2006;11(3):279–287.
20. Nagachinta T, Cortese M, Roper M, et al. Chapter 13: Tetanus. Manual for the Surveillance of Vaccine-Preventable Diseases. 3rd ed. Wharton M, Hughes H, and Reilly M. Centers for Disease Control and Prevention, eds, 2002. http://www.cdc. gov/nip/publications/surv-manual/default.htm; Accessed 8/25/2006.
21. Perl D. Image 3377. In: Public Health Image Library, Centers for Disease Control and Prevention, www.phil.cdc.gov; 1971.

CHAPTER 103

Common Antibiotics

Risa M. Webb

OBJECTIVES

- To describe the blood–brain barrier and its effect on antibiotic delivery to the central nervous system
- To explain the effect of meningeal inflammation on the ability of different antibiotic classes to cross the blood–brain barrier
- To discuss the significant central nervous system and peripheral nervous system adverse drug events associated with commonly used antibiotics
- To describe the common drug interactions between neurologic drugs and antibiotics

CASE VIGNETTE

A 76-year-old-man, with a prior seizure disorder, presented to his primary care physician with nausea and vomiting for the past 24 hours. His family reported he had had increasing headache and lethargy for the past 3 weeks. Current medications included phenytoin for his seizure disorder. Computed tomographic (CT) scan showed a right frontal lobe abscess. Surgical excision and drainage was done. Cultures were positive for *Bacteroides fragilis*, *Escherichia coli*, and *Staphylococcal aureus*. The patient had a history of a severe penicillin type I allergy. He was treated initially with intravenous vancomycin, trimethoprim-sulfamethoxazole, and metronidazole. His headache, systemic symptoms, and lethargy resolved. Dilantin level on day 7 was noted to be elevated and the dosage was reduced. After 14 days, he was discharged on intravenous vancomycin with oral trimethoprim-sulfamethoxazole and metronidazole. On day 21 of treatment, he presented with mild confusion and a mild glove-and-stocking distribution dysethesia. Phenytoin level was therapeutic (18 μg/mL). Attempts were made to continue metronidazole, but symptoms worsened. On examination, the patient was oriented to self and time, but not place. He was unable to differentiate pinprick sensation below the midcalf and showed a loss of muscle stretch reflexes in the lower extremities. Metronidazole was discontinued. The confusion resolved and the peripheral neuropathy gradually abated.

This patient illustrates the importance of familiarity with antibiotic pharmacodynamics in patients with neurologic infections and disorders. Utilization of antibiotics to which the etiologic agents are susceptible must be coupled with the agent's ability to achieve therapeutic concentrations at the infection site. In this case, the antibiotic must both cross the blood–brain barrier (BBB) and penetrate into the abscess to reach bactericidal levels. Further, the choice of antibiotics must take into account potential toxicities and avoid neurologic drug interactions. This chapter focuses on the pharmacodynamics of antibiotics used in the treatment of central nervous system (CNS) infections. Additionally, the recognized neurologic toxicities and common drug interactions that these antibiotics have with neurologic treatments are also briefly discussed.

PHARMACODYNAMICS OF ANTIBIOTICS AND THE NERVOUS SYSTEM

Cerebrospinal fluid (CSF) is formed in the choroid plexus by both filtration and active transport. Reabsorption of CSF occurs in the arachnoid villi, which are located in the superior sagittal and intracranial venous sinuses. Normally, the arachnoid villi only allow one-way transport of CSF into blood. The term BBB actually refers to two physiologic barriers that prevent the entry of fluids, electrolytes, and other substances, such as antibiotics, from the blood into the CSF (blood CSF barrier) or brain tissue (blood tissue barrier). An understanding of the anatomic and morphologic considerations related to the BBB complements the knowledge of an antibiotic's ability to reach therapeutic concentrations in the CNS.

The compartments of the CNS that might be infected include the CSF, where most studies of antibiotic concentration are done; the extracellular space of the nervous tissue; and the intracellular space of the neurons, glial cells, and leucocytes (1). The barrier to these compartments confronting antibiotics is found anatomically in two places (Fig. 103-1). Whereas the blood vessels throughout most of the body have fenestrated endothelial cells, the endothelial cells of the blood vessels in the CNS have tight junctions that prohibit or impede many antibiotics from crossing to the CSF and other compartments of the brain. The blood CSF barrier occurs in the choroid plexus. Although the endothelial cells are fenestrated, the epithelial cells of the choroid plexus have very tight junctions and it is the epithelial cells that contribute to the blood CSF barrier in the choroid plexus (2). Also, a brain CSF barrier occurs in the pia mater, which is mediated by the layer of astrocytes that cover the basement membrane of cells in the pia mater. Antibiotics with a low molecular weight, lipophilicity, and low protein binding more readily cross the cells and tight

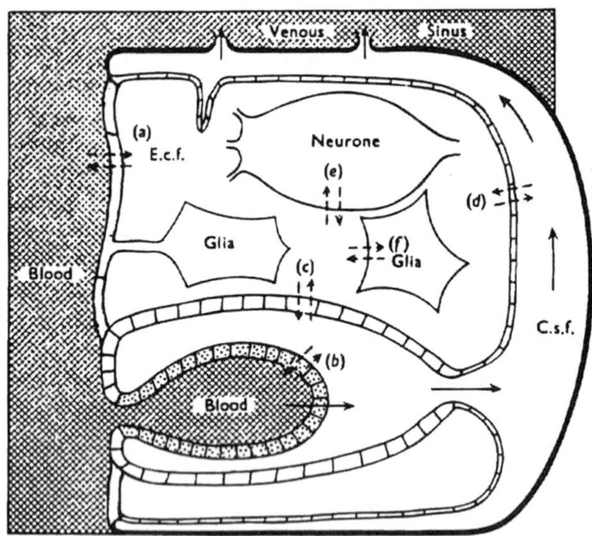

FIGURE 103-1. Blood–Brain Barrier and Blood Cerebrospinal Fluid Barrier. (Reprinted from Dawson H, Segal MB. *Physiology of the CSF and Blood Brain Barriers.* Boca Raton, FL: CRC Press, 1996, with permission.)

junction of these anatomic and functional barriers. Infection or inflammation loosens the tight junctions of both endothelial cells and epithelial cells that then allows the antibiotics to cross these barriers and achieve bactericidal levels at the site of infection (Fig. 103-1).

The treatment of CNS infections is also complicated by the relative lack of host defenses in the CNS. Specific antibody and complement may not be present, thus leading to decreased phagocytosis (3). This lack of opsonins in the CSF requires a rapid bactericidal drug action once antibiotics cross the barrier. Drug concentrations at least 10 to 20 times the normal minimal inhibitory concentration (MIC) are needed to assure bactericidal activity in the CSF (4). The combination of the BBB and the need for bactericidal levels often requires the highest level of antibiotic dosing for CNS infections. As inflammation resolves, the BBB is restored as the endothelial and epithelial tight junctions are repaired. Because therapeutic drug levels must be sustained to ensure eradication of infection, continued high doses of antibiotics are required even as the patient improves (4–9). Because of these concerns, multiple studies were conducted regarding the use of dexamethasone to decrease inflammation and thereby result in a decrease in antibiotic penetration into the CNS. Penetration of antibiotics into brain abscesses also occurs at the site of the abscess because of destruction of the capillaries at that site, allowing greater entrance of antibiotics (10).

Several other factors should be considered in the treatment of neurologic infections. The clinical significance of these, however, is not well documented. The most important is the recognition that antibiotic levels are not the same throughout the CNS compartments. Ventricular fluid antibiotic levels, when checked, are usually less than concentrations in the lumbar CSF (11–13). In severe ventriculitis, this can translate to the need for direct intraventricular dosing. Second, high-level dosing of antibiotics that leads to rapid bactericidal action also leads to increased proinflammatory products as the bacteria are lysed.

Some studies have tested less bacteriolytic drugs to determine if their use and the evidence of a decreased proinflammatory response result in better outcomes (14,15). Next, the bactericidal activity of many antibiotics is reduced by the acid environment seen in brain abscesses and in the CSF of patients with meningitis. Examples of antibiotics shown to be less effective in eradication of bacteria in an acidic environment include the aminoglycosides, macrolides, and quinolones (16,17). Although not well documented, an acidic pH of the CSF can also lead to greater diffusion of antibiotics from the CSF back into the blood (18,19). Varied transport systems also exist for rapid removal of antibiotics from the CNS, including the probenecid efflux transport system and the P-glycoproteins that can be variably expressed. As a result, antibiotics that easily penetrate the BBB, such as quinolones, are also readily transported out by these systems (18). Bacterial properties can also have an adverse effect on the ability of an antibiotic to result in cure. Further, high bacterial counts in the CSF can result in high concentrations of β-lactamase within the CSF which, in turn, reduces the active concentrations of β-lactam antibiotics. Also, bacteria replication can be slowed by the depletion of substrates in the heavily infected brain abscess or CSF. Those antibiotics, which are inhibitors of cell wall synthesis (e.g., β-lactam antibiotics), are less effective if replication is not ongoing.

ANTIBIOTICS

The choice of antibiotics for the treatment of CNS infection can be discussed in a variety of ways. The most practical for the physician is to group antibiotics by their ability to cross the BBB in the presence or absence of inflammation (Table 103-1) (20,21). These categories are based on animal models of meningitis and drug levels found in human CNS, but are also tempered by clinical experience (17,18). Recommended regimens for specific microbiologic causes of CNS infections are discussed in Parts 12, 20, and 21.

ANTIBIOTICS THAT CROSS THE BLOOD–BRAIN BARRIER WITH INFLAMMATION

β-Lactams, Carbapenems, and Monobactams

β-Lactam antibiotics are generally hydrophilic and have a high molecular weight. As noted above, the larger, less lipophilic drugs have more difficulty in crossing the endothelial and epithelial barriers with their tight junctions. As with other drugs in this category, however, the presence of inflammation leads to loosening of these tight cellular junctions and high doses of penicillins or selected cephalosporins cross the BBB and achieve therapeutic levels. Because of their inherent low toxicity, these agents are well tolerated even when administered in high doses. Antibiotic dosing is given to reach a target CSF antibiotic concentration of ten times the MIC and five times the minimum bactericidal concentration (MBC) of the susceptible pathogens. These concentrations will result in a rapid bactericidal effect (17,18). In particular, high doses of penicillin can be used to treat penicillin susceptible *S. pneumoniae* and meningococcal disease. Nafcillin crosses the BBB and achieves concentrations in the CSF that are effective for the treatment of methicillin susceptible *S. aureus.* Other semisynthetic penicillins cross the BBB similarly and, if susceptibilities dictate, can

TABLE 103-1. Antibiotic Penetration Across the Blood Brain Barrier

ANTIBIOTICS THAT PENETRATE THE BLOOD–BRAIN BARRIER WITH INFLAMMATION
Penicillins (high doses)
Cephalosporins (high doses)
Ceftriaxone
Cefotaxime
Cefepime
Ceftazidime
Vancomycin (high doses for ventriculitis)
Tetracycline
Clindamycin
Erythromycin
Ethambutol
Imipenem
Meropenem
Amphotericin B
Caspofungin
ANTIBIOTICS THAT HAVE GOOD PENETRATION ACROSS THE BLOOD–BRAIN BARRIER
Chloramphenicol
Isoniazid
Pyrazinamide
Rifampin
Ethionamide
Trimethoprim-sulfamethoxazole (TMP-SMX)
Fluoroquinolones
Minocycline > Doxycycline
Linezolid
Flucytosine
Fluconazole
Voriconazole
Zidovudine
Stavudine
Lamivudine
Indinavir
Vidarabine
Nevirapine
Efavirenz
Acyclovir
Foscarnet

(Adapted from Ziglam H, Finch R. Bacterial infection of the central nervous system. In: Finch R, Greenwood D, Norrby S, et al. *Antibiotic and Chemotherapy Anti-Infective Agents and Their Use in Therapy.* Churchill Livingstone; 2003; and Cunha B. *Antibiotic Essentials.* Physicians Press; 2002, with permission.)

be used for treatment. Often used with penicillins are clavulanic acid and sulbactam. Clavulanic acid does not penetrate well, even in the presence of inflammation. Sulbactam does reach therapeutic concentrations in the CSF and may aid in treatment with ampicillin (17).

Third generation cephalosporins in high doses have been shown in multiple trials to successfully treat common causes of meningitis. Multiple randomized trials have shown their equivalency and, in some cases, benefit is comparable to penicillins and cefuroxime (20). In meningitis trials comparing cefuroxime and ceftriaxone, time to negative CSF cultures and hearing loss was greater in the group placed on cefuroxime. Cefotaxime has also been studied extensively in susceptible CNS infections with good results. If *pseudomonas* is suspected, ceftazidime and cefepime cross the BBB when inflammation is present. Ceftazidime, however, should not be used for treatment of *S. pneumonia* meningitis. Cefepime was shown in one study to have an increased risk of seizures and encephalopathy when higher doses were used (20). Imipenem, meropenem, and azactam have all shown ability to cross the BBB and reach elevated MIC levels when inflammation is present. Seizures may prohibit the higher doses of imipenem and it is usually avoided in CNS infections (17). Again, high doses of all β-lactam antibiotics must be maintained after clinical improvement as their ability to cross the BBB diminishes.

Glycopeptides

Vancomycin and teichoplanin have a high molecular mass. At least 55% of vancomycin is protein bound and this may be one reason for its decreased penetration (17,18). Protein binding in teicoplanin is even greater and it is not recommended in the treatment of meningitis (18). Vancomycin reaches therapeutic levels in the CSF when given at doses of 15 mg/kg every 6 hours (22). Nephrotoxicity usually precludes dosing above 2 gm/day. Some experts recommend intrathecal or intraventricular administration. Although clinical trials have not been done, intrathecal or intraventricular dosing can be considered in a patient with methicillin-resistant *S. aureus* infection or with renal toxicity when not responding to vancomycin (particularly if an Ommaya reservoir is in use) (18–20,22,23).

Other Antibiotics Crossing the Blood–Brain Barrier with Inflammation

Clindamycin can achieve therapeutic levels at its usual dose when inflammation of the CNS is present. It is most often used in toxoplasma encephalitis. It has been shown in animal and one small clinical study to reduce proinflammatory release after treatment in *S. pneumonia* meningitis. Further study would be required before this could be recommended to provide neurologic protection (14,15). Tetracycline is the least lipid soluble of its drug class and cannot be relied on to cross the BBB unless meningitis is present. Macrolides have a high molecular weight and increased protein binding, predictors of their lowered CSF penetration. Their use in legionella with neurologic symptoms can be enhanced with the addition of rifampin (18). They are bacteriostatic against *S. pneumonia* in the CSF. Although *in vitro* studies have been done with quinupristin/dalfopristin, it likely penetrates poorly unless the meninges are inflamed. A small number of successful case studies have been reported (24,25). Ethambutol reaches 25% to 40% of plasma levels and can be used for treatment in tubercular (TB) meningitis with other appropriate drugs (17,18).

Despite being the drug of choice for many fungal CNS infections, amphotericin B has less than 5% penetration as compared with serum levels. In animal data, however, meningeal and brain levels may be higher than CSF levels (26,27). Liposomal formulations of amphotericin B do not reach higher levels than nonliposomal amphotericin. Caspofungin is hydrophilic and has a high molecular weight and high protein binding. It has little penetration without inflammation. It must be noted, however, that in a murine models and in a few reported human cases, this agent has cleared candidal meningitis and an CNS aspergillus infection (28,29).

Indinavir is the only protease inhibitor shown to cross the BBB but at a CSF:plasma ratio of only 0.11 (30). Larger molecular weight and high protein binding decrease the ability of protease inhibitors to cross the blood brain barrier (31). Some more current studies show a decrease in CSF human immunodeficiency virus (HIV) viral loads with highly active antiretroviral therapy (HAART) inclusive of other protease inhibitors (32,33). Ganciclovir reaches the CSF at levels attaining 24% to 67% of the serum level, which are adequate for cytomegalovirus (CMV) meningitis or encephalitis (17).

ANTIBIOTICS THAT ACHIEVE CEREBROSPINAL FLUID LEVELS AT USUAL DOSING WITH LESS EFFECT BY INFLAMMATION

Several antibiotics can be relied on to achieve therapeutic concentrations with their usual doses and routes. Metronidazole, even given orally, reaches levels in the CSF similar to plasma levels within 90 minutes of administration. Chloramphenicol is likely the drug with the greatest history in this grouping and has been relied on in the past when other options were not available. Minocycline is more lipid soluble than doxycycline, but both agents can reach the CSF compartment. The fluoroquinolones have no postantibiotic effect in the CSF, but do have high lipid solubility and can easily attain therapeutic concentrations (17). Moxifloxacin has been shown to reach 50% to 80% of the plasma level. Ciprofloxacin has been proved to reach 50% of serum levels and has been used successfully in treating *Pseudomonas meningitis.* Trimethoprim concentrations in the CSF are about 50% of those achieved in plasma. Sulfonamides reach therapeutic concentrations in the CSF. Trimethoprim-sulfmethoxisole can be used if resistance is not present (17). Several case reports of linezolid use for CNS infection have been published, including a case series of 10 patients. Linezolid penetrates CSF well and can theoretically be expected to be effected in the treatment of resistant gram-positive infections and possibly for mycobacteria (33).

The mycobacterial drugs for the treatment of TB meningitis that reach therapeutic concentrations at standard dose include isoniazid, ethionamide, rifampin, and pyrazinamide. Pyrazinamide readily penetrates the BBB and should be included if at all possible (17).

Fluconazole penetrates at 50% to 60% of the serum levels and at even higher levels in meningitis. Levels of flucytosine in the CSF approach 75% of that in serum. Voriconazole CSF levels have been measured at 50% of serum levels. Itraconazole levels are less than those of fluconazole or voriconazole and should be used for maintenance therapy only (27). Acyclovir, foscarnet, and antiinfluenza compounds all cross the BBB with good penetration (17). Efavirenz, zidovudine, nevirapine, stavudine, saquinavir, didanosine, and ritonavir have all been shown to penetrate the BBB (17,20,31). In one severe combined immunodeficiency (SCID) HIV-infected mouse model, zidovudine, lamivudine, and indinavir were reported to decrease neuroanatomic changes (34).

ANTIBIOTICS THAT DO NOT RELIABLY CROSS THE BLOOD–BRAIN BARRIER

Antibiotics that do not cross the BBB and should not be used include the first generation cephalosporins, erythromycin, polymyxin, and fusidic acid. Intravenous aminoglycosides cannot be relied on to reach therapeutic levels in the CNS.

ADVERSE NEUROLOGIC EVENTS OF COMMONLY USED ANTIBIOTICS

When treating either a primary neurologic infection or a nonneurologic infection, the ability of an antibiotic to cross the BBB may be indicative of their ability to result in CNS toxicity, and peripheral neuropathy (Table 103–2). For example, penicillins are generally well tolerated even in high doses used for CNS infections. In patients who are uremic, however, the organic acids compete for the transport of penicillin out of the CNS. This can result in very high penicillin concentrations that can cause seizures. Imipenem has an especially high incidence of seizures and should be avoided with patients who have a history of prior seizures, head trauma, or stroke. Meropenem is better tolerated and is the carbapenem of choice when needed with patients at high risk of seizures. Quinolones have known adverse neurologic events even when used for nonneurologic infections. Adverse events include encephalopathy, confusion, depression, seizures, and hallucinations. These severities are thought to be caused by blockade of γ-aminobutyric acid. Minocycline has caused benign intracranial hypertension, dizziness, ataxia, vertigo, and tinnitus. These events have occurred more commonly in women. Trimethoprim can lead to a hypersensitivity reaction and an aseptic meningitis, although this is rare. Isoniazid can cause hallucinations and psychotic episodes. Encephalopathy in renal patients has also been reported. Peripheral neuropathy has been noted with isoniazid, although this is rare when pyridoxine levels are sufficient. Metronidazole can lead to confusion and peripheral neuropathy, particularly with intravenous administration, as described in the case vignette. Headache, dizziness, syncope, ataxia, and seizures have all been associated with intravenous metronidazole treatment. Oral treatment has been associated with irritability, depression, insomnia, vertigo, and incoordination. Symptoms usually disappear if the dose is discontinued or markedly reduced.

Aminoglycosides can cause neuromuscular blockade. Although uncommon, the greatest risk is in patients receiving muscle relaxants or anesthetics or who have myasthenia gravis. The blockade can be reversed with neostigmine. Similar effects have also been described in the gastrointestinal tract and the uterus. These effects can be reversed by calcium. A single

TABLE 103-2. Common Antibiotics Used in Neurologic Infections and Their Neurotoxicities

Antibiotic	*Neurotoxicity*
Penicillins, cephalosporins, carbapenems	Seizures
Quinolones	Encephalopathy, confusion, depression, seizures, hallucinations
Minocycline	Benign intracranial hypertension, dizziness, ataxia, vertigo, tinnitus
Isoniazid	Hallucinations, psychotic episodes, encephalopathy, peripheral neuropathy
Metronidazole	Peripheral neuropathy, headache, dizziness, syncope, ataxia, confusion, seizures, irritability, depression, insomnia
Aminoglycosides	Neuromuscular blockade

report exists of neuromuscular blockade with an overdose of intravenous clindamycin (17).

ANTIBIOTICS INTERACTIONS WITH CENTRAL NERVOUS SYSTEM DRUGS

The choice of specific antibiotics for the treatment of CNS and non-CNS infections may result in serious drug–drug interactions that can enhance toxicity or reduce the efficiency of either of the drugs. The primary interactions are with the seizure medications phenytoin, phenobarbital, and carbamazepine. These agents are inducers of the hepatic CYP-450, 3A4 metabolic pathway. Clinical failures have been noted in patients treated with any of these seizure medications and the azoles antifungal drugs (e.g., itraconazole, fluconazole, voriconazole). Serum levels should be monitored in these patients to assure clinical efficacy and reduce toxicity. Many of the antiretrovirals agents also affect the CYP-450,3A4 pathway. Some of these agents enhance whereas others inhibit this important metabolic drug pathway. Other interactions include phenobarbital with doxycycline, itraconazole, and voriconazole; phenytoin with isoniazid, oxacillin, penicillin, caspofungin, ciprofloxacin, fluconazole, itraconazole, trimethoprim, and voriconazole; and carbamazepine with caspofungin, isoniazid, itraconazole, and voriconazole (31). Of note, the concurrent administration of nonsteroidal anti-inflammatory drugs (NSAID) and quinolones can increase the risk of CNS seizures (31). Trimethoprim-sulfamethoxazole can commonly cause of over anticoagulation in patients treated with coumadin. For detail information regarding drug–drug interaction the reader is referred to Thomson MICROMEDEX health care series (http//www.micromedex.com).

CLINICAL RECOMMENDATIONS OF THE VIGNETTE

The choice of therapy for the patient was based on the ability of the specific antibiotics to cross the BBB and blood CSF barrier. The ability to penetrate into the abscess cavity and to be active in an acid pH were important consideration.

The CNS has a paucity of host defenses. As such, bactericidal antibiotics should be used for treatment. High-dose intravenous therapy is usually required to achieve bactericidal concentrations. Knowledge of neurologic adverse events by the commonly used antibiotics resulted in the early identification and treatment of the peripheral neuropathy caused by metronidazole seen in this patient.

SUMMARY

The BBB limits the penetration of many antibiotics into the CSF and brain tissue. In general, inflammation or infection breaks down the BBB and allows penetration of most antibiotics into the CSF and brain tissue. Higher doses of antibiotics are required to treat CNS infections, owing to the difficulty of crossing the BBB. Recommended dosing should be followed to achieve bactericidal levels and maintained continued till treatment is completed. Many of the common antibiotics have associated neurologic adverse events and patients treated with these agents should be carefully observed for the development of neurotoxicity (Table 103-2). Significant drug–drug interactions have been reported between antibiotics and drugs used for the treatment of neurologic diseases, especially antiseizure medicines. Serum levels of these medications must be carefully monitored and dosage adjusted to assure effective treatment.

REFERENCES

1. Nabeshima S, Reese TS, Landis DMD, et al. Junctions in the meninges and marginal glia. *J Comp Neurol.* 1975;164:127–170.
2. Zwahlen A, Nydegger UE, Vaudaux P, et al. Complement-mediated opsonic activity in normal and infected human cerebrospinal fluid: Early response during bacterial meningitis. *J Infect Dis.* 1982;145:635–646.
3. Tauber MG, Hoshino K, Hohmura M, et al. Antibacterial activity of beta-lactam antibiotics in experimental meningitis due to Streptococcus pneumonia. *J Infect Dis.* 1984;149: 568–574.
4. Tunkel AR. *Bacterial Meningitis.* Philadelphia: Lippincott Williams & Wilkins; 2001.
5. Nu R, Schmidt T, Kaye K, et al. Quinolone antibiotics in therapy of experimental pneumococcal meningitis in rabbits. *Antimicrob Agents Chemother.* 1995;39:593–597.
6. Schaad UB, McCracken GH, Loock CA, et al. Pharmacokinetics and bacteriological efficacy of moxalactam, cefotaxime, cefoperazone and rocephin in experimental bacterial meningitis. *J Infect Dis.* 1981;143:156–163.
7. Strausbaugh LJ, Sande MA. Factors influencing the therapy of experimental Proteus mirabilis in rabbits. *J Infect Dis.* 1978;137:251–260.
8. Scheld WM, Sande MA. Bactericidal versus bacteriostatic antibiotic therapy of experimental pneumococcal meningitis in rabbits. *J Clin Invest.* 1983;71:411–419.
9. Wispelwey B, Dacey RG, Scheld WM. Brain abscess. In: Scheld WM, Whitley RJ, Durack DT, eds. *Infections of the Central Nervous System,* 2nd ed. Philadelphia: Lippincott Raven; 1997:463–493.
10. Wellman WE, Dodge HW, Heilman FR, et al. Concentrations of antibiotics in the brain. *J Lab Clin Med.* 1954;43:275–279.
11. Wise BL, Perkins RK, Stevenson E, et al. Penetration of C14 labeled mannitol from serum into cerebrospinal fluid and brain. *Exp Neurol.* 1964;10:264–270.
12. Nau R, Prange HW, Muth P, et al. Passage of cefotaxime and ceftriaxone into cerebrospinal fluid of patients with uninflamed meninges. *Antimicrob Agents Chemother.* 1993;37:1518–1524.
13. Spreer A, Kerstan H, Bottcher T, et al. Reduced release of pneumolysin by Streptococcus pneumonia in vitro and in vivo after treatment with nonbacteriolytic antibiotics in comparison to ceftriaxone. *Antimicrob Agents Chemother.* 2003;47:2649–2654.
14. Bottcher T, Ren H, Goiny M, et al. Clindamycin is neuroprotective in experimental Streptococcus pneumonia meningitis compared with ceftriaxone. *J Neurochem.* 2004;91:1450–1460.
15. Schmidt T, Froula J, Tauber MG. Clarithromycin lacks bactericidal activity in cerebrospinal fluid in experimental pneumococcal meningitis. *J Antimicrob Chemother.* 1993;32: 627–632.
16. Nau R, Sorgel F, Prange HW. Clinical Pharmacokinietic Optimisation of the Treatment of Bacterial Central Nervous System Infections. *Clinical Pharmacokinetics.* 1998; 35(3):223–246.
17. Tanaka M, Hoshino K, Hohmura M, et al. Effect of growth conditions on antimicrobial activity of DU-6859a and its bactericidal activity determined by the killing curve method. *J Antimicrob Chemother.* 1996;37:1091–1102.
18. Finch R, Greenwood D, Norrby S, et al. *Antibiotic and Chemotherapy: Anti-Infective Agents and Their Use in Therapy.* Churchill Livingstone; 2003.
19. Ziglam H, Finch R. Bacterial infection of the central nervous system. In: Finch R, Greenwood D, Norrby S, et al., eds. *Antibiotic and Chemotherapy: Anti-Infective Agents and Their Use in Therapy.* Churchill Livingstone; 2003.
20. Cunha B. *Antibiotic Essentials.* Physicians Press; 2002.
21. Reesor C, Chow AW, Kureishi A, et al. Kinetics of intraventricular vancomycin in infectious of cerebrospinal fluid shunts. *J Infect Dis.* 1988;158:1142–1143.
22. Albanèse J, Léone M, Bruguerolle B, et al. Cerebrospinal fluid penetration and pharmacokinetics of vancomycin administered by continuous infusion to mechanically ventilated patients in an intensive care unit. *Antimicrob Agents Chemother.* 2000;44:1356–1358.
23. Williamson JC, Glazier SS, Peacock JE, Jr. Successful treatment of ventriculostomy-related meningitis caused by vancomycin-resistant Enterococcus with intravenous and intraventricular quinupristin/dalfopristin. *Clin Neurol Neurosurg.* 2002;104(1):54–56.
24. Dever LL, Smith SM, Dejesus D, et al. Treatment of vancomycin-resistant Enterococcus faecium infections with an investigational streptogramin antibiotic (quinupristin/dalfopristin): A report of fifteen cases. *Microb Drug Resist.* 1996;2(4):407–413.
25. Perfect JR, Durack DT. Chemotactic activity of cerebrospinal fluid in experimental cryptococcal meningitis. *Sabouraudia.* 1985;23(1):37–45.
26. Mattiuzzi G, Giles FJ. Management of intracranial fungal infections in patients with haematological malignancies. *Br J Haematol.* 2005;131:(3)287–300.
27. Liu KH, Wu CJ, Chou CH, et al Refractory candidal meningitis in an immunocompromised patient cured by caspofungin. *J Clin Microbiol.* 2004;42(12):5950–5953.
28. Colombo AL, Rossas RC. Successful treatment of an aspergillus brain abscess with caspofungin. *Eur J Clin Microbiol Infect Dis.* 2003;22(9):575–576.
29. Rupprecht TA, Pfister HW. Clinical experience with linezolid for the treatment of central nervous system infections. *Eur J Neurol.* 2005;12:536–542.
30. Piscitelli S, Rodvold K. *Drug Interactions in Infectious Disease.* Totowa, NJ: Humana Press; 2005.
31. Cook JE, Dasagupta S, Middaugh LD, et al. Highly active antiretroviral therapy and human immunodeficiency virus encephalitis. *Ann Neurol.* 2005;57(6):795–803.

CHAPTER 104

Opiates

Michael A. Sloan

OBJECTIVES

- To discuss the classes of opiate receptors and their effects
- To describe the various opiates, opioids, and opiate antagonists
- To explain the protean neurologic complications of opiate addiction, specifically heroin
- To describe an approach to diagnosis and treatment of neurologic complications of opiate use
- To discuss the approach to management of opiate withdrawal

CASE VIGNETTE

A 48-year-old man with a history of hypertension, cigarette smoking, intravenous heroin abuse, and recent difficulty walking was brought to the emergency department after being found poorly responsive at home. His temperature was 99.6°F, blood pressure was 110/70 mm Hg, pulse was 66 beats per minute, and respirations were 10 per minute and shallow. Skin examination showed needle tracks at both antecubital fossae with fresh blood on the left. Pupils were 1 mm; reactivity was sluggish. Oculocephalic maneuver demonstrated normal eye movements. A subtle decrease was noted in right facial grimace with supraorbital pressure. On pinch stimulation, there were semipurposeful movements on both sides, left greater than right, and arms greater than legs. Bilateral hyperreflexia and Babinski signs, right greater than left were noted. After the administration of 2 mg of naloxone, the patient became more alert. A few moments later, he developed hypertension, tachycardia, yawning, irritability, agitation, lacrimation, and sweating. The neurologic asymmetries became less marked, but persisted.

DEFINITION AND PHARMACOLOGY

Opiates, opioids, and opiate antagonists are classes of drugs that act on specific receptors to produce a variety of clinical effects, especially sedation and analgesia. Opiates are alkaloid agents derived directly from the opium poppy. Opiates are a broader class of drugs that either produce opiumlike effects or bind to opioid receptors. A semisynthetic opioid (e.g., heroin, oxycodone) is created by chemical modification of an opiate. A synthetic opiate is a nonopioid compound that binds to an opioid receptor and can produce opioid clinical effects. For the purposes of this discussion, the term *opioid* encompasses opiates and opioids (1,2).

Three major classes of opioid receptors exist, each with multiple subtypes, with diverse clinical effects (Table 104-1). All opioid receptor subtypes are members of a superfamily of membrane-bound receptors that are coupled to G-proteins, which are involved in signaling of receptor activation and initiation of cellular effects via specific effector systems. Clinical effects of opioids are summarized in Table 104-2. Specific agents can be agonists, agonist-antagonists, or antagonists at opioid receptors. The clinical effects of opioids differ according to whether the agent serves as an agonist, agonist-antagonist, or antagonist at specific receptor types. The characteristics and potency of the various opiates are shown in Table 104-3. Mu receptors are responsible for most of the analgesic effects of morphine. The highest concentrations of these receptors are located in the periaqueductal gray, nucleus raphe magnus, locus ceruleus, and medial thalamus. Activation of these supraspinal receptors leads to enhancement of inhibitory outflow, with dampening of nociceptive transmission from spinal cord sensory nuclei. Activation of Mu-Delta receptors in the ventral tegmental area of the mesolimbic system promotes dopamine release, with resulting euphoria. Most adverse or toxic effects from opioids are predictable, although some compounds produce agent-specific responses. Despite variations in clinical manifestations attributable to activation of different receptor subtypes, the classic elements of the syndrome of opioid poisoning include mental status depression, hypoventilation, miosis, and reduced bowel motility (1). Minor molecular modifications convert an opiate agonist into an opiate antagonist. Naloxone, naltrexone, and nalmefene are derivatives of oxymorphone and are pure competitive antagonists at Mu receptors.

EPIDEMIOLOGY

The history and epidemiology of opiate use and addiction, especially heroin, has recently been reviewed (3). Historically, the sources of opium production include Mexico, Turkey, Iran, Afghanistan, Southeast Asia, and some South American countries. In the 1990s, the price of heroin dropped, resulting in an increased frequency of heroin use, particularly among adolescents and young adults, which was associated with an increase in morbidity and mortality in the United States. In 1996, the cost of heroin addiction in the United States was estimated to be $21.9 billion (3). According to the 2001 US National Household

TABLE 104-1. Opioid Receptors and Clinical Effects

1996 Conventional Name	*Important Clinical Effects*
Mu-1 Receptor	Supraspinal analgesia Peripheral analgesia Sedation Euphoria Prolactin release
Mu-2 Receptor	Spinal analgesia Respiratory depression Physical dependence Gastrointestinal dysmotility Pruritis Bradycardia Growth hormone release
Kappa-1 Receptor	Spinal analgesia Miosis Diuresis
Kappa-2 Receptor	Psychotomimesis Dysphoria
Kappa-3 Receptor	Supraspinal analgesia
Delta Receptor	Spinal and supraspinal analgesia Modulation of Mu-receptor function Inhibition of dopamine release
Nociception/Orphanin FQ Receptor	Anxiolysis Analgesia

(From Nelson LS. Opioids. In: Flomenbaum NE, Goldfrank LR, Hoffman RS, et al., eds. *Goldfrank's Toxicologic Emergencies*, 8th ed. New York: McGraw-Hill; 2006:590–613, with permission.)

Survey on Drug Abuse (4), the estimated number of heroin users was 200,000, with 67,000 between the ages of 18 and 25 years. The number of intermittent or 'controlled' users, however, may be substantially higher (3). In 2002, Afghanistan became the major source of the world's heroin with a 19 times increase in opium production when the ban on poppy cultivation, processing, and trafficking became unenforceable (3). A case-control study at Harlem Hospital Center showed that past and current heroin use was a risk factor for new-onset seizures, independent of overdose, head injury, infection, stroke, or use of alcohol or other illicit drugs (5).

TABLE 104-2. Clinical Effects of Opioids

Organ System	*Clinical Effect*
Cardiovascular	Peripheral vasodilation (histamine release) Orthostatic hypotension Bradycardia Dysrhythmias (ion channel effects)
Pulmonary	Respiratory depression (Mu-2) Bronchospasm (histamine release) pulmonary edema
Ophthalmic	Miosis
Neurologic	Sedation, coma Analgesia Euphoria Seizures (meperidine, propoxyphene) Antitussive
Dermatologic	Flushing (histamine release) Pruritus
Gastrointestinal	Reduced motility Reduced gastric acid secretion Increased biliary tract pressure Increased anal sphincter tone
Endocrinologic	Reduced antidiuretic hormone release Reduced gonadotropin release

(Modified from R Nelson LS. Opioids. In: Flomenbaum NE, Goldfrank LR, Hoffman RS, et al., eds. *Goldfrank's Toxicologic Emergencies*, 8th ed. New York: McGraw-Hill; 2006:590–613, with permission.)

ETIOLOGY, PATHOGENESIS, CLINICAL MANIFESTATIONS, AND SPECIAL SITUATIONS

Numerous case reports and case series have demonstrated that the neurologic manifestations of opiate (specifically heroin) are protean (3,6–12), as summarized in Table 104-4. In general, the clinical syndromes can be caused by the toxic effects of heroin, adulterant(s), an infectious complication, such as human immunodeficiency virus (HIV), another systemic factor, or some combination of all of these. In this section, specific categories of neurologic manifestations will be discussed. In addition, the management of opioid intoxication and withdrawal will be covered.

GENERAL CEREBRAL

Seizures are an unusual feature of heroin or morphine overdose. In this setting, seizures are most likely attributable to hypoxia. In patients with focal neurologic findings, a structural lesion should be sought. Meperidine, via its metabolite normeperidine, however, will lower the seizure threshold in a dose-related manner. Seizures should be anticipated in cases of propoxyphene and tramadol toxicity. Except for neonatal withdrawal in cases of dependence developed in utero, seizures are not a feature of opiate withdrawal (1,9).

Spongiform encephalopathy was first described in 47 Dutch heroin smokers practicing the presumably safer technique of "chasing the dragon," or inhaling the vapor of heroin heated on metal foil (13). In the first stage, motor restlessness, ataxia, and soft speech were very common. Over 2 to 4 weeks, about two thirds of patients progressed to the second stage with worsening cerebellar dysfunction, gait disorder, pyramidal tract findings, tremor, and jerking; 15 had some degree of improvement. The condition in eleven patients progressed further to pyrexia, perceptual alteration, respiratory depression, and death. Computed tomographic (CT) scanning showed cerebellar and, to a lesser degree, cerebral white matter changes. Necropsy showed spongiform degeneration in the white matter. Spinal cord dysfunction in a pattern mimicking subacute combined degeneration has been described (14). Potential etiologic factors include triethyl tin in the aluminum foil or a toxin produced by pyrolysis of an adulterant (Beuhler M, personal communication November 15, 2006).

INFECTIONS

The heroin user is at risk for a wide variety of infections that affect the brain, meninges, spine, and spinal cord. These infections can be associated with heroin use per se via contiguous or hematogenous spread or result from immunosuppression, such as with HIV infection. Cerebral infections include bacterial cerebritis caused by septic embolization from acute or subacute bacterial endocarditis, diverse forms of meningitis, viral encephalitis, various mycobacterial, and fungal infections as might occur in an

TABLE 104-3. Opioids: Classification, Characterization

Opioid	Analgesic Dose (mg) *Type*	*~10 mg Morphine SC*	*Comments*
NATURAL			
Codeine	Agonist	120 mg po	Demethylation by CYP2D6 to morphine
Morphine	Agonist	10 mg SC/IM	
Paregoric (Parepectolin)	Agonist	25 mL po	Tincture of opium (4 mg/mL)
SEMISYNTHETIC			
Dextromethorphan (Robitussin)	?	Nonanalgesic 10–30 mg	Antitussive; Agonism Mu-2, Kappa Psychotomimetic (Sigma, NMDA)
Heroin (Diamorph)	Agonist	5 mg SC	Diacetylmorphine
Nalbuphine (Nubain)	Agonist/antagonist	10 mg IM	
Levorphanol (Levodromoran)	Agonist	2 mg SC/IM	
Hydrocodone (Vicodin)	Agonist	10 mg po	
Hydromorphone (Dilaudid)	Agonist	1.3 mg SC	
Oxycodone (Percocet, Oxycontin)	Agonist	10 mg po	Oxycontin-sustained release 'Hillbilly heroin'
Oxymorphone (Numorphan)	Agonist	1 mg SC	
Butorphanol (Stadol)	Agonist/antagonist	2 mg IM	
Buprenorphine (Buprenex)	Partial agonist; Agonist/antagonist	0.4 mg IM	Opioid substitution rx 6–16 mg/day
Nalorphine	Agonist/antagonist	15 mg IM	Historically an antagonist
Pentazocine (Talwin)	Agonist/antagonist	50 mg SC	Psychotomimetic or dysphoria (Kappa or Sigma)
Naloxone (Narcan)	Antagonist	Nonanalgesic 0.1–0.4 mg IV/IM	Short-acting (0.5 h)
Nalmefene (Revex)	Antagonist	Nonanalgesic 0.1 mg IM	Long acting (4–6 h)
Naltrexone (Trexan)	Antagonist	Nonanalgesic 50 mg po	Very long acting (24 h)
SYNTHETIC			
Propoxyphene(Darvon)	Agonist	65 mg po	Seizures, dysrhythmias (QT prolongation)
Tramadol (Ultram)	Agonist	50–100 mg po	Seizures
Meperidine (Demerol)	Agonist	75 mg SC/IM	Seizures due to metabolite accumulation
Methadone (Dolophine)	Agonist	10 mg IM	Very long acting (24 h); QT prolongation
Fentanyl (Sublimaze, Duragesic)	Agonist	0.125 mg IM	Very short acting (<1 h)
Alpha-methylfentanyl	Agonist		'China White'
3-methylfentanyl	Agonist	.001–.01 mg	'Tango and Cash'
Diphenoxylate (Lomotil)	Agonist	Nonanalgesic 2.5 mg po	Antidiarrheal, combined with atropine
Loperamide (Imodium)	Agonist	Nonanalgesic 2 mg po	Antidiarrheal

Agonist, full agonist at Mu-1, Mu-2, and Kappa receptors; agonist/antagonist, Kappa receptor agonist, Mu receptor antagonist; antagonist, full antagonist at Mu-1, Mu-2, and Kappa receptors; partial agonist, agonist at Mu-1 and M-2 receptors, antagonist at Kappa receptors.
Notes: Agonist-antagonists, partial agonists, and antagonists can cause withdrawal in tolerant individuals. Duration of therapeutic clinical effect is 3 to 6 hours, unless otherwise stated.
SC, subcutaneously; po, oral; IM, intramuscular; NMDA, *N*-methyl-d-aspartate.
(Modified from Nelson LS. Opioids. In: Flomenbaum NE, Goldfrank LR, Hoffman RS, et al., eds. *Goldfrank's Toxicologic Emergencies,* 8th ed. New York: McGraw-Hill; 2006:590–613, with permission.)

TABLE 104-4. Neurologic Manifestations of Opiate (Primarily Heroin) Addiction

Category	*Specific Disorder or Clinical Finding*
GENERAL/CEREBRAL	
Acute intoxication	Analgesia, euphoria, miosis, drowsiness, coma, suppression of REM sleep, respiratory depression
Withdrawal	Irritability, anxiety, seizures, muscle spasms, myalgia, mydriasis, yawning. Associated findings: Fever, hypertension, tachycardia, tachypnea, productive coughing, sweating, abdominal cramps, nausea, vomiting, diarrhea, piloerection, lacrimation, rhinorrhea, hot flashes
Seizures	Partial, partial complex, generalized
Spongiform encephalopathy	Apathy, bradyphrenia, cerebellar dysarthria and ataxia, spastic hemi- or quadriparesis, tremor, chorea, myoclonus, pseudobulbar palsy, blindness
INFECTIOUS	
Endocarditis	Septic embolization with infarction, brain or spinal cord abscess, vasculitis, mycotic aneurysm with or without subarachnoid hemorrhage. Organisms: *Staphylococcus aureus, Pseudomonas aeruginosa, Candida albicans*
Vertebral osteomyelitis/epidural abscess	Back or neck pain, radiculopathy, spinal cord compression. Organisms: *S. aureus, P. aeruginosa, C. albicans*
Encephalitis/encephalopathy	Herpes simplex, herpes zoster, hepatitis C.
Clostridial	Tetanus ('skin poppers'), botulism ("Black tar heroin"), gas gangrene, wound infections
Anthrax	Meningitis, septic shock
Malaria	FUO, rapidly evolving stupor and coma
Tuberculosis	Tuberculoma, brain abscess, meningitis
Fungal	Cerebral mucormycosis, intravertebral candidiasis, nocardia brain abscess, brainstem chromoblastomycosis
HIV infection	Meningitis, encephalopathy (AIDS-dementia complex), toxoplasmosis, tuberculosis (tuberculoma, brain abscess, meningitis), syphilis (meningitis, meningovascular), cryptococcus (meningitis, granuloma), other fungi (e.g., candida, mucor, nocardia), virus (herpes simplex, herpes zoster, cytomegalovirus), stroke (nonbacterial thrombotic endocarditis, cerebral vasculitis, intracranial hemorrhage), progressive multifocal leukoencephalopathy, lymphoma, vacuolar myelopathy, Guillain-Barré syndrome, painful sensory neuropathy
VASCULAR	
Cerebral	Ischemic stroke, hemorrhagic stroke
Spinal	Anterior spinal arterylike syndrome, vasculitis, borderzone infarct
MOVEMENT DISORDERS	
Cerebellar	Ataxia, dysmetria
Extrapyramidal	Chorea, dyskinesias, dystonia, oculogyric crisis, parkinsonism (MPTP, meperidine), tremor
Other	Myoclonus, tics, coprolalia
OCULAR	
Ophthalmic	Quinine amblyopia, dyschromatopsias
SPINAL CORD	
Acute myelopathy	Anterior spinal arterylike syndrome with hypotension, immune-mediated or hypersensitivity myelitis-like syndrome
Subacute-Chronic Myelopathy	Subacute combined degenerationlike syndrome, epidural abscess, spongiform encephalopathy
NEUROMUSCULAR	
Peripheral nerve	Peripheral nerve injury (direct needle injection), direct neurotoxicity, peripheral nerve compression, compartment syndrome, brachial plexitis, lumbar plexitis, Guillain-Barré syndrome, cranial neuropathy
Muscular	Rhabdomyolysis, myoglobinuria, fibrotic myositis
RENAL DISEASE	
Nephropathy/uremia	Malignant hypertension, hypertensive encephalopathy, intracerebral hemorrhage

REM, rapid eye movement; FUO, fever of unknown origin; HIV, human immunodeficiency virus; AIDS, acquired immunodeficiency syndrome; MPTP, methyl-phenyl-tetrahydropyridine.
(Adapted from Brust JCM. Opioids. In: Brust JCM. *Neurological Aspects of Substance Abuse,* 2nd ed. Philadelphia: Elsevier Butterworth Heinemann; 2004:43–103; Brust JCM. Abused agents: Acute effects, withdrawal, and treatment. In: Brust JCM, ed. *Neurologic Complications of Substance Abuse,* ***CONTINUUM,*** American Academy of Neurology; 2004;10:14–47; Britton CB. Infections of the nervous system complicating alcoholism and illicit drug abuse. In: Brust JCM, ed. *Neurologic Complications of Substance Abuse,* ***CONTINUUM,*** American Academy of Neurology; 2004;10:48–76; Williams O. Movement disorders and substance abuse. In: Brust JCM, ed. *Neurologic Complications of Substance Abuse,* ***CONTINUUM,*** American Academy of Neurology, 2004;10:77–87; Williams O. Substance abuse and seizures. In: Brust JCM, ed. *Neurologic Complications of Substance Abuse,* ***CONTINUUM,*** American Academy of Neurology; 2004;10:88–99; Sloan MA, Kittner SJ, Price TR. Stroke and illicit drug use. In: Ginsburg MD, Bogousslavsky J, eds. *Cerebrovascular Disease: Pathophysiology, Diagnosis and Management.* Vol. II. Cambridge: Blackwell Science; 1998:1589–1609; Williams O. Stroke and substance abuse. In: Brust JCM, ed. *Neurologic Complications of Substance Abuse.* ***CONTINUUM,*** American Academy of Neurology; 2004;10:100–114; and Welmer LH. Spinal and neuromuscular complications of substance abuse. In: Brust JCM, ed. Neurologic Complications of Substance Abuse. ***CONTINUUM,*** American Academy of Neurology; 2004;10:115–143, with permission.)

immunocompromised host. Spine or spinal cord infections include osteomyelitis, discitis, and epidural and intramedullary abscesses. Systemic processes, such as clostridial (tetanus, botulism), anthrax, and malaria, may have both central nervous system and peripheral neuromuscular manifestations. In the patient with heroin addiction and HIV, the neurologic manifestations of infection may be caused by primary HIV involvement (primary meningitis, encephalopathy or acquired immunodeficiency syndrome [AIDS] dementia complex, vacuolar myelopathy, Guillain-Barré, sensory neuropathy) or from effects in an immuno-compromised host (toxoplasmosis, herpes infections, mycobacterial and fungal infections, JC virus, and progressive multifocal leukoencephalopathy [PML] and lymphoma) (1,3,7,10,12).

VASCULAR

Stroke (ischemia:hemorrhage: 2 to 3:1) occurs in about 20% of endocarditis cases. Ischemic stroke can occur via a variety of mechanisms: Embolism of partially crushed particulate matter; refractile particles, such as magnesium silicate (talc) and microcrystalline cellulose and cocoa butter in a suppository; hypoperfusion leading to borderzone ischemia (hypotension or large vessel stenoocclusive disease); allergic vasculitis associated with diverse systemic immunologic aberrations; and toxic vasculitis. Spinal cord infarction can result from embolism, with resultant anterior spinal artery syndrome borderzone ischemia. Mechanisms of intracranial hemorrhage include coagulopathy caused by hepatic failure with reduced clotting factors, use of anticoagulant adulterants, hypertension, and ruptured mycotic aneurysms or arteriovenous malformations (3,10,11).

MOVEMENT DISORDERS

Occult attempts to synthesize meperidine analogs led to the creation of 1-methyl-4-phenyl-1,2,3,6-tetrahydropyridine (MPTP) which, when converted by monoamine oxidase to methyl-phenylpyridium ion, is neurotoxic in a dose-dependent manner to nigral dopaminergic neurons, leading to parkinsonism. Myoclonus has been associated with use of meperidine (normeperidine), morphine, hydromorphone, and methadone, as well as withdrawal from fentanyl. Tremor and choreiform movements have been reported in patients on methadone maintenance therapy. Dyskinesias have been reported in patients treated with fentanyl. Nasal inhalation of heroin has been associated with dystonia and oculogyric crisis. A woman with Tourette syndrome developed coprolalia and motor tics after smoking heroin (3,8).

SPINAL CORD

A uniform clinical syndrome is lacking. Direct involvement of the spinal cord may be caused by opiate overdose with coma and hypotension leading to recognition of myelopathy on awakening or naloxone reversal or anterior spinal artery syndrome. The spinal cord can also be affected by a toxic effect from drug or adulterant or from embolism of particulate matter. In addition, an immune-mediated hypersensitivity reaction leading to myelopathy has been observed following renewed heroin use following a period of abstinence. Finally, infectious complications, such as intramedullary abscess and cord compression from epidural compression, can occur at various spinal locations (3,7,10,12).

NEUROMUSCULAR DISORDERS

Although described in case reports, a causal link between heroin injection and Guillain-Barré syndrome has not been established. Peripheral neuropathic syndromes associated with heroin abuse include mononeuropathies caused by direct compression (coma with muscle injury and compartment syndrome), direct trauma (needle injury), direct neurotoxicity, or hypersensitivity reaction. Brachial and lumbar plexitis, either mimicking idiopathic disease or caused by involvement from a septic aneurysm or local abscess have been described. Primary drug-induced rhabdomyolysis has been reported and must be distinguished from direct muscle injury from coma or prolonged immobility. It is unclear if the effect is caused by heroin or an adulterant. Fibrotic myositis occurs with chronic intramuscular injection of heroin, meperidine, and pentazocine.

MANAGEMENT OF INTOXICATION AND WITHDRAWAL

Tolerance to the effects of opiates develops rapidly with respect to euphoria, sedation, and respiratory depression, but develops to a lesser extent with respect to pupillary and smooth muscle effects. The clinical manifestations of opiate intoxication and withdrawal are shown in Table 104-4. Pure opioid antagonists produce no clinical effects in the nonopioid-dependent, nonstressed patient. In tolerant individuals, antagonists lead to withdrawal reactions (1,2). These reactions can also include an overshoot phenomenon, with potentially dangerous agitation, hypertension, tachycardia, and myocardial ischemia. Patients who present with profound hypoventilation or hypoxia are at risk for development of acute lung injury or posthypoxic encephalopathy. Often, patients abuse multiple drugs; in such cases, use of naloxone may unmask the effects of other drugs.

Treatment of opiate overdose includes respiratory (mechanical ventilation) and blood pressure support (intravenous fluids, rarely vasopressors) and the use of opiate antagonists, such as naloxone (Table 104-5). Opioids impair brainstem carbon dioxide sensitivity, so oxygen should be given cautiously. The goal of naloxone therapy is not complete arousal but the restitution of adequate spontaneous ventilation. Precipitation of withdrawal is often unpredictable and potentially detrimental, so the lowest practical dose should be used initially, with dose escalation as clinically warranted. Most patients respond to 0.05 mg of naloxone intravenously, although the requirement for ventilatory assistance may be prolonged because the onset of action may be slower than with larger doses. The dose can then be increased to 0.4 mg, 2 mg, and then 10 mg. If the patient has no response to 10 mg, then an opioid is likely not responsible for the respiratory depression. This approach may avoid the need for endotracheal intubation, and allows timely identification of nonopioid causes of the patient's clinical condition and avoids precipitation of acute opioid withdrawal (1,2). Evaluation for the return of sedation and respiratory depression should be monitored continuously. The duration of monitoring for recurrence of sedation and respiratory depression should be 2 hours for an intravenous opiate overdose and extended for an oral opiate overdose. Patients with recurrence of sedation or respiratory depression can be treated with repeat of the effective dose of naloxone or a repeated bolus followed by a continuous infusion. Two thirds of the effective bolus dose, when given hourly, usually maintains the desired effect. Patients should be hospitalized for close observation and to

TABLE 104-5. Treatment of Opioid Overdose

*Ventilatory support

*If hypoventilation does not respond to ventilation, use intravenous isotonic fluids (vasopressors rarely necessary)

*Consider prophylactic intubation

*Use of naloxone: Titrate dose: 0.05 mg, 0.4 mg, 2 mg, 10 mg
Dose preparation for naloxone 0.4 mg/mL:
Draw up 3 mL of 0.9% normal saline in a 5 mL syringe
Draw up 1 mL of 0.4 mg/mL
Mix, creating 0.4 mg naloxone in 4 ml saline, which is equivalent to 0.05 mg in 0.5 mL saline.
Dose preparation for continuous naloxone infusion:
Multiply effective bolus dose by 6.6
Add that quantity to 1000 mL of normal saline
Infuse solution at 100 mL/h

*Hospitalization and close observation. Watch for signs of intoxication from other drugs. Substance abuse counseling. Referral for detoxification or maintenance therapy program.

(Adapted from Nelson LS. Opioids. In: Flomenbaum NE, Goldfrank LR, Hoffman RS, et al., eds. *Goldfrank's Toxicologic Emergencies,* 8th ed. New York: McGraw-Hill; 2006:590–613; Howland MA. Opioid antagonists. In: Flomenbaum NE, Goldfrank LR, Hoffman RS, et al., eds. *Goldfrank's Toxicologic Emergencies,* 8th ed. New York: McGraw-Hill; 2006:614–619; and Brust JCM. Abused agents: Acute effects, withdrawal, and treatment. In: Brust JCM, ed. *Neurologic Complications of Substance Abuse, **CONTINUUM:*** American Academy of Neurology; 2004;10:14–47, with permission.)

begin substance abuse counseling, detoxification, or maintenance therapy, as appropriate (1,2,6).

DIAGNOSTIC APPROACH

For cases of opioid intoxication or overdose syndrome, patients and family or friends, if available and feasible, should be questioned about which drug(s) the patient may have taken. The history is notoriously unreliable, so urine toxicology screens are needed to identify the substance(s) taken. The drug assay results, however, must be viewed in the clinical context. Commercial opioid assays will not detect most semisynthetic and synthetic opioids. Oxycodone, hydrocodone, and other common morphine derivatives have variable detectability by various opioid screens (1). Diagnostic testing, including brain and spine neuroimaging, vascular imaging, lumbar puncture, laboratory tests, microbiology, polymerase chain reaction tests, neurophysiology, biopsy, and so forth for other neurologic syndromes should be designed according to acceptable clinical indications. Patients with neurologic syndromes and who have an immunocompromised status or HIV infection will likely require a more intensive diagnostic evaluation to look for evidence of HIV-specific disorders and opportunistic infections. The history and physical examination may also indicate that the patient has multiple concurrent neurologic disease processes. In these cases, evaluation for each disorder may be appropriate.

TREATMENT

Therapy for specific disorders is determined by establishing the cause(s) of symptoms, although evidence-based guidelines specifically pertaining to opiate-related neurologic syndromes are lacking. Ideally, the patient will take advice and cease using opiates. Seizures are treated with withdrawal of the offending agent, antiepileptic drugs, or both, depending on the clinical setting. No effective treatment exists for spongiform encephalopathy. Infections are treated with appropriate antibacterial, antitubercular, antiviral, and antifungal agents, as well as surgery or drainage for cranial and spinal abscesses, as appropriate. HIV should be treated with antiretroviral therapy and antimicrobial prophylaxis, as appropriate. Vascular disease should be treated according to the underlying stroke mechanism. Movement disorders can be treated with pharmacologic agents with presumed efficacy for the specific manifestation. Spinal and neuromuscular syndromes can be treated with medication, physiotherapy, and surgical decompression, as appropriate. With evidence of drug-associated inflammation or vasculitis, the patient can be treated with short- or long-term steroids or immunosuppressive agents, as appropriate.

CLINICAL RECOMMENDATIONS OF THE VIGNETTE

The patient has several neurologic issues to address. He had ongoing withdrawal and required hospitalization and observation for complications. After treatment for opiate intoxication and withdrawal, his blood pressure rose to 170/90 mm Hg. The neurologic examination suggests at least two lesions: One in the left side of the brain and the other in or affecting the spinal cord. CT scan of the brain showed cerebral atrophy, leukoencephalopathy, and an old left basal ganglia lacune. Magnetic resonance scan of the cervical and thoracic spine showed vacuolar myelopathy in the mid thoracic spine. HIV testing was positive. Vitamin B_{12}, folate, thyroid-stimulating hormone (TSH), and antinuclear antibody (ANA) were negative. He was treated with hydrochlorothiazide (25 mg) and aspirin (81 mg) for stroke prevention, multivitamins, antiretroviral therapy, and physical therapy.

SUMMARY

The pharmacology of opiate drugs is complex. Opiates are in wide clinical usage for purposes of analgesia and sedation. These drugs are subject to abuse, however. The opiate user or abuser is at risk to develop intoxication, overdose, and a wide variety of neurologic disorders. Careful management of intoxication and overdose will help avoid complications. Neurologic manifestations, which are protean, can result from the effects of the drug, adulterants, or accompanying illnesses, including HIV. A detailed neurologic examination and evaluation will lead to accurate diagnosis and management.

REFERENCES

1. Nelson LS. Opioids. In: Flomenbaum NE, Goldfrank LR, Hoffman RS, et al., eds. *Goldfrank's Toxicologic Emergencies,* 8th ed. New York: McGraw-Hill; 2006:590–613.
2. Howland MA. Opioid antagonists. In: Flomenbaum NE, Goldfrank LR, Hoffman RS, et al., eds. *Goldfrank's Toxicologic Emergencies,* 8th ed. McGraw-Hill; 2006:614–619.
3. Brust JCM. Opioids. In: Brust JCM. *Neurological Aspects of Substance Abuse,* 2nd ed. Philadelphia: Elsevier Butterworth Heinemann; 2004:43–103.
4. Substance Abuse and Mental Health Services Administration. *Results from the 2001 National Household Survey on Drug Abuse.* Vol. 1. Summary of National Findings. Rockville, MD: Office of Applied Studies, NHSDA Series H-17, US Department of Health and Human Services; 2002. Publication SMA 02-3758.

5. Ng SKC, Brust JCM, Hauser WA, et al. Illicit drug use and the risk of new onset seizures: Contrasting effects of heroin, marijuana, and cocaine. *Am J Epidemiol.* 1990;132:47–57.
6. Brust JCM. Abused agents: Acute effects, withdrawal, and treatment. In: Brust JCM, ed. *Neurologic Complications of Substance Abuse,* ***CONTINUUM:*** American Academy of Neurology; 2004;10:14–47.
7. Britton CB. Infections of the nervous system complicating alcoholism and illicit drug abuse. In: Brust JCM, ed. *Neurologic Complications of Substance Abuse,* ***CONTINUUM:*** American Academy of Neurology; 2004;10:48–76.
8. Williams O. Movement disorders and substance abuse. In: Brust JCM, ed. *Neurologic Complications of Substance Abuse,* ***CONTINUUM:*** American Academy of Neurology, 2004;10:77–87.
9. Williams O. Substance abuse and seizures. In: Brust JCM, ed. *Neurologic Complications of Substance Abuse,* ***CONTINUUM:*** American Academy of Neurology; 2004;10:88–99.
10. Sloan MA, Kittner SJ, Price TR. Stroke and illicit drug use. In: Ginsburg MD, Bogousslavsky J, eds. *Cerebrovascular Disease: Pathophysiology, Diagnosis and Management.* Vol. II. Cambridge: Blackwell Science; 1998:1589–1609.
11. Williams O. Stroke and substance abuse. In: Brust JCM, ed. *Neurologic Complications of Substance Abuse.* ***CONTINUUM:*** American Academy of Neurology; 2004;10:100–114.
12. Welmer LH. Spinal and neuromuscular complications of substance abuse. In: Brust JCM, ed. *Neurologic Complications of Substance Abuse.* ***CONTINUUM:*** American Academy of Neurology; 2004;10:115–143.
13. Wolters ECH, Van Winjungaarden GK, Stam FC, et al. Leukoencephalopathy after inhaling "heroin pyrolysate." *Lancet.* 1982;II:1233–1237.
14. McCreary M, Emerman C, Hanna J, et al. Acute meyelopathy following intranasal insufflation of heroin: A case report. *Neurology.* 2000;55:316–317.

CHAPTER 105

Amphetamines and Over-the-Counter Sympathomimetics

Michael A. Sloan

OBJECTIVES

- To describe the various amphetamines and over-the-counter sympathomimetics
- To discuss the neurologic complications of use and abuse of amphetamines and over-the-counter sympathomimetics
- To explore the approach to the diagnosis and treatment of neurologic complications of amphetamine use
- To describe the approach to management of amphetamine withdrawal

CASE VIGNETTE

A 24-year-old woman with no previous medical history was brought to the emergency department after becoming agitated, having a generalized tonic–clonic seizure, and remaining poorly responsive at a dance club. She was delirious, agitated, variably lethargic or hypervigilant, hallucinating, and had paranoid ideation. Her temperature was 102.6°F, blood pressure was 170/110 mm Hg, pulse was 108 beats per minute, and respirations were 18 per minute. Skin was diaphoretic but showed no needle track marks. Neck was supple. Glasgow Coma Scale score was E2M5V2 = 9. Mental status examination revealed orientation to person only, left hemispatial neglect, and denial of deficits. Speech was dysarthric. Cranial nerve examination demonstrated 6 mm and sluggish pupils, right gaze preference, left visual field extinction, left central facial paresis, and tongue deviation to the left. Motor examination demonstrated semipurposeful movements on both sides, right greater than left, bilateral hyperreflexia and a left Babinski sign.

DEFINITION AND PHARMACOLOGY

Amphetamine refers to *racemic beta-phenylisopropylamine or alpha-methylphenylethylamine* and belongs in the family of phenylethylamines. Amphetamine was first synthesized in 1887, and was later rediscovered in the 1920s. Methamphetamine, or d-phenylisopropylmethylamine hydrochloride, was synthesized about that time. Amphetamine was initially marketed as Benzedrine inhaler, a nasal decongestant, and also used as a treatment for narcolepsy, but was it banned by the US Food and Drug Administration (FDA) in 1959. Propylhexedrine, a less potent form of amphetamine, was marketed as Benzedrex inhaler in 1949. The term amphetamine refers to amphetamine analogs. Amphetaminelike drugs (i.e., over-the-counter sympathomimetic drugs, such as phenylpropanolamine, ephedrine, pseudoephedrine, phentermine, phendimetrazine, and so forth), have been marketed as nasal decongestants and anorectic agents.

The primary mechanism of action of amphetamines is to increase the release of catecholamines, particularly dopamine and norepinephrine (and serotonin to a lesser extent) from presynaptic nerve terminals. For example, with increasing doses of amphetamine, the drug diffuses through the presynaptic terminal membrane and interacts with the neurotransmitter transporter, causing exchange release of dopamine into the cytoplasm, alkalinizing the storage vesicles, and permitting release of dopamine from the vesicles and delivery to the synapse by reverse transport. Amphetamines can also block catecholamine reuptake by competitive inhibition (1). As a result, the main clinical effects of amphetamines are cardiovascular, neurologic, and psychiatric.

Structure-activity relationships for these compounds have been described (1-4). Table 105–1 describes some of these agents. Amphetamines are structurally similar, nonhydrazine amine-derivative monoamine oxidase inhibitors, such as phenelzine and tranylcypromine. Amphetamines differ from catecholamines in that they lack the catechol structure (hydroxyl groups at the 3 and 4 positions of the phenyl ring) and are resistant to metabolism by catechol-O-methyltransferase (COMT). The α-methyl group confers chirality to the molecule. Except for certain analogs (e.g., methylenedioxymethamphetamine or MDMA and certain MDMA analogs), the *d*-enantiomers are much more potent (typically four to ten times) than the *l*-enantiomer. Compounds devoid of –OH groups tend to cross the blood–brain barrier and have enhanced central nervous system (CNS) activity. Substitution at the α-carbon blocks oxidation by monoamine oxidase (MAO), whereas β-carbon substitution increases agonist activity at α- and β-adrenergic receptors and reduces CNS stimulant action. Compounds with α-methyl substitution, such as amphetamine and methamphetamine, possess strong stimulant, cardiovascular and anorectic properties. Large

TABLE 105-1. Amphetamine, Over-the-Counter Sympathomimetics, and 'Designer Drugs'

Generic Name	*Trade Name*	*Street Names*
2-amino-5-phenyl-oxazoline or aminorex		
Amphetamine	Benzedrine	Uppers, ups, bennies, black beauties, dexies, pep pills, jelly beans
Amphetamine and dextroamphetamine	Biphetamine	
Benzphetamine	Didrex	
Benzylketoamphetamine	Cathinone	Khat
Dexfenfluramine	Redux—withdrawn	
Dextroamphetamine	Dexedrine	
4-bromo-2,5-dimethoxy-amphetamine	DOB	
4-bromo-2,5-methoxyphenyl-ethylamine	2CB, MFT	"nexus"
Diethylpropion	Tenuate, Tepanil	
Ephedrine	Withdrawn	
Ephedra alkaloids		Ma huang, cloud 9, herbal ecstasy, ultimate euphoria, up your gas
Fenfluramine	Pondimin(R)—withdrawn	
Mazindol	Sanorex, Mazanor	
Methcathinone		Cat, Jeff, khat, ephedrone
4-methyl-2,5-dimethoxyamphetamine	DOM/STP	serenity, peace, tranquility
3,4-methylenedioxyamphetamine	MDA	Love drug
3,4-methylenedioxyethamphetamine	MDEA	Eve
3,4-methylenedioxymethamphetamine	MDMA	Ecstasy, Adam, XTC, M&M, the Yuppie drug, essence, clarity, venus, zen, doctor
MDMA and lysergic acid diethylamide (LSD)		Candy flipping
MDMA and ethanol, marijuana, other psychoactive agents		Staking
Methamphetamine	Methedrine, Desoxyn, Fetamin	Speed, yaba, crack, go
Methamphetamine and amphetamine		Crank, tina
Methamphetamine high purity, crystalline form		Ice
Methamphetamine and coffee		Biker's coffee
Methylphenidate	Ritalin	Vitamin R, skippy, poor man's cocaine, smart drug
Naphalozine	Privine nasal solution Naphcon ophthalmic solution	
Oxymetazoline	Afrin nasal solution Ocular ophthalmic solution	
para-Chloroamphetamine		
para-Methoxyamphetamine	PMA	
Pemoline	Cylert	
Phendimetrazine	Plegine, Bontril	
Phenylpropanolamine	Propadrine, Propagest Nasal decongestants, diet pills—withdrawn	
Phenmetrazine	Preludin, Prelu-2	
Phentermine	Ionamin, Wilpo, Adipex-P, Fastin	
Propylhexadrine	Benzedrex nasal inhaler	
Pseudoephedrine	Tightly regulated	
Tetrahydrozoline	Tyzine nasal solution Visine ophthalmic solution	
2,4,5-Trimethoxyamphetamine		

(From Chiang WK. Amphetamines. In: Flomenbaum NE, Goldfrank LR, Hoffman RS, et al., eds. *Goldfrank's Toxicologic Emergencies*, 8th ed. New York: McGraw-Hill; 2006:1118–1132; Brust JCM. Amphetamines and other psychostimulants. In: Brust JCM. *Neurological Aspects of Substance Abuse*, 2nd ed. Philadelphia: Elsevier Butterworth Heinemann; 2004:105–138; and Brust JCM. Abused agents: Acute effects, withdrawal, and treatment. In: Brust JCM, ed. *Neurologic Complications of Substance Abuse.* ***CONTINUUM***, American Academy of Neurology; 2004;10:14–47, with permission.)

group substitutions at the α-carbon reduces stimulant and cardiovascular effects, but retains the anorectic properties (e.g., phentermine). Substitution at the para-position of the phenyl ring enhances hallucinogenic or serotonergic effects (e.g., DOB, parachloroamphetamine, paramethoxyamphetamine, and MDMA). Drugs with stimulant and hallucinogenic properties, such as MDMA and methyldiethanolamine (MDEA), are called *entactogens* (Latin: "to be moved," Greek: "within"). Typical clinical effects are shown in Table 105-2. There is tolerance to the anorectic, cardiovascular, hyperthermic, and lethal effects, but sensitization (reverse tolerance) to dyskinesias, psychotomimetic effects and seizures (1,2).

Resistance to COMT and MAO permit better oral availability and longer duration of action. Amphetamines are eliminated via diverse hepatic transformations (*N*-dealkylation and demethylation primarily via CYP2D6 and CYP3A4, hydroxylation) and renal elimination. Depending on the particular compound, active metabolites of secondary amphetamines and ephedrine derivatives can be formed. Amphetamines are strong bases with a typical pKa range (the pH at which the concentrations of the ionized and ionized forms are equal) from 9 to 10, with renal elimination depending on urine pH. Renal elimination is substantial for amphetamine (30%), methamphetamine (40% to 50%), MDMA (65%), and phentermine (80%). The half-lives of selected drugs are amphetamine 8 to 0 hours, methamphetamine 12 to 34 hours, MDMA 5 to 10 hours, methylphenidate 2.5 to 4 hours, phentermine 19 to 24 hours, and para-methoxyamphetamine 16 to 38 hours. Repetitive administration during binge use leads to drug accumulation, with prolonged half-life and duration of action (1).

EPIDEMIOLOGY

The history and epidemiology of amphetamine use and addiction has recently been reviewed (1,2,5,6). Historically, the source of amphetamines has been discovery by pharmaceutical companies, but most amphetamine use is nonprescription or illicit (1,2). The Controlled Substance Act of 1970 placed amphetamines into Schedule II to regulate diversion of amphetamines for nonmedicinal uses, with resultant decrease in amphetamine use in the 1970s. From the late 1980s to 1990s, a dramatic resurgence in methamphetamine use occurred, because of the availability of high purity crystalline methamphetamine or 'ice.' From 1991 to 1994, the number of deaths attributable to methamphetamine tripled, particularly in Los Angeles, San Diego, San Francisco, and Phoenix. Since the late 1990s, the ease and low cost of methamphetamine production, often from pseudoephedrine, has facilitated the spread of this drug, mostly via synthesis of the powder in clandestine laboratories, to every state, particularly in the midwestern and western United States. According to the 2001 US National Household Survey on Drug Abuse (5), it was estimated that 7 million people had used 'psychotherapeutic drugs,' including stimulants and hallucinogens. Most European methamphetamine is supplied in pills made in Southeast Asia.

Since the 1980s, more than 200 so-called *designer drugs*, mostly methylenedioxy derivatives of amphetamine, metamphetamine, and methamphetamine, have been synthesized to circumvent existing regulations (1,2). The best known of these agents are MDMA and MDEA. In 1986, the legal standard changed to include any agent that was used as a stimulant, hallucinogen, or anorectic. Despite this, the use of MDMA became, and remains, the most widely used amphetamine by teenagers, college students, and at parties, dance clubs, and 'rave' or 'techno' parties. According to the 2001 US National Household Survey on Drug Abuse (5), the estimated prevalence of current (within 30 days) MDMA use was 8.1 million. By 2003, use within the past year declined to 2.1 million (7).

Khat (*Catha edulis*) is a shrub indigenous to East Africa and the Arabian peninsula that contains cathinone, or benzylketoamphetamine. Individuals in these world regions chew fresh khat leaves for their stimulant, euphoric, and anorexant effects. Methcathinone (ephedrane) is the methyl derivative of cathinone, which is synthesized from ephedrine. It has potency similar to methamphetamine. The drug has been widely abused in the former Soviet Union and, more recently, midwestern United States.

Cardiac (8–14), pulmonary (15–17), and neurologic (18,19) complications have been described in patients taking appetite suppressants, such as phentermine, fenfluramine, and dexfenfluramine (8–17) and nasal decongestants or ephedra alkaloids (18,19). In patients taking appetite suppressants, the prevalence of cardiac valvular abnormalities ranged from 0.14% to 32% (1). In a meta-analysis (14), a 12% prevalence of valvular regurgitation (mostly aortic) was seen with >90 days use in the exposed group compared with 5.9% in the unexposed group. The highest risks were for patients taking combination fenfluramine-phentermine, and for those who used the drug for >4 months. Serial echocardiography shows that the valvular dysfunction typically improves following cessation of therapy. A substantially increased risk (up to 23-fold) of pulmonary hypertension exists in patients taking appetite suppressant drugs for >3 months, particularly with fenfluramine (17). In the Hemorrhagic Stroke Project (18), phenylpropanolamine has been associated with a 16.5 times increased risk of hemorrhagic stroke in women (95% confidence interval = 1.51–182.21, $P = 0.02$). An analysis of US Food and Drug Administration (FDA) MedWatch reports on use of dietary supplements containing ephedra alkaloids (ma huang) (19) revealed that 31% of 140 reported adverse events, including 10 strokes and 7 seizures, were definitely or probably related to the use of the supplements. In the United States, fenfluramine, dexfenfluramine, phenylpropanolamine, and ephedrine have been withdrawn from the market, and pseudoephedrine has been more tightly regulated.

ETIOLOGY, PATHOGENESIS, CLINICAL MANIFESTATIONS, AND SPECIAL SITUATIONS

Numerous case reports and case series have demonstrated that the acute and chronic neurologic manifestations of amphetamine use are protean (2,6,18–29), as summarized in Table 105-3. In general, the clinical syndromes can be caused by toxic effects of amphetamines, adulterant(s), an infectious complication (e.g., human immunodeficiency virus [HIV], another systemic factor, or some combination. In this section, specific categories of neurologic manifestations are discussed. In addition, the management of amphetamine intoxication and withdrawal will be covered.

GENERAL CEREBRAL

Seizures are a not an uncommon feature of amphetamine toxicity or withdrawal, with an estimated prevalence of 3% to 22%

TABLE 105-2. Clinical Effects of Amphetamines

Organ System	*Clinical Effect*	*Agents*
CARDIOVASCULAR	Hypertension	Various
	Tachycardia	
	Dysrhythmias	
	Myocardial ischemia/infarction	
	Valvular regurgitation	Fenfluramine, dexfenfluramine, phentermine
OTHER SYMPATHETIC	Diaphoresis	Various
	Tachypnea	
	Mydriasis	
	Tremor	
	Nausea	
NEUROLOGIC	Hyperthermia	Various
	Euphoria	
	Anorexia	
	Headache	
	Lethargy	
	Coma	
	Seizures	
	Nystagmus	MDMA
	Hyperreflexia	
	Choreoathetoid movements	
	Parkinsonism	MDMA
	Bruxism	
	Myoclonus	MDMA
	Muscle rigidity	
	Dystonia	
	Tourette syndrome	
	Rhabdomyolysis	
PSYCHIATRIC	Agitation	Various
	Violence, including suicide and homicide	
	Psychosis-like paranoid schizophrenia	
	Compulsive, repetitive behaviors	
	Flashbacks	MDMA
	Hallucinations: Visual, tactile	DOM, MDA, MDMA, MDEA
DERMATOLOGIC	Flushing	
	Diaphoresis	
OTHER SYSTEMIC	Vasculitis	Various
	Aortic dissection	
	Cardiomyopathy: Acute and chronic	
	Acute lung injury (noncardiogenic pulmonary edema)	
	Pulmonary hypertension	Fenfluramine
	Pneumomediastinum	Amphetamine
	Ischemic colitis	
	Pancreatitis	
	Acute renal failure	
	Disseminated intravascular coagulation	
LABORATORY ABNORMALITIES		
	Hyponatremia	Various
	Hypernatremia	
	Hyperglycemia	
	Hypoglycemia	
	Elevated liver enzymes	
	Leukocytosis	
	Elevated creatine kinase (CK)	
	Myoglobinuria	
	Renal insufficiency	

MDMA, methylenedioxymethamphetamine; DOM, 4-bromo-2,5-dimethoxy-amphetamine; MDA, 3,4-methylenedioxyethamphetamine; MDEA, 3,4-methylenedioxyethamphetamine.
(Modified from Chiang WK. Amphetamines. In: Flomenbaum NE, Goldfrank LR, Hoffman RS, et al., eds. *Goldfrank's Toxicologic Emergencies*, 8th ed. New York: McGraw-Hill; 2006:1118–1132; Brust JCM. Amphetamines and other psychostimulants. In: Brust JCM. *Neurological Aspects of Substance Abuse*, 2nd ed. Philadelphia: Elsevier Butterworth Heinemann; 2004:105–138; and Brust JCM. Abused agents: Acute effects, withdrawal, and treatment. In: Brust JCM, ed. *Neurologic Complications of Substance Abuse.* ***CONTINUUM***: American Academy of Neurology; 2004;10:14–47, with permission.)

TABLE 105-3. Neurologic Manifestations of Amphetamine Use or Addiction

Category	*Specific Disorder or Clinical Finding*
GENERAL OR CEREBRAL	
Acute Intoxication	Alertness, hypervigilance, lethargy, coma, euphoria, increased motor activity, hyperthermia, hypertension, tachycardia, arrhythmias, tachypnea, mydriasis, agitation, depression, psychosis, headache, seizures, movement disorders, suppression of REM sleep
Withdrawal	Fatigue, depression, excessive sleep, drug craving, dysphoria, suicidal ideation
Seizures	Partial, partial complex, generalized
Cognitive impairment	Inattention, memory loss
Spongiform encephalopathy	Apathy, bradyphrenia, cerebellar dysarthria and ataxia, spastic hemi/quadriparesis, tremor, chorea, myoclonus, pseudobulbar palsy, blindness
PSYCHIATRIC	
Psychosis	Auditory, visual, olfactory, haptic/cutaneous
Schizophrenia	Paranoia, delusions, violence
INFECTIOUS	
Endocarditis	Septic embolization with infarction, brain/spinal cord abscess, vasculitis, mycotic aneurysm with or without subarachnoid hemorrhage. Organisms: *Staphylococcus aureus, Pseudomonas aeruginosa, Candida albicans*
Vertebral osteomyelitis/ Epidural abscess	Back or neck pain, radiculopathy, spinal cord compression Organisms: S. aureus, P. aeruginosa, C. albicans
Encephalitis/encephalopathy	Herpes simplex, herpes zoster, hepatitis C
Clostridial	Tetanus ('skin poppers'), botulism ("Black tar heroin"), gas gangrene, wound infections
Tuberculosis	Tuberculoma, brain abscess, meningitis
Fungal	Cerebral mucormycosis, intravertebral candidiasis, Nocardia brain abscess, brainstem chromoblastomycosis
HIV infection	Meningitis, encephalopathy (AIDS-dementia complex), toxoplasmosis, tuberculosis (tuberculoma, brain abscess, meningitis), syphilis (meningitis, meningovascular), cryptococcus (meningitis, granuloma), other fungi (candida, mucor, nocardia, etc.), virus (herpes simplex, herpes zoster, cytomegalovirus), stroke (nonbacterial thrombotic endocarditis, cerebral vasculitis, intracranial hemorrhage), progressive multifocal leukoencephalopathy, lymphoma, vacuolar myelopathy, Guillain-Barré syndrome, painful sensory neuropathy
VASCULAR	
Cerebral	Ischemic stroke, hemorrhagic stroke
Spinal	Anterior spinal arterylike syndrome, Brown-Sequard syndrome
MOVEMENT DISORDERS	
Cerebellar	Ataxia, dysmetria
Extrapyramidal	Chorea, dyskinesias, dystonia
Other	Myoclonus, bruxism, tics
OCULAR	
Ophthalmic	Retinal artery branch occlusion (phenoxazoline, oxymetazoline)
SPINAL CORD	
Acute myelopathy	Anterior spinal arterylike syndrome
Muscular	Rhabdomyolysis, myoglobinuria
RENAL DISEASE	
Nephropathy/uremia	Malignant hypertension, hypertensive encephalopathy, intracebral hemorrhage

REM, rapid eye movement; HIV, human immunodeficiency virus; AIDS, acquired immunodeficiency syndrome.

(Adapted from Chiang WK. Amphetamines. In: Flomenbaum NE, Goldfrank LR, Hoffman RS, et al., eds. *Goldfrank's Toxicologic Emergencies,* 8th ed. New York: McGraw-Hill; 2006:1118–1132; Brust JCM. Amphetamines and other psychostimulants. In: Brust JCM. *Neurological Aspects of Substance Abuse,* 2nd ed. Philadelphia: Elsevier Butterworth Heinemann; 2004:105–138; and Brust JCM. Abused agents: Acute effects, withdrawal, and treatment. In: Brust JCM, ed. *Neurologic Complications of Substance Abuse.* ***CONTINUUM***: American Academy of Neurology; 2004;10:14–47; Britton CB. Infections of the nervous system complicating alcoholism and illicit drug abuse. In: Brust JCM, ed. *Neurologic Complications of Substance Abuse.* ***CONTINUUM***: American Academy of Neurology; 2004;10:48–76; Williams O. Movement disorders and substance abuse. In: Brust JCM, ed. *Neurologic Complications of Substance Abuse,* ***CONTINUUM***: American Academy of Neurology; 2004;10:77–87; Williams O. Substance abuse and seizures. In: Brust JCM, ed. *Neurologic Complications of Substance Abuse.* ***CONTINUUM***: American Academy of Neurology; 2004;10:88–99; Sloan MA, Kittner SJ, Price TR. Stroke and illicit drug use. In: Ginsburg MD, Bogousslavsky J, eds. *Cerebrovascular Disease: Pathophysiology, Diagnosis and Management.* Vol. II. Cambridge: Blackwell Science; 1998:1589–1609; Williams O. Stroke and substance abuse. In: Brust JCM, ed. *Neurologic Complications of Substance Abuse.* ***CONTINUUM***: American Academy of Neurology; 2004;10:100–114, with permission.)

(22). In this setting, seizures can be attributable to a direct neurotoxic effect, underlying structural lesion, or hypoxia. In patients with focal neurologic findings, a structural lesion should be sought. Chronic experimental administration of amphetamines, particularly amphetamine, methamphetamine, and MDMA, may be neurotoxic to dopaminergic and serotonergic nerve terminals. These agents can also lead to functional metabolic abnormalities, including cortical underactivity, in the absence of structural abnormalities on magnetic resonance imaging (MRI) studies. Autopsy studies in human methamphetamine users demonstrate reduced striatal levels of dopamine and dopamine transporter. Impaired memory and cognitive performance have been described in chronic MDMA users (2). Spongiform encephalopathy, similar to the entity observed in users of pyrolized heroin (see Chapter 106), has been described in one daily khat user, but use of other drugs was denied (2).

PSYCHIATRIC

Amphetamine produces positive schizophrenic symptoms (paranoia, hallucinations) without negative symptoms (emotional withdrawal, motor retardation). Paranoia can lead to violence, homicide, and suicide. Psychosis can occur after a single 'run' or emerge after months. Premorbid psychopathology is common in chronic users, but psychosis can occur in apparently normal subjects. Psychosis can recur, even after prolonged abstinence. Stereotyped, repetitive behavior can last for hours (1,2).

INFECTIONS

The amphetamine user is at risk for a wide variety of infections that affect the brain, meninges, spine, and spinal cord. These infections can be associated with amphetamine use *per se* via contiguous or hematogenous spread or than can be caused by immunosuppression, such as with HIV infection. Cerebral infections can result from bacterial cerebritis caused by septic embolization from acute or subacute bacterial endocarditis, diverse forms of meningitis, viral encephalitis, and from various mycobacterial and fungal infections that might occur in an immunocompromised host. Spine or spinal cord infections include osteomyelitis, discitis, and epidural and intramedullary abscesses. Systemic processes, such as clostridial (tetanus, botulism) and malaria, may have CNS and peripheral neuromuscular manifestations. In the patient with amphetamine addiction and HIV, the neurologic manifestations of infection may be caused by primary HIV involvement (primary meningitis, encephalopathy or acquired immunodeficiency syndrome [AIDS] dementia complex, vacuolar myelopathy, Guillain-Barré syndrome, sensory neuropathy), or from effects in an immunocompromised host (toxoplasmosis, herpes infections, mycobacterial and fungal infections, JC virus, and progressive multifocal leukoencephalopathy (PML) and lymphoma (2,20).

SYSTEMIC VASCULOPATHY

Amphetamine abuse is associated with necrotizing vasculitis (1,2,23–25). The vasculitis is a direct effect of amphetamines, and can involve multiple organ systems, including CNS, cardiovascular system, and gastrointestinal and renal systems.

Systemic manifestations include aortic dissection, myocardial infarction, acute and chronic cardiomyopathy, noncardiogenic pulmonary edema, ischemic colitis, pancreatitis, and acute renal failure.

VASCULAR

Stroke has most frequently been reported to complicate the use of amphetamine, methamphetamine, methylphenidate, ephedrine, pseudoephedrine, phenylpropanolamine, and MDMA (1,2,18,19,23–28). Ischemic and hemorrhagic stroke (ischemia:hemorrhage, 2 to 3:1) occurs in about 20% of endocarditis cases. Widespread angiographic beading of cerebral arteries, with occlusion of arterioles, has been reported in intravenous methamphetamine users (24). In MDMA users, low cortical 5-HT2 receptor densities were associated with low cerebral blood vessel volumes (implying vasoconstriction) and high cortical 5-HT2 receptor densities with high cerebral blood vessel volumes (implying vasodilatation) in specific brain regions have been observed (27). Ischemic stroke can occur via a variety of mechanisms: Embolism of partially crushed particulate matter; refractile particles, such as magnesium silicate (talc) and microcrystalline cellulose; or direct inadvertent injection into an artery; hypoperfusion leading to borderzone ischemia (hypotension or large vessel stenoocclusive disease) and toxic vasculitis. Spinal cord infarction can result from embolism with resultant anterior spinal artery syndrome borderzone ischemia or a Brown-Sequard syndrome. Mechanisms of intracranial hemorrhage, both intracerebral and subarachnoid, include hypertension, vasculitis, or ruptured berry aneurysms, mycotic aneurysms, or arteriovenous malformations (1,2,23–27).

MOVEMENT DISORDERS

Theoretically, parkinsonism can be induced because of methamphetamine-associated reduction in striatal dopamine and dopamine transporter. It is unclear, however, if these findings increase the risk of Parkinson disease with advancing age (2). Lower extremity myoclonus has been associated with use of MDMA. Choreoathetoid movements and bruxism have uncommonly been reported in patients with acute and chronic amphetamine use. Tourette syndrome has been exacerbated or precipitated by use of amphetamine, methylphenidate, and pemoline (2).

NEUROMUSCULAR DISORDERS

Primary amphetamine-induced rhabdomyolysis and myoglobinuria have been reported in patients using intravenous amphetamines, MDMA and MDEA. These agents have also produced serotonin syndrome, which has been linked to muscle ischemia and myoglobinuria. These effects must be distinguished from direct muscle injury from coma or prolonged immobility. If hyperthermia is present, heat stroke and malignant hyperthermia must be considered (1,2).

MANAGEMENT OF INTOXICATION AND WITHDRAWAL

Tolerance to the effects of amphetamines develops rapidly with respect to euphoria, 'rush,' and cardiovascular effects, but not

TABLE 105-4. Treatment of Amphetamine Overdose

Reduce excitement:	Verbal communication in a quiet, lighted room
Protect against injury:	Physical restraint as necessary
Ventilatory support:	As appropriate
Intravenous isotonic fluids	
Intravenous glycemic control:	D50W for hypoglycemia Insulin for hyperglycemia Thiamine 100 mg
Hyponatremia:	3% Hypertonic saline
Antihypertensive agents:	Alpha blocker – phentolamine Nitroprusside
Hyperthermia:	External cooling with ice packs ?Intravascular techniques
Sedation:	Benzodiazepines
Antiepileptic drugs:	Diazepam, valproate
Hospitalization and close observation	
Watch for signs of intoxication from other drugs	
Substance abuse counseling	
Referral for detoxification program	

(Adapted from Chiang WK. Amphetamines. In: Flomenbaum NE, Goldfrank LR, Hoffman RS, et al., eds. *Goldfrank's Toxicologic Emergencies,* 8th ed. New York: McGraw-Hill; 2006:1118–1132; Brust JCM. Amphetamines and other psychostimulants. In: Brust JCM. *Neurological Aspects of Substance Abuse,* 2nd ed. Philadelphia: Elsevier Butterworth Heinemann; 2004:105–138; and Brust JCM. Abused agents: Acute effects, withdrawal, and treatment. In: Brust JCM, ed. *Neurologic Complications of Substance Abuse.* ***CONTINUUM***: American Academy of Neurology; 2004;10:14–47, with permission.)

the psychiatric effects. The clinical manifestations of amphetamine intoxication and withdrawal are shown in Table 105-3. Often, patients abuse multiple drugs; in such cases, clinical evaluation and laboratory testing may be useful to distinguish between various pharmacologic agents. The usual fatal dose of amphetamine in a nontolerant adult is 20 to 25 mg/kg. Death most commonly results from hyperthermia, cardiac dysrhythmias, and intracerebral hemorrhage, although acidosis, renal failure, or coagulopathy may contribute (1,2).

Treatment of amphetamine overdose (Table 105-4) usually begins with reducing excitement and protecting against injury. General medical therapy includes mechanical ventilation, as appropriate; blood pressure control with antihypertensives, such as phentolamine or nitroprusside, intravenous fluids, intravenous glucose (D50W), or thiamine (100 mg), as appropriate; control of hyperthermia with external cooling; control of agitation with benzodiazepines (sometimes up to 100 mg of diazepam); and antiepileptic drugs, such as diazepam and valproate. Intravenous fluids should be given to maintain urine output of 1 to 2 mL/kg/hour. Although urinary acidification can significantly increase the elimination and decrease the half-lives of amphetamine and methamphetamine, this pH manipulation can increase the risk of renal compromise and acute tubular necrosis from rhabdomyolysis by precipitating ferrihemate in the renal tubules. Patients with acute renal failure, academia, and hyperkalemia will likely require urgent dialysis. Antipsychotic agents are not ideal for control of agitation or psychosis, because they can lower the seizure threshold, alter temperature regulation, and cause acute dystonia and cardiac dysrhythmias. Hyponatremia can be treated with 3% normal saline in standard fashion to avoid complicating central pontine myelinolysis. As with cocaine users, 'body packers' with suspected leakage of amphetamine-containing packets require surgical intervention (1,2).

GENERAL DIAGNOSTIC APPROACH

For cases of amphetamine intoxication or overdose syndrome, patients and family or friends, if available and feasible, should be questioned about which drug(s) the patient may have taken. The history is notoriously unreliable, so urine toxicology screens are needed to identify the substance(s) taken. Drug assay results, however, are not drug-specific, nor are they valuable in the acute overdose setting. Commercial amphetamine immunoassays will cross-react with cold preparations containing pseudoephdrine. Selegiline, a MAO B inhibitor used for treatment of Parkinson disease, is metabolized to amphetamine and methamphetamine, and will result in a false–positive test results. Most immunoassays do not react with all amphetamines, and thus will lead to false–negative results. MDMA frequently goes unrecognized. The reference standard, gas chromatography-mass spectrometry, can misidentify isomeric substances, such as *l*- for *d*-amphetamine, if performed by inexperienced personnel. The prevalence of amphetamine abuse in the local geographic region should heighten suspicion of amphetamine toxicity in patients with an appropriate clinical presentation (1).

Diagnostic testing, including brain and spine neuroimaging; vascular imaging, lumbar puncture, laboratory tests, microbiology, polymerase chain reaction tests, neurophysiology, biopsy, and so on, for other neurologic syndromes should be designed according to acceptable clinical indications. Hyponatremia should specifically be suspected for any patient with altered sensorium and suspected MDMA usage. Patients with neurologic syndromes and an immunocompromised status or HIV infection will likely require a more intensive diagnostic evaluation to look for evidence of HIV-specific disorders and opportunistic infections. The history and physical examination may also indicate that the patient has multiple concurrent neurologic disease processes. In these cases, evaluation for each disorder may be appropriate.

TREATMENT

Therapy for specific disorders is determined by establishing the cause(s) of symptoms, although evidence-based guidelines specifically pertaining to amphetamine-related neurologic syndromes are lacking. Metabolic disorders, such as extremes of glycemic control or sodium homeostasis, should be treated accordingly. Ideally, the patient will take advice and cease using amphetamines. Seizures are treated with withdrawal of the offending agent, antiepileptic drugs, or both, depending on the clinical setting. No effective treatment exists for spongiform encephalopathy. Infections are treated with appropriate antibacterial, antitubercular, antiviral, and antifungal agents, as well as surgery or drainage for cranial and spinal abscesses, as appropriate. HIV should be treated with antiretroviral therapy and antimicrobial prophylaxis, as appropriate. Vascular disease should be treated according to the underlying stroke mechanism. Movement disorders can be treated with pharmacologic agents with presumed efficacy for the specific manifestation. Spinal and neuromuscular syndromes can be treated with medication, physiotherapy, and surgical decompression, as appropriate. With evidence of drug-associated inflammation or vasculitis, the patient can be treated with short- or long-term steroids or immunosuppressive agents, as appropriate.

CLINICAL RECOMMENDATIONS OF THE VIGNETTE

The patient had several medical and neurologic issues that needed to be addressed. She had seizure activity that required treatment with diazepam and valproate. Hypertension was treated with nitroprusside. Serum sodium was 112 mEq/L, and 3% hypertonic saline was administered, ultimately correcting to 132 mEq/L at 24 hours. The neurologic examination also suggested a right brain lesion. Computed tomographic (CT) scan of the brain showed a 3.3 × 2.4 × 3.6 cc *3 hemorrhage centered in the lateral right basal ganglia, with extension to the ventricular system and mild ventriculomegaly. Neurosurgical evaluation recommended follow-up CT scan the next day, which revealed no hydrocephalus. She was treated with nitroprusside for 2 days, and then was weaned from them. She then became normotensive. Several days after admission, she admitted to MDMA use, and substance abuse counseling was instituted. With rehabilitation, physical and occupational therapy, her nondominant syndrome and left hemiparesis improved. She was left with minimal neurologic residual.

SUMMARY

The pharmacology of amphetamine drugs is complex. Amphetamines are in wide usage for nonmedicinal purposes and are subject to abuse. The amphetamine user or abuser is at risk to develop intoxication, overdose, and a wide variety of life-threatening medical and neurologic disorders. Careful management of intoxication and overdose will help avoid complications. Neurologic manifestations are protean and can result from the effects of the drug, adulterants, or accompanying illnesses, including HIV. A detailed neurologic examination and evaluation will lead to accurate diagnosis and management.

REFERENCES

1. Chiang WK. Amphetamines. In: Flomenbaum NE, Goldfrank LR, Hoffman RS, et al., eds. *Goldfrank's Toxicologic Emergencies*, 8th ed. New York: McGraw-Hill; 2006:1118–1132.
2. Brust JCM. Amphetamines and other psychostimulants. In: Brust JCM. *Neurological Aspects of Substance Abuse*, 2nd ed. Philadelphia: Elsevier Butterworth Heinemann; 2004:105–138.
3. Weiner N. Norepinephrine, epinephrine, and the sympathomimetic amines. In: Gilman AG, Goodman LS, Rall TN, et al., eds. *The Pharmacologic Basis of Therapeutics*, 7th ed. New York: Macmillan; 1980:145–180.
4. Goodman L, Gilman A, Rall TW, et al., eds. *The Pharmacologic Basis of Therapeutics*. Elmsford, NY: Pergamon; 1990:210–214.
5. Substance Abuse and Mental Health Services Administration. *Results from the 2001 National Household Survey on Drug Abuse*. Vol. 1. Summary of national findings. Rockville, MD: Office of Applied Studies, NHSDA Series H-17, US Dept of Health and Human Services; 2002. Publication SMA 02-3758.
6. Brust JCM. Abused agents: Acute effects, withdrawal, and treatment. In: Brust JCM, ed. *Neurologic Complications of Substance Abuse*. **CONTINUUM**: American Academy of Neurology; 2004;10:14–47.
7. Substance Abuse and Mental Health Services Administration (SAMHSA). *2003 National Household Survey on Drug Abuse: Results*. Rockville, MD: Office of Applied Studies, US Department of Health and Human Services; 2004.
8. Centers for Disease Control and Prevention (CDC). Cardiac valvulopathy associated with exposure to fenfluramine or dexfenfluramine: US Department of Health and Human Services interim public health recommendations, November, 1997. *MMWR Morb Mort Wkly Rep*. 1997;46:1061–1066.
9. Connolly HM, Crary JL, McGoon MD, et al. Valvular heart disease associated with fenfluramine-phentermine. *N Engl J Med*. 1997;337:581–588.
10. Khan MA, Herzog CA, St. Peter JV, et al. The prevalence of cardiac valvular insufficiency assessed by transthoracic echocardiography in obese patients treated with appetite-suppressant drugs. *N Engl J Med*. 1998;339:713–718.
11. Jick H, Vasilakis C, Weinrauch LA, et al. A population-based study of appetite-suppressant drugs and the risk of cardiac-valve regurgitation. *N Engl J Med*. 1998;339:719–724.
12. Weissman NJ, Tighe JF, Jr., Gottdeiner JS, et al. An assessment of heart-valve abnormalities in obese patients taking dexfenfluramine, sustained-release dexfenfluramine, or placebo. *N Engl J Med*. 1998;339:725–732.
13. Gardin JM, Schumacher D, Constantine G, et al. Valvular abnormalities and cardiovascular status following exposure to dexfenfluramine and phentermine/fenfluramine. *JAMA*. 2000;283:1703–1709.
14. Sachdev M, Miller WC, Ryan T, et al. Effects of fenfluramine-derivative diet pills on cardiac valves: A meta-analysis of observational studies. *Am Heart J*. 2002;144:1065–1073.
15. Kringsholm B, Christofferson P. Lung and heart pathology in fatal drug addiction. *Forensic Sci Int*. 1987;34:39–41.
16. Schaiberger PH, Kennedy TC, Miller FC, et al. Pulmonary hypertension associated with long-term inhalation of "crank" methamphetamine. *Chest*. 1993;104:614–616.
17. Abenhaim L, Moride Y, Brenot F, et al. Appetite-suppressant drugs and the risk of primary pulmonary hypertension. *N Engl J Med*. 1996;335:609–615.
18. Kernan WN, Viscoli CM, Brass LM, et al. Phenylpropanolamine and the risk of hemorrhagic stroke. *N Engl J Med*. 2000;343:1826–1832.
19. Haller CA, Benowitz NL. Adverse cardiovascular and central nervous system events associated with dietary supplements containing ephedra alkaloids. *N Engl J Med*. 2000;343: 1833–1838.
20. Britton CB. Infections of the nervous system complicating alcoholism and illicit drug abuse. In: Brust JCM, ed. *Neurologic Complications of Substance Abuse*. **CONTINUUM**: American Academy of Neurology; 2004;10:48–76.
21. Williams O. Movement disorders and substance abuse. In: Brust JCM, ed. *Neurologic Complications of Substance Abuse*, **CONTINUUM**: American Academy of Neurology; 2004;10:77–87.
22. Williams O. Substance abuse and seizures. In: Brust JCM, ed. *Neurologic Complications of Substance Abuse*. **CONTINUUM**: American Academy of Neurology; 2004;10:88–99.
23. Citron BP, Halpern M, McCarron M, et al. Necrotizing angiitis associated with drug abuse. *N Engl J Med*. 1970;283:1003–1011.
24. Rumbaugh CL, Bergeron RT, Fang HCH, et al. Cerebral angiographic changes in the drug abuse patient. *Radiology*. 1971;101:335–344.
25. Sloan MA, Kittner SJ, Price TR. Stroke and illicit drug use. In: Ginsburg MD, Bogousslavsky J, eds. *Cerebrovascular Disease: Pathophysiology, Diagnosis and Management*. Vol. II. Cambridge: Blackwell Science; 1998:1589–1609.
26. Williams O. Stroke and substance abuse. In: Brust JCM, ed. *Neurologic Complications of Substance Abuse*. **CONTINUUM**: American Academy of Neurology; 2004;10:100–114.
27. Reneman L, Habraken JBA, Majoie CBL, et al. MDMA ("Ecstasy") and its association with cerebrovascular accidents: Preliminary findings. *AJNR Am J Neuroradiol*. 2000;21: 1001–1007.
28. McEvoy AW, Kitchen ND, Thomas DGT. Intracerebral haemorrhage and drug abuse in young adults. *Br J Neurosurg*. 2000;14:449–454.
29. Welmer LH. Spinal and neuromuscular complications of substance abuse. In: Brust JCM, ed. *Neurologic Complications of Substance Abuse*. **CONTINUUM**: American Academy of Neurology; 2004;10:115–143.

CHAPTER 106

Cocaine

John Kashani

OBJECTIVES

- To describe the history and epidemiology of cocaine
- To outline the pharmacology of cocaine and its metabolites
- To describe the effects of cocaine on various body systems
- To discuss the role of diagnostic testing with cocaine abuse
- To explore the management of the cocaine intoxicated patient

CASE VIGNETTE

A 26-year-old previously healthy man developed a severe headache, slurred speech, and left-sided hemiparesis shortly after drinking alcohol and using cocaine intranasally. He was brought to the emergency department via emergency medical services. His vital signs were a heart rate of 125 beats per minute, blood pressure was 148/92 mm Hg, temperature 98.6°F, and a respiratory rate of 20 per minute. On examination, the patient was lethargic and was noted to have nuchal rigidity, left-sided hemiparesis, and a left sided hemisensory deficit.

A computerized tomographic (CT) scan of the head showed a large, right temperoparietal intracerebral hematoma with mass effect. A right carotid angiogram demonstrated an aneurysm of the right middle cerebral artery with dye extravasation.

HISTORY

The cocaine shrub, *Erythroxulum coca*, grows in numerous places, including Central America and Indonesia. Ceramic pottery illustrating the harvesting and chewing of cocaine leaves appeared in Peru and Bolivia over 1,200 years ago. Coca leaves were used in various religious and social traditions by the Inca Indians, and were given as tokens of appreciation.

In 1854 Pizzi, a laboratory director at La Paz in Bolivia, extracted the alkaloid form of cocaine from the coca leaf. It was not until 1860 that the alkaloid was termed *cocaine*. The anesthetic effects of cocaine were soon realized and it was used to relieve laryngeal pain in England and America. Shortly thereafter, cocaine was introduced as a topical ophthalmologic anesthetic by Carl Koller. William Halsted was the first surgeon to report the use of cocaine to produce nerve blocks. The combination of anesthetic and vasoconstrictive properties made cocaine an ideal agent for use in surgical procedures. The reports of toxicity from cocaine also began with the advent of its use for surgical procedures. In addition to the complications arising from the use of cocaine in surgical procedures, the recreational use of cocaine became rampant.

By 1902, it was reported that only 5% of cocaine sold in New York and other metropolitan areas was used for medicinal use, the rest presumably diverted for recreational purposes. In 1914, the Harrison Narcotics Act was passed in an attempt to regulate the distribution of cocaine. Nationwide efforts to prevent the recreational use of cocaine are ongoing, but its use for this purpose remains a problem today.

EPIDEMIOLOGY

The 2005 the National Survey on Drug Use and Health estimates that there were 2.4 million regular cocaine users aged 12 years and older (http://oas.samhsa.gov/nsduh/2k5nsduh/2k5Results.htm#5.3). The Drug Abuse Warning Network (https://dawninfo.samhsa.gov/default.asp) reports that cocaine was involved in 383,350 emergency department visits in 2004 and cocaine alone accounted for 83,816 such visits. Additionally, 11% of patients presenting to an emergency department for a suicide attempt tested positive for cocaine and 46% of patients presenting to the emergency department for detoxification tested positive for cocaine. The Toxic Epidemiologic Surveillance System (TESS), a reporting system used by poison centers, reports 7,077 exposures to cocaine in 2005 with 124 associated deaths (1). It is likely that the reported estimates of cocaine abuse underestimate its true prevalence.

ETIOLOGY, DEFINITIONS, AND PATHOGENESIS

Cocaine is extracted from the *Erythroxylum coca* plant by using a hydrocarbon. The cocaine is converted to the hydrochloride salt and extracted into an aqueous base leaving cocaine hydrochloride. Cocaine hydrochloride can be ingested, injected, insufflated, and pyrolyzed, although smoking of cocaine is inefficient because of the decomposition of most of the cocaine.

Freebase cocaine refers to the base form of cocaine, a less-soluble (in water), but more volatile form of the drug, meaning it can be smoked without destruction of most of the drug. Crack cocaine is an easy to prepare form of freebase cocaine made by dissolving cocaine hydrochloride in water, adding a weak base (baking soda), and filtering or drying the product. This type of cocaine makes a cracking sound when heated; hence the name "crack."

Cocaine is rapidly absorbed through all routes of exposure, with injection and smoking the freebase form of cocaine having the fastest onset of effect (<1 minute) and ingestion taking the longest amount of time for onset (up to an hour). Application of cocaine to mucous membranes can delay the absorption because of the vasoconstrictive properties.

METABOLISM

Most cocaine metabolism is to benzoylecgonine, an inactive metabolite. Cocaine is also metabolized by esterases (serum and liver) to ecgonine methyl ester, a metabolite with less activity than the parent compound. Liver disease can prolong the duration of cocaine's effect secondary to decreased synthesis of cholinesterases. Additionally, compounds that inhibit serum esterases, such as organophosphates, can theoretically prolong cocaine's activity by inhibiting this metabolic pathway.

Cocaine undergoes a minor demethylation metabolic conversion by the liver to norcocaine, an inactive metabolite (2). Methylecgonidine is a metabolite that has only been found with patients that smoke cocaine and, therefore, may be used to differentiate pyrolysis of cocaine versus other routes of exposure (3). Cocaethylene is produced with the concurrent consumption of alcohol and cocaine, and it is believed that cocaethylene is responsible for the enhanced euphoric effect with concomitant exposure to cocaine and ethanol, but its exact role in pathogenesis is uncertain (4).

PHARMACOLOGY

Cocaine blocks the reuptake of norepinephrine, epinephrine, dopamine, and serotonin. The relative contribution and susceptibility of the various reuptake transporters has been investigated in both the animal and human model, but is not well defined (5). Accepted, however is that the inhibition of the reuptake of the various biogenic amines is responsible for most of the pathophysiology of cocaine toxicity. Increases in norepinephrine and epinephrine cause an increase in heart rate, blood pressure, and glycogenolysis and can have variable effects on cognition. The increase in serotonin neurotransmission has diverse effects, both centrally and peripherally. Serotonin is involved in platelet aggregation, gastrointestinal motility, behavior, and feelings of well being. Excess dopaminergic transmission can effect body movement, cognition, and temperature regulation. Choreoathetosis or involuntary movements that occur secondary to excess dopamine, is well described in cocaine use and is sometimes called *crack dancing*. The rewarding and, thus, addictive properties of cocaine are thought to be mediated through excess dopamine and serotonin (6,7).

CLINICAL MANIFESTATIONS

The clinical manifestations that are seen with cocaine intoxication are largely the result of an increased sympathetic activity, although some direct drug effect occurs on sodium channels and platelets (8). Vital sign abnormalities include hypertension, tachycardia, and tachypnea, with the potential development of hyperthermia with severe toxicity. On physical examination, varying degrees of mydriasis, alterations in cognition, agitated behavior, and diaphoresis may be present. The neurologic manifestations of cocaine are largely dose dependent. At low doses, the pleasurable effects (e.g., hypersexuality) and increased alertness may be experienced. As the dose is increased, untoward effects (e.g., agitation, confusion, and hallucinations) can occur. Seizures can occur with a potential increased rate occurring with concomitant brain injury or in a person with previous seizure disorder. Multiple and focal seizures may be indicative of brain injury (9). The repeated exposure to cocaine may predispose the user to seizures as a result of a kindling process (10).

The diverse cerebrovascular manifestations of cocaine abuse have recently been summarized (11). The rapid rise in blood pressure that occurs as a result of cocaine use has a significant risk of causing hemorrhagic strokes (12–14). Hemorrhage can result from rupture of arterioles, disruption of normal autoregulation by the increased blood pressure and perfusion of ischemic brain tissue. Although cocaine users with unrecognized structural vascular lesions would be at greatest risk for central nervous system (CNS) hemorrhage, it can occur in patients without anatomic abnormalities.

Ischemic strokes have been well described in the setting of cocaine use (15). The pathogenesis leading to ischemic strokes with cocaine is poorly defined. Vasospasms in combination with hypertension and platelet effects of cocaine are likely contributing factors.

A pancerebellar syndrome, occurring after a hyperthermic insult with cocaine use, has been described as well (16). Cerebral vasculitis, as a delayed presentation of cocaine use, occurred in a 22-year-old man in the absence of other potential causes for vasculitis (17). Small vessel vasculitis has also been described in a 32-year-old man with an intracranial hemorrhage temporally related to cocaine use (18). Cocaine was believed to be the etiological agent for the vasculitis because other causes were ruled out. The contribution of the vasculitis to the development of the intracranial hemorrhage is unknown and may have occurred as an independent process.

Cocaine has been implicated in causing intestinal infarction, presumably as a result of vasoconstriction with subsequent decrease in perfusion of segments of colon (19,20). Perforated ulcers are commonly described in cocaine users as well (21). The high metabolic requirements of the liver and kidneys may predispose them to ischemic injury from cocaine-induced infarction (22,23). The contribution of a hepatotoxic metabolite of cocaine metabolism is not well defined; however, it may have contributory effects compounded with ischemic injury (24). Body packers (see special situations below) may present with various abdominal complaints, including obstruction, as a result of mechanical effect of drug packages, but rupture of the packets is the much more dangerous situation.

Cocaine induces a myriad of effects on the cardiovascular system. The vasoconstriction caused by cocaine in combination with an elevated heart rate causes an imbalance between myocardial oxygen supply and demand. Additionally, cocaine can cause myocardial hypertrophy in response to increased wall stress. Autopsy results of the heart weights of cocaine users are on an average 10% greater than mean predicted weights (25). Although cocaine has also been implicated in accelerating atherosclerosis, the systematic study of cocaine's effect on atherosclerosis is limited because of the difficulty making the distinction between a natural atherosclerotic process and one induced or accelerated by cocaine use. *In vitro* experiments have shown that cocaine induces apoptosis in aortic vascular smooth muscle cells (26) and coronary artery endothelial cells (27). Morphologically, the changes in the myocardium on autopsy from pheochromocytoma and chronic cocaine exposure are similar (28).

At high concentrations, cocaine can cause blockade of fast sodium channels on myocardial cells, decreasing sodium entry into the myocyte and resulting in a widened QRS. Cocaine also affects the repolarization of myocardial cells by blocking potassium efflux. Pulmonary insult can occur through various mechanisms with the use of cocaine. In an attempt to increase exposure, cocaine users may use the Valsalva maneuver while smoking. This can increase intrathoracic pressure and cause rupture of a pleural bleb, resulting in pneumothoraces and pneumomediastinum (29). It should be noted that this does not occur from a direct effect of cocaine, rather it is a mechanical effect from the abuse behavior pattern.

Cocaine can exacerbate lung disease and cause new onset bronchospasm in a person not previously diagnosed with reactive airway disease (30). Bronchospasm can occur from cocaine's vasoconstrictive properties, contaminants, and thermal injury. The contribution of each is not known. Additionally, hemorrhagic alveolitis (crack lung), eosinophilia, pruritis, and elevated IgE levels have been described (31).

Musculoskeletal injury from cocaine is usually secondary to trauma. Cocaine metabolites were found in 22% of patients admitted to an orthopedic trauma unit (32). Cocaine can also produce muscle injury, with a resulting rise in creatine phosphokinase, even in the absence of vigorous body activity (33). The reason for muscle injury in this setting is unknown, however, a direct myotoxic effect of cocaine is presumed.

SPECIAL SITUATIONS

BODY PACKERS

A body packer is a person who attempts to smuggle drug packets concealed in the digestive tract to be retrieved after the person reaches a specific destination. The leakage or rupture of drug packets containing cocaine are particularly worrisome and have resulted in fatalities (34). Management of these patients when symptomatic will most likely require surgical intervention to remove drug packets. These patients have very high morbidity and require aggressive early treatment.

BODY STUFFERS

A person who hastily ingests packets of drugs to hide evidence when confronted by law enforcement is a body stuffer. The packets are often intended for sale and, therefore, are not as securely packaged as those in body packers. Most cocaine body stuffers do not develop symptoms suggestive of cocaine toxicity; however, deaths have been reported and so conservative treatment is warranted for all of these patients (35).

PREGNANCY

The use of cocaine during pregnancy can result in chronic effects as well as acute catastrophic events. The vasonconstrictive nature of cocaine can result in a decrease in uterine blood flow and at extremes can result in placental abruption. Exposures that occur over time can produce repetitive insults to the developing fetus, possibly causing developmental problems (36).

ACUTE CORONARY SYNDROME

Chest pain is a common complaint with patients presenting to the emergency department after cocaine use. In addition to the anatomic considerations mentioned in the pulmonary section, vasospasm with or without predisposing atherosclerotic heart disease can cause cardiac ischemia. It must be noted that the ECG in cocaine users, even in the setting of myocardial infarction, is often nondiagnostic. The management approach in the setting of cocaine chest pain, for the most part, is the same as in the setting of chest pain without cocaine use. The notable exceptions are the use of benzodiazepines in the initial management and the contraindication to the use of β-blocking agents. Verapamil and nitroglycerin have been shown to alleviate cocaine-induced coronary vasoconstriction and, thus, are recommended in the management of an acute coronary event induced by cocaine. If an antihypertensive agent is to be used, the alpha antagonist phentolamine is one of the preferred agents.

DIAGNOSTIC APPROACH

Although cocaine and its metabolites can be detected in blood, hair, saliva, and meconium, these tests are expensive and not readily available. The most widely used test for exposure to cocaine is the urine drug of abuse screen. Cocaine is rapidly eliminated and within a few hours of use benzylecgonine (metabolite) can be detected in the urine for 2 to 3 days. With the chronic use of cocaine, a urine test may remain positive considerably longer, up to 5 to 7 days. It is important to understand the limitations of the use of the urine drug abuse screen. A positive screen is highly suggestive of exposure, but cannot determine if it is from recent use. Additionally, a urine cocaine drug screen test may be negative if the urine is too dilute or benzylecgonine is not yet present in the urine. If recent cocaine use is highly suspected, it may be prudent to repeat the urine screen if the initial screen was negative.

TREATMENT

Although cocaine is bound by activated charcoal in both an acidic and alkaline environment, the role of activated charcoal is limited (except for body stuffers or packers, see below) in that most cocaine is insufflated or smoked (37). Supportive and anticipatory management is usually all that is needed when managing a cocaine intoxicated patient. A few exceptions are seen, such as a patient with a cocaine-induced acute coronary syndrome or stroke. In these settings, benzodiazepines are considered a first-line agent and the use of β-blocking agents is contraindicated because of coronary vasoconstriction. Give serious thought before ever prescribing a β-blocker to a patient known to use cocaine, even if that person is not currently symptomatic.

If endotracheal intubation is being considered, caution should be used when choosing a paralytic agent. Both succinylcholine and cocaine are metabolized by plasma cholinesterase and, theoretically, a risk exists of prolonging the toxicity of cocaine or paralysis. Additionally, in the setting of hyperkalemia caused by muscle injury, the rise in potassium with the use of succinylcholine can precipitate arrhythmias. It is important to note that vigorous body activity or seizures need not be present for muscle injury and hyperkalemia to occur with cocaine use.

In the setting of a cocaine body stuffer, administration of activated charcoal and observation is all that is needed. As mentioned, most body stuffers do not develop signs or symptoms suggestive of cocaine toxicity, but observation for 8 hours after ingestion is what is believed to be a safe amount of time. Patients should be monitored closely and should not be medically cleared if they have an unexplained increase in heart rate or blood pressure. Rupture of a package of cocaine in a body packer can result in disastrous consequences. Rupture is an indication for surgical intervention to remove packets. In the absence of rupture, management can include the use of whole bowel irrigation, activated charcoal, and benzodiazepines. The use of abdominal radiographs or CT may help identify packets of drugs in both a body stuffer and packer.

A widened QRS interval occurs secondary to blockage of myocardial sodium channels. Hypotension and arrhythmias can develop if sodium channel blockade becomes sufficiently profound. Administration of sodium bicarbonate is indicated in the setting QRS widening, 1 to 2 mEq/kg bolus with a repeat ECG shortly after can result in a decrease in the sodium channel blockade and narrowing of the QRS interval with possible hemodynamic improvement.

The clinician should aggressively treat hyperthermia occurring in the setting of cocaine intoxication. Mechanical restraints should be avoided because of the potential heat generation with a patient fighting against the restraints. Initial mechanical restraints may be necessary, however, to gain control of a patient's agitation and to safely administer chemical restraint agents. Avoid using haloperidol or other antipsychotics for primary control agents of their agitation because this has been shown to increase morbidity in a rodent model (37). After controlling the patient's agitation, a detailed examination and search should be conducted looking for any additional pathology, such as rhabdomyolysis, organ infarction (stroke, renal infarcts), or trauma.

CLINICAL RECOMMENDATIONS OF THE VIGNETTE

The patient was brought immediately to the operating room where a right temperoparietal craniotomy was done. The intracerebral hematoma was evacuated and the arterial aneurysm was clipped. The patient did well postoperatively with almost complete resolution of his aphasia and moderate improvement of his hemiparesis.

SUMMARY

This case exemplifies the catastrophic events that could occur with the use of cocaine. The combination of the presence of an arteriovenous malformation and the surge in blood pressure with the use of cocaine is a deadly combination. Cocaine and its metabolites exert a myriad of effects on various body systems, the most dramatic occurring on the nervous and cardiovascular system. Most cocaine-intoxicated patients can be managed with supportive and anticipatory management alone, but vigilance must be maintained for the rare but devastating complications.

REFERENCES

1. 2005 Annual Report of the American Association of Poison Control Centers' National Poisoning and Exposure Database. *Clinical Toxicology.* 2006;(44)6–7:912.
2. Maurer HH, Sauer C, Theobald DS. Toxicokinetics of drugs of abuse: Current knowledge of the isoenzymes involved in the human metabolism of tetrahydrocannabinol, cocaine, heroin, morphine and codeine. *Ther Drug Monit.* 2006;(28)3:447–453.
3. Scheidweiler KB, Plessinger MA, Shojaie J, et al. Pharmacokinetics and pharmacodynamics of methylecgonidine, a crack cocaine pyrolyzate. *Journal of Pharmacology & Experimental Therapeutics.* 2003;307:1179–1187.
4. Hearn W, Flynn D, Hime G, et al. Cocaethylene: A unique cocaine metabolite displays high affinity for the dopamine transporter. *J Neurochem.* 1991;56:697–701.
5. Han DD, Gu HH. Comparison of monoamine transporters from human and mouse in their sensitivities to psychostimulant drugs. *BMC Pharmacology.* 2006;6:6.
6. Hummel M, Unterwald E. D1 dopamine receptor: A putative neurochemical and behavioral link to cocaine action. *J Cell Physiol.* 2002;191:17–27.
7. Matgozata F, Matgozata F, Zaniewska AG, et al. The serotinergic system and its role in cocaine addiction. *Pharmacology Reports.* 2005;57:685–700.
8. Callahan K, Malinin A, Atar D, et al. Platelet activation as a universal trigger in the pathogenesis of acute coronary events after cocaine abuse. *Swiss Med Wkly.* 2001;131:487–489.
9. Pascual-Leone A, Dhuma A, Altafullah I, et al. Cocaine-induced seizures. *Neurology.* 1990; 40:404–407.
10. Stripling JS, Hendricks C. Effect of cocaine and lidocaine on the expression of kindled seizures in the rat. *Pharmacology, Biochemistry & Behavior.* 1981;14(3):397–403.
11. Sloan MA, Kittner SJ, Price TR. Stroke and illicit drug use. In: Ginsburg MD, Bogousslavsky J, eds. *Cerebrovascular Disease: Pathophysiology, Diagnosis and Management.* Volume II. Cambridge: Blackwell Science; 1998:1589–1609.
12. Lehman LB. Intracerebral hemorrhage after intranasal cocaine use. *Hospital Physician.* 1987;July:69–70.
13. Lichtenfeld PJ, Rubin DB, Feldman RS. Subarachnoid hemorrhage precipitated by cocaine snorting. *Arch Neurol* 1984;41(2):223–224.
14. Kaku D, Lowenstein D. Emergency of recreational drug abuse as a major risk factor for stroke in young adults. *Ann Intern Med.* 1990;113:821–827.
15. Daras M, Tuchman A, Marks S. Central nervous system infarction related to cocaine abuse. *Stroke.* 1991;22:1320–1325.
16. Tenvetyanon T, Dissin J, Selcer U. Hyperthermia and chronic pancerebellar syndrome after cocaine abuse. *Arch Intern Med.* 2001;161:608–610.
17. Kaye B, Finstat M. Cerebral vasculitis associated with cocaine abuse. *JAMA.* 1987;258: 2104–2106.
18. Harris N, McNeely W, Sheppard JA, et al. Case 27-1993: A 32-year old man with the sudden onset of a right-sided headache and left hemiplegia and hemianesthesia. *N Engl J Med.*1993;329:117–124.
19. Herrine SK, Park PK, Wechsler RJ. Acute mesenteric ischemia following intranasal cocaine use. *Dig Dis Sci.* 1998 Mar;43(3):586–589.
20. Freudenberger RS, Cappell MS, Hutt DA. Intestinal infarction after intravenous cocaine administration. *Ann Intern Med.* 1990;113(9):715–716.
21. Yahchouchy E, Debet A, Fingerhut A. Crack cocaine-related prepyloric perforation treated laparoscopically. *Surg Endosc.* 2002;16(1):220.
22. Radin DR. Cocaine-induced hepatic necrosis; CT demonstration. *J Comput Assist Tomogr.* 1992;16(1):155–156.
23. Bemanian S, Motallebi M, Nosrati SM. Cocaine-induced renal infarction: Report of a case and review of the literature. *BMC Nephrology.* 2005;6:10.
24. Boelsterli UA, Goldlin C. Biomechanisms of cocaine-induced hepatocyte injury mediated by the formation of reactive metabolites. *Arch Toxicol.* 1991;65(5):351–360.
25. Kitzman DW, Scholz DG, Hagen PT, et al. Age-related changes in normal human hearts during the first 10 decades of life. Part II (Maturity): A quantitative anatomic study of 765 specimens from subjects 20 to 99 years old. *Mayo Clin Proc.* 1988; 63:137–146.
26. Su J, Li J, Li W, et al. Cocaine induces apoptosis in primary cultured rat aortic vascular smooth muscle cells: Possible relationship to aortic dissection, atherosclerosis, and hypertension. *Int J Toxicol.* 2004;23(4):233–237.
27. He J, Xia Y, Zhang L. Cocaine induces apoptosis in human coronary artery endothelial cells. *J Cardiovasc Pharmacol.* 2000;35(4):572–580.
28. Karch SB, Billingham ME. Myocardial contraction bands revisited. *Hum Pathol.* 1986;17(1):9–13.
29. Maeder M, Ullmer E. Pneumomediastinum and bilateral pneumothorax as a complication of cocaine smoking. *Respiration.* 2003;70(4):407.
30. Osborn HH, Tang M, Bradley K, et al. New-onset bronchospasm or recrudescence of asthma associated with cocaine abuse. *Acad Emerg Med.* 1997;4(7):689–692.
31. Kissner DG, Lawrence WD, Selis JE, et al. Crack lung: Pulmonary disease caused by cocaine abuse. *Am Rev Respir Dis.* 1987;136(5):1250–1252.
32. Levy RS, Herbert CK, Munn BG, et al. Drug and alcohol use in orthopedic trauma patients: A prospective study. *J Orthop Trauma.* 1996;10(1):21–27.
33. Counselman FL, McLaughlin EW, Kardon EM, et al. Creatine phosphokinase elevation in patients presenting to the emergency department with cocaine-related complaints. *Am J Emerg Med.* 1997;15(3):221–223.
34. Wetli CV, Mittleman RE. The "body packer syndrome"—Toxicity following ingestion of illicit drugs packaged for transportation. *Journal of Forensic Sciences.* 1981;26(3):492–500.
35. June R, Aks S, Keys N, et al. Medical outcome of cocaine bodystuffers. *J Emerg Med.* 2000;18(2):221–224.
36. Codero R, Medina C, Helfgott A. Cocaine body packing in pregnancy. *Ann Emerg Med.* 2006;48(3):323–325.
37. Witkin JM, Goldberg SR, Katz JL. Lethal effects of cocaine are reduced by the dopamine-1 receptor antagonist SCH 23390 but not by haloperidol. *Life Sci.*1989;44(18):1285–1291.

CHAPTER 107

Hallucinogens

Robert Schwaner

OBJECTIVES

- To provide a brief historical review of hallucinogens
- To categorize nonamphetamine serotonergic hallucinogens
- To explore the physiology responsible for hallucinogenic potential
- To review the common and serious side effects of serotonergic hallucinogens
- To explain how to clinically recognize and appropriately treat a patient exposed to a hallucinogen

CASE VIGNETTE

Friends brought a 16-year-old boy to the emergency department (ED) after he was noted to be behaving strangely while at a party. Earlier in the day, he had revealed to friends that he was going to "trip" later that day. He initially told friends that he was scared because everybody looked distorted. The lights, in particular, frightened him, as did the loud music that was playing. His friends initially decided to just keep a close watch of him, but after multiple episodes of vomiting they became frightened and brought him to the ED.

Physical examination in the ED revealed an agitated, apprehensive male with a look of fear on his face. Vomitus was present on his clothes and his shirt was ripped. His vital signs were as follows: Blood pressure, 160/95 mm Hg; pulse, 115 beats per minute; respiratory rate, 30 breaths per minute; temperature, 100.7°F (38.2°C); and pulse oximetry, 99% on room air. His blood glucose registered 106 mg/dL. His skin was moist and pale. Pupils measured 6 mm and were slowly reactive to light bilaterally. No nystagmus was noted. He exhibited a fine tremor of his hands, but had an otherwise unremarkable neurologic examination. The remaining head, eyes, ears, nose, and throat examination was unremarkable. Lungs were clear to auscultation bilaterally. Heart sounds were unremarkable. His abdomen was soft and nontender, with mildly increased bowel sounds. He described visualizing spoken words coming out of the mouths around him. He did understand where he was, but he was extremely agitated and expressed irrational thoughts.

DEFINITION

Hallucinogens are a heterogeneous group of compounds capable of altering perception and thoughts without completely altering mental status. A *hallucination* can be described as a false perception that does not arise from any external perceptional input. An example would be a patient seeing snakes in a room. In contrast, an *illusion* arises from perceptual distortion of the environment. An example would be a patient observing the walls pulsating and moving. Hallucinogens are capable of producing both hallucinations and illusions, but illusions are much more common. Other terms are used to describe some of the bizarre sensory misinterpretations and experiences that occur when exposed to hallucinogens (Table 107-1) (1).

EPIDEMIOLOGY

Plant and fungally derived hallucinogens have been used predominately for religious experiences for thousands of years. Soma, a deity and hallucinogenic substance used for entheogenic ceremonies, was a construct of early Indian religion and is believed by some to be the origin for the spread of hallucinogen use during entheogen ceremonies to other cultures throughout Eurasia (2). The Aztecs also used hallucinogens during religious ceremonies. They employed both teonanacatl (psilocybin-containing mushrooms known to the Aztecs as 'flesh of the gods') and a substance known as ololiuqui (found within morning glory seeds and structurally similar to lysergic acid diethylamide [LSD]). Evidence exists that Mayan priests and shamans used multiple hallucinogenic materials, including toads, mushrooms, and water lilies, for healing and religious ceremonies (3). During the middle ages, fungally derived ergots ingested with wheat and rye caused epidemics resulting in thousands of deaths—illness marked by significant hallucinations. In fact, ergotism has been implicated as recently as 1692 during the bizarre events surrounding the Salem Witch Trials of Salem, Massachusetts (4).

Within the last century, an explosion has occurred in the hallucinogenic world. In 1938, the Swiss chemist Albert Hoffman synthesized a compound known as LSD-25. Hoffman inadvertently exposed himself to the substance and realized the potential for hallucinogenic compounds to be synthesized. Afterward, LSD was marketed for use during psychotherapy with the belief that it would encourage the patient to reveal repressed thoughts or feelings. During the 1960s, recreational use of LSD began (5). It was during this time that Timothy Leary introduced the phrase "Tune in, Turn on, Drop out" (6). Shortly afterward, federal laws prohibited the use of LSD because of public health and safety concerns.

TABLE 107-1. Hallucinogens–Category of Sensory Misinterpretations

Term	*Definition*
Synesthesia	The coupling of two bodily senses
Grapheme-color synesthesia	The perception of numbers and letters are coupled with color
Psychotomimetic	Producing psychosis
Entheogen	Generating a religious experience
Oneirogen	Producing dreams

Since the federal ban of LSD, its use had slowly dipped through the 1970s and 1980s. During the 1990s, however, the use of LSD among the US population was increasing and peaked in the mid 1990s. Ever since this time, however, LSD use has steadily declined. Many attribute this change to decreased availability as a result of federal arrests of key LSD production chemists. Regardless of the cause, surveys as recent as 2004 show a continued decline in LSD use with just 10% of citizens above the age of 12 years reporting LSD use (7,8). Despite this decline, hallucinogens are still considered widely available for recreational use.

CATEGORIES OF SEROTONERGIC HALLUCINOGENS

As mentioned previously, the hallucinogenic amphetamine derivatives (as well as the tetrahydrocannabinoids) will not be included in this review. The serotonergic hallucinogens discussed can be divided into two major structural classes, the indolealkylamines or tryptamines, and lysergamides. Figure 107-1 shows the structural similarity of common hallucinogens to serotonin. Please see Table 107-2 for dosing and effect information for hallucinogens discussed in this chapter.

Indolealkylamines and Tryptamines

Psilocybin-containing mushrooms are widely distributed throughout the world and can be found in six of seven continents (9). Psilocybin is broken down in the body to psilocin. In 1958, Albert Hoffman identified these two substances as being responsible for the hallucinogenic potential of these mushrooms (10). Different species contain varying percentages of these substances. Even mushrooms within the same species within subsequent flushes (crops) possess varying amounts of the hallucinogens (11). *Psilocybe cubensis* and *Psilocybe semilanceata* are two of the more common species consumed. Slang terms used for these mushrooms include *shrooms* or *magic mushrooms.* Dosing depends on the amount of psilocybin and psilocin contained within them and the intensity of hallucination desired; this often ends up being based on what the user can keep down without vomiting. These mushrooms are typically eaten and produce effects lasting approximately 6 hours (12).

Ibogaine is an indole alkaloid obtained from the African shrub, *Tabernanthe iboga.* Indigenous tribes used its hallucinogenic potential during religious ceremonies. During the 1960s, its recreational potential was realized within the United States. It was later classified as a schedule I substance by the US Food and Drug Administration (FDA). Ibogaine is typically ingested and possesses two phases of effect. The first is an intense hallucination phase that occurs 4 to 8 hours after ingestion. This is followed by a second stage of intellectual evaluation of these hallucinations lasting 8 to 24 hours. Intense sleep typically follows. Oddly, ibogaine has been used as a substance withdrawal adjunct for other illicit drugs, including opiates and cocaine. After using ibogaine, many people describe a decreased urge to use their drug of abuse and feel that they have gained insight into the destructive nature of their addictive behavior. The side effects inherent to hallucinogens have limited ibogaine's use in this capacity (13).

N,N-Dimethyltryptamine (DMT) is an extremely potent and short-acting tryptamine that is found in *Psychotria viridis,* but its source for abuse historically has been synthetic. This plant grows in the Amazon River basin and is used locally by shaman to make a hallucinogenic infusion known as "Spirit Vine." DMT is one of the few hallucinogens not absorbed from the gastrointestinal tract. Instead, it is classically smoked, snorted, injected, or used as snuff. To be orally active, it is combined with an herbal source of a monoamine oxidase inhibitor (MAOI). As with other smoked or snorted drugs, DMT's onset of action is extremely fast in hallucinogenic terms and occurs within 5 or 10 minutes. This rapid onset of action is coupled with an extremely short duration of action. Effects are typically gone within an hour. Together, these qualities displayed by DMT

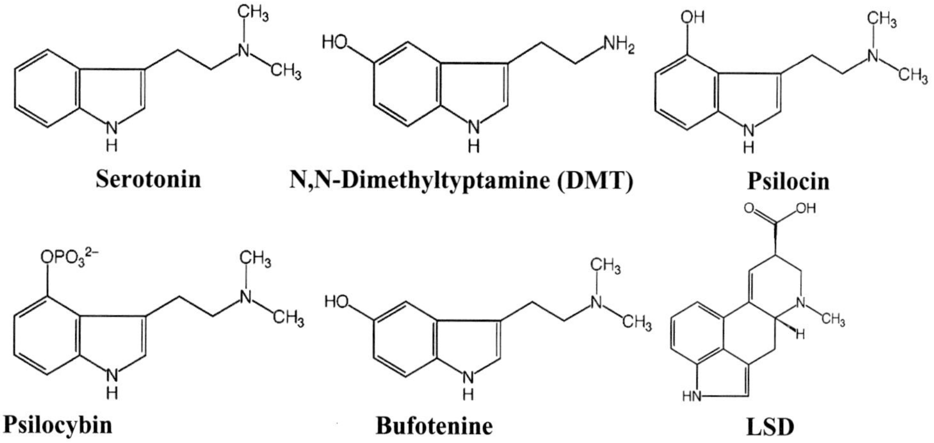

Serotonin N,N-Dimethyltyptamine (DMT) Psilocin

Psilocybin Bufotenine LSD

FIGURE 107-1. Structural similarity of common hallucinogens to serotonin.

TABLE 107-2. Hallucinogens—Dosing and Effect

Hallucinogen	*Dose*	*Delivery*	*Onset*	*Peak Effect*	*Duration*
DMT	10–60 mg	IV, smoked	1–15 min	5–30 min	10–60 min
Psilocybin	0.25–5 g	Ingested	10–60 min	1–3 h	6 h
Mescaline	100–600 mg	Ingested	30–60 min	~3 h	4–8 h
LSD	25–400 μg	Ingested	30–60 min	3–5 h	8–12 h
Ibogaine	400–1,000 mg	Ingested	2–4 h	4–8 h	18–24 h

DMT, N,N-Dimethyltyptamine; LSD, lysergic acid diethylamide; IV, intravenous.

have caused it to be referred to as "the businessman's trip." As a hallucinogen, it would be attractive to someone who would not be able to invest the amount of time inherent to using most other longer acting hallucinogens (14).

Bufotenine, a schedule I compound, is a naturally occurring tryptamine obtained from skin secretions of the *Bufo* genus of toads. Controversy exists concerning whether it is a true hallucinogen (15), but recent evidence supports its appropriate classification as such. In contrast, 5-methoxy-N,N-dimethyltryptamine (5-MeO-DMT) does cross the blood–brain barrier and is known to produce intense hallucinations. It is also derived from toads of the genus *Bufo,* but from only one species, *Bufo alvarius,* the Colorado River toad (16). It is these hallucinogens that have prompted some to lick the backs of toads in an effort to hallucinate. This practice is dangerous, with deaths occurring not from the bufotenine, but from the digoxinlike substances (bufodienolides) that are secreted by this genus of toads. Patients poisoned in this manner have been successfully treated with digoxin-specific Fab fragments (17). Abuse of synthetic 5-MeO-DMT is rare because the experiences are described as powerful and unsettling and the drug is not active orally.

Hundreds of tryptamines exist, but two others worthy of mention include 5-methoxydiisopropyltyptamine ("foxy methoxy") and α-methyltrytptamine (AMT), both recently (2004) placed into schedule I by the US Drug Enforcement Agency (DEA). AMT has its roots as an antidepressant used during the 1960s in the former Soviet Union. Foxy methoxy, in contrast, has much more recent roots after first being synthesized for use in the late 1990s. Both of these tryptamines are potent hallucinogens that have recently gained popularity at raves and other types of dance clubs. Seizures had been regarded as their main negative effect. Recently, however, fatal overdoses have been reported with the use of AMT (18). They have both been associated with producing the most feared side effect of the serotonergic hallucinogens, serotonin syndrome. This syndrome will be discussed in further detail later in the chapter.

Lysergamides

The structural class of lysergamides includes the synthetic ergot alkaloid derivative LSD and naturally occurring lysergic acid hydroxyethylamide (found in several species of morning glory and the Hawaiian baby woodrose). LSD exhibits about ten times the potency of lysergic acid hydroxyethylamide, and 25 μg of LSD will produce effects (19). It is typically provided as a colorless, tasteless, odorless liquid on a small piece of paper referred to as a "blotter" or "microdot." Its potency means that, with rare exception, when patients say they have ingested a piece of paper with the drug on it, most likely it is going to be LSD because its potency and oral activity stands out from the other hallucinogens. In contrast, hundreds of morning glory seeds are needed to provide the Aztecs with ololiuqui, the hallucinogenic substance used for their religious ceremonies. These seeds need to be crushed and pulverized because their intact husks would prevent any gastrointestinal absorption from occurring.

Mescaline

Mescaline is a phenylethylamine more closely related to methylenedioxymethamphetamine (MDMA) (ecstasy). Mescaline, however, will be discussed as its effect is closer to the other hallucinogens than to the amphetamines. Mescaline is derived from the peyote cactus (*Lophophora williamsii*). This is a small and spineless cactus found in southwestern United States and Mexico. In these areas, mescaline is still used by many Native American churches for religious ceremonies. In fact, it is one of the few hallucinogens still legal to use within the United States, but only for this purpose (20). It is typically eaten in units referred to as *buttons*—disc sized pieces of cactus sliced from the top of the cactus that contain most of the mescaline. Typically, five to ten buttons are eaten to produce hallucinogenic effects. Notable to mescaline, ingestion produces nausea, vomiting, and diaphoresis before producing its psychological effects (21).

PHARMACOLOGY

Recent evidence supports a similar mechanism demonstrated by the above hallucinogens. Alteration of the serotonin system is believed to be responsible for both the hallucinogenic and psychological properties of these substances. Serotonin (5-hydroxytryptamine or 5-HT) is found throughout the body and has many functions. Within the brain, serotonin acts as a neurotransmitter involved with many physiologic and psychological processes. Multiple serotonin receptors subtypes exist, with most authors agreeing that there are seven major subtypes (5-HT_1 through 5-HT_7). Stimulation of the 5-HT_2 receptor is associated with hallucination modulation. 5-HT_2 receptors are found throughout the cerebral cortex and midbrain (22,23). Of note, 5-HT_{2A} receptors are believed to be responsible for the serotonin syndrome.

The serotonergic system is responsible for modulating sleep, mood, appetite, some motor functions, thermoregulation, and sexual activity. It is important to realize, however, that these hallucinogens tend to be nonselective in nature and act at many of these subtypes in addition to other neurotransmitter receptors. For example, recent work has demonstrated that the lysergamides are capable of stimulating dopaminergic receptors as well (24). Therefore, despite the extensive work demonstrating the serotonergic activity hallucinogens possess, their end effects may result from complex interactions between multiple neurotransmitter and receptor systems.

Although many of the hallucinogens produce similar effects, an enormous variation is demonstrated among them regarding their times to onset of action, peak effect, and duration of action (Table 107-2). A broad spectrum of onset and duration of effect exists among the hallucinogens. Some of this variation in onset or duration can be attributed to difference in modes of delivery. Other reasons include differences in the rate of elimination as well as variations in receptor affinity.

As the most studied of the hallucinogens, LSD provides many of the answers to questions pertaining to tolerance, dependence, and withdrawal. In fact, some degree of tolerance occurs among habitual users of LSD. This tolerance, however, quickly dissipates over a few days after terminating use. No evidence, however, exists for any physiologic dependence or withdrawal syndromes occurring from hallucinogen use (25). On the contrary, ibogaine, as mentioned previously, has been used as an adjunct to aid other withdrawal syndromes.

CLINICAL MANIFESTATIONS

The primary effects of the serotonergic hallucinogens are to the perceptual system. The type of experience that an individual has while under the influence depends on his or her mindset, emotional stability, surroundings, and accompanying individuals (sitters). Individuals who are depressed, agitated, or in an unfamiliar environment are more likely to have an adverse reaction. For this reason, panic attacks are by far the most commonly experienced adverse psychiatric effect (26). Other adverse psychiatric effects include psychosis, true hallucinations, and dysphoric reactions that tend to be depressive.

The physiologic changes produced by hallucinogens are typically mild and tend to occur before any of the psychological effects manifest. These physiologic effects may caused by a direct receptor-mediated effect of the hallucinogenic substance or by increased central sympathetic outflow secondary to psychiatric disturbance. The sympathetic effects often include tachycardia, hypertension, diaphoresis, hyperthermia, tachypnea, and mydriasis. Other effects seen include nausea, vomiting, ataxia, shivering, decreased muscle tone, hyperactivity, altered mental status, coma, and, occasionally, piloerection. Compared with substances such as cocaine, amphetamines, and the arylcyclohexylamines (phencyclidine [PCP] and ketamine), the sympathetic effects of the hallucinogens are much less prominent. Hallucinogenic amphetamines (MDMA [ecstasy] and PMA [paramethoxyamphetamine]), however, can cause significant sympathomimetic effects. A key difference used to distinguish other drugs from the nonamphetamine serotonergic hallucinogens is the presence or absence of an altered mental status.

The hallucinogens covered in this chapter typically do not produce delirium. In fact, most people who use hallucinogens are fully aware that they are under the influence of a drug. In contrast, substance such as cocaine, amphetamines, and PCP rarely produce hallucinations in combination with a preserved sensorium. Of course, the approach to any patient with an altered mental status is to consider infectious, toxic-metabolic, organic, and structural disease as potential causes. For this reason, when the patient cannot provide a clear history documenting the recent use of a hallucinogen, it is important to consider explore these other causes. The threshold for imaging and cerebrospinal fluid analysis must remain low (27). As stated, these patients often retain insight to their present state and can provide the history confirming that they have recently used a hallucinogen.

The most serious side effect produced by serotonergic hallucinogens is serotonin syndrome. Serotonin syndrome is often described as a clinical triad of altered mental status combined with neuromuscular and autonomic hyperactivity. Contributions from each of the triad vary from case to case and occur on a continuum from mild and typically unrecognized symptoms of slight hypertension, tremor, and diarrhea to extreme autonomic instability and death, if left untreated. Serotonin syndrome develops from a dose-related phenomenon of excess serotonergic activity within the CNS and periphery. Activity at all serotonergic receptor subtypes is felt to contribute. Stimulation at some of these receptor subtypes, however, is believed to contribute more to this syndrome than others. The two subtypes most commonly implicated for this greater effect are the 5-HT_{2A} and 5-HT_{1A} subtypes. The excess stimulation typically results from multiple serotonergic drug interactions, but single agents (e.g., these hallucinogens) have been implicated.

Although fairly common, the diagnosis is often unappreciated by clinicians. Some of the confusion surrounding the diagnosis stems from historical attempts to capture the syndrome within specific and strict diagnostic criteria (28). Newer diagnostic criteria have been established and tend to capture a greater number of these patients on the continuum of this syndrome. Any patient with rapidly developing (minutes to hours) tremor, hyperreflexia, and clonus (typically more pronounced in the lower extremities) in the setting of exposure to a serotonergic agonist should have the diagnosis considered (29).

DIAGNOSTIC APPROACH

As with other diseases, the history is crucial and often provides much that is needed to treat the patient. Once a history of hallucinogen use is obtained, other important historical data to gather include the specific hallucinogen used, amount used, time of use, concomitant use of other medications or hallucinogens, and if others using the same hallucinogen(s) at the time experienced any ill effects. Failure historically to determine the specific agent(s) involved should not change management for any of the hallucinogens discussed in this chapter. A careful history combined with classic physical examination findings generally provides all the information needed to appropriately diagnose and treat these patients.

Physical examination of these patients often confirms the diagnosis. Most striking within these patients are their pupils. Often described as "saucers," the mydriasis observed frequently measures 5 or 6 mm. This finding combined with affect changes including anxiety, a feeling of lost control, and self-awareness of the situation is highly suggestive of hallucinogen exposure. Mild tachycardia, hypertension, and diaphoresis are often present. A mild tremor is also common. Timely laboratory analysis targeted for specific hallucinogenic agents is not currently available from most laboratories. Even if available, these tests would not alter the management of such cases. The only utility of routine laboratory analysis during management is to provide information for end-organ damage and information to reveal (or exclude) any comorbidity unattained from the history.

TREATMENT

Despite the general feeling that nonamphetamine hallucinogens are relatively safe in comparison to other mind-altering substances such as cocaine, amphetamines, and PCP, these substances are still capable of considerable harm to the patient and have resulted in death. Many patients using hallucinogens have an increased chance of harming themselves as a result of risky behavior that they engage. Using a sitter may prove life saving. Of the patients who present to the hospital, the harm they typically experience is caused by altered mental status and resultant psychomotor agitation. Seizures have been reported with LSD and other hallucinogens (30,31), but most of the harm with these toxins is either from serotonin syndrome, extreme psychomotor agitation, or a combination of the two. These pathways, when untreated, typically lead to hyperthermia, rhabdomyolysis with resultant renal failure, hepatic necrosis, disseminated intravascular coagulopathy, and ultimately death (32).

Supportive care is the mainstay of treatment. As with the case in the vignette, simply providing a small dose of benzodiazepines, in addition to a quiet and dark environment, is typically all that is needed. Paramount to caring for the patient with extreme psychomotor agitation is rapidly obtaining vital signs, including temperature and blood glucose. Hyperthermia must be treated with aggressive cooling to prevent further decline. In the setting of psychomotor agitation, temperatures above 105°F (40.6°C) require aggressive cooling. This ideally would be accomplished by returning the patient's temperature to 101°F as rapidly as possible. Placing a cooling blanket under the patient with wet sheets above while fans are running can be effective. Care must be taken to avoid overcooling the patient. Removing the agitation must be addressed simultaneously, which is most often accomplished with the use of benzodiazepines. The use of phenothiazines and the 5-HT$_{2A}$ receptor antagonist risperidone has been discouraged in the setting of LSD use because of a potential for producing a disorder known as *hallucinogen-persisting perception disorder* (HPPD) (33,34). HPPD is more commonly referred to, and known as, *flashbacks*. Debate exists whether HPPD is a real phenomenon. Regardless, this potential side effect serves as an additional reminder that benzodiazepines are well tolerated and highly effective for relieving any anxiety or agitation and, therefore, should be thought of as first-line treatment among patients exposed to hallucinogens.

The hyperthermia produced by psychomotor agitation is a result of excessive muscle use and, therefore, it is inadvisable to place the patient in any physical restraints or environments that can increase the level of agitation. Aggressive hydration for increased insensible losses, cooling when needed, and benzodiazepines to decrease central sympathetic outflow are usually adequate to stabilize most patients who presents with agitation and hyperthermia caused by hallucinogenically derived psychomotor agitation. In the case of serotonin syndrome, in addition to removing the offending agent(s), cyproheptadine can be used. It is an oral 5-HT$_{2A}$ antagonist that has been shown to be effective in animal models, but human data are lacking. Most generally agree that cyproheptadine should be a part of treating serotonin syndrome. It is dosed at 12 to 24 mg over a 24-hour period (reduce the dose in the pediatric population); however, remember that serotonin syndrome uncommonly lasts for more than 12 hours. Management of serotonin syndrome and significant hyperthermia must occur over minutes and not hours. On rare occasion, the extremes of agitation and temperature may necessitate intubation and muscle paralysis, in addition to the above measures, to stabilize the patient. Finally, the newer 5-HT$_{3A}$ serotonin antagonist agents (e.g., ondansetron, dolasetron) have been shown to be particularly effective for treating persistent vomiting and show fewer side effects than other antiemetics.

CLINICAL RECOMMENDATIONS OF THE VIGNETTE

Resolution of the case presented in the vignette illustrates a few of the salient management points. An intravenous line was placed and 15 mg of diazepam administered slowly. He also received normal saline and 4 mg of ondansetron for his vomiting. A dark, quiet room was provided for observation. Approximately 4 hours later, he was alert and oriented and no longer experiencing any hallucinations. Repeated vital signs and his examination normalized, except for some mild persistent mydriasis. He admitted to ingesting hallucinogenic mushrooms earlier that day. The temporal course (≈4 hour duration) and clinical picture (hallucinations, vomiting) corroborate this history and suggest against LSD as the cause. No role was seen for further testing because his gastrointestinal symptoms resolved and the risk of a concurrent hepatotoxic mushroom ingestion appeared remote. Drug counseling was offered and he was discharged shortly thereafter to family members with no apparent sequelae.

SUMMARY

Hundreds of hallucinogens exist, which come from a myriad of sources (plants, fungi, animals, and the laboratory). They all share a common mechanism of altering the serotonergic system to produce their desired effects. Although generally safe to use (comparing them with many other illicit substances), these substances are still capable of considerable morbidity and mortality. Most patients who present to the hospital require only simple supportive care: A quiet, dark room and perhaps a small dose of benzodiazepines. Patients who present near death because of hallucinogen use usually are suffering from either extreme psychomotor agitation or serotonin syndrome. Stabilizing resuscitative measures include external cooling, aggressive hydration, and the administration of benzodiazepines. As with any other cause of psychomotor agitation, when unable to obtain a clear history for hallucinogenic use, other causes must be considered and explored. The continued use of hallucinogens requires practitioners to familiarize themselves with their history, uses, and effects.

REFERENCES

1. Strassman RJ. Hallucinogenic drugs in psychiatric research and treatment. *J Nerv Ment Dis.* 1995;183:127–138.
2. Spess DL. *Soma: The Divine Hallucinogen.* Rochester VT: Park Street Press; 2000.

3. de Rios MD, Alger N, Crumrine NR, et al. The influence of psychotropic flora and fauna on Maya religion. *Current Anthropology.* 1974;15:147–164.
4. Caporeal LR. Ergotism: The satan loosed in Salem? *Science.* 1976;192:21–26.
5. Stevens J. *Storming Heaven.* New York: Harper and Row; 1987.
6. Leary T. *Turn on, Tune in, Drop out.* Berkeley CA: Ronin Publishing; 1999.
7. Substance Abuse and Mental Health Services Administration. *2004 National Survey on Drug Use & Health: National Findings.* [online] 2005 [accessed 2006 Nov 3] Available from: URL: http://www.oas.samhsa.gof/nsduh.htm.
8. Erowid E, Erowid F. Erowid visitors on LSD: The results of eight LSD-related surveys conducted on erowid between OCT 2005 and JAN 2006. *Erowid Extracts.* 2006;10:4–8.
9. Gaston G, Allen JW, Gartz J. A worldwide geographical distribution of the neutrotropic fungi, an analysis and discussion. *Annali Del Museo Civico Di Rovereto.* 1998;14:189–280.
10. Hofmann A, Troxler F. Identification of psilocin. *Experientia.* 1959;15:101–102.
11. Bigwood J, Beug MW. Variation of psilocybin and psilocin levels with repeated flushes (harvests) of mature sporocarps of *Psilocybe cubensis* (earle) singer. *J Ethnopharmacol.* 1982;5:287–291.
12. Erowid E, Erowid F. Erowid Vaults: Mushrooms. [online] 1995 [accessed 2006 Dec 1] Available from: http://www.erowid.org/plants/mushrooms/mushrooms.shtml.
13. Erowid E, Erowid F. Erowid Vaults: Ibogaine. [online] 1995 [accessed 2006 Nov 28] Available from: URL: http://www.erowid.org/chemicals/ibogaine/ibogaine.shtml.
14. Blackledge RD, Taylor CM. *Psychotria viridis*—A botanical source of dimethyltyptamine (DMT). *Microgram Journal.* 2003;1:18–22.
15. Lyttle T, Goldstein D, Gartz J. Bufo toads and bufotenine: Fact and fiction surrounding an alleged psychedelic. *J Psychoactive Drugs.* 1996;28:267–290.
16. Weil AT, Davis W. *Bufo alvarius*: A potent hallucinogen of animal origin. *J Ethnopharmacol.* 1995;41:1–8.
17. Brubacher JR, Lachmanen D, Ravikumar PR, et al. Efficacy of digoxin-specific Fab fragments (Digibind) in the treatment of toad venom poisoning. *Toxicon.* 1999;37:931–942.
18. Boland DM, Andollo W, Hime GW, et al. Fatality due to acute α-methyltryptamine intoxication. *J Anal Toxicol.* 2005;29:394–397.
19. Kulig K. LSD. *Emerg Med Clin North Am.* 1990;8:551–558.
20. Bullis RK. Swallowing the scroll: Legal implications of the recent Supreme Court peyote cases. *J Psychoactive Drugs.* 1990;22:325–332.
21. Schultes RE, Hoffman A. *Plant of the Gods.* Rochester VT: Healing Art Press; 1992.
22. Nichols DE, Lloyd DH, Johnson MP, et al. Synthesis and serotonin receptor affinities of a series of enantiomers of α-methyltryptamines: Evidence for the binding conformation of tryptamines at serotonin 5-HT_{1B} receptors. *J Med Chem.* 1988;31:1406–1412.
23. Glennon RA, Chaurasia C, Titeler M. Binding of indolylalkylamines at 5-HT_2 serotonin receptors: Examination of a hydrophobic binding region. *J Med Chem.* 1990;33:2777–2784.
24. Giacomelli S, Palmery M, Romanelli L, et al. Lysergic acid diethylamide (LSD) is a partial agonist of D2 dopaminergic receptors and it potentiates dopamine-mediated prolactin secretion in lactrotrophs in vitro. *Life Sci.* 1998;63:215–222.
25. Blaho K, Merigan K, Windberry S, et al. Clinical pharmacology of lysergic acid diethylamide: Case reports and review of the treatment of intoxication. *Am J Ther.* 1997;4:211–221.
26. Kulick AR, Ahmed I. Substance-induced organic mental disorders: A clinical and conceptual approach. *Gen Hosp Psychiatry.* 1986;8:168–172.
27. Sternbach H. The serotonin syndrome. *Am J Psychiatry.* 1991;148:705–713.
28. Boyer EW, Shannon M. The serotonin syndrome. *N Engl J Med.* 2005;352:1112–1120.
29. Leikin JB, Krantz AJ, Zell-Kanter M, et al. Clinical features and management of intoxication due to hallucinogenic drugs. *Med Toxicol Adverse Drug Exp.* 1989;4:324–350.
30. Fisher DD, Ungerleider JT. Grand mal seizures following ingestion of LSD. *Calif Med.* 1967;106:210–211.
31. McCawley EL, Brummett RE, Dana GW. Convulsions from psilocybe mushroom poisoning. *Proc West Pharmacol Soc.* 1962;5:27–33.
32. Klock JC, Boemer U, Becker CE. Coma, hyperthermia, and bleeding associated with massive LSD overdose. *West J Med.* 1973;120:183–188.
33. Abraham HD, Mamen A. LSD-like panic from risperidone in post-LSD visual disorder. *J Clin Pharmacol.* 1996;16:238–241.
34. Abraham HD. Visual phenomenology of the LSD flashback. *Arch Gen Psychiatry.* 1983; 40:884–889.

CHAPTER **108**

Alcohol

Kathy L. Ferguson • Gar Ming Chan

OBJECTIVES

- To describe the signs and symptoms of alcohol dependence
- To explain the signs and symptoms of alcohol withdrawal
- To discuss the complications of acute and chronic alcohol use
- To explore effective treatments for alcohol withdrawal

CASE VIGNETTE

A 53-year-old man with a history of alcoholism presented to the emergency department (ED) for surgical repair of an eyebrow laceration after a fall. He denied loss of consciousness, vomiting, or headache, and was alert and oriented but tremulous. His vital signs were as follows: Blood pressure 151/91 mm Hg; heart rate 111 beats per minute; respirations 16 breaths per minute; and temperature 36.2°C. The patient's laceration was surgically repaired and he was discharged. Fifteen minutes later, the patient had a generalized tonic–clonic seizure. He was postictal when brought back to the ED and then had a second generalized tonic–clonic seizure during his ED evaluation. His tonic–clonic seizures responded to two separate doses of intravenous lorazepam (2 mg). He was given parenteral thiamine, folate, and a multivitamin. A chest radiograph revealed bilateral lobar pneumonia. He was given intravenous antibiotics and admitted to the medical intensive care unit (MICU) for management of alcohol withdrawal and pneumonia.

DEFINITIONS

Alcohol addiction describes the physiologic or psychological desire to obtain and consume alcohol, often in a compulsive manner. *Alcohol abuse* involves the misuse of alcohol, either habitually or in a "binge-type" fashion, to the extent that it interferes with a patient's social functioning and responsibilities. It frequently leads to the development of alcohol dependence. *Alcohol dependence* is a physiologic state in which the body has adapted to chronic alcohol consumption. Characteristic withdrawal symptoms will manifest with alcohol cessation that can be relieved by resumption of drinking. Alcohol-dependent patients develop tolerance to alcohol with chronic exposure over time. This tolerance involves changes in neurotransmitter receptor levels within the central nervous system (CNS) resulting in decreased CNS effects with similar doses. Patients will often increase dose, frequency, or both to achieve the desired effects. Additionally, tolerant individuals can develop signs and symptoms of alcohol withdrawal at alcohol levels that would be inebriating to alcohol-naïve patients. *Alcoholism* is the chronic disease state resulting from alcohol dependence. *Alcohol withdrawal*, as defined by the fourth edition of the *Diagnostic and Statistical Manual of Mental Disorders* (DSM-IV), involves the cessation of alcohol intake after prolonged or heavy use, in conjunction with two or more of the following: Autonomic hyperreactivity, increased hand tremor, insomnia, nausea or vomiting, transient hallucinations or illusions, psychomotor agitation, anxiety, or grand mal seizures (1). The symptoms must cause significant distress in the patient's functioning, and must not be caused by a general medical condition or mental disorder.

EPIDEMIOLOGY

Alcohol abuse affects the social or occupational functioning of almost 14 million Americans at a given time. Alcoholism outweighs all other diseases in the United States in terms of morbidity and mortality. The economic burden of alcohol abuse and dependence in the United States is staggering. In 1998 alone, the estimated economic cost from alcohol abuse was over $184 billion (2). In the 2005 National Survey on Drug Use and Health (NSDUH), 51.8% of Americans over age 12 reported having at least one drink within the past month (3). This corresponds to 126 million people, a figure that is 5 million higher than the 2004 survey estimate. In addition, almost 23% of responders over age 12 reported binge drinking at least once in the prior month. Heavy alcohol use was reported by 6.6% of responders in 2005, representing an estimated number of 16 million people. The effects of alcohol abuse and dependence do not only have an impact on the drinker, they also have an impact on the drinker's family, friends, and community. Greater than 50% of American adults have a close family member who abuses alcohol (2). Almost one fourth of violent crimes in the United States are committed by individuals who have consumed alcohol. In 2005, motor vehicle collisions involving alcohol abuse killed more than 16,000 Americans (4). Alcohol and alcohol-related events are the number one cause of mortality in young adults.

ETIOLOGY AND PATHOGENESIS

Alcoholism has been linked to both genetic and environmental factors (5). Studies have shown that children adopted by alcoholic parents do not have a higher tendency to become alcoholics than the rest of the population. On the other hand, children with biological alcoholic parents, even when reared away from home, have a higher tendency to become alcoholics (6). A three- to fivefold increased prevalence of alcoholism is found among immediate biological family members of alcoholics. In addition to genetic influences, many authors believe that certain personality traits and environmental factors may play a role in the development of alcoholism.

The etiology and pathogenesis of alcohol withdrawal is complex and not completely understood. γ-aminobutyric acid (GABA) is the major inhibitory neurotransmitter in the brain. Alcohol exerts its sedative effects by GABA-(subtype A) receptor agonism. Chronic alcohol use leads to downregulation of these inhibitory GABA-A receptors. This downregulation is thought to be partially responsible for the phenomenon of tolerance. Over time, alcoholics need to drink more to experience the same effect. In addition to GABA-A downregulation, evidence suggests that excitatory NMDA (N-methyl-d-aspartate) receptors become upregulated with chronic alcohol use (7). Alcohol withdrawal manifests as hypersympathetic activity from the combination of loss of GABA inhibition coupled with increased NMDA excitation. This can lead to hypertension, tachycardia, fever, tremors, agitation, hallucinations, and seizures (8).

PATHOLOGY

Alcohol is rapidly absorbed from the gastrointestinal tract. Most of the absorbed alcohol is metabolized by two major enzymes in a step-wise fashion. First, alcohol dehydrogenase (ADH), which is present in both the gastric mucosa and the liver, oxidizes alcohol to form acetaldehyde. Next, aldehyde dehydrogenase (ALDH) further oxidizes acetaldehyde to form acetic acid, which is used to form acetylcoenzyme-A (acetyl-CoA) which enters the Krebs cycle. The required cofactor needed for the pyruvate dehydrogenase complex to convert acetic acid to acetyl-CoA is thiamine (vitamin B_1).

In alcohol-naïve patients, ADH and ALDH serve as the primary means of metabolizing alcohol. In chronic drinkers, however, the cytochrome P-450 microsomal enzyme, CYP2E1, in the liver becomes upregulated and effectively functions as ADH, converting alcohol to acetaldehyde. The acetaldehyde then undergoes oxidation in the mitochondria by ALDH. The induced CYP2E1 enzymes, as part of the microsomal ethanol oxidizing system (MEOS), function to increase the rate of alcohol metabolism (9). This change in metabolism and brain receptors results in tolerance requiring the alcoholic to drink greater amounts of alcohol to achieve its desired effects.

Alcoholism leads to a wide array of nutritionally depleted states. Thiamine deficiency causes two distinct clinical syndromes: "Wet" beriberi and "dry" beriberi. Wet beriberi is manifested as high-output cardiac failure from arteriovenous fistula formation. Dry beriberi is also known as Wernicke encephalopathy (WE). WE is manifested by a triad of symptoms: Ataxia, ophthalmoplegia, and confusion. Korsakoff psychosis is a more progressive manifestation of thiamine deficiency and WE. It involves the additional symptoms of short-term memory loss and confabulation. Korsakoff psychosis is irreversible, whereas WE can be reversed with thiamine replacement. Together, the two syndromes may coexist as Wernicke-Korsakoff psychosis. In addition to WE and Korsakoff psychosis, alcoholics can also develop *pellagra* from nutritional depletion of niacin and tryptophan. This manifests traditionally as the "4D's": Diarrhea, dermatitis, dementia, and death. Pellagra is reversible with niacin repletion. Over time, nutritionally deficient alcoholics who abuse tobacco can develop *tobacco-alcohol amblyopia,* characterized by central scotoma, decreased color vision, and papillomacular bundle damage. Tobacco-alcohol amblyopia is also referred to as *toxic-nutritional optic neuropathy* (10).

Other CNS effects result from long-term changes in neuronal structure. Studies have shown that over time alcoholics develop cerebellar atrophy, specifically in the Purkinje cells of the anterior and superior cerebellar vermis (11,12). This atrophy more commonly is found in alcoholics with WE (13). *Alcoholic cerebellar degeneration* can lead to ataxia and gait difficulty. In addition, demyelination of the corpus callosum can result in the rare *Marchiafava-Bignami disease* (MBD), which in its mild form can manifest as unilateral apraxia and agraphia with contralateral hemineglect. In its severe form, MBD can lead to severe alterations in consciousness, mutism, and seizures (14). *Central pontine myelinolysis* (CPM) is seen in chronic alcoholics, often in the setting of rapidly corrected hyponatremia. CPM involves white matter demyelination and its clinical manifestations depend on the site of the lesion (e.g., corticospinal tract demyelination can lead to paraparesis) (15). *Alcoholic dementia* is a controversial entity. Over time, alcoholics develop defects in cognition, which some believe to be secondary to direct neurotoxic effects of alcohol on cortical neurons in the brain (15,16). It may be difficult to distinguish the cognitive impairments of alcoholic dementia from other causes related to alcoholism, such as WE. In addition, alcoholics tend to sustain repeated traumatic head injuries secondary to their states of intoxication which, in combination with nutritional deficiency states and possible direct neurotoxicity of ethanol, can lead to worsened cognition and a dementialike picture.

Alcohol very commonly affects the peripheral nervous system in alcoholics. In fact, peripheral polyneuropathy is the most common neurologic complication (15). It is unclear whether *alcoholic polyneuropathy* is caused by direct neurotoxicity, nutrient depletion, or both. The peripheral neuropathy of alcoholism can affect sensory, motor, and autonomic nerves. It develops slowly and progressively over time. The sensory neuropathy involves initial numbness mainly of the distal aspects of the lower extremities, which then progresses proximally ("dying-back neuropathy"). The numbness can progress to paresthesias and become severely painful. In the upper extremities, it begins in the fingertips and spreads proximally as well. This leads to a stocking-and-glove type pattern of sensory loss. The motor form of alcoholic neuropathy causes weakness of distal muscles and eventual wasting. In addition, deep tendon reflexes are decreased to absent. Autonomic neuropathies are relatively rare, but when present they can manifest as sympathetic or parasympathetic dysfunction. *Alcoholic myopathy* can be either acute or chronic. Acute alcoholic myopathy occurs after a drinking binge over several days. Patients often develop muscle pain, weakness, and rhabdomyolysis with myoglobinuria and increased creatine kinase levels. Acute alcoholic myopathy can be severe, and can become life-threatening from renal failure and hyperkalemia-induced dysrhythmias. Chronic alcohol myopathy is a progressive, insidious, painless sydrome involving weakness of proximal muscles with eventual atrophy. The myopathy can be worsened by the coexistence of alcoholic polyneuropathy. Myopathies have been noted to occur in well-nourished alcoholics, so evidence suggests that alcohol or its metabolites can cause a direct toxic insult to the muscles themselves (15).

Many other organ systems are also affected by chronic alcohol intake. In the liver, chronic alcohol use can lead to fatty change, which can be reversible with the discontinuation of alcohol. With further drinking, however, it can lead to alcoholic cirrhosis and liver failure. Cardiovascular effects of alcoholism include dilated cardiomyopathy with potential cardiac failure. Gastritis and pancreatitis can result from alcohol. Alcoholics can develop chronic pancreatitis, which can result in nutritional deficiencies from malabsorption. Chronic alcohol use has also been linked to increased risk of certain cancers, namely within the upper gastrointestinal tract and liver (17).

CLINICAL MANIFESTATIONS AND SPECIAL SITUATIONS

The clinical manifestations of acute alcohol intoxication are manifested mainly within the CNS. Sedation, respiratory depression, and cerebellar effects predominate. Clinically, an acutely intoxicated patient exhibits slurring of speech, horizontal nystagmus, slowing of mentation, loss of inhibitions, and ataxia. In addition to CNS and cognitive effects, the patient may experience gastrointestinal upset, ranging from nausea and vomiting to acute gastritis. Alcohol-induced hypoglycemia occurs mostly in children and the malnourished from reduced glycogen stores. Alcohol metabolism causes a change in the redox state of the patient, forcing conversion of pyruvate to lactate and interfering with gluconeogenesis, which contributes to hypoglycemia (18).

Alcoholic ketoacidosis (AKA) is a special situation that occurs in the chronic alcoholic after a period of binging drinking, without other forms of caloric intake. The patient is often volume depleted secondary to vomiting associated with gastritis, pancreatitis, hepatitis, or other acute illness (19). In AKA, a high anion gap metabolic acidosis is present without a concurrent elevated lactate. The treatment of AKA is centered on fluid resuscitation with crystalloids, glucose administration, and nutritional supplementation with thiamine. The acidosis of AKA is mainly from the presence of ketoacids, similar to a starvation state. The serum laboratory test for ketones may not always test positive, because most hospital laboratories test for acetone or acetoacetate and in AKA much of the ketonemia exists in the form of β-hydroxybutyrate. With treatment of AKA, the β-hydroxybutyrate is converted to acetoacetate potentially resulting in a false–positive increase in ketones when clinical improvement of the patient is occurring. AKA itself is not usually life-threatening, however clinicians should search for possible underlying precipitating disorders, such as occult infection.

Alcohol withdrawal involves a spectrum of disease-state manifestations that can be divided into four distinct clinical categories: Alcoholic tremulousness, alcoholic hallucinosis, alcoholic withdrawal seizures, and delirium tremens (20). *Alcoholic tremulousness* manifests as tremor, agitation, and autonomic instability, which can develop within several hours of cessation of drinking. Patients will often self-medicate by drinking more alcohol to relieve the symptoms. *Alcoholic hallucinosis* involves the development of hallucinations (usually visual or tactile) in a non delirious patient. Patients experiencing alcoholic hallucinosis remain oriented to person, time, and place in contrast to patients with delirium tremens. *Alcohol withdrawal seizures* (also known as 'rum fits') are generalized, tonic–clonic seizures with a brief postictal state, which rarely progress to status epilepticus (21). They can occur in up to 10% of patients exhibiting signs of alcohol withdrawal (20). Although not all patients who seize will progress to delirium tremens, the occurrence of alcohol withdrawal seizures can be an indicator of risk. *Delirium tremens (DT)* is a life-threatening manifestation of alcohol withdrawal that usually begins after 2 to 3 days of abstinence from alcohol, and can last for up to 2 weeks (22). It involves the characteristic signs and symptoms of alcoholic tremulousness and hallucinosis, but with increased severity and in conjunction with an altered sensorium. The autonomic instability is severe in DT and patients can die from the effects of uncontrolled sympathetic hyperactivity. The severity of alcohol withdrawal appears to increase with repeated episodes. This is the phenomenon known as *kindling* (23,24). With each episode of alcohol withdrawal, the subsequent episode of withdrawal appears more severe, often leading to the development of alcohol withdrawal seizures. With repeated episodes, those seizures can become relatively resistant to benzodiazepine administration (25).

Perhaps the most disturbing effects of alcoholism are seen in the *fetal alcohol syndrome* (FAS). Alcohol is a known teratogen with an unclear mechanism of teratogenicity. FAS occurs when a pregnant woman chronically abuses alcohol during her pregnancy. Children with FAS have developmental delays, emotional and cognitive problems, mental retardation, and physical deformities. Physical developmental anomalies in FAS include microcephaly, dysmorphic facies, skeletal joint abnormalities, and cardiovascular anomalies.

DIAGNOSTIC APPROACH

The diagnosis of acute intoxication with alcohol can be achieved using various clinical and laboratory data. Clinical signs of acute alcohol intoxication include ataxia, dysmetria, nystagmus, slurred speech, and CNS depression. Blood alcohol levels can be measured in a hospital laboratory. Breath alcohol analyzers ("breathalyzers") have been shown to be accurate at predicting true blood alcohol concentrations (26). Blood alcohol levels, however, correlate poorly with actual clinical degree of intoxication. This is because of alterations in CNS neurotransmitter receptors involved in tolerance. For example, an alcohol-naïve patient may be impaired with a blood alcohol level of 80 mg/dL (legally intoxicated level), but a similar level in an alcoholic can produce withdrawal symptoms and even seizures.

The diagnosis of chronic alcoholism is more difficult, especially early on. Two main screening tools are used to identify those with alcoholism. The CAGE questionnaire is a set of four questions asked of an individual suspected of alcohol abuse. The questions ask if the patient has ever felt the need to cut down on drinking, has been annoyed by others when questioned about their drinking, has felt guilty about their drinking, or whether or not they have needed an early morning "eye-opener" to relieve stress or treat a hangover. If the individual answers yes to two or more of the four questions, the diagnosis of alcoholism is likely. The Brief Michigan Alcoholism Screening Test (MAST) is a set of ten yes or no questions similar to, but more comprehensive than, the CAGE questionnaire. A point value is given to certain answers of "yes" or "no," and a score of six or greater means a probable diagnosis of alcoholism.

The diagnosis of alcohol withdrawal is mainly clinical, focusing on the patient's mental status and vital signs. Patients withdrawing can be tremulous, agitated, or delirious. Hemodynamically, they can be hypertensive, tachycardic, and may have low-grade fever from their hypersympathetic states. Alcohol withdrawal, in the form of DT, can be life-threatening. Patients suspected of alcohol withdrawal should be admitted to an intensive care unit for close monitoring for the development of DT. The Clinical Institute Withdrawal Assessment of Alcohol, Revised (CIWA-Ar) scale is a clinical tool designed for hospital staff to assess the severity of alcohol withdrawal (Table 108-1). It consists of a scored set of subjective criteria based on clinical observation of the patient, with a maximal achievable score of 67. The CIWA-Ar should be measured frequently for progression of withdrawal.

TREATMENT

Treatment of the acutely alcohol-intoxicated patient involves airway and breathing assessment, fluid hydration, electrolyte replacement, and management of the complications associated with acute intoxication (e.g., pancreatitis, AKA, trauma). If chronic alcoholism is suspected, nutritional supplementation with thiamine is recommended. Folate and multivitamins are often given as well. Magnesium should be supplemented if the patient's serum level is low. The potential for hypoglycemia should be investigated early, especially in children.

Besides counseling and support groups, medications have been used to help treat alcohol addiction. Disulfiram inhibits the action of ALDH, thus inhibiting the conversion of acetaldehyde to acetic acid. When ethanol is ingested, the resultant increase in acetaldehyde creates unpleasant effects, the so-called *disulfiram-alcohol reaction.* Symptoms include flushing, urticaria, nausea, vomiting, abdominal pain, chest pain, and dyspnea. These symptoms may appear as early as 15 minutes after drinking alcohol in a patient who has taken disulfiram. Although temporarily debilitating, these symptoms are rarely fatal, but disulfiram is not without other side effects, and does nothing for alcohol withdrawal. Other medications that have been used are opiod antagonists, serotonin agonists, and lithium (27).

Treatment of a patient with alcohol withdrawal can be complex. Clinicians should search for the underlying cause of drinking cessation. Often, patients will have an occult infection that could go untreated if not sought-after and recognized. There exists tremendous individual variability among patients in terms of severity of the withdrawal response. Patients can progress from one state of withdrawal to the next in an unpredictable manner. For example, some patients will develop alcohol withdrawal seizures before the onset of tremor, hypersympathetic state, or hallucinations (22). The mainstay of therapy for alcohol withdrawal is benzodiazepines. Some consider diazepam the benzodiazepine of choice in alcohol withdrawal, because of is extended half-life and active metabolite, desmethyldiazepam (28). Several studies have demonstrated the superiority of "symptom-triggered therapy" for alcohol withdrawal (29–31) in that it decreases the amount of medication needed to treat withdrawal, decreases length of stay, and decreases the occurrence of DT. Symptom-triggered therapy involves intravenous (IV) push doses of benzodiazepines in response to withdrawal symptoms. Withdrawal symptoms can range from tremor and agitation, to tachycardia, hypertension, fever, hallucinations, and seizures. IV push doses of benzodiazepines are given on an as-needed basis with frequent vital sign and CIWA-Ar score checks. This regimen is opposed to standing order regimens of benzodiazepines, which may oversedate or undertreat patients.

Management of alcohol withdrawal seizures, in particular, deserves special mention. No beneficial role appears to exist for traditional antiepileptic drugs in the primary or secondary prevention of alcohol withdrawal seizures (32). Once termed *alcoholic epilepsy,* the seizures of alcohol withdrawal do not appear to share similar pathophysiology with idiopathic epilepsy. Unlike idiopathic epilepsy, alcohol withdrawal seizures occur from global uninhibited NMDA excitation coupled with loss of GABA-A inhibition, secondary to alcohol cessation. Several studies have demonstrated no benefit, and possibly increased risks, by acutely or chronically treating alcohol withdrawal seizures with phenytoin or other antiepileptic drugs (33,34).

Other adjunctive medications can be used in severe cases of alcohol withdrawal when benzodiazepines alone fail. As stated, alcohol withdrawal symptoms occur from loss of GABA agonism coupled with unopposed NMDA excitatory activity. Phenobarbital, as a GABA agonist, can be used in conjunction with benzodiazepines to enhance GABAergic transmission (35). Propofol (a GABA agonist with different binding properties) can also be used in the treatment of severe alcohol withdrawal (36,37). It is administered as a continuous IV infusion and has the advantage of a very fast onset of action. It can lead to hypotension and excessive CNS depression, however. Many patients treated with propofol are intubated for airway control and protection. Propofol has a relatively short duration of action, and its effects are usually reversed after several minutes of stopping the infusion.

An intubated, sedated patient in alcohol withdrawal might exhibit only subtle signs of withdrawal, such as hypertension, tachycardia, and fever. The sedated patient will not appear anxious and delirious, and evaluation of mental status is difficult. Because of kindling, each episode of withdrawal should be aggressively controlled so that future episodes are not at risk of becoming more severe. The vital sign abnormalities in alcohol withdrawal are best treated with increased use of benzodiazepines, possibly in conjunction with phenobarbital or propofol. Any attempt to mask vital sign abnormalities (e.g., β-blockers) may alleviate anxiety in the clinician, but does not treat the underlying pathology. Vital sign abnormalities in alcohol withdrawal result from excessive CNS stimulation with loss of GABA inhibition. Medications used for alcohol withdrawal should target withdrawal at the level of the CNS, not just peripheral receptors.

CLINICAL RECOMMENDATIONS OF THE VIGNETTE

In the MICU, the patient developed two additional seizures, both of which responded to intravenous lorazepam. He

TABLE 108-1. Clinical Institute Withdrawal Assessment of Alcohol Scale, Revised (CIWA-Ar)

Patient:________________________ **Date:** ______________ **Time:** _____________ (24 hour clock, midnight = 00:00)

Pulse or heart rate, taken for one minute:______________________ **Blood pressure:**______

NAUSEA AND VOMITING—Ask "Do you feel sick to your stomach? Have you vomited?" Observation.
0 no nausea and no vomiting
1 mild nausea with no vomiting
2
3
4 intermittent nausea with dry heaves
5
6
7 constant nausea, frequent dry heaves and vomiting

TREMOR—Arms extended and fingers spread apart. Observation.
0 no tremor
1 not visible, but can be felt fingertip to fingertip
2
3
4 moderate, with patient's arms extended
5
6
7 severe, even with arms not extended

PAROXYSMAL SWEATS—Observation.
0 no sweat visible
1 barely perceptible sweating, palms moist
2
3
4 beads of sweat obvious on forehead
5
6
7 drenching sweats

ANXIETY—Ask "Do you feel nervous?" Observation.
0 no anxiety, at ease
1 mild anxious
2
3
4 moderately anxious, or guarded, so anxiety is inferred
5
6
7 equivalent to acute panic states as seen in severe delirium or acute schizophrenic reactions

AGITATION—Observation.
0 normal activity
1 somewhat more than normal activity
2
3
4 moderately fidgety and restless
5
6
7 paces back and forth during most of the interview, or constantly thrashes about

TACTILE DISTURBANCES—Ask "Have you any itching, pins and needles sensations, any burning, any numbness, or do you feel bugs crawling on or under your skin?" Observation.
0 none
1 very mild itching, pins and needles, burning or numbness
2 mild itching, pins and needles, burning or numbness
3 moderate itching, pins and needles, burning or numbness
4 moderately severe hallucinations
5 severe hallucinations
6 extremely severe hallucinations
7 continuous hallucinations

AUDITORY DISTURBANCES—Ask "Are you more aware of sounds around you? Are they harsh? Do they frighten you? Are you hearing anything that is disturbing to you? Are you hearing things you know are not there?" Observation.
0 not present
1 very mild harshness or ability to frighten
2 mild harshness or ability to frighten
3 moderate harshness or ability to frighten
4 moderately severe hallucinations
5 severe hallucinations
6 extremely severe hallucinations
7 continuous hallucinations

VISUAL DISTURBANCES—Ask "Does the light appear to be too bright? Is its color different? Does it hurt your eyes? Are you seeing anything that is disturbing to you? Are you seeing things you know are not there?" Observation.
0 not present
1 very mild sensitivity
2 mild sensitivity
3 moderate sensitivity
4 moderately severe hallucinations
5 severe hallucinations
6 extremely severe hallucinations
7 continuous hallucinations

HEADACHE, FULLNESS IN HEAD—Ask "Does your head feel different? Does it feel like there is a band around your head?" Do not rate for dizziness or lightheadedness. Otherwise, rate severity.
0 not present
1 very mild
2 mild
3 moderate
4 moderately severe
5 severe
6 very severe
7 extremely severe

ORIENTATION AND CLOUDING OF SENSORIUM—Ask "What day is this? Where are you? Who am I?"
0 oriented and can do serial additions
1 cannot do serial additions or is uncertain about date
2 disoriented for date by no more than 2 calendar days
3 disoriented for date by more than 2 calendar days
4 disoriented for place/or person

Total **CIWA-Ar** Score _____
Rater's Initials _____
Maximum Possible Score 67

The **CIWA-Ar** is not copyrighted and may be reproduced freely. This assessment for monitoring withdrawal symptoms requires approximately 5 minutes to administer. The maximum score is 67 (see instrument). Patients scoring less than 10 do not usually need additional medication for withdrawal.
From Sullivan JT, Sykora K, Schneiderman J, et al. Assessment of alcohol withdrawal: The revised Clinical Institute Withdrawal Assessment for Alcohol scale (**CIWA-Ar**). *British Journal of Addiction* 84:1353-1357, 1989.

developed visual hallucinations and became combative. Because of his altered sensorium, the patient was intubated to control his withdrawal and behavior. A lorazepam infusion was initiated and maintained for several days. He did not develop additional seizures. He was given metoprolol for the treatment of hypertension and tachycardia. Three days after extubation, he returned to a normal mental status. Before discharge, the patient admitted to having a productive cough for several days before admission and abstained from alcohol use because he felt "too sick to drink."

The case illustrates several important points about alcohol withdrawal. First, the patient initially presented with tremor and mildly abnormal vital signs. Clinicians must be vigilant in recognizing the subtle signs of alcohol withdrawal. In the ICU, he was given β-blockers to control his hypertension and tachycardia, but these symptoms would have been better treated by increased symptom-triggered benzodiazepine administration targeting the underlying pathology. Such therapy likely would have controlled both his central and peripheral hypersympathetic states. Finally, although the reason for presentation was that the patient was status postseizure, he also had an underlying bilateral pneumonia. This reiterates the importance of searching for, and treating, a possible occult medical cause of alcohol cessation.

SUMMARY

Alcoholism is a significant public health problem that places an enormous economic and social burden on the public. It should be recognized early and attempts at stopping its progression should be initiated through counseling, support groups, and possibly medications. Alcoholism causes various deleterious physical effects on both the individual, and on an unborn fetus. Alcohol withdrawal should be aggressively managed and controlled, to prevent possible progression to life-threatening delirium tremens.

REFERENCES

1. American Psychiatric Association. *Diagnostic and Statistical Manual of Mental Disorders*, 4th ed. Text Revision. Washington, DC; 2000.
2. National Institute on Alcohol Abuse and Alcoholism, US Department of Health and Human Services. *10th Special Report to the US Congress on Alcohol and Health.* June 2000 [accessed November 28, 2006]. Available at http://pubs.niaaa.nih.gov/publications/10report/intro.pdf.
3. Substance Abuse and Mental Health Services Administration, US Department of Health and Human Services. *2005 National Survey on Drug Use and Health: National Findings.* (Formerly known as the National Household Survey on Drug Abuse) [accessed November 30, 2006]. Available at http://www.oas.samhsa.gov/nsduh.htm.
4. National Highway Traffic and Safety Administration, National Center for Statistics and Analysis. *Traffic Safety Facts, Crash-Stats 2005* [accessed November 15, 2006]. Available at: http://www-nrd.nhtsa.dot.gov/pdf/nrd-30/NCSA/RNotes/2006/810644.pdf.
5. Cloninger CR. Neurogenetic adaptive mechanisms in alcoholism. *Science.* 1987;236(4800):410–416.
6. Cloninger CR, Bohman M, Sigvardsson S. Inheritance of alcohol abuse. Cross-fostering analysis of adopted men. *Arch Gen Psychiatry.* 1981;38(8):861–868.
7. Haugbol SR, Ebert B, Ulrichsen J. Upregulation of glutamate receptor subtypes during alcohol withdrawal in rats. *Alcohol Alcohol.* 2005;40(2):89–95.
8. Isbell H, Fraser HF, Wikler A, et al. An experimental study of the etiology of "rum fits" and delirium tremens. *Quarterly Journal of Studies on Alcohol.* 1955;16:1–33.
9. Lieber CS. Microsomal ethanol oxidizing system (MEOS): The first 30 years (1968–1998)—A review. *Alcohol Clin Exp Res.* 1999;23(6):991–1007.
10. Behbehani R, Sergott RC, Savino PJ. Tobacco-alcohol amblyopia: A maculopathy? *Br J Ophthalmol.* 2005;89(11):1543–1544.
11. Torvik A, Lindboe CF, Rogde S. Brain lesions in alcoholics. A neuropathological study with clinical correlations. *J Neurol Sci.* 1982;56(2–3):233–248.
12. Torvik A, Torp S. The prevalence of alcoholic cerebellar atrophy. A morphometric and histological study of an autopsy material. *J Neurol Sci.* 1986;75(1):43–51.
13. Baker KG, Harding AJ, Halliday GM, et al. Neuronal loss in functional zones of the cerebellum of chronic alcoholics with and without Wernicke's encephalopathy. *Neuroscience.* 1999:91(2):429–438.
14. Berek K, Wagner M, Chemelli AP, et al. Hemispheric disconnection in Marchiafava-Bignami disease: Clinical, neuropsychological and MRI findings. *J Neurol Sci.* 1994; 123(1–2): 2–5.
15. Diamond I, Messing RO. Neurologic effects of alcoholism. *West J Med.* 1994;161(3): 279–287.
16. Charness ME. Brain lesions in alcoholics. *Alcohol Clin Exp Res.* 1993;17(1):2–11.
17. Cotran RS, Kumar V, Collins T. *Robbins Pathologic Basis of Disease*, 6th ed. Philadelphia: WB Saunders; 1999:410–412.
18. Hoffman RS, Golfrank LR. Ethanol-associated metabolic disorders. *Emerg Med Clin North Am.* 1989;(4):943–961.
19. Fulop M. Alcoholic ketoacidosis. *Endocrinol Metab Clin North Am.* 1993;22(2):209–219.
20. Gold J, and Nelson LS. Ethanol Withdrawal. In: Flomenbaum NE, Goldfrank LR, Hoffman RS, et al. eds. *Goldfrank's Toxicologic Emergencies*, 8th ed. New York: McGraw-Hill; 2006: 1168–1169.
21. Victor M, Braush C. The role of abstinence in the genesis of alcoholic epilepsy. *Epilepsia.* 1967;8(1):1–20.
22. Victor M, Adams RD. The effect of alcohol on the nervous system. *Research Publications–Association for Research in Nervous and Mental Disease.* 1953;32:526–573.
23. Becker HC, Hale RL. Repeated episodes of ethanol withdrawal potentiate the severity of subsequent withdrawal seizures: An animal model of alcohol withdrawal "kindling." *Alcohol Clin Exp Res.* 1993;17(1):94–98.
24. Brown ME, Anton RF, Malcolm R, et al. Alcohol detoxification and withdrawal seizures. Clinical support for a kindling hypothesis. *Biol Psychiatry.* 1988;23(5):507–514.
25. Woo E, Greenblatt DJ. Massive benzodiazepine requirements during acute alcohol withdrawal. *Am J Psychiatry.* 1979;136(6):821–823.
26. Wenzel J, McDermott FT. Accuracy of blood alcohol estimations obtained with a breath alcohol analyzer in a casualty department. *Med J Aust.* 1985;142:627–628.
27. Yip L. Ethanol. In: Flomenbaum NE, Goldfrank LR, Hoffman RS, et al. eds. *Goldfrank's Toxicologic Emergencies*, 8th ed. New York: McGraw-Hill; 2006:1157.
28. Wretlind M, Pilbrant A, Sundwall A, et al. Disposition of three benzodiazepines after single oral administration in man. *Acta Pharmacologica et Toxicologica.* 1977;40[Suppl 1](1): 28–39.
29. Daeppen JB, Gache P, Landry U, et al. Symptom-triggered vs fixed-schedule doses of benzodiazepine for alcohol withdrawal: A randomized treatment trial. *Arch Intern Med.* 2002;162(10):1117–1121.
30. Jaeger TM, Lohr RH, Pankratz VS. Symptom-triggered therapy for alcohol withdrawal syndrome in medical inpatients. *Mayo Clin Proc.* 2001;76(7):695–701.
31. Saitz R, Mayo-Smith MF, Roberts MS, et al. Individualized treatment for alcohol withdrawal: A randomized double-blind controlled trial. *JAMA.* 1994;272(7):519–523.
32. Hillbom M, Pieninkeroinen I, Leone M. Seizures in alcohol-dependent patients: Epidemiology, pathophysiology and management. *CNS Drugs.* 2003;17(14):1013–1030.
33. Allredge BK, Lowenstein DH, Simon RP. Placebo-controlled trial of intravenous diphenylhydantoin for short-term treatment of alcohol withdrawal seizures. *Am J Med.* 1989;87 (6):645–648.
34. Rathlev NK, D'Onofrio G, Fish SS, et al. The lack of efficacy of phenytoin in the prevention of recurrent alcohol-related seizures. *Ann Emerg Med.* 1994;23(3):513–518.
35. Ives TJ, Mooney AJ III, Gwyther RE. Pharmacokinetic dosing of phenobarbital in the treatment of alcohol withdrawal syndrome. *South Med J.* 1991;84(1):18–21.
36. Coomes TR, Smith SW. Successful use of propofol in refractory delirium tremens. *Ann Emerg Med.* 1997;30(6):825–828.
37. McCowan C, Marik P. Refractory delirium tremens treated with propofol: A case series. *Crit Care Med.* 2000;28(6):1781–1784.

CHAPTER **109**

Solvents

William J. Holubek

OBJECTIVES

- To describe the approach a patient with a solvent exposure
- To discuss specific solvents that have unique toxicities
- To discuss the wide spectrum of clinical presentations For solvent exposure
- To explore the controversial areas of management and treatment

CASE VIGNETTE

A 14-year-old boy complains of numbness and muscle weakness of his left foot for 3 weeks, muscle weakness of his right foot for 1 day, and nonthreatening visual and auditory hallucinations. He admits to sniffing unleaded gasoline about 20 times a day for 15 to 20 minute intervals for the past 10 weeks. He has no medical problems, takes no medications, and is developmentally appropriate for his age.

Physical examination indicated normal mental status. Cranial nerves were intact. Motor and sensory examination of both upper extremities was intact. In the lower extremities, dorsiflexion and foot eversion strength was 0/5 on the left and 3/5 on the right. The left ankle reflex was hypoactive and the right ankle reflex was absent. Sensation to pinprick, light-touch, and temperature was decreased bilaterally in a stocking distribution. Also decreased focal sensation was noted along the lateral aspect of the left leg below the knee.

DEFINITIONS

Hydrocarbons are compounds made primarily of carbon and hydrogen atoms, which can be divided into two broad classes, *aliphatic* (straight or branched chain of carbon atoms) and *cyclic* (closed ring of carbon atoms). Hydrocarbons with short chain lengths exist as gases (e.g., methane), intermediate chain lengths exist as liquids (e.g., kerosene), and long chain lengths exist as solids (e.g., tar). *Aromatic* hydrocarbons are cyclic hydrocarbons that contain a benzenelike ring structure (e.g., benzene and toluene). *Halogenated* hydrocarbons contain one or more halogen atoms (e.g., chloroform and trichloroethylene). Countless substitutions and additions can be made to hydrocarbon molecules that alter its physical properties and toxicity. Physical properties of hydrocarbons that can influence its toxicity include *viscosity* (a measure of a fluids resistance to flow), *surface tension* (a measure of the force of attraction between molecules), and *volatility* (a measure of how easily a liquid becomes a gas).

A *solvent* is a class of chemicals that is used to dissolve other compounds. Water is a commonly used industrial solvent, and the primary solvent for biochemical processes. *Organic* solvents contain at least one carbon atom, and many of the solvents used in industry are hydrocarbons. The main commercial source of hydrocarbons is obtained from the distillation of petroleum, or from crude oil. These extraction processes often result in products that contain a mixture of different hydrocarbon compounds. Those hydrocarbons with high volatility, called *volatile* hydrocarbons, are contained in a wide variety of commercial products. Volatile hydrocarbons are commonly abused for their potential euphoric effects via sniffing, huffing, and bagging. *Sniffing* involves inhalation directly from a source (e.g., sniffing glue or a marker pen). *Huffing* involves soaking a rag or towel with a hydrocarbon and inhaling deeply, whereas *bagging* refers to depositing a solvent inside of a bag and then breathing the air from the bag.

EPIDEMIOLOGY

In 2005, the Toxic Exposure Surveillance System (TESS) database of the American Association of Poison Control Centers (AAPCC) reported 53,889 exposures to hydrocarbons, of which 17,685 were reported in children <6 years of age. Thirteen deaths were also reported to be associated with hydrocarbons (1). The Drug Abuse Warning Network (DAWN) in 2004 reported an estimated 9,275 emergency department visits related to inhalants (2).

ETIOLOGY AND PATHOLOGY

Hydrocarbons can be absorbed through oral, inhalational, and dermal exposure routes. Most small, low-molecular weight hydrocarbons and solvents are well absorbed by inhalation and ingestion, with aromatic compounds being generally absorbed better than aliphatic compounds. The amount of hydrocarbon absorbed through the skin is highly variable, depending on the exact molecular functional groups as well as the area of skin exposed. The high lipid solubility of hydrocarbons can cause dissolution of fatty tissues and allow penetration of cell membranes. Once absorbed, hydrocarbons have a wide variety of distribution, but commonly accumulate in fatty tissues. Hydrocarbons are eliminated either unchanged or through metabolism to more polar compounds.

The most common effect from hydrocarbon inhalation is central nervous system (CNS) depression. Halogenated hydrocarbons are frequently used by anesthesiologists as inhalational anesthetics to induce general anesthesia (e.g., *halothane*). The potency of different agents is compared using their *minimal alveolar concentration* (MAC). MAC is the concentration of vapor within the alveoli that produces loss of nociception in 50% of patients. The Meyer-Overton hypothesis suggests an inverse relationship between MAC and lipid solubility; in other words, very lipid-soluble agents can penetrate the CNS easily and, thus, have a lower MAC. This hypothesis, however, does not account for a compound's effect on specific neurotransmitters and receptors, such as stimulation of γ–aminobutyric acid ($GABA_A$) receptors by *trichloroethane.* The mechanism of hydrocarbon-induced CNS depression is complex and cannot be explained by a single process.

Peripheral sensorimotor polyneuropathy has been reported with solvent exposures. This is a toxic axonopathy that initially affects the distal portion of the largest or longest axons, and progresses proximally (3). See specific compounds below.

Pulmonary injury from aspiration is the most likely organ system associated with serious solvent toxicity. Hydrocarbons with low viscosity tend to be the ones that are easily aspirated. The exact mechanism of solvent-induced pulmonary injury is not known, but likely involves dissolution of the lipid surfactant layer and damage to tissues resulting in inflammation, alveolar edema, and hemorrhage, as well as bronchial injury.

GENERAL CLINICAL MANIFESTATIONS

The most common effect from acute hydrocarbon inhalation and ingestion is CNS depression. This manifests as ataxia, dizziness, headache, nausea, reduced inhibitions, and lethargy. The desired effect by individuals who abuse solvents is a general sense of euphoria. CNS excitation can occur, but is usually transient. Patients with chronic exposure to solvents can develop irreversible CNS damage, which is best described with toluene (see below), but can occur with other solvents. Peripheral sensorimotor polyneuropathy has also been described with solvent exposure (see specific compounds below).

The *solvent syndrome* is a controversial diagnosis proposed to exist in individuals with chronic (usually at least 9 years) low-level solvent exposure causing symptoms including memory loss, personality changes, fatigue, irritability, depression, dizziness, and incoordination (3). Thus far, current scientific literature does not support this diagnosis (4).

Pulmonary injury, which is usually caused by aspiration, is heralded by symptoms including vomiting, choking, and coughing. Patients with hydrocarbon pneumonitis can develop tachycardia, tachypnea, bronchospasm, hypoxia, fever, and radiographic findings, usually within 6 hours of exposure (7).

Symptoms from cardiac toxicity can include palpitations, shortness of breath, and syncope. Electrocardiographic (ECG) findings can include atrial fibrillation, premature ventricular contractions, QTc prolongation, and U waves. *Sudden sniffing death* is a term that is used to describe the many reports of witnessed sudden death of inhalant abusers (6). The mechanism is unclear; however, it is proposed that hydrocarbons (particularly halogenated hydrocarbons) prolong repolarization, thus "sensitizing the myocardium" to develop dysrhythmias in response to a catecholamine surge (5). A typical scenario involves a patient inhaling a solvent, who immediately performs exertion (e.g., running), and then loses consciousness, likely as a result of a fatal ventricular dysrhythmia.

Other organ systems can be affected by hydrocarbons. Gastrointestinal toxicity manifests as nausea and vomiting. Vomiting appears to be associated with an increased risk of developing pneumonitis. Methanol is known to cause pancreatitis. Halogenated hydrocarbons have been associated with hepatotoxicity (see specific compounds below). Nephrotoxicity, including acute renal failure and distal renal tubular acidosis, have also been associated with ingestion of halogenated hydrocarbons (e.g., chloroform, carbon tetrachloride, ethylene dichloride, tetrachloroethane). Dermal exposure to hydrocarbons can result in a wide spectrum of findings from contact dermatitis and blistering to full-thickness dermal damage. Chronic inhalational abuse of volatile hydrocarbons can produce dry, cracked skin around the mouth and nose, known as *huffer's eczema,* which can assist with the diagnosis of huffing. *Chloracne* is a condition caused by halogenated hydrocarbons (e.g., dioxins, polychlorinatedbiphenyls) resulting in severe, disfiguring scarring.

Fetal solvent syndrome (FSS) has been proposed based on the self-reported "heavy" or "daily" abuse of inhalants. Features are very similar to fetal alcohol syndrome (FAS) and include facial dysmorphia, growth retardation, and microcephaly.

GENERAL DIAGNOSTIC APPROACH

A detailed history of the route of exposure, specific hydrocarbon, and clinical presentation of the patient is very helpful in guiding an approach. An altered mental status may be the desired effect by solvent abusers; however, it is important to have an elevated suspicion for other causes (e.g., head trauma and infection), especially with persistent alteration. Chronic solvent effects on the CNS usually show up on neuroimaging as nonspecific cerebral volume loss. Specific neurodiagnostic tests (e.g., electromyograms [EMG], nerve conduction velocity (NVC) measurements, electroencephalograms [EEG], computerized tomography [CT] brain scans, and magnetic resonance imaging [MRI]) may be helpful and should be obtained on an individual basis (8).

Patients presenting with hydrocarbon ingestions and inhalations are at risk for pulmonary toxicity. An initial assessment of respiratory function is mandatory, including respiratory effort, respiratory rate, lungs sounds, and oxygen saturation. Radiographic evidence of hydrocarbon pneumonitis can take up to 4 to 6 hours to develop. Findings on chest radiograph (CXR) with aspiration can include perihilar infiltrates, increased bronchovascular markings, and bibasilar infiltrates. Abdominal radiographs in cases with large solvent ingestions may reveal the *double-bubble* sign (which represents the interface between air, hydrocarbon, and gastric fluid) or radiopaque material (e.g., chloroform, chloral hydrate) (9,10).

In general, blood levels of solvents are not available in real time to assist the clinician; even if they were available in most cases, it would not alter management, with some notable exceptions. Methanol should be measured on suspected exposures because treatment decision can be based on this level. Carbon monoxide levels should be drawn on patients exposed to methylene chloride.

GENERAL TREATMENT

Solvents, a diverse group of compounds, have a wide spectrum of toxicities that influence management strategies. After initial stabilization of the patient, options for decontamination must be considered. Because many solvents can be absorbed from dermal exposure, skin decontamination with soap and water may be necessary. Protection of medical personnel is of utmost importance, especially for the more toxic solvents or mixtures.

Gastrointestinal decontamination with gastric lavage remains controversial because of the risk of aspiration. Some solvents, however, contain toxic hydrocarbons and harmful xenobiotics, and the benefit of gastric lavage may exceed the risk of aspiration. The use of activated charcoal is also controversial because of its relative inability to adsorb many solvents, and its predisposition to cause vomiting. Consultation with a medical toxicologist is recommended.

Treatment of solvent ingestion is mostly supportive. Management should begin with assessment for electrolyte and acid-base abnormalities, hypoxia, and hypotension. The prophylactic use of antibiotics for pneumonitis is generally discouraged, and corticosteroid use is controversial. Patients with severe hydrocarbon pneumonitis requiring mechanical ventilation may benefit from the use of elevated positive end-expiratory pressure (PEEP), high-frequency jet ventilation (HFJV), or extracorporeal membrane oxygenation (ECMO). Cyanosis in an otherwise well-appearing patient should raise the concern for methemoglobinemia, which can be caused by other additives contained in the solvent (e.g., nitrites and aniline dyes). Hypotension probably does not result from the solvent itself, but potentially from co-ingested compounds (e.g., nitrites), reduced cardiac output from dehydration, or pulmonary injury. The use of α-adrenergic catecholamines should be minimized because of the potential for cardiac sensitization shown by several hydrocarbons and the potential to cause cardiac dysrhythmias. The involvement of pulmonary and critical care specialists is recommended for these patients.

In the setting of acute hydrocarbon ingestion with witnessed syncope and ventricular fibrillation, treatment with a β-adrenergic antagonist may be beneficial, as additional catecholamines (e.g., epinephrine) would further stimulate the already sensitized myocardium. The involvement of pulmonary and critical care specialists is recommended for these patients (11).

Peripheral neuropathies caused by solvents are managed primarily by removing the source of exposure, after which symptoms usually resolve over weeks to months.

SPECIFIC COMPOUNDS

Benzene

Benzene is an aromatic hydrocarbon that is widely used as an intermediate in making other chemicals. It can be found in many commercial products, including rubber materials, lubricants, dyes, detergents, and pesticides. Benzene, a known hematotoxin, is associated with hemolysis, aplastic anemia, and acute myelogenous leukemia. Currently, no convincing evidence links benzene exposure and the development of multiple myeloma. Given its carcinogenic risk, benzene-based products were removed from the US market, but many solvents (including gasoline) today still contain small amounts of benzene (5).

Carbon Tetrachloride

Carbon tetrachloride (CCl_4) was widely used in dry cleaning solvents, and as a refrigerant, in fire extinguishers and a pesticide until its use was restricted because of it known hepatotoxicity and nephrotoxicity. Encephalopathy can occur in the setting of hepatotoxicity, along with jaundice and right upper quadrant pain. Current evidence suggests benefits of N-acetylcysteine in cases of hepatotoxicity caused by CCl_4, and some animal models have reported benefit from hyperbaric oxygen therapy (6).

Dichloroacetylene

Dichloroacetylene (DCA) is a contaminant decomposition product of *trichloroethylene* (TCE), a halogenated hydrocarbon. TCE is found in typewriter correction fluid, paint strippers, degreasing agents, rug cleaning solvents, and spot removers. TCE is highly lipid soluble and well absorbed through the gastrointestinal and pulmonary system. As is common with most halogenated hydrocarbons, inebriation and CNS depression are common initial symptoms. DCA is of particular interest because it has been associated with visual field abnormalities, ataxia, and cranial neuropathies, particularly in the sensory nucleus of the trigeminal nerve. Symptoms can be delayed for up to 24 hours and can last for years. Somatosensory-evoked potential testing may be useful in making this diagnosis (12,13). Other case reports have suggested an association of TCE with the development of dilated cardiomyopathy and centrilobular hepatic necrosis.

Hexane and Methyl-n-Butyl Ketone

Hexane, an aliphatic hydrocarbon commonly used as a solvent in the shoe manufacturing, furniture restoration, and automobile industries, can be found in gasoline, rubber cement, glues, spray paints, and brake-cleaning fluids. Methyl-n-butyl-ketone (MnBK) is also a commonly used solvent in plastic resins, inks, and cleaning products. These two solvents share a common neurotoxic intermediate metabolite, 2,5-hexanedione, that has been reported to cause peripheral sensorimotor polyneuropathies from long-term occupational exposures. Clinically, this manifests as numbness and parasthesias initiating in the distal extremities, which progress proximally. Patients can also present with generalized muscle weakness that can eventually lead to muscle atrophy. This is classically described as a "dying-back" neuropathy, and its presentation is often confused with Guillain-Barré Syndrome (GBS), NCV show a slowing of motor conduction velocities and increased distal latencies, whereas EMG show muscle denervation. Somatosensory-evoked potential testing may show abnormalities as well.

Peripheral neuropathies caused by n-hexane and MnBK are managed primarily by removing the source of exposure, after which symptoms usually resolve over weeks to months. In some situations, symptoms may progress before improvement, despite intervention; this phenomenon is referred to as *coasting*.

Methanol

Methanol, a hydrocarbon with an added hydroxyl group, is commonly referred to as a *toxic alcohol*. It can be found in carburetor cleaners, cooking fuel (Sterno cans), model airplane fuel, windshield washer fluid, photocopying fluid, perfumes, and gasoline antifreeze. Significant methanol levels can be obtained by oral ingestion or inhalation (14). The initial clinical manifestations are inebriation and CNS depression, but its toxicity arises from its metabolite. Methanol is ultimately metabolized to formic acid, which causes an elevated anion-gap metabolic acidosis. Retinal pigmented epithelial cells and optic nerve cells appear to be uniquely sensitive to formic acid, resulting in hyperemia and pallor of the optic disc and papilledema. Clinically, patients can develop visual impairment ranging from blurry vision and "snowfield vision" to complete blindness. Severely methanol poisoned patients have also shown bilateral basal ganglia lesions (most commonly in the putamen) on brain CT and MRI.

The decision to treat and the modality of treatment for methanol toxicity is controversial and is usually based on the severity of acidosis, serum methanol level, and end-organ effects. Visual impairments have been reported in patients with methanol concentrations >50 mg/dL. As a safety margin, some experts recommend treating patients who have serum methanol levels >25 mg/dL. Treatment modalities include ethanol, fomepizole, and hemodialysis. Alcohol dehydrogenase (ADH) is the first enzyme in the metabolism of both methanol and ethanol. Because ADH has a higher affinity for ethanol, it is protective against the metabolism of methanol. Fomepizole (4-methylpyrazole) is a competitive ADH inhibitor that blocks the formation of formic acid. Fomepizole has been used in children and is pregnancy category C (5). As an adjunctive therapy, folic acid will enhance the clearance of formate, although this has not been shown to affect clinical outcome in humans. Involvement of a medical toxicologist in management of inhalational methanol exposures can help to optimize resources.

Methylene Chloride

Methylene chloride, a halogenated hydrocarbon commonly found in degreasing agents and paint strippers, is also used as an aerosol spray propellant. Exposure is usually oral ingestion or inhalation. Metabolism of methylene chloride produces carbon monoxide (CO), which can lead to CO poisoning. Some controversy exists over the use of hyperbaric oxygen therapy as a treatment modality for CO poisoning, and so consultation with a medical toxicologist or poison center is recommended in these cases (5).

Toluene

Toluene is a common solvent used in many products including paint, paint thinners, printing inks, and glues. It is commonly contained in solvents abused by huffers. Initial acute effects include euphoria and excitement, however higher doses can cause confusion, headache, nausea, ataxia, and tremors.

The effects of chronic exposure to solvents are best described in painters who were chronically overexposed to toluene. Chronic toluene abuse has been shown to cause white matter degeneration (leukoencephalopathy) that can be irreversible. These patients developed a leukoencephalopathic syndrome (white matter dementia) characterized by ataxia, dysarthria, tremor, and dementia (15). This syndrome can occur in "heavy" or "daily" abusers of toluene. The extent to which these symptoms are reversible depends on the duration and severity of abuse. EEG have been reported to show mild, diffuse slowing; brain CT scans show cerebellar and cortical atrophy; and MRI show signs of white matter disease with loss of gray or white matter differentiation on T2-weighted images (16). Autopsy and neuroimaging of toluene abusers have shown multifocal involvement, diffuse demyelination of the subcortical white matter, and peripheral axonopathy.

A sensorimotor polyneuropathy has been reported with chronic toluene abuse. These patients typically present with distal parasthesias and muscle weakness, which progresses proximally, in a classic "dying-back" neuropathy. Patients have been reported to present with isolated muscle weakness (quadriparesis) and no sensory deficits, making the distinction from GBS difficult (17); however, it is suspected that the solvent abused by these patients may have also contained hexane or MnBK.

Chronic toluene exposure also causes a syndrome similar to a distal renal tubular acidosis; however, the metabolite of toluene (hippuric acid) produces an acidosis that complicates this diagnosis. Other reported effects associated with toluene exposure are dilated cardiomyopathy, hypokalemia, rhabdomyolysis, and transient elevation in liver enzymes. A toluene withdrawal syndrome has been proposed that includes sleep disturbances, tremor, nausea, and irritability (5).

Toluene embryopathy is a fetal solvent syndrome described from cases of infants born to mothers who reported inhalant abuse of toluene. The teratogenic effects of toluene appear similar to those of alcohol, including small palpebral fissure, thin upper lip, and midfacial hypoplasia. Craniofacial features that appear unique to toluene embryopathy include micrognathia, ear anomalies, narrow bifrontal diameter, and a large fontanelle (18).

CLINICAL RECOMMENDATIONS OF THE VIGNETTE

In the patient, the NCV demonstrated findings consistent with bilateral peroneal neuropathies. A right median neuropathy at the wrist was also evident, as well as a mild length-dependent sensorimotor polyneuropathy. A left sural nerve biopsy 2 weeks after presentation was normal.

The patient stopped sniffing gasoline. Four weeks after symptoms onset, he no longer described visual or auditory hallucinations. Dorsiflexion and foot eversion strength normalized in the left, but now was 2/5 on the right. By 12 weeks, the patient regained full strength and sensation (19).

SUMMARY

Solvents comprise a massive number of compounds to which individuals are exposed on a daily basis. The patient in the case vignette demonstrates the variability of clinical presentation and the wide spectrum of neurologic toxicities caused by solvents. A careful and thorough history must include information about recreational practices and occupational exposures. A solid understanding of the potential toxicities of specific solvents and the treatment modalities available will improve patient care and outcome.

REFERENCES

1. Lai MW, Klein-Schwartz W, Rodgers GC, et al. 2005 annual report of the American Association of Poison Control Centers' national poisoning and exposure database. *Clinical Toxicology.* 2006;44(6):803–932.

2. Drug Abuse Warning Network, 2004: National estimates of drug-related emergency department visits. [online] 2004 [cited 2006 Dec 12]. Available from https://dawninfo.samhsa.gov/pubs/edpubs/
3. Bleecker ML, Bolla KI, Agnew J, et al. Dose-related subclinical neurobehavioral effects of chronic exposure to low levels of organic solvents. *Am J Ind Med.* 1991;19:715–728.
4. Sullivan JB, Krieger GR, eds. *Clinical Environmental Health and Toxic Exposures,* 2nd ed. Philadelphia: Lippincott Williams & Wilkins; 2001.
5. Flomenbaum NE, Goldfrank LR, Hoffman RS, et al., eds. *Goldfrank's Toxicological Emergencies,* 8th ed. New York: McGraw-Hill; 2006.
6. Bass M. Sudden sniffing death. *JAMA.* 1970;212(12):2075–2079.
7. Chenoweth MB. Ventricular fibrillation induced by hydrocarbons and epinephrine. *Journal of Industrial Hygiene and Toxicology.* 1946;28(4):151–158.
8. Linz DH, de Garmo PL, Morton WE, et al. Organic solvent-induced encephalopathy in industrial painters. *J Occup Environ Med.* 1986;28(2):119–125.
9. Dally S, Garnier R, Bismuth C. Diagnosis of chlorinated hydrocarbon poisoning by X ray examination. *Br J Indust Med.* 1987;44:424–425.
10. Daffner RH, Jimenez JP. The double gastric fluid level in kerosene poisoning. *Radiology.* 1973;106:383–384.
11. Nelson LS. Toxicologic myocardial sensitization. *J Toxicol Clin Toxicol.* 2002;40:867–879.
12. Szlatenyi CS, Wang RY. Encephalopathy and cranial nerve palsies caused by intentional trichloroethylene inhalation. *Am J Emerg Med.* 1996;14(5):464–466.
13. Baker EL, Fine LJ. Solvent neurotoxicity: The current evidence. *J Occup Environ Med.* 1986;28(2):126–129.
14. Frenia ML, Schauben JL. Methanol inhalation toxicity. *Ann Emerg Med.* 1993;22(12): 151–155.
15. Knox JW, Nelson JR. Permanent encephalopathy from toluene inhalation. *N Engl J Med.* 1966;275(26):1494–1496.
16. Filley CM, Heaton RK, Rosenberg NL. White matter dementia in chronic toluene abuse. *Neurology.* 1990;40:532–534.
17. Steicher HZ, Gabow PA, Moss AH, et al. Syndromes of toluene sniffing in adults. *Ann Intern Med.* 1981;94:758–762.
18. Pearson MA, Hoyme E, Seaver LH, et al. Toluene embryopathy: Delineation of the phenotype and comparison with fetal alcohol syndrome. *Pediatrics.* 1994;93:211–215.
19. Burns TM, Shneker BF, Juel VC. Gasoline sniffing multifocal neuropathy. *Pediatr Neurol.* 2001;25:419–421.

CHAPTER 110

Marijuana

David C. Lee

OBJECTIVES

- To describe the epidemiology of marijuana usage
- To discuss the clinical manifestation of marijuana toxicity
- Explain the long term ramifications of chronic marijuana usage
- Describe the "endocannabinoid system"

CASE VIGNETTE

A 19-year-old man with a history of depression is admitted to the psychiatric ward with a diagnosis of new onset schizophrenia. His family states that he had complained of auditory hallucinations and inability to sleep. He has a history of alcohol and illicit recreational drug use. On presentation, he appears withdrawn, uncooperative, and answers questions intermittently with a flat affect. Other than his mental status, his physical examination is normal. Findings from a medical workup performed in the emergency department consisting of a routine laboratory tests, lumbar puncture, and a computed axial tomographic (CAT) scan of the head are reported as normal. A urine drug screen is reported the next day to be positive for delta-9-tetrahydrocannabinol (THC). There is a debate whether to transfer this patient to the medical service for a workup of delirium.

DEFINITION

The cannabis plant has often been referred to as the hemp plant. Its commercial and medicinal use has been well described over thousands of years. The first written use of cannabis as a medicinal was in 2327 BC in China. In the United States, it was commonly used until it was banned by the 1937 Marijuana Tax Act (1).

Many plant species have been described as cannabis. The plant that contains the psychotropic compounds known as cannabinoids has been established as *Cannabis sativa.* Marijuana refers to products of the *Cannabis sativa* plant that is used for its psychotropic effects. Other commonly used terms referring to marijuana products include *hashish,* referring to the resin obtained from *Cannabis sativa*; *sinsemilla,* referring to the seedless or unpollinated plants; *joints,* referring to the cigarette-shaped vehicles that contain marijuana; *blunts* referring to the cigar-shaped vehicles that contain marijuana that is often mixed with tobacco or other substances.

EPIDEMIOLOGY

Marijuana is the most frequent illegal substance abused in the United States. Several national studies have reported approximately between 4% and 6% of the US population has used marijuana in the last 30 days and, in 2000, more than 25% of all teenagers had admitted to using marijuana within the last 30 days (2–4). It has been estimated that approximately 20 million people use marijuana weekly and 3 million use it daily. Marijuana has often been perceived as a "soft drug," where the use has limited personal and societal harm. It has also been perceived as a *gateway* drug or as a *stepping stone* to drugs of greater lethality and consequence (5).

With an increasing popularity and demand for marijuana, growers have developed cannabis plants that have higher concentrations of THC, the main psychoactive ingredient in marijuana. Before the 1970s, most confiscated marijuana had THC concentrations of <1%. Presently, marijuana plants have been identified with concentrations of >30%. In 2002, the average confiscated marijuana contained THC concentrations of 5% in the United States (2). In the Netherlands, where marijuana use is socially tolerated, the average concentration of THC in Dutch grown marijuana was approximately 20% in 2004. Hashish produced in the Netherlands averaged 40% (6). Concentrations of THC can be manipulated by controlling light, moisture, nutrients, soil type, and growing environments (1).

ETIOLOGY, PATHOGENESIS, AND PATHOLOGY

Over the past two decades, there has been great interest in a newly described neurotransmission system labeled the *endocannabinoid system.* Endocannabinoids are a newly identified type of naturally occurring lipids that include amides, esters, and ethers of long chain polyunsaturated fatty acids. Two such encocannabinoids that have been relatively well studied include 2-arachidonolyl-glycerol and ananadamide. These endogenous ligands are released from lipid membranes and bind to cannabinoid receptors and are able to mimic the active compounds of marijuana, THC. They then undergo cellular uptake and hydrolysis (7).

Cannabinoid receptors are G-protein–mediated receptors. Two types of receptors have so far been identified. Cannabinoid receptor-1 (CB1) is predominantly found in the brain and spinal cord. These receptors are particularly abundant in the basal ganglia, hippocampus, cortex, and cerebellum (8). At the cellular level, these receptors are most often located at nerve terminal where they prevent neurotransmitter release (9). In mice, modulation of the CB1 receptor in the amygdala affects the interaction between stress and anxiety (10). In rats, the euphoric effects of marijuana have been associated with CB1 and dopamine type 2 receptors in the nucleus accumbens. Effects of locomotor function have been associated with CB1 receptors in the rat cerebellum (11). There have been case reports of hypotension and vasodilatation and these affects have also been attributed to CB1 receptors (12). Cannabinoid receptor-2 is predominantly found in the peripheral nerves and immune tissues. The endocannabinoid system has also been suggested to be involved with mechanisms determining alcohol abuse, schizophrenia, and depression (13). It is even less clear how this system interacts with the immune system.

Acute and chronic use has been shown to interact with dopaminergic activity, specifically in the mesolimbic system. This has been theorized to affect the body's "reward system." Tolerance and withdrawal syndromes have been described with chronic use. At the cellular level, tolerance develops as the CB1 receptor is downregulated and the receptor is uncoupled from its secondary messenger systems. Withdrawal symptoms include irritability, anxiety, craving, nausea, vomiting, and decreased quantity and quality of sleep (14,15). In one study of chronic users, approximately 17% described withdrawal symptoms.

CLINICAL MANIFESTATIONS AND SPECIAL SITUATIONS

Marijuana most commonly is smoked. Smoking has affects within a few seconds as compared with ingestion, which can have variable affects because of delayed absorption secondary to coingestion and acidity of the stomach. Approximately 10% to 50% of THC is absorbed via inhalation versus 3% to 6% via ingestion (1).

Marijuana produces a variety of characteristic effects: Locomotor, sensory, and psychoactive. It induces a loss of internal control and causes cognitive impairment, which includes perseveration, mental inflexibility, reduced learning ability, and shortened attention spans. Motor effects include decreased ability to track, and impaired motor coordination with complex tasks (8,16). Marijuana users have often described the use of it for purposes of relaxation, anxiolysis, euphoria, sense of well-being, and enhancements of differing sensations. Marijuana users have described it causing alterations in time and space perception. These affects can linger days after the acute intoxication (17,18).

As with most recreational and mood-altering drugs, the danger of these substances stems from impairment of the user's psychomotor skills and judgment. Marijuana use is associated with increased risk-taking behavior and increased rates of traumatic injuries (3,19). It is the most common illicit substances detected in drivers involved in motor vehicle accidents. Many studies investigating culpability of motor vehicle accidents and drivers with THC-positive urine screens are contradictory. Because urinary THC may reflect prior use (in certain circumstances, months prior to the time of the accident), urinary THC concentrations, however, may not reflect acute toxicity. Studies that utilize serum THC concentrations suggest that drivers with THC detected in serum are three to seven times more likely to be responsible for a motor vehicle accident (20).

Another physiologic effect of marijuana is hypotension, although this effect is highly variable (12). Conjunctival injection and increased appetite are well-publicized effects of cannabis use. Chronic lung injury has been associated with frequent users. Smoking a marijuana cigarette has been associated with greater inhalation of carbon monoxide and particulate matter as compared with smoking a commercial tobacco cigarette.

It remains controversial whether marijuana can cause acute psychosis and schizophrenia. Although multiple case reports exist of marijuana users developing acute psychosis, and many authors have suggested that marijuana use may have unmasked underlying mental illnesses (21–24). It remains unclear whether chronic marijuana users have a higher propensity to develop these mental illnesses (vulnerability hypothesis) or whether persons predisposed to these illnesses have a higher propensity to use marijuana (self-medication hypothesis) (25–27).

Chronic users have been reported to have subtle impairments in cognition and brain function, which include attention span, multitasking, and short- and long-term memory. Increasing duration and frequency of use has been associated with increasing impairment. Brain imaging studies have supported these views by demonstrating altered function, metabolism, and vascular supply in heavy users (17).

MEDICAL USES

Great interest has been expressed in developing marijuana and its by-products into accepted medicinals. They have been shown to be useful as an antiemetic and appetite stimulant. In the United States, one cannabinoid, THC, (Dronabinol, commercially known as Marinol) has been approved to treat nausea, vomiting, and anorexia. In animals, cannabinoids have been shown to affect lower esophageal sphincter tone via mechanisms within the CNS and the vagal nerve; however, in humans, it has also been shown to delay gastric emptying (28,29). The exact mechanism of its antiemetic properties remains unclear.

Cannabinoids are presently being studied to treat multiple sclerosis. It is hypothesized that cannabinoids alter various cytokines and T-helper cells via the CB2 receptor, which may prove beneficial in multiple sclerosis (30,31). Several trials, however, have reported minimal or no significant efficacy in treating the major symptoms of multiple sclerosis, balance and motor control (32). Nor have these studies described any differences in targeted immune function with the addition of cannabinoids (33). Other trials have described improvements in bladder function, improved pain scores, and reduced sleep disturbance in patients with multiple sclerosis using cannabinoids (34,35).

Cannabis has been touted to combat glaucoma, but its efficacy in glaucoma has been debated (36). Cannabinoids have varying effects on intraocular pressure (37). It is hypothesized that its affect is mediated by CB1 receptors in the ciliary body (38).

Cannabinoids have also been suggested to aid in the treatment of seizures, parkinsonism, and asthma (39). Its clinical efficacy remains controversial, however. No definitive large, randomized control studies have investigated cannabinoids in these disease states.

DIAGNOSTIC APPROACH

Multiple commercial products use standard immune assay for detection of THC in urine. Because THC is lipid soluble and is concentrated in fat stores, THC can be detected in urine for several days after a single use (one cigarette) and up to 70 days for heavy chronic users.

TREATMENT

The mainstay of therapy for acute marijuana poisoning is supportive care. No deaths from isolated marijuana poisoning have been reported. Trauma and risk taking behavior are the main mechanisms of injury from acute exposure. In patients presenting with acute psychosis, benzodiazepines and antipsychotics are the mainstays of treatment (21). Long-term effects may include increase risks for mental illness and long-term impairments in higher brain function.

CLINICAL RECOMMENDATIONS OF THE VIGNETTE

Chronic cannabis use is associated with higher rates of mental illness. It is highly unlikely that the patient is suffering from delirium and it would be highly unlikely that acute cannabis use would cause a delirium that persisted more than 24 hours. Furthermore, a positive marijuana screen does not reflect acute intoxication. The patient should remain on the psychiatry service to complete his evaluation and treatment.

SUMMARY

Marijuana and by-products of *Cannabis sativa* are commonly used. Acute manifestations of toxicity include cognitive and locomotor impairment. The long-term effects of chronic use are still unclear, although many investigators have noted long-term cognitive impairments and predisposition for mental illness with chronic users. With recent discoveries of the function of the endocannabinoid system, the biochemical and cellular mechanism of THC, the active ingredient of marijuana, has been better clarified.

REFERENCES

1. Selden BS, Clark RF, Curry SC. Marijuana. *Emerg Med Clin North Am.* 1990;8:527–539.
2. Compton WM, Grant BF, Colliver JD, et al. Prevalence of marijuana use disorders in the United States: 1991–1992 and 2001–2002. *JAMA.* 2004;291:2114–2121.
3. Kann L, Kinchen SA, Williams BI, et al. Youth risk behavior surveillance—United States, 1999. *MMWR CDC Surveill Summ.* 2000;49:1–32.
4. Khalsa JH, Genser S, Francis H, et al. Clinical consequences of marijuana. *J Clin Pharmacol.* 2002;42:7S–10S.
5. Raphael B, Wooding S, Stevens G, et al. Comorbidity: Cannabis and complexity. *J Psychiatr Pract.* 2005;11:161–176.
6. Pijlman FT, Rigter SM, Hoek J, et al. Strong increase in total delta-THC in cannabis preparations sold in Dutch coffee shops. *Addict Biol.* 2005;10:171–180.
7. Paradisi A, Oddi S, Maccarrone M. The endocannabinoid system in ageing: A new target for drug development. *Curr Drug Targets.* 2006;7:1539–1552.
8. Sim-Selley LJ. Regulation of cannabinoid CB1 receptors in the central nervous system by chronic cannabinoids. *Crit Rev Neurobiol.* 2003;15:91–119.
9. Pertwee RG. The pharmacology of cannabinoid receptors and their ligands: An overview. *Int J Obes (Lond).* 2006;30[Suppl 1]:S13–S18.
10. Patel S, Cravatt BF, Hillard CJ. Synergistic interactions between cannabinoids and environmental stress in the activation of the central amygdala. *Neuropsychopharmacology.* 2005;30:497–507.
11. Casu MA, Pisu C, Sanna A, et al. Effect of delta-9-tetrahydrocannabinol on phosphorylated CREB in rat cerebellum: An immunohistochemical study. *Brain Res.* 2005;1048:41–47.
12. Gorelick DA, Heishman SJ, Preston KL, et al. The cannabinoid CB1 receptor antagonist rimonabant attenuates the hypotensive effect of smoked marijuana in male smokers. *Am Heart J.* 2006;151:754.e1–754.e5.
13. Vinod KY, Hungund BL. Endocannabinoid lipids and mediated system: Implications for alcoholism and neuropsychiatric disorders. *Life Sci.* 2005;77:1569–1583.
14. Haney M. The marijuana withdrawal syndrome: Diagnosis and treatment. *Curr Psychiatry Rep.* 2005;7:360–366.
15. Budney AJ, Hughes JR, Moore BA, et al. Review of the validity and significance of cannabis withdrawal syndrome. *Am J Psychiatry.* 2004;161:1967–1977.
16. Lundqvist T. Cognitive consequences of cannabis use: Comparison with abuse of stimulants and heroin with regard to attention, memory and executive functions. *Pharmacol Biochem Behav.* 2005;81:319–330.
17. Solowij N, Stephens RS, Roffman RA, et al. Cognitive functioning of long-term heavy cannabis users seeking treatment. *JAMA.* 2002;287:1123–1131.
18. Pope HG, Jr., Yurgelun-Todd D. The residual cognitive effects of heavy marijuana use in college students. *JAMA.* 1996;275:521–527.
19. Macdonald S, Anglin-Bodrug K, Mann RE, et al. Injury risk associated with cannabis and cocaine use. *Drug Alcohol Depend.* 2003;72:99–115.
20. Ramaekers JG, Berghaus G, van Laar M, et al. Dose related risk of motor vehicle crashes after cannabis use. *Drug Alcohol Depend.* 2004;73:109–119.
21. Leweke FM, Gerth CW, Klosterkotter J. Cannabis-associated psychosis: Current status of research. *CNS Drugs.* 2004;18:895–910.
22. Verdoux H, Gindre C, Sorbara F, et al. Effects of cannabis and psychosis vulnerability in daily life: An experience sampling test study. *Psychol Med.* 2003;33:23–32.
23. Phillips LJ, Curry C, Yung AR, et al. Cannabis use is not associated with the development of psychosis in an 'ultra' high-risk group. *Aust N Z J Psychiatry.* 2002;36:800–806.
24. Nunez LA, Gurpegui M. Cannabis-induced psychosis: A cross-sectional comparison with acute schizophrenia. *Acta Psychiatr Scand.* 2002;105:173–178.
25. Barnes TR, Mutsatsa SH, Hutton SB, et al. Comorbid substance use and age at onset of schizophrenia. *Br J Psychiatry.* 2006;188:237–242.
26. Semple DM, McIntosh AM, Lawrie SM. Cannabis as a risk factor for psychosis: Systematic review. *J Psychopharmacol.* 2005;19:187–194.
27. Henquet C, Krabbendam L, Spauwen J, et al. Prospective cohort study of cannabis use, predisposition for psychosis, and psychotic symptoms in young people. *BMJ.* 2005;330:11. Epub 2004 Dec 1.
28. McCallum RW, Soykan I, Sridhar KR, et al. Delta-9-tetrahydrocannabinol delays the gastric emptying of solid food in humans: A double-blind, randomized study. *Aliment Pharmacol Ther.* 1999;13:77–80.
29. Partosoedarso ER, Abrahams TP, Scullion RT, et al. Cannabinoid1 receptor in the dorsal vagal complex modulates lower oesophageal sphincter relaxation in ferrets. *J Physiol.* 2003;550:149–158.
30. Ehrhart J, Obregon D, Mori T, et al. Stimulation of cannabinoid receptor 2 (CB2) suppresses microglial activation. *J Neuroinflammation.* 2005;2:29.
31. Malfitano AM, Matarese G, Bifulco M. From cannabis to endocannabinoids in multiple sclerosis: A paradigm of central nervous system autoimmune diseases. *Curr Drug Targets CNS Neurol Disord.* 2005;4:667–675.
32. Smith PF. The safety of cannabinoids for the treatment of multiple sclerosis. *Expert Opinions in Drug Safety.* 2005;4:443–456.
33. Katona S, Kaminski E, Sanders H, et al. Cannabinoid influence on cytokine profile in multiple sclerosis. *Clin Exp Immunol.* 2005;140:580–585.
34. Rog DJ, Nurmikko TJ, Friede T, et al. Randomized, controlled trial of cannabis-based medicine in central pain in multiple sclerosis. *Neurology.* 2005;65:812–819.
35. Freeman RM, Adekanmi O, Waterfield MR, et al. The effect of cannabis on urge incontinence in patients with multiple sclerosis: A multicentre, randomised placebo-controlled trial (CAMS-LUTS). *International Urogynecological Journal of Pelvic Floor Dysfunction.* 2006;17:636–641. Epub 2006 Mar 22.
36. Kalant H. Medicinal use of cannabis: History and current status. *Pain Res Manag.* 2001;6:80–91.
37. Tomida I, Azuara-Blanco A, House H, et al. Effect of sublingual application of cannabinoids on intraocular pressure: A pilot study. *J Glaucoma.* 2006;15:349–353.
38. Porcella A, Maxia C, Gessa GL, et al. The synthetic cannabinoid WIN55212-2 decreases the intraocular pressure in human glaucoma resistant to conventional therapies. *Eur J Neurosci.* 2001;13:409–412.
39. Killestein J, Uitdehaag BM, Polman CH. Cannabinoids in multiple sclerosis: Do they have a therapeutic role? *Drugs.* 2004;64:1–11.

CHAPTER 111

PCP/Ketamine

D. Adam Algren

OBJECTIVES

- To review the history and epidemiology of phencyclidine and ketamine use
- To describe the pharmacology of phencyclidine and ketamine
- To explain the clinical manifestations of phencyclidine and ketamine intoxication
- To review the management of phencyclidine and ketamine intoxication

CASE VIGNETTE

A 25-year-old man was transported by emergency medical services to the emergency department (ED) for injuries sustained while attempting to evade police capture. Bystanders called police because the patient was displaying bizarre and inappropriate behavior. On police confrontation, the patient attempted to flee by jumping off a 25-foot wall, but on landing, sustained an open fracture-dislocation of his right ankle.

In the ED his vital signs were temperature 100.2°F, pulse 128 beats per minute, blood pressure 150/100 mm Hg. The physical examination demonstrated an open fracture-dislocation of the right ankle, an intact neurovascular examination, and no evidence of other injuries. The neurologic examination was remarkable for rotary nystagmus and fluctuating behavior. He alternated between an agitated and aggressive state to a calm demeanor in which he appeared to "zone out" and not respond to verbal or physical stimuli yet remained alert.

DEFINITION AND EPIDEMIOLOGY

Phencyclidine (PCP) [1-(1-phenylcyclohexyl) piperdine] is a dissociative agent with analgesic and psychotropic effects. PCP was developed as a human anesthetic in the 1950s and was marketed under the trade name Sernyl (1). Sernyl could produce anesthesia and analgesia with minimal respiratory or cardiovascular depression (2). Its use was quickly abandoned, however, and it was withdrawn from the market in 1963 after numerous postanesthetic emergence reactions (delirium, agitation, hallucinations, and seizures) were reported (3). PCP continued to be distributed as a veterinary anesthetic (Sernylan) until 1978 when all legal manufacturing was terminated (1). Currently, PCP is listed as a schedule II drug under the Controlled Substances Act.

Illicit use of PCP was first reported in Los Angeles in 1965. Subsequently, the *PeaCe Pill* appeared on the streets of San Francisco in 1967 and drug users rapidly acknowledged that it was associated with a high incidence of emergence reactions and other side effects (1,3). Although popularity waned for PCP, its low cost and ease of production combined with increased knowledge and ability to titrate its effects resulted in a resurgence of PCP use (1). By the mid-1970s, PCP use had spread nationwide. Data from the Drug Abuse Warning Network (DAWN) suggest that PCP continues to enjoy regional popularity in the United States and a steady increase is seen in the number of PCP-related emergency department visits over the past decade. In 2004, DAWN reported 8,928 PCP-related emergency department visits; whereas the number of exposures reported to the American Association of Poison Control Centers Toxic Exposure Surveillance System (AAPCC-TESS) has remained constant (approximately 500/year) over the last decade (4–6).

Ketamine, an analog of PCP, shares similar pharmacologic properties as an anesthetic and analgesic. It was developed for use as an anesthetic in 1962 after significant adverse effects (see above) were noted with PCP (7). The ability of ketamine to produce dissociative and psychotropic effects with fewer emergence reactions led to experimentation among drug users. Currently, ketamine is used to induce sedation and analgesia for painful procedures, as well as an induction agent for endotracheal intubation. Ketamine continues to be a common veterinary anesthetic and this widespread availability in veterinary clinics allows for the diversion of ketamine for illegitimate use (8). Ketamine was classified as a schedule III drug in 1999.

Reports of illicit ketamine use appeared shortly after its introduction. Ketamine was reported to have a lower incidence of emergence reactions and "bad trips" compared with PCP. Its decreased potency and shorter half-life allowed for a more predictable "high," resulting in an increased popularity of ketamine among drug users. Over the last decade, an increasing number of reports have highlighted the illicit use of ketamine (8,9). This drug has become particularly popular among adolescents and the rave subculture (10–12). Drug use is common with ravers as they seek sensory augmentation to heighten their experience (12). Ketamine has also gained notoriety as being a drug used to facilitate sexual assaults. Confirmed cases of ketamine being used for this purpose are uncommon, however; ketamine accounted for <1% of drugs detected in a series that examined toxicologic findings in victims of drug-facilitated sexual assault (13). DAWN reported 227 ED visits for ketamine in 2004 and this is consistent with the number of yearly cases reported over the past decade (14). The AAPCC-TESS reported 161 exposures and 1 death from ketamine in 2005 (6). The number of ketamine exposures reported has remained constant since the AAPCC began specifically reporting ketamine exposures in 2003 (15). Estimating the prevalence of both PCP and ketamine use within the drug-using population is difficult. Both DAWN and AAPCC-TESS data are subject to reporting (and other) biases and, therefore, likely underestimate the true prevalence of use.

PHARMACOLOGY

PCP is available in several formulations and can be ingested, smoked, insufflated, or, rarely, injected parenterally. Smoking is the most common method of using PCP (2,16). PCP powder can be added to tobacco or marijuana cigarettes, or cigarettes can be dipped into a solution of PCP which facilitates diffusion of PCP throughout the cigarette (2). PCP has many street or slang names that can make exact identification difficult (Table 111-1). Knowledge of local names can be helpful to the practitioner when evaluating an intoxicated patient or when obtaining history from family or friends.

PCP has a large volume of distribution (6.2 L/kg) and is extremely lipid soluble (2). It is rapidly distributed to the brain and accumulates in adipose tissue. The liver is the primary site of metabolism of PCP. Following hydroxylation, inactive metabolites are excreted by the kidneys. A small amount of PCP (<10%) is excreted unchanged in the urine (2,3). Clinical effects are noted within 2 to 5 minutes, and peak effects occur within 15 minutes of smoking or insufflating PCP. Ingestion results in a slower onset of action of 15 to 30 minutes. The duration of major effects is generally 4 to 6 hours with complete resolution within 24 to 48 hours (1,2,17). Prolonged effects, including psychosis and mania, lasting days to weeks have been reported in chronic PCP users (1–3,17).

Ketamine is usually found as a crystalline powder. It is typically insufflated, but can be ingested, smoked, or injected parenterally. As with PCP, ketamine also is known by a variety of street names (Table 111-1). Ketamine is highly lipid soluble with a large volume of distribution (18). Most of the parent drug is metabolized in the liver by cytochrome P450 enzymes CYP 3A4, 2B6, and 2C9 to norketamine, an active metabolite. Less than 4% of ketamine is excreted unchanged into the urine (18). The onset of clinical effects depends on the route of administration. With injection, smoking, or insufflation, a rapid onset of action occurs within 15 seconds to 1 minute. After ingestion, ketamine is poorly absorbed and undergoes first-pass metabolism to norketamine. This results in clinical effects that are slower in onset (within 30 minutes), but more prolonged in duration compared with other routes of administration (18). Clinical effects typically last 1 to 3 hours, but may be prolonged following repeated ingestion or chronic use (19,20).

PCP and ketamine are arylcyclohexylamines with similar chemical structures (Fig. 111-1), which explains why they demonstrate similar clinical effects. Both PCP and ketamine have complex mechanisms of action and affect multiple neurotransmitter systems. The major action of both drugs involves noncompetitive antagonism of the N-methyl-d-aspartate (NMDA) receptor (18,21–23). NMDA receptors are glutamate receptors. Glutamate is the major excitatory neurotransmitter in the brain. After binding to a site within the NMDA receptor complex, PCP and ketamine prevent calcium influx into the neuron and, thus, have an inhibitory effect (22). By interfering with glutamate neurotransmission, these drugs serve to dissociate somatosensory input from the higher cognitive centers in

TABLE 111-1. Street Names of Phencyclidine and Ketamine

Phencyclidine	*Ketamine*
Angel dust	Cat valium
Angel hair	Green
Angel mist	Jet
Animal tranquilizer	K
Cadillac	Kit-kat
C.J.	Mean green
Crystal joint	Special K
Dust	Super acid
Elephant tranquilizer	Super K
Embalming fluid	Vitamin K
Goon	
Gorilla biscuits	
Hog	
Horse tranquilizer	
K.J.	
Killer weed	
Mist	
Monkey dust	
Ozone	
Peace	
Rocket fuel	
Scuffle	
Sheets	
Stardust	
Super grass	
Super weed	
Tic tac	
Water	
Wet	
Whack	
Whacky weed	
Zombie dust	

From Young T, Lawson GW, Gacono CB. Clinical aspects of phencyclidine (PCP). *Int J Addict.* 1987;22(1):1–15; Dove HW. Phencyclidine: Pharmacologic and clinical review. *Psychiatric Medicine.* 1984;2(2): 189–209; Freese TE, Miotto K, Reback CJ. The effects and consequences of selected club drugs. *J Subst Abuse Treat.* 2002;23(2):151–156; Smith KM, Larive LL, Romanelli F. Club drugs: Methylenedioxymethamphetamine, flunitrazepam, ketamine hydrochloride and γ-hydroxybutyrate. *Am J Health Syst Pharm.* 2002;59(11):1067–1076; Pradhan SN. Phencyclidine (PCP): Some human studies. *Neurosci Biobehav Rev.* 1984;8(4):493–501; and Wolff K, Winstock AR. Ketamine from medicine to misuse. *CNS Drugs.* 2006;20(3):199–218, with permission.)

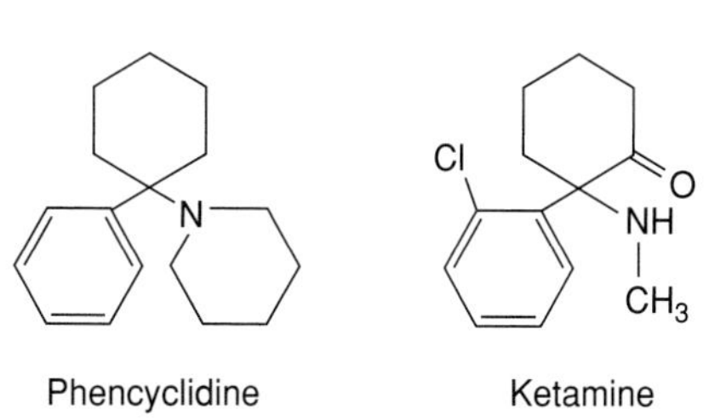

Phencyclidine Ketamine

FIGURE 111-1. Chemical structures of phencyclidine and ketamine

the brain. Ketamine differs from PCP in that it has approximately 10% of PCP's affinity for this receptor (22). This decreased potency is responsible for the decreased incidence of adverse effects noted with ketamine.

These drugs, as well as other NMDA antagonists, can induce a clinical syndrome identical to schizophrenia (21). This has allowed PCP and ketamine intoxication to serve as a clinical model for facilitating research into the pathogenesis of schizophrenia. Unlike other psychostimulants that tend only to reproduce the positive symptoms of schizophrenia, PCP and ketamine also induce negative symptoms in addition to severe cognitive dysfunction (24). Subanesthetic doses of ketamine have been demonstrated to induce psychosis in healthy volunteers and cause an exacerbation of symptoms in patients with previously well-controlled schizophrenia (25–27). Decreased expression of NMDA receptors in the brains of patients with schizophrenia has been documented (28). Animal models have also confirmed that PCP administration can produce metabolic and electrophysiologic dysfunction that is manifested clinically as a syndrome indistinguishable from schizophrenia (29,30). Thus, glutamate hypoactivity can be a contributing factor in the development of schizophrenia.

Cognitive dysfunction induced by these drugs is related to the development of altered neurotransmission in the prefrontal cortex. Healthy individuals have been noted to develop increased metabolic activity in the prefrontal cortex following a single administration of ketamine (31), whereas chronic users are reported to have an upregulation of dopamine receptors in the prefrontal cortex (32). This suggests that chronic use leads to decreased activation and function of cortical areas responsible for memory and higher-order thought processes. Decreased blood flow and activation of the prefrontal cortex have also been observed in chronic PCP users, resemblings findings reported in schizophrenia (21).

PCP and ketamine increase tyrosine levels in the brain, which could theoretically modulate brain norepinephrine and dopamine levels (3). Both drugs also act to increase biogenic amine levels by acting as weak inhibitors of norepinephrine and dopamine reuptake (3). This may be responsible for the sympathomimetic (tachycardia, hypertension) and psychomotor effects that occur following their use. PCP has both agonist and antagonistic effects on central acetylcholine neurotransmission, which could account for the abnormal muscular activity observed during intoxication (3). At higher doses, PCP and ketamine bind to the sigma and mu opioid receptors, although they display less affinity for these compared with the NMDA receptor (3,18). Agonism at these receptors could contribute to the analgesia and dysphoria associated with significant intoxication (18).

Seizures and status epilepticus have been reported with severe intoxication (1–3,16,17). The cause of the seizures is incompletely understood, but likely is multifactorial. Excessive agonism or antagonism of central nicotinic or muscarinic acetacholine receptors, as well as elevated levels of norepineprine and dopamine, could result in seizures. NMDA receptor antagonism does not appear to potentiate seizure development and has been shown to be protective against the development of seizures (33). Other factors, including concomitant drug use or hypoxia, could lower the seizure threshold.

CLINICAL MANIFESTATIONS

The clinical presentation of PCP and ketamine intoxication can be quite variable. Multiple factors, including dose, route of administration, associated drug use, and acute versus chronic use, influence what signs and symptoms develop.

The neuropsychiatric manifestations of PCP and ketamine intoxication can be very dramatic and are typically what prompts an individual to present for medical evaluation (8,16,34–36). At lower doses, PCP users often experience inebriation, depersonalization, and spatial disorientation (17,34). As doses increase, patients begin to demonstrate the dissociative effects of PCP. Delirium and psychosis can occur and patients can become agitated and display bizarre behavior. Catatonia, mutism, and unusual posturing or mannerisms have all been described (1–3,17,22). PCP intoxication can produce a psychosis that is clinically identical to schizophrenia. At high doses, seizures and coma can occur (1–3,17). The clinical course can wax and wane as patients alternate between catatonia and agitation; however, symptoms typically resolve over 4 to 6 hours. Chronic use is associated with prolonged symptoms, including psychosis that may require days to weeks to resolve. Individuals with underlying psychiatric illness, especially schizophrenia, are at higher risk of developing prolonged psychosis, even following a single dose of PCP (1,3,17,22). Establishing a correct diagnosis can be difficult without a history of PCP use because this clinical syndrome is often impossible to differentiate from schizophrenia.

Strokes have been reported following PCP use, but they are rare. In a retrospective review of 116 strokes, 11 were associated with illicit drug use (37). Two of these cases were temporally related to PCP use. Also been isolated reports are found of subarachnoid hemorrhage, intracerebral hemorrhage, and cerebral vasospasm (38–40). Several factors, including increased levels of catecholamines, could result in hypertension that contributes to vasospasm or hemorrhage. Animal studies also support the existence of distinct PCP receptors within the cerebral vasculature that contribute to the vasospasm (41,42).

Agitation and violence are common with acute PCP intoxication because individuals are dissociated from their environment and misinterpret external stimuli. Patients are also at risk for self-harm and other traumatic complications (35,43,44). The analgesic effect of PCP can result in patients remaining unaware of significant trauma, and a thorough physical examination is required to detect occult injuries (2,3).

Nystagmus, a common finding, was present in 57% of cases in a large clinical series, and is often described as rotary. Mydriasis was noted in 6% of patients, whereas only 2% were reported to have miosis (16). Adrenergic findings of hypertension and tachycardia were present in 57% and 30%, respectively. Hyperthermia is uncommon, but mandates aggressive treatment (16). Other motor findings that have been reported include generalized rigidity, dystonias, choroathetosis, and myoclonus (1–3,17), which can result from excess central cholinergic or dopaminergic stimulation. Peripheral cholinergic finding are also uncommon, but include vomiting, bronchospasm, and hypersalivation (2,3,16,36).

Ketamine intoxication shares many of the same features of PCP intoxication; however, the symptoms tend to be milder and resolve more quickly. Its use has been most popular with adolescents who use it to alter sensory interpretation to enhance their social activities. Users commonly describe being down in a "K hole" (8,18). This has been described as an out-of-body experience that can range from having a "pleasant journey" to a near death experience in which individuals feel that they are traveling in a dark tunnel at high speed while experiencing intense visual stimulation (18). In an emergency department case series of ketamine users, only 25% required benzodiazepines for treatment of agitation. Most individuals had mild symptoms that resolved within 5 hours of presentation. Tachycardia, the most common clinical finding, was noted in 60% of cases. Interestingly, nystagmus was present in only 15% of cases (45). Frequent use of ketamine is associated with residual cognitive dysfunction and memory impairment that can last several days (19,20).

DIAGNOSIS AND LABORATORY ANALYSIS

The diagnosis is often suggested in individuals who present with the characteristic neuropsychiatric effects. The clinical manifestations, however, can be variable. Other drugs or syndromes that should be considered in the differential diagnosis of PCP and ketamine intoxication include sympathomimetics (e.g., cocaine, amphetamine), anticholinergics, hallucinogens, alcohol or sedative-hypnotic withdrawal, and serotonin syndrome. Several clinical features can help differentiate PCP intoxication from other psychostimulant intoxications. PCP intoxication often produces nystagmus and negative symptoms (e.g., catatonia, mutism, bizarre behaviors) that are not associated with other drug intoxications. The adrenergic signs (tachycardia, hypertension) associated with PCP tend to be less severe when compared with those resulting from sympathomimetics, such as cocaine.

Diagnostic testing should be individualized to each patient and the severity of the patient's clinical signs and symptoms. A rapid blood glucose should be obtained in those individuals with altered mental status. A serum creatine kinase (CK) should be checked in most intoxicated individuals because rhabdomyolysis is common, up to 70% in one series (16,36). Other laboratory testing, although nonspecific, can be helpful in ruling out other coexistent conditions. A head computed tomographic (CT) scan should be obtained in patients with focal neurologic findings and in those who fail to demonstrate an improvement in mental status following a period of observation.

Most laboratories can perform a qualitative urine immunoassay for PCP. These results should never influence clinical management of an intoxicated patient, however, because other medical or traumatic conditions could also be present and should be excluded. Dextromethorphan and venlafaxine have both reported to result in qualitative urine immunoassay testing that is falsely positive for PCP (46–48). Thus, a positive urine immunoassay that is performed in an area of low prevalence of PCP use is highly likely to represent a false–positive finding. A situation where this generates anxiety is when a child tests positive for PCP; unnecessary concern is raised when the most likely reason is a false-positive test from dextromethorphan. Conversely, a urine sample could be falsely negative if collected shortly after use or if the urine is extremely alkaline, which theoretically could decrease excretion of PCP (1,2). Quantitative serum PCP testing is not widely available or helpful in the clinical management of intoxicated patients.

Ketamine does not have a widely available immunoassay. Gas chromatography or mass spectroscopy can be used to detect ketamine when confirmation of use is required. Conflicting evidence exists regarding the ability of ketamine to cross-react with PCP urine immunoassays (45,49).

TREATMENT AND CLINICAL MANAGEMENT

Treatment of PCP and ketamine intoxication is supportive and focuses on controlling agitation and diagnosing medical or traumatic complications that have contributed to, or resulted from, intoxication.

Acutely agitated and delirious patients demand aggressive interventions to prevent harm to themselves and others. Physical restraints may be necessary initially, but should be quickly replaced with pharmacologic sedation. Benzodiazepines are the agents of choice in controlling agitation. High doses may be required to treat highly aggressive or agitated patients. Hyperthermia should be treated rapidly with active cooling and sedation. The sole use of psychotropic medications, such as haloperidol, to control acute agitation is not recommended. Neuroleptics can be helpful in treating the symptoms of persistent psychosis, however, they do not appear shorten its duration (1,17).

Hypertension and tachycardia are usually self-limited and often respond to benzodiazepines and gaining control of the patient's agitation. Severe hypertension associated with PCP has been associated with intracranial hemorrhage, thus significant, persistent elevations of blood pressure require treatment (2,36,40).

Rhabomyolysis is treated with intravenous hydration to ensure adequate urine output. Use of sodium bicarbonate can be considered to alkalinize the urine and decrease the precipitation of myoglobin in the renal tubules. Urinary acidification is not recommended because, although it theoretically enhances the excretion of PCP, it places the patient at high risk for myoglobin-induced renal injury (1,2).

Recent research has focused on the development of vaccines and other immunotherapies for the treatment of drug intoxication and addiction. Several studies have shown promising results in the ability to treat acute PCP intoxication, as well as passively immunize animals against the development of PCP intoxication (50,51).

CLINICAL RECOMMENDATIONS OF THE VIGNETTE

The patient did not complain of any pain from his injury and did not require any pain medication while in the ED. He was placed in restraints, had an intravenous line established, and was given 1 L of normal saline. Room air oxygen saturation and bedside glucose testing were normal. Intravenous antibiotics and benzodiazepines were administered. Laboratory studies were remarkable for a white blood cell count of 15,000 and CK of 4,000; urine drug immunoassay was positive for PCP. Orthopedic surgery was consulted, and the patient was taken to the operating room for reduction and fixation of his fracture. Internal medicine was consulted for management of his intoxication.

Postoperatively, the patient's mental status returned to normal and he admitted to occasional PCP use. His CK peaked at 22,000 for which he received intravenous fluids and urine alkalinization with intravenous sodium bicarbonate. His serum creatinine remained normal. Psychiatry was consulted regarding his drug abuse; he was offered, but declined counseling and rehabilitation. He was discharged home 4 days later.

SUMMARY

PCP and ketamine are drugs that act as antagonists at NMDA glutamate receptors to dissociate the somatosensory cortex of the brain from the higher cognitive centers. By altering sensory integration these agents produce a clinical syndrome that resembles schizophrenia. Ketamine is less potent than PCP; however, both agents are associated with dramatic neuropsychiatric manifestations. Chronic use can result in memory and cognition impairment that resolves over days to weeks. PCP and ketamine intoxication are managed with supportive care after excluding coexistent medical or traumatic complications.

REFERENCES

1. Young T, Lawson GW, Gacono CB. Clinical aspects of phencyclidine (PCP). *Int J Addict.* 1987;22(1):1–15.
2. Baldridge EB, Bessen HA. Phencyclidine. *Emerg Med Clin North Am.* 1990;8(3):541–550.
3. Dove HW. Phencyclidine: Pharmacologic and clinical review. *Psychiatric Medicine.* 1984;2(2):189–209.
4. Drug Abuse Warning Network. *2004: National Estimates of Drug-related Emergency Department Visits.* Available at *ehttps://dawninfo.samhsa.gov/files/DAWN2k4ED.htm. Accessed December 1, 2006.*
5. Litovitz TL, Felberg L, White S, et al. 1995 Annual Report of the American Association of Poison Control Centers Toxic Exposure Surveillance System. *Am J Emerg Med.* 1996;14(5):487–537.
6. Lai MW, et al. 2005 Annual Report of the American Association of Poison Control Centers' National Poisoning and Exposure Database. *Clin Toxicol.* 2006;44(6–7):803–932.
7. Jansen KLR. A review of the nonmedical use of ketamine: Use, users, and consequences. *J Psychoactiv Drugs.* 2000;32(4):419–433.
8. Freese TE, Miotto K, Reback CJ. The effects and consequences of selected club drugs. *J Subst Abuse Treat.* 2002;23(2):151–156.
9. Wu LT, Schlenger WE, Galvin DM. Concurrent use of methamphetamine, MDMA, LSD, ketamine, GHB, and flunitrazepam among American youths. *Drug Alcohol Depend.* 2006;84(1):102–113.
10. Weir E. Raves: A review of the culture, the drugs, and the prevention of harm. *CMAJ.* 2000;162(13):1843–1848.
11. Ricaurte GA, McCann UD. Recognition and management of complications of new recreational drug use. *Lancet.* 2005;365(9477):2137–2145.
12. Smith KM, Larive LL, Romanelli F. Club drugs: Methylenedioxymethamphetamine, flunitrazepam, ketamine hydrochloride and γ-hydroxybutyrate. *Am J Health Syst Pharm.* 2002;59(11):1067–1076.
13. Scott-Ham M, Burton FC. Toxicological findings in cases of alleged drug-facilitated sexual assault in the United Kingdom over a 3 year period. *J Clin Forensic Med.* 2005;12(4): 175–186.
14. Drug Abuse Warning Network. The DAWN report: Club Drugs 2002 Update. Available from https://dawninfo.samhsa.gov/old_dawn/pubs_94_02/shortreports/files/DAWN_tdr_club_drugs02.pdf. Accessed December 1, 2006.
15. Watson WA, Litovitz TL, Klein-Schwartz W, et al. 2003 Annual Report of the American Association of Poison Control Centers Toxic Exposure Surveillance System. 2004:22(5):335–404.
16. McMarron MM, Schulze BW, Thompson GA, et al. Acute phencyclidine intoxication: Incidence of clinical findings in 1,000 cases. *Ann Emerg Med.* 1981;10(5):237–242.
17. Pradhan SN. Phencyclidine (PCP): Some human studies. *Neurosci Biobehav Rev.* 1984;8(4): 493–501.
18. Wolff K, Winstock AR. Ketamine from medicine to misuse. *CNS Drugs.* 2006;20(3):199–218.
19. Curran HV, Monaghan L. In and out of the K-hole: A comparison of the acute and residual effects of ketamine in frequent and infrequent users. *Addiction.* 2001;96(5):749–760.
20. Curran HV, Morgan C. Cognitive, dissociative and psychotogenic effects of ketamine on recreational users on the night of drug use and 3 days later. *Addiction.* 2000;95(4):575–590.
21. Jentsch JD, Roth RH. The neuropsychopharmacology of phencyclidine: From NMDA receptor hypofunction to the dopamine hypothesis of schizophrenia. *Neuropsychopharmacology.* 1999;20(3):201–225.
22. Javitt DC, Zukin SR. Recent advances in the phencyclidine model of schizophrenia. *Am J Psychiatry.* 1991;148(10):1301–1308.
23. Morris BJ, Cochran SM, Pratt JA. PCP: From pharmacology to modeling schizophrenia. *Curr Opin Pharmacol.* 2005;5(1):101–106.
24. Krystal JH, Perry EG Jr, Gueorguieva R, et al. Comparative and interactive human psychopharmacologic effects of ketamine and amphetamine: Implications for glutamatergic and dopaminergic model psychoses and cognitive function. *Arch Gen Psychiatry.* 2005;62(9):985–994.
25. Micallef J. Effects of subanesthetic doses of ketamine on sensorimotor information processing in healthy subjects. *Clin Neuropharmacol.* 2002;25(2):101–106.
26. Lahti AC, Weiler MA, Michaelidis T, et al. Effects of ketamine in normal and schizophrenic volunteers. *Neuropsychopharmacology.* 2001;25(4):455–467.
27. Lahti AC, Koffel B, LaPorte D, et al. Subanesthetic doses of ketamine stimulate psychosis on schizophrenia. *Neuropsychopharmacology.* 1995;13(1):9–19.
28. Noga JT, Hyde TM, Herman MM, et al. Glutamate receptors in the postmortem striatum of schizophrenic, suicide, and control brains. *Synapse.* 1997;27(3):168–176.
29. Cochran SM, Steward LJ, Kennedy MB, et al. Induction of metabolic hypofunction and neurochemical deficits after chronic intermittent exposure to phencyclidine: Differential modulation by antipsychotic drugs. *Neuropsychopharmcology.* 2003;28(2):265–275.
30. Maxwell CR, Ehrlichman RS, Liang Y, et al. Ketamine produces lasting disruptions in encoding of sensory stimuli. *J Pharmacol Exp Ther.* 2006;316(1):315–324.
31. Brier A, Malhotra AK, Pinals DA, et al. Association of ketamine-induced psychosis with focal activation of the prefrontal cortex in healthy volunteers. *Am J Psychiatry.* 1997;154(6): 805–811.
32. Narendran R, Frankle WG, Keefe R, et al. Altered prefrontal dopaminergic function in chronic recreational ketamine users. *Am J Psychiatry.* 2005;162(12):2352–2359.
33. National Institute on Drug Abuse. Research Monograph. Phencyclidine: An update. *NIDA Res Monogr.* 1986;64:1–260.
34. Nicholi AM, Jr. Phencyclidine hydrochloride (PCP) use among college students: Subjective and clinical effects, toxicity, diagnosis, and treatment. *J Am Coll Health.* 1984;32(5): 197–200.
35. McCarron MM, Schulze BW, Thompson GA, et al. Acute phencyclidine intoxication: Clinical patterns, complications, and treatment. *Ann Emerg Med.* 1981;10(6):290–297.
36. Barton CH, Sterling ML, Vaziri ND. Phencyclidine intoxication: Clinical experience in 27 cases confirmed by urine assay. *Ann Emerg Med.* 1981;10(5):243–246.
37. Sloan MA, Kittner SJ, Rigamonti D, et al. Occurrence of stroke associated with use/abuse of drugs. *Neurology.* 1991;41(9):1358–1364.
38. Boyko OB, Burger PC, Heinz ER. Pathological and radiological correlation of subarachnoid hemorrhage in phencyclidine abuse. Case report. *J Neurosurg.* 1987;67(3):446–448.
39. Crosley CJ, Binet EF. Cerebrovascular complications in phencyclidine intoxication. *J Pediatr.* 1979;94(2):316–318.
40. Bessen HA. Intracranial hemorrhage associated with phencyclidine abuse. *JAMA.* 1982;248(5):585–586.
41. Altura BT, Quirion R, Pert CB, et al. Phencyclidine ("angel dust") analogs and sigma opiate benzomorphans cause cerebral arterial spasm. *Proc Natl Acad Sci U S A.* 1983;80(3): 865–869.
42. Lu YF, Sun FY, Zhang LM, et al. Phencyclidine receptors in porcine cerebral arteries. *Zhongguo Yao Xue Bao.* 1989;10(6):508–511.
43. Burns RS, Lerner SE. Phencyclidine deaths. *JACEP.* 1978;7(4):135–141.
44. Poklis A, Graham M, Maginn D, et al. Phencyclidine and violent deaths in St. Louis, Missouri: A survey of medical examiners' cases from 1977 through 1986. *Am J Drug Alcohol Abuse.* 1990;16(3–4):265–274.
45. Weiner AL, Vieira L, McKay CA, et al. Ketamine abusers presenting to the emergency department: A case series. *J Emerg Med.* 2000;18(4):447–451.
46. Schier J, Diaz JE. Avoid unfavorable consequences: Dextromethorphan can bring about a false-positive phencyclidine urine drug screen. *J Emerg Med.* 2000;18(3):379–381.
47. Sena SF, Kazimi S, Wu AHB. False-positive phencyclidine immunoassay results caused by venlafaxine and o-desmethylvenlafaxine. *Clin Chem.* 2002;48(4):676–677.
48. Bond GR, Steele PE, Uges DR. Massive venlafaxine overdose resulted in a false positive Abbott AxSYM urine immunoassay for phencyclidine. *J Toxicol Clin Toxicol.* 2003;41(7): 999–1002.
49. Shannon M. Recent ketamine administration can produce a urine toxic screen which is falsely positive for phencyclidine. *Pediatr Emerg Care.* 1988;14(2):180.
50. Haney M, Kosten TR. Therapeutic vaccines for substance dependence. *Expert Rev Vaccines.* 2004;3(1):11–18.
51. Meijler MM, Matsushita M, Wirshing P, et al. Development of immunopharmacotherapy against drugs of abuse. *Curr Drug Discov Technol.* 2004;1(1):77–89.

CHAPTER **112**

Other Intoxicants

Michael C. Beuhler

OBJECTIVES

- To discuss the neurologic sequelae of nitrous oxide exposure
- To review the proper workup and treatment of a patient with nitrous oxide neuropathy
- To describe the clinical presentation and management of γ-hydroxybutyrate (GHB) intoxication
- To explain the mechanism and clinical presentation of *Salvia divinorum* intoxication

CASE VIGNETTE

A frantic mother brought her 2-year-old child into the emergency department. The child ingested a "small" amount of an industrial cleaner and rapidly became unconscious. On presentation, the child was lethargic and minimally responsive to painful stimuli. His vital signs were: pulse, 85 beats per minute; respiration, 24 breaths per minute; blood pressure, 95/60 mm Hg; and temperature, 36.5°C. Initial glucose was 103 mg/dL. On examination, the child had pupils of 3 mm, normal oropharyngeal mucosa, soft abdomen, and normal bowel sounds, but had globally decreased muscle tone. The unlabeled bottle contained a viscous clear liquid without any smell that had a neutral pH.

DEFINITION

In this chapter are discussed several divergent toxins that have minimal relationship to each other beyond being potentially abused and, thus, this chapter is arranged differently than the previous substance abuse chapters. Nitrous oxide (N_2O) is an anesthesia gas used for dental and conscious sedation procedures that can cause significant neurological sequella. GHB is a simple four-carbon molecule, with several analogues that can induce coma and apnea. *Salivia divinorium* is a plant that contains salvanorin A, a powerful nonalkaloid hallucinogen.

NITROUS OXIDE

N_2O is an anesthesia gas used to induce analgesia and conscious sedation; true surgical anesthesia cannot be accomplished using nitrous oxide alone because sufficiently high alveolar concentrations of N_2O (minimal alveolar concentration [MAC]) cannot be achieved without hypoxia (1). It has a low solubility in blood, allowing for rapid onset and offset. Besides medicinal gas cylinders, N_2O is available as gas mini-cylinders, which the abuser can open into balloons (using a "cracker"), or released into a whipped cream dispenser, allowing for the controlled inhalation of the gas. N_2O is used extensively in dentistry, and abuse is not uncommon in that occupation. But even with legitimate use in dentistry, it is difficult to minimize the ambient contamination by N_2O during dental operations and the resulting low levels of exposure can cause subtle illness in some individuals (2,3).

N_2O can result in neurologic injury through two mechanisms. One is by inducing asphyxia (with resulting hypoxic encephalopathy) when the user is exposed to N_2O without adequate oxygen. This is more common with a continuous medical gas source, but could happen with other devices. Head trauma is a potential risk from syncope resulting from inhalation while standing. The other injury is a sensorimotor polyneuropathy with spinal cord involvement.

N_2O causes oxidization of the cobalt (I) (B_{12s}) to cobalt (II) (B_{12r}) in the bound vitamin B_{12} cofactor (methylcobalamin) of methionine synthetase, producing a reactive oxygen species and damaging the enzyme (4,5). This irreversible inhibition of methionine synthetase traps folate as 5-methyltetrahydrofolate. This causes a relative folate deficiency, resulting in bone marrow suppression and megaloblastic anemia. The neuropathy is most likely caused by the inhibition of methionine synthetase and subsequent lack of methionine. Animals chronically exposed to N_2O demonstrate ataxia and tremor with corresponding spinal degeneration; supplementation with methionine reduced these changes. Humans have involvement of posterior columns and corticospinal tracts. N_2O does not affect the vitamin B_{12} cofactor (deoxyadenosylcobalamin) found with methylmalonyl CoA mutase (6). Global depletion of vitamin B_{12} will likely occur, however, with chronic exposure.

Exposure to N_2O for as few as 2 hours can initiate megaloblastic bone marrow changes in susceptible patients, especially those with reduced vitamin B_{12} levels, but usually periods of up to 6 hours of N_2O exposure are safe (7,8). Humans with underlying cobalamin deficiency are at increased risk of developing B_{12}-related illness from N_2O exposure (9). Animal studies have shown pathologic effects within 6 hours of N_2O exposure; however, animals demonstrate a more rapid onset of methionine synthetase inhibition than humans (10). The shunting of folate to 5-methyl tetrahydrofolate at the expense of purine metabolism would be expected to cause early megaloblastic anemic changes with the neurologic changes potentially taking several days to weeks to manifest.

Inhalation of nitrous produces a euphoric state lasting a few seconds. Untoward reactions, including claustrophobia, apprehension, and hallucinations have been reported. The hallucinatory experience occasionally has manifested as delusions of sexual molestation (11). Acute symptoms resolve rapidly after removal from the N_2O source.

With chronic abuse, symptoms of clumsiness in extremities, weakness, dizziness, delusions, and gait disturbances have been reported (3,12,13). Paresthesias are common, initially in the feet or knees and spreading to encompass the entire lower extremity; upper extremity numbness can develop in the shoulders or the fingertips (14). An electric shocklike sensation from the toes upward to back of the neck on flexion has been reported (reverse Lhermitte sign) (3). Commonly reported clinical findings are a glove and stocking-glove distribution loss of light touch, vibration, and position sense. Additionally, decreases in reflexes and minimal loss of motor strength are reported (15). Even chronic low levels of N_2O, such as ambient levels in dental offices, have been associated with complaints of numbness, weakness, and paresthesias.

Diagnosis is based on history, which may not be forthcoming regarding the abuse. A manual peripheral blood smear analysis may reveal megaloblastic (macrocytosis with increased mean corpuscular volume and hypersegmentation) changes (16). Vitamin B_{12} levels in patients exposed to N_2O can be normal, but low vitamin B_{12} levels may suggest a coexisting vitamin deficiency unmasked by the N_2O toxicity. Serum homocysteine levels may be increased (17). Electromyography and motor nerve conduction velocities may be normal or near normal. Magnetic resonance imaging (MRI) of the cervical and thoracic spine may demonstrate changes in the posterior column, which resolve with treatment (15).

Early diagnosis and counseling to halt the abuse is the most important intervention because cessation of N_2O exposure results in clinical improvement. Vitamin B_{12} supplementation should be conducted immediately on recognition of the abuse, but if the exposure is not halted, the supplemented vitamin B_{12} will be inhibited. Oral methionine would be expected to provide benefit as well. The benefit of methionine (the product of the inhibited enzyme) would be expected to be more rapid in onset than vitamin B_{12} replacement would provide. Additionally (although not recommended) methionine may even benefit patients who do not halt their abuse (although this will *not* fix the vitamin B_{12} global depletion). Neither folic nor folinic acid supplementation will be effective nor should they be performed without adequate vitamin B_{12} replacement because of the potential for exacerbating the neurologic symptoms.

GAMMA HYDROXYBUTERATE

GHB is a simple four-carbon molecule not dissimilar from γ-aminobutyric acid (GABA). GHB is naturally found in human brain at low levels (18). It had some limited use as an anesthetic in Europe for a number of years, but side effects have limited its use. The popularity of GHB began in the 1980s when it was demonstrated to cause an increase in growth hormone following ingestion. This factoid was latched onto by the bodybuilding culture and abuse began to develop. Now GHB abuse has spread to the club scene as well as being an agent for sexual assault. It has many slang names (see Table 112-1) (19). GHB was made schedule I in the United States in 2000, but sodium oxybate (the sodium salt of GHB) is available as a schedule III drug (Xyrem) with stringent regulations on its use.

TABLE 112-1. Street Names for γ-hydroxybutyrate (GHB)

Cherry menth
Easy lay
Everclear (Also 95% ethanol)
Fantasy
Gamma-oh
Georgia home boy
Goop
Great hormones at bedtime
G-riffick
Grievous bodily harm
Hydro (also slang for Marijuana)
Jib
Jolt
Liquid E
Liquid X
Organic quaalude
Salty water
Scoop
Sleep-500
Soap
Vita-g
Water

(From Micromedex. Thomson MICROMEDEX. Vol. 130 accessed 12/15/2006, with permission.)

Several molecules are metabolized to GHB, including γ-butyrolactone (GBL) and 1,4 butanediol (20). Previously, GBL was converted to GHB using a strong alkali and subsequent neutralization; this appears to be unnecessary because GBL is internally metabolized by lactonases to GHB. 1,4 butanediol is rapidly metabolized by alcohol dehydrogenase to GHB, but this pathway can be temporarily inhibited by ethanol (or fomepazole), delaying onset of symptoms. Sources of 1,4 butanediol include cleaners, printer ink cartridges, and makeup (mascara), all of which have been consumed for their intoxicating effects. There are also analogues that clinically behave as GHB, but do not necessarily become metabolized to GHB, such as γ-valerolactone (21) GHB is rapidly metabolized to succinate semialdehyde with an elimination half life of 30 to 60 minutes (22,23).

The mechanism of central nervous system (CNS) effects of GHB is still being determined. At low endogenous levels, it binds to its own GHB receptor; at high levels, however, it demonstrates agonistic effects at $GABA_B$ receptors (24). Additionally, it has effects on decreasing dopaminergic neuronal activity. (25,26) The dose causing sedation is approximately 30 to 40 mg/kg (23).

GHB intoxication is characterized by lethargy, ataxia, vomiting, mild hypotension, mild bradycardia, coma, and apnea (27,28). Myoclonic jerking is occasionally noted. The coma from GHB is relatively short lived when compared with many other CNS depressants, so much so that it is rare to hospitalize a GHB intoxicated patient who does not have any other comorbidity (e.g., trauma or aspiration). Often the period of ventilator support does not last more then a few hours with the patient going from comatose to awake fairly rapidly.

Diagnosis of acute toxicity is usually made by the history and physical examination. Abuse in the club scene is not uncommon; alternatively it is abused by the bodybuilding community. Notable clinical characteristics are the rapid onset of coma as well as the rapid recovery to a lucid state, usually within 2 to 3 hours (29). Examination may reveal apnea, periods of agitation, dysconjugate gaze, flaccidity, occasional myoclonus, and hypothermia (27,29). Seizures (rather than just myoclonus) occasionally occur with GHB ingestion, but some controversy exists about their true existence (28,30–32). Electrocardiographic (ECG) changes of U waves have been reported; their exact cause and frequency are unknown (27).

Laboratory assessment is limited; GHB levels can be determined (urine is usually the best matrix for testing), although they are not routinely available. One reason for obtaining such levels might be in a sexual assault case, but otherwise they are clinically irrelevant. Levels in urine are transient, and will often be lost within 24 hours of the ingestion (33). Ethanol levels and a urine drug screen can be useful to evaluate for other causes of the altered mental status. Although several drugs have been touted as possible chemical submission ("date rape") agents, GHB appears to be the one most likely to be used, based on its lack of significant taste and analysis done of urine from sexual assault victims (34).

Management of acute GHB toxicity is primarily supportive. Airway is the first step in management. Many GHB intoxicated patients have alternating episodes of marked agitation followed by apnea. These agitation episodes can be triggered by attempts to intubate. Because of the short duration of the drug's effect, some choose to support with bag valve mask ventilation only, but this would depend on the degree of apnea, presence of gag reflex, and available manpower. If intubation is chosen for definitive airway support, rapid sequence intubation should be used because of the often violent response to laryngeal stimulation (27). If sedation is needed, short-acting sedatives, such as propofol or midazolam, should be used. Use of these sedation agents is preferred because the patient can be extubated in a controlled manner after 2 to 3 hours, avoiding the (common) complication of self-extubation. Decontamination should not be conducted for GHB alone, because it is rapidly absorbed and of relatively low toxicity. Activated charcoal will not adsorb GHB, and lavage would be highly unlikely to remove any clinically relevant amount of drug given its rapid absorption. If decontamination measures are performed (potentially for a coingestion), the patient's airway should be secured. Neither phenytoin nor valproate is recommended for "seizure" activity because, theoretically, they could potentate toxicity (32,35,36).

GHB withdrawal can be difficult to manage. Symptomatically, is similar to ethanol withdrawal (see Chapter 108, Alcohol), but with some notable differences. GHB withdrawal often begins within just a few hours after the last dose, which is much faster then ethanol withdrawal. Symptoms include agitation, tachycardia, diaphoresis, tremor, and hypertension. Additionally, many patients present with hallucinations, psychosis, and delirium without significant physiologic withdrawal symptoms or before any such symptoms begin. Although alcohol withdrawal can produce hallucinations before the severe physiologic derangements develop, this phenomenon seems to be more characteristic with GHB withdrawal. Treatment is with large amounts of benzodiazepines, usually diazepam, using a symptom-triggered regimen. Other agents, such as phenobarbital and pentobarbital, have been added to the benzodiazepine withdrawal regimen with some success (37–39).

SALVIA DIVINORUM (SALVANORIN A)

Salvia divinorum is a plant originally from the Sierra Mazatec region of Mexico. It has the potential for wide cultivation because it has minimal environmental requirements (unlike *Erythroxylon coca*). Salvinorin A was historically used as a divinatory or spiritual tool by native American (Mexican) shaman. The active compound is salvinorin A, which is a nonalkaloid (nonnitrogen containing) neoclerodane diterpene. It is one of the most potent natural hallucinogens known.

Salvinorin A is an agonist at kappa opioid receptors. The mu opioid receptors (Chapter 104, Opiates) are responsible for respiratory depression, euphoria, and analgesia, whereas the kappa opioid receptors have psychotomimetic, dysphoric and some analgesic effects (1,40). Salvinorin A is very specific in its activity, not having any activity at mu opioid, serotonin $5HT_1$, $5HT_2$, dopamine, or muscarininc receptors, nor any activity at the dopamine, serotonin, or norepinephrine transporters (41). Little to no organ toxicity was observed in an extremely high dose rat model (42).

A dose of 500 μg will cause human intoxication, although under typical situations it is impossible to determine an accurate dose. Salvia is often sold as crushed leaf extract, where the salvinorin has been extracted and concentrated onto the remaining plant material using a solvent. Although labeled as 5× and 10×, these products have no quality control and have been demonstrated to have vastly different amounts of salvinorin A (usually much less than claimed) as well as other contaminants (43).

Salvinorin A undergoes extensive first pass metabolism. Therefore, typical exposure routes are smoking, vaporization, and buccal. Clinically, intoxication with salvinorin A causes intense hallucinations and depersonalization. Other symptoms reported are ataxia, alterations in perception, amnesia, delirium, and coma (44,45). The duration is usually one half hour for inhalation and 2 hours for ingestion. The hallucinations from salvinorin A are often described as unpleasant; many who use the herb never do so again. Rat studies have demonstrated it causes a decrease in brain dopamine levels, unlike the addictive drugs (46). Humans with drug abuse histories given kappa agonists report that they did not like the drug (47). These facts suggest that chronic abuse will not occur in humans. There are reports of *Salvia divinorum* acting as an antidepressant in a substantial number of users (45,48), but no reports of it causing prolonged mental illness.

The diagnosis of salvinorin A intoxication must be made based on the clinical history, because no specific clinical finding will suggest the diagnosis, and no way exists to routinely test for salvinorin. Treatment for salvinorin A overdose would be similar to the treatments for hallucinogen intoxication (Chapter 107, Hallucinogens). Differences include a much shorter time of symptoms such that unless the salvinorin was ingested, symptoms should be resolving by the time they are evaluated by the health care provider. Also, serotonin syndrome is a risk for some of the tryptamine hallucinogens, but it is not a risk from salvinorin ingestion. It is important to investigate and comorbidity, such as trauma, if a patient presents with delirium; also, if the delirium does not clear within 1 hour, other etiological possibilities should be explored.

CLINICAL RECOMMENDATIONS OF THE VIGNETTE

Continuous pulse oximeter monitoring was done and intravenous fluids were initiated. The patient's electrolytes were normal, the urine drug screen was negative, head computed tomographic (CT) scan was normal and the volatile or toxic alcohol screen (ethanol, methanol, isopropanol, and ethylene glycol) was negative. The patient woke up within a few hours and behaved normally; he was subsequently discharged (after consultation with child protective service). Gas chromatography or mass spectroscopy analysis of the solvent revealed the presence of 99%+ 1,4 butanediol. In retrospect, the need for the head CT scan was questionable; however, with the rapid onset of coma there was concern for potential oxygen emboli arising from ingestion of concentrated hydrogen peroxide. No need was seen to monitor the patient following the return to a normal mental status; although GHB (and its analogues) do cause waxing and waning of symptoms, they do not cause recurrence of coma once a patient becomes completely lucid or awake.

SUMMARY

The astute clinician should be cognizant of the symptoms associated with some of the less commonly abused substances. These symptoms include a neuropathy from nitrous oxide abuse similar to vitamin B_{12} deficiency, profound but short-lived sedation from abuse of GHB (and its analogues), and atypical hallucinogenic effects from the abuse of *Salvia divinorum*.

REFERENCES

1. Hardman JG, Limbird LE, eds. *Goodman & Gillman's The Pharmacological Basis of Therapeutics*, 10th ed. New York: McGraw-Hill; 2001.
2. Brodsky JB, Cohen EN, Brown B, et al. Exposure to nitrous oxide and neurologic disease among dental professionals. *Anesth Analg.* 1981;60:297–301.
3. Layzer RB, Fishman RA, Schafer JA. Neuropathy following abuse of nitrous oxide. *Neurology.* 1978;28:504–506.
4. Banks RGS, Henderson RJ, Pratt JM. Reactions of gases in solution. Part III. Some reactions of nitrous oxide with transition-metal complexes. *J Chem Soc (A).* 1968;2886–2888.
5. Drummond JT, Matthews RG. Nitrous oxide degradation by cobalamin-dependent methionine synthase: Characterization of the reactants and products in the inactivation reaction. *Biochemistry.* 1994;33:3732–3741.
6. Deacon R, Lumb M, Perry J, et al. Selective inactivation of vitamin B12 in rats by nitrous oxide. *Lancet.* 1978;2(8098):1023–1024.
7. O'Sullivan H, Jennings F, Ward K, et al. Human bone marrow biochemical function and megaloblastic hematopoiesis after nitrous oxide anesthesia. *Anesthesiology.* 1981;55:645–649.
8. Nunn JF, Chanarin I, Tanner AG, et al. Megaloblastic bone marrow changes after repeated nitrous oxide anaesthesia. *Br J Anaesth.* 1986;58:1469–1470.
9. Schilling RF. Is nitrous oxide a dangerous anesthetic for vitamin b12-deficient subjects? *JAMA.* 1986;255(12):1605–1606.
10. Scott JM, Dinn JJ, Wilson P, et al. Pathogenesis of subacute combined degeneration: A result of methyl group deficiency. *Lancet.* 1981;August 15:334–337.
11. Jastak JT, Malamet SF. Nitrous oxide sedation and sexual phenomena. *J Am Dent Assoc.* 1980;101:38–40.
12. Hadzic A, Krzysztof G, Sanborn KV, et al. Severe neurologic deficit after nitrous oxide. *Anesthesia.* 1995;83:863–866.
13. Sethi NK, Mullin P, Torgornick J, et al. Nitrous oxide "whippit" abuse presenting with cobalamin responsive psychosis. *Journal of Medical Toxicology.* 2006;2(2):71–74.
14. Flippo TS, Holder WD. Neurological degeneration associated with nitrous oxide anesthesia in patients with vitamin b12 deficiency. *Arch Surg.* 1993;128:1391–1395.
15. Pema PJ, Horak HA, Wyatt RH. Myelopathy caused by nitrous oxide toxicity. *AJNR Am J Neuroradiol.* 1998;19:894–896.
16. Amess JAL, Burman JF, Rees GM, et al. Megaloblastic haemopoiesis in patients receiving nitrous oxide. *Lancet.* 1978;August 12:339–342.
17. Ermens AAM, Refsum H, Rupreht J, et al. Monitoring cobalamin inactivation during nitrous oxide anesthesia by determination of homocysteine and folate in plasma and urine. *Clin Pharmacol Ther.* 1991;49:385–393.
18. Roth RH, Giarman NJ. Natural occurrence of gamma-hydroxybutyric acid in mammalian brain. *Biochem Pharmacol.* 1970;18:247–250.
19. Micromedex. Thomson MICROMEDEX. Vol. 130. Accessed December, 15, 2006.
20. Zvosec DL, Smith SW, McCutcheon R, et al. Adverse events, including death, associated with the use of 1,4-butanediol. *N Engl J Med.* 2001;344(2):87–94.
21. Tancredi DN, Shannon MW. Case30-2003: A 21 year old man with sudden alteration of mental status. *N Engl J Med.* 2003;349:1267–1275.
22. Roth RH, Giarman NJ. Conversion in vivo of γ-aminobutyric acid to γ-hydroxybutyric acid in the rat. *Biochem Pharmacol.* 1969;18:247–250.
23. Lingenhoehl K, Brom B, Heid J, et al. Gamma-hydroxybutyrate is a weak agonist at recombinant $GABA_B$ receptors. *Neuropharmacology.* 1999;38:1667–1673.
24. Howard SG, Feigenbaum JJ. Effect on gamma-hydroxybutyrate on central dopamine release in vivo. *Biochem Pharmacol.* 1997;53:103–110.
25. Roth RH, Doherty JD, Walters JR. Gamma-hydroxybutyrate: A role in the regulation of central dopaminergic neurons? *Brain Res.* 1980;189:556–560.
26. Package Insert, Xyrem® [Sodium Oxybate] Revised 11/2005.
27. Li J, Stokes SA, Woeckener A. A tale of novel intoxication: Seven cases of γ-hydroxybutyric acid overdose. *Ann Emerg Med.* 1998;31(6):723–727.
28. Shannon M, Quang L. Gamma-hydroxybutyrate, gamma-butyrolactone and 1,4 butanediol: A case report and review of the literature. *Pediatr Emerg Med.* 2000;16(6):435–440.
29. Sporer K, Chin RL, Dyer JE, et al. γ-hydroxybutyrate serum levels and clinical syndrome after severe overdose. *Annals of Emergency Medicine.* 2003;42(1):3–8.
30. Entholzner E, Mielke L, Pichlmeier R, et al. EEG changes during sedation with γ-hydroxybutyric. *Anesthetist.* 1995;44:345–350.
31. Cisek J, Holstege C, Rose R. Seizure associated with butanediol ingestion. *J Toxicol Clin Toxicol.* 1999;37(5):650 (abst).
32. Sneed OC, III. Ontogeny of γ-hydroxybutyric acid. II. Electroencephalographic effects *Brain Res.* 1984;317:89–96.
33. Brenneisen R, El Sohly MA, Murphy TP, et al. Pharmacokinetics and excretion of gamma-hydroxybutyrate (GHB) in healthy subjects. *J Anal Toxicol.* 2004;28:625–630.
34. El Sohly MA, Salamone SJ. Prevalence of drugs used in cases of alleged sexual assault. *Journal of Analytical Toxicology.* 1999;23:141–146.
35. Snead OC, Bearden LJ, Pegram V. Effect on acute and chronic anticonvulsant administration on endogenous gamma-hydroxybutyrate in rat brain. *Neuropharmacology.* 1980;12: 47–52.
36. Hechler V, Ratomponirina C, Maitre M. γ-hydroxybutyrate conversion into GABA induces displacement of $GABA_B$ binding that is blocked by valproate and ethosuximide. *J Pharmacol Exper Ther.* 1997;281;281:753–760.
37. Schneir AB, Ly BT, Clark RF. A case of withdrawal from the GHB precursors gamma-butyrolactone and 1,4-butanediol. *J Emerg Med.* 2001;21(1):31–33.
38. Sivilotti MLA, Burns MJ, Aaron CK, et al. Pentobarbital for severe γ-butyrolactone withdrawal. *Ann Emerg Med.* 2001;38(6):660–665.
39. Rosenberg MH, Deerfield LJ, Baruch EM. Two cases of severe γ-hydroxybutyrate withdrawal delirium on a psychiatric unit: Recommendations for management. *The American Journal of Drug and Alcohol Abuse.* 2003;29(2):487–496.
40. McCurdy CR, Sufka KJ, Smith GH, et al. Antinociceptive profile of salvinorin a, a structurally unique kappa opioid receptor agonist. *Pharmacology, Biochemistry and Behaviour.* 2006;83(1):109–113.
41. Roth BL, Baner K, Westkaemper R, et al. Salvinorin A: A potent naturally occurring non-nitrogenous k opioid selective agonist. *Proceedings of the National Academy of Sciences.* 2002;99(18):11934–11939.
42. Mowry M, Mosher M, Briner W. Acute physiologic and chronic histologic changes in rats and mice exposed to the unique hallucinogen salvinorin A. *J Psychoactive Drugs.* 2003;35(3): 379–382.
43. Wolowich W, Cienki JJ, Perkins AM. Salvia: Concentrations and contaminants. *J Toxicol Clin Toxicol.* 2004;42(5):759(abst).
44. Valdes LJ. Salvia divinorum and the unique diterpene hallucinogen, Salvinorin A. *J Psychoactive Drugs.* 1994;26(3):277–283.
45. Carlezon WA, Jr., Beguin C, Di Nieri JA, et al. Depressive-like effects of the kappa-opioid receptor agonist Salvinorin A on behavior and neurochemistry in rats. *Journal of Pharmacology & Experimental Therapeutics.* 2006;316(1):440–447.
46. Walsh SL, Geter-Douglas B, Strain EC, et al. Enadoline, a selective kappa opioid agonist: Comparison with butorphanol and hydromorphone in humans. *Psychopharmacology.* 2001;157:151–162.
47. Baggott M, Erowid E, Erowid F. A survey of Salvia divinorum users. E*rowid Extracts.* 2004;6:12–14.
48. Hanes KR. Antidepressant effects of the herb Salvia divinorum: A case report. *J Clin Psychopharmacol.* 2001;21(6):634–635.

CHAPTER 113

Hypothermia

Galen V. Henderson

OBJECTIVES

- To define and review hypothermia: primary (accidental) and secondary
- To discuss the physiologic changes associated with hypothermia
- To review induced hypothermia in ischemic stroke, cardiac arrest, traumatic brain injury
- To discuss control of intracranial hypertension
- To explore potential complications of induced hypothermia

CASE VIGNETTE

On a cold winter night, a 62-year-old homeless man was transported to the emergency department by emergency medical services (EMS) after being found on the sidewalk and unable to stand. The patient's friends noted that over the last 6 hours he became progressively confused, agitated, and then lethargic. His speech was slow and his gait became progressively unstable. EMS noted that his temperature was 34.1°C; heart rate, 42 beats per minute; and blood pressure was normal. While being transported to hospital, the patient suffered a cardiac arrest and required cardiopulmonary resuscitation (CPR). The patient was found to have ventricular fibrillation (VFIB) arrest and was eventually resuscitated in the ambulance. On arrival to the emergency department, his examination was consistent with a coma. Remarkable laboratory data included normal coagulation studies and low platelets of 71 K/mm^3. His K+ was 4.8, blood urea nitrogen (BUN) 46, and creatinine 1.4.

DEFINITION

Hypothermia occurs when core temperature is below 35°C (95°F). Primary hypothermia (accidental) is the result of the direct exposure of a previously healthy individual to the cold. Secondary hypothermia has a much higher mortality rate because it is seen as with other serious systemic disorders. Also induced hypothermia is a possible neuroprotective option to improve neurologic outcomes in several disease states. Regardless of how the patient becomes hypothermic, many of the compensatory physiologic mechanisms to conserve heat begin to fail.

Accidental hypothermia is usually, but not always, geographically and seasonally pervasive. Multiple variables may make individuals more susceptible (Table 113-1 and Table 113-2).

The elderly have a diminished thermal perception and are more vulnerable to immobility, malnutrition, and many systemic illnesses that interfere with heat generation or conservation. Neonates have high rates of heat loss because much of their heat is lost from the skull; they have increased skull surface-to-body mass ratio and lack an effective shivering and adaptive behavioral response. Malnutrition can contribute to heat loss because of diminished subcutaneous fat and because of its association with depleted energy stores used for thermogenesis. Individuals who have hobbies or occupations, such as hunters, sailors, military personnel, hikers, ice fishers, skiers, and climbers, are also are at great risk of exposure to cold.

Toxic exposure with agents, such as ethanol, causes vasodilatation, which increases heat loss and reduces thermogenesis and gluconeogenesis and can impair judgment or lead to confusion or a decreased level of consciousness. Other medications, such as phenothiazines, barbiturates, tricyclic antidepressants, benzodiazepines, and others can affect centrally mediated vasoconstriction.

Several types of endocrine dysfunction can lead to hypothermia. Severe hypothermia reduces the metabolic rate and impairs thermogenesis and behavioral responses. Hypopituitarism or adrenal insuffiency can also increase the susceptibility to hypothermia.

Neurologic injury from stroke, trauma, cerebral hemorrhage, or any hypothalamic lesions increases susceptibility of hypothermia. This is probably more commonly seen in acute spinal cord injury, which disrupts the autonomic pathways that lead to shivering and prevents the cold-induced reflex vasoconstrictive responses.

CLINICAL PRESENTATION

In many cases of hypothermia the diagnosis is straightforward because a history of exposure to environmental factors, such a prolonged exposure to the outdoors without adequate clothing. Presentations, however, are more difficult and subtle in other situations, such as toxin exposures or psychiatric disorders. The physical examination can be changed by hypothermia. For example, a patient with hypothermia can be confused or agitated, or even comatose. The classic example of maladaptive behavior in patients with hypothermia is paradoxic undressing, which involves the inappropriate removal of clothing in response to the stress of cold. A cold

TABLE 113-1. Risk Factors for Hypothermia

AGE EXTREMES	ENDOCRINE RELATED
Elderly	Hypoglycemia
Neonates	Hypothyroidism
	Adrenal insufficiency
	Hypopituitarism
OUTDOOR EXPOSURE	**NEUROLOGIC DISORDERS**
Occupational	Stroke
Sports-related	Hypothalamic disorders
Inadequate clothing	Parkinson's disease
	Spinal cord injury
DRUGS AND INTOXICANTS	**MULTISYSTEM**
Ethanol	Malnutrition
Phenothiazines	Sepsis
Barbiturates	Shock
Anesthetics	Hepatic or renal failure
Neuromuscular blockers	
	OTHERS
	Burns and exfoliative dermatologic disorders
	Immobility or debilitation

(Adapted from Danzl DF, Pozos RS. Accidental hypothermia. *N Engl J Med.* 1994;331(26):1756–1760, with permission.)

induced ileus and abdominal rectus spasm may be present, which can mimic the presentation of an acute abdomen. For patients having survived severe hypothermia, the neurologic examination can be confused with that fulfilling the criteria for brain death.

TABLE 113-2. Mechanism of Heat Loss

Radiation	Transfer of heat between the separated surfaces of two objects with the different temperatures via electromagnetic (infrared) radiation, without direct contact between the objects and without heat transfer medium. Accounts for 50% to 70% of heat loss in awake patients.
Conduction	Direct transfer of heat from one surface to a second, adjacent surface. Amount of heat loss is closely related to contact surface; in standing, a patient's heat loss through conduction is negligible, but this increased in the sitting or lying position.
Convection	Transfer of heat from a surface to the surrounding air. Accounts for 20% to 30% of heat loss at room temperature in the absence of wind.
Evaporation	Heat loss derived from the evaporation of water from skin and lungs. Accounts for ±15% of heat loss (5% from skin, 10% from the lungs) under nonsweating circumstances.

(Adapted from Polderman KH. Application of therapeutic hypothermia in the intensive care unit. Opportunities and pitfalls of a promising treatment modality. Part 2: Practical aspects and side effects. *Intensive Care Med.* 2004;30(5):757–769, with permission.)

Once hypothermia has been confirmed, the patient should be continuously monitored by measurements of the core temperature. Changes in rectal and bladder temperatures often lag behind fluctuations in the core temperature, such as from a pulmonary artery (PA) catheter, and esophageal readings can be elevated during the inhalation of heated air. Reliance on infrared tympanic thermography should await the results of further studies in patients with hypothermia (1).

Hypothermia shifts the oxyhemoglobin-dissociation curve to the left, resulting in decreased oxygen release from hemoglobin into the tissues at a lower partial pressure of oxygen. For example, at 27°C, the saturation of hemoglobin is 100% at a partial pressure of oxygen of 59 mm Hg. Vasoconstriction and increased blood viscosity are additional impediments to tissue oxygenation. Metabolic causes of acidosis include lactate generation from shivering and decreased tissue perfusion, coupled with impaired hepatic metabolism and acid excretion. Dehydration from cold-induced diuresis and fluid sequestration after a lengthy exposure to the cold can be seen. Gastric and bladder catheterization are indicated because ileus and fluid shifts are commonly encountered in patients who present with a body temperature below 32°C (1).

The hematocrit increases 2% per 1°C decline in temperature. Hypothermia masks potassium-induced changes in the electrocardiogram, therefore, the potassium level should be checked frequently. Empiric potassium supplementation, therefore, can produce a toxic reaction once the patient is rewarmed. Hyperkalemia can be particularly dangerous in a patient with metabolic acidosis, rhabdomyolysis, or renal failure. Persistent hyperglycemia suggests pancreatitis or diabetic ketoacidosis (1).

Coagulopathies often develop in patients with hypothermia despite the presence of normal levels of clotting factor. These normal recordings occur because prothrombin time or activated partial-thromboplastin measurements are routinely performed only at 37°C. As the body temperature decreases, platelet activity declines because the production of thromboxane B_2 by platelets is temperature dependent. This impaired platelet function can further exacerbate the cold-induced thrombocytopenia that results from direct suppression of bone marrow and hepatosplenic sequestration. Hypercoagulability also occurs and can result in thromboembolism (1). Table 113-3 lists the physiologic changes seen with hypothermia.

NORMAL TEMPERATURE REGULATION

The preoptic anterior hypothalamus normally orchestrates thermoregulation by the autonomic nervous system that includes the cascade of (*a*) an afferent thermal sensing, (*b*) central regulation, and (*c*) efferent responses working together to maintain the normal core body temperature. The responses to hypothermia include the release of norepinephrine, increased muscle tone, and shivering, leading to thermogenesis and an increase in basal metabolic rate. Cutaneous cold thermoreception causes direct reflex vasoconstriction to conserve heat. The core temperature can be reliably measured in the pulmonary artery or distal esophagus (2). For clinical purposes, the core temperature can also be adequately estimated on the basis of rectal or bladder temperature (3).

TABLE 113-3. Physiologic Changes Associated with Hypothermia

Severity	*Body Temperature*	*Central Nervous System*	*Cardiovascular*	*Respiratory*	*Renal and Eendocrine*	*Neuromuscular*
Mild	35°C (95°F)–32.2°C (90°F)	Linear depression of cerebral metabolism; amnesia; apathy; dysarthria; impaired judgment; maladaptive behavior	Tachycardia, then progressive bradycardia; cardiac-cycle prolongation; vasoconstriction; increase in cardiac output and blood pressure	Tachypnea, then progressive decrease in respiratory minute volume; declining oxygen consumption; bronchorrhea; bronchospasm	Diuresis; increase in catecholamines, adrenal steroids, triiodothyronine and thyroxine; increase in metabolism with shivering	Increased preshivering muscle tone, then fatigue shivering induced thermogenic ataxia
Moderate	<32.2°C (90°F)–28°C (82.4°F)	Electroencephalogram (EEG) abnormalities; progressive depression of level of consciousness; pupillary dilatation; paradoxical undressing; hallucinations	Progressive decrease in pulse an cardiac output; increased atrial and ventricular arrhythmias; nonspecific and suggestive ECG changes; prolonged asystole	Hypoventilation; 50% decrease in carbon dioxide production per 8°C drop in temperature; absence of protective airway reflexes; 50% decrease in oxygen consumption	50% increase in renal blood flow; renal autoregulation intact; impaired insulin action	Hyporeflexia; diminishing shivering induced thermogenicity; rigidity
Severe	<28°C (82.4°F)	Loss of cerebrovascular autoregulation; decline in cerebral blood flow; coma; loss of ocular reflexes; progressive decrease in EEG	Progressive decreases in blood pressure, heart rate and cardiac output; reentrant dysrhythmias; decreased ventricular arrhythmia threshold; asystole	Pulmonary congestion and edema; 75% decrease in oxygen consumption; apnea	Decrease in renal blood flow parallels decrease in cardiac output; extreme oliguria; poikilothermia; 80% decrease in basal metabolism	No motion; decreased nerve conduction velocity; peripheral areflexia

(Adapted from Danzl DF, Pozos RS. Accidental hypothermia. *N Engl J Med.* 1994;331(26):1756–1760, with permission.)

EVALUATION OF INDUCED HYPOTHERMIA FOR POSSIBLE NEUROPROTECTION

Induced hypothermia has been studied in a wide variety of illnesses, both ischemic and nonischemic, hopefully to improve neurologic outcomes (4–6). These studies have include traumatic brain injury, status epilepticus (7), arrhythmia, sepsis, and the ischemic illnesses of myocardial infarction, stroke (6), and cardiac arrest (8). In this chapter are discussed potential clinical applications for possible neuroprotection. Physicians working in emergency departments and intensive care units should have some knowledge regarding the evidence supporting the clinical applications, physiologic consequences, and side effects that can develop when patients are treated with induced hypothermia.

Although the exact pathophysiologic mechanisms of neuroprotection of hypothermia are not completely worked out beyond its ability to reduce metabolic demand for oxygen and glucose, additional potential benefits are as follows:

- Suppression of inflammatory response (9,10)
- Decreased release of excitotoxic neurotransmitters (11,12)
- Inhibition of production and release of oxygen free radicals
- Stabilization of the blood–brain barrier(13) and cerebral edema (14)

HYPOTHERMIA IN ACUTE ISCHEMIC STROKE

Stroke is the second most common cause of death in the world, and the leading cause of disability in patients over 65 years of age (15). A few advances in acute stroke care have improved the general outcome of the disease (16), other than treatment with recombinant tissue plasminogen activator (rtPA) within 3 hours of ischemic stroke onset (17). Because core body temperature has been suggested to be an independent predictor of outcome in patients with acute stroke (18), other options for outcome improvement, such as induced hypothermia, must be investigated.

Induced hypothermia in the setting of stroke remains experimental, but data exist to support its use (19,20). To date, several uncontrolled clinical trials have assessed the feasibility of induced hypothermia in patients with stroke (21–24). These studies mostly included patients with middle cerebral artery territory infarctions. Most of these trials were small and the largest one included only 50 patients (22). The use of hypothermia was reported to be feasible and with limited side effects (22). Hypothermia decreased intracranial pressure (ICP) in all of these studies and Schwab et al. (21,22) reported increased survival among hypothermic patients compared with historical controls. Mortality rates of middle cerebral artery territory infarction can be as high as 80% in cases secondary to cerebral edema, intracranial hypertension, and cerebral herniation (24). In contrast, mortality in the largest study by Schwab et al. (22) was only 38%. Many of the deaths occurred during rewarming after rebound increases in ICP. A subsequent study by the same group demonstrated that these increases in ICP could be prevented by slower and controlled rewarming (25). The time intervals between onset of ischemic stroke and initiation of hypothermia were relatively long, 22 ± 9 hours with a range of 4 to 75 hours in the largest study (22). Average time required to achieve temperatures ≤33°C was 6.5 hours, and ranged from 3.5 to 11 hours. In most published studies, this period ranged from 24 to 72 hours, averaging 55 hours in the largest study (22). The optimal duration of cooling is also unknown. Following induced hypothermia treatment, passive or active rewarming can induce rebound effects on ICP; therefore, rates of rewarming are probably a key in preserving any beneficial effects of hypothermia.

In summary, hypothermia for acute stroke treatment is a promising area for development and preliminary clinical studies suggest that mild hypothermia can be feasible and beneficial for the treatment of acute stroke (21,23,26,27). Data for standardization of induced hypothermia for the treatment of ischemic stroke, however, are insufficient to recommend it at this time (28). Although the induction of hypothermia after ischemic stroke requires additional refinement, aggressive prevention of hyperthermia is clearly indicated. Presently, it is probably more important to know that modest elevations in temperature increase stroke severity and patient mortality (29,30). A clinical investigation using these measures demonstrated significant mortality risk reduction (31). Antipyretic medications in combination with either forced-air cooling or cooling blankets are sufficient to maintain core temperatures to a goal of 37°C.

HYPOTHERMIA IN CARDIAC ARREST

Cardiac arrest outside the hospital is a major cause of unexpected death in developed countries. Commonly associated with extensive brain damage, it often results in pervasive cognitive deficits, specifically memory deficits, for those who survive. Experimental use of moderate hypothermia in animal models of cardiac arrest and in other brain-injury paradigms has demonstrated significant neuroprotective effects, and clinical studies have shown hypothermia to be feasible and safe for ischemic brain injury after cardiac arrest.

To date, the most convincing data to support induced hypothermia come from two randomized trials. In a multicenter, randomized trial from the Hypothermia after Cardiac Arrest Study Group, mild therapeutic hypothermia (32°C to 34°C for 24 hours) was compared with normothermia in 275 patients who were successfully resuscitated after cardiac arrest caused by ventricular fibrillation, but who remained comatose. At 6 months, the 137 patients who were treated with hypothermia had significantly better neurologic outcomes and overall survival than did the 138 patients in the normothermia group. A favorable neurologic outcome (good recovery or moderate disability on a five-point category scale) occurred in 55% of the hypothermia group compared with 39% of the normothermia group (risk ratio, 1.40; number needed to treat (NNT) to prevent one unfavorable outcome, six). Six-month mortality rates were 41% in the hypothermia group and 55% in the normothermia group (risk ratio, 0.74; NNT to prevent one death, seven). Rates of unfavorable outcomes among surviving patients were low in both groups (hypothermia, 7%; normothermia, 13%). Infection and bleeding complications were not significantly higher in the hypothermia group (32).

In a smaller study with a similar design and similar inclusion criteria, Bernard et al. (33) randomized 77 patients with cardiac arrest to treatment with hypothermia (33°C for 12 hours) or to normothermia. A good neurologic outcome at discharge occurred in 49% of patients who were hypothermic patients and 26% of those who were normothermic.

Although the two groups in the Hypothermia After Cardiac Arrest Group study had differences (the normothermic group having more patients with diabetes and coronary artery disease, but also more who received bystander basic life support), the risk ratio did not change significantly after adjustment for baseline variables. With the additive benefits of mild therapeutic hypothermia, as shown by Bernard et al. (32), more compelling evidence now indicated starting implementation of cooling protocols for survivors of cardiac arrest.

In the first study, a longer period was needed to achieve target temperature (8 hours, vs. 2 hours, respectively), but also had a therapeutic benefit. Hypothermia seemed to have a greater impact on mortality than on favorable outcome among survivors.

As a result of this and related information, unconscious adult patients with spontaneous circulation after out-of-hospital cardiac arrest should be cooled to 32°C to 34°C for 12 to 24 hours when the initial cardiac rhythm is ventricular fibrillation. Cooling may also be beneficial for other cardiac rhythms or in-hospital cardiac arrest (34). In the future, it is hoped that investigations will explore brain temperature estimation, optimal cooling methods (external versus endovascular), duration of cooling, therapeutic window for induction of hypothermia, and the rewarming period.

INDUCED HYPOTHERMIA TO CONTROL REFRACTORY INTRACRANIAL HYPERTENSION

The best method for treating patients with massive hemispheric strokes that have been refractory to traditional medical therapy, such as intermittent hyperventilation, hyperosmolar therapy, sedation, and head-of-bed elevation remains unclear. In selected patients, decompressive craniectomy allows the brain to herniate outward instead of inward, potentially resulting in dramatic resolution of midline shift and reduced mortality. Although this approach is increasingly accepted, randomized evidence is lacking, patient selection for the procedure can be problematic, and the long-term clinical outcomes are unknown.

Els et al. (35) randomized 25 consecutive patients with "malignant" middle cerebral artery territory infarcts to either decompressive craniectomy followed by hypothermia (35°C) maintained for 48 hours or craniectomy alone. Inclusion criteria were age <65 years, severe stroke (National Institutes of Health Stroke Scale [NIHSS] score >20 for left-sided infarcts and >15 for right-sided ones), and infarct involving more than two thirds of the middle cerebral artery (MCA) territory with no diffusion—perfusion mismatch with magnetic resonance imaging (MRI) of the brain. Immediate postsurgical mortality did not differ between the two groups, nor did length of stay or duration of mechanical ventilation. At 6 months, the combination-therapy group had a trend toward better outcomes compared with the surgery-only group (mean Barthel index, 81 vs. 70). The combination-therapy group required higher mean doses of norepinephrine to maintain blood pressure during hypothermia (1.3 mg/hour vs. 0.9 mg/hour; $P = 0.05$). The authors concluded that, given the trend toward improved outcome with combination therapy, this approach should be considered as "an additional treatment option" for these patients (35).

Although hemicraniectomy plus hypothermia to control intracranial hypertension is feasible, it warrants further study. Larger randomized, controlled trials are needed to define the risks and benefits of decompressive surgery alone, hypothermia alone, as well as the two combined. Therefore, recommending it as a standard of care for ischemic stroke care in treating patients who are refractory in traditional measures, would be premature.

TRAUMATIC BRAIN INJURY

Traumatic brain injury (TBI) is the most common cause of death and disability in young people in western countries. In the United States, TBI is responsible for approximately 270,000 hospital admissions, 52,000 deaths, and 80,000 patients with permanent neurologic disabilities (36). All neurologic damage does not occur at the time of injury, but develops over hours to days (37). The two phases of injury are described as *primary injury* (at the time of injury) and *secondary injury* (hours to days after the event).

In TBI, secondary injury includes swelling of the brain and cerebral edema formation within hours, which can lead to a rise in ICP brain tissue shifts causing cerebral herniation or additional vascular compromise causing strokes and increasing morbidity and chances of death. Local hyperthermic areas are found in the damaged brain and temperatures are up to 2°C higher than core temperature (38,39).

In 2001, Clifton et al. (40) published the results of a large multicenter trial that included 392 patients in 11 centers, and observed no benefits in survival or neurologic outcome of induced hypothermia in TBI. The only subgroup that appeared to benefit from hypothermia were patients with hypothermia already present at admission (40). The debate regarding use of hypothermia in TBI had apparently been settled by this study; however, in the past year the results of two large new clinical trials have been published, both of which reported significant improvements in neurologic outcome and survival in patients with TBI treated with hypothermia (41,42). Polderman et al. (41) showed significant benefits of hypothermia in neurologic outcome and survival in a group of 136 patients, despite that hypothermia was used only as an option of last therapeutic option. Zhi et al. (42) showed rates of good neurologic outcome of 38.8 versus 19.7%; for moderate disability; 22.7 versus 18.2%; and death, 25.7 versus 36.4% for hypothermia patients versus controls, respectively.

Overall, results from animal experiments overwhelmingly support the use of induced hypothermia in TBI. Clinical trials have provided conflicting results, however; therefore, the routine usage of hypothermia in TBI currently cannot be recommended. Hypothermia is clearly effective in controlling intracranial hypertension, but a lower ICP has not improved outcomes.

TREATMENT OF POTENTIAL COMPLICATIONS OF INDUCED HYPOTHERMIA

Despite the benefits of induced hypothermia, it is not without risk. As the body cools, a series of physiologic changes take place, including shivering, alterations in the clotting cascade, immunologic suppression, and cardiac membrane changes that increase the risk of arrhythmias.

SHIVERING

Shivering, a common occurrence during the induction of hypothermia, can serve to counteract cooling by increasing metabolic rates and myocardial oxygen demands. Medications used to control shivering include opioid and neuroleptic medications. To help control shivering, the combination of meperidine and buspirone should be considered because of their synergistic effects and reducing shivering (43). Warming the arms and legs during central cooling has demonstrated some reduction in shivering as well, supporting the notion that an increase in peripheral to central temperature gradient may be responsible for triggering a shivering response (44). In ventilated patients, this can be counteracted by the administration of sedatives and analgesics or the administration of muscle paralyzers. When using paralyzers, opiates, or both is deemed undesirable, alternatives to treat shivering include the administration of clonidine, neostigmine, and ketanserine (45). Care should be taken, however, to avoid adverse effects; for example, clonidine can aggravate hypothermia-induced bradycardia (45).

ELECTROLYTE ABNORMALITIES

With potential electrolyte abnormalities that may be seen, induced hypothermia also induces a diuresis, which can develop significant hypokalemia, hypomagnesemia, or hypophosphatemia (46) because of the significant amount of fluid loss. Any beneficial effects of hypothermia may be lost because of side effects if not treated aggressively. The diuresis usually occurs during induction of hypothermia, These problems are much less evident, however, in other categories of patients, such as those with postanoxic coma following CPR (45).

INFECTIONS

Evidence from clinical and in vitro studies shows that hypothermia can impair immune function. Hypothermia inhibits the release of various proinflammatory cytokines (47) and suppresses chemotactic migration of leukocytes and phagocytosis (48). Hypothermia-induced insulin resistance and hyperglycemia can further increase infection risks.

In a study of stroke patients, the risk of pneumonia was increased with hypothermia and this was consistent with the results cardiac arrest studies (21). It is unclear whether the immune system is globally suppressed by hypothermia or whether some pulmonary-specific mechanism is responsible for this increased pneumonia risk. Induced hypothermia does not seem to lead to a significantly increased risk of bacteremia, urinary tract infection, or other infectious complications. Whether patients who are having induced hypothermia should be treated prophylactically with antibiotics is unclear.

CARDIAC ARRHYTHMIAS

Hypothermia is initially associated with sinus tachycardia and then followed by bradycardia. Although cardiac arrhythmias are a risk of induced hypothermia, human studies in which the target mild hypothermia temperatures were above 32°C did not have result in significant arrhythmia. Therefore, no additional clinical precautions need be taken when hypothermia to 32°C to 34°C is performed. When the temperature is below 30°C, the arrhythmia is usually atrial fibrillation and may be followed by the increased risk of ventricular flutter or fibrillation. In addition, arrhythmias in deeply hypothermic patients are difficult to treat because the myocardium becomes less responsive to defibrillation and antiarrhythmic drugs (45).

CLINICAL RECOMMENDATIONS OF THE VIGNETTE

For this patient, it was difficult to determine the cause for the subacute mental status change. After the patient developed VFIB arrest and was resuscitated, his neurologic examination was extremely poor. In an attempt to decrease the degree of neurologic injury, induced hypothermia must be considered. Induced hypothermia can be an effective mode of neuroprotection in postischemic injury following CPR, at least in selected categories of patients. Although the ideal temperature and time for induced hypothermia is not known, most experts believe that cooling to 32°C to 34°C and for a minimum of 24 hours is optimal. After this period, rapid rewarming may have adverse effects that may negate any benefits derived from cooling. Therefore, rewarming should be done slowly, approximately 18 hours after target temperature is reached (or 24 hours of total cooling). Many aim for <1°C per hour over 6 hours. For clinicians using external cooling, passive rewarming and active rewarming is usually done after <36°C after 12 hours. It is important also to be cognizant of the physiologic changes that occur during the cooling and rewarming, such as the changes in volume status and potassium homeostasis.

SUMMARY

This chapter defines primary hypothermia (accidental) hypothermia, and diseases states that places patients at risk for the development of secondary hypothermia. Reviewed were the physiologic changes associated with hypothermia which change as the depth of hypothermia increases. Also evaluated were induced hypothermia in the treatment of ischemic stroke, TBI, control of intracranial hypertension, cardiac arrest, and the potential complications of such treatment.

REFERENCES

1. Danzl DF, Pozos RS. Accidental hypothermia. *N Engl J Med.* 1994;331(26):1756–1760.
2. Cork R, Vaughan R, Humphrey L. Precision and accuracy of intraoperative temperature monitoring. *Anesth Analg.* 1983;62(2):211–214.
3. Sessler DI. Mild perioperative hypothermia. *N Engl J Med.* 1997;336(24):1730–1737.
4. Bernard S. Induced hypothermia in intensive care medicine. *Anaesthia Intensive Care.* 1996;24(3):382–388.
5. Colbourne F, Sutherland G, Corbett D. Postischemic hypothermia. A critical appraisal with implications for clinical treatment. *Mol Neurobiol.* 1997;14(3):171–201.
6. Eisenburger P, Stertz F, Holzer M, et al. Therapeutic hypothermia after cardiac arrest. *Curr Opin Crit Care.* 2001;7(3):184–188.
7. Orlowski JP, Erenberg G, Lueders H, et al. Hypothermia and barbiturate coma for refractory status epilepticus. *Crit Care Med.* 1984;12(4):367–372.
8. Leonov Y, Sterz F, Safar P, et al. Moderate hypothermia after cardiac arrest of 17 minutes in dogs. Effect on cerebral and cardiac outcome. *Stroke.* 1990;21(11):1600–1606.
9. Wang GJ, Deng HY, Maier CM, et al. Mild hypothermia reduces ICAM-1 expression, neutrophil infiltration and microglia/monocyte accumulation following experimental stroke. *Neuroscience.* 2002;114(4):1081–1090.
10. Deng H, Han HS, Cheng D, et al. Mild hypothermia inhibits inflammation after experimental stroke and brain inflammation. *Stroke.* 2003;34(10):2495–2501.
11. Xu L, Yenari MA, Steinberg GK, et al. Mild hypothermia reduces apoptosis of mouse neurons in vitro early in the cascade. *Cereb Blood Flow Metab.* 2002;22(1):21–28.
12. Baker AJ, Zoronow MH, Grafe MR, et al. Hypothermia prevents ischemia-induced increases in hippocampal glycine concentrations in rabbits. *Stroke.* 1991;22(5): 666–673.
13. Huang ZG, Xue D, Preston E, et al. Biphasic opening of the blood–brain barrier following transient focal ischemia: Effects of hypothermia. *Can J Neurol Sci.* 1999;26(4):298–304.
14. Clasen RA, Pandolfi S, Russell J, et al. Hypothermia and hypotension in experimental cerebral edema. *Arch Neurol.* 1968;19(5):472–486.
15. Kaste M, Fogelholm R, Rissanen A. Economic burden of stroke and the evaluation of new therapies. *Public Health.* 1998;112(2):103–112.
16. DeGraba TJ, Pettigrew LC. Why do neuroprotective drugs work in animals but not humans? *Neurol Clin.* 2000;18(2):475–493.
17. Kwiatkowski TG, Libman RB, Frankel M, et al. Effects of tissue plasminogen activator for acute ischemic stroke at one year. National Institute of Neurological Disorders and Stroke Recombinant Tissue Plasminogen Activator Stroke Study Group. *N Engl J Med.* 1999;340(23):1781–1787.
18. Reith J, Jorgensen HS, Pedersen PM, et al. Body temperature in acute stroke: Relation to stroke severity, infarct size, mortality, and outcome. *Lancet.* 1996;347(8999):422–425.
19. Feigin VL, Anderson CS, Rodgers A, et al. The emerging role of induced hypothermia in the management of acute stroke. *J Clin Neurosci.* 2002;9(5):502–507.
20. Hanley DF. Review of critical care and emergency approaches to stroke. *Stroke.* 2003;34(2):362–364.
21. Schwab S, Schwarz S, Bertram M, et al. Moderate hypothermia in the treatment of patients with severe middle cerebral artery infarction. *Stroke.* 1998;29(12):2461–2466.
22. Schwab S, Georgiadis D, Berouschot J, et al. Feasibility and safety of moderate hypothermia after massive hemispheric infarction. *Stroke.* 2001;32(9):2033–2035.
23. Krieger DW, De Georgia MA, Abou-Chebel A, et al. Cooling for acute ischemic brain damage (COOL AID): An open pilot study of induced hypothermia in acute ischemic stroke. *Stroke.* 2001;32(8):1847–1854.
24. Berrouschot J, Sterker M, Bettin S, et al. Mortality of space-occupying ('malignant') middle cerebral artery infarction under conservative intensive care. *Intensive Care Med.* 1998;24(6):620–623.
25. Steiner T, Friede T, Aschoff A, et al. Effect and feasibility of controlled rewarming after moderate hypothermia in stroke patients with malignant infarction of the middle cerebral artery. *Stroke.* 2001;32(12):2833–2835.
26. Hammer MD, Krieger DW. Hypothermia for acute ischemic stroke: Not just another neuroprotectant. *Neurologist.* 2003;9(6):280–289.
27. Kasner SE, Wein T, Piriyawat P, et al. Acetaminophen for altering body temperature in acute stroke: A randomized clinical trial [Editorial Comment: A Randomized Clinical Trial.] *Stroke.* 2002;33(1): 130–135.
28. Adams H, Adams R, Del Zoppo G, et al. Guidelines for the early management of patients with ischemic stroke: 2005 guidelines update a scientific statement from the Stroke Council of the American Heart Association/American Stroke Association. *Stroke.* 2005;36(4):916–923.
29. Wang Y, Lim LL, Levi C, et al. Influence of admission body temperature on stroke mortality. *Stroke.* 2000;31(2):404–409.
30. Hajat C, Hajat S, Sharma P. Effects of poststroke pyrexia on stroke outcome: A meta-analysis of studies in patients. *Stroke.* 2000;31(2):410–414.
31. Kammersgaard LP, Rasmussen BH, Jorgensen HS, et al. Feasibility and safety of inducing modest hypothermia in awake patients with acute stroke through surface cooling: A case-control study: The Copenhagen Stroke Study. *Stroke.* 2000;31(9):2251–2256.
32. The Hypothermia after Cardiac Arrest Study Group. Mild therapeutic hypothermia to improve the neurologic outcome after cardiac arrest. *N Engl J Med.* 2002;346(8):549–556.
33. Bernard SA, Gray TW, Buist MD, et al. Treatment of comatose survivors of out-of-hospital cardiac arrest with induced hypothermia. *N Engl J Med.* 2002;346(8):557–563.
34. Nolan JP, Morley PT, Vanden Hoek TL, et al. Therapeutic hypothermia after cardiac arrest: An advisory statement by the Advanced Life Support Task Force of the International Liaison Committee on Resuscitation. *Circulation.* 2003;108(1):118–121.
35. Els T, Oehm E, Voigt S, et al. Safety and therapeutical benefit of hemicraniectomy combined with mild hypothermia in comparison with hemicraniectomy alone in patients with malignant ischemic stroke. *Cerebrovasc Dis.* 2006;21(1–2):79–85. Epub 2005 Nov 28.
36. Sosin DM, Sniezek JE, Thurman DJ. Incidence of mild and moderate brain injury in the United States, 1991. *Brain Inj.* 1996;10(1):47–54.
37. Ghajar J. Traumatic brain injury. *Lancet.* 2000;356(9233):923–929.
38. Mellergard P, Nordstrom CH. Intracerebral temperature in neurosurgical patients. *Neurosurgery.* 1991;28(5):709–713.
39. Schwab S, Spranger M, Aschoff A, et al. Brain temperature monitoring and modulation in patients with severe MCA infarction. *Neurology.* 1997;48(3):762–767.

40. Clifton GL, Miller ER, Choi SC, et al. Lack of effect of induction of hypothermia after acute brain injury. *N Engl J Med.* 2001;344(8):556–563.
41. Polderman KH, Tjong Tjin Joe R, Peerdeman SM, et al. Effects of therapeutic hypothermia on intracranial pressure and outcome in patients with severe head injury. *Intensive Care Med.* 2002;28(11):1563–1573.
42. Zhi D, Zhang S, Lin X. Study on therapeutic mechanism and clinical effect of mild hypothermia in patients with severe head injury. *Surg Neurol.* 2003;59(5):381–385.
43. Mokhtarani M, Mahqoub AN, Moriska N, et al. Buspirone and meperidine synergistically reduce the shivering threshold. *Anesth Analg.* 2001;93(5):1233–1239.
44. Sund-Levander M, Wahren LK. Assessment and prevention of shivering in patients with severe cerebral injury. A pilot study. *J Clin Nurs.* 2000;9(1):55–61.
45. Polderman KH. Application of therapeutic hypothermia in the intensive care unit. Opportunities and pitfalls of a promising treatment modality. Part 2: Practical aspects and side effects. *Intensive Care Med.* 2004;30(5):757–769.
46. Polderman KH, Peerdeman SM, Girbes AR. Hypophosphatemia and hypomagnesemia induced by cooling in patients with severe head injury. *J Neurosurg.* 2001;94(5): 697–705.
47. Kimura A, Sakurada S, Okhuni H, et al. Moderate hypothermia delays proinflammatory cytokine production of human peripheral blood mononuclear cells. *Crit Care Med.* 2002;30(7):1499–1502.
48. Salman H, Bergman M, Bessler H, et al. Hypothermia affects the phagocytic activity of rat peritoneal macrophages. *Acta Physiol Scand.* 2000;168(3):431–436.

CHAPTER 114

Hyperthermia

Deborah M. Green

OBJECTIVES

- To distinguish fever and hyperthermia
- To discuss the significance of hyperthermia in brain injury
- To describe the early signs of heat stroke and its pathophysiology
- To describe the signs of malignant hyperthermia and its treatment
- To explain ways to avoid neuroleptic malignant syndrome and how to treat it when it does occur

CASE VIGNETTE

A 37-year-old man with no medical history was hiking on a hot, humid day when he complained of dizziness and headache. En route to the emergency room he was agitated, and on arrival he had a generalized tonic–clonic seizure. His skin was dry and hot, and he was found to have a temperature of 41°C. He remained unresponsive and hypotensive and had to be intubated and placed on an intravenous infusion of norepinephrine. A computed tomographic (CT) scan of his brain showed no abnormalities. Lumbar puncture demonstrated normal cerebrospinal fluid (CSF) with no evidence of meningitis. Laboratory testing showed elevated serum creatinine level of 2.5 mg/dL, blood urea nitrogen (BUN) level of 33 mg/dL, and creatine kinase (CK) level of 5,024 IU/L. The prothrombin time (PT) was elevated with an international normalized ratio (INR) of 1.6. A comprehensive toxicology screen was negative.

Fever and Hyperthermia

Hyperthermia is a distinct entity from fever. Fever is generally defined as a body temperature >38.3°C and is the result of an increased hypothalamic temperature set point caused by an infectious or inflammatory illness. This results from hypothalamic prostaglandin E synthesis stimulated by systemic inflammatory pyrogens. Hyperthermia, on the other hand, refers to clinical conditions where the body temperature exceeds the hypothalamic set point (1). This can occur when an exogenous or an endogenous source of heat production overwhelms the heat-dissipating mechanisms of the body. An example of an exogenous source would be "classic" heat stroke, whereas examples of an endogenous source include "exertional" heat stroke, malignant hyperthermia, and neuroleptic malignant syndrome.

The differential diagnosis for hyperthermia also includes such conditions as thyrotoxicosis, pheochromocytoma, meningitis, drug reaction, and "central fever." Certain drugs can impair thermoregulation leading to hyperthermia. This list includes amphetamines, cocaine, opiates, antihistamines, serotonin reuptake inhibitors, beta blockers, and diuretics. *Central fever* is a controversial diagnosis and some advocate eliminating this term. It has been described in patients with an unexplained high, refractory temperature usually after a large intracranial hemorrhage, particularly with an anterior communicating artery aneurysm rupture. It is not clear, however, whether this reflects fever (hypothalamic set point elevation) or hyperthermia. Direct damage to the preoptic region, disinhibition of thermogenesis at the lower midbrain level, and prostaglandin production have each been a suggested mechanism (1,2).

Hyperthermia is toxic to ischemic neurons and is known to be associated with a poor outcome in stroke and traumatic brain injury (TBI). In animal studies of both stroke and TBI, 1 to 2 degrees of hyperthermia leads to worsened outcome (3,4). A prospective study of 183 patients found that those having a temperature 38°C or greater within a week of stroke onset were more likely to have a poor outcome (5). Hyperthermia has also been associated with larger infarct volume and worse outcome when occurring within 24 hours of stroke onset (6). Other studies of ischemic stroke confirm higher rates of worse outcome and mortality with hyperthermia (7,8). Poor outcome has also been associated with hyperthermia in intracerebral hemorrhage, aneurysmal subarachnoid hemorrhage (SAH), and after cardiac arrest (9–11). Hyperthermia is specifically associated with higher intracranial pressure in both SAH and TBI (12).

Heat Stroke

DEFINITION

Heat stroke is defined by a core body temperature >40°C with central nervous system (CNS) and multiorgan dysfunction resulting from environmental heat (*classic*) or strenuous exercise (*exertional*).

EPIDEMIOLOGY

In one study of an urban area in the United States during a heat wave, 17 to 26 cases per 100,000 people were reported, mostly among the very young or elderly without air conditioning (13). This also tends to occur in young people who exercise for a prolonged time in a hot environment. In Saudi Arabia, the incidence of heat stroke can run as high as 1,800 per 100,000 population (14).

ETIOLOGY AND PATHOGENESIS

Heat stroke is thought to be the result of thermoregulatory failure combined with an exaggerated acute phase response from either high environmental temperature or strenuous exercise (14). Normally, a rise in the temperature of blood by $<1°C$ leads to activation of peripheral and hypothalamic heat receptors that signal the hypothalamic regulatory center. This results in increased delivery of heated blood to the body surface by sympathetic cutaneous vasodilation. Body temperature elevation causes tachycardia, increased cardiac output, increased minute ventilation, and increased sweating, resulting in greater salt and water loss. Dehydration and salt loss can lead to impaired thermoregulation. Inability to increase cardiac output because of salt and water loss or cardiovascular disease or medications can increase susceptibility to heat stroke.

As blood is shunted to the body surface, there is diminished perfusion to the viscera. This can lead to intestinal ischemia resulting in increased generation of reactive oxygen and nitrogen species that, in turn, can increase intestinal permeability. This can be followed by leakage of endotoxins from the intestine to the circulation, enhancing the acute phase inflammatory response with increased production of cytokines and nitric oxide. The potential final result is thermal dysregulation, hypotension, and heat stroke (14).

Systemic inflammation is induced via IL-1 and a number of cytokines. Nearly all cells respond to heating by producing heat-shock proteins. Heat-shock proteins can protect cells by binding to partially folded or misfolded proteins, preventing their denaturation (14). Another suggested mechanism is that the heat-shock proteins regulate the baroreceptor response to heat, thereby lessening the hypotension and bradycardia and conferring cardiovascular protection (15). Aging and genetic polymorphisms can be associated with a low level of expression of heat-shock proteins. Thermoregulatory failure, exaggeration of the acute phase response, and change in expression of heat shock proteins, thus, can be the contributing factors to progression to heat stroke.

The multiorgan dysfunction that occurs with heat stroke is the result of the direct cytotoxicity of heat, the exaggerated inflammatory response, and also from the coagulopathic response. As heat stroke occurs, coagulation factors are activated with decreased levels of proteins C and S and antithrombin. Fibrinolysis is also activated, leading to vascular endothelial damage, microthrombosis, disseminated intravascular coagulation, and, finally, multiorgan damage.

PATHOLOGY

In individuals subjected to heat stress, there is enhanced expression of heat shock proteins in muscle and blood.

CLINICAL MANIFESTATIONS AND SPECIAL SITUATIONS

Heat exhaustion, a more common, milder illness than heat stroke, consists of hyperthermia (between 37°C and 40°C), dehydration, and oliguria, with the patient complaining of thirst, weakness, fatigue, muscle cramping, and paresthesias, which can progress to headaches, delirium, incoordination, and dizziness. It is not known why some people progress from heat exhaustion to heat stroke. Those at highest risk for heat stroke are the elderly, infants, and young people who exercise excessively in the heat.

Heat stroke in its early phase consists of hot and dry skin, headache, somnolence, confusion, and agitation, which can progress in its later stages to seizures, focal neurologic deficits, pinpoint pupils, coma, and even death. Initial signs can be as subtle as inappropriate behavior or impaired judgment. Seizures can occur, particularly during cooling. Anhidrosis usually occurs and the skin appears dry and hot. Vomiting, diarrhea, tachycardia, hypotension, and tachypnea (often with a P_{CO_2} of <20 mm Hg) are common. Respiratory alkalosis occurs in classic heat stroke and a mixed respiratory alkalosis and lactic acidosis occurs in exertional heat stroke. Initial hypophosphatemia, hypokalemia, and hypercalcemia convert to hyperphosphatemia, hyperkalemia, and hypocalcemia with cooling. Rhabdomyolysis can occur with exertional heat stroke. Acute renal failure, adult respiratory distress syndrome, myocardial infarction, intestinal ischemia and infarction, liver damage, and disseminated intravascular coagulation with severe thrombocytopenia are all sequelae of heat stroke.

DIAGNOSTIC APPROACH

Diagnosis of heat stroke is based on the clinical manifestations occurring in the setting of either exertional or environmental heat.

TREATMENT

Patients with heat stroke should be cooled immediately and supported in terms of their multiorgan dysfunction. Normalizing the core temperature inhibits fibrinolysis but, as in sepsis, activation of the coagulation cascade continues. Cooling can be accomplished with conduction (decreased room temperature), evaporation (ice and cold water), and convection (fan). Intravascular cooling devices are now being utilized as well. Shivering can be avoided with use of warmer water and hot moving air. Dantrolene was found not to be useful in one study of heat stroke (16). Studies in animals have found IL-1-receptor antagonists, endotoxin antibodies, and corticosteroids were associated with improved survival (17–19). Recombinant activated protein C replacement, used to attenuate the coagulation and inflammation in severe sepsis, can also help in heat stroke (14,20).

Ideally, the best treatment is prevention. Education includes recommendations to decrease physical activity and increase salt and water intake during heat waves. Those who are at highest risk, including the very young, the elderly, and people on medications, such as diuretics and anticholinergic agents that impair sweating, should be advised to maximize their time in air-conditioned environments. Future research may look at other methods of prevention. Partial, although not excessive, upregulation of heat shock proteins may enhance tolerance of heat and protect cells. Salicylates and nonsteroidal anti-inflammatory medications induce transcription and translation of heat-shock proteins, and their use had been suggested for this purpose (14,21). Oral glutamine enhanced heat-shock protein expression and was associated with lower mortality in a rat model of heat stroke (22). Further research is needed to determine if these are efficacious methods for prevention of heat shock in humans.

Heat stroke is a preventable condition and knowledge of its early signs and its treatment can help reduce risk of progression to multiorgan failure and death.

Malignant Hyperthermia

DEFINITION

Malignant hyperthermia (MH) is an inherited skeletal muscle disorder first described in 1960 and characterized by rapidly rising body temperature, rigidity, and hypermetabolism occurring shortly after receiving general anesthesia (23).

EPIDEMIOLOGY

MH occurs in 1 of every 10,000 to 50,000 patients receiving either inhalational anesthesia (e.g., halothane, isoflurane) or succinylcholine (24). The mean age of occurrence is 15 years, but can occur at any age, including infants and the elderly. It is most common in whites of northern European descent.

ETIOLOGY AND PATHOGENESIS

MH is a metabolic polymyopathy inherited as an autosomal dominant trait. With MH, calcium is released from the sarcoplasmic reticulum at an excessively high rate, leading to sustained hypermetabolism. Enhanced metabolism leads to increased lactate production, increased adenosine triphosphate (ATP) and oxygen consumption, and increased carbon dioxide (CO_2) and heat production. Uncoupling of oxidative phosphorylation with excess metabolic breakdown likely contributes to activation of the sympathetic nervous system and release of catecholamines (25). In its later stages, ATP production stops, resulting in failure of membrane pumps, with electrolyte, CK, and myoglobin leakage causing arrhythmias, end-organ damage, and death. It has been suggested that halothane can cause release of calcium from the sarcoplasmic reticulum and prevent its reaccumulation, thus impairing muscle relaxation. The putative defect is in the ryanodine receptor or another receptor that controls the structure of the calcium channel (26). Hyperthermia can be caused by muscle activation or be a direct effect of the anesthetic on the thermoregulatory centers.

PATHOLOGY

If the patient dies shortly after MH occurs, the muscle may appear normal under light microscopy. If the patient survives for several days, the muscle biopsy may show segmental necrosis and phagocytosis of sarcoplasm without signs of inflammation. Regenerative activity and rhabdomyolysis cores are also noted (26).

CLINICAL MANIFESTATIONS AND SPECIAL SITUATIONS

MH usually starts within 1 hour of induction of anesthesia, but can occur up to several hours postoperatively. An early sign of MH is a rapid rise in end tidal CO_2. Arterial CO_2 may >100 mm Hg and blood pH may drop to 7 (26). Other clinical signs of MH are generalized rigidity, especially of the masseter muscle, hyperthermia (although not always), tachycardia, tachypnea, cyanosis, rhabdomyolysis, acidosis, hyperkalemia, elevated CK level (usually >20,000 U/L), and myoglobinuria. Disseminated intravascular coagulopathy, pulmonary edema, and cerebral edema can occur later. Neurologic and renal failure can occur up to several days after the onset of MH. Hyperkalemia can lead to cardiac arrest. The mortality rate for MH has dropped from 70% to 80% in 1960 to about 5% to 10% today (24,27).

DIAGNOSTIC APPROACH

The diagnosis of MH is based on the clinical setting and manifestations. Certain patients have different gene mutations on chromosome 19 for the skeletal muscle ryanodine (calcium release channel) receptor. This can help predict susceptibility in some patients. The caffeine-halothane contracture test involves a muscle biopsy at one of the MH diagnostic centers in the United States. This can be utilized for definitive diagnosis of a patient and other family members. Some susceptible individuals may have certain phenotypic features, such as short stature, ptosis, high-arched palate, and kyphoscoliosis, known as *King-Denborough syndrome.* Two disorders involving the ryanodine receptor, Duchenne-Becker muscular dystrophy and central core myopathy, are associated with MH (26).

TREATMENT

Immediate treatment of MH is to stop the anesthetic agent and hyperventilate the patient with 100% oxygen. Hyperkalemia is treated with intravenous bicarbonate (1 to 2 mg/kg), insulin (10 U with dextrose), or both. Cooling measures are introduced, as needed. Arrhythmias need to be treated accordingly, avoiding calcium channel blockers. Electrolytes, arterial blood gases, myoglobin, CK, and coagulation studies should be monitored. Urine output should be kept >2 mL/kg/hour to avoid renal failure. Recommendations are to monitor the patient in the intensive care unit (ICU) a minimum of 36 hours after onset.

Dantrolene, a skeletal muscle relaxant, inhibits the release of calcium from the sarcoplasmic reticulum and has an onset of action of 2 to 3 minutes when given intravenously and a half-life of 5 to 12 hours. The Malignant Hyperthermia Association of the United States (MHAUS) recommends an initial loading dose of intravenous dantrolene (2.5 mg/kg) with repeated doses as needed up to a total of 10 mg/kg. This is followed by 1 mg/kg every 4 to 6 hours for 24 to 72 hours (24).

Halothane, succinylcholine, and other volatile anesthetic agents should be avoided in any future surgeries for these patients. Nitrous oxide, thiopental, fentanyl, or local anesthesia should be used. Intravenous dantrolene (2.5 mg/kg) is given over 1 hour before anesthesia to help prevent MH.

Careful history-taking to determine whether any family history of MH exists should be done before anesthesia induction. After induction, a rapid rise in end tidal CO_2 should be an early indicator and prompt treatment should be initiated. Discussions with the patient and family regarding obtaining a muscle biopsy for definitive diagnosis at an approved MH testing facility and registering with the North American Malignant Hyperthermia Registry should occur.

Neuroleptic Malignant Syndrome

DEFINITION

Neuroleptic malignant syndrome (NMS), also known as *parkinsonism-hyperpyrexia syndrome,* consists of severe hyperthermia and rigidity in patients either receiving dopamine-2 receptor blocking agents or those who have recently decreased or stopped their dopaminergic medication.

EPIDEMIOLOGY

NMS occurs in 0.2% to 1.5% of patients receiving dopamine-2 receptor blocking drugs (28). It usually occurs in young males and especially in patients who are dehydrated, agitated, or who have had previous electroconvulsive therapy (29,30). NMS is more common with rapid and parenteral administration of the drug, a rapid increase in dosing, and simultaneous use of two or more neuroleptics (31). It also can occur in patients with Parkinson disease, particularly those with moderate to advanced disease, after a decrease in dose or discontinuation of their dopaminergic medication. Without early recognition and treatment, the mortality rate is 15% to 30% (32).

ETIOLOGY AND PATHOGENESIS

NMS occurs as an idiosyncratic reaction to neuroleptic agents. An acute blockade of nigrostriatal and hypothalamic dopamine pathways occurs in NMS. Decreased dopamine signaling is the result of introduction of agents that block dopamine signaling or sudden withdrawal of dopamine agents. The sympathetic nervous system is also involved because patients with NMS have been shown to have markedly elevated blood and cerebrospinal fluid (CSF) catecholamine levels (25). Some suggest NMS is partially the result of direct effects on skeletal muscle (31). As in MH, susceptibility to NMS is likely a genetic factor.

PATHOLOGY

On muscle biopsy, diffuse myonecrosis is seen (32).

CLINICAL MANIFESTATIONS AND SPECIAL SITUATIONS

The onset of NMS is usually within a month of starting a dopamine receptor blocking drug or of increasing the dosage. Up to 16%, however, occur within the first 24 hours and 30% occur within 2 days (28). The clinical manifestations evolve over 24 to 72 hours and include severe hyperthermia (usually much >38°C), profuse sweating, catatonic rigidity (usually axial), and delirium. Although rigidity is usually present, dystonia, chorea, or a parkinsonian appearance are sometimes seen. The patient may progress to become stuporous and develop autonomic instability with tachycardia, tachypnea, labile blood pressure, diaphoresis, and incontinence. In 70% of 340 cases in one study, mental status changes occurred first, followed by rigidity, hyperthermia, and autonomic dysfunction (33). Hypoxic brain injury can occur because of hypotension and shock.

DIAGNOSTIC APPROACH

The diagnosis of NMS is based on the clinical setting and typical manifestations. A brain imaging study, either magnetic resonance imaging (MRI) or CT, and a lumbar puncture should be considered to rule out other possible causes for mental status changes. Included in the differential diagnosis of NMS is serotonin syndrome, which can occur after serotonergic antidepressant use. One distinguishing feature is that serotonin syndrome cases typically present within 24 hours of patients starting their medication, whereas NMS can occur at any time in the drug course, with peak symptoms taking days to occur. Also, vomiting, diarrhea, clonus, hyperreflexia, and myoclonus are commonly reported with serotonin syndrome and, rarely, reported with NMS (25).

The CK level in NMS is quite elevated and can range from 10,000 to >70,000 IU/L and the white blood cell count is often elevated without bandemia. Renal failure can occur owing to myoglobinuria. Low serum iron levels have been described in patients with NMS and have been thought possibly to be a precipitant (34).

TREATMENT

Initial treatment is immediate discontinuation of the causative dopamine blocking agent or, in the case of patients with Parkinson disease, to restart or increase the dose of a recently discontinued or decreased dosage of a dopaminergic drug. The patient should be kept well hydrated and cooling measures should be instituted emergently. Any anticholinergic agent that can inhibit heat dissipation should be tapered (to avoid rebound rigidity) and discontinued. Supportive care should include deep venous thrombosis prophylaxis.

Bromocriptine (a central dopamine agonist) can be given orally at 2.5 to 10 mg every 4 hours, being careful to avoid hypotension. The dose can be increased to as much as 50 mg/day. Other potential side effects are dyskinesia and erythematous, tender lower extremities (25). Subcutaneous apomorphine is an alternative dopamine agonist that can give a rapid response. In cases of significant hyperthermia, dantrolene (a skeletal muscle relaxant) can be administered intravenously (1 to 3 mg/kg every 8 hours) or orally (a dose of 100 to 400 mg/day divided four times a day) (25). Liver toxicity is a potential side effect of dantrolene and it should not be administered to patients with liver disease. Amantadine has been used at times for NMS. A retrospective review of more than 700 NMS cases found that bromocriptine, dantrolene, or amantadine reduced mortality more than supportive care alone (35). Benzodiazepines have also been used for the anxiety and catatonia associated with NMS. Reports in the literature describe the efficacy of methylprednisolone (Solu-Medrol) and of plasmapheresis in these patients (36,37). Electroconvulsive therapy has been utilized in medically refractory cases because it is thought to facilitate brain dopamine activity, although controlled studies are lacking (38).

Treatment should be continued for at least 10 days after resolution of symptoms to avoid recurrence. Recovery usually occurs over 1 to 2 weeks, but neuropsychologic symptoms can last for weeks to months (39). Recurrence when a dopamine receptor blocking drug is reintroduced occurs in <15% of cases. The putative agent, however, should be avoided in the future. Although the more highly potent neuroleptic medications are more likely to be associated with NMS, even the less-potent antiemetics, such as Promethazine, and the newer atypical antipsychotic drugs can be associated with NMS (32,40,41).

A high clinical suspicion of NMS is needed for rapid diagnosis, which can be life-saving. NMS can be avoided by slowly increasing dosages of neuroleptic medications and by not abruptly withdrawing dopaminergic drugs.

CLINICAL RECOMMENDATIONS OF THE VIGNETTE

The 37-year-old man described in the case vignette was diagnosed with exertional heat stroke. Cooling measures were promptly instituted with cooling the room temperature and body surface cooling using cooling blankets, ice water, and fans. Acetaminophen was administered via nasogastric tube with a goal of normalizing the core body temperature to 37°C. His rhabdomyolysis was treated with aggressive intravenous fluid administration and diuretics to maintain a urine output of >200 mL/hour. Aggressive cooling measures had to be maintained for several days to normalize the body temperature. He began to awaken after 2 days, renal function improved over 5 days, and he was extubated 1 week after admission with no neurologic sequelae.

SUMMARY

Hyperthermia, whether induced by environmental or exertional heat, or by toxins such as anesthetics or neuroleptic medications, can rapidly result in brain injury and multiorgan damage, making the recognition of its cause and its treatment crucial in avoiding further morbidity and mortality. All of these conditions consist of a disturbance of normal thermoregulation resulting in activation of the hypothalamus and sympathetic nervous system coupling heat generation with impaired heat dissipation. Cooling measures are the common treatment for each of these conditions, but some differences in treatment require careful history-taking and physical examination for an accurate diagnosis. Improving our understanding of the pathophysiology of these syndromes may help further research on targeted treatments to reduce the persistently high morbidity and mortality rates.

REFERENCES

1. Fever and infections in the neurological intensive care unit. In: Ropper AH, et al. Neurological and Neurosurgical Intensive Care. Fourth Edition. Philadelphia: Lippincott Williams & Wilkins, 2004;113–114.
2. Shibata M. Hyperthermia in brain hemorrhage. *Med Hypoth.* 1998;50:185–190.
3. Kim Y, Busto R, Dietrich WD, et al. Delayed postischemic hyperthermia in awake rats worsens the histopathologic outcome of transient forebrain ischemia. *Stroke.* 1996;27:2274–2281.
4. Dietrich WD, Alonso O, Halley M, et al. Delayed posttraumatic brain hyperthermia worsens outcome after fluid percussion brain injury: A light and electron microscopic study in rats. *Neurosurgery.* 1996;38:533–541.
5. Azzimondi G, Bassein L, Nonino F, et al. Fever in acute stroke worsens prognosis. A prospective study. *Stroke.* 1995;26:2040–2043.
6. Castillo J, Davalos A, Marrugat J, et al. Timing for fever-related brain damage in acute ischemic stroke. *Stroke.* 1998;29:2455–2460.
7. Wang Y, Lim LL-Y, Levi C, et al. Influence of admission body temperature on stroke mortality. *Stroke.* 2000;31:404–409.
8. Hajat C, Hajat S, Sharma P. Effects of post-stroke pyrexia on stroke outcome. A meta-analysis of studies on patients. *Stroke.* 2000;31:410–414.
9. Schwarz S, Häfner K, Aschoff A, et al. Incidence and prognostic significance of fever following intracerebral hemorrhage. *Neurology.* 2000;54:354–361.
10. Oliveira-Filho J, Ezzeddine MA, Segal AZ, et al. Fever in subarachnoid hemorrhage. Relationship to vasospasm and outcome. *Neurology.* 2001:56:1299–1304.
11. Zeiner A, Holzer M, Sterz F, et al. Hyperthermia after cardiac arrest is associated with an unfavorable neurologic outcome. *Arch Intern Med.* 2001;161:2007–2012.
12. Rossi S, Roncati Zanier E, Mauri I, et al. Brain temperature, body core temperature, and intracranial pressure in acute cerebral damage. *J Neurol Neurosurg Psychiatry.* 2001;71: 448–454.
13. Jones TS, Liang AP, Kilbourne EM, et al. Morbidity and mortality associated with the July 1980 heat wave in St. Louis and Kansas City, Mo. *JAMA.* 1982;247:3327–3331.
14. Bouchama A, Knochel J. Heat stroke. *N Engl J Med.* 2002;346:1978–1988.
15. Li PL, Chao YM, Chan SH, et al. Potentiation of baroreceptor reflex response by heat shock protein 70 in nucleus tractus solitarii confers cardiovascular protection during heatstroke. *Circulation.* 2001;103:2114–2119.
16. Bouchama A, Cafege A, Devol EB, et al. Ineffectiveness of dantrolene sodium in the treatment of heatstroke. *Crit Care Med.* 1991;19:176–180.
17. Lin MT, Liu HH, Yang YL. Involvement of interleukin-1 receptor mechanisms in development of arterial hypotension in rat heatstroke. *J Physiol.* 1997;273: H2072–H2077.
18. Gathiram P, Wells MT, Brock-Utne JG, et al. Antilipopolysaccharide improves survival in primates subjected to heat stroke. *Circulation Shock.* 1987;23:157–164.
19. Liu CC, Chien CH, Lin MT. Glucocorticosteroids reduce interleukin-1 concentration and result in neuroprotective effects in rat heatstroke. *J Physiol.* 2000;27:333–343.
20. Bernard GR, Vincent J-L, Laterre P-F, et al. Efficacy and safety of recombinant human activated protein C for severe sepsis. *N Engl J Med.* 2001;344:699–709.
21. Polla BS, Bachelet M, Elia G, et al. Stress proteins in inflammation. *Ann NY Acad Sci.* 1998;851:75–85.
22. Singleton KD, Wischmeyer PE. Oral glutamine enhances heat shock protein expression and improves survival following hyperthermia. *Shock.* 2006;25:295–299.
23. Denborough MA, Lovel RH. Anesthetic deaths in a family. *Lancet.* 1960;2:45.
24. McCarthy EJ. Malignant hyperthermia. Pathophysiology, clinical presentation, and treatment. *American Association of Critical-Care Nurses—Clinical Issues.* 2004;15: 231–237.
25. Rusyniak DE, Sprague JE. Toxin-induced hyperthermic syndromes. *Med Clin N Am.* 2005;89:1277–1296.
26. The hereditary myotonias and periodic paralyses (the channelopathies). In: Victor M, Ropper AH, eds. *Adams and Victor's Principles of Neurology.* Seventh edition. New York: McGraw-Hill, 2001:1563.
27. Denborough M. Malignant hyperthermia. *Lancet.* 1998;91:352:1131–1136.
28. Caroff SN, Mann SC. Neuroleptic malignant syndrome. *Psychopharm Bull.* 1988;24: 24–29.
29. Sachdev P, Mason C, Hadzi-Pavlovic D. Case-control study of neuroleptic malignant syndrome. *Am J Psychiatry.* 1997;154:1156–1158.
30. Naganuma H, Fujii I. Incidence and risk factors in neuroleptic malignant syndrome. *Acta Psych Scand.* 1994;90:424–426.
31. Bhanushali MJ, Tuite PJ. The evaluation and management of patients with neuroleptic malignant syndrome. *Neurol Clin N Am.* 2004;22:389–411.
32. Disorders of the nervous system due to drugs and other chemical agents. In: Victor M, Ropper AH, eds. *Adams and Victor's Principles of Neurology.* Seventh edition. New York: McGraw-Hill, 2001:1265.
33. Velamoor VR, Norman RM, Caroff SN, et al. Progression of symptoms in neuroleptic malignant syndrome. *J Nerv Mental Dis.* 1994;182:168–173.
34. Rosebush PI, Mazurek MF. Serum iron and neuroleptic malignant syndrome. *Lancet.* 1991;338:149–151.
35. Rosebush PI, Stewart T, Mazurek MF. The treatment of neuroleptic malignant syndrome. Are dantrolene and bromocriptine useful adjuncts to supportive care? *Br J Psych.* 1991;159:709–712.
36. Sato Y, Asoh T, Metoki N, et al. Efficacy of methylprednisolone pulse therapy on neuroleptic malignant syndrome in Parkinson's disease. *J Neurol Neurosurg Psychiatry.* 2003;74: 574–576.
37. Gaitini L, Fradis M, Vaida S, et al. Plasmapheresis in neuroleptic malignant syndrome. *Anaesthesia.* 1997;52:165–168.
38. Davis JM, Janicak PG, Sakkas P, et al. Electroconvulsive therapy in the treatment of the neuroleptic malignant syndrome. *Convulsive Therapy.* 1991;7:111–120.
39. Adityanjee A, Sajatovic M, Munshi KR. Neuropsychiatric sequelae of neuroleptic malignant syndrome. *Clin Neuropharm.* 2005;28:197–204.
40. Ananth J, Parameswaran S, Gunatilake S, et al. Neuroleptic malignant syndrome and atypical antipsychotic drugs. *J Clin Psych.* 2004;65:464–470.
41. Filice GA, McDougall BC, Ercan-Fang N, et al. Neuroleptic malignant syndrome associated with olanzapine. *Annals of Pharmacotherapy.* 1998;32:1158–1159.

CHAPTER **115**

Disorders Associated with Diving, Decompression, and Gas Bubbles

James T. Boyd • Kenneth M. LeDez

OBJECTIVES

- To distinguish clinically the key disorders related to decompression and gas embolism
- To describe the at risk populations and risk factors associated with decompression illness and gas embolism
- To discuss the diagnostic approach to suspected cases
- To explain how to determine the necessity for hyperbaric oxygen therapy
- To explain the institution of appropriate hyperbaric oxygen or other treatment

CASE VIGNETTE

The cases summarized in Table 115-1 illustrate four different patients seen at the Centre for Offshore and Remote Medicine (MEDICOR), Faculty of Medicine, Memorial University of Newfoundland.

DEFINITION

Decompression disorders have been classically divided into three categories (1,2): *type 1* (minor—musculoskeletal, skin, lymphatic, fatigue); *type 2* (serious—neurologic, cardiorespiratory ("chokes"), audiovestibular, shock); and *arterial gas embolism.* This categorization has significant limitations and does not adequately guide treatment or reflect the common patterns of injury. A consensus exists among hyperbaric physicians (1,2) to describe these disorders in terms of: *Evolution* (progressive, static, spontaneously resolving, and relapsing); *manifestations* (pain—limb or girdle), cutaneous, neurologic, audiovestibular, pulmonary, lymphatic, and constitutional); *time of onset, gas burden, and evidence of barotraumas.*

Although some debate the appropriate terminology, essentially two key entities exist: *Decompression sickness* (1) (commonly called the "bends") is caused by gas coming out of solution and the bubbles then enlarging as ambient pressure decreases (Henry's (3) and Boyle's Laws (4), respectively). Bubbles can be intravascular (usually venous) or form within tissues (autochthonous) (5). During time spent at increased pressure, excess gas is taken up by tissues, which are then super saturated once a pressure reduction occurs (6). *Arterial gas embolism* refers to the situation whereby gas bubbles enter the arterial circulation and cause obstruction of flow and complex secondary effects (7). In some cases, it may not be possible to distinguish whether the clinical findings are caused by decompression sickness (DCS), arterial gas embolism (AGE), or mixed etiology; in this setting, the encompassing term "decompression illness" is generally preferred (1).

EPIDEMIOLOGY

The population at risk ranges from recreational, technical, occupational, and military divers; to persons working under increased pressure environments and to patients having routine medical procedures. Knowledge of the technical and operational aspects of each situation facilitates diagnosis and management. Dysbaric events are most likely to occur among recreational SCUBA divers (who number approximately 5 million in the United States) (8). Occupational and military divers are fewer in number, although typically have greater exposure (higher "gas load"), thus increasing their relative risk of decompression illness (DCI). Divers Alert Network (DAN) observational data reports an incidence of 2 to 3 cases of DCI per 10,000 dives (9). Possible factors associated with an increased risk of DCI include the depth and pattern of the dive, dehydration or hemoconcentration before diving, patent foramen ovale (PFO), poor physical fitness, personal history of DCI, high body fat content, advanced age, and female gender (2,10). The later two are speculated to indirectly result from greater body fat composition, and resultant increased nitrogen storage capacity (5). PFO appears to be an independent risk factor for all subsets of neurologic DCI, with increasing risk with greater PFO size (11–13).

TABLE 115-1. Four Clinical Cases

	Case A	*Case B*	*Case C*	*Case D*
Patient	Healthy male recreational diver: age early 30s	Healthy teenage female: first open-water SCUBA training dive	A 3-month infant with complex cyanotic congenital heart disease	Healthy young male dive instructor, no difficulty equalizing ears
Symptoms and signs	Paraplegia progressing to quadriplegia, uncooperative during treatment	Unconscious underwater, breathing regulator out of her mouth	Seizure, loss of conscious ness, hemodynamic instability	Vertigo, nausea soon after a recreational dive
Etiology	Rapid ascent from 85 FSW (but just within dive tables) assisting dive buddy who was out of air	10-foot jump into the ocean (depth was <18 FSW). CPR on the beach, rapid transport for HBOT	Infusion and flushing double lumen femoral venous catheter (*in situ* after second stage of cardiac surgery)	Dive tables exceeded; diagnosed as unrelated to dive (ER), then as oval or round window trauma (ENT).
Diagnosis	Spinal cord plus cerebral decompression illness	Cerebral air embolism (lung barotraumas) complicated by near drowning	Cerebral air embolism in an infant with a right-to-left shunt	Inner ear decompression illness
Special tests	After initial treatments: CT spinal cord, SSEP	After completing hyperbaric treatments: MRI, EEG	Three cerebral air emboli on CT, resolved after HBOT	Audiograms
Treatment	HBOT at 165 FSW (USN Table 6A with extensions); repeated HBOT at 45 FSW for 28 days	HBOT at 165 FSW (USN Table 6A with extensions); two further HBOT at 45 FSW	Modified HBOT after further delay	None (never referred for hyperbaric opinion: self referred 2 weeks later)
Response	Ambulatory, chronic bladder dysfunction, no cognitive deficit	Ventilated 1 week for pulmonary complications; complete recovery	Apparent cognitive recovery with mild hemiparesis	Some resolution but permanent disability

FSW, feet of seawater; CT, computed tomography; SSEP, somatosensory evoked potentials; USN, United States Navy; HBOT, hyperbaric oxygen treatment; MRI, magnetic resonance imaging; EEG, electroencephalogram; ER, emergency room; ENT, ear, nose and throat.

DCI can arise in caisson and compressed air tunnel workers (elevated pressures are used to keep water out of the worksite); hyperbaric chamber staff; high-altitude aviators and astronauts; employees in pressure vessels in a variety of industrial applications and disabled submarine evacuation (10). Patients with right-to-left shunts from any cause are at increased risk of AGE from peripheral or central venous catheters. AGE can also arise from chest injuries and various invasive and surgical procedures (e.g., bronchoscopy and cardiopulmonary bypass) (14,15).

ETIOLOGY AND PATHOGENESIS

The general perception that decompression illness is caused by diving "too deep, too long or coming up too quickly" is essentially correct (10). Published dive tables are based on empiric observations, statistical studies of divers, experimental dives with determination of venous bubble counts using Doppler ultrasound, and on mathematical modeling (6,10). Examples of dive tables include those of the United States Navy (USN), Defence and Civil Institute for Environmental Medicine (DCIEM) Canadian tables, and Royal Navy (UK) (16,17). The purpose of these tables is to define reasonably safe depth-time profiles taking into account the particular breathing gas used because this affects inert gas uptake, distribution, elimination, and gas-phase separation (10). Adherence to dive tables and the use of diving computers reduces, but does not eliminate, DCI risk.

Multiple different theoretic "tissue compartments" take up and eliminate inert gas at different rates according to tissue solubility and perfusion. Inert gas accumulation occurs most readily in lipid-rich tissues (6). A "safe" dive profile is one that avoids excessive supersaturation of any tissue compartment during or after the dive (10). Because oxygen is actively metabolized and carbon dioxide is relatively soluble, these gases can be expected to readily deplete from bubbles, leaving mainly inert gas (nitrogen when air or nitrox is used, helium when heliox is used), which is poorly soluble and not metabolized (6). The extended persistence of such bubbles can also be partially explained by complex interactions at the gas–tissue interface resulting in a relative "diffusion block" (6).

Gas super-saturation is not necessary for AGE, which most commonly arises because of airway obstruction during decompression resulting in expansion and rupture of alveoli (7,18). Pulmonary barotrauma, right-to-left cardiopulmonary shunting, and extensive venous bubbling sufficient to overcome the pulmonary "filter" are the mechanisms by which gas can be introduced into the systemic arterial system (7). Arterial anatomy and a vertical posture during ascent result in arterial bubbles being distributed primarily to the brain (18).

The causes of neurologic decompression illness have not been fully elucidated, but the hypotheses proposed include (*a*) arterial bubble embolism; (*b*) solid emboli; (*c*) bubble-related venous infarction; (*d*) activation of complement; and (*e*) autochthonous (*in situ*) bubble formation. These theories have been extensively reviewed (5). Various tissues of the nervous system are affected with differing times of onset and rates of symptom progression. No single mechanism is sufficient to account for the pathologic findings and range of neurologic disorders associated with diving. Dysbaric disorders affecting the brain are most likely caused by arterial bubble emboli. Autochthonous bubble formation most probably accounts for spinal cord decompression illness of very rapid onset associated with dives deeper than 82 feet of seawater (FSW), although some spinal cord cases may be caused by venous infarction or be of mixed cause. Vestibulochochlear DCI is suspected to result from autochthonous bubble formation within the endolymph or arterial bubbles (5,19). Systemic manifestations of decompression illness are most likely attributable to the inflammatory response that occurs because of the gas–tissue interface including, activation of the complement or kinin systems and neutrophil activation with elaboration of cytokines (1,20).

PATHOLOGY

Human pathologic series in neurologic DCI are limited. Most divers are young and most diving accidents are not fatal. Postmortem evaluations of acute fatal dysbaric events are often confounded by simultaneous anoxia because of drowning. Massive arterial gas embolism can occur during underwater rescue of unconscious divers. Intra- and extravascular bubble formation occurs during and in the first few hours after (18) corpse recovery from depth (Boyle's Law) (4). Resuscitation efforts can distribute bubbles even postmortem (18). Although the autopsy on divers should be conducted by a pathologist with expertise in such investigations (4), in practice this infrequently occurs. Published advice on conducting autopsies and diving fatality investigations is available (18,21,22). A key issue is the presence and nature of pathologic findings in the brain and spinal cord of persons at risk for DCI and whether there is documentation of any episodes of DCI.

Observed acute cerebral postmortem changes include dilated empty vessels (arterial and venous), vacuolation of myelin, and small foci of cortical necrosis (23). Chronic histopathologic changes include diffuse white matter perivascular lacunae and vessel wall hyalinization, despite the absence of known hypertension (23). Observed acute spinal cord degeneration in divers has revealed distended empty vasculature, including meninges, roots, and white matter tracts; evidence of vasogenic edema with perivascular proteinaceous globules; and, occasionally, perivascular hemorrhages (24). Pathologic findings of spinal cord damage—even in cases with good functional recovery from an episode of DCI—suggest that even minor residual clinical findings can be associated with extensive pathology. This casts doubt on the appropriateness of continued diving when residua exist (25).

CLINICAL MANIFESTATIONS AND SPECIAL SITUATIONS

The clinical manifestations of decompression illness can be considered as either tissue- or organ-specific or systemic or constitutional. Neurologic DCI can involve the brain, spinal cord, vestibulocochlear apparatus, or peripheral nerves, either individually or in combination.

ONSET AND PRESENTATION

Most neurologic DCI manifest rapidly. More than 50% become symptomatic within 10 minutes of resurfacing and 85% within 1 hour (26). In general, the faster the onset of symptoms after surfacing, the more serious the DCI is likely to be. The extent of neurologic dysfunction can be greater than first apparent (27) and a thorough neurologic examination is mandatory. Initially, this should be relatively brief to enable prompt therapeutic recompression. At least 50% of DCI involves the nervous system (9,28). Of DCI, 35% presents with pain (nearly all upper extremities) (9) that, in some cases, can represent an additional manifestation of nervous system involvement. Delayed presentation is common, mainly because of uncertainty to the cause of symptoms and reluctance to accept the diagnosis (29). Delayed onset DCI can be precipitated by the reduction in ambient pressure associated with air travel (30–32,10). Not all neurologic symptoms occurring in divers and persons exposed to altered-pressure environments are caused by decompression illness or arterial gas embolism. Table 115-2 outlines the potential diagnostic considerations in neurologic disorders associated with diving, decompression, and gas bubbles.

Cerebral Arterial Gas Embolism

AGB generally presents with dramatic symptoms within seconds or several minutes on ascent from depth (16). Acute loss of consciousness occurs in >40% of victims (29). Obstruction of cerebral vessels (with associated loss of perfusion) results in both diffuse and focal neurologic deficits, comparable to thrombotic and thromboembolic events. Consequences include encephalopathy, hemiparesis or hemiplegia, hemisensory disturbance, aphasia, visual disturbance, and ataxia (14,29). Bihemispheric or brainstem involvement can result in persistent stupor or coma (14,29,33). Early spontaneous improvement from unconsciousness can be seen with a subsequent gradual accumulation of focal dysfunction over hours. When a diver is found unconscious immediately after surfacing, the presumptive diagnosis should be cerebral AGE or cardiopulmonary arrest. Air embolism can occur when ascending just 4 feet while breath-holding (7). Seizures can be the initial manifestation of cerebral AGE, suggesting involvement of distal cortical vessels (14,29).

Cerebral Decompression Illness

Cerebral DCI without cerebral AGE is a less well-defined clinical and pathologic entity. Symptoms can include somnolence, confusion, disorientation, personality changes, apathy, and headache. Onset can be vague, gradually escalating over minutes to hours (usually, <1 hour) after surfacing (28,1).

Spinal Cord Decompression Illness

Spinal cord DCI is the most common subset of neurologic involvement. The most severe cases develop symptoms promptly after surfacing, and frequently within <10 minutes (27,34,26). Symptoms, however, can manifest minutes to hours following the dive and progress or fluctuate in severity. Pain and paresthesias generally occur after 60 to 90 minutes (9). Spinal DCI tends to involve the dorsal columns and lateral spinothalamic tracts of the middle and lower thoracic cord. Spinal involvement is not limited to these tracts and levels, however, and is frequently multilevel and patchy in nature (24,28,34). Common signs and symptoms include single or

TABLE 115-2. Diagnostic Considerations in Potential Neurologic Bubble-Related Disorders

External Factors	*Medical and Personal Factors*
EQUIPMENT OR BREATHING GAS SUPPLY • Breath hold dive (hypoxia, hypercarbia) • Bronchospasm, increased gas density • Hyperventilation • Empty breathing tank or entrapment underwater or equipment malfunction • Carotid sinus syndrome (compression by dive suits)	**SINGLE NERVE COMPRESSION** • Cranial nerves V or VII **DECOMPRESSION ILLNESSES** • Decompression illness caused by increased gas load in tissues • Mixed decompression sickness or gas embolism • Arterial gas embolism caused by pulmonary barotrauma
COMPOSITION OF BREATHING GAS • Carbon monoxide or other breathing gas contaminants • Hypoxic breathing mixture • Hyperoxic seizures • Nitrogen narcosis • Counter-diffusion DCI	**VERTIGO OR BALANCE DISTURBANCE** • Cerebellar decompression illness • Inner ear decompression illness • Oval or round window trauma • Alternobaric vertigo • Ruptured tympanic membrane (caloric stimulation)
EXOGENOUS CIRCULATORY GAS • Medical misadventure (central lines, surgery, cardiopulmonary bypass) • Trauma (especially pulmonary)	**PRE-EXISTING OR COINCIDENTAL MEDICAL CONDITIONS** • Seizure disorders, diabetes, hypoglycemia, cerebral aneurysm, tumors, myocardial ischemia or infarction, arrhythmias, stroke, and so on
TOXIN EXPOSURE • Venomous marine life • Contaminated environments	**NEAR DROWNING** • Hypoxic brain injury (may complicate any diving emergency) • Vomiting or aspiration
HIGH PRESSURE NERVOUS SYNDROME (HPNS) • Depths >300 to 500 FSW • Rapid rate of compression	**PSYCHOLOGICAL OR PSYCHIATRIC** • Drug and alcohol abuse • Panic • Psychiatric disorders or drug effects

DCI, decompression illness; FSW, feet of seawater.

multiple dermatomal band(s) of tightness, pain, or paresthesia or anesthesia about the thorax, or anesthetic sensory level; monoparesis, paraparesis, or quadraparesis with associated long tract signs; gait ataxia without evidence of vestibulopathy; and urinary retention (27,34). Unlike other forms of myelopathy that produce a well-demarcated sensory level, anesthesia can be irregular and interspersed with intact sensation. Spinal cord involvement should be considered in all instances of post-dive pain or altered sensation.

Vestibulocochlear Decompression Illness

Vestibulocochlear DCI can produce acute vertigo, nystagmus, nausea or emesis, tinnitus, hearing loss, and truncal or gait ataxia. Mixed vestibulocochlear dysfunction is most commonly followed by isolated vertigo (35,36). Symptoms can begin minutes to hours after surfacing, with the mean time of onset at approximately 1 hour (9). Although most commonly associated with helium mixed-gas diving, vestibulocochlear DCI does occur in recreational and occupational divers breathing air or nitrox (35). Evidence should be sought of coexistent brainstem or cerebellar findings suggesting cerebral DCI. Such findings will not alter the ultimate decision to treat, but could influence treatment schedules and assessment of treatment response.

Auditory Barotrauma

Auditory barotraumas, particularly rupture of the round or oval window or the tympanic membrane, can present similarly to vestibulocochlear DCI, but is usually distinguished by a history of forcible attempts to equalize ear pressures. Hyperbaric oxygen treatment (HBOT) is avoided in such cases because it is unnecessary and potentially harmful. Ear barotrauma symptoms typically begin during descent; they are associated with ear pain and fullness and otoscopic evidence of tympanic membrane injury may be present (37). Alternobaric vertigo is a different clinical entity caused by asymmetric middle ear pressure equilibration during either increasing or decreasing ambient pressure (37,38). Symptoms are generally brief and may resolve with repeated attempts at equilibration (38). Symptoms, however, occasionally persist for 1 or 2 days before resolving spontaneously.

Mononeuropathy

Mononeuropahty in a limb has been reported as a symptom of DCI, but would be considered rare (39–41). Unilateral dysfunction of the fifth and seventh cranial nerves is more common in association with elevated pressures in the maxillary sinus or middle ear (42). Such cases of neuropraxia may be related to diving or even failure to equalize adequately on commercial flights. Because this is not a form of DCI, hyperbaric therapy is not indicated and spontaneous recovery occurs (42). Decongestants may be of value.

Constitutional Symptoms

Constitutional symptoms, such as fatigue, are common after dives and are associated with an accumulated gas load ("decompression stress") and are thought to be caused by the aforementioned systemic inflammatory effects of bubbles (5).

Near Drowning

Near drowning can be expected to complicate any situation where a diver becomes unconscious or incapacitated in the water. The presence of near drowning should not be interpreted as the primary cause of altered consciousness unless decompression illness and AGE can be positively excluded. (Further information can be found in chapter 116, Drowning.)

Chronic Cognitive and Psychological Sequelae

Chronic cognitive and psychological sequelae are a postulated as consequences of frequent occupational or recreational exposure to increased pressures even without a history of DCI, but available data are conflicting (25,45). Evidence of mild cognitive impairment on psychometric testing has been reported in divers and compressed air workers, with and without a history of DCI (25,43–47).

DIAGNOSTIC APPROACH

The diagnosis of DCI or AGE requires familiarity and experience with dive tables (determination whether the patient has an accumulated gas load); detailed analysis of the circumstances (information from the victim, witnesses, dive instruments); and clinical examination (48) Preexisting or coincidental conditions can confound the situation (48).

Key points to be sought on history include the following (16):

1. Presenting complaint (if pain, character and location)
2. Timing of most recent dive and total dives in the preceding day(s)
3. Characteristics of the dive profile (maximal depth, bottom time, activities or work performed, any unusual circumstances during the dive)
4. Problems occurring during the dive to victim or other divers (e.g., difficulty equalizing, out-of-air, uncontrolled ascent)
5. Onset of symptoms in relation to the dive (before, during, after); if onset during the dive (during descent, ascent or on the bottom)
6. Intensity and progression of symptoms
7. Previous history of DCI
8. Similar symptoms previously with or without diving
9. Any preexisting or new medical conditions

The clinical examination should seek evidence of barotrauma (pneumothorax, subcutaneous emphysema, tympanic membrane) and neurologic abnormalities (48). The *sharpened Romberg sign* (performed with the feet in tandem) has a reported high sensitivity for postural instability because of spinal proprioceptive or vestibular symptoms of DCI (49,50). Erect evaluation of posture and gait, however, should be deferred until during, or after, recompression if AGE is suspected because of the potential for reembolization (18). Urinary retention or loss of rectal tone is relatively common in the presence of other spinal cord dysfunction.

Laboratory tests do not assist in confirming a diagnosis of DCI, but can aid subsequent management. Hemoconcentration (increased endothelial permeability), elevated creatine kinase, transaminases, and lactate dehydrogenase (LDH) have been reported (52,53). Electrocardiogram (ECG) and cardiac enzymes may be considered because myocardial infarction and ischemia can be a primary or secondary occurrence in diving accidents. A chest x-ray study should be performed before recompression in victims with dyspnea, hemoptysis, or suspected pulmonary barotrauma.

A noncontrasted cerebral computed tomographic (CT) scan may be considered to exclude alternative causes and may demonstrate intravascular air in AGE. A normal CT scan does not exclude DCI or AGE and neither CT nor magnetic resonance imaging (MRI) is recommended before initial HBOT to avoid delays. Brain and spinal cord MRI before HBOT, therefore, have not been rigorously assessed. Sensitivity appears low in brain and greater in spinal cases, and both are often normal despite significant deficits (54–56). A higher frequency of T2 and T2 fluid-attenuated inversion recovery (FLAIR) hyperintense cerebral lesions have been seen in acute AGE relative to DCS. Subcortical parietal lesions were most common, but abnormalities were seen diffusely in both white and gray matter structures (57). Mixed data exist regarding the prevalence of accumulated white matter T2 lesions in divers without a DCI history (58–62). Documented cord syndromes with corresponding T1 hypointense and T2 hyperintense white matter lesions have been reported (56). Improvement or resolution of cerebral and spinal imaging abnormalities with associated clinical improvement are reported in conjunction with HBOT (63,64).

Cerebral single-photon emission computed tomography (SPECT) studies have revealed perfusion defects in both asymptomatic and symptomatic divers (65,66). Electroencephalographic (EEG) studies have shown both increased slow wave activity and temporal sharp waves, but have low sensitivity and specificity (54,60,67). Somatosensory evoked potential latencies are frequently abnormal in spinal DCI, but appear no more sensitive than clinical examination in detecting acute or chronic cord dysfunction (68,69). The diagnostic studies above have all demonstrated abnormalities in acute and chronic DCI, but because of a lack of specificity and definitive prognostic value, they are of little utility in the acute situation.

TREATMENT

HBOT is the primary therapy for all forms of DCI and AGE and, therefore, transfer to a hyperbaric facility is essential (48,70). Delays are associated with a worse outcome (71). A hyperbaric medicine physician should be involved in any transportation decisions. Air transportation has the potential to cause serious or fatal deterioration because of decreased cabin pressure and bubble expansion (Boyle's Law) (4). A helicopter must fly below 800 feet altitude (48,70). A fixed wing aircraft must be capable of maintaining sea level cabin pressure at the altitude required for the flight (48,70).

The mechanisms of action of HBOT include reduction in bubble size with increased ambient pressure (Boyle's Law) (4); enhanced elimination of inert gas from bubbles and tissues (Fick's Law of diffusion) (72) because of increased concentration gradient when the inert gas is eliminated from inspired gas; elevated partial pressures of oxygen with increased dissolved oxygen (Henry's Law) (3) enabling oxygenation of ischemic penumbra; also, controlled decompression allows better off-gassing and helps to prevent recurrence of symptoms that have resolved in the chamber. HBOT has other physiologic effects (e.g., altered neutrophil-endothelial adherence, effects on a variety of enzyme systems), but it is unclear whether these play a therapeutic role in decompression disorders.

Most treated patients will achieve some recovery; 40% to 79% complete recovery, about 30% improve, and <10% achieve no recovery (9,27). In practice, a significant number of patients who achieve a good result with hyperbaric oxygen appear to relapse. For this reason, it is common for follow-up or "tailing" hyperbaric treatments to be given. Although no controlled trial of this approach has been conducted, residual symptoms frequently resolve with these additional hyperbaric treatments and relapse appears to be much less common.

Multiplace hyperbaric chambers should be used for treating decompression disorders. Although monoplace hyperbaric chambers have been used, they have limited depth capabilities and hands-on care is not possible. Supportive care, including intubation and positive pressure ventilation where needed, is an important aspect of management. Maintenance of blood pressure in spinal cord decompression illness is as essential as it is in other forms of spinal injury.

The complications of HBOT include all the risks of diving plus those associated with hyperoxia. Tympanic membrane barotrauma is usual in patients who are intubated or who have altered consciousness. Opinions vary regarding the appropriateness of myringotomy by a nonspecialist versus accepting inevitable middle ear barotraumas in these cases (73,74). Hyperoxic seizures respond to temporary cessation of oxygen and benzodiazepines or other antiepileptic medication and are not an indication for the premature termination of HBOT (75,76). Mild pulmonary oxygen toxicity manifesting clinically as retrosternal discomfort and limitation of deep breathing is commonplace after exposure to USN treatment Tables 6 or 6A. These symptoms usually resolve within days. Health care personnel accompanying the patient inside the chamber receive lesser oxygen exposure, but are at some risk of DCI.

CLINICAL RECOMMENDATIONS OF THE VIGNETTE

Many factors determine the best approach to managing patients with these disorders. The decision to utilize a deep treatment depth such as 6 ATA (USN Table 6A involving initial compression to 165 FSW) for bubble shrinkage has major implications for both patient and staff. Cases A and B were treated initially using USN 6A. Both of these critically injured patients had good outcomes. This is a prolonged schedule that can take approximately 11 hours. Interrupting this schedule risks serious decompression illness in health care personnel and, therefore, the patient is relatively inaccessible. Many hyperbaric physicians, however, favor such deep treatment depths for AGE and severe neurologic DCI. Abbreviated HBOT at a lesser pressure was utilized for case C because this small infant was critically unstable and little published information was available regarding treatment risks and responses in infants with complex cyanotic heart disease (77).

In case D, vertigo and nausea began after surfacing from a dive exceeding no decompression limits indicating DCI rather than round or oval window rupture (no forcible attempts were made to equalize and symptoms did not begin while underwater). Prompt HBOT (within 6 to 12 hours) is usually effective for audiovestibular DCI, but this patient was not referred for recompression.

SUMMARY

Diagnosis is clinical, based on analysis of circumstances and examination of the patient, particularly neurologic status in conjunction with detailed appreciation of dive tables and the equipment and operational procedures. Promptness of treatment determines outcome.

REFERENCES

1. James T, Francis R, Mitchell SJ. Manifestations of decompression disorders. In: Brubakk A, Neumann T, eds. *Bennett and Elliott's Physiology and Medicine of Diving,* 5th ed. Philadelphia: WB Saunders (Elsevier); 2003:578–599.
2. Walker R. Decompression sickness: Clinical. In: Edmonds C, Lowry C, Pennefather J, et al., eds. *Diving and Subaquatic Medicine,* 4th ed. London: Oxford University Press; 2002: 137–150.
3. Davis PD, Kenny GNC. Solubility. In: *Basic Physics and Measurement in Anaesthesia,* 5th ed. London: Butterworth–Heinemann; 2005:65–74.
4. Davis PD, Kenny GNC. The gas laws. In: *Basic Physics and Measurement in Anaesthesia,* 5th ed. London: Butterworth–Heinemann; 2005:37–49.
5. James T, Francis R, Mitchell SJ. Pathophysiology of decompression sickness. In: Brubakk A, Neumann T, eds. *Bennett and Elliott's Physiology and Medicine of Diving,* 5th ed. Philadelphia: Saunders (Elsevier); 2003:530–556.
6. Tikuisis P, Gerth WA. Decompression theory. In: Brubakk A, Neumann T, eds. *Bennett and Elliott's Physiology and Medicine of Diving,* 5th ed. Philadelphia: Saunders (Elsevier); 2003: 419–454.
7. Neuman TS. Arterial gas embolism and pulmonary barotraumas. In: Brubakk A, Neumann T, eds. *Bennett and Elliott's Physiology and Medicine of Diving,* 5th ed. Philadelphia: Saunders (Elsevier); 2003:557–577.
8. Hardy KR. Diving-related emergencies. *Emerg Med Clin North Am.* 1997;15(1):223–240.
9. Vann RD, Caruso J, Denoble P, et al. Divers Alert Network. *Annual Diving Report.* Durham, NC: 2006.
10. Hamilton RW, Thalmann ED. Decompression practice. In: Brubakk A, Neumann T, eds. *Bennett and Elliott's Physiology and Medicine of Diving,* 5th ed. Philadelphia: Saunders (Elsevier); 2003:455–500.
11. Cantais E, Louge P, Suppini A, et al. Right-to-left shunt and risk of decompression illness with cochleovestibular and cerebral symptoms in divers: Case control study in 101 consecutive dive accidents. *Crit Care Med.* 2003;31:84–88.
12. Torti SR, Billinger M, Schwerzmann M, et al. Risk of decompression illness among 230 divers in relation to the presence and size of patent foramen ovale. *Eur Heart J.* 2004;25(12):1014–1020.
13. Wilmshurst P, Bryson P. Relationship between the clinical features of neurological decompression illness and its causes. *Clin Sci (Lond).* 2000;99(1):65–75.
14. Muth CM, Shank ES. Gas embolism. *N Engl J Med.* 2000;342(7):476–482.
15. Murphy BP, Harford FJ, Cramer FS. Cerebral air embolism resulting from invasive medical procedures. Treatment with hyperbaric oxygen. *Ann Surg.* 1984;201(2):242–245.
16. U.S. Navy Diving Manual. Flagstaff, AZ: Best Publishing Company; 2006. Available at http://www.supsalv.org/manuals/diveman5/divManual5.htm
17. *DCIEM Diving Manual.* Defense and Research Development Canada. North York, Ontario; 1992.
18. Walker R. Pulmonary barotraumas. In: Edmonds C, Lowry C, Pennefather J, et al., eds. *Diving and Subaquatic Medicine,* 4th ed. London: Oxford University Press; 2002:55–71.
19. Klingmann C, Benton PJ, Ringleb PA, et al. Embolic inner ear decompression illness: Correlation with a right-to-left shunt. *Laryngoscope.* 2003;113(8):1356–1361.
20. Ersson A, Walles M, Ohlsson K, et al. Chronic hyperbaric exposure activates proinflammatory mediators in humans. *J Appl Physiol.* 2002;92(6):2375–2380.
21. Teather RG. *Encyclopedia of Underwater Investigations.* Flagstaff, AZ: Best Publishing Company; 1994.
22. Caruso JL. Pathology of diving accidents. In: Brubakk A, Neumann T, eds. *Bennett and Elliott's Physiology and Medicine of Diving,* 5th ed. Philadelphia: Saunders (Elsevier); 2003: 729–743.
23. Palmer AC, Calder IM, Yates PO. Cerebral vasculopathy in divers. *Neuropathol Appl Neurobiol.* 1992;18(2):113–124.
24. Palmer AC, Calder IM, et al. Spinal cord degeneration in divers. *Lancet.* 1987;2(8572): 1365–1366.

25. Dutka AJ, Long term effects on the central nervous system. In: Brubakk AO, Newman TS (editors). *Bennet and Elliott's Physiology and Medicine of Diving*. Philadelphia: Elsevier, 2003:680–699.
26. Francis TJ, Pearson RR, Robertson AG, et al. Central nervous system decompression sickness: Latency of 1070 human cases. *Undersea Biomedical Research.* 1988;15(6):403–417.
27. Aharon-Peretz J, Adir Y, Gordon CR. Spinal cord decompression sickness in sport diving. *Arch Neurol.* 1993;50(7):753–756.
28. Barratt DM, Harch PG, Van Meter K. Decompression illness in divers: A review of the literature. *The Neurologist.* 2002;8(3):186–202.
29. Dick AP, Massey EW. Neurologic presentation of decompression sickness and air embolism in sport divers. *Neurology.* 1985;35(5):667–671.
30. Eberhardt O, Nagele T, Dichgans J. Delayed spinal decompression sickness after air flight. *J Neurol.* 2005;252(11):1414–415. Epub 2005 August 17.
31. Freiberger JJ, Denoble PJ, Pieper CF, et al. The relative risk of decompression sickness during and after air travel following diving. *Aviat Space Environ Med.* 2002;73(10):980–984.
32. Allan GM, Kenny D. High-altitude decompression illness: Case report and discussion. *CMAJ.* 2003;169(8):803–807.
33. Gillen HW. Symptomatology of cerebral gas embolism. *Neurology.* 1968;18(5):507–512.
34. Mastaglia FL, McCallum RI, Walder DN, et al. Myelopathy associated with decompression sickness: A report of six cases. *Clin Exp Neurol.* 1983;19:54–59.
35. Nachum Z, Shupak A, Spitzer O, et al. Inner ear decompression sickness in sport compressed-air diving. *Laryngoscope.* 2001;111(5):851–856.
36. Farmer JC, Thomas WG, Youngblood DB, et al. Inner ear decompression sickness. *Laryngoscope.* 1976;86(9): 1315–1327.
37. Hunter SE, Farmer JC. Ear and sinus problems in diving. In: Bove A, ed. *Bove and Davis' Diving Medicine*, 4th ed. Philadelphia: Saunders (Elsevier); 2004.
38. Uzun C, Yagiz R, Tas A, et al. Alternobaric vertigo in sport SCUBA divers and the risk factors. *J Laryngol Otol.* 2003;117(11):854–860.
39. Greer HD, Massey EW. Neurological consequences of diving. In: Bove A, ed. *Bove and Davis' Diving Medicine.* Philadelphia: WB Saunders; 2004:461–473.
40. Isakov AP, Broome JR, Dutka AJ. Acute carpal tunnel syndrome in a diver: Evidence of peripheral nervous system involvement in decompression illness. *Ann Emerg Med.* 1996;28(1):90–93.
41. Sanders HW. Mononeuropathy of the medial branch of the deep peroneal nerve in a scuba diver. *J Peripher Nerv Syst.* 1999;4(2):134–137.
42. Molvaer OI, Eidsvik S. Facial baroparesis: A review. *Undersea Biomedical Research.* 1987;14(3): 277–295.
43. Curley MD, Schwartz HJ, Zwiingleberg KP. Neuropsychologic assessment of cerebral decompression sickness and gas embolism. *Undersea Biomedical Research.* 1988;15(3): 223–236.
44. Calder I. Does diving damage your brain? *Occup Med (Lond).* 1992;42(4):213–214.
45. Cordes P, Keil R, Bartsch R, et al. Neurologic outcome of controlled compressed-air diving. *Neurology* 2000;55(11):1743–1745.
46. Tetzlaff K, Friege L, Hutzelmann A, et al. Magnetic resonance signal abnormalities and neuropsychological deficits in elderly compressed-air divers. *Eur Neurol.* 1999;42(4): 194–199.
47. Rozsahegyi I. Late consequences of the neurological forms of decompression sickness. *Br J Ind Med.* 1959;16:311–317.
48. LeDez KM. Guide to safe diving and diving emergencies. WHSCC-Newfoundland and Labrador; 1999. Available at http://www.whscc.nf.ca/pubs/pdf/brochures/DivingBooklet.pdf. [Accessed 2006].
49. Lee CT. Sharpening the sharpened Romberg. *South Pacific Underwater Medicine Society.* 1998;28(3):125–132.
50. Fitzgerald B. A review of the sharpened Romberg test in diving medicine. *SPUMS J.* 1996;26(3):142–146.
51. Walker R. Pulmonary barotraumas. In: Edmonds C, Lowry C, Pennefather J, eds. *Diving and Subaquatic Medicine*, 4th ed. London: Oxford University Press; 2002:55–71.
52. Boussuges A, Blanc P, Molenat F, et al. Haemoconcentration in neurological decompression illness. *Int J Sports Med.* 1996;17(5):351–355.
53. Smith RM, Neuman TS. Elevation of serum creatine kinase in divers with arterial gas embolization. *N Engl J Med.* 1994;330(1):19–24.
54. Gronning M, Risberg J, Skerdsvoll H, et al. Electroencephalography and magnetic resonance imaging in neurological decompression sickness. *Undersea Hyperb Med.* 2005;32(6):397–402.
55. Gorman D, Sames C, Drewry A, et al. A case of type 3 DCS with a radiologically normal spinal cord. *Intern Med J.* 2006;36(3):193–196.
56. Hierholzer J, Tempka A, Stroszczynski C, et al. MRI in decompression illness. Neuroradiology. 2000;42(5):368–370.
57. Reuter M, Tetzlaff K, Hutzelmann A, et al. MR imaging of the central nervous system in diving-related decompression illness. *Acta Radiol.* 1997;38(6):940–944.
58. Reul J, Weis J, Jung A, et al. Central nervous system lesions and cervical disc herniations in amateur divers. *Lancet.* 1995;345(8962):1403–1405.
59. Rinck PA, Svihus R, de Francisco P. MR imaging of the central nervous system in divers. *J Magn Reson Imaging* 1991;1(3):293–299.
60. Sipinen SA, Ahovuo J, Halonen JP. et al. Electroencephalography and magnetic resonance imaging after diving and decompression incidents: A controlled study. *Undersea Hyperb Med.* 1999;26(2):61–65.
61. Warren LP, Jr., Djang WT, Moon RE. Neuroimaging of scuba diving injuries to the CNS. *AJR Am J Roentgenol.* 1988;151(5):1003–1008.
62. Hutzelmann A, Tetzlaff K, Reuter M, et al. Does diving damage the brain? MR control study of divers' central nervous system. *Acta Radiol.* 2000;41(1): 18–21.
63. Mitchell SJ, Benson M, Vladamudi L, et al. Cerebral arterial gas embolism by helium: An unusual case successfully treated with hyperbaric oxygen and lidocaine. *Ann Emerg Med.* 2000;35(3):300–303.
64. Sparacia G, Banco A, Sparacia B, et al. Magnetic resonance findings in scuba diving-related spinal cord decompression sickness. *Magma (New York, NY).* 1997;5(2):111–115.
65. Hodgson M, Smith DJ, Mcleod MA. Case control study of cerebral perfusion deficits in divers using 99Tcm hexamethylpropylene amine oxime. *Undersea Biomed Res.* 1991;18(5–6): 421–431.
66. Shields TG, Duff PM, Evans SA, et al. Correlation between 99Tcm-HMPAO-SPECT brain image and a history of decompression illness or extent of diving experience in commercial divers. *Occup Environ Med.* 1997;54(4):247–253.
67. Todnem K, Skeidsvoll H, Svihus R, et al. Electroencephalography, evoked potentials and MRI brain scans in saturation divers. An epidemiological study. *Electroencephalogr Clin Neurophysiol.* 1991;79(4):322–329.
68. Murrison A, Glasspool E, Francis J, et al. Somatosensory evoked potentials in acute neurological decompression illness. *J Neurol.* 1995;242(10):669–676.
69. Murrison AW. The contribution of neurophysiologic techniques to the investigation of diving-related illness. *Undersea Hyperb Med.* 1993;20(4):347–373.
70. Macdonald RD, O' Donnell C, Michael Allan G, et al. Interfacility transport of patients with decompression illness: Literature review and consensus statement. *Prehosp Emerg Care.* 2006;10(4):482–487.
71. Ball R. Effect of severity, time to recompression with oxygen, and re-treatment on outcome in forty-nine cases of spinal cord decompression sickness. *Undersea Hyperb Med.* 1993;20(2):133–145.
72. Davis PD, Kenny GNC. Diffusion and osmosis. In: *Basic Physics and Measurement in Anaesthesia*, 5th ed. London: Butterworth–Heinemann; 2005:75–85.
73. Kidder T. Myringotomy. In: Kindwall EP, Whelan HT, eds. *Hyperbaric Medicine Practice*, 2nd ed. Flagstaff (AZ): Best Publishing Company; 1999:355–363.
74. Presswood G, Zamboni WA, Stephenson LL, et al. Effect of artificial airway on ear complications from hyperbaric oxygen. *Laryngoscope.* 1994;104(11Pr 1);1383–1384.
75. Clark JM, Thom SR. Oxygen under pressure. In: Brubakk A, Neumann T, eds. *Bennett and Elliott's Physiology and Medicine of Diving*, 5th ed. Philadelphia: WB Saunders (Elsevier); 2003:358–418.
76. Clark J, Whelan H. Oxygen toxicity. In: Kindwall EP, Whelan HT, eds. *Hyperbaric Medicine Practice*, 2nd ed. Flagstaff (AZ): Best Publishing; 1999:69–82.
77. LeDez KM, Zbitnew G. Hyperbaric treatment of cerebral air embolism in an infant with cyanotic congenital heart disease. *Can J Anaesth.* 2005;52(4):403–408.

CHAPTER **116**

Drowning

Mark Gorman

OBJECTIVES

- To discuss the pathophysiology of drowning
- To describe the pathophysiology of brain damage in drowning
- To explain the principles of resuscitation
- To discuss the prognosis of patients who survive drowning

CASE VIGNETTE

A 14-year-old boy was swimming with his friends in a local lake and they had a competition to determine who could swim the farthest underwater. Later in the day, it was noticed that he was not with the group. A quick search finds him face down in the lake water, very pale and mottled and not breathing. Two older boys pull him from the water and an ambulance is summoned. No one knows how to do cardiopulmonary resuscitation (CPR) and it takes approximately 8 minutes for emergency medical service (EMS) to arrive at the scene. When EMS arrived, the boy had a thready pulse; his blood pressure (BP) was 46/palpable and he was apneic. CPR was instituted immediately and he was intubated at the scene. Sinus tachycardia was observed when the paddles were placed on the chest and initial temperature was recorded at 32°C. Fluid resuscitation was begun with normal saline. Initially unresponsive, with unreactive pupils, by the time of arrival in the local emergency department (ED) his pupils react and he has what appears to be a tonic–clonic seizure. No one at the scene is certain of how long he was in the water, but he was thought to have been with the group about 25 minutes before being found. What could have been done for him at the scene, how should he be managed at the hospital, and what is his prognosis for recovery?

DEFINITION

Drowning is defined as a primary respiratory impairment resulting from immersion or submersion in a liquid medium, typically involving aspiration of the fluid (1,2). It can result in death or the victim may survive (formerly, near drowning). Other definitions and terminology, such as *near, dry, wet,* and *secondary* drowning have been rejected in the International Liaison Committee on Resuscitation (ILCOR) Advisory Statement representing the opinions of leaders in the field as well as several important organizations (1).

EPIDEMIOLOGY AND ETIOLOGY

Asphyxia is divided into several methodologic categories: Chemical asphyxia, drowning, strangulation, and suffocation. Drowning accounts for about one third of asphyxial deaths, with 90% involving males (3). Accidents accounted for 78.1%, suicides for 17.1%, and the rest homicides.

Drowning is a significant cause of mortality, accounting for more than 500,000 deaths annually worldwide (1) and occurring in a variety of circumstances, depending on the age of the victim. For infants and young children, sites in the home are typically the bathtub (where inadequate supervision, bathing with siblings, and use of infant bath seats have been contributory) and outside are generally swimming pools and freshwater lakes and streams (4). Toddlers' physical and cognitive immaturity limits their ability to extricate themselves from water, whereas adolescent drowning is often related to intoxication or risk-taking behavior. Hyperventilation before underwater swimming has been implicated in some cases. Although this is known by many children to increase the length of time that can be spent submerged because of suppression of the ventilatory drive, at times hypoxemia can result in loss of consciousness while underwater, resulting in reflex breathing and aspiration (5). Adult drowning falls into one of several categories: (*a*) recreational or accidental (alcohol intoxication is a huge factor—nearly half of the cases in one large study (6); (*b*) medical-related (either a seizure or cardiac arrest); (*c*) suicide and homicide. Drowning survival is estimated at two to twenty times more frequent than death by drowning, although it is difficult to estimate because of perceived underreporting (5).

PATHOGENESIS

Inherent to the definition of drowning is a gas or liquid interface at the level of the larynx that results in suffocation. This interface blocks the person's ability to inhale gas, resulting in progressive hypoxemia and hypercarbia. The organs most vulnerable to hypoxemia are the brain and the heart. Victims conscious at the time of submersion may hold their breath initially, but the progressive hypoxemia will soon result in unconsciousness with involuntary inhalation of fluid. Large amounts of fluid are typically swallowed as well. In approximately 7% to 10% of drowning victims, little or no fluid is aspirated into the lungs because of induction of severe laryngospasm (formerly "dry" drowning), whereas the rest aspirate fluid (1,7).

The final common pathophysiology of drowning is hypoxemia and acidosis related to hypoventilation and lactic acidosis. Hypoxemia remains a significant problem after resuscitation (because of the poor capillary–alveolar interface and atelectasis), whereas acidosis usually improves with adequate ventilation. Mitigating circumstances include the temperature of the drowning medium (very cold water can have a temporary ameliorating effect) and the type of fluid aspirated (salt, fresh, or polluted water all create different pathophysiologic issues). The lungs are the primary organ injured in aspiration and the type of injury depends on the liquid aspirated.

Fresh water inhalation results in rapid absorption of a large hypotonic fluid load and initial hypervolemia. Redistribution of this fluid, however, can lead to rapid hypovolemia and should be anticipated in the resuscitation process (5). Although rarely do significant electrolyte disorders occur, hyponatremia can be found in fresh water, hypernatremia in salt water drowning (unusual cases need to be taken individually, such as Dead Sea drowning, which results in abnormalities of serum magnesium, calcium, and phosphorus, but not sodium (8). Salt-water aspiration results in an osmotic load to the alveoli and net movement of fluid from the vasculature to the airspaces, with resultant intravascular volume depletion and poor air exchange because of shunting.

Fluid aspiration of any sort causes a certain amount of mechanical trauma and reduces the amount of surfactant. Additional injury can occur from aspiration of gastric contents. Without surfactant, alveoli collapse and, depending on the degree of injury, acute respiratory distress syndrome (ARDS) can ensue within hours for those who survive (5). Endothelial barrier interruption leads to edematous capillary or alveolar membrane impeding gas exchange and increasing shunting. At times, this can be a striking event in a patient who has apparently nearly fully recovered from the drowning episode and then rapidly develops pulmonary decompensation (formerly, "secondary" drowning) (9).

Other injuries can occur, depending on the fluid aspirated. Pneumonia is most commonly documented to occur with drowning in polluted water and can include rare infections, such as with the fungus *Scedosporium apiospermum* (10). At times, particulate matter has been reported to cause lung injury (7). Pneumonia is an uncommon complication, presenting days after resuscitation and, unless aspiration of polluted water is documented, prophylactic antibiotics are not recommended (7).

Central nervous system (CNS) pseudallescheriasis (*Pseudallescheria boydii*) is a fungal infection, with more than one third of the reported cases resulting from drowning (presumably aspiration, followed by hematogenous dissemination from the lungs) (10–12). CNS pseudallescheriasis generally occurs in children and young adults (10). It occurs in immunocompetent drowning victims, and is clinically heralded by unexplained fevers or neurologic abnormalities, often months after the near-drowning experience. It was found to be 75% fatal in a recent review (12). A high degree of suspicion, resulting in rapid diagnosis and aggressive management may ameliorate the associated poor prognosis (11,12).

With severe hypoxemia, the brain and the heart are most quickly and severely affected. Myocardial contractility becomes depressed and the workload increases initially because of increased sympathetic tone (tachycardia and hypertension) and pulmonary hypertension. Arrhythmias ensue, further reducing the efficiency of the myocardium and, with prolonged hypoxemia, the inevitable consequence is cardiac arrest. Electrolyte disturbances are rarely clinically significant during resuscitation or immediately afterward (13). Other organ systems, such as kidney (hypoxemia results in acute tubular necrosis) and liver, can be affected, but are not usually of concern in the immediate period (perhaps 24 hours) after rescue and resuscitation.

CLINICAL MANIFESTATIONS AND PATHOLOGY

BRAIN INJURY IN DROWNING

In a typical pediatric drowning case, submersion and aspiration result in progressive hypoxemia and respiratory acidosis, with initially intact circulation. As the hypoxemia progressively affects the heart with attendant myocardial dysfunction, cerebral hypoperfusion and ischemia develop until complete cardiac arrest occurs (14). The brain suffers rapid hypoxic damage, with loss of consciousness occurring within minutes and permanent damage following shortly thereafter. The parts of the brain to suffer first are those most sensitive to hypoxic damage. Supratentorial structures seem most at risk, with the parietal and occipital lobes slightly more susceptible to anoxia than the frontal lobes, and the globus pallidus, hippocampus, and dentate nucleus, which are also particularly at risk (15). Hypoperfusion adds in watershed zone ischemia (between the major arterial branches as well as between deep and superficial arterial territories). Impaired brainstem auditory evoked responses in pediatric drowning survivors with cardiac arrest indicate that damage may have occurred to the upper brainstem and supratentorial structures (16). Neuroimaging in drowning shows differential changes as the brain ages. In young children, initial diffusion changes are visible in the posterior lateral lentiform and ventrolateral thalamic nuclei; later changes involve the entire thalami, basal ganglia, and the perirolandic and visual cortex (16).

Although the most significant prognostic factor appears to be down-time (period of time with inadequate circulation and oxygenation), even a prolonged period of hypoxemia can still yield a good outcome in selected cases (17–19). In most cases not involving cardiopulmonary arrest, the patient recovers well (14,20).

SPECIAL SITUATION: COLD WATER DROWNING

Because of the rapid equilibration of heat that occurs in a fluid medium (depending on the temperature of the fluid and the degree of insulation of the clothes worn), most drowning victims, even in warm water are hypothermic. Mild hypothermia results in slowing of breathing commensurate with reduced metabolic demand. More significant hypothermia results in hypoventilation with concomitant hypercapnea and respiratory acidosis. Hypothermia results in neurologic dysfunction and can contribute to the rapidity of drowning in someone who is conscious in cold water.

Cold water immersion causes a severe response characterized by hyperventilation, hypertension, tachycardia, peripheral vasoconstriction, and rapid hypothermia (21). This so-called "cold shock response" reaches a maximum within 3 minutes and seems to be a result of a profound sympathetic overdrive. This sympathetic response can also lead to cardiac dysrhythmias (predominantly supraventricular and junctional dysrythmias), and with them, a potential compromise of circulation.

Significant hypothermia can be both neuroprotective and can cause reversible neurologic dysfunction. Hypothermia reduces cerebral oxygen consumption and thereby its demand. A group of 15 relatively young victims of severe hypothermia (core temperature <28°C, 5 <20°C) and cardiopulmonary arrest (none were drowning victims) were all initially comatose with fixed, dilated pupils; when rewarmed rapidly with cardiopulmonary bypass and appropriate supportive care, however, all survived without permanent neurologic dysfunction (22). Because of this and similar case reports (18), recommendations are for full resuscitative efforts even in prolonged cold water drowning.

DIAGNOSTIC APPROACH

Predictions of neurologic outcome in those who, at least temporarily, are resuscitated has proved difficult. In a review of 93 pediatric warm-water drowning victims, consistent predictors of severe neurologic impairment or death were unreactive pupils, absence of a perfusing cardiac rhythm on ED arrival, or requirement for cardiotonic medications (either at the scene or in the ED) to enhance perfusion. Age, gender, estimated submersion times, and acidosis on arrival were not reliable outcome predictors (23). The Glasgow Coma Scale (GCS) was applied retrospectively to a group of drowning victims and found a score of 5 or less to delineate a high risk group (containing most patients who eventually died or retained permanent neurologic injury, but a few who had normal outcomes). The authors suggest that the GCS be used to identify a lower risk group who are likely to do well (24). A retrospective application of the Pediatric Risk of Mortality (PRISM) Score, a numeric scale assigned to 14 physiologic variables and 23 variable ranges, to 50 drowning patients found that all with PRISM scores (obtained in the ED) of <25 survived neurologically intact and all who had ≥25 died or survived with severe neurologic impairment (25).

TREATMENT

In general, drowned individuals who arrive at the hospital with a pulse survive and do well. Death or poor outcome is largely in those drowning victims who also have cardiac arrest. Most of the reported studies link survival to the application of early bystander resuscitation. Victims found pulseless and not breathing at the scene have rarely survived without immediate resuscitative efforts. Because little is available clinically that is conclusively predictive of outcome, recommendations are to attempt CPR immediately at the scene and make arrangements for transfer to an appropriate facility via ambulance as quickly as possible.

The Heimlich maneuver or other attempts to clear the airways of fluid are not recommended unless mechanical obstruction by a solid object is suspected because little evidence suggests that the Heimlich maneuver results in expulsion of fluid from the lungs and it can cause regurgitation and aspiration of gastric contents and delay in resuscitation (5). A swipe of the hand through the mouth if evidence is seen of obstructive debris is usually adequate before initiation of mouth-to-mouth resuscitation. Jaw thrust alone is the preferred method of maintaining airway patency because, although a relatively small percentage of drowning victims have cervical cord injury (26) (typically found only in diving, surfing, and severe boating accidents), this will be somewhat preventive of secondary injuries (5). A head board is not generally recommended (unless diving was involved and cervical spine injury suspected) because this will also delay other resuscitative efforts (27).

Standard advanced cardiac life support protocols should be instituted until restoration of spontaneous circulation occurs. Initial efforts frequently revolve around maintaining adequate oxygenation and organ perfusion, given the myocardial dysfunction and dehydration that generally are present (more so in salt water drowning). Electrocardiographic monitoring will help to identify dysrhythmias and echocardiography delineates poorly functioning myocardium. Fluid resuscitation will be necessary in many cases and invasive monitoring can be used if doubt exists to its adequacy or if myocardial dysfunction is suspected. Frequently, mechanical ventilation will be necessary, and may be prolonged, depending on the severity of lung injury and subsequent infections. Aspiration of gastric contents may have occurred in the process of resuscitation (and also because of the typical swallowing of large volume of water while drowning) and contribute to pulmonic injury. Positive end expiratory pressure (PEEP) or continuous positive airway pressure (CPAP) have been shown to be effective in maintenance of adequate oxygenation in situations of impaired gas exchange and should be used (7,13).

CEREBRAL RESUSCITATION

Limiting secondary hypoxic injury by paying attention to cerebral perfusion and maximizing the efficiency of oxygenation would seem reasonable initial therapeutic goals for drowning victims. Increased intracranial pressure (ICP) may become an issue for those with severe hypoxic-ischemic encephalopathy, but usually not until the subacute period of injury. The use of ICP monitoring has not been shown to be uniformly beneficial (likely because the edema occurs as the result of significant cerebral injury) and decisions regarding its use should be individualized. Jugular bulb monitoring of cerebral oxygenation has been reported helpful in a case (28). Because life-threatening drowning is a complex issue and the numbers of subjects available for study are limited, the progress of research specifically with regard to drowning has been slow (29). Much of our current understanding and therapeutic approach, by necessity, is extrapolated from similar situations of global hypoxic-ischemic injury and increased ICP. Specific techniques that can influence cerebral resuscitation include induced hypothermia and rewarming via cardiopulmonary bypass.

Induced Hypothermia

An early study utilizing invasive procedures including hypothermia, barbiturate-induced coma, pharmacologic paralysis, and ICP monitoring did not show benefit from induced hypothermia (31°C to 33°C for a minimum of 24 to 36 hours after drowning). This particular effort, while ICP were well controlled, did not mention cerebral perfusion pressures and treated a number of children who, in retrospect, may have been destined to die or to have poor outcome (some with resuscitation times up to 90 minutes following the period of drowning) (30). Selected cases have demonstrated a beneficial outcome following even prolonged hypoxemia after drowning when induced hypothermia has been applied (17). More recent articles showed benefit of induced mild to moderate hypothermia (32°C to 34°C) for neurologic outcome following cardiac arrest (31,32). These articles have perhaps limited applicability to the subject of this chapter, because they did not include anyone under 18 years of age; they were all victims of ventricular fibrillation-related cardiac arrest and in one of the studies body temperature at entry had to be >30°C (32). Despite these differences, these two studies offer some hope that induced hypothermia may be beneficial for drowning victims if tested with an appropriate approach.

Cardiopulmonary Bypass

Cardiopulmonary bypass (CPB) is the most well-known rapid method of rewarming in severe hypothermia and has the advantage of providing circulatory support during the process. Patients with deep hypothermia (<28°C) with circulatory arrest may benefit from rapid core rewarming with CPB (18), and current recommendations include CPB for a core temperature of <30°C (33). This has the advantage of warming the core of the body (heart, brain, lungs) to allow oxygenation of vital structures before peripheral warming, which can result in high oxygen demand, acidosis, and vasodilatory shock. If the patient cannot be oxygenated adequately or perfusion is still impaired, switching to extracorporeal membrane oxygenation (ECMO) may be life-saving (34).

CLINICAL RECOMMENDATIONS OF THE VIGNETTE

The patient was likely the victim of one of two circumstances. Either he developed hypoxemia resulting in loss of consciousness while submerged following hyperventilation or he developed a seizure while swimming (or both). No history of seizures is presented, so it is unclear if the witnessed seizure is primary or secondary to the physiologic abnormalities incurred in drowning. No one performed CPR at the scene, which has been associated with improved outcomes. Overall, his long-term outcome is likely fairly good because, although almost certainly hypoxic, his ischemia was likely brief and mild. Mechanical ventilation with PEEP and intensive care management should result in rapid resolution of his hypoxemia and other physiologic abnormalities. Serial neurologic examinations will help to monitor progress. Magnetic resonance imaging (MRI) may be helpful to assess severity of damage and degree of edema. If his examination result is very poor or he needs to be sedated, electroencephalogram (EEG) should be performed, and consideration given to ICP or jugular venous oxygen saturation monitoring.

SUMMARY

Preventive measures are documented to reduce the incidence of drowning and should be promoted whenever possible (27). Neurologic injury is mediated primarily by hypoxemia and is more severe when cardiac arrest ensues. Immediate bystander cardiopulmonary resuscitation enhances survival. Initial resuscitation efforts revolve around restoring adequate blood flow and oxygenation. The degree of cerebral injury varies, neurologic outcome is difficult to predict, and cases of full recovery after prolonged submersion (20 to 60 minutes) have been reported, seemingly justifying heroic measures. Hypothermia complicates many cases; it may provide cerebral protection and rapid core rewarming is recommended for severe cases. Induced hypothermia has never been comprehensively studied for drowning, but represents a potential avenue of future research aimed to improve neurologic outcome in cases of drowning.

REFERENCES

1. Idris AH, Berg RA, Bierens J, et al. ILCOR Advisory Statement. Recommended guidelines for uniform reporting of data from drowning: The "Utstein style." *Resuscitation.* 2003;59: 45–57.
2. Papa L, Hoelle R, Idris A. Systematic review of definitions for drowning incidents. *Resuscitation.* 2005;65:255–264.
3. Azmak D. Asphyxial deaths. A retrospective study and review of the literature. *Am J Forensic Med Pathol.* 2006;27(2):134–144.
4. Somers GR, Chiasson DA, Smith CR. Pediatric drowning. A 20-year review of autopsied cases: III. Bathtub drownings. *Am J Forensic Med Pathol.* 2006;27(2):113–116.
5. Weinstein MD, Krieger BP. Near-drowning: Epidemiology, pathophysiology, and initial treatment. *J Emerg Med.* 1996;14(4):461–467.
6. Levy DT, Mallonee S, Miller TR, et al. Alcohol involvement in burn, submersion, spinal cord, and brain injuries. *Med Sci Monit.* 2004;10(1):CR17–CR24.
7. Modell JH. Drowning. *N Engl J Med.* 1993;328(4):253–256.
8. Saidel-Odes LR, Almog Y. Near-drowning in the dead sea: A retrospective observational analysis of 69 patients. *Isr Med Assoc J.* 2003;5:856–858.
9. Milne S, Cohen A. Secondary drowning in a patient with epilepsy. *BMJ.* 2006;332: 775–776.
10. Buzina W, Feierl G, Haas D, et al. Lethal brain abscess due to the fungus Scedosporium apiospermum (teleomorph Pseudallescheria boydii) after a near-drowning incident: Case report and review of the literature. *Med Mycol.* 2006;44:473–477.
11. Kowacs PA, Soares Silvado CE, Monteiro de Almeida S, et al. Infection of the CNS by Scedosporium apiospermum after near drowning. Report of a fatal case and analysis of its confounding factors. *J Clin Pathol.* 2004;57:205–207.
12. Panichpisal K, Nugent K, Sarria JC. Central nervous system pseudallescheriasis after near-drowning. *Clin Neurol Neurosurg.* 2006;108:348–352.
13. Orlowski JP, Szpilman D. Drowning. Rescue, resuscitation and reanimation. *Pediatr Clin North Am.* 2001;48(3):627–646.
14. Jacinto SJ, Gieron-Korthals M, Ferreira JA. Predicting outcome in hypoxic-ischemic brain injury. *Pediatr Clin North Am.* 2001;48(3):647–660.
15. Kaga K, Ichimura K, Kitazumi E, et al. Auditory brainstem responses in infants and children with anoxic brain damage due to near-suffocation or near-drowning. *Int J Pediatr Otorhinolaryngol.* 1996;36:231–239.
16. Grant PE, Yu D. Acute injury to the immature brain with hypoxia with or without hypoperfusion. *Radiol Clin North Am.* 2006;44(1):63–77.
17. Varon J, Marik PE. Complete neurological recovery following delayed initiation of hypothermia in a victim of warm water near-drowning. *Resuscitation.* 2006;68:421–423.
18. Bolte RG, Black PG, Bowers RS, et al. The use of extracorporeal rewarming in a child submerged for 66 minutes. *JAMA.* 1988;260(3):377–379.
19. Modell JH, Idris AH, Pineda JA, et al. Survival after prolonged submersion in freshwater in Florida. *Chest.* 2004;125(5):1948–1951.
20. Meyer RJ, Theodorou AA, Berg RA. Childhood drowning. *Pediatr Rev.* 2006;27(5): 163–169.
21. Datta A, Tipton M. Respiratory responses to cold water immersion: Neural pathways, interactions, and clinical consequences awake and asleep. *J Appl Physiol.* 2006;100: 2057–2064.
22. Walpoth BH, Walpoth-Aslan BN, Mattle HP, et al. Outcome of survivors of accidental deep hypothermia and circulatory arrest treated with extracorporeal blood warming. *N Engl J Med.* 1997;337:1500–1505.
23. Nichter MA, Everett PB. Childhood near-drowning: Is cardiopulmonary resuscitation always indicated? *Crit Care Med.* 1989;17(10):993–995.
24. Dean JM, Kaufman ND. Prognostic indicators in pediatric near-drowning: The Glasgow coma scale. *Crit Care Med.* 1981;9(7):536–539.
25. Zuckerman GB, Gregory PM, Santos-Damiani SM. Predictors of death and neurologic impairment in pediatric submersion injuries. *Arch Pediatr Adolesc Med.* 1998;152: 134–140.
26. Hwang V, Shofer FS, Durbin DR, et al. Prevalence of traumatic injuries in drowning and near drowning in children and adolescents. *Arch Pediatr Adolesc Med.* 2003;157:50–53.
27. 2005 American Heart Association Guidelines for Cardiopulmonary Resuscitation and Emergency Cardiovascular Care. Part 10.3: Drowning. *Circulation.* 2005;112[24 Suppl]: IV133–IV135.

28. Hermon MM, Golej J, Burda G, et al. Monitoring of cerebral oxygen saturation with a jugular bulb catheter after near-drowning and respiratory failure. *Wein Klin Wochenschr.* 2003; 115(3–4):128–131.
29. Bierens JJLM, Knape JTA, Gelissen HPMM. Drowning. *Curr Opin Crit Care.* 2002;8:578–586.
30. Bohn DJ, Biggar WD, Smith CR, et al. Influence of hypothermia, barbiturate therapy, and intracranial pressure monitoring on morbidity and mortality after near-drowning. *Crit Care Med.* 1986;14(6):529–534.
31. Bernard SA, Gray TW, Buist MD, et al. Treatment of comatose survivors of out-of-hospital cardiac arrest with induced hypothermia. *N Engl J Med.* 2002;346(8):557–563.
32. The Hypothermia after Cardiac Arrest Study Group. Mild therapeutic hypothermia to improve the neurologic outcome after cardiac arrest. *N Engl J Med.* 2002;346(8): 549–556.
33. 2005 American Heart Association Guidelines for Cardiopulmonary Resuscitation and Emergency Cardiovascular Care. Part 10.4: Hypothermia. *Circulation.* 2005;112[24 Suppl]: IV136–IV138.
34. Eich C, Brauer A, Kettler D. Recovery of a hypothermic drowned child after resuscitation with cardiopulmonary bypass followed by prolonged extracorporeal membrane oxygenation. *Resuscitation.* 2005;67:145–148.

CHAPTER 117

Carbon Monoxide Poisoning

Monica Simionescu • Rima M. Dafer

OBJECTIVES

- To identify the potential causes of carbon monoxide toxicity
- To discuss the pathogenesis of carbon monoxide toxicity
- To review the acute and delayed neurologic manifestations of carbon monoxide intoxication
- To discuss the management of carbon monoxide toxicity

CASE VIGNETTE

A 55-year-old man was found by hunting friends unconscious in his cabin beside a coal-heating oven. His medical history was remarkable for arterial hypertension controlled on lisinopril, and for cigarette smoking. On examination, he was comatose with a Glasgow Coma Scale (GCS) of 4 of 15. He had no nuchal rigidity. He had cyanosis of the skin and mucous membranes. Heart rate was 120 beats per minute, blood pressure was 90/50 mm Hg, rectal temperature was 36.5°C, and respiratory rate was 25 breaths per minute. Pupils were 2 mm and reacted to light bilaterally. He blinked to visual threat. Corneal reflexes were present. Face appeared symmetric. He had a good cough and gag reflexes. Generalized limb flaccidity was noted bilaterally. He could move all extremities to painful stimuli. Muscle stretch reflexes were depressed. Plantar responses were flexor bilaterally. Initial arterial blood gases (ABG) on room air showed a pH 7.37, $PaCO_2$ 96 mm Hg, Pao_2 44 mm Hg, and oxygen saturation of 75%. The patient was intubated and transferred to the medical intensive care unit for further management. Ancillary studies, including blood count, complete metabolic profile, thyroid function tests, and toxicology screening were unremarkable. Chest X-ray (CXR) and initial head computed tomographic (CT) scan were normal. An electrocardiogram (ECG) showed changes consistent with inferior wall myocardial ischemia. Carboxyhemoglobin (COHb) blood level was 26.4% (normal, 3%). A diagnosis of carbon monoxide poisoning was made.

DEFINITION

Carbon monoxide (CO), a colorless, odorless, and nonirritating gas, results from incomplete combustion of organic matter under conditions of restricted oxygen supply preventing the complete oxidation to carbon dioxide.

EPIDEMIOLOGY

CO poisoning is responsible for more then half of all fatal poisoning worldwide (1). CO poisoning accounts for an estimated 40,000 emergency room visits per year in the Unites States. CO poisoning remain the most common cause of death in combustion-related inhalation injuries, with approximately 5,000 to 6,000 annual fatalities in the Unites States, and an overall mortality rate up to 30% (2–4). Intentional poisoning is approximately ten times higher than accidental poisoning, with an observed peak during the winter months and in cold climates (5). The highest incidence of occult CO poisoning has been reported in South Korea (5.4% to 8.4%) because of the household use of charcoal briquettes for heating and cooking (6). Morbidity and mortality depend on the amount of CO inhaled and duration of exposure. Delayed neurocognitive impairment is observed in approximately 40% of survivors (4).

ETIOLOGY

Common sources of CO include smoke inhalation in house fires, furnaces, heating systems, wood-burning stoves, motor vehicle exhausts in closed spaces, and propane-powered equipment (7). Suicide attempts are often related to inhalation of cooking gas or automobile exhaust. CO poisoning can also complicate scuba diving (8). An increased incidence of CO exposure has also been reported in the aftermath of hurricanes (9). CO is produced endogenously in small amounts as a byproduct of heme catabolism. Elevated endogenous CO production can be observed in cases of hemolytic anemia and severe sepsis (10,11). Under normal conditions, the levels of COHb do not exceed 3%.

PATHOGENESIS

Tissue hypoxia results from a reduced oxygen content in the blood (hypoxemic hypoxia), the inability of tissues to properly utilize oxygen because of inhibition of mitochondrial enzymes (histotoxic hypoxia), or an inadequate supply of oxygenated blood (stagnant hypoxia). All three types of tissue hypoxia (hypoxemic, histotoxic, stagnant) have been implicated in CO poisoning. Hypoxemic hypoxia is the main mechanism related to COHb formation. Cytochrome binding with subsequent inhibition of mitochondrial enzymes produces histotoxic hypoxia. Cardiac complications, such as systemic hypotension or cardiac arrest, result in stagnant hypoxia. Selective neuronal vulnerability to hypoxia is responsible for the unique pathophysiologic aspects of CO intoxication. The pathophysiology and clinical manifestations of CO poisoning result from the hypoxemic effects at the cellular levels (12–14). Inhaled CO diffuses rapidly across the alveolo-capillary membranes. It binds to the iron moiety of heme and other porphyrins, with 250 times the affinity of oxygen to form COHb. The result is an allosteric change of the hemoglobin molecule that greatly diminishes the ability of the other three oxygen-binding sites to deliver oxygen to the tissues. The oxygen-hemoglobin dissociation curve is distorted and shifted to the left. The arterial and tissue oxygen tensions decrease secondary to the low oxygen content and the presence of carboxyhemoglobin, ultimately contributing to tissue hypoxia (15). Although the direct intracellular effects of CO remain incompletely understood, various mechanisms of CO poisoning have been suggested, including (*a*) direct cellular toxicity caused by binding to heme-containing proteins other than hemoglobin, such as cytochromes, myoglobin, and guanylyl cyclase; (*b*) inactivation of mitochondrial enzymes, leading to disruption of cellular respiration and free radical formation (16); (*c*) myoglobin binding, resulting in reduced oxygen availability to cardiac and skeletal muscles, leading to cardiac arrhythmias, rhabdomyolysis, and acute renal failure (17,18); (*d*) binding to guanylyl cyclase and generation of guanylyl monophosphate, resulting in cerebral vasodilatation causing loss of consciousness (19,20); (*e*) nitric oxide (NO) release from endothelium and platelets, also leading to cerebral vasodilatation (21,22); (*f*) immune-mediated mechanisms caused by antigenic changes of myelin basic protein (MBP) (23); (*g*) glutamate-mediated neuronal injury (24,25); (*h*) increased atherogenesis (26); and (*i*) apoptosis (24).

PATHOLOGY

The neuropathologic changes associated with CO poisoning have long been known. The basal ganglia are most often affected. There is selective vulnerability of pallidal neurons, followed by the cerebral white matter, hippocampi, and cerebellum. This selective vulnerability of the pallidal neurons has been attributed to arterial hypotension and hypoperfusion in the arterial territory of pallidal branches of the anterior choroidal artery and to the relatively high iron content of the pallidum. Acute, severe CO toxicity also may be associated with cerebral edema and petechial hemorrhages. Reversible cerebral demyelination and infarction in *watershed* areas can occur. Delayed toxicity is associated with pallidal necrosis, delayed diffuse white matter demyelination with relative sparing of axons, and foci of cerebellar ischemia (27). Microscopic foci of ischemic or hemorrhagic necrosis usually involve the anterior portion of the inner segments of the pallidum (28). CO poisoning can cause delayed postanoxic demyelination, also known as *Grinker's myelinopathy*, characterized by discrete or confluent multiple small necrotic foci involving the deep central white matter and corpus callosum. These lesions tend to preserve axons in the deep periventricular white matter (27). A delayed effect of CO on the cerebral microcirculation associated with a marked increase in venous pressure has been proposed as a possible mechanism (29). In general, no direct correlation exists between the pathologic lesions, clinical status, and outcome (27).

CLINICAL MANIFESTATIONS

CO is a silent killer. Clinical manifestations are protean and depend on the amount of inhaled CO concentration, duration of exposure, individual susceptibility, and underlying comorbidity. General manifestations include headaches, malaise, nausea, and generalized weakness. Cardiovascular manifestations include arterial hypotension, tachycardia, cardiac arrhythmias, myocardial ischemia, pulmonary edema, and, in extreme cases, cardiac arrest (30,31). Noncardiogenic pulmonary edema and cutaneous blisters have also been described (32,33). The classic "cherry red" skin discoloration is seldom encountered in clinical practice (33). Rhabdomyolysis leading to acute renal failure can occur (34). Neurologic compromise involvement is common. Acutely, patients commonly present with headaches, disorientation, dizziness, malaise, fatigue, and flulike symptoms. Nausea and vomiting can occur. With prolonged and more severe exposure, hyperactivity, syncope, seizures, acute strokelike syndromes, cerebral edema, and coma can develop (3,14,35,36). Retinal hemorrhages may be present. Delayed neuropsychiatric manifestations vary widely, and are reported in 3% to 44% of cases (37,38). The delayed neuropsychiatric manifestations can appear within weeks following exposure, and include apathy, aphasia, amnesia, apraxia, dementia, akinetic mutism, personality changes, psychosis, cortical blindness, chorea, parkinsonism, sphincteric incontinence, and peripheral neuropathies (35,37,38). Because CO easily crosses the placenta and fetal COHb eliminates slower than maternal COHb, a potential risk exists of fetal malformations and serious neurologic sequelae (39–41). Spontaneous recovery, however, often occurs within 1 month in nearly 100% of patients after mild CO exposures. Conversely, symptoms of severe CO exposure tend to resolve gradually, only after many months from exposure, and only in approximately 75% of cases. The acute and delayed neurologic manifestations of CO poisoning are summarized in Tables 117-1 and 117-2.

DIAGNOSTIC APPROACH

A high clinical suspicion is required because history of exposure may be lacking, particularly in cases associated with severe neurologic dysfunction. Clinicians must be aware that, although endogenous and environmental exposure to CO in a nonsmoker is expected to give a baseline COHb level <3%, smokers often

TABLE 117-1. Acute Neurologic Manifestations of Carbon Monoxide Poisoning

Coma
Cerebral edema
Headaches
Nausea and vomiting
Irritability
Visual disturbances
Dizziness
Seizures
Ataxia
Cerebral infarction

TABLE 117-2. Delayed Neurologic Manifestations of Carbon Monoxide Poisoning

Cognitive impairment or memory loss
Amnesia
Depression
Psychosis
Akinetic mutism
Cortical blindness
Chorea
Parkinsonism
Peripheral neuropathy

have elevated baseline levels up to 10%. Detailed clinical neurologic and cardiac assessment, complete metabolic panel, cardiac enzymes, ABG, COHb level, ECG, CXR, and CT scan or brain magnetic resonance imaging (MRI) are required. Pulse oxymetry is often unreliable, because it can overestimate the true fraction of arterial oxygen saturation. Conversely, direct spectroscopic measurement of COHb level in blood is reliable helping to differentiate abnormal hemoglobins by wavelength. Increased metabolic demands and hypoxia are responsible for the presence of metabolic acidosis and elevated serum lactate levels. Elevated cardiac enzymes, nonspecific ECG changes or evidence of acute myocardial ischemia, and CXR findings suggestive of pulmonary edema may be present. Prolonged CO exposures can also cause polycytemia. Markers of brain damage, such as neuron-specific enolase, or the S-100B protein may have prognostic value (42). CO-exposed pregnant women require fetal monitoring.

CT of the brain may be normal on initial clinical presentation. The presence of areas of low attenuation in both globus pallidus can be delayed for several days. MRI may show decreased signal intensity on T1-weighted images, and increased signal intensities on T2-weighted images in both globus pallidus and substantia nigra, as well as white matter hyperintensities on T2-weighted images (35). As observed with the neuropathologic data, often no correlation exists between the severity of CO poisoning and the degree of MRI changes. The delayed neurologic sequelae (DNS) occasionally observed with CO intoxication have been correlated to functional compromise in the temporo-parieto-occipital watershed cortical areas (43). Neuropsychological testing is a useful adjunct tool in the assessment of these patients. Electroencephalogram (EEG), single photon emission computed tomography (SPECT), positron emission tomography (PET), and quantitative MRI (QMRI) can be used as adjunctive studies to asses the extent of brain damage in these patients.

TREATMENT

Mainstay of treatment consists of the immediate administration of 100% oxygen until normalization of the COHb level. Complications, such as metabolic acidosis, seizures, pulmonary edema, and cardiac arrhythmias, should be promptly identified and treated. Patients require cardiac monitoring, and may need transfer to a hyperbaric oxygen (HBO) chamber when hemodynamically stable. Cognitive sequelae can develop in the setting of mild to moderate CO poisoning and early treatment (6 hours) with HBO is often associated with better outcomes (44). Likewise, a reduced risk of developing DNS is associated with HBO administration within 24 hours from exposure (45). Currently, however, a concensus is lacking regarding who will benefit from HBO. HBO is usually considered for patients presenting with coma, myocardial ischemia, severe metabolic acidosis, or those presenting with levels of COHb >15%; and pregnant women with evidence of fetal compromise. Benefits of HBO include enhancement of COHb elimination, improvement of tissue oxygenation, improvement of mitochondrial function, inhibition of platelet adhesion, and inhibition of CNS lipid peroxidation. Potential side effects of HBO include barotrauma and oxygen toxicity manifestations, such as seizures, reversible myopia, chest tightness, cough, and reversible decline in pulmonary function. Untreated pneumothorax is an absolute contraindication to HBO (35).

No class I studies exist to support the use of HBO in the treatment of CO poisoning. Six prospective clinical trials compared HBO with normobaric oxygen administration in patients with acute CO poisoning. Four of these studies showed better outcomes among HBO treated patients. A recent Cochrane Review concluded that not sufficient evidence yet supports the routine use of HBO in CO poisoning to decrease long-term neurologic sequelae (46). The potential role of radical scavengers, monoamine oxidase inhibitors, and *N*-methyl-d-aspartate (NMDA) blockers is under active investigation (47).

CLINICAL RECOMMENDATIONS OF THE VIGNETTE

The patient received 100% oxygen and was transferred for HBO treatment. He received daily HBO treatment for 5 consecutive days, showing remarkable improvement on his level of consciousness. At 3 months follow-up, he had evidence of mild residual memory deficits, mild resting tremor, and minimal bradykinesia.

SUMMARY

Public awareness and education of the danger of CO poisoning are keys to primary prevention. Early recognition of CO toxicity, rapid administration of oxygen therapy, and, if possible, HBO are necessary to avoid substantial neurocognitive morbidity.

REFERENCES

1. Raub JA, Mathieu-Nolf M, Hampson NB, et al. CO poisoning—A public health perspective. *Toxicology.* 2000;145:1–14.
2. Tomaszewski C. Carbon monoxide. Goldfrank LR, Flomenbaum NE, Lewin NA, et al. (eds). *Goldfrank's Toxicologic Emergencies,* 7th ed. New York: McGraw-Hill; 2002:1478–1497.
3. Ernst A, Zibrak JD. CO poisoning. *N Engl J Med.* 1998;339:1603–1608.
4. Tibbles PM, Perrotta PL. Treatment of CO poisoning: A critical review of human outcome studies comparing normobaric oxygen with hyperbaric oxygen. *Ann Emerg Med.* 1994;24: 269–276.
5. Unintentional non-fire-related carbon monoxide exposure-United States, 2001–2003. *MMWR Morb Mortal Wkly Rep.* 2005;54:36.
6. Cho SH, Lee DH, Yeun DR, Incidence of carbon monoxide intoxication. *J Korean Med Assoc.* 1986;29:1233–1244.
7. Thomassen O, Brabetto G, Rostrup M. Carbon monoxide poisoning while using a small cooking stove in a tent. *Am J Emerg Med.* 2004;22:204.
8. Chang YL, Yang CC, Deng JF, et al. Diverse manifestations of oral methylene chloride poisoning: Report of 6 cases. *J Toxicol Clin Toxicol.* 1999;37:497.
9. Monitoring poison control center data to detect health hazards during hurricane session-Florida 2003–2005. *MMWR Morb Mortal Wkly Rep.* 2006;55:426.
10. Naik JS, O'Donaughy TL, Walker BR. Endogenous carbon monoxide is an endothelial-derived vasodilator factor in the mesenteric circulation. *Am J Physiol Heart Circ Physiol.* 2003;284:H838–H845.

11. Zegdi R, Perrin D, Burdin M, et al. Increased endogenous carbon monoxide production in severe sepsis. *Intensive Care Med.* 2002;28:793–796.
12. Rottman SJ. Carbon monoxide screening in the ED. *Am J Emerg Med.* 1991;9:204–205.
13. Norkool DM, Kirkpatrick JN. Treatment of acute CO poisoning with hyperbaric oxygen: A review of 115 cases. *Ann Emerg Med.* 1985;14:1168–1171.
14. Myers RA. CO poisoning. *J Emerg Med.* 1984;1:245–248.
15. Roughton FJW, Darling RC. The effect of carbon monoxide on the oxyhemoglobin dissociation curve. *Am J Physiol.* 1944;141:17–31.
16. Hardy KR, Thom SR. Pathophysiology and treatment of CO poisoning. *J Toxicol Clin Toxicol.* 1994;32:613–629.
17. Florkowski CM, Rossi ML, Carey MP, et al. Rhabdomyolysis and acute renal failure following CO poisoning: Two case reports with muscle histopathology and enzyme activities. *J Toxicol Clin Toxicol.* 1992;30:443–454.
18. Wolff E. CO poisoning with severe myonecrosis and acute renal failure. *Am J Emerg Med.* 1994;12:347–349.
19. Richardson RS, Noyszewski EA, Saltin B, et al. Effect of mild carboxy-hemoglobin on exercising skeletal muscle: Intravascular and intracellular evidence. *Am J Physiol.* 2002;283: R1131–R1139.
20. Verma A, Hirsch DJ, Glatt CE, et al. Carbon monoxide: A putative neural messenger. *Science.* 1993;259:381–384.
21. Meyer-Witting M, Helps S, Gorman DF. Acute carbon monoxide exposure and cerebral blood flow in rabbits. *Anaesth Intensive Care.* 1991;19:373–377.
22. Sinha AK, Klein J, Schultze P, et al. Cerebral regional capillary perfusion and blood flow after carbon monoxide exposure. *J Appl Physiol.* 1991;71:1196–1200.
23. Thom SR, Kang M, Fisher D, et al. Release of glutathione from erythrocytes and other markers of oxidative stress in CO poisoning. *J Appl Physiol.* 1997;82:1424–1432.
24. Piantadosi CA, Zhang J, Levin ED, et al. Apoptosis and delayed neuronal damage after CO poisoning in the rat. *Exp Neurol.* 1997;147:103–114.
25. Penney DG, Chen K. NMDA receptor–blocker ketamine protects during acute CO poisoning, while calcium channel–blocker verapamil does not. *J Appl Toxicol.* 1996;16: 297–304.
26. Thom SR, Fisher D, Xu YA, et al. Role of nitric oxide-derived oxidants in vascular injury from carbon monoxide in the rat. *Am J Physiol.* 1999;276:H984–H992.
27. Jain KK. Neurological aspects of carbon monoxide poisoning. *Medlink Neurology.* Clinical Summary. www.medlinkneurology.com, 2006.
28. Schochet SS, Gray F. Acquired metabolic disorders. Chapter 9. In: Gray F, De Girolami U, Poirier J. *Escourolle & Poirier Manual of Neuropathology,* 4th ed. Philadelphia: Butterworth Heinemann; 2004:197–217.
29. Leestma JE. Forensic Aspects of Neurotoxicology. Chapter 9. In: *Forensic Neuropathology.* New York: Raven Press; 1988:357–395.
30. Hardy KR, Thom SR. Pathophysiology and treatment of CO poisoning. *J Toxicol Clin Toxicol.* 1994;32:613–629.
31. Yanir Y, Shupak A, Abramovich A, et al. Cardiogenic shock complicating acute CO poisoning despite neurologic and metabolic recovery. *Ann Emerg Med.* 2002;40:420–424.
32. Myers RA, Snyder SK, Majerus TC. Cutaneous blisters and CO poisoning. *Ann Emerg Med.* 1988;30:28–30.
33. Thom SR. Smoke inhalation. *Emerg Med Clin North Am.* 1989;7:371–387.
34. Herman GD, Shapiro AB, Leikin J. Myonecrosis in CO poisoning. *Vet Hum Toxicol.* 1998;16: 429–432.
35. Kao LW, Nanagas KA. Toxicity associated with carbon monoxide. *Clin Lab Med.* 2006;26(1): 99–125.
36. Herman LY. CO poisoning presenting as an isolated seizure. *J Emerg Med.* 1998;16: 429–432.
37. Min SK. A brain syndrome associated with delayed neuropsychiatric sequelae following acute carbon monoxide intoxication. *Acta Psychiatr Scand.* 1986;73:80–86.
38. Choi IS. Delayed neurologic sequelae in carbon monoxide intoxication. *Arch Neurol.* 1983;40:433–435.
39. Foster M, Goodwin SR, Williams C, et al. Recurrent acute life-threatening events and lactic acidosis caused by chronic CO poisoning in an infant. *Pediatrics.* 1999;104:e34.
40. Crocker PJ, Walker JS. Pediatric carbon monoxide toxicity. *J Emerg Med.* 1985;3:443–448.
41. Caravati EM, Adams CJ, Joyce SM, et al. Fetal toxicity associated with maternal CO poisoning. *Ann Emerg Med.* 1988;17:714–717.
42. Brvar M, Mozina H, Osredkar J, et al. S100B protein in CO poisoning: A pilot study. *Resuscitation.* 2004;61:357–360.
43. Gale SD, Hopkins RO, Weaver LK, et al. MRI, quantitative MRI, SPECT, and neuropsychological findings following CO poisoning. *Brain Inj.* 1999;13:229–243.
44. Thom SR, Taber RL, Mendiguren II, et al. Delayed neuropsychologic sequelae after CO poisoning: Prevention by treatment with hyperbaric oxygen. *Ann Emerg Med.* 1995;25: 474–480.
45. Weaver LK, Hopkins RO, Chan KJ, et al. Hyperbaric oxygen for acute CO poisoning. *N Engl J Med.* 2002;347:1057–1067.
46. Juurlink DN, Buckley NA, Stanbrook MB, et al. Hyperbaric oxygen for carbon monoxide poisoning. *Cochrane Database Syst Rev.* 2005;(1):CD002041.
47. Ishimaru H, Katoh A, Suzuki H, et al. Effects of NMDA receptor antagonists on carbon monoxide-induced brain damage in mice. *J Pharmacol Exp Ther.* 1992;261:349–352.

CHAPTER 118

The Evaluation and Management of Lightning Injuries

Bruce Crookes

The neurologic and systemic sequelae that result from lightning injuries are diverse, and range from transient to permanent. The rarity of the entity, coupled with the diversity of its implications, make lightning injuries extremely difficult to characterize with definitive accuracy. In this chapter lightning injuries are characterized and some guidelines provided for those clinicians (neurologists, critical care physicians, and trauma surgeons) who will come into contact with these injuries.

OBJECTIVES

- To delineate the epidemiology of lightning injuries
- To discuss the basic pathophysiology of lightning injuries
- To identify the possible range of the sequellae of lightning injuries, as well as define the categories of injury that can occur
- To discuss the treatment of these injuries

CASE VIGNETTE

A 27-year-old man is struck by lightning while standing on a golf course. Several onlookers immediately called for help after witnessing the lightning strike. While the patient was amnestic to the event, onlookers reported that he did not lose consciousness. The patient is found to be somnolent and lethargic on arrival at the hospital. On physical examination, the patient is noted to have an entrance wound located over the left scalp, with exit wounds located over the right lower leg, medial malleolus, and instep. He is noted to have deep, full-thickness burns around the entrance and exit wound sites, consistent with a 7% total body surface area (TBSA) burn. His lower extremities are blue, mottled, cold, and pulseless. He appears to have a lower extremity paralysis.

The patient is electively intubated and aggressively resuscitated using normal saline. Lower extremity compartment pressures were measured, and found to be within normal limits. After 4 hours of resuscitation, the patient is noted to have spontaneous resolution of the mottling of his lower extremities, with easily palpable dorsalis pedis and posterior tibialis pulses bilaterally. On hospital day 2 (HOD-2), the patient is brought to the operating room for a right lower extremity débridement; on HOD-6, the patient is brought back to the operating room for a tangential excision of his burns, with subsequent split-thickness skin graft. His immediate postoperative course was uneventful, and the patient was extubated on HOD-8. A completely thorough neurologic evaluation notes a paralysis of the right common peroneal nerve, as well as memory loss and some difficulties with simple problem-solving. In addition, the patient complains of fatigue and joint pains. On HOD-12, the patient was discharged to a neurorehabilitation hospital that included both physical and traumatic brain injury programs.

DEFINITION

Lightning can be defined as a transient, high-current electric discharge, whose path length can be measured in kilometers (1). Injury occurs when a portion of the human body completes an electrical circuit, with the extent of the injury being determined by the current of the shock, and the duration of the exposure (2). Although the scope of lightning injuries can vary widely, the two most common organ systems that are damaged are the cardiovascular and central nervous systems (CNS).

EPIDEMIOLOGY

By all indicators, lightning strikes are relatively uncommon events within the United States; the Centers for Disease Control estimates that approximately 0.23 deaths per million persons are caused by lightning, with most of these events occurring in the southern and midwestern United States (3). Lightning-related deaths are estimated to be the second most common mechanism of weather-related injury, accounting for 100 deaths and 200 to 300 injuries per year in the United States (4–6). This represents an estimation, however, because currently no mandated central agency exists to track lightning injuries; most data are collected from the National Oceanic and Atmospheric Administration's (NOAA) "Storm Data" (6). This database is dependent on media reports of lightning-related injuries and, thus, the under-reporting rate is unknown (5,6). Because pf the infrequency of these injuries, relatively few series of lightning injuries have been published; in fact, most reports consist of sporadic cases, with the largest case series in the literature consisting of a single center's experience with 13 cases over a 10-year period (7).

ETIOLOGY AND PATHOGENESIS

Lightning can injure its victims through a variety of mechanisms, ranging from a direct strike to blast effects. Although lightning strikes can carry voltages ranging from 100 million to 2 billion volts (8,9), the flow of current takes place over a thousandth of a second. The type and degree of injury that the victim incurs depend on the amount of current, the time of its passage, the path of the current, and the resistance of the tissue in the pathway (7). Generally, current reaches the injured through one of four mechanisms:

1. Direct strike: This mechanisms usually occurs when the victim is standing out in the open (5), and is struck by lightning directly. Usually fatal, the rare survivors appear to have devastating neurologic sequellae, ranging from anoxic encephalopathy to cerebellar syndrome (8).
2. Side flash of *splash*: These injuries occur when lightning strikes a nearby object (e.g., a tree) and, following the path of least resistance, arcs to a victim standing close to the object.
3. Stride current: Lightning strikes the ground or a nearby object, and disseminates and diminishes as it moves outward. As humans are composed primarily of salt water, they may offer a lower resistance conductor than the ground. A human stride results in a potential difference between the two legs and, thus, current preferentially flows up one leg and down another.
4. Blunt trauma: One of two mechanisms cause blunt trauma. First, the musculature of the victim contracts diffusely, causing the victim to be thrown away from the electrical strike. Second, the concussive forces from the shockwave of the lightning strike can throw the victim for long distances, and can result in tympanic membrane rupture and blunt force trauma to the central nervous system (CNS) (e.g., traumatic brain injuries) and internal organs (e.g., liver, spleen). This cluster of injuries is similar to that encountered in blast injuries (9,10).

Although lightning strikes impart massive electrical energy to the victim, the duration of the energy burst is relatively short. As a result, little of the energy is transferred internally to the victim, with most of it flowing over the external surface of the victim's body. This phenomenon is known as "flash over."

PATHOLOGY

As electrical energy passes through a conductor, it is converted to heat; this transition occurs as a function of Joule's law, which states that the heat that is generated is proportional to the square of the strength of the current, the duration of the flow of the current, and the resistance of the conductor:

$$P = I^2 \times R \times T$$

where P = *energy*, I = *current*, R = *resistance, and* T = *time*

Body tissues vary in their ability to conduct electricity, based on their fluid and electrolyte content; nerves conduct electricity the best, followed in decreasing order by blood vessels, muscle, skin, tendon, tendon, fat, and bone (11), Thus, when a current is applied across a human body, bone, fat, and tendon have a tendency to generate large amounts of heat, resulting in coagulation necrosis (2,11,12). The more heat that is generated, the more tissue damage ensues.

Lightning injuries are typically different from other types of electrical injuries, because of the relatively brief duration of the exposure. When lightning strikes a person, the current is initially conducted internally, after which the skin breaks down, resulting in an external "flashover." This event can cause water on the skin surface to vaporize, resulting in a blast effect that can blow the clothes and shoes off of the victim (5). Lightning injuries rarely result in significant deep tissue destruction, because the internal flow of current is rarely as prolonged as it is in major electrical burns.

CLINICAL MANIFESTATIONS AND SPECIAL SITUATIONS

A lightning strike can induce a broad spectrum of injuries and, thus, a thorough physical examination is mandatory for these patients. Virtually every organ system can be affected, ranging from integument injuries (i.e., partial or full thickness burns) (5,13) to ophthalmologic injuries (transient blindness) (14), to renal injuries (e.g., myoglobinuria) (5), to blunt soft tissue injuries resulting from the blast effect. Sufficient energy can flow internally to "short-circuit" multiple electrical systems, including the heart, respiratory center of the brain, and the autonomic nervous system (9). Lightning has been noted to cause asystole, rather than ventricular fibrillation. Although the duration of the aystolic event can be brief, with a return of cardiac rhythm, the prolonged respiratory arrest can cause the development of secondary, refractory arrhythmias (5). As a result of the broad spectrum of organ systems that can be affected, as well as the variations in the amount of energy that is transferred to the victim, patients injured in lightning strikes can have a cluster of injuries that range from minor to severe.

Minor injuries can include dystesthesias in an extremity that was struck by lightning, confusion, transient amnesia, temporary deafness, temporary blindness, and muscle pain. Major injuries can include motor paralysis, spinal shock with associated hypotension, and seizures. Severe injuries can include ventricular fibrillation, cardiac standstill, and anoxic brain injury (5). It appears clear, however, that the neurologic injuries have the most profound effect on the survivors of lightning strikes. As with the previously mentioned system of categorizing injuries, neurologic injuries can be divided into four categories.

CATEGORY I

Category I injuries are immediate and transient, lasting for only a few days after the lightning strike (8,15). Loss of consciousness appears to occur in most of these patients, as does amnesia and confusion (12). Keraunoparalysis (KP), a transient paralytic state unique to lightning injuries, can occur in up to two thirds of patients (2,5). This syndrome appears to have been first described by Charcot, although he was not the first author to apply the term KP to the injury complex (15). The syndrome is characterized by transient motor weakness that is greater in the upper limbs than in the lower limbs; pale skin, paresthesias, and decreased pulses (8); and can be the result of sympathetic instability and vascular spasm (5). The cause of the symptom remains unclear, with various theories implicating the effects of lightning on the spinal cord, the peripheral nerves, or the autonomic nervous system (2). The duration of these symptoms last from several minutes to several hours, and always resolve without intervention (5,8,15).

CATEGORY II

Category II injuries are immediate and they can be prolonged or permanent. Lightning-related posthypoxic encephalopathy is the result of cardiac arrest secondary to a cardiac event, and carries an extremely poor prognosis. Whereas recovery is possible in rare instances, most cases are fatal. Intracranial hematomas can include both intracerebral and subarachnoid hemorrhages; whereas some of the lesions in these patients can result from the associated trauma, victims of lightning strikes typically have lesions in the basal ganglia and in the brainstem (15). Cerebral infarction is an uncommon finding (15). Peripheral nerve lesions are relatively uncommon with lightning strikes, unlike in electrical injuries (2,15). Myelopathy, however, is much more common and typically has devastating long-term effects; paralysis, autonomic dysfunction, spasticity, and chronic pain can result. Pathologic examination of the spinal cord in these patients shows selective degeneration of myelin without inflammation (8,16). Autonomic dysfunction, ranging from cardiac arrhythmias, to cold intolerance, to dysphagia has been reported (15,17). Neurobehavioral and psychological problems are not infrequent, with symptoms ranging from personality changes, to emotional lability, to memory deficits, to chronic headaches and fatigue (15,18). The behavioral changes seen in the victims of lightning strikes often resemble those seen in patients who have had a traumatic brain injury (19,20). Neurobehavioral deficits gathered under the term "post-lightning shock syndrome" include attention deficits, impaired concentration, impaired initiation, easy fatigability, slowed information processing, poor problem-solving, myofascial and joint pains, tinnitus, visual focusing difficulties, dizziness, headaches, sleep disturbances, depression, and mood lability (20).

CATEGORY III

Category III includes delayed neurologic injuries, whose onset occurs weeks or months after the lightning strike (8,15). Amyotrophic lateral sclerosis (ALS), parkinsonism, chronic epilepsy, and delayed tics have all been reported in the literature, although their link to the original insult is controversial (8,15). Cognitive changes have been reported to appear 1 to 2 years after the initial accident (18).

CATEGORY IV

Injuries that are the result of complications from the lightning strike itself comprise category IV: falls from a height, blunt injuries suffered as the result of being struck by debris, or effects from the blast. Tympanic membrane examination may provide an early indicator of a more severe blast injury, with rupture indicating a patient who merits a more extensive evaluation for internal injuries (10).

DIAGNOSTIC APPROACH

The differential diagnosis of lightning injuries can be difficult, because the initial insult may have been not been witnessed. This leads to a list of differential diagnoses that includes seizures, cerebrovascular accident, closed head injury, cardiac arrhythmias, and myocardial infarction. The presence of a classic lightning burn pattern may be helpful in making the diagnosis: linear burns in areas in which sweat usually accumulates (down the chest or back, in the axillae), "feathering burns," or punctate burns, which are discrete and geometrically circular may be noted on the victim (5,12).

The initial management of the lightning victim is complex because of the spectrum of conditions with which patients present, as well as the multiple organ systems that can be injured. Initial resuscitation of the victim should proceed in accordance with standard Advanced Trauma Life Support (ATLS) guidelines (21), paying special attention to the identification of cardiac arrhythmias during the initial resuscitation; arrhythmias should be treated as they arise. Once completing the initial primary survey, attention should be turned toward a thorough physical examination of the patient, in an attempt to emergently identify category IV injuries. Special attention should be paid to the tympanic membrane which, if intact, would appear to rule out significant blast injury to the victim (10).

A careful and thorough physical examination will help to identify superficial burns, and initial treatment with topical agents (i.e., silver sulfadine) should be carried out once the patient as been stabilized. KP should be identified through the physical examination findings of transient motor weakness that is greater in the upper limbs than in the lower limbs, pale skin, paresthesias, and decreased pulses. Caution must be taken not to confuse KP with lower extremity compartment syndrome, which requires emergent surgical intervention, and carries with it many of the same clinical findings. Careful measurement of lower extremity compartment pressures will easily differentiate between the two syndromes. Ophthalmologic evaluation and documentation should be carried out, because of the possibility of developing cataracts (14).

Acutely, imaging of the CNS via computed tomographic (CT) scan is indicated to evaluate the patient for the presence of an intracranial hematoma (8,12). Spinal cord injuries can result from fractures of the cervical, thoracic, or lumbar spine, and can be evaluated with either plain films or via CT. A chest X-ray study may help to identify the presence of pulmonary contusions (12). Injuries to hollow visceral organs have not been reported as a direct result of lightning injury, but they may be present as the result of blunt trauma. Thus, CT scans of the abdomen are not mandatory, but should be ordered with the presence of an associated indicator of large kinetic energy blunt trauma (i.e., multiple rib fractures, large abdominal wall contusions, abdominal pain on physical examination).

Laboratory evaluation of the patient depends on the extent of the injury. All patients who have had a significant insult should have a complete blood count (CBC), electrolyte panel, blood urea nitrogen (BUN), creatinine level, and a urinalysis with a myoglobin level. If blunt abdominal trauma is suspected, liver function tests, as well as serum amylase and lipase, should be requested. Serial blood gases should be performed in intubated patients to assess systemic ventilation and oxygenation, as well as in patients with significant burns, to follow their systemic base deficit and gauge the adequacy of the ongoing resuscitation. In patients with suspected myoglobinuria, serial measurements of creatinine kinase (CK) should be conducted.

All patients should have an electrocardiogram (ECG), and should be placed on telemetry for at least the duration of their emergency room stay. Any patient who complains of chest pain should be evaluated for a myocardial infarction with cardiac isoenzymes.

Multiple services and clinicians can be involved in the acute care of these patients, ranging from trauma and burn surgeons, to cardiologists and neurologists. Any patient who has significant burns should be admitted to a regional burn center, and patients with significant blunt trauma should be admitted to the hospital under the care of a trauma surgeon. Cardiology consultations are mandatory for any patient who has had a cardiac arrest or who has arrhythmias on initial examination.

TREATMENT

Treatment of lightning injuries can be broken down by the category of injury. Because category I injuries are immediate and transient, no specific treatment is required. Amnesia and confusion will spontaneously resolve, as will KP. The symptoms of KP will last from several minutes to several hours, and always resolve without intervention (5,8,15).

Category II injuries, which occur immediately and are prolonged or permanent, represent a far greater challenge. Lightning-related posthypoxic encephalopathy is the result of cardiac arrest secondary to a cardiac event, and carries an extremely poor prognosis. Treatment required does not differ from that of any other form of anoxic brain injury—good neurocritical care services. Survivors of these events who are not in a permanent vegetative state at 3 months have a small chance of recovery, but have an ultimate life expectance of 2 to 5 years (20). Intracerebral and subarachnoid hemorrhages require neurosurgical consultations, with surgical outcome dependent on the time to evacuation (22). Myelopathy can be devastating and require the involvement of a neurorehabilitation specialist. These patients can face many long-term issues, ranging from skin sores to neurogenic bowel and bladder problems, to deep venous thrombosis, to the conversion of a flaccid paralysis into a spastic paralysis. All of these issues are more commonly addressed in the setting of spinal cord injuries, and the outcome for these patients appears to mirror that patient population: most individuals with complete tetraplegia will require attendant care at discharge, whereas most paraplegics can live independently (20). Neurobehavioral deficits gathered under the term "post lightning shock syndrome" include attention deficits, impaired concentration, impaired initiation, easy fatigability, slowed information processing, poor problem-solving, myofascial and joint pains, tinnitus, visual focusing difficulties, dizziness, headaches, sleep disturbances, depression, and mood lability (20). Successful management of postlightning shock syndrome requires the involvement of a neurorehabilitation specialist, and should involve a broad-based program of rehabilitation, education, and psychological counseling (20).

Category III injuries, because of their delay in presentation, might be difficult to attribute directly to the lightning strike itself. Regardless, treatment of these sequelae does not vary from the methods commonly used in treating these conditions in the absence of a prior history of lightning strike. Evaluation and treatment by a neurologist is mandatory for this class of injuries.

Category IV injuries consist of injuries that are the result of complications from the lightning strike itself: falls from a height, blunt injuries caused by being struck by debris, or effects from the blast. The treatment of these injuries is beyond the scope of this text. Evaluation and management by a trauma surgeon of these injuries is mandatory, and should be performed in the acute setting, preferably within the first hour of the patient's arrival at the hospital.

CLINICAL RECOMMENDATIONS OF THE VIGNETTE

The patient who was struck by lightning must be treated aggressively in the acute setting. Initial resuscitation and evaluation should be carried out according to ATLS guidelines, and the patient must be carefully evaluated for category IV injuries in the acute setting. Great care must be taken not to mistake the findings of KP with compartment syndrome, especially in the setting of myoglobinuria and burns. Such a patient must have a thorough physical examination, as well as cognitive testing to identify subtle category II deficits that could ultimately lead to lifelong debilitation. The involvement of a neurorehabilitation specialist is warranted in such patients to obtain the best possible long-term outcomes.

SUMMARY

Lightning strikes, which are relatively uncommon, result in a broad spectrum of injuries, which can present acutely or in a delayed fashion. Whereas some injuries are unique to lightning strikes, none require unique management strategies. The involvement of multiple specialties, including neurologists, trauma and burn surgeons, and neurorehabilitation specialists, is required to obtain an optimal outcome.

REFERENCES

1. Krider EP, Uman MA. Cloud-to-ground lightning: Mechanisms of damage and methods of protection. *Semin Neurol.* 1995;15(3):227–232.
2. Wilbourn AJ. Peripheral nerve disorders in electrical and lightning injuries. *Semin Neurol.* 1995;15(3):241–255.
3. Adekoya N, Nolte KB. Struck-by-lightning deaths in the United States. *J Environ Health.* 2005;67(9):45–50, 58.
4. Lightning-associated injuries and deaths among military personnel—United States, 1998–2001. *MMWR Morb Mortal Wkly Rep.* 2002;51(38):859–862.
5. O'Keefe Gatewood M, Zane RD. Lightning injuries. *Emerg Med Clin North Am.* 2004;22(2): 369–403.
6. Cherington M. Lightning injuries. *Ann Emerg Med.* 1995;25(4):517–519.
7. Cherington M, Yarnell PR, London SF. Neurologic complications of lightning injuries. *West J Med.* 1995;162(5):413–417.
8. Cherington M. Central nervous system complications of lightning and electrical injuries. *Semin Neurol.* 1995;15(3):233–240.
9. Whitcomb D, Martinez JA, Daberkow D. Lightning injuries. *South Med J.* 2002;95(11): 1331–1334.
10. DePalma RG, Burris DG, Champion HR, et al. Blast injuries. *N Engl J Med.* 2005;352(13): 1335–1342.
11. Fontanarosa PB. Electrical shock and lightning strike. *Ann Emerg Med.* 1993;22(2 Pt 2): 378–387.

12. Cooper MA. Emergent care of lightning and electrical injuries. *Semin Neurol.* 1995;15(3):268–278.
13. Garcia Gutierrez JJ, Melendez J, Torrero JV, et al. Lightning injuries in a pregnant woman: A case report and review of the literature. *Burns.* 2005;31(8):1045–1049.
14. Grover S, Goodwin J. Lightning and electrical injuries: Neuro-ophthalmologic aspects. *Semin Neurol.* 1995;15(4):335–341.
15. Cherington M. Spectrum of neurologic complications of lightning injuries. *NeuroRehabilitation.* 2005;20(1):3–8.
16. Kleinschmidt-DeMasters BK. Neuropathology of lightning-strike injuries. *Semin Neurol.* 1995;15(4):323–328.
17. Silbergleit AK, Trenkner SW. Dysphagia following lightning strike. *Dysphagia.* 1988;2(4):228–229.
18. Reisner AD. A case of lightning injury with delayed-onset psychiatric and cognitive symptoms. *Brain Inj.* 2006;20(10):1093–1097.
19. Primeau M, Engelstatter GH, Bares KK. Behavioral consequences of lightning and electrical injury. *Semin Neurol.* 1995;15(3):279–285.
20. Yarnell PR, Lammertse DP. Neurorehabilitation of lightning and electrical injuries. *Semin Neurol.* 1995;15(4):391–396.
21. Alexander RH, Proctor HJ; American College of Surgeons. Committee on Trauma. *Advanced Trauma Life Support Program for Physicians: ATLS,* 5th ed. Chicago, IL: American College of Surgeons; 1993.
22. Seelig JM, Becker DP, Miller JD, et al. Traumatic acute subdural hematoma: Major mortality reduction in comatose patients treated within four hours. *N Engl J Med.* 1981;304(25):1511–1518.

CHAPTER 119

High Altitude Illness

Adam D. Quick

OBJECTIVES

- To describe the three primary forms of high altitude illness and discuss their clinical features
- To explain the factors leading to high altitude illness and the ways to prevent it
- To discuss the fundamental tenets of treatment that are effective in all forms of high altitude illness
- To discuss the physiology underlying the development of acute mountain sickness and high altitude cerebral edema
- To discuss the chronic diseases that can lead to increased susceptibility for high altitude illness

CASE VIGNETTE

A physically active 34-year-old man from New York City traveled to Nepal to hike with his friends who had already spent several weeks in the area. At an altitude of 3,000 m, he initially felt well, but as evening approached, he developed an intense, pulsatile headache with associated nausea and withdrew from social activities. After a restless night, he felt worse the next morning and decided to take the next 2 days to relax. That evening his symptoms began to improve and his second night of sleep was more restful. Near the end of the second day, he was nearly symptom free and the following morning headed out on a trek into the mountains with his friends.

During the hike, the group gained another 1,500 m of altitude in the first 2 days. At this point, despite his high level of physical fitness, he began to tire quickly and required frequent breaks, but decided to continue onward. A dry cough developed and a few hours later he was tachycardic and short of breath even while at rest. When the cough worsened and audible chest congestion evolved, he was brought to a nearby high-altitude aid post where he made a full recovery with appropriate treatment.

DEFINITION

High altitude illness is the term used to describe several clinical syndromes that occur shortly after ascent to a high altitude. It classically consists of (*a*) acute mountain sickness (AMS), which is distressing but relatively benign; (*b*) the severe, potentially life-threatening conditions of high-altitude pulmonary edema (HAPE); and (*c*) high-altitude cerebral edema (HACE). High-altitude headache, an important component of AMS, can occur in isolation from other symptoms and is sometimes listed as a distinct entity (1,2). Neurologic symptoms are predominant in AMS and HACE. Although HAPE involves the pulmonary system most significantly, it is discussed here because its occurrence can coincide with and exacerbate AMS or HACE.

The definition of high altitude itself is variable, but is best categorized by associated physiologic effects. At high altitude, 1,500 to 3,500 m (4,921 to11,483 ft), there is decreased exercise performance and increased ventilation, but only minor decrease in arterial oxygen saturation. Very high altitudes of 3,500 to 5,500 m (11,483 to 18,045 ft) produce more significant decreases in oxygen saturation and are associated with the more severe clinical syndromes. Extreme altitudes of 5,500 to 8,850 m (18,045 to 29,035 ft) are above the level of highest permanent human inhabitation and result in progressive deterioration in physiologic functions (3,4).

In any discussion of high altitude illness, it is useful to include the concept of acclimatization. This physiologic process involves responses by various organ systems. Acclimatization allows an individual to tolerate the hypoxic environment of high altitude by maintaining the partial pressure of oxygen in tissues near sea level values, despite the decrease in environmental partial oxygen pressure. The most important aspect of acclimatization is increased ventilation mediated by the carotid body that occurs in the setting of acute hypoxia. This is termed the *hypoxic ventilatory response* (HVR) that results in a respiratory alkalosis, which is compensated for by the kidney via elimination of bicarbonate. Hematologic changes in acclimatization are well known and include increased hemoglobin concentration, number of red blood cells, and affinity of hemoglobin for oxygen. On initial ascent, cardiac output increases, but as acclimatization progresses, it returns to sea level values. Pulmonary vascular resistance also increases, which slightly improves ventilation-perfusion matching, but leads to pulmonary hypertension. Norepinephrine levels rise and typically remain elevated. Vasodilatation and an increase in cerebral blood flow occur in the central nervous system (CNS) (5).

EPIDEMIOLOGY

The advent of modern automobile and air transportation has made it increasingly easier for people to ascend to high altitudes in a short period of time. Consequently, more individuals are able to access high altitude areas without having adequate time for acclimatization, thus increasing the likelihood of developing acute altitude illness. Rate of ascent, sleeping altitude, and final altitude are important factors in determining the risk for developing high altitude illness. Additionally, several environmental factors, such as temperature and barometric pressure, play significant roles in patient outcomes (3).

A study of mountaineers during expedition style climbs of Mt. Aconcagua (6,962 m) found the incidence of AMS to be 39% (6). In the Mt. Cook region of New Zealand (2,042 to 3,754 m) and the Jade Mountain area of Taiwan (3,952 m), the incidence of AMS was 26% and 28%, respectively (7,8). A large study in the United States found a 25% incidence of AMS among 3,158 visitors to conferences and resorts in the Rocky Mountain region of Colorado at elevations of 1,920 to 2,957 m (9). A smaller study of visitors to the same region found a similar incidence at elevations of about 2,000 m (10). The incidences of HAPE and HACE are more difficult to study and less well defined than those for AMS. Approximately 0.2% to 6% of people may develop HAPE at altitudes of 4,500 m and between 2% and 15% at 5,500 m (11). The incidence of HACE appears lower at 2% to 3% at altitudes greater than or equal to 5,500 m (12).

Despite the inherent difficulties in performing epidemiologic studies of high altitude illness, several clear trends emerge. The rate of ascent and total altitude obtained both correlate well with increased rates and severity of illness (3,11,13–15). In addition, previous history of high altitude illness is correlated with increased risk, indicating differences in individual susceptibility (14,16). Individuals who live at higher altitudes have a relatively lower risk than those who live at sea level (9,10). Interestingly, older individuals seem less susceptible to high altitude illness and the incidence of symptoms seems to decrease progressively with increasing age (9,17). Physical fitness does not appear to be protective and exercise on arrival at high altitude can exacerbate hypoxemia and promote the development of high altitude illness (18,19). Findings are conflicting to whether men or women are more susceptible to illness at high altitudes (3,9). It is well known that higher sleeping altitude results in an increased incidence of illness (20,21).

ETIOLOGY AND PATHOGENESIS

The exact mechanism underlying the development of high altitude illness remains unknown. In the latter part of the 19th century, it became clear that hypoxia rather than decreased atmospheric pressure is the principal causative factor. This was determined through the work of the French physiologist Paul Bert. Using decompression chambers, he demonstrated that administering supplementary oxygen could reduce or reverse the effects of a low pressure environment (22).

AMS and HACE are generally considered to be the results of a similar pathophysiologic process representing different ends of a disease spectrum. Much recent research has focused on the CNS aspects of these disorders. Evidence from early neuroimaging studies have demonstrated the presence of cerebral edema in severe AMS and HACE (23,24). Magnetic resonance imaging (MRI) studies in patients with HACE have shown that the edema is vasogenic in nature, resulting from breakdown of the blood–brain barrier and confined to the cerebral white matter. Interestingly, the edema seems to affect the splenium of the corpus callosum primarily with some extension into the centrum semiovale (25). The reasons for this predilection are not fully understood. The edema completely resolves in follow-up imaging after patients have recovered from the acute symptoms (Fig. 119-1), a finding that is consistent with that seen in other causes of vasogenic edema (25,26). Despite the convincing finding of vasogenic edema in HACE, its presence in early AMS has been questioned. Studies on this are limited, but one report did not find evidence of any type of cerebral edema in patients with moderate to severe AMS using T2, fluid-attenuated inversion recovery (FLAIR), and diffusion-weighted imaging (DWI) sequences (27). The reason for the discrepancy between this and earlier reports may be the duration to which subjects were exposed to the high altitude environment.

The development of vasogenic edema in HACE can be related to both mechanical and biochemical factors. Cerebral blood flow (CBF) is elevated in response to acute hypoxia and can produce mechanical stress on vessels. A number of studies have suggested that in the setting of hypoxic vasodilation, cerebral vascular autoregulation is altered, resulting in elevated

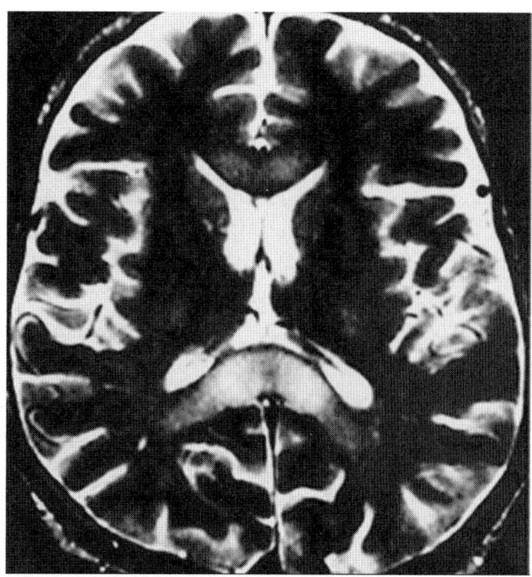
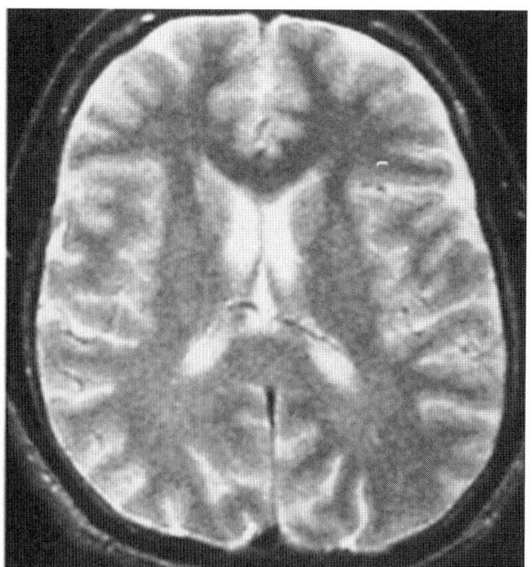

FIGURE 119-1. Axial T2-weighted images of a patient who developed high-altitude cerebral edema (HACE). On the **left** is the initial scan showing hyperintense signal in the splenium of the corpus callosum extending into the centrum semiovale. On the **right** is a follow-up scan performed after the patient had recovered, demonstrating resolution of the abnormal signal. (From Hackett PH, Yarnell PR, Hill R, et al. High-altitude cerebral edema evaluated with magnetic resonance imaging: Clinical correlation and pathophysiology. *JAMA.* 1998;280:1924, with permission.)

cerebral capillary pressure and culminating in vasogenic edema (28,29). Animal models of elevated CBF and cerebral capillary pressure without accompanying hypoxia did not produce significant edema. This suggests that cerebral vasodilation and increased capillary pressures alone are likely not sufficient (24). A variety of biochemical factors have been implicated as causes for the increased vascular permeability, including free radical-mediated damage, nitric oxide (NO) production, and elevated levels of vascular endotheliae growth factor. Research in these areas has yielded inconsistent results and definitive conclusions about the importance of these factors in the development of HACE are difficult to make (30–34).

Other considerations in the pathophysiology of AMS or HACE have included the significance of brain swelling (with or without edema) related to increased CBF in the setting of hypoxia. The idea of this *tight fit* hypothesis is that the development of AMS may depend on the ability of the brain to buffer increases in volume via movement of cerebrospinal fluid (CSF) out of the intracranial space through the foramen magnum (24). This would help explain why older individuals who have age-related atrophy seem less susceptible to AMS. Multiple MRI studies have demonstrated that, indeed, a detectable increase in brain volume occurs during exposure to high altitude. No correlate, however, exists between changes in brain volume and symptoms of AMS (32,35,36). This does not necessarily refute the *tight fit* hypothesis, because individual variation may exist in the ability to accommodate changes in brain volume, with some people able to tolerate larger changes than others without developing symptoms.

Some studies have specifically examined the role of increased CBF in the pathophysiology of AMS. Using both transcranial Doppler and radioactive xenon, significant increases in CBF have been seen in association with ascent to high altitude, but no differences were seen between individuals who developed AMS and those who did not (37–39).

Given the finding of increased brain volume on ascent to high altitude, the possibility of elevated intracranial pressure (ICP) as a cause for the symptoms in AMS has been studied. CSF pressure measured using a lumbar catheter during a simulated ascent to 5,000 m found a slight asymptomatic increase when subjects were at rest and, with exertion, CSF pressures increased more profoundly. As noted, exertion is a risk factor for the development of AMS. Interventions that reduce ICP, such as hyperventilation and breathing supplemental oxygen, improve symptoms and support this concept (24).

Higher sleeping altitudes can contribute to the development of acute altitude illness. Periodic breathing occurs in almost everyone who travels to high altitude. Sleep eliminates much of the cortical influence on respiration, leaving hypoxemia at carotid chemoreceptors as the primary drive for respiration. Combined with the lower partial pressures of carbon dioxide in the blood and CSF from hyperventilation, control of respiration is unstable. This leads to oscillatory periods of apnea followed by hyperventilation. The result is significant drops in arterial oxygen saturation during sleep and worsened hypoxemia (40).

Outside of the CNS, a variety of mechanisms are thought to contribute to the development of AMS. A vigorous increase in ventilation on ascent to high altitude is protective, and relative hypoventilation and impaired gas exchange in the lungs have both been found in symptomatic patients (41), which is likely caused by occult pulmonary edema (42). Some studies have found that individuals with a lower sea level HVR are at increased risk for developing AMS (43). Others have found that people who failed to increase their HVR on ascent were more susceptible to becoming ill (44). Studies of subjects who develop AMS have shown relatively higher degrees of fluid retention secondary to decreased urine output and resulting in lower plasma sodium concentrations. The reason for this appears to be higher levels of antidiuretic hormone in those with AMS (45). Additional hormonal changes seen in people who develop AMS include elevated norepinephrine and aldosterone levels (45,46).

HAPE is a form of noncardiogenic pulmonary edema. The pathophysiology underlying its development likely involves both increased capillary pressure and permeability. Ascent to high altitude is associated with pulmonary hypertension resulting from hypoxic pulmonary vasoconstriction. This appears to be exaggerated in those who develop HAPE (47). Studies using functional MRI of pulmonary blood flow have demonstrated that regional blood flow in HAPE-susceptible subjects becomes more heterogeneous with exposure to hypoxia. This was not seen in those who did not have a history of HAPE. Heterogeneity in pulmonary blood flow is thought to result in elevated pressures in areas of higher flow, leading to traumatic breaks in the basement membranes of alveolar capillaries and leakage of highly cellular and proteinaceous fluid. Those capillary beds that are distal to areas of more pronounced vasoconstriction are thought to be relatively protected (48,49). People with congenital and acquired abnormalities in the pulmonary circulation are more susceptible to the development of HAPE (50,51). Endothelial dysfunction has also been implicated in the development of HAPE. Exaggerated hypoxic pulmonary vasoconstriction is associated with impaired synthesis of NO, an important endothelium-derived vasodilatory factor (41). Increased sympathetic activity can play a role in HAPE by contributing to excessive pulmonary hypertension. Higher levels of plasma and urinary norepinephrine levels are found in affected individuals (11). Recent work using brochoalveolar lavage early in the clinical course has shown that inflammation is not a cause, but is a secondary factor, counter to historical theory (49). An additional element thought to be important in the pathophysiology of HAPE is impaired alveolar fluid clearance. Hypoxia appears to inhibit apical membrane epithelial Na channels and the basement membrane Na/K adenosine triphosphatase (ATPase) decreasing transepithelial Na transport and, thus, the reabsorption of fluid from the alveoli (11).

PATHOLOGY

Relatively few autopsy reports are found of individuals who have died of high altitude illness. Most fatalities occur in harsh conditions that necessitate survivors leaving those who have died behind. The few pathologic studies that are available in cases of HACE have shown generalized cerebral edema occasionally accompanied by tonsillar herniation, petechial hemorrhages, subarachnoid hemorrhage, and venous thrombosis (52). MRI findings in mountain climbers who did not use supplemental oxygen have shown evidence of diffuse cortical atrophy and enlargement of Virchow-Robin spaces, regardless of whether acute altitude illness developed or not. A less-frequent finding was the presence of subcortical white matter lesions (53). In

HAPE, characteristic pathologic findings include diffuse edema with leukocytic infiltration, alveolar hemorrhages, and thrombi in capillaries and arterioles. Pulmonary infarction was infrequently encountered, but right ventricular dilatation was often present (54).

CLINICAL MANIFESTATIONS AND SPECIAL SITUATIONS

The first descriptions of AMS come from Chinese sources and date to between 37 and 32 BC. Here, a Chinese official described how, ". . . men's bodies become feverish, they lose their color and are attacked with headache and vomiting," during his trip across the Karakoram Range (5). This account accurately conveys the potentially debilitating nature of AMS, but also illustrates the nonspecific character of the illness. In the context of recent ascent to high altitude in an unacclimatized individual, AMS should always be at the top of the differential diagnosis until another cause is found.

Headache, the most constant and consistent symptom of exposure to high altitude, can occur in isolation or in concert with other AMS symptoms. It usually begins a few hours following ascent and typically worsens following a night of sleep. The most common features are moderate to severe intensity, holoacranial location, and a pulsatile quality that worsens with exercise and improves with rest. The headache evolves in an oscillating manner, and concurrent symptoms in many individuals include anorexia, irritability, and anxiety (1). Other symptoms include nausea, vomiting, fatigue, weakness; or general malaise, dizziness, and lightheadedness; insomnia; and shortness of breath (12,47,55). Heart rate is increased and patients may feel cold (56). Individuals with AMS often wish to be left alone and may withdraw from planned social activities or athletic endeavors. The first few days of a vacation to high altitude locations become somewhat miserable. At moderate altitudes, symptoms begin to remit gradually over a period of 2 to 4 days and the individual is able to resume normal activities (10).

HACE is thought to represent the end stage of AMS. It is a neurologic syndrome that develops over the course of hours to days in people with AMS or HAPE (3). HACE is the least common, but most severe, form of high altitude illness with a high potential for mortality if not treated in an urgent manner. The onset of HACE is characterized by the presence of truncal and gait ataxia with altered consciousness. The altered consciousness is usually a global encephalopathy, with drowsiness followed by progression to stupor, coma, and finally death from herniation (47). Other findings can include visual and auditory hallucinations, seizures, diplopia, blurred vision, irrational behavior, and focal neurologic signs, including cranial nerve palsies and hemiparesis (57). Other examination findings include papilledema and hyperreflexia.

High-altitude retinopathy is often present on funduscopic examination. This condition, which is seen commonly above 5,000 m, is characterized by the presence of increasingly dilated retinal veins and arteries. Hemorrhages are seen in the preretinal or intraretinal areas and are usually located peripherally, but occasionally are seen in the macula. Vitreous hemorrhage, papillary hemorrhage, peripapillary hyperemia, and papilledema may be seen in more severe cases (58). Unlike HACE, high-altitude retinopathy is a relatively benign condition that is usually asymptomatic and resolves without sequela unless there is macular involvement.

HAPE is the most frequent cause of death because of its higher incidence and occurrence at somewhat lower altitudes than HACE. The initial symptoms of HAPE usually begin during the first 2 to 4 days after arrival at altitudes >2,500 m, most often on the second night (41). HAPE can occur independent of AMS symptoms. Cold and exertion are significant risk factors and males appear to be more frequently affected (59). Increased dyspnea on exertion, dry cough, chest tightness, and fatigue are the earliest manifestations, followed by tachycardia, tachypnea at rest, low-grade fever, and worsened cough, which may produce frothy, pink sputum as the disease progresses. In end-stage HAPE, the patient is more likely to develop concomitant HACE. On physical examination, rales or wheezing and cyanosis may be noted. Chest X-ray stuffy reveals a patchy infiltrate that is limited to the right lung initially, but then becomes generalized. An electrocardiogram (ECG) may show evidence of right-sided heart strain (47).

Patients with a variety of chronic illnesses worsened by hypoxia are susceptible to exacerbation when exposed to high altitude. Ascent is contraindicated in several disorders, including uncompensated congestive heart failure, pulmonary hypertension, sickle cell anemia, and moderate to severe chronic obstructive pulmonary disease (COPD). A variety of other conditions require caution with exposure to altitude, but are not contraindications. These include cardiac arrhythmias, compensated congestive heart failure, cerebrovascular and cardiovascular disease, mild COPD, sleep apnea syndrome, and those with high-risk pregnancy. Asthmatics may actually do better at higher altitude because of decreased air density and lower numbers of airborne allergens, with the caveat that cold exposure may still induce bronchospasm. Women with uncomplicated pregnancies may ascend without increased risk to around 4,000 m.

DIAGNOSTIC APPROACH

The diagnosis of all high altitude illnesses is clinical and the differential diagnosis is extensive (Table 119-1). A high index of suspicion should be maintained until a definitive diagnosis is made. A consensus statement regarding the diagnostic criteria for AMS, HACE, and HAPE was adopted at the 1991 International Hypoxia Symposium at Lake Louise in Alberta, Canada. AMS is defined as the presence of headache with at least one of the following: gastrointestinal symptoms (nausea, vomiting, or anorexia), insomnia, fatigue or weakness, and dizziness or lightheadedness. Symptoms must occur in an unacclimatized individual who has recently arrived at altitude >2,500 m, although, rarely, symptoms may occur at lower altitudes. HACE is defined as the presence of ataxia, mental status change, or both in a person with AMS. HAPE can be diagnosed in the setting of recent altitude gain with the presence of at least two symptoms of dyspnea at rest, cough, weakness or decreased exercise performance, and chest tightness or congestion, plus two signs of crackles or wheezing in at least one lung field, central cyanosis, tachypnea, and tachycardia (60).

TREATMENT

Effective treatment in all altitude-related illnesses are descent and administration of supplemental oxygen. In mild cases, this is not necessary, whereas in severe cases, it may be necessary

TABLE 119-1. Differential Diagnosis of High Altitude Illnesses

ACUTE MOUNTAIN SICKNESS
Carbon monoxide poisoning
Dehydration
Exhaustion
Gastroenteritis
Hangover
Hypothermia
Hyponatremia
Hypernatremia
Migraine or other tension headache
Viral or bacterial meningitis
Viral infections
HIGH ALTITUDE CEREBRAL EDEMA
Cerebral vein thrombosis
Concussion
Intracerebral hemorrhage
Migraine
Psychosis
Seizure
Stroke
Transient ischemic attack
HIGH ALTITUDE PULMONARY EDEMA
Asthma exacerbation
Bronchitis
Congestive heart failure
Myocardial infarction
Pneumonia
Pulmonary embolism

but impossible. AMS is generally self-limited and usually resolves with acclimatization. When mild AMS is present, further ascent should be halted until adequate time for rest and acclimatization is allowed. Respiratory depressant drugs (e.g., alcohol and narcotics) should be avoided and adequate hydration encouraged. When symptoms resolve, an individual may continue to ascend cautiously. The Himalayan Rescue Association recommends that >3,000 m, sleeping altitude be no higher than 300 to 500 m greater than the previous day. Also, every second or third day should be devoted to rest while ascending (61). Ibuprofen, naproxen, aspirin, and acetaminophen have all been shown to be beneficial for symptomatic relief of AMS, particularly for the headache (62–64). Antiemetics (e.g., metoclopramide, promethazine, prochlorperazine) are also helpful for the nausea accompanying AMS. Prochlorperazine is particularly beneficial because it can increase HVR (65). For moderate or severe cases of AMS, descent is the treatment of choice. Even an altitude decrease of a few hundred meters can result in marked improvement. Supplemental oxygen administration is also useful, when available. Dexamethasone given in doses of 4 mg every 6 hours with or without an 8-mg initial dose is a mainstay of treatment when descent is not possible (23,66). Patients should not continue to ascend despite relief of AMS with dexamethasone unless there is no recurrence of symptoms for several days after the drug is stopped (59). Acetazolamide is useful in the acute treatment of AMS, but is particularly beneficial for prevention when taken 24 to 48 hours both before and following ascent (59,67). As a carbonic anhydrase inhibitor, the drug induces bicarbonate diuresis and metabolic acidosis. This stimulates ventilation and speeds the process of acclimatization. It also helps reduce periodic breathing and improves nocturnal oxygen saturation (47). The typical dose is between 125 and 500 mg twice daily (68–70). Dexamethasone at doses of 2 mg every 6 hours has also been shown to be beneficial as a prophylactic agent, but should be used with caution because of the potential for rebound of symptoms with discontinuation of the medication, a problem that is not encountered with acetazolamide (59,71–73).

In contrast to AMS, HACE and HAPE represent medical emergencies, and descent with possible evacuation to an appropriate medical center should be the focus. Because this is not immediately possible in many situations, a variety of temporizing strategies may be useful until descent is feasible. For HACE, 8 mg of dexamethasone initially, followed by 4 mg every 6 hours is recommended. Supplemental high flow oxygen or the use of a portable hyperbaric chamber may be lifesaving. Intubation may be necessary, but excessive hyperventilation should be avoided because patients are already hypocapnic. Oxygen administration via the endotracheal tube is sufficient to decrease excessive cerebral blood flow, blood volume, and intracranial pressure (3).

Treatment of HAPE should place a high priority on increasing alveolar oxygen content. Breathing supplemental oxygen reduces the pulmonary artery pressure resulting from hypoxemic vasoconstriction and can lead to rapid improvement. The goal should be to maintain arterial oxygen saturation above 90% (47). Because exertion and cold air exacerbate symptoms, the patient should be kept warm and relaxed. Similar to HACE, use of a portable hyperbaric chamber can be an important temporizing measure until descent is possible. Medical therapy with nifedipine at doses of 10 mg every 4 hours or 30 mg of an extended release preparation two to three times a day can result in improved oxygenation, reduction of pulmonary artery pressure, and clearing of alveolar edema (74). Slow release preparations of nifedipine (at doses of 20 mg every 8 hours) can help prevent HAPE in individuals known to be susceptible (75). Recently, sildenafil has been shown to normalize pulmonary artery pressure and improve gas exchange during ascent to high altitude (76,77).

CLINICAL RECOMMENDATIONS OF THE VIGNETTE

The patient experienced symptoms of AMS shortly after his arrival at high altitude. Although he did not seek medical treatment for this, he appropriately decided to rest for 2 days, allowing acclimatization to occur. During this time, ibuprofen or aspirin and prochlorperazine would likely have been effective symptomatic treatments. Alternatively, he could have taken acetazolamide for 24 to 48 hours before and after his arrival and possibly avoided AMS altogether. As he trekked into the higher elevations, decreased exercise tolerance and dry cough developed, heralding the onset of HAPE. At this point, the patient made a critical mistake and continued onward when descent of just a few hundred meters would have resulted in improvement. As his clinical picture worsened, he sought aid at a local medical station. Here, supplemental oxygen given to keep arterial saturation above 90% and oral nifedipine would likely lead to recovery within a few hours. If the patient had not sought medical attention, it is possible that his condition would have progressed to life-threatening HACE.

SUMMARY

High altitude illness is the term used to describe the three clinical syndromes of AMS, HACE, and HAPE. The pathophysiology underlying these disorders is complex and prominently involves the CNS as well as multiple other organ systems. The symptoms of AMS are nonspecific and a high index of suspicion must be maintained in anyone who has recently ascended to high elevations. Although AMS is unpleasant, it is usually self-limited and relatively benign. In contrast, HACE and HAPE are severe, life-threatening medical emergencies. Descent and administration of supplemental oxygen are effective treatments in all forms of high altitude illness and are mandatory in the management of HACE and HAPE. Slow ascent rates, avoidance of overexertion, and allowing adequate time for rest and acclimatization are effective means of prevention.

REFERENCES

1. Serrano-Duenas M. High altitude headache. A prospective study of its clinical characteristics. *Cephalalgia.* 2005;25(12):1110–1116.
2. Silber E, Sonnenberg P, Collier DJ, et al. Clinical features of headache at altitude: A prospective study. *Neurology.* 2003;60(7):1167–1171.
3. Gallagher SA, Hackett PH. High-altitude illness. *Emerg Med Clin North Am.* 2004;22(2): 329–355, viii.
4. West JB. Highest permanent human habitation. *High Alt Med Biol.* 2002;3(4):401–407.
5. Ward M, Milledge JS, West JB. *High Altitude Medicine and Physiology,* 3rd ed. London New York: Arnold; copublished by Oxford University Press; 2000.
6. Pesce C, Leal C, Pinto H, et al. Determinants of acute mountain sickness and success on Mount Aconcagua (6962 m). *High Alt Med Biol.* 2005;6(2):158–166.
7. Murdoch DR, Curry C. Acute mountain sickness in the Southern Alps of New Zealand. *N Z Med J.* 1998;111(1065):168–169.
8. Kao WF, Kuo CC, Hsu TF, et al. Acute mountain sickness in Jade Mountain climbers of Taiwan. *Aviat Space Environ Med.* 2002;73(4):359–362.
9. Honigman B, Theis MK, Koziol-McLain J, et al. Acute mountain sickness in a general tourist population at moderate altitudes. *Ann Intern Med.* 1993;118(8):587–592.
10. Montgomery AB, Mills J, Luce JM. Incidence of acute mountain sickness at intermediate altitude. *JAMA.* 1989;261(5):732–734.
11. Bartsch P, Mairbaurl H, Maggiorini M, et al. Physiological aspects of high-altitude pulmonary edema. *J Appl Physiol.* 2005;98(3):1101–1110.
12. Klocke DL, Decker WW, Stepanek J. Altitude-related illnesses. *Mayo Clin Proc.* 1998;73(10): 988–992; quiz 92–93.
13. Rashid H, Hashmi SN, Hussain T. Risk factors in high altitude pulmonary oedema. *J Coll Physicians Surg Pak.* 2005;15(2):96–99.
14. Schneider M, Bernasch D, Weymann J, et al. Acute mountain sickness: Influence of susceptibility, preexposure, and ascent rate. *Med Sci Sports Exerc.* 2002;34(12):1886–1891.
15. Maggiorini M, Buhler B, Walter M, et al. Prevalence of acute mountain sickness in the Swiss Alps. *BMJ.* 1990;301(6756):853–855.
16. Bartsch P, Mairbaurl H, Swenson ER, et al. High altitude pulmonary oedema. *Swiss Med Wkly.* 2003;133(27–28):377–384.
17. Roach RC, Houston CS, Honigman B, et al. How well do older persons tolerate moderate altitude? *West J Med.* 1995;162(1):32–36.
18. Roach RC, Maes D, Sandoval D, et al. Exercise exacerbates acute mountain sickness at simulated high altitude. *J Appl Physiol.* 2000;88(2):581–585.
19. Honigman B, Read M, Lezotte D, et al. Sea-level physical activity and acute mountain sickness at moderate altitude. *West J Med.* 1995;163(2):117–121.
20. Burgess KR, Johnson P, Edwards N, et al. Acute mountain sickness is associated with sleep desaturation at high altitude. *Respirology.* 2004;9(4):485–492.
21. Barash IA, Beatty C, Powell FL, et al. Nocturnal oxygen enrichment of room air at 3800 meter altitude improves sleep architecture. *High Alt Med Biol.* 2001;2(4):525–533.
22. Houston CS, Zeman EJ. *Going Higher: Oxygen, Man and Mountains,* 5th ed. Seattle: The Mountaineers Books; 2005.
23. Levine BD, Yoshimura K, Kobayashi T, et al. Dexamethasone in the treatment of acute mountain sickness. *N Engl J Med.* 1989;321(25):1707–1713.
24. Roach RC, Hackett PH. Frontiers of hypoxia research: Acute mountain sickness. *J Exp Biol.* 2001;204(Pt 18):3161–3170.
25. Hackett PH, Yarnell PR, Hill R, et al. High-altitude cerebral edema evaluated with magnetic resonance imaging: Clinical correlation and pathophysiology. *JAMA.* 1998;280(22): 1920–1925.
26. Lamy C, Oppenheim C, Meder JF, et al. Neuroimaging in posterior reversible encephalopathy syndrome. *J Neuroimaging.* 2004;14(2):89–96.
27. Fischer R, Vollmar C, Thiere M, et al. No evidence of cerebral oedema in severe acute mountain sickness. *Cephalalgia.* 2004;24(1):66–71.
28. Lassen NA. Increase of cerebral blood flow at high altitude: Its possible relation to AMS. *Int J Sports Med.* 1992;13[Suppl 1]:S47–S48.
29. Van Osta A, Moraine JJ, Melot C, et al. Effects of high altitude exposure on cerebral hemodynamics in normal subjects. *Stroke.* 2005;36(3):557–560.
30. Bailey DM, Davies B. Acute mountain sickness; prophylactic benefits of antioxidant vitamin supplementation at high altitude. *High Alt Med Biol.* 2001;2(1):21–29.
31. Bailey DM, Kleger GR, Holzgraefe M, et al. Pathophysiological significance of peroxidative stress, neuronal damage, and membrane permeability in acute mountain sickness. *J Appl Physiol.* 2004;96(4):1459–1463.
32. Bailey DM, Roukens R, Knauth M, et al. Free radical-mediated damage to barrier function is not associated with altered brain morphology in high-altitude headache. *J Cereb Blood Flow Metab.* 2006;26(1):99–111.
33. Tissot van Patot MC, Leadbetter G, Keyes LE, et al. Greater free plasma VEGF and lower soluble VEGF receptor-1 in acute mountain sickness. *J Appl Physiol.* 2005;98(5): 1626–1629.
34. Mark KS, Burroughs AR, Brown RC, et al. Nitric oxide mediates hypoxia-induced changes in paracellular permeability of cerebral microvasculature. *Am J Physiol Heart Circ Physiol.* 2004;286(1):H174–H180.
35. Bartsch P, Bailey DM, Berger MM, et al. Acute mountain sickness: Controversies and advances. *High Alt Med Biol.* 2004;5(2):110–124.
36. Hackett PH. High altitude cerebral edema and acute mountain sickness. A pathophysiology update. *Adv Exp Med Biol.* 1999;474:23–45.
37. Lysakowski C, Von Elm E, Dumont L, et al. Effect of magnesium, high altitude and acute mountain sickness on blood flow velocity in the middle cerebral artery. *Clin Sci (Lond).* 2004;106(3):279–285.
38. Baumgartner RW, Spyridopoulos I, Bartsch P, et al. Acute mountain sickness is not related to cerebral blood flow: A decompression chamber study. *J Appl Physiol.* 1999;86(5): 1578–1582.
39. Jensen JB, Wright AD, Lassen NA, et al. Cerebral blood flow in acute mountain sickness. *J Appl Physiol.* 1990;69(2):430–433.
40. Mason RJ, Murray JF, Nadel JA, eds. *Murray and Nadel's Textbook of Respiratory Medicine.* 2005. [Electronic book available in HTML format] [cited; 4th] Available from: http://home.mdconsult.com/das/book/51114597-2/view/1288.
41. Basnyat B, Murdoch DR. High-altitude illness. *Lancet.* 2003;361(9373):1967–1974.
42. Ge RL, Matsuzawa Y, Takeoka M, et al. Low pulmonary diffusing capacity in subjects with acute mountain sickness. *Chest.* 1997;111(1):58–64.
43. Moore LG, Harrison GL, McCullough RE, et al. Low acute hypoxic ventilatory response and hypoxic depression in acute altitude sickness. *J Appl Physiol.* 1986;60(4):1407–1412.
44. Bartsch P, Swenson ER, Paul A, et al. Hypoxic ventilatory response, ventilation, gas exchange, and fluid balance in acute mountain sickness. *High Alt Med Biol.* 2002;3(4):361–376.
45. Loeppky JA, Icenogle MV, Maes D, et al. Early fluid retention and severe acute mountain sickness. *J Appl Physiol.* 2005;98(2):591–597.
46. Milledge JS. Salt and water control at altitude. *Int J Sports Med.* 1992;13[Suppl 1]:S61–S63.
47. Hackett PH, Roach RC. High-altitude illness. *N Engl J Med.* 2001;345(2):107–114.
48. Hopkins SR, Levin DL. Heterogeneous pulmonary blood flow in response to hypoxia: A risk factor for high altitude pulmonary edema? *Respir Physiol Neurobiol.* 2006;151(2–3):217–228.
49. Swenson ER, Maggiorini M, Mongovin S, et al. Pathogenesis of high-altitude pulmonary edema: Inflammation is not an etiologic factor. *JAMA.* 2002;287(17):2228–2235.
50. Hackett PH, Creagh CE, Grover RF, et al. High-altitude pulmonary edema in persons without the right pulmonary artery. *N Engl J Med.* 1980;302(19):1070–1073.
51. Naeije R, De Backer D, Vachiery JL, et al. High-altitude pulmonary edema with primary pulmonary hypertension. *Chest.* 1996;110(1):286–289.
52. Clarke C. High altitude cerebral oedema. *Int J Sports Med.* 1988;9(2):170–174.
53. Fayed N, Modrego PJ, Morales H. Evidence of brain damage after high-altitude climbing by means of magnetic resonance imaging. *Am J Med.* 2006;119(2):168e1–168e6.
54. Hultgren HN, Wilson R, Kosek JC. Lung pathology in high-altitude pulmonary edema. *Wilderness Environ Med.* 1997;8(4):218–220.
55. Harris MD, Terrio J, Miser WF, et al. High-altitude medicine. *Am Fam Physician.* 1998;57(8): 1907–1914.
56. Loeppky JA, Icenogle MV, Maes D, et al. Body temperature, autonomic responses, and acute mountain sickness. *High Alt Med Biol.* 2003;4(3):367–373.
57. Basnyat B. Isolated facial and hypoglossal nerve palsies at high altitude. *High Alt Med Biol.* 2001;2(2):301–303.
58. Wiedman M, Tabin GC. High-altitude retinopathy and altitude illness. *Ophthalmology.* 1999;106(10):1924–1927.
59. Zafren K, Honigman B. High-altitude medicine. *Emerg Med Clin North Am.* 1997;15(1):191–222.
60. Thomas E, Dietz M. *The High Altitude Medicine Guide.* [online] 1995 [cited 2006 August 25] Available from URL: http://www.high-altitude-medicine.com.
61. Himalayan Rescue Association [online] cited 2006 August 25. Available from URL: http://www.himalayanrescue.org/hra/index.php.
62. Harris NS, Wenzel RP, Thomas SH. High altitude headache: Efficacy of acetaminophen vs. ibuprofen in a randomized, controlled trial. *J Emerg Med.* 2003;24(4):383–387.
63. Broome JR, Stoneham MD, Beeley JM, et al. High altitude headache: Treatment with ibuprofen. *Aviat Space Environ Med.* 1994 Jan;65(1):19–20.
64. Burtscher M. [High altitude headache: Epidemiology, pathophysiology, therapy and prophylaxis]. *Wien Klin Wochenschr.* 1999;111(20):830–836.
65. Olson LG, Hensley MJ, Saunders NA. Augmentation of ventilatory response to asphyxia by prochlorperazine in humans. *J Appl Physiol.* 1982;53(3):637–643.
66. Keller HR, Maggiorini M, Bartsch P, et al. Simulated descent v dexamethasone in treatment of acute mountain sickness: A randomised trial. *BMJ.* 1995;310(6989):1232–1235.
67. Grissom CK, Roach RC, Sarnquist FH, et al. Acetazolamide in the treatment of acute mountain sickness: Clinical efficacy and effect on gas exchange. *Ann Intern Med.* 1992; 116(6):461–465.
68. Chow T, Browne V, Heileson HL, et al. Ginkgo biloba and acetazolamide prophylaxis for acute mountain sickness: A randomized, placebo-controlled trial. *Arch Intern Med.* 2005; 165(3):296–301.

69. Carlsten C, Swenson ER, Ruoss S. A dose-response study of acetazolamide for acute mountain sickness prophylaxis in vacationing tourists at 12,000 feet (3630 m). *High Alt Med Biol.* 2004;5(1):33–39.
70. Basnyat B, Gertsch JH, Johnson EW, et al. Efficacy of low-dose acetazolamide (125 mg BID) for the prophylaxis of acute mountain sickness: A prospective, double-blind, randomized, placebo-controlled trial. *High Alt Med Biol.* 2003;4(1):45–52.
71. Basu M, Sawhney RC, Kumar S, et al. Glucocorticoids as prophylaxis against acute mountain sickness. *Clin Endocrinol (Oxf).* 2002;57(6):761–767.
72. Johnson TS, Rock PB, Fulco CS, et al. Prevention of acute mountain sickness by dexamethazone. *N Engl J Med.* 1984;310(11):683–686.
73. Hackett PH, Roach RC, Wood RA, et al. Dexamethasone for prevention and treatment of acute mountain sickness. *Aviat Space Environ Med.* 1988;59(10):950–954.
74. Oelz O, Maggiorini M, Ritter M, et al. Nifedipine for high altitude pulmonary oedema. *Lancet.* 1989;2(8674):1241–1244.
75. Bartsch P, Maggiorini M, Ritter M, et al. Prevention of high-altitude pulmonary edema by nifedipine. *N Engl J Med.* 1991;325(18):1284–1289.
76. Perimenis P. Sildenafil for the treatment of altitude-induced hypoxaemia. *Expert Opin Pharmacother.* 2005;6(5):835–837.
77. Richalet JP, Gratadour P, Robach P, et al. Sildenafil inhibits altitude-induced hypoxemia and pulmonary hypertension. *Am J Respir Crit Care Med.* 2005;171(3):275–281.

CHAPTER 120

Ciguatera Poisoning

Hrayr P. Attarian

OBJECTIVES

- To discuss the prevalence and the geographic distribution of ciguatera poisoning
- To highlight the clinical features of ciguatera poisoning
- To discuss the diagnostic issues associated with ciguatera poisoning
- To discuss the different treatment methods available for patients with ciguatera poisoning

CASE VIGNETTE

A 28-year-old woman had distal dysesthesias of all four limbs following a bout of severe, self-limiting gastrointestinal upset characterized by nausea, vomiting, and diarrhea. She had just returned from a Caribbean vacation. She had no other illnesses, and claimed that the discomfort waxed and waned, and primarily involved her hands and feet. Peanuts, almonds, and alcohol made her dysesthesias worse. She also complained of a rather particular and uncomfortable hot feeling when her feet touched cold tile floors. In addition, she had occasional tingling of her gums. Her neurologic examination was unremarkable.

DEFINITION

Ciguatera is the most common non-bacterial form of seafood poisoning in North America and Europe.

EPIDEMIOLOGY

Serious, although rarely fatal (0.1%) (1), the mortality rate of ciguatera poisoning in one single outbreak reached 20% (2,3). Annually, approximately 50,000 cases of ciguatera poisoning are reported worldwide (4). Ciguatera poisoning is epidemic in certain areas of the Caribbean, Florida, Hawaii, Australia, and the South Pacific (4). In recent years, two major outbreaks also occurred in Hong Kong (5). Travelers from endemic areas (6–9) and imported seafood (10) have led to multiple case reports from nonendemic areas. Ciguatera is prevalent where there are recent blooms of algae harboring the toxic dinoflagellate. Sewage outfall, global warming, coral bleaching, and recent construction of dams and seawalls have produced conditions favorable to the proliferation of these toxic microorganisms (11,12). Geographic differences of the implicated toxins exist, as well as symptoms related to toxin exposure (13).

ETIOLOGY AND PATHOGENESIS

Ciguatera is contracted by eating any of a large number of species of fish containing ciguatoxin. Common offenders include barracuda, grouper jacks, hogfish, kingfish, moray eel, parrotfish, rock hind, certain sharks, snappers, surgeonfish, and triggerfish (Fig. 120-1) (14).

The likelihood of a fish containing significant toxin increases with the size of the fish. The risk of ciguatera poisoning also increases with the consumption of visceral organs and gonads (e.g., sea urchin) (15). Consumption of deep-water fish, shellfish, and cold water fish outside tropical areas, with rare exceptions, is generally safe(14,15). The toxin or toxins originate from a variety of dinoflagellates (unicellular flagellated organisms) (*Gambierdiscus toxicus*) (14,16) dwelling in the tropical bottom algae. These are ingested by bottom-feeding fish, that in turn, are eaten by larger fish, which despite bearing the toxin, appear healthy and, therefore, are consumed by humans.

The toxin, a tasteless, colorless, and odorless lipid-soluble polyether, is not removed or inactivated by any known cleaning method or storage condition.

In addition to ciguatoxin, many other toxins are found in dinoflagellates, including scaritoxin, maitotoxin, palytoxin, okadaic acid, and subvariants of these toxins (14,17,18). These toxins are known to cause an axonal channelopathy. Maitotoxin, acts at the calcium channel (19–21). Other adverse effects of these toxins include interference with a number of enzyme systems, hemolysis (22,23), as well as cholinergic and adrenergic side effects (14,24).

PATHOLOGY

Neuronal excitability is increased by ciguatoxin by a voltage shift of the activation of tetrodotoxin-sensitive Na+ channels to more negative potentials (25,26). Certain subtypes of ciguatoxin also act on tetrodotoxin-resistant Na+ channels at the level of the dorsal root ganglia (27). Other poorly understood cellular mechanisms are also involved in the pathogenesis of ciguatoxin toxicity (28,29). Gambierol, a toxin similar to ciguatoxin has been shown to cause systemic congestion of internal organs, primarily the lungs. Cyatoxin also causes gastrointestinal (GI) trace ulcerations (30). Neuronal nodal swelling and changes in internodal length and volume have been shown in experiments with *in vitro* ciguatoxins (31–33). This may

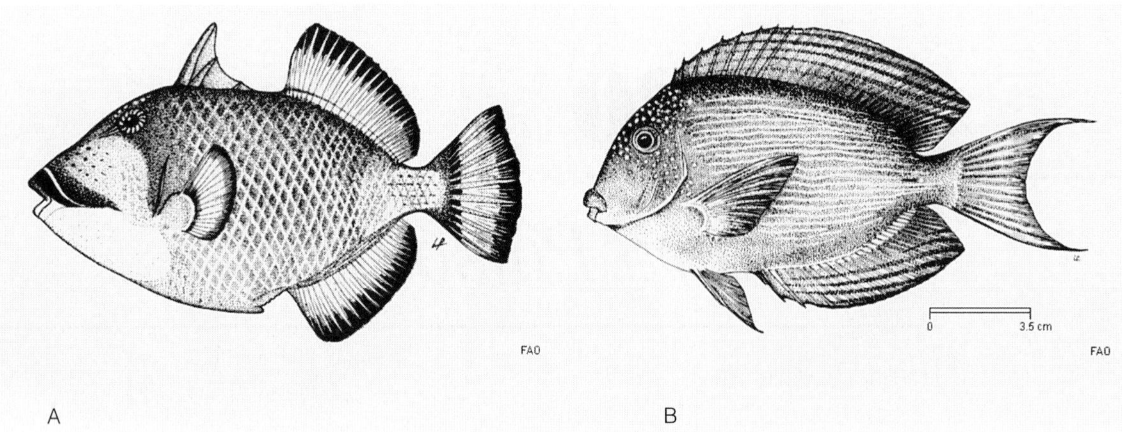

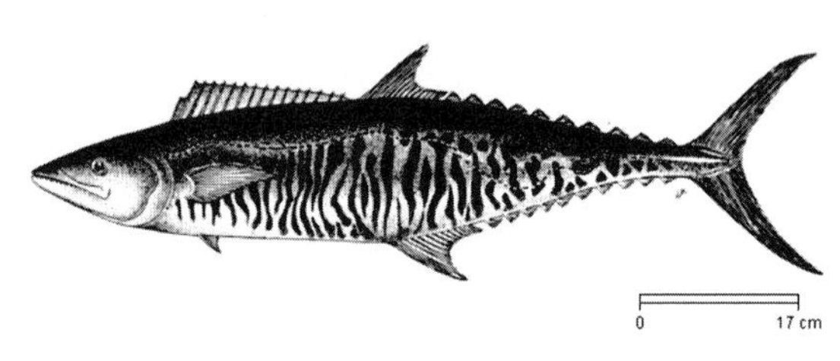

A: Triggerfish
B: Surgeonfish
C: Kingfish

FIGURE 120-1. Three types of fish commonly associated with ciguatera. (From Food and Agricultural Organization of the United Nations, Rome, Italy, with permission.)

account for the significantly slowed sensory and motor nerve conduction velocities and F-wave latencies found on electrophysiologic testing (34,35).

CLINICAL MANIFESTATIONS

The diverse symptomatology of ciguatera poisoning reflects its multiorgan involvement. Symptoms usually start 15 to 30 minutes following consumption of affected fish, but it can take up to 12 hours for the clinical manifestations to develop.

NEUROLOGIC

A unique feature of marine toxins, is the occurrence of an inverted sensory phenomenon, where "hot" feels "cold" and vice versa (14,36,37). Other sensory complaints include numbness, burning, itching, prickling, and other dysesthesias primarily affecting the limbs. These sensory complaints are usually made worse by alcohol consumption. Other neurologic symptoms include dizziness, headaches, perioral numbness, dry mouth, tooth pain, a metallic taste, fatigue, and diffuse muscular pain and stiffness. The more serious and rare neurologic symptoms (Table 120-1) tend to occur later in the course of the disease (14,38).

After the acute phase has subsided, symptoms associated with ciguatera poisoning can become chronic, lasting months to years. This stage is often characterized by fatigue, malaise, depression, muscle and joint aches, sensitivity to cold, and a variety of sensory symptoms, including pruritus after alcohol consumption (14,36,42). Rare cases of polymyositis have been reported months to years after the other manifestations of ciguatera have completely subsided (43,44).

DIAGNOSTIC APPROACH

No physical findings are characteristic of ciguatera poisoning nor do any confirmatory diagnostic laboratory tests exist. A retrospective history is often the only tool for diagnosis. As a result, ciguatera poisoning remains underdiagnosed, unless a high index of suspicion is present.

TABLE 120-1. Ciguatera Poisoning: Neurologic Manifestation

Cranial nerve palsies	Delirium and other behavioral problems
Areflexia	Stupor
Trismus	Generalized convulsions
Meningismus	Respiratory failure
Incoordination	Death
Carpopedal spasm	
Muscle weakness-flaccid paralysis	

(From Ting JY, Brown AF. Ciguatera poisoning: A global issue with common management problems. *Eur J Emerg Med.* 2001;8(4):295–300, with permission.)

TABLE 120-2. Ciguatera Poisoning: Other Symptoms by Body System Involved

Gastrointestinal	*Dermatologic*	*Genitourinary*[a]	*Cardiovascular*
Nausea/vomiting	Diffuse erythematous rash	Dysuria	CHF
Hypersalivation	Hair loss	Dyspareunia	Arrhythmias
Abdominal cramps		Pain with breastfeeding	Hypertension
Diarrhea			Hypotension
			Pulmonary edema

[a]Sexual, placental and breast milk transmission.
(From Ting JY, Brown AF. Ciguatera poisoning: A global issue with common management problems. *Eur J Emerg Med.* 2001;8(4):295–300; Lange WR. Ciguatera fish poisoning. *Am Fam Physician.* 1994;50(3): 579–584; Lange WR, Lipkin KM, Yang GC. Can ciguatera be a sexually transmitted disease? *J Toxicol Clin Toxicol.* 1989;27(3):193–197; and Blythe DG, de Sylva DP. Mother's milk turns toxic following fish feast. *JAMA.* 1990;264(16):2074, with permission.)

Multisystem symptomatology (Table 120-2) in a remarkably uncomfortable patient, in the context of a history of suspicious fish consumption, should raise the possibility of ciguatera poisoning. Occasionally, only GI or neurologic symptoms may be present.

Differential diagnosis includes, among others, sea food allergy and self-limiting bacterial infections from sea food consumption. Those with potentially serious consequences are *Vibrio* infection (42), botulism, and other selective seafood poisonings, including pufferfish and shellfish poisonings (4). A worsening of the condition can occur after reexposure (14).

Methods to detect the affected fish vary from the "folkloric" to sophisticated highly technical methodology. Some fishermen in tropical regions of the world, rub fish organs on their gums. In the case that the fish is affected, they would experience tingling in their gums (45). Others lay out suspected fish on the sand; if ants seem attracted to it, then the fish is felt to be fit for consumption(46). On the other hand, radioimmunoassay, enzyme immunoassay, high-performance liquid chromatography with mass spectrometry, and hapten-specific antibodies are available to detect toxin in affected fish (47–52).

TREATMENT

No antidote is available for ciguatera poisoning. Treatment remains supportive, including cardiopulmonary monitoring and mechanical respiratory support and cardiac pacing if needed, as well as correction of fluid and electrolyte imbalance associated with severe dehydration (14,53). If vomiting has not occurred within 6 to 8 hours after fish ingestion, gastric lavage, emetics, or both can be administered.

Traditionally, intravenous administration of mannitol has been first-line treatment in acute cases seen within 24 hours of poisoning. Use of mannitol after the first 24 hour period is less effective. Retreatment if symptoms persist, can be useful (54–57). A potential adverse effect of mannitol treatment includes severe dehydration. Mannitol increases water efflux to the extracellular space, hence reducing nodal swelling (55–60). A recent study, however, showed mannitol to be of equal efficacy to normal saline, but with more side effects in the first 24 hours of administration (61) As a preventative measure, lactated ringer solutions are often used (14).

Many case reports discuss the use of various other medications for symptomatic relief (Table 120-3), including calcium channel blockers, chlorpromazine, diphenhydramine, H2 receptor blockers, mexiletine, neostigmine, tramadol, vitamin B complex, and vitamin B_{12}. A serotonin-sparing diet (without seafood, nuts, seeds, alcohol, chocolate, fungi, and mayonnaise) is advocated, not only during the acute phase, but also up to 6 months following resolution of symptoms (14,62).

CLINICAL RECOMMENDATIONS OF THE VIGNETTE

The patient had an electromyogram (EMG). The nerve conduction velocity (NCV) study that followed showed a mild delay in F-waves in both upper and lower limb. A diagnosis of ciguatera poisoning was made and she was advised to avoid alcohol, nuts and nut oils, and seafood for 6 months after exposure.

TABLE 120-3. Ciguatera Poisoning Symptomatic Management

Symptoms	*Medication(s)*
Symptomatic bradycardia	Intravenous (IV) atropine
Prolonged hypotensive episodes	Dopamine infusion
Hypocalcemia (ciguatoxin competitively inhibits calcium)	IV calcium gluconate
Agitation	Benzodiazepines[a]
Seizures	Benzodiazepines/phenytoin[b]
Pain and dysesthesias	NSAID/acetaminophen/ steroids/gabapentin/lidocaine
Pruritus	Cyproheptadine Lidocaine
Fatigue and malaise	Amitriptyline Fluoxetine

[a]Opiates can cause hypotension, and therefore are generally avoided.
[b]Barbiturates can cause hypotension, and therefore are generally avoided.
NSAID, nonsteroidal anti-inflammatory drugs.
(From Stommel EW. Ciguatera. In: Gilman S, ed. *MedLink Neurology.* San Diego: MedLink; 2006; Sims JK. A theoretical discourse on the pharmacology of toxic marine ingestions. *Ann Emerg Med.* 1987;16(9): 1006–1015; Perez CM, Vasquez PA, Perret CF. Treatment of ciguatera poisoning with gabapentin. *N Engl J Med.* 2001;344(9):692–693; and Berlin RM, King SL, Blythe DG. Symptomatic improvement of chronic fatigue with fluoxetine in ciguatera fish poisoning. *Med J Aust.* 1992; 157(8):567, with permission.)

Symptomatic treatment of paresthesias was to be accomplished with gabapentin or amitriptyline.

SUMMARY

Ciguatera poisoning is a relatively common, but often underdiagnosed seafood toxicity associated with multisystem involvement. Symptoms are often nonspecific. A pathognomonic symptom is a reversal of temperature sensation. Treatment is mainly symptomatic. Opiates and barbiturates should be avoided. During the recovery phase, alcohol, nuts, and fish should be avoided.

Prevention is primarily accomplished by avoiding consumption of tropical reef fish, primarily those at the top of the food chain (fish >2 kg), as well as avoidance of consuming gonads and visceral organ meat.

REFERENCES

1. Lange WR. Ciguatera toxicity. *Am Fam Physician.* 1987;35(4):177–182.
2. Glaziou P, Legrand AM. The epidemiology of ciguatera fish poisoning. *Toxicon.* 1994;32(8): 863–873.
3. Habermehl GG, Krebs HC, Rasoanaivo P, et al. Severe ciguatera poisoning in Madagascar: A case report. *Toxicon.* 1994;32(12):1539–1542.
4. Ting JY, Brown AF. Ciguatera poisoning: A global issue with common management problems. *Eur J Emerg Med.* 2001;8(4):295–300.
5. Wong CK, Hung P, Lee KL, et al. Study of an outbreak of ciguatera fish poisoning in Hong Kong. *Toxicon.* 2005;46(5):563–571.
6. Payne CA, Payne SN. Ciguatera in Puerto Rico and the Virgin Islands. *N Engl J Med.* 1977;296(16):949–950.
7. Puente Puente S, Cabrera Majada A, Lago Nunez M, et al. [Ciguatera: Eight imported cases]. *Rev Clin Esp.* 2005;205(2):47–50.
8. Raikhlin-Eisenkraft B, Finkelstein Y, Spanier E. Ciguatera-like poisoning in the Mediterranean. *Vet Hum Toxicol.* 1988;30(6):582–583.
9. Blume C, Rapp M, Rath J, et al. [Ciguatera poisoning. Growing differential diagnostic significance in the age of foreign tourism]. *Med Klin (Munich).* 1999;94(1):45–49.
10. Pilon P, Dion R, Jochem K, et al. Ciguatera food poisoning linked to the consumption of imported barracuda—Montreal, Quebec, 1998. *Can Commun Dis Rep.* 2000;26(9):73–76.
11. Hokama Y, Wachi KM, Shiraki A, et al. The biological assessment of flora and fauna as standards for changes in the near-shore ocean environment: A study of Barbers Point Harbor. *J Nat Toxins.* 2001;10(1):57–68.
12. Lehane L. Ciguatera update. *Med J Aust.* 2000;172(4):176–179.
13. Lewis RJ. The changing face of ciguatera. *Toxicon.* 2001;39(1):97–106.
14. Stommel EW. Ciguatera. In: Gilman S, ed. *MedLink Neurology.* San Diego: MedLink; 2006.
15. Pottier I, Vernoux JP, Lewis RJ. Ciguatera fish poisoning in the Caribbean islands and Western Atlantic. *Rev Environ Contam Toxicol.* 2001;168:99–141.
16. Bagnis R, Chanteau S, Chungue E, et al. Origins of ciguatera fish poisoning: A new dinoflagellate, Gambierdiscus toxicus Adachi and Fukuyo, definitively involved as a causal agent. *Toxicon.* 1980;18(2):199–208.
17. Kodama AM, Hokama Y, Yasumoto T, et al. Clinical and laboratory findings implicating palytoxin as cause of ciguatera poisoning due to Decapterus macrosoma (mackerel). *Toxicon.* 1989;27(9):1051–1053.
18. Tosteson TR. The diversity and origins of toxins in ciguatera fish poisoning. *Puerto Rico Health Science Journal.* 1995;14(2):117–129.
19. Yamaoka K, Inoue M, Miyahara H, et al. A quantitative and comparative study of the effects of a synthetic ciguatoxin CTX3C on the kinetic properties of voltage-dependent sodium channels. *Br J Pharmacol.* 2004;142(5):879–889.
20. Gutmann L, Gutmann L. Axonal channelopathies: An evolving concept in the pathogenesis of peripheral nerve disorders. *Neurology.* 1996;47(1):18–21.
21. Butera R, Prockop LD, Buonocore M, et al. Mild ciguatera poisoning: Case reports with neurophysiological evaluations. *Muscle Nerve.* 2000;23(10):1598–1603.
22. Ohizumi Y. [Pharmacological studies on toxins from marine organisms that act on ion channels]. *Yakugaku Zasshi.* 1987;107(7):471–484.
23. Wu CH, Narahashi T. Mechanism of action of novel marine neurotoxins on ion channels. *Annu Rev Pharmacol Toxicol.* 1988;28:141–161.
24. Escalona De Motta G, Mercado JA, Tosteson TR, et al. Modulation of acetylcholine receptor channel by a polar component isolated from toxic Ostreopsis lenticularis extracts. *Bull Soc Pathol Exot.* 1992;85(5 Pt 2):489–493.
25. Hogg RC, Lewis RJ, Adams DJ. Ciguatoxin (CTX-1) modulates single tetrodotoxin-sensitive sodium channels in rat parasympathetic neurones. *Neurosci Lett.* 1998;252(2):103–106.
26. Hogg RC, Lewis RJ, Adams DJ. Ciguatoxin-induced oscillations in membrane potential and action potential firing in rat parasympathetic neurons. *Eur J Neurosci.* 2002;16(2): 242–248.
27. Strachan LC, Lewis RJ, Nicholson GM. Differential actions of pacific ciguatoxin-1 on sodium channel subtypes in mammalian sensory neurons. *J Pharmacol Exp Ther.* 1999;288(1): 379–388.
28. Dechraoui MY, Naar J, Pauillac S, et al. Ciguatoxins and brevetoxins, neurotoxic polyether compounds active on sodium channels. *Toxicon.* 1999;37(1):125–143.
29. Dechraoui MY, Tiedeken JA, Persad R, et al. Use of two detection methods to discriminate ciguatoxins from brevetoxins: Application to great barracuda from Florida Keys. *Toxicon.* 2005;46(3):261–270.
30. Ito E, Suzuki-Toyota F, Toshimori K, et al. Pathological effects on mice by gambierol, possibly one of the ciguatera toxins. *Toxicon.* 2003;42(7):733–740.
31. Benoit E, Juzans P, Legrand AM, et al. Nodal swelling produced by ciguatoxin-induced selective activation of sodium channels in myelinated nerve fibers. *Neuroscience.* 1996;71(4): 1121–1131.
32. Mattei C, Benoit E, Juzans P, et al. Gambiertoxin (CTX-4B), purified from wild Gambierdiscus toxicus dinoflagellates, induces Na(+)-dependent swelling of single frog myelinated axons and motor nerve terminals in situ. *Neurosci Lett.* 1997;234(2–3):75–78.
33. Mattei C, Dechraoui MY, Molgo J, et al. Neurotoxins targeting receptor site 5 of voltage-dependent sodium channels increase the nodal volume of myelinated axons. *J Neurosci Res.* 1999;55(6):666–673.
34. Cameron J, Flowers AE, Capra MF. Electrophysiological studies on ciguatera poisoning in man (Part II). *J Neurol Sci.* 1991;101(1):93–97.
35. Cameron J, Flowers AE, Capra MF. Effects of ciguatoxin on nerve excitability in rats (Part I). *J Neurol Sci.* 1991;101(1):87–92.
36. Bagnis R, Kuberski T, Laugier S. Clinical observations on 3,009 cases of ciguatera (fish poisoning) in the South Pacific. *Am J Trop Med Hyg.* 1979;28(6):1067–1073.
37. Cameron J, Capra MF. The basis of the paradoxical disturbance of temperature perception in ciguatera poisoning. *J Toxicol Clin Toxicol.* 1993;31(4):571–579.
38. Angibaud G, Rambaud S. Serious neurological manifestations of ciguatera: Is the delay unusually long? *J Neurol Neurosurg Psychiatry.* 1998;64(5):688–689.
39. Lange WR. Ciguatera fish poisoning. *Am Fam Physician.* 1994;50(3):579–584.
40. Lange WR, Lipkin KM, Yang GC. Can ciguatera be a sexually transmitted disease? *J Toxicol Clin Toxicol.* 1989;27(3):193–197.
41. Blythe DG, de Sylva DP. Mother's milk turns toxic following fish feast. *JAMA.* 1990;264(16): 2074.
42. Eastaugh J, Shepherd S. Infectious and toxic syndromes from fish and shellfish consumption. A review. *Arch Intern Med.* 1989;149(8):1735–1740.
43. Stommel EW, Jenkyn LR, Parsonnet J. Another case of polymyositis after ciguatera toxin exposure. *Arch Neurol.* 1993;50(6):571.
44. Stommel EW, Parsonnet J, Jenkyn LR. Polymyositis after ciguatera toxin exposure. *Arch Neurol.* 1991;48(8):874–847.
45. Caplan CE. Ciguatera fish poisoning. *CMAJ.* 1998;159(11):1394.
46. Irving AM. Ciguatera fish poisoning. *CMAJ.* 1999;160(8):1127.
47. Boydron-Le Garrec R, Benoit E, Sauviat MP, et al. [Detection of ciguatoxins: Advantages and drawbacks of different biological methods]. *J Soc Biol.* 2005;199(2):115–125.
48. Hokama Y, Asahina AY, Shang ES, et al. Evaluation of the Hawaiian reef fishes with the solid phase immunobead assay. *J Clin Lab Anal.* 1993;7(1):26–30.
49. Hokama Y, Nishimura K, Takenaka W, et al. Simplified solid-phase membrane immunobead assay (MIA) with monoclonal anti-ciguatoxin antibody (MAb-CTX) for detection of ciguatoxin and related polyether toxins. *J Nat Toxins.* 1998;7(1):1–21.
50. Lewis RJ, Jones A, Vernoux JP. HPLC/tandem electrospray mass spectrometry for the determination of sub-ppb levels of Pacific and Caribbean ciguatoxins in crude extracts of fish. *Anal Chem.* 1999;71(1):247–250.
51. Park DL. Evolution of methods for assessing ciguatera toxins in fish. *Rev Environ Contam Toxicol.* 1994;136:1–20.
52. Pottier I, Vernoux JP, Jones A, et al. Analysis of toxin profiles in three different fish species causing ciguatera fish poisoning in Guadeloupe, French West Indies. *Food Addit Contam.* 2002;19(11):1034–1042.
53. Currie BJ. Marine antivenoms. *J Toxicol Clin Toxicol.* 2003;41(3):301–308.
54. Mattei C, Molgo J, Marquais M, et al. Hyperosmolar D-mannitol reverses the increased membrane excitability and the nodal swelling caused by Caribbean ciguatoxin-1 in single frog myelinated axons. *Brain Res.* 1999;847(1):50–58.
55. Palafox NA, Jain LG, Pinano AZ, et al. Successful treatment of ciguatera fish poisoning with intravenous mannitol. *JAMA.* 1988;259(18):2740–2742.
56. Pearn JH, Lewis RJ, Ruff T, et al. Ciguatera and mannitol: Experience with a new treatment regimen. *Med J Aust.* 1989;151(2):77–80.
57. Purcell CE, Capra MF, Cameron J. Action of mannitol in ciguatoxin-intoxicated rats. *Toxicon.* 1999;37(1):67–76.
58. Swift AE, Swift TR. Ciguatera. *J Toxicol Clin Toxicol.* 1993;31(1):1–29.
59. Williams RK, Palafox NA. Treatment of pediatric ciguatera fish poisoning. *Am J Dis Child.* 1990;144(7):747–748.
60. Blythe DG, De Sylva DP, Fleming LE, et al. Clinical experience with i.v. Mannitol in the treatment of ciguatera. *Bull Soc Pathol Exot.* 1992;85(5 Pt 2):425–426.
61. Schnorf H, Taurarii M, Cundy T. Ciguatera fish poisoning: A double-blind randomized trial of mannitol therapy. *Neurology.* 2002;58(6):873–880.
62. Sims JK. A theoretical discourse on the pharmacology of toxic marine ingestions. *Ann Emerg Med.* 1987;16(9):1006–1015.
63. Perez CM, Vasquez PA, Perret CF. Treatment of ciguatera poisoning with gabapentin. *N Engl J Med.* 2001;344(9):692–693.
64. Cameron J, Flowers AE, Capra MF. Modification of the peripheral nerve disturbance in ciguatera poisoning in rats with lidocaine. *Muscle Nerve.* 1993;16(7):782–786.
65. Bowman PB. Amitriptyline and ciguatera. *Med J Aust.* 1984;140(13):802.
66. Calvert GM, Hryhorczuk DO, Leikin JB. Treatment of ciguatera fish poisoning with amitriptyline and nifedipine. *J Toxicol Clin Toxicol.* 1987;25(5):423–428.
67. Davis RT, Villar LA. Symptomatic improvement with amitriptyline in ciguatera fish poisoning. *N Engl J Med.* 1986;315(1):65.
68. Berlin RM, King SL, Blythe DG. Symptomatic improvement of chronic fatigue with fluoxetine in ciguatera fish poisoning. *Med J Aust.* 1992;157(8):567.

CHAPTER 121

Venomous Snakebites in the US

Christopher Commichau

OBJECTIVES

- To dispel many of the common phobias surrounding snakes
- To describe the real risk posed by venomous snakes in the US
- To discuss the basic field measures in case of envenomation
- To describe the signs and symptoms of envenomation and the need for urgent medical attention

CASE VIGNETTE

A 32-year-old man was brought to a local emergency room after being bitten by a rattlesnake above the left ankle. His friends witnessed the bite and shot the snake. Initially, the patient walked to his truck until the pain in his leg became severe. He was then carried by his friends and was placed in the back of his truck and covered with blankets. The incident occurred 35 minutes before his arrival in the emergency room. On initial evaluation, he was diaphoretic, tachycardic, and tachypneic. He complained of nausea, a tingling scalp, and a metallic taste. He also complained of severe pain in his leg and was mildly confused. His temperature was 99.1°F and his blood pressure was 98/66 mm Hg. He had swelling of the left leg 6 inches above visible puncture wounds, one of which had a superimposed crude incision that was oozing. He had ecchymotic areas on the left calf. Additional history obtained from his friends revealed that he had two shots of tequila to help with the pain en route. His friends also smelled of alcohol.

Two 18 gauge intravenous lines were placed and normal saline was infused at 200 mL/hour. He was administered morphine for pain. Laboratory values came back with a prolonged prothrombin time of 13.9 s, a platelet count of $129 \times 10^3/\text{mm}^3$ and fibrinogen of 190 mg/dL. His blood alcohol level was 0.198.

Antivenin was reconstituted by the medical team and given when it was ready for use (approximately 45 minutes after his arrival). He required a second dose of antivenin before his laboratory values, vital signs, and clinical examination normalized. He spent 8 days in the hospital and required débridement of the skin over the puncture sites. He did not require skin grafting.

DEFINITION

Little else in the natural world has so captivated our collective psyche as have snakes. They are the subject of our most virulent phobias and wreak havoc on our cinematic nerves. We are fascinated by them, yet understand them little. In reality, very few pose any real danger to inhabitants of the United States. Several poisonous snake species, however, do account for serious envenomations in the United States. Approximately 25% of snake species native to the United States are venomous (1). Most are members of the crotalid family that includes rattlesnakes, cottonmouths, and copperheads. The crotalids are also known as pit vipers, a descriptive that refers to the heat-seeking apparatus (pits) located on their triangular heads. crotalids are also characterized by their elliptical pupils. Rattlesnakes are widespread throughout the United States and the largest is the eastern diamondback species, which can easily reach 6 feet in length or greater. The elapid family accounts for the only other venomous species in the United States, the coral snakes. Coral snakes are colorful, slender snakes that tend to be shy and reclusive, striking only when handled. Their color pattern places a red band directly next to a yellow band. Other, nonvenomous species can be mistaken for coral snakes, but have red bands contiguous with black bands. This distinction has given rise to the saying "red on black-friend of Jack, red on yellow-kill a fellow."

EPIDEMIOLOGY

Estimates of snakebites vary, ranging from 6,000 to 45,000 annually in the United States (2,3). Bites from venomous snakes are approximately 3,000 to 8,000 annually. Interestingly, all states in the continental United States, except Maine, have indigenous rattlesnake populations (3). Deaths are almost certainly fewer than 10 per year (4,5). Deaths are more likely in the very young and very old or those with significant comorbid medical conditions. Fundamentalist group members that include snake handling as part of their religious practice may be at increased risk of sustaining significant envenomation. Young white men are the demographic group most likely to sustain a bite. Venomous bites are more likely to occur in the southern states with a trend toward the southwest (6). The expansion of population in the southwest is placing humans and snakes in closer proximity, whereas eastern snake populations seem to be declining as habitat disappears. Alcohol plays a role in many preventable envenomations (7). The summer months see the highest rates of snakebite. Increasingly, nonnative snakes, including venomous species, are being kept as pets and account for a number of serious bites (1).

ETIOLOGY AND PATHOGENESIS

The danger of snakebite lies in the delivery of the venom. The delivery system ultimately ends with the fangs, but includes venom glands and ducts. It is thought that the heat-sensing pits on vipers can regulate the amount of venom delivered, depending on the size of prey or perceived threat (8). The size of the snake has an important relation to the amount of venom delivered (9,10). A quarter of humans bitten result in no delivery of venom for various reasons (11,12). Severe envenomations occur even less commonly. The fangs of vipers are relatively large, retractable, fragile, and act as hypodermic needles. The fangs of coral snakes are smaller and are fixed in the jaw (unlike those of pit vipers) and require the snake to "chew" to inject sufficient venom. Snake venom is complex and can vary substantially in composition from species to species, between individuals of the same species, and from samples taken from the same individual (5,13). Environmental factors, such as temperature, diet, and age, can influence the composition of venom (14). Most venoms are a mixture of several different proteins possessing enzymatic activity. The action of the enzymes leads to tissue damage and systemic morbidity. Venom tends to be stable, resistant to deactivation, a fact that has implications for treatment as toxic effects can be seen for days (15). The list of proteins that have been isolated from North American snake venom is impressive and includes transaminases, phospholipases, collegenases, acetylcholinesterase, endonucleases, and other proteolytic enzymes, such as metalloproteinase (16). As has been pointed out by others, labeling venoms under a single category, such as a *myotoxin*, *neurotoxin*, or other, is simply misleading and fails to recognize the biologic diversity of these substances (17). Pit viper venom damages capillary endothelium eventually leading to leakage of plasma and red cells into tissue, which then serves as substrate for other enzymatic activity (18). The loss of circulating volume can lead to significant edema and can precipitate circulatory collapse and shock. The most deleterious effects of venom seem to be on the hematologic, cardiac, respiratory, and nervous systems (15). Myonecrosis can be prominent (19). The hematologic effects are often prominent and affect capillaries preferentially resulting in petechiae. Thrombinlike proteins can interfere with fibrinogen and produce unstable clots, which are subsequently lysed. Endothelial damage can lead to platelet aggregation and thrombosis causing organ damage and a consumptive coagulopathy. Populations of Mojave rattlesnakes and timber rattlesnakes have been shown to contain more neurotoxic substances in their venom (20,21). Neurotoxic effects can be through presynaptic blockade of acetylcholine and interruption of neurotransmission leading to paralysis (22,23). Myokymia is seen particularly with timber rattlesnake venom and is thought to be mediated through calcium channel interruption (24). Neuromuscular effects are prominent with elapid venom and are thought to result from postsynaptic blockade of acetylcholine in the neuromuscular junction (25). This venom also contains significant proteolytic enzymes allowing for rapid spread of venom through tissue. A mature coral snake carries toxins sufficient to kill five adults (26).

PATHOLOGY

Because death from snakebite is rare, few autopsy series exist for pathologic reports. Most pathologic findings mirror the effects of the venom. Myonecrosis is reported in autopsy cases (27). Laboratory abnormalities include increased creatine kinase (CK) and potassium. Erythrocytes can appear misshapen because of altered membrane function. Levels of fibrinogen and platelets can be low. The prothrombin time can be prolonged and the partial thromboplastin time abnormal. Disseminated intravascular coagulation has been reported and can give rise to thrombosis in many organ systems (5). Hemorrhagic blebs and underlying tissue necrosis is often seen. White blood cell counts and glucose levels may be elevated. The hematocrit can be elevated if significant plasma has been lost or it can be low in cases of frank hemorrhage. Serum creatinine can rise if renal failure is present. The urinalysis, electrocardiogram, and chest X-ray study may all show abnormalities.

CLINICAL MANIFESTATIONS

The exact progression of symptoms after an envenomation is hard to anticipate because venom varies in composition and potency. Pain and swelling are early and common symptoms in crotalid bites. Pain is usually present early and prominently at the bite site. Edema formation begins shortly thereafter and is a sign of ongoing capillary damage. Ecchymoses and lymphangitis are other local symptoms. Systemic findings include nausea and vomiting. A metallic taste or other gustatory sensation can be present (11). A general sense of weakness pervades as may a sense of doom. Whether this is a direct effect of the toxins or a psychogenic response is not clear. Early, there may be tachycardia with tachypnea and hypertension followed later, in serious envenomation, by hypotension and shock as the intravascular volume is depleted. Consumptive coagulopathy can lead to systemic bleeding, including bleeding in the central nervous system. Respiratory distress can ensue because of neurotoxins or pulmonary edema. Neuromuscular paralysis and parasthesias, along with fasciculations and myokymia, may be present. Neurotoxic effects are often prominent in coral snake bites. Symptoms can be delayed as venom progresses through tissue before significant neurologic effects are evident. Altered mental status is common and can present as euphoria (28). Cranial nerve abnormalities, which are often seen, include ptosis, dysarthria, and dysphagia. Neuromuscular respiratory failure is particularly worrisome.

Snakebite in pregnancy raises additional concerns and, in general, focus should be on the mother. In cases with significant hematologic effects, placental abruption and preterm labor have been documented (29). Children and the elderly are especially at risk for serious envenomations because of size and comorbidity.

DIAGNOSIS

It is important to identify the species administering the venom and, when possible, the animal should be safely transported for knowledgeable identification. Care must be taken even with dead snakes because the bite reflex persists well after death (11). Puncture sites should be identified and can often help in determining venomous from nonvenomous bites. Lacking positive identification, signs and symptoms can often suggest a likely species.

TREATMENT

Care of the snakebite victim begins immediately and in the field. Immobilization of the stricken limb at or below the level of the heart is ideal. Transport to the nearest facility staffed by skilled personnel is paramount. Folk treatments heard through the years should not be attempted and may worsen injury. This includes incisions, suction, tourniquets, ice packs, and heat packs (6,30). The principles of ABC (airway, breathing and circulation) should rule. If the victim must walk, the limb should be splinted and any jewelry removed in anticipation of swelling (15). The leading edge of tissue swelling should be marked and timed. There may be benefit to pressure immobilization for elapid bites (13,28). Once in a health care facility, vital signs are monitored closely; a history and a baseline examination should be documented and laboratory studies are drawn. Crystalloid solutions should be started. In the absence of serious symptoms, patients with cortaid bites should be monitored at least 8 hours and elapid bite patients a minimum of 24 hours because of the high neurotoxicity and delayed onset of effects (15). Pain control should be achieved; however, caution should be used in administering sedation and opioids in coral snake bites and certain rattlesnake bites because of their neurotoxic venoms (15). Medications effecting coagulation should be limited. Antibiotics are not routinely used. Tetanus status should be up-to-date. Historically, fasciotomy was used commonly to relieve pressure in edematous tissue. Elevated compartment pressures more likely stem from direct effect on muscle by toxin and may respond to antivenin alone. Fasciotomy is reserved for elevated compartment pressures with neurovascular compromise in patients who have already received antivenin (31,32). Significant envenomations should be treated with antivenin. Currently, two commercially available crotalid antivenins in the United States are Antivenin Crotalidae Polyvalent (ACP) made by Wyeth-Ayerst Laboratories (Philadelphia) and CroFab made by Protherics (Brentwood, Tennessee), which was approved by the US Food and Drug Administration (FDA) in 2000. Antivenin is also available for coral snakes envenomations. All antivenin preparations carry the risk of allergic reaction, including anaphylaxis. The risk appears lower with the newer agent (33). In general, antivenin is used for moderate envenomations, with any sign of rapid progression of local effects, neurologic, hematologic, or cardiac derangement. Initial dosages vary depending on the suspected severity of envenomation. Repeated doses may be necessary. If coral snakebite is suspected, antivenin is given immediately because the neurologic effects can be delayed and are difficult to reverse once initiated (15). If possible, the facility receiving the patient should be alerted before arrival to have the antivenin reconstituted and ready for use. Patients receiving antivenin need to be monitored closely until clinical and laboratory signs return to normal. Patients need to be counseled on the signs and symptoms of delayed serum sickness. Tissue injury often needs surgical attention for débridement.

Regional poison control centers and zoos can be extremely helpful in guiding appropriate therapy when there is uncertainty in the offending species or when antivenin is needed.

CLINICAL RECOMMENDATIONS OF THE VIGNETTE

The patient presented highlights several key issues in responding to venomous snakebite. His friends should have transported the patient to a vehicle with his leg immobilized rather than allowing him to walk. It would have been ideal for someone to have called 911 or called ahead to the hospital so that antivenin could have been reconstituted before arrival.

The practice making incisions over the puncture sites to extract venom has no basis because it likely causes more tissue injury and is not effective in removing venom. Little should be done in the field other than assisting the victim with comfort and removal from the field. The most important element in immediate care is early transport to an appropriate facility. the patient was appropriately kept calm and warm on transport to the hospital. On arrival, he had systemic signs of envenomation and was immediately given fluid resuscitation. His laboratory values suggested coagulation abnormalities. His vital signs suggested volume depletion. Antivenin was indicated and given as soon as it was reconstituted. He required an extended stay because of tissue damage, but eventually recovered. He required a tetanus shot because his immunization status was unknown. It may have been helpful for his friends to have brought in the snake for species identification.

SUMMARY

Snakebites in the United States rarely result in death. Serious consequences, however, can result from envenomation by many species indigenous to the United States. Prompt initiation of measures in the field that limit the rapid circulation of venom can be helpful. The patient should be immobilized and kept calm and warm. Rapid transport to the nearest facility equipped to treat the injury is crucial to good outcome. Basic life support measures should be instituted to support the circulatory and respiratory systems. The use of antivenin has proved to be efficacious and lifesaving, despite potential risks of allergic reaction.

Clearly, prevention is the best strategy because many encounters resulting in snakebite can be avoided. When traveling in an area populated by venomous snakes, it is prudent to know the location of the nearest medical center as well as the number to the nearest poison control center.

REFERENCES

1. Gold BS. Bites and stings. In: Beers MH, Berlow R, ed. *The Merck Manual of Diagnosis and Therapy*, 17 ed. New York: John Wiley & Sons; 1999:2644.
2. Watson WA, Litovitz TL, Klein-Schwartz W, et al. 2003 annual report of the American Association of Poison Control Centers Toxic Exposure Surveillance System. *Am J Emerg Med.* 2004;22:335.
3. Parrish HM. Incidence of treated snakebites in the United States. *Public Health Rep.* 1966;81:269–276.
4. Langley RL, Morrow WE. Deaths resulting from animal attacks in the United States. *Wilderness Environ Med.* 1997;8:8–16.
5. Singletary EM, Rochman AS, Bodmer JCA, et al. Envenomations. *Med Clin North Am.* 2005;89:1195–1224.
6. Gold BS, Wingert WA. Snake venom poisoning in the United States: A review of therapeutic practice. *South Med J.* 1994;87:579–589.
7. Wingert WA, Chin L. Rattlesnake bites in southern California and rationale for recommended treatment. *West J Med.* 1988;148:37–44.

8. Wingert WA, Wainschel J. Diagnosis and management of envenomation by poisonous snakes. *South Med J.* 1975;68:1015–1026.
9. Hayes WK. Ontogeny of striking, prey-handling and envenomation behavior of prairie rattlesnakes, Crotalus v. viridis. *Toxicon.* 1991;29:867–875.
10. Klauber LM. *Rattlesnakes: Their Habits, Life Histories, and Influence on Mankind,* 2 ed. Berkeley: University of California Press; 1997.
11. Russell FE. *Snake Venom Poisoning.* New York: Scholium International; 1983.
12. Parrish HM, Goldner JC, Silberg SL. Poisonous snakebites causing no venomation. *Postgrad Med.* 1966;39:265–269.
13. Norris RL, Bush SP. North American venomous reptile bites. In: Auerbach, ed. *Wilderness Medicine,* 4th ed. St. Louis: Mosby; 2001.
14. Glenn JL. Geographical variation in Crotalus scutulatus scutulatus (Mojave rattlesnake) venom properties. *Toxicon.* 1983;21:119–130.
15. Gold BS, Barish RA, Dart RC. North American snake envenomation: Diagnosis, treatment, and management. *Emerg Med Clin North Am.* 2004;22:423–443.
16. Bjarnason JB, Fox JW. Hemorrhagic metalloproteinases from snake venoms. *Pharmacol Ther.* 1994;62:325–372.
17. Russell FE. Snake venom poisoning in the US. *Annu Rev Med.* 1980;31:247–259.
18. Obrig TG, Louise CB, Moran TP, et al. Direct cytotoxic effects of hemorrhagic toxins from Crotalus ruber ruber and Crotalus atrox on human endothelial cells. *Microvasc Res.* 1993;46:412–416.
19. Ownby CL, Colberg TR, White SP. Isolation, characterization and crystallization of a phospholipase A2 myotoxin from the venom of the prairie rattlesnake. *Toxicon.* 1997;35:111–124.
20. Clark RFL, Williams SR, Nordt SP, et al. Successful treatment of crotalid-induced neurotoxicity with a new polyspecific crotalid Fab antivenom. *Ann Emerg Med.* 1997;30:54–57.
21. Jansen PW, Perkin RM, Van Stralen D. Mojave rattlesnake envenomation: Prolonged neurotoxicity and rhabdomyolysis. *Ann Emerg Med.* 1992;21:322–325.
22. Valdes JJ, Thompson RG, Wolff VL, et al. Inhibition of calcium channel dihydropyridine receptor binding by purified Mojave toxin. *Neurotoxicol Teratol.* 1989;11:129–133.
23. Hodgson WC, Wickramaratna JC. In vitro neuromuscular activity of snake venoms. *Clin Exp Pharmacol Physiol.* 2002;29(9):807–814.
24. Lewis RL, Gutman L. Snake venoms and the neuromuscular junction. *Semin Neurol.* 2004;24(2):175–179.
25. Chang CC. The action of snake venoms on nerve and muscle. In: Lee CY, ed. *Snake Venoms.* New York: Springer-Verlag; 1979.
26. Fix JD. Venom yield of the North American coral snake and its clinical significance. *South Med J.* 1980;73:737–738.
27. Carroll RR, Hall EL, Kitchens CS. Canebrake rattlesnake envenomation. *Ann Emerg Med.* 1997;30:45–48.
28. McCollough NC, Gennaro JF. Treatment of venomous snakebite in the United States. *Clin Toxicol.* 1970;3:483–500.
29. Zugaib M, de Barros AC, Bittar RE, et al. Abruptio placentae following snakebite. *Am J Obstet Gynecol.* 1985;151:754–755.
30. Gold BS, Dart RC, Barish RA. Bites of venomous snakes. *N Engl J Med.* 2002;347(5):347–356.
31. Tanen DA, Danish DC, Grice GA, et al. Fasciotomy worsens the amount of myonecrosis in a porcine model of crotaline envenomation. *Ann Emerg Med.* 2004;44:99–104.
32. Hall El. Role of surgical intervention in the management of crotaline snake envenomations. *Ann Emerg Med.* 2001;37:175–180.
33. Dart RC, McNally J. Efficacy, safety, and use of snake antivenoms in the United States. *Ann Emerg Med.* 2001;37:181–188.

PART XV Dermatological Diseases

CHAPTER 122

Skin Neoplasms

Betsy B. Love • Charles W. Love

OBJECTIVES

- To identify skin neoplasms (benign and malignant) that are associated with neurologic findings
- To define the neurologic complications of skin neoplasms
- To address diagnosis and management of the skin neoplasms and the central nervous system (CNS) sequelae

CASE VIGNETTE

A 40-year-old woman presents with a 2-week history of headaches and a 1-week history of mild weakness of her left arm and leg. She has no history of medical illnesses and she is not taking any medications. Her general examination shows an irregularly pigmented, black, irregularly bordered nodule on her left calf, and palpable lymph nodes in the left inguinal region. Neurologic examination is notable for no evidence of papilledema, intact cranial nerves, mild (4/5) strength of the left arm and leg, and hyperreflexia on the left. What is the likely etiology of her signs and symptoms?

DEFINITION

Skin neoplasms are simply defined as abnormal growth of tissue in the skin. Skin neoplasms can be benign or malignant. A benign skin neoplasm is defined as an abnormal, but not harmful, new growth of skin tissue. A malignant skin neoplasm is characterized by the proliferation of anaplastic cells that can invade surrounding tissues and can metastasize to other body sites. Certain skin neoplasms are associated with neurologic complications through their association as part of a syndrome, by metastasis of a malignant neoplasm, or rarely, by remote effects, such as with paraneoplastic disorders. Neoplasms to be discussed include malignant melanoma and associated syndromes, Merkel cell carcinoma, nevoid basal cell carcinoma, and hemangiomas. Sturge-Weber syndrome and epidermal-nevus syndrome are discussed in Chapter 123).

Melanoma

Melanoma is a skin neoplasm caused by a proliferation of transformed melanocytes, the pigment-producing cells of neural crest origin. Melanocytes are found primarily in the skin, but can also arise in other tissues where pigment cells are found. Melanoma is the most lethal form of skin cancer, and it ranks only behind lung cancer and breast cancer as a cause of CNS metastases. Neurologic complications include brain metastases resulting from hematogenous spread from melanoma of the skin, and leptomeningeal melanocytosis, which is primarily seen in congenital melanocytic nevus syndrome. Rarely, intracranial melanoma arises directly from the leptomeninges or dura mater.

EPIDEMIOLOGY

The incidence of melanoma is increasing dramatically, at a rate faster than any other cancer (1). Melanoma is the sixth most common cancer in Americans (1). The probability of developing melanoma during a lifetime is currently 1 of 52 for males and 1 of 77 for females (1). The latest statistics predict 62,200 new cases of melanoma and 7,910 deaths from invasive malignant melanoma this year (1). Brain or leptomeningeal metastases are present at autopsy in 50% to 75% of persons who die of melanoma (2,3).

ETIOLOGY AND PATHOGENESIS

A number of the risk factors for the development of melanoma are listed in Table 122-1. Several syndromes or congenital conditions that increase the risk for melanoma will be discussed briefly.

Atypical or dysplastic nevus syndrome is characterized by multiple clinically and histologically atypical nevi. These nevi are generally asymmetric, irregularly pigmented or dark in color, irregularly bordered, and >5 mm in diameter (4). Although controversy exists about the precise histologic criteria for atypical or dysplastic nevi, their clinical occurrence is a significant marker for increased risk of melanoma.

Large congenital melanocytic nevi (LCMN), also referred to as congenital pigmented nevi and giant hairy nevi, are pigmented lesions of the skin noted in 1 in 20,000 births (Fig. 122-1) (5). The lifetime risk of developing melanoma in patients with LCMN is 4.5% to 8.5% (6–9). Persons with LCMN are at risk for development of neurocutaneous melanocytosis (NCM). This is a rare neurologic complication characterized by benign or malignant proliferation of melanocytes in the CNS. Most cases occur in those 3 years of age and younger (10). Signs and symptoms of NCM are caused by the proliferation of melanocytes blocking the cisternal pathways and by obliteration of arachnoid villi resulting in symptoms of increased

TABLE 122-1. Risk Factors for Melanoma

New mole or changes in an existing mole
Atypical nevus syndrome
Large congenital melanocytic nevi
Dysplastic, multiple or atypical nevi
Personal or family history (first-degree) of melanoma
Lentigo maligna
Xeroderma pigmentosa
Psoralen-UV-A treatment
Tanning bed use, regularly
Immunosuppression
Sun-sensitive skin type
Frequent sunburns (more than 2/year) before age 40
Nonmelanoma skin cancer

cerebrospinal fluid (CSF) pressure and hydrocephalus (10). Nearly half of patients with NCM develop primary CNS melanomas (10). LCMN in posterior axial locations, associated with satellite melanocytic nevi are at the highest risk for the development of NCM (11,12). The diagnosis is made presumptively with magnetic resonance imaging (MRI) of the brain revealing meningeal infiltrates and other associated structural abnormalities. CSF cytology may be positive for melanocytes. Chemotherapy and radiation do not significantly alter the prognosis of this disorder. The prognosis in NCM is poor, with >90% of patients dying from benign or malignant CNS involvement (10).

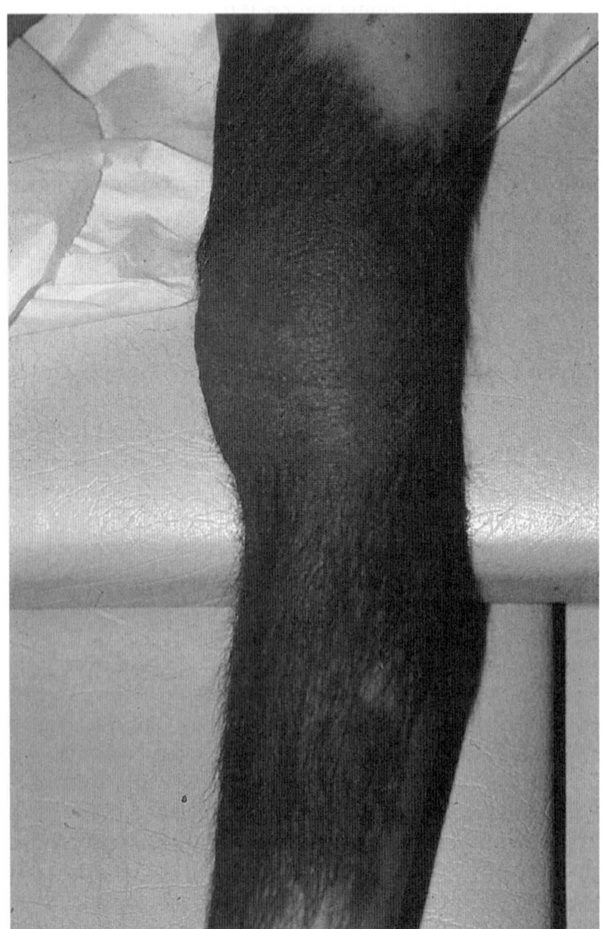

FIGURE 122-1. Large cutaneous melanocytic nevus of the lower limb.

Xeroderma pigmentosa (XP) is an autosomal recessive disorder that involves an inability of the skin to repair DNA damage from UV light. Neurologic abnormalities that can be present in some types of XP include mental retardation, developmental delay, microcephaly, deafness, dysarthria, poor coordination, spasticity, neuropathy, and short stature. An excess risk of melanoma is found in patients with XP, estimated to be >1,000 times the normal rate in persons under age 20 (13).

PATHOLOGY

The histologic diagnosis of melanoma of the skin is based on the presence of malignant melanocytes, usually characterized by cytologic atypia with pronounced cellular enlargement, nuclear variability, enlarged nuclei, and increased nuclear to cytoplasmic ratios. Each specific type of melanoma has characteristic histologic features.

Parenchymal brain metastases are well-circumscribed nodules of various sizes that can be solid or partially cystic. They are surrounded by marked edema and can be filled with hemorrhage or necrotic debris. Typical histologic features include poorly defined clusters of large, eosinophilic epithelioid cells with prominent nucleoli. Immunohistochemical studies further assist in the diagnosis.

CLINICAL MANIFESTATIONS

CUTANEOUS

The five subtypes of primary malignant melanomas of the skin with different clinical manifestations are discussed below.

Lentigo maligna melanoma (LMM) arises in lentigo maligna lesions and represents approximately 5% of melanomas. Lentigo maligna is an irregularly pigmented macular lesion occurring most frequently on the sun-exposed areas in elderly, actinically damaged patients. Histologically, melanoma *in situ* is noted. LMM shows invasive melanoma in a lesion similar to lentigo maligna. The incidence of progression of lentigo maligna to lentigo maligna melanoma is not known.

Superficial spreading malignant melanoma (SSMM) is the most common type of melanoma, representing 70% of all cases. Although SSMM can occur on any part of the skin, it occurs most frequently on the trunk in men and on the legs in women. The most frequent age of onset is in the fourth and fifth decades of life. SSMM usually is an irregularly pigmented, black, irregularly bordered nodule or macule (Fig. 122-2).

Nodular melanomas, representing 15% to 30% of all melanomas, are characterized by a vertical growth phase resulting in a rapidly growing nodule, which is usually black or blue-black in color.

Acral lentiginous melanomas, representing 2% to 8% of all melanomas, are similar in appearance to SSMM but are confined to the palms, soles, nail beds, mucous membranes, and penis (Fig. 122-3). Not all melanomas in these locations necessarily are categorized into this subgroup of melanoma. Notably, this type of melanoma is the most common subtype of melanoma in darker skinned races.

Amelanotic melanomas usually present as an asymptomatic, nonpigmented, erythematous macule with irregular and indistinct borders. They account for <5% of all melanomas.

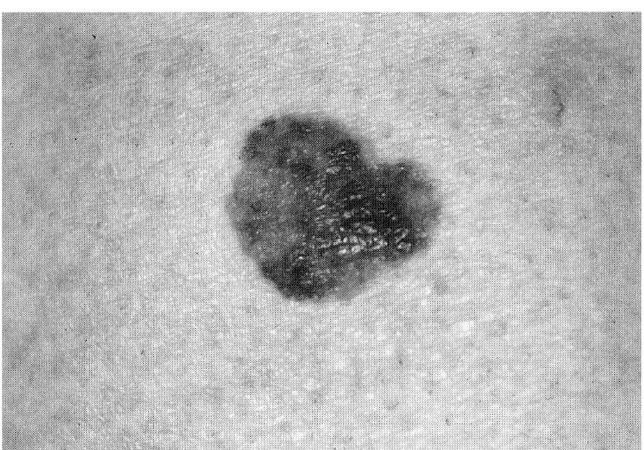

FIGURE 122-2. Melanoma of the skin with irregular margins and irregular pigmentation.

NEUROLOGIC

Melanoma with spread to the brain is frequently associated with multiple intracranial metastases. Clinical features, therefore, depend on the number and location of the lesion(s) (14). Signs and symptoms that are suggestive of CNS metastases include headache, nausea and vomiting, visual changes, focal neurologic deficits, seizures, confusion, or personality changes. Patients may have sudden neurologic deterioration because of the propensity of these lesions to hemorrhage. Symptoms of headache, mental status alterations, radicular back pain, seizures, nausea, and vomiting can be found with leptomeningeal disease. Signs of leptomeningeal involvement are variable, depending on the extent of brain and spinal involvement. Abnormal mental status, cranial nerve abnormalities, papilledema, nuchal rigidity, lower motor neuron weakness, dermatomal sensory loss, or absent reflexes may be present (15).

SPECIAL CONSIDERATIONS: PREGNANCY

The impact of pregnancy on melanoma is a subject of controversy in the literature. Many reports have suggested that pregnancy, because of high circulating hormones, yielded thicker tumors or a worse prognosis and that melanoma was more common in pregnancy. Several case-controlled studies and a growing body or literature has tended dispel these concerns, however (16,17).

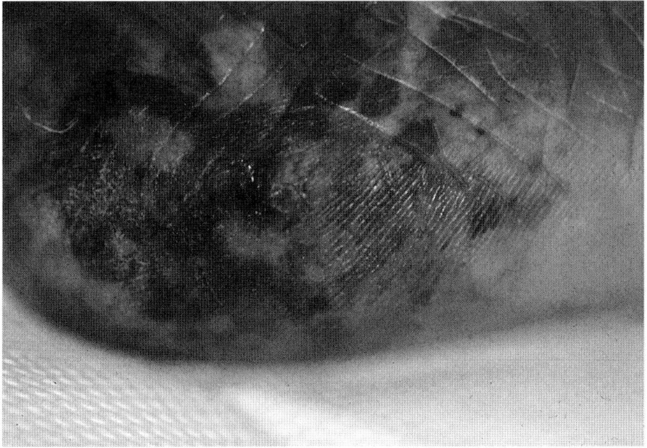

FIGURE 122-3. Acral lentiginous melanoma on the heel.

DIAGNOSTIC APPROACH

Because of the great disparity in the prognosis of early versus advanced melanomas, the early diagnosis of melanoma is critically important to the proper care of patients. If the disease is detected early, it is highly curable. In contrast, 5-year survival rates for stage IV melanoma, which includes intracranial metastases, is <5% (18,19).

The initial diagnosis is usually made by an excisional biopsy of the skin lesion. A complete excision is best because it allows a more definitive diagnosis by the pathologist and because it contains the full thickness of the lesion, making measurement of the degree of invasion possible. The pathology report will give an indication of tumor thickness (Breslow's measurement) and the level of invasion (Clark's level), the subtype of melanoma, the margin characteristics, and whether ulceration is present.

According to guidelines published by the American Joint Committee on Cancer in 2001, staging of primary cutaneous melanomas is based on the depth of invasion measured in millimeters, the presence and number of nodes involved, and the presence of local or distant metastases (20). The risk of melanoma recurrence and death is highly dependant on the stage at presentation.

Further testing, including a chest radiograph and a liver profile, is indicated as a baseline and to evaluate for evidence of metastases. Computed tomography (CT) or MRI of the brain may be indicated to evaluate for brain metastases, which are often multiple (Fig. 122-4). MRI of the brain, with contrast enhancement, is the most sensitive imaging method to detect brain metastases and to evaluate for leptomeningeal spread. Other tests, including chest and abdominal CT may be indicated based on the clinical situation.

TREATMENT

The management of primary malignant melanoma of the skin is generally limited to a wide local excision of the lesion with adequate margins. Recommended margins range from 5 mm for melanoma *in situ* to 20 mm for melanomas of >2 mm of invasion (21).

Patients with brain metastases from melanoma may be symptomatically managed with corticosteroids, such as dexamethasone. In the presence of seizures, anticonvulsant therapy is used. Overall, the diagnosis of brain metastases confers a very poor prognosis in melanoma, with mean survival ranging from 2.75 to 4.0 months after diagnosis (22–25). Certain favorable prognostic indicators have been identified, however, including solitary brain metastasis, controlled primary tumor, younger age (<60 to 65 years), absence of systemic metastases, and good performance status (19,26–29). In favorable prognosis, patients with limited or no extracranial disease, and a single or limited number of brain metastases, surgical resection may be considered. In other patients, stereotactic radiosurgery (SRS) may be indicated when the metastases are located in surgically inaccessible or eloquent brain areas. Whole brain radiation

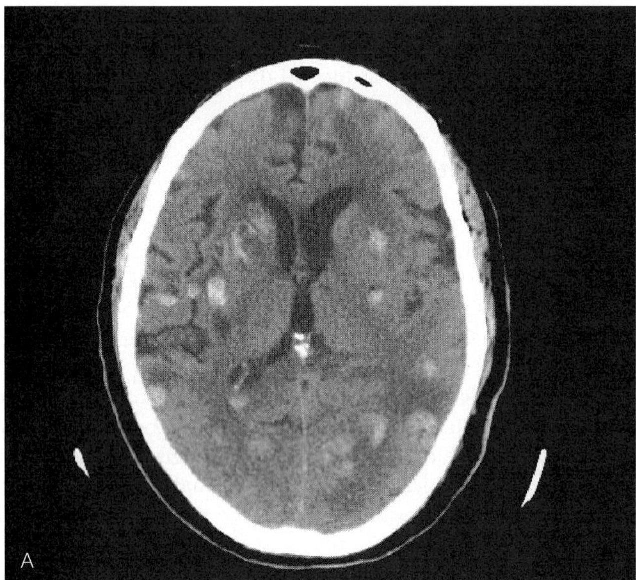

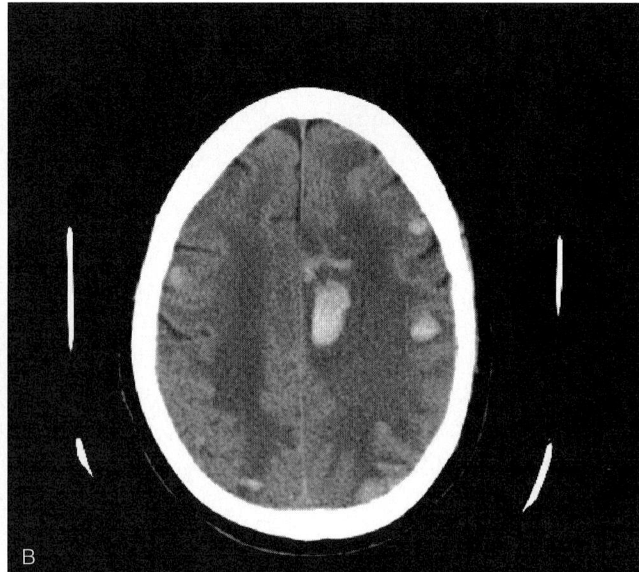

FIGURE 122-4. Noncontrast computed tomographic (CT) scan of the brain in a patient with diffuse metastatic melanoma at the level of the midventricles (**A**) and the corona radiata (**B**) shows multiple hemorrhagic metastases ranging in size from a few millimeters to 1.5 cm. Note: most of these lesions are in the gray–white junction and some involve the deep white matter.

therapy (WBRT) can be used for palliative treatment of multiple brain metastases (30). There is no indication that WBRT increases survival after surgery (30). Chemotherapy and immunotherapy have been used in patients with stage IV melanoma, but must be considered experimental at this time.

Merkel Cell Carcinoma

Merkel cell carcinoma (MCC), also known as trabecular cell carcinoma, neuroendocrine cancer of the skin, or small-cell carcinoma of the skin, is an uncommon, aggressive skin cancer that has been associated with neurologic involvement, including metastasis to the brain, and rarely, leptomeningeal carcinomatosis and Lambert-Eaton myasthenic syndrome (LEMS).

EPIDEMIOLOGY

MCC is an uncommon skin neoplasm, but it is the second most common cause of nonmelanoma skin cancer death (31). The incidence of MCC is reported to have risen threefold since 1986, with an incidence of 0.44 per 100,000 person-years in 2001 (31). The incidence of MCC is notably higher in whites, males, and in persons >65 years of age (32). A clear association with aging is seen, with 95% of cases occurring in persons >50 years of age (32). To obtain a relative perspective regarding the incidence of MCC in whites, it should be noted that for every 1 case of MCC, there are 65 cases of melanoma (32).

ETIOLOGY AND PATHOGENESIS

The exact cause of MCC is unclear. MCC has been associated with sun exposure (32). This association is supported by the predilection of MCC to occur in sun-exposed areas and by case reports of MCC in patients with psoriasis who have been treated with psoralin and UVA radiation. Another possible factor in some cases of MCC is an impaired immune system, such as with iatrogenic immunosuppression with organ transplantation, human immunodeficiency virus (HIV) infection or neoplasia (33). Patients with first primary MCC have a significantly increased risk, particularly in the first year after diagnosis, of developing a subsequent cancer, especially cancers of the salivary gland, biliary tree (other than liver and gallbladder), and non-Hodgkin lymphoma (34). Diagnosis of MCC as a second primary malignancy was elevated three- to sevenfold following the diagnosis of multiple myeloma, chronic lymphocytic leukemia, and malignant melanoma (34). Although these associations may be related to increased surveillance, the increased reciprocal risk may suggest that MCC shares etiologic influences with other malignancies (34).

On a molecular level, some evidence indicates that some patients with MCC have deletions in chromosome Ip35-36, the same location that has been suspected for genetic changes in pheochromocytoma, neuroblastoma, and melanoma (35).

MCC of the skin metastasizes to the regional lymph nodes and then to higher nodal groups. Approximately 10% to 30% of patients present with regional lymph node involvement (36,37). Less than 5% of patients have distant metastases at presentation, but 50% or more may subsequently develop them. MCC can spread to secondary skin sites, liver, lung, bone, and brain (38). Leptomeningeal carcinomatosis has been described rarely (39,40,41). Finally, LEMS has been reported in a patient with parenchymal and leptomeningeal metastases from MCC. Its association is not surprising because MCC is a type of extrapulmonary small cell carcinoma (41).

PATHOLOGY

Merkel cells are small cutaneous mechanoreceptors in the basal epidermis that contain dense-core neurosecretory granules.

The discovery of similar neurosecretory granules within tumor cells in the dermis led to identification of this tumor, which was initially described as *trabecular cell carcinoma*, as MCC (42). MCC is considered an adult small cell neuroendocrine tumor. MCC arises in the dermis, with frequent extension into the subcutaneous fat.

Microscopically, the tumor is composed of small blue cells with hyperchromatic nuclei minimal cytoplasm, frequent mitoses, and widespread apoptosis (33). Lymphovascular invasion is often present. Three histologic subtypes are noted (intermediate, small cell, and trabecular). The small cell variant is histologically identical to other small cell carcinomas and must be distinguished from metastatic small cell carcinoma of the lung by its immunocytochemical profile (33,41).

CLINICAL MANIFESTATIONS

CUTANEOUS

Patients typically present with a single, painless, flesh-colored, red, purple, or blue, firm, nontender dermal nodule or indurated plaque that has grown rapidly over a few weeks to months. Ulceration may be present. MCC can occur in any cutaneous or mucosal site, but is most frequent in sun-exposed skin, with 50% of tumors occurring on the face or neck and 40% involving the extremities (33). Tumor size may range from 2 to 200 mm, but is usually <20 mm (33).

NEUROLOGIC

Clinical features of parenchymal brain involvement with MCC depend on the location of the metastasis. In general, symptoms of intracranial mass lesions are headache, transient visual obscurations or diplopia, changes in mental status, nausea, and vomiting. Patients may have papilledema or unilateral or bilateral sixth nerve palsy on ocular examination. Seizures can be present. In the presence of hydrocephalus caused by blockage of CSF flow, loss of memory, gait ataxia, balance disturbance, and urinary incontinence may occur.

Clinical signs and symptoms of leptomeningeal carcinomatosis can include headache, meningismus, mental status changes, encephalopathy, nausea, vomiting, cranial nerve palsies, spinal nerve involvement, strokelike episodes or limb weakness, or seizures.

Clinical features of LEMS can include dry mouth and other autonomic symptoms, dysphagia, dysarthria, ptosis, proximal greater than distal muscle weakness, especially in the lower limbs, and diminished or absent deep tendon reflexes. Strength may improve after exercise, and then weaken as activity is sustained.

DIAGNOSTIC APPROACH

MCC is best diagnosed with a thorough clinical examination and a biopsy of the lesion. After histologic diagnosis, patients should have a CT of the chest, abdomen, and pelvis. Staging using lymphoscintigraphy and sentinel lymph node biopsy may be indicated in selected patients. MRI of the brain is indicated if neurologic involvement is suspected. CSF analysis may be indicated if leptomeningeal carcinomatosis is suspected. In rare cases of suspected paraneoplastic neuromuscular involvement with LEMS, tensilon testing, paraneoplastic antibody testing, acetylcholine receptor antibodies, repetitive nerve stimulation studies, needle electromyography, and single-fiber electromyography may be considered.

TREATMENT AND PROGNOSIS

Surgical excision using Mohs micrographic surgery or wide surgical margins should be performed. Because of the rare occurrence of MCC, no prospective clinical studies assessing various treatment modalities have been undertaken. A commonly used staging system categorizes patients based on clinical presentation: stage I, localized skin disease (stage IA ≤2 cm, IB >2 cm); stage II, regional lymph node disease; and stage III, metastatic disease (43). Stage I and II disease is usually treated surgically and with adjuvant radiation therapy. Stage III disease is usually treated with radiation therapy and chemotherapy. Some recent reviews examine treatment recommendations in detail (31,33). The 5-year relative survival rate is 75% for localized, 59% for regional, and 25% for distant MCC (44). Positive predictors of survival are female sex, limb presentation, localized disease, and younger age (44).

Nevoid Basal Cell Carcinoma Syndrome

Nevoid basal cell carcinoma syndrome (NBCCS), also known as Gorlin syndrome or Gorlin-Goltz syndrome, is a rare, autosomal dominant disorder associated with multiple developmental anomalies and malignant systemic tumors, including multiple nevoid basal-cell carcinomas and medulloblastoma (45).

EPIDEMIOLOGY

The estimated prevalence of NBCCS is between 1 of 57,000 and 1 of 164,000 (46–48). The incidence of NBCCS in patients with medulloblastoma is estimated to be between 1% and 2% overall and between 4% and 5% in patients <5 years of age (49).

ETIOLOGY AND PATHOGENESIS

NBCCS is caused by germline mutations in the human homolog of the patched (PTCH) tumor suppressor gene located on chromosome 9q22.3 (50).

PATHOLOGY

The multiple basal cell carcinomas (BCC) that develop in this syndrome are indistinguishable from ordinary BCC, even when they occur in the early nevoid stage. *Nevoid* refers to the pigmented early lesions of this disease that appear like melanocytic nevi. These lesions, at biopsy, reveal histology typical for BCC with nests or strands of basophilic staining cells with peripheral palisading and stromal retraction.

CLINICAL MANIFESTATIONS

Major clinical manifestations include (*a*) early development of multiple BCC; (*b*) keratocysts of the bone, especially the jaw; (*c*) palmoplantar pits; (*d*) ectopic intracranial calcification; and (*e*) family history of nevoid basal cell carcinoma syndrome (NBCCS). Minor criteria include (*a*) craniofacial anomalies (macrocephaly, frontal bossing, hypertelorism); (*b*) bifid ribs; (*c*) early onset medulloblastomas; (*d*) cardiac or ovarian fibromas, often bilateral; (*e*) lymphomesenteric cysts; and (*f*) congenital malformation (cleft lip or palate, polydactyly, colobomas, cataracts and glaucoma) (51).

CUTANEOUS

BCC in this syndrome appear as multiple tan-brown papules, most frequently on sun-exposed areas. These can appear as acrochordons (skin tags) in children, but at biopsy, these lesions actually represent BCC (52). Other skin disorders include milia, epidermoid cysts, chalazia, and palmar or plantar pits (53).

NEUROLOGIC

The desmoplastic subtype of medulloblastoma is associated most commonly with NBCCS (54). The most common early symptoms of medulloblastoma are caused by increased intracranial pressure related to mass effect from the cerebellar tumor or related to obstruction of the fourth ventricle. Patients may have lethargy, headaches, papilledema, and vomiting. Cranial nerve dysfunction (VI, VII, VIII) may be present. Cerebellar symptoms, including ataxia of the trunk and appendages, usually are present. Presentation in the very young patient may be more nonspecific, with failure to thrive, irritability, anorexia, macrocephaly, spread sutures with a bulging fontanel, and paralyzed upgaze. Symptomatic leptomeningeal disease is rare, but can include, seizures, focal neurologic symptoms, motor weakness, or spinal cord compression.

DIAGNOSTIC APPROACH

Suspicious skin lesions should be biopsied. An initial cranial CT is helpful to evaluate for intracranial calcification, hydrocephalus, and agenesis or dysgenesis of the corpus callosum. Because of the desire to limit radiation exposure, an annual MRI of the brain is recommended for screening for medulloblastoma in persons <8 years of age. Depending on symptoms, other testing, including radiography of the jaw, skull, and neck; echocardiography; and ultrasonography of the pelvis, are indicated, and are often used for screening purposes.

TREATMENT

Sun exposure should be avoided. Patients need to be monitored very closely for skin changes. Early identification of BCC and treatment when the lesions are small and curable are paramount. BCC can be treated with simple excision or Mohs micrographic surgery. Topical treatments, including 5-fluorouracil, retinoids, and imiquimod, have been used to treat superficial lesions (53,55).

Treatment for medulloblastoma depends on disease stratification after surgical resection, and can include radiation, chemotherapy, or both. Treatment is complicated in these patients, because radiation should be minimized or avoided because of the development of extensive and invasive BCC in the radiation field. If BCC are treated early and no other malignancies develop, these patients can have a normal life expectancy. Overall 5-year, disease-free survival for children with medulloblastoma ranges between 50% and 60% (56).

Cutaneous Vascular Lesions

Several cutaneous vascular neoplasms of the skin are associated with neurologic abnormalities. These include hemangiomas and angiokeratomas. Hemangiomas of the skin are common benign tumors of the vascular endothelium. Angiokeratomas are vascular ectasias in the papillary dermis.

EPIDEMIOLOGY

The incidence of hemangiomas is 1.0% to 2.6% in all newborns, but can be as high as 10% among whites (57). They are four times more frequent in females than in males and are especially common in premature infants (57). The exact incidence of angiokeratomas is not known.

ETIOLOGY AND PATHOGENESIS

Hemangiomas are typically characterized by phases of proliferation and involution. The exact cause of these changes is unknown. Angiokeratomas are telangiectasias of preexisting vessels. The mechanism of these changes is unknown.

CLINICAL MANIFESTATIONS

Hemangiomas located over the lumbar or sacral spine can be associated with spinal dysraphism, such as a tethered cord. The most worrisome lesions are those that span the midline and are flat or telangiectatic in appearance (57).

Two syndromes with hemangiomas deserve special mention. PHACES syndrome is a syndrome in infants consisting of *p*osterior fossa malformations, *h*emangiomas (especially, large, plaquelike, facial lesions), *a*rterial anomalies, *c*ardiac anomalies, and coarctation of the aorta, *e*ye abnormalities, and *s*ternal cleft or supraumbilical raphe (58).

The syndrome of *p*olyneuropathy, *o*rganomegaly, *e*ndocrinopathy, *M* protein, and *s*kin changes (POEMS) is a multisystem syndrome that can be associated with plasma cell dyscrasias. The skin changes noted include hyperpigmentation, hypertrichosis, hyperhidrosis, skin thickening, and hemangiomas. A particular type of hemangioma, glomeruloid hemangioma, is seen exclusively in POEMS and is a diagnostic marker for the disorder (59).

Angiokeratomas may be seen in several syndromes with neurologic findings. Fabry disease (angiokeratoma corporis diffusum) is an X-linked recessive disorder caused by defective activity of α-galactosidase A with angiokeratomas, pain crises, cerebrovascular, cardiovascular, and renal involvement. Angiokeratomas are also seen with Cobb syndrome, a rare, noninherited disorder involving spinal angiomas or arteriovenous malformations with congenital, cutaneous vascular lesions in the same dermatome, port-wine stains, angiomas, angiokeratomas, angiolipomas, and lymphangioma circumscriptum. Angiokeratomas and hemangiomas may also be seen with Klippel-Trenaunay syndrome, which is a congenital disorder characterized by skin vascular abnormalities, underlying venous varicosities, and underlying soft tissue or bony hypertrophy. Seizures, arterial thromboembolic events, and mental deficiency are other neurologic symptoms that may be present.

PATHOLOGY

Congenital hemangiomas are characterized by greatly dilated capillaries and ectatic vessels. Angiokeratomas seen with Cobb and Klippel-Trenaunay syndromes are characterized by dilated capillary spaces in the papillary and reticular dermis, with varying degrees of hyperkeratosis, papillomatosis, and irregular acanthosis.

DIAGNOSTIC APPROACH AND TREATMENT

Diagnosis is usually based on the clinical findings. Biopsy of the skin lesions is confirmatory. In the presence of hemangiomas or angiokeratomas grouped over the spine in a newborn or infant, an MRI of the spine is indicated to exclude spinal dysraphism or Cobb syndrome. The skin lesions do not require any special treatment. Patients with associated syndromes often require a multidisciplinary approach to management.

CLINICAL RECOMMENDATIONS OF THE VIGNETTE

The patient is an individual with an abnormal skin examination and neurologic findings. A leading consideration in this case is malignant melanoma with metastases to the brain. The skin lesion should be completely excised and submitted for pathologic diagnosis. The presence of lymph node enlargement in the inguinal region suggests the need for further staging tests. Because of both focal and diffuse neurologic findings, an MRI of the brain with contrast enhancement would be indicated. If the clinical diagnosis is confirmed to be malignant melanoma with multiple metastases to the brain, the prognosis is guarded. Palliative WBRT, SRS, or immunotherapy may be considered.

SUMMARY

Skin neoplasms can be associated with important neurologic sequelae and syndromes. It is important for physicians to be aware of these important associations for optimal patient management.

REFERENCES

1. Jemal A, Siegel R, Ward E, et al. Cancer statistics, 2006. *CA Cancer J Clin.* 2006;56:106–130.
2. de la Monte SM, Moore GW, Hutchins GM. Patterned distribution of metastases from malignant melanoma in humans. *Cancer Res.* 1983;43:3427–3433.
3. Patel JK, Didolkar MS, Pickren JW, et al. Metastatic pattern of malignant melanoma: A study of 216 autopsy cases. *Am J Surg.* 1978;135:807–810.
4. Hussein MR. Melanocytic dysplastic naevi occupy the middle ground between benign melanocytic naevi and cutaneous malignant melanomas: Emerging clues. *J Clin Pathol.* 2005;58:453–456.
5. Caslla EE, Dutra MDG, Oriolo-Parreiras IM. Epidemiology of congenital pigmented naevi. *Br J Dermatol.* 1981;35:529–538.
6. Egan CL, Oliveira SA, Elenitsas R, et al. Cutaneous melanoma risk and phenotypic changes in large congenital nevi: A follow-up study of 46 patients. *J Am Acad Dermatol.* 1998;39: 923–932.
7. Swerdlow AJ, English JSC, Qiao Z. The risk of melanoma in patients with congenital nevi: Clinical, histopathologic, and therapeutic considerations. *J Pediatr.* 1992;120:906–911.
8. Quaba AA Wallace AF. The incidence of malignant transformation in giant pigmented nevi. *Plast Reconstr Surg.* 1986;78:174–179.
9. Lorentzen M, Pers M, Bretteville-Jensen G. The incidence of malignant transformation in giant pigmented nevi. *Scand J Plast Reconstr Surg.* 1977;11:163–167.
10. Bittencourt AA, Marghoob AA, Kopf AW, et al. Large congenital melanocytic nevi and the risk for development of melanoma and neurocutaneous melanocytosis. *Pedatrics.* 2000;106:736–741.
11. DeDavid M, Orlow SJ, Provost N, et al. Neurocutaneous melanosis: Clinical features of large congenital melonocytic nevi in patients with manifest central nervous system melanosis. *J Am Acad Dermatol.* 1996;35:529–538.
12. Marghoob AA, Dusza S, Oliveria S, et al. Number of satellite nevi as a correlate for neurocutaneous melanocytosis in patients with large congenital melanocytic nevi. *Arch Dermatol.* 2004;140:171–175.
13. Kramer KH, Lee MM, Andrews AD, et al. The role of sunlight and DNA repair in melanoma and nonmelanoma skin cancer. *Arch Dermatol.* 1994;130:1018–1021.
14. Johnson JD, Young B. Demographics of brain metastasis. *Neurosurg Clin N Am.* 1996;7: 337–344.
15. Posner JB. Leptomeningeal metastases. In: Posner JB. *Neurologic Complications of Cancer.* Philadelphia; FA Davis; 1995:143–171.
16. Driscoll MS, Grin-Jorgensen CM, Grant-Kels JM. Does pregnancy influence the prognosis of malignant melanoma? *J Am Acad Dermatol.* 1993;29:619–630.
17. O'Meara AT, Cress R, Xing G, et al. Malignant melanoma in pregnancy. A population-based evaluation. *Cancer.* 2005;103:1217–1226.
18. McWilliams RR, Brown PD, Buckner JC, et al. Treatment of brain metastases from melanoma. *Mayo Clin Proc.* 2003;78:1529–1536.
19. Tarhini AA, Argawala SS. Management of brain metastases in patients with melanoma. *Curr Opin Oncol.* 2004;16:161–166.
20. Balch CM, Buzaid AC, Soong SJ, et al. Final version of the American Joint Committee on Cancer staging system for cutaneous melanoma. *J Clin Oncol.* 2001;19:3635–3648.
21. Sober A, Chuang T, Duvic M, et al. Guidelines of care for primary cutaneous melanoma. *J Am Acad Dermatol.* 2001;45:579–586.
22. Amer MH, AlSarraf M, Baker LH, et al. Malignant melanoma and central nervous system metastases: Incidence, diagnosis, treatment and survival. *Cancer.* 1978;42:660–668.
23. Byrne TN, Cascino TL, Posner JB. Brain metastasis from melanoma. *J Neurooncol.* 1983;1:313–317.
24. Budman DR, Camacho E, Wittes RE. The current causes of death in patients with malignant melanoma. *Eur J Cancer.* 1978;14:327–330.
25. Einhorn LH, Burgess MA, Vallejos C, et al. Prognostic correlations and response to treatment in advanced metastatic malignant melanoma. *Cancer Res.* 1974;34:1995–2004.
26. Sampson JH, Carter JH, Jr., Friedman AH, et al. Demographics, prognosis, and therapy in 702 patients with brain metastases from malignant melanoma. *J Neurosurg.* 1998;88:11–20.
27. Sahs S, Meyer M, Krememtz ET, et al. Prognostic evaluation of intracranial metastasis in malignant melanoma. *Ann Surg Oncol.* 1994;1:38–44.
28. Lagerwaard FJ, Levendag PC, Nowak PJ, et al. Identification of prognostic factors in patients with brain metastases: A review of 1292 patients. *Int J Radiat Oncol Biol Phys.* 1999;43:795–803.
29. Gaspar L, Scott C, Rotman M, et al. Recursive partitioning analysis (RPA) of prognostic factors in three Radiation Therapy Oncology Group (RTOG) brain metastases trials. *Int J Radiat Oncol Biol Phys.* 1997;37:745–751.
30. Wronski M, Arbit E. Surgical treatment of brain metastases from melanoma: A retrospective study of 91 patients. *J Neurosurg.* 2000;93:9–18.
31. Alam M. Management of Merkel cell carcinoma. What we know. *Arch Dermatol.* 2006;142:771–774.
32. Miller RW, Rabkin CS. Merkel cell carcinoma and melanoma: Etiological similarities and differences. *Cancer Epidemiol Biomarkers Prev.* 1999;8:153–158.
33. Goessling W, McKee PH, Mayer RJ. Merkel cell carcinoma. *J Clin Oncol.* 2002;20:588–598.
34. Howard RA, Dores GM, Curtis RE, et al. Merkel cell carcinoma and multiple primary cancers. *Cancer Epidemiol Biomarkers Prev.* 2006;15:1545–1549.
35. Voetmeyer AO, Merino MJ, Boni R, et al. Genetic changes associated with primary Merkel cell carcinoma. *Am J Clin Pathol.* 1998;109:565–570.
36. Yiengpruksawan A, Coit DG, Thaler HT, et al. Merkel cell carcinoma: Prognosis and management. *Arch Surg.* 1991;126:1514–1519.
37. Hitchcock CL, Bland KI, Laney RG III, et al. Neuroendocrine (Merkel cell) carcinoma of the skin: Its natural history, diagnosis, and treatment. *Ann Surg.* 1988;207:210–207.
38. Medina-Franco H, Urist MM, Fiveash J, et al. Multimodality treatment of Merkel cell carcinoma: Case series and literature review of 1024 cases. *Ann Surg Oncol.* 2001;8:204–208.
39. Snodgrass SM, Landy H, Markoe AM, et al. Neurologic complications of Merkel cell carcinoma. *J Neurooncol.* 1994;22:231–234.
40. Chang DT, Mancuso AA, Riggs CE, et al. Merkel cell carcinoma of the skin with leptomeningeal metastases. *Am J Otolaryngol.* 2005;26:210–213.
41. Eggers SDZ, Salomao DR, Dinapoli RP, et al. Paraneoplastic and metastatic neurologic complications of Merkel cell carcinoma. *Mayo Clin Proc.* 2001;76:327–330.
42. Toker C. Trabecular carcinoma of the skin. *Arch Dermatol.* 1972;105:107–110.
43. Yiengpruksawan A, Coit DG, Thaler HT, et al. Merkel cell carcinoma: Prognosis and management. *Arch Surg.* 1991;126:1514–1519.
44. Agelli M, Clegg LX. Epidemiology of primary Merkel cell carcinoma in the United States. *J Am Acad Dermatol.* 2003;49:832–841.
45. Rahbari H, Mehregan AH. Basal cell epithelioma (carcinoma) in children and teenagers. *Cancer.* 1982;49:350–353.

46. Cohen MM, Jr. Nevoid basal cell carcinoma syndrome: Molecular biology and new hypotheses. *Int J Oral Maxillofac Surg.* 1999;28:216–223.
47. Fardon PA, Del Mastro RG, Evans DGR, et al. Location of gene for Gorlin syndrome. *Lancet.* 1992;339:581–582.
48. Shanley S, Ratcliffe J, Hockey A, et al. Nevoid basal cell carcinoma syndrome: Review of 118 affected individuals. *Am J Med Genet.* 1994;50:282–290.
49. Evans DGR, Farndon PA, Burnell LD, et al. The incidence of Gorlin syndrome in 173 consecutive cases of medulloblastoma. *Br J Cancer.* 1991;5:643–646.
50. Hahn H, Wicking C, Zaphiropoulous PG, et al. Mutations of the human homolog of Drosophila patched in the nevoid basal cell carcinoma syndrome. *Cell.* 1996;14;85: 841–851.
51. Kimonis VE, Goldstein AM, Pastakia B, et al. Clinical manifestations in 105 persons with nevoid basal cell carcinoma syndrome. *Am J Med Genet.* 1997;69:299–308.
52. Chiritescu E, Maloney ME. Acrochordons as a presenting sign of nevoid basal cell carcinoma syndrome. *J Am Acad Dermatol.* 2001;44:789–794.
53. Gorlin RJ. Nevoid basal-cell carcinoma syndrome. *Medicine.* 1987;66:98–113.
54. Amiashi SFA, Riffaud L, Brassier G, et al. Nevoid basal cell carcinoma syndrome: Relation with desmoplastic medulloblastoma in infancy. A population-based study and review of the literature. *Cancer.* 2003;98:618–624.
55. Sterry W, Ruzicka T, Herrera E, et al. Imiquimod 5% cream for the treatment of superficial and nodular basal cell carcinoma: Randomized studies comparing low-frequency dosing with and without occlusion. *Br J Dermatol.* 2002;147:1227–1236.
56. David KM, Casey AT, Hayward RD, et al. Medulloblastoma: Is the 5-year survival rate improving? *J Neurosurg.* 1997;86:13–21.
57. Metry DW, Hebert AA. Benign cutaneous vascular tumors of infancy. When to worry, what to do. *Arch Dermatol.* 2000;136:905–914.
58. Metry DW, Dowd CF, Barkovich AJ, et al. The many faces of PHACE syndrome. *J Pediatr.* 2001;139:117–123.
59. Weimer T, Norton A, Gutmann L. Glomeruloid angiomas: A marker for POEMS. *Neurology.* 2006;66:453–454.

CHAPTER 123

Phakodermatoses and Other Genetic Conditions with Dermatologic Manifestations

Terrence M. Brogan • Beth L. Brogan • Robert M. Pascuzzi

OBJECTIVES

- To identify the cutaneous and systemic findings of the most common phakodermatoses, or neurocutaneous syndromes, including the earliest clinical diagnostic clues and the full clinical spectrum of cutaneous and neurologic disease
- To demonstrate the range of neurologic abnormalities and clinical and radiologic findings observed in tuberous sclerosis and neurofibromatosis, the most common neurocutaneous syndromes
- To identify the gene defects found in these disorders, including their inheritance patterns, pathophysiology, and relationship to clinical findings
- To provide a brief overview of other, less common, neurocutaneous syndromes

CASE VIGNETTE

A 10-year-old girl with a history of generalized seizure disorder and developmental delay presents with new violaceous papules growing around her nose and lips. Her mother, who accompanies her, has had similar skin lesions since adolescence. At birth, the girl was noted to have hypopigmented macules scattered over her skin as well as smaller "confetti" macules over her shins. At 2 years of age, she developed a 6 cm, yellow, rubberlike plaque on her lower back. In addition, the girl's mother exhibits flesh-colored 4 and 6-mm papules located on the periungual region of several of her fingers.

DEFINITION

Congenital or genetic disorders involving both the nervous system and the skin are collectively referred to as *neurocutaneous syndromes*, or *phakomatoses*.

Tuberous Sclerosis

DEFINITION

Tuberous sclerosis complex (TSC), or Bourneville disease, is an autosomal dominant multisystem tumor syndrome characterized by the development of hamartomas of the nervous system and skin as well as internal organs, such as heart, lung, and kidneys.

EPIDEMIOLOGY

Tuberous sclerosis complex affects an estimated 1 of 6,000 individuals.

ETIOLOGY AND PATHOGENESIS

TSC results from an autosomal-dominant mutation in one of two tumor suppressor genes, *TSC1* and *TSC2* (1). *TSC1* on chromosome 9q34 encodes for hamartin, whereas *TSC2* on chromosome 16p13 encodes for tuberin. The two gene products form a complex that ultimately appears to regulate the cell cycle. Loss of function of the inherited gene product, along with a "second hit" mutation, is thought to explain tumor formation (2). The complementary action of gene products in a complex may explain the similarity in clinical disease findings between patients with different gene mutations. Approximately two thirds of cases are the result of new mutations. Numerous studies have shown that disease resulting from mutations in *TSC1* is less severe than disease resulting from *TSC2* mutations (3).

PATHOLOGY

A shagreen patch is a collagenous plaque that histologically shows increased bundles of collagen. Adenoma sebaceum are actually angiofibromas or benign fibrous vascular tumors, and are not related to the sebaceous glands.

Cortical tubers and subependymal nodules are hamartomas. White matter abnormalities histologically show dysmyelinated or dysplastic white matter. Subependymal giant cell astrocytoma is a central nervous system (CNS) astrocytoma with spindle cell morphology and rare mitotic figures. Despite the designation as an astrocytoma, the prognosis with surgical resection is favorable (4).

CLINICAL MANIFESTATIONS

The cutaneous manifestations of TSC include hypomelanotic patches, shagreen plaques, periungal fibromas, and facial angiofibromas. Hypomelanotic patches are usually present at birth and seen in 90% of patients with TS, although they are also seen in healthy individuals. They may present as several centimeter patches, classically in the shape of an ash leaf, or as speckled "confetti" macules, often on the shins. The shagreen plaque appears in 20% to 30% of patients as a yellow to flesh-colored rubbery dermal plaque that is most often found on the trunk. Facial angiofibromas are vascular papules presenting during school years in 70% patients, usually in the malar and nasolabial region (Fig. 123-1). Periungual fibromas are fleshy, pea-sized papules that present around the nail margin in about 20% of patients.

The neurologic manifestations of TS include mental retardation, epilepsy, and behavioral abnormalities. Epilepsy occurs in 62% of patients and presents with various forms of seizures, including infantile spasms, focal motor, generalized, and complex partial (5). Of patients with infantile spasms, 25% have underlying TS and a high association with mental retardation (6). The structural CNS abnormalities include white matter abnormalities, cortical tubers, subependymal nodules, and subependymal giant cell astrocytomas (Figs. 123-2 and 123-3). Subependymal giant cell tumors occur near the foreman of Monro intraventricularly and can cause obstructive hydrocephalus. Computed tomographic (CT) imaging is potentially useful if the cortical tubers have calcified, but magnetic resonance imaging (MRI) is better for migrational abnormalities, noncalcified CNS lesions, and giant cell astrocytomas.

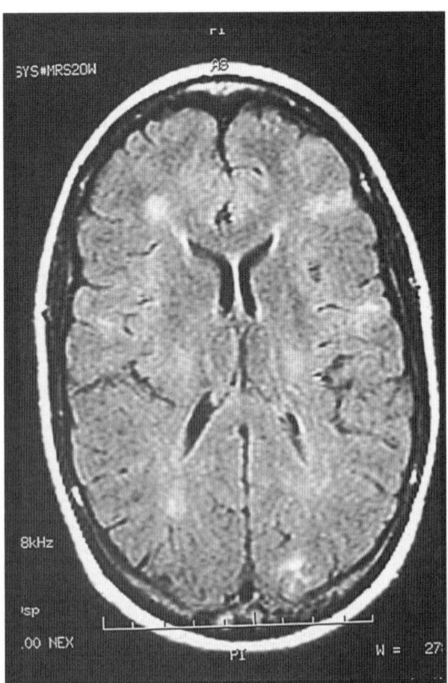

FIGURE 123-2. Magnetic resonance imaging (MRI) of tuberous sclerosis showing cortical tubers.

Systemic features include retinal hamartomas, renal angiomyolipomas, pulmonary lymphangiomyomatosis, dental pits, and bone cysts. Cardiac rhabdomyomas are seen in a few infants with TS, but they are most often asymptomatic and usually spontaneously regress (7).

DIAGNOSTIC APPROACH

The diagnosis of TSC rests on major and minor diagnostic criteria (Table 123-1) (8). Prenatal diagnosis may be suspected with intracardiac tumors seen on ultrasound, and experimental prenatal genetic testing is currently available (9). The

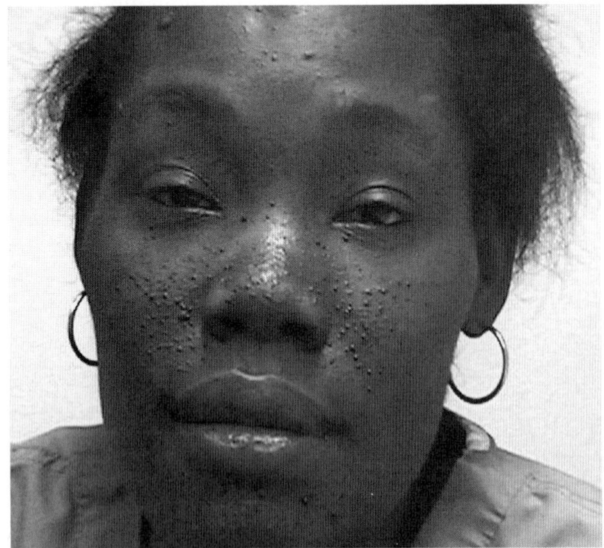

FIGURE 123-1. Typical angiofibroma in a patient with tuberous sclerosis.

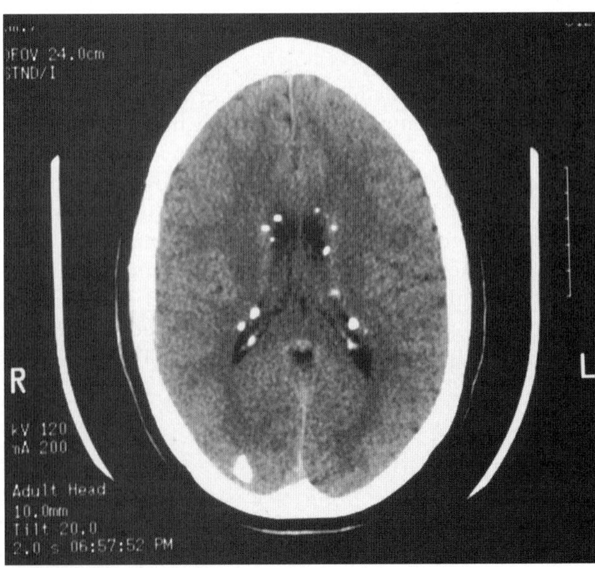

FIGURE 123-3. Computed tomographic (CT) scan of tuberous sclerosis showing subependymal nodules.

TABLE 123-1. Criteria for the Diagnosis of Tuberous Sclerosis Complex (TSC)

Two major features or one major feature plus two minor features are required for a definite clinical diagnosis of TSC.

MAJOR CRITERIA

Facial angiofibroma
Ungual fibroma
Shagreen patch
Hypomelanotic macule
Cortical tuber
Subependymal nodule
Subependymal giant-cell tumor
Retinal hamartoma
Cardiac rhabdomyoma
Renal angiomyolipoma
Lymphangiomyomatosis

MINOR CRITERIA

Multiple pits in dental enamel
Hamartomatous rectal polyps
Bone cysts
Cerebral white-matter radial migration lines
Gingival fibromas
Retinal achromic patch
Confetti skin lesions
Multiple renal cysts

hypopigmented macules present at birth are often subtle; therefore, the neurologic manifestations often precede the search for cutaneous findings.

TREATMENT

Treatment consists of antiepileptic medications for epilepsy. Surgical intervention is occasionally possible for selective patients. Genetic counseling is recommended for families. Pulsed-dye laser provides a good cosmetic outcome for facial angiofibroma.

Neurofibromatosis

DEFINITION

Neurofibromatosis (NF) is a neurocutaneous disease composed of two distinct syndromes. NF-1 is a syndrome of predominately cutaneous and ocular findings, whereas NF-2 exhibits bilateral acoustic schwannomas. A recent secondary subset of NF-2 called *schwannomatosis*, consisting of multiple deep painful schwannomas, has also been described (10).

EPIDEMIOLOGY

NF-1 is the most common neurocutaneous disorder with an incidence of 1 of 3,000. In comparison, NF-2 occurs in 1 of 50,000.

ETIOLOGY AND PATHOGENESIS

NF-1 results from an autosomal-dominant mutation in the *NF-1* gene, a tumor suppressor gene found on chromosome 17q that codes for *neurofibromin*. Neurofibromin is a guanosine triphosphatase (GTPase)-activating protein that regulates products of the *ras* protooncogene. A mutation in NF-1, therefore, leads to dysregulation of cell growth. Of NF-1 cases, 50% are caused by spontaneous mutations. Segmental, somatic, and gonadal mosaicism is also possible (11).

NF-2 results from an autosomal-dominant mutation in the *NF-2* gene found on chromosome 22. The NF-2 protein *schwannomin* acts as a tumor suppressor protein.

PATHOLOGY

On dermatopathology, a cutaneous neurofibroma is a round, nonencapsulated, well-circumscribed dermal nodule composed of spinal cells, mostly schwann cells and fibroblasts. A plexiform neurofibroma, which is pathognomonic for NF, is similar but with a more complex wormlike fasicular growth pattern (12). The optic glioma is considered a low-grade astrocytoma, and astrocytoma is the major type of CNS tumor in NF-1 (13).

CLINICAL MANIFESTATIONS

Neurofibromatosis, or von Recklinghausen disease, is characterized by cutaneous neurofibromas and CNS tumors. The cutaneous features include café au lait macules, axillary freckling, neurofibromas, and plexiform neurofibromas. Café au lait spots are hyperpigmented oval macules of a size that varies with age. Neurofibromas are soft papules and nodules that are located in the dermis and arise from the peripheral nerves (Fig. 123-4). Plexiform neurofibromas occur in 25% to 30% of patients and arise from large nerve roots, often located deep in the body, occurring on the face and can lead to disfigurement. A 5% lifetime risk exists for malignant transformation.

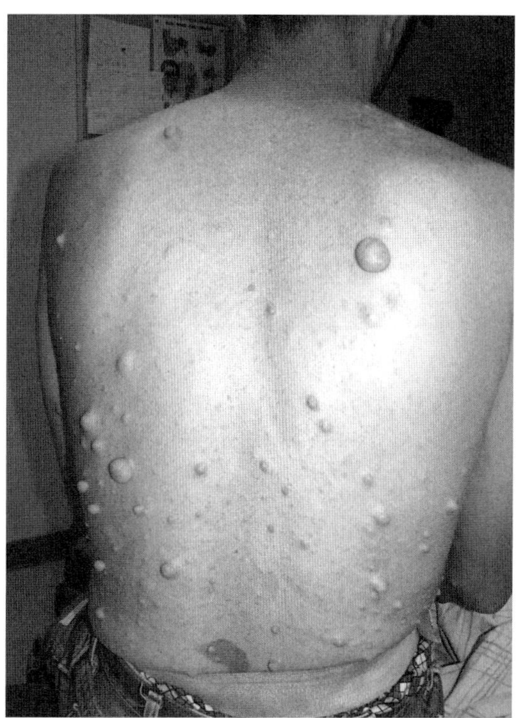

FIGURE 123-4. Neurofibromatosis. Multiple neurofibromas and café au lait macules.

Other systemic findings include Lisch nodules, which are pigmented iris hamartomas that are also pathognomonic for NF. They develop in teenage years and are found in 90% of patients. Patients with NF-1 are at risk of developing CNS tumors, although less than patients with NF-2. Optic gliomas are the most common tumor, occurring in 15% of patients, either unilaterally or bilaterally. Presenting signs include optic atrophy and progressive vision loss followed by pain. Other CNS tumors include mostly low-grade gliomas, medulloblastomas, or ependymomas, often arising in atypical sites. MRI of the head reveals that approximately 60% of patients have radiographic evidence of white matter abnormalities in the basal ganglia, thalamus, brainstem, and cerebellum. The cause of these lesions is unknown (4). Many patients with NF-1 have learning disabilities and most have low-average intelligence. Finally, orthopedic complications, including spinal deformities from interforamen neurofibromas, scoliosis, and congenital tibial dysplasia, may arise (10).

Patients with NF-2 have few cutaneous lesions. The hallmark of the disease is the development of bilateral acoustic neuromas. Complaints with large acoustic neuromas include hearing loss, tinnitus and vertigo, and facial weakness. Smaller lesions can cause only hearing loss. Other CNS tumors include ependymomas, meningiomas, and astrocytomas. The signs and symptoms of these disorders mainly result from the location of the primary tumor. A variant of NF-2 exists with the development of multiple schwannomas without vestibular tumors. These tumors produce intractable pain and have limited expression of disease confined to just a single limb or single segment (14).

DIAGNOSIS

The diagnosis of neurofibromatosis is made by meeting well-defined clinical criteria (Table 123-2). Gene testing is also available to detect protein truncation which is detected in 60% to 70% of NF-1 mutations. Direct DNA sequencing is also able to detect mutations in 95% of individuals.

TABLE 123-2. Criteria for the Diagnosis of Neurofibromatosis

NIH Consensus Criteria for Diagnosis for NF-1: 1987

NEED TWO OR MORE OF THE FOLLOWING FEATURES

Six or more café au lait macules >5 mm in greatest diameter in prepubertal individuals and >15 mm in greatest diameter in postpubertal individuals
Two or more neurofibromas of any type or one plexiform neurofibroma
Freckling in the axillary or inguinal regions
Optic glioma
Two or more Lisch nodules
A distinctive osseous lesion, such a sphenoid dysplasia, or thinning of long bone cortex with or without pseudoarthrosis
A first degree relative with NF-1 by the above criteria

NIH, National Institutes of Health; NF-1, neurofibromatosis, type 1.

TREATMENT

Genetic counseling is indicated. Comprehensive clinical referrals are indicated for developmental pediatricians, neurologists, ophthalmologists, dermatologists, and orthopedic surgeons.

Sturge-Weber Syndrome

DEFINITION

Sturge Weber syndrome (SWS) is a congenital syndrome consisting of a unilateral or bilateral facial capillary malformation, or port wine stain, and ipsilateral leptomeningeal and brain angiomatosis, resulting in a constellation of neurologic findings.

EPIDEMIOLOGY

The estimated frequency of SWS is 1 per 50,000.

ETIOLOGY AND PATHOGENESIS

The cause of SWS is unknown. The disorder is sporadic and there is no known genetic or environmental cause. Stasis in the leptomeningeal angiomatosis results in underlying ischemia leading to calcification and necrosis (15). Glaucoma can be caused by increased episcleral venous pressure from arteriovenous shunts or perhaps secondary to anterior chamber angle abnormalities (1).

PATHOLOGY

Histopathology of the skin shows a collection of widely dilated thin-walled venules in the dermis (15). In the brain, calcifications are seen in meningeal arteries and cortical and subcortical veins. Cortical necrosis, neuronal loss, and gliosis can also occur (15).

CLINICAL MANIFESTATIONS

The primary cutaneous feature is a facial capillary malformation, or port-wine stain, that is present at birth. The most clinically significant malformation involves the ophthalmic portion of cranial nerve V with involvement of the superior eyelid. In patients with these findings, 10% to 20% will have CNS involvement. The leptomeningial angioma occur ipsilateral to the facial angioma in 85% of the patients, but can occur bilaterally (Figs. 123-5 and 123-6).

Epilepsy occurs in up to 90% of patients with SWS and involves mostly focal and generalized tonic–clonic seizures, but infantile spasms, and myoclonic and atonic seizures also occur (15,16). Epilepsy usually is correlated to focal structural abnormalities. Neurologic deficits, such as visual field deficits, are usually a consequence of the location of the leptomeningial angiomata, such as the occipital region. Developmental abnormalities and mental retardation are present in 50% of patients. Other clinical manifestations include contralateral hemiparesis, contralateral hemiatrophy, and homonymous hemianopia. Studies have shown as high as 71% of patients with SWS have elevated intraocular pressures or glaucoma, with many cases occurring before 2 years of age.

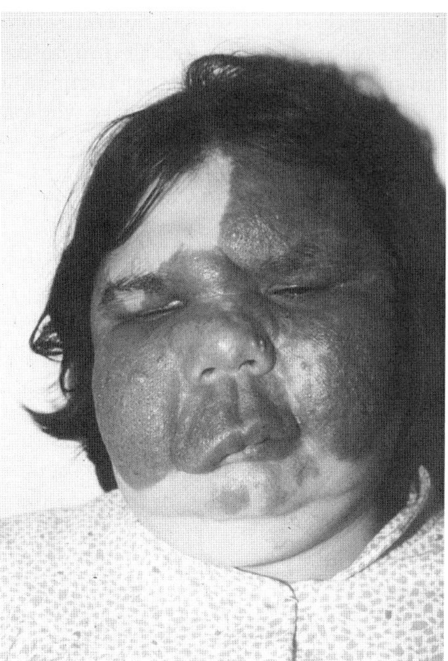

FIGURE 123-5. Bilateral capillary malformations in V_1 and V_2 distribution in a patient with Sturge-Weber syndrome.

DIAGNOSIS

Clinical examination at birth reveals a port-wine stain, and imaging evaluates for intracranial disease. Plain skull films can evaluate for intracranial calcification, but are rarely helpful in the neonatal period. CT imaging may evaluate for subtle atrophy, but MRI is currently the preferred imaging technique to evaluate for intracranial involvement.

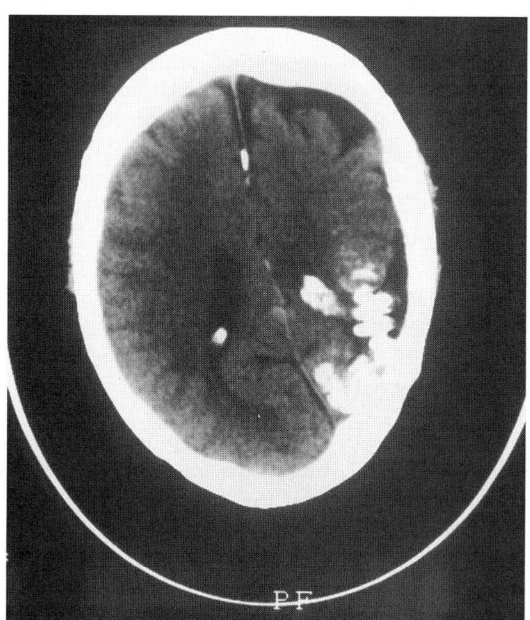

FIGURE 123-6. Computed tomography (CT) findings of the patient in Figure 123-5.

TREATMENT

Treatment usually involves symptomatic control of the epilepsy. Studies have shown that 50% of patients will obtain seizure control and 39% have partial control. For those with refractory seizures, surgery (e.g., focal surgical resection or hemispherectomy) is an option. Annual ophthalmologic screening is recommended. Treatment of the port-wine stain for cosmetic purposes is performed with a pulsed-dye laser.

Ataxia: Telangiectasia Syndrome

DEFINITION

Ataxia telangiectasia (AT) is a neurodegenerative disorder characterized by a slowly progressive ataxia combined with the development of cutaneous telangiectasias, immunodeficiency, a predisposition to cancer, and a hypersensitivity to radiation.

EPIDEMIOLOGY

The prevalence is estimated between 1 of 40,000 to 500,000 individuals, with an increased incidence in populations with a high percentage of inbreeding (17).

ETIOLOGY AND PATHOGENESIS

AT is an autosomal recessive disorder. The ataxia telangiectasias mutated (ATM) gene is a large gene located on chromosome 11q22-23, and >400 mutations have been discovered. The gene is thought to have a role in DNA repair, particularly through cell cycle regulation allowing for repair (18). The ataxia is attributable to a progressive loss of Purkinje cells in the cerebellum. The sensory ataxia may be caused by the involvement of a large fiber sensory neuropathy. The increased incidence of malignancy and immunodeficiency are also attributable to ineffective DNA repair.

PATHOLOGY

The cerebellum shows severe Purkinje loss, particularly in the cerebellum (18). Changes can also be seen in the spinal cord with demyelination of the posterior columns and degeneration of the posterior columns and anterior horn cells.

CLINICAL MANIFESTATIONS

The cutaneous features include telangiectasias that develop in early childhood around age 5 years. The classic locations include the ocular sclerae, earlobes, and bridge of the nose. Other associated cutaneous findings are extensor arm hypertrichosis and poikiloderma.

Ataxia begins around age 2 years. Initially, truncal ataxia is the dominant feature making sitting and gait difficult, but eventually ataxia involves the limbs. Strength remains normal, but movement disorders can develop, including myoclonus, choreoathetosis, and intention tremors. Most children are wheelchair bound by the age of 12 years. The other constant feature is ocular motility difficulties. Oculomotor apraxia presents with limitations of upgaze and voluntary smooth pursuit.

Adults may exhibit a distal muscular atrophy with fasciculation and large fiber sensory neuropathy.

Some studies have shown a 10% to 15% chance of developing a lymphoid malignancy in early childhood. Most commonly, T-cell leukemia and lymphomas arise. Other nonlymphoid tumors account for 20% of malignancies and include dysgerminoma, retinoblastoma, and pancreatic carcinoma. Females are at increased risk for ovarian and uterine cancers. The increased risk for malignancies is seen in nonaffected female family members with a five times increased risk of breast cancer. In addition to the increased risk for malignancy, there is also an increased risk for infections. The most common infection is chronic sinopulmonary disease.

DIAGNOSIS

Clinical findings may precipitate laboratory investigation. Patients will have elevated α-fetoprotein levels. The immunoglobin levels will show a pan decrease with a larger selective deficiency in the IgG2 subclass. Cellular features include a shortened cell life span and increased hypersensitivity to ionizing radiation.

TREATMENT

Physical therapy and the use of assistive devices are the mainstay of treatment of the ataxia. If radiation therapy is used for lymphoma treatment, it should be with small fractionated doses. Sunscreens and protective clothing are used for cutaneous protection.

Ehlers-Danlos Syndrome

DEFINITION

Ehler-Danlos syndrome (EDS) is a spectrum of disorders of hyperelastic skin, hyperextensible joints, vascular lesions, and excessive scarring after injury. Seven subsets of disease exist, but 80% are within the classic and hypermobility types. The vascular type, formerly known as *type IV*, is the most common with neurologic complications.

EPIDEMIOLOGY

The incidence is approximately 1 of 10,000 births (20).

ETIOLOGY AND PATHOGENESIS

Vascular type EDS is inherited as an autosomal-dominant disorder. The gene defect is in COL3A1 that encodes for a missense mutation in α_1 chain in type III collagen.

CLINICAL MANIFESTATIONS

The neurologic findings are mainly the result of vascular complications, although rare associated peripheral neuropathies are seen (21). The vascular defects consist of intracranial aneurysms, carotid-cavernous fistulas, and arterial dissections. Aneurysms most often occur in the carotid artery near the cavernous sinus resulting in a carotid cavernous fistula. A carotid-cavernous fistula can also arise spontaneously or after mild head trauma. Possible symptoms include proptosis, chemosis, diplopia, and pulsatile tinnitus. Another complication is arterial dissection, which can lead to focal stroke syndromes.

DIAGNOSIS

The history and clinical features are helpful in classifying patients with EDS. To confirm the diagnosis, a skin biopsy may be performed for protein analysis for collagens type I, III, and V. Molecular analysis for COL3A1 can also be performed (22).

TREATMENT

Genetic counseling should be given to an individual of childbearing potential. In patients with vascular EDS, a two-dimension echocardiogram is recommended to evaluate the ascending aortic root.

Epidermal Nevus Syndrome

DEFINITION

Epidermal nevus syndrome is a collection of disorders characterized by epidermal nevi and neurologic manifestations. They are classified according to the predominate tissue contained within the epidermal nevus: nevus verrucosus (containing keratinocytes), nevus sebaceous (containing sebaceous glands), or nevus comedonicus (containing hair follicles). Some feel this is not a distinct disorder, but rather a collection of disorders including Shimelpenning- Feurestein-Mims syndrome, proteus syndrome, CHILD (congenital hemidysplasia with ichthyosiform erythroderma) syndrome, nevus comedonicus syndrome and phakomatosis pigmentokeratotica.

EPIDEMIOLOGY, ETIOLOGY, AND PATHOGENESIS

Isolated epidermal nevi are common but are rarely associated with syndromes. The epidermal nevi syndromes are extremely rare disorders that occur spontaneously. The common genetic trait is mosaicism, and they may represent a lethal disorder that is rescued by mosaicism (23).

PATHOLOGY

The pathology depends on the specific subtype of epidermal nevus within the syndrome.

CLINICAL MANIFESTATIONS

The common cutaneous feature is the epidermal nevus, which presents at birth or in infancy as linear, raised, verrucous plaques, which are often on the head and neck and follow Blaschko lines. The nevi can be inflamed or associated with cutaneous malignancies, such as keratoacanthoma, basal cell or squamous cell carcinoma, or Spitz nevus (24).

Neurologic features include cognitive deficits, epilepsy, and intracranial and cerebrovascular malformations. The epilepsies are mostly focal, with associated focal slowing. The neurologic examination may show focality with hemiparesis and cranial nerve deficits. Intracranial malformations include unilateral hemimegalencephaly and other neuronal migrational abnormalities (25). The cerebrovascular abnormalities consist of dysplastic and occluded arteries.

Other systemic features include an increase in malignancy, and skeletal, ocular, cardiovascular, and genitourinary abnormalities.

DIAGNOSIS

MRI is the most sensitive technique for evaluating for structural and migrational abnormalities. Intracranial imaging most commonly reveals megalencephaly ipsilateral to the facial epidermal nevus.

TREATMENT

Appropriate symptomatic treatment is indicated. If other organ systems are involved, appropriate referrals are indicated.

Hypomelanosis of Ito

DEFINITION

Hypomelanosis of Ito is a systemic disorder that affects the skin with whorled hypopigmentation, and variably causes brain, eye, skeleton, and other organ abnormalities.

ETIOLOGY AND PATHOGENESIS

Hypomelanosis of Ito is an extremely rare disorder affecting males and females, thus differentiating it from incontinetia pigmenti. It is a sporadic disorder without a recognized gene defect, but it likely represents a form of chromosomal mosaicism.

PATHOLOGY

Cutaneous biopsies taken from within the hypopigmented regions show decreased numbers of melanocytes.

CLINICAL FEATURES

Cutaneous features are characterized by hypopigmented whorls, streaks, and patches following Blaschko lines that are present at birth or in infancy. The hypopigmentation can involve the trunk and extremities and be unilateral or bilateral. Woods lamp can be used to detect lesions in fair-skinned individuals. Affected individuals can also display café au lait macules, nevus of Ota, trichorrhexis (fragile hair), and nail dystrophy.

Neurologic features occur in approximately 50% to 80% of cases. Deficits can consist of epilepsy, mental retardation, or developmental abnormalities. Structural abnormalities of cerebral and cerebellar hypoplasia, hemimegalencephaly, and lissencephaly are possible.

Systemic findings can potentially affect every organ system. Ocular findings include iridis, dacryostenosis, pannus, corneal opacities, cataracts, and retinal abnormalities. Musculoskeletal defects of hemihypertrophy, cleft palate, and butterfly vertebrae can occur. Dental abnormalities, including cleft lip and palate, hypoplastic dental enamel; and cardiac defects, including tetralogy of Fallot, pulmonary stenosis, and septal defects are all possible.

DIAGNOSIS

A clinical diagnosis is achieved based on compatible history, physical examination, and radiologic findings.

TREATMENT

Symptomatic treatment is indicated.

Neurocutaneous Melanosis

DEFINITION

Neurocutaneous melanosis, a congenital disorder of melanotic cell development, increases the numbers of melanocytes that most commonly involves the skin and leptomeninges.

ETIOLOGY AND PATHOGENESIS

Neurocutaneous melanosis is a rare disorder with an unknown incidence, but it is not a hereditary disorder. Melanocytes are derived from the ectoderm and are normally found in the skin and meninges. Congenital melanocytic nevi do not necessarily have CNS involvement and CNS melanosis does not always require cutaneous involvement.

PATHOLOGY

Neurocutaneous melanosis is a disorder of migration in melanocytes. Histopathologically, there are increased numbers of normal-appearing melanocytes. Abnormal proliferation of the melanocyte leads to melanoma.

CLINICAL MANIFESTATIONS

The cutaneous features include hyperpigmented macules, plaques, and patches. Congenital nevi are often giant hairy nevi located in the bathing trunk distribution or on the upper back as a cape nevus. Several satellite nevi may be present on other portions of the body and 20% of cases do not have giant nevi. Potential diagnostic criteria have been proposed including large or multiple congenital nevi with a size >20 cm in adults, >9 cm on an infant scalp, or >6 cm on the body of an infant. Patients must not have primary cutaneous or meningeal melanoma that could explain a metastatic melanocytic lesion (26). The lifetime risk of developing a melanoma within a lesion is estimated between 10% and 25%.

Neurologic abnormalities result from complications from melanocytes or from malformations. Complications from the melanocytes include leptomeningeal melanosis or intracranial melanoma. CNS malformations include cerebral or spinal malformations. Neurologic symptoms usually present around age 2 years. Leptomeningeal melanosis usually occurs at the ventral brainstem, or upper cervical or ventral lumbosacral cord. It can be associated with hydrocephalus. In some studies, nevi located on back have been shown to correlate with a higher incidence of disease.

DIAGNOSIS

The diagnosis is supported by laboratory and radiologic testing. The CSF may reveal rounded cells with dark brown cytoplasmic vesicles and irregular fingers projecting from the cell bodies. Neuroimaging documents abnormalities in 50% of patients with cutaneous disease. MRI of the head reveals hyperintensity abnormalities in T1-weighted imaging, most often in anterior temporal lobes along the basilar meninges. Less often, the pons, medulla, thalamus, and the base of the frontal lobes are involved. CNS melanoma is difficult to diagnose by MRI and is best performed by comparing serial studies. Focal signs of CNS melanoma include the presence of necrosis, perilesional edema, contrast enhancement, or hemorrhage.

TREATMENT

The decision made early in life to surgically resect the congenital nevus often depends on the extent of CNS involvement. Long-term, close follow-up examinations are required to monitor for changes in the cutaneous melanocytic lesions. Any suspicious change in a cutaneous lesion should be biopsied, examining for melanoma. In addition, patients should have repeat neurologic imaging if a new neurologic deficit occurs to evaluate for CNS melanoma or increased intracranial pressure (27).

Xeroderma Pigmentosum

DEFINITION

Xeroderma pigmentosum is a group of neurocutaneous disorders with an increased susceptibility to malignancy caused by UV or chemical injury because of a defect in nuclear excision repair. The skin, and the ocular and nervous systems are most often involved.

EPIDEMIOLOGY

The incidence is estimated to be 1 of 30,000 to 250,000 individuals.

ETIOLOGY AND PATHOGENESIS

The disease is transmitted through an autosomal recessive pattern. The genetic defect is an abnormality in DNA nucleotide excision repair. Photo-induced injury explains the cutaneous features of the disorder, but has difficulty explaining the degenerative neurologic features. It is speculated that the neurologic injury is caused by damage from reactive oxygen species. The genetics of xeroderma pigmentosa involves complementation groups, which represent different proteins involved in DNA repair. Seven different complementation groups exist that have overlapping phenotypic features labeled as XP-A through XP-G. XP–A, XP-C, and XP-D are the most common. Similar gene mutations occur in Cockayne syndrome, trichothiodystrophy, and DeSanctisCacchione syndrome

PATHOLOGY

The neurologic deficits represent a widespread primary degeneration of the nervous system. Cortical atrophy leads to dementia, whereas basal ganglia involvement leads to movement disorders and cerebellum involvement leads to ataxia (28).

The cutaneous malignancies all have characteristic dermatopathology features to help classify the tumors. Melanoma is an atypical proliferation of the melanocytes. Squamous cell carcinoma and keratoacanthomas are proliferations of keratinocytes and basal cell carcinoma is a proliferation of basal layer keratinocytes.

CLINICAL MANIFESTATIONS

The cutaneous features are marked photosensitivity, with burning, hyperpigmentation, xerosis, and atrophy. As a result of the chronic UV light damage, there is a predisposition to cutaneous malignancy, including actinic keratosis, basal cell carcinoma, squamous cell carcinoma, and melanoma. The median onset is at approximately 1 to 2 years of age. The initial cutaneous problems involve freckling, erythema, and blistering after sun exposure. As damage from chronic sun exposure continues, the skin becomes atrophic and xerotic, with overlying telangiectasias. The risk of cutaneous malignancy is increased 1,000 times compared with healthy individuals.

Common ocular features are damage to the cornea and conjunctiva, also from UV light. Keratitis and conjunctivitis occur with sun exposure. Chronic changes include scarring, loss of eyelashes, entropion, and ectropion. An increased risk also exists of cutaneous malignancies, including and surrounding the eye.

Neurologic features are present in 20% of patients, mostly seen with the XP-A, XP-B, XP-D, and XP-G variants (29). The neurologic features consist of a progressive dementia, sensorineural hearing loss, movement disorders, and ataxia. The onset of neurologic symptoms starts with memory loss in early school years, followed by cerebellar dysfunction and hearing loss occurring around age 10 years. Most of these children have lost muscle stretch reflexes by the age of 6 years.

DIAGNOSIS

The diagnosis is made by having compatible clinical features. The fibroblast survival test after UV irradiation can support the diagnosis (30).

TREATMENT

Treatment consists of UV radiation avoidance. UV radiation exposure can be reduced with use of sunscreen and protective clothing. Routine cancer screening by a dermatologist is required. Cases have been reported of medication used to prevent cutaneous malignancy, such as topical retinoids, local interferon injection, and topical prokaryotic DNA repair enzyme. Systemic gene therapy is a future potential treatment that has been studied in xeroderma pigmentosum with some success in skin fibroblasts (31).

Other Disorders with Dermatologic and Neurologic Manifestations

Incontinentia pigmenti (IP), or *Bloch-Sulzberger syndrome*, is an X-linked dominant disorder that is lethal in prenatal males. The cutaneous signs occur in four classic stages, all in a Blascko pattern distribution. The skin disease begins perinatally with intensely inflammatory vesicles, followed by verrucous patches around 2 to 6 weeks of life, hyperpigmented whorls around 3 to 6 months of age, and finally, scarring in the second to third decade (Fig. 123-7). Recurrence of vesicles, even into adolescence is not uncommon. The neurologic signs of IP, which occur in about 30% of patients, include seizures, mental retardation, and spastic paraparesis. Anodontia and peg teeth, dystrophic nails, alopecia, and retinal vascular abnormalities, possibly leading to blindness are additional clinical findings. The gene defect in IP is in Nuclear Factor κ β Essential Modifier (NEMO), which is required for the activation of the transcription factor (nuclear factor-kappa B [NF-κB]) (32). NF-κB plays an important role in the initiation of inflammation, either through impaired activation, as in IP, or through over activation (33).

Kinky hair syndrome, also known as *Menkes disease*, is an X-linked disorder of neural and connective tissue caused by a defect in the ATP7a copper-transporting gene leading to an abnormality in copper metabolism and a decrease in the activity of numerous copper-requiring enzymes. It has been suggested that copper has a role in activity-dependent modulation of synaptic activity (34). The frequency ranges from 1 of 100,000 to 300,000 individuals. Hypotonia is apparent in infants, within the first few months, and gradually the hypotonia evolves into spastic quadriparesis. Epilepsy is common, with partial and generalized seizures and an increased incidence of myoclonic seizures. Less commonly, children can present with later onset disease with milder symptoms, but the disorder is slowly progressive. Children exhibit failure to thrive and die in early childhood. The pathognomonic dermatologic feature is pili torti, which clinically presents as kinky, twisted hair and microscopically shows hair which is twisted 180 degrees. The skin is often redundant and described as "doughy" in nature. MRI usually shows scattered cerebral white matter lesions suggestive of demyelination and torturous intracranial vessels. Treatment with replacement copper histidine may be promising, but long-term results are still pending (35).

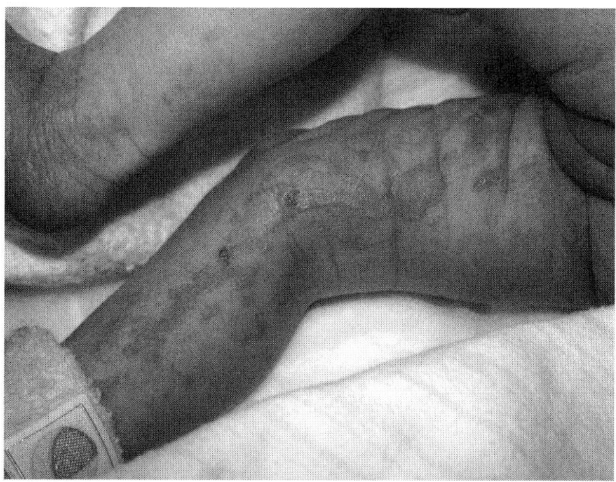

FIGURE 123-7. The vesicular stage of incontinentia pigmenti.

Von Hippel-Lindau disease is a multisystem syndrome associated with various benign and malignant tumors of the CNS and visceral organs. The incidence is estimated at 1 or 36,000. The syndrome is caused by an autosomal-dominant mutation in the *VHL* tumor suppressor gene on chromosome 3. The most common tumor is a hemangioblastoma that may arise in the retina or the CNS. The cutaneous findings occur in <5% of patients and consist of a capillary malformation, usually of the head and neck. Tumors of the kidneys, adrenal glands, pancreas, and reproductive organs are also possible and can include renal cell carcinoma, pheochromocytoma, pancreatic neuroendocrine tumors, and epididymal and broad ligament cystadenomas (36).

Fabry's disease, or *angiokeratoma corporis diffusum*, is an X-linked recessive disorder caused by defective activity of α-galactosidase A. The defect leads to an accumulation of neutral glycosphingolipids preferentially in vascular endothelium, resulting in ischemia and infarction. The incidence is 1 of 40,000 males and variable expression is seen in female carriers. The primary neurologic manifestation is the development of pain crises, which are most severe in the hands and feet, but can extend proximally. They can be precipitated by exercise, fever, or stress. Cerebrovascular accidents and persistent acroparesthesias can also develop. The angiokeratoma is the dominant cutaneous finding, but hypohidrosis is also a consistent finding later in life. The angiokeratoma is a red to violaceous papule with overlying hyperkeratosis, usually located on the lower trunk and extremities. Premature death usually results from renal and cardiovascular involvement. Antiepileptic drugs, such as low-dose phenytoin, may help the pain crises. Enzymatic replacement is available and has shown benefit to symptomatic patients (37).

CLINICAL RECOMMENDATIONS OF THE VIGNETTE

A multidisciplinary approach is recommended. The patient and her mother should have genetic counseling and should be informed of the 50% risk of passing the disorder to any future offspring. The patient's siblings should also be screened by a dermatologist and, depending on those findings, their examination should include an MRI of the head.

A developmental pediatrician is beneficial in caring for this patient, and may help coordinate care. The patient should have an MRI of the brain approximately every 1 to 2 years until puberty to assess for tuber formation and obstructive hydrocephalus. A baseline echocardiogram and electrocardiogram are recommended to assess for rhabdomyomas and arrhythmias. Routine renal ultrasounds should be done every 2 to 5 years throughout adulthood to assess for renal angiomyolipomas. A neurologist should provide ongoing management of the seizure disorder as well as conduct frequent neurologic examinations. Facial angiofibromas are routinely treated with pulsed-dye laser and periungual fibromas may be surgically removed.

SUMMARY

Phakomatoses and other neurocutaneous syndromes are a diverse group of inherited and congenital syndromes with features of neurologic disease and wide spectrum of cutaneous findings. When a patient presents with a neurologic disorder, cutaneous findings may be outward and recognizable signs to aid in diagnosis. Conversely, skin findings may be the first sign of disease, leading to an appropriate search for a neurologic pathology. Most of the disorders discussed here require a multidisciplinary approach involving neurologists, dermatologists, geneticists, and other specialists.

REFERENCES

1. Povey S, Burley MW, Attwood J, et al. Two loci for tuberous sclerosis: One on 9q13 and one on 16p13. *Annals of Human Genetics.* 1994;58:107–127.
2. Rosner M, Freilinger A, Hengstschlager M. The tuberous sclerosis genes and regulation of the cyclin-dependent kinase inhibitor p27. *Mutat Res.* 2006;613:10–16.
3. Hung CC, Su YN, Chien SC, et al. Molecular and clinical analyses of 84 patients with tuberous sclerosis complex. *BMC Medical Genetics.* 2006;7:72.
4. Chow CW, Klug GL, Lewis EA. Subependymal giant cell astrocytoma in children: An unusual discrepancy between histological and clinical features. *Neurosurgery.* 1988;68:880–883.
5. Webb DW, Fryer AE, Osborne JP. On the incidence of fits and mental retardation in tuberous sclerosis. *Am J Med Genet.* 1991;28:395–397.
6. Pampiglione G, Pugh E. Infantile spasms and subsequent appearance of tuberous sclerosis. *Lancet.* 1975;2:1046.
7. Crino PB, Nathanson KL, Henske EP. The tuberous sclerosis complex. *N Engl J Med.* 2006;355:1345–1356.
8. Roach ES, Gomez MR, Northrup H. Tuberous sclerosis complex consensus conference: Revised clinical diagnostic criteria. *J Child Neurol.* 1998;13:624–628.
9. Milunsky A, Shim SH, Ito M, et al. Precise prenatal diagnosis of tuberous sclerosis by sequencing the TSC2 gene. *Prenat Diagn.* 2005;25(7):582–585.
10. Crawford A, Schorry E. Neurofibromatosis update. *J Pediatr Orthop.* 2006;26(3):413–423.
11. Niiyama S, Satoh K, Kaneko S, et al. Segmental neurofibromatosis. *Acta Derm Venereol.* 2005;85:448–449.
12. Argenyi ZB. Neural and neuroendocrine tumors. In: Barnhill RL, Crowson AN, eds. *Textbook of Dermatopathology.* New York: McGraw-Hill; 2004:893–914.
13. Ruggieri, M, Huson SM. The neurofibromatoses. An overview. *Italian Journal of Neurological Sciences.* 1999;20:89–108.
14. MacCollin M, Willett C, Heinrich B, et al. Familial schwannomatosis. *Neurology.* 2003;60: 1968–1974.
15. Thomas-Sohl KA, Vaslow DF, Maria BL. Sturge-Weber syndrome: A review. *Pediatr Neurol.* 2004;30:303–310.
16. Hunt SJ, Santa Cruz DJ, Barnhill RL. Vascular tumors. In: Barnhill RL, Crowson AN, eds. *Textbook of Dermatopathology.* New York: McGraw-Hill; 2004:825.
17. Zaroff CM, Isaacs K. Neurocutaneous syndromes: Behavioral features. *Epilepsy and Behavior.* 2005;7:133–142.
18. Spacey SD, Gatti RA, Bebb G. The molecular basis and clinical management of ataxia telangiectasia. *Can J Neurol Sci.* 2000;27:184–191.
19. Taylor AMR, Byrd PJ. Molecular pathology of ataxia telangiectasia. *J Clin Pathol.* 2005;58:1009–1015.
20. Germain DP. Clinical and genetic features of vascular Ehlers-Danlos syndrome. *Ann Vasc Surg.* 2001;16:391–397.
21. Galan E, Kousseff BG. Peripheral neuropathy in Ehlers-Danlos syndrome. *Pediatr Neurol.* 1995;12:242–245.
22. Malfait F, Hakim AJ, De Paepe A, et al. The genetic basis of the joint hypermobility syndromes. *Rheumatology.* 2006;45:502–507.
23. Happle R. Mosaicism in human skin. *Arch Dermatol.* 2003;129:1460–1470.
24. Kishida E, Silva M, Pereira F, et al. Epidermal nevus syndrome associated with adnexal tumors, spitz nevus and hypophosphatemic vitamin D rickets. *Pediatr Dermatol.* 2005;22:48–54.
25. Zhang W, Simos P, Ishibashi H, et al. Neuroimaging features of epidermal nevus syndrome. *American Journal of Neuroradiology.* 2003;24:1468–1470.
26. Kadonaga IN, Frieden U. Neurocutaneous melanosis: Definition and review of the literature. *J Am Acad Dermatol.* 1991;24(5 Pt 1):747–755.
27. Plikaitis C, David L, Argenta L. Neurocutaneous melanosis: Clinical presentations. *Journal of Craniofacial Surgery.* 2005;16-5:921–925.
28. Rapin I, Lindenbaum Y, Dickson DW, et al. Cockayne syndrome and xeroderma pigmentosum. *Neurology.* 2002;55:1442–1449.
29. Sidwell RU, Sandison A, Wing J, et al. A novel mutation in the XPA gene associated with unusually mild clinical features in a patient who developed a spindle cell melanoma. *Br J Dermatol.* 2006;155:81–88.
30. Woods CG. DNA repair disorders. *Arch Disease Child.* 1998;78:178–184.
31. Zeng L, Quiliet X, Chevallier-Lagente O, et al. Retrovirus-mediated gene transfer corrects DNA repair defect of xeroderma pigmentosum cells of complementation groups A, B, C. *Gene Ther.* 1997;4:1077–1084.
32. Smahi A, Courtois G, Vabres P, et al. Genomic rearrangement in *NEMO* impairs NF-κB activation and is a cause of incontinentia pigmenti. *Nature.* 2000;405:466–472.
33. Sebban H, Courtois G. NF-kB and inflammation in genetic disease. *Biochem Pharmacol.* 2006;72:1153–1160.
34. Schlief ML, West T, Craig AM, et al. Role of Menkes copper-transporting ATPase in NMDA receptor-mediated neuronal toxicity. *Proc Natl Acad Sci U S A.* 2006;106:12919–12924.
35. Kaler SG. Metabolic and molecular bases of Menkes disease and occipital horn syndrome. *Pediatr Dev Pathol.* 1998;1:85–98.
36. Lonser RR, Glenn GM, Walther M, et al. von Hippel-Lindau disease. *Lancet.* 2003;361: 2059–2067.
37. Eng CM, Germain DP, Banikazemi M, et al. Fabry disease: Guidelines for the evaluation and management of multi-organ system involvement. *Genet Med.* 2006;8(9):539–548.

CHAPTER **124**

Neuro-Dermatological Presentations of Systemic Illness

Lawrence A. Mark • James D. Fleck

OBJECTIVES

- To describe the dermatologic manifestations of several diseases with neurologic involvement
- To explain the appropriate workup to verify the cause of these diseases
- To discuss the initial treatment and management of the conditions presented
- To provide knowledge about when and when not to suspect anticonvulsant hypersensitivity syndrome

CASE VIGNETTE

A 23-year-old female veterinary student with a 2-week history of retroorbital headache, treated with amoxicillin for a suspected sinusitis, now presents with lethargy and decreased mental status. On examination, she is febrile and has an obvious petechial rash (Figs. 124-1 and 124-2). She becomes progressively less responsive.

DEFINITION

The integument is the largest and most readily visible organ of the human body. Because of its visibility, skin findings can be a clinician's earliest clue to the cause of a systemic illness. Furthermore, changes in skin findings often correlate well with changes in the internal condition it represents. This is particularly true for systemic neurologic illness, because the nervous system is intimately and complexly associated with the skin, providing it support, growth stimulation, and sensation. With this framework in mind, the following illnesses that most often or primarily affect skin and the nervous system will be discussed: sarcoidosis, syphilis, herpes simplex virus, Rocky Mountain spotted fever, and Lyme disease. Additionally, no discussion of neuro-dermatologic disease would be complete without mention of the anticonvulsant drug hypersensitivity syndrome (ADHS).

EPIDEMIOLOGY

Sarcoidosis can have a protean presentation, most often affecting the lungs, but also can be seen in the skin in 25% of cases, and in the central nervous system (CNS) in 5% of cases. A genetic predisposition to developing sarcoidosis has been postulated because of its higher incidence in certain ethnic backgrounds; in particular, it is up to 20 times more prevalent among blacks than whites and vanishingly rare among Native Americans. In the United States, sarcoidosis has an incidence of about 10 to 40 cases per 100,000 persons.

Syphilis, another protean disease, remains an important health risk in America despite ongoing public education and health department efforts. Unrecognized, it is a progressively debilitating disease and especially devastating in the congenital form. The incidence reached a low in the 1940s after the advent of penicillin, but had a resurgence in the 1980s. Centers for Disease Control (CDC) figures from 2004 show an incidence of 2.7 per 100,000 person, mostly affecting women aged 20 to 24 years and men aged 35 to 39 years, representing a particular increase in men having sex with men.

Herpes simplex virus (HSV) is a very common infection. It is estimated that by age 12 years, >72% of the US population has circulating antibodies to HSV-1, HSV-2 or both (1). It is a significant condition because of its ability to cause devastating neurologic sequelae in newborns.

Rocky Mountain spotted fever (RMSF) has its highest incidence in children aged 5 to 9 years from the southern Atlantic US states, but the overall average incidence of RMSF is 0.22 per 100,000 persons (2).

For Lyme disease, nearly 17,000 new cases were reported in 1998. Most cases were from the north-central and northeastern United States, with the highest incidence in children aged 5 to 9 years (3).

Anticonvulsant drug hypersensitivity syndrome is seen only in the setting of a patient who has recently been placed on aromatic ring-containing antiepileptic medication; phenytoin, carbamazepine, oxcarbazepine, phenobarbital, or lamotrigine.

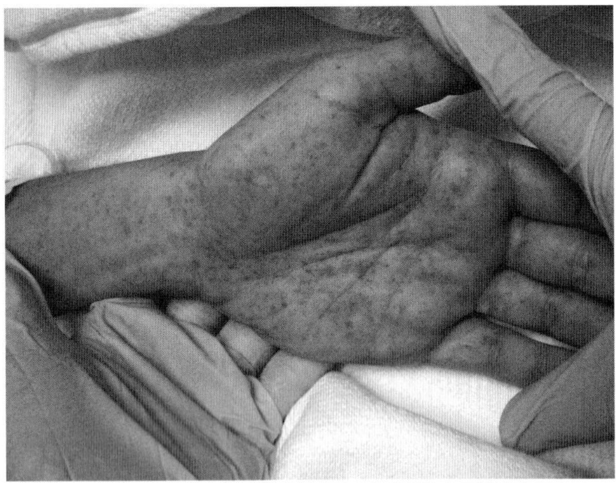

FIGURE 124-1. Petechial rash located on hands and wrists.

Data regarding the incidence of severe reactions to these medications are lacking, but phenytoin has been associated with some type of skin eruption in 5% to 10% of patients (4).

ETIOLOGY AND PATHOGENESIS

Sarcoidosis has an idiopathic etiology and is best considered an autoimmune disease. Evidence points to an environmental trigger in the setting of a genetic susceptibility to disease development, but no one trigger has been yet identified. The basic element of disease is the formation of noncaseating, epithelioid, granulomatous infiltrates in target tissues, which can then interfere with target tissue structure and function.

The etiologic agent in syphilis is the spirochete, *Treponema pallidum*, a bacterial agent essentially unknown in Europe until the discovery of the New World. It can spread by sexual contact, prenatal transmission, and accidental direct inoculation. Disease is caused by both the inflammatory reaction to the bacteria and bacterial infiltration of target tissues. Intrauterine infection is particularly important for its association with TORCH syndrome (toxoplasmosis; other infections—namely hepatitis B, syphilis, and herpes zoster; rubella; cytomegalovirus; and herpes simplex virus), and numerous congenital sequelae.

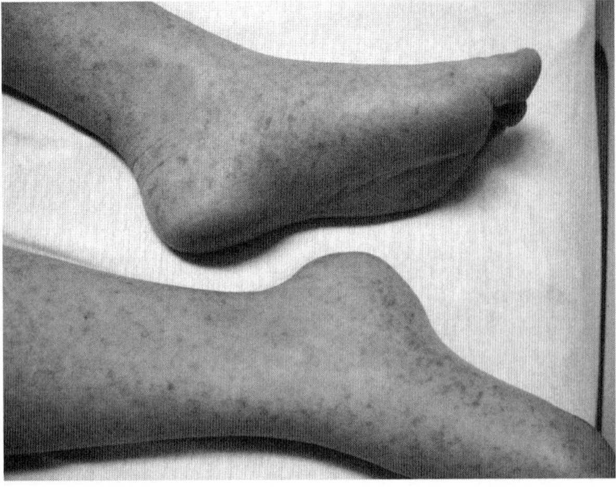

FIGURE 124-2. Petechial rash on feet and ankles.

HSV, a double-stranded DNA (ds-DNA) virus, is spread via skin or mucosal contact with infected integument that is actively shedding virus. The most virulent eruption occurs in primary infection and is the result of intracellular replication of virus particles. Once neutralizing antibodies are formed, however, the virus may remain latent in nerves for years until such time as host immunity sufficiently declines to allow reactivation. During primary or reactivation infection, it can readily infect the newborn as it passes through the birth canal, leading to neural tissue infection in a relatively immunoincompetent host, and resulting in a life-threatening viral encephalitis.

Fever, headache, and a vasculitis are characteristics of RMSF infection caused by the rickettsial spirochete, *Rickettsia rickettsii*. The disease is spread through the tick vectors *Dermacentor variabilis* (American dog tick, *Dermacentor andersoni*), Rocky Mountain wood tick, or *Rhipicephalus sanguineus* (common brown dog tick). When the tick bites and feeds for several hours, it may regurgitate, infecting the host in the process. Infection is unlikely if the tick has been present for <6 hours. After inoculation, bacteria locate to vascular endothelium where they replicate intracellularly for approximately a week before symptoms occur. Symptoms are the result of subsequent vascular damage affecting multiple organs, most notably skin, CNS, and liver.

Lyme disease is caused by infection with the spirochete, *Borrelia burgdorferi*, and the body's immune response to the infection. The field mouse appears to be the reservoir for the spirochete, but disease transmission to humans is through the *Ixodes* tick, or deer tick, which has fed on the mouse in the nymph or adult stages of its life cycle. A tick must then attach to a person to feed for at least 24 hours to effectively pass on the infection. The inflammatory response to *B. burgdorferi* is probably the cause of erythema chronicum migrans, pseudolymphoma, and meningoencephalitis; however, systemic inflammatory cytokine release likely contributes to Lyme arthritis.

Anticonvulsant drug hypersensitivity syndrome occurs in the setting of aromatic ring-containing antiepileptic medication administration. It is postulated that the syndrome results from production of toxic drug metabolites that accumulate because of deficient epoxide hydrolase activity needed for complete degradation of this drug class. Variability in epoxide hydrolase activity is thought to result from genetic polymorphisms found in the population. The formed metabolites then lead to an immune reaction resulting in fever, hepatitis, and eosinophilia characteristic of this disease.

PATHOLOGY

Microscopic examination of sarcoidal nodules most characteristically reveals what is termed a "naked" granuloma caused by granulomatous foci of multinucleated giant cells and histiocytes that have relatively few infiltrating lymphocytes at the periphery. Lymphocyte-rich and interstitial-patterned granulomatous variants exist, however. These must be histologically distinguished from other granulomatous diseases, such as tuberculosis, leprosy, and Crohn disease. Laboratory abnormalities can include serum calcium and angiotensin-converting enzyme (ACE) levels that can be elevated in up to 15% and 60% of cases, respectively. Elevated ACE levels are not typically useful for diagnosis; however, an elevated ACE level can be followed for disease activity and is typically associated with lung involvement. In addition, hilar lymphadenopathy or lung disease is present in up to 90% of cases and can be diagnosed via chest X-ray studies and pulmonary function tests.

Syphilis can be diagnosed through tissue biopsy, which reveals spirochetes and a mixed-cell inflammatory response in primary and tertiary lesions, but will have relatively few (if any) identifiable organisms in secondary disease. Secondary lesions will have a nonspecific mixed inflammatory response, but may have a more characteristic plasma cell component to the infiltrate.

HSV lesions show typical keratinocyte necrosis, cytoplasmic ballooning, nuclei with steel gray coloration, nucleoplasm margination, and multinucleate formation on hematoxylin and eosin stain. Tzank smears can also be done that show the typical multinucleate giant cells of herpes virus that can be seen in HSV, Varicella-zoster virus (VZV), and cytomegalovirus (CMV) infections.

RMSF histology is typically of a nonspecific lymphocytic small vessel vasculitis variety. Special stains using Warthin-Starry method poorly reveal organisms, but antibodies against the spirochete for confirmatory diagnosis are available at specialized and research institutions.

In Lyme disease, erythema chronicum migrans biopsy likewise will show an unspecific superficial and deep perivascular and interstitial lymphocytic infiltrate with plasma cells and possibly eosinophils. Warthin-Starry staining may be positive in up to 50% of specimens.

Skin biopsy in ADHS typically reveals a superficial perivascular lymphocytic infiltrate that may or may not contain eosinophils. It is not specific, however, unless correlated with the clinical presentation of a morbilliform eruption. Liver biopsy likewise will reveal a perivascular and interstitial liver parenchyma lymphocytic infiltrate indistinguishable from autoimmune hepatitis unless a significant eosinophilic component is present.

CLINICAL MANIFESTATIONS

As mentioned, sarcoidosis has a protean presentation owing to the many organ systems it can affect. Because it most often affects lung and skin, the most typical presentation consists of waxy erythematous to skin-colored papules and nodules on the head (oronasopharyngeal passageways), neck, and upper extremities. A history of dry cough and worsening shortness of breath will accompany significant lung parenchymal infiltration or pulmonary fibrosis.

Neurologic symptoms are highly variable and essentially any level of the nervous system can be affected. Examples would include cranial neuropathies, aseptic meningitis, endocrine abnormalities (e.g., pituitary insufficiency and diabetes insipidus), seizures, strokes, neuropathy, and myopathy. Special, well-described sarcoidal presentations also exist. *Lupus pernio* consists of violaceous nodular lesions on the face or extremities, especially on the nose. *Löfgren syndrome* is characterized by erythema nodosum, bilateral hilar adenopathy, and arthritis. The constellation of arthritis, uveitis, and parotiditis with facial nerve involvement is known as *Heerfordt-Waldenstrom syndrome.*

Untreated, syphilis classically evolves through three stages: primary, secondary, and tertiary; additionally, it can have a latency phase. Also, not all cases will progress through each stage, and the stages can overlap. Primary syphilis is characterized by the formation of a relatively painless chancre at the site of inoculation approximately 3 weeks after initial contact. Regional, firm, painless adenopathy can accompany the chancre. The ulcer will spontaneously heal over 4 to 6 weeks, with scarring. Secondary syphilis follows the primary phase within 1 to 3 months and can last up to a year or more. It presents with flulike illness, lymphadenopathy, and a myriad of cutaneous eruptions. The cutaneous lesions can include a papulosquamous eruption of pityriasis rosealike or psoriasislike plaques, "moth-eaten" alopecia, generalized maculopapular eruptions, including ham-colored "copper pennies" of the palms and soles and "nickels and dimes" of other glabrous skin (Fig. 124-3), split-papules of the oral commissures and ears, mucous patches of oral mucosa, and verrucous appearing *condyloma lata* of the intertriginous zones. In addition, patients may manifest iritis, optic neuritis, neural deafness, meningitis, inflammation of the periosteum, nephrotic syndrome, nephritis, and hepatitis. Latency is marked by the lack of signs or symptoms of active disease. During early latent syphilis, up to 2 years from the time of infection, the patient remains infectious. Late latent syphilis is defined as existing 2 years or longer from the time of infection, and the inability to infect others. Untreated, one third of cases will develop into tertiary syphilis after a latency of 3 to 25 years. Tertiary syphilis has cardiovascular, cutaneous, and neurologic presentations. Panarteritis of the ascending aorta can result in aortic aneurism, valve insufficiency, and coronary artery stenosis. At this stage, annular plaques and erythematous nodules on the trunk, face, mucosa, scalp, and arms are known as *cutaneous gummas.* Neurosyphilis can be categorized as asymptomatic neurosyphilis, symptomatic meningitis, meningovasculitis, parenchymatous (e.g., tabes dorsalis), and gummatous neurosyphilis. Early congenital syphilis is manifest by an acral vesiculobullous eruption in the newborn, flulike symptoms, lymphadenopathy, hepatosplenomegaly, papulosquamous or maculopapular skin eruption, and neurosyphilis. Late congenital syphilis (after 2 years of age) is characterized by

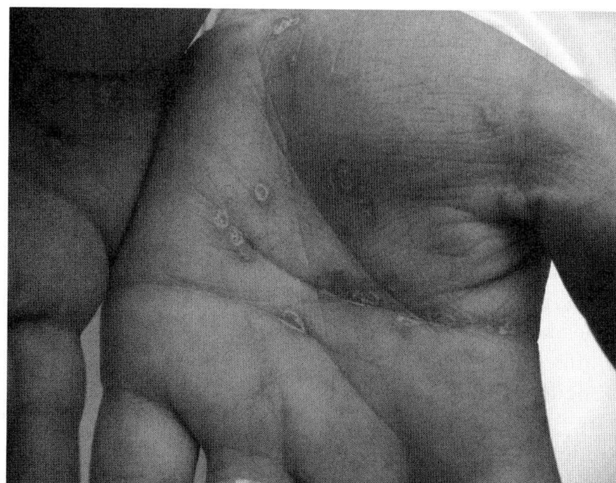

FIGURE 124-3. "Copper pennies" of secondary syphilis. (Courtesy of Mindi Morris, MD.)

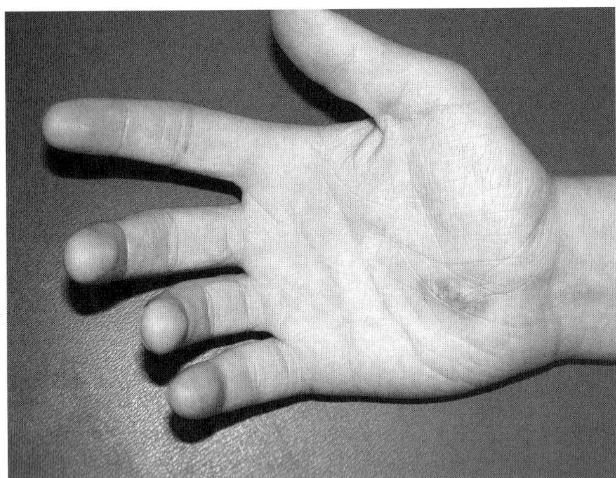

FIGURE 124-4. Primary herpes simplex virus (HSV) eruption. (Courtesy of Matthew C. Reeck, MD.)

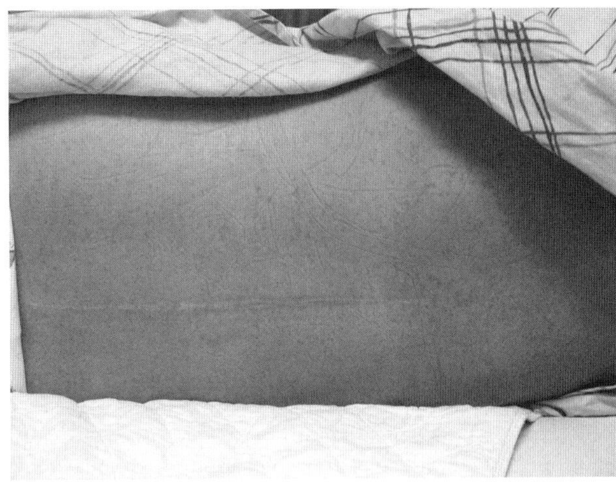

FIGURE 124-5. Morbilliform eruption of drug hypersensitivity syndrome caused by carbamazepine.

neurosyphilis, gummas, keratitis, iridocyclitis, deafness, frontal bossing, saddle-nose deformity, high arched palate, mulberry molars, peg-shaped incisors with notched enamel (*Hutchinson's teeth*), sternoclavicular thickening, saber shins, rhagades, and pseudoparalysis caused by osteochondritis. *Hutchinson's triad* consists of interstitial keratitis, peg-shaped upper incisors, and cochlear nerve deafness (5).

Primary HSV presents with fever, malaise, and a painful, crusted or hemorrhagic vesicular eruption that can take 2 to 3 weeks to resolve (Fig. 124-4). This can be significantly prolonged in the immunocompromised host. Newborns, because of their relative immunocompromised state, may have involvement of the CNS, leading to long-term neurologic damage, including mental retardation, paralysis, blindness, and even death. The vesicular eruptions of secondary HSV have an onset typically preceded by low-grade fever and parasthesias at the site of outbreak within several hours before the first identifiable signs of clinical disease occur. The reactivation disease course generally only lasts 5 to 7 days, however. Both HSV-1 and HSV-2 viruses can cause meningitis and HSV-1 is the most common viral cause of acute sporadic encephalitis. It is not common, however, for patients with HSV-related meningitis or encephalitis to manifest a dermatologic abnormality.

Clinical manifestations of RMSF usually include fever, headache, malaise, myalgias, vomiting, decreased mental status, and a cutaneous vasculitis that starts on the hands and feet, with centripetal spread to the head and trunk.

Lyme disease will present as a centrifugal spread of erythema and pruritus (*erythema migrans*) from the site of initial inoculation, the tick bite. Subsequent development of arthritis may follow within a month of inoculation. Other associated clinical findings include a nodule of reactive lymphoid tissue within the skin termed *pseudolymphoma* or *lymphocytoma cutis.* Lyme disease can affect both the peripheral nervous system and CNS. Cranial neuropathies, especially facial nerve palsies, commonly occur. A painful radiculoneuritis, brachial and lumbar plexopathies, mononeuropathies, and polyneuropathies have also been described (6). The most common CNS manifestation is lymphocytic meningitis. A multifocal encephalomyelitis can also occur.

Patients with ADHS generally start with a morbilliform eruption accompanied by low-grade fever (Figs. 124-5 and 124-6). As the disease progresses, high-grade fever, pruritus, signs of hepatitis, arthritis, myocarditis, glomerulonephritis, and obtundation may ensue. No skin or mucosal sloughing occurs. Onset will generally be within 10 to 21 days of anticonvulsant initiation. If the rash occurs outside of this time frame, ADHS becomes less likely and the differential diagnosis becomes much broader, including viral exanthems, other forms of drug reaction, rheumatic disease, bacterial infection, and so forth.

DIAGNOSTIC APPROACH

With only skin manifestations and no significant positive findings on review of systems, consideration only for obtaining a chest X-ray study and pulmonary function tests would be expected in sarcoidosis. Skin biopsy should be performed, however, to verify the diagnosis and rule out other granulomatous

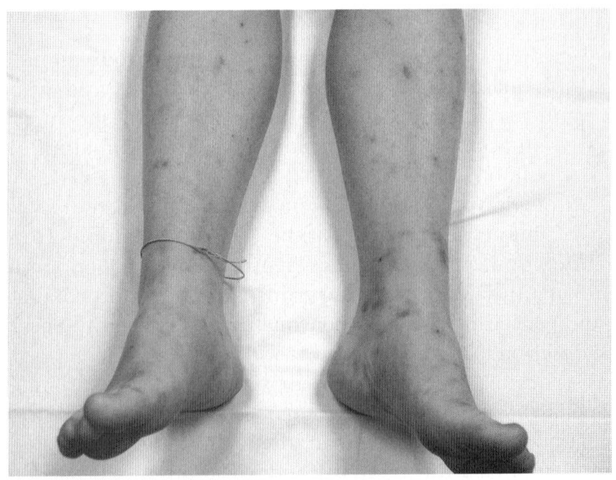

FIGURE 124-6. Morbilliform drug eruption to carbamazepine.

entities such as tuberculosis (TB), leprosy, or other atypical mycobacteria and deep fungal infections. With focal neurologic deficits of otherwise unidentifiable cause, consideration for neurosarcoidosis should be given and imaging studies may be helpful. An elevated serum ACE level can be seen in those with systemic disease. Tissue sampling, however, is the gold standard for diagnosis.

Syphilis is best diagnosed with appropriate history-taking and measurement of rapid plasma regain (RPR) or VDRL test followed by the confirmatory fluorescent treponemal antibody (FTA) assay if either preliminary test is positive. With treatment, the RPR should be expected to decrease by half every couple of weeks. Be aware that, once positive, FTA will always remain positive. Cerebrospinal fluid (CSF) analysis should be done in anyone suspected of having neurosyphilis. The most common abnormality would be a mononuclear pleocytosis with a mildly elevated protein content. The CSF VDRL test is a very specific, but not very sensitive, test for neurosyphilis. On the other hand, the CSF FTA is a fairly sensitive test, but not very specific test for neurosyphilis.

Diagnosis of HSV is usually based on clinical history, but can be confirmed with tissue biopsy, viral culture, or direct immunofluorescence of an active lesion, if necessary. Measurement of HSV-1 and HSV-2 IgM or IgG antibodies is rarely (if ever) clinically indicated, unless done in the newborn period as confirmation of exposure.

Clinical suspicion and history are most important for making the diagnosis of RMSF. Additionally, response to tetracycline antibiotic therapy is helpful in establishing the diagnosis. Skin biopsy may be helpful to show the typical leukocytoclastic vasculitis that accompanies this disease. Antibodies to the spirochete may not be clinically useful in the first few days because they generally take too long to be reported before the need for medical intervention, especially in severe cases. They can be used, however, as a confirmatory test after initiation of appropriate antibiotic therapy is already underway or completed. CSF analysis in patients with RMSF usually shows a lymphocytic or polymorphonuclear pleocytosis, an increased protein concentration, and a normal glucose concentration.

Likewise, Lyme titers are not always useful because findings may be falsely negative in up to 50% of cases. This is a disease diagnosed on clinical grounds and good history-taking. A typical rash with headache or arthritis is diagnostic.

Suspicion of ADHS should be followed by discontinuation of the offending agent. Once again, clinical history, appropriate timing of rash eruption, and physical examination are most useful in establishing the diagnosis. Recommended additional tests include skin biopsy to rule out other causes, serial liver function tests to follow trends in hepatocellular damage, urinalysis for eosinophiluria and proteinuria or hematuria, and complete blood count (CBC) with differential to follow eosinophilia. It is important to watch for signs of associated myocarditis or nephritis.

TREATMENT

Sarcoidosis can be treated with oral hydroxychloroquine if isolated to skin; however, involvement of pulmonary, neurologic, or other vital systems requires systemic therapy with glucocorticoids. Once in remission, systemic steroids can be tapered very slowly. Other immunosuppressants, such as methotrexate, azathioprine, or cyclophosphamide, have been tried to spare patients some of the side effects of systemic corticosteroids or for those with refractory disease.

The favored treatment of all forms of syphilis is benzathine penicillin, tailored in dose and duration to the stage of syphilis being treated. Alternative therapeutic choices include doxycycline and tetracycline; however, it is recommended that patients allergic to penicillin instead be desensitized to allow safe treatment with penicillin when at all possible. Neurosyphilis should be treated with aqueous penicillin intravenously for 10 to 14 days or procaine penicillin intramuscularly once daily plus probenecid for 10 to 14 days.

Standard therapy for HSV is acyclovir, in either oral form or for neonatal and complicated cases, the intravenous formulation. Caution for renal tubular precipitation must be taken when using the intravenous form. Oral valacyclovir and famciclovir are alternative choices for uncomplicated cases, but patients with human immunodeficiency virus (HIV) should avoid high-dose valacyclovir because of reports of drug-associated thrombotic thrombocytopenic purpura and hemolytic uremic syndrome occurring in this population. Patients with strains of herpes virus resistant to this thymidine kinase class of antivirals may respond to foscarnet.

The treatment of choice for RMSF remains doxycycline for at least 2 days after the patient is no longer febrile. For pregnant patients, children <8 years of age, or those who are tetracycline allergic, chloramphenicol is the alternative choice.

Early Lyme disease is ideally treated with doxycycline for up to 21 days. Alternative antibiotics include amoxicillin.

In ADHS, the cornerstone of therapy is discontinuation of the offending agent. Otherwise, supportive care is indicated. For complicated cases involving significant hepatocellular damage, high fever, and myocarditis or nephritis, prednisone (starting at 1 mg/kg, tapered off slowly, over approximately 6 weeks) is needed to suppress the hypersensitivity reaction and avoid a rebound phenomenon associated with premature withdrawal of immunosuppressive therapy.

CLINICAL RECOMMENDATIONS OF THE VIGNETTE

The patient presented with recent onset of headache, decreased mental status, a petechial rash, and fevers. History revealed that she was a student in a veterinarian school. Suspicion for RMSF should be high in this setting, even without incontrovertible knowledge of a tick bite. Although punch biopsy and serology for rickettsial antibodies can be obtained, early institution of doxycycline therapy for the presumptive diagnosis is imperative to avoid long-term neurologic sequelae. Additionally, a head computed tomographic (CT) scan and lumbar puncture should be part of the workup to rule out viral, autoimmune, or other causes.

SUMMARY

We have discussed diseases that have both dermatologic and neurologic manifestations. Sarcoidosis, syphilis, and Lyme disease can present with a variety of signs and symptoms and often recognizing the dermatologic signs is the first step in obtaining a correct diagnosis and initiating appropriate treatment. The identification of the rash associated with RMSF would allow for the prompt treatment of an infection that could lead to significant morbidity and mortality if not recognized. Evaluating a patient with a rash who is taking an anticonvulsant is a common clinical problem. Recognizing when a patient does or does not have ADHS is important in limiting morbidity or perhaps directing attention to other medications that can also cause a rash. Our goal was to provide both important clinical information and awareness of the classic skin manifestations of these disorders.

REFERENCES

1. Xu F, Schillinger JA, Sternberg MR, et al. Seroprevalence and coinfection with herpes simplex virus type 1 and type 2 in the United States, 1988–1994. *J Infect Dis.* 2002;185(8):1019–1024.
2. Treadwell TA, Holman RC, Clarke MJ, et al. Rocky Mountain spotted fever in the United States, 1993–1996. *Am J Trop Med Hyg.* 2000;63(1–2):21–26.
3. Orloski KA, Hayes EB, Campbell GL, et al. Surveillance for Lyme disease—United States, 1992–1998. *MMWR Surveill Summ.* 2000;49(3):1–11.
4. Silverman AK, Fairley J, Wong RC. Cutaneous and immunologic reactions to phenytoin [Review]. *J Am Acad Dermatol.* 1988;18(4 Pt 1):721–741.
5. Goens JL, Janniger CK, De WK. Dermatologic and systemic manifestations of syphilis [Review]. *Am Fam Physician.* 1994;50(5):1013–1020.
6. Halperin JJ. Lyme disease. In: Roos KL, ed. *Principles of Neurologic Infectious Diseases.* New York: McGraw-Hill; 2005:233–240.

CHAPTER 125

Commonly Used Dermatological Drugs

Terrence M. Brogan • Beth L. Brogan

OBJECTIVES

- To provide an overview of commonly prescribed dermatologic medications
- To highlight specific neurologic side effects of drugs used in dermatology
- To provide a brief overview of drug mechanisms as they pertain to pathophysiology of dermatologic disease
- To discuss additional more common side effects of these medications

CASE VIGNETTE

A 17-year-old obese young man with cystic scarring acne presents to the emergency department with new onset headache. He has no history of headache and is otherwise healthy. In the past his acne was resistant to treatment with topical retinoids and oral minocycline. One month earlier his dermatologist initiated isotretinoin (40 mg daily) for his acne. He describes a generalized headache without aura, but associated with pulsatile tinnitus. Pain is exacerbated by movement, and he had a transient visual loss. On examination, he had inflamed cysts, scarring, and open comedones over both cheeks. On neurologic examination, funduscopy showed blurred optic disc margins bilaterally. Visual fields to confrontation findings were normal. Visual acuity was 20/20 OU. Pupils were 3 mm in diameter and reactive to light and near. No relative afferent papillary defect was noted. Color vision was unremarkable. Extraocular movements were full. No nystagmus was found and the remainder of the neurologic examination was normal.

DEFINITION

Dermatology, as with all fields of medicine, uses a wide range of medications to treat its various disorders. One of its distinguishing features is that a number of treatments are topically applied. Because of the low systemic absorption of topically applied medications, most of them have a low frequency of systemic or neurologic side effects. A number of oral medications used in dermatology, however, can be associated with neurologic side effects. In addition, in rare instances, topically applied medications to a large surface area can promote absorption and systemic side effects. Because a number of drugs commonly used in dermatology are also used in other fields of medicine, special attention is paid here to those medications unique to dermatology and those with unique neurologic side effects.

EPIDEMIOLOGY

Acne vulgaris ranges from minor, cosmetically bothersome breakouts to severe, painful, scarring cysts as seen in the patient in the case vignette above. Acne is perhaps the most common dermatologic disease, affecting at least 50% of adolescents and more than 10% of adult women (1,2) and leading to countless dermatologic prescriptions for topical and oral medications. Another disease commonly encountered by dermatologists is psoriasis, which is estimated to affect 2% of the US population. Although most dermatologists are also trained as surgeons, most routinely prescribe medications to nearly every medical patient examined.

ETIOLOGY AND PATHOGENESIS

Etiology and pathogenesis for skin diseases is diverse. Autoimmunity, type I and type IV hypersensitivity, and lymphocytic dysregulation account for a number of dermatologic conditions, such as lupus, alopecia areata, urticaria, eczema, drug hypersensitivity, and psoriasis. Dermatologists also encounter infectious diseases, including bacterial, fungal, and viral. Neoplasia is commonly treated in dermatology. Pharmaceuticals are used in all of these areas of dermatology.

PATHOLOGY

The dermatopathology for the dermatologic conditions treated with pharmaceuticals is complex and assorted. The skin biopsy is a useful tool to dermatologists and is frequently used to guide treatment plans.

CLINICAL MANIFESTATIONS

Dermatology is unique among medical specialties because of the visual nature of the examination. The dermatologic patient varies widely from the teenager with cystic acne, such as the patient in the vignette, to the middle-aged woman with thick psoriatic plaques, the infant with a crusted eczematous eruption, or the elderly farmer with an eroded tumor on the scalp. The unifying feature of the dermatologic patient is the presence of visible skin disease. The examination, therefore, is paramount in determining medical, pharmaceutical, and surgical intervention.

DIAGNOSTIC APPROACH

All areas of medicine, history, and particularly, the physical examination, are essential in diagnosing skin disease. Clinical appearance is perhaps the most important aspect of diagnosis, but clinical and pathologic correlation is also significant. Unlike other fields of medicine, in dermatology the skin is readily accessible for biopsy, a helpful diagnostic tool.

TREATMENT

Treatment plans and the choice of drugs in dermatology vary between diseases and between practitioners. Many treatment options are based on evidence-based medicine; however, off-label use of medications in dermatology is common (3). The remainder of the chapter provides an overview of these medications.

RETINOIDS

The retinoids are vitamin A derivatives that can be used topically or systemically. The most commonly used systemic retinoid is isotretinoin, which is an extremely effective medication for severe acne vulgaris. Acitretin, another systemic retinoid, is most commonly used for psoriasis, but can also be used off label for other dermatologic conditions, such as cutaneous lupus erythematosus, lichen planus, and in skin cancer prevention. Bexarotene, a third generation retinoid available topically or orally, is used exclusively to treat cutaneous T-cell lymphoma.

Isotretinoin is strictly regulated by the US Food and Drug Administration (FDA) and can be prescribed only by physicians, mostly dermatologists, who are registered in the iPLEDGE program. The regulations are the result of isotretinoin's severe teratogenicity, seen in 30% of pregnancies that occur while a patient is on isotretinoin. Fetal defects include central nervous system (CNS) defects, and craniofacial and cardiac abnormalities. Patients taking isotretinoin are also registered and female patients are required to use two forms of birth control. Monthly pregnancy tests are mandatory throughout the treatment course, which generally lasts 5 to 8 months, depending on the patient's weight and the dosage. Because of the long half-life of acitretin and its possible accumulation in fat stores, it is generally not prescribed to women of future child bearing potential.

The patient in the vignette exhibits the classic findings of *idiopathic intracranial hypertension*, or *pseudotumor cerebri*, an uncommon side effect of systemic retinoids (4,5). The symptoms include headache, transient visual obscurations, and papilledema. The risk is greatly increased by the concomitant use of tetracyclines, and their combination with retinoids is contraindicated. The pathogenesis of pseudotumor is controversial, but obesity and female sex are risk factors. Symptoms resolve slowly on discontinuation of the medication.

Other more common side effects of retinoids are myalgias, reported in approximately 15% of patients, and dry skin, lips, and eyes, which are experienced by most patients. A more controversial side effect of oral retinoids is depression and suicidal ideation. Isotretinoin has ranked in the top ten of the FDA's adverse events reporting system for reports of depression and suicide (6). Causality has not been established, however, and prospective cohort studies have shown no increase in depression or suicide with isotretinoin use (7). Despite a lack of strong clinical evidence, monthly screening for depression is recommended in patients receiving isotretinoin. Finally, a well-known side effect of the retinoids is the elevation of triglycerides and cholesterol, with a conversion of high-density lipoprotein (HDL) to low-density lipoprotein (LDL). Of patients on isotretinoin, 20% to 30% will have an increase in their HDL-to-LDL ratio or triglyceridemia, and the abnormalities are more exaggerated with bexarotene. Although the elevated ratio can be a significant vascular risk factor in older patients with long-term use of acitretin or bexarotene, it is unlikely to cause stroke in young people with short-term use of isotretinoin. Nonetheless, monthly or bimonthly screening lipid panels are recommended with any retinoid use.

Retinoids are commonly prescribed topically. Tretinoin and adapalene are commonly used for acne, whereas tazarotene is also approved for psoriasis. In addition, topical retinoids improve the appearance of photoaging and can reduce precancerous skin changes. The topical applications can cause local dryness and irritation, but systemic absorption is minimal with normal use. Topical tazarotene is pregnancy category X, given its use over larger body surface areas.

ANTIBIOTICS

Tetracyclines

The tetracyclines are broad-spectrum antibiotics, such as tetracycline, minocycline, and doxycycline, which inhibit bacterial protein synthesis, but also exhibit anti-inflammatory properties even at subantimicrobial doses. Dermatologists most commonly use the tetracyclines to treat acne vulgaris and acne rosacea, but they also have a role as a steroid-sparing medication in inflammatory conditions, such as bullous pemphigoid, and other autoimmune disorders, such as lupus erythematosus. Recently, they have become an important antimicrobial to treat skin infections caused by community-acquired methacillin-resistant *Staphylococcus aureus*, which is often sensitive to tetracycline (8). Treatment regimens range from 100 mg twice daily for severe acne or skin infection to 30 mg daily or every other day. Minocycline is generally considered to be the superior medication in the group, but with the greatest potential for side effects.

The most frequent neurologic side effect of the tetracyclines is vertigo, reportedly affecting up to 10% of recipients. The effect is most pronounced with minocycline, which can cause neurologic symptoms of lightheadedness, unsteadiness, or vertigo in up to 75% of patients with short-term use and 3.4% with long-term use. A more severe association with tetracyclines has been with the condition of pseudotumor cerebri. Several case reports and series are found regarding the association between the drug and the disorder. Most patients develop symptoms within the first 4 weeks of therapy, but some had been on therapy for months. On discontinuing the tetracycline, the symptoms resolved within a few weeks to a month, but a few patients have had permanent vision loss (9).

Commonly, nonneurologic side effects include gastrointestinal intolerance, particularly with tetracycline which is taken without a meal, and photosensitivity, which occurs with all tetracyclines. A unique long-term side effect of minocycline is blue-black pigment deposition in the skin in either a diffuse or localized pattern.

Dapsone

Dapsone is the treatment of choice for the dermopathy associated with gluten-sensitive enteropathy, or dermatitis herpetiformis. Dermatitis herpetiformis is characterized by intensely pruritic vesicles located on extensor surfaces of the extremities in patients with gluten sensitivity. Treatment can include the avoidance of gluten, but the diet is strict and difficult to follow. Dapsone is extremely effective in treating the eruption and the pruritus and few alternative medical treatments exist. Dapsone is also used in dermatology to treat many disorders mediated by neutrophils, such as Sweet syndrome, cutaneous lupus erythematosus, and bullous diseases (e.g., bullous pemphigoid). As an antimicrobial, it is the drug of choice for Hansen disease. The dose of dapsone ranges from 25 mg daily to 100 mg twice daily.

A neurologic complication of dapsone is the development of a motor neuropathy. The clinical scenario is the progressive development of distal weakness, particularly after high-dose, short-term or low-dose, long-term use of the drug. The neuropathy is axonal and caused by injury to the soma and axons of the motor neurons. Electromyographic (EMG) findings show axonal degeneration. Prognosis for recovery after stopping dapsone is good, but can be slow, taking months to years. Because of the extreme nature of the pruritus associated with dermatitis herpetiformis, it is often difficult to convince patients to stop dapsone despite the neuropathy.

Another side effect of dapsone is a dose-dependant hemolytic anemia and the development of methemoglobinema. These effects are severe in patients with G6PD deficiency, and complete blood counts are carefully monitored in all patients receiving dapsone. Idiopathic agranulocytosis and liver damage are uncommon side effects.

Topical Antibiotics

Topical antibiotics, such as clindamycin, sodium sulfacetamide, and metronidazole, are frequently used to treat acne vulgaris and acne rosacea. In acne vulgaris, they are generally used in conjunction with topical retinoids. They are well tolerated with few side effects.

ANTIFUNGALS

Griseofulvin

Griseofulvin is approved to treat tinea infections of the hair, skin, and nails and is most commonly administered to children with tinea capitis. Treatment is generally prescribed at doses of 20 mg/kg for 6 to 8 weeks, and has a low risk of hepatocellular damage and neurologic side effects when used for this length of time. It is rarely used for nail infection because more effective treatments are available.

Terbinafine

Terbinafine is an allylamine antifungal medication that is used topically and systemically in dermatology to treat dermatophyte infections of the skin and nails. A common treatment regimen is 250 mg daily for 6 weeks for fingernails and 12 weeks for toenail disease. Topical terbinafine is available over the counter and has few side effects. A common neurologic side effect of oral terbinafine is headache. Hepatic dysfunction is rare, but screening laboratory results are generally obtained during therapy. Another rare, but significant, side effect is drug-induced lupus, particularly of the subacute cutaneous subtype.

Imidazoles

The imidazole antifungals are widely used in dermatology in treating cutaneous and deep fungal infections. The mechanism of action is by inhibiting P450 enzyme lanosterol 14-alpha demethylase. This eliminates the conversion of lanosterol to ergosterole, the primary sterol in fungal cell membranes. The imidazoles are well known to inhibit the hepatic enzyme P450 and, therefore, a number of drug interactions are possible (10).

Itraconazole is commonly used in onychomycosis and deep fungal infections. It is better absorbed with a full meal and has extensive distribution within fat tissues. It is metabolized through the liver and can cause hepatic damage, so routine screening laboratory studies are indicated with prolonged use. CNS side effects include frequent headache and, less commonly, dizziness, tremor, and vertigo. Fluconazole can also be used for deep or systemic infections, but in dermatology is most commonly used for mucocutaneous yeast infections. A one-time dose of 150 mg is indicated for vulvovaginal candidiasis and can also be used for tinea versicolor. Fluconazole is significant for less protein binding and, predominately, renal secretion than other imidazoles.

Topical Antifungals

Topical terbinafine and topical imidazoles, such as clotrimazole, miconazole, and ketoconazole, are commonly used to treat superficial tinea infections (e.g., tinea pedis) or superficial candidal infections. Many of these agents are available over the counter and are considered safe and effective. Ketoconazole is available as a shampoo and is commonly used in seborrheic dermatitis. Nystatin is a unique antifungal that is used to treat cutaneous and mucocutaneous candidal infections. It is available as a cream, powder, mouthwash, or oral pastille; even when taken by mouth, it has no systemic absorption.

ANTIHISTAMINES

Sedating

Antihistamines are widely used in dermatology to treat urticaria and pruritus, or itching. First-generation antihistamines have CNS effects because of their lipophilic state and their ability to cross the blood–brain barrier. They almost uniformly cause sedation, but occasionally lead to excitability or impairment of cognitive function. Many dermatologists consider sedation beneficial in patients who have difficulty sleeping or relaxing because of pruritus. The most commonly used sedating antihistamines are hydroxyzine and doxepin. Doxepin is also used as a tricyclic antidepressant, usually prescribed at higher doses. Doxepin is also available in a topical formulation that generally has few side effects, but through systemic absorption can cause sedation or even an anticholinergic syndrome as reported in one elderly individual (11).

The second-generation antihistamines are not lipophilic and, therefore, have much less CNS toxicity, sedation, and neuropsychiatric side effects. Their primary use in dermatology is to treat urticaria, often in combination with sedating antihistamines, and H2 receptor blockers. The most commonly used nonsedating antihistamines are loratidine, which is available over the counter, fexofenadine, and cetirizine, which is the most sedating of these agents.

IMMUNOSUPPRESSANT MEDICATIONS

Corticosteroids

Corticosteroids are perhaps the most common topical medication used in dermatology. Topical corticosteroids are indicated in the treatment of a vast number of skin disorders not limited to psoriasis, eczema, and dermatitis. A classification system provides a guide to potency and ranks topical steroids by their ability to constrict cutaneous vasculature (Table 125-1). Potency depends both on the type of corticosteroid and on its formulation. Ointments, which are composed of primarily greases (e.g., petroleum jelly), are the most occlusive and tend to be more potent. Creams and lotions, which contain an emulsion that includes water, are likely to be less potent. Topical corticosteroids are common in a variety of formulations, including ointment, cream, lotion, oil, gel, foam, solution, and impregnated tape.

Class I, or superpotent, topical corticosteroids are the most potent, but also have the highest potential for side effects. A serious local side effect is irreversible thinning of the skin, including translucency, atrophy, and stretch marks. Because these side effects are more common with higher potency steroids, their use is primarily limited to the trunk, scalp, and extremities for a finite treatment period, such as 3 weeks. Midpotency topical corticosteroids can be used over larger body surface areas, and lower potency steroids are used in areas of delicate skin, such as intertriginous areas, groin, and face. Other local side effects of topical corticosteroids include acne, rosacea, and contact allergy. Topical steroids used in areas of infection (e.g., tinea or scabies) will exacerbate these infections; for this reason, most dermatologists avoid the use of combination products containing corticosteroids and antifungal agents. With prolonged use over large body surface areas, particularly with higher potency steroids, systemic side effects are also possible. Children have a higher body surface-to-weight ratio as well as thinner, more penetrable skin, all of which make pituitary axis suppression a concern in their treatment.

TABLE 125-1. Potency Ranking of Frequently Prescribed Topical Corticosteroids

CLASS I (SUPERPOTENT)	Betamethasone dipropionate ointment 0.05% Clobetasol propionate cream, ointment 0.05% Halobetasol propionate cream, ointment 0.05%
CLASS II (POTENT)	Amcinonide ointment 0.1% Betamethasone dipropionate cream 0.05% Desoximetasone cream, gel, ointment 0.25% Fluocinonide cream, gel, ointment, solution 0.05% Halcinonide cream 0.1% Mometasone furoate ointment 0.1%
CLASS III (POTENT)	Amcinonide cream, lotion 0.1% Betamethasone valerate ointment 0.01% Fluticasone propionate ointment 0.005% Halcinonide ointment, solution 0.1%
CLASS IV (MIDSTRENGTH)	Betamethasone valerate lotion 0.01% Fluocinolone acetonide ointment 0.25% Flurandrenolide ointment 0.05% Mometasone furoate cream, lotion 0.1% Triamcinolone acetonide ointment 0.1%
CLASS V (MIDSTRENGTH)	Bethamethasone dipropionate lotion 0.05% Betamethasone valerate cream 0.01% Flucinolone acetonide cream 0.025% Hydrocortisone butyrate cream, ointment, solution 0.1% Hydrocortisone valerate cream, ointment 0.2% Triamcinolone acetonide lotion 0.1%
CLASS VI (MILD)	Alcometasone dipropionate cream, ointment 0.05% Betamethasone valerate lotion 0.01% Desonide cream 0.05% Flucinolone acetonide cream, solution 0.01% Prednicarbate 0.1%
CLASS VII (LEAST POTENT)	Dexamethasone cream 0.1% Hydrocortisone 0.05%, 1% (OTC), 2.5%

Dermatologists commonly use systemic glucocorticoids as well. Prednisone is often prescribed in short-term courses at a dose of 1 mg/kg of body weight, tapering over 3 weeks to treat acute dermatitis. Long-term regimens with much slower tapers are used to treat bullous dermatoses (e.g., pemphigus vulgaris or connective tissue disorders (e.g., dermatomyositis).

The complete side effect profile of oral glucocorticoids is beyond the scope of this chapter. Of note, steroid use can also be associated with pseudotumor cerebri, especially during a withdrawal of the dosage, and the diagnosis should be considered when patients present with the symptom complex of headache, nausea, and impaired vision. Behavioral changes, even as considerable as psychosis, can occur with high doses, and sleep disturbance is common. Depression can be a side effect during steroid use or withdrawal. Other common nonneurologic side effects include gastroesophageal reflux, glucose intolerance, and hypertension.

Methotrexate

Methotrexate is a chemotherapeutic agent used at low doses in dermatology, most commonly to treat psoriasis. Methotrexate is a dihydrofolate reductase inhibitor, thereby inhibiting purine synthesis and inducing immunosuppression. It is also very effective in the treatment of psoriatic arthritis, lupus, and severe atopic dermatitis. Methotrexate is most commonly prescribed in doses of 10 to 25 mg once weekly. One of the most serious side effects of methotrexate is liver injury, and careful hepatic enzyme monitoring and even infrequent liver biopsy is indicated. Frequent monitoring for bone marrow suppression is also recommended. More common side effects are headache, flulike symptoms, and gastrointestinal intolerance, particularly on the day the methotrexate is dosed. To counteract these side effects and perhaps lend protection against severe bone marrow suppression, folic acid is prescribed in conjunction with methotrexate without compromising its benefits (12).

Cyclosporine

Cyclosporine is used mainly in dermatology for immunomodulating effects, particularly in psoriasis. The drug selectively inhibits T lymphocytes and suppresses the early immune response to antigenic and regulatory stimuli. Because of the risk of renal toxicity, short-term (<1 year), and low (2 to 3 mg/kg) doses are commonly used in dermatology. At these doses, the most common neurologic side effect is tremor. With higher or elevated levels, a potential toxicity is a posterior reversible leukoencephalopathy, which usually presents with visual, autonomic, and mental status changes, with possible new onset seizures (13).

Antimalarial Agents

Hydroxychloroquine is the most commonly used antimalarial agent in dermatology, with chloroquine and quinacrine less frequently prescribed. Hydroxychloroquine is FDA approved to treat lupus erythematosus, but is commonly used in dermatology for sarcoidosis, dermatomyositis, and other photosensitive dermatoses. The exact mechanism of action of antimalarial agents is not understood, but they are thought to act in an anti-inflammatory manner. The most common dose of hydroxychloroquine used is 200 mg twice daily.

Rare neurologic side effects of seizure and psychosis have been reported with hydroxychloroquine (14,15). Complaints of tinnitus, headache, and vertigo are also uncommon side effects. Perhaps the most concerning side effect of the antimalarial drugs is retinopathy. Baseline and semiannual ophthalmologic examinations for patients receiving hydroxychloroquine are recommended by dermatologists to prevent irreversible retinopathy; however, recent literature indicates that the risk to patients receiving <6.5 mg/kg for <6 years is minimal (16). The risk of retinopathy is greater with chloroquine use, and is not seen with quinacrine use.

The antimalarial medications can induce a hemolytic anemia, particularly in patients with G6PD deficiency, and can damage the liver. Most dermatologists perform routine screening laboratory tests throughout treatment with these drugs.

Topical Immunosuppressants

In addition to topical corticosteroids, two nonsteroidal immunosuppressants are commonly prescribed in dermatology. Pimecrolimus cream (1%) and tacrolimus ointment (0.03% and 0.1%) are indicated for mild to moderate and moderate to severe atopic dermatitis, respectively. In practice, however, they are commonly used to treat other skin diseases, such as lichen planus, contact dermatitis, and seborrhea. These unique topical medications act by inhibiting calcineurin, thereby inducing local immunosuppression. They are useful as second-line agents when the risks of topical corticosteroids, including skin thinning and systemic absorption, preclude their use. They are highly effective in reducing local inflammation, particularly in areas of delicate skin (e.g., the eyelid).

Local side effects include burning and stinging, particularly with tacrolimus, and a concern exists for cutaneous viral infection, such as herpes simplex virus, in children who are already predisposed to such infections because of their atopy. More concerning than local side effects, however, is the theoretic risk of systemic side effects, including the development of lymphoma. Despite numerous studies showing little or no systemic absorption of these medications in normal use, the FDA has issued a *black box warning* for the topical calcineurin inhibitors regarding their potential for increased malignancy, largely based on animal studies. Limiting treatment duration and application sites, restricting use to children aged 2 years and older, and the prudent use of sunblock are recommended (17).

BIOLOGICS

Biologic medications are proteins produced *in vitro* and made through recombinant DNA techniques. In dermatology, they are primarily used to treat psoriasis.

The pathogenesis of psoriasis starts with T-cell activation, with a greater involvement from TH1 cells. T cells are activated by either antigen-presenting cells or macrophages and migrate to the skin. In the skin, the activated TH1 cells secrete cytokines, including IL2 and IFN-γ, causing local reactive response from keratinocytes, which secrete tumor necrosis factor-α (TNF-α) and IL-8. The culmination of this inflammatory pathway's response is the production of psoriasis (18). Biologic proteins are used *in vivo* to block certain steps in this inflammatory pathway.

With all immunomodulating agents, including the biologic medications, concern for immunosuppression exists, thus predisposing to viral and bacterial infections and reactivation of tuberculosis. In addition, a theoretic risk is seen for increasing the incidence of certain malignancies, particularly lymphomas.

Etanercept

Etanercept is used in dermatology to treat psoriasis and psoriatic arthritis. It is a combination of human antibody fused with a TNF receptor. The proposed mechanism of action is by binding to naturally occurring TNF-α, thereby rendering it inactive. Etanercept's activity occurs in keratinocytes, and endothelial and inflammatory cells (19).

The dosage most commonly used for psoriasis is 50 mg injected subcutaneously twice weekly for 3 months, followed by a maintenance therapy of 50 mg weekly or 25 mg twice weekly. Additional dosing options include starting doses of 25 mg or 50 mg/week (8).

A possible side effect of etanercept is CNS demyelinating and cases have been reported of transverse myelitis, optic neuritis, multiple sclerosis, and new onset or exacerbation of seizure disorders (20). Despite the lack of a clear causal relationship between etanercept and demyelinating disorders, its use in patients with known multiple sclerosis is contraindicated. Another side effects reported with etanercept is an associated increased incidence in heart failure (21). Positive antinuclear antibody (ANA) values in some patients displaying symptoms of drug-induced lupus have been reported. Finally, an increased risk exists for serious infection, including the reactivation of tuberculosis. All patients on etanercept must have a negative purified protein derivative (PPD) test before initiating therapy.

Efalizumab

Efalizumab is used in dermatology to treat psoriasis, but has not been shown to be beneficial in psoriatic arthritis. It is a humanized monoclonal antibody against CD11a. CD11a is a subunit of the leukocyte function-associated antigen involved in T-cell activation.

The dosing of efalizumab starts at 0.7 mg/kg injected subcutaneously weekly for the first week, with an increase to 1 mg/kg subcutanously weekly and a maximum of 200 mg per dose. Efalizumab is generally well tolerated, but when initiating the medication, a first dose reaction complex composed of headache, fever, chill, nausea, and myalgia is common, usually starting within the first 2 days (22). The headache may be the most prominent side effect and may occur after the first several doses before subsiding. During therapy, some patients experienced transient localized pustular eruptions and others experienced rebound symptoms after discontinuing the medications (23).

Initial trials with efalizumab have not shown an increased rate of infections, especially tuberculosis, or rates of lymphoproliferative malignancy. Isolated cases of thrombocytopenia have been seen, and laboratory monitoring is indicated.

Alefacept

Alefacept is also used to treat psoriasis. It is a recombinant protein that binds to CD2 on memory-effector T cells to inhibit their activation and reduce the number of memory effector T cells. Alefacept is the only biologic that is intended for pulse therapy and it may induce a remission even while the patient is off medication.

Dosing for alefacept is 7.5 mg intramuscularly once weekly for 12 weeks. A potential side effect of alefacept is the severe lowering of systemic T cells, particularly CD4 cells. During therapy, repeated T-cell counts are obtained before continued dosing, although generally a small decrease is expected. Alefacept is generally well tolerated and no major side effects have yet been reported. Initial studies have not shown an increase in rate of infections, especially tuberculosis, or rates of lymphoproliferative malignancy (24).

Interferons

Interferons (IFN) act by blocking key components of the activating factors in the inflammation system. Their use in dermatology is limited, but includes metastatic melanoma and life-threatening infantile hemangioma. The most common side effects include flulike symptoms of fever, chills, muscular pain, headaches, and arthralgia. Rare neurologic side effects include diffuse encephalopathy and psychomotor dysfunction. A rare pediatric side effect includes spastic diplegia. Seizures can occur with IFN-α exposure in both adults and children, but may be more common in young children.

Imiquimod is a unique topical medication used to induce local IFN production. Although not an IFN itself, imiquimod is used topically to treat viral papillomas and precancerous and superficial cancerous neoplasms by inducing local production of IFN-α and IFN-γ, as well as TNF, a number of interleukins, and granulocyte-stimulating factors. It is approved to treat genital condyloma for which it is applied thinly three times weekly. It is also approved to treat actinic keratoses and superficial basal cell carcinoma for which it is applied two to five times weekly. The side effects include local inflammation and irritation and, only rarely, involve flulike symptoms similar to systemic IFN use.

MISCELLANEOUS AGENTS

Botulinum Toxin A

Botulinum toxin is used in dermatology for cosmetic treatment of rhytids and the treatment of hyperhidrosis. Botulinum toxin A is one of eight exotoxins produced by *Clostridium botulinum*. The exotoxins are all neurotoxic and include A, B, C1, D, E, F, and G, with A being the most potent (25). Botulinum toxin A acts to block motor nerve activation at the presynaptic level. It attaches to the cholinergic receptor site on the presynaptic motor nerve end plate, and the nerve cell invaginates the toxin–receptor complex. The botulinum molecule then binds to synaptosome-associated protein 25 (SNAP-25), which prevents the fusion of acetylcholine vesicles to the presynaptic membrane, thereby preventing the release of acetylcholine and, thus, motor transmission (26). The body has to remake SNAP-25, which is the time-limiting factor for the effectiveness of muscle paralysis.

Cosmetically botulinum toxin is used to paralyze small muscles of the face, thereby greatly decreasing mimic lines and wrinkles, frown lines, glabellar lines, and crow's feet. Typically, 3 to 20 U of botulinum toxin are injected into given facial areas with a 30-gauge needle. The paralysis lasts for 3 to 6 months. Side effects are rare, but include headache and ptosis. Other indications for botulinum toxin A are palmar hyperhidrosis and axillary hyperhidrosis (25).

Contraindications to use include pregnancy and lactation. Botulinum toxin is also not recommended for use in patients with neuromuscular diseases, such as myasthenia gravis, Lambert-Eaton syndrome, or amyotrophic lateral sclerosis. It should not be used in conjunction with aminoglycoside because of interference with the metabolism of the medication and prolongation of its half-life (27).

Lindane

Lindane is infrequently used in dermatology to treat scabies and head lice. The mechanism of action is by inhibiting neurotransmission of these parasites. It is supplied as a 1% lotion or shampoo to be applied topically. Although toxicity is rare and primarily associated with ingestions or improper application of the medication, the feared complication is seizures (28).

Thalidomide

The uses of thalidomide in dermatology include inflammatory disorders, such as erythema nodosum leprosum, actinic prurigo, discoid lupus erythematosus, recurrent apthosis, and Jessner lymphocytic infiltration of the skin. Thalidomide mechanism of action is complex, but includes inhibition of TNF-α and the suppression of IL-12. Severe teratogenicity, including limb defects, is perhaps thalidomide's most well-known side effect. Appropriate contraceptive methods and strict FDA regulations, including a prescriber registry (System for Thalomide Education and Prescribing Safety [S.T.E.P.S.]), are allowing for a resurgence of the medication's use. Neurologic complications are the limiting factor in thalidomide use. The drug uniformly causes sedation, which is often dose limiting. It also causes a painful, symmetric, distal, sensory axonal neuropathy. The incidence is between 1% and 70%, depending on the clinical use (29,30).

CLINICAL RECOMMENDATIONS OF THE VIGNETTE

The patient highlights the importance of a rare association with a commonly prescribed dermatologic agent. Isotretinoin has been associated in the literature as causing pseudotumor cerebri. Diagnosis usually is made by detailed neuroophthalmologic examination and measurement of cerebrospinal fluid (CSF) opening pressure. Initial treatment includes acetazolamide, removal of the offending medication, and weight loss. The level of further treatment usually is dictated by the degree of visual field involvement. The patient was started on acetazolamide and had the isotretinoin discontinued. The headaches resolved within 1 month of initiating treatment.

SUMMARY

Dermatology, as with all fields of medicine, has a diverse group of disorders that are treated with an equally diverse set of medications. Many of these medications are well tolerated and associated with few side effects. A few medications with significant side effects, however, do affect the neurologic system. This chapter provides a brief introduction to several medications prescribed by dermatologist that may be significant in a neurologist's evaluation or that may have a specific neurologic side effect.

REFERENCES

1. Smithard A, Glazebrook C, Williams HC. Acne prevalence, knowledge about acne and psychological morbidity in mid-adolescence: A community-based study. *Br J Dermatol.* 2001;145(2):274–279.
2. Goulden V, Stables GI, Cunliffe WJ. Prevalence of facial acne in adults. *J Am Acad Dermatol.* 1999;41(4):577–580.
3. Abeni D, Girardelli CR, Masini C, et al. What proportion of dermatological patients receive evidence-based treatment? *Arch Dermatol.* 2001;137(6):771–776.
4. Lee GL. Pseudotumor cerebri after treatment with tetracycline and isotretinoin for acne. *Cutis.* 1995;55:165.
5. Roytman M, Frumkin A, Bohn T. Pseudotumor cerebri caused by isotretinoin. *Cutis.* 1998;42:399.
6. Wysowski D, Pitt M, Beitz J. An analysis of reports of depression and suicide in patients treated with isotretinoin. *J Am Acad Dermatol.* 2001;45:515–519.
7. Chia C, Lane W, Chibnall J, et al. Isotretinoin therapy and mood changes in adolescents with moderate to severe acne: A cohort study. *Arch Dermatol.* 2005;141(5):557–560.
8. Tenover FC, McDougal LK, Goering RV, et al. Characterization of a strain of community-associated methicillin-resistant *Staphylococcus aureus* widely disseminated in the United States. *J Clin Microbiol.* 2006;44(1):108–118.
9. Cleach LL, Bocquet H, Roujeau J-C. Reactions and interactions of some commonly used systemic drugs in dermatology. *Dermatol Clin.* 1998;16(2):421–428.
10. Zhang W, Ramamoorthy Y, Kilicarslan T, et al. Inhibition of cytochromes P450 by antifungal imidazole derivatives. *Drug Metab Dispos.* 2002;30(3):314–318.
11. Jones ME. Systemic adverse effects from topical doxepin cream. *Ann Pharmacother.* 2001;35:505.
12. Strober BE, Menon K. Folate supplementation during methotrexate therapy for patients with psoriasis. *J Am Acad Dermatol.* 2005;53(4):652–659.
13. Chang SH, Lim CS, Low TS, et al. Cyclosporine-associated encephalopathy: A case report and literature review. *Transplant Proc.* 2001;33;3700.
14. Malcangi G, Fraticelli P, Palmieri C, et al. Hydroxychloroquine-induced seizure in a patient with systemic lupus erythematosus. *Rheumatol Int.* 2000;20(1):31–33.
15. Ward WQ, Walter-Ryan WG, Shehi GM. Toxic psychosis: A complication of antimalarial therapy. *J Am Acad Dermatol.* 1985;12(5 Pt 1):863–865.
16. Mavrikakis I, Sfikakis PP, Mavrikakis E, et al. The incidence of irreversible retinal toxicity in patients treated with hydroxychloroquine: A reappraisal. *Ophthalmology.* 2003;110(7):1321–1326.
17. Berger TG, Duvic M, Van Voorhees AS, et al. American Academy of Dermatology Association Task Force. The use of topical calcineurin inhibitors in dermatology: Safety concerns. Report of the American Academy of Dermatology Association Task Force. *J Am Acad Dermatol.* 2006;54(5):818–823.
18. Nicholoff BJ. The immunologic and genetic basis psoriasis. *Arch Dermatol.* 1999;135:1104.
19. Goldsmith DR, Wagstaff AJ. Etanercept: A review of its use in the management of plaque psoriasis and psoriatic arthritis. *Am J Clin Dermatol.* 2005;6(2):121–136.
20. Immunex Corporation. Enbrel (Etanercept): Package insert (US). Available from http://www.wyeth.com [accessed April 25, 2007]
21. Kwon HJ, Cote TR, Cuffe MS, et al. Case reports of heart failure after therapy with a tumor necrosis factor antagonist. *Ann Intern Med.* 2003;138:807.
22. Scheinfeld N. Efalizumab: A review of events reported during clinical trials and side effects. *Expert Opinion on Drug Safety.* 2006;5(2):197–209.
23. Carey W, Glazer S, Gottlieb AB, et al. Relapse, rebound, and psoriasis adverse events: An advisory group report. *J Am Acad Dermatol.* 2006;54[4 Suppl 1]:S171–S181.
24. Weinberg JM. An overview of infliximab, etanercept, efalizumab, and alefacept as biologic therapy for psoriasis. *Clin Ther.* 2003;25(10):2487–2505.
25. Wollina U, Konrad H. Managing adverse events associated with botulinum toxin type A: A focus on cosmetic procedures. *Am J Clin Dermatol.* 2005;6(3):141–150.
25. Said S, Meshkinpour A, Carruthers A, et al. Botulinum toxin A: Its expanding role in dermatology and esthetics. *Am J Clin Dermatol.* 2003;4(9):609–616.
27. Glogau RG. Review of the use of botulinum toxin for hyperhidrosis and cosmetic purposes. *Clin J Pain.* 2002;18[6 Suppl]:S191–S197.
28. Boffa MJ, Brough PA, Ead RD. Lindane neurotoxicity. *Br J Dermatol.* 1995;133:1013.
29. Ochonisky S, Verroust J, Bastuji-Garin S, et al. Thalidomide neuropathy incidence and clinicoelectrophysiologic findings in 42 patients. *Arch Dermatol.* 1994;130:66.
30. Basuji-Garin S, Ochoinisky S, Bouche P, et al. Incidence and risk factors for thalidomide neuropathy: A prospective study of 135 dermatologic patients. *J Invest Dermatol* 2002;119(5):1020–1026.

PART XVI Critical Care

CHAPTER 126

Coma (Non-traumatic) and Brain Death

Michael J. Schneck • Vikram C. Prabhu

OBJECTIVES

- To identify the cardinal semiotics of coma
- To explore the possible etiologic categories for coma and determine a diagnostic paradigm for rapid evaluation of comatose patients
- To identify prognostic factors for adverse outcomes from coma
- To describe criteria for patients with cessation of neurologic function ('brain-death')

CASE VIGNETTE

A 60-year-old man with a history of arterial hypertension, hyperlipidemia, and diabetes mellitus had uneventful left hip surgery. Following surgery, he was doing well on a general medical–surgical floor awaiting transfer to an inpatient rehabilitation facility when he was found unresponsive and bradycardiac with a weak pulse. He did not open his eyes to voice or noxious stimuli. Pupils were 3 mm in diameter and minimally reactive bilaterally, but corneal and oculocephalic reflexes were preserved. Breathing was irregular and laborious. He did not move spontaneously and localized sluggishly to stimulus bilaterally. Muscle stretch reflexes were symmetric. Plantar responses were equivocal bilaterally. The patient was intubated and transferred to the intensive care unit (ICU). He was not hypoglycemic. He did not awake following administration of naloxone for possible narcotic overdose. Blood tests demonstrated a large troponin leak. Following stabilization, a computed tomographic (CT) scan was obtained that showed only nonspecific, old, small subcortical white matter ischemic changes. Electroencephalography (EEG) showed diffuse slowing. After 3 days, he still had no eye opening. Pupils were symmetric and sluggishly reactive to light bilaterally. Noted were minimal flexion response of the upper extremities and extension of the lower extremities to noxious stimulus.

DEFINITION

Coma is a deep state of unconsciousness (1). The critical elements of consciousness are (*a*) the level of wakefulness or alertness and (*b*) the level of awareness of self or the environment. Coma is a prolonged state of unconsciousness characterized by a total lack of both wakefulness and awareness. Comatose patients have no spontaneous eye opening, speech, or spontaneous movement, and the response to noxious stimulus is typically reflexive; and speech production is at best limited to meaningless sounds on noxious stimulation. In the comatose patient, sleep–wake cycles are absent.

Coma, in a sense, however, is a transitional state. Patients in coma can recover with no or varying degrees of residual brain injury, including a *minimally conscious state*. After a certain amount of time, arbitrarily a minimum of 1 month, some patients may fall into the category of *persistent vegetative state*. These patients may have preserved sleep–wake cycles and apparent spontaneous movements, but they never regain cognition and never achieve any awareness of environment or response to stimuli. Another subset of patients will lose all hemispheric and brainstem function and, at that point, with cessation of brain function, can be declared dead.

EPIDEMIOLOGY

The epidemiology of coma is not well defined in the literature. Although data regarding severe head injury exist in regional trauma data banks, actually very little data is available about the incidence of nontraumatic coma. Data suggest that postsurgical comatose states are uncommon (2). Elsewhere, Ropper (3) has suggested that "altered levels of unconsciousness," including a comatose state, are not uncommon in the emergency department setting. In a pediatric study from England, the incidence of nontraumatic coma was 30.8 per 100,000 children under age 16 years annually; the age-specific incidence was higher in the first year of life at 160 per 100,000 per year. In infants, most presentations were with nonsystemic signs. Central nervous system (CNS)-specific presentations were more common with older children. Infection was the most common cause, comprising 38% of cases (4).

PATHOPHYSIOLOGY AND PATHOGENESIS

The reticular activating system (RAS) originates in the midbrain and pontine tegmentum and projects to subcortical and cortical structures. Impairments in wakefulness occur with derangements of the RAS and alterations of awareness occur with global derangements of the cerebral cortex and its connections to subcortical structures, including the basal ganglia, thalamus, and hypothalamus (1,5).

The cause of coma is diverse. Mechanistically, coma can derive from direct structural injury to hemispheric and midbrain or pontine structures. Primary injury to the hemispheres must either involve both sides, as occurs with global hypoxic-ischemic injury following cardiac arrest, or must be sufficiently large to cause herniation syndromes, as may be seen with traumatic brain injuries, tumors or large hemorrhagic or ischemic strokes. Focal lesions of the brainstem or diencephalon may not be as large, but must involve bilateral injury (e.g., bilateral thalamic lesions). Coma can also occur as a secondary manifestation of systemic insults, including toxic (e.g., drug overdose), metabolic insults, as well as systemic infections through ill-defined alteration in brain metabolism and neuronal function (5).

CLINICAL MANIFESTATIONS AND EXAMINATION

The approach to the comatose patient first requires basic ABC (airway, breathing, circulation) of stabilization (3,5,6). The overwhelming majority of these patients will probably require intubation for airway protection and may have issues of hemodynamic stability requiring pressor support or antihypertensive therapy. Acute respiratory failure can simply reflect the comatose state. Depending on where the damage has initiated, abnormal breathing patterns may be seen before intubation, which may help localize the initial location or severity of coma. When the initial damage is in the cerebral hemispheres, the initial abnormality typically seen is hyperpnea alternating with periods of apnea (Cheyne-Stokes breathing). As coma worsens to involve midbrain structures, a central reflex hyperpnea (neurogenic pulmonary edema) may be seen, followed by very irregular patterns of breathing as pontine and then medullary structures are involved (apneustic, clustering, ataxic, and gasping patterns) (1). Elevated blood pressure can suggest drug overdoses, hypertensive encephalopathy, elevated intracranial pressure (ICP) (especially when the patient is bradycardic—a phenomenon known as *Cushing's response*), or an acute stroke. Low blood pressure reflects shock or other circulatory derangements. Consideration of occult trauma in patients who are found unconsciousness and then brought to the emergency department may necessitate neck immobilization pending clinical and imaging evaluation of the cervical spine.

A rapid, but thorough, neurologic examination, including an overall assessment of the level of consciousness, assists in determination of severity of the comatose state and possibly prognosis. It also guides the diagnostic evaluation for the underlying cause of coma. The examination includes evaluation of the head and neck for occult trauma. The examination should also include evaluation for meningismus or otitis that may suggest an infectious process. The skin should be examined for rashes and inflammation related to infection, emboli, or collagen-vascular disorder. The fundi should be examined for papilledema as a sign of cerebral edema and subhyaloid hemorrhages as a possible sign of subarachnoid hemorrhage. Findings on examination for retinal emboli may suggest a patient at high risk for atheroembolic stroke or global hypoxic-ischemic injury from atheroma, fat, air, and other embolic sources. The neurologic survey includes assessment of the cranial nerves and motor response to help localize lesions in the brainstem, as well as identify any lateralizing abnormalities that might suggest an intracranial structural process. For example, normal pupillary and preserved oculocephalic responses suggest that brainstem structures are relatively preserved. Decorticate posturing, manifested by flexion and adduction of the upper extremities and extension of the lower extremities, suggests sparing of midbrain and caudal structures, whereas extensor posturing, manifested by extension of both the upper and lower extremities, indicate injury of the midbrain or pons.

For the assessment of consciousness, the Glasgow Coma Scale (GCS) is the best known and most widely used assessment tool for comatose patients. Scores range from 3 to 15, with a score of 13 or higher correlating to mild injury, a score of 9 to 12 moderate injury; and a score of 8 or less corresponding to severe brain injury. The elements of the GCS are found in Table 126-1 below. The prognostic value of the GCS is well established in traumatic head injury. It has also been shown to have prognostic value in meningitis, intracerebral hemorrhage, and subarachnoid hemorrhage and is also a component of other prognostic scales of CNS injury (7). The FOUR (*f*ull *o*utline of *unr*esponsiveness) score is a new coma scale, recently developed at the Mayo Clinic, which addresses some of the scoring limitations of the GCS for intubated patients. The FOUR Scale uses a 0 to 4 scale for four distinct domains: respiration, brainstem reflexes, eye response, and motor response. This new scale, however, lacks the familiarity and the extensive time-tested validation of the GCS (8).

TABLE 126-1. Glasgow Coma Scale

Points	*Eye Opening*	*Best Verbal Response*	*Best Motor Response*
6	**Not scored**	**Not scored**	Obeys commands
5	**Not scored**	oriented	Localizing response to pain
4	Spontaneous	confused	Withdrawal response to pain
3	Responds to verbal commands	Inappropriate words	Flexion to pain
2	Responds to pain	Incomprehensible sounds	Extension to pain
1	No eye opening	No verbal response	No motor response

DIAGNOSTIC APPROACH

The diagnostic evaluation is geared to rapid identification of the underlying causes of the comatose state (3,5,6). Immediate testing of the comatose patient should include a blood glucose level; when the cause of coma is unclear or possibly due to hypoglycemia, immediate treatment of patient with dextrose and thiamine 100 mg intravenously should occur. With any question of opiate overdose, especially if the patient has pinpoint pupils, intravenous naloxone hydrochloride must be immediately given intravenously or flumazenil for possible benzodiazepine overdose. Flumazenil should be used with caution if any suspicion of seizure history exists because this drug can precipitate status epilepticus. Other routine blood studies to investigate metabolic or infectious causes should include a metabolic panel, liver enzyme profile, and perhaps an ammonia level; and complete blood cell count with differential and coagulation parameters. All patients should have an arterial blood gas; pulse oximetry is insufficient to assess blood pH and P_{CO_2}. A urine drug screen and alcohol level should be considered in all patients presenting to the emergency department and possibly for some hospitalized patients as well. A hypoadrenal state or myxedema coma must be considered in patients without other structural or metabolic abnormalities and thyroid profiles and serum cortisol levels may be appropriate in selected patients.

Neuroimaging with either CT or magnetic resonance imaging (MRI) is a critical component in the investigation of structural intracranial processes, including focal mass lesions, focal or global ischemic injury, and elevated ICP secondary to either displacement or shift from focal lesions, enlargement of the ventricles owing to hydrocephalus, or diffuse cerebral edema. MRI provides far greater information about the brainstem and also greater detail about cerebral ischemia and, therefore, should be the preferred diagnostic modality. Because MRI may be less readily available, particularly for unstable patients, CT of the brain is often the initial diagnostic imaging study.

EEG can provide diagnostic information about patients with nonconvulsive status epilepticus, which can be present in upward of 10% of comatose patients. Also, particular focal slow wave EEG patterns, such as periodic lateralizing epileptiform discharges (PLED), may be associated with viral encephalitides, such as herpes encephalitis. Diffuse slow wave abnormalities can be seen in the context of acute toxic or metabolic encephalopathies; although not pathognomonic, a triphasic slow wave pattern is suggestive of hepatic or renal encephalopathy. By contrast, diffuse, rapid EEG patterns may be seen in drug overdoses or diffuse cerebral ischemia. EEG may also be prognostic. Burst-suppression or severe generalized slowing portends a worse outcome.

Cerebrospinal fluid (CSF) examination is appropriate whenever an infectious or inflammatory cause of coma is being considered, although if a mass lesion or cerebral edema is a concern, neuroimaging should be first obtained. Regardless, antibiotic therapy, if indicated, should never be delayed while awaiting brain imaging and lumbar puncture. In some circumstances, ICP monitoring or ventricular CSF drainage may be helpful. Guidelines suggest ICP monitoring in traumatic brain injury when the GCS <8. Additionally, ICP monitoring can be of use in cases of hepatic coma, especially those cases with hyperammonemia associated with acetaminophen overdose.

TREATMENT

Management of the comatose patient is generally supportive in nature and is otherwise directed at the underlying cause of coma, if possible. Measures for reduction of elevated ICP, including judicious hyperventilation, mannitol, and ventricular CSF drainage are appropriate in selected patients, especially those with herniation as a result of mass lesions or hydrocephalus and certain instances of diffuse cerebral edema (e.g., hepatic coma). These measures are less useful in patients with brain swelling as a result of global hypoxic-ischemic injury. Anticonvulsants should be used in cases of suspected nonconvulsive status, but the data for empiric seizure prophylaxis in the comatose patient are ill-defined.

PROGNOSIS AND OUTCOME

Outcome from coma is determined by a number of factors (9). The severity of the initial coma injury as measured by the GCS is important, but other more critical determinants include the underlying cause and severity of neurologic damage as well as the extent and location of the initial insult. Patients in deep coma as a result of drug overdose or metabolic derangements may recover with no residual deficits, whereas patients with structural damage resulting from hypoxic-ischemic injury (i.e., from massive stroke, hemorrhage, or cardiac arrest) may never regain consciousness. The chance of meaningful recovery after a sustained comatose state is negligible and, although anecdotal reports exist of patients waking up after prolonged states of impaired consciousness, close examination of these cases typically do not meet criteria for either a comatose or vegetative state.

The indicators of outcome have been best defined for patients following hypoxic-ischemic arrest, including after cardiopulmonary arrest (10). Factors include an absent pupillary light response, or corneal reflexes, and extensor or no motor response to pain after 3 days of observation. The presence of the myoclonic form of status epilepticus is also a poor prognostic factor. Prognosis cannot be based on circumstances of cardiopulmonary resuscitation (CPR) or elevated body temperature. Bilateral absent cortical responses on somatosensory-evoked potential studies recorded 3 days after CPR also predicted poor outcome. Additionally, burst suppression or generalized epileptiform discharges on EEG predict poor outcomes, but with insufficient prognostic accuracy. Among biochemical markers predicting outcome, serum neuron-specific enolase >33 pg/L might predict poor outcomes. Whereas diffuse anoxic-ischemic injury on brain imaging (CT or MRI) describes the degree of structural damage in these patients, the role of brain imaging in predicting outcome has not been adequately studied in cardiac arrest patients.

SPECIAL CIRCUMSTANCES: BRAIN DEATH

In patients for whom brain function ceases, death can be determined if strict criteria are followed (11). These include clinical, imaging evidence of a major neurologic event consistent with an etiologic determination of irreversibility, or both; exclusion of confounding variables to clinical assessment, including hypothermia, drug intoxications (illicit or iatrogenic), and corrected metabolic parameters. The neurologic examination must be consistent with absent cortical or brainstem function, including the comatose state. Brainstem findings must include (*a*) absent pupillary light responses, (*b*) corneal reflexes, (*c*) oculocephalic (Doll's) *and* oculovestibular (caloric) responses, (*d*) absent motor responses (except for possible spinal reflexes), (*e*) absent gag or cough, including to deep pharyngeal stimulation; and (*f*) a positive apnea test. A positive apnea test requires an absence of respiratory movement, despite a rise in the $PACO_2$ to value of >20 mm Hg above baseline values in otherwise well-oxygenated but nonventilated comatose patients. Some experts have argued that a waiting period between two separate examinations is unnecessary. However, in some instances, especially in the case of children and younger adult patients, a waiting period between two separate examinations may be desirable and may particularly help provide assurance to the patient's family that a considered and precise determination of 'brain death' has occurred. Although a well-done clinical evaluation by skilled practitioners of neurologic assessment is sufficient for determination of death, in some instances ancillary diagnostic tests are needed. This may include infants for whom the clinical assessment is more difficult, patients in whom cranial nerves cannot be adequately examined (i.e., because of head trauma), or patients in whom the apnea test cannot be completed because of hemodynamic instabilities. Among the ancillary testing options are electrophysiologic tests (EEG, evoked potentials) and brain blood flow tests (nuclear medicine single-photon emission computed tomography [SPECT] studies, transcranial Doppler and cerebral angiography). The Wijdick (11) review discusses the respective advantages and disadvantages of the different studies.

CLINICAL RECOMMENDATIONS OF THE VIGNETTE

The patient exemplifies coma resulting from global hypoxic-ischemic injury following an acute in-hospital myocardial infarction. Subsequent MRI revealed bilateral cortical and watershed areas of infarction in both hemispheres. In such instances, prognosis for meaningful recovery is poor and discussion with family of ongoing cardiopulmonary support is critical.

SUMMARY

The comatose state reflects either structural injury to the brain or systemic derangements that cause bilateral impairment to the cerebral cortex, diencephalon, or the brainstem and the connections between these structures. The evaluation of the patient in coma is focused on diagnosis and treatment of the underlying cause. Although coma can be reversible, patients with more prolonged or severe comatose states have a much less favorable outcome.

REFERENCES

1. Plum F, Posner JB, eds. *The Diagnosis of Stupor and Coma*, 3rd ed. Philadelphia: FA Davis; 1982.
2. Gamil M, Fanning A. The first twenty four hours after surgery. A study of complications after 2153 consecutive operations. *Anaesthesia.* 1991;46:712–715.
3. Ropper AH. Coma in the emergency room. In: Earnest MP, ed. *Neurologic Emergencies.* New York: Churchill Livingstone; 1983:79–715.
4. Wong CP, Forsyth RJ, Kelly TP, et al. Incidence, aetiology and outcome of non-traumatic coma: A population based study. *Arch Dis Child.* 2001;84(3):193–199.
5. Stevens RD, Bhardwaj A. Approach to the comatose patient. *Crit Care Med.* 2006;34(1): 31–41.
6. Bateman, DE. Neurological assessment of coma. *J Neurol Neurosurg Psychiatry.* 2001; 71[Suppl1]:13–17.
7. Teasdale G, Jennet B. Assessment of coma and impaired consciousness. A practical scale. *Lancet.* 1974;2:81–84.
8. Widjick EF, Bamlet WR, Maramattom BV, et al. Validation of a new coma scale: The FOUR score. *Ann Neurol.* 2005;58(4):585–593.
9. Bates D. The prognosis of medical coma. *J Neurol Neurosurg Psychiatry.* 2001;71[Suppl i]: i20–i23.
10. Wijdicks EFM, Hijdra A, Young GB, et al. Practice parameter: Prediction of outcome in comatose survivors after cardiopulmonary resuscitation (an evidence-based review): Report of the Quality Standards Subcommittee of the American Academy of Neurology. *Neurology.* 2006;67:203–210.
11. Wijdicks, EFM. The diagnosis of brain death. *N Engl J Med.* 2001;344:1215–1221.

CHAPTER 127

Shock

Ankush Gosain • Fred A. Luchette

INTRODUCTION

Cardiovascular failure can be either the end result of multisystem organ failure (MSOF) or a precursor to shock and MSOF. Most often, cardiovascular failure will manifest itself with clinical signs and symptoms of pump failure. The most common cause of cardiovascular failure is hypovolemic shock, which results in decreased preload or decreased right ventricle filling volumes. It manifests as tachycardia and hypotension. Cardiogenic shock, resulting from the heart's inability to pump a normal volume or loss of myocardial contractility, and septic shock, characterized by failure of the heart to overcome decreased vascular tone, are also commonly seen in the critically ill patient. Neurogenic shock results from loss of sympathetic innervation to the arterioles, leading to increased capacitance of both the arterial and venous systems.

Cardiovascular failure and shock are generally amenable to treatment if the underlying cause is promptly identified and therapy instituted in a timely fashion. Therapy to support the failing cardiovascular system is directed at the cause of the shock state; it includes fluid resuscitation (preload) as well as pharmacologic modulation of vascular tone (afterload), contractility (with inotropes), and heart rate (with chronotropes).

OBJECTIVES

- To examine the cause and pathogenesis of shock
- To review the diagnostic and treatment approach to shock

CASE VIGNETTE

A 58-year-old woman is admitted to the intensive care unit (ICU) postoperatively following an elective abdominal aortic aneurysm (AAA) repair. The operating surgeon reports episodic hypotension intraoperatively, with systolic blood pressure (BP) of 50 to 70 mm Hg. The patient's medical history is remarkable for tobacco use, diabetes mellitus, hyperlipidemia, and coronary artery disease. Her vital signs are (BP) 90/50 mm Hg, heart rate (HR) 110 beats per minute, respiratory rate (RR) 14 breaths per minute, and temperature 36.6°C. On arrival to the ICU, physical examination demonstrates that she is intubated but awake, and is moving only her right hemibody. Results from laboratory analysis include a hemoglobin of 6.4 g/dL.

DEFINITIONS, ETIOLOGY, AND PATHOGENESIS

Cardiac output (CO) is defined as the quantity of blood ejected into the aorta by the heart each minute and is calculated as HR multiplied by stroke volume (SV) (CO = HR × SV). This is the quantity of blood that flows through the circulation and is responsible for oxygen and nutrient transport to the tissue beds. The primary determinants of cardiac output are preload (the venous return to the right atrium), afterload (the resistance against which the left ventricle contracts), contractility (the extent to which the myocardial cells contract), and HR. The quantity of blood returning to the right atrium each minute is the venous return, or preload. The primary determinant of cardiac output is the filling of the heart and the ability to pump that volume effectively. Most therapeutic modalities are aimed at augmenting cardiac output focus on restoring filling pressures and augmenting ineffective myocardial contractility.

Cardiac output varies with the level of activity of the body, and is influenced by level of metabolism, exercise state, age, size of the individual, and other factors. In females, cardiac output is generally stated as being 10% to 20% lower than in men. When correcting for age, the average cardiac output for adults is approximated as 5 L/min. Laboratory and clinical research have demonstrated that cardiac output increases in proportion to increasing body surface area. Variation in cardiac output between individuals because of a difference in body habitus is standardized by correcting for body surface area (cardiac output/body surface area) and is the cardiac index.

PRELOAD

Preload is the force that stretches myocardium before contraction. The concept of preload is derived from laboratory experiments in which strips of muscle are stretched with weight (preload) before initiating contraction. Contraction is initiated by electrical stimulation and a transducer determines the resultant force. Both *in vitro* experiments and *in vivo* correlates have revealed that increasing sarcomere length to a maximum of 0.2 μm by the addition of weight results in increased force of contraction. With additional lengthening, the myocardial contractility decreases. This is referred to as the *Frank-Starling relationship,* and was first described in amphibian hearts by Otto Frank in 1884. In 1914, Ernest Starling repeated these experiments with mammalian hearts. The mechanisms linking preload and contractile force are still incompletely understood. Although initially it was thought that increased myocardial stretch optimized the overlap of contractile actin and myosin leading to increased force of contraction, more recent research indicates that contractile force is also dependent on sensitivity of the myocyte to ionized calcium gradients, as determined by sarcomere length (1–3).

The Frank-Starling relationship provides a paradigm by which the cardiovascular system and its derangements can be approached. By increasing preload, the volume of intraventricular blood during systole (stroke volume) is increased. Therefore, the most important clinical determinant of preload is intravascular volume. Hypovolemia, or decreased preload, is the result of decreased blood volume resulting from internal or external fluid losses. An additional factor affecting preload is vascular tone of the venous system. Changes in venous capacitance are often unwanted side effects of pharmacologic agents. It also occurs with neurogenic shock.

Together, intravascular volume and venous return determine left ventricular end diastolic volume (LVEDV), which determines the force of ventricular contraction. The Swan-Ganz catheter is used to measure the pulmonary arterial wedge pressure (PAWP), which approximates left ventricular end diastolic pressure (LVEDP). Assuming unaltered ventricular compliance, LVEDP theoretically approximates the LVEDV. In the setting of critically ill patients, factors such as myocardial ischemia, heart failure, myocardial edema, endotoxemia, cardiac hypertrophy and circulating tumor necrosis factor (TNF) can decrease ventricular compliance, rendering measurement of PAWP as a surrogate for LVEDV unreliable. In these situations, normal or elevated PAWP may not eliminate inadequate preload as a cause of low cardiac output.

Aside from changes in venous capacitance, venous return to the heart can be compromised by increased intrathoracic pressure. This is most evident with tension pneumothorax, when the shock state is immediately reversed by decompression of the pleural space. Additionally, in the mechanically ventilated patient, the use of positive-pressure ventilation coupled with positive end-expiratory pressure (PEEP) can impair venous return to the heart. In this patient population, when intravascular volume is low, the adverse effects of increased intrathoracic pressure on preload predominate and cardiac output is diminished. It is important to remember that placing an under-resuscitated patient on positive-pressure ventilation, can lead to cardiovascular collapse. In the reverse scenario, patients with normal to high intravascular volume may benefit from the afterload-reducing effects of elevated intrathoracic pressure seen with positive-pressure ventilation. Synchronization of positive-pressure ventilation with the cardiac cycle has been described as a method of afterload reduction and cardiac output augmentation (4–6). It is not surprising that patients in cardiogenic shock arrest from sudden cardiovascular collapse when ventilatory support is removed.

AFTERLOAD

Cardiovascular failure caused by a reduction in afterload is referred to as *distributive shock*, and it has multiple subtypes: septic shock, neurogenic shock, and anaphylactic shock. Afterload is the force that opposes ventricular contraction. Similar to preload, the concept of afterload is derived from *in vitro* experiments. These studies have established that increasing afterload decreases the speed and force of contraction. Clinically, vascular impedance appears to be the best *in vivo* correlate of ventricular afterload. Vascular impedance is not a readily assessed clinical quantity, and the clinician must rely on systemic vascular resistance (SVR) as a surrogate. SVR is calculated using the hemodynamic equivalent of Ohm's law:

$$SVR = (MAP - CVP)/CO$$

In this equation, MAP is the mean arterial blood pressure, CVP is the central venous pressure, and CO is the cardiac output. This equation provides an approximation of vascular impedance with the assumption of nonpulsatile flow. It is important, therefore, to realize that measuring afterload or SVR with data from the Swan-Ganz catheter actually provides a calculated value. Finally, because SVR is inversely proportional to cardiac output, rather than treating an abnormally high SVR, it is important first to treat the low cardiac output with fluid administration to maximize preload.

CONTRACTILITY

Contractility, also known as *inotropic state*, is the force with which myocardial contraction occurs. The inotropic state of the myocardium and the stroke work performed, can be visualized by the construction of a left ventricular pressure-volume loop. This loop is bounded by the four phases of the cardiac cycle: isovolemic relaxation, diastolic filling, isovolemic contraction, and systolic ejection. Stroke work is defined as the area bounded by this loop.

Instantaneous pressure-volume curves provide a more elegant approach to understanding the inotropic state of the myocardium (7). Using this approach, LVEDP is plotted against left ventricular volume for a range of loading conditions. The slope of the line connecting these points is equal to end systolic elastance. Elastance, the reciprocal of compliance, approximates the stiffness of the ventricle and, therefore, characterizes the intrinsic contractility of the myocardium.

Presently, the use of pressure-volume curves in patient care is limited to centers using newer generation pulmonary artery (PA) catheters that measure ventricular volume as well as pressure (8). More commonly, clinicians rely on Frank-Starling curves to determine myocardial performance and estimate contractility. Contractility can be estimated by angiographic or echocardiographic determination of ventricular ejection fraction, but this method is highly sensitive to changes in afterload, and may be less reliable.

HEART RATE

Heart rate is a key determinant of CO. In the setting of constant stroke volume, increasing the number of cardiac contractions per unit time results in increased CO. In addition, increasing the HR increases contractility, a phenomenon known as the *Bowditch effect.* In the setting of cardiac failure, however, it is not uncommon to observe HR sufficiently high that ventricular filling is compromised, resulting in decreased CO. Rapid ventricular rates that impair cardiac filling are most commonly seen in patients with preexisting or evolving myocardial ischemia. In this setting, rate control becomes paramount in ensuring matched oxygen delivery and utilization.

MYOCARDIAL DYSFUNCTION

Myocardial dysfunction can be defined on the basis of perturbed preload, afterload, contractility, or HR. Systemic hypovolemia (e.g., inadequate preload), secondary to hemorrhage or third space losses, is the most common cause in the patient after surgery or the trauma patient. Other causes of decreased CO can arise from failing or decreased contractile function of the heart. Evolving ischemia can lead to areas of myocardium that lose their ability to contract, leading to decreased CO. The myocardial contractility can also become altered following any insult that disrupts intrinsic cellular metabolism. This typically occurs in the settings of sepsis, after cardiac arrest, or after cardiopulmonary bypass. Direct physical injury to the myocardium, as occurs following blunt chest injury, can produce contused cardiac muscle, which can lead to contractile dysfunction and decreased CO.

DIAGNOSTIC APPROACH

CENTRAL VENOUS PRESSURE

Invasive monitoring of the CVP has been used for more than four decades. This allows assessment of right ventricular filling pressure or right-sided heart preload. The catheter is typically placed percutaneously into the superior vena cava and is used to guide volume status during resuscitation. In healthy individuals, the CVP is between 0 and 4 mm Hg. In contrast, in critically ill patients with myocardial dysfunction, the CVP may need to be as high as 12 to 18 mm Hg for optimal myocardial function. A low CVP usually indicates hypovolemia, whereas an elevated CVP (>18 mm Hg) may be evidence of volume overload. Increases or decreases in CO or index may be further used in conjunction with CVP to assess volume status as evidenced by the Frank-Starling curve. CVP and PAWP correlate well in the normal functioning heart (ejection fraction [EF] >50%), but this correlation is not maintained in patients with cardiac impairment (EF <40%) (9). CVP measurement has its limitations and is affected by multiple variables, which can cause an inadequate assessment of intravascular volume. Malplacement of the catheter, congestive heart failure (right- or left-sided), pneumothorax, venomotor tone, pulmonary embolus, cardiac tamponade, and increased intrathoracic and intraabdominal hypertension can all lead to a false elevation in CVP readings.

PULMONARY ARTERY CATHETERS

Pulmonary artery catheters (PAC) or Swan-Ganz catheters, first introduced for clinical use in 1970, have been widely accepted as the standard for invasive monitoring of both volume status and cardiac function by measurement and approximation of left ventricular pressures during diastole. Measurement of the PAWP is used as an indirect determination of LVEDP, which is assumed to correlate with LVEDV. These measurements, however, often show poor correlation (10,11). Continuous monitoring of cardiac output or index, along with other information provided by newer PAC, allows early identification of compromised oxygen delivery or increased oxygen consumption. Commercially available PAC currently incorporate multiple calculations to derive other indices of cardiac function and tissue perfusion, such as mixed venous oxygen saturation (S_VO_2), SVR, oxygen delivery (DO_2), and consumption (VO_2). This real-time information at the bedside allows the clinician to quickly respond.

ECHOCARDIOGRAPHY

Transthoracic and transesophageal echocardiography has gained wide acceptance for evaluation of cardiac function. Both are effective tools in the ICU as a guide to resuscitation and fluid status and cardiac performance. In addition, information about structural abnormalities of the heart, aorta, and main pulmonary arteries can be obtained by this method, along with assessment of ventricular dysfunction, ventricular filling, valvular abnormalities, ventricular hypertrophy, and pulmonary embolus. Transesophageal echocardiography can give accurate measurements of both right- and left-sided filling volumes of the heart and may provide a better assessment of myocardial preload when compared with CVP or PA catheter measurements (12). Placed in the esophagus, Doppler probes can accurately predict CO using the diameter of the aorta and measurements of blood flow velocity.

MIXED VENOUS OXYGEN SATURATION

The difference between DO_2 and VO_2 is the extraction ratio and correlates with the S_VO_2. Fiberoptic probes within PAC allow measurement of the oxygen saturation in the pulmonary artery with normal values ranging between 75% and 80%. Continuous measurement of S_VO_2 serves as a monitor of systemic oxygen utilization, with decreasing values of S_VO_2 indicating increased consumption by tissues or decreased delivery to the tissues. This measurement can also serve as an ongoing assessment of the DO_2/VO_2 ratio, therefore guiding optimization and the titration of specific treatments. During the septic state, the cell's inability to utilize delivered oxygen can increase S_VO_2. Cellular destruction from prolonged ischemia or cellular metabolic poisoning following carbon monoxide inhalation often yield normal or increased S_VO_2 despite inadequate end-organ perfusion because of an inability to utilize the oxygen delivered.

TREATMENT

PRELOAD AUGMENTATION AND REWARMING

Myocardial dysfunction is frequently caused by intravascular volume loss. Before the development of hypotension, most adult patients will demonstrate a decrease in urine output, indicative of end-organ hypoperfusion. Prompt restoration of intravascular volume will augment preload and reverse this dysfunction. Depending on the degree of volume loss, most patients respond to simple crystalloid solutions. If severe or ongoing hemorrhage is present, and the patient is not responding to crystalloid administration, transfusion of blood products may be necessary. Normalization of HR and BP and adequate urine output are simple and effective measurements of adequate volume restoration.

During resuscitation, attention must be given to the patient's temperature to avoid hypothermia. Both systolic and diastolic left ventricular function are impaired in the hypothermic patient (13). Infusion of warmed fluids during resuscitation reduces the rate of heat loss and preserves left ventricular diastolic function, whereas recovery of systolic function is prolonged (14,15), likely because of long-lasting effects of hypothermia on the excitation-contraction coupling of the actin-myosin interaction.

PHARMACOLOGIC

A multitude of pharmacologic agents are available for the management of myocardial dysfunction. Selection of the appropriate agent(s) should be tailored to the specific clinical situation. The agents can be classified into those that effect afterload by vasodilatation or constriction and ones that augment cardiac contractility. Selected agents have multiple mechanisms of action.

Dopamine

Dopamine, a naturally occurring catecholamine, has several cardiovascular effects. These include increased HR, increased contractility, and peripheral vasoconstriction. It acts on α- and β-adrenoreceptors as well as dopamine (DA)1 and DA2 receptors. The specific receptor activated is dose dependent. Dopamine is used primarily for inotropic support to maintain brain, heart, and kidney perfusion. The greatest clinical utility is as a cardiac β-adrenoreceptor agonist, which occurs at a moderate dose (3 to 5 μg/kg/min). This dose increases myocardial contractility and thus cardiac output.

It has long been thought that low dose dopamine (1 to 3 μg/kg/min), also known as *renal-dose* dopamine, increases renal blood flow and maintains diuresis via the DA1 and DA2 receptors (16). More recent, rigorous investigation has revealed that individual variation in the pharmacokinetics of dopamine typically results in poor correlation between blood levels and administered dose. Dopamine also acts as a proximal tubular diuretic and increases sodium delivery to tubular cells, increasing their oxygen demands and causing naturesis (17). Finally, two meta-analyses and a large prospective, double-blinded randomized, controlled trial failed to demonstrate that dopamine alters renal function in critically ill patients with acute renal failure (18–20). For these reasons, insufficient evidence exists to support the use of low-dose dopamine to maintain renal perfusion.

At higher doses of dopamine (10 μg/kg/min), peripheral vasoconstrictive effects from stimulation of α-adrenergic receptors predominate. This can result in significant coronary vasoconstriction, resulting in angina, vasospasm, and increased PAWP (21). Additionally, increasing afterload from vasoconstriction, coupled with an increased HR seen at this dose, results in increased myocardial oxygen consumption and demand (22).

Dopamine, at any administered dose, can result in tachyarrhythmias, which can lead to increased myocardial oxygen demand and worsening cardiovascular failure. Because of the variable effects of dopamine, the dosage ranges used to define specific receptor effects are to be used as broad guidelines only, with the awareness that dopamine can have the unwanted effects at any of the dose ranges described above with an individual patient.

Dobutamine

Dobutamine is a synthetic catecholamine with primarily β-adrenergic effects, although it does possess some α_1-adrenergic properties. It is an inotrope, increasing contractility with minimal chronotropic effects (23). Dobutamine also possesses mild β_2-adrenoreceptor activity, producing peripheral vasodilatation. The combination of increased contractility and reduced afterload results in improved left ventricular function and an increase in cardiac output without an increase in myocardial oxygen consumption (24). Because of the vasodilatory effects of dobutamine, afterload may also be reduced. This combination of responses makes dobutamine ideally suited for use in low-output cardiac states. It should be considered the inotrope of choice for patients with low cardiac output in the presence of adequate preload (25). Two large prospective trials, however, failed to demonstrate a benefit to raising oxygen delivery to supranormal levels with the use of dobutamine (26,27), likely because of an inability of the peripheral tissues to utilize the additional oxygen delivered (28).

Epinephrine

Epinephrine is an endogenous catecholamine with α- and β-adrenergic activity. At low doses, epinephrine exerts primarily β-adrenergic effects, increasing contractility and reducing SVR. Despite this, little evidence indicates that epinephrine is superior to dobutamine in the treatment of low cardiac output states (e.g., myocardial infarction). The increases in stroke volume and CO seen with epinephrine have the potential of decreasing BP in patients with an increased preload. In patients with septic shock who have been resuscitated, epinephrine increases HR and SV (and, therefore, CO) and systemic oxygen delivery without altering afterload (pulmonary vascular resistance [PVR] and SVR) (29). At higher rates of infusion, epinephrine exerts primarily α-adrenergic effects, increasing SVR and BP and is indicated for patients with ventricular dysfunction refractory to dopamine or dobutamine.

Care must be exercised when using high doses of epinephrine, because renal vasoconstriction, cardiac arrhythmias, and increased myocardial oxygen consumption and demand may result. Additionally, metabolic abnormalities are common, including dyskalemias, hyperglycemia, and ketoacidosis (30,31). Finally, epinephrine increases blood lactate levels in patients recovering from cardiopulmonary bypass or those with septic shock, likely through increases in tissue oxygen extraction in the absence of adequate delivery (32–34).

Norepinephrine

Norepinephrine, an endogenous sympathetic neurotransmitter, acts on both α- and β-adrenergic receptors. At high doses, the α-adrenergic receptor effect predominates, resulting in increased SVR and BP. This potent vasoconstrictor effect is generally reserved for patients who are refractory to both volume resuscitation and other inotropic agents (35,36). At low doses, however, the β-adrenergic actions of norepinephrine predominate, resulting in increased HR and contractility. Specifically, in the setting of right ventricular failure, low-dose norepinephrine improves cardiac function without adversely affecting visceral perfusion (37). As an aside, norepinephrine is widely used in the care of the patient with head injury. The vasoconstrictive effects of norepinephrine do not extend to the cerebral vasculature, making it an ideal agent for maintaining cerebral perfusion pressure (38,39).

Amrinone and Milrinone

Synthetic bipyridines, amrinone and milrinone are phosphodiesterase inhibitors and demonstrate both positive inotropic and vasodilatory actions. Although these agents inhibit intracellular phosphodiesterase III, leading to intracellular cyclic adenosine monophosphate (cAMP), their positive inotropic effects are likely related to downstream increases in intracellular calcium (40).

Both drugs have the theoretic advantage of dual mechanisms of action: augmenting cardiac output while reducing cardiac work by positive inotropic actions and peripheral vasodilatation (40). Amrinone and milrinone have demonstrated clinical utility in multiple low cardiac output states; however, as single-agent therapy, neither amrinone nor milrinone have proved superior to single inotropes (e.g., dobutamine) for improving cardiac performance. An additional advantage of dobutamine is its short half-life, which allows minute-to-minute titration for effect, whereas amrinone and milrinone both have prolonged half-lives.

In selected situations, an additive effect in myocardial function is observed when dobutamine and either amrinone or milrinone are combined. For example, the phosphodiesterase inhibitors can be used as single-agent therapy in patients with isolated systolic heart failure, but are more commonly used as secondary agents (in addition to dobutamine) in cases of refractory heart failure. In this scenario, the beneficial effects on cardiac output are additive because the phosphodiesterase inhibitors do not act via the adrenergic receptors. An unwanted effect of the bipyridines results from their potent vasodilatory action is hypotension in patients who are hypovolemic.

Vasopressin

Arginine vasopressin, a potent vasoconstrictor, has gained popular acceptance as a treatment for septic shock that is refractory to volume resuscitation and conventional pressor agents. The supply of endogenous vasopressin production by the posterior pituitary is quickly exhausted in septic shock. Restoration of this deficiency is beneficial in weaning norepinephrine and other pressor agents. It also imparts a short-term survival benefit in this group of patients. When vasopressin is combined with norepinephrine, outcome in the treatment of catecholamine-resistant cardiovascular failure caused by septic shock is superior to therapy with norepinephrine alone (41).

Vasopressin has also emerged as a therapy for cardiac arrest and acute resuscitation (42). Current guidelines for CPR recommend vasopressin as an alternative to epinephrine for shock-resistant ventricular fibrillation. It is superior to epinephrine for restoring cardiac rhythm in the asystolic patient, but is equivalent to epinephrine alone in the treatment of ventricular fibrillation and pulseless electrical activity (43). In the postoperative treatment of a patient after coronary artery bypass, vasopressin significantly reduces HR and the need for both pressor and inotropic support, with no adverse effect on the myocardium. A significant reduction was seen in cardiac enzyme levels and rate of cardioversion for arrhythmias with the initial use of vasopressin (44). Patients having cardiopulmonary bypass often experience hemodynamic instability similar to that seen with septic shock, with characteristics of peripheral vasodilatation and hypotension, and a diminished response to conventional pressor agents. Vasopressin has been shown to correct vasodilatory shock following cardiopulmonary bypass, regardless of normal circulating vasopressin levels (45).

Nitrovasodilators

The nitrovasodilators are useful agents for reducing vascular tone, thus allowing manipulation of both preload and afterload. The most common indication for their use is in states of elevated SVR. Sodium nitroprusside acts primarily on arteriolar smooth muscle, reducing afterload. The onset of action of sodium nitroprusside is rapid, and its effects cease almost instantly once the infusion is discontinued. When titrating the dose of sodium nitroprusside, SVR will decrease with a concomitant increase in CO, thereby maintaining a relatively constant systemic arterial pressure. Whereas the effects of sodium nitroprusside favor arterial dilatation, it does have mild venous dilatory effects that can lead to an increase in venous capacitance and decreased preload.

With high doses ($>10\ \mu g/kg/min$ or infusion for several days) of sodium nitroprusside, cyanide toxicity is a known side effect. This results from the ferrous iron contained in sodium nitroprusside reacting with sulfhydryl-containing compounds in erythrocytes, producing cyanide. Toxicity results when the rate of production exceeds the capacity of the liver to metabolize cyanide to thiocyanate. Toxicity manifests as an unexplained rise in mixed venous oxygen tension as a result of reduced oxygen consumption. Treatment is with sodium nitrite and it is aimed at providing an alternate substrate for the cyanide ion. Sodium nitrite also converts hemoglobin to methemoglobin, producing a ferric ion that competes with the ferric ion in the cytochrome system for the cyanide ion. Finally, methylene blue can be administered to treat the methemoglobinemia that results from sodium nitrite toxicity.

Nitroglycerin, a potent arteriolar and venous smooth muscle dilator, is a useful agent when both preload and afterload are elevated. The effects of nitroglycerin are dose dependent, with low doses primarily increasing venous capacitance and higher doses relaxing arterial tone. Side effects are generally the result of an overly rapid reduction in venous or arterial tone, and are readily reversed by cessation of the medication.

Steroids

The use of steroids as replacement therapy for insufficient adrenal production has reduced mortality in patients with cardiovascular collapse. The use of steroids for hemodynamic support in septic shock has gained renewed interest. New data suggest that in adrenal-insufficient patients, low-dose glucocorticoid replacement therapy is beneficial (46).

In addition to their use as a replacement therapy, steroids are known anti-inflammatory agents. Cardiopulmonary bypass produces an inflammatory response because of the production of oxygen-free radicals. These byproducts have been associated with hypotension and arrhythmias. The use of steroids to temper the production of free oxygen radicals in patients after bypass has been studied. In a prospective, randomized trial, no difference was found in the incidence of cardiac arrhythmias in patients receiving steroids (47). Therefore, the use of steroids in the treatment of cardiovascular collapse secondary to sepsis in non–adrenal-insufficient patients or as an anti-inflammatory agent in cardiopulmonary bypass patients cannot be recommended.

Intraaortic Balloon Pump Counterpulsation

When myocardial failure has an underlying, surgically correctable, anatomic cause (e.g., acute mitral regurgitation, intraventricular septal defect, high-grade coronary artery stenosis) and pharmacologic methods have been ineffective in augmenting CO, the use of intraaortic balloon counterpulsation (IABP) is indicated. IABP involves placement of a balloon catheter into the proximal descending aorta (distal to the origin of the left subclavian artery) via a femoral arterial approach. A mechanical pumping device inflates the balloon during diastole and deflates during systole. Balloon inflation displaces approximately 40 mL of blood retrograde into the coronary arterial circulation and antegrade into the descending aorta. The balloon is abruptly deflated at the beginning of systole, allowing the left ventricle to eject its stroke volume. These dual functions augment coronary arterial flow while decreasing afterload, thereby reducing myocardial oxygen consumption.

CLINICAL RECOMMENDATIONS OF THE VIGNETTE

The 58 year-old patient is admitted to the ICU for resuscitation following elective AAA repair. Her initial laboratory studies demonstrates anemia, most likely from acute blood loss intraoperatively. Additionally, the operating surgeon relays a history of hypotensive episodes intraoperatively and the patient demonstrates a focal neurologic deficit. The constellation of findings points to a patient in hemorrhagic shock and in need of aggressive resuscitation. Multiple diagnostic adjuncts are available for use in this patient, including CVP monitoring, close monitoring of the urine output, and the use of a PAC to guide resuscitation. Following an appropriate clinical response and normalization of her hemodynamics, a CT of the brain is warranted as an initial step to evaluate for possible ischemic infarct. The possibility of a watershed infarct occurring in the border zone between adjacent perfusion beds should be considered.

SUMMARY

Appropriate management of myocardial dysfunction involves optimization of intravascular volume (preload), systemic vascular resistance (afterload), and myocardial contractility. Cardiovascular failure in the critically ill patient most often is caused by hypovolemia, and volume resuscitation should be initiated before pharmacologic measures. Following resuscitation, determination of impaired myocardial function or altered vascular tone using the diagnostic techniques detailed in this chapter should be undertaken, and appropriate therapy initiated. Finally, cardiovascular failure is rarely the single cause of mortality in critically ill patients. In this setting, cardiac failure is most frequently a component of MSOF and the clinician must maintain concern for the entire physiology of the patient, not just an isolated organ system.

REFERENCES

1. McDonald KS, Field LJ, Parmacek MS, et al. Length dependence of Ca2+ sensitivity of tension in mouse cardiac myocytes expressing skeletal troponin C. *J Physiol.* 1995;483(Pt 1):131–139.
2. McDonald KS, Moss RL. Strongly binding myosin crossbridges regulate loaded shortening and power output in cardiac myocytes. *Circ Res.* 2000;87(9):768–773.
3. McDonald KS, Wolff MR, Moss RL. Sarcomere length dependence of the rate of tension redevelopment and submaximal tension in rat and rabbit skinned skeletal muscle fibres. *J Physiol.* 1997;501(Pt 3):607–621.
4. Pinsky MR, Marquez J, Martin D, et al. Ventricular assist by cardiac cycle-specific increases in intrathoracic pressure. *Chest.* 1987;91(5):709–715.
5. Pinsky MR, Summer WR. Cardiac augmentation by phasic high intrathoracic pressure support in man. *Chest.* 1983;84(4):370–375.
6. Pinsky MR, Summer WR, Wise RA, et al. Augmentation of cardiac function by elevation of intrathoracic pressure. *J Appl Physiol.* 1983;54(4):950–955.
7. Sagawa K, Suga H, Shoukas AA, et al. End-systolic pressure/volume ratio: A new index of ventricular contractility. *Am J Cardiol.* 1977;40(5):748–753.
8. Chang MC, Mondy JS, 3rd, Meredith JW, et al. Clinical application of ventricular end-systolic elastance and the ventricular pressure-volume diagram. *Shock.* 1997;7(6):413–419.
9. Mangano DT. Monitoring pulmonary arterial pressure in coronary-artery disease. *Anesthesiology.* 1980;53(5):364–370.
10. Calvin JE, Driedger AA, Sibbald WJ. Does the pulmonary capillary wedge pressure predict left ventricular preload in critically ill patients? *Crit Care Med.* 1981;9(6):437–443.
11. Raper R, Sibbald WJ. Misled by the wedge? The Swan-Ganz catheter and left ventricular preload. *Chest.* 1986;89(3):427–434.
12. Madan AK, UyBarreta VV, Aliabadi-Wahle S, et al. Esophageal Doppler ultrasound monitor versus pulmonary artery catheter in the hemodynamic management of critically ill surgical patients. *J Trauma.* 1999;46(4):607–611; discussion 611–612.
13. Fischer UM, Cox CS, Laine GA, et al. Mild hypothermia impairs left ventricular diastolic but not systolic function. *J Invest Surg.* 2005;18(6):291–296.
14. Tveita T, Ytrehus K, Myhre ES, et al. Left ventricular dysfunction following rewarming from experimental hypothermia. *J Appl Physiol.* 1998;85(6):2135–2139.
15. Tveita T, Mortensen E, Hevroy O, et al. Experimental hypothermia: Effects of core cooling and rewarming on hemodynamics, coronary blood flow, and myocardial metabolism in dogs. *Anesth Analg.* 1994;79(2):212–218.
16. McDonald RH, Jr., Goldberg LI, McNay JL, et al. Effect of dopamine in man: Augmentation of sodium excretion, glomerular filtration rate, and renal plasma flow. *J Clin Invest.* 1964;43:1116–1124.
17. Friedrich AD. The controversy of "renal-dose dopamine." *International Anesthesiology Clinics.* 2001;39(1):127–139.
18. Bellomo R, Chapman M, Finfer S, et al. Low-dose dopamine in patients with early renal dysfunction: A placebo-controlled randomised trial. Australian and New Zealand Intensive Care Society (ANZICS) Clinical Trials Group. *Lancet.* 2000;356(9248):2139–2143.
19. Kellum JA. Use of dopamine in acute renal failure: A meta-analysis. *Crit Care Med.* 2001;29(8):1526–1531.
20. Marik PE. Low-dose dopamine: A systematic review. *Intensive Care Med.* 2002;28(7):877–883.
21. Crea F, Chierchia S, Kaski JC, et al. Provocation of coronary spasm by dopamine in patients with active variant angina pectoris. *Circulation.* 1986;74(2):262–269.
22. Fowler MB, Alderman EL, Oesterle SN, et al. Dobutamine and dopamine after cardiac surgery: Greater augmentation of myocardial blood flow with dobutamine. *Circulation.* 1984;70(3 Pt 2):I103–I111.
23. Tanaka H, Tajimi K, Nakatani T, et al. Changes in hemodynamics and myocardial metabolism following discontinuation of a dopamine or dobutamine infusion. *J Cardiothorac Vasc Anesth.* 1990;4(6):695–703.
24. Ko W, Zelano JA, Fahey AL, et al. The effects of amrinone versus dobutamine on myocardial mechanics and energetics after hypothermic global ischemia. *J Thorac Cardiovasc Surg.* 1993;105(6):1015–1024.
25. Dellinger RP, Carlet JM, Masur H, et al. Surviving sepsis campaign guidelines for management of severe sepsis and septic shock. *Crit Care Med.* 2004;32(3):858–873.
26. Gattinoni L, Brazzi L, Pelosi P, et al. A trial of goal-oriented hemodynamic therapy in critically ill patients. SvO2 Collaborative Group. *N Engl J Med.* 1995;333(16):1025–1032.
27. Hayes MA, Timmins AC, Yau EH, et al. Elevation of systemic oxygen delivery in the treatment of critically ill patients. *N Engl J Med.* 1994;330(24):1717–1722.
28. Hayes MA, Yau EH, Timmins AC, et al. Response of critically ill patients to treatment aimed at achieving supranormal oxygen delivery and consumption. Relationship to outcome. *Chest.* 1993;103(3):886–895.
29. Moran JL, O'Fathartaigh MS, Peisach AR, et al. Epinephrine as an inotropic agent in septic shock: A dose-profile analysis. *Crit Care Med.* 1993;21(1):70–77.
30. Craig AB, Jr., Honig CR. Hepatic metabolic and vascular responses to epinephrine: A unifying hypothesis. *Am J Physiol.* 1963;205:1132–1138.
31. Ellis S, Beckett SB. Mechanism of the potassium mobilizing action of epinephrine and glucagon. *J Pharmacol Exp Ther.* 1963;142:318–326.
32. Bourgoin A, Leone M, Delmas A, et al. Increasing mean arterial pressure in patients with septic shock: Effects on oxygen variables and renal function. *Crit Care Med.* 2005;33(4):780–786.
33. Meier-Hellmann A, Reinhart K, Bredle DL, et al. Epinephrine impairs splanchnic perfusion in septic shock. *Crit Care Med.* 1997;25(3):399–404.
34. Totaro RJ, Raper RF. Epinephrine-induced lactic acidosis following cardiopulmonary bypass. *Crit Care Med.* 1997;25(10):1693–1699.
35. Martin C, Papazian L, Perrin G, et al. Norepinephrine or dopamine for the treatment of hyperdynamic septic shock? *Chest.* 1993;103(6):1826–1831.

36. Levy B, Bollaert PE, Charpentier C, et al. Comparison of norepinephrine and dobutamine to epinephrine for hemodynamics, lactate metabolism, and gastric tonometric variables in septic shock: A prospective, randomized study. *Intensive Care Med.* 1997;23(3): 282–287.
37. Angle MR, Molloy DW, Penner B, et al. The cardiopulmonary and renal hemodynamic effects of norepinephrine in canine pulmonary embolism. *Chest.* 1989;95(6):1333–1337.
38. Johnston AJ, Steiner LA, Chatfield DA, et al. Effect of cerebral perfusion pressure augmentation with dopamine and norepinephrine on global and focal brain oxygenation after traumatic brain injury. *Intensive Care Med.* 2004;30(5):791–797.
39. Steiner LA, Johnston AJ, Czosnyka M, et al. Direct comparison of cerebrovascular effects of norepinephrine and dopamine in head-injured patients. *Crit Care Med.* 2004;32(4): 1049–1054.
40. Alousi AA, Johnson DC. Pharmacology of the bipyridines: Amrinone and milrinone. *Circulation.* 1986;73(3 Pt 2):III10–III24.
41. Dunser MW, Mayr AJ, Ulmer H, et al. Arginine vasopressin in advanced vasodilatory shock: A prospective, randomized, controlled study. *Circulation.* 2003;107(18):2313–2319.
42. Guidelines 2000 for Cardiopulmonary Resuscitation and Emergency Cardiovascular Care. Part 6: Advanced cardiovascular life support: Section 1: Introduction to ACLS 2000: Overview of recommended changes in ACLS from the guidelines 2000 conference. The American Heart Association in collaboration with the International Liaison Committee on Resuscitation. *Circulation.* 2000;102[8 Suppl]:I86–I89.
43. Wenzel V, Krismer AC, Arntz HR, et al. A comparison of vasopressin and epinephrine for out-of-hospital cardiopulmonary resuscitation. *N Engl J Med.* 2004;350(2):105–113.
44. Dunser MW, Mayr AJ, Stallinger A, et al. Cardiac performance during vasopressin infusion in postcardiotomy shock. *Intensive Care Med.* 2002;28(6):746–751.
45. Forrest P. Vasopressin and shock. *Anaesth Intensive Care.* 2001;29(5):463–472.
46. Annane D, Sebille V, Charpentier C, et al. Effect of treatment with low doses of hydrocortisone and fludrocortisone on mortality in patients with septic shock. *JAMA.* 2002;288(7): 862–871.
47. Volk T, Schmutzler M, Engelhardt L, et al. Effects of different steroid treatment on reperfusion-associated production of reactive oxygen species and arrhythmias during coronary surgery. *Acta Anaesthesiol Scand.* 2003;47(6):667–674.

CHAPTER 128

Sepsis

John M. Santaniello

OBJECTIVES

- To define sepsis, severe sepsis, and inflammatory response syndrome
- To discuss the epidemiology of sepsis
- To discuss the cause of sepsis
- To describe the pathophysiology of sepsis
- To discuss the diagnostic approach to the septic patient
- To discuss treatment options and new therapies in sepsis

CASE VIGNETTE

A 55-year-old man involved in a motor vehicle collision was brought to the hospital after sustaining a closed head injury with a subarachnoid hemorrhage (SAH). The Glasgow Coma Score was 7 on arrival. He was intubated for respiratory insufficiency. Further tests revealed multiple rib fractures with a flail chest on the left, a left lung contusion, and a severe pelvic fracture. He received lactated Ringer's solution and blood products for tachycardia and hypotension. Abdominal examination was negative for an intraabdominal injury. The patient was brought to the intensive care unit (ICU) for further monitoring and resuscitation. In the ICU, he received an intracranial pressure (ICP) monitor, a central venous access catheter, an arterial line, and a Foley catheter.

Over the course of his ICU stay, his head injury stabilized without evidence of further central nervous system (CNS) bleeding. The intracranial pressure (ICP) normalized. He was on minimal ventilator support with an FIO_2 of 50%, and positive end-expiratory pressure (PEEP) of 5, breathing spontaneously. His pelvic fracture was operatively repaired. On postoperative day 7, he spiked a temperature to 39°C, became tachycardic and his blood pressure dropped to 80/40 mm Hg. Urine output has also dwindled to 10 to 15 mL/hour for the past 3 hours. He also had an increase in his oxygen requirements to 90% FIO_2 to maintain his SaO_2 about 92%.

DEFINITION

Strict definitions of sepsis are relatively new within the last decade. Patients with signs and symptoms are routinely classified as being *septic*. Because of wide variations in definitions, however, it is often impossible to compare patients from different regions and centers when analyzing sepsis research.

Whereas the septic patient usually requires an infectious source to meet criteria for sepsis, newer definitions recognize the inflammatory response as an integral part of sepsis. Thus, in 1992, the American College of Chest Physicians (ACCP) and the Society of Critical Care Medicine (SCCM) (1) officially adopted the term *systemic inflammatory response syndrome* (SIRS). SIRS refers to activation of the innate inflammatory response, which can be caused by either infectious or noninfectious sources, such as burns, noninfectious peritonitis, and multiple system traumas. It is important to realize that a routine surgical procedure or identical insults in different patients may produce markedly different inflammatory responses. Therefore, SIRS is defined as having more than one of the following findings: (*a*) temperature >38°C or >36°C; (*b*) heart rate >90 beats/min; (*c*) respiratory rate >20 breaths/min; and (*d*) leukocytosis or leukopenia with white blood cell count (WBC) >12,000 or <4,000.

Sepsis is defined as clinical manifestations of SIRS with infection, whereas infection is defined as invasion of a normally sterile tissue.

Although documented infection is a standard criterion for sepsis, other signs and symptoms can also be used to diagnose early sepsis, because infection is often difficult to prove. These include altered hemodynamic variables, such as high cardiac output with decreased systemic vascular resistance, hyper- or hypoglycemia, coagulation abnormalities, and intolerance to enteral feeding (2). Although these are nonspecific signs, clinicians should be aware of them as being early warning clues that the inflammatory response has suddenly progressed to sepsis, despite no microbiologic data to support it.

Severe sepsis is defined as sepsis associated with organ dysfunction, as defined by a number of organ dysfunction scoring systems in use today (3,4). Septic shock refers to sepsis with arterial hypotension despite adequate fluid resuscitation. Standard definition of arterial hypotension is that of a systolic blood pressure of 90 mm Hg or less, or a mean arterial blood pressure of <70 mm Hg. In chronic hypertensive patients, relative hypotension can be present, despite a normal-appearing blood pressure, and this must be taken into account when evaluating these patients because a decrease in systolic blood pressure of >40 mm Hg from baseline is considered in the hypotensive range. Once adequately fluid resuscitated, if vasopressors are still required to increase the blood pressure, the patient is still classified as being in septic shock despite a normal blood pressure that is being augmented by pharmacologic vasopressor agents.

EPIDEMIOLOGY

The epidemiology of sepsis has changed over the years. As definitions change and heterogeneous group of patients are compared, no clear consensus on the epidemiology of sepsis has yet been reached. Most studies are conducted at large academic tertiary care centers and, therefore, definite conclusions about the true incidence of sepsis cannot accurately be made. The incidence of septicemia was shown to have increased from 73.6/100, 000 population in 1979, to 175.9/100,000 in 1989 in a large study conducted by the Centers for Disease Control (CDC) (5). Other large studies have defined occurrence rates, but have failed to describe incidence owing to lack of data on the general population. In one study, the authors found an occurrence of 26% meeting the ACCP/SCCM consensus criteria for sepsis (6). Other large studies have shown occurrence rates on admission to ICU for sepsis ranging from approximately 5% to 10 % (7,8).

Attempts have been made to define risk factors associated with mortality in patients with the sepsis. Recurrent risk factors for mortality included presence of shock, type and dosages of antibiotics used, comorbid conditions, and use of vasopressor agents (9). Microbiologic differences in attributable mortality suggest that infections with *Candida* and *Enterococcus* organisms have a mortality of 30% to 40%, whereas mortality is about 15% to 20% associated with coagulase-negative *Staphylococci* organisms (10). Recent studies also suggest that the specific microbiology may also influence response to certain interventions (11), emphasizing that when comparing groups of patients with sepsis no assumption can be made that one species of gram-negative or gram-positive organism will respond to treatments in a similar fashion as others will. Genetic predispositions have also been studied as risk factors for adverse outcomes in patients with sepsis, particularly tumor necrosis factor (TNF) polymorphisms (12). Likewise, studies on gender differences have found the incidence of sepsis and septic shock to be lower among women (13).

Decreased mortality in septic patients has gone from 31% in 1979 to 25.3% in 1989 (5). Recent studies have shown overall mortality rates to be approximately 50%, ranging between 40% and 80% (14). Although comparison of these studies is difficult, the one constant observation is that, as severity of illness increases, so does mortality. Therefore, if patients progress from SIRS to sepsis, to severe sepsis, then, mortality increases accordingly (8).

ETIOLOGY AND PATHOGENESIS

Organisms associated with severe infections and sepsis have evolved. Whereas gram-negative organisms predominated early on in the 1960s and 1970s, gram-positive organisms are the source of half the cases of severe sepsis over the past two decades, with recent studies showing gram-positive organisms as the leading source of sepsis. Although *Candida* species have emerged as the most common organism associated with fungal sepsis, the incidence of fungal sepsis is only 5% (15–17). Because evidence of an infectious organism is the hallmark of sepsis, the importance of correctly identifying the microbiologic flora is of paramount importance. With ever-increasing resistance patterns of organisms, the identification of an organism and its antibiotic susceptibilities is not only of importance from a research and epidemiologic standpoint, but if a correct treatment regimen is to be started early, the correct identification of the offending organism should be one of the main treatment goals in patients with sepsis.

The most common offending gram-negative organisms associated with gram-negative sepsis are *Escherichia coli*, *Klebsiella* spp. and *Pseudomonas* spp. Gram-negative sepsis is caused by binding of bacterial lipopolysaccharides, located in the outer cell membrane, to the host's lipopolysaccharide-binding protein. Recently, toll-like receptor 4 has also been identified as a lipopolysaccharide co-receptor.

The most common gram-positive organisms associated with sepsis include *Staphylococcus aureus* and coagulase-negative staphylococcus, along with streptococci species, including *Streptococcus viridans*, *S. pneumoniae*, and *S. pyogenes*. Usually associated with indwelling intravascular catheters, and skin and soft tissue infections, bacteremia, and pulmonary infections can also occur. Gram-positive organisms produce sepsis by secretion of exotoxins, which bind to antigen-presenting cells and go on to stimulate large amounts of cytokines when presented to T cells. Stimulation of the innate immune system is the other mechanism Gram-positive organisms produce sepsis. This mechanism does not use exotoxins and is believed to be similar to mechanisms of gram-negative sepsis-induced shock.

PATHOPHYSIOLOGY

Whereas a number of insults can produce a systemic inflammatory response, sepsis is usually an orderly and well-characterized reaction to infectious stimuli. The cytokine system, with both inflammatory (TNF-α, IL-1, IL-6, and IL-8) and anti-inflammatory (TNF-soluble receptor, IL-1 receptor antagonists, and IL-10) components, plays a key role in the systemic response to infection. When an infectious source is localized, local release of inflammatory cytokines plays a key role in containment and destruction of the source, by amplification of the inflammatory response. Almost simultaneously, anti-inflammatory cytokines are released in response to inflammatory cytokines. Therefore, normal defense mechanisms rely on a balance between the inflammatory and anti-inflammatory cytokines both to control infectious sources and to contain the increased inflammatory response initiated by these cytokines. This balance is overwhelmed by inflammatory cytokines leading to sepsis and its classic response, most notably, activation of complement, coagulation, and kinin systems. Neutrophils seem to play a key role by causing a secondary injury by the production of oxygen-free radicals, and byproducts of phagocytosis of infectious organisms. Both leukocyte and endothelial cell-derived cytokines can be implicated in sepsis and sepsis syndromes. The physiologic derangements seen among patients with sepsis are reproducible in both animal and human experiments. With onset of the inflammatory cascade secondary to infection, patients with sepsis often exhibit an increased cardiac output and decreased systemic vascular resistance, resulting in arterial hypotension. Although cardiac output can be elevated, systolic and diastolic function is decreased, as evidenced by increased end diastolic and end systolic volumes (18,19). In patients not adequately resuscitated with fluids, a hypodynamic state can occur, with a low to normal cardiac output. Recovering patients normalize their cardiac function, whereas cardiac function remains depressed despite inotropic support among the nonsurvivors (20,21). Decreased intravascular volume seen among patients with sepsis is often multifactorial. Sepsis produces relative hypovolemia because of increase in venous capacitance, increased vascular permeability, and intracellular fluid shifts in addition to redistribution of blood flow and increases in insensible losses. Increased vascular permeability and capacitance are thought to occur secondary to nitric oxide production. Changes in cell membrane permeability have been linked to increases in cell wall permeability to sodium. Some inflammatory cytokines may play a role in increasing cell membrane permeability by inducing changes in the cells ion permeable channels (22,23).

Despite an increase in cardiac output, blood flow is not distributed in a normal or even manner during sepsis. Although some studies vary in their findings, a consistent derangement is a decrease in splanchnic blood flow. More specifically, a decrease in mucosal blood flow leading to acidosis and hypoxia of the mucosa, and possibly increased permeability, which can be linked to bacterial translocation (24,25).

Despite an increase in cardiac output, along with increased oxygen delivery, the utilization of oxygen delivered is dysfunctional. Whereas normal venous oxygen saturation (SVo_2) of 75% is seen among healthy individuals, derangements at the cellular level often produce decreased utilization of delivered oxygen resulting in an increased SVo_2. Therefore, the once believed treatment of supranormal oxygen delivery to increase survival in critically ill surgical patients (26) has been virtually abandoned because oxygen use is independent of delivery.

DIAGNOSTIC APPROACH

Confirming the diagnosis of sepsis continues to present difficult challenges, even to the most experienced clinicians, because most of the clinical signs of sepsis are nonspecific, and can be similar to those observed with other noninfectious disease states, as well as to those seen with the normal physiologic response to injury or postoperatively. Once a diagnosis of sepsis has been entertained, ruling out noninfectious sources is paramount. The possible sources of the responses seen in sepsis and other disease states must be approached in a stepwise manner. Fever or hypothermia, leukocytosis or leucopenia, tachycardia, and hypotension can also be found in response to multiple trauma, hypovolemia, and endocrine abnormalities (e.g., thyroid storm, adrenal insufficiency).

Patients presenting with SIRS or suspected sepsis have often been mismanaged in the early stages of this disease, and progress to full-blown severe sepsis or septic shock occurs in a matter of hours after presentation. In patients presenting with two or more SIRS criteria and a documented or suspected infection, the diagnosis of sepsis is made and prompt treatment should be initiated. Recent studies have shown that delay in treatment of the patient with sepsis leads to increased mortality and utilization of hospital resources (27,28). Patients presenting with hypotension are treated with volume resuscitation and normalization of vital signs; however, the clinician must be aware, that 10% to 15% of patients in shock will have physiologically compensated and present with normal vital signs (29). Therefore, other signs of tissue hypoperfusion must be sought to diagnose and treat sepsis sufficiently early to make a difference.

No one laboratory test exists to establish a diagnosis of sepsis. Several serum markers have been used in combination or alone to help guide resuscitation and make the probability of sepsis more likely. Serum lactate of ≥4 mmol/L at presentation or inability to clear lactate levels at 6 hours have both been shown to be associated with higher morbidity and mortality (30–32). Serum base deficit and bicarbonate concentrations have also been shown to correlate with decreased tissue perfusion (33). It is important be aware, however, that other factors can spuriously alter these values (i.e., use of illicit drugs, hypothermia, hyperchloremia) and must be considered. C-reactive protein (CRP), a marker of inflammation, has been shown to be elevated in sepsis. At what level it differentiates sepsis from inflammation has been debated, however, with lower CRP values being more sensitive, but less specific. Procalcitonin, also a marker of inflammation, has been shown to increase faster and clear quicker at onset and resolution of inflammation (34). In a study of patients in the ICU, procalcitonin levels of ≥1.5 ng/mL were 100% sensitive and 72% specific in identifying sepsis (35). IL-6 and endotoxin have also been studied as markers to aid in the early detection of sepsis. IL-6, although elevated in sepsis, is nonspecific and is also elevated in many noninfectious disease states. Therefore, IL-6 levels are more useful to study as trends over time rather than as a single assay. Endotoxin has been shown to be specific for gram-negative infection and outcomes (36). Newer assays for endotoxin have been shown in preliminary work to have a high negative predictive value to rule out gram-negative infection (37).

It, therefore, seems that, despite many efforts to come up with a single test to diagnose sepsis, a high index of suspicion along with other clinical signs will continue to be used in conjunction with assays and technology until newer and better markers of sepsis are discovered.

SPECIAL SITUATIONS

SEPTIC ENCEPHALOPATHY

Deterioration or change in mentation in the patient with sepsis can be multifactorial. Hypoxia, medication, perfusion abnormalities, and metabolic sequelae have all been found to be causes of mental dysfunction in such patients. Once these more common factors have been remedied and ruled out as a source of encephalopathy, septic encephalopathy should be sought as the cause. Described by Hippocrates and Galen, septic encephalopathy is not a new phenomenon. Septic encephalopathy has been reported to occur in approximately 10% to 70% of patients with sepsis (38,39). The true incidence is probably not known, however, because of the masking of mental function secondary to medication or sedation and paralytics, in addition to the wide variation in definitions used.

Septic encephalopathy is usually divided into *early* (before onset of other organ failure) or *late* (after onset of other organ failure). Once thought to be caused by the bacteremia of sepsis' effect on the brain, encephalopathy is also seen when no identifiable source of bacteremia is found. More likely, it is the systemic inflammation seen in sepsis or sepsis syndromes that causes septic encephalopathy.

TNF-α and interferon-γ have been shown to increase the permeability of human cerebral endothelial cells by promoting pinocytosis without affect on the intracellular tight junctions (40). Oxygen-free radicals produced by activated leukocytes have been shown to reduce the deformability of erythrocytes, which may lead to decreased circulation in the microvasculature and increase cerebral hypoperfusion (41,42).

Alteration of the blood–brain barrier has also been implicated in the pathogenesis of septic encephalopathy. Both endogenous and exogenously administered vasoactive drugs have been shown to increase the vascular resistance in the cerebral circulation.

Direct damage to astrocytes by inflammatory mediators has also been implicated as a cause of septic encephalopathy. Possessing receptors for inflammatory mediators, direct damage to astrocytes can exacerbate neuronal damage by causing dilatation of local blood vessels, reduce synaptic activity, and increase permeability of the blood–brain barrier (43–66).

Increased levels of amino acids have also been implicated as the cause of septic encephalopathy; however, secondary dysfunction of both the hepatic and renal systems may also contribute to the abnormalities seen. Increased levels of tryptophan, tyrosine, and phenylalanine, both in the plasma and in the brain, may contribute to alterations in neurotransmission and the severity of septic encephalopathy has been predicted by the concentration of these aromatic compounds (38,47).

To summarize, septic encephalopathy is multifactorial. Although many mechanisms are described, no one has been found to be *the* causative factor. Treatment is largely supportive of the ongoing septic insult seen in these patients, however long-term neurologic sequelae in surviving patients must be addressed in the ongoing treatment of sepsis and its complications.

PREGNANCY

The occurrence of sepsis in pregnancy has declined from 0.6% to 0.3% from 1979 to 2000 (17). Whereas gram-positive organisms are on the rise as etiologic factors in sepsis, the gravid population is still predominantly infected with gram-negative organisms (48). The physiologic state of the pregnant patient increases the risk of infection, which may include pneumonia secondary to decreased functional residual capacity of the lungs, chorioamnionitis and septic abortion, and pyelonephritis. The cardiovascular derangements seen in pregnancy often mimic those of sepsis, with an increased cardiac output and decreased blood pressure and systemic vascular resistance. The myocardial dysfunction associated with sepsis, therefore, may be particularly harmful because it is the physiologic increase in heart rate and cardiac output that helps maintain arterial blood pressure during pregnancy. Peripartum cardiomyopathy can also be exacerbated by the cardiac dysfunction associated with sepsis (49). Multiple coagulation abnormalities exist in the pregnant patient and these can also play a role in the development of organ dysfunction and disseminated intravascular coagulation (DIC) as seen in sepsis.

Decreased plasma colloid-osmotic pressure in pregnancy can also predispose to the development of acute lung injury and acute respiratory distress syndrome (ARDS) secondary to increased pulmonary edema and decreased capacity and compliance (50).

Treatment of the septic pregnant patient centers on the mother, because maternal well-being has the highest impact on fetal survival. Broad-spectrum antibiotic coverage should be initiated, based on both a presumed or documented infection and institution sensitivities and organisms. When treating pregnant patients, particular attention must be paid to the choice of antibiotics, especially in the first trimester when organogenesis is taking place. Tetracycline and chloramphenicol should be avoided. Other therapies aimed at the treatment of sepsis will be covered later in this chapter.

SEPSIS AND MALIGNANCY

With better and more toxic chemotherapeutic and surgical treatments, patients with cancer are surviving longer. This, along with the immunocompromised state of patients with cancer, makes them highly susceptible to infection and sepsis. Patients with cancer are 10 times more likely to acquire sepsis than those patients without cancer. Cancer is an independent risk factor for death among patients with sepsis (51). Causes for increased mortality are multifactorial, perhaps stemming from the fact that patients with cancer are immunocompromised from drugs and are often be malnourished. Patients with pancreatic cancer were found to be at highest risk for the development of sepsis, and those with breast cancer at the lowest risk (51).

TREATMENT STRATEGIES

Over the years, sepsis has continued to have high mortality rates despite advances in therapy. Recent advancements have led to new treatments that may have begun to open the door to increased survival of the patient with sepsis. Currently, activated protein C, tight blood glucose control, early goal-directed therapy, and vasopressin and corticosteroid administration have all been used with some success in treating sepsis. These therapies will be briefly discussed.

ACTIVATED PROTEIN C

Because of the dysregulation of the coagulation system in sepsis, as evidenced by increased levels of activated coagulation factors in patients with sepsis, along with autopsy reports of microvascular thrombi in these patients, various treatments targeting this system have been used. Activated protein C (aPC), which targets both the inflammatory pathway and the coagulation cascade, has shown a small improvement in survival, significantly decreasing mortality from 30.8% to 24.7% in patients with severe sepsis (52). This study, however, was in a select patient population at high risk of death based on the number of organ systems in failure. A subsequent study has shown no benefit in survival, and an increased risk of bleeding complications in the patient with sepsis at low risk of death (53). The use of antithrombin III (AT-III) has also been studied as a possible pathway to target in the coagulation cascade to increase survival. To date, AT-III has not shown a benefit in survival of for patients with sepsis (54). Therefore the use of anticoagulation therapies has shown some benefit with aPC in severe sepsis with patients at high risk of death. The success of aPC and the failure of other anticoagulant therapies may lie in the fact that, whereas AT-III and other anticoagulation treatments targets only one aspect of the systemic dysregulation seen in patients with sepsis (i.e., the coagulation cascade), aPC acts both as an anti-inflammatory agent and as an anticoagulant.

GLUCOSE CONTROL

Hyperglycemia in hospitalized patients has often been left untreated until levels have reached approximately 220 mg/dL, using the rationale that, at this level, patients began to spill glucose into the urine, which can lead to hypovolemia secondary to an osmotic diuresis. Whereas insulin resistance is the mechanism for hyperglycemia in sepsis, patients often have elevated blood sugars without a history of diabetes. New onset hyperglycemia has been shown to be an early marker of infection and sepsis. Recent studies to obtain tight blood glucose control in sepsis have shown decreased mortality in both surgical and medical patients in the ICU. Tight glycemic control achieved by intravenous insulin therapy to achieve blood glucose levels between 80 and 110 mg/dL has been shown to significantly decrease mortality from 8% to 4.6% in surgical patients on mechanical ventilation (55). In patients in the medical ICU with length of stays longer than 3 days, intensive insulin therapy was shown to significantly decrease in hospital mortality from 52.5% to 43% (56). Whereas tight glycemic control has shown benefits in reducing mortality in patients with sepsis, it is important always to take into account the dangers of possible episodes of hypoglycemia and its complications, especially in the patient with head injury. In addition, moderate glycemic control between the ranges of 110 and 200 mg/dL have not been studied and this less-strict control may also have the benefits of tighter control with the theoretic decreased risk of causing severe hypoglycemia.

EARLY GOAL-DIRECTED THERAPY

Once the diagnosis of sepsis is made, prompt treatment aimed at specific goals or endpoints has proved of benefit. Patients presenting to emergency rooms often spend hours waiting to be seen by the proper physician, which often results in time spent with ongoing hemodynamic abnormalities and worsening end-organ hypoxia. A study carried out on emergency room patients looked at early treatment of these patients presenting with signs of sepsis or shock. An algorithmic approach was undertaken to guide treatment based on hemodynamic parameters, volume resuscitation, inotropic support, and end-organ perfusion to optimize therapy in the first 6 hours. Patients presenting with signs of sepsis or septic shock were monitored with the use of central venous catheters, blood pressure monitors, and measurement of SVo_2 as a guide to end-organ perfusion. Once sufficient preload was administered in the form of crystalloid to a central venous pressure (CVP) of 8 to 12 mm Hg, the blood pressure then guided therapy. Mean arterial pressures (MAP) of <65 mm Hg were then treated with vasoactive agents (dopamine, norepinephrine, vasopressin, or phenylephrine). SVo_2 was then measured once a MAP of ≥65 mm Hg was reached. SVo_2 of <70% was then treated with administration of packed red blood cells to a hematocrit level of 30%. If SVo_2 remained <70% at this point, inotropic support would be initiated to achieve the desired SVo_2 of ≥70%. If goals of SVo_2 of ≥70% and MAP ≥65 mm Hg were not achieved at this point, therapies to decrease oxygen consumption, in the form of intubation, sedation, analgesics, and control of hyperpyrexia, were undertaken. This algorithmic, stepwise approach within the first 6 hours of presentation significantly reduced mortality by 16% (57).

VASOPRESSIN

Arginine vasopressin (AVP) has been found to be of some benefit in the treatment of septic shock that is unresponsive to other vasopressor medication or in cases of catecholamine-resistant septic shock. Patients with vasodilatory shock that is unresponsive to other agents are thought to have an AVP deficiency (58). In patients with sepsis compared with patients in cardiogenic shock, AVP levels have been shown to be decreased, despite similar hypotension (59). AVP acts directly on V1 receptors of the endothelium to stimulate contraction, thereby reversing the vasodilatory effects of nitric oxide and other inflammatory mediators. Low doses of vasopressin (0.04 U/min) in catecholamine-resistant shock increases systemic blood pressure without increasing pulmonary vascular resistance or pulmonary artery pressure (60). At higher doses, the vasoconstrictive effects of vasopressin have been shown to decrease splanchnic and renal circulation, in addition to decreasing cardiac index, oxygen delivery, and oxygen uptake (61,62).

The use of vasopressin, therefore, has shown benefits in increasing blood pressure and earlier withdrawal of other vasoactive medications in patients with sepsis. However, no long-term survival benefit has been found with its use in sepsis.

CORTICOSTEROIDS

In patients with septic shock who are unresponsive to fluid therapy and vasopressors, adrenal insufficiency should suggest the diagnosis. Originally thought to be the *magic bullet* of sepsis treatment, early studies of high-dose steroids for the treatment of septic shock showed no benefit and worse outcomes secondary to increased infectious complications (63–66). Recent studies have focused on low-dose or physiologic-dose corticosteroid treatment for severe sepsis and septic shock. Whereas patients with septic shock, who are unresponsive to conventional treatments, focusing on fluid resuscitation and pressor therapy have shown some improved survival when adrenal insufficiency or relative adrenal insufficiency has been discovered and treated. In patients not showing evidence of adrenal insufficiency by laboratory testing, however, no survival benefit was shown and, in fact, mortality from this therapy may have increased (67).

Therefore, low-dose corticosteroid treatment for refractory septic shock has shown benefit when patients were found to be adrenal insufficient; however, corticosteroids should not be used in patients without evidence of adrenal insufficiency.

CLINICAL RECOMMENDATIONS OF THE VIGNETTE

The patient has undergone multiple procedures and has had a prolonged ventilator requirement. Whether he classifies as septic or not remains to be seen. That he was doing well, but has had abrupt change in his vital signs and ventilator requirements should prompt a search for a source of infection and treat it accordingly. If the patient requires >1 to 2 L of fluid to correct the hypotension and tachycardia, a central venous line should be inserted, if not already in place, and CVP assessed; further information can also be gathered by using a pulmonary artery catheter. Vasopressors may be needed as a temporary treatment or a *stop gap* while fluids are infusing to keep the blood pressure at an acceptable range. With the need for multiple indwelling catheters, the search for an infected line or urinary tract infection should be addressed and all central venous catheters should be changed and moved to a new site, if still required. The patient's increasing FIO_2 requirements should be investigated with an X-ray study and bronchial lavage performed to rule out pneumonia as a source, while remembering that acute lung injury and ARDS may also present in the same manner. The abdominal examination findings initially were negative. In patients with history of pelvic fixation, however, an intraabdominal source must also be ruled out. Questions should center on what was done during the operation: Was the peritoneum entered? If the patient is unable to say that he has increased abdominal pain or discomfort, then a CT scan should be obtained. Other intraabdominal causes unrelated to the operation must be entertained (e.g., acalculous cholecystitis, ulcer disease, bowel ischemia, retroperitoneal sources, appendicitis).

SUMMARY

Whereas the diagnosis and classification of sepsis remains somewhat cryptic at times, prompt initiation to restore physiologic parameters, along with a high index of suspicion and a complete differential diagnosis is the key to successful management of these complex patients.

REFERENCES

1. Members of the American College of Chest Physicians/Society of Critical Care Medicine Consensus conference Committee: American College of Chest Physicians/Society of Critical Care Medicine Consensus Conference: Definitions for sepsis and organ failure and guidelines for the use of innovative therapies in sepsis. *Crit Care Med.* 1992;20:864–874.
2. Levy MM, Fink MP, Marshall JC, et al. 2001 SCCM/ESICM/ACCP/ATS/SIS International Sepsis Definitions Conference. *Crit Care Med.* 2003;31:1250–1256.
3. Marshall JC, Cook DJ, Chritou NV, et al. Multiple organ dysfunction score: A reliable descriptor of a complex clinical outcome. *Crit Care Med.* 1995;23:1638–1652.
4. Ferreira FL, Bota DP, Bross A, et al. Serial evaluation of the SOFA score to predict outcome in critically ill patients. *JAMA.* 2002;286:1754–1758.
5. Center for Disease Control. Increase in national hospital discharge survey rates for septicemia: United States, 1979–1987. *MMWR Morb Mortal Wkly Rep.* 1990;39:31–34.
6. Rangel-Frausto MS, Pittet D, Costigan M, et al. The natural history of systemic inflammatory response syndrome (SIRS): A prospective study. *JAMA.* 1995;273:117–123.
7. Brun-Buisson C, Doyon F, Carlet J, et al. Incidence, risk factors, and outcome of severe sepsis and septic shock in adults: A multicenter prospective study in intensive care units. *JAMA.* 1995;274:968–974.
8. Salvo I, de Cian W, Musicco M, et al. The Italian SEPSIS study: Preliminary results on the incidence and evolution of SIRS, Sepsis, severe sepsis and septic shock. *Intensive Care Med.* 1995;21:S244–S249.
9. Barriere SL, Lowry SF. An overview of mortality risk prediction in sepsis. *Crit Care Med.* 1995;23:376–393.
10. Rangel-Frausto MS. The epidemiology of bacterial sepsis. *Infect Dis Clin North Am.* 1999; 13:299–312.
11. Opal SM, Cohen J. Clinical Gram-positive sepsis: Does it fundamentally differ from Gram-negative bacterial sepsis? *Crit Care Med.* 1999;27:1608–1616.
12. Mira JP, Cariou A, Grall F, et al. Association of TNF2, a TNF-α promoter polymorphism, with septic shock susceptibility and mortality: A multicenter study. *JAMA.* 1999;282: 561–568.
13. Wichmann MW, Inthorn D, Andress H-J, et al. Incidence and mortality of severe sepsis in surgical intensive care patients: The influence of patient gender on disease process and outcome. *Intensive Care Med.* 2000;26:167–172.
14. Angus DC, Linde-Zwirble WT, Lidicker J, et al. Epidemiology of severe sepsis in the United States: Analysis of incidence, outcome, and associated costs of care. *Crit Care Med.* 2001;29: 1303–1310.
15. Bochud PY, Glauser MP, Calandra T. Antibiotics in sepsis. *Intensive Care Med.* 2001;27[Suppl 1]:S33–S48.
16. Marchetti O, Calandra T. Infections in neutropenic cancer patients. *Lancet.* 2002;359: 723–725.
17. Martin GS, Mannino DM, Eaton S, et al. The epidemiology of sepsis in the United States from 1979 through 2000. *N Engl J Med.* 2003;348:1546–1554.
18. Ognibene FP, Parker MM, Natanson C, et al. Depressed ventricular performance: Response to volume in fusion in patients with sepsis and septic shock. *Chest.* 1988;93:903–910.
19. Suffredini AF, Fromm RE, Parker MM, et al. The cardiovascular response of normal humans to the administration of endotoxin. *N Engl J Med.* 1989;321:280–287.
20. Parker MM, Shelhamer JH, Natanson C, et al. Serial cardiovascular variables in survivors and nonsurvivors of septic shock: Heart rate as an early predictor of prognosis. *Crit Care Med.* 1987;15:923–929.
21. Metrangolo L, Fiorillo M, Friedman G, et al. Early hemodynamic course of septic shock. *Crit Care Med.* 1995;23:1971–1975.
22. James JH, Fang CH, Schrantz SJ, et al. Linkage of aerobic glycolysis to sodium–potassium transport in rat skeletal muscle: Implications for increased muscle lactate production in sepsis. *J Clin Invest.* 1996;98:2388–2397.
23. Kagan BL, Baldwin RL, Munoz D, et al. Formation of ion permeable channels by tumor necrosis factor-alpha. *Science.* 1992;255:1427–1430.
24. Ziegler TR, Smith RJ, O'Dwyer ST, et al. Increased intestinal permeability associated with infection in burn patients. *Arch Surg.* 1988;123:1313–1319.
25. O'Dwyer ST, Mitchie HR, Ziegler TR, et al. A single dose of endotoxin increases intestinal permeability associated with infection in burn patients. *Arch Surg.* 1988;123:1459–1464.
26. Shoemaker WC, Appel PL, Kram HB, et al. Prospective trial of supranormal values of survivors as therapeutic goals in high risk surgical patients. *Chest.* 1988;94:1176–1186.
27. Lundberg JS, Perl TM, Wiblin T, et al. Septic shock: An analysis of outcomes for patients with onset on hospital wards versus intensive care units. *Crit Care Med.* 1998;26:1020–1024.
28. Engoren M. The effect of prompt physician visits on intensive care unit mortality and cost. *Crit Care Med.* 2005;33:727–732.
29. Donnino M, Nguyen H, Jacobsen G, et al. Cryptic septic shock: A sub-analysis of early goal directed therapy. *Chest.* 2003;124:S90.
30. Aduen J, Bernstein WK, Khaastgir T, et al. The use and clinical importance of a substrate specific electrode for rapid determination of blood lactate concentrations. *JAMA.* 1994;272:1678–1685.
31. Shapiro NI, Howell MD, Talmor D, et al. Serum lactate as a predictor of mortality in emergency department patients with infection. *Ann Emerg Med.* 2005;45:524–528.
32. Nguyen HB, Rivers EP, Knoblich BP, et al. Early lactate clearance is associated with improved outcome in severe sepsis and septic shock. *Crit Care Med.* 2004;32:1637–1642.
33. Eachempati SR, Reed RL II, Barie PS. Serum bicarbonate concentration correlates with arterial base deficit in critically ill patients. *Surgical Infections.* 2003;4:193–197.
34. Luzzani A, Polati E, Dorizzi R, et al. Comparison of procalcitonin and C reactive protein as markers of sepsis. *Crit Care Med.* 2003;31:1737–1741.
35. de Werra I, Jaccard C, Corradin SB, et al. Cytokines, nitrite/nitrate, soluble tumor necrosis factor receptors, and procalcitonin concentrations: Comparisons in patients with septic shock, cardiogenic shock, and bacterial pneumonia. *Crit Care Med.* 1997;25:607–613.
36. van Langevelde P, Joop K, van Loon J, et al. Endotoxin, cytokines, and procalcitonin in febrile patients admitted to the hospital: Identification of patients at high risk of mortality. *Clin Infect Dis.* 2000;31:1343–1348.
37. Marshall JC, Foster B, Vincent JL, et al. Diagnostic and prognostic implications of endotoxemia in critical illness: Results of the MEDIC study. *J Infect Dis.* 2004;190:527–534.
38. Sprung CL, Peduzzi PN, Shatney CH, et al. Impact of encephalopathy on mortality in the sepsis syndrome. *Crit Care Med.* 1990;18:474–479.
39. Pine RW, Wertz MJ, Lennard ES, et al. Determinants of organ malfunction or death in patients with intra-abdominal sepsis. *Arch Surg.* 1983;118:242–249.
40. Huynh HK, Dorovini-Zis K. Effects of interferon-gamma on primary cultures of human brain microvessel endothelial cells. *Am J Pathol.* 1993;142:1265–1278.
41. Bowton DL, Bertels NH, Prough DS, et al. Cerebral blood flow is reduced in patients with sepsis syndrome. *Crit Care Med.* 1989;17:399–403.
42. Maekawa T, Fujii Y, Sadamitsu D, et al. Cerebral circulation and metabolism in patients with septic encephalopathy. *Am J Emerg Med.* 1991;9:139–143.
43. Landis DMD. Brain as a tissue: The interacting cell populations of the central nervous system. In: Ransohoff RM, Benveniste EN, Eds. *Cytokines and the CNS.* Boca Raton: CRC Press; 1996:63–83.
44. Paulson OB, Newman EA. Does the release of potassium ions from astrocyte endfeet regulate cerebral blood flow? *Science.* 1987;237:896–898.
45. Tsacopoulos M, Magistretti PJ. Metabolic coupling between glia and neurons. *J Neurosci.* 1996;16:877–885.
46. Janzer RC, Raff MC. Astrocytes induce blood–brain barrier properties in endothelial cells. *Nature.* 1987;325:253–257.
47. Freund H, Atamian S, Holroyd J, et al. Plasma amino acids as predictors of the severity and outcome of sepsis. *Ann Surg.* 1979;190:571–576.
48. Maupin RT. Obstetric infectious disease emergencies. *Clin Obstet Gynecol.* 2002;45:393–404.
49. Stamler J, Horowitz SF, Goldman ME, et al. Peripartum cardiomyopathy: A role for cardiac stress determinants other than pregnancy? *Mt Sinai J Med.* 1989;56:285–289.
50. Clark SL, Cotton DB, Lee W, et al. Central hemodynamic assessment of normal term pregnancy. *Am J Obstet Gynecol.* 1989;161:1439–1442.

51. Danai PA, Moss M, Mannino DM, et al. The epidemiology of sepsis in patients with malignancy. *Chest.* 2006;129:1432–1440.
52. Bernard GR, Vincent JL, Laterre PF, et al. Efficacy and safety of recombinant human activated protein C for severe sepsis. *N Engl J Med.* 2001;344:699–709.
53. Abraham E, Laterre PF, Garg R, et al. Drotrecogin alfa (activated) for adults with severe sepsis and a low risk of death. *N Engl J Med.* 2005;353:1332–1341.
54. Warren BL, Eid A, Singer P, et al. Caring for the critically ill patient: High dose antithrombin III in severe sepsis–a randomized controlled trial. *JAMA.* 2001;286:1869–1878.
55. Van Den Berghe G, Wouters P, Weekers F, et al. Intensive insulin therapy in critically ill patients. *N Engl J Med.* 2001;345:1359–1367.
56. Van Den Berghe G, Wilmer A, Hermans G, et al. Intensive insulin therapy in the medical ICU. *N Engl J Med.* 2006;449–461.
57. Rivers E, Nguyen B, Havstad S, et al. Early goal directed therapy in the treatment of severe sepsis and septic shock. *N Engl J Med.* 2001;345:1368–1377.
58. Reid IA. Role of vasopressin deficiency in the vasodilatation of septic shock. *Circulation.* 1997;95:1108–1110.
59. Landry DW, Levin HR, Gallant EM, et al. Vasopressin deficiency contributes to the vasodilation of septic shock. *Circulation.* 1997;95:1122–1125.
60. Tsuneyoshi I, Yamada H, Kakihana Y, et al. Hemodynamic and metabolic effects of low-dose vasopressin infusions in vasodilatory septic shock. *Crit Care Med.* 2001;29:487–493.
61. Malay MB, Ashton JL, Dahl K, et al. Heterogeneity of the vasoconstrictor effect of vasopressin in septic shock. *Crit Care Med.* 2004;32:327–331.
62. Klinzing S, Simon M, Reinhart K, et al. High–dose vasopressin is not superior to norepinephrine in septic shock. *Crit Care Med.* 2003;31:2646–2650.
63. Cronin L, Cook DJ, Carlet J, et al. Corticosteroid treatment for sepsis: A critical appraisal and meta-analysis of the literature. *Crit Care Med.* 1995;23:1430–1439.
64. Lefering R, Neugebauer EA. Steroid controversy in sepsis and septic shock: A meta-analysis. *Crit Care Med.* 1995;23:1294–1303.
65. Bone RC, Fisher CJ, Clemmer TP, et al. A controlled clinical trial of high-dose methylprednisolone in the treatment of severe sepsis and septic shock. *N Engl J Med.* 1987; 317:653–658.
66. Sprung Cl, Caralis PV, Marcial EH, et al. The effects of high-dose corticosteroids in patients with septic shock: A prospective, controlled study. *N Engl J Med.* 1984;311:1137–1143.
67. Annane D, Sebille V, Charpentier C, et al. Effect of treatment with low doses of hydrocortisone and fludrocortisone on mortality in patients with septic shock. *JAMA.* 2002;288: 862–871.

CHAPTER 129

Mechanical Ventilation

Bruce Kleinman • Kere Frey

OBJECTIVES

- To discuss the situations that require mechanical ventilation
- To describe the physiologic consequences of mechanical ventilation
- To explain the parameters defining a positive pressure breath
- To describe the modes of ventilation
- To explore application of the above concepts to those patients with critical neurologic disease.

CASE VIGNETTE

A 32-year-old woman is brought into the emergency room (ER) unconscious. A family member reports that just before becoming unconscious, she complained of double vision and the worst headache of her life. Presently, her respiratory rate (RR) is 34 breaths per minute. She has bibasilar rales. A recent arterial blood gas on a non-rebreather oxygen mask shows a pH of 7.50, PCO_2 of 28 mm Hg, and PO_2 of 52 mm Hg.

INTRODUCTION

The principles of ventilatory support can be broadly applied to any patient in ventilatory failure, irrespective of the patient's underlying disease process. Patients with neurologic disease, in either acute ventilatory failure or impending ventilatory failure who require mechanical ventilation, however, need special considerations. Along these lines, it is important to remember that mechanical ventilators can do only three things. They can (*a*) provide the power to breathe, (*b*) can manipulate the breathing pattern, and (*c*) control the airway pressure.

DEFINITION AND BASIC PRINCIPLES

Although patients can be ventilated without an endotracheal tube, most patients in need of mechanical ventilatory support will need tracheal intubation. There are four reasons for tracheal intubation in the critical care unit (1).

1. Ventilation
2. Tracheal bronchial toilet
3. Airway obstruction
4. Airway protection

Ventilation, in regard to a patient, refers to one who needs to have his or her breathing supported or assisted with mechanical ventilation; for instance, a patient with an acute lung injury (ALI) or acute respiratory distress syndrome (ARDS). Tracheal bronchial toilet refers to a procedure used for patient who cannot cough up secretions, but who may be breathing spontaneously. A prototypal example would be a patient who has just had a stroke. An endotracheal tube allows the nurse to safely pass a suction catheter into the trachea and give supplemental oxygen before and after each catheter pass. A child with acute epiglottitis best exemplifies airway obstruction. Passage of a tracheal tube is a life-saving event. Finally, airway protection refers to that used in a patient who is at risk for pulmonary aspiration of gastric contents. A cuffed tracheal tube, although not providing a perfect seal, will protect the patient from aspiration of large particulate matter. The classic example is the patient presenting to the ER with an altered level of alertness from an intracranial hemorrhage. While that patient may be breathing, he or she is at risk for pulmonary aspiration of gastric contents.

Likewise, three reasons exist for instituting mechanical ventilation in the critical care unit (1). They are as follows:

1. Apnea
2. Acute ventilatory failure
3. Impending ventilatory failure

Apnea is self-evident for the need for mechanical ventilation. Patient who are apneic are not breathing. Acute ventilatory failure, also known as *acute respiratory acidosis*, is defined as an acutely decreasing pH in the presence of increasing PCO_2. In this regard, it is important to understand that ventilation is always defined in terms of PCO_2: A high PCO_2 is defined as *hypoventilation*; a low PCO_2 is defined as *hyperventilation*. If the underlying cause cannot be quickly reversed then, the patient will die from an acute respiratory acidosis. Finally, impending ventilatory failure is a clinical judgment. The patient, in fact, may have an alkalemia, but be diaphoretic, tachypneic, and tachycardic. This is frequently how patients with ALI or ARDS present. A clinical judgment must be made whether to institute mechanical ventilation and to electively relieve the work of breathing now, rather than emergently later, either because of acute ventilatory failure or cardiopulmonary arrest. Some include hypoxemia as an indication for the initiation of mechanical ventilatory support. We do not for the following reasons. First, the practitioner can treat hypoxemia with oxygen therapy. Second, those patients with refractory hypoxemia will often have acute restrictive lung disease, such as ALI or ARDS. The work of breathing in these disease states is so high such that these patients will meet the criteria for impending ventilatory failure. Hence, in the reason for instituting mechanical ventilation is impending ventilatory failure and not necessarily hypoxemia.

When thinking about instituting mechanical ventilatory support, consider the following three phases (2).

1. Commitment
2. Maintenance
3. Discontinuance (or weaning)

Commitment occurs when the decision is made to institute mechanical ventilation. Typically, this will involve tracheal intubation followed by positive pressure ventilation. It is important to anticipate potential hemodynamic instability caused by medications used to secure the airway. Virtually all short-acting anesthetics used for sedation are potent vasodilators. Additional consideration includes that positive pressure ventilation will often decrease venous return. Therefore, it is important to be prepared for profound hypotension and ready to volume resuscitate or administer vasopressors as needed through appropriate intravenous access. Once the patient is hemodynamically stable and mechanically ventilated, the maintenance phase begins. This phase involves administering sedation and an appropriate mode of ventilation (see *Modes of Ventilation*). Acute discontinuation of mechanical ventilation is reasonable when indications for assisted ventilation are no longer present. Very ill patients who recover from an insult that required prolonged ventilatory support may not be able to have their mechanical ventilation acutely discontinued, however, because of nutritional deficits, respiratory muscle weakness or discoordination. These patients will have to have classic weaning trials (3).

VENTILATORS

Today, one type of ventilator is typically available in the intensive care setting that functions with high-generated pressures and, therefore, can deliver a constant tidal volume at variable airway pressures. These volume-limited (or volume-preset) machines permit adjustment (through dials on the control panel) such that the machine can function as a pressure generator. The ventilator will then deliver breaths at constant airway pressure, but variable tidal volume (pressure limited or pressure preset).

COMPRESSION VOLUME

If a positive pressure breath is volume limited (volume preset), the *effective* tidal volume is determined by the relative compliance of the patient's lungs. The compliance of the ventilator circuit tubing is usually 3 mL/cm H_2O of airway pressure. For example, if the peak airway pressure is 20 cm H_2O, and the tidal volume is 1,000 mL, 960 mL is delivered to the patient's lungs and 40 mL is compressed or trapped in the machine circuit. If the patient's lungs become stiff (ARDS) and proximal airway pressure increases to 100 cm H_2O, then 700 mL is delivered to the patient's lungs and 300 mL is compressed in the ventilator circuit. Because the tidal volume is usually measured on the expiratory side of the circuit, under both conditions, the tidal volume reading will be 1,000 mL, although the effective tidal volume differs significantly between the two conditions.

CLASSIFICATION OF POSITIVE PRESSURE BREATHS

Different parameters are used to describe any positive pressure breath (4). The first parameter describes who or what initiates or triggers the positive pressure breath. If the patient initiates or triggers the positive pressure, then the breath is called *an assisted breath.* If time initiates or triggers the positive pressure breath, then the breath is called a *control breath.* Assisted breaths are initiated by the ventilator sensing changes in airway pressure or flow. Mandatory ventilator breaths or control breaths are initiated or triggered by time (i.e., if the respiratory rate is set at 10, that means a mandatory positive pressure breath will be initiated every 6 seconds). If the patient or the ventilator can initiate a breath, then an assist control breath ensues. In summary, assisted breaths are initiated by changes in pressure (P) or flow (F). Control breaths are initiated by time (T).

The second parameter describes what is constant or limited. This is usually pressure (P), volume (V), or flow (F).

The third parameter describes how the positive pressure breath is terminated or cycled. Cycling is either by volume (V), time (T), pressure (P), or flow (F). Therefore, V, T, P, F, or any combination thereof can stipulate this parameter.

The last, or fourth, parameter signifies whether the ventilator permits unassisted spontaneous breathing (either between positive pressure breaths or during positive pressure breaths). This is either Y for yes or O for no. For example, a positive pressure breath in pressure control mode would be described as control, pressure limited, time-cycled, with no allowance for unassisted spontaneous breathing (T-P-T-O). During pressure support mode, the same breath would be described as assist, pressure-limited, flow-cycled, with no allowance for unassisted spontaneous breathing (P-P-F-O).

MODES OF VENTILATION

Volume Control

Historically, volume is one of the first modes of ventilation. Typically, a time trigger initiates the tidal volume; hence, the machine initiates the breath; this, by definition, is control. Because the patient cannot breathe spontaneously, no circuit exists to permit unassisted, spontaneous ventilation and neuromuscular blockers have often been used. The positive pressure breath is volume limited (fixed tidal volumes, variable airway pressures), and either time or volume cycled (T-V-TV-O) (Fig. 129-1A).

Assist Control

If a patient could not breathe spontaneously during classic volume control mode, he or she had to be heavily sedated and often paralyzed with neuromuscular blockers. This led to the development of machines known as *assistors,* where the positive pressure breath could be triggered or initiated by the patient's spontaneous breath. Typically, the positive pressure breath was

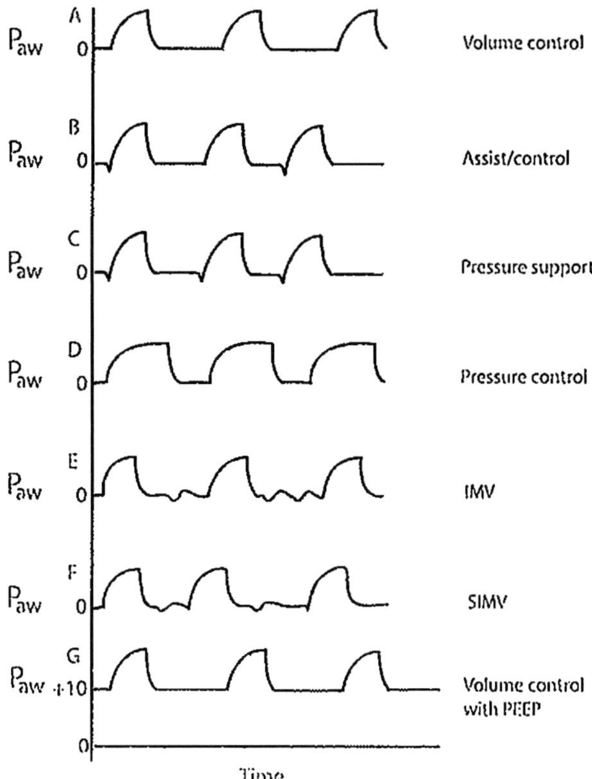

FIGURE 129-1. Airway pressure tracings (Paw) vs. time during common modes of ventilatory support. See text for details.

volume limited (hence, airway pressures were variable) and time or volume cycled. A time trigger would ensure that a minimal respiratory rate would be delivered if the patient became apneic. These time-triggered breaths are *controlled breaths*, hence the designation *assist control* (PFT-V-VT-O) (Fig. 129-1B).

Pressure Support

Pressure support is an assist mode. A positive pressure breath is delivered each time the patient spontaneously breathes. Tidal volumes vary, depending whether the patient takes a *deep* or *shallow* breath, but airway pressures are constant. Inspiration ends when a preset flow rate is reached—pressure initiated, pressure limited, flow cycled. This mode can be used to overcome the resistive work of breathing inherent in the ventilator circuit and endotracheal tube or it can be used to provide full ventilatory support. This is an assist mode, however; if the patient stops breathing, no backup control mode (P-P-F-O) exists (Fig. 129-1C).

Pressure Control

Pressure control is analogous to volume control, except that the positive pressure breath is pressure limited (tidal volumes vary, airway pressures are constant) and time cycled—time initiated, pressure limited, time cycled. No allowance exists for unassisted, spontaneous breathing. A possible advantage in using this mode is the ability to limit the amount of airway pressure and, therefore, limit potential barotrauma (T-P-T-O) (Fig. 129-1D).

Intermittent Mandatory Ventilation

Because advantages to spontaneous breathing (see next section) exist, anesthesiologists designed ventilatory circuits that permitted patients to breathe spontaneously if they chose to do so. The intermittent mandatory ventilation (IMV) circuit was essentially a parallel breathing circuit to the ventilator from which the patient could breathe spontaneously unassisted. A positive pressure breath from a ventilator with an IMV circuit was typically time initiated (i.e., control), volume limited, and volume or time cycled. This mode has largely been replaced by SIMV (T-V-VT-Y) (Fig. 129-1E).

Synchronized Intermittent Mandatory Ventilation

The synchronized intermittent mandatory ventilation (SIMV) (5) mode was designed to permit the patient to breathe spontaneously and also allow the positive pressure breath to be delivered in a coordinated fashion with the patient's spontaneous breath. Because positive pressure breaths in the IMV mode were not *coordinated* or *synchronized* with the patient's spontaneous breath, physicians believed certain undesirable physiologic effects might occur. Among these, was *breath stacking*: The positive pressure breath occurs when the patient has already taken a maximal spontaneous breath. Whereas classic assist control delivers a positive pressure breath with every spontaneous effort, SIMV would limit the delivered positive pressure breath to a specific timing window. In this window, a spontaneous breath would trigger a positive pressure breath (just as in assist) and if the spontaneous breath did not occur, then a mandatory controlled positive pressure breath would be delivered (just as in control). Outside the timing window, the patient breathes in an unassisted spontaneous manner. Positive pressure breaths in SIMV are time (control), pressure, or flow (assist) initiated; volume limited, volume or time cycled, with provision for unassisted spontaneous breathing (TPF-V-VT-Y) (Fig. 129-1F).

Contemporary ventilators expand on the historical designation of the above modes of ventilation. For instance, assist control, historically involved volume-limited ventilation. Assist control can now be delivered with pressure-limited ventilation—pressure, flow, time initiated (assist control), pressure limited, and time cycled. Likewise SIMV, which historically was volume limited can also now be pressure limited—pressure, flow, time initiated, pressure limited, and time cycled.

POSITIVE END-EXPIRATORY PRESSURE AND CONTINUOUS POSITIVE AIRWAY PRESSURE

Historically, positive end expiratory pressure (PEEP) was used with patients receiving full ventilatory support from volume control ventilation (Fig. 129-1G). PEEP increases the functional residual capacity and, therefore, is particularly useful in patients with acute restrictive lung disease such as ARDS. The benefit of PEEP in these situations is to improve PaO_2 and, therefore, decrease the required FIO_2. Also, potential deleterious effects exist, such as decreased cardiac output and decreased total oxygen delivery, alveolar overdistention, and increased intracranial pressure (ICP). The optimal *dose* of PEEP is subject to much speculation. Levels of PEEP have ranged from 5 cm H_2O to as high as 50 cm H_2O, the so-called *super PEEP.* Only recently completed large, randomized trials have suggested that no difference is seen in outcome in patients with ARDS receiving low PEEP (8 cm H_2O) versus high PEEP (13 cm H_2O) (6). Applying PEEP to spontaneously breathing patients is known as continuous positive airway pressure CPAP.

PHYSIOLOGIC EFFECTS OF POSITIVE PRESSURE BREATHING

Positive pressure breathing typically decreases cardiac output (by decreasing venous return) and increases dead space ventilation (7–9). These disadvantages of positive pressure breathing have led to the increased use of modes of ventilation that enable patients to breathe spontaneously—intermittent mandatory ventilation (IMV) and synchronized intermittent mandatory ventilation (SIMV)—and reap the benefits of unassisted spontaneous breathing.

Large Tidal Volumes Versus Small Tidal Volumes

As stated, positive pressure breathing is associated with physiologic imbalances. These adverse consequences of positive pressure breathing have led to practices designed to limit positive pressure ventilation. The first strategy was to permit the patient to do some of the spontaneous work of breathing (by utilizing IMV or SIMV circuits). The second strategy was to use relatively low ventilator rates. To provide the appropriate minute ventilation—as well as the appropriate alveolar ventilation—large tidal volumes (twice normal) were used (i.e., 12 mL/kg). The concern with using large tidal volumes, particularly in the face of acute lung injury, was whether this approach resulted in an increase in barotrauma and volutrauma. After much controversy and inconclusive small studies, a large cooperative study showed a 9% absolute decrease in mortality (31% versus 40%) in those patients ventilated with low tidal volumes (6 mL/kg) at low airway pressures (plateau pressure <30 cm/H_2O versus those ventilated with large tidal volumes of 12 mL/kg (10). Both groups were ventilated in the assist control mode.

Fraction of Inspired Oxygen—the FIO_2

The FIO_2 is typically adjusted to maintain oxygen saturation of 90% or above. In patients with primary lung injuries, such as those with ALI or ARDS, high FIO_2 are toxic (11). Therefore, it is important to try to keep the FIO_2 at 0.5 or less. This can be accomplished by the judicious use of PEEP.

CONCERNS IN THE PATIENT WITH NEUROLOGIC DISEASE

Patients with acute cerebrovascular events, for instance aneurysmal subarachnoid hemorrhage (SAH), or acute head trauma, may need tracheal intubation and ventilatory support because of acute or impending ventilatory failure. With acute ventilatory failure, the acutely increasing PCO_2 can cause cerebral vasodilatation and thereby lead to increased ICP and decreased cerebral perfusion.

Patients in impending ventilatory failure may be alkalemic and hyperventilating. Ventilatory support is indicated to electively relieve the high work of breathing in these patients (12). Hopes are that this early intervention will prevent a cardiopulmonary arrest.

MANAGING ACUTE LUNG INJURY IN PATIENTS WITH ACUTE NEUROLOGIC DISEASE

Some patients with acute intracerebral events may be in pulmonary edema. The therapeutic goal is to augment oxygen delivery to the brain by maintaining cardiac output, cerebral perfusion pressure, and oxygenation. Initiation of ventilatory support is frequently associated with a decrease in cardiac output. This decrease in cardiac output is largely caused by a decrease in venous return. Administering a fluid bolus, using vasoconstrictors, or both can counter this. If cerebral autoregulation is still present, which may not be so in severe brain injures, avoiding severe hypotension and reducing increased ICP by using hyperventilation can maintain perfusion pressure. Hyperventilation will transiently reduce elevated ICP. The lower PCO_2 will cause cerebral vasoconstriction, thereby decreasing intracerebral volume and, thereby, ICP as well. Too much hyperventilation can cause too much vasoconstriction, thereby decreasing brain perfusion. This ventilatory strategy is based on the fact that the injured brain may still be CO_2 responsive. In addition, no study has shown that hyperventilation in this setting improves outcome (13). Even less evidence or rationale supports the use of prolonged hyperventilation (13). After approximately 4 to 6 hours, the pH of the cerebral spinal fluid normalizes (by decreasing bicarbonate), so that a vasoconstriction response to continued hyperventilation will not occur. Therefore, in general, the goal of prolonged ventilatory support should be to maintain eucapnia.

Frequently, because of the associated ALI, many patients with acute neurologic injury will be hypoxemic. In these situations, PEEP use may be indicated. The concern in these patients as opposed to patients with ALI in the absence of an acute intracerebral process is that some of the PEEP can be transmitted to the cranium, thereby increasing ICP and decreasing cerebral perfusion. As the lungs become more and more noncompliant in the setting of ALI, less and less of the PEEP is transmitted to the vascular space and the brain. PEEP has been used in patients with acute brain injury without adverse effect (14). ICP monitoring might be required in those patients with brain injury who require levels of PEEP >15 cm/H_2O.

CLINICAL RECOMMENDATIONS OF THE VIGNETTE

The patient has had a catastrophic neurologic event, likely a SAH. The rales and the hypoxemia suggest pulmonary edema, probably neurogenic in origin. This is not an uncommon finding in patients with a subarachnoid bleed. The pulmonary edema is caused by the enormous catecholamine discharge that accompanies these catastrophic events, leading to postalveolar capillary vasoconstriction and, therefore, very high alveolar capillary pressures. This patient needs to be intubated and mechanically ventilated. The reason for mechanical ventilation is impending ventilatory failure. The patient's blood pH is alkalemic. This is not an uncommon finding in patients with ALI or ARDS from any cause. By definition, she is hyperventilating. Given the pulmonary edema (which would cause decreased lung compliance) and that her respiratory rate is high, clinical judgment is that her oxygen cost of breathing is also high. From a teleologic viewpoint, patients with acutely stiff lungs try to minimize the work of breathing by breathing at low tidal volumes (and thereby minimize transpulmonary pressures), but at high rates. Given the case scenario, if allowed to continue to breathe as she is doing, she will eventually develop acute ventilatory failure or cardiopulmonary arrest. Therefore, clinical judgment is to intervene early and electively relieve the work of breathing. Once the patient is committed to mechanical ventilation, an assist control mode of ventilation is recommended.

The four reasons for this recommendation are as follows. First, this mode would still permit spontaneous efforts by the patient, yet provide almost full ventilatory support—spontaneous breathing via an SIMV mode might result in too high a work of breathing in a patient such as this. Two, this mode would obviate the need for neuromuscular blockers and their subsequent adverse consequences. Three, the classic assist control mode would ensure constant tidal volumes (albeit at variable airway pressures). And finally, assist control was the mode used in the largest study showing the benefit of small tidal volumes versus large tidal volumes in patients with ALI and ARDS. Specifically, we would set tidal volumes at 6 mL/kg and keep plateau pressures <30 cm/H_2O. An attempt should be made to raise the PO_2 by the judicious use of PEEP and lower the FIO_2 if possible to 0.5 or less. If arterial blood pressure is maintained (either by volume administration or vasoactive medications), then PEEP in the range of 8 to 13 cm/H_2O can be safely used without monitoring ICP. If the patient remains alkalemic, recommendation is to use sedatives (i.e., morphine) to decrease her respiratory drive and strive for eucapnic ventilation.

SUMMARY

The numerous individual clinical entities requiring mechanical ventilatory support can be divided into three broad categories. Mechanical ventilation has profound benefits, but is also accompanied by profound pathophysiologic consequences. Three parameters are necessary to define a positive pressure breath. Once these parameters are understood, the common modes of ventilation are easily understood as well. Finally, these principles can be applied to the patient who is in impending ventilatory failure secondary to a major intracranial bleed.

REFERENCES

1. Shapiro BA, Harrison RA, Walton JR. *Clinical Application of Blood Gases,* 2nd ed. Chicago: Year Book Medical Publishers; 1977:213–218.
2. Shapiro BA, Harrison RA, Trout CA. *Clinical Application of Respiratory Care,* 2nd ed. Chicago: Year Book Medical Publishers; 1979:239–241.
3. Andrés Esteban A, Frutos F, Tobin MJ, et al., for The Spanish Lung Failure Collaborative Group. A comparison of four methods of weaning patients from mechanical ventilation. *N Engl J Med.* 1995;332:345–350.
4. Shapiro BA. A historical perspective on ventilator management. *New Horizons.* 1994;2: 8–18.
5. Shapiro BA, Harrison RA, WaltonRJ. Intermittent demand ventilation (IDV): A new technique for supporting ventilation in critically ill patients. *Respir Care.* 1976;21:521–525.
6. The National Heart, Lung, and Blood Institute ARDS Clinical Trials Network. Higher versus lower positive end-expiratory pressures in patients with the acute respiratory distress syndrome. *N Engl J Med.* 2004;351:327–336.
7. Cournand A, Motley HL,Werko L, et al. Physiological studies of the effects of intermittent positive pressure breathing on cardiac output in man. *Am J Physiol.* 1948:152:162–174.
8. Watson WE. Observations on physiologic dead space during intermittent positive pressure respirations. *Br J Anaesth.* 1962;34:502–508.
9. Froese AB, Bryan A. Effects of anesthesia and paralysis on diaphragmatic mechanics in man. *Anesthesiology.* 1974;41:242–255.
10. The Acute Respiratory Distress Syndrome Network. Ventilation with lower tidal volumes as compared with traditional tidal volumes for acute lung injury and the acute respiratory distress syndrome. *N Engl J Med.* 2000;324:1301–1308.
11. Witschi HR, Haaschek WM, Klein-Szanto AJ. Potentiation of diffuse lung damage by oxygen: Determining variables. *Am Rev Respir Dis.* 1981;123:98–103.
12. Tobin MJ. Advances in mechanical ventilation. *N Engl J Med.* 2001;344:1986–1995.
13. Brian JE. Carbon dioxide and the cerebral circulation. *Anesthesiology.* 1998;88(5): 1365–1386.
14. Georgiadis D, Schwarz S, Baumgartner RW, et al. Influence of positive end-expiratory pressure on intracranial pressure and cerebral perfusion pressure in patients with acute stroke. *Stroke.* 2001;32:2088–2092.

CHAPTER **130**

Acid–Base Disorders

Carol R. Schermer • Ellen C. Omi

OBJECTIVES

- To discuss the mechanisms of acid–base balance
- To discuss the categories of acid–base disturbances, their causes and treatment
- To explore how to recognize and diagnose simple and mixed acid–base disorders

CASE VIGNETTE

A 28-year-old man with a history of juvenile (type I) diabetes mellitus was brought to the emergency department by ambulance because he was experiencing lethargy, vomiting, and tachycardia. His mother who is with him, states that he has not been feeling well for the last 24 hours. He has been home from work with a fever and a productive cough. Physical examination demonstrates a young thin man who is arousable, but lethargic. He is able to follow some commands and answer simple questions, but his speech is slurred. The patient has no lateralizing neurologic deficits. His breath smells of fruit and his mucous membranes are dry. Laboratory examination shows a white blood count (WBC) of 16,000, sodium 132 mEq/L, potassium 4.7 mEq/L, chloride 96 mEq/L, bicarbonate 11 mEq/L, glucose of 520 mg/dL, and arterial pH of 7.21. Urinalysis reveals large amount of ketones. Chest radiograph demonstrates a right lower lobe infiltrate.

DEFINITION

Homeostasis is determined by the plasma pH. Normal plasma pH is 7.40, but can range from 7.35 to 7.45. The pH in plasma is determined by the amount of CO_2 and bicarbonate dissolved in it. *Acidemia* is defined as a plasma pH <7.35 (or a hydrogen ion concentration above the normal range of 36 to 44 nmol/L). *Alkalemia* is defined as a plasma pH >7.45 (or a hydrogen ion concentration below the normal range of 36 to 44 nmol/L). The suffix *osis* refers to a primary disorder that would result in acidemia or alkalemia if uncompensated.

A number of processes occur in the intensive care unit (ICU) that both cause an acid–base disorder and alter the patient's ability to cope with acid–base disorders. The metabolic composition of the body can have drastic effects on the function of the central nervous system (CNS). This is a logical interaction, because the CNS relies on the flux of ions through specialized channels on the cell membrane for conduction of nerve impulses, release of hormones, and autoregulation of the environment in which it exists. In contrast, the CNS can contribute to the acid–base disturbance or compensation seen in patients by altering the buffering system of the body in the form of the respiratory drive and hormonal regulation.

EPIDEMIOLOGY

Acid–base disorders in the hospitalized patient, and especially the critically ill patient, are very common and are usually the result of the severity of some underlying illness causing the patient to seek medical care. Because acid–base disorders are not primary diagnoses, but result from underlying illnesses and pathology, it is impossible to quantify their epidemiology. The incidence of the effects of acid–base disorders on the neurologic status of patients has not been quantified, but they are associated with nearly all critical illnesses that require ICU admission. The presence of severe acid–base disorders can be predictive of patient outcomes and severity of disease.

ETIOLOGY, PATHOGENESIS, AND PATHOPHYSIOLOGY

In the ICU, underlying disorders are more likely to cause metabolic acid–base disorders than they are to cause respiratory disorders. In general, metabolic acidosis is caused by a gain of acids above their excretion rate or loss of bicarbonate faster than its rate of regeneration. Acid–base disorders can be thought of as either too much acid or base going in (poisonings), too much being generated (ketones and lactate), too much base being excreted (diarrhea), or too little being excreted (renal mechanisms). Metabolic acidoses are generally caused by a generation of organic anions (lactate and ketones), loss of cations (e.g., diarrhea), or an abnormal handling of ions within the kidney. Acid handling by the kidney is mostly mediated through chloride balance. Bicarbonate represents 75% to 80% of the extracellular buffering capacity. The extra hydrogen ions can also combine with phosphate, serum proteins, and hemoglobin.

The major homeostatic mechanism of acid–base control is the carbonic acid–bicarbonate buffering system. This is accomplished by the lungs, via CO_2 elimination, and the kidneys, with the conservation of bicarbonate and excretion of hydrogen ion. Although in the human body many compounds affect acid–base status (e.g., phosphoric acid, proteins, and amino acids), the carbonic acid–bicarbonate buffering system is most commonly used because it is easy to measure and accounts for 80% of buffering capacity. In general, the body makes approximately 1 mEq/Kg/day of acid, primarily from metabolism leading to production of sulfuric acid, phosphoric acid, and other organic acids. To maintain acid–base equilibrium, the body must excrete the endogenously produced or exogenously administered acid, minus any exogenously administered base. This is primarily accomplished by renal excretion of fixed acids in the form of phosphates and ammonia. The kidney can directly influence acid excretion by three mechanisms: excretion of phosphate, synthesis of ammonia, and control of bicarbonate directional flow. Hydrogen ions are excreted via both acceptance by phosphate and ammonia functioning as proton acceptors. The carbonic anhydrase system results in generation of hydrogen and bicarbonate from CO_2 and results in reabsorption of bicarbonate to regenerate the bicarbonate pool and excretion of hydrogen ion.

CLINICAL MANIFESTATIONS

Abnormalities of acid–base status affect how well oxygen is delivered and how well the heart and blood vessels respond to vasopressor medications. Compensation for a metabolic acidosis can cause such profound minute ventilation requirements that respiratory failure may ensue. Certain clinical settings in the ICU are commonly associated with mixed acid–base disorders, including cardiorespiratory arrest, sepsis, drug intoxications, diabetes, and organ failure. The therapy of mixed acid–base disorders, however, is similar to simple acid–base disorders in that it is aimed at reversing the etiologic components.

RESPIRATORY ACIDOSIS AND ALKALOSIS

Respiratory alkalosis, a very common acid–base disturbance, results from alveolar ventilation in excess of CO_2 production. This is usually due to some form of central nervous system overstimulation. Table 130-1 lists common respiratory acidoses and alkaloses. Treatment is directed at correcting the underlying disease.

A reduction in the arterial partial pressure of CO_2 leads to a rapid reduction in cerebral blood flow (CBF). Despite continuing hypocapnia, however, secondary recovery of CBF occurs over time as a result of increases in lactic acid production. Hypocapnia reduces intracranial pressure (ICP) and has been used by clinicians during treatment of acute traumatic brain injury, acute intracranial hemorrhage, and acutely expanding brain tumors or other intracranial space-occupying lesions.

Hyperventilation lowers ICP by the induction of cerebral vasoconstriction, with a subsequent decrease in cerebral blood volume. The downside of hyperventilation, however, is that cerebral vasoconstriction can decrease cerebral blood flow to ischemic levels. Because of this risk-to-benefit relationship, hyperventilation should be considered only in patients with raised ICP under specific monitoring conditions and for very short periods of time. Controversy exists on specific indications, timing, depth, and duration of hypocapnia.

In addition, profound alkalemia can impair oxygen delivery because of stronger hemoglobin-oxygen affinity, vasoconstriction, and alterations in the redox potential of cytochrome c. Increased oxygen demands ($\dot{V}O_2$), for example during physical activity, results in a rapid compensatory increase in cardiac output and redistribution of blood flow to the appropriate skeletal muscles. These cardiovascular changes are matched by suitable ventilatory increments.

ANION GAP ACIDOSIS

Anion gap acidoses (Table 130-2) result from unmeasured anions. Unmeasured anions can be *organic*: lactate, keto acids, albumin; *inorganic*: phosphate, sulfate; *exogenous*: salicylate, formate, nitrate, penicillins, and *others*: paraldehyde, acetate, ethylene glycol, methanol, salicylates, urea, and glucose. For a simple anion gap metabolic acidosis, the increment in the anion gap, defined as the *delta gap*, should equal the decrement in the bicarbonate, defined as the *delta bicarbonate*. When the delta bicarbonate is greater than the delta gap, a mixed high anion gap and hyperchloremic acidosis is present. When the delta HCO_3 is less than the delta gap, a mixed metabolic alkalosis and acidosis is often present.

Lactic acidoses caused by decreased oxygen delivery or defective oxygen utilization are associated with high mortality. The treatment of lactic acidosis is controversial. The use of bicarbonate to increase pH is rarely successful and, by generating PCO_2, it may worsen outcome. Ketoacidosis is usually secondary to diabetes or alcohol. Treatment is aimed at turning off ketogenesis and repairing fluid and electrolyte

TABLE 130-1. Common Causes of Respiratory Acid–Base Disorders

Respiratory Acidosis	*Respiratory Alkalosis*
Airway obstruction	Anxiety
Respiratory center depression (e.g., narcotics)	Fever
Neuromuscular defects	Salicylate intoxication
Restrictive lung diseases	Central nervous system (CNS) disorders
Smoke inhalation	Hypoxemia
Inadequate mechanical ventilation	Hepatic insufficiency
	Gram-negative sepsis
	Pregnancy
	Mechanical hyperventilation

TABLE 130-2. Types of Metabolic Acidosis

Anion Gap	*Hyperchloremic (Normal or Low Anion Gap)*
Renal failure	Renal tubular acidosis
Diabetic ketoacidosis	Carbonic anhydrase inhibitor therapy
Lactic acidosis	Diarrhea
Salicylates	Ureteral diversions
Toxins, including methanol, paraldehyde, and ethylene glycol	Early renal failure
	Added HCL (NH4CL, arginine, lysine)
	Adrenal insufficiency, hypoaldosteronism
	Gastrointestinal fistulae (pancreatic)

TABLE 130-3. Definitions and Expected Compensation for Primary Acid–Base Disorders

Primary Disorder	*Definition*	*Expected Compensation*
Acute respiratory acidosis	P_{CO_2} >45	HCO_3^- = {(P_{CO_2}−40)/10} + 24 Or 1 mmol increase for each 10 mm Hg P_{CO_2} increase >40 mm Hg
Acute respiratory alkalosis	P_{CO_2} <35	HCO_3^- + 24 − {(40 − P_{CO_2})/10} Or 2 mmol decrease for each 10 mm Hg P_{CO_2} decrease under 40 mmHg
Metabolic acidosis	HCO_3^- <22 mEq/L	P_{CO_2} = (1.5 × HCO_3^-) + 8 ± 2
Metabolic alkalosis	HCO_3^->26 mEq/L	P_{CO_2} = 0.6 × (24 − serum HCO_3^-)
Chronic respiratory acidosis	P_{CO_2} >45	4 mmol increase for each 10 mm Hg P_{CO_2} increase >40 mm Hg
Chronic respiratory alkalosis	P_{CO_2} <35	5 to 7 mmol decrease for each 10 mm Hg P_{CO_2} decrease <40 mm Hg

abnormalities. Methanol, ethylene glycol, and salicylates are responsible for most toxin-induced anion gap acidoses. Both methanol and ethylene glycol are associated with severe acidoses and elevated osmolar gaps. Treatment of both is alcohol infusion to decrease formation of toxic metabolites and dialysis to remove toxins. Salicylate toxicity usually is associated with a mild metabolic acidosis and a respiratory alkalosis. Uremia is associated with a mild acidosis secondary to decreased ammonia secretion and an anion gap caused by the retention of unmeasured anions.

As a general rule, high anion gap acidoses are often owing to generation and accumulation of organic acids. Hence, correction of anion gap acidosis usually requires correction of the associated, causal metabolic abnormality. Because plasma proteins are nonbicarbonate buffers, serum albumin participates in the acid–base status by carrying a negative charge and acts as a nonvolatile weak acid. The decrease in the weak acid (albumin) may offset and hide an excess of unmeasured anions, such as lactate or keto acids. Hence, hypoalbuminemia causes errors in calculation of the anion gap.

A decrease in serum albumin by 1 g/dL decreases the base excess (BE) by 3.7 mEq/L and the anion gap (AG) by 2.75 mEq/L. If the base excess method is used to calculate anion gaps, a high P_{CO_2} may also result in a falsely low anion gap because the total CO_2 used in the AG calculation is not the same as the standard bicarbonate value used to identify metabolic acidosis by the BE method.

NONANION GAP METABOLIC ACIDOSIS

As opposed to anion gap acidosis, nonanion gap acidoses (Table 130-2) are generally caused by loss of bicarbonate or inability to excrete hydrogen ion, administration of HCl or NH_4Cl, or failure to regenerate the bicarbonate pool. Hence, treatment of nonanion gap acidosis requires attention to where the bicarbonate losses are occurring. Losses of the bicarbonate pool can come from the gastrointestinal tract and include duodenal and pancreatic fistulae, diarrhea, and ureterosigmoidostomies. Intrinsic renal losses occur most commonly from renal tubular acidosis, but they can also occur from interstitial nephritis; adrenal insufficiency, including hypoaldosteronism; and acetazolamide therapy. Treatment of nonanion gap acidosis requires correction of the acidosis plus administration of bicarbonate therapy, except in type 4 renal tubular acidosis. To replete the lost bicarbonate, the bicarbonate deficit can be calculated as follows:

$$HCO_2 - \text{deficit} = 0.3 \times \text{weight (kg)} \times (24\text{-}HCO_2^-)$$

In general, only half of the corrected deficit is given over 24 hours to avoid overcorrection.

METABOLIC ALKALOSIS

The fundamental abnormality in metabolic alkalosis is an absolute or relative base excess, generally in the form of bicarbonate. Although the excess tends to be offset by a decrease in minute ventilation, the respiratory response to metabolic alkalosis is not as predictable as it is to metabolic acidosis. In general, the P_{CO_2} will not rise above 45 in a compensatory fashion. The underlying mechanisms of metabolic alkalosis are loss of hydrogen ion (along with chloride), gain of exogenous base, or extracellular fluid contraction (Table 130-4). Gain of exogenous base can be masked as citrate in transfused blood and plasma or infusion of Ringer's lactate solution.

Similar to metabolic acidosis, metabolic alkalosis can be divided into two categories: chloride responsive and chloride resistant. The definition is based on measurement of the urine chloride, which if low (>10 to 15 mEq/L) is said to be chloride *responsive* and if high (urine Cl >30 mEq/L) is said to be *chloride resistant.* Chloride responsive alkaloses are generally associated with volume depletion (e.g., aggressive diuresis, gastric acid losses) and respond to sodium chloride administration. If

TABLE 130-4. Types of Metabolic Alkalosis

Chloride Responsive	*Chloride Resistant*
Vomiting, high nasogastric (NG) output	Administration of exogenous base: (lactate and acetate as intravenous fluid bicarbonate)
Volume depletion (especially, if associated with low K or low CL)	Citrate conversion after large volume blood transfusion
Post-hypercapnic states	Adrenal cortical hormone excess
Diuretic therapy	Hepatic coma Severe K depletion

they are severe (pH >7.60), they need treatment with 0.1 N HCl. In cases of hypochloremic alkalosis losses because of loss of voluminous gastric contents, chloride reabsorption in the kidney is done at the expense of potassium or hydrogen ion to maintain volume. This results in a *paradoxic aciduria.* The primary treatment of chloride responsive alkalosis is administration of normal saline.

Chloride-resistant alkaloses suggest a renal origin or a hormone- or drug-related effect on the kidney, such as hyperaldosteronism, increased corticosteroids, or licorice ingestion. They are also associated with administration of excess base, such as citrate and lactate. If the metabolic alkalosis results in significant CO_2 retention, a renal tubular acidosis can be induced with acetazolamide to correct the abnormality.

DIAGNOSTIC APPROACH

Acid–base disorders need to be approached in a systematic way to help determine the cause of the disorder and the therapeutic interventions. Clues about the underlying disorder are obtained from the history and physical examination. Assessment of the pH, PCO_2, and HCO_2^- allow determination of whether the primary disorder is metabolic or respiratory. Calculation of the predicted compensatory response then suggests whether a simple or mixed disorder is present. A mixed disorder is suggested if the compensation is not appropriate. Calculation of the serum and urine anion gaps and the delta gap are helpful in determining a differential diagnosis of metabolic acidosis.

A number of published methods exist for diagnosing metabolic acid–base disorders, including relying on the plasma bicarbonate concentration and anion gap (1), the base excess or deficit, and the strong ion difference method (2,3). This chapter uses the plasma bicarbonate and anion gap method. Identification of acid–base disorders can provide a clue to the underlying disorder. After obtaining a complete history and physical examination, a systematic analytic approach is required, which includes the following (4):

1. Assessing accuracy via the Henderson-Hasselbalch equation
2. Examining the serum electrolytes and additional laboratory data
3. Calculating the serum anion gap and whether it needs correcting
4. Identifying the primary acid–base disturbance
5. Determining whether a simple or mixed disturbance is present
6. Measuring the urine pH and electrolytes to calculate the urine anion and osmolal gaps

Acid–base disorders can be either metabolic or respiratory in origin. Respiratory alkalosis refers to a PCO_2 of <35 and respiratory acidosis refers to a PCO_2 of >45. Metabolic alkalosis is defined by a plasma HCO_3^- concentration of >26 mEqL and metabolic acidosis to a plasma CO_3^- concentration of <22 mEqL. Other definitions of acid–base disorders are based on the standard base excess that is outside of the −3 to +3 mEq/L range.

Carbon dioxide affects the hydrogen ion concentration by the following reversible reaction:

$$CO_2 + H_2O = H_2CO_3 = H^+ + HCO_3^-$$

This equation demonstrates that alterations in PCO_2 caused by respiratory derangements can cause major changes in hydrogen ion concentration. Because the relationship of alveolar ventilation and PCO_2 is simple, changes in alveolar ventilation should directly fix the respiratory acidosis or alkalosis. For each change of 10 in PCO_2, the pH changes by 0.07 to 0.08 in the opposite direction (this relationship, however, is nonlinear for extreme changes). Similarly, to calculate the expected respiratory changes for metabolic acidosis, an easy rule of thumb is that for each decrease in the pH by 0.1 unit, the compensatory decrease in PCO_2 is by 7 mm Hg. At pH <7.1, the compensation no longer occurs and the respiratory compensation becomes less effective. See Table 130-3 for definitions and expected compensations.

Interpretation of arterial blood gases is important in the assessment of the acid–base balance in a patient. First and foremost, any laboratory test is subject to error and misinterpretation. PCO_2 will decrease in a sample over time and, hence, should be measured promptly. In addition, ongoing cellular metabolism in a sample can affect the pH. Interpretation of blood gases in patients who are hypothermic is problematic because the blood sample is warmed to 37°C and, hence, does not reflect values at low temperatures.

The body has normal compensatory mechanisms for acid–base disorders. If the compensated value is not where it should be, the patient may have a mixed or complex disorder. Table 130-3 shows the usual compensations that should occur for a given disorder.

The initial determination should be whether the patient is acidemic or alkalemic, and the second step should be a determination of whether the disorder is metabolic or respiratory. As discussed above, if the primary component is respiratory, changes in minute ventilation need to occur to correct the disorder. The two main categories of metabolic acidosis are *anion gap* and nonanion gap.

Important equations to consider in the calculations of the acid–base disorder are as follows:

$$\text{Anion gap} = \{(Na + K) - (Cl + HCO_3)\}$$

$$\text{Adjusted anion gap} = \text{AG observed} + 0.25\ (\text{normal albumin} - \text{observed albumin})$$

$$\text{Base excess caused by albumin changes} = 3.4 * (4.5 - \text{albumin})$$

Henderson-Hasselbalch equation:

$$pH = 6.10 + \log\left[(HCO_3^-) / PCO_2 * 0.03\right]$$

The anion gap is calculated by subtracting the anions (HCO_3 and Cl) from the cations (Na and K). The *gap* refers to unmeasured anions. Common types of metabolic acidosis seen in the ICU are in Table 130-1. A normal anion gap is typically <12. Similarly, metabolic alkalosis is categorized according to its anion (Cl) depletion into chloride responsive and chloride resistant alkaloses.

TREATMENT

Treatment for the various acid–base disorders is targeted at the underlying disorder causing the imbalance as described above. In addition, any neurologic consequences of the acid–base imbalance will also be alleviated with the treatment of the underlying pathology. The treatment for all causes of acid–base disturbances is beyond the scope of this chapter.

CLINICAL RECOMMENDATIONS OF THE VIGNETTE

The patient has evidence of diabetic ketoacidosis (DKA). The calculated anion gap is 20.7 [(132+4.7) − (96+11)], so the patient has an anion gap metabolic acidosis. The excess acid is from the ketones that are produced in this condition and is evident in this patient because of the fruity smell on his breath.

The mainstay of therapy for this patient is correction of the underlying problem that led him to this state. With the history of productive cough, fever, and a right lower lobe infiltrate on chest radiograph, the patient likely has pneumonia. In the scenario of the insulin-dependent diabetic patient who presents to the Emergency Department with DKA, it is often precipitated by an underlying infection. It is the role of the practitioner to identify an occult infection in this type of patient. The infection causes the hyperglycemia and the ketoacidosis is from the lack of insulin driving the glucose into cells. In this situation, the treatment would include culture and administration of antibiotic for pneumonia, hydration, correction of electrolyte abnormalities, and administration of insulin. With the resolution of the ketoacidosis and the pneumonia, the patient's lethargy will resolve. Patients with the diagnosis of DKA are profoundly dehydrated and, in extreme cases, can present with focal neurologic deficits as a result. Cerebral edema can be seen in patients with DKA, especially children, during resuscitative therapy. The key is to avoid hypotonic solutions while restoring intravascular volume (5).

SUMMARY

Acid–base disorders are common in patients in an intensive care unit. The body has specific compensatory mechanisms to attempt to minimize the impact of the pH change on necessary physiologic reactions. Knowledge of expected pH and compensatory changes is essential to determine the cause of the disorder and whether a mixed disorder exists and to facilitate treatment. Correction should be aimed at the underlying disorder that results in the disturbance.

REFERENCES

1. Fall PJ. A stepwise approach to acid–base disorders. Practical patient evaluation for metabolic acidosis and other conditions. *Postgrad Med.* 2000;107(3):249–250.
2. Fencl V, Jabor A, Kazda A, et al. Diagnosis of metabolic acid-base disturbance in critically ill patients. *Am J Respir Crit Care Med.* 2000;162:2246–2251.
3. Moviat M, van Haren F, van der Hoeven H. Conventional or physicochemical approach in intensive care unit patients with metabolic acidosis. *Crit Care.* 2003;7(3):R41–R45.
4. Kraut JA, Madias NE. Approach to patients with acid-base disorders. *Respir Care.* 2001;46 (4):392–440.
5. Larsen PR, ed. *Williams Textbook of Endocrinology*, 10th ed. Philadelphia: WB Saunders; 2003:chapter 30. pp. 1485–1504.

CHAPTER **131**

Fluid and Electrolyte Disorders

Ankush Gosain • Fred Luchette

INTRODUCTION

Disorders of serum electrolytes are common clinical entities that have a broad array of presenting symptomatology. Serum sodium plays a key role in osmotic balance between the intracellular and extracellular spaces and is central to the pathogenesis of cerebral edema. Disorders of serum calcium have both central nervous system (CNS) and peripheral nervous system (PNS) manifestations, reflecting the key role of this cation in stabilization of the cell membrane. Although disorders of serum magnesium and phosphorus are less common, they often coexist with other electrolyte imbalances, and prompt recognition and treatment is key to the prevention of morbidity. Finally, whereas both hypokalemia and hyperkalemia are common electrolyte abnormalities found in hospitalized and critically ill patients, their primary symptomatology is related to the cardiac system and discussion of these entities is beyond the scope of this chapter.

OBJECTIVES

- To examine the cause and pathogenesis of commonly encountered electrolyte abnormalities, with a special emphasis on CNS and PNS manifestations
- To review the diagnostic and treatment approach to the most commonly encountered electrolyte abnormalities

CASE VIGNETTE

A 68-year-old male nursing home resident is found lying on the floor and "convulsing" by the staff. On arrival in the emergency room, he is confused and oriented only to person. His medical history is remarkable for alcoholic cirrhosis and diabetes mellitus. His vital signs are blood pressure (BP) 110/70 mm Hg, heart rate (HR) 55 beats per minute, respiratory rate (RR) 18 breaths per minute, and temperature 37.6°C. On physical examination, he is somnolent and bradycardic. His abdomen is moderately distended. He is poorly cooperative with the neurologic examination, but muscle stretch reflexes are noted to be brisk and symmetric. Results from laboratory analysis include serum sodium of 110 mmol/L, calcium of 8.0 mg/dL, magnesium of 1.4 mEq/L, and creatinine of 1.8 mg/dL. He is admitted to the intensive care unit (ICU) for further evaluation and treatment.

Sodium Disorders

DEFINITION

Disorders of serum sodium, the most common electrolyte abnormality in clinical medicine, manifest predominantly as CNS dysfunction (1). Hypernatremia is defined as a serum sodium concentration >145 mmol/L and is always reflective of hypertonic plasma. In contrast, hyponatremia is defined as a serum sodium concentration <136 mmol/L and may reflect low, normal, or high tonicity.

EPIDEMIOLOGY, ETIOLOGY, PATHOGENESIS, AND PATHOLOGY

Serum sodium concentration is a function of water homeostasis, which is controlled by thirst, arginine vasopressin, and the kidneys. Hypernatremia results from a deficit of water in relation to the total body water, most frequently as a consequence of net water loss (2). Alternatively, hypernatremia can result from the gain of total body sodium as a result of clinical intervention or sodium loading (e.g., hypertonic saline). Importantly, hypernatremia always reflects a hypertonic state. In the hospitalized patient, hypernatremia most often develops as an iatrogenic condition. Other causes of net water loss include diabetes insipidus, osmotic diuresis, hypercalcemia, hypokalemia, and intrinsic renal disease. Additionally, extrarenal sources of water loss can lead to hypernatremia, including excessive sweating, diarrhea, and thirst disorders. In infants, hypernatremia is most frequently the result of diarrhea. In elderly patients, it can result from febrile illness or thirst impairment (3). The elderly are at particular risk because of diminished thirst response and reduced urinary concentrating capacity. Mortality from hypernatremia is high, ranging from 20% in children to 50% in adults (1). Additionally, considerable morbidity is associated with hypernatremia, with permanent brain damage resulting in a third of patients (4).

Hyponatremia, which represents an excess of total body water relative to total body sodium, results in a hypoosmolal state. Hyponatremia is further subdivided based on extracellular fluid (ECF) volume into hypovolemic, normovolemic, and hypervolemic subtypes. Patients at high risk for developing hyponatremia include postoperative patients (25% of all cases of hyponatremia), patients with acquired immunodeficiency syndrome (AIDS), syndrome of inappropriate antidiuretic hormone (SIADH), adrenal insufficiency, and patients with isotonic fluid losses (e.g., diarrhea, emesis). In surgical patients, hyponatremia is commonly seen following the use of large volumes of hypotonic or low sodium irrigation solutions (e.g., transurethral prostatectomy) (5). SIADH is the most common cause of hyponatremia in the hospitalized patient. CNS causes include malignancies, bleeds, infections, and trauma, all of which cause SIADH through the excessive release of ADH. It is important to distinguish SIADH from cerebral salt wasting syndrome (CSWS), which is also characterized by a natriuresis, but results in hypovolemia hyponatremia.

The pathophysiologic manifestations of hypo- and hypernatremia result from changes in intracellular fluid (ICF) and ECF water balance. The cell membrane serves as a semipermeable barrier to fluid shifts between the ECF and ICF, which normally exist in a ratio of approximately 1 to 2. When an osmolal gradient develops between these two compartments, water moves passively from the area of lower osmolality to the area of higher osmolality, thereby restoring equilibrium. In the case of hypernatremia, water shifts from the intracellular space to the extracellular space, resulting in cerebral dehydration. In hyponatremia, the reverse situation is present, and fluid shifts to the intracellular space, resulting in cerebral edema. The brain possesses a number of mechanisms to address changes in sodium balance, including the Na^+/K^+- adenosine triphosphatase (ATPase) pump. Interestingly, women tend to experience greater permanent morbidity in the form of brain damage from hyponatremia because of inhibition of the Na^+/K^+-ATPase pump by endogenous sex hormones (6).

CLINICAL MANIFESTATIONS

Hypernatremia manifests as CNS dysfunction (2). Generally, symptomatology is worse when changes in serum sodium are great and occur rapidly (7). When hypernatremia is slow to develop, the brain is partially able to compensate for the deleterious osmolal gradient by increasing the influx of electrolytes across the cell membrane to increase intracellular osmolality and avoid water loss (8). In infancy, typical signs include hyperpnea, muscle weakness, restlessness, high-pitched crying, insomnia, lethargy, and coma. In elderly patients, however, symptoms rarely manifest until the serum sodium rises >160 mmol/L. Initially, intense thirst is present as a compensatory mechanism, but disappears as hypernatremia persists. Convulsions are typically absent unless rapid sodium loading has occurred (usually iatrogenic) (9). Orthostatic hypotension and tachycardia are reflective of underlying hypovolemia. Additionally, rapid brain dehydration can result in tearing of the bridging veins with resultant subdural hemorrhage.

Patients with hyponatremia have high intracellular osmolality, resulting in fluid shifts from the intravascular space to the intracellular space. At serum sodium levels >125 mEq/L, gastrointestinal (GI) symptoms predominate, including nausea, vomiting, and anorexia. At lower levels of serum sodium, typically <115 mEq/L, acutely symptomatic hyponatremia manifests as CNS disturbances (e.g., encephalopathy) because of cerebral edema. The degree of CNS depression ranges from mild confusion to coma, depending on the degree of cerebral edema, magnitude of hyponatremia, and the rapidity of onset (10). With severe hyponatremia, convulsions can manifest. Findings of opisthotonic posturing, respiratory arrest, and fixed and dilated pupils suggest profound cerebral edema and herniation of the brainstem. Peripheral neurologic symptoms, primarily muscle twitching and increased muscle stretch reflexes, result from alterations in ion conductance in peripheral nerves (11). Additionally, in hypervolemic hyponatremia, signs of volume overload, such as hypertension and bradycardia, may be present. Alternatively, in hyponatremia with a total body sodium deficit (rather than water excess), hypotension and oliguria leading to acute renal failure and cirrhosis are typical presentations. Finally, in the setting of SIADH, impaired excretion of renal free water leads to a hyponatremic state with normal total body sodium (12). In this setting, urinary sodium is high, with concentrated urine (>100 mOsm/L).

DIAGNOSTIC AND TREATMENT APPROACH

The initial step in diagnosis for hypernatremia is a careful assessment of volume status, because hypovolemia, isovolemia, or hypervolemia may be present (2). Patients with hypovolemic hypernatremia typically have a total body sodium deficit. This results from excessive fluid losses from the GI tract (emesis or nasogastric suction, diarrhea), genitourinary (GU) tract (osmotic diuresis or diuretic administration), cutaneous losses (burns, sweating), or peritoneal losses (peritonitis, prolonged operations). Treatment includes the administration of isotonic saline or lactated Ringer's solution. Administration of intravenous free water is contraindicated, because this results in rapid lowering of plasma osmolality at the infusion site and results in massive hemolysis. Hypervolemic hypernatremia is generally an iatrogenic condition, and is readily treated with diuretics and water replacement. In correcting acute hypernatremia, a rate of correction of up to 1 mEq/L/hour can be used, because the brain cells can extrude accumulated electrolytes. In chronic hypernatremia, the water deficit should be corrected over a 48-hour period and no faster than 0.5 mEq/L/hour to avoid seizures or cerebral edema. Finally, focal neurologic findings in patients with hypernatremia can result from subdural, intraparenchymal, or subarachnoid hemorrhage, and computed tomography (CT) of the brain is indicated.

Neurogenic diabetes insipidus (DI) represents a condition with normal total body sodium in the presence of a pure water deficit (13). This disease process, a result of impaired renal water conservation, results in extensive loss of urine that is almost completely devoid of solutes. Polyuria and urine osmolarity <200 mOsm/L are characteristic of this diagnosis. Treatment includes the administration of vasopressin and replacement of free water. The total body free water deficit should be calculated and half of this deficit replaced over 24 hours, with the remainder given over the next 1 to 2 days. Rapid replacement can result in cerebral coma (14).

The diagnosis of hyponatremia can be made in error, often by phlebotomy proximal to a hypotonic fluid infusion. Additionally, hyponatremia can be artifactual secondary to elevated circulating levels of other osmotically active substances, such as mannitol or glucose (11). Hyperglycemia, for example, will lower serum sodium concentrations by 1.6 mEq/L for every 100 mg/dL rise above normal and should be considered when calculating serum sodium concentration. Following confirmation of true hyponatremia, an accurate assessment of volume status should be performed and serum electrolytes, blood urea nitrogen, creatinine level, and osmolality obtained. Serum osmolality should be calculated and compared with measured osmolality to rule out the presence of unidentified serum osmoles (e.g., mannitol).

The treatment approach to hyponatremia varies, depending on the chronicity and severity of symptoms. In the treatment of chronic, mild hyponatremia, when serum sodium is >120 mEq/L and the patient is euvolemic, free water restriction is the primary treatment measure. Acute hyponatremia is accompanied by massive cerebral edema and is highly morbid and potentially mortal if not rapidly treated (5,9). In these patients, isotonic saline is used to replace volume deficit in the setting of alkalosis and lactated Ringer's solution in those patients with acidosis. Patients with hyponatremia-induced seizures should be placed in a monitored setting and started on hypertonic saline infusion. In this situation, serum sodium should not be raised by more than 12 mEq/L during the first 24 hours. Pulmonary edema can develop from rapid intravascular volume expansion during hypertonic fluid administration, but is readily treated with diuresis (4). Hypertonic infusion should be discontinued once the patient is asymptomatic or serum sodium has risen >120 to 125 mEq/L.

Central pontine myelinolysis (CPM) was first described in 1959 among patients with alcoholism or malnutrition who developed spastic quadriplegia, pseudobulbar palsy, and varying degrees of encephalopathy or coma from acute, noninflammatory demyelination that centered within the basis pontis (15). Although CPM has been described most commonly among patients with alcoholism and Wernicke-Korsakoff syndrome, other groups of patients can be affected. These include those with severe liver damage (including, those status post-orthotopic liver transplantation), malnutrition, anorexia, and severe burns. Ongoing research in the pathogenesis of CPM has led investigators to propose that in regions of compact interdigitation of white and gray matter, cellular edema, which is caused by fluctuating osmotic forces, results in compression of fiber tracts and induces demyelination. Prolonged hyponatremia followed by rapid sodium correction results in edema. During the period of hyponatremia, the concentration of intracellular charged protein moieties is altered and reversal cannot parallel a rapid correction of electrolyte status (16). Additionally, this series of changes is not necessarily confined to the pons, and the term *osmotic myelinolysis* is more appropriate than *central pontine myelinolysis* for demyelination occurring in extrapontine regions after the correction of hyponatremia (17). Typically, T2-weighted magnetic resonance images (MRI) demonstrate hyperintense or bright areas where demyelination has occurred caused by relatively increased water content in those regions (18). Recently, investigators have demonstrated that CPM does not result from rapid correction of acute hyponatremia, and is more likely related to delays in initiation of therapy, overcorrection of serum sodium, or superimposed hypoxic events (9).

Calcium Disorders

DEFINITION

Disorders of calcium homeostasis are also clinically common and often reflect iatrogenic causes (19). Hypocalcemia is defined as a serum calcium level <8.0 to 8.5 mg/dL (2.0 to 2.1 mmol/L). Hypercalcemia is defined as serum calcium level >10.5 mg/dL (3.0 mmol/L) and is considered severe when >14 mg/dL (3.5 mmol/L).

EPIDEMIOLOGY, ETIOLOGY, PATHOGENESIS, AND PATHOLOGY

Severe hypercalcemia typically is caused from either underlying malignancy or from parathyroid disease and almost half of all patients with hypercalcemia will develop neurologic manifestations (20). Malignancy, the most common underlying diagnosis in the hospitalized patient, is most often reflective of bone metastases from lung, breast, ovarian, renal, hematologic, head and neck, or GI cancers. In ambulatory patients, primary hyperparathyroidism is the most frequent diagnosis. Medications can also be the source of hypercalcemia; thiazide diuretics prevent the loss of calcium from the renal tubule. In all of these cases, hypercalcemia develops when entry of calcium into the serum from bone and GI resorption exceed loss by the kidneys.

Hypocalcemia, often the result of vigorous hydration of malnourished hospital patients, is generally asymptomatic. Symptomatic hypocalcemia is more frequently the result of thyroid or parathyroid operations with damage to, or removal of, the parathyroid gland (21). Additionally, hyperphosphatemia and decreased synthesis of 1,25-dihydroxycholcalciferol in chronic renal failure can cause hypocalcemia and decreased synthesis of parathyroid hormone. Because ionized calcium is responsible for stabilization of nerve and muscle cell membranes and regulates presynaptic neurotransmitter release, hypocalcemia has both PNS and CNS manifestations.

CLINICAL MANIFESTATIONS

The signs and symptoms of hypercalcemia span many organ systems and are often nonspecific (20). GI symptoms are common, including vague abdominal pain, often associated with increased gastric acid secretion and pancreatitis. CNS symptoms are often present as well, including depression, lethargy, fatigue, and clouded consciousness. The severity of these changes is directly proportional to the serum calcium. In profound hypercalcemia, proximal muscle weakness, stupor, and coma can develop. Hypercalcemia impairs the urinary concentrating ability of the renal tubules, resulting in a state similar to diabetes insipidus (13). Finally, cardiovascular symptoms can result from decreased HR and shortened ventricular systolic times because of alterations in myocardial electrical conductance.

Manifestations of hypocalcemia include perioral paresthesias and tetany (19). Paresthesias result from instability of neuromuscular membranes, whereas tetany results from repetitive generation of nerve action potentials secondary to spontaneous depolarization caused by hypocalcemia. Provocative testing may be required to elicit tetany; Chvostek sign is contraction of the ipsilateral facial muscles in response to light percussion over the facial nerve (17). Trousseau sign is carpal spasm in response to ischemia from application of a blood pressure cuff maintained above systolic for at least 3 minutes. Severe tetany does not require provocative testing and can manifest as lower extremity spasm and laryngeal stridor. CNS manifestations of hypocalcemia are nonspecific and include irritable mood, depression, delirium, hallucinations, and dementia. Seizures can result if the onset of hypocalcemia is rapid.

DIAGNOSTIC APPROACH AND TREATMENT

Severe hypercalcemia should be approached as a medical emergency (19,20). Patients should be placed in a monitored setting, with Foley catheter insertion to assess renal function, as well as central venous pressure monitoring for volume status. The first maneuver in the treatment of hypercalcemia is rehydration with normal saline. The volume administered varies with the degree of hypercalcemia, ranging from 3 L/day for mild cases up to 10 L/day for severe cases. Loop diuretics should be used as an adjunct with this large volume infusion for diuresis and also to promote renal excretion of calcium.

Following hydration and loop diuresis, if hypercalcemia persists, calcitonin can be used (22). Calcitonin, the most rapidly acting anticalcemic agent available, inhibits bone resorption and promotes renal excretion of calcium. Long-term therapy includes the use of bisphosphonate agents, which require approximately 2 days to become effective. Corticosteroids can also be useful agents in the long-term treatment of hypercalcemia, but have no role in the acute management phase. Attention must also be paid to the other electrolytes during treatment for hypercalcemia, because massive volume infusion and diuretic therapy can cause disturbances in serum sodium, potassium, and magnesium. Following normalization of serum calcium, attention may be returned to the underlying cause.

Treatment of hypocalcemia is variable, based on severity of symptomatology (23). Asymptomatic patients require only a search for the cause of hypocalcemia. Mildly symptomatic patients, such as those with perioral and extremity paresthesias, can be given oral calcium supplementation. Those patients with severe symptoms, such as tetany and carpopedal spasm, however, require emergent therapy with intravenous agents. Calcium gluconate or calcium chloride can be used; the latter is more likely to cause venous irritation because of its high osmolarity.

Magnesium Disorders

DEFINITION

Disorders of serum magnesium are often overlooked because magnesium is not included in the standard panel of electrolytes at most hospitals (24). Hypomagnesemia is defined as a serum level <1.5 mEq/L and hypermagnesemia is present when levels >4 mEq/L.

EPIDEMIOLOGY, ETIOLOGY, PATHOGENESIS, AND PATHOLOGY

Hypermagnesemia is seen only in patients with renal insufficiency who are receiving exogenous magnesium, often as a part of a dietary supplement (25). Elevated levels of magnesium block presynaptic calcium channels, limiting calcium influx to the cell during depolarization and resulting in decreased release of acetylcholine from nerve terminals and symptoms of neuromuscular depression.

Deficits of serum magnesium can result from dilution caused by fluid therapy, GI tract losses through diarrhea or fistulas, malnutrition from alcoholism or other causes, diabetic ketoacidosis, use of loop diuretics, and primary hyperaldosteronism (26). Additionally, patients with steatorrhea (e.g., from pancreatic exocrine insufficiency) develop hypomagnesemia from chelation of magnesium by fat in the GI tract.

CLINICAL MANIFESTATIONS

Signs and symptoms of hypermagnesemia are rare until levels exceed 4 mEq/L; they include drowsiness and lethargy, nausea, vomiting, and diaphoresis. The primary symptom is muscular weakness or paralysis from blockade of acetylcholine release at the neuromuscular junction. Cardiac manifestations appear earlier than neurologic manifestations, with hypotension seen at serum levels >3 mEq/L (26). Severe neurologic manifestations can occur, with diminished muscle stretch reflexes and ataxia at levels between 7 and 10 mEq/L, and coma above 10 to 15 mEq/L. These levels are accompanied by respiratory depression and further cardiac embarrassment.

Mild hypomagnesemia often presents as hypokalemia that is refractory to replacement therapy (26). Additionally, it can present concurrently with hypocalcemia and its attendant symptomatology of paresthesias and tetany. Severe cases of hypomagnesemia often present with seizures, neuromuscular excitability, and cardiac arrhythmias.

DIAGNOSTIC APPROACH AND TREATMENT

Hypermagnesemia is a rare entity, generally confined to patients with renal insufficiency (27). Treatment includes cessation of magnesium-containing oral supplements and hydration. If the patient is nonoliguric, treatment with furosemide promotes natriuresis, which is accompanied by urinary magnesium excretion. If signs of magnesium toxicity are present (e.g., hyporeflexia and cardiac conduction abnormalities), intravenous calcium (90 to 180 mg) can be used to transiently stabilize the cardiomyocytes, but hemodialysis with a magnesium-free dialysate is often necessary for definitive treatment.

Treatment for hypomagnesemia includes both oral and intravenous replacement (28). In severe hypomagnesemia with life-threatening manifestations (e.g., seizures and arrhythmias), rapid infusion of magnesium sulfate 16 to 32 mEq over 10 to 15 minutes is warranted. In patients who are clinically stable but demonstrate depressed serum magnesium levels, more moderate amounts of intravenous magnesium combined with oral magnesium gluconate tablets are recommended. Treatment of concomitant hypokalemia or hypocalcemia should be undertaken as well.

Phosphorous Disorders

DEFINITION

Phosphorous is necessary to produce adenosine triphosphate (ATP) and is critical for bone mineralization, cellular structure, genetic coding, and energy metabolism (26). In the adult, 80% to 90% of total body phosphorous is mineralized within the bone, 10% to 14% is intracellular, and approximately 0.1% to

1% is extracellular. The normal range for serum phosphorous is 2.5 to 4.5 mg/dL (0.81 to 1.45 mmol/L). Hyperphosphatemia is considered significant above 5 mg/dL in adults and 7 mg/dL in children. Hypophosphatemia is defined as mild (2 to 2.5 mg/dL), moderate (1 to 2 mg/dL), or severe (<1 mg/dL) (29). Mild to moderate hypophosphatemia is generally asymptomatic, with clinical symptomatology becoming evident with severe hypophosphatemia. Because such a low fraction of total body phosphorous is extracellular, serum phosphorous levels may be poorly indicative of true phosphorous status.

EPIDEMIOLOGY, ETIOLOGY, PATHOGENESIS, AND PATHOLOGY

Phosphorous homeostasis is normally tightly regulated through a balance of GI absorption and renal excretion, both of which are under the hormonal control of parathyroid hormone. Because serum phosphorous is filtered by the proximal tubule, hyperphosphatemia generally results in patients with renal insufficiency. Elevated serum phosphate is an independent risk factor for cardiovascular disease and patients with chronic phosphate levels (>6.5 mg/dL) have a 20% to 40% greater mortality rate compared with those with normal serum levels.

Hypophosphatemia results from decreased dietary intake, decreased intestinal absorption, increased urinary excretion, and a shift from the extracellular to intracellular space (30). Decreased dietary intake is rare outside of patients with eating disorders or profound chronic alcoholism with minimal solid food intake. Decreased intestinal absorption is seen in patients with malabsorption syndromes, chronic diarrhea, or prolonged emesis or nasogastric suctioning. Hypophosphatemia is a common finding in patients with primary and secondary hyperparathyroidism because of increased urinary excretion of phosphate by the kidney in response to parathyroid hormone. Additionally, proximal tubule diuretics interfere with the ability to reabsorb phosphorus. Finally, respiratory alkalosis is the primary cause of hypophosphatemia seen in the ICU. Respiratory alkalosis activates phosphofructokinase to stimulate intracellular glycolysis, shifting phosphate into the cells to be consumed in the production of phosphorylated glucose precursors.

CLINICAL MANIFESTATIONS

Patients with hyperphosphatemia generally manifest CNS or cardiovascular symptoms. The CNS symptoms include altered mental status, delirium, obtundation, coma, convulsions and seizures, muscle cramping or tetany, neuromuscular excitability, and paresthesias (31). It is important to note that most of these symptoms are caused by secondary hypocalcemia, and the initial treatment is aimed at correcting this electrolyte abnormality. Cardiac manifestations include prolonged QT interval, hypotension, and heart failure.

Hypophosphatemia presents as a weakness of skeletal or smooth muscle, and is often found in patients in the ICU who are presenting with difficulty in weaning from the ventilator (32,33). Rhabdomyolysis can result from hypophosphatemia secondary to ATP depletion and the inability of muscle cells to maintain membrane integrity. Cardiac dysfunction results from impaired cardiac contractility, and is rapidly improved on correction of serum phosphate. Finally, neurologic manifestations such as confusion, seizures, and coma can result from hypophosphatemia. A syndrome similar to Guillain-Barré can result, including peripheral neuropathy and ascending motor paralysis.

DIAGNOSTIC APPROACH AND TREATMENT

Along with measurement of serum phosphate levels, workup of hypo- and hyperphosphatemia must include an evaluation of potential associated abnormal electrolytes, such as calcium and magnesium. Hypomagnesemia and hypercalcemia are associated with hypophosphatemia, whereas the reverse is true with hyperphosphatemia. An electrocardiogram is warranted in patients with arrhythmias, and may demonstrate QT prolongation in hyperphosphatemia.

Hyperphosphatemia is associated with secondary hypocalcemia, and this is the cause of most symptoms and clinical sequelae (29). The initial management goal is correction of serum calcium, as outlined above. Following this, reduction of serum phosphate <5.5 mg/dL should be initiated. Oral phosphate binders (e.g., sevelamer hydrochloride, lanthanum carbonate) are given to decrease the gastrointestinal absorption of phosphorus. Additionally, proximal tubule diuretics (e.g., acetazolamide) can be used to increase urinary excretion of phosphate. Finally, hemodialysis can be useful in patients with severe, refractory hyperphosphatemia. As with all electrolyte abnormalities, treatment of the underlying cause should be undertaken.

Treatment of hypophosphatemia includes correction of the underlying cause and replacement of phosphate stores. The route of replacement depends on the severity of depletion, with both oral and intravenous options available. Patients with mild to moderate symptoms generally benefit from correction of the underlying cause alone, but may require oral supplementation with elemental phosphorus daily (2 to 3 g). Patients with severe hyperphosphatemia require intravenous replacement (34). Caution must be taken to avoid precipitating a hypocalcemic state from overcorrection of phosphate.

CLINICAL RECOMMENDATIONS OF THE VIGNETTE

The patient, a 68-year-old man with alcohol dependence, is admitted to the ICU for further care following a seizure at the nursing home. His initial laboratory work demonstrates hyponatremia, borderline hypocalcemia, and hypomagnesemia. Additionally, this patient demonstrates characteristics of alcoholic cirrhosis on examination, and may have volume overload, given his impaired renal function and the presence of bradycardia. The underlying cause in this situation is likely hypervolemia hyponatremia from alcohol use, a setting in which it is common to have multiple electrolyte abnormalities. Although the patient is acutely symptomatic, his electrolyte imbalances are likely chronic. The initial approach to this patient should include treatment with hypertonic saline to raise serum sodium above 120 mEq/L, as well as intravenous calcium and magnesium therapy. Additionally, diuretic therapy will help correct the hypervolemia and avoid volume overload associated with hypertonic saline infusion. Based on his clinical response, invasive monitoring to determine central venous pressure may become necessary.

SUMMARY

Disorders of the serum electrolytes are commonly found in the clinical setting and have myriad manifestations. Both central and peripheral nervous system manifestations are common, and reflect the broad role that these molecules play in basic physiology. It is important to be cognizant of the full range of manifestations of these imbalances, as well as their appropriate treatment. Detailed here is the general approach to patients manifesting serum electrolyte abnormalities, which are often multiple. Finally, it is important to re-emphasize that, whereas the acute management of these disorders is geared toward minimizing morbidity and mortality, the true goal should be elucidation of the underlying disease process and institution of appropriate therapy.

REFERENCES

1. Kumar S, Berl T. Sodium. *Lancet.* 1998;352(9123):220–228.
2. Adrogue HJ, Madias NE. Hypernatremia. *N Engl J Med.* 2000;342(20):1493–1499.
3. Palevsky PM, Bhagrath R, Greenberg A. Hypernatremia in hospitalized patients. *Ann Intern Med.* 1996;124(2):197–203.
4. Berl T. Treating hyponatremia: Damned if we do and damned if we don't. *Kidney Int.* 1990;37(3):1006–1018.
5. Hahn RG. Fluid absorption in endoscopic surgery. *Br J Anaesth.* 2006;96(1):8–20.
6. Arieff AI. Influence of hypoxia and sex on hyponatremic encephalopathy. *Am J Med.* 2006;119[7 Suppl 1]:S59–S64.
7. Andrews BT. Fluid and electrolyte disorders in neurosurgical intensive care. *Neurosurg Clin N Am.* 1994;5(4):707–723.
8. Pullen RG, DePasquale M, Cserr HF. Bulk flow of cerebrospinal fluid into brain in response to acute hyperosmolality. *Am J Physiol.* 1987;253(3 Pt 2):F538–F545.
9. Ayus JC, Krothapalli RK, Arieff AI. Treatment of symptomatic hyponatremia and its relation to brain damage. A prospective study. *N Engl J Med.* 1987;317(19):1190–1195.
10. Han DS, Cho BS. Therapeutic approach to hyponatremia. *Nephron.* 2002;92[Suppl 1]:9–13.
11. Adrogue HJ, Madias NE. Hyponatremia. *N Engl J Med.* 2000;342(21):1581–1589.
12. Decaux G. Is asymptomatic hyponatremia really asymptomatic? *Am J Med.* 2006; 119[7 Suppl 1]:S79–S82.
13. Blevins LS, Jr., Wand GS. Diabetes insipidus. *Crit Care Med.* 1992;20(1):69–79.
14. Gullans SR, Verbalis JG. Control of brain volume during hyperosmolar and hypoosmolar conditions. *Annu Rev Med.* 1993;44:289–301.
15. Adams R, Victor M, Mancall E. Central pontine myelinolysis: A hitherto undescribed disease occurring in alcoholic and malnourished patients. *Arch Neurol Psychiatry.* 1959;81:154–156.
16. Murase T, Sugimura Y, Takefuji S, et al. Mechanisms and therapy of osmotic demyelination. *Am J Med.* 2006;119[7 Suppl 1]:S69–S73.
17. Riggs JE. Neurologic manifestations of fluid and electrolyte disturbances. *Neurol Clin.* 1989;7(3):509–523.
18. DeWitt LD, Buonanno FS, Kistler JP, et al. Central pontine myelinolysis: Demonstration by nuclear magnetic resonance. *Neurology.* 1984;34(5):570–576.
19. Bushinsky DA, Monk RD. Electrolyte quintet: Calcium. *Lancet.* 1998;352(9124):306–311.
20. Bilezikian JP. Management of acute hypercalcemia. *N Engl J Med.* 1992;326(18):1196–1203.
21. Gourgiotis S, Moustafellos P, Dimopoulos N, et al. Inadvertent parathyroidectomy during thyroid surgery: The incidence of a complication of thyroidectomy. *Langenbecks Arch Surg.* 2006;391(6):557–560.
22. Pecherstorfer M, Brenner K, Zojer N. Current management strategies for hypercalcemia. *Treatments in Endocrinology.* 2003;2(4):273–292.
23. Reber PM, Heath H, 3rd. Hypocalcemic emergencies. *Med Clin North Am.* 1995;79(1): 93–106.
24. Wong ET, Rude RK, Singer FR, et al. A high prevalence of hypomagnesemia and hypermagnesemia in hospitalized patients. *Am J Clin Pathol.* 1983;79(3):348–352.
25. Clark BA, Brown RS. Unsuspected morbid hypermagnesemia in elderly patients. *Am J Nephrol.* 1992;12(5):336–343.
26. Weisinger JR, Bellorin-Font E. Magnesium and phosphorus. *Lancet.* 1998;352(9125): 391–396.
27. Massry SG, Seelig MS. Hypomagnesemia and hypermagnesemia. *Clin Nephrol.* 1977;7(4): 147–153.
28. al-Ghamdi SM, Cameron EC, Sutton RA. Magnesium deficiency: Pathophysiologic and clinical overview. *Am J Kidney Dis.* 1994;24(5):737–752.
29. Thatte L, Oster JR, Singer I, et al. Review of the literature: Severe hyperphosphatemia. *Am J Med Sci.* 1995;310(4):167–174.
30. Gaasbeek A, Meinders AE. Hypophosphatemia: An update on its etiology and treatment. *Am J Med.* 2005;118(10):1094–1101.
31. Berner YN, Shike M. Consequences of phosphate imbalance. *Annu Rev Nutr.* 1988;8: 121–148.
32. Gluck EH. Predicting eventual success or failure to wean in patients receiving long-term mechanical ventilation. *Chest.* 1996;110(4):1018–1024.
33. Aubier M, Murciano D, Lecocguic Y, et al. Effect of hypophosphatemia on diaphragmatic contractility in patients with acute respiratory failure. *N Engl J Med.* 1985;313(7):420–424.
34. Charron T, Bernard F, Skrobik Y, et al. Intravenous phosphate in the intensive care unit: More aggressive repletion regimens for moderate and severe hypophosphatemia. *Intensive Care Med.* 2003;29(8):1273–1278.

CHAPTER **132**

Hemodynamic Control: Pressors and Antihypertensive Agents

Michael H. Whiteley • W. Scott Jellish

OBJECTIVES

- To discuss the considerable controversy concerning optimal management of blood pressure in patients with acute stroke, traumatic brain injury, and other neurologic emergencies
- To describe the neurologic emergencies requiring either support of blood pressure or immediate reduction and control of blood pressure
- To discuss the hypotensive agents producing the optimal reduction and control of blood pressure
- To explain the potential side effects and complications of drug-induced hypertension in these patient.

CASE VIGNETTE

A 67-year-old man with a history of hypertension, hypercholesterolemia, and coronary artery disease is brought to the emergency room (ER) by family members after an extended episode of left-sided weakness. He has had a history of transient ischemic attacks (TIA) and has been on appropriate treatment. This episode, however, is not remitting. He has been treated for hypertension with beta-blockers and calcium channel blockers. On admission to the ER, his blood pressure (BP) is noted initially to be 137/87 mm Hg. After several hours, the patient's BP has fallen to 90/60 mm Hg. This drop in blood pressure is associated with a worsening of the patient's neurologic symptoms.

DEFINITION

Neurologic critical care emergencies that may be amenable to manipulation of systemic BP with either vasopressor medications or vasodilators include ischemic stroke, traumatic brain injury, spinal cord injury and subarachnoid hemorrhage with associated vasospasm. Stroke or brain attack is defined as the abrupt onset of a focal neurologic deficit attributable to a focal vascular cause (1). Therefore, the diagnosis of stroke is made by clinical criteria. Laboratory studies, such as neuroimaging, are used to support the diagnosis.

ETIOLOGY

Strokes are either hemorrhagic or ischemic. Approximately 80% are ischemic, triggered by either a thrombus or embolus lodging in an artery in the brain causing hypoxia with ischemia, injury, or infarction to the area distal to the occlusion. Hemorrhagic stroke occurs when a blood vessel ruptures and blood enters the cerebral tissue, ventricles, or subarachnoid space.

Not only stroke, but also traumatic brain injury (TBI) is associated with decreased cerebral perfusion. This is well documented both in clinical and experimental studies (2). TBI is usually the result of some blunt trauma: motor vehicle crash, assault, falls, and so on. Decreased cerebral blood flow (CBF) in these cases is associated with unfavorable outcomes.

Acute spinal cord injury (SCI) can be the result of trauma or compromise of blood supply that might occur after major vascular surgery. Evidence indicates that acute SCI leaves tissue susceptible to secondary injury in the presence of hypotension and inadequate perfusion of the spinal cord (3).

Although relatively little direct evidence suggests that hypertension definitively contributes to rebleeding after aneurysmal subarachnoid hemorrhage (SAH), most centers control systolic blood pressure (SBP) to 160 mm Hg or less before surgical or endovascular treatment.

TREATMENT

Many neurologic emergencies, specifically those mentioned above, involve both a direct insult to the nerve tissue and the possibility of extension of injury to adjacent tissues that are at risk. The specific mechanisms of decreased blood flow after ischemic or traumatic injury are not completely understood, but many possibilities have been proposed. The release of vasoconstrictive agents, such as endothelin and serotonin, may be involved.

The metabolic demands of the brain and, by extension, the rest of the central nervous system (CNS), are met by the flow of blood defined by the cerebral (or spinal cord) perfusion pressure. Cerebral perfusion pressure (CPP) is calculated as mean arterial blood pressure (MABP) minus intracranial pressure (ICP) or central venous pressure (CVP), whichever is greater. Cerebrovascular autoregulation refers to the brain's ability to maintain a constant CBF over a wide range of CPP. This range is understood to be from 50 to 150 mm Hg of CPP (4). It is well accepted that acute neurologic diseases, such as ischemic stroke, TBI, SCI, and SAH with vasospasm can disable cerebral autoregulation in the zones of injury and lead to blood flow becoming entirely related to CPP.

Astrup et al. (5) in 1981 introduced the term *ischemic penumbra* to describe an area of the brain surrounding a stroke in which normal electroencephalogram (EEG) signal was disrupted, but cell death associated with ion pump failure had not yet occurred. They concluded that this penumbra region can be rescued to some extent by increasing CPP, thereby potentially improving outcome after ischemic stroke.

PATHOLOGY

It remains unclear whether acute hypertension is causally associated with stroke morbidity and mortality. Some retrospective analyses have reported associations between elevated admission BP and poor outcome, whereas others have found no association. More recent observations have reported a U-shaped relationship where poor outcome was associated with especially low or high BP (6). Also, a spontaneous decline of BP within the first 4 to 48 hours after stroke is associated with impaired outcome.

Increasing MABP in stroke or TBI by using pressor agents, in theory, should improve CPP and potentially lead to improved outcome after these injuries. Some potentially harmful effects of these agents are found, however. Pressor agents (e.g., dopamine) can produce local cerebral vasoconstriction if the blood–brain barrier is compromised. Increased MABP could also lead to increased ICP if autoregulation is impaired, especially if fluid infusion is included in a regimen to elevate the MABP. The combination of increased MABP, fluid infusion, and presssor agent use could contribute to the exacerbation of brain edema and subsequent increases in ICP (7). Elevations in BP or heart rate can also increase the workload on the myocardium, leading to increased oxygen demand, which can also lead to exacerbations of myocardial ischemia in those patients who have a history of coronary artery disease.

DIAGNOSTIC APPROACH

Elevated BP during and after acute stroke is thought to be a compensating mechanism to improve cerebral circulation to the ischemic brain. As a result, it has been a common practice to reduce or withhold BP treatment until the clinical condition stabilizes. No large clinical studies exist on which to base definite recommendations for lowering BP. The American Stroke Association, however, has provided guidelines: If SBP is >220 mm Hg or diastolic blood pressure (DBP) is 120 to 140 mm Hg, a cautious reduction in BP by 10% to 15% is recommended (8). If DBP is >140 mm Hg, sodium nitroprusside could be used to decrease BP by 10% to 15%. Sodium nitroprusside is usually avoided, however, because of severe drops in BP and the possibility of increased ICP. Nitroprusside is a direct-acting, nonselective peripheral vasodilator that causes relaxation of arterial and venous smooth muscle. Onset of action is immediate, and its duration of action is short lived, requiring a continuous infusion.

Nitroprusside produces nitric oxide, which activates the enzyme guanylate cyclase, producing increased concentrations of cyclic guanosine monophosphate in smooth muscle leading to vasodilation. Metabolism of nitroprusside yields unstable nitroprusside radicals. This molecule breaks down releasing cyanide, which reacts with methemoglobin to form cyanmethemoglobin. Thus, the patient on nitroprusside could develop cyanide toxicity and be resistant to the hypotensive affects of the drugs. Nitroprusside should be administered on the basis of total dose and not on the BP effect that is achieved. The usual infusion rate is 0.5 to 2 $\mu g \cdot kg^{-1} \cdot min^{-1}$ intravenously. Hypotension produced by nitroprusside is followed by increased receptor sensitivity, which contributes to the subsequent increased dose requirements needed to maintain BP at reduced levels.

Optimal management of BP during acute ischemic stroke with the use of intravenous thrombolysis is better understood. Because diastolic hypertension has been identified as a risk factor for intracerebral hemorrhage (ICH) in pilot studies of intravenous tissue plasminogen activator (tPA), BP exclusion criteria exist. Within the first 3 hours of symptoms, if a computed tomographic (CT) scan does not demonstrate hemorrhage, short-acting parenteral antihypertensives should be given for a SBP of >185 and DBP >110 mm Hg (9). During and after infusion of intravenous tPA, BP control is tighter. Targets for BP decreases are 5 mm Hg less for both the SBP and DBP.

Therapy for BP reduction during acute stroke often uses labetalol or nicardipine as the preferred agents (Table 132-1). Labetalol exhibits selective α_1 and nonselective β_1 and β_2 antagonism. In humans, the ratio of α-to-β receptor blockade is estimated to be 1:7 after intravenous administration. Metabolism of labetalol is by conjugation to glucuronic acid with <5% of the drug unchanged. Administration of intravenous labetalol (0.1 to 0.5 mg/kg) over 2 minutes acutely lowers BP by decreasing systemic vascular resistance. The maximal BP-lowering effect of intravenous labetalol is preset after 5 to 10 minutes. Additional doses can be injected every 10 minutes or, alternatively, a continuous intravenous infusion (0.5 to 2 mg $\cdot$ min^{-1}) can be initiated.

Nicardipine is a dihydropyridine calcium channel blocker that inhibits influx of Ca^{2+} into vascular smooth muscle with minimal affects on the heart. The BP-lowering effect is caused by relaxation of vascular smooth muscle with associated vasodilation and reduction in BP, owing to a decline in systemic vascular resistance. Parenteral administration is by continuous infusion because of the short half-life. Nicardipine dosing begins with an initial bolus of 5 μg/kg/min with a decrease to 1 to 3 μg/kg/min after the target BP is achieved.

Esmolol infusions can also be titrated to effect. Esmolol is a rapid-onset, short-acting selective β_1 receptor antagonist. These characteristics make esmolol useful for treating adverse BP and heart rate increases that occur. A bolus of esmolol (80 mg)

TABLE 132-1. Antihypertensives

Drug	*Mechanism*	*Dose*	*Onset*	*Duration*	*Common Adverse Effects*
Labetalol	α-1, β-1, β-2-antagonist	20 to 80 mg bolus every 10 min, up to maximum 300 mg; 0.5 to 2 mg/min infusion	5 to 10 min	3 to 6 h	Bradycardia (heart block), dizziness, nausea, vomiting, scalp tingling, bronchospasm, orthostatic hypotension, hepatic injury
Esmolol	β-1-antagonist	500 μg/kg bolus, 50 to 300 μg/kg/min infusion	1 to 2 min	10 to 30 min	Bradycardia (heart block), hypotension, nausea, bronchospasm
Nicardipine	L-type CCB (dihydropyridine)	5 to 15 mg/h infusion	5 to 10 min	30 min to 4 h	Reflex tachycardia, headache, nausea, flushing, local phlebitis
Enalaprilat	ACE inhibitor	0.625 mg bolus, then 1.25 to 5 mg every 6 h	15 to 30 min	6 to 12 h	Variable response, precipitous fall in blood pressure in high-renin states, headache, cough
Fenoldopam	DA-1 agonist	0.1 to 0.3 μg/kg/min infusion	5 to 15 min	30 min to 4 h	Tachycardia, headache, nausea, dizziness, flushing
Nitroprusside	Vasodilator (arterial and venous)	0.25 to 10 μg/kg/min infusion	Immediate	1 to 4 min	Nausea, vomiting, muscle twitching, sweating, thiocyanate and cyanide intoxication

CCB, calcium channel blocker; ACE, angiotensin-converting enzyme; DA, dopamine; μ, microgram.
(From Rose JC, Mayer SA. Optimizing blood pressure in neurological emergencies. *Neurocritical Care.* 2004;1:287–299, with permission.)

intravenously, followed by a continuous intravenous infusion (12 mg/min^{-1}) lowers heart rate and BP in adults. The short duration of the drug results from its rapid metabolism in blood by hydrolysis of the methyl ester. The principal contraindication of administration of beta antagonists is preexisting atrioventricular heart block or cardiac failure. Beta antagonists should also not be administered to patients with chronic obstructive airway disease. In many instances, therapy using labetalol or esmolol work well, especially if the patient is tachycardic. Nicardipine is the preferred agent if the patient is bradycardic. Fenoldopam, a short-acting dopamine receptor agonist and vasodilator decreases BP while increasing renal blood flow and glomerular filtration rate. It is used to lower BP in hypertensive neurologic emergencies accompanied by acute hypertensive nephropathy. The plasma half-life of fenoldopam is approximately 4 minutes. During continuous infusion, a steady state is achieved within 20 minutes and the plasma levels are proportional to the dose once steady state has been achieved. The pharmacologic effect of fenoldopam is dose related, with proportional increases in renal blood flow, diuresis, fractional execution of sodium, and filtration fraction. Renal vasodilation is maximal at 0.5 μg/kg/min and, at greater doses, generalized peripheral vasodilation occurs. Therefore, a dose-related reduction in total vascular resistance and systemic BP occurs as well.

Angiotensin-converting enzyme (ACE) inhibitors (e.g., ramipril) have also been used to reduce BP after strokes. Studies have demonstrated that its therapeutic use reduced the incidence of nonfatal stroke by 24% and fatal stroke by 61% (10). Blockade of the angiotensin system may have beneficial effects on stroke. This class of drugs inhibits the activity of ACE, resulting in decreased levels of angiotensin II and aldosterone. They are most affective in treating arterial hypertension secondary to high renin production. Except for enalaprilat, all of the ACE inhibitors are administered orally. Many of the ACE inhibitors are designed as prodrugs to enhance their oral availability. ACE inhibition can also stabilize atherosclerotic plaques by reducing oxidative stress as well as inflammatory and proliferative processes. The concern behind not treating elevated BP is that such action could promote edema formation, increase hemorrhagic transformation and risk, or contribute to endothelial damage.

Maximizing perfusion pressure after TBI to areas of nerve tissue at risk has been accomplished several ways. Previously in the treatment of these neurologic emergencies, the effort to improve CPP was aimed primarily at reducing ICP. Later data have shown the adverse effects of systemic hypotension on outcome after TBI (11). In addition, it was shown that inadequate CBF is a very common occurrence after acute CNS injury (12). Subsequently, more attention has been paid to the maintenance or even augmentation of systemic BP as a means of overcoming the posttraumatic uncoupling of cerebral autoregulation. Several vasoactive drugs have been used with this in mind. These include phenylephrine, dopamine, and norepinephrine (Table 132-2).

In 1999, Cherian et al. (13) induced severe cortical impact injury in rats to compare the therapeutic effects of phenylephrine with L-arginine (a substrate for nitric oxide synthase). The infusion of saline was used in a third group as a control. The goal was to test a potential cerebral vasodilatory agent against the traditional means of raising CBF with a pressor agent. They found that the immediate response to injury was an increase in ICP and a decrease in MABP, CPP, and laser Doppler flow. Infusion of both phenylephrine and L-arginine resulted in increased CBF back to near baseline. Phenylephrine increased CBF by increasing CPP and L-arginine increased CBF without changing CPP. The improvement in CBF in both cases was accompanied by a decrease in neurologic injury as determined after the subject animals were killed.

In the clinical setting, dopamine is often used to increase MABP and, therefore, improve CPP. The use of dopamine, however, does carry potential adverse effects. The infusion of dopamine at 2 to 6 μg/kg/min significantly increased CBF, higher doses of dopamine (7 to 20 μg/kg/min), however,

TABLE 132-2. Vasopressors

Drug	*Mechanism*	*Dose*	*Onset*	*Duration*	*Common Adverse Effects*
Phenylephrine	α-1 agonist	40 to 180 μg/min	Immediate	20 to 40 min	Headache, myocardial ischemia, tachycardia, nausea, dyspnea
Dopamine	DA-1 agonist α-1, DA-1 agonist α-1, β-1, DA-1 agonist	1 to 2.5 μg/kg/min 2.5 to 10 μg/kg/min >10 μg/kg/min	1 to 2 min	<10 min	Headache, tachycardia, nausea, chest pain, dyspnea, ischemic limb necrosis
Norepinephrine	α-1, β-1, agonist	2 to 40 μg/min	Immediate	<10 min	Tachycardia, infusion site necrosis, limb ischemia
Dobutamine	β-1, β-2, agonist	2 to 20 μg/kg/min	1 to 2 min	10 to 15 min	Headache, tachycardia, nausea, dyspnea, cardiac ectopy

CCB, calcium channel blocker; ACE, angiotensin-converting enzyme; DA, dopamine. (From Rose JC, Mayer SA. Optimizing blood pressure in neurological emergencies. *Neurocritical Care.* 2004;1:287–299, with permission.)

decreased CBF (14,15). A biphasic effect of dopamine was also found in the rat pial arteriole (16). Exacerbation of posttraumatic vasogenic edema is also a concern. This could potentially lead to increased ICP, decreased CPP, and worsening ischemic injury.

Kroppenstedt et al. (2) evaluated the potential adverse effect of dopamine in the treatment of TBI. They found that, after trauma, the cortical CBF was decreased by 46% in the region of the cortical contusion. Infusions of saline or dopamine (10 to 12 μg/kg/min) did not change the MABP or the cortical CBF. An infusion of dopamine at 40 to 50 μg/kg/min elevated MABP from 89 to 120 mm Hg and increased the posttraumatic CBF in and around the cortical contusion by 35%. Hemispheric swelling, water content, and cerebrospinal fluid (CSF) concentrations of glutamate and hypoxanthine were not affected. They found no evidence for dopamine-mediated cerebral vasoconstriction, nor was their evidence of exacerbation of edema or increases in the tested CSF markers for tissue injury.

Episodes of hypotension have been associated with worsening neurologic outcome in head injury, ischemic stroke, and spinal cord injury (3). An increase in SBP could logically improve perfusion of at risk tissue. Indeed, many clinical reports support this idea. Weiss et al. (17) reported the onset of flaccid paralysis and paraplegia to the T10 dermatome 45 minutes after arrival in the ICU of a patient who underwent abdominal aortic aneurysm (AAA) repair. The onset of symptoms was associated with a drop in MABP from 78 to 48 mm Hg. Treatment with volume expansion, dopamine and phenylephrine to raise MABP to 75 mm Hg, and placement of a lumbar drain led to a reversal of the symptoms within 1 hour (17). Ackerman and Traynelis (18) reported on six patients having thoracoabdominal aneurysm repair with rapidly progressing motor and sensory loss in the lower extremities. Hypotensive events had immediately preceded the onset of the deficits in the postsurgical patients. The patients were treated with volume expansion and vasopressors to keep the MABP >70 mm Hg. Four of the patients also received a lumbar CSF drain. Two patients received CSF drainage after a delay of several hours and did not improve. The four patients who received BP support and prompt CSF drainage showed marked neurologic improvement.

In many instances of diminished CNS perfusion, BP elevation will be beneficial for neurologic outcome. In other neurologic emergencies, however, BP elevation might precipitate hemorrhagic stroke with accompanying ICH or hypertensive encephalopathy. Such hypertensive emergencies are characterized by severe elevation in BP (>180/120 mm Hg) complicated by evidence of impending or progressive target organ dysfunction. If an intracerebral bleed occurs from hypertension, the pressure and degree of acute hypertension can affect outcome after ICH. Several reports have demonstrated an increased risk of deterioration, death, or dependency with increased admission BP after ICH (19–20). Other studies, however, have noted that a rapid BP decline after ICH was associated with increased mortality (21). Current guidelines recommend that MABP be maintained at 130 mm Hg or less for patients with ICH who have a history of hypertension and that MABP be maintained at 100 mm Hg or less in all patients who have had a craniotomy to remove an intracerebral hematoma (22).

Hypertensive encephalopathy arises from SBP elevation sufficient to regionally overwhelm the upper limit of cerebrovascular autoregulation. Pressure and volume overload on the cerebral circulation leads to endothelial dysfunction, blood–brain barrier disruption, hydrostatic vasogenic edema, petechial hemorrhages, and a characteristic pattern of edema primarily involving the posterior circulation. The BP can be extremely high (>250/150 mm Hg), but the rate of rise and the baseline BP may be more important clinical determinates than the actual peak BP reached. Untreated, hypertensive encephalopathy can lead to seizures, cortical blindness, frank intracranial hemorrhage, coma, or death. Few clinical trial findings exist to support treatment methodology. These patients should be admitted to an intensive care unit (ICU) or acute stroke care unit, for continuous monitoring of BP and parenteral administration of an appropriate agent. The initial goal of therapy is to reduce MABP by no more than 25%. Then, if stable, to 160/100 to 110 mm Hg within the next 2 to 6 hours (23). Excessive falls in blood pressure that can precipitate renal, cerebral, or coronary hypoperfusion should be avoided. For this reason, nifedipine is no longer considered an acceptable therapy in the initial treatments of hypertensive emergencies. Nifedipine can be administered only by the oral sublingual route (10 to 30 mg). It has a relatively rapid onset (within 20 minutes with a peak effectiveness in 1 to 1.5 hours. Short-acting parenteral antihypertensives (e.g., labetalol, nicardipine, or enalaprilat) should be given initially. Nitroprusside, which could cause cerebral vasodilation and increased ICP, is also avoided.

BP reduction can also be important in the hypertensive patient who has an aneurysmal SAH. The annual incidence of aneurysmal SAH is approximately 10 per 100,000. Almost 1 of 6 patients with an aneurysmal SAH will die immediately. Of patients who survive to be admitted to the hospital, about 25% will still die and only approximately 50% will recover completely. The rate and volume of bleeding are the fundamental determinates of outcome.

Little evidence shows that uncontrollable hypertension definitely increases the risk of bleeding. Nevertheless, most physicians actively control elevated BP to an SBP of 160 mm Hg or less before surgical or endovascular treatment. A recent study reported a positive linear correlation between very early rebleeding and increased BP (24). Extremes in BP on admission to the ICU (MABP >130 or <70) have also been associated with poor outcome after SAH.

The specific BP target and agents used to treat acute hypertension vary between centers and clinicians. Some physicians advocate not treating unless the MABP is >130 mm Hg, whereas others maintain SBP less than or equal to 140 to 160 mm Hg. The current American Heart Association management guidelines state that antihypertensive therapy alone is not recommended to prevent rebleeding, but is frequently used in combination with monitored bedrest (25). If elevated BP is treated, an arterial catheter is recommended and a short-acting parenteral agent that has minimal adverse cardiovascular and ICP effects is desirable. Labetalol, esmolol, and nicardipine meet these criteria. In most instances, these medications are given as an infusion and titrated to effect.

Cerebral vasospasm associated with SAH is a significant contributor to morbidity, even after definitive treatment of aneurysmal bleeding. *Triple H* therapy is common practice in an effort to ameliorate the risk of cerebral vasospasm. Triple H therapy consists of aggressive infusion of colloid and crystalloid to reach a CVP of 8 mm Hg or higher, a pulmonary diastolic pressure of 14 mm Hg or higher, and vasopressor administration (4). Although controlled trials demonstrating the safety and efficacy of this practice have not been reported (4), it is the practice of many intensivists to maintain hypertension up to a maximum of about 200 mm Hg until a resolution of the neurologic deficits (4).

Finally, eclampsia is a disease state that also produces a hypertensive neurologic crisis. It produces a particular form of hypertensive encephalopathy that occurs in the setting of pregnancy-induced hypertension. It is associated with microvascular and endothelial damage and, because of this, neurologic manifestations can occur at much lower BP values. In these instances, management of BP is considerably more complicated than in *routine* cases of hypertensive encephalopathy. In eclampsia, the physiology of pregnancy can alter drug metabolism. Furthermore, two circulations are to be considered, and certain antihypertensive agents are strictly contraindicated based on adverse fetal effects (ACE inhibitors and angiotensin II receptor blockers) and MABP in eclampsia should be maintained between 105 and 125 mm Hg. Magnesium sulfate (2 g/hour) intravenously reduces the risk of recurrent seizures and lowers BP. It should be administered to all preeclamptic and eclamptic patients. As with other neurologic hypertensive emergencies, initial control of BP with a fast-acting, easily titratable agent (e.g., labetalol or nicardipine) is recommended.

CLINICAL RECOMMENDATIONS OF THE VIGNETTE

In many neurologic emergencies, hemodynamic control is the key to a good outcome with reduced morbidity. In some instances, BP reduction reduces the risk of hemorrhage from loss of cerebral autoregulation. In other instances, however, BP support may improve both perfusion to an ischemic penumbra and outcome. In some studies, a spontaneous reduction in BP within the first 4 to 48 hours after stroke was associated with an improved outcome. Other reports, however, have found a worse outcome with increasing BP decline. The symptoms in the patient had worsened with a spontaneous fall in BP, and decreased cerebral perfusion to penumbral areas is a possibility. An infusion of phenylephrine (60 μg/min) was begun and titrated to a MABP of 75 to 80 mm Hg with associated symptomatic improvement.

SUMMARY

BP variability is often associated with many neurologic emergencies. Control of BP is important either to improve perfusion to ischemic areas or to prevent autoregulatory breakthrough with associated hemorrhage destruction. Precise BP control is accomplished with short-acting pressors (e.g., phenylephrine, dopamine, dobutamine, and norepinephrine) or BP lowering agents (e.g., labetalol, esmolol, nicardipine, and ACE inhibitors). Clinical presentation and type of neurologic injury will dictate the therapeutic hemodynamic manipulation to be utilized.

REFERENCES

1. Kasper DL, Braunwald E, Fauci A, et al., eds. *Harrison's Principles of Internal Medicine*, 16th ed. Vol. 2. St. Louis: McGraw-Hill, 2005:2372.
2. Kroppenstedt, SN, Stover JF, Unterberg AW. Effects of dopamine on post-traumatic cerebral blood flow, brain edema, and cerebrospinal fluid glutamate and hypoxanthine concentrations. *Crit Care Med.* 2000;28:3792–3798.
3. Hadley MN. Blood pressure management after acute spinal cord injury. *Neurosurgery.* 2002;50(3)[Suppl]:S58–S62.
4. Rose JC, Mayer SA. Optimizing blood pressure in neurological emergencies. *Neurocritical Care.* 2004;1:287–299.
5. Astrup J, Siesjo BK, Symon L. Thresholds in cerebral ischemia: the ischemic penumbra. *Stroke.* 1981;12:723–725.
6. Christensen H, Meden P, Overguard K, et al. The course of blood pressure in acute stroke is related to the severity of neurologic deficits. *Acta Neurol Scand.* 2002;106:142–147.
7. DeWitt DS, Prough DS. Should pressors be used to augment cerebral blood flow after traumatic brain injury? *Crit Care Med.* 2000;28:3933–3934.
8. Adams HP, Adams RJ, Brott T, et al. Guidelines for the early management of patients with ischemic stroke: A scientific statement from the Stroke Council of the American Stroke Association. *Stroke.* 2003;34:1056–1083.
9. Furlan A, Higashida R, Wechsler L, et al. Intraarterial pro-urokinase for acute stroke: The PROACT II study: A randomized controlled trial. *JAMA.* 1999;282:2003–2011.
10. Yusufs S, Sleight P, Pogue J, et al. Effects of an angiotensin-converting enzyme inhibitor, ramipril on cardiovascular events in high-risk patients. The Heart Outcomes Prevention Elevation Study Investigators. *N Engl J Med.* 2000;342:145–153.
11. Chestnut RM, Marshall SB, Piek J, et al. Early and late systemic hypotension as a frequent and fundamental source of cerebral ischemia following severe brain injury in the Traumatic Coma Data Bank. *Acta Neurochir.* 1993;50:121–125.
12. Bouma GJ, Muizelaar JP, Choi SC, et al. Cerebral circulation and metabolism after severe traumatic brain injury: The elusive role of ischemia. *J Neurosurg.* 1991;78:685–693.
13. Cherian L, Chacko G, Goodman JC. Cerebral hemodynamic effects of phenylephrine and L-arginine after cortical impact injury. *Crit Care Med.* 1999;27:2512–2517.
14. von Essen C, Zervas NT, Brown DR, et al. Local cerebral blood flow in the dog during intravenous infusion of dopamine. *Surg Neurol.* 1980;13:181–188.
15. von Essen C, Kistler JP, Lees RS, et al. Cerebral blood flow and intracranial pressure in the dog during intravenous infusion of nitroglycerin alone and in combination with dopamine. *Stroke.* 1981;12:331–338.

16. Altura BM, Gebrewold A, Lassoff S. Biphasic responsiveness of rat pial arterioles to dopamine: Direct observations on the microcirculation. *Br J Pharmacol.* 1980;69:543–544.
17. Weiss SJ, Hogan MS, McGarvey ML, et al. Successful treatment of delayed onset paraplegia after suprarenal abdominal aortic aneurysm repair. *Anesthesiology.* 2002;97:504–506.
18. Ackerman LL, Trayhelis VC. Treatment of delayed onset neurological deficit after aortic surgery with lumbar cerebrospinal fluid drainage. *Neurosurgery.* 2002;51:1414–1422.
19. Hemphill JC, Bonovich DC, Besmertis L, et al. The ICH Score: A simple, reliable grading scale for intracerebral hemorrhage. *Stroke.* 2001;32:891–897.
20. Fogelholm R, Avikainen S, Murros K. Prognostic value and determinants of first-day mean arterial pressure in spontaneous supratentorial intracerebral hemorrhage. *Stroke.* 1997;28:1396–1400.
21. Qureshi AI, Bliwise DL, Bliwise NG, et al. Rate of 24 hour blood pressure decline and mortality after spontaneous intracerebral hemorrhage: A retrospective analysis with a random effects regression model. *Crit Care Med.* 1999;30:2025–2032.
22. Schellinger PD, Fiebach JB, Hoffmann K, et al. Stroke MRI in intracerebral hemorrhage: Is there a perihemorrhagic penumbra? *Stroke.* 2003;34:1674–1679.
23. Vidt DG. Emergency room management of hypertensive urgencies and emergencies. *J Clin Hypertens.* 2001;3:158–169.
24. Wijdicks EFM. *Aneurysmal Subarachnoid Hemorrhage in the Clinical Practice of Critical Care Neurology*, 2nd ed. Oxford: Oxford University Press; 2003:185–220.
25. Ohkuma H, Tsurutani H, Suzuki S. Incidence and significance of early aneurysmal rebleeding before neurosurgical on neurological management. *Stroke.* 2001;32:1176–1180.

CHAPTER **133**

Sedation and Analgesia in the Neurological Intensive Care Unit

Steven B. Edelstein • Kurt Baker-Watson

OBJECTIVES

- To provide a better understanding of the varying degrees of sedation when dealing with patients in the neurologic intensive care unit (ICU)
- To discuss the different sedation scales used
- To describe the tools used to assess sedation
- To explain the pharmacokinetics and pharmacodynamics of agents commonly used in sedation of patients in the ICU

CASE VIGNETTE

A 58-year-old man was admitted to the ICU after having a large left hemispheric stroke. His medical history was remarkable for hypertension, seizures, coronary artery disease, and diabetes mellitus.

During his admission intake, the patient was noted to be progressively agitated and at times lethargic. After evaluation by the ICU team, a decision was made to institute mechanical ventilation to protect his airway from possible aspiration. The nursing staff requested orders regarding sedation protocol, including goals, agents, and assessment tools.

DEFINITION

IMPORTANCE OF SEDATION AND ANALGESIA

When managing cases of critically ill patients, sedation plays an important role to the overall medical management. Undertreatment of pain has many adverse effects. Notably, significant increases occur in the levels of catecholamines because of sympathetic nervous system stimulation and persistence of the catabolic state. In addition, poorly controlled sedation increases the incidence of hypercoagulability and leads to immunosuppression (1). Prolongation of pain also leads to severe anxiety and delirium. Without sedation, patients are noted to have increased complications, such as extubations, removal of invasive lines, and increase myocardial oxygen consumption (2).

In addition, oversedation has its own set of problems. Complications of oversedation (respiratory depression, prolonged time requiring mechanical ventilation, increased costs, unrecognized cerebral insults) could be prevented by the proper use of a sedation protocol that includes the frequent assessment of sedation level (3).

To formulate a cohesive sedation plan for case management of the adult patient in the intensive care unit (ICU), it is important to understand some of the definitions surrounding sedation. Overall, the goal of therapy is to promote anxiolysis, provide hypnosis, and deliver amnesia. Brief definitions of these terms include the following (4):

1. Anxiolysis: a decrease in response, and implying a calm and tranquil state
2. Hypnosis: a state of minimal motor activity that appears similar to sleep
3. Amnesia: impairment of memory attributable to alteration in attention, arousal, or mood

A need exists for a common terminology regarding the different types of sedation. Because a large number of nonanesthesia providers are involved in nonoperating room sedation, the American Society of Anesthesiologists, via practice guidelines (5), has developed a definition of the terms *minimal sedation or anxiolysis, moderate sedation or conscious sedation, deep sedation or analgesia,* and *general anesthesia* as they apply to responsiveness, airway, spontaneous ventilation, and cardiovascular function (Table 133-1).

DIAGNOSTIC APPROACH

To manage these cases appropriately, an appropriate assessment needs to be made of the tools for sedation. As mentioned, undersedation and oversedation are both problematic. Active and ongoing research is underway to find the ideal sedation assessment tool that would be easy to apply and interpret, and have both construct validity and reliability.

One of the first, and most widely used, sedation assessment tools was the Ramsay Scale (6). This scale enables providers to

TABLE 133-1. Continuum of Depth of Sedation: Definition of General Anesthesia and Levels of Sedation or Analgesia

	Minimal Sedation ("Anxiolysis")	*Moderate Sedation/ Analgesia ("Conscious Sedation")*	*Deep Sedation or Analgesia*	*General Anesthesia*
Responsiveness	Normal response to verbal stimulation	Purposeful (not reflex withdrawal) response to verbal or tactile stimulation	Purposeful (not reflex withdrawal) response following repeated or painful stimulation	Unarousable, even with painful stimulation
Airway	Unaffected	No intervention required	Intervention may be required	Intervention often required
Spontaneous ventilation	Unaffected	Adequate	May be inadequate	Frequently inadequate
Cardiovascular function	Unaffected	Usually maintained	Usually maintained	May be impaired

(From Gross J, Bailey P, Connis R, et al. Practice guidelines for sedation and analgesia by non-anesthesiologists. *Anesthesiology.* 2002;96:1004–1017, with permission.)

have a common language regarding levels of sedation. It is composed of six gradations that stretch from awake to asleep levels (Table 133-2). Problems, however, exist in that this scale has to be modified if muscle relaxants are used, no consensus exist to what level is appropriate, and finally it can be confounded by analgesic requirements (4).

The Observers' Assessment of Alertness/Sedation Scale (OAA/S) has been shown to be both valid and reliable and was initially used with midazolam sedation models (7). Components include both verbal and physical stimuli that assist in quantifying the level and quality of sedation provided (Table 133-3).

The Harris Scale (8) has been used to determine levels of sedation in patients receiving propofol while having hemofiltration in the ICU setting. It differs from the Ramsay Scale in that it focuses more on compliance with mechanical ventilation and responses to endotracheal suctioning (Table 133-4).

Riker et al. (2) developed a more recent and detailed assessment tool. The study (2) is known as the *Sedation-Agitation Scale*, this tool has proved to be valid and reliable via a single center study. It also adds to the Ramsay Scale by providing additional stratification that is essential when dealing with complex cases in the ICU (Table 133-5).

ROLE OF BISPECTRAL INDEX MONITORING

The bispectral index (BIS) can be useful as a tool to measure the level of consciousness by processing and analyzing the electroencephalograph (EEG) signals via proprietary algorithms. A number is generated that reportedly correlates with the patient's level of consciousness. The scale ranges from 100 for fully awake patients, 85 to 65 for light to deep sedation, 65 to 40 for general anesthesia, and <40 for deep hypnotic states (9). This tool has been used to a degree some ICU settings to help assess levels of sedation. Problems have arisen, however, regarding electromyographic interference and other issues in this complex patient population (10–13). Currently, further studies are underway, and the utility of BIS has yet to be determined.

TABLE 133-2. Ramsay Sedation Scale

AWAKE LEVELS	1	Anxious, agitated, restless, or all three
	2	Cooperative, oriented, and tranquil
	3	Respond to commands only
ASLEEP LEVELS	4	Brisk response to light glabellar tap or loud auditory stimulus
	5	Sluggish response to light glabellar tap or loud auditory stimulus
	6	No response to light glabellar tap or loud auditory stimulus

(From Ramsay M, Savage T, Simpson B, et al. Controlled sedation with alphaxalone-alphadolone. *BMJ.* 1974;2:656–659, with permission.)

TABLE 133-3. Responsiveness Scores of the Modified Observers' Assessment of Alertness/Sedation Scale (OAA/S)

Responsiveness	*Score*
Responds readily to name spoken in normal tone	5 (alert)
Responds lethargically to name spoken in normal tone	4
Responds only after name is called loudly and/or repeatedly	3
Responds only after mild prodding or shaking	2
Responds only after painful trapezius squeeze	1
Does not respond to painful trapezius squeeze	0

(From Chernik DA, Gillings D, Laine H, et al. Validity and reliability of the observers' assessment alertness/sedation scale: Study with intravenous midazolam. *J Clin Psychopharmacol,* 1990;10:244–251, with permission.)

TABLE 133-4. Harris Scale

A. General Condition
1. Confused and uncontrollable
2. Anxious and agitated
3. Conscious, oriented, and calm
4. Asleep, but arousable to speech and obeys command
5. Asleep, but responds to loud auditory stimulus or sternal pressure
6. Unarousable

B. Compliance with Mechanical Ventilation
1. Unable to control ventilation
2. Distressed, fighting ventilator
3. Coughing when moved, but tolerating ventilation for most of the time
4. Tolerating movement

C. Response to Endotracheal Suctioning
1. Agitation, distress, prolonged coughing
2. Coughs, distressed, rapid recovery
3. Coughs, not distressed
4. No cough

(From Harris CE, O'Donnell C, MacMillian RR, et al. Use of propofol by infusion for sedation of patients undergoing haemofiltration on the level of sedation and on blood propofol concentration. *J Drug Dev.* 1991;4[Suppl 3]:37–39, with permission).

TREATMENT

A considerable gap in knowledge exists, stemming from the greater need for additional research and study concerning the pathophysiology and the altered pharmacology peculiar to patients in the ICU, and how these perturbations affect the pharmacology of sedatives and analgesic agents in various subpopulations. The presence of multifactorial insults, end-organ failure, drug–drug interactions, and diverse comorbidity often contribute to some of the uncertainties in the care of these complex patients. The basic pharmacology of popular sedatives, and issues pertinent to specific subpopulations is reviewed in Table 133-6.

MECHANISM OF ACTION

Most drugs used for sedation act by binding to and increasing the neuroinhibitory effects of γ-aminobutyric acid (GABA) receptors. Additionally, these drugs all maintain physiologic coupling of cerebral blood flow and cerebral metabolic oxygen requirements by causing a reduction in both.

Benzodiazepines

The most frequently used drugs include the highly lipid-soluble and albumin-bound diazepam, lorazepam, and midazolam. Midazolam is the most frequently used agent overall because of its ease of titration and it is uniquely appropriate for intramuscular absorption in that the drug is water soluble in the acidic solution in which it is packaged. Midazolam ultimately undergoes a conformational change in its structure to become lipophilic at physiologic pH. Diazepam, however, is difficult to use for intramuscular injections secondary to its prolonged effects and slow onset time.

Clinical action of benzodiazepines terminates by redistribution after a single bolus or by hepatic metabolism when infusions are used. The oxidative pathway of diazepam and its half-life can be prolonged by factors affecting hepatic function, including liver failure, advanced age, and the use of oxidation-inhibiting drugs (e.g., cimetidine). The degradative pathways of midazolam and lorazepam are largely unaffected by the aforementioned factors, although the half-life of midazolam can be prolonged with inhibitors of the cytochrome P-450 system (e.g., erythromycin). The metabolites of all three agents depend on renal excretion. Midazolam and diazepam have active metabolites that can accumulate with renal dysfunction.

Among the variety of uses for benzodiazepines are amnesia, decreasing intracranial pressure (ICP) while maintaining cerebral perfusion pressure (CPP), elevation of seizure threshold, skeletal muscle relaxation, therapy for alcohol withdrawal, and decreasing opioid requirements (14). A valuable feature of benzodiazepines when used for sedation is a relatively mild respiratory and cardiovascular depression when compared with other sedatives. Benzodiazepines have not been shown to

TABLE 133-5. Riker Sedation-Agitation Scale

7	Dangerous agitation	Pulling endotracheal tube, removing catheters, climbing over rail, striking staff, thrashing side-to-side
6	Very agitated	Does not calm, despite verbal reminding of limits; requires physical restraints; biting endotracheal tube
5	Agitated	Anxious or mildly agitated, attempts to sit up, calms with verbal instruction
4	Calm and cooperative	Calm, awakens easily, follows commands
3	Sedated	Difficult to arouse, awakens to verbal stimulation or gentle shaking, but drifts off again; follows simple commands
2	Very sedated	Arouses to physical stimuli, but does not communicate or follow commands; may move spontaneously
1	Unarousable	Minimal or no response to noxious stimuli; does not communicate

(From Riker R, Picard JT, Fraser GL. Prospective evaluation of sedation-agitation scale for adult critically ill patients. *Crit Care Med.* 1999;27(7):1325–1329, with permission.)

TABLE 133-6. Agents for Sedation

Agent	*Onset (sec)*	*Peak (min)*	*Elimination Half-life (h)*	*Sedative Bolus Dose (mg/kg)*	*General Anesthesia Dose (mg/kg)*	*Maintenance Dosing*
Midazolam	30 to 60	6	1 to 4	0.05 to 0.10	0.10 to 0.20	0.25 to 1.0 μg/kg/min
Lorazepam	60 to 120	30 to 40	10 to 20	0.025 to 0.050	0.1	0.02 mg/kg bolus only
Diazepam	30 to 60	10	21 to 37	0.125 to 0.2	0.3 to 0.5	0.1 mg/kg bolus only
Methohexital	60	1.5 to 3	4	0.1 to 0.5	1 to 1.5	50 to 150 μg/kg/min
Thiopental	60	1.5 to 3	12	0.25 to 0.75	3 to 5	1 to 4 mg/kg/h
Propofol	30 to 60	2	0.5 to 1.5	0.5 to 1	2 to 3	25 to 100 μg/kg/min for sedation, 50 to 300 μg/kg/min for general anesthesia
Etomidate	30 to 60	2 to 3	2 to 5	Not applicable	0.2 to 0.3	5 to 8 μg/kg/min for sedation, 10 μg/kg/min for general anesthesia
Dexmedetomidine (therapeutic dose 0.5 to 1.0 ng/mL)	5 to 10 min	10 min bolus infusion	2 to 3	2.5 to 6.0 μg/kg/h over 10 min as load	Maintenance only: 170 ng/kg/min over 10 min then 10 ng/kg/min	0.1 to 1.0 μg/kg/h

provide an isoelectric EEG (15) or to be neuroprotective during ischemic events to the degree established with the use of barbiturates (16).

Flumazenil, a competitive inhibitor at the GABA receptor site, is available as a reversal agent. Because of its short duration of action, midazolam is the most readily reversible agent. Flumazenil has a rapid onset of about 1 minute, with peak effects seen by 3 minutes. Benzodiazepine reversal can precipitate seizures in susceptible patients. Furthermore, the antagonism achieved by flumazenil usually is outlasted by the clinical action of the three benzodiazepines. Therefore, an infusion of flumazenil may be necessary.

Disadvantages of benzodiazepines include a potential for paradoxic agitation, development of tolerance over minutes to hours, and physical dependence. Midazolam has been shown to inhibit neutrophils and the implication of this feature in the patient in the ICU is of some debate (17).

Propofol

Propofol, a substituted isopropylphenol, is a highly lipid-soluble and highly protein-bound compound. Consequently, it also has a rapid onset of clinical effects. Whether using bolus dosing or infusions, termination of its clinical action is mediated by both redistribution and metabolism. Hepatic conjugation is the primary route of degradation. Extrahepatic metabolism, however, occurs in the intestines and kidneys. Inactive metabolites are excreted in urine. Cumulative effects and the context-sensitive half-life of agents are of particular concern in patients with hepatic or renal dysfunction.

The rapid (within minutes) return of consciousness among patients sedated with propofol infusions is because the drug is redistributed within its large volume of distribution. It is clinically possible to establish a prolonged context-sensitive half-life of propofol, however, through the administration of a large amount over a short period of time, resulting in the saturation of most of the binding sites within that volume of distribution. Under this circumstance, the cessation of clinical action depends on the slower processes of hepatic metabolism and excretion over hours.

The benefits of propofol include minimal cumulative effects with routine clinical management, minimal residual depression of mental status on return of consciousness, reduction of ICP, reduction of intraocular pressure, elevation of seizure threshold, ability to produce an isoelectric EEG, and neuroprotective, antiemetic, and antipruritic activity. A neuroprotective effect of propofol can be associated with the antioxidant qualities and inhibition of *N*-methyl-d-aspartate (NMDA) glutamate receptors (18). Concerns with propofol use include pain on injection, hyperlipidemia, and increased caloric intake because of its lipid-based formulation. Dose-dependent decreased cardiac output from vasodilatation and myocardial depression are also produced. The potential for a decrease in CPP exists from this cardiovascular depression in patients with increased ICP.

Instances of bradycardia and asystole have also been seen with bolus dosing, as have both green discoloration of the urine from phenol metabolites and the propofol infusion syndrome that is characterized by severe unexplained metabolic acidosis (19–21). Also a potential risk exists for bacterial contamination and sepsis. Thus, opened vials must be discarded after 6 hours, and infusion lines changed after 12 hours. Other complications include allergic reactions to the sulfa-based preservatives, myoclonus, and tolerance with chronic use.

Barbiturates

Barbiturates available for sedative use include thiopental and methohexital. They are less plasma protein bound than the preceding agents discussed. The lipophilic barbiturates display rapid clinical effects, with short onset times, approximately 60 seconds. Drug–drug interactions that interfere with albumin-barbiturate transport can increase the free concentrations of barbiturates. Termination of clinical action for bolus dosing depends primarily on redistribution rather than hepatic metabolism. Barbiturate hepatic metabolism is relatively unaltered by all but the most profound end-stage liver disease. Thiopental

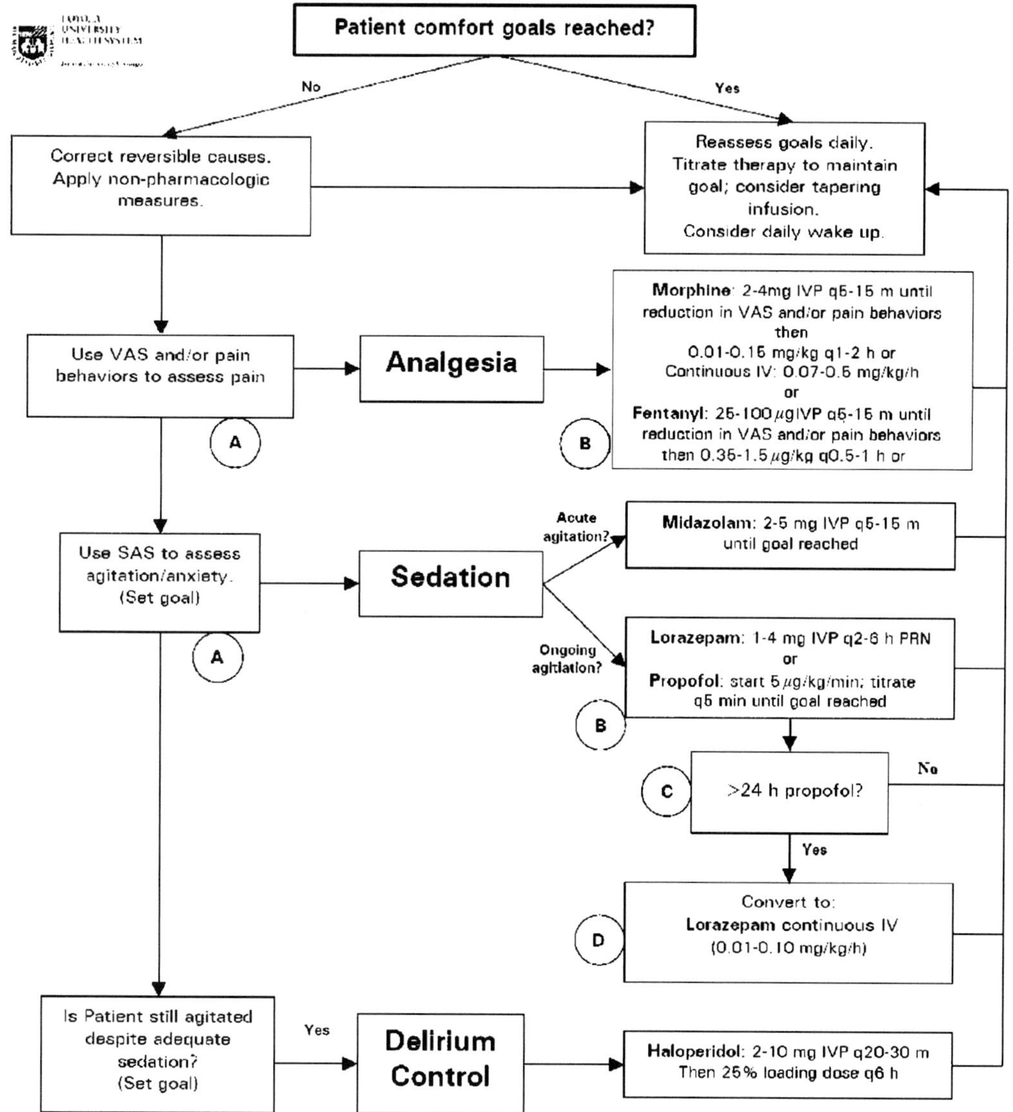

FIGURE 133-1. Analgesia and Sedation Protocol. (From Loyola University Health System Department of Medicine, Maywood, Illinois; October 2003, with permission.)

and methohexital metabolites have little to no activity and are excreted in urine.

Methohexital infusions have been associated with seizures and are currently not recommended (22). Thiopental infusions have been used for prolonged barbiturate-induced coma and burst suppression, and to control cases of refractory status epilepticus.

Barbiturates reduce ICP and intraocular pressure while preserving CPP. Side effects include hypotension, tachycardia, respiratory depression, allergic reactions, myoclonus, depression of neutrophil-mediated immune function, induction of hepatic microsomal enzymes after prolonged therapy with altered metabolism of other drugs (23), tolerance within days of extended use, and physical dependence.

Etomidate

Etomidate is a highly lipid-soluble carboxylated imidazole compound, with moderate binding to albumin. Etomidate's free fraction can increase with hypoalbuminemia because of its hepatic metabolism. Its clearance depends on hepatic blood flow and hepatic microsomal enzymes and plasma esterases hydrolyze etomidate. The resulting inactive metabolite is mostly excreted in the urine and, to some extent, in bile. The offset of clinical action occurs mostly by redistribution rather than metabolism.

Etomidate, a direct cerebral vasoconstrictor provides an isoelectric EEG, lowers ICP and intraocular pressure, increases the seizure threshold, and provides some neuroprotection (24). When used in routine concentrations, etomidate has minimal cardiovascular depression and minimal effects on renal blood flow. Etomidate, however, can cause moderate respiratory depression. Other concerns with the use of etomidate include adrenocortical suppression, pain on injection, and myoclonic activity.

Dexmedetomidine

Dexmedetomidine is a lipid-soluble, *centrally-acting* α-2 receptor agonist, and a highly protein-bound compound. Its primary advantages are α-2 receptor-mediated sedation through the locus ceruleus and spinal cord and analgesia (25). An added benefit is the minimal respiratory depression. Side effects include hypertension during the bolus dose, and hypotension, bradycardia, and dry mouth from the infusion. Dexmedetomidine undergoes hepatic metabolism and is primarily excreted by the kidneys. Its context-sensitive half-life varies significantly with the duration of the infusion from <10 minutes to several hours.

FUTURE AGENTS FOR SEDATION

Research continues on numerous sedative agents. Volatile anesthetic gases, such as isoflurane, desflurane, and xenon, have been studied. Xenon has potential because of its sedative and analgesic effects, minimal cardiovascular depression; its excretion via exhalation with minimal metabolism, makes it useful among patients with hepatic or renal failure (26). Concerns with its use include high cost and pollution of the ICU environment, with possible effects on health care workers. The other gases have a similar risk-to-benefit profile. Isoflurane, however, is a potent vasodilator, whereas desflurane can cause tachycardia.

CLINICAL RECOMMENDATIONS OF THE VIGNETTE

Many factors come into play when clinicians undertake the task of sedating patients in the ICU. A fine balance must be obtained between the underlying disease states, interaction with multiple drugs with varying pharmacokinetic and pharmacodynamic properties, and assessment tools. Currently, multiple approaches to sedation in the ICU settings fall within the practice guidelines set forth by the Society of Critical Care Medicine (27), and are composed of algorithmic approaches to this complex problem.

Our algorithm depends on the Sedation-Agitation Scale (SAS) (Fig. 133-1) (28). Others use different assessment tools that can be easily found on the internet (e.g., www.icudelirium.org sponsored by Vanderbilt University, Nashville, TN).

SUMMARY

Management of sedation in the ICU setting can be significantly complex. A detailed knowledge of basic pharmacologic principles and selection of appropriate assessment tools facilitates the administration of an appropriate sedation schema. Although many approaches are described, a single *best practice* model has yet to be determined. Flexibility and titration are important when dealing with these complex issues.

REFERENCES

1. Lewis K, Whipple J, Michael K, et al. Effect of analgesic treatment on physiological consequences of acute pain. *American Journal of Hospital Pharmacy.* 1994;51:1539–1554.
2. Riker R, Picard J, Fraser GL. Prospective evaluation of sedation-agitation scale for adult critically ill patients. *Crit Care Med.* 1999;27(7):1325–1329.
3. Ramsay MAE. Measuring levels of sedation in the intensive care unit [Letter]. *JAMA.* 2000;284(4):441–442.
4. Young C, Knudsen N, Hilton A, et al. Sedation in the ICU. *Crit Care Med.* 2000;28(3):854–866.
5. Gross J, Bailey P, Connis R, et al. Practice guidelines for sedation and analgesia by non-anesthesiologists. *Anesthesiology.* 2002;96:1004–1017.
6. Ramsay M, Savage T, Simpson B, et al. Controlled sedation with alphaxalone-alphadolone. *BMJ.* 1974;2:656–659.
7. Chernik DA, Gillings D, Laine H, et al. Validity and reliability of the observers' assessment alertness/sedation scale: Study with intravenous midazolam. *J Clin Psychopharmacol.* 1990;10:244–251.
8. Harris CE, O'Donnell C, MacMillian RR, et al. Use of propofol by infusion for sedation of patients undergoing haemofiltration on the level of sedation and on blood propofol concentration. *Journal of Drug Development.* 1991;4[Suppl 3]:37–39.
9. Johansen JW, Sebel PS. Development and clinical application of electroencephalographic bispectrum monitoring. *Anesthesiology.* 2000;93:1336–1344.
10. Mondello E, Siliotti R, Noto G, et al. Bispectral index in ICU: Correlation with Ramsay Score on assessment of sedation level. *J Clin Monit Comput.* 2002;17(5):271–277.
11. Tonner PH, Wei C, Bein B, et al. Comparison of two bispectral index algorithms in monitoring sedation in postoperative intensive care patients. *Crit Care Med.* 2005;33(3):580–584.
12. Roustan JP, Valette S, Aubas P, et al. Can electroencephalographic analysis be used to determine sedation levels in critically ill patients? *Anesth Analg.* 2005;101(4):1141–1151.
13. LeBlanc JM, Dasta JF, Kane-Gill SL. Roles of the bispectral index in sedation monitoring in the ICU. *Ann Pharmacother.* 2006;40(3):490–500.
14. White P. Intravenous nonopioid anesthesia. *Seminars in Anesthesia and Perioperative Medicine and Pain.* 2005;24(2):101–107.
15. Mirski M, Muffelman B, Ulatowski J, et al. Sedation for the critically ill neurologic patient. *Crit Care Med.* 1995;23(12):2038–2053.
16. Nugent M, Artru A, Michenfelder J. Cerebral metabolic, vascular and protective effects of midazolam maleate. *Anesthesiology.* 1982;56:172–176.
17. Stevenson G, Hall S, Rudnick S. The effect of anesthetic agents on the human immune response. *Anesthesiology.* 1990;72:542–552.
18. Bayona N. Propofol neuroprotection in cerebral ischemia and its effects on low-molecular-weight antioxidants and skilled motor tasks. *Anesthesiology.* 2004;100(5):1151–1159.
19. Vasile B. The pathophysiology of propofol infusion syndrome: A simple name for a complex syndrome. *Intensive Care Med.* 2003;29(9):1417–1425.
20. Liolios A. Propofol infusion syndrome associated with short-term large-dose infusion during surgical anesthesia in an adult. *Anesth Analg.* 2005;100(6):1804–1806.
21. Hanna J. Rhabdomyolysis and hypoxia associated with prolonged propofol infusion in children. *Neurology.* 1998;50(1):301–303.
22. Rockoff M, Goudsouzian N. Seizures induced by methohexital. *Anaesthesia.* 1981;54:333–335.
23. Angelini G. Use of propofol and other nonbenzodiazepine sedatives in the intensive care unit. *Crit Care Clin.* 2001;17(4):863–880.
24. Cheng M. Intravenous agents and intraoperative neuroprotection. Beyond barbiturates. *Crit Care Clin.* 1997;13(1):185–199.
25. Maze M. New agents for sedation in the intensive care unit. *Crit Care Clin.* 2001;17(4):881–897.
26. Bedi A, Murray J, Dingley J, et al. Use of xenon as a sedative for patients receiving critical care. *Crit Care Med.* 2003;31(10):2470–2476.
27. Jacobi J, Fraser GL, Coursin DB, et al. Clinical guidelines for sustained use of sedatives and analgesics in the critically ill adult. *Crit Care Med.* 2002;30(1):119–141.
28. Loyola University Medical Center Department of Medicine. Available at http://147.126.98.11/ClinicalProtocol/Docs/Analgesia-Sedation%20Protocol.pdf. Accessed July 19, 2006.

CHAPTER 134

Critical Illness Polyneuropathy and Myopathy

Jasvinder P.S. Chawla

OBJECTIVES

- To explore the ways that critical illness polyneuropathy and myopathy have been associated most often with sepsis and multiorgan dysfunction syndrome
- To identify common signs and symptoms associated with critical illness polyneuropathy and myopathy
- To identify treatment options available for the disorder
- To show how to determine prognosis based on illness severity

CASE VIGNETTE

A 45-year-old man, previously healthy, was brought to the hospital with severe right lower quadrant pain, nausea, and fever. He was found to have a ruptured appendix, and had an appendectomy. He developed sepsis from postoperative peritonitis, however. Respiratory insufficiency ensued, requiring prolonged mechanical ventilation. Thrombocytopenia and anemia developed, requiring multiple transfusions of blood products. He remained hemodynamically unstable and developed *Staphylococcus epidermidis septicemia.* A tracheostomy was performed 2 weeks after endotracheal intubation. His condition stabilized around the third week of hospitalization, and he was weaned off all sedatives. He then complained of limb numbness, and was found to have a flaccid quadriparesis.

On examination, all four extremities were flaccid, with marked weakness of both upper and lower extremities. Muscle stretch reflexes were absent. Sensation was reduced to pinprick in both hands and feet. Serum vitamin B_{12}, folate, and thyrotropin were normal. As he could not be weaned off the ventilator, an electromyography and nerve conduction study (EMG/NCS) was done 3 weeks after surgery. The study revealed markedly reduced motor amplitudes, with preserved latencies and conduction velocities. EMG findings were consistent with acute denervation involving multiple muscles tested of both upper and lower extremities. Findings were consistent with a severe, diffuse acute sensory-motor axonal polyneuropathy.

DEFINITION

Critical illness polyneuropathy (CIP) is the most common acquired neuromuscular condition in the intensive care unit (ICU setting) (1). Bolton et al. first reported CIP in critically ill patients in the early 1980s (1). The entity was found primarily among survivors of severe sepsis and multi-organ dysfunction syndrome (MODS) (2–4). Recent literature has emphasized the involvement of muscle that has variously been termed as *acute quadriplegic myopathy, acute necrotizing myopathy of intensive care, thick filament myopathy,* and *critical illness myopathy* (CIM) (5). CIP has also been described in terms of the systemic inflammatory response syndrome (SIRS) that occurs in more than half the patients who have been on mechanical ventilation for >1 week and sepsis lasting >2 weeks (6). Onset of CIP can occur as early as 3 days following onset of sepsis or SIRS. CIP and CIM, singly or in combination, can occur commonly in these patients and present as generalized limb weakness as well as difficulty in weaning from the ventilator (6).

EPIDEMIOLOGY

Polyneuropathies associated with critical illness have been described in patients with prolonged sepsis, anoxic coma after cardiac arrest, metabolic crises, severe burns, as well as with use of medications such as gentamicin and pancuronium bromide (7,8). The predominance of either CIP or CIM in an individual patient probably varies, depending on the previous use of neuromuscular blocking agents or corticosteroids. Thus, in an ICU setting where these medications were often used in posttransplant recipients, the incidence of CIM was significantly high (9), whereas in another ICU where there were no posttransplant recipients, and neuromuscular blocking agents or corticosteroids were rarely used, the incidence of CIM was low (4). The range of severity of combined CIP and CIM may be significantly marked. CIP has also been reported in children, but the incidence is considerably less than in adults because of a much lower incidence of SIRS in the pediatric population in the ICU (10).

ETIOLOGY AND PATHOGENESIS

The pathogenesis of CIP remains unknown. CIP is characterized by an axonal distal degeneration of sensory and motor fibers (11). In 1996, Bolton (12) proposed that axonal degeneration may be caused by factors attributed to sepsis, such as the presence of tumor necrosis factor (TNF), histamine, arachidonic acid metabolites, local free radical formation, and activation of the complement and cell adhesion systems. Microcirculatory disturbance of the peripheral nerves was also considered a possible pathophysiologic mechanism (13). Besides sepsis and MODS, CIP has also been associated with other conditions, including prolonged mechanical ventilation (14–16), malnutrition, vitamin deficiencies (17), immunologic disorder (3), Guillain-Barré syndrome (GBS) (18), toxin-producing bacteria, coagulopathies (3), use of gentamicin or other neuromuscular blocking agents (pancuronium bromide) (19), hyperosmolality or changes in osmolality (20), and hypotension (21).

Use of neuromuscular blocking agents and corticosteroids have accounted for a high incidence of myopathy (9). Sepsis may be the only underlying factor in some patients who have never received these drugs (22). Lacomis et al. (22) have proposed various entities associated with pure muscle weakness be labeled as CIM. CIP can occur in settings other than the ICU (23). Patients with end-stage renal failure can develop severe and rapidly developing axonal, predominantly motor, polyneuropathy. Similarly, patients with chronic liver disease can have a mild, predominantly demyelinating motor and sensory polyneuropathy, but the SIRS occurring in this setting rarely induces a CIP (2).

PATHOLOGY

Nerve biopsy studies demonstrate fiber loss and primary axonal degeneration, with no evidence of inflammation, and predominant involvement of distal nerve segments. Peripheral axonal degeneration is represented by central chromatolysis of the anterior horn cells, as well as by moderate loss of dorsal root ganglion cells. Muscle pathology demonstrates acute and chronic denervation with occasional myopathic changes (24). Primary axonal degeneration of the phrenic nerves and denervation atrophy of respiratory muscles may explain the respiratory insufficiency (25).

CLINICAL MANIFESTATIONS

CRITICAL ILLNESS POLYNEUROPATHY

CIP and CIM can both occur significantly in the same patients (17). Often, typical signs and symptoms of CIP and CIM requiring neurologic consultation are difficulty weaning from mechanical ventilation and severe generalized muscle weakness (26). Neuromuscular clinical manifestations may be occult in 50% of cases (18). Findings on physical examination usually include intact cranial nerve function (25), diffuse muscular atrophy, flaccid quadriparesis, and reduced to absent muscle stretch reflexes (15). Muscle stretch reflexes, however, can be normal in one third of patients with CIP (15,17), or even hyperactive in patients with associated central nervous system (CNS) lesions (15).

CIP is often preceded by septic encephalopathy, which can create certain difficulties with a detailed neuromuscular examination in these patients. Thus, the polyneuropathy may not easily be identified clinically in half of the patients (18). Sensory testing is often unreliable in patients who are encephalopathic, but evidence of distal loss to pain, temperature, and vibration may be observed among more responsive patients (11).

CRITICAL ILLNESS MYOPATHY

An acute myopathy affecting critically ill patients has been identified by different terms, including acute quadriplegic myopathy or CIM. Limb weakness develops after onset of a critical illness. A diffuse flaccid weakness involves all limb muscles, neck flexors, and, frequently, the facial muscles and diaphragm. Unlike inflammatory myopathies, myalgias are less commonly seen in CIM. Examination could be challenging in patients who are encephalopathic who have received neuromuscular blocking agents. Three main subtypes of CIM are recognized (12).

Thick Filament Myopathy

Thick filament myopathy is mainly observed in patients with severe asthma often requiring ventilator support, high-dose corticosteroids, or neuromuscular blocking agents. Serum creatine kinase (CK) levels are mildly elevated. Muscle biopsy shows destruction of thick myosin filaments.

Acute Necrotizing Myopathy

Often precipitated by multiple causes of myoglobinuria, the serum CK levels in acute necrotizing myopathy are markedly elevated. Myoglobulinuria is present and electrophysiologic studies demonstrate a severe myopathy. Muscle biopsies show widespread necrosis of muscle fibers.

Cachectic Myopathy

Also known as disuse atrophy, cachectic myopathy is responsible for marked wasting and weakness of muscles. Laboratory studies are generally nonspecific. Muscle biopsy may show type 2 fiber atrophy. Cachectic myopathy remains a diagnosis of exclusion.

DIFFERENTIAL DIAGNOSIS

GBS and acute pure axonal motor neuropathy are the major differential diagnoses (12). Ancillary studies may assist in their differentiation. Findings favoring the diagnosis of CIP include normal cerebrospinal fluid (CSF) protein levels, electrophysiologic findings of axonal neuropathy, and nerve biopsy showing absence of inflammatory changes (11,27). The axonal variant of GBS characteristically occurs before presentation to the ICU setting, and is often associated with *Campylobacter jejuni* infection (28).

DIAGNOSTIC APPROACH

Patients intubated, sedated, and receiving neuromuscular blocking agents, with or without superimposed encephalopathy, require a detailed neurologic examination to accurately identify these disorders. Both the identification and characterization of polyneuropathy or myopathy require the appropriate interpretation of a comprehensive neurologic examination, electrophysiologic studies, and determination of serum CK levels. Diagnostic criteria for critical illness polyneuropathy and myopathy have been outlined by Bolton (29).

Major criteria include a critical illness (sepsis, multiple organ failure, SIRS), difficulties with ventilator weaning, possible limb weakness, and electrophysiologic evidence of axonal motor-sensory polyneuropathy. Phrenic nerve conduction studies and needle EMG of the diaphragm can also assist establishing CIP as the possible cause of failure to wean from the ventilator (30). NCS show low-amplitude compound motor and sensory action potentials. Fibrillation potentials and positive sharp waves are present in both CIM and CIP. In CIM, the motor unit potentials are of low amplitude and short duration, with increased recruitment of motor unit potentials (18).

Other laboratory testing should at least include determination of serum CK levels. Markedly elevated levels suggest a necrotizing myopathy, whereas in other types of CIM, serum CK elevations are not as elevated and may be delayed for 10 days or more after administration of corticosteroids. Conversely, in CIP, serum CK levels are either normal or only mildly elevated (12). Muscle biopsy is occasionally indicated to differentiate critical illness myopathy from other myopathies or from critical illness polyneuropathy. Muscle biopsy should be considered for the exact treatment as well as prognosis (12). Muscle biopsy in CIM may show atrophy or necrosis, with clearly absent inflammatory changes. Atrophy is typically seen in type 2 fibers, but may involve type 1 fibers, or even a combination of both the fibers (31).

TREATMENT

GENERAL

No specific treatment exists for CIN and CIM (32). Management is focused in treating the underlying critical illness. Specific treatment for CIN and CIM is supportive, including psychological support for patients and families, analgesics if needed, and frequent neurologic assessments (15). Treatments need to be individualized, depending on illness severity and underlying comorbidy. Adequate prevention of decubitus ulcers, prophylaxis of deep vein thrombosis, and aggressive physical therapy is mandatory.

Management of Critical Illness Polyneuropathy

CIP requires proper treatment of sepsis, multiorgan dysfunction syndrome, and careful management of ventilation, physical therapy, and rehabilitation. Airway, breathing, and circulation should be maintained, with concomitant management of septic shock. Despite these and other measures, the mortality rate in sepsis and multiple organ failure in the ICU is still approximately 30% to 50%. With early institution of proper and aggressive treatment, CIP often improves in a matter of weeks in mild cases, or months in severe cases (12,25). Administration of intravenous immunoglobulin (IVIgG) has been attempted without significant benefit (33).

Management of Critical Illness Myopathy

Because corticosteroids and neuromuscular blocking agents can contribute to CIM, they are best avoided or used in the lowest possible dosages, and only for a short period of time (24).

PROGNOSIS

For either CIP or CIM, prognosis depends on the extent of axonal damage. Full recovery often occurs in mild to moderate cases. In severe cases, recovery can be longer or incomplete. Severe cases are still associated with a high mortality rate (4,24). Severe forms of CIP and the necrotizing myopathy of intensive care can have a poor prognosis for recovery (5).

CLINICAL RECOMMENDATIONS OF THE VIGNETTE

The patient was discharged to a rehabilitation center and remained on ventilator support for almost 2 months after surgery; then, he was successfully extubated. Hemodynamic functions slowly improved with supportive management as well as aggressive physical therapy. He subsequently recovered fully from the polyneuropathy after months of intense rehabilitation.

SUMMARY

CIP and CIM are among the most common neuromuscular complications in critically ill patients. Signs and symptoms of CIP and CIM must be recognized early and proper measures taken to allow the best possible recovery after sepsis or MODS.

REFERENCES

1. Bolton C, Gilbert J, Hahn A, et al. Polyneuropathy in critically ill patients. *J Neurol Neurosurg Psychiatry.* 1984;47:1223–1231.
2. Bolton C. Neuromuscular manifestations of critical illness. *Muscle Nerve.* 2005;32:140–163.
3. Zifko U. Long-term outcome of critical illness polyneuropathy. *Muscle Nerve Suppl.* 2000;9:S49–S52.
4. Fletcher S, Kennedy D, Ghosh I, et al. Persistent neuromuscular and neurophysiologic abnormalities in long-term survivors of prolonged critical illness. *Crit Care Med.* 2003; 31:1012–1016.
5. Dalton H. Critical illness polyneuropathy and myopathy. *Critical Care Med.* 2001;29: 2388–2390.
6. Bolton C, Young B, Zochodne D. The neurological complications of sepsis. *Ann Neurol.* 1993;33:94–100.
7. Garnacho-Montero J, Madrazo-Osuna J, Garcia-Garmendia JL, et al. Critical illness polyneuropathy: Risk factors and clinical consequences. A cohort study in septic patients. *Intensive Care Med.* 2001;27:1288–1296.
8. Henderson BL, Koepke GH, Feller I. Peripheral polyneuropathy among patients with burns. *Arch Phys Med Rehabil.* 1971;52:149–151.
9. Lacomis D, Petrella JT, Giuliani MJ. Causes of neuromuscular weakness in the intensive care unit: A study of ninety-two patients. *Muscle Nerve.* 1998;21:610–617.
10. Geller TJ, Kaiboriboon K, Fenton GA, et al. Vecuronium-associated axonal motor neuropathy: A variant of critical illness polyneuropathy? *Neuromuscul Disord.* 2001;11:579–582.
11. Zochodne DW, Bolton CF, Wells GA, et al. Critical illness polyneuropathy. A complication of sepsis and multiple organ failure. *Brain.* 1987;110:819–842.
12. Bolton C. Sepsis and the systemic inflammatory response syndrome: Neuromuscular manifestations. *Crit Care Med.* 1996;24:1408–1416.
13. Bone RC. Sepsis syndrome. New insights into its pathogenesis and treatment. *Infect Dis Clin North Am.* 1991;5(4):793–805.
14. Hund E, Fogel W, Kreiger D, et al. Critical illness polyneuropathy: Clinical findings and outcomes of a frequent cause of neuromuscular weaning failure. *Crit Care Med.* 1996;24:1328–1333.
15. van Mook W, Hulsewe-Evers R. Critical illness polyneuropathy. *Curr Opin Crit Care.* 2002; 8:302–310.
16. Hund E, Genzwurker H, Bohrer H, et al. Predominant involvement of motor fibres in patients with critical illness polyneuropathy. *Br J Anaesth.* 1997;78:274–278.
17. Hund E. Critical illness polyneuropathy. *Curr Opin Neurol.* 2001;14:649–653.
18. Bolton CF, Laverty DA, Brown JD, et al. Critically ill polyneuropathy: Electrophysiological studies and differentiation from Guillain-Barre syndrome. *J Neurol Neurosurg Psychiatry.* 1986;49:563–573.
19. de Letter M, Schmitz P, Visser L, et al. Risk factors for the development of polyneuropathy and myopathy in critically ill patients. *Crit Care Med.* 2001;29:2281–2286.
20. Waldhausen E, Keser G, Schulz B, et al. Weaning failure due to acute neuromuscular disease. *Crit Care Med.* 1989;17:594–595.
21. Rivner MH, Kim S, Greenberg M, et al. Reversible generalized paresis following hypotension: A new neurological entity. *Neurology.* 1983;33:164–165.
22. Hoke A, Rewcastle NB, Zochodne DW. Acute quadriplegic myopathy unrelated to steroids or paralyzing agents: Quantitative EMG studies. *Can J Neurol Sci.* 1999;26:325–329.
23. Lacomis D, Zochodne DW, Bird SJ. Critical illness myopathy. *Muscle Nerve.* 2000;23: 1785–1788.
24. Bolton CF, Gilbert JJ, Hahn AF, et al. Polyneuropathy in critically ill patients . *J Neurol Neurosurg Psychiatry.* 1984;47:1223–1231.

25. Hund E. Neurological complications of sepsis: Critical illness polyneuropathy and myopathy. *J Neurol.* 2001;248:929–934.
26. Zifko UA, Zipko HT, Bolton CF. Clinical and electrophysiological findings in critical illness polyneuropathy. *J Neurol Sci.* 1998;159:186–193.
27. Op de Coul A, Lambregts P, Koeman J, et al. Neuromuscular complications in patients given Pavulon (pancuronium bromide) during artificial ventilation. *Clin Neurol Neurosurg.* 1985;87:17–22.
28. Kupfer Y, Namba T, Kaldawi E, et al. Prolonged weakness after long-term infusion of vecuronium bromide. *Ann Intern Med.* 1992;117:484–486.
29. Bolton CF. Electrophysiologic studies of critically ill patients. *Muscle Nerve.* 1987;10:129–135.
30. Bolton CF. Clinical neurophysiology of the respiratory system. *Muscle Nerve.* 1993;16:809–818.
31. Showalter CJ, Engel AG. Acute quadriplegic myopathy: Analysis of myosin isoforms and evidence for calpain-mediated proteolysis. *Muscle Nerve.* 1997;20:316–322.
32. Hund E. Critical illness polyneuropathy. *Curr Opin Neurol.* 2001;14:649–653.
33. Wijdicks EF, Fulgham JR. Failure of high dose intravenous immunoglobulins to alter the clinical course of critical illness polyneuropathy. *Muscle Nerve.* 1994;17:1494–1495.

CHAPTER **135**

ICU Psychosis

Harold W. Goforth • Murali S. Rao

OBJECTIVES

- To describe how to recognize delirium as a common presentation in acute inpatient care
- To distinguish between delirium and other comorbidity (dementia, depression)
- To describe the pathophysiology of delirium
- To discuss the management of common delirious states

CASE VIGNETTE

A 42-year-old man was admitted to the intensive care unit (ICU) after sustaining 40% second-degree burns, and 10% third-degree burns to his body after a boiler explosion. After 4 days in the ICU setting, the patient became hyperactive and attempted to self-discontinue intravenous lines. When examined, his attention span was fluctuating and he appeared to be mumbling to himself as though he was interacting with someone. He was clearly disorientated and believed he was in a school. An electroencephalogram (EEG) demonstrated diffuse slowing in the 2 Hz range. His white blood count (WBC) was elevated at 16,000, with 85% neutrophil band forms. Blood cultures showed growth of methycillin-resistant staphylococcus aureus (MRSA).

DEFINITION

Intensive care unit (ICU) psychosis is a common subtype of delirium historically ascribed to the ICU environment and accompanying stressors, such as impaired sleep, isolation from sunlight and disruption of circadian rhythm, and sensory overload. More recent data, however, dispute these environmental roles, and underlying causes are similar to other forms of delirium. Essential features of delirium include a disturbance of consciousness, attention, and perception, which arises over a relatively short period of time and fluctuates over the course of the day. The disturbance in consciousness is most frequently manifest by deficits in the ability to focus, sustain, and shift attention, but also frequently involves reduced awareness of the surrounding environment, disorientation, secondary memory, language impairments (e.g., dysnomia and dysgraphia), and visuoconstructional impairment representing a diffuse cerebral process. Perceptual disturbances are common as well, and can include misinterpretations, illusions, delusions, and hallucinations (1).

Delirium must not be better accounted for by a preexisting dementia, and it represents an acute and significant decline in functioning. Delirium in the *Diagnostic and Statistical Manual of Mental Disorders*, fourth edition, text revision (DSM-IV-TR) is attributable to a general medical condition, substance-induced delirium, multiple causes, or not otherwise specified (1). Identification of the underlying cause of delirium is paramount in importance and will be the mainstay of treatment as well as influence treatment of the delirious process. Other terms used for delirium that are generally synonymous with it include ICU psychosis, ICU syndrome, encephalopathy, acute confusional state, organic brain syndrome, toxic psychosis, and acute brain failure.

EPIDEMIOLOGY

Delirium is widely prevalent in inpatient settings, and estimates suggest that 10% of all inpatients will develop delirium over the course of their hospitalization. This figure increases considerably in special populations, including those with dementia (75%), hospitalized patients with acquired immunodeficiency syndrome (AIDS), patients in the ICU (30%), and burn patients (20%). Hepatic encephalopathy has been noted in up to 70% of patients with cirrhosis, and debilitating symptoms, including coma, are experienced by approximately 30% of patients with end-stage liver disease (2).

Delirium is one of the most frequent hospital complications in elderly patients (2 to 3 million patients per year), and its presence significantly prolongs hospital and ICU stays, with an estimated $4 billion increase in hospitalization costs (3). Delirium is also a highly distressing experience for caregivers and nurses involved in patient care. Prompt recognition and treatment of delirium is critically important, however, and has been demonstrated to reduce both suffering and distress (1).

ETIOLOGY AND PATHOGENESIS

The causes of delirium and ICU psychosis are varied, and it is important to determine the primary cause because treatment of the underlying condition is central to the resolution of delirium. General medical conditions are the most common cause of this syndrome, and underlying conditions associated with it include central nervous system (CNS) disorders, metabolic disorders, cardiopulmonary disease, and systemic illness (Table 135-1) (2). One of the more common causes for ICU delirium includes medications, and it is important to perform a thorough and accurate review of all medications in such patients. Offending medications often have significant anticholinergic potential, and serum anticholinergic load has been linked to the development of acute confusional states. Table 135-2 lists common medications associated with delirium (4).

Various substances and withdrawal syndromes can also precipitate confusion in the ICU setting, but the most common offending agents include alcohol and benzodiazepines. Other agents, including cocaine, hallucinogens, and narcotics, must be considered in this class as well. Withdrawal syndromes vary between agents, but alcohol and benzodiazepine withdrawal are especially important, given the substantial risk of death resulting from uncontrolled withdrawal from these agents in a medically or surgically ill patient (2).

Delirium from multiple causes is especially common in the critically ill and hospitalized elderly populations such that Francis and Kapoor (5) found that 46% of delirium cases in the elderly had an average of 2.8 causes per patient (5). It is important to perform a complete review of a patient's medical record to eliminate additive factors that may be responsible for the delirious process, including combinations of infections, metabolic disturbances, iatrogenic causes, and underlying compromised neurologic states. Other risk factors for the development of acute confusional states include use of physical restraints, use of three or more medications, malnutrition, use of a bladder catheter, and any iatrogenic event (4).

PATHOLOGY

All subtypes of delirium are manifestations of neuronal dysfunction, and areas of particular involvement include the cortex and deep brainstem structures responsible for regulation of consciousness, such as the reticular activating system. It is clear, however, that delirium can result from both excessive neurotransmitter release and electrophysiologic dysfunction (6).

Acetylcholine has been clearly linked to the development of delirium in both animal and clinical studies, and an anticholinergic medication is one of the most common causative factors for the development of delirium in compromised individuals such as the elderly and those with dementia. Serum anticholinergic activity has also been linked to delirium, which strengthens the role of this neurotransmitter in precipitating confusional states. Dopamine is another neurotransmitter with strong links to the development of delirious states, and may play an intermediary role through acetylcholine, given that these two neurotransmitters are linked in a reciprocal relationship. High-potency neuroleptic medications (e.g., haloperidol) with little anticholinergic capacity have long been the mainstay of delirium treatment, and these agents offer substantial symptomatic relief (6).

Although acetylcholine and dopamine have been the two neurotransmitters most closely linked with the development of delirium, serotonin may also play a role, given that hallucinogens, such as lysergic acid diethylamide (LSD), frequently produce delirium and act as serotonergic agonists. Recent data have also linked inflammatory cytokines to the development of delirium, including IL-1, IL-6, and tumor necrosis factor-alpha (TNF-α). The putative role of these substances, however, has not yet been well characterized. Other topics of interest include the roles potentially played by cortisol, β-endorphins, and amino acids acting as false neurotransmitters (6).

The pathophysiology of hepatic encephalopathy as a subtype of ICU psychosis or acute confusional state deserves special mention and is postulated to be derived from neurotoxic substances, including ammonia and manganese, which obtain entry into the CNS during times of hepatic insufficiency and result in swollen astrocytes and neuronal dysfunction. Other possibilities include upregulation of peripheral-type benzodiazepine receptors, which may result in γ-aminobutyric acid (GABA)ergic predominance and impaired neurotransmission and neurotoxins, such as short-chain fatty acids and mercaptans, but the role of these substances is not currently well understood (7).

Neurophysiologic alterations are common in delirium, and EEG studies frequently demonstrate evidence of global cerebral

TABLE 135-1. Underlying Diseases Associated with Delirium and Acute Confusional States

Endocrinopathies, especially thyroid or parathyroid
Fecal impaction or urinary retention
Hepatic or renal insufficiency or failure
Hypo- or hyperglycemia
Hypoperfusion, including dehydration
Hypoxia
Infection
Medication-induced delirium, especially anticholinergic medications
Metabolic abnormalities
Nutritional deficiency, especially thiamine and cyanocobalamin
Pain
Seizures
Structural abnormalities of brain
Substance withdrawal, especially alcohol, sedative-hypnotic agents

TABLE 135-2. Medications Associated with Delirium

Anesthetics, especially ketamine; occasionally inhalational agents
Antiarrhythmics: digoxin, beta-blockers, others
Antibiotics, especially fluoroquinolones
Anticonvulsants, especially barbiturates
Antidepressants, especially tricyclic medications, even in small doses
Antihistamines: first generation
Antihypertensives: beta-blockers, diuretics, ACE inhibitors
Antiparkinsonian agents, especially anticholinergic compounds
Antipsychotics, especially phenothiazines and sedating compounds
H2-blockers, cimetidine
Mood stabilizers: lithium
Motion sickness medications: scopolamine, dimenhydrinate
Pain medications, especially meperidine, other narcotics; occasionally NSAID
Sedative-hypnotic agents

ACE, angiotensin-converting enzymes; NSAID, nonsteroidal anti-inflammatory drugs.

dysfunction in the form of generalized slowing. Classic EEG changes associated with hepatic encephalopathy include high-amplitude, low-frequency waves and triphasic waves; however, these are not specific for hepatic causes and may be observed in other metabolic derangements (8).

CLINICAL MANIFESTATIONS

The clinical manifestations of ICU psychosis typically develop over the course of several hours to days, and fluctuate in severity during the course of the illness. The acute onset and fluctuating nature of delirium is helpful in distinguishing this disorder from dementia, although dementia remains a powerful risk factor for delirium with upwards of 75% of demented individuals demonstrating delirium over the course of a lifetime. Thus, the two disorders often coexist in susceptible individuals. In contrast to dementia, however, delirium typically clears in the days or weeks following correction of the underlying medical illness (1).

Delirium can present in hypoactive, hyperactive, and mixed states, which complicates the differential diagnosis during the initial assessment. Hypoactive delirium can present with features similar to depression, such as withdrawal, refusal of self-care, tearfulness, and despair with associated mood-congruent delusions. Yet, in contract to depressive disorders, individuals with hypoactive delirium manifest global cerebral dysfunction across multiple cognitive spheres with a worsened outcome similar to other subtypes of delirium (9).

Psychomotor agitation is the most common reason for consultations for hyperactive and mixed delirium, and agitation often leads to an inability to provide appropriate medical care because of the patient's refusal of care, violence, or self-discontinuation of medical care, such as removing intravenous lines or catheters. Consultations for capacity evaluation are common also in this environment when patients are less physically agitated, but their confusion is sufficient to prompt refusal of medical care or threats to leaving the treating facility. Any capacity evaluation in an inpatient hospital setting must evaluate the presence of delirium, because this will be a key determinant in allowing proper medical care to proceed.

Sleep–wake cycle disturbances are common, and the architecture of sleep is commonly disturbed with periods of random sleep or a reversal of existing sleep architecture. Also, visual hallucinations are common during delirium, and these can become frightening, which can lead to agitation and combative behavior. Psychosis of any modality can occur such as tactile, olfactory, and auditory hallucinations; illusions; delusions; and disorganized thought processes. Delirium remains high in the differential diagnosis of any evaluation of new-onset psychosis in an inpatient setting (1).

Cognitive impairment, which can be profound, affects diffuse cortical areas, leading to disorders in the ability to focus, sustain, and shift attention; secondary memory impairment; and dysnomia, apraxia, and dysarthrias. These deficits can be most easily elicited by routine clinical testing of forward–backward digit spans, serial sevens, object recall, clock-drawing test, and trials of repetition. In cases of mild delirium, evidence of objective cognitive impairment may only be noted with administration of standardized clinical scales, which illustrates the importance of a thorough evaluation of these patients (1).

TABLE 135-3. Common Diagnostic Workup of Delirium

LABORATORY STUDIES

Arterial blood gas
Complete blood count with differential diagnosis
Electrolytes and glucose
Renal function testing
Liver function testing
Thyroid profile
Urinalysis with culture and sensitivities
Urine or serum drugs of abuse screen
Sedimentation rate, if indicated

IMAGING AND PROCEDURAL STUDIES

Chest x-ray
Electrocardiography (ECG)
Electroencephalography (EEG)
Head computed tomography (CT)
Lumbar puncture (LP), if indicated

DIAGNOSTIC APPROACH

The diagnosis of delirium is a clinical one, and no specific medical test exists that is sensitive or specific for this diagnosis. Laboratory tests may be confirmatory and supportive, but cannot replace clinical acumen in making this diagnosis—especially in cases of mild delirium where clinical symptoms are less forthcoming. Selected laboratory tests are listed in Table 135-3. Although it is easier to diagnose delirium in the context of a hyperactive or mixed presentation, it is important to identify hypoactive delirium as well in that it has a worsened impact on prognosis, recovery, and rehabilitation than other more noticeable forms (9).

Several validated rating scales have been developed for delirium, and routine use of one of these scales is encouraged during both initial assessment and follow-up examinations to better monitor the disease course and response to treatment. The *Confusional Assessment Method* (CAM) has been validated under a variety of circumstances for delirium screening, and a positive response to the CAM suggests the presence of delirium. The *Memorial Delirium Assessment Scale* (MDAS) and the *Delirium Rating Scales* (DRS, DRS-98) have been validated as both screening instruments and as being useful for tracking changes in the severity of delirium (10) The Folstein *Mini-Mental Status Examination* (MMSE) is commonly used clinically for delirium, but it is of limited use clinically because it has not been validated for use in delirious states. It may be helpful, however, in that it covers a wide variety of cortical domains, and fluctuating scores can suggest the presence of a delirious process.

TREATMENT

The goal of treating delirium is to identify and correct the underlying cause while managing the cognitive and behavioral aspects of the syndrome to maximize patient comfort and enable neurobehavioral recovery. Serial examinations using a validated assessment tool, such as the MDAS or the DRS, will assist in monitoring improvement, decline, and response to particular interventions. Furthermore, discontinuing medications that are not essential to the medical care of the patient may improve cognitive functioning, independent of treating the underlying disorder. Beyond these measures, the appropriate interventions may best be divided into behavioral and pharmacologic categories.

Behavioral interventions include correcting perceptual deficits experienced by the patient (e.g., poor vision and poor hearing). These sensory deficits have been documented to increase the prevalence of delirium, and interventions, such as ensuring the patient has access to corrective lenses and hearing aids, can do much to minimize the misinterpretation of existing stimuli and reduce the occurrence of illusions during the hospitalization process. Also, minimizing the degree of unnecessary stimuli around a delirious patient will serve well to help reduce the degree of behavioral agitation. The presence of comforting and familiar items (e.g., blankets, photographs, and family) around the patient will also reduce the impact from environmental factors (11).

Pharmacologic interventions can be effective, both in treating the delirium and in reducing distress and shortening hospitalizations when used appropriately. Intravenous use of haloperidol has been the standard treatment of delirium because of its virtual freedom from anticholinergic effects as well as reduced incidence of extrapyramidal effects when used intravenously. Intravenous haloperidol is generally safe from a cardiovascular profile, with the exception of a small risk of torsades de point when used in the setting of metabolic abnormalities—especially hypokalemia and hypomagnesemia (12). It has little deleterious effect on the respiratory drive of critically ill individuals who may require mechanical ventilation, and has a wide margin of safety as evidenced by reports of use of up to 1,200 mg daily. Although case reports support a wide safety range with this agent, typical starting doses of haloperidol for agitated delirium are recommended to be 0.5 to 3 mg given intravenously every 4 to 6 hours on a scheduled basis, and then titrated to effect until appropriate control of the delirium has been achieved (13).

Other traditional neuroleptic agents have been reported to be successful in treating delirium, but low-potency agents, such as chlorpromazine, should generally be avoided because of their heavy anticholinergic profiles and the potential to worsen delirium in those who are susceptible. Atypical neuroleptic agents are used increasingly from a clinical standpoint to treat delirium; however, the data supporting their use are generally less than that for haloperidol. Risperidone is the atypical agent most similar to haloperidol, and a comparative study has shown equal efficacy with haloperidol in treating delirium (14).

Treatment of refractory agitation in delirious patients poses a special challenge to the practitioner, and agents used to augment the effects of haloperidol or atypical medications include benzodiazepines and opiates. Intravenous or intramuscular lorazepam is reliable, effective, and synergistic with haloperidol in the treatment of behavioral agitation associated with delirium. Typical intervention strategies include intravenous lorazepam (1 to 2 mg) every 4 to 6 hours on an as needed or scheduled basis, depending on the degree of agitation, and given in conjunction with a scheduled haloperidol dosing strategy. Also, intravenous narcotics (e.g., hydromorphone) can play an important role in calming agitation in cases of severe agitation unresponsive to a neuroleptic–benzodiazepine combination or in delirium exacerbated by untreated pain complaints (15).

Benzodiazepines rarely have a primary role in delirium or ICU psychosis except used in conjunction with neuroleptic therapy unless the confusional state is secondary to alcohol, benzodiazepine, or barbiturate withdrawal. In these special cases, the appropriate use of benzodiazepines is both a standard of care as well as a life-saving intervention. No single benzodiazepine agent has been documented to be of superior efficacy over other agents, but the most commonly used agents for purposes of withdrawal include chlordiazepoxide, diazepam, lorazepam, and oxazepam (16).

Patients with a history of delirium caused by alcohol or sedative-hypnotic withdrawal ("delirium tremens") should be prophylactically treated with a benzodiazepine taper before the emergence of delirium under ideal circumstances. Patients already experiencing delirium from these causes must be treated aggressively to avert the high incidence (25%) of mortality associated with unchecked withdrawal from these substances. Frequent use of substance withdrawal rating scales, such as the Clinical Institute Withdrawal Assessment of Alcohol Scale (CIWA), can assist in providing guidance for proper dosing, but scheduled oral chlordiazepoxide (50 mg) or its equivalent every 4 hours can serve as a point of initiation when beginning treatment. Chlordiazepoxide (50 mg) every 1 to 2 hours on an as required dosing basis should be provided in addition to the scheduled dose for those in severe withdrawal for agitation, confusion, and elevated autonomic indices. High-dose thiamine (100 to 300 mg daily), folate, and multivitamin combinations should be administered routinely in this high-risk population to prevent or minimize the effect of Wernicke syndrome and malnutrition (16).

Delirium secondary to hepatic encephalopathy is based on decreasing colonic bacteria and lowering serum ammonia levels with such agents as lactulose, neomycin, or rifaximin. Typically, lactulose is dosed initially at 30 mL orally twice daily, and titrated to achieve three to four loose stools per daily. Agents, such as neomycin can be dosed at 250 mg two to four times daily to reduce colonic bacteria, but continued use of the aminoglycosides can be complicated by ototoxicity and nephrotoxicity owing to mild systemic absorption. Rifaximin, which is a nonabsorbable derivative of rifampin, is currently approved as an orphan drug for the treatment of hepatic encephalopathy and has comparable efficacy to lactulose, and comparable tolerability to placebo (17). Cost considerations, however, have prevented it becoming a first-line agent at many centers.

CLINICAL RECOMMENDATIONS OF THE VIGNETTE

A screening using CAM was suggestive for delirium. The patient was diagnosed with delirium, and was treated with vancomycin and haloperidol (1 mg) intravenously twice daily, while nonessential stimulation was minimized. The patient became more alert, attentive, and rational in his verbal responses over the next 7 days, and haloperidol was discontinued after resolution of his bacteremia. Screening for delirium, particularly for the hypoactive type, with a screening instrument such as CAM-ICU or DRS is recommended for all cases of altered mental status in the ICU setting because (*a*) of its fluctuating course; (*b*) at its most subtle level, delirium is a deficit in attention; and (*c*) detection and treatment can help reduce morbidity and mortality.

SUMMARY

Delirium is often a marker of medical decline in affected patients, and it commonly presents in the ICU settings. It is associated with significant morbidity and mortality up to 1 year after discharge from the inpatient unit. Accurate recognition and treatment of this disorder are important in reducing morbidity and mortality in affected patients. Treatment must address both the underlying medical cause and minimize the neurobehavioral sequelae of this disorder.

REFERENCES

1. Practice guideline for the treatment of patients with delirium. American Psychiatric Association. *Am J Psychiatry.* 1999;156[5 Suppl]:1–20.
2. Fann JR. The epidemiology of delirium: A review of studies and methodological issues. *Semin Clin Neuropsychiatry.* 2000;5(2):64–74.
3. Franco K, Litaker D, Locala J, et al. The cost of delirium in the surgical patient. *Psychosomatics.* 2001;42(1):68–73.
4. Alagiakrishnan K, Wiens CA. An approach to drug induced delirium in the elderly. *Postgrad Med J.* 2004;80:388–393.
5. Francis J, Kapoor WN. Delirium in hospitalized elderly. *J Gen Intern Med.* 1990;5:65–79.
6. Trzepacz PT. Delirium. Advances in diagnosis, pathophysiology, and treatment. *Psychiatr Clin North Am.* 1996;19:429–448.
7. Butterworth RF. Pathophysiology of hepatic encephalopathy: A new look at ammonia. *Metab Brain Dis.* 2002;17:221–227.
8 . Jacobson S, Jerrier H. EEG in delirium. *Semin Clin Neuropsychiatry.* 2000;5:86–92.
9. O'Keeffe ST, Lavan JN. Clinical significance of delirium subtypes in older people. *Age and Ageing.* 1999;28:115–119.
10. Schuurmans MJ, Deschamps PI, Markham SW, et al. The measurement of delirium: Review of scales. *Research Theory in Nursing Practice.* 2003;17:207–224.
11. Inouye SK, Bogardus ST, Charpentier PA, et al. A multicomponent intervention to prevent delirium in hospitalized older patients. *N Engl J Med.* 1999;340:669–676.
12. Menza MA, Murray GB, Holmes VF, et al. Decreased extrapyramidal symptoms with intravenous haloperidol. *J Clin Psychiatry.* 1987;48:278–280.
13. Wise MG, Trzepacz PT. Delirium (confusional states). In: Rundell JR, Wise MG, eds. *Textbook of Consultation-Liaison Psychiatry.* Washington, DC: American Psychiatric Publishing; 1996:258–274.
14. Schwartz TL, Masand PS. The role of atypical antipsychotics in the treatment of delirium. *Psychosomatics.* 2002;43:171–174.
15. Stern TA, Cassem NH, Fricchione G. *Massachusetts General Hospital Handbook of General Hospital Psychiatry,* 5th ed. Philadelphia: Elsevier; 2004.
16. Galanter M, Kleber HD. *The American Psychiatric Publishing Textbook of Substance Abuse Treatment,* 3rd ed. Washington, DC: American Psychiatric Publishing; 2004.
17. Festi D, Vestito A, Mazzela G, et al. Management of hepatic encephalopathy: Focus on antibiotic therapy. *Digestion.* 2006;73[Suppl 1]:94–101.

CHAPTER 136

Orbital Diseases

Michael P. Merchut • Amjad Ahmad

OBJECTIVES

- To describe the signs and symptoms typical with orbital disease
- To explain how extraocular muscle dysfunction can occur, either from orbital (muscle) or retroorbital (oculomotor, trochlear or abducens cranial nerve) lesions
- To discuss features of thyroid eye disease, the most common cause of unilateral or bilateral proptosis in adults
- To discuss features of an acutely painful, swollen eye, which is usually caused by orbital cellulitis or an inflammatory pseudotumor syndrome, if local trauma is excluded

CASE VIGNETTE

A 60-year-old woman has a 2-month history of trouble focusing her eyes. Whenever her vision blurs, it improves by covering one eye. She feels pressure in her left eye, which feels as if it is "moving outwards." On examination, the left eye appears proptotic as compared with the right, with mild limitation of lateral gaze and upgaze. The left upper eyelid is retracted above the cornea and the eye appears injected. Both pupils react briskly to light with normal optic discs.

DEFINITION

The orbits are pyramidal-shaped cavities within the skull, each containing the eye (globe), lids, and lacrimal gland. The optic nerve and ophthalmic artery enter the orbit posteriorly at its apex through the optic canal, surrounded by a cone-shaped array of extraocular muscles attached to the globe. These muscles are innervated by the oculomotor (III), trochlear (IV), and abducens (VI) cranial nerves, which pass through the superior orbital fissure. Paranasal sinuses intimate with the orbit are the ethmoid (medially), the maxillary (inferiorly), and the sphenoid (posteriorly). Paranasal infections and tumors can spread into the orbits causing functional deficits in motility and vision.

EPIDEMIOLOGY

The most common cause of proptosis in children is orbital cellulitis, because of their propensity to acquire ethmoid sinusitis. The distribution of orbital diseases is shown in Table 136-1 (1).

In middle-aged adults, thyroid orbitopathy affects women four to five times more often than men, with a more equal incidence occurring in later adult life. More severe thyroid eye disease usually occurs with an acute onset over weeks, rather than over 4 to 5 months or longer, accompanied by hyperthyroidism of recent onset, which is often difficult to control. Severe visual loss from thyroid eye disease is rare, but tends to occur in older men who currently smoke (2). Orbital inflammatory syndromes are more often idiopathic (orbital pseudotumor) than secondary to systemic disorders such as sarcoidosis or Wegener's granulomatosis (3).

ETIOLOGY AND PATHOGENESIS

Usually, thyroid orbitopathy is temporally related to clinical hyperthyroidism, occurring within 18 months of the onset of Graves' disease, but it can also develop in patients who are hypothyroid or euthyroid. An autoimmune process appears to link Graves' disease, often with accompanying pretibial myxedema, and thyroid orbitopathy. In thyroid orbitopathy, extraocular muscles, and perhaps orbital fat and fibrous tissue, are infiltrated by mononuclear, T-cell predominant infiltrates. The specifically targeted receptors may be those for thyrotropin (thyroid-stimulating hormone [TSH]). A complex cytokine inflammatory response is manifested by orbital fibroblasts and adipocytes. Production of cytokines, along with oxygen free radicals, can be further enhanced by patients currently smoking cigarettes, who tend to have more severe thyroid orbitopathy (4). The proliferation of orbital fat and asymmetric swelling of orbital muscle not only limits ocular motility, but also impairs venous or lymphatic drainage, causing local pain, proptosis, periorbital edema, and other signs of orbital congestion. Extensive swelling and crowding within the orbit can cause compression of the optic nerve at the orbital apex, leading to visual loss. If significant scarring occurs after the initial inflammatory phase, ocular motility may remain limited. Overall, severe disease only occurs in about 10% to 15% of patients, with many cases resolving spontaneously. In patients with Graves' disease, 90% may have abnormalities on orbital imaging studies (e.g., enlarged extraocular muscles), but only 50% have obvious clinical findings (2).

Primary orbital tumors originate from orbital neural elements, muscles, lacrimal glands, eyelids, and soft tissue. Optic nerve gliomas are part of the neurofibromatosis (NF) syndrome. NF-1, autosomal dominant, involves chromosome 17, and appears to lack the tumor suppressor gene. Multiple cutaneous neurofibromas are typical, although clinical manifestations are

TABLE 136-1. Orbital Diseases[a]

Thyroid Orbitopathy	*Neoplastic*	*Congenital and Traumatic*	*Inflammatory and Infectious*	*Vascular*	*Degenerative*	*Other*
52%	18%	12%	9%	4%	2%	3%
Fourth to sixth decades	**	Dermoid or epidermoid cysts, mucoceles	Sinusitis, pseudotumor syndrome	Arteriovenous fistulae, lymphatic malformations	Fat prolapse, post-irradiation changes	

[a]Patients (N = 3,919) at the University of British Columbia Orbital Clinic, 1976–1999; percentages rounded to add up to 100%.
**Common in children: capillary hemangiomas, optic nerve gliomas, neurofibromas, rhabdomyosarcomas; common in adults: lymphomas, cavernous malformations, schwannomas, metastases.
(From Rootman J, Chang W, Jones D. Distribution and differential diagnosis of orbital disease. In: Rootman J, ed. *Diseases of the Orbit,* 2nd ed. Philadelphia: Lippincott Williams & Wilkins; 2003:53–84, with permission.)

variable. NF-2, which is less common, is typically associated with multiple neurofibromas, meningiomas, and gliomas of the brain and spinal cord, and, most classically, bilateral acoustic neuromas. Secondary orbital tumors can invade from the paranasal sinuses and temporalis fossa, or from distant systemic malignancies (5).

Orbital trauma can cause ocular injury, retrobulbar hematomas, or optic nerve damage. Fracture of the medial or inferior orbit can entrap an extraocular muscle, limiting motility and causing diplopia. Decreased motility in the traumatized orbit can also occur from local muscle edema or paresis from nerve injury. Traumatic rupture of an internal carotid artery into the surrounding cavernous (venous) sinus creates an abnormal arteriovenous fistula, leading to engorged scleral and retinal veins, periorbital swelling, proptosis, ocular bruit, and a pulsatile globe.

PATHOLOGY

The prominent feature in thyroid eye disease is infiltration of the extraocular muscles, especially the medial and inferior recti. This initial lymphocytic infiltration and mucopolysaccharide deposition can be followed by fibrosis and fatty replacement of atrophic muscle fibers (2,4). Noninfectious granulomatous infiltrates of the orbit prompt a systemic evaluation for sarcoidosis or Wegener granulomatosis, whereas lymphocytic involvement of the lacrimal glands is typical of Sjögren's syndrome (6). Orbital pseudotumor refers to a spectrum of poorly understood, painful disorders where mononuclear infiltrates involve the orbit anywhere from the conjunctivae and eyelid to the orbital apex. A vague orbital mass (pseudotumor) or swollen extraocular muscles may be evident on computed tomography (CT) or magnetic resonance imaging (MRI), but either condition resolves quickly after corticosteroid therapy (3).

Orbital neural tumors arising from peripheral nerve elements include neurofibromas and the more encapsulated schwannomas. Optic nerve tumors arise from the nerve itself (gliomas) or its dural sheath (meningiomas). Patients with either of these tumors should be evaluated for NF-1 (cutaneous café au lait spots or neurofibromas, Lisch nodules of the iris, axillary freckling) or NF-2 (deafness from vestibular schwannomas [acoustic neuromas]). Orbital lymphomas, usually B-cell in type, can now be distinguished from inflammatory pseudotumors by immunostaining or flow cytometry. Systemic lymphoma can secondarily involve the eyelids or lacrimal glands.

Tumors arising from orbital structures include hemangiomas, rhabdomyosarcomas, various fibromas and sarcomas, lacrimal adenomas and dysplasia, or tumors of bone or cartilage. Nasopharygeal tumors and distant metastases can involve the orbit (5). Only 1% to 3% of orbital pathology is caused by metastases, usually in patients with known systemic cancer; in 25% of cases, however, the primary site is not known. A primary breast cancer is most common, followed by lung, prostate, and melanoma. Breast cancer typically spreads to orbital soft tissues, whereas prostate cancer tends to involve the bony orbit (5,7).

Orbital cellulitis, often bacterial and more common in children, typically spreads from an adjacent sinusitis or other facial infection. Although overall rare, fungal infections from *Mucor* and *Aspergillus* species are typically aggressive and often fatal in patients who are immunocompromised or diabetic. Either fungus can invade blood vessels; the ischemic inflammation from *Mucor* organisms produces a typical black eschar (6).

CLINICAL MANIFESTATIONS

Signs of orbital congestion (swollen lids, chemosis, conjunctivitis, dilated scleral vessels, local pain) accompanied by proptosis most strongly suggest an orbital lesion, whereas ophthalmoplegia, visual impairment, and facial sensory loss may be caused by orbital or retroorbital (cavernous sinus, superior orbital fissure) lesions. *Proptosis,* or bulging of the eye, can appear symmetric or toward one direction. Inferior displacement of the eye from a lacrimal gland tumor will also be more inward, whereas inferior displacement of the eye from a frontal sinus mucocele moves the eye more outward. A medial subperiosteal abscess from ethmoidal sinusitis will displace the eye laterally, whereas upward displacement would occur from a similar process in the maxillary sinus. Proptosis, with other orbital signs, is usually bilateral, although asymmetric, in Graves' disease, with lid lag or retraction (Fig. 136-1). *Ptosis,* however, tends to occur from orbital inflammatory syndromes or cellulitis, which are usually unilateral in adults. *Diplopia,* improved by covering either eye, indicates an ocular motility problem, ranging from clinically subtle to overtly severe. Diplopia is caused by restriction of extraocular muscles; by infiltration, inflammation, or mass effect; or by a lesion involving cranial nerves III,

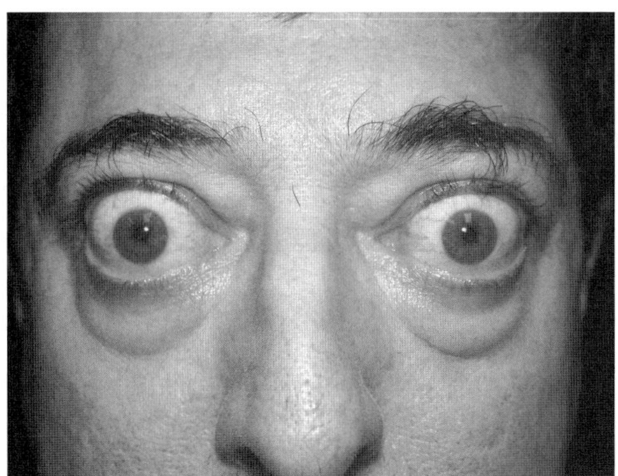

FIGURE 136-1. Thyroid orbitopathy: proptosis, lid retraction, and mild periorbital swelling.

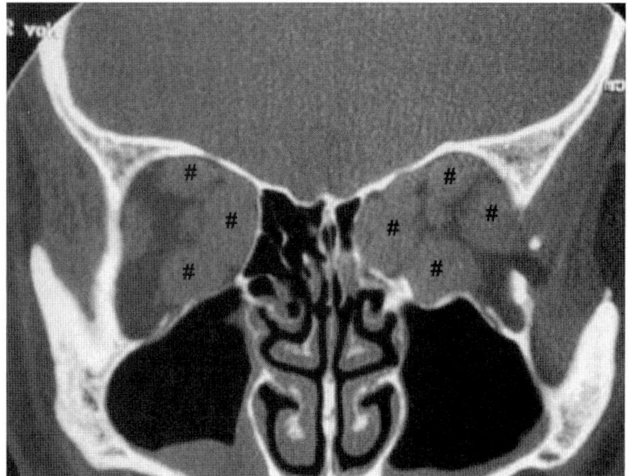

FIGURE 136-2. Thyroid orbitopathy: coronal computed tomographic (CT) scan of orbits, showing enlarged extraocular muscles (#) surrounding the optic nerves.

IV, or VI. A restrictive pathology is favored by resistance to forced duction testing (attempted passive movement of the globe after topical anesthesia), whereas a freely movable globe occurs with a neurogenic lesion. Severe orbital muscle edema from Graves' disease not only impairs ocular motility, but also compresses the optic nerve. In the absence of anterior inflammation or opacity of the eye, patchy loss of vision (scotomas) or graying out (impaired color vision) implies involvement of the optic nerve, which appears swollen or pale. This occurs with tumor infiltrating or compressing the optic nerve, or other inflammatory or infiltrative processes, particularly at the orbital apex posteriorly.

Symptom evolution within hours suggests an orbital hemorrhage or severe inflammatory process, whereas more gradual development is typical of lower grade inflammation or tumor infiltration. Episodic symptoms can be provoked by certain head positions, where a mass effect through a skull defect can occur; or, during the Valsalva maneuver, where venous drainage is transiently impaired, as in a vascular malformation (2,8).

An acutely painful eye, with photophobia and signs of inflammation (proptosis, conjunctivitis, periorbital and lid edema) may signal orbital cellulitis or an idiopathic, inflammatory pseudotumor syndrome. The strictly unilateral involvement and rapid onset are unusual for thyroid orbital disease. A fever, leukocytosis, and any signs of recent infection of the sinuses, face, or nasopharynx support the diagnosis of orbital cellulitis. Eye movement abnormalities, ptosis, or a unilateral visual deficit can occur with either orbital cellulitis or pseudotumor. The idiopathic pseudotumor syndrome includes a spectrum of inflammatory disorders, located more anteriorly (lacrimal gland or lid edema, scleritis), or posteriorly (myositis, optic perineuritis). The Tolosa-Hunt syndrome refers to an inflammatory pseudotumor at the superior orbital fissure or orbital apex, with painful ophthalmoplegia and numbness over the forehead (ophthalmic branch of the trigeminal nerve) (6).

DIAGNOSTIC APPROACH

Obviously, a thorough systemic evaluation of the patient with orbital disease may uncover significant clues to the presence of cancer, recent head trauma, bleeding disorder, or neurofibromatosis. Serum thyroid function tests and perhaps autoantibodies (TSH receptor antibodies) are indicated in undiagnosed Graves' disease.

A detailed ophthalmologic examination should include visual acuity, visual fields, pupillary responses, measurement of ocular motility and proptosis, dilated fundoscopy, and intraocular pressure readings. Substantial increases in intraocular pressure measurements during sustained upgaze or during forced duction testing occur from extraocular muscle swelling (2). Axial and coronal CT scan images of the orbits (Fig. 136-2) serve to further localize the lesion (e.g., orbital walls or apex, extraocular muscles); its type (e.g., abscess, tumor, hemorrhage, or inflammation); and, perhaps, origin (e.g., from the ethmoid sinus or sphenoid bone). The contrasting density or signal of orbital fat helps to sharply delineate the optic nerve, extraocular muscles, and globe from any lesions therein. Both CT and MRI scans also visualize any associated lesions in the adjacent retroorbital area, paranasal sinuses, skull, or brain. Echography, or orbital ultrasound, in the hands of the ophthalmologist, can also provide useful images, especially to guide needle biopsy of anteriorly located lesions.

In most cases of orbital disease, the diagnosis can be made with the history, clinical findings, and appropriate imaging. Occasionally, surgery is required both to explore the orbit and to obtain tissue for pathologic diagnosis.

TREATMENT

Mild thyroid orbitopathy may only require lubrication to prevent exposure keratitis, or head elevation in bed, to avoid the morning periorbital swelling from reclining while asleep. Early and effective control of hyperthyroidism may or may not lessen the orbitopathy, but it is usually recommended by initially using thyroid suppressive drugs (methimazole, propylthiouracil), followed by thyroidectomy or radioactive iodine, although the latter seems associated with more severe orbital disease. Patients can be given a 4- to 6-week trial of oral prednisone (30 to 40 mg) daily to decrease acute inflammation, although the effects may be transient and must be weighed against the risks of corticosteroids. Patients with loss of vision secondary to compressive optic neuropathy should be treated aggressively with initial oral doses of prednisone (80 to 100 mg) daily. Intravenous pulse methylprednisolone has fewer systemic side-effects, and can be given as 1 g boluses three times a week, and repeated every 4 to 6 weeks as clinically necessary for severe visual loss. Patients who are not responding to steroids or who cannot tolerate them should be sent for either orbital decompression or orbital radiation. Surgery consists of removal of the orbital bones, usually the medial and inferior walls, to allow the edematous orbital tissues to expand into the adjacent sinuses. Orbital radiotherapy (20 Gy per eye, in 10 fractions over 2 weeks) usually improves periorbital swelling or optic nerve compression after 4 to 6 weeks, but not ocular dysmotility from fibrosis. Patients with diabetic or ischemic retinopathy should not receive orbital radiation, because it can accelerate vasculopathy. For steroid nonresponders or those with diabetes avoiding steroids, other immunosuppressive medications have been tried, such as oral azathioprine (100 to 150 mg) daily, oral methotrexate (5 to 25 mg) weekly, oral cyclosporine (50 to 200 mg) twice daily, oral cyclophosphamide (100 to 200 mg) daily (or, 0.5 to 1.0 g intravenous pulses every 1 to 2 months). The role of plasmapheresis, octreotide (somatostatin analogs), and intravenous high-dose gammaglobulin therapy remains uncertain. Future early treatment may involve cytokine antagonists to counteract the initial inflammatory phase of this disorder. The acute inflammatory phase of thyroid eye disease usually burns out within 1 to 2 years. Once patients enter the chronic or fibrotic stage, surgical rehabilitation is planned to repair their ocular deviation and eyelids (2,4).

Orbital cellulitis must always be considered with the presentation of an acutely painful, swollen eye. Urgent CT or MRI of the orbit is critical, to determine the site of involvement, the presence of an abscess cavity and any adjacent sinusitis, as well as to exclude the presence of a neoplastic or other process. Culturing of the infected area, perhaps by an endoscopic approach, and initial broad-spectrum antibiotic coverage is required. In the absence of fever, and an obvious site of infection, an acutely painful, swollen eye can also be caused by an inflammatory pseudotumor syndrome. The pain and swelling of the latter typically respond within 24 to 48 hours with corticosteroid therapy (e.g., oral prednisone 60 to 80 mg daily). The daily prednisone dose can be decreased by 5 mg weekly, with dose increases for symptomatic flare-ups. Oral steroid nonresponders, or those with initially severe visual loss, could be treated with pulse 1 g doses of intravenous methylprednisolone. As with the treatment for thyroid orbitopathy, those unable to take corticosteroids may benefit from orbital radiation, or the other immunosuppressive agents mentioned above. Orbital pseudotumor can recur, but a poor therapeutic response or a persistent or progressive orbital lesion may signify a different cause and requires a biopsy for a definitive diagnosis (3,6).

The role of surgical biopsy or resection of an orbital tumor will vary, based on its extent, location, and invasiveness within the orbit, as well as the age and condition of the patient. Discovery of any metastatic lesion prompts a search and staging of its primary source, with further treatment (chemotherapy, radiation) based on those findings.

CLINICAL RECOMMENDATIONS OF THE VIGNETTE

The patient has unilaterally impaired ocular motility, proptosis, lid retraction, and mild orbital inflammation of subacute to chronic onset. These findings should be further assessed or quantified by a complete ophthalmologic examination, complemented by a CT or MRI scan of the orbits and brain, with and without contrast. Given the likelihood of Graves' disease, thyroid functions should be tested, with achievement of a euthyroid state.

SUMMARY

Hyperthyroidism (Graves' disease) is the most common cause of orbital disease overall. Such patients require endocrinology and ophthalmology input both to stabilize systemic thyroid disease and to manage any ocular complications, which range from minor irritation to severe visual loss. Orbital cellulitis must be excluded in the presentation of an acutely, painful, swollen eye, which alternatively may be caused by an inflammatory orbital pseudotumor. The latter readily responds to oral corticosteroids, with alternative therapies, including orbital radiation and other immunosuppressive agents. Primary orbital tumors present at different ages, with orbital metastases more common in middle to late adulthood. The presence of systemic findings, such as neurofibromatosis, or a diagnosed malignancy, offer clues to the nature of a subacute to chronic orbital mass. CT and MRI of the orbit also helps shed light on the orbital pathology, as well as on its exact location and extent.

REFERENCES

1. Rootman J, Chang W, Jones D. Distribution and differential diagnosis of orbital disease. In: Rootman J, ed. *Diseases of the Orbit,* 2nd ed. Philadelphia: Lippincott Williams & Wilkins; 2003:53–84.
2. Rootman J, Dolman PJ. Thyroid orbitopathy. In: Rootman J, ed. *Diseases of the Orbit,* 2nd ed. Philadelphia: Lippincott Williams & Wilkins; 2003:169–212.
3. Jacobs D, Galetta S. Diagnosis and management of orbital pseudotumor. *Curr Opin Ophthalmol.* 2002;13:347–351.
4. Bartalena L, Wiersinga WM, Pinchera A. Graves' ophthalmopathy: State of the art and perspectives. *J Endocrinol Invest.* 2004;27:295–301.
5. Rootman J. Neoplasia. In: Rootman J, ed. *Diseases of the Orbit,* 2nd ed. Philadelphia: Lippincott Williams & Wilkins; 2003:213–384.
6. Rootman J. Inflammatory diseases. In: Rootman J, ed. *Diseases of the Orbit,* 2nd ed. Philadelphia: Lippincott Williams & Wilkins; 2003:455–506.
7. Goldberg RA, Rootman J, Cline RA. Tumors metastatic to the orbit: A changing picture. *Surv Ophthalmol.* 1990;35:1–24.
8. Rootman J. An approach to diagnosis. In: Rootman J, ed. *Diseases of the Orbit,* 2nd ed. Philadelphia: Lippincott Williams & Wilkins; 2003:85–96.

CHAPTER 137

Ocular Infections and Inflammation

Anuradha Khanna • Michael P. Merchut

OBJECTIVES

- To describe some of the common clinical patterns and possible systemic associations with ocular infections and inflammation
- To explain how vision can be threatened in monocular pain and inflammation caused by hyperacute conjunctivitis, corneal ulceration, acute angle-closure glaucoma, uveitis, or scleritis

CASE VIGNETTE

A 34-year-old black woman awakens with a painful, blurry right eye, without trauma, fever, or infection. She had received prednisone for a left peripheral facial palsy 6 months ago. At times, she feels breathless climbing two flights of stairs. She is difficult to examine because of photophobia, but has a visual acuity of 20/50 OD, and 20/20 OS. The right pupil (2 mm, irregular) constricts poorly to light, whereas the left pupil (4 mm, regular) reacts briskly. A subtle, reddish injection is noted around the right limbus, whereas the rest of the external examination and extraocular movements are normal. A limited view of the optic discs and retina uncovers nothing abnormal.

DEFINITION

Inflammation can occur in various parts of, or around, the eye, whether primarily immune mediated or caused by allergy, trauma, or infection. *Conjunctivitis* involves the mucous membrane, which is the innermost layer of the eyelids, and the outermost layer of the ocular globe. *Episcleritis* is inflammation of the episclera, which is the loose connective tissue between the conjunctiva and the sclera, whereas *scleritis* (Fig. 137-1) pertains to the inflammatory process extending to the sclera itself, the dense, collagenous white layer of the globe. *Keratitis* refers to inflammation of the cornea, normally clear and transparent, whereas *blepharitis* pertains to the eyelids. Several of these conditions might coexist. The uvea, or uveal tract, consists of the iris, ciliary body, and choroid, and is basically the vascularized layer between the retina and sclera. Generally, *uveitis* refers to inflammation of these structures, with more specifically localized inflammation described as iritis, cyclitis, choroiditis, or combinations thereof. The ciliary body produces aqueous humor, which flows across the anterior lens, through the pupil and into the anterior chamber of the eye, entering the trabecular meshwork and exiting via the canal of Schlemm. Any obstruction of this pathway can acutely elevate intraocular pressure and impair vision by means of optic nerve damage. *Acute angle-closure glaucoma* is created by apposition or adherence of the iris to the trabecular meshwork, and is clinically manifested as a painful red eye with impending visual loss, mimicking some of the inflammatory conditions discussed above (1,2).

EPIDEMIOLOGY

Common ocular problems in general ophthalmology and primary care medicine include conjunctivitis, traumatic keratitis, and "dry eyes," although precise incidence and prevalence data are lacking. Episcleritis and, especially, scleritis are comparatively infrequent (3). An abruptly painful red eye can be caused by acute angle-closure glaucoma, with a prevalence of 0.04% to 0.9%—more rare than primary open-angle glaucoma (4). Uveitis tends to affect all age groups, yet the incidence appears to increase with patient age. Based on the findings of the Northern California Epidemiology of Uveitis Study (5), the incidence of anterior uveitis is 37 cases per 100,000 person-years. It is estimated that uveitis is responsible for 30,000 new cases of blindness annually, and up to 10% of all the cases of blindness in the United States. A systemic disease association is seen in about 50% of patients with uveitis. Sarcoidosis-related uveitis is more common in blacks, whereas Native American Indians usually have uveitis from Vogt-Koyanagi-Harada (VKH) syndrome. Behçet disease tends to occur in Asian or Middle Eastern people.

ETIOLOGY AND PATHOGENESIS

Conjunctivitis can be viral, allergic, or bacterial. Viral conjunctivitis, commonly caused by adenovirus, is highly contagious and associated with an upper respiratory infection in the patient or in close contacts. Individuals who are atopic typically develop allergic conjunctivitis, often in the company of sinusitis or rhinitis. Bacterial conjunctivitis is usually caused by gram-positive organisms. None of these conditions leads to visual

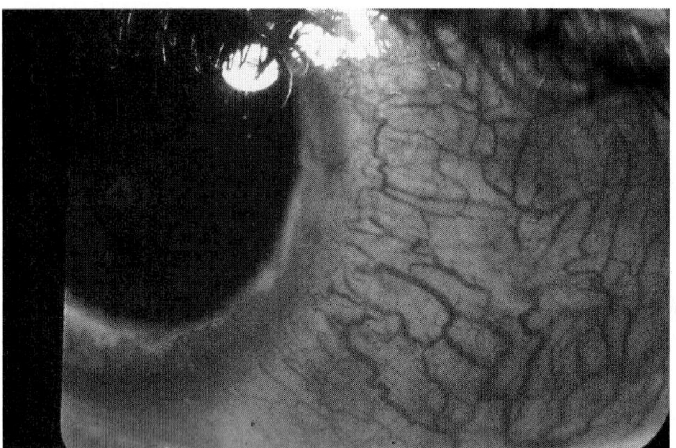

FIGURE 137-1. Diffuse, anterior scleritis.

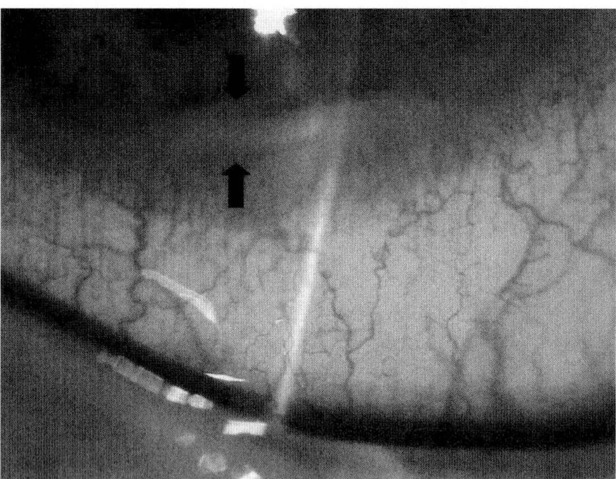

FIGURE 137-2. A hypopyon (**between the arrows**) is seen in the inferior anterior chamber between the iris and the posterior cornea. It consists of leukocytes layering out in the anterior chamber.

deficits, although sexually active patients with gonorrhea can develop a more severe hyperacute conjunctivitis which, if untreated, can progress to corneal ulceration and visual loss. Chlamydial inclusion conjunctivitis is also sexually transmitted, but rarely seen in the United States. *Staphylococci* and *Streptococci* organisms cause keratitis, which also occurs from pseudomonas in contact-lens wearers. Keratitis can also result from trauma, foreign bodies, or chronically dry eyes (1,2).

Episcleritis is self-limited and often recurrent, which is suggestive of an autoimmune process, whereas scleritis often appears related to a systemic inflammatory or vasculitic disorder (3). A subconjunctival hemorrhage appears as a focal or restricted lesion, distinct from these other inflammations, often precipitated by minor trauma, coughing, or sneezing in patients with bleeding disorders or hypertension.

The abnormal apposition of iris to trabecular meshwork in acute angle-closure glaucoma tends to occur in anatomically susceptible patients, such as farsighted individuals with a shorter globe length, and elderly patients with a thicker lens, which pushes the iris forward. An attack is often triggered in the dimmer light of evening, when the pupil normally dilates. The abruptly elevated intraocular pressure not only impairs the iris sphincter but eventually the optic nerve, if untreated (1).

Uveitis can have an infectious, autoimmune, or idiopathic cause. Infectious causes of uveitis include toxoplasmosis, cat scratch disease, toxocariasis, histoplasmosis, Lyme disease, syphilis, cytomegalovirus (CMV), herpes, tuberculosis, and leprosy. Connective tissue diseases associated with uveitis include rheumatoid arthritis, systemic lupus erythematosus, polyarteritis nodosa, and Wegener granulomatosis. Systemic syndromes associated with ocular inflammation include Behçet disease, reactive arthritis (Reiter syndrome), VKH syndrome, and Kawasaki disease.

Localized ocular diseases can cause uveitis in the absence of a systemic disorder. *Sympathetic ophthalmia* occurs when trauma or surgery affects one eye, and uveitis develops "sympathetically" in the other, perhaps as a result of a triggered autoimmune response. *Birdshot choroidopathy* describes multiple yellowish spots ("birdshot") in the retinal pigment epithelium of middle-aged women. *Pars planitis* involves inflammation of the ciliary body, an "intermediate" uveitis possibly associated with multiple sclerosis , Lyme disease, or sarcoidosis.

Various systemic inflammatory diseases can manifest as uveitis. Anterior uveitis, particularly iritis, occurs in men with ankylosing spondylitis and an HLA-B27 antigen type, and can reoccur. Iritis and HLA-B27 are also associated with reactive arthritis (formerly Reiter syndrome), psoriatic arthritis, and inflammatory bowel disease. Sarcoidosis causes an anterior as well as posterior uveitis, with a chronic, bilateral, or recurrent course. A more chronic, painless, anterior uveitis can occur in young girls with juvenile idiopathic arthritis (formerly juvenile rheumatoid arthritis), remaining asymptomatic until scarring and visual loss develop. Behçet disease can be associated with a chronic, bilateral panuveitis that involves both anterior and posterior ocular segments with hypopyon (Fig. 137-2) and retinal vasculitis being prominent features. VKH syndrome involves an autoimmune attack on melanocytes, thereby causing bilateral panuveitis, hearing loss, and aseptic meningitis. Uveitis is also associated with lupus or adult-onset rheumatoid arthritis (6).

PATHOLOGY

Superficial conjunctival blood vessels are diffusely dilated in conjunctivitis. Any purulent discharge is usually bacterial in nature. Because the cornea has richer innervation than the conjunctivae, keratitis is a more painful condition. Corneal ulcerations can occur in gonococcal conjunctivitis, with perforation leading to visual impairment. A dendritic corneal ulcer can occur from herpes simplex virus and herpes zoster, accompanied by a painful, vesicular facial eruption. IgE hypersensitivity to various airborne antigens causes allergic conjunctivitis (1,2). In episcleritis, the radially oriented episcleral blood vessels can be dilated and inflamed more segmentally, rather than diffusely over the eye. Topical 2.5% phenylephrine will constrict, or blanch, the dilated blood vessels of the conjunctivae and, to some extent, the episcleral vessels, but not those in the sclera, which is a distinguishing feature. In scleritis, the presence of granulomas favors sarcoidosis, tuberculosis, syphilis, or leprosy as the cause. Local vasculitis and scleral necrosis can also occur. Bluish areas often indicate scleral thinning (3).

The hallmark of anterior uveitis (iridocyclitis) is inflammatory cells and increased protein ("flare") in the anterior chamber of the affected eye, best seen by slit-lamp examination. The character of keratitic precipitates, which are collections of inflammatory cells on the inner surface of the cornea, such as the granulomatous type in sarcoidosis, may be a diagnostic aid for the ophthalmologist. Glaucoma can occur from impaired flow of aqueous humor owing to accumulating leukocytes or subsequent scarring. Scar tissue also causes irregular pupils and cataracts. Posterior uveitis is the inflammation of any combination of choroid, retina, or vitreous body, where retinal atrophy, retinal detachment, or macular edema can lead to visual loss.

CLINICAL MANIFESTATIONS

Infectious conjunctivitis begins with a diffuse hyperemia ("red eye") and variable lid swelling in one eye, spreading to the other within a few days. Patients have irritation ("foreign body sensation") and a discharge, which tends to be more purulent if bacterial, matting the eyelashes together on awakening. Blepharitis can further increase local irritation. A risk of rapid loss of vision exists in hyperacute gonococcal conjunctivitis, wherein occurs a copious, purulent discharge, painful swelling of eyelids and conjunctivae, and frequent preauricular adenopathy. Allergic conjunctivitis affects both eyes simultaneously, with prominent itching, often related to seasonal pollen or animal dander exposure. A subconjunctival hemorrhage is readily distinguished from conjunctivitis; it consists of a bright red, small, painless, focal hemorrhage obscuring the underlying sclera, without adjacent inflammation or pain, and usually self-resolving in its course (1,2).

Episcleritis consists of an acute, patchy, or segmental hyperemia. There is irritation more than actual pain, with spontaneous resolution but possible recurrences. Scleritis manifests with segmental or global redness in one or both eyes, typically with a deep pain in the globe. Overlying conjunctival and episcleral vessels can also be inflamed, whereas photophobia can signify simultaneous iridocyclitis. Scleral necrosis and perforation lead to visual loss. Symptoms can last months, often heralding systemic inflammatory or vasculitic disorders such as rheumatoid arthritis, Wegener granulomatosis, lupus, or inflammatory bowel disease, especially Crohn disease (3).

Severe, acute ocular pain, even accompanied by nausea and vomiting, occurs in acute angle-closure glaucoma. There is corneal haziness, causing the patient typically to see haloes around lights. A key clinical finding is a mid-dilated pupil, unreactive to light. Visual loss can become permanent because optic atrophy develops within hours of sustained, elevated intraocular pressure (1,2).

Acute, anterior uveitis involves inflammation of the iris and ciliary body (iridocyclitis), causing pain, blurred vision, and photophobia. The redness is more intense at the limbus, with a characteristically irregular shape of the pupil owing to iris adhesion to the lens, and a sluggish pupillary reaction to light. If inflammation is severe, leukocytes layering out in the anterior chamber can be observed, without a slit-lamp, as a whitish fluid level in front of the iris (hypopyon). Other patients with a chronic or insidious onset of anterior uveitis can be asymptomatic until scarring leads to cataracts and retinal edema resulting in visual impairment. The affected eye can have minimal pain in posterior uveitis. Here, symptoms include hazy vision, "blind spots" or "floaters," and flashing lights from retinal involvement (6).

Particular nonocular signs and symptoms may reveal a systemic disease associated with uveitis. Patients who are HLA-B27 antigen positive can have ankylosing spondylitis, with sacroiliitis and limited spinal mobility, or reactive arthritis (Reiter syndrome), with urethritis, arthritis, and conjunctivitis. Sarcoidosis often involves the lungs (dyspnea, cough, hilar adenopathy), and can cause parotitis, lymphadenopathy, or erythema nodosum; however, the finding of noncaseating granulomas is needed to confirm the diagnosis. Juvenile idiopathic arthritis (juvenile rheumatoid arthritis) affects children <16 years of age, involving few or many joints, with or without fever and rash. Behçet disease is manifest by painful orogenital ulcers and vasculitis. Other conditions that initially appear to be uveitis, but truly are not, include B-cell lymphoma, melanoma, or metastatic carcinoma confined to the eye (6).

DIAGNOSTIC APPROACH

Geriatric patients often complain of dry eyes, but a significant sicca syndrome may indicate Sjögren syndrome. A careful history helps determine whether conjunctivitis is infectious or allergic, itching being a significant symptom in allergic conjunctivitis. All patients with "red eye" should have a corneal ulceration ruled out by fluorescein staining, done first in the unaffected eye to avoid cross-contamination. Corneal ulcers, usually painful, should be evaluated by an ophthalmologist. Acute angle-closure glaucoma, an ocular emergency, always needs to be ruled out in the presence of an abrupt, very painful, diffusely injected, red eye. Measurement of intraocular pressure by tonometry is helpful here, as well as in uveitis, where glaucoma can secondarily develop. Significant pain, photophobia, or visual impairment also requires ophthalmologic consultation to rule out scleritis or uveitis, either of which can lead to permanent visual loss. Slit-lamp and dilated funduscopic examinations are crucial, in addition to testing visual fields, visual acuity, pupillary responses, extraocular movements, and examination of the eyelids and external orbit.

Clinical clues for an associated systemic inflammatory or vasculitic disorder in the patient with scleritis should be sought, which includes rheumatoid arthritis, Wegener granulomatosis, polyarteritis nodosa, lupus, relapsing polychondritis, and Crohn disease. Screening can include an erythrocyte sedimentation rate (ESR) or C-reactive protein (CRP), antinuclear antibody (ANA) and antineutrophil cytoplasmic antibody (ANCA) titers, rheumatoid factor (RF), and rapid plasmin reagin (RPR) or venereal disease research laboratory (VDRL) serology. In suspected cases, further evaluation for tuberculosis or sarcoidosis may be necessary (3).

If uveitis is present, further history, signs and symptoms, or work-up is necessary to determine if it is caused by an infection, localized ocular inflammation, or is a manifestation of a systemic disease. Thoracic computed tomographic (CT) scanning for hilar adenopathy is worthwhile if sarcoidosis is suspected, whereas HLA-B27 antigen testing and sacroiliac X-ray studies are useful in patients with iritis and spondylosis. The history or presence of orogenital ulcers supports the diagnosis of Behçet disease, whereas lumbar puncture may be needed to document the aseptic meningitis found in VKH syndrome. Screening blood tests are similar to those for scleritis, including an ESR or CRP, RPR, or VDRL serology and perhaps an ANA titer in selected patients with arthritis, given the rarity of lupus-related uveitis (6).

TREATMENT

Elderly patients with "dry eyes" may only require artificial tears. Viral conjunctivitis is generally mild and self-limited, perhaps only requiring symptomatic therapy with lubricant eyedrops. Strict handwashing and ocular hygiene help prevent spreading this infection. Because topical corticosteroids can worsen herpetic keratitis or lead to secondary bacterial infections, these should be avoided, especially in the presence of eyelid or facial vesicles. Topical acyclovir could be given if a dendritic corneal ulcer from herpes simplex virus is found, but topical therapy is ineffective for herpes zoster, where oral acyclovir (800 mg five times daily for 7 to 10 days) or another antiviral, is given. Allergic conjunctivitis could be treated with antihistamine eyedrops, or topical ketotifen or olopatadine. Bacterial cultures can guide specific therapy for a more severe conjunctivitis with purulent discharge. Topical antibacterial agents include ciprofloxacin or other fluoroquinolones, sulfacetamide, or trimethoprim–polymyxin. In addition to topical therapy, systemic treatment of gonorrhea is needed in hyperacute gonococcal conjunctivitis (1,2).

Episcleritis is usually self-limited, but topical non-steroidal anti-inflammatory drug (NSAID) eyedrops may help reduce pain. Mild to moderate scleritis is also treated with an NSAID, whereas more severe cases require corticosteroid therapy (oral prednisone 1 mg/kg daily, or 0.5 to 1 g intravenous methylprednisolone daily for 3 days, then an oral prednisone taper) followed by steroid-sparing agents such as methotrexate. Other immunosuppressant agents have been used as well (azathioprine, mycophenolate, cyclosporine, chlorambucil, or cyclophosphamide), with various associated side effects or toxicity (3).

Specific antiviral or antimicrobial medications are used to treat infectious retinitis from herpes, CMV, syphilis, or toxoplasmosis. Corticosteroids are used to treat noninfectious uveitis, with the dose and route dictated by the severity of the inflammation. Anterior uveitis (iridocyclitis) can benefit from topical corticosteroids, but posterior uveitis requires systemic therapy. As with scleritis, other immunosuppressant agents have been used as well. Topical mydriatic or cycloplegic drugs help prevent scarring or adhesions between lens and iris, as well as reduce painful ciliary spasms and photophobia (6).

CLINICAL RECOMMENDATIONS OF THE VIGNETTE

Clinically, this patient appears to have an anterior uveitis. Because of the pain and photophobia, a corneal ulcer should be ruled out. Although the pupil is small, rather than mid-dilated, tonometry could definitively exclude acute angle-closure glaucoma. The ophthalmologist's slit-lamp examination would be most helpful here, in addition to a detailed funduscopic examination to rule out any retinal involvement. The patient's respiratory symptoms suggest that she may have sarcoidosis, which should be further evaluated.

SUMMARY

The ophthalmologist's examination of the patient with an ocular infection or inflammation helps refine the diagnosis, unveils helpful clues to the cause, and suggests therapy. The internist or neurologist can evaluate the patient for systemic diseases often associated with uveitis or scleritis.

REFERENCES

1. Leibowitz HM. The red eye. *N Engl J Med.* 2000;343:345–351.
2. Roscoe M, Landis T. How to diagnose the acute red eye with confidence. *Journal of the American Academy of Physicians' Assistants.* 2006;19:24–30.
3. Goldstein DA, Tessler HH. Episcleritis, scleritis and other scleral disorders. In: Yanoff M, Duker JS, eds. *Ophthalmology,* 2nd ed. St. Louis: Mosby; 2004:511–519.
4. Fraser S, Wormald R. Epidemiology of glaucoma. In: Yanoff M, Duker JS, eds. *Ophthalmology,* 2nd ed. St. Louis: Mosby; 2004:1413–1417.
5. Gritz DC, Wong IG. Incidence and prevalence of uveitis in northern California. The Northern California Epidemiology of Uveitis Study. *Ophthalmology.* 2004;111(3):491–500.
6. Hajj-ali RA, Lowder C, Mandell BF. Uveitis in the internist's office: Are a patient's eye symptoms serious? *Cleve Clin J Med.* 2005;72:329–339.

CHAPTER 138

Optic Neuritis and Retinal Vascular Disorders

Felipe De Alba • Michael P. Merchut

OBJECTIVES

- To enhance awareness that acute, partial, or complete nontraumatic monocular visual loss requires emergency ophthalmologic evaluation for a retinal or optic nerve disorder
- To explain that optic neuritis typically occurs subacutely in the younger adult, with a diffuse or partial monocular deficit, impaired color vision, and orbital pain, often related to multiple sclerosis or other systemic inflammatory or immune-mediated diseases
- To discuss ischemic disorders of the retina or optic nerve and explore the ways they tend to occur in older adults, causing sudden monocular blindness or altitudinal deficits, usually related to cardiovascular disease and emboli, hypertension, or temporal arteritis

CASE VIGNETTE

A 70-year-old hypertensive man is seen in the emergency room because of sudden, painless blindness of his right eye while watching television 3 hours earlier. He sees only hand motion with his right eye and his left eye has a corrected visual acuity of 20/30. Shining a penlight in the left pupil produces brisk constriction, but pupillodilation occurs when the light is moved to the right pupil. A dilated funduscopic examination demonstrates attenuated, small-caliber retinal vessels on the right, with yellow-orange luminescent material in the central retinal artery, a normal right optic disc, and diffuse retinal pallor, creating a prominent macular "cherry red spot." The left retina and optic disc are unremarkable, with normal external examination findings and extraocular movements.

DEFINITION

Exiting axons of the retinal ganglion cells coalesce into the optic nerve, which can be viewed funduscopically as the optic disc in the nasal retina. Blurred margins or apparent elevation of the optic disc are the nonspecific clinical signs of a *swollen disc.* A unilateral, acutely swollen disc results from local inflammation, compression, or infiltration, and is termed *optic neuritis* or *papillitis.* If such optic nerve pathology occurs a few millimeters more posteriorly, a similar visual deficit may be produced, but the optic disc may not appear swollen to the examiner (retrobulbar neuritis). Bilaterally swollen discs are typically caused by diffuse elevation of intracranial pressure (ICP), termed *papilledema.*

Retinal arteries and veins appear to pierce the normal optic disc, forming longer, superior and inferior temporal arcades, as well as shorter, superior and inferior nasal arcades. The central retinal artery, which perfuses the retina, and the posterior ciliary arteries, which supply the optic nerve and choroid, are all branches of the ophthalmic artery, which originates from the internal carotid artery.

EPIDEMIOLOGY

Optic neuritis usually occurs in young (20 to 50 years of age) adults, more commonly in women (67% to 75% cases), at an incidence of approximately 5 cases per 100,000 per year. After 10 years of follow-up, 31% of patients have had another episode of optic neuritis, and 38% were diagnosed with multiple sclerosis (MS) (1,2).

Ischemic optic neuropathy (ION) occurs at about 2 to 10 cases per 100,000 annually, in patients >50 years, and it affects men and women equally. Arteritic ION is rarer still, involving an even older age group (3). Retinal artery occlusions are diagnosed in 10 or fewer cases per 100,000 annual outpatient visits, with men outnumbering women about 2 to 1. Likewise, the chronic ocular ischemic syndrome (OIS) also favors older men, but is infrequent (4).

ETIOLOGY AND PATHOGENESIS

As it branches from the ophthalmic artery, the central retinal artery pierces the optic nerve, continuing longitudinally within the nerve, parallel to the nerve fibers, until it reaches the optic disc, where it subdivides to supply the retina. This fairly linear flow pattern makes it easier for arterial emboli to reach and occlude the central retinal artery or one of its branches. The posterior ciliary arteries also arise from the ophthalmic artery, but branch out abruptly at approximately 90° angles to supply the optic nerve itself, perpendicular to the nerve fibers. This nonlinear flow pattern makes it unlikely for emboli to cause ischemic optic neuropathy, which is typically related to thrombosis or hypoperfusion of the posterior ciliary arteries (3).

Any of these acute ischemic syndromes of the retina or optic nerve tend to occur in patients with atherosclerotic risk factors, including arterial hypertension, diabetes, coronary artery disease, hyperlipidemia, cigarette smoking, and a family history of cardiovascular disease. A retinal embolus is visible funduscopically in about 60% of branch retinal artery occlusions, but only in about 20% of central retinal artery occlusions, because emboli are harder to see at the optic disc. Emboli are composed of cholesterol (Hollenhorst plaque), calcium, or fibrin, originating from the ipsilateral arterial system (aortic arch, common or internal carotid arteries), cardiac endothelium, and heart valves. Nonatherosclerotic sources of emboli include carotid artery dissection, fibromuscular dysplasia, cardiac myxoma, temporal arteritis, systemic lupus erythematosus (SLE), and various hypercoagulable states (4,5).

Arteritic ION is attributed to posterior ciliary artery thrombosis from vasculitis, which is most commonly temporal (giant cell or cranial) arteritis. Less common vasculitides include Wegener granulomatosis, SLE, and vasculitis associated with inflammatory bowel disease. The pathogenesis of nonarteritic ION varies and is only weakly linked to hypertension and diabetes. Contributing factors include systemic hypotension (e.g., acute bleeding, antihypertensive drugs, or phosphodiesterase-5 inhibitors for erectile dysfunction), anemia, an anatomically "crowded disc" (small cup-to-disc ratio) at risk for vascular compression, local vasospasm from migraine or sympathomimetic drugs, and rarely, hypercoagulable states (3).

The OIS involves a chronic state of decreased flow to both the central retinal artery and posterior ciliary arteries from ophthalmic artery hypoperfusion. Ipsilateral internal carotid artery occlusion or high-grade stenosis was noted in 76% of OIS cases, where external carotid collateral flow can pass retrograde through the ophthalmic artery and, thus, may also contribute to retinal and optic nerve ischemia as a "steal syndrome" (5).

Because the optic nerve is actually part of the central nervous system (CNS), its myelinated fibers often become a target of the immune-mediated inflammation from MS, occasionally as its first manifestation. Other causes of optic neuritis involve other immune-mediated or vasculitic diseases (e.g., SLE, inflammatory bowel disease), viral infections (e.g., childhood measles, mumps, or varicella), nerve infiltration (e.g., sarcoid granulomas, lymphoma), or local pressure (e.g., thyroid orbitopathy, optic nerve sheath meningioma) (2).

PATHOLOGY

A unilateral blurred optic disc, with relatively abrupt visual loss, signifies an optic nerve lesion. Optic neuritis from MS consists of varying degrees of mononuclear cell inflammation, edema, myelin loss, and gliosis (2). In arteritic ION from temporal arteritis, posterior ciliary arteries are thrombosed by infiltrating lymphocytes and multinucleated giant cells, with fragmentation of the internal elastic lamina (3). Except for a few reported cases of bilateral, simultaneous optic neuritis in children, the finding of bilateral disc swelling raises concern about papilledema from increased ICP. Early visual loss does not occur in papilledema, although headache, nausea, and vomiting can reflect increased ICP. Causes of papilledema include an intracranial mass, cerebral venous thrombosis, severe encephalitis, or idiopathic intracranial hypertension (pseudotumor cerebri). Both optic discs become edematous, primarily because of transmitted elevated pressure via the adjacent subarachnoid (cerebrospinal fluid) space, thereby impairing axoplasmic flow in the optic nerve. In both untreated optic neuritis and papilledema, optic nerve fiber atrophy ensues, with chronic visual impairment and a clinically pale, white optic disc on funduscopic examination.

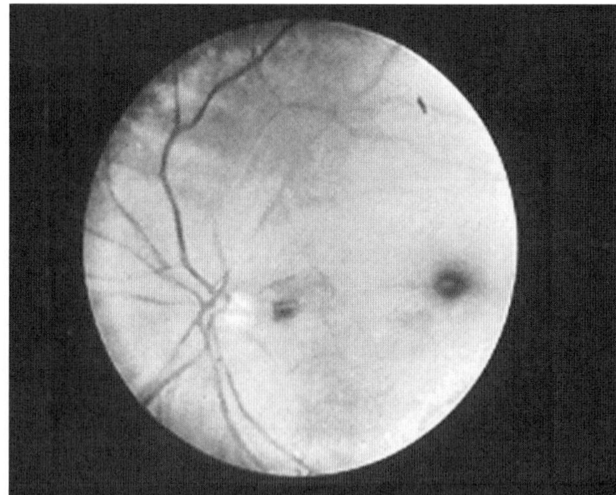

FIGURE 138-1. Central retinal artery occlusion (CRAO) of left eye with diffuse retinal pallor. Attenuated vessels and dark "cherry red spot" macula, seen at R.

In central (CRAO) or branch retinal arterial occlusions (BRAO), the ischemic segment of inner retina undergoes coagulative necrosis, with edematous retinal cells creating the gray-white retinal pallor seen clinically. Retinal pallor with attenuated vessels may be diffuse with CRAO, or an area of segmental ischemia in the setting of a BRAO. The cherry red spot seen in CRAO corresponds to the normal red-colored fovea (macula) perfused by the choroid, in contrast to the surrounding pale retina (Figs. 138-1, and 138-2). The emboli observed in retinal

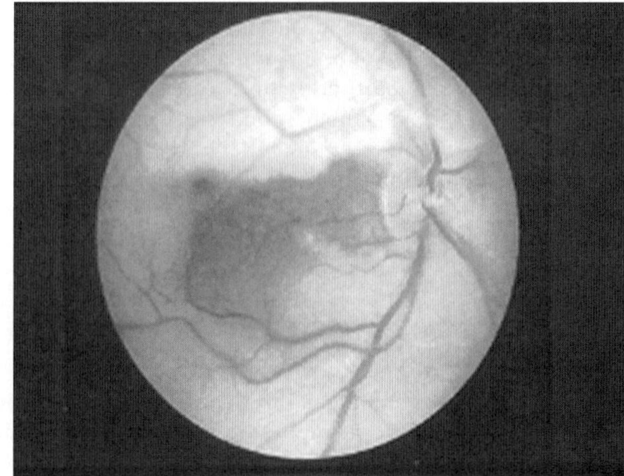

FIGURE 138-2. Central retinal artery occlusion (CRAO), of right eye with greater pallor and vessel attenuation superiorly, and preserved cilioretinal perfusion, seen as darker segment between optic disc (R) and macula (L).

arteries can consist of fibrin, calcium, or cholesterol. The latter (Hollenhorst plaque) appears as a luminescent, fiery yellow-orange particle lodged within a retinal artery, some of which are asymptomatic and nonobstructive to flow because of their thin, flakelike configuration (4,5).

In OIS, the neovascularization induced by chronic ischemia may be seen in the optic disc, midretina, and iris. Characteristic neovascular glaucoma occurs after vascular proliferation in the angle of the iris, raising the intraocular pressure, which can further compromise retinal perfusion (5).

CLINICAL MANIFESTATIONS

Patients with substantial, acute visual loss from optic neuritis, ION, or CRAO usually have an abnormal pupillary response. Often, pupilloconstriction to light is sluggish to absent in the affected eye, yet normally brisk for both pupils with light shined in the normal eye. Thus, if a penlight is "swung" from one pupil to the other, the affected pupil appears to dilate with the penlight in front of it (relative afferent pupillary defect). In ION, the visual loss is more acute, often present on awakening, and painless (Table 138-1). An altitudinal visual loss (the upper or lower visual field of that eye) strongly favors a vascular cause (ION or even retinal artery occlusion), because of the superior and inferior branching of the retinal vessels. Splinter hemorrhages around a swollen optic disc support the diagnosis of ION. The older patient with ION may have temporal arteritis, with achiness, fever, anorexia, weight loss, malaise, jaw claudication, headache, and palpably tender or pulseless temporal arteries. The visual loss is often more severe in arteritic ION, with an increased risk of involving the other eye (3).

Optic neuritis evolves over hours to days, often impairing color vision, with a diffuse, partial, or even altitudinal visual field defect. Orbital pain, particularly with eye movement, is common. The typically younger patient with optic neuritis may have signs and symptoms of MS, or other systemic inflammatory disorders such as SLE. Overall, the prognosis for visual recovery is far better for optic neuritis than for ION (1).

Patients with retinal artery occlusion may have had previous episodes of transient monocular blindness (amaurosis fugax), because both are related to emboli. The sudden, painless loss of vision is more global with a CRAO, with acuity reduced to finger counting or worse. Obviously, visual loss is segmental or partial with a BRAO. The typical retinal findings were described previously.

Transient monocular blindness can also occur in older patients with OIS, where visual loss develops slowly over weeks to months, often with orbital pain. A history of stroke deficit or the presence of focal neurologic findings may heighten the suspicion of severe atherosclerotic carotid disease ipsilateral to the blind eye. With very tenuous retinal perfusion, the vision may fade by merely rubbing or blinking the eye. Externally, the affected eye appears red or swollen, with findings of conjunctivitis and corneal edema, whereas cataracts, dilated retinal veins, and retinal blot hemorrhages may also be seen (5).

DIAGNOSTIC APPROACH

Acute monocular blindness may be the first symptom of undiagnosed hypertension, diabetes, or latent atherosclerosis, so a thorough cardiovascular evaluation should be performed in all of these patients. Important factors to investigate in younger or atypical patients include the use of sympathomimetic drugs or oral contraceptives, hypercoagulable states, nonatherosclerotic vasculopathies, or vasculitis.

A complete, but urgent, eye examination should include testing of visual acuity, color vision, pupillary responses, extraocular movements, confrontational visual fields; external examination of the eyelids, orbit, and anterior segment, as well as a dilated funduscopic examination. Visual defects could be serially monitored with automated Humphrey or manual Goldmann visual field testing. Fluorescein angiography may be needed in selected cases. Obviously, the ophthalmology consultant plays an important role here, but the internist or neurologist needs to act urgently, when required on clinical grounds, such as ordering a sedimentation rate (ESR) and corticosteroid therapy when temporal arteritis is highly suggested. The visual loss in nonarteritic ION can be reduced if any systemic hypotension is found and corrected.

Basic blood tests for patients with monocular visual loss include a complete blood count (CBC) (to reveal polycythemia or an anemia from temporal arteritis), ESR, or C-reactive protein and antinuclear antibody (ANA) titer (to screen for temporal arteritis or other systemic inflammatory disorders, such as SLE), lipid profile, blood glucose or glycosylated hemoglobin, and prothrombin time (PT), and activated partial thromboplastin time (aPTT) (to screen for a coagulopathy). Other hypercoagulable blood tests (e.g., cardiolipin antibodies) should be ordered selectively in patients with few or no atherosclerotic risk factors. Although uncommon now, syphilis serology (rapid plasma

TABLE 138-1. Optic Neuritis and Retinal Vascular Disorders

	Optic Neuritis	*ION*	*CRAO/BRAO*	*OIS*
Age, gender	Younger, F > M	Older, M = F	Older, M > F	Older, M > F
Onset	Subacute (hours to days)	Acute	Acute	Chronic (weeks to months)
Typical visual defect	Diffuse, partial or altitudinal	Altitudinal	Altitudinal or central scotoma	Global
Orbital pain	+	− (arteritic if +)	−	+
Swollen disc	+ (unless retrobulbar)	+	−	−
Common associations	MS	Arteritic: TA; Nonarteritic: HTN, DM, acute hypotension, others	Cardiovascular emboli	Ipsilateral ICA stenosis or occlusion

ION, ischemic optic neuropathy; CRAO/BRAO, central or branch retinal artery occlusion; OIS, ocular ischemic syndrome; MS, multiple sclerosis; TA, temporal arteritis; HTN, hypertension; DM, diabetes mellitus; ICA, internal carotid artery.

reagin, [RPR], fluorescent treponemal antibody absorption [FTA-ABS] test) should be checked in unusual cases of optic neuritis (2).

An evaluation for embolic sources is required in patients with CRAO or BRAO, and perhaps selected cases of ION. Magnetic resonance angiography (MRA) or computed tomographic (CT) angiography provides imaging from the aortic arch throughout the carotid arterial system, whereas carotid ultrasound limits the evaluation to the cervical portion of that artery. A transesophageal, rather than a transthoracic, echocardiogram is more sensitive in detecting sources of cardiac emboli and it also provides some imaging of the aortic arch. Because of the high association of ipsilateral, high-grade carotid stenosis or occlusion with OIS, carotid imaging studies are essential. A temporal artery biopsy is needed to confirm arteritic ION as well as in elderly patients highly suspected of having temporal arteritis causing their retinal artery occlusion. If a temporal artery biopsy finding is normal, yet the clinical suspicion of temporal arteritis is high, the contralateral temporal artery could also be biopsied. In this situation, however, the diagnostic yield remains low (3). In patients having optic neuritis without a diagnosis of MS, an MRI of the brain and orbits—with and without contrast—would help to further investigate that possibility.

TREATMENT

Despite an overall poor therapeutic response, patients with CRAO of <24 hours duration merit some intervention in an attempt to improve their vision. Multiple therapies exist, without a preferred first choice, but all aim to dislodge or fragment the embolus so retinal perfusion is improved. Ten to 15 seconds of ocular massage may physically fragment the embolus. Inhalation of Carbogen (95% oxygen, 5% carbon dioxide) can cause retinal arterial dilatation, with distal propagation of the embolus. Retinal oxygenation may also be improved with Carbogen or hyperbaric oxygen therapy. Clot propagation may also be enhanced by lowering the intraocular pressure, using anterior chamber paracentesis, topical timolol, or intravenous acetazolamide. More aggressive measures have yet to be proved effective in larger, controlled trials, although intravenous or selective intraarterial thrombolytic therapy appears promising. After acute therapy is begun, or if the patient has sought medical attention beyond 24 hours, evaluation for an embolic source or for nonatherosclerotic causes is undertaken. Given the partial visual loss with better prognosis in BRAO, only conservative therapy (e.g., ocular massage) is usually undertaken, although the vascular workup must still be pursued (4,5).

In patients with nonarteritic ION, no effective acute therapy exists, with the possible exception of rapid recognition and reversal of systemic hypotension. In patients with OIS, laser panretinal photocoagulation may help promote regression of their neovascularization. Carotid endarterectomy should be considered in patients with OIS who are surgical candidates, or carotid angioplasty or stenting in those who are not (5). Those with OIS with complete carotid occlusion, and progressive or refractory ocular symptoms, may potentially benefit from extracranial-intracranial vascular bypass surgery.

In patients suspected of arteritic ION, urgent steroid therapy should be started before a temporal artery biopsy, given the possibility of visual loss in the opposite eye. The findings of vasculitis will still be present, even after 7 days of steroid treatment. Therapy is often begun with intravenous methylprednisolone (250 to 500 mg) every 6 hours for 3 to 5 days, followed by daily oral prednisone, or initially with oral prednisone alone. Daily prednisone can be started at 40 to 80 mg/day, and tapered by 5 to 10 mg every 1 to 2 weeks, according to clinical response, with treatment duration often lasting several months. The efficacy of nonsteroid immunosuppressant therapy is currently uncertain (3).

The Optic Neuritis Treatment Trial (ONTT), published in 1992, compared initial intravenous steroids followed by oral steroids (intravenous methylprednisolone 250 mg every 6 hours for 3 days, then 1 mg/kg oral prednisone for 11 days, tapered off over 4 days) versus treatment with oral steroids alone (1 mg/kg oral prednisone for 14 days, tapered off over 4 days) (6). With initial intravenous methylprednisolone, visual recovery improved faster, although eventual visual outcome at 1 year and beyond was the same for either therapy. The risk of developing MS within 2 years after intravenous methylprednisolone was reduced, compared with oral prednisone or placebo, but this benefit did not persist beyond 2 years of follow-up. Subjects receiving only oral prednisone had a greater risk of recurrent optic neuritis within the next 2 years. For all these reasons, then, the current recommendation is to treat acute optic neuritis initially with intravenous methylprednisolone. Patients with optic neuritis without prior neurologic deficits appear to have a greater risk of developing MS in the presence of two or more periventricular, ovoid white matter lesions on brain MRI scan. This risk can be reduced, however, if IFN-β therapy is begun within 1 to 3 months of the presenting optic neuritis (1,2).

CLINICAL RECOMMENDATIONS OF THE VIGNETTE

The patient has a right central retinal arterial occlusion (CRAO). His cardiovascular status and possible embolic sources should be evaluated. Because of his age, an ESR should be ordered to screen for temporal arteritis, which may occasionally cause a CRAO. A temporal artery biopsy may be indicated if the ESR is very elevated, or clinical suspicion is high. Acute ocular therapy should be started immediately, under guidance of an ophthalmologist, because his symptoms are <24 hours in duration.

SUMMARY

Patients presenting with acute, monocular visual loss should be referred urgently to an ophthalmologist, who will confirm the diagnosis and recommend therapy to optimize recovery. The long-term prognosis for these patients also depends on recognition and management of the associated systemic disorders (cardiovascular disease and its risk factors, hypercoagulable states, immune-mediated disease) or CNS disease (MS) causing the visual symptoms.

REFERENCES

1. Balcer LJ. Optic neuritis. *N Engl J Med.* 2006;354:1273–1280.
2. Balcer LJ, Beck RW. Inflammatory optic neuropathies and neuroretinitis. In: Yanoff M, Duker JS, eds. *Ophthalmology*, 2nd ed. St. Louis: Mosby; 2004:1263–1267.
3. Purvin V. Ischemic optic neuropathy. *Semin Cerebrovasc Dis Stroke.* 2004;4(1):18–38.
4. Duker JS. Retinal arterial obstruction. In: Yanoff M, Duker JS, eds. *Ophthalmology*, 2nd ed. St. Louis: Mosby; 2004:854–861.
5. Santiago ME, Wafapoor H, Corbett JJ. Ocular ischemic syndrome, central retinal artery obstruction, and branch retinal artery obstruction. *Seminars in Cerebrovascular Disease and Stroke.* 2004;4(1):39–52.
6. Beck RW, Cleary PA, Anderson MM Jr., et al. A randomized, controlled trial of corticosteroids in the treatment of acute optic neuritis. *N Engl J Med.* 1992;326:581–588.

CHAPTER 139

Head, Neck, and Skull Base Neoplasms

Chad Zender • Sam J. Marzo • John P. Leonetti • Athena Kostidis • Rima M. Dafer

OBJECTIVES

- To describe a group of neoplasms that frequently presents with various cranial neuropathies
- To identify subtle factors in presentation that can be helpful in differentiating a benign from a malignant process
- To present a standardized approach to evaluating these patients
- To help clarify when and what type of imaging and diagnostic test are most useful in the patient evaluation

CASE VIGNETTE

A 26-year-old right-handed woman presents with a history of voice changes developing over 3 weeks. She notes that her voice is not as strong as it once was. She also notes occasional difficulty swallowing, as well as a pulsating sound in the right ear, with slightly muffled hearing. She denies any recent history of trauma, neck surgery, infections, or other diseases. Her medical history is unremarkable. She saw her primary care physician 2 weeks ago and was diagnosed as having laryngitis and otitis media. She was placed on 10 days of oral penicillin, vocal rest, and told to drink fluids. Her symptoms have not improved.

On examination, she is a well-developed woman with normal facial strength and symmetry. Examination of the nasal cavity is unremarkable. No lesions are seen on the oral cavity examination. Palatal movement appears normal on the left, but the right side appears weak and does not move well. No auricular lesions are noted. Otoscopy examination finding is normal on the left; on the right, an inferiorly based reddish mass is present behind an intact tympanic membrane. No cervical lymphadenopathy is noted. Flexible laryngoscopy reveals pooling of secretions in the right pyriform sinus, and a weak, flaccid right true vocal cord. The remainder of the neurologic and head and neck examination is unremarkable.

INTRODUCTION

The head and neck, as well of the junction of these two areas (which is often referred to as the *skull base*), contain many critical neurovascular structures. Neoplasms of this area can often present with subtle signs and symptoms. Accurate and timely diagnosis is important for treatment, to minimize complications and to improve the patient's quality of life. Often the diagnosis is not made until the patient presents with cranial nerve deficits. The posterior cranial fossa and the neurovascular structures traversing this area into the ear and neck are a common site of skull base neoplasms. This chapter contains an approach to patients with tumors in this area, highlighted by the above case vignette.

Skull base neoplasms can present intracranially, extracranially, or with extension into both areas. The most common intracranial skull base tumor is the vestibular schwannoma. It typically presents with unilateral aural symptoms, including tinnitus, aural pressure, hearing loss, and, occasionally, a mild balance disturbance. The tumor begins on the vestibular nerve and can extend into the internal auditory canal or into the cerebellopontine angle (CPA). Other types of tumors that can present within the CPA are meningiomas, lipomas, schwannomas of the seventh nerve, and metastatic tumors. Anterosuperior to the internal auditory canal is the fifth cranial nerve. Meningiomas and schwannomas are common tumors in this area. Most present with unilateral fifth nerve findings. Metastatic lesions are also possible. Posteroinferior to the internal auditory canal is the jugular foramen, through which traverse the jugular venous system and cranial nerves IX, X, and XI. The most common tumor in this area is the glomus jugulare tumor, which is a paraganglioma that begins along glomus bodies of the jugular bulb. Schwannomas of the lower cranial nerves can also occur as well as meningiomas, chondromas, chondrosarcomas, and metastatic tumors. Pain and rapidly progressive cranial neuropathies are suggestive of malignant neoplasms.

DEFINITION

Paragangliomas of the head and neck include glomus jugulare, glomus tympanicum, glomus vagale, and carotid body tumors. Paragangliomas in other sites, including the larynx and nasal cavity, have been described, but these are rare. A glomus tympanicum tumor begins along glomus bodies along the middle ear, near a branch of the ninth cranial nerve, called *Jacobsen's nerve.* These tumors are limited to the middle ear cleft, but can also extend into the mastoid. Glomus jugulare tumors begin in glomus bodies along the jugular bulb, and are typically more extensive then glomus tympanicum tumors. They can have extension along multiple pathways, including intracranially. Carotid body tumors develop in glomus bodies along the vagus nerve, presenting with a painless pulsatile neck mass. Because paraganglioma are the most common temporal bone neoplasms, the remainder of the discussion will focus on these lesions.

EPIDEMIOLOGY

Glomus tumors have a frequency of 1 per 1.3 million people (1). A familial variant of paragangliomas has been described with varying degrees of penetrance. Of paragangliomas, 15% to 25% are now considered to be familial (2,3). These tumors are three times more common in females and may be multicentric in 22% of cases, with bilateral carotid body tumors being the most common combination (4).

ETIOLOGY AND PATHOGENESIS

Paraganglioma develop from neural crest cells, more specifically from the diffuse neuroendocrine system, and thus can secrete neuropeptides and catecholamines (5). These cells are found throughout the head and neck, including the vagus nerve (glomus vagale), the carotid body (carotid body tumor), Jacobson's nerve in the middle ear (glomus tympanicum), and the jugular foramen (glomus jugulare) in addition to other less common areas (e.g., larynx). Less than 5% of paragangliomas secrete catecholamines, and patients with paragangliomas typically have symptoms of hypertension, tachycardia, palpitations, headaches, and flushing (6).

PATHOLOGY AND CLINICAL MANIFESTATIONS

Paragangliomas of the head and neck are usually slow-growing neoplasms, with an average growth rate of approximately 1 mm per year (7). These lesions are usually benign and present with mass effect symptoms. Temporal bone erosion can occur, especially with glomus jugulare tumors. Involvement of the mastoid segment of the facial nerve can result in facial paresis or paralysis. The lower cranial nerves can be involved as the tumor destroys the jugular foramen. The bony labyrinth, which includes the cochlea and semicircular canals, is usually preserved, except in very large glomus jugulare neoplasms.

Malignant paragangliomas are rare, with a reported incidence of approximately 5% (8). The diagnosis is typically not possible by analysis of the primary neoplasm. Diagnosis in this case requires the identification of locoregional (cervical lymph node) or distant metastasis.

The symptoms of glomus tumors vary, depending on the location. Carotid body tumors typically present as a painless anterolateral neck mass. Glomus tympanicum tumors present with unilateral pulsatile tinnitus and a conductive hearing loss from involvement of the ossicular chain. The tumor is reddish on otoscopy and limited to the middle ear. Glomus jugulare tumors also present with pulsatile tinnitus and a conductive hearing loss, but are typically more extensive than glomus tympanicum tumors. Approximately 38% of glomus jugular tumors present with a cranial neuropathy (9). The signs and symptoms can include hoarseness from involvement of the vagus; dysphagia from involvement of the glossopharyngeal or vagus nerves; shoulder dysfunction and trapezius wasting from involvement of the spinal accessory nerve; and hemitongue atrophy from involvement of the hypoglossal nerve. Facial paresis is possible as the tumor erodes the mastoid segment of the facial nerve canal. Computed tomographic (CT) scan imaging is necessary to determine the extent of the tumor and to differentiate this tumor from a glomus tympanicum, which can have the identical appearance on physical examination.

Because paraganglioma and other neoplasms of the head and neck can present with cranial nerve findings, a complete history and physical examination are necessary to accurately stage these tumors and counsel the patient about treatment options. Flexible laryngoscopy is usually necessary to document function of the vagus nerve. Tuning fork testing and audiometric testing can help quantify the degree and nature of hearing loss. Finally, in the review of systems, questions concerning symptoms of catecholamine secretion can be elucidated and treated.

DIAGNOSTIC APPROACH

Imaging studies are extremely helpful in the evaluation of any patient with a suspected head and neck neoplasm. CT is best in demonstrating the extent of the tumor within the confines of the temporal bone, as well as any bony erosion. Glomus tympanicum tumors usually present as a mass on the promontory or middle wall of the ear. They can fill the entire middle ear cleft; however, by definition, they are limited to the middle ear and mastoid. Glomus jugulare tumors begin along the jugular bulb and, with growth, will erode and involve the jugular foramen.

Magnetic resonance imaging (MRI) is useful in delineating the soft tissue extent of glomus jugulare tumors. MRI is not usually necessary for evaluation of glomus tympanicum tumors. These tumors are very vascular and will enhance with contrast. Figure 139-1 shows the typical MRI appearance of a glomus

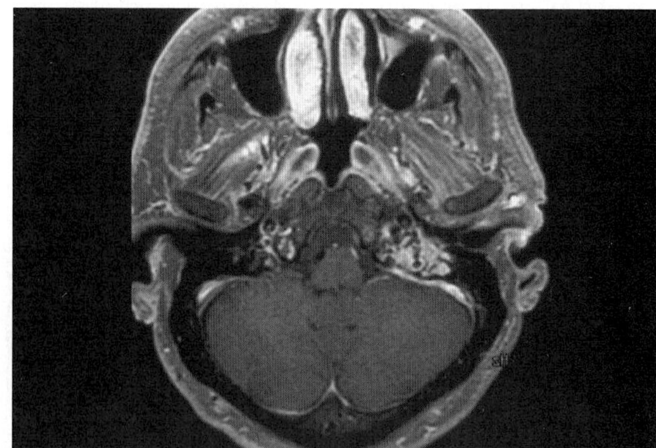

FIGURE 139-1. Axial magnetic resonance imaging (MRI) of left glomus jugulare lesion, showing enhancing lesion with multiple flow voids.

jugulare tumor. MRI is also excellent for identifying any intracranial extension, as well as extension along the petrous carotid artery. Carotid body tumors, typically, show a splaying of the internal and external carotid artery. This can be helpful in differentiating this tumor from a glomus vagale tumor, which causes anterior displacement of the cervical carotid artery, and is more likely to be associated with vagal nerve paralysis (10).

Angiography is very important, both diagnostically and therapeutically, in the modern day management of paraganglioma. The arterial phase will demonstrate feeder vessels, which can be ligated endovascularly preoperatively. The venous phase will identify the patency of the jugular bulb, as well as the ipsilateral and contralateral venous drainage patterns, which are important in treatment planning. Angiography may also help identify small synchronous paragangliomas not seen on CT or MRI (11).

Biopsy of paraganglioma to confirm the diagnosis is to be condemned, because these tumors are very vascular, any biopsy can cause significant hemorrhage. The accurate diagnosis of paraganglioma (and many skull base neoplasms), thus, depends on history, clinical findings, and radiographic imaging.

TREATMENT

Treatment of paraganglioma and skull base neoplasms generally depends on multiple factors, including the symptomatology, age, and overall health of the patient, as well as the perceived growth rate, stage, and potential complications of the neoplasm. Treatment, thus, is tailored to the individual patient. Because, by nature, paraganglioma are slow growing, benign tumors, elderly patients and patients with multiple comorbid conditions and minimal symptomatology might be better served with observation only. Radiotherapy would be an option in such patients if the tumors become symptomatic.

Younger patients, in general, are best treated with surgical therapy. Over a typical lifespan, the tumors in such patients likely will continue to grow and eventually may cause further symptoms. Surgical therapy is the only treatment that can result in a cure. Table 139-1 lists a classification system of paragangliomas of the head, neck, and skull base, as well as preferred surgical approaches (12). Carotid body and glomus vagale tumors can be treated with a transcervical excision with proximal and distal vascular control. Glomus tympanicum tumors, which are confined to the middle ear and mastoid, can be resected through a transcanal or transmastoid approach, which has little morbidity. Glomus jugulare neoplasms are generally treated through a postauricular infratemporal fossa approach. The main morbidities of this approach are a maximal unilateral conductive hearing loss (from resection of the external auditory canal, tympanic membrane, and ossicular chain) as well as transient, occasionally permanent facial weakness (from anterior mobilization of the facial nerve, which is directly lateral to the jugular foramen), and lower cranial nerve dysfunction (from tumor compression or invasion).

Rehabilitation of cranial nerve deficits after skull base therapy can significantly improve a patient's functional recovery and minimize postoperative morbidity. The treatment of the conductive hearing loss can be accomplished with a bone anchored hearing aid (13), which vibrates the mastoid bone and, thus, the cochlea, bypassing the external auditory canal and middle ear. Lower cranial nerve paralysis (cranial nerves IX and X) can be improved with a vocal cord medialization procedure, as well as speech and swallowing therapy (14).

TABLE 139-1. Paraganglioma Classification and Surgical Approaches

Classification	*Surgical Approach*
Vagale, carotid body	Transcervical
Glomus tympanicum	Transcanal, transmastoid
Glomus jugulare	
Jugular bulb	Mastoid neck, with limited facial nerve rerouting
Carotid artery	Infratemporal fossa or subtemporal
Transdural	Infratemporal fossa or intracranial

(From Brackman DE, Arriga MA. Surgery for glomus and jugular foramen tumors. In: Brackman DE, Shelton CF, Arriga MA, eds. *Otologic Surgery*, 2nd ed. Philadelphia: WB Saunders; 2001:478–492, with permission.)

CLINICAL RECOMMENDATIONS OF THE VIGNETTE

The patient has muffled hearing, pulsatile tinnitus, a middle ear mass, and weakness of the right palate and right true vocal cord (representing involvement of the glossopharyngeal and vagus nerve). The most likely diagnosis is a glomus jugulare tumor. A glomus tympanicum tumor is unlikely because the patient has a lower cranial nerve neuropathy. Complete otolaryngologic and cranial nerve examinations are important to document any preoperative cranial nerve deficits, as is evident in this patient.

Other preoperative studies are indicated, including audiometry. This will demonstrate the degree and type of hearing loss, as well as document normal function of the contralateral left ear. This is important, especially because surgical treatment for the patient will result in a unilateral maximal conductive hearing loss. Other essential studies are CT, which documentes destruction of the jugular bulb, as well as MRI, which shows that the tumor did not extend intracranially. Once these tests were performed, the patient was counseled regarding treatment options. In view of her youth, preoperative cranial nerve deficits, and absence of comorbid conditions, the patient opted for surgical therapy. Discussed with her at length were the goals and objectives of treatment, as well as potential complications and available rehabilitation techniques.

Preoperatively, on the day before surgery, she had a diagnostic and therapeutic angiogram. This study showed no involvement of the carotid artery, occlusion of the ipsilateral jugular bulb, and an adequate contralateral venous drainage system. At the end of the angiogram, feeding vessels to the tumor (usually the ascending pharyngeal artery and its tributaries) were taken endovascularly. This technique has been shown to reduce intraoperative blood loss (15).

Surgical therapy was performed the following day via a postauricular infratemporal fossa approach. At the time of surgery, the vagus and glossopharyngeal nerves were compressed, but not involved with the tumor. These nerves were anatomically spared and complete tumor resection was performed. An abdominal fat graft was used to obliterate the dead space resulting from the surgical resection. Her postoperative course was unremarkable and she was discharged home on postoperative day 4. Because her vocal cord dysfunction did not improve postoperatively, she was treated with a medialization procedure. She also had successful speech and swallowing therapy postoperatively. She later had implantation of a bone-anchored hearing aid for rehabilitation of her conductive hearing loss.

SUMMARY

Neoplasms of the head, neck, and skull base can present with subtle symptoms and, occasionally, cranial neuropathies. A complete history, otolaryngologic examination, and cranial nerve testing are necessary. Adjunctive studies, including audiometry, CT, MRI, and angiography are often necessary for staging and treatment planning. Diagnosis is made via a combination of preoperative clinical findings and imaging studies. Biopsy is often not possible until definitive surgical resection. Most neoplasms in this area are benign, but can be aggressive, however, especially in younger patients. In healthy symptomatic young patients, surgical therapy is the best option, whereas elderly patients or patients with multiple comorbidity might be better managed with observation. Collaboration between multiple disciplines is necessary for the optimal treatment of these patients.

REFERENCES

1. Moffat DA, Hardy DG. Surgical management of large glomus jugulare tumors: Infra- and trans-temporal approach. *J Laryngol Otol.* 1989;103:1167–1180.
2. Oosterwijk JC, Jansen JC, van Schothorst EM, et al. First experiences with genetic counseling based on predictive DNA diagnosis in hereditary glomus tumors (paragangliomas). *J Med Genet.* 1996;33:379–383.
3. Baysal BE, van Schothorst EM, Farr JE: Repositioning the hereditary paraganglioma critical region on chromosome band 11q23. *Hum Genet.* 1999;104:219–225.
4. Sykes J, Ossoff R. Paragangliomas of the head and neck. *Otolaryngol Clin North Am.* 1986;19:755–767.
5. Farr HW. Carotid body tumors: A 40-year study. *Cancer.* 1980;30:260–265.
6. Schwaber M, Glasscock ME, Nissen AJ, et al. Diagnosis and management of catecholamine secreting glomus tumors. *Laryngoscope.* 1984;94:1008–1015.
7. Jansen JC, van den Berg R, Kuiper A, et al. Estimation of growth rate in patients with head and neck paragangliomas influences the treatment proposal. *Cancer.* 2000;88:2811–2816.
8. Manolidis S, Shohet J, Jackson C, et al. Malignant glomus tumors. *Laryngoscope.* 1999; 109:30–34.
9. Ogura J, Spector G, Gado M. Glomus jugulare and vagale. *Ann Otol Rhinol Laryngol.* 1978;87:622–629.
10. Rao AB, Koeller KK, Adair CF. Paragangliomas of the head and neck: Radiologic-pathologic correlation. *Radiographics.* 1999;19:1605–1632.
11. Lasjaunias P, Berenstein A. *Surgical Neuro-Angiography: Endovascular Treatment of Craniofacial Lesions.* Vol 2. New York: Springer-Verlag; 1987.
12. Brackman DE, Arriaga MA. Surgery for glomus and jugular foramen tumors. In Brackman DE, Shelton CF, Arriaga MA, eds. *Otologic Surgery*, 2nd ed. Philadelphia: WB Saunders; 2001:478–492.
13. Tjellstrom A. Osseointegrated systems and their application in the head and neck. *Adv Otolaryngol Head Neck Surg.* 1989;3:39–70.
14. Netterville JL, Jackson CG. Rehabilitation of lower cranial nerve deficits after neurotologic skull base surgery. *The American Journal of Otolaryngology.* 1993;14:460–465.
15. Murphy TP, Brackman DE. Effects of preoperative embolization on glomus jugulare tumors. *Laryngoscope.* 1989;99:1244–1247.

CHAPTER **140**

ENT Infections and Inflammation

Joseph M. Scianna • James A. Stankiewicz • Adriana Rodriguez Quiñónez

OBJECTIVES

- To review signs and symptoms of common otolaryngologic diseases: otitis media and sinusitis
- To review common bacteria resulting in otolaryngologic infections
- To describe the relative anatomy of the paranasal sinuses and the temporal bone and its relation to neurologic symptomotology
- To discuss the indications for both medical and surgical treatment in complications from otitis media and sinusitis
- To review the inflammatory condition of Wegener granulomatosis and its otolaryngologic and neurologic manifestations

The field of otolaryngology, head and neck surgery encompasses a wide variety of local and systemic diseases that can present with neurologic symptoms. The anatomy of the ear and temporal bone allows for bacteriologic access to the middle cranial fossa and surrounding structures, such as the sigmoid sinus, internal carotid artery, and facial nerve. The paranasal sinuses are housed beneath the anterior cranial fossa, medial to the orbital musculature, extend posteriorly to the optic chiasm and abut the cavernous sinus. Infections and inflammatory processes that extend into these areas can result in multiple orbital neuropathies, trigeminal nerve deficits, and mental status changes (1,2).

CASE VIGNETTE

A 3-year-old girl is brought into the emergency room after becoming progressively more obtunded. The family had recently been traveling out of the country when the child complained of an earache. While outside of the country, the child was given a medication that the family believes was an antibiotic. However, the family is uncertain of the type of antibiotic and the exact dose. The patient continued to complain of right-sided otalgia over the next week with occasional fevers. Over the last 12 hours the child has become progressively less responsive. Physical examination demonstrates a somnolent child with minimal responsiveness. The patient responds to painful stimuli and winces when pressure is applied behind the right auricle. Otologic examination reveals opacification of the right tympanic membrane. The membrane is intact. No nuchal rigidity or meningeal signs are noted.

EPIDEMIOLOGY

Acute otitis media is an infection of the middle ear defined by acute onset, presence of middle ear effusion, and signs of middle ear inflammation. Acute otitis media most commonly occurs in children and is the most frequent specific diagnosis in children who are febrile. Recurrent otitis media is defined as three episodes of acute otitis media within 6 months or four or more episodes within 1 year. In the United States, otitis media is commonplace, with nearly 50% of children having an episode during the first year of life and 80% of children under the age of 3 years having had at least one episode (1,3). An estimated $3 to $4 billion is spent each year on care of patients with acute otitis media and related complications. Boys are slightly more affected than girls, although the exact reason for this is unknown (3). Native American Indians have a higher incidence of otitis media and patients with a cleft palate invariably have recurrent otitis media secondary to anatomic eustachian tube dysfunction (1).

Sinusitis represents an inflammation of the lining of the paranasal sinuses caused by bacterial overgrowth in a closed cavity. Sinusitis represents the single most common diagnosis in adults treated with antibiotics in an ambulatory care setting. By definition, acute sinusitis symptoms last <3 weeks, subacute sinusitis symptoms last 21 to 60 days, and chronic sinusitis symptoms last >60 days (1,4). An estimated 30 million Americans develop sinusitis each year, with approximately 16 million physician office visits per year. More than $2 billion are spent on purchasing over-the-counter medications to treat the symptoms of sinusitis (4). Sinusitis can occur in all age groups and does not have any particular race or sex predilection.

Wegener granulomatosis (WG) is a disease of unknown cause, which is characterized by necrotizing granulomatous vasculitis of the upper and lower respiratory tract, glomerulonephritis, and a variable degree of small-vessel vasculitis. WG occurs with a frequency of approximately 1 case per 30,000 individuals. WG is primarily a disease among the white population, with men having a slightly higher incidence of the disease. The typical age at diagnosis is approximately 45 years (5,6).

ETIOLOGY AND PATHOGENESIS

Acute otitis media and sinusitis are common otorhinolarynogologic diseases seen in the primary care setting. Acute otitis media has been linked to abnormalities of eustachian tube function related to its developmental anatomy. In the child, an abnormally patent, not obstructed, eustachian tube with a shallow angle of ascent from the nasopharynx to the middle ear allows for bacterial entry into the normally sterile middle ear environment. The three most common bacterial causes of acute otitis media are *Streptococcus pneumoniae, Haemophilus influenza,* and *Branhamella catarrhalis* (3,7).

The cause of sinusitis, acute or chronic, is less clear. The prevailing theory in sinusitis is that inflammation of the mucosa surrounding the natural ostia of the paranasal sinuses allows for outflow obstruction, with subsequent accumulation of mucus and sinus debris. The inciting inflammatory event can be multifactorial. Allergy, fungal debris, and viral upper respiratory disease can all lead to mucosal inflammation and secondary bacterial suprainfection. Primary bacterial infection can also lead to similar inflammation (4). Again *S. pneumonaie* and *H. influenzae* are primary bacterial pathogens. *Staphylococcus aureus,* anaerobes, and gram-negative rods have also been identified as bacterial pathogens. Spread into the brain is most often vascular, through the veins of Breschet, which penetrate the posterior wall of the frontal sinus (8). In the patient with chronic sinusitis or the previously operated patient, *Pseudomonas aeruginosa* has been found to be a typical pathogen. Whereas fungal disease itself can result in mucosal inflammation, invasive fungal disease is generally relegated to the immunocompromised individual.

WG has an unknown cause, but the presence of antineutrophil cytoplasmic antibodies (ANCA) suggests that WG represents an autoimmune disease (5). The exact cause of the formation of the ANCA in WG is unclear; however, a mainstay of treatment continues to be immunosuppressive and anti-inflammatory medication (5,6).

PATHOLOGY

The neurologic sequelae of otitis media and sinusitis are related to the surrounding anatomic structures. Infectious spread from the ear and temporal bone can cause intracranial complications. Spread of infection can occur through direct extension, thrombophlebitis, and hematogenous dissemination. Extracranial complications result from localized acute or chronic inflammation. The complications of otitis media include the following: postauricular abscess, facial nerve paresis, labyrinthitis, labyrinthine fistula, mastoiditis, temporal lobe abscess, petrositis, intracranial abscess, meningitis, otic hydrocephalus, sigmoid sinus thrombosis, encephalocele, and cerebrospinal fluid (CSF) leak (3,9,10).

With acute sinusitis, the most severe complications are related to direct spread of infection into surrounding structures. Orbital cellulitis and orbital abscess can result from an ethmoid sinus infection, with direct spread through the paper-thin lamina papyracea or through a small dehiscence in this structure (11). Acute infection of the anterior ethmoids of the frontal sinus can also spread hematogenously to create a frontal lobe abscess with meningitis. In addition, veins present in the mucosa of the frontal sinus communicate with the dura and the diploe of the cranium. Spread of infection through these veins can then lead to the development of a subdural or brain abscess (8). Lastly, inflammation in the posterior ethmoid and sphenoid sinus can result in secondary thrombophlebitis of the intracranial cavernous sinus and subsequent cavernous sinus thrombosis. The valve-less venous system of the ptyergoid plexus allows for the posterior extension of disease, whereas an anterior ethmoid or maxillary sinusitis can spread into the cavernous sinus via the ophthalmic vein (12,13).

WG can result in a number of neurologic sequelae. Peripheral and cranial neuropathies are commonplace. Peripheral neuropathy most often manifests as acute mononeuritis multiplex. Direct vasculitic injury, compression, extension of granulomatous disease from adjacent sinuses, or cavernous sinus thrombosis, can result in multiple cranial neuropathies. Cortical injury can occur from direct effects of inflammation, secondary tissue ischemia, or compressive forces from the granulomatous disease or related edema. Few patients present with evidence of WG-induced meningitis (5).

CLINICAL MANIFESTATIONS

The clinical manifestations of the complications from otitis media, sinusitis, and WG result from the primary infection or site of inflammation. The typical patient with otitis media will present with otalgia that is progressive in nature. The associated middle ear effusion will result in a conductive hearing loss in the affected ear. As the disease progresses and a secondary complication of the otitis media occurs, the symptomotology changes significantly. Although evidence of middle ear effusion persists, local effects of infection can result in a facial nerve paresis or complete paralysis. This is thought to be secondary to bacterial endotoxins and nerve inflammation within its encasement in the temporal bone (10). Similarly a labyrinthitis, with resultant vertigo, may also be present. A typical infectious labyrinthitis will result in peripheral vertigo lasting days to weeks, with gradual resolution as the infection clears. Temporal bone osteitis can result in mastoiditis, coalescence of mastoid air cells, and the formation of a subperiosteal abscess. This will typically present as a swollen erythematous mass behind the auricle, overlying the mastoid tip. With extension of the disease through the temporal bone into the middle cranial fossa, subsequent meningeal symptoms may become evident. Lethargy and an obtunded nature are not uncommon. Temporal lobe abscesses can result in a number of central processing and language disorders, depending on the location of the disease (7).

Typical signs for a sigmoid sinus thrombosis are less specific than those of a cavernous sinus thrombosis. Low-grade or picket fence-type fevers can occur. Neck tenderness, torticollis, or muscular inflammation resembling nuchal rigidity can occur. Papilledema and swelling over the occiput can occur. A jugular foramen syndrome can develop, with progressive paresis of cranial nerves (CN) IX, X, and XII. Progression of the thrombosis can result in a palpable cord of the internal jugular vein on the affected side. CSF pressure may be increased (7,9).

Signs of an advanced acute sinusitis typically begin with development of a periorbital cellulitis, with subsequent periorbital edema and erythema. Tenderness is also typically present. Initially, ophthalmologic examination is normal with no limitation of extraocular movements and no increase in intraocular pressure. Development of an orbital abscess along the lamina papyracea will result in impairment of the medial rectus on the affected side and subsequent diplopia with medial gaze. An elevation of intraocular pressure can also occur (11).

Cavernous sinus thrombosis typically develops from a primary orbital cellulitis secondary to a sinusitis, although, as discussed, direct extension into the cavernous sinus can occur through a sphenoid sinusitis and the ptyergoid venous plexus. Cavernous sinus thrombosis represents a severe intracranial complication that can rapidly progress to bilateral orbital involvement. All nerves within the cavernous sinus may be impaired: CN III, IV, and VI, with resultant opthalmoplegia, and VI and VII with resultant sensory impairment. Severe progressive chemosis can develop with retinal engorgement from ophthalmic vein compression. Very high fevers, meningitis, and death have been reported as a result of cavernous sinus thrombosis (12).

Frontal lobe abscess or meningitis secondary to acute sinusitis can also develop. Meningeal signs will be present and evidence of increased intracranial pressure may also be noted. Lethargy, headache, intractable vomiting, and a progressive obtunded nature should be seriously investigated in a patient with sinusitis (8).

Many clinical manifestations may be present with WG. From an otolaryngologic standpoint, this diagnosis is suggested when a patient presents with chronic sinusitis, nasal ulceration, upper respiratory tract symptoms or lower respiratory symptoms of hemoptysis, dyspnea, or chronic cough. An unexplained saddle nose deformity is pathopneumonic for WG (5). Progression of the disease into the eustachian tube or the middle ear can result in a conductive hearing loss, with effusion. A sensorineural hearing loss has also been associated with WG, which is thought to be caused vasculitis of the cochlea (6). Constitutional symptoms (e.g., fever, weight loss, and anorexia) may suggest systemic disease. Ocular symptoms are common and related to vasculitis. Physical examination may reveal proptosis, episcleritis, optic neuropathy secondary to cavernous sinus thrombosis, corneoscleral ulcers, dacrocysitis, uveitis, and retinal occlusion. Seizures, strokes, altered cognition, and focal motor and sensory deficits may be present secondary to cerebritis. Acute, chronic, or stepwise deterioration resulting from parenchymal or meningeal inflammation or scarring may also be seen.

DIAGNOSTIC APPROACH

The diagnostic approach always begins with a complete history and physical examination. Specific to the head and neck examination, pneumatic otoscopy, microscopic otoscopy, or both allows for clear visualization of the tympanic membrane and determination of the presence or absence of middle ear effusion. Perform Weber and Rinne tests, using a 512 Hz tuning fork, to determine if a conductive or sensorineural hearing loss is present. In the nonacute setting, an audiogram with tympanogram alternatively can be done.

A complete cranial nerve examination must occur. Documentation of the status of ocular motility and vision are essential. Aid from the ophthalmologist may be required for detailed retinal examination. Documentation of facial sensation and facial movement should occur as well as evaluation of glossopharyngeal nerve (CN IX), vagus nerve (CN X) via laryngoscopic evaluation of vocal cord function, spinal accessory nerve (CN XI), and hypoglossal nerve (CN XII) function.

Intranasal examination with identification of nasal polyps, nasal crusting, ulceration, or pus should be performed. Augmentation to the intranasal examination can include transnasal endoscopy, with either a flexible or rigid telescope. This will aid in the diagnosis of sinusitis and can provide the opportunity for biopsy in the case of WG or obtain intranasal cultures in the case of sinusitis.

Manual palpation of the neck will identify the presence or absence of lymphadenopathy or the presence of an internal jugular vein cord. If a lumbar drain is present, compression of the contralateral jugular vein should result in an increase in the CSF pressure, whereas compression of the ipsilateral thrombosed jugular vein will not result in change in the CSF pressure.

Laboratory evaluation should include a complete blood count to determine the presence of leukocytosis. If WG is suspected, a basic metabolic panel should be added to evaluate for renal function. In addition, an erythrocyte sedimentation rate, a C-reactive protein and a c-ANCA should be ordered. The cytoplasmic-antineutrophilic cytoplasmic antibody (c-ANCA) can be followed serially to determine the status of the condition.

One of the mainstays of sinus evaluation continues to be a screening computed tomographic (CT) scan of the sinuses (14). A screening scan, without contrast, can quickly determine the presence or absence of a sinus condition. Opacification of the sinuses may be evident as well as a subperiosteal or orbital abscess. If the presence of an orbital abscess is unclear, an orbital CT scan may help further delineate its existence. CT scan of the temporal bone without contrast will be diagnostic of a middle ear effusion and should delineate the presence of a subperiostal abscess or mastoid air cell coalescence. A head CT with contrast is a better study to determine the presence of a temporal or frontal lobe abscess (2,14).

Magnetic resonance imaging (MRI) can be an adjunctive test for diagnosis of sinusitis or mastoiditis. A T2-weighted image will help differentiate fluid within the paranasal sinuses from a mass or other pathology. An MRI with contrast may also help determine a cerebral abscess. Typical MRI findings include a ring-enhancing lesion with uniform wall thickness, central low T1 signal and a high T2 signal. Cerebritis can present amorphous high signal area of brain on T2 or T1 with FLAIR (fluid-attenuated inversion recovery) and no ring enhancement is seen with contrast. Subperiosteal abscess will present with a low central T1 signal and an increased T2 signal centrally. Cavernous sinus thrombosis or sigmoid sinus thrombosis can present with an enlarged, heterogeneous-enhancing, cavernous sinus with lack of a signal flow void. The extraocular muscles can also become swollen and enlarged secondary to venous engorgement. In addition, magnetic resonance venography (MRV) can be performed to aid in the evaluation of a cavernous sinus thrombosis or a lateral sinus thrombosis. Cerebral angiography with venous run-off may need to be performed to diagnose venous thrombosis definitively in cases of contraindication to MRV or proposed endovascular intervention (2).

TREATMENT

For acute otitis media with neurologic complications, treatment is aimed at resolution of the inciting infection. In the cases of labyrinthitis, facial nerve paresis or paralysis, and conductive hearing loss secondary to effusion, wide myringotomy with or without polyethylene tube placement will allow for drainage of the effusion and culture of the middle ear. Intravenous antibiotics can be given and should be directed toward common organisms. Close followup is used initially to ensure responsiveness to the therapy (1,3).

If complications, such as subperiosteal abscess, mastoid opacification with meningitis, or temporal lobe abscess develop, more aggressive surgical intervention can be considered. Simple mastoidectomy, with drainage of a subperiosteal abscess, provides adequate culture and release of the abscess. A transmastoid craniotomy can be performed to drain an intracranial abscess through the tegmen of the middle ear. A meningeal empyema can be drained in a similar fashion. For sigmoid sinus thrombosis, treatment with anticoagulation may aid in the resolution of the thrombosis and prevent its progression (7,9).

For complications of acute sinusitis, early recognition and treatment with intravenous antibiotics is a mainstay. As with complications related to acute otitis media, antibiotics should be aimed at common sinonasal organisms. In addition to appropriate antibiotic administration, intranasal decongestants (e.g., oxymetazoline) can be used to decrease nasal inflammation and allow for natural drainage of the sinuses. Nasal saline rinses and intranasal steroids can be used to aid in the clearance of the paranasal sinuses (4).

Development of orbital complications is a clear indication to operate (11). Decompression of the lamina papyracea can be done to preserve ocular function. Drainage of the maxillary, ethmoid, and sigmoid sinuses can provide for a quicker resolution of the acute infection. Presence of an anterior cranial fossa abscess or frontal lobe abscess is a clear indication for surgical drainage of the sinuses. Surgical drainage should be aimed at creating widely patent natural ostia of the sinuses to prevent reaccumulation or recurrent disease (8). Cultures should be taken to allow for appropriate antibiotic administration. As in sigmoid sinus thrombosis, anticoagulation can be given to prevent progression of the thrombus and aid in its resolution (9,13).

Treatment of WG can achieve a remission rate of 70%, but relapses are common (1). Later neurologic involvement can be lessened with aggressive treatment of pulmonary and renal involvement at the time of initial diagnosis. Multiple steroid dosing regimens have been used to decrease the prevalence of relapses. Cyclophosphamide, azathioprine, and methotrexate are all immunosuppressant drugs that can be used to control the disease process. None of the immunosuppressant therapies are considered safe during pregnancy. Frequent otolaryngologic follow up with sinonasal débridement will aid in maintenance of a healthy nasal cavity (5,6).

CLINICAL RECOMMENDATIONS OF THE VIGNETTE

The patient was evaluated in the emergency room and a CT of the temporal bones revealed an extradural abscess in the floor of the middle cranial fossa or tegmen of the middle ear. The patient was brought to the operating room where a simple mastoidectomy was performed. The tegmen was removed and extradural pus was evacuated and sent for culture. Culture-driven intravenous antibiotics were continued for a total of 6 weeks.

SUMMARY

Acute otitis media and sinusitis are common infections that potentially can result in severe neurologic complications. Early recognition and treatment of these infections can help prevent the development of devastating neurologic sequelae. A multidisciplinary approach, with input from the otolaryngologist, opthamologist, neurologist, neurosurgeon, and infectious disease specialist, can best allow for rapid diagnosis and treatment. WG represents a systemic vasculitis that can also produce a variety of neurologic sequelae. A high index of suspicion and early diagnosis can allow for immunosuppressive therapy to be delivered in a timely fashion. Thorough examination, proper laboratory and radiologic evaluation, and aggressive treatment, both medically and, if indicated, surgically, can provide the best opportunity to avoid these devastating neurologic complications.

REFERENCES

1. Cummings CW. *Otolaryngology Head and Neck Surgery*, 3rd ed. St. Louis: Mosby-Year Book; 1998.
2. Harnsberger HR, Hudgins P, Wiggins R, et al. *Diagnostic Imaging of the Head and Neck*. Salt Lake City, UT: Amirsys; 2004.
3. Bluestone CD. Studies in otitis media: Children's Hospital of Pittsburgh-University of Pittsburgh progress report—2004. *Laryngoscope*. 2004;114(11 Pt 3)[Suppl 105]:1–26.
4. Benninger MS, Ferguson BJ, Hadley JA, et al. Adult chronic rhinosinusitis: Definitions, diagnosis, epidemiology, and pathophysiology. *Otolaryngol Head Neck Surg*. 2003;129[3 Suppl]:S1–S32.
5. Bucolo S, Torre V, Montemagno A, et al. Wegener's granulomatosis presenting with otologic and neurologic symptoms: Clinical and pathological correlations. *J Oral Pathol Med*. 2003;32(7):438–440.
6. Takagi D, Nakamaru Y, Maguchi S, et al. Otologic manifestations of Wegener's granulomatosis. *Laryngoscope*. 2002;112(9):1684–1690.
7. Oestreicher-Kedem Y, Raveh E, Kornreich L, et al. Complications of mastoiditis in children at the onset of a new millennium. *Ann Otol Rhinol Laryngol*. 2005;114(2):147–152.
8. Fountas KN, Duwayri Y, Kapsalaki E, et al. Epidural intracranial abscess as a complication of frontal sinusitis: Case report and review of the literature. *South Med J*. 2004;97(3): 279–282.
9. Bradley DT, Hashisaki GT, Mason JC. Otogenic sigmoid sinus thrombosis: What is the role of anticoagulation? *Laryngoscope*. 2002;112(10):1726–1729.
10. Gaio E, Marioni G, de Filippis C, et al. Facial nerve paralysis secondary to acute otitis media in infants and children. *Journal of Paediatrics & Child Health*. 2004;40(8):483–486.
11. Howe L, Jones NS. Guidelines for the management of periorbital cellulitis/abscess. *Clin Otolaryngol*. 2004;29(6):725–872.
12. Bhatia K, Jones NS. Septic cavernous sinus thrombosis secondary to sinusitis: Are anticoagulants indicated? A review of the literature. *J Laryngol Otol*. 2002;116(9):667–676.
13. Younis RT, Lazar RH, Anand VK. Intracranial complications of sinusitis: A 15-year review of 39 cases. *Ear Nose Throat J*. 2002;81(9):636–638, 640–642, 644.
14. Younis RT, Anand VK, Davidson B. The role of computed tomography and magnetic resonance imaging in patients with sinusitis with complications. *Laryngoscope*. 2002;112(2): 224–229.

CHAPTER 141

Vertigo

Rita Schuman • Sam J. Marzo • John P. Leonetti •
Athena Kostidis • Rima M. Dafer

OBJECTIVES

- To define vertigo
- To discuss the epidemiology and various etiologies
- To discuss the clinical presentation
- To present a logical approach to diagnosis
- To discuss the medical and surgical treatments options

CASE VIGNETTE

A 31-year-old woman presents to her otolaryngologist with complaints of dizziness and dysequilibrium. She notes that for the last 6 months she has had several episodes in which she felt as if the room was spinning. She denies syncope or loss of vision, but notes that the episodes were accompanied by nausea and once with emesis. On most days, she feels off balance. She denies any previous history of vertigo and has not experienced any hearing loss, tinnitus, or otalgia. Otherwise, she is healthy with no significant medical or surgical history. Current medications include an oral contraceptive.

On further questioning, the patient admits to a history of frequent severe headaches that seemed to increase in intensity with her menstrual cycle. Both her mother and sister have similar problems with headaches. She has observed that her dysequilibrium worsens after she has a headache. She currently takes over-the-counter analgesics, with only slight relief of her pain. Her head and neck examination, including a neurologic evaluation, reveals no abnormalities and an audiogram shows normal hearing bilaterally. Her Dix-Hallpike test findings were negative.

DEFINITION

Patients use a myriad of terms to describe vertigo, including *dizziness, lightheadedness, off balance,* or *dysequilibrium.* It is important to have patients describe their symptoms using terms other than those listed to determine if they have indeed experienced true vertigo. Vertigo is defined as "an illusory sense of motion of either oneself or one's surroundings (1)." It is the sensation that the environment or the patient is in motion. Vertiginous episodes can last from seconds to weeks and are often accompanied with pallor, diaphoresis, nausea, and vomiting. Vertigo is frequently incapacitating, often resulting in emergency room visits and frequent office consultations.

EPIDEMIOLOGY

Both primary care physicians and many subspecialists deal with the vertiginous patient every day. It is estimated that >90 million patients in the United States present to their physician with the chief complaint of dizziness every year (2). Within the general population, dizziness affects approximately 20% of people (3). It affects people of all ages and races and both men and women alike. It is the most common presenting complaint of patients >75 years of age (4), but this is not a disorder restricted to adults. In 1998, it was estimated that 15% of school-aged children experienced at least one episode of vertigo (5). Because these cases can be very complex, it is essential to have a thorough understanding of the cause and pathophysiology of vertigo and the latest treatment recommendations to provide effective care for these patients.

ETIOLOGY AND PATHOGENESIS

The peripheral vestibular system, composed of the vestibular labyrinth and the vestibular nerve, the proprioceptive organs, and the visual system, all combine to present information to the central vestibular neurons in the brainstem essential to maintaining balance. Efferents from the central processing centers help to maintain a person's balance and compensation to motion (6). Abnormal processing of any of these individual components can cause patients to sense imbalance or dizziness.

PATHOLOGY AND CLINICAL MANIFESTATIONS

Numerous causes exist for vertigo of both peripheral and central origin, including vertebrobasilar ischemia, space-occupying lesions, multiple sclerosis and other demyelinating disorders, degenerative neurologic disorders, perilymphatic fistulas, and vestibulotoxicity are just some of the many examples. It is important to keep in mind that the differential diagnosis is lengthy and, therefore, only the most common of these conditions will be discussed here in greater detail: benign paroxysmal peripheral vertigo, vestibular migraine, Ménière's disease, vestibular neuritis, and traumatic brain injury.

The most common cause of vertigo, and perhaps the least understood, is vestibular migraine. Migraines are estimated to affect 15% to 25% of women and 5% to 8% of men (7,8). Within that population of migraine sufferers, it has been found that episodic vertigo occurs in up to 25% (9). Conversely, a significantly higher prevalence of migraine has been seen in patients presenting with dizziness as compared with matched controls (38% versus 24%) (8,9).

Recent research suggests that vertigo, dizziness, and imbalance can all be manifestations of migraine and occur before, during, or after headaches (or all of those) and, in a select group of patients, may be the only symptom of a migraine attack. A personal or family history of headaches or migraines may not be initially volunteered by patients for what they may perceive as irrelevant to their complaint of vertigo, but is now known to be an essential part of the patient's medical history. Knowledge of the International Headache Society (IHS) classification of migraine can help in the diagnosis of those patients who have not been previously aware of their condition. According to the IHS, vertigo is a migrainous symptom within the context of basilar migraine and migraine variants, including benign paroxysmal vertigo of childhood, although current research has demonstrate that vertigo can be a symptom in all types of migraine. Recurrent attacks of vertigo can last from 5 to 60 minutes, with or without a headache or other common migraine symptoms (e.g., nausea, vomiting, photophobia), especially in the setting of a positive personal or a family history of migraine, which supports the diagnosis of vestibular or vertiginous migraine.

Although the pathophysiology of migraine-related vertigo is not presently fully understood, migraine headache is believed to result from the sensitization of the trigeminovascular system., whereas the migraine-related visual aura is thought to be caused by cortical spreading depression. Migraine variants, such as hemiplegic migraine, have been linked to abnormal voltage-dependent P/Q-type calcium channel α_{1A}.

Treatment of these patients is twofold: one is to address the underlying cause (i.e., to treat the migraine headaches with oral medication both symptomatically and prophylactically) and the other is to help prevent the recurrence via avoidance of certain foods and behaviors that may act as migraine triggers (e.g., caffeine, foods with tyramine, and stress). Ergotamines and triptans, which are frequently used to abort a migraine headache, have failed to stop the attacks of vertigo. Beta blockers, calcium-channel blockers, antiepileptic agents, and tricyclic amines have all been used to treat these patients with intention to reduce the number or severity of headaches and the other neurootologic manifestations as well.

Benign paroxysmal positional vertigo (BPPV) is thought to be one of the most common causes of peripheral vertigo, with published incidences varying between 11 and 64 cases per 100,000 patients (10,11). Patients typically present with a history of acute onset vertigo or dizziness brought about by rapid changes in head position. One of the most common scenarios reported is vertigo that occurs after rolling over in bed. Patients also note difficulty with looking upward and bending over. The vertigo and imbalance that these patients experience tends to last only for seconds to less than 1 minute and, as its name suggests, is episodic in nature. Typically, these patients have an accompanying nystagmus that is both torsional and vertical. It is thought that BPPV is caused by free-floating particulate matter, otoliths arising from the vestibular labyrinth, found within the endolymph of the posterior semicircular canal (12).This has often been referred to as *canalithiasis.* BPPV has also been associated with other conditions, such as head trauma and vestibular neuritis (13).

The diagnosis of BPPV is suggested by both the history and physical examination, but is confirmed by performance of the Dix-Hallpike test done in the office or at the bedside. This maneuver involves rapid head movements with induction of the combined torsional and vertigo nystagmus. Classic findings demonstrate a 1- to 2-second latency, with the nystagmus lasting for approximately 10 to 20 seconds, ultimately fatiguing over the next 20 to 30 seconds. Although the condition improves spontaneously in many patients, requiring no treatment, others may require treatment that consists of specific canalith repositioning maneuvers intended to dislodge the debris from the posterior semicircular canal into the utricle. The Epley maneuver, perhaps the most popular of these techniques, has been found to be of benefit (14).

Ménière's disease, first described by Prosper Ménière in 1861, is an incapacitating disorder estimated to affect approximately 45,000 new patients every year, with >615,000 people living with this condition currently in the United States, according to the National Institute on Deafness and Other Communication Disorders 2001 (15). This disorder is characterized by the "presence of recurrent, spontaneous episodic vertigo; hearing loss; aural fullness; and tinnitus." The vertigo must be rotational and must have two episodes lasting at least 20 minutes to make the diagnosis, although the vertigo frequently lasts for several hours (16,17). The hearing loss is fluctuant and sensorineural in nature, typically affecting the lower frequencies.

Endolymphatic hydrops causing dilation of the endolymphatic labyrinth in the cochlea and vestibule, which was first noted on temporal bone histologic sections in 1938, is the pathophysiologic mechanism of Ménière's disease (18). Because Ménière's disease causes incapacitating vertigo that can last for hours and is often accompanied by nausea and vomiting, initial therapy is aimed at symptomatic control, with vestibular suppressants (e.g., meclizine and diazepam) and antiemetics (e.g., Promethazine). With the understanding of the above described pathophysiology, both medical and surgical therapy is aimed at addressing the endolymphatic hydrops. Patients are instructed to adhere to a low-salt diet and most are placed on a diuretic as well. Avoidance of caffeine, smoking, stress, and alcohol is also recommended. If conservative measures are not effective, however, then intratympanic gentamicin can be used to perform a chemical labyrinthectomy. Surgical therapy is reserved for patients with medically refractory vertigo. For patients with good hearing, an endolymphatic sac decompression or vestibular neurectomy can be beneficial. For patients with poor hearing, a labyrinthectomy is recommended. These procedures, however, are not without potential morbidity and patients must be made aware of the risks and benefits before proceeding with such procedures.

Vestibular neuritis describes a syndrome of peripheral vertigo of acute onset thought to be the result of a viral infection that causes vestibular nerve inflammation. A number of different terms are used to describe this syndrome, including *labyrinthitis, vestibular neuronitis*, and *neurolabrynthitis* (19). The diagnosis depends on a history of vertigo that is spontaneous, prolonged, and consistent with a peripheral origin and the absence of other neurologic signs or symptoms. Vestibular testing is not necessary if the history and physical examination are consistent. Testing, if done, would confirm a peripheral cause of the vertigo. Imaging is typically not deemed necessary if the patient's history and physical examination are consistent with this process and the patient shows some improvement within 48 hours (20). Despite the suspected viral causes, treatment is aimed at symptomatic relief. In the acute setting, these patients receive intravenous and oral vestibular suppressants. They typically continue to experience imbalance and dizziness; however, for the next several weeks, some cases need vestibular rehabilitation. It is important that patients refrain from vestibular suppressants during their rehabilitation such that they have the ability to learn to compensate. No studies have yet demonstrated a benefit to the use of antiviral medications and oral steroids in this setting (21).

When approaching a patient with vertigo, as with any medical complaint, the history is of utmost importance. A history of trauma, a fall, or head injury is critical to determining the cause of the patient's complaint of vertigo. Traumatic vestibulopathy is not uncommon after a traumatic brain injury. Up to 15% of patients with a mild traumatic brain injury have symptoms of postconcussive syndrome, of which vertigo is one (22). These cases are often difficult to manage because the symptoms of imbalance and dysequilibrium are chronic and frequently associated with other psychological and cognitive impairments. These patients typically present with normal head and neck examination findings and may or may not have abnormal audiograms and vestibular testing findings. After ruling out other possible causes, including perilymphatic fistula, which may necessitate surgical intervention, these patients should be referred for vestibular rehabilitation to help them learn to compensate (23). It is important, however, that these patients be made aware that they may still be left with imbalance, making it difficult to return to certain occupations and activities. Objective scales and vestibular tests have been created to help assist physicians and patients determine the level recovery likely, but they have limitations and should be individualized for each patient (24). Because of the difficult nature of treating these patients, a multidisciplinary approach should be used consisting of neurologists, otolaryngologists, psychiatrists, and audiologists, as needed.

DIAGNOSTIC APPROACH

It is important first to understand the appropriate workup of these patients. As with any aspect of medicine, the history is of utmost importance. The onset, duration, and concomitant symptomatology help to create an appropriate differential diagnosis. Associated symptoms of headache, visual changes, hearing loss or other neurologic abnormalities, as well a history of stroke, traumatic brain injury, or recent neuroontologic procedure can help to determine the cause of the vertigo and help to differentiate whether it is of central or peripheral origin. The physical examination must be complete, including a thorough neurologic examination and a Dix-Hallpike test. Eye movement can be evaluated with Frensel glasses as well. Patients with vertigo should also have an audiologic examination. Imaging is not essential for all patients, but should be considered in certain situations. Abnormalities of the temporal bone, including fracture and cholesteotoma, warrant computed tomographic (CT) scans of the temporal bone. Magnetic resonance imaging (MRI) is considered in patients in whom mass lesions are suspected or in patients with a history of head injury (25).

Vestibular testing can be performed to confirm diagnostic suspicion. Electronystagmography (ENG) consists of a battery of tests that investigate both the vestibular and oculomotor components of the balance system. These tests include evaluation of spontaneous gaze and positional nystagmus; the fistula test and bithermal caloric tests; pursuit system, saccadic system, and optokinetic and fixation system. The rotary chair and dynamic posturography complete the battery of testing. ENG testing helps the clinician differentiate and confirm whether the vertigo is of central or peripheral origin. The following findings are typical of a central disorder: spontaneous or positional nystagmus with normal calorics, direction-changing nystagmus, failure of fixation suppression, abnormal saccade or pursuit results, and hyperactive caloric responses. Vertigo of peripheral origin, on the other hand, often has the following ENG findings: unilateral caloric weakness, bilateral caloric weakness with history of ototoxic medication usage, fatiguing positional nystagmus, intact fixation suppression, and direction-fixed nystagmus (26).

TREATMENT

Effective treatment and symptomatic control is critical in the management of the vertiginous patient. The goal of treatment is both to rid the patient of current symptoms of dysequilibrium and imbalance and to prevent futures episodes and attacks. Both medical and surgical options are available, some of which have been described above. In the acute setting, it is often necessary to treat patients with vestibular suppressants, including meclizine and benzodiazepines, to control their symptoms. It is important to keep in mind that these patients should not be on these medications long term, because they need to learn to compensate for the vestibular loss. Also important, is to treat concomitant symptomatology, such as nausea and vomiting, with antiemetics. Addressing and treating the underlying condition to prevent further attacks is essential. For example, canalith repositioning maneuvers can be helpful in BPPV and adequately treating a patient for migraine headaches with oral medication and dietary and behavior modifications can be of benefit. Patients with Meniere's disease may benefit from a low-salt diet and a diuretic. Finally, certain patients will continue to experience chronic imbalance, and they can benefit from vestibular rehabilitation in which the patient works with a therapist learning different exercises and techniques to compensate for the loss of vestibular function. This is particularly important in patients with traumatic brain injury.

Procedural and surgical options are available for those with Meniere's disease. In considering several of the available options, it is important to address the risks of the surgical procedure, including possible permanent hearing loss. Intratympanic gentamicin therapy is perhaps the least invasive and technically simple procedure available. This procedure typically preserves hearing and has a vertigo control rate of

75% to 90% (27,28). Endolymphatic sac decompression is a surgical option with variable results. Although this procedure intends to preserve hearing and has a relatively quick recovery period, long-term control of vertigo is approximately 50%, although a larger percentage of patients may have short-term success (29). Patients with intractable vertigo may elect for a vestibular neurectomy in which the vestibular nerve is sectioned at the brainstem. Although it appears that excellent control of vertigo is achieved via this procure, a far greater morbidity and potential risk exist as compared with the other alternatives described (30). Finally, in patients with poor hearing, a labyrinthectomy can be performed in which both the vestibular and hearing mechanisms are destroyed on the affected side with the highest control rate; long-term results vary, however (31).

CLINICAL RECOMMENDATIONS OF THE VIGNETTE

The patient with vertigo who initially presented to her otolaryngologist with complaints of vertigo and imbalance was diagnosed with vestibular migraine. She was educated regarding the possible triggers of her headaches and was given a handout on dietary recommendations to help reduce the frequency of her attacks. Finally, the patient was subsequently evaluated by a migraine specialist who placed her on appropriate medication. The patient was to be reevaluated and would be offered vestibular rehabilitation if her symptoms of disequilibrium persisted.

SUMMARY

Vertigo is a common problem that physicians of many specialties must diagnose and treat. It affects people of all ages and races and is frequently incapacitating. It is essential to have a clear understanding of the various causes and the appropriate diagnostic workup of these often complicated cases. Not only is that essential in selecting the most effective treatment, but it is critical in differentiating benign causes from those more serious potentially life-threatening causes that may require urgent treatment. Correct diagnosis and treatment can drastically improve the quality of life for these patients.

REFERENCES

1. Furman J, Cass S. Benign paroxysmal positional vertigo. *N Engl J Med.* 1999;341:1590.
2. Task Force on the National Strategic Research Plan. *Balance and the Vestibular System.* Bethesda, MD: National Institute of Health; 1989.
3. Kroenke K, Price RK. Symptoms in the community. Prevalence, classification, and psychiatric comorbidity. *Arch Intern Med.* 1993;153:2474–2480.
4. Kroenke K, Arrington ME. The prevalence of symptoms in medical outpatients and the adequacy of therapy. *Arch Intern Med.* 1990;150:1685.
5. Russell G, Abu-Arafeh I. Paroxysmal vertigo in children: An epidemiological study. *Int J Pediatr Otorhinolaryngol.* 1999;49:S105–S107.
6. Minor L, Zee DS. Evaluation of the dizzy patient. In: Cummings et al. *Otolaryngology Head and Neck Surgery*, 3rd ed. St. Louis:Mosby; 1998:2623–2671.
7. Stewart WF, Simon D. Population variation in migraine prevalence: A meta-analysis. *J Clin Epidemiol.* 1995;48:269–280.
8. Neuhauser H, Leopold M. The interrelations of migraine, vertigo, and migrainous vertigo. *Neurology.* 2001;56:436–441.
9. Kayan A, Hood JD. Neuro-otological manifestations of migraine. *Brain.* 1984;107: 1123–1142.
10. Froehling DA, Silverstein MD. Benign paroxysmal vertigo: Incidence and prognosis in a population-based study in Olmsted County, Minnesota. *Mayo Clin Proc.* 1991;66:596–601.
11. Mizukoshi K, Watanbe Y. Epidemiological studies on benign paroxysmal positional vertigo in Japan. *Acta Otolaryngol Suppl.* 1988;447:67–72.
12. Furman JM, Cass SP. Benign paroxysmal positional vertigo. *N Engl J Med.* 1999;341: 1590–1596.
13. Baloh RW, Honrubia V. Benign positional vertigo: Clinical and oculographic features in 240 cases. *Neurology.* 1987;37(3)371–378.
14. Hilton M, Pinder D. The Epley (canalith repositioning) manoeuvre for benign paroxysmal positional vertigo. *Cochrane Database Syst Rev.* 2005;4.
15. Ervin SE. Ménière's disease: Identifying classic symptoms and current treatments. *American Association of Occupational Health Nurses.* 2004;52:156–158.
16. Committee on Hearing and Equilibrium guidelines for the diagnosis and evaluation of therapy in Ménière's disease. *Otolaryngol Head Neck Surg.* 1995;113:181–185.
17. Mizukoshi K, Watanabe Y. Preliminary guidelines for reporting treatment results in Ménière's disease conducted by The Committee of the Japanese Society for Equilibrium Research, 1993. *Acta Otolaryngol Suppl.* 1995;519:211–215.
18. Shambaugh GE, Wiet RJ. The endolymphatic sac and Ménière's disease. *Otolaryngol Clin North Am.* 1980;13:585–588.
19. Baloh RW. Vestibular neuritis. *N Engl J Med.* 2003;348:1027–1032.
20. Hotson JR, Baloh RW. Acute vestibular syndrome. *N Engl J Med.* 1998;339;680–685.
21. Stokroos RJ, Albers FWJ. Antiviral treatment of idiopathic sudden sensorineural hearing loss: A prospective, randomized, double-blind clinical trial. *Acta Otolaryngol.* 1998;118:488–495.
22. Paniak C, Toller-Lobe G. A randomized trial of two treatments for mild traumatic brain injury: 1 year follow-up. *Brain Inj.* 2000;14:219–226.
23. Marzo, SJ, Leonetti JP. Diagnosis and management of post-traumatic vertigo. *Laryngoscope.* 2004;114:1720–1723.
24. Gottshall K, Drake A. Objective vestibular tests as outcome measures in head injury patients. *Laryngoscope.* 2003;113:1746–1749.
25. Konrad HR, Bauer CA. Peripheral vestibular disorders. *Head and Neck Surgery-Otolaryngology*, 3rd ed. Philadelphia: Lippincott Williams & Wilkins; 2001:1975–1976.
26. Driscoll CL, Green JD. Balance function tests. *Head and Neck Surgery-Otolaryngology*, 3rd ed. Philadelphia: Lippincott Williams & Wilkins; 2001:1651–1658.
27. Marzo SJ, Leonetti JP. Intratympanic gentamicin therapy for persistent vertigo after endolymphatic sac surgery. *Otolaryngol Head Neck Surg.* 2002;126:31–33.
28. Cohen-Kerem R, Kisilevsky V. Intratympanic gentamicin for Ménière's disease: A meta-analysis. *Laryngoscope.* 2004;114:2085–2091.
29. Durland WF, Pyle GM. Endolymphatic sac decompression as a treatment for Ménière's disease. *Laryngoscope.* 2005;115:1454–1457.
30. Silverstein H, Wanamaker HH. Vestibular neurectomy. In: Jackler RK, Brackman DE, eds. *Neurotology.* St. Louis: Mosby; 1994:945.
31. Levine SC, Glasscock M. Long-term results of labyrinthectomy. *Laryngoscope.* 1990;100: 125–127.

CHAPTER 142

Preeclampsia and Eclampsia

John G. Gianopoulos

OBJECTIVES

- To review the pathogenesis of preeclampsia and eclampsia
- To review diagnostic criteria for the diagnosis of both mild and severe preeclampsia and eclampsia
- To highlight the strategy for conservative management remote from term in severe preeclampsia
- To discuss therapeutic interventions for hypertension and seizure prevention in preeclampsia
- To review the use of magnesium sulfate for seizure treatment and prophylaxis
- To discuss clinical strategies for diagnosis and intervention in eclampsia

CASE VIGNETTE

An 18-year-old woman, gravida 1 para 0 at 38 weeks, 7 days gestation presents to the emergency room with a 3-hour history of a severe throbbing frontal headache. She has seen white spots before her eyes for the last hour. She also has felt anxious and "jumpy" for the last several hours. To date, her pregnancy has been uncomplicated. She has had significant swelling in both legs and hands over the last week, however. She has received regular prenatal care, with her last visit 2 weeks ago. She reported at that visit "everything was fine." She has been concerned that she has been gaining 3 to 4 pounds each week and is worried that she is "retaining water." Her fetus is "not moving very much today." She has an uncomplicated medical history.

On examination, her blood pressure is 160/110 mm Hg. She has hyperreflexia with 4+ muscle stretch reflexes in all four extremities and bilateral ankle clonus. Funduscopic examination shows a heightened light reflex, with marked arterial vasospasm. She has +3 pedal edema, and edema of her hands and face. Her urine dipstick shows +4 protein in her urine. Fetal monitoring demonstrates decreased fetal heart rate variability, without decelerations. While in the emergency department, the patient suddenly has a generalized tonic–clonic seizure.

DEFINITIONS

The patient described in the case vignette highlights a significant problem faced by both obstetricians and neurologists. Hypertension related to pregnancy complicates 8% to 10% of all pregnancies. Despite modern management, it remains a significant cause of maternal and fetal morbidity and mortality (1).

During pregnancy, hypertension is classified as (*a*) preexisting hypertension, (*b*) preeclampsia or eclampsia, (*c*) chronic hypertension with superimposed preeclampsia or eclampsia, and (*d*) gestational hypertension.

Preeclampsia is defined as proteinuric hypertension after the 20th week of gestation. A patient must demonstrate a sustained blood pressure of 140/90 mm Hg to be classified as hypertensive in pregnancy. Proteinuria must exceed 300 mg in 24 hours or demonstrate +1 on urine dipstick at least twice in 6 hours (1,2). A patient who has a tonic–clonic seizure in the presence of preeclampsia is classified as eclamptic, in the absence of other neurologic conditions. Gestational hypertension is defined as hypertension originating in pregnancy (140/90 sustained) without proteinuria (1,3).

EPIDEMIOLOGY

Preeclampsia complicates 8% to 10% of all pregnancies. Its incidence is higher in nonwhite women, patients from lower socioeconomic strata of society, primigravidas, and patients with preexisting hypertension, renal disease, or diabetes. Eclampsia complicates 1 of 2,000 to 3,000 pregnancies. The peak incidence of preeclampsia or eclampsia occurs at the ends of the reproductive spectrum, with teens and women >35 years of age having a higher incidence (4,5).

ETIOLOGY AND PATHOGENESIS

The etiology for preeclampsia and eclampsia remains a medical enigma. Many theories, ranging from placental toxins to helminthic infestations, have been proposed. Despite centuries of inquiry into the cause of preeclampsia and eclampsia, nature continues to hide this secret.

Much is known, however, regarding its underlying pathophysiology. Arteriolar vasospasm with intravascular volume depletion is the primary pathologic alteration leading to preeclampsia. Precipitating pathologic factors include failure of prostacyclin-mediated vasodilatation, endothelial damage leading to release of endothelins, and thromboxane and vasoactive proteins (6–8). These intravascular changes lead to the loss of catecholamine insensitivity of normal pregnancy and angiotensin hypersensitivity, leading to vasospasm and hypertension. Changes in vascular endothelin growth factor (VEGF) and placental growth factor (PGF) have been associated with aberrant trophobalstic implantation and may be integral in the pathogenesis of the preeclampsia and eclampsia syndrome. The disruption of placental angiogenesis can be related to onset of this disease (9–13). As vascular resistance increases, blood flow to vital organs decreases and microangiopathy ensues. As proteinuria increases, blood albumin levels drop, decreasing plasma oncotic pressure. When paired with endothelial damage, this leads to generalized edema. Renal blood flow is decreased; renal endothelial cells swell, leading to an impaired filtration function allowing large molecules (e.g., proteins) to filter (14–16).

The pathophysiology of eclamptic seizures is not well understood. Hypertensive encephalopathy, cerebral vasospasm, cerebral edema, microinfarctions, and hemorrhages have all been theorized as potential mechanism (17).

CLINICAL MANIFESTATIONS

Preeclampsia is defined as either mild or severe. Criteria that define severe preeclampsia are blood pressure 160/110 mm Hg, neurologic hyperreactivity (headaches, hyperreflexia, scotomata), oliguria, proteinuria of >5 g in 24 hours, renal failure, epigastric pain, elevated liver enzymes, thrombocytopenia, pulmonary edema, disseminated intravascular coagulation (DIC), hemolysis, fetal compromise, oligohydramnios, and fetal growth restriction. Mild preeclampsia includes those patients with the disease, but without clinical features characteristics of the severe form (1). Before seizure onset, patients may complain of occipital-frontal headaches, epigastric pain, blurred vision, photophobia, and altered mental state. At least 50% to 75% of patients with eclampsia will have one of these symptoms before seizure onset (Table 142-1). Occipital-frontal headache is the most common prodromal symptom, occurring in 60% to 80% of patients who have an eclamptic seizure (17,19). Any patient complaining of a severe occipital frontal headache in the presence of preeclampsia must be immediately treated or a significant risk exists of a seizure ensuing.

A syndrome of *h*emolysis, *e*levated *l*iver enzymes, and *l*ow *p*latelet count has been identified as a severe preeclamptic variant. This syndrome has been termed the *HELLP syndrome* (20). This constellation of symptoms may be seen in 2% to 12% of patients with preeclampsia; as many as 30% to 50% of these patients may not manifest hypertension or proteinuria. This syndrome is a severe form of preeclampsia and is life threatening. The exact pathogenesis is unknown; vasospasm, endothelial damage, and microangiopathic hemolysis may be contributing factors. The HELLP syndrome can progress to eclampsia and needs to be treated immediately. Platelet consumption and fibrin deposition in the liver can lead to areas of necrosis. Rarely, a subcapsular hematoma or even hepatic rupture can occur in these patients (20).

TABLE 142-1. Prodromal Symptoms in Eclampsia

Clinical Symptoms	*Incidence (%)*
Headaches	50 to 70
Visual disturbances	19 to 32
Epigastric pain (right upper quadrant pain)	12 to 19
Hyperreflexia	30 to 70
At least one symptom	60 to 70

(From Sibai BM. Diagnosis, prevention, and management of eclampsia. *Obstet Gynecol.* 2005;150:402, with permission.)

Any patient with the preeclampsia syndrome can become eclamptic. A patient with severe disease has a greater risk of seizure, but even cases of mild disease can develop into eclampsia without the patient manifesting any signs or symptoms of severe disease. Therefore, patients with preeclampsia must always be viewed as a medical emergency. Appropriate intervention must be undertaken to prevent disease progression (21).

An eclamptic seizure can begin as a focal motor seizure and progress to a generalized tonic–clonic seizure. Peripheral feedback from the myoneural junction is needed for the overall progression to a generalized tonic–clonic seizure. Seizures are self-limited as peripheral myoneural junctions depolarize (18). Patients who have had a seizure are at risk for intracranial bleeding, and each successive seizure increases the risk of this potentially fatal complication. Most seizures (~50%), occur in the intrapartum period; however, 25% occur antepartum and 25% occur postpartum (19,22). Most postpartum seizures occur in the first 48 hours, although patients have been reported to have had seizes as late as 23 days postpartum. Almost all cases of eclampsia occur after 28 weeks' gestation (~90%). Approximately 8% occur between 21 and 27 weeks of gestation. It is rare to have eclampsia before 20 weeks' gestation, unless throphoblastic disease is present (23).

DIAGNOSTIC APPROACH

No specific biochemical or biophysical marker exists to identify patients with this syndrome. Clinical signs and symptoms are used to establish the diagnosis. All prenatal patients during the last month of pregnancy are screened weekly for blood pressure, proteinuria, and unusual increases in weight. Once the disease is suspected, careful assessment for possible end-organ involvement is critical. Assessment of renal and hepatic function, coagulation status, hematologic parameters, neurologic function, and fetal status should be undertaken. Reliable patients with mild disease can be treated as an outpatient when remote from term. Twice weekly visits, with both close maternal and fetal surveillance, are necessary. If any progression of the disease occurs, admission and hospital evaluation is warranted. Patients at term or with severe disease require hospitalization and evaluation (24,25). Initial evaluations should include assessment for hepatomegaly; pulmonary status with chest examination; cardiac and neurologic examination (focusing on detailed sensory examination, muscle stretch reflexes, funduscopic examination); extremity examination; pregnancy assessment (evaluation of gestational age, and fetal well-being with biophysical assessment, ultrasound, and fetal heart rate monitoring); and status of the cervix for possible induction of labor. Laboratory assessment includes complete blood count (CBC) with platelet count; blood urea nitrogen (BUN); creatinine, serum uric acid, serum alanine aminotransferase (ALT), aspartate amniotransferase (AST), and lactic acid dehydrogenase (LDH); in addition, a 24-hour urine

TABLE 142-2. Differential Diagnosis of Eclampsia

Hypertensive encephalopathy
Epilepsy
Metabolic disease
Brain tumor
Thrombotic thrombocytopenic purpura
Cerebral vasculitis
Stroke
Ruptured cerebral aneurysm

(From Sibai BM. Diagnosis, prevention, and management of eclampsia. *Obstet Gynecol.* 2005;150:402, with permission.)

for protein and creatinine clearance and coagulation studies, (prothrombin time [PT], partial thromboplastin time [PTT], fibrinogen).

Patients with eclampsia require medical stabilization and preparation for delivery. These patients should have neuroimaging studies done because intracranial bleeding can occur in these patients (26). Cranial computed tomography (CT) or magnetic resonance imaging (MRI) studies have shown areas of cerebral edema or small infarctions within the subcortical white matter and adjacent gray matter in approximately 40% to 50% of cases of eclampsia (26–28). Patients need to be assessed in a similar manner to those with preeclampsia, paying particular attention to hepatic, renal, and coagulation status. These patients often become thrombocytopenic or have decrements in renal function. Fetal surveillance is critical, as with each seizure an approximate 20% to 30% risk is seen for fetal death. Fetal surveillance with ultrasonic biophysical parameters and fetal heart rate monitoring is indicated. Once stabilized, patients should undergo delivery. Induction of labor is the preferred route, if the cervix is favorable and the fetal status is stable. Cesarean section should be undertaken for usual obstetrical indications (29).

Differential diagnosis of preeclampsia includes systemic lupus erythematosus (SLE) glomerulonephritis, hemolytic uremic syndrome, thrombotic thrombocytopenic purpura, and primary renal disease. Eclampsia is the most common cause of convulsions in pregnancy or the immediate postpartum period in association with hypertension. Many medical conditions have similar presenting symptoms and clinical findings. The differential diagnosis for eclampsia is outlined in Table 142-2 (17).

Eclampsia is also associated with an increased rate of maternal morbidity, including abruptio placenta (7% to 10%), acute renal failure (5% to 9%), pulmonary edema (3% to 5%), DIC (7% to 11%), aspiration pneumonia (2% to 3%), and cardiopulmonary arrest (2% to 5%). Eclampsia also remains a significant cause of maternal mortality in developing countries (14%). The mortality in the developed world is only 0 to 1.8% (18,22,29).

TREATMENT

The only definitive treatment for preeclampsia and eclampsia is delivery of the fetus. Patients with mild disease and remote from term can be treated conservatively with very close maternal and fetal surveillance. Patients at or near term (or once fetal maturity status is documented) should have delivery effected. Patients with severe disease at term or near term must be hospitalized, evaluated, and stabilized, and infant delivered. Patients who are remote from term with severe disease pose a significant clinical dilemma. Previously, the dogma was delivery regardless of gestational age. Several randomized studies have shown, however, that in selected patients with severe preeclampsia remote from term, conservative management in a tertiary care environment may be undertaken (25,30–32). Less than 28 weeks gestation, patients can be given corticosteroids for fetal lung maturity, transferred to a tertiary care setting, and treated conservatively. Close monitoring for maternal decompensation must be undertaken in these patients. Laboratory studies and fetal surveillance as outlined in the previous section must be done. Arterial hypertension must be treated. Between 28 weeks and 34 weeks gestation, patients with severe disease receive corticosteroids (intramuscularly, either betamethasone 12 mg every 24 hours for two doses or dexamethasone 6 mg every 12 hours for 48 hours), with close maternal and fetal surveillance and reassessment after 48 hours (33,34). If severe parameters still persist, delivery should then be undertaken. Between 32 and 34 weeks and beyond, patients should be stabilized and the infant delivered. All patients with eclampsia require delivery after initial stabilization. Any potential fetal benefit from delaying delivery does not outweigh the risk of significant maternal decompensation.

Magnesium sulfate is the agent of choice to prevent and treat eclamptic seizures. Two large randomized trials have demonstrated the superiority of magnesium sulfate over phenytoin in the prevention of eclampsia and the prevention of recurrent seizures in eclampsia (35–37). The World Health Organization (WHO), the International Society for the Study of Hypertension in Pregnancy, and the American College of Obstetricians and Gynecologists (ACOG) have all recommended magnesium sulfate as the therapy of choice to prevent and treat eclamptic seizures (38–42). Magnesium sulfate may be administered intravenously or intramuscularly. The most common administration protocol is to give a loading dose of 2 to 4 g of a dilute solution (20%) intravenously over 15 to 20 minutes. This is to be followed with a maintenance dose of 2 g/hour. Magnesium levels can become toxic, leading to respiratory or cardiac arrest. These patients require intensive monitoring of their respiratory and cardiovascular functions and neurologic status. As magnesium is renally cleared, adequate urine output must be maintained. If patients manifest oliguria, decrease or discontinuation of magnesium is indicated. Magnesium toxicity is directly related to serum levels. Muscle stretch reflexes are lost at 8 to 10 mEq/L; respiratory arrest occurs at 10 to 15 mEq/L; and cardiac arrest may occur at levels of 20 to 25 mEq/L (40–42). If magnesium toxicity is manifest, it may be reversed with administration of intravenous calcium (10 mL of a 10% solution of calcium gluconate given slowly over 5 to 10 minutes). This calcium rescue must be given slowly, because too rapid administration could precipitate a fatal cardiac arrhythmia. Close monitoring is required of maternal respiratory status and reflexes (41).

Most eclamptic seizures are self-limited. Magnesium sulfate is given to prevent subsequent seizures. The dose and route of administration are as described above. In cases unresponsive to magnesium, benzodiazepines may be used. Diazepam (0.1 to 0.5 mg/kg) or midazolam (0.02 to 0.1 mg/kg) is often used. Rarely, patients remain unresponsive. The next agent of choice is intravenous phenytoin (10 to 20 mg/kg over 20 minutes). In severe, unresponsive cases, intravenous sodium amobarbitol is given in 50 mg increments to a total dose of 250 mg. In cases where none of the above agents are effective, the patient must have muscle paralysis with general anesthesia and ventilatory support (17,43). Patients with severe preeclampsia and eclampsia have all been shown to benefit from magnesium therapy. Controversy still exists, however, on the use in magnesium in patients with mild preeclampsia. No randomized trial yet has shown a clear benefit. The use of magnesium sulfate in patients with mild preeclampsia must be individualized. The WHO recommends the use of magnesium sulfate for prevention of seizure in mild disease in developing countries. ACOG recognizes that no clear consensus exists regarding the use of magnesium in patients with mild preeclampsia and recommends individualization based on patients presentation (21,39,40). The exact mechanism of action of magnesium to prevent eclamptic seizure is unknown. Magnesium sulfate has a mild central sedative effect; it is an osmotic diuretic and reduces cerebral edema; and it relaxes smooth muscle and has a mild vasodilatory effect. It is theorized that magnesium sulfate may work peripherally at the myoneural junction, decreasing muscle contractions and breaking the feedback loop needed to sustain these seizures.

In patients with preeclampsia or eclampsia, hypertension should be treated when the systolic blood pressure exceeds 160 mm Hg or the diastolic pressure exceeds 110 mm Hg (1). Preservation of the fetal circulation must be considered when treating these conditions. Hydralazine has been recommended for the acute management of hypertension in patients with preeclampsia or eclampsia. A test intravenous dose of 5 mg is administered, followed by 10 mg doses every 15 minutes. Some recent data show that labetalol may be a superior antihypertensive in these acute situations, because it does not increase maternal pulse rate. A 10 mg test dose is given. This is followed by an intravenous 20 mg dose in 10 minutes. If no response is observed in blood pressure, the dose may be increased to 40 mg. If no response is observed in 20 minutes, the dose is increased to 80 mg. If no response is observed in 20 minutes, a second 80 mg dose is given. The total dose is not to exceed 300 mg (1,44–46). Rarely, continuous labetalol is needed (intravenous dose of 2 to 4 mg/min). In more chronic conditions nifedipine may be used. The patient must be well hydrated, however, because the fetal circulation can be compromised if maternal hypotension is paradoxically produced. Because of the intravascular volume depletion in most patients with preeclampsia or eclampsia, this agent is not used (47). Nitroprusside should be avoided, if possible. This agent is converted in the fetal circulation to sodium thiocyanide and the fetus lacks the necessary hepatic cytochrome system to metabolize this metabolic byproduct. In hypertensive crisis unresponsive to other agents, it may be used with extreme caution. Angiotensin-converting enzyme inhibitors (ACE) and angiotensin receptor blockers (ARB) are contraindicated in pregnancy. In the first trimester, they have been shown to be teratogenic and lead to fetal death in the second and third trimesters of pregnancy (48,49).

Anesthesia for delivery or cesarean section is best accomplished with regional techniques (epidural or spinal). The patient must be well hydrated and closely monitored to avoid hypotension (50).

CLINICAL RECOMMENDATIONS OF THE VIGNETTE

The patient should be promptly stabilized. Her airway was secured with a nasopharyngeal airway, oxygen was administered, intravenous magnesium sulfate was given, blood pressure was controlled with intermittent doses of labetalol, and laboratory assessment undertaken. Once the maternal condition was stabilized, the patient was admitted to labor and delivery and fetal status determined. Ultrasonic biophysical parameters were performed and fetal heart rate monitoring assessed. The fetal and maternal status was stable, so labor was induced with very close maternal and fetal surveillance. Because the maternal status was stable, a CT was done of the maternal cranial anatomy to assess for intracranial bleeding. Cesarean section should be done only if the fetal status is not reassuring or other obstetric indications exist. The patient will be maintained on magnesium sulfate for 24 hours after delivery as seizure prophylaxis.

SUMMARY

Cases of patients with preeclampsia or eclampsia require intensive medical and obstetric management. Most patients require hospital admission and physiologic and laboratory assessment of physiologic function, renal, hepatic, cardiovascular, hematologic, and neurologic status. At or near term, after stabilization, delivery of the fetus is the treatment of choice. Remote from term in mild disease, conservative observation may suffice. Management of severe cases must be individualized. Patients with eclampsia at any gestational age are best treated with stabilization and delivery. Magnesium sulfate is the agent of choice to treat and prevent eclamptic seizures. Blood pressure should be controlled if above 160/110 mm Hg. Close fetal surveillance, with ultrasound and fetal heart rate monitoring, is indicated. Given these interventions, maternal and perinatal mortality and morbidity have been significantly reduced.

REFERENCES

1. Working group report on high blood pressure in pregnancy. Washington, DC: National Institute of Health; 2000.
2. Sibai BM. Pitfalls in diagnosis and management of pre-eclampsia. *Am J Obstet Gynecol.* 1988;159:1.
3. Milne F, Redman C, Walker J, et al. The pre-eclampsia community guideline (PRECOG): How to screen for and detect onset of pre-eclampsia in the community. *BMJ.* 2005;330: 576–580.
4. Mogren I, Hogberg U, Winkvist A, et al. Familial occurrence of preeclampsia. *Epidemiology.* 1999;10:518.
5. Lie RT, Rasmussen S, Brunborg H, et al. Fetal and maternal contributions to risk of pre-eclampsia: Population based study. *BMJ.* 1998;316(7141):1343–1347.
6. Everitt RB, Worlij RJ, MacDonald J, et al. Effect prostaglandin synthetic inhibitors on pressor response to angiotensin II in human pregnancy. *J Clin Endocrinal Metab.* 1978;46: 1007–1010.
7. Gant NF, Chand S, Whalley PG, et al. The nature of pressor responsiveness to angiotensin II in human pregnancy. *Obstet Gynecol.* 1974;43:854–859.
8. Mastrogiannis DS, O'Brien WF, Krammer K, et al. Potential role of endothelial in normal and hypertensive pregnancies. *Am J Obstet Gynecol.* 1997;165:1771–1775.
9. Lain KY, Roberts JM. Contemporary concepts of the pathogenesis and management of preeclampsia. *JAMA.* 2002;287:3183–3186.
10. Zhou Y, Damsky CH, Fisher SJ. Preeclampsia is associated with failure of human cytotrophoblasts to mimic a vascular adhesion phenotype. One cause of defective endovascular invasion in this syndrome? *J Clin Invest.* 1997;99:2152–2157.
11. Chambers JC, Fusi L, Malik IS, et al. Association of maternal endothelial dysfunction with preeclampsia. *JAMA.* 2001;285(12):1607–1612.
12. Maynard SE, Min JY, Merchan J, et al. Excess placental soluble fms-like tyrosine kinase 1 (sFit1) may contribute to endothelial dysfunction, hypertension, and proteinuria in preeclampsia. *J Clin Invest.* 2003;111:649–658.

13. Zhou Y, McMaster M, Woo K, et al. Vascular endothelial growth factor ligands and receptors that regulate human cytotrophoblast survival are dysregulated in severe pre-eclampsia and hemolysis, elevated liver enzymes, and low platelets syndrome. *Am J Pathol.* 2002;160: 1405–1410.
14. Vuorela P, Helske S, Hornig C, et al. Amniotic fluid-soluble vascular endothelial growth factor receptor-1 in preeclampsia. *Obstet Gynecol.* 2000;95:353–355.
15. Levine RJ, Maynard SE, Qian C, et al. Circulating angiogenic factors and the risk of preeclampsia. *N Engl J Med.* 2004;350:672–676.
16. Meyer NL, Mercer BM, Freidman SA, et al. Urinary dipstick protein: A poor predictor of absent or severe proteinuria. *Am J Obstet Gynecol.* 1994;170(1):137–141.
17. Sibai BM. Diagnosis, prevention, and management of eclampsia. *Obstet Gynecol.* 2005;150: 402–410.
18. Katz VL, Farmer R, Kuller J. Preeclampsia into eclampsia: Toward a new paradigm. *Am J Obstet Gynecol.* 2000;182:1389–1396.
19. Chames MC, Livingston JC, Invester TS, et al. Late postpartum eclampsia: A preventable disease? *Am J Obstet Gynecol.* 2002;186:1174–1177.
20. Weinstein L. Syndrome of hemolysis, elevated liver enzymes and low platelet count a severe consequence of hypertension in pregnancy. *Am J Obstet Gynecol.* 1982;142:159–163.
21. Alexander JM, McIntire D, Leveno K, et al. Selective magnesium sulfate prophylaxis for the prevention of eclampsia in women with gestational hypertension. *Obstet Gynecol.* 2006; 108(4):826–832.
22. Douglas KA, Redman CW. Eclampsia in the United Kingdom. *BMJ.* 1994;309:1395–1400.
23. Mattar F, Sibai BM. Eclampsia. VIII. Risk factors for maternal morbidity. *Am J Obstet Gynecol.* 2000;182:307–312.
24. Sibai BM. Treatment of hypertension in pregnant women. *N Engl J Med.* 1996;335: 257–260.
25. Odendaal HJ, Pattenson RC, Bam R, et al. Aggressive of expectant management for patients with severe preeclampsia between 28–34 weeks' gestation: Randomized controlled trial. *Obstet Gynecol.* 1990;76:818–822.
26. Belfort MA, Grunewald C, Saade GR, et al. Preeclampsia may cause both overperfusion and underperfusion of the brain. *Acta Obstet Gynecol Scand.* 1999;78:586–591.
27. Dahmus MA, Barton JR, Sibai BM. Cerebral imaging in eclampsia: Magnetic resonance imaging versus computed tomography. *Am J Obstet Gynecol.* 1992;167:935–941.
28. Sibai BM, Sarinoglu C, Mercer BM. Eclampsia. VII. Pregnancy outcome after eclampsia and long-term prognosis. *Am J Obstet Gynecol.* 1992;166:1757–1763.
29. Coppage KH, Polzin WJ. Severe preeclampsia and delivery outcomes: Is immediate cesarean delivery beneficial? *Am J Obstet Gynecol.* 2002;186:921–923.
30. Sibai BM, Mercer BM, Schiff E, et al. Aggressive versus expectant management of severe preeclampsia at 28 to 32 weeks' gestation: A randomized controlled trial. *Am J Obstet Gynecol.* 1994;171:818–822.
31. Chari RS, Friedman SA, O'Brien JM, et al. Daily antenatal testing in women with severe preeclampsia. *Am J Obstet Gynecol.* 1995;173:1207–1210.
32. Sibai BM, Barton JR, Aki S, et al. A randomized prospective comparison of nifedipine and bed rest versus bed rest alone in the management of preeclampsia remote from term. *Am J Obstet Gynecol.* 1992;167:879–885.
33. Effect of antenatal steroids for fetal maturation on perinatal outcomes. NIH Consensus Statement 1994;12:1.
34. American College of Obstetricians & Gynecologists. Antenatal corticosteroid therapy for fetal maturation. ACOG Committee Opinion No. 210. Washington, DC: American College of Obstetricians & Gynecologists; 1998.
35. Which anticonvulsant for women with eclampsia? Evidence from the Collaborative Eclampsia Trial. *Lancet.* 1995;345:1455–1461.
36. Lucas MJ, Leveno KJ, Cunningham FG. A comparison of magnesium sulfate with phenytoin for the prevention of eclampsia. *N Engl J Med.* 1995;333:201–208.
37. Witlin AG, Sibia BM. Magnesium sulfate therapy in preeclampsia and eclampsia. *Obstet Gynecol.* 1998;92:883–886.
38. Roberts JM, Villar J, Arulkumaran S. Preventing and treating eclamptic seizures. *BMJ.* 2002;325:609–612.
39. Sibai BM. Magnesium sulfate prophylaxis in preeclampsia: Lessons learned from recent trials. *Am J Obstet Gynecol.* 2004;190:1520–1526.
40. American College of Obstetricians & Gynecologists. Diagnosis and management of preeclampsia and eclampsia. ACOG Practice Bulletin #33. *Obstet Gynecol.* 2002;99:159–162.
41. Belfort MA, Anthony J, Saade GR, et al. A comparison of magnesium sulfate and nimodipine for the prevention of eclampsia. *N Engl J Med.* 2003;348:304–309.
42. Do women with pre-eclampsia, and their babies, benefit from magnesium sulphate? The Magpie Trial: A randomized placebo-controlled trial. *Lancet.* 2002;359:1877–1881.
43. Witlin AG, Sibai B. Magnesium sulfate therapy in preeclampsia and eclampsia. *Obstet Gynecol.* 1998;92:883–889.
44. Magee LA, Ornstein MP, von Dadelszen P. Fortnightly review: Management of hypertension in pregnancy. *BMJ.* 1999;318:1332–1338.
45. Magee LA, Cham C, Waterman EJ, et al. Hydralazine for treatment of severe hypertension in pregnancy: Meta-analysis. *BMJ.* 2003;327:955–960.
46. Duley L, Henderson-Smart DJ. Drugs for treatment of very high blood pressure during pregnancy. *Cochrane Database Syst Rev.* 2002; CD001449.
47. Impey L. Severe hypotension and fetal distress following sublingual administration of nifedipine to a patient with severe pregnancy induced hypertension at 33 weeks. *Br J Obstet Gynecol.* 1993;100:959–962.
48. Friedman JM. ACE inhibitors and congenital anomalies. *N Engl J Med.* 2006;354: 2498–2500.
49. Cooper WO, Hernandez-Diaz S, Arbogast PG, et al. Major congenital malformations after first-trimester exposure to ACE inhibitors. *N Engl J Med.* 2006;354:2443–2451.
50. Wallace DH, Leveno KJ, Cunningham FG, et al. Randomized comparison of general and regional anesthesia for cesarean delivery in pregnancies complicated by severe preeclampsia. *Obstet Gynecol.* 1995;86:193–199.

CHAPTER **143**

Headaches in Pregnancy

Richard E. Besinger • Robert M. Abrams

OBJECTIVES

- To provide an understanding of the different causes of headaches in pregnancy
- To differentiate among the three types of primary headaches
- To list a hierarchic differential diagnosis of new-onset headaches in pregnancy
- To describe the different diagnostic modalities available in the evaluation of pregnant patients with headaches
- To discuss medications that may be used to treat headaches in pregnancy

CASE VIGNETTE

A 35-year-old gravida 1, para 0, at 37 weeks' gestation had a history of severe migraine headaches. During this pregnancy, the frequency of her migraines has been markedly decreased. When she has a migraine headache, it is often controlled with acetaminophen and relaxation techniques. Her pregnancy has been uncomplicated to this point. She presents to the labor and delivery department with a bifrontal headache rated as "8/10" on the visual analog scale (VAS) for pain assessment. The headache began the night before and has progressively worsened. It is described as "different" from her usual migraines. She has no history of visual aura, photophobia, phonophobia, osmophobia, diplopia, transient visual obscurations, numbness, nausea, vomiting, anxiety, or depression. She cannot relate any precipitating factor. She took acetaminophen the previous night with no resolution of the headache.

She states that fetal movements are good. She has had no contractions, vaginal bleeding, or leakage of amniotic fluid, and no history of abdominal pain, visual changes, or dizziness. Her blood pressure is 140/90 mm Hg. Physical examination, including detailed funduscopy, is unremarkable except for 2+ pretibial edema. Neurologic examination showed brisk muscle stretch reflexes. Her fundal height measures 34 cm. Fetal heart monitor tracing is reassuring, and she is not having contractions. Laboratory study is significant for 3+ proteinuria in the urinalysis.

The resident on duty formulates an extensive differential diagnosis that includes exacerbation of migraine headache, new-onset cluster or tension headache, preeclampsia, arteriovenous malformation, pseudotumor cerebri, subarachnoid hemorrhage, brain tumor, and cerebral venous thrombosis.

DEFINITION

During childbearing years, approximately 80% of women have headaches (1). Thus, headaches are very common during pregnancy. Two broad categories of headaches have been classified by the International Headache Society as primary and secondary headache disorders (2) (Table 143-1). Primary headaches are defined as those headaches not associated with an underlying pathology—the illness is the headache itself. Secondary headaches are caused by pathology, which may stem from extracranial, intracranial, or systemic disorders.

Primary headaches are further categorized as migraine (with or without aura), tension type, and cluster. These headaches account for >90% of headaches in pregnancy.

Migraine headaches are usually characterized as a severe, throbbing, unilateral headache. Oftentimes, photophobia, phonophobia, nausea, and vomiting accompany these headaches, which can last for several days.

Tension-type headaches are frequently described as a tight band around the head. The pain is often bilateral and moderate in intensity. The pain generally lasts no longer than several hours, although it can last as long as 1 week (2).

Cluster headaches are far more common in men than women and, therefore, are seldom seen in pregnant patients. The classic presentation of a cluster headache is a sharp, unilateral periorbital pain that lasts, on average, 30 to 90 minutes (3). The headache is also accompanied by concurrent symptoms, such as conjunctional injection, lacrimation, nasal conjection, facial or forehead sweating, miosis, and eyelid ptosis.

The etiology, pathogenesis, and treatment of each of these headache types are reviewed in this chapter.

Secondary headaches during pregnancy are much less common than primary headaches. Many obvious clinical conditions can contribute to secondary headaches, such as trauma, substance abuse, infections, psychiatric disorders, and vascular disorders.

ETIOLOGY AND PATHOGENESIS

Headaches are one of the most common complaints during pregnancy. Because the prevalence of migraines is highest in reproductive-aged women, they are frequently the reason for acute clinical visits.

TABLE 143-1. New International Headache Society classification (2004)

PRIMARY HEADACHE DISORDERS

Migraine
Tension-type headache
Cluster headache and other trigeminal autonomic cephalalgias
Other primary headaches

SECONDARY HEADACHE DISORDERS

Headache attributed to the following:
 Head or neck trauma
 Cranial or cervical vascular disorders
 Nonvascular intracranial disorders
 A substance or its withdrawal
 Infection
 A disorder of homeostasis
 A psychiatric disorder
Headache or facial pain attributed to a disorder of cranium, neck, eyes, ears, nose, sinuses, teeth, mouth, or other facial or cranial structures
Cranial neuralgias and central causes of facial pain
Other headache, cranial neuralgia, central or primary facial pain

(Adapted from Headache Classification Committee. *The International Classification of Headache Disorders*, 2nd ed. *Cephalgia.* 2004;24:1–160, with permission.)

A proposed etiology of migraine headaches is based on fluctuating serum hormone levels of estrogen. Maternal progesterone has not been proved to affect the frequency or severity of migraine headaches significantly. Most women who have migraines experience an improvement in symptoms during pregnancy because of the high estrogen levels (4). This is not always the rule, however, and despite the elevated estrogen, some women experience worsening of their migraines. This theory proves true in the postpartum period, because migraine headaches usually worsen in association with a rapid decline of estrogen levels.

The cause of tension-type headaches does not appear to be hormonally related, which potentially differentiates it from migraines. Previously, it was believed that muscle contraction in the head and neck caused vasoconstriction leading to headaches (5). More recent research has linked tension-type headaches to the trigeminal neurovascular system and instability of the serotonergic neurotransmitters (6). Hence, tension-type headaches do not correlate with hormonal changes during pregnancy.

The pathophysiology of cluster headaches is not completely understood. When hypothesizing a cause, the model must explain the main characteristics of a cluster headache, which are trigeminal distribution of the pain, episodic pattern of attacks, and ipsilateral cranial autonomic features (7). Likely, a combination of neuronal dysfunction leading to excitation of the trigeminovascular system and involvement of the hypothalamus results in the symptoms of cluster headaches. Recent research is linking cluster headaches with a genetic component in its etiology (8). Other risk factors for cluster headaches include smoking and alcohol use. Therefore, much as with tension-type headaches, the hormonal contribution of pregnancy to cluster headaches is felt to be negligible.

CLINICAL MANIFESTATIONS AND SPECIAL SITUATIONS

PREGNANCY

Pregnancy poses an additional problem in the diagnosis of headaches, because multiple clinical circumstances exist of which the practitioner must be aware that are unique to pregnancy.

Preeclampsia can present with headaches. A patient who complains of severe headaches in pregnancy (especially in the third trimester) should warrant a thorough evaluation and preeclampsia must be considered. A headache may be the only presenting complaint of a woman with severe preeclampsia (9). If left untreated, an eclamptic seizure can ensue. Other signs and symptoms of preeclampsia include hypertension (>140/90 mm Hg), proteinuria (>300 mg/dL), right-upper quadrant pain, and visual disturbances. Blood pressure elevation must be sustained over a 6-hour period as well as persistent proteinuria.

Another consideration of a patient presenting with a severe headache is an aneurysmal subarachnoid hemorrhage (SAH). The incidence of SAH is approximately 10 of 100,000 pregnancies (10). Pregnancy itself does not increase the risk for SAH; however, a large increase is seen in the risk at 6 weeks' postpartum (6). The classic presentation is a patient complaining of "the worst headache" ever experienced. Nontraumatic SAH often results from rupture of an intracranial aneurysm or arteriovenous malformation.

As more research is being done in genetics, pregnant women with adverse pregnancy outcomes are being evaluated for mutations that can increase their risk for thrombotic events, known as *inheritable thrombophilias.* Because pregnancy is a hypercoagulable state in and of itself, women with thrombophilic states are at a much higher risk for cerebral venous thrombosis. Specifically, women with factor V Leiden mutation, prothrombin gene (G20210A) mutation, and protein C and S deficiencies are most at risk. Diagnosis can be difficult because of the high frequency of headaches during pregnancy. Certain clues that may aid in considering cerebral venous thrombosis in the differential include a patient's history of thrombotic events, a family history of thrombosis, or prior poor obstetrical outcome. If a patient presents with a severe headache and concomitant neurologic signs, further imaging studies must be done to rule out this type of ischemic stroke.

Women who delivered with assistance of a labor epidural or who had a cesarean delivery with regional anesthesia are at risk of postdural puncture headaches. Postdural puncture headaches occur when an iatrogenic leakage of cerebrospinal fluids (CSF) occurs. The subarachnoid space contracts and the pain-sensitive intracerebral veins subsequently expand (11). Patients complain of severe headaches when raising their head above a nonsupine position. Resolution of a postdural puncture headache usually occurs with conservative measures, such as bedrest, caffeine, and intravenous fluid. If these modalities do not result in cessation of the headache, an autologous epidural blood patch may be placed (12).

Another important cause of secondary headaches to be considered among pregnant women presenting with headaches is *idiopathic intracranial hypertension* (pseudotumor cerebri). This is most common among reproductive-aged, obese women (13). In this condition, headaches start as a mild ache and progressively worsen in intensity and increase in frequency. A clue to this diagnosis is that headaches often worsen on increasing the intraabdominal pressure by coughing or straining. Diagnosis is made by lumbar puncture (LP) demonstrating an elevated CSF opening pressure. Conservative treatment consists of acetaminophen. To decrease the amount of CSF production, acetazolamide, a carbonic anhydrase inhibitor, can be used. Rarely, serial LP may be needed, but this approach is painful and often difficult. A lumboperitoneal shunt can also be difficult for pregnant patients. Before delivery, consideration must be given to exteriorize the shunt to avoid infection from a possible cesarean delivery. Optic nerve sheath decompression may be the preferred approach to save vision.

DIAGNOSTIC APPROACH

The evaluation of a pregnant patient who presents with a headache requires a well-organized, systematic approach that will enable the provider to exclude the most critical of diagnoses. As with any presenting complaint, the most important initial clinical tool is a detailed history and thorough physical examination. When a pregnant patient presents for evaluation of a headache, it is important to characterize the headache as detailed as possible. The character of onset, duration, severity, and location of the headache should be carefully assessed. Other contributing symptoms that may lead to diagnosis are visual disturbances, numbness, or vomiting. A medical history should be taken to evaluate the patient's history of headaches (migraine, tension type, or cluster), medication history, personal and family history of thrombosis, and diet history as causes for the headache. Many women in pregnancy decide to limit their caffeine intake, and this withdrawal is a common reason for headaches during pregnancy. Social history should elicit any use of drugs or history of depression or other psychiatric disorders as confounding factors. Of course, if the patient is postpartum, it is important to know if she received regional anesthesia to evaluate for postdural puncture headache.

After a detailed clinical history is obtained, physical examination should focus on the mother's health and fetal well-being. If the fetus is at a gestational age of viability (usually, 24 weeks), the patient should be placed on a fetal monitor to ensure that the fetus is well oxygenated. Vital signs, neurologic assessment, and thorough physical examination oftentimes lead to the identification of the cause for the patient's headache. With any concern for preeclampsia, it would be appropriate to send a complete blood count (CBC), urinalysis to assess for protein, and liver enzymes to eliminate the possibility of *h*emolysis, *e*levated *l*iver enzymes, and *l*ow *p*latelet count (HELLP syndrome).

If a clinical diagnosis cannot be formulated after a history, physical examination, and laboratory studies are collected, further investigations using radiologic studies are warranted. Also, acute-onset headaches, trauma, focal neurologic findings, or neck stiffness suggestive of meningitis necessitate central nervous system (CNS) imaging (14).

A general axiom in radiologic examinations of pregnant women is that a missed or delayed diagnosis is usually far worse than the risk of radiation to either the patient or her fetus. The American College of Obstetricians and Gynecologists (ACOG), however, still does not recommend use of radiologic studies in the first trimester because of theoretic teratology risks (15). No adverse fetal effects (anomalies or pregnancy loss) have been demonstrated with radiation exposure <0.05 Gy. To put this in perspective, a computed tomographic (CT) scan of the head exposes the uterus to a mere 1 millirad, which is well below the critical exposure. Magnetic resonance imaging (MRI) does not use ionizing radiation and, thus, poses no risk to the developing fetus.

In emergent conditions, a noncontrast CT is the best initial study to obtain. Situations where this would be appropriate include a patient presenting with "the worst headache of my life" or a headache of sudden onset and extreme severity. These subjective findings may be suggestive of cerebral edema secondary to preeclampsia, intracranial hemorrhage, or large tumor. Severe headache with absence of focal neurologic findings should raise the possibility of an impending eclamptic seizure in late gestation.

MRI is a better modality to use if nonhemorrhagic pathology is suspected, such as tumor, inflammation, or infection. Magnetic resonance angiography (MRA) is useful to detect arterial vascular lesions using gadolinium as contrast material. Gadolinium does cross the placenta, however, the fetal kidneys excrete this contrast with no adverse effects yet reported. Magnetic resonance venogram (MRV) is the gold standard for diagnosing cerebral venous thrombosis, in which timely diagnosis is crucial. Despite its known safety, the National Radiological Protection Board still advises to avoid MRI imaging in the first trimester because only limited data assessing its effect on organogenesis exist.

If idiopathic intracranial hypertension is suspected, an LP is indicated after neuroimaging studies exclude a structural lesion or hydrocephalus. Other indications for LP during pregnancy include assessing for infections (meningitis) and ruling out SAH in suspicious cases with normal CT findings. Of course, timely consultation with a neurologist, or if necessary, a neurosurgeon may be indicated.

TREATMENT

A major concern of medication use during pregnancy is the risk of teratology and late toxicity to the fetus. The US Food and Drug Administration (FDA) places medications into five separate categories, based on the safety of their use in pregnancy (Table 143-2). This system was introduced in 1979 and has been recently criticized, because it does not accurately communicate what is known about the human effects of a medication. Rather, it relies primarily on animal studies. The separation into different categories does not effectively guide the practitioner about what clinical action to take. For example, a category X medication might be assigned to a drug that does not cause reported human birth defects, but it does not have any conceivable use in pregnancy. Oral contraceptive pills are an example of this. In 1994, the Teratology Society issued a recommendation that the *category system* be abandoned in favor of a plain text explanation of the available information on toxicity during development. Multiple human-based data sources are now available, which may be better resources for learning about the safety of medications in pregnancy. REPROTOX is one example of such source.

TABLE 143-2. US Food and Drug Administration Pregnancy Risk Factor Definitions

Category A:	Controlled studies in women who fail to demonstrate a risk to the fetus in the first trimester, and the possibility of fetal harm appears remote
Category B:	Either animal-reproduction studies have not demonstrated a fetal risk, but there are no controlled studies in pregnancy women or animal-reproduction studies have shown an adverse effect that was not confirmed in controlled studies in women
Category C:	Either studies in animals have revealed adverse effects on the fetus and there are no controlled studies in women or studies in women and animals are not available
Category D:	There is positive evidence of human fetal risk, but the benefits from use in pregnant women may be acceptable despite the risk
Category X:	Studies, adequate well-controlled or observational, in animals or pregnant women have demonstrated positive evidence of fetal abnormalities. The use of the product is contraindicated in women who are or may become pregnant.

Most medications used to treat headaches in pregnancy are generally considered safe, however. Of course, all medication use during pregnancy should be limited and only used if conservative measures are not effective.

Treatment of primary headaches during pregnancy can be classified into two categories: acute treatment and preventive treatment. Avoidance of all medication, if possible, in the first trimester is recommended because of minor concerns for teratogenesis.

As stated, migraine headaches resolve during pregnancy in most women. For those patients whose migraines persist throughout pregnancy, however, treatment is essential. Nonpharmacologic treatments are the first-line treatments. These include avoidance of trigger factors, biofeedback, and relaxation training (16). First-line pharmacologic treatment of acute migraines is acetaminophen. Nonsteroidal anti-inflammatory drugs (NSAID) can also be used in early pregnancy and for short treatments only. In the third trimester, NSAID should not be used, because concern exist of oligohydramnios and premature closure of the ductus arteriosus. Opiods (e.g., oxycodone, morphine, codeine) can be safely added if acetaminophen alone is not sufficient. The above-mentioned medications are categorized as category B and considered safe to use during pregnancy. The remote potential exists, however, for neonatal withdrawal syndrome from the opioids.

If conservative measures and first-line pharmacologic treatments do not cause abatement of the migraine headaches, the next step would be the selective serotonin agonists. These include sumatriptan, zolmitriptan, and naratriptan. No increase in birth defects or adverse pregnancy outcomes has been ascertained, although these medications are classified as category C because of limited human controlled studies. Other migraine-specific medications that can be used in the nonpregnant state, the ergot alkaloids, are absolute contraindications during pregnancy. The ergots are potent vasoconstrictors and can cause uterine artery constriction and uterine contractions, which might lead to pregnancy loss. Because of this, ergot alkaloids are classified as FDA category X. In refractory cases of migraines, prednisone may be useful (17).

Preventive treatment of migraine headaches is indicated if the patient has multiple episodes per month that are refractive to acute treatment. Behavioral techniques should be attempted first before medications are added. Useful medications that are frequently used include β-blockers, calcium channel blockers, and tricyclic antidepressants. β-blockers (atenolol, metoprolol, propranolol) are category D medications because of the small theoretic risk of fetal growth restriction (<10th percentile) in the third trimester. Because of the possibility of fetal bradycardia and other symptoms of β-blockade, use of these medications is reserved for those patients whose migraines are not controlled with the other modalities that are available.

Tension-type headaches oftentimes can be treated with acetaminophen alone. As with migraine headaches, behavioral therapy should be tried first, which includes relaxation techniques, and biofeedback. Caffeine may be of some help in relieving these headaches.

Cluster headaches are difficult to treat because of the short-lived nature of these headaches. If these headaches are severe, inhalation of 100% oxygen has been shown to be effective (18).

Treatment of secondary headaches generally aims at treating the underlying cause. In the pregnancy-related cause of headache from severe preeclampsia, treatment is delivery of the fetus. Remember, headaches caused by preeclampsia can be associated with an unremarkable neurologic examination, but brisk reflexes and clonus are common findings in the patient with preeclampsia. The cause of the headache is unknown, but some studies have postulated that it is caused by cerebral edema or ischemia secondary to vasoconstriction (19). Patients with severe preeclampsia who have headaches as the presenting complaint must have their fetus delivered, regardless of gestational age, which can lead to delivering a very premature fetus with long-term neurologic sequelae. If possible, administration of corticosteroids for 24 to 48 hours may hasten fetal lung maturity before the need for delivery.

Patients whose headaches can be attributed to a postdural puncture recover many times with the previously described conservative measures. Those who do not get relief may benefit from a blood patch, which the anesthesiologist may place. The CSF leak is essentially plugged by using the patient's blood as a sealant. Immediate relief is usually the outcome.

Treatment for idiopathic intracranial hypertension (pseudotumor cerebri) may be with medications, such as acetazolamide (500 to 2,000 mg) as previously described. Serial LP, shunting, or optic nerve sheath decompression can be used in cases of vision loss.

Alternative therapies for headaches are gaining acceptance in the western world, and these applications have been emerging in treating pregnant women. The obvious benefits are that medication use is avoided and, thus, eliminates any concern over teratogenic effects and untoward fetal outcomes. Acupuncture, biofeedback, and relaxation techniques may be incorporated in the management of headaches in pregnant women, although further studies are needed to assure their safety and efficacy.

CLINICAL RECOMMENDATIONS OF THE VIGNETTE

The patient presented to the labor and delivery unit because of new onset headache. Because of her history of migraine headaches, a common error would be to attribute her headache to exacerbation of the migraine. It is important to understand all causes of headaches in pregnancy, including those that are exclusive to the pregnant state. Because of her elevated blood pressure, brisk muscle stretch reflexes, and otherwise normal neurologic examination findings, diagnosis should be a serious consideration of preeclampsia. Important in the patient's history is the description of the headache in that it differed from her typical migraine.

It is important to ascertain the cause of her headache and formulate an effective treatment plan that is beneficial both to her and to her fetus. In this specific case, a workup for preeclampsia would include a formal urinalysis, liver enzymes, and frequent blood pressure monitoring. In general, as the gestational age increases, the threshold for delivery decreases. Because this patient is at 37 weeks' gestation and presents with a severe headache and elevated blood pressure, preeclampsia would be the most likely diagnosis, and treatment would include induction of labor and administration of magnesium sulfate for seizure prophylaxis.

SUMMARY

Because headaches in pregnancy are so common, it is imperative for the health care provider to understand the multitude of different causes. Primary headaches improve or are unchanged during pregnancy in most cases. For those women whose migraines worsen, care must be taken in managing these pregnancies and comanagement with a neurologist is preferable. Although concern of taking medications during pregnancy always exists, most pharmacologic modalities are considered safe with judicious use and may be helpful in alleviating the patient's symptoms.

If a patient presents during her pregnancy with a new-onset headache, special considerations must be undertaken to eliminate diagnoses that may be directly related to the hypercoagulable state, such as CNS thrombosis. If concern exists for an intracerebral hemorrhage, radiologic imaging should not be withheld because of concern for fetal toxicity. Preeclampsia must also be considered in any pregnant patient who presents with complaints of a headache, especially in the third trimester.

Accurately diagnosing the cause of headaches in the pregnant patient will potentially optimize outcomes for both the patient and her fetus. A multidisciplinary team, consisting of the obstetrician, internist, and neurologist, may be necessary to ensure that the patient's headaches are appropriately treated.

REFERENCES

1. Waters WE, O'Connor PJ. Epidemiology of headache and migraine in women. *J Neurol Neurosurg Psychiatry.* 1971;34:148.
2. Headache Classification Committee. *The International Classification of Headache Disorders,* 2nd ed. *Cephalalgia.* 2004;24:1–160.
3. Silberstein SD. Headaches in pregnancy. *Neurol Clin.* 2004;22:727–756.
4. Marcus DA. Interrelationships of neurochemicals, estrogen, and recurring headache. *Pain.* 1995;62:129.
5. Rollnik JD, Karst M, Fink M, et al. Botulinum toxin type A and EMG: A key to the understanding of chronic tension-type headaches? *Headache.* 2001;41:985.
6. Bartleson JD. Transient and persistent neurological manifestations of migraine. *Stroke.* 1984;15:383.
7. May A. Cluster headache: Pathogenesis, diagnosis, and management. *Lancet.* 2005; 366:843.
8. Russell MB. Epidemiology and genetics of cluster headache. *Lancet Neurol.* 21004;3:279.
9. American College of Obstetricians and Gynecologists. Hypertension in pregnancy. *ACOG Ttechnical Bbulletin No 219.* Washington, DC: American College of Obstetricians and Gynecologists, Washington, DC; 1996.
10. Kittner SJ, Stern BJ, Feeser BR, et al. Pregnancy and the risk of stroke. *N Engl J Med.* 1996;335:768–774.
11. Ponder TM. Differential diagnosis of postdural puncture headache in the parturient. *Clinical Forum of Nurse Anesthetists.* 1999;10:145–154.
12. Duffy PJ, Crosby ET. The epidural blood patch. Resolving the controversies. *Can J Anaesth.* 1999;46:878.
13. Martin SR, Foley M. Approach to the pregnant patient with headache. *Clin Obstet Gynecol.* 2005;48:2–11.
14. Von Wald T, Walling AD. Headache during pregnancy. *Obstet Gynecol Surv.* 2002;57:179–185.
15. American College of Obstetricians and Gynecologists. Guidelines for diagnostic imaging during pregnancy. ACOG Committee Opinion 158. Washington, DC: American College of Obstetricians and Gynecologists; 1995.
16. Scharff L, Marcus DA, Turk DC. Maintenance of effects in the nonmedical treatment of headaches during pregnancy. *Headache.* 1996;36:285–290.
17. Solomon GD, Cady RK, Klapper JA, et al. Standards of care for treating headache in primary care practice. National Headache Foundation. *Cleve Clin J Med.* 1997;64:373.
18. Fogan L. Treatment of cluster headache. A double blind comparison of oxygen vs. air inhalation. *Arch Neurol.* 1985;42:362.
19. Belfort, MA, Saade GR, Grunewald, C, et al. Association of cerebral perfusion pressure with headache in women with preeclampsia. *Br J Obstet Gynaecol.* 1999;106:814.

CHAPTER **144**

Epilepsy in Pregnancy

Jorge J. Asconapé

OBJECTIVES

- To review the effects of pregnancy on epilepsy
- To describe the effects of epileptic seizures on the mother and fetus
- To explore the effects of pregnancy on the pharmacokinetics of antiepileptic drugs (AED)
- To provide guidelines for the management of epilepsy during pregnancy

CASE VIGNETTE

A 22-year-old woman with a history of complex partial seizures is referred for neurologic evaluation because of a recent unexplained worsening of her seizures. She has recently become pregnant despite being on oral contraceptives. Before the pregnancy, the seizures were well controlled on carbamazepine monotherapy.

DEFINITION

Epilepsy is a chronic condition of the central nervous system (CNS) characterized by recurrent seizures. A seizure is the manifestation of abnormal and excessive synchronized discharge of a group of cerebral neurons.

EPIDEMIOLOGY

Seizures are one of the most common neurologic problems in clinical practice. The incidence of epilepsy is approximately 80 per 100,000 persons per year; the point prevalence is about 5 to 10 cases per 1,000 persons; and the cumulative incidence is between 3% and 5%. About 50 live births per 1,000 women of childbearing age with epilepsy occur each year.

ETIOLOGY AND PATHOGENESIS

The cause of epilepsy varies among the different age groups and geographical locations. Congenital and genetic disorders are the main cause in childhood and adolescence. In young adults, trauma, hippocampal sclerosis, tumors, vascular malformations, and alcohol and drug abuse are the most frequent causes.

The risk of epilepsy is not increased during pregnancy, but occasionally, it can start during pregnancy. In such cases, lowering of the seizure threshold by hormonal mechanisms may activate a latent epileptic condition. The term **gestational epilepsy** refers to cases where the seizures occur exclusively during pregnancy.

The most common causes of seizures are observed with increased frequency during pregnancy or puerperium include eclampsia, cerebral infarct, venous sinus occlusion, thrombotic thrombocytopenic purpura, subarachnoid and intracerebral hemorrhage, chorion carcinoma, and amniotic fluid embolism.

CLINICAL MANIFESTATIONS

The treatment of epilepsy during pregnancy has vastly improved in recent years because of a number of advances in diagnostic techniques and AED therapy. In this era, most women with epilepsy can expect to become pregnant and bear normal children, but an increased risk exists of complications. A spectrum of management issues needs to be addressed by the treating physician to minimize those risks.

EFFECTS OF EPILEPSY ON PREGNANCY

More than 90% of pregnancies in women with epilepsy have good outcomes. Epilepsy, however, has been reported to increase the risk of common obstetrical complications. Adverse obstetric outcomes include vaginal bleeding, hyperemesis gravidarum, preeclampsia, premature labor and delivery, induced labor, forceps or vacuum-assisted delivery, cesarean section, stillbirth, miscarriage or perinatal death, neonatal hemorrhage, low birthweight, and feeding difficulties (1). Recent studies indicate that, with appropriate care during preconception, pregnancy, delivery, and puerperium, the risk of obstetric complications can be virtually reduced to those of the general population (2).

Seizures during pregnancy can have serious complications (3). Traumatic injuries are a frequent indirect consequence of seizures. Maternal and fetal trauma, including placental abruption, is a serious concern. Trauma is the leading cause of nonobstetrica death in pregnancy. Generalized tonic–clonic seizures can increase the risk of hypoxia and acidosis. Stillbirth has been observed following a single generalized tonic–clonic seizure or status epilepticus. Maternal seizures during gestation have been linked to cognitive deficits in the offspring (4). Intracranial hemorrhage in utero has been reported following a maternal seizure (5). Status epilepticus is rare during pregnancy, but is associated with a high risk of maternal and fetal death. Generalized tonic–clonic seizures complicate about 1% to 3.5% of the deliveries in women with epilepsy and have been associated with profound effects on fetal cardiac rate, neonatal hypoxia, and low Apgar scores.

The effects of nonconvulsive seizures on the fetus have not been properly assessed, but appear to be less deleterious. A strong, prolonged uterine contraction, followed by 3.5 minutes of fetal heart deceleration, was reported in a woman experiencing a complex partial seizure during labor (6). One study has shown that maternal seizures of all types during the first trimester were associated with higher malformation rates in the offspring (7). This finding, however, has not been replicated in other studies.

Therefore, convulsive seizures during pregnancy can have potentially serious consequences, and continuation of AED therapy during pregnancy is justified in most women.

EFFECTS OF PREGNANCY ON EPILEPSY

Most women with epilepsy will not experience a significant change in seizure control during pregnancy. In a recent series, 56% of women experienced no change in seizure frequency, 27% a reduction, and only 18% a worsening of seizure control (8). Results from a large European pregnancy registry showed that 78.2% of women with epilepsy maintained good seizure control with AED monotherapy throughout the pregnancy, thus reducing the risk of teratogenicity and poor neurocognitive outcome in the offspring (9). In that same series, only 17.3% of women had worsening of their seizures, whereas 15.9% had a decrease in seizure frequency. Status epilepticus was noted in only 1.8% of the women, with approximately a third of those cases being of the convulsive type (9). The risk of increased seizure frequency during pregnancy appears to be unrelated to the type of seizures or the duration of the epilepsy. Seizure frequency in prior pregnancies has no predictive value.

Proposed mechanisms of increased seizure frequency in pregnancy include hormonal effects on seizure threshold, water and sodium retention, decreased AED serum levels, medication noncompliance, stressors, and sleep deprivation. Low serum concentrations of AED are frequently observed during pregnancy, but they have not been necessarily associated with increased seizure frequency (8).

Self-discontinuation of AED is a very common situation that can lead to loss of seizure control. A study using AED concentrations in hair showed that 15% of pregnant women had stopped their medication without informing their physician (10). Proper patient education about the potential risks of seizures is essential to prevent this situation.

ANTIEPILEPTIC DRUGS IN PREGNANCY

The numerous physiologic changes that occur during pregnancy markedly affect the pharmacokinetics of the AED (11). Rarely, drug absorption can be decreased with a resulting reduction in the bioavailability of certain drugs, such as phenytoin. The distribution of AED is affected by increases in total body water and extracellular fluid. An increase in fat stores leads to a decreased elimination of lipid soluble drugs. A decrease in the plasma concentrations of albumin and α_1-glycoprotein alters the protein binding, leading to an increase in the free fraction of drugs, such as phenytoin, valproate, tiagabine, or carbamazepine. Enzymatic induction of the cytochrome P450 system by increased endogenous steroids results in increases in the clearance of many AED. Increased cardiac output and renal flow contributes to the increased elimination of AED.

As a result of the physiologic changes mentioned above, tendency is for a decline in plasma concentration of the AED during pregnancy (Table 144-1) (11). In the case of highly protein

TABLE 144-1. Antiepileptic Drug (AED) Pharmacokinetic Characteristics and Alterations of Clearance During Pregnancy

AED	*Major Metabolic Route*	*Protein Binding (%)*	*Reported Increases in Clearance (%)*	*Reported Decreases in Total Plasma Concentrations (%)*	*Reported Decreases in Free Plasma Concentrations (%)*
Phenytoin	CYP 2C9, 2C19	90	20 to 100	55 to 61	18 to 31
Carbamazepine	CYP 3A4	80	0 to 20	0 to 42	0 to 28
Valproate	Glucuronide conjugation (50%), β-oxidation (40%), CYP 2A6, 2C9	90	35 to 183	50	29
Phenobarbital	CYP 2C9, 2C19	50	—	55	50
Lamotrigine	Glucuronidation by UGT enzymes (70% to 90%)	55	65 to 350	—	—
Oxcarbazepine	MHD: glucuronide conjugation, renal excretion	40 (MHD)	64	36	—
Topiramate	Renal excretion (50% to 80%)	13 to 17	No data available	—	—
Gabapentin	Renal excretion (100%)	None	No data available		
Zonisamide	CYP 3A4 (50%), acetylation (15%)	40	No data available		
Levetiracetam	Renal excretion (66%), hydrolysis of acetamide group (not CYP450-dependent)	<10	No data available		
Pregabalin	Renal excretion (100%)	None	No data available		

(Modified from Pennell PB. Antiepileptic drug pharmacokinetics during pregnancy and lactation. *Neurology*. 2003;61[Suppl 2]:S35–S42, with permission.)

bound drugs, such as valproate and phenytoin, the decline in the total plasma concentration is more dramatic than that of the free fraction, making free levels more accurate for monitoring.

Both the timing and rate of decline of plasma concentrations are unpredictable, but tend to be maximal in the last half of the pregnancy. It is also quite variable among the different AED, given their different pharmacokinetic properties and elimination routes. AED with glucuronidation as their major metabolic rate are especially susceptible to increases in their clearance during pregnancy. Such is the case with lamotrigine and oxcarbazepine where marked increases in the total daily dose are often required to maintain constant plasma concentrations (9).

Lamotrigine clearance steadily increases throughout pregnancy until the 32nd week, reaching an average peak of >350% of the baseline clearance (12). The clearance then slowly trends downward and returns to preconception levels within 2 to 3 weeks of delivery. These findings, however, showed marked interindividual differences, suggesting that frequent plasma level determinations (i.e., monthly) are especially important with this drug.

Oxcarbazepine is a prodrug that is rapidly metabolized into the active metabolite 10-hydroxycrbamazepine (MHD). MHD undergoes glucuronidation and direct renal excretion as its main route of elimination. Results from a large pregnancy registry showed that oxcarbazepine use during pregnancy was associated with a higher risk of seizures and more frequent dose increments compared with other AED (9). In a recent study, the clearance of MHD was increased during pregnancy, with a reduction of plasma concentrations of about 36% in the third trimester (13). Compared with prepregnancy baseline, mean dose-corrected MHD levels were 72% in the first trimester, 74% in the second trimester, and 64% in the third trimester. Therefore, frequent plasma level determinations appear to be also advisable for oxcarbazepine use during pregnancy.

BREAST-FEEDING AND ANTIEPILEPTIC DRUGS

Breast-feeding is generally safe in term infants, and the benefits are thought to outweigh the small risk of adverse events. Throughout pregnancy, the fetus is constantly exposed to the AED taken by the mother. Umbilical cord plasma concentrations of AED are very similar to maternal plasma concentrations at the time of birth, indicating extensive transplacental transfer. Exposure to AED in the neonate can continue via breast-feeding. The concentration of a given AED in breast milk is inversely proportional to its protein binding. For most AED, the concentrations in breast milk are lower than in maternal serum. Therapeutic serum concentrations, however, have been found in neonates. Newborns have immature enzymatic metabolic systems with prolonged elimination half-lives compared with the adult, which could lead to higher steady-state plasma concentrations of the AED (Table 144-2) (11). AED in breast milk can result in excessive sedation and feeding difficulties in the infant. Withdrawal symptoms have also been observed, especially with phenobarbital, other barbiturates, or benzodiazepines.

Most AED have a low risk for adverse effects in breast-fed infants. Of the traditionally AED, phenobarbital, primidone, and ethosuximide have a higher risk of adverse events. Of the newer agents, lamotrigine can potentially accumulate given the immaturity of the glucuronidation mechanisms in the neonate.

TABLE 144-2. Antiepileptic Drug (AED) Exposure Through Breast-Feeding

AED	*Breast Milk Maternal Concentration*	*Adult Half-life (hours)*	*Neonatal Half-life (hours)*
Carbamazepine	0.4 to 0.6	8 to 25	8 to 28
Phenytoin	0.18 to 0.4	12 to 50	15 to 105
Phenobarbital	0.36 to 0.6	75 to 126	45 to 500
Ethosuximide	0.8 to 0.9	32 to 60	32 to 40
Primidone	0.7 to 0.9	4 to 12	7 to 60
Valproate	0.01 to 0.10	6 to 18	30 to 60
Lamotrigine	0.6	—	Prolonged
Topiramate	0.69 to 0.86	—	—
Zonisamide	0.41 to 0.93	63	61 to 109
Levetiracetam	0.24 to 1.34	—	—

(Modified from Pennell PB. Antiepileptic drug pharmacokinetics during pregnancy and lactation. *Neurology.* 2003;61[Suppl 2]:S35–S42, with permission.)

These drugs should be used with caution, and careful monitoring of the infant is recommended.

ANTIEPILEPTIC DRUGS AND NEONATAL HEMORRHAGE

Infants of mothers with epilepsy are at increased risk for hemorrhage during the early neonatal period. The bleeding occurs internally during the first 24 hours after birth and has been associated with greater than 30% mortality. The maternal coagulation study findings are typically normal, whereas the neonate shows prolonged prothrombin and partial thromboplastin times. The incidence of this condition is not known but appears to be rare.

The pathophysiology is not completely understood, but the bleeding may result from a deficiency of vitamin K-dependent clotting factors II, VII, IX, and X. This deficiency is presumably secondary to induction of the fetal cytochrome P450 by the AED, resulting in increased metabolism of vitamin K. A prothrombin precursor, protein induced by vitamin K absence (PIVKA), has been found in the maternal plasma (2). More recent studies indicate that vitamin K deficiency in pregnant women on enzyme-inducing AED is common. The presence of PIVKA is less so, but neonatal hemorrhage is rare. The use of vitamin K supplementation is further complicated by the fact that AED have a warfarinlike effect, inhibiting the transplacental transfer of vitamin K. Large doses of vitamin K, however, can overcome this effect.

It is generally agreed that, until this condition is better understood, pregnant women on AED should receive vitamin K supplementation (10 mg orally) during the last month of pregnancy. Furthermore, the infant should receive 1 mg of vitamin K intramuscularly or intravenously at birth. If bleeding occurs, fresh frozen plasma intravenously has been recommended.

DIAGNOSTIC APPROACH

In most pregnant patients, the diagnosis of epilepsy has been established before conception and no diagnostic tests are usually necessary. In general, when the onset of the epilepsy is during pregnancy, the diagnostic evaluation is not different from that of seizures outside of pregnancy.

The type of epilepsy syndrome needs to be established for proper management. It is important to determine whether the patient has idiopathic generalized epilepsy, which is genetically determined, or symptomatic partial epilepsy, possibly secondary to a brain lesion. In most cases, electroencephalograms (EEG) show specific epileptiform discharges and help differentiate between partial and generalized epilepsy. A magnetic resonance imaging (MRI) of the brain is the neuroimaging procedure of choice for the evaluation of epilepsy. An MRI is necessary in practically all cases of partial seizures and in generalized seizures unless a clear genetically determined syndrome can be established. Computed tomographic (CT) scan is usually indicated in the acute management of seizures.

Neuroimaging procedures are sometimes deferred until the completion of the pregnancy if the patient is clinically stable. MRI, however, is considered safe to use during pregnancy and a CT scan can be performed with the proper precautions.

TREATMENT

Treatment of the pregnant woman with epilepsy is based on the careful balance between the need to prevent seizures while minimizing the exposure to AED. A number of guidelines and evidence-based parameters have been published (14–21).

The potential consequences of uncontrolled seizures are so severe that withdrawing AED is not practical for most patients. If withdrawal of medication is recommended, it should be completed at least 6 months before conception.

If AED therapy is needed, use monotherapy if possible, at the lowest effective dosage. Because no completely safe AED exists, choose the most effective for the epileptic syndrome or seizure type. Whenever possible, avoid valproate or phenobarbital. Optimization of AED therapy should be done before conception. If convulsive seizures are poorly controlled, pregnancy should be deferred.

Preconception planning is an essential step and should include education of the patient and the family of the risks of AED therapy, the risks of seizures and of self-cessation of therapy, and the possible effects of pregnancy on seizures. Because many pregnancies are unplanned, patients should be counseled about the interaction of oral contraceptives with AED and folic acid supplementation. The Centers for Disease Control and Prevention (CDC) recommends that all women of childbearing age take 0.4 mg of folic acid to prevent neural tube defects. For women with epilepsy, doses of 1 to 4 mg have been recommended.

Management of pregnancy in women with epilepsy requires a collaborative team effort, including an experienced neurologist and an obstetrician experienced in treating patients at high risk. With adequate monitoring, the risks of obstetric complications can be minimized. Prenatal screening for major malformations is recommended (see Chapter 145).

AED plasma concentrations should be monitored regularly throughout the pregnancy, and doses should be adjusted to maintain therapeutic levels. Lamotrigine and oxcarbazepine may require more careful monitoring.

Vitamin K needs to be properly supplemented for the last month of pregnancy. The newborn should receive vitamin K at birth.

Most infants of women with epilepsy can be breast-fed without complications. Infants exposed to phenobarbital, primidone, ethosuximide, or lamotrigine should be monitored more closely.

CLINICAL RECOMMENDATIONS OF THE VIGNETTE

It became evident that the patient had stopped the carbamazepine therapy after learning that she was pregnant. She was very concerned about the potential teratogenic effects. Although other possible mechanisms of seizure exacerbation need to be considered during pregnancy, self-cessation of medication is very common. Discontinuing medication once the pregnancy is detected is too late to prevent the occurrence of major malformations (see Chapter 146). Once this was explained to the patient and the potential risks of seizures were discussed, she was willing to resume carbamazepine therapy.

The unexpected pregnancy that the patient experienced can be explained by the interaction between carbamazepine and hormonal contraceptives. AED, such as phenytoin, carbamazepine, phenobarbital, and primidone, are potent enzyme inducers that decrease the efficacy of oral contraceptives. AED that have an intermediate, dose-dependent risk include oxcarbazepine, topiramate, and felbamate. Drugs considered safe include gabapentin, lamotrigine, levetiracetam, pregabalin, tiagabine, valproate, and zonisamide.

SUMMARY

Pregnancy presents unique challenges to the treatment of women with epilepsy. Adequate management begins with extensive preconceptional planning. Counseling about the effects of pregnancy on epilepsy and the risks of AED therapy needs to be done as early as possible. Discontinuation or optimization of AED therapy should be done before conception.

With modern medical care, most women with epilepsy will have a normal pregnancy. If seizure control is reasonable, women should not be discouraged from considering pregnancy.

Most women will require continuing AED therapy during pregnancy. The use of monotherapy at the lowest effective dose reduces the risk of major malformations. Because the information on the differential teratogenicity of the individual AED is limited, the AED that best controls the seizures should be used. As results from ongoing pregnancy registries become available, the selection of an AED may become more specific.

A team approach with a neurologist with expertise in epilepsy and an obstetrician experienced in caring for patients at high risk is ideal for optimal management of these patients. Periodic monitoring of AED levels is important in maintaining seizure control. Adequate supplementation of folic acid and vitamin K should be administered. Breast-feeding is possible in most cases without untoward effects.

REFERENCES

1. Zahn C. Neurologic care of pregnant women with epilepsy. *Epilepsia.* 1998;39[Suppl 8]: S26–S31.
2. Richmond JR, Krishnamoorthy P, Andermann E, et al. Epilepsy and pregnancy: An obstetric perspective. *Am J Obstet Gynecol.* 2004;190:371–379.

3. Yerby MS, Kaplan P, Tran T. Risks and management of pregnancy on women with epilepsy. *Cleve Clin J Med.* 2004;71[Suppl 2]:S25–S37.
4. Leonard G, Andermann E, Schopflocker C. Cognitive effects of antiepileptic drug therapy during pregnancy on school-age offspring. *Epilepsia.* 1997;38[Suppl 3]:170.
5. Minkoff H, Schaffer RM, Delke I, et al. Diagnosis of intracranial hemorrhage in utero after a maternal seizure. *Obstet Gynecol.* 1985;65[Suppl]:S22–S24.
6. Nei M, Daly S, Liporace J. A maternal complex partial seizure in labor can affect fetal heart rate. *Neurology.* 1998;51:904–906.
7. Lindhout D, Omtzigt JG, Cornell MC. Spectrum of neural-tube defects in 34 infants prenatally exposed to antiepileptic drugs. *Neurology.* 1992;42[Suppl 5]:111–118.
8. Viinikainen K, Heinonen S, Eriksson K, et al. Community-based, prospective, controlled study of obstetric and neonatal outcome of 179 pregnancies in women with epilepsy. *Epilepsia.* 2006;47:186–192.
9. EURAP Study Group. Seizure control and treatment in pregnancy: Observations from the EURAP Epilepsy Pregnancy Registry. *Neurology.* 2006;66:354–360.
10. Williams J, Myson V, Steward S, et al. Self-discontinuation of antiepileptic medication in pregnancy: Detection by hair analysis. *Epilepsia.* 2002;43:824–831.
11. Pennell PB. Antiepileptic drug pharmacokinetics during pregnancy and lactation. *Neurology.* 2003;61[Suppl 2]:S35–S42.
12. Pennell P, Montgomery J, Clements S, et al. Lamotrigine clearance markedly increases during pregnancy. *Epilepsia.* 2002;45[Suppl 7]:234–235.
13. Christensen J, Sabers A, Sidenius P. Oxcarbazepine concentrations during pregnancy: A retrospective study in patients with epilepsy. *Neurology.* 2006;67:1497–1499.
14. Commission on Genetics, Pregnancy, and the Child, International League Against Epilepsy. Guidelines for the care of epileptic women of childbearing age. *Epilepsia.* 1989;30: 409–410.
15. Commission on Genetics, Pregnancy, and the Child. International League Against Epilepsy. Guidelines for the care of epileptic women of childbearing age with epilepsy. *Epilepsia.* 1993;34:588–589.
16. Committee on Educational Bulletins of the American College of Obstetricians and Gynecologists: ACOG Educational Bulletin. Seizure disorders in pregnancy. *Int J Gynaecol Obstet.* 1997;56:279–286.
17. Quality Standard Subcommittee of the American Academy of Neurology. Practice parameter: Management issues for women with epilepsy (summary statement). *Neurology.* 1998;51: 944–948.
18. Crawford P, Appleton R, Betts T, et al. The Women with Epilepsy Guidelines Development Group: Best practice guidelines for the management of women with epilepsy. *Seizure.* 1999;8:201–217.
19. SIGN. Diagnosis and management of epilepsy in adults: A national clinical guideline recommended for use in Scotland. Available from http://www.sign.ac.uk. Edinburgh: Scottish Intercollegiate Guidelines Network. Accessed October 2005.
20. NHS. Newer drugs for epilepsy in adults. Available from http://www.nice.org.uk/pdf/TA076fullguidance.pdf. London: National Institute of Clinical Excellence, 2004. Accessed March 2004.
21. Delgado-Escueta AV, Janz D. Consensus guidelines: preconception counseling, management, and care of the pregnant woman with epilepsy. *Neurology.* 1992;42[Suppl 5]:149–160.

CHAPTER 145

Teratogenicity of Antiepileptic Drugs

Jorge J. Asconapé

OBJECTIVES

- To review the incidence of birth defects associated with the prenatal exposure to antiepileptic drugs (AED)
- To delineate the most common patterns of major malformations and minor anomalies associated with AED
- To review the potential neurocognitive deficits in children exposed to AED during pregnancy
- To discuss different strategies to minimize the risk of congenital malformations

CASE VIGNETTE

A 26-year-old woman presents with a history of complex partial and secondarily generalized tonic–clonic seizures secondary to a head injury. Initially, she was experiencing three to four complex partial seizures per month and two to three secondarily generalized tonic–clonic seizures per year. She had a poor response to carbamazepine and phenytoin. Her best results were on valproate monotherapy, and she has remained seizure free for the past 5 years on a dose of 1,000 mg twice a day. Her most recent valproate serum concentration was 93 μg/mL.

She presents sooner than expected after finding out that she is pregnant. Her last menstrual period was 6 weeks ago. She is very concerned about the potential teratogenic effects of valproate and is wondering if the medication could be stopped or replaced.

DEFINITIONS

A major congenital malformation is defined as a physical defect that is present at birth resulting in significant impairment of function and requiring major medical or surgical intervention. Dysmorphisms or minor anomalies consist of deviations from normal morphology that do not impair function or require specific treatment. The term *fetal anticonvulsant syndrome* includes combinations of the following features: minor anomalies, major malformations, intrauterine growth retardation, cognitive dysfunction, microcephaly, and infant mortality (1).

EPIDEMIOLOGY

Epilepsy is one of the most common chronic neurologic conditions, affecting 0.6% to 1% of the general population. In the United States, approximately 24,000 children are born to mothers with epilepsy every year. Because epileptic seizures are potentially dangerous, both for the mother and the fetus, most women with epilepsy need to continue therapy with AED during pregnancy. When other indications are included, such as bipolar illness or neuropathic pain, close to 45,000 children are exposed to AED in utero every year in the United States.

Use of AED during pregnancy has been associated with intrauterine growth retardation, microcephaly, major congenital malformations, dysmorphisms, postnatal developmental delay, and infant mortality.

Infants of mothers with epilepsy exposed to AED in utero have a two- to threefold risk of major malformations. Major malformation rates in the general population range from 1.6% to 3.2%, whereas the rates in infants exposed to AED in utero have been estimated at 4% to 8%. Although multiple factors, such as socioeconomic status, heredity, or maternal seizures, could contribute, it has been shown that AED are largely responsible for the increased risk (2). The offspring of epileptic women not taking AED during pregnancy or of epileptic fathers appear to have a malformation risk similar to that of the general population. Recently reported malformation rates in monotherapy exposures to AED range from 3.3% to 10.5% (Table 145-1) (3–12), whereas polytherapy rates range from 6.5% to 18.8%, essentially doubling or tripling the monotherapy risk (1,3).

Data on the differential risks for individual AED monotherapy regimens are incomplete at present and available mostly for the classic AED and lamotrigine, whereas it remains very limited for the newer AED (Table 145-2) (2,4,6–9,11–26). In general, these individual risks appear to be similar for phenytoin, carbamazepine, and lamotrigine. Valproic acid, on the other hand, has shown a consistent trend toward higher major malformation rates than other AED.

The risk of congenital malformations seems to increase with higher daily doses and peak serum concentrations of the individual AED (27). Minimizing peak concentrations through the

TABLE 145-1. Most Recent Major Malformation Rates for Antiepileptic Drug In Utero Monotherapy Exposures

Reference	*Country*	*Monotherapy Exposures (N)*	*Malformation Rate (%, 95% CI)*
Samrén et al., 1997 (4)	Germany, Finland, Netherlands Italy	709	8.0 (6.0 to 10.1)
Canger et al., 1999 (5)	Canada, Italy, Japan	313	10.5 (7.4 to 14.5)
Kaneko et al., 1999 (6)	Netherlands	500	7.8 (5.6 to 10.5)
Samrén et al., 1999 (7)	USA	899	3.3 (2.3 to 4.7)
Holmes et al., 2001 (8)	Finland	223	4.3 (2.2 to 8.1)
Kaaja et al., 2003 (9)	Australia	594	3.3 (2.3 to 8.7)
Vajda et al., 2003 (10)	Denmark	206	8.7 (5.3 to 13.5)
Sabers et al., 2004 (11)	United Kingdom	109	3.7 (1.0 to 9.1)
Morrow et al., 2005 (12)		3,609	3.7 (0.5 to 2.19)

(Modified from Tomson T, Perucca E, Battino D. Navigating toward fetal and maternal health: The challenge of treating epilepsy in pregnancy. *Epilepsia.* 2004;45:1171–1175, with permission.)

use of the lowest possible doses and extended-release formulations or three or four times daily dosing may reduce the risk.

PATHOLOGY

MAJOR MALFORMATIONS

Virtually all AED currently in use have been associated with a major malformation, and none can be considered absolutely safe. The birth defects most commonly observed with AED exposure include oral clefts (cleft lip and cleft palate), congenital heart defects (ventricular septal defect), neural tube defects (myelomeningocele and anencephaly), and urogenital defects (hypospadeas). Facial clefts account for approximately 30% of the malformations observed in these infants (28).

Most of these drugs have not been linked to any specific malformation pattern; however, some exceptions are shown in Table 145-3 (29). Valproate and carbamazepine have been associated

TABLE 145-2. Reports of Major Malformation Rates by Specific In Utero Exposures

Type of In Utero Exposure	*Percentages of Major Malformation Rates (95% Confidence Interval)*	*OR or RR (95% Confidence Interval) for Major Malformations*
No AED, general population	1.62% (2); 1.8% (8); 2.34% (13); 3.2% (14)	
No AED, women with epilepsy	0.8% (9); 1.7% (15); 3.5% (1.8% to 6.8%); (12); 3.1% (6)	OR, 0.99 (0.92 to 4.00) (16)
All AED exposures	3.1% (11); 3.8% (9); 4.5% (15); 6.0% (17); 9.0% (6)	OR, 1.86 (1.42 to 2.44) (18); RR 2.2 to 2.5 (1.2 to 5.0) (19); OR, 3.26 (2.15 to 4.93) (16)
Polytherapy	6.0% (4.8% to 8.8%) (12); 6.5% (15); 8.6% (8); 10% (17); 15% (20); 15.6% (21); 18.8% (13)	OR, 5.1 (1.0 to 21.1) (8)
Monotherapy	2.34%[a] (22); 3.7% (3.0% to 4.5%) (12); 4.2% (15); 4.5% (8); 4.7% (17); 5% (20); 6.5% (21); 7.8% (6)	OR, 2.6 (0.8 to 8.3) (8)
Phenobarbital	4.7% (8); 5.1% (6); 6.5% (2.1% to 14.5%) (2)	OR, 2.7 (0.6 to 16.4) (8); RR 4.2 (1.5 to 9.4) (2)
Phenytoin	0.7% (0.02% to 3.6%) (7); 3.4% (8); 3.7% (1.3% to 10.2%) (12); 9.1% (4.8% to 15.3%) (6)	OR, 1.9 (0.3 to 9.2) (8)
Primidone	14.3% (6)	OR, 5.3 (6)
Carbamazepine	2.2% (1.4% to 3.4%) (12); 2.3% (1.4% to 3.7%) (23); 3.0% (15); 4.9% (1.3% to 18.0%) (4); 5.2% (8); 5.28% (13); 5.7% (6)	OR, 2.21 (1.44 to 3.39) (13); RR 2.24 (1.1 to 4.56) (24); OR, 2.5 (1.0 to 6.0) (9); OR, 3.0 (0.6 to 16.0) (8); RR 4.9 (1.3 to 18.0) (4)
Valproate	5.9% (23); 6.2% (4.6% to 8.2%) (12); 6.7% (11); 10% (15); 10.7% (22); 11.1% (6); 16.0% (25)	OR, 4.1 (1.5 to 11) (9); RR, 4.9 (1.6 to 15) (4); OR, 4.0 (6); RR, 5.0 (2.9 to 8.6) (22); OR, 2.51 (1.43 to 4.68) compared with carbamazepine monotherapy (18)
Lamotrigine	2.0% (11); 2.1% (23); 3.2% (2.1% to 4.9%) (12); 2.9% (1.6% to 5.1%) (26)	

AED, antiepileptic drug; OR, odds ratio; RR, relative risk; CI confidence interval.
[a]For AED monotherapies other than valproate.
(From Pennell PB. Using current evidence in selecting antiepileptic drugs for use during pregnancy. *Epilepsy Currents.* 2005;5(2):45–51, with permission.)

TABLE 145-3. Relative Timing and Developmental Pathology of Certain Malformations

Tissues	*Malformations*	*Interval after First Day of Last Menstrual Period*
Central nervous system	Myelomeningocele	28 days
Face	Cleft lip	26 days
	Cleft palate	10 weeks
Heart	Ventricular septal defect	6 weeks

(Modified from Delgado-Escueta AV, Janz D. Consensus guidelines: Preconception counseling, management, and care of the pregnant woman with epilepsy. *Neurology*. 1992;42[Suppl 5]:149–160, with permission.)

with a specific risk for neural tube defects, primarily myelomeningocele and anencephaly. The reported incidence of neural tube defects with valproate ranges from 1% to 5.4%, compared with 0.06% in the general population (7,30,31). The risk appears especially high for the offspring of women receiving doses >1.000 mg/day or with serum concentrations >70 μg/mL (6,7,25). Carbamazepine has been associated with a 0.5% to 1% risk of spina bifida (32). Folic acid supplementation has been shown to reduce the risk of neural tube defects in women without epilepsy or in those at high risk because of a family history of dysraphism. In epileptic women treated with AED, however, studies have failed to demonstrate a protective effect of periconceptional folic acid use against neural tube defects or other major malformations (25,33). Despite these findings, women of childbearing age with epilepsy should receive a daily dose of 1 to 4 mg of folic acid routinely.

An elevated risk of nonsyndromic facial clefts with fetal exposure to lamotrigine was reported recently by the North American Antiepileptic Drug Pregnancy Registry (34). This finding, however, has not been observed in other registries, and its significance is still unclear.

DYSMORPHISMS

Dysmorphisms or minor anomalies have been reported in 10% to 15% of children exposed to AED in utero, as opposed to 4% of children in the general population. Dysmorphic features include hypertelorism, epicanthal folds, upturned nose, broad or flat nasal bridge, long philtrum, full lips, distal phalange hypoplasia, nail bed hypoplasia, and abnormal dermatoglyphics. These dysmorphic features, often associated with mental retardation, have been known in the medical literature as the *fetal AED syndrome* and have been reported with all the classic AED.

NEURODEVELOPMENTAL OUTCOME

Studies of cognitive function in children of women with epilepsy show an increased risk of mental deficiency. Cognitive deficits are observed in 1.4% to 6% of these children, compared with 1% in the general population (1). Among many possible factors, AED appear to play an important role. The risk appears to be higher with phenobarbital and valproate, and exposure during the third trimester of pregnancy appears to be the most detrimental (1).

DIAGNOSTIC APPROACH

Ultrasound at 11 to 13 weeks is used to detect neural tube defects (anencephaly) and possibly other major anomalies. Anatomic ultrasound at 18 to 22 weeks can be used to detect neural tube defects, cardiac defects, and facial clefts. A fetal echocardiogram at 18 to 22 weeks can be used to check for cardiac abnormalities. Maternal α-fetoprotein can be given at 16 weeks for neural tube defects. Perform amniocentesis if α-fetoprotein or ultrasound findings are suspicious. Ultrasound can be used every 2 to 3 weeks, starting at 28 weeks, to monitor intrauterine growth.

TREATMENT

The decision to use AED during pregnancy is based on the careful weighing of potential harmful effects of uncontrolled seizures to the mother or fetus against the risks of major malformations or neurodevelopmental deficits. Ideally, the selection of the proper AED should be done early during the woman's reproductive years and before pregnancy occurs. If medication changes are recommended as part of a prepregnancy planning, a minimum of 6 months should be allowed to assess the effects of those changes on seizure control.

Because data on the specific teratogenic effects of the individual AED are still insufficient to recommend a specific drug, the AED that best controls the seizures is generally the one to be used. The classic AED valproate, phenytoin, phenobarbital, and carbamazepine are rated by the US Food and Drug Administration (FDA) as category D (teratogenic effects have been demonstrated in animals and humans), whereas all the newer AED are rated as category C (teratogenic effects in animals, but no adequate studies have been done in humans).

Accepted treatment strategies include AED monotherapy at the lowest effective dose and folic acid supplementation. Whenever possible, valproate or AED polytherapy should be avoided.

CLINICAL RECOMMENDATIONS OF THE VIGNETTE

The patient presented with a history of frequent generalized tonic–clonic seizures, so the risks of stopping valproate clearly outweigh the benefits of stopping the drug. Given that the patient is already pregnant, changing to an alternative AED is not advisable because it would be too late to prevent the occurrence of spina bifida (the posterior neuropore closes by the end of the fourth week). Furthermore, the process of switching to an alternative AED will expose the patient to the risks of polytherapy and could result in breakthrough seizures.

For this patient, a valproate serum level of 93 μg/mL is rather high and may increase the risk of neural tube defects. Had the patient had the benefit of prepregnancy planning, a gradual reduction of the valproate dose, aiming for serum concentrations close to 50 μg/mL (low therapeutic range), and switching to an extended-release formulation would have been warranted.

SUMMARY

AED have a mild but definite teratogenic effect. Given the potential risk of epileptic seizures, their use is justified in most of women with epilepsy. There appears to be no completely safe AED. The risk is similar for most of the AED, except for valproate, which is associated with a higher risk. Information is very limited with the newer AED. Polytherapy and high serum levels increase the risk.

The incidence of neurocognitive deficits is increased in children exposed to AED during pregnancy. This risk is higher with phenobarbital and valproate. Exposure in the third trimester may carry the highest risk.

REFERENCES

1. Pennell PB. Using current evidence in selecting antiepileptic drugs for use during pregnancy. *Epilepsy Currents.* 2005;5(2):45–51.
2. Holmes LB, Wyszynski DF, Lieberman E. The AED (antiepileptic drug) pregnancy registry: A 6-year experience. *Arch Neurol.* 2004;61:673–678.
3. Tomson T, Perucca E, Battino D. Navigating toward fetal and maternal health: The challenge of treating epilepsy in pregnancy. *Epilepsia.* 2004;45:1171–1175.
4. Samren EB, van Duijn CM, Koch S. Maternal use of antiepileptic drugs and the risk of major congenital malformations: A joint European prospective study of human teratogenesis associated with maternal epilepsy. *Epilepsia.* 1997;38:981–990.
5. Canger R, Battino D, Canevini MP, et al. Malformations in the offspring of women with epilepsy: A prospective study. *Epilepsia.* 1999;40:1231–1236.
6. Kaneko S, Battino D, Andermann E. Congenital malformations due to antiepileptic drugs. *Epilepsy Res.* 1999;33:145–158.
7. Samren EB, van Duijn CM, Christiaens GC, et al. Antiepileptic drug regimens and major congenial abnormalities in the offspring. *Ann Neurol.* 1999;46:739–746.
8. Holmes LB, Harvey EA, Coull BA, et al. The teratogenicity of antiepileptic drugs. *N Engl J Med.* 2001;344:1132–1138.
9. Kaaja E, Kaaja A, Hiilesmaa V. Major malformations in the offspring of women with epilepsy. *Neurology.* 2003;60:575–579.
10. Vajda FJ, O'Brien TJ, Hitchcock A, et al. The Australian registry of anti-epileptic drugs in pregnancy: Experience after 30 months. *J Clin Neurosci.* 2003;10:543–549.
11. Sabers A, Dam M, Rogvi-Hansen B, et al. Epilepsy and pregnancy: Lamotrigine as main drug used. *Acta Neurol Scand.* 2004;109:9–13.
12. Morrow J, Russell A, Guthrie E, et al. Malformation risks of antiepileptic drugs in pregnancy: A prospective study from the UK Epilepsy and Pregnancy Register. *J Neurol Neurosurg Psychiatry.* 2005;77:193–198.
13. Matalon S, Schechtman S, Goldzweig G, et al. The teratogenic effect of carbamazepine: A meta-analysis of 1255 exposures. *Reprod Toxicol.* 2002;16:9–17.
14. Honein MA, Paulozzi LJ, Cragan JD, et al. Evaluation of selected characteristics of pregnancy drug registries. *Teratology.* 1999;60:356–364.
15. Isojarvi J, Artama M, Auvinen A. Pregnancy outcomes in women with epilepsy treated with oxcarbazepine. *Epilepsia.* 2003;44[Suppl 9]:277–278.
16. Fried S, Kozer E, Nulman I, et al. Malformation rates in children of women with untreated epilepsy: A meta-analysis. *Drug Saf.* 2004;27:197–202.
17. Tomson T, Battino D, Bonizzoni E, et al. Collaborative EURAP Study Group. EURAP: An international registry of antiepileptic drugs and pregnancy. *Epilepsia.* 2004;45:1463–1464.
18. Wide K, Winblah B, Kallen B. Major malformations in infants exposed to antiepileptic drugs in utero, with emphasis on carbamazepine and valproic acid: A nation-wide, population-based register study. *Acta Paediatr.* 2004;93:174–176.
19. Hernández-Díaz S, Werler MM, Walker AM, et al. Neural tube defects in relation to use of folic acid antagonists during pregnancy. *Am J Epidemiol.* 2001;153:961–968.
20. Dravet C, Julian C, Legras C, et al. Epilepsy, antiepileptic drugs, and malformations in children exposed to antiepileptic drugs before birth: A French prospective cohort study. *Neurology.* 1992;42[Suppl 5]:75–82.
21. Kaneko S, Otani K, Fukushima Y, et al. Teratogenicity of antiepileptic drugs: Analysis of possible risk factors. *Epilepsia.* 1988;29:459–467.
22. Holmes LB, Wyszynski DF. The AED (antiepileptic drug) pregnancy registry: A seven-year experience. *Epilepsia.* 2004;45[Suppl 7]:187.
23. Morrow J. Which antiepileptic drug is safest in pregnancy? *Epilepsia.* 2003;44[Suppl 8]:60.
24. Diav-Citrin O, Schechtman S, Arnon J, et al. Is carbamazepine teratogenic? A prospective controlled study of 210 pregnancies. *Neurology.* 2001;57:321–324.
25. Vajda FJ, O'Brien TJ, Hitchcock A, et al. Critical relationship between sodium valproate dose and human teratogenicity: Results of the Australian register of antiepileptic drugs in pregnancy. *J Clin Neurosci.* 2004;11:854–858.
26. GlaxoSmithKline. International Lamotrigine Pregnancy Registry, interim report, March 31, 2006.
27. Battino D, Binelli S, Caccamo ML, et al. Malformations in offspring of 305 epileptic women: A prospective study. *Acta Neurol Scand.* 1992;85:204–207.
28. Yerby MS, Kaplan P, Tran T. Risks and management of pregnancy in women with epilepsy. *Cleve Clin J Med.* 2004;71[Suppl 2]:S25–S37.
29. Delgado-Escueta AV, Janz D. Consensus guidelines: Preconception counseling, management, and care of the pregnant woman with epilepsy. *Neurology.* 1992;42[Suppl 5]:149–160.
30. Lindhout D, Omtzigt JG, Cornell MC. Spectrum of neural-tube defects in 34 infants prenatally exposed to antiepileptic drugs. *Neurology.* 1992;42[Suppl 5]:111–118.
31. Lindhout D, Schmidt D. In-utero exposure to valproate and neural tube defects. *Lancet.* 1986;1:1392–1393.
32. Rosa F. Spina bifida in infants of women treated with carbamazepine during pregnancy. *N Engl J Med.* 1991;324:674–677.
33. Nambisan M, Wyszynski DF, Holmes LB. No evidence of a protective effect due to periconceptional folic acid (PCFA) intake on risk for congenital anomalies in the offspring of mothers exposed to antiepileptic drugs (AEDs). *Birth Defects Research.* 2003;67:75.
34. Holmes LB, Wyszynski DF, Baldwin EJ, et al. Increased risk for non-syndromic cleft palate among infants exposed to lamotrigine during pregnancy. *Clinical and Molecular Teratology.* 2006;76:318.

CHAPTER 146

Pregnancy-Related Neuropathies

Jasvinder P.S. Chawla

OBJECTIVES

- To name the nerves affected and the peripheral nerve disorders occurring during pregnancy
- To describe the most common symptoms and associated signs with various neuropathies
- To discuss the most useful diagnostic tests to confirm various neuropathies
- To discuss the most common treatments for neuropathies in pregnancy

CASE VIGNETTE

A 28-year-old right-handed woman during her 36-week gestational period had a 3- to 4-week history of progressively worsening pain and numbness in both hands and bilateral arm pain. Symptoms were worse at right, disturbing her sleep. Symptoms were also made worse with repetitive activities such as working on her computer and doing household activities with her hands, as well as lifting her other child, who is 1 year of age. Symptoms were most pronounced on the thumb, index, and middle fingers.

On examination, she had a positive Tinel's sign and a positive Phalen's maneuver. No associated atrophy or weakness of median innervated muscles was noted. Muscle stretch reflexes were symmetric and sensory examination findings were normal.

DEFINITION

Neuropathies associated with pregnancy, delivery, and the puerperium period are considered pregnancy-related neuropathies. Neuropathies can be caused by various factors, broadly divided into acquired and familial (1). Several physiologic as well as pathologic conditions predispose to the development of these neuropathies. Incidence can vary, depending on the existence of prepregnancy neuropathic conditions.

EPIDEMIOLOGY

Acquired peripheral nerve disorders are further classified into traumatic, inflammatory, toxic, metabolic, and those associated with systemic diseases (1). Socioeconomic factors, including quality of prenatal care, as well as comorbidity also play a significant role. Nerve damage can be localized to a single nerve (mononeuropathies), such as nerve involvement in carpal tunnel syndrome (CTS), or in the case of meralgia paresthetical, with isolated involvement of the lateral femoral cutaneous nerve. Multiple nerves can be involved symmetrically and, at the same time and in an acute fashion such as in Gullain-Barré syndrome, or involvement may take place in a more chronic fashion, such as in cases of chronic inflammatory demyelinating polyneuropathy. Multiple nerves can be involved asymmetrically, as in mononeuropathy multiplex associated with systemic lupus erythematosus (SLE), other connective tissue disorders, certain diabetic neuropathies, leprosy, and in some paraneoplastic neuromuscular syndromes (1).

ETIOLOGY AND PATHOGENESIS

As discussed, multiple causes have been proposed, but no obvious one is found in approximately one fifth of patients (2). Trauma to the nerves can be mild, moderate, or severe. Degree of recovery depends on degree of initial nerve damage. Mild damage can be clinically unrecognized at the time of initial insult. Repetitive mild trauma, such as a pudendal nerve lesion resulting from repeated mild traumatic compression during multiple pregnancies, ultimately may become manifest clinically (3).

With partial lesions, a full functional recovery in a shorter time is usually the case. More than 50% of fiber loss or complete lesions, however, cause, immediate functional loss and long, drawn-out recovery. Different focal mononeuropathies result from different delivery techniques, especially forceps delivery. Compression is the most common underlying cause, which can be complicated by prolonged or obstructed labor. Cesarean section has a small incidence of associated nerve injuries (4).

PATHOLOGY

Pathology depends whether nerve involvement is traumatic or nontraumatic. Traumatic nerve injuries can be characterized by neurapraxia (mild), axonotmesis (moderate), or neurotmesis (severe). *Neurapraxia* refers to nerve injury without any loss of anatomic continuity of either nerve or axons and carries an excellent prognosis. Neurapraxia is recognized electrophysiologically by the presence of a conduction block across the lesion. Neurapraxia is clinically manifested by weakness. Repeated trauma or prolonged nerve compression can result in axonal damage. Nerve trauma with distal axonal degeneration, which can cause damage to the axons, is called *axonotmesis* (5). This type of lesion requires regeneration of axons from the lesion site to the target before full recovery can be expected. N*eurotmesis* involves the entire nerve, including its sheaths and usually carries a poor prognosis for full recovery (5).

Nontraumatic nerve lesions can be predominantly *axonal* or *demyelinating,* and further classified as acute, chronic, or relapsing-remitting (6). Most inflammatory-related neuropathies are demyelinating. Most toxic neuropathies are axonal.

Clinically, neuropathies are further classified into large and small fiber neuropathies. The A fiber group represents myelinated somatic fibers, further subdivided into α, β, γ, and δ, from largest to smallest, respectively. The B fiber group represents preganglionic autonomic fibers. The C fibers are unmyelinated. A δ fiber, together with unmyelinated fibers, represents a small fiber group. This distinction is clinically very important because most painful neuropathies and the autonomic neuropathies present as small-fiber dysfunction (7).

CLINICAL MANIFESTATIONS

NEUROPATHIES INVOLVING THE FACE

Idiopathic Peripheral Facial Nerve Palsy: Bell's Palsy

The incidence of the idiopathic form of peripheral facial palsy (Bell's palsy) in pregnancy has varied in different studies. In the Copenhagen Facial Nerve Study of 2,500 patients that included 46 pregnant patients, peripheral facial nerve palsy was 19 times less commonly seen in pregnant patients compared with the general population of women with facial palsy. It usually occurs during the third trimester of pregnancy, or in the postpartum period. Clinically, it appears as an acute onset of asymmetric lower motor neuron type of facial palsy with an inability to close an eye. Most cases have a good prognosis, because it involves a demyelinating type injury. Recovery may be prolonged and incomplete in cases with axonal damage (8,9).

NEUROPATHIES INVOLVING THE UPPER EXTREMITY, BRACHIAL PLEXUS AND INTERCOSTAL NERVES

Carpal Tunnel Syndrome

The most frequent neuropathy during pregnancy is CTS. It is reported in up to 50% of pregnancies (10). CTS typically presents during the third trimester, with numbness, tingling, and pins and needles of the thumb, index, and middle fingers. Patients often shake their hands in an attempt to alleviate symptoms, which are usually worse during the night or morning hours and frequently awaken the patients. Symptoms are often bilateral, although rarely symmetric. In approximately 10% of patients with hand symptoms, the distribution of paresthesias develops primarily in the ulnar nerve, and rarely the entire hand (11).

CTS can also appear for the first time during the puerperium, and is usually seen in primiparae who are breast-feeding. It also appears in older primiparae, but no clear explanations exist for the cause, because edema is not a feature in these women as it is in women with CTS during pregnancy. Combinations of hormonal changes with local swelling and possible exacerbation of compression by handling of infants, as well as certain repetitive activities of daily living are most likely causes (10–13). CTS can be confirmed by electrophysiologic testing, which should include transcarpal nerve conduction study.

Brachial Plexopathy: Parsonage-Turner Syndrome

Brachial plexopathy or Parsonage-Turner syndrome is most commonly idiopathic and typically associated with severe arm pain. It is associated with atrophy of proximal shoulder muscles and slow recovery (14). The recurrent kind of brachial plexopathy is often the result of a hereditary form of tomaculous neuropathy, and recurs frequently during pregnancy (15,16).

Intercostal Neuralgia

Multiple causes for neuropathic thoracic pain during pregnancy have been reported, including problems at the level of the nerve roots, nerve trunk, and even at the spinal cord level. Patients may develop symptoms resembling thoracic radiculopathy or intercostal neuropathy. Electromyograph (EMG) study may slow resting denervation activity with fibrillation potentials or positive waves in thoracic paraspinal muscles. Compression on the nerve roots or the intercostal nerves during pregnancy is the proposed mechanism. A major differential diagnosis remains with intraabdominal pathology, which needs to be excluded in these patients (17).

NEUROPATHIES INVOLVING THE LOWER EXTREMITY AND LUMBOSACRAL PLEXUS

Lateral Femoral Cutaneous Neuropathy: Meralgia Paresthetica

Meralgia paresthetica is a pure sensory neuropathy localized to the upper and middle lateral aspect of the thigh. Patients complain of burning thigh pain and unpleasant sensations of pins and needles. It is believed to be the result of compression of the lateral femoral cutaneous nerves under the lateral part of the inguinal ligament. Clinical diagnosis is usually straightforward, but electrophysiologic studies can be used for diagnosis confirmation. Swelling during pregnancy and major change in the patient's weight has been postulated as a cause of compression (18,19).

Obturator Nerve Lesions

The obturator nerve runs under the psoas muscle, with the anterior motor branch supplying the obturator, pectineus, adductor longus, brevis, and gracilis muscles. The sensory branch innervates the upper medial thigh. The fetal head along the lateral pelvic wall may compress the obturator nerve before entering the obturator canal. The lesion is often incomplete, and functional recovery is typically good. Severe obturator nerve lesions can result in a chronic upper medial thigh pain (20,21).

Femoral Nerve Lesions

The femoral nerve passes through the psoas muscle and then exits the thigh under the inguinal ligament. It innervates the quadriceps femoris and sartorius muscles and, to some extent, the iliopsoas. It provides sensory distribution to the anterior and medial thigh as well as to the medial calf via the terminal saphenous branch. Femoral neuropathy can be unilateral or bilateral. It is associated with numbness involving the anterior thigh as well as weakness of hip flexion and knee extension. Prolonged labor, cephalopelvic disproportion, and the lithotomy position can cause femoral neuropathy (22).

Peroneal Nerve Lesions

Peroneal neuropathy most commonly occurs during the postpartum period. Although it usually occurs from pelvic compression, lesions at the knee level can also occur if improper position of legs and leg holders during delivery takes place, or excessive hand pressure over the lateral knee and fibular head by the patient during the later stages of delivery. Foot drop can also result from compression of the lumbosacral trunk when the peroneal nerve fibers are predominantly involved (23). The foot drop can be unilateral or bilateral, and sensory loss may involve the dorsum of the foot and lateral aspect of the leg (24).

Lumbosacral Plexus Lesions

The lumbosacral plexus is formed from the L4-S2 roots. A postpartum foot drop may be the presenting clinical manifestation. This is commonly accompanied by a deficit in the distribution of the peroneal nerve. Sensory and motor deficit could also occur in the distribution of any other nerve involved (single or multiple nerves distribution). Short built primigravidas are at risk, especially if the baby is large. Forceps delivery is another risk, as are a narrow pelvis and occipitoposterior rotation. Nerve conduction studies can assess the extent and amount of axonal damage (23).

Pudendal Nerve Lesions

The pudendal plexus is formed from the S2-S4 nerve roots. It exits the pelvis through the infrapiriform foramen. It provides sensation to the perineal skin, labia majora, and clitoris, and motor supply to the levator ani, coccygeus, external anal and urethral sphincters, transversal perineal muscles, and superficial pelvic floor-bulbocavernosus muscle. Compression from prolonged fetal head pressure can cause tissue necrosis and result in nerve damage. Large episiotomies can result in local nerve damage with sensory loss as well as possible anal sphincter disturbances. These disorders are more common in women with multiple pregnancies. Symptoms do not appear immediately postpartum, and can develop years later as a result of repeated pudendal plexus trauma (3).

GENERALIZED NEUROPATHIES

Metabolic Neuropathies

Metabolic neuropathies during pregnancy include diabetic neuropathies as well as those caused by certain vitamin deficiencies. Diabetic neuropathy in pregnancy is seen in cases of juvenile-onset diabetes mellitus. It can involve small fibers, large fibers, or a combination of these. Large fiber involvement can cause combined axonal and demyelinating neuropathies. It can be asymptomatic with mild fiber loss, but can be very painful in cases with predominant small-fiber involvement. Pregnancy can also accelerate neuropathy in the short term, but it does not lead to long-term diabetic complications (25). The most dangerous form is diabetic autonomic neuropathy, which can lead to blood pressure fluctuations. Intractable vomiting with gastroparesis may be a contraindication for continuing pregnancy in view of the risk to both mother and fetus (26). Malnutrition and porphyria, especially the acute intermittent form, may appear for the first time during pregnancy (27). With better prenatal care and easy access to vitamins, these disorders now rarely occur during pregnancy. Neuropathy resulting from deficiency of vitamins B_{12} and folate is predominantly an axonal neuropathy and can easily be prevented with vitamin supplements.

Acute Inflammatory Demyelinating Neuropathy: Guillain-Barré Syndrome

Guillain-Barré syndrome (GBS) is an acute autoimmune disorder, with rapidly ascending weakness. It usually does not interfere with pregnancy because it does not involve smooth uterine muscles. Rarely, more severe forms require ventilatory assistance, which can interfere with pregnancy. Overall, risk of GBS is lower during pregnancy, but recent evidence points toward a higher incidence in puerperium (28). Diagnosis is made on the basis of a characteristic cerebrospinal fluid (CSF) albuminocytologic dissociation as well as early absence of F-waves in nerve conduction studies with focal slowing of nerve conduction velocities seen diffusely.

Chronic Inflammatory Demyelinating Polyneuropathy

Chronic inflammatory demyelinating polyneuropathy (CIDP) is another autoimmune peripheral nerve disorder characterized by diffuse asymmetric weakness. In patients diagnosed with CIDP, McCombe et al. (29) reported a significant increase in the number of relapses during the year of pregnancy and a propensity for symptoms to worsen during the third trimester or immediate postpartum period. The slightly higher incidence in pregnancy was suggested from alteration in the immune system during pregnancy (29).

Multifocal Motor Neuropathy

Chaudhary et al. (30) reported three women with multifocal motor neuropathy (MMN) who became weaker during pregnancy and regained their prepregnancy strength after delivery. Thus, pregnancy may worsen underlying MMN (30). Nerve conduction studies revealed involvement of motor nerves with conduction block.

DIAGNOSTIC APPROACH

A detailed history and physical examination are key to proper diagnosis. In addition to clinical evaluation, the diagnosis of neuropathy may require extensive metabolic testing, neurophysiologic tests, and, in some cases, nerve biopsy.

Nerve conduction studies (NCS) and EMG are usually adequate to document the extent and type of lesion (e.g., axonal versus demyelinating) (6). NCS and EMG are also indicated to determine prognosis. It usually takes 2 to 3 weeks for full denervation to develop, depending on the distance of the muscle from the nerve involved. NCS and EMG predominantly evaluate large fiber functions. Tests, such as quantitative sensory testing (QST) or quantitative sudomotor axon reflex test (QSART), are required to assess small fiber function (31). Other specific tests are outlined under the topics mentioned above. Occasionally, the diagnosis can be confirmed only by nerve biopsy, which is usually not considered during pregnancy.

TREATMENT

Management of nontraumatic neuropathies primarily involves removing the offending agent(s) and treating the underlying metabolic or inflammatory abnormality. No specific medications are used to treat neuropathy, and vitamins are useful only if the neuropathy is caused by a specific vitamin deficiency. Treatment of traumatic neuropathies depends on cause and severity of nerve damage. In pregnancy, because the inciting cause is generally short term, usually resulting from compression and swelling, most causes are managed conservatively. Most neuropathies during delivery are almost always incomplete and, therefore, have a good prognosis without surgical intervention. Specific treatment for various neuropathies is discussed below.

NEUROPATHIES INVOLVING THE FACE

Treatment of Bell's palsy is usually symptomatic and protection of cornea. Copenhagen Facial Nerve Study revealed that no treatment, including prednisone, was able to give a better prognosis (8,9).

NEUROPATHIES INVOLVING THE UPPER EXTREMITY, BRACHIAL PLEXUS AND INTERCOSTAL NERVES

CTS in pregnancy is usually reversible within 2 weeks after delivery (11). Conservative treatment for CTS in pregnancy includes wrist splints, physical therapy, and low-salt diet. Conservative management with neutral wrist splints, worn every night, is the most effective treatment as has been shown with improvement seen in sensory and motor nerve conduction studies (12,13). Steroid injections were ineffective based on clinical as well as electrophysiologic findings (13). Medications should be avoided during pregnancy and if the symptoms are persistent after puerperium and do not respond to conservative treatment, surgery might be indicated (4,10,32).

Brachial plexopathy or Parsonage-Turner syndrome is managed mainly with physical therapy (14,15). As in neuralgic amyotrophy, corticosteroid treatment may diminish pain in patients with brachial plexopathy (16). Patients with intercostal neuralgia have a good prognosis with frequent relief of symptoms after delivery. Topical lidocaine patches for thoracic neuralgia can be tried as used in patients with postherpetic neuralgia (17).

NEUROPATHIES INVOLVING THE LOWER EXTREMITY AND LUMBOSACRAL PLEXUS

Patients with meralgia paresthetica require supportive management during pregnancy. They should be counseled for weight reduction and avoidance of local trauma, such as wearing tight underwear. In intractable cases with persistent neuropathic symptoms during pregnancy, local application of lidoderm patches (pregnancy category B), low-dose amitriptyline (pregnancy category C), or local anesthetic injection at the level of the inguinal ligament can be tried. Anticonvulsants as pain prophylaxis are usually pregnancy category C or D and, thus, are relatively contraindicated (18,19).

Chronic pain from obturator neuropathy is usually eased by an obturator nerve block, which is sometimes indicated for both diagnosis and treatment (20). Complications of pudendal nerve block include a compressing hematoma at the area of the obturator foramen (21).

Most cases of femoral neuropathy have a good prognosis and require no specific therapy. Even complete femoral nerve compressions have excellent prognosis (22).

If a lumbosacral plexus compression is expected, then cesarean section is the delivery method of choice because the lesion is very proximal with incomplete recovery. Severe axonal lesions carry a poor prognosis with minimal chance of complete recovery. Physical therapy and ankle foot orthosis may be required in some patients (23).

GENERALIZED NEUROPATHIES

Patients with GBS often have a fair prognosis with almost complete recovery in a few weeks. Because an early aggressive treatment must be instituted, early diagnosis is extremely important, as mentioned earlier. GBS in pregnancy is treated no differently than in any other clinical situation, including early and, if necessary, repeated plasmapheresis, repeated administration of intravenous immune gamma globulin (IVIgG), or both (29). Patients with CIDP may require plasmapheresis or IVIgG during acute exacerbation of patient's symptoms. Patients with MMN have also been successfully treated with IVIgG during pregnancy (30). Plasmapheresis and IVIgG are by and large safe therapies in pregnancy and have been used in the abovementioned conditions (33).

Pregnancy does not exacerbate underlying diabetic neuropathy. Strict blood glucose control remains the treatment of choice. Some patients may require symptomatic treatment with pain prophylactic medications, such as low-dose tricyclic antidepressants. Autonomic function should be assessed in pregnant women with diabetes because of the potential complications. Acute intermittent porphyria has been treated initially with concentrated glucose solution. If the symptoms remain persistent for 2 to 4 days, however, hematin is next in line (27). Similarly, hypothyroid neuropathy can occur during pregnancy; however, it is usually mild and does not require any special treatment other than control of thyroid functions.

CLINICAL RECOMMENDATIONS OF THE VIGNETTE

The patient was advised to have a wrist splint at a neutral position worn most of the times while awake and during sleep. While counseling the patient, she was also given reassurance that the problem would most likely resolve after delivery. If this regimen failed, however, then other treatment options were also discussed as a back-up plan. Other treatment options included referral for surgical decompression. The role of steroid injections (controversial) was also discussed with the patient.

Patient was advised to have a follow-up visit to the clinic after the delivery of her child. The patient returned to the clinic 4 weeks after she delivered her child with almost complete resolution of her symptoms. No further testing was done and patient, thus, was advised to continue to use her hand splint for another 2 to 4 weeks till she achieves complete recovery. No further follow-ups were to be made unless any new symptoms or the present symptoms worsen.

SUMMARY

Peripheral neuropathies are among the most common neuromuscular complications during pregnancy. The signs and symptoms of the common peripheral nerve disorders, as well as generalized neuropathies, should be recognized. Measures must be taken to allow for the best possible recovery. Periodic follow-up examinations on all patients during pregnancy, delivery, and puerperium who develop signs and symptoms suggestive of neuropathy are advisable. Because compressive neuropathies have a higher incidence during pregnancy, proper counseling and reassurance need to be provided. Although physiologic, rather than pathologic, causes would be more commonly expected, health care professionals should stay vigilant for any possible pathologic or disabling peripheral nerve disorders during this time period and consider treatment if warranted.

REFERENCES

1. Brown WF, Bolton CF, Aminoff MJ. *Neuromuscular Function and Disease*, 1st ed. Philadelphia: WB Saunders; 2002.
2. Mabie WC. Peripheral neuropathies during pregnancy. *Clin Obstet Gynaecol*, 2005;48:57-66.
3. Snooks SJ, Swash M, Mathers SE, et al. Effect of vaginal delivery on the pelvic floor: A 5-year follow-up. *Br J Surg.* 1990;77:1358–1360.
4. Graham JG. Neurological complications of pregnancy and anaesthesia. *Clin Obstet Gynaecol.* 1982;9:333–350.
5. Seddon JH. Three types of nerve injury. *Brain.* 1943;66:237–288.
6. Kimura J. *Electrodiagnosis in Diseases of Nerve and Muscle: Principles and Practice*, 3rd ed. New York: Oxford University Press; 2001.
7. Low PA, Vernino S, Suarez G. Autonomic dysfunction in peripheral nerve disease. *Muscle Nerve.* 2003;27:646–661.
8. Peitersen E. Bell's palsy: The spontaneous course of 2,500 peripheral facial nerve palsies of different etiologies. *Acta Otolaryngol Suppl.* 2002;(549):4–30. Review.
9. Gilden DH. Bell's palsy. *N Engl J Med.* 2004;351:1323–1331.
10. Stolp-Smith KA, Pascoe MK, Ogburn PL, Jr. Carpal tunnel syndrome in pregnancy: Frequency, severity, and prognosis. *Arch Phys Med Rehabil.* 1998;79:1285–1287.
11. Padua L, Aprile I, Caliandro P, et al. Carpal tunnel syndrome in pregnancy. Multiperspective follow-up of untreated cases. *Neurology.* 2002;59:1643–1646.
12. Turgut F, Cetinsahinahin M, Turgut M, et al. The management of carpal tunnel syndrome in pregnancy. *J Clin Neurosci.* 2001;8:332–334.
13. Sevin S, Dogu O, Camdeviren H, et al. Long-term effectiveness of steroid injections and splinting in mild and moderate carpal tunnel syndrome. *Neurol Sci.* 2004;25(2):48–52.
14. Parsonage MJ, Turner JWA. Neuralgic amytotrophy: The shoulder-girdle syndrome. *Lancet.* 1948;1:973–978.
15. Geiger LR, Mancall EL, Penn AS. Familial neuralgia amyotrophy. Report of three families with review of the literature. *Brain.* 1974;97:87–102.
16. Klein CJ, Dyck PJB, Friedenberg SM, et al. Inflammation and neuropathic attacks in hereditary brachial plexus neuropathy. *J Neurol Neurosurg Psychiatry.* 2002;73:45–50.
17. Skeen MB, Eggleston M. Thoraconeuralgia gravidarum. *Muscle Nerve.* 1999;22:779–780.
18. Wiezer MJ, Franssen H, Rinkel GJ, et al. Meralgia paraesthetica: Differential diagnosis and follow up. *Muscle Nerve.* 1996;19:522–524.
19. Devers A, Galer BS. Topical lidocaine patch relieves a variety of neuropathic pain conditions: An open-label study. *Clin J Pain.* 2000;16:205–208.
20. Hopf HC. Obturator nerve paralysis during parturition. *J Neurol.* 1974;207:165–166.
21. Wong CA, Scavone BM, Dugan S, et al. Incidence of postpartum lumbosacral spine and lower extremity nerve injuries. *Obstet Gynecol.* 2003;101:279–282.
22. al Hakim M, Katirji B. Femoral mononeuropathy induced by the lithotomy position: A report of 5 cases with a review of literature. *Muscle Nerve.* 1993;16:891–895.
23. Feasby TE, Burton SR, Hahn AF. Obstetrical lumbosacral plexus injury. *Muscle Nerve.* 1992;15(8):937–940.
24. Colahis SC, 3rd, Pease WS, Johnson EW. A preventable cause of foot drop during childbirth. *Am J Obstet Gynecol.* 1994;171:270–272.
25. Hemachandra A, Ellios D, Lloyd CE, et al. The influence of pregnancy on IDDM complications. *Diabetes Care.* 1995;18:950–954.
26. Macleod AF, Smith SA, Snoksen PH, et al. The problem of autonomic neuropathy in diabetic pregnancy. *Diabet Med.* 1990;7:80–82.
27. Isenschmid M, Konig C, Fassli C, et al. Acute intermittent porphyria in pregnancy: Glucose or hematin therapy? *Schweiz Med Wochenschr.* 1992;122(46):1711–1715.
28. Jiang GX, de Pedro-Cuesta J, Strigard K, et al. Pregnancy and Guillain-Barré syndrome: A nationwide register cohort study. *Neuroepidemiology.* 1996;15:192–200.
29. McCombe PA, MaManis PG, Frith JA et al. Chronic inflammatory demyelinating polyradiculoneuropathy associated with pregnancy. *Ann Neurol.* 1987;21:102–104.
30. Chaudhry V, Escolar DM, Cornblath DR. Worsening of multifocal motor neuropathy during pregnancy. *Neurology.* 2002;59(1):139–141.
31. Low PA. Laboratory evaluation of autonomic failure. In: Low PA, ed. *Clinical Autonomic Disorders: Evaluation and Management.* Rochester, NY: Little, Brown and Company; 1993.
32. Stahl S, Blumenfeld Z, Yarnitsky D. Carpal tunnel syndrome in pregnancy: Indications for early surgery. *J Neurol Sci.* 1996;136:182–184.
33. Yamada H, Noro N, Kato EH, et al. Massive intravenous immunoglobulin treatment in pregnancy complicated by Guillain-Barré syndrome. *Eur J Obstet Gynecol Reprod Biol.* 2001;97:101–104.

CHAPTER 147

Movement Disorders in Pregnancy

Federico E. Micheli

Physiological changes occurring during pregnancy and puerperium cam adversely affect the central nervous system (CNS), complicate the management of preexisting neurologic conditions, induce the development of new disorders, or even trigger preexisting, but asymptomatic, movement disorders.

This chapter focuses on movement disorders typically occurring during pregnancy, such as chorea gravidarum (CG), and those occurring or often exacerbated during pregnancy, such as the restless legs syndrome (RLS). Other movement disorders presenting during pregnancy or puerperium are beyond the scope of this review.

OBJECTIVES

- To describe the most common movement disorders in pregnancy
- To explain how to detect (diagnose) the underlying cause of the movement disorder
- To describe the pathophysiology of each movement disorder
- To explore the therapeutic strategies for this conditions

CASE VIGNETTE

A 29-year-old, gravida 1, para 0, at 7 weeks' gestation, had a rapid and progressive onset of facial grimacing and writhing movements of the right side of her body. At age 13, she had an episode (lasting 2 months) of involuntary movements, involving mainly the left side of her body. She also had a history of recurrent episodes of sore throat as a youngster. No family history of neurologic disorders was uncovered. On examination, random movements were mainly choreic, but some ticlike movements and myoclonic jerking were also evident to involve facial and limb muscles, mainly on the right side. The movements abated during sleep, improved when relaxed, and worsened when stressed. Mild limb hypotonia was also evident.

Ancillary investigations for autoimmune disorders (systemic lupus erythematosus [SLE]), Wilson disease, Hashimoto thyroiditis, and neuroacanthocytosis were negative. Two-dimensional echocardiography was normal.

DEFINITION

Movement disorders encompass a wide array of disorders of muscle tone and involuntary movements of a diverse nature and etiology. Whereas physicians are familiar with the most common expression of these disorders (i.e., tremor), unusual presentations or a perceived "peculiar" phenomenology can be overlooked or even misdiagnosed as psychogenic. Some of these movements occur almost in isolation (essential tremor, primary dystonia). Others, present as a manifestation of a progressive neurodegenerative disorder (Huntington's disease), or secondary to an acute and potentially life-threatening neurologic event (brain hemorrhage). Conversely, others may only account for some *cosmetic* inconveniences. Some of these movement disorders are transient; others, however, are persistent, permanent, or even progressive.

Pregnancy may unmask a preexisting potential for CG, or induce or exacerbate RLS, but generally, pregnancy has a limited effect on most other movement disorders (1).

CHOREA GRAVIDARUM

CG refers to chorea occurring during pregnancy. Recognized causes of chorea with onset at this time of life, include hereditary, immune, and vascular factors, and drugs, among others.

That CG is less commonly reported than previously is probably a reflection of a lower incidence of rheumatic fever (Sydenham chorea) caused by the widespread use of antibiotics.

CG is characterized by the presence of choreic movements, involving mainly one half of the body (hemichorea), during pregnancy.

RESTLESS LEGS SYNDROME

Diagnostic criteria for RLS include the following: (*a*) desire to move the limbs usually associated with paresthesias or dysesthesias; (*b*) motor restlessness; (*c*) worsening of symptoms at rest with at least partial and temporary relief by activity; and (*d*) worsening of symptoms in the evening or at night (2,3).

EPIDEMIOLOGY

Movement disorders are uncommon among women of childbearing age. As a consequence, epidemiologic data, and management guidelines are very limited (4). The two most commonly observed movement disorders in pregnancy are RLS and CG (4). Chronic conditions affecting young people, such as essential tremor (ET) and, occasionally, Huntington disease (HD) and Parkinson disease (PD), can also be seen in pregnancy.

CHOREA GRAVIDARUM

Choreiform and athetoid movements presenting during pregnancy are rare. CG, the term used for chorea of any cause occurring during pregnancy, was first described as early as in 1661 in the works of Hortius (5). Scarce information is available on the epidemiology of CG in modern literature, and even the initial descriptions report small case series, showing that this has always been an uncommon disorder. Recently, Cardoso from Brazil reported that in his center, where a large number of patients with Sydenham chorea are seen, CG accounts for 3.6% of all the cases (6).

RESTLESS LEGS SYNDROME

A relatively common, but frequently unrecognized disorder, RLS has a prevalence ranging from 2.5% to 15% of the general population, increasing with age and with a female preponderance (7–9) and is certainly the most frequent movement disorder in pregnancy. Pregnancy is considered a risk factor for the development or worsening of RLS; prevalence increases up to 26% among pregnant women. Women are usually affected by a benign self-limited form known as *transient RLS* during pregnancy. The disease seems to be strongly related to the third trimester of pregnancy, and tends to disappear near the time of delivery. Affected women present lower values of hemoglobin and mean corpuscular volume when compared with healthy controls (10,11). Women affected by preexisting RLS often complain of worsening of symptoms during pregnancy, with the highest degree of severity also peaking in the third trimester (11).

ETIOLOGY AND PATHOGENESIS

CHOREA GRAVIDARUM

CG is composed of a heterogeneous group of disorders. Etiologic factors include rheumatic fever, chorea minor, hormonal, psychic, and autoimmune disorders as well as cerebrovascular diseases, among others. A recent review of the literature on chorea gravidarum suggests that SLE may be a more common cause than previously reported (12). Regarding poststreptococcal CNS syndromes, pathologic data are limited to a few postmortem studies. Because of their life-threatening nature, they possibly represent the most severe end of the spectrum and may not be representative of the average pathologic findings. The immunopathogenesis of poststreptococcal CNS syndromes is not fully understood. It is hypothesized that group A streptococcal infection induces an immune response that cross-reacts with the brain. No evidence, however, suggests that streptococcal organisms directly enter the brain. Recent experiments have shown that activated lymphocytes or antibodies are capable of entering the CNS without disrupting the blood–brain barrier (13). If lymphocytes recognize antigens in the CNS, immune activation can occur with consequent neural dysfunction or damage.

RESTLESS LEGS SYNDROME

RLS is generally idiopathic, with a familial component in 40% to 60% of the cases and may be inherited with an autosomic-dominant transmission. It may also be a symptom of associated conditions (secondary forms), such as peripheral neuropathies, uremia, iron deficiency (with or without anemia), diabetes, PD, and pregnancy. Based on the presence of associated conditions, such as iron deficiency, uremia, peripheral neuropathy, and pregnancy, RLS could be classified as idiopathic or symptomatic.

It is unknown what causes the association between RLS and pregnancy. Several hypotheses have been put forward, including iron and folate deficiency; hormonal influences related to the increase of prolactin, progesterone, and estrogens during late pregnancy; and the changing motor habits and psychological state of pregnant women. The importance of folate and iron supplementation during pregnancy in the prevention of RLS, however, is still unclear. Although RLS is clinically well characterized, the underlying pathology has not been elucidated; however, several indicators suggest that the dopaminergic system, particularly the central nigrostriatal system, may play a role (14–16).

Response to dopaminergic drugs and the aggravation of symptoms under dopamine antagonists or antipsychotic agents indicate that dopamine receptors play a role.

Although much progress has been made in diagnosis and treatment in the last decade, more is needed to fully describe the etiology and pathophysiology of RLS (17).

CLINICAL MANIFESTATIONS AND SPECIAL SITUATIONS

CHOREA GRAVIDARUM

CG features involuntary movements, lack of coordination, slurred speech, and psychic disorders. The neurologic state is normal, except for a loss of muscle tone. CG begins after the first trimester in half of the patients, spontaneously abates in approximately one third before delivery, and in most cases resolves spontaneously after 2 to 3 months. The severity of the chorea typically decreases as the pregnancy progresses. Approximately one of five women experience CG recurrence with subsequent pregnancies (18) and, in some cases, psychoses is also likely to occur. Usually, CG is not a life-threatening disorder, although in some cases it may represent an emergency situation in pregnancy (19). Mortality has declined and lies below 1%; nevertheless, when severe, CG can cause hyperthermia, rhabdomyolysis, myoglobinuria, and, eventually, death.

RESTLESS LEGS SYNDROME

RLS is a sensory-motor disorder characterized by discomfort and an urge to move the legs, primarily during rest or inactivity, with partial or total relief with movement and worsening in the evening. RLS in pregnant women is frequently misdiagnosed; pregnant women are often worried about the symptoms, but doctors do not usually provide good explanations (11).

RLS is often associated with nocturnal periodic limb movements featuring stereotyped repetitive movements most often described as an extension of the big toe with a flexion of the leg at the ankle, knee, and hip (20).

DIAGNOSTIC APPROACH

CHOREA GRAVIDARUM

Previously, rheumatic disease was generally the cause of CG, but today, collagen vascular disease should also be considered (21,22). Certain disorders, such as transient ischemic attacks (TIA) and CG, appear to be related to antiphospholipid (aPLA). It is important to recognize pregnant women with aPLA so they can be appropriately treated to avoid fetal loss and thromboembolic events (23). Three of 50 (6%) patients with chorea and the aPLA syndrome have been reported to develop chorea gravidarum (24).

RESTLESS LEGS SYNDROME

Sleep disturbances are so frequent in pregnancy that RLS is easily overlooked as a cause of significant morbidity. Some sleep disorders often manifest for the first time in pregnancy, but this can be taken as normal. The diagnosis is clinical, but polysomnography is useful to determine its impact on sleep (difficulties in sleep onset, maintaining sleep during the night, and sleep fragmentation) and to confirm periodic leg movements during sleep and waking hours. RLS is generally idiopathic, but laboratory and neurophysiologic studies to rule out secondary cases, such as those caused by peripheral neuropathies, uremia, iron deficiency (with or without anemia), and diabetes, are required.

TREATMENT

CHOREA GRAVIDARUM

When symptoms are mild or well tolerated, pharmacologic treatment is not necessary because CG is usually a self-limited condition and movements tend to abate as pregnancy progresses. Drug treatment is recommended for those patients in whom symptoms are so severe to adversely affect either their health or the fetus if they remain untreated. Treatment includes neuroleptic agents (category C) for symptomatic relief (25) and therapies targeted toward the underlying pathology.

No prospective studies in pregnant women have been carried out and the decision to treat is based on case reports, case series, and retrospective studies(26). Oral contraceptives are not recommended because they can trigger episodes of severe chorea (27,28). Cases of recurrent chorea induced by a topical vaginal cream that contained conjugated estrogens have also been reported (29).

RESTLESS LEGS SYNDROME

In some cases of secondary RLS, an etiologic treatment can be instituted. When it is associated with iron deficiency anemia, replacement is advocated (30). Earley (31) recommends 325 mg ferrous sulfate with 100 mg vitamin C (to enhance absorption) three times daily. Iron deficiency is defined as ferritin levels 18 μg/L or iron saturation <16%. Supplementation should be continued until ferritin levels are at or above 50 μg/L and the iron saturation >20%. Supplementation with folate, based on studies that find lower folate levels in pregnant patients who have RLS, has also been proposed, but this association needs further study. Currently in the United States, many pregnant women are already taking folate to prevent neural tube defects and, by law, all cereal products sold (after 1998) are fortified with folate. In most cases, no cause other than pregnancy can be found and treatment remains symptomatic. In this case, treatment options include dopamine agonists and levodopa (category D); opiates (propoxyphene [category D], oxycodone [category D], and methadone [category D]); anticonvulsants (gabapentin [category C], carbamazepine [category D]), and benzodiazepines (clonazepam [category D]) (31) (Fig. 147-1). In general, dopamine agonists are first-line agents in the treatment of RLS (32,33). Most of the available data on the safety of these agents are from animal studies. No controlled trials are available for RLS during pregnancy.

RECOMMENDATIONS

An accurate diagnosis should be made as early as possible. In most instances complete information of the nature of a

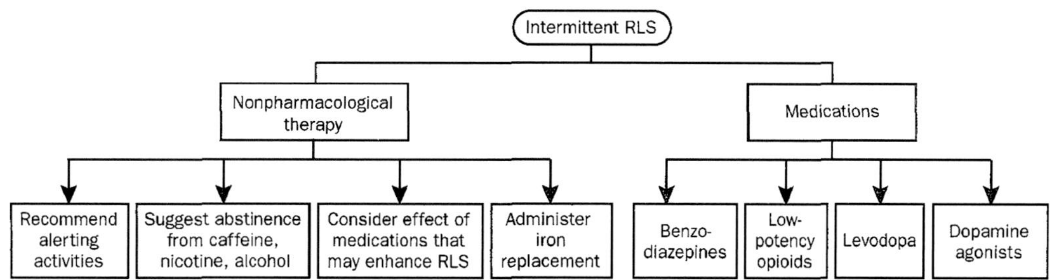

FIGURE 147-1. Algorithm for the management of intermittent restless legs syndrome (RLS).

disorder which is benign and self-limited is sufficient to control anxiety awaiting a spontaneous recovery. When symptoms are severe, however, pharmacologic treatment may be necessary. Both conditions are benign in nature, but on rare occasions CG can be a life-threatening disorder

CLINICAL RECOMMENDATIONS OF THE VIGNETTE

After discussing potential therapeutic options and because of the mild severity of the patient's involuntary movements, she decided to remain untreated. Her involuntary movements gradually decreased during the second trimester, and completely subsided before delivery. She delivered a healthy full-term baby by cesarean section. Magnetic resonance imaging (MRI) of the brain obtained after delivery was unremarkable.

SUMMARY

Movement disorders in pregnancy are uncommon. An unmet need exists for additional epidemiologic data and refined guidelines on how to best manage these cases. Until this information becomes available, physicians will have to weigh the potential pros and cons on an individual basis, and make their choices based on case reports, animal studies, or even on their own experience.

REFERENCES

1. Golbe LI. Pregnancy and movement disorders. *Neurol Clin.* 1994;12:497–508.
2. Walters AS. Toward a better definition of the restless legs syndrome. The International Restless Legs Syndrome Study Group. *Mov Disord.* 1995;10:634–642.
3. Allen RP, Picchiotti D, Hening WA, et al. Restless legs syndrome: Diagnostic criteria, special considerations, and epidemiology. A report from the restless legs syndrome diagnosis and epidemiology workshop at the National Institutes of Health. *Sleep Med.* 2002;4:101–119.
4. Smith MS, Evatt ML. Movement disorders in pregnancy. *Neurol Clin.* 2004;22:783–798.
5. Willson P, Preece AA. Chorea gravidarum. *Arch Intern Med.* 1932;49:471–533.
6. Cardoso F, Vargas AP, Cunningham MCQ, et al. Chorea gravidarum: New lessons from an old disease. *Neurology.* 1999;52[Suppl 2]:A121.
7. Rothdach AJ, Trenkwalder C, Haberstock J, et al. Prevalence and risk factors of RLS in an elderly population. MEMO Study. *Neurology.* 2000;54:1064–1068.
8. Lavigne GJ, Montplaisir JY. Restless legs syndrome and sleep bruxism. Prevalence and association among Canadians. *Sleep.* 1994;17:739–43.
9. Chokroverty S, Jankovic J. Restless legs syndrome: A disease in search of identity. *Neurology.* 1999;52:907–910.
10. Manconi M, Govoni V, De Vito A, et al. Restless legs syndrome and pregnancy. *Neurology.* 2004;63:1065–1069.
11. Manconi M, et al. Pregnancy as a risk factor for restless legs syndrome. *Sleep Medicine.* 2004;5:305–308.
12. Wolf RE, McBeath JG. Chorea gravidarum in systemic lupus erythematosus. *J Rheumatol.* 1985;12:992–993.
13. Knopf PM, Harling-Berg CJ, Cserr HF, et al. Antigen-dependent intrathecal antibody synthesis in the normal rat brain: Tissue entry and local retention of antigen-specific B cells. *J Immunol.* 1998;161:692–701.
14. Turjanski N, Lees AJ, Brooks DJ. Striatal dopaminergic function in restless legs syndrome. 18F-dopa and 11C-raclopride PET studies. *Neurology.* 1999;52:932–937.
15. Wetter TC, Stiasny K, Winkelmann J, et al. randomized controlled study of pergolide in patients with restless legs syndrome. *Neurology.* 1999;52:944–950.
16. Wetter TC, Pollmacher T. Restless legs and periodic leg movements in sleep syndromes. *J Neurol.* 1997;24[Suppl]:37–45.
17. Zucconi M, Ferini-Strambi L. Epidemiology and clinical findings of restless legs syndrome. *Sleep Medicine.* 2004;5:293–299.
18. Ghanem Q. Recurrent chorea gravidarum in four pregnancies. *Can J Neurol Sci.* 1985;12: 136–138.
19. Austin DA. Neurologic emergencies in pregnancy. NAACOGS. *Clinical Issues in Perinatal and Women's Health Nursing.* 1992;3:491–497.
20. Thorpy MJ, ed. *ICSD—International Classification of Sleep Disorders: Diagnostic and Coding Manual.* Rochester, MN: American Sleep Disorders Association; 1990.
21. Dike GL. Chorea gravidarum: A case report and review. *Maryland Medical Journal.* 1997;46:436–439.
22. Agrawal BL, Foa RP. Collagen vascular disease appearing as chorea gravidarum. *Arch Neurol.* 1982;39:192–193.
23. Branch DW. Antiphospholipid antibodies and pregnancy: Maternal implications. *Semin Perinatol.* 1990;14:139–146.
24. Cervera R, Asherson RA, Font J, et al. Chorea in the antiphospholipid syndrome. Clinical, radiologic, and immunologic characteristics of 50 patients from our clinics and the recent literature. *Medicine (Baltimore).* 1997;76:203–212.
25. Donaldson JO. Control of chorea gravidarum with haloperidol. *Obstet Gynecol.* 1982;59: 381–382.
26. Grover S, Avasthi A, Sharma Y. Psychotropics in pregnancy: Weighing the risks. *Indian J Med Res.* 2006;123(4):497–512.
27. Omdal R, Roalso S. Chorea gravidarum and chorea associated with oral contraceptives diseases due to antiphospholipid antibodies? *Acta Neurol Scand.* 1992;86:219–220.
28. Jutz P, Clavadetscher P, Ketz E, et al. Chorea minor under ovulation inhibitors. *Schweiz Med Wochenschr.* 1976;106:803–805.
29. Caviness JN, Muenter MD. An unusual cause of recurrent chorea. *Mov Disord.* 1991;6: 355–357.
30. Smith MS, Evatt ML. Movement disorders in pregnancy. *Neurol Clin.* 2004;22:783–798.
31. Earley CJ. Restless legs syndrome. *N Engl J Med.* 2003;348:2103–2109.
32. Hening W, Allen R, Earley C, et al. The treatment of restless legs syndrome and periodic limb movement disorder: An American Academy of Sleep Medicine review. *Sleep.* 1999;22: 970–999.
33. Chesson AL, Jr., Wise M, Davila D, et al. Practice parameters for the treatment of restless legs syndrome and periodic limb movement disorder: An American Academy of Sleep Medicine report. *Sleep.* 1999;22:961–968.

PART XX Pediatrics

CHAPTER 148

Diphtheria

Wendy L. Hobson-Rohrer • James F. Bale, Jr.

OBJECTIVES

- To describe the clinical manifestations of diphtheria
- To explain the appropriate diagnostic testing for suspected diphtheria
- To show how to initiate appropriate management of cases of suspected or proven diphtheria
- To explore appropriate surveillance and management of exposed contacts

CASE VIGNETTE

Malaise, low-grade fever, and sore throat developed in a 41-year-old laboratory technician. She was seen 1 day later in an emergency room with shortness of breath; pharyngeal swelling, white membrane over the right tonsil and soft palate, adenopathy, and cervical swelling were noted. A presumptive diagnosis of diphtheria was made; tracheotomy was performed immediately. The patient was treated with intravenous benzyl penicillin G (600,000 U every 12 hours for 10 days) and diphtheria antitoxin (100,000 U for 3 days). *Corynebacterium diphtheriae* were cultured from a tonsillar swab obtained before antibiotic treatment (1).

DEFINITION

Diphtheria is a localized or systemic disorder caused by toxigenic or nontoxigenic strains of the gram-positive, pleomorphic bacillus, *Corynebacterium diphtheriae.*

EPIDEMIOLOGY

Diphtheria results from human-to-human transmission of *C. diphtheriae* (2). The bacterium spreads by direct contact with infected respiratory droplets or skin lesions. Respiratory transmission occurs more commonly during the winter months, whereas infections linked to skin wounds occur more commonly in summer. In rare instances, *C. diphtheriae* are transmitted by fomites, raw milk, or milk products (2). Diphtheria is uncommon in immunized populations, although immunized persons can serve as asymptomatic carriers of the organism.

In the 1990s, a massive epidemic of diphtheria among unimmunized persons living in the former Soviet Union caused death and severe disease (3). The epidemic began in the Russian Federation and spread to the Ukraine in 1991 and to 12 new independent states (NIS) during 1993–1994 (4). Reported cases of diphtheria in the NIS ranged from 839 in 1989 to 47,802 in 1994. In 1994, 1,746 persons died from diphtheria; case-fatality rates ranged from 2.8% (Russian Federation) to 23.0% (Lithuania and Turkmenistan) (4). A substantial proportion of the adult population lacks protective immunity against *C. diphtheriae* (5,6), even in nations with compulsory immunization.

PATHOGENESIS

Nontoxigenic strains of *C. diphtheria* cause pharyngitis or invasive disease via direct bacterial infection (2). Following oropharyngeal or cutaneous infection, toxigenic strains produce a circulating exotoxin that suppresses protein synthesis in several tissues, including the myocardium, kidney, and cranial or peripheral nerves. The pathologic process in cranial or peripheral nerves consists of a demyelinating neuropathy, whereas myocardial damage results from the direct effect of the toxin on muscle cells (7).

CLINICAL MANIFESTATIONS

After an incubation period of 2 to 7 or more days, infected persons experience low-grade fever and cutaneous or respiratory symptoms (2). Diphtheric oropharyngeal membrane can affect up to 50% of infected persons and cause acute, life-threatening airway obstruction (8,9). Neurologic complications occur in approximately 10% of persons with signs of pharyngeal diphtheria (7–9). These consist of acute cranial motor nerve palsies, affecting cranial nerves III, VI, VII, IX, or X, or a disorder similar to Guillain-Barré syndrome, affecting the distal extremities (9). Cranial neuropathies tend to occur within 2 weeks after the onset of respiratory symptoms, whereas peripheral neuropathies can occur up to 8 weeks later (8,9). In rare instances, diphtheria can produce a toxic encephalopathy associated with chorea, coma, and convulsions (10).

DIAGNOSTIC APPROACH

The diagnosis of diphtheria can be made by detecting the bacterium in nasal, nasopharyngeal, or cutaneous lesions (2) or by culturing pharyngeal membranes. The organism requires special medium; toxigenic strains can be identified by state or reference laboratories. *C. diphtheriae* isolates should be forwarded to the Centers for Disease Control and Prevention (CDC) (2). The CDC case definition is an upper respiratory illness characterized by sore throat, low-grade fever, and an adherent membrane of the tonsils, pharynx, or nose without other apparent cause; isolation of *C. diphtheriae* confirms the diagnosis.

TREATMENT

Management of diphtheria consists of antibiotic therapy to eradicate *C. diphtheriae* and antitoxin administration to block the effects of circulating toxin. Antitoxin, an equine product, should be given intravenously when diphtheria is clinically suspected. Because 5% to 20% of the population manifests allergic reactions to horse serum, patients suspected of having diphtheria should undergo scratch and intradermal tests with a 1:1,000 dilution of antitoxin in saline before intravenous therapy. Desensitization is required should reactions occur (2).

The dose of antitoxin should be tailored to the severity of the patient's symptoms and signs; patients with pharyngeal disease of short duration (≤48 hours) require 20,000 to 40,000 U, whereas those with extensive, prolonged disease (≥3 or more days) should receive 80,000 to 120,000 U (2). The role for antitoxin in cutaneous disease is unclear (2). Antibiotic therapy should consist of oral or parenteral erythromycin or intramuscular or intravenous penicillin G. Two sequential negative cultures obtained 24 hours apart should be obtained to confirm eradication of *C. diphtheriae.*

Carriers of diphtheria require immunization and antibiotic therapy with erythromycin or penicillin (2). Cultures should be obtained thereafter to confirm eradication of the organism. Hospitalized patients with diphtheria require droplet precautions, as well as standard precautions. Close contacts require surveillance, cultures for *C. diphtheriae,* and antibiotic prophylaxis with erythromycin (40 to 50 mg/kg/day for 10 days ; maximum of 2 g/day) or a single injection of penicillin G benzathine (600,000 U for children weighing <30 kg and 1.2 million U for children >30 kg and adults) (2). Asymptomatic contacts who were previously immunized require booster immunization with the appropriate diphtheria toxoid vaccine (2). In addition, diphtheria booster immunization should be provided to adults and children in combination with tetanus toxoid during routine, periodic immunization, or wound management (2).

CLINICAL RECOMMENDATIONS OF THE VIGNETTE

The patient experienced mild myocarditis, that resolved within 2 weeks, and also had local paralysis of the soft palate and posterior pharyngeal wall. Two weeks after the onset of her illness, a peripheral neuropathy with paresthesias and weakness of the right arm developed. The weakness resolved completely over the subsequent year.

SUMMARY

Although uncommon among immunized populations, diphtheria remains a potentially life-threatening disease among persons not immunized. This threat is illustrated by the high rates of death during the outbreak in the former Soviet Union (3). Suspected diphtheria requires urgent management, as illustrated by the case. Even with appropriate management, however, neurologic complications can ensue.

REFERENCES

1. Geiss HK, Kiehl W, Thilo W. A case report of laboratory-acqired diphtheria. *Euro Surveill.* 1997;2(8):67–68.
2. American Academy of Pediatrics. Diphtheria. In: Pickering LK, Baker CJ, Long SS, et al., eds. *Red Book: 2006 Report of the Committee on Infectious Diseases,* 27th ed. Elk Grove Village, IL: American Academy of Pediatrics; 2006:277–281.
3. Vitek CR. Diphtheria. *Curr Top Microbiol Immunol.* 2006;304:71–94.
4. CDC. Diphtheria epidemic—New Independent States of the Former Soviet Union, 1990–1994. *Morb Mortal Wkly Rep MMWR.* 1995;44;177–181.
5. Volzke H, Kloker KM, Kramer A, et al. Susceptibility to diphtheria in adults: Prevalence and relationship to gender and social variables. *Clin Microbiol Infect.* 2006;12(10):961–967.
6. Crossley K, Irvine P, Warren JB, et al. Tetanus and diphtheria immunity in urban Minnesota adults. *JAMA.* 1979;242:2298–3000.
7. Dobie RA, Tobey DN. Clinical features of diphtheria of the respiratory tract. *JAMA.* 1979;242:2197–2201.
8. Bowman CG, Bonventre PF. Studies on the mode of action of diphtheria toxin. III. Effect on subcellular components of protein synthesis from the tissues of intoxicated guinea pigs and rats. *J Exp Med.* 1970;131:659–674.
9. Benson CA, Harris AA. Acute neurologic infections. *Med Clin North Am.* 1986;70:987–1011.
10. Gupta OK, Saksena PN, Gupta NN. A clinical study of 856 patients with diphtheria. *Indian J Pediatr.* 1975;40:93–101.

CHAPTER 149

Pertussis

April E. Kilgore • Charlotte T. Jones

OBJECTIVES

- To describe the common presentation of *B. pertussis* infections, their management and sequelae
- To understand the epidemiology and pathophysiology of *Bordetella pertussis* infections
- To describe the neurologic complications associated with *B. pertussis* infections
- To describe the long-term neurologic sequelae of *B. pertussis* infections

CASE VIGNETTE

A 2-month-old infant presents to the emergency department with a 2-week history of cough. His parents describe that at the onset of illness, he had rhinorrhea and a mild nonproductive cough. Over the past few days, he has developed worsening cough; at times having coughing spells lasting approximately 30 seconds followed by a gasping sound. He has been afebrile. Parents report decreased oral intake secondary to cough and rhinorrhea. The child's father has been ill with a mild cough over the past 3 weeks. Further history reveals that the patient has not yet received any immunizations. On examination, he initially is resting comfortably without signs of respiratory distress. He develops paroxysms of cough, however, that last 20 to 30 seconds, associated with hypoxemia. A complete blood count (CBC) shows an elevated white blood count (WBC) with a lymphocytosis and chest X-ray study reveals right upper lobe atelectasis. The patient is admitted for further care. On hospital day 3, he is noted to be increasingly fussy and is difficult to console. He then develops episodes of apnea and generalized seizures.

DEFINITION

Pertussis, or whooping cough, is an infection primarily of the upper respiratory tract caused by the gram-negative bacilli *Bordatella pertussis* and *B. parapertussis.*

EPIDEMIOLOGY

The incidence of pertussis in the postvaccine era in estimated to be 0.5 to 1.0 per 100,000 population (1). These reported cases may only represent 15% to 25% of infections (1), however, because of the atypical presentation in adolescents and adults. Despite vaccination, pertussis epidemics occur every 2 to 5 years (1,2). Routine vaccination has changed which population is most affected by the disease. In the prevaccine era, 85% of cases occurred in patient ages 1 to 9 years. In the postvaccine era, 41% of cases are patients <1 year of age and 28% are patients >10 years of age (1).

EPIDEMIOLOGY OF NEUROLOGIC MANIFESTATIONS

Because of routine vaccination, most of what is known about the neurologic manifestations of pertussis is based on data and case reports from the 1950s and 1960s. The number of children with neurologic problems may be different today than reported in these older articles. Medical care has changed and more aggressive treatment of hypoxia may improve long-term outcome. Additionally, improved diagnostic techniques (genetic and radiologic) may allow children previously thought to suffer from pertussis effects to now have other causes identified. A chart review performed in 1966 in Sydney, Australia looked at the incidence of neurologic complications of pertussis infections in 632 patients admitted over a period of 11.5 years. The authors found that seizures occurred in 1.74% of patients and meningoencephalitis in 0.79% (3). The authors note, however, that only patients with severe infection were admitted and, thus, the incidence in the general population may be less than that of the study. Incorpora et al. (4) performed a similar review of 340 cases in Sicily and report seizures in 4.1% of patients and encephalopathy in 1.2%. The estimated incidence of neurologic complications in pertussis infections are seizures in 1.9% and encephalopathy in 0.3% (5); however, no good studies have evaluated this. Rare complications of pertussis infections include subdural hematoma and syndrome of inappropriate antidiuretic hormone (SIADH).

ETIOLOGY AND PATHOGENESIS

Pertussis, or whooping cough, is caused by *Bordatella pertussis,* a gram-negative aerobic bacillus, and, less frequently *Bordatella parapertussis. B. pertussis* exclusively infects humans. *B. bronchiseptica* typically causes disease in animals, but can cause a pertussislike illness in humans (1).

B. pertussis causes disease by attaching to the epithelium of the respiratory tract. Clinical manifestations are caused by local effects on the respiratory tract and toxin production. The organism does not cause a disseminated disease (2). Toxins produced by the organism act to aid in attachment (pertussis toxin, filamentous hemagglutinin, pertactin), cause local tissue damage (tracheal cytotoxin and pertussis toxin), and impede bacterial clearance and host immune function (adenylate cyclase toxin and dermonecrotic toxin) (2).

PATHOGENESIS OF NEUROLOGIC MANIFESTATIONS

The pathogenesis of neurologic manifestations is less clear. Seizures, the most common neurologic sequelae of pertussis infections, can result from hypoxia secondary to the paroxysms of cough or can be toxin mediated (5,6). Woolf and Caplan (6) describe a case of a child with known pertussis infection who developed meningoencephalitis and seizures and subsequently died. Autopsy findings showed evidence of meningoencephalitis and anoxic injury. It was unclear, however, whether the anoxic injury was the result of coughing paroxysms or status epilepticus (6). Endotoxin, released through bacterial lysis, has been postulated as a potential inducer of encephalopathy; however, no studies have confirmed this speculation (5). Eckman et al. (7) demonstrated that infusion of gram negative bacterial endotoxin can cause alterations in the blood–brain barrier and increase permeability (8). Furthermore, it is felt that CO_2 retention may disturb cerebral vascular autoregulation, disturbing the blood–brain barrier and creating an entry point for bacterial toxins (5). In addition, a study looking at cytokine production following pulmonary infection with pertussis showed increased levels of inflammatory cytokines in the brain, particularly the hippocampus and hypothalamus (9).

SIADH has been seen in pertussis infections. Mathern et al. (9) describes two cases in which SIADH developed during pertussis infection and were further complicated by hyponatremic seizures. It is postulated that SIADH in pertussis infections is caused by increased intrathoracic pressure, resulting in increased resistance to pulmonary blood flow and decreased left atrial filling. Stretch receptors sense hypovolemia and stimulate release of ADH (11).

Although uncommon, subdural hematomas have been reported in patients with pertussis. A case is described of an 8-month-old male infant with confirmed pertussis infection who develops bilateral subdural hematomas (11). It is postulated that increased intracranial pressure secondary to coughing was the cause (2,11).

PATHOLOGY

At autopsy, infiltration of the mucosa by lymphocytes and polymorphonuclear cells is noted. Inflammatory debris is found in the lumen of the bronchus. Initially, peribronchial lymphoid hyperplasia is seen. Later, necrosis of the midzonal and basilar layers of the bronchial epithelium is seen (1).

NEUROPATHOLOGY

Autopsy reports have described lymphocytic perivascular cuffing, with some extension into the perivascular cerebral tissue, and a lymphocytosis of the subarachnoid space (7). Areas of focal degeneration, consistent with anoxic injury were noted in the cerebral cortex; however, the cause of the anoxic injuries was unclear (7). Litvak et al. (11) describes pathology findings in 39 patients as involving cerebral edema, congestion, and multiple punctuate hemorrhages. An additional case report describes a normal brain biopsy in a patient with a pertussis-related encephalopathy (12).

CLINICAL MANIFESTATIONS

Whooping cough classically presents as an illness divided into three stages: catarrhal, paroxysmal, and convalescent, with the duration anywhere from 6 to 8 weeks. During the catarrhal stage, mild cough, rhinorrhea, and conjunctivitis are the predominant symptoms (2). The patient is usually afebrile. This stage persists for 1 to 2 weeks, gradually worsening until paroxysms of cough develop. The paroxysmal stage is characterized by repetitive coughs occurring in a series. This is sometimes followed by a large inspiratory effort, creating the characteristic whooping sound (1). Cyanosis resulting from the paroxysms is fairly common (85%) (2); additional symptoms include bulging eyes, neck vein distention, and salivation (1). During the attacks, the child may be ill-appearing and exhausted because of the effort involved; however, between attacks the patient may appear well (1). Sneezing, yawning, eating, or drinking can trigger the cough (1). Complications of this stage include pneumonia (may be secondary bacterial infection), conjuctival hemorrhage, emphysema, pneumothorax, and umbilical and inguinal hernias (2).

The paroxysmal stage is followed by the convalescent stage. This stage can last 1 to 2 weeks and is characterized by persistent cough. During this time, the severity of disease gradually decreases (1).

Atypical illness can be seen in vaccinated adults and teens, which is characterized by a persistent cough that is refractory to treatment (6). These patients may be the source of disease in nonimmunized infants, who typically have a severe course.

NEUROLOGIC MANIFESTATIONS

Neurologic manifestations typically occur during the paroxysmal phase. Generalized tonic–clonic seizures have been reported in patients with pertussis infections, as well as a meningoencephalopathy (3, 6). Subdural hematomas, SIADH, and spinal epidural hematoma can also be seen (10,11). Encephalopathy typically presents with lethargy and altered level of consciousness (6). In addition, headache and vomiting may also be seen (4). Seizures may also be a presenting sign of meningoencephalitis (6). Focal neurologic signs have been reported, including strabismus, hyperreflexia, and hemiparesis (6,11,13).

Subdural hematomas may present with focal neurologic signs and altered level of consciousness. In neonates, a bulging anterior fontanel and macrocephaly may also be seen (10,11).

The initial presenting sign of SIADH may be seizures caused by hyponatremia (14). This highlights the importance of monitoring serum electrolytes in patients with pertussis infections (9). Patients with spinal epidural hematomas may present initially with progressive ataxia and paraparesis (15).

Infants may not present with classic disease, but instead with other nonspecific symptoms, such as apnea (16). Up to one third of cyanotic episodes in patients with pertussis may be caused by apneic episodes (16). It has been speculated that

B. pertussis infection can be a cause of sudden infant death syndrome (1). The characteristic whoop typically is not present in infants (1).

DIAGNOSTIC APPROACH

The gold standard in diagnosing pertussis infections is culture of a nasopharyngeal swab. Culture results may be falsely negative, however, if the sample was not transported rapidly to the laboratory or improper transport medium are used. It is important to inform laboratory staff of possible pertussis infection so the proper medium, Bordet-Gengou, can be obtained. Other factors include sample collection >2 weeks into the illness, before immunization and antibiotic treatment can decrease the likelihood of a positive culture (1). For this reason, the use of polymerase chain reaction (PCR) has become the preferred methodology for detection. Acute and convalescent titers can also be used to diagnose infection, but again may be falsely negative, depending on the time line of disease (1). Leukocytosis with lymphocytosis in a symptomatic child or infant with apnea is highly suggestive of pertussis infection (6). Diagnosis of pertussis encephalopathy is clinical. Cerebrospinal fluid (CSF) study findings typically are normal or have a mild pleocytosis as are those of imaging studies.

Other illnesses can present similarly and must be included in the differential diagnosis. These include *Chlamydia pneumoniae, Mycoplasma pneumoniae,* C. trachomatis, and adenovirus. Bronchiolitis, bacterial pneumonia, cystic fibrosis, and tuberculosis can also mimic pertussis infection (1). Thus, additional laboratory testing should be aimed at distinguishing pertussis infection from these other causes.

TREATMENT

Treatment of pertussis is largely supportive. Use of erythromycin in the early stages of disease may shorten the course. Treatment with erythromycin during any stage of the illness will reduce bacterial shedding. The recommended dose of erythromycin in children is 50 mg/kg/day divided every 6 hours for 2 weeks. Trimethoprim-sulfamethoxazole can be used as an alternative in erythromycin allergic patients (1). Supportive care involves maintaining adequate hydration, nutrition, and supplemental oxygen, as needed (1). Close contacts of infected patients should be treated with erythromycin as well, and the patient should be kept in respiratory isolation. Because SIADH can occur, serum electrolytes should be closely monitored. If a patient develops a fluctuating level of consciousness or focal neurologic deficits, evaluation for possible encephalopathy or subdural hematoma should occur.

Prevention of disease is most important, and routine vaccination with the acellular vaccine is recommended. Whole cell vaccines continue to be used in some parts of the world. Much research and debate has revolved around the possible neurologic adverse effects of the whole cell vaccine. This is discussed in the vaccine section of this text.

Few studies have looked at the long-term neurologic sequelae of patients with pertussis infections. Researchers in Great Britain followed a group of patients after an epidemic of pertussis in 1977–1979. They specifically looked at children who were <5 years of age and had neurologic complications with infections, such as seizures and encephalopathy. The authors used a case-control study designed to evaluate effects on IQ and development. Researchers found statistically significant deficiencies in multiple areas, including nonverbal reasoning, reading, comprehension, and spelling (17). In addition, Berg (13) described mental retardation following pertussis illness complicated by apnea and seizures, in a previously healthy child.

CLINICAL RECOMMENDATIONS OF THE VIGNETTE

The patient was treated acutely with lorazepam and transferred to the pediatric intensive care unit. A head computed tomographic (CT) scan was performed and finding was normal. A lumbar puncture showed a white blood cell count of 1, red blood cell count of 150, protein 45, and glucose of 80. Serum glucose at the time of the examination was 110. CSF and blood specimens were sent for culture and Gram stain. The patient was started on ampicillin and cefotaxime empirically, pending culture results. The patient had no further seizure activity, and cultures remained negative. He continued to improve clinically, both from a respiratory and neurologic standpoint. On discharge, he had no subsequent neurologic impairment. It was explained to the parents that, although the examination finding was normal, up to one third of patients with encephalopathy secondary to pertussis infection may experience intellectual impairment and learning disabilities (13,17). The patient was discharged home on hospital day 10.

SUMMARY

Despite routine vaccination, pertussis infections and outbreaks continue to occur. Atypical disease in adults and adolescents is thought to be a reservoir for the disease and is becoming increasingly more recognized and reported. Although classic disease continues to occur, it must be recognized that other nonspecific presentations occur as well, particularly in infants. Neurologic manifestations occur in 2% to 3% of those infected, with seizures being the most common. Other sequelae include encephalopathy, subdural hematoma, and SIADH. Encephalopathy can be fatal in one third of patients, and an additional one third may have long-term deficits, including learning disabilities. The remaining one third are normal (11). Treatment consists of antibiotic therapy with erythromycin and supportive measures, addressing complications as they arise (18). Close contacts of the patient should be treated prophylactically as well. The mainstay of defense against the disease continues to be vaccination. Current vaccines in the United States are acellular and carry a low risk of adverse effects. Whole cell vaccines, however, continue to be used in other parts of the world. The association of vaccine and neurologic disorders is described more fully in another chapter in this text.

REFERENCES

1. Cherry JD, Heininger U. Pertussis and other Bordetella infections. In: Feigin RD and Cherry JD. *Textbook of Pediatric Infectious Disease,* 4th ed. Philadelphia: WB Saunders; 1988:1423–1439.
2. Fenichel GM. Pertussis: The disease and the vaccine. *Pediatr Neurol.* 1988:4(4):201–206.
3. Celermajer JM, Brown J. The neurological complications of pertussis. *Med J Aust.* 1966;1(25):1066–1069.
4. Incorpora G, Pavone L, Parano E, et al. Neurological complications in hospitalized patients with pertussis: A 15-year Sicilian experience. *Child Nerv Syst.* 1996;12(6):332–335.

5. Menkes JH, Kinsbourne M. Workshop on neurologic complications of pertussis and pertussis vaccination. *Neuropediatrics.* 1990;21(4):171–176.
6. Woolf A, Caplan H. Whooping cough encephalitis. *Arch Dis Child.* 1956;31(156):87–91.
7. Eckman P, King W, Brunson J. Studies on the blood brain barrier. *Am J Pathol.* 1958;34(4): 631–643.
8. Loscher C, Donnelly S, Lynch M, et al. Induction of *I*nflammatory *C*ytokines in the brain following respiratory infection with Bordatella pertussis. *J Neruoimmunol.* 2000;102(2): 172–181.
9. Mathern P, Matson J, Marks MI. Pertussis complicated by the syndrome of inappropriate antidiuretic hormone secretion. *Clin Pediatr.* 1986;25(1):46–48.
10. Watts CC, Acosta C. Pertussis and bilateral subdural hematomas. *Am J Dis Child.* 1969;118(3):518–519.
11. Litvak AM, Gibel H, Rosenthal S, et al. Cerebral complications in pertussis. *J Pediatr.* 1948;32:357–379.
12. Davis LE, Burstyn DG, Manclark CR. Pertussis encephalopathy with a normal brain biopsy and elevated lymphocytosis promoting factor antibodies. *Pediatr Infect Dis.* 1984;3(5): 448–451.
13. Berg J. Neurological sequelae of pertussis with particular reference to mental defect. *Arch Dis Child.* 1959;34:322–324.
14. Abe Y, Watanabe T. Pertussis pneumonia complicated by a hyponatremic seizure. *Pediatr Emerg Care.* 2003;19(4):262–264.
15. Jackson F. Spontaneous spinal epidural hematoma coincident with whooping cough. *J Neurosurg.* 1963;20:715–717.
16. Southall DP, Thomas MG, Lambert HP. Severe hypoxaemia in pertussis. *Arch Dis Child.* 1988;63(6):598–605.
17. Williams W. Study of intellectual performance of children in ordinary schools after certain serious complications of whooping cough. *BMJ.* 1987;295(6605):1044–1047.
18. Committee on Infectious Diseases American Academy of Pediatrics. *Red Book.* 2003: 472–485.

CHAPTER 150

Measles

Hannah Klein de Licona • Daniel J. Bonthius

OBJECTIVES

- To identify the ways in which measles can be transmitted
- To discuss the pathogenesis of classic measles virus infection
- To explain the clinical presentation of measles virus infection and its complications
- To compare and contrast primary measles encephalitis, measles-associated acute disseminated encephalomyelitis, and subacute sclerosing panencephalitis
- To identify diagnostic tests for measles virus infection
- To discuss treatment options for patients infected with measles virus

CASE VIGNETTE

A 13-year-old-boy was referred to the pediatric neurology clinic for evaluation of cognitive decline and a movement disorder. He was of Thai descent and had spent the first 4 years of life in an orphanage in Thailand before he was adopted by an American family. No history of measles was reported at the time of adoption, nor did he ever have an illness resembling measles after the adoption. As a child, he had mild attention deficits, for which he was successfully treated with methylphenidate. He remained healthy until the age of 13 years, when he developed irritability and worsened attention problems. Several months later, he developed myoclonic jerking movements of the extremities. The boy's psychiatric symptoms worsened, and he began to fail academically. His movement disorder evolved into drop attacks, which caused him to fall to the floor multiple times per day.

On examination, the boy appeared healthy and was cooperative, but reticent to speak and had difficulty following commands that his adoptive mother said he could easily have followed previously. Cranial nerve examination was remarkable for saccadic pursuit movements of gaze, and the motor examination revealed cogwheeling in the upper extremities. Most notable were intermittent shocklike dipping movements of the head and shoulders with no evident change in level of consciousness.

Magnetic resonance imaging (MRI) of the brain revealed a single focus of increased T2 signal intensity in the subcortical white matter of the left frontal lobe (Fig. 150-1). Electroencephalogram (EEG) revealed high amplitude bursts of periodic slow-wave complexes, accompanied clinically by generalized myoclonic spasms (Fig. 150-2). Cerebrospinal fluid (CSF) glucose, total protein, and cellular content were normal, but the CSF immunoglobulin G (IgG) was abnormally high at 16.3 mg/dL (normal, 0.5 to 5.9 mg/dL). Furthermore, rubeola (measles) IgG antibody titers were markedly elevated in the CSF at 1:160 (normal, <1:5) and in the serum at 1:5120. In contrast, IgM antibodies for measles were undetectable in CSF or serum. Both the EEG and CSF abnormalities were pathognomonic for subacute sclerosing panencephalitis (Bonthius et al., 2000).

DEFINITION

Measles is an acute disease caused by infection with the highly communicable measles virus. *Measles* means "little spots" and derives its name from the Dutch word *maese*, meaning "spot" or "stain" (1), which describes the disease's characteristic exanthem. Measles virus is associated with significant childhood morbidity and mortality worldwide, despite the availability of the live attenuated measles vaccine (2,3).

Measles virus, also known as *rubeola*, is a *Morbillivirus* and a member of the *Paromyxovirus* family that includes mumps, respiratory syncytial virus, parainfluenza virus, and human metapneumovirus. It is a single-stranded RNA virus that has a lipid envelope and a diameter that varies between 120 and 250 nm (4,5).

EPIDEMIOLOGY

Measles occurs globally in temperate, tropical, and arctic climates. Humans are the only natural host of the measles virus. Measles is the most communicable of childhood exanthems and is transmitted by the respiratory route. In temperate climates, such as the United States, measles has a peak incidence between the months of March and May. This corresponds with the end of winter—a time when many children have been crowded indoors—providing an ideal environment for human-to-human transmission. Before the vaccine era, most cases of measles in developed countries occurred in preschool and young school-aged children. Epidemics occurred in two to three year cycles, as pools of susceptible children were exhausted by viral spread, and a new pool of susceptible children emerged from new births (1).

Following introduction of the live attenuated vaccine in 1963, the incidence of measles has decreased by more then 99% in the United States. From 1989 to 1991, however, the incidence of measles increased because of low immunization rates in preschool-aged children (6). The incidence dropped again in 1991 and has remained low ever since (7). Currently, most

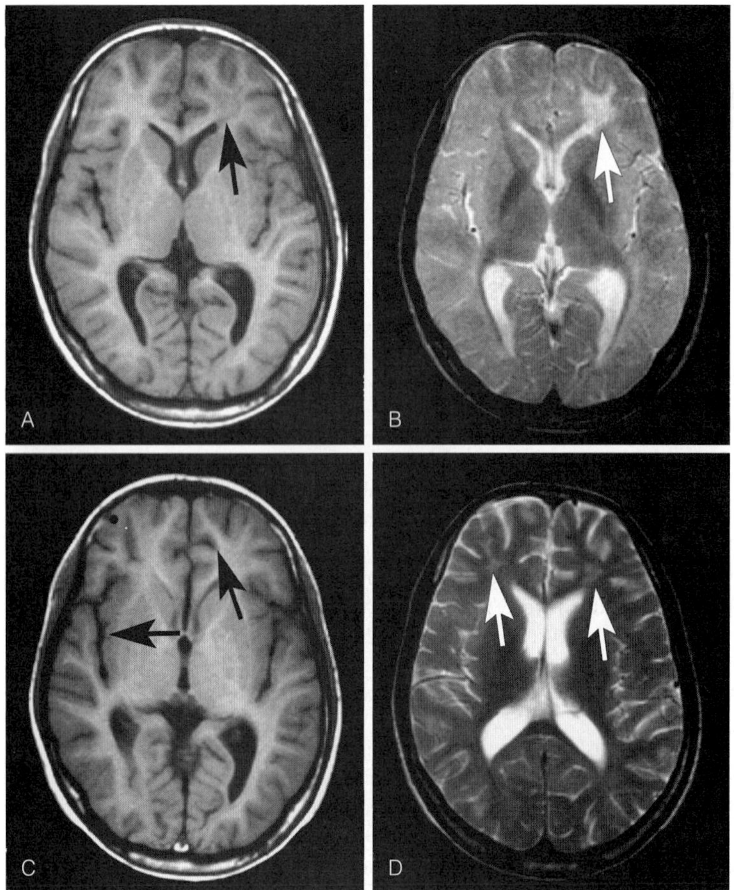

FIGURE 150-1. Magnetic resonance imaging (MRI) scans of the brain in a patient with subacute sclerosing panencephalitis (SSPE). (**A,B**) Obtained at the time of presentation. (**C,D**) Obtained 3 months later. (**A,C**) T1-weighted images. (**B,D**) T2-weighted images. The initial MRI scan (**A** and **B**) reveals a focal lesion in the subcortical white matter of the left frontal lobe, manifesting as a hypointense signal on the T1-weighted image (*arrow* in **A**) and a hyperintense signal on the T2-weighted image (*arrow* in **B**). The follow-up scan reveals progression of the disease with substantial and diffuse cortical atrophy, signified by prominent sulci (*arrows* in **C**) and white matter abnormalities, which had initially been unilateral and are now bilateral (*arrows* in **D**).

measles cases in the United States originate from hosts who acquired it internationally (8,9). In 2000, leaders in the field concluded that measles is no longer endemic to the United States (10).

Although the measles vaccine has led to a drastic decrease in measles in developed countries, the infection remains a serious disease, with high mortality and morbidity worldwide. In 1997, measles was the eighth most common cause of childhood death worldwide (3) and in 2002 was responsible for 5% of all deaths in children <5 years of age (2). Before the introduction of the vaccine, 7 to 8 million children died annually from measles infection. In 2001, the World Health Organization (WHO) reported 30 million cases and nearly 800,000 measles-related deaths (2).

Patients with measles are most contagious 1 to 2 days before onset of symptoms and 3 to 5 days before onset of rash. This corresponds to the end of the asymptomatic incubation period. Risk of contagion drastically decreases 48 hours after the exanthem appears. Patients, however, remain infectious for at least 3 days after exanthem onset (11).

ETIOLOGY AND PATHOGENESIS

Measles is a systemic infection caused by the measles virus. Acute infection usually involves the skin, lymphatic and respiratory systems, and, less often, the brain. In some patients, especially malnourished children, measles can induce croup, pneumonia, diarrhea, encephalitis, hemorrhagic rashes, and keratitis with scarring and blindness (12). In rare situations, measles virus can persist asymptomatically for years with a low level of replication and eventually cause a neurodegenerative disease, subacute sclerosing panencephalitis (SSPE) (13).

Measles virus is transmitted by direct contact with infectious droplets or by airborne spread. The virus gains access through the nose, oropharynx, or conjunctival mucosa and, initially, replicates in the epithelium of the upper respiratory tract (13). The virus may first infect immune cells. Macrophages from the initial site of infection deliver the virus to local lymph nodes, where further replication and infection of other mononuclear cells occur (15). A transient viremia, in which the virus is carried by monocytes, transports the virus to the spleen, lymph nodes, and other organs of the reticuloendothelial system (14). This leads to a second phase of replication, through infection of macrophages, lymphocytes, and dendritic cells of the reticuloendothelial system. A secondary viremia then disseminates the virus to the skin, conjunctiva, kidney, gut, respiratory mucosa, and other organs (16). The virus infects these organs by infiltrating within macrophages and lymphocytes or by infecting the epithelial or endothelial surfaces (15).

These steps of infection take place primarily during the asymptomatic incubation period. By the time symptoms appear, the virus is actively replicating in the skin, gut, and respiratory mucosa. Viral-specific cellular immunity leads to the rash and initiates viral clearance from the blood and tissues (17).

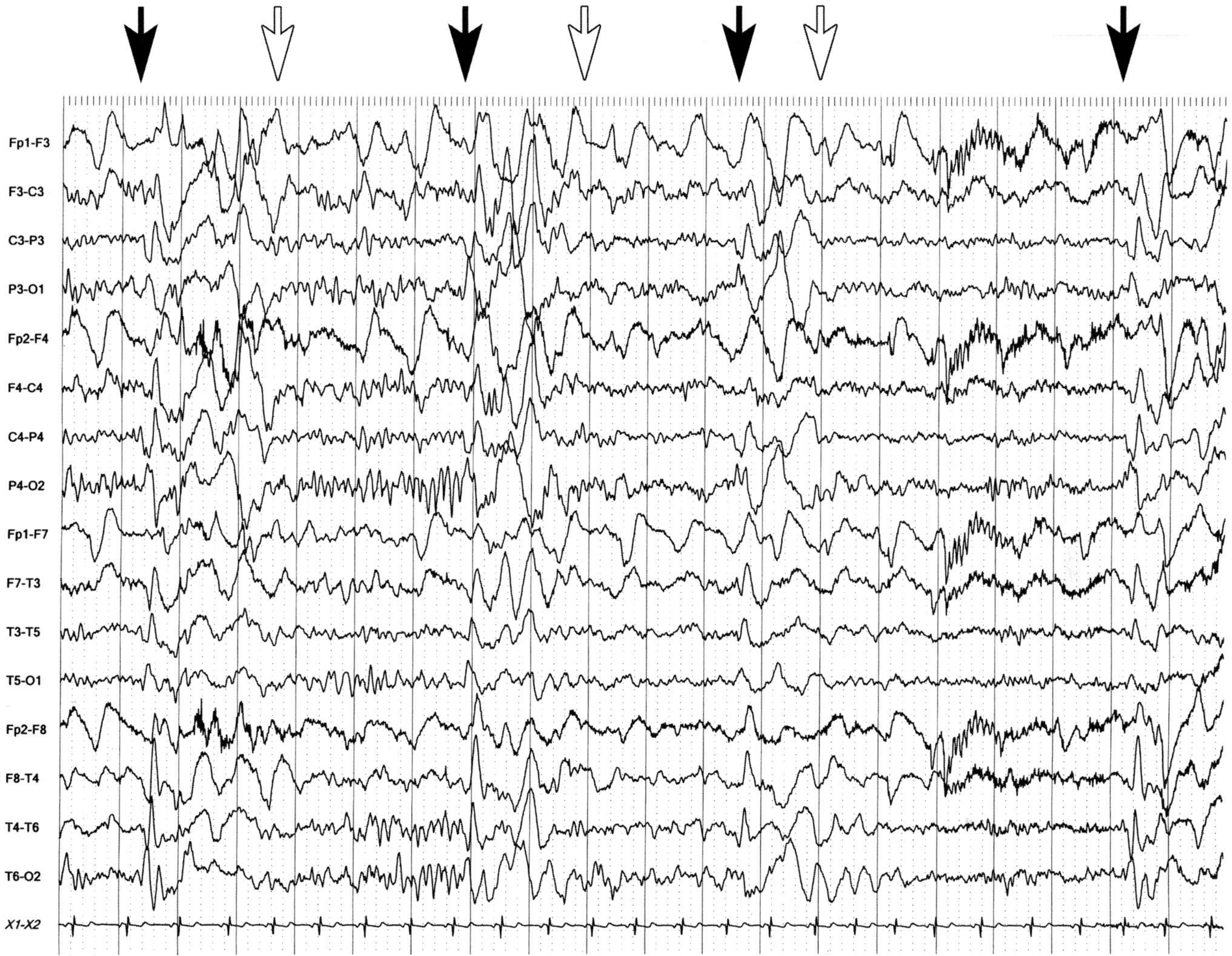

FIGURE 150-2. Electroencephalogram (EEG) in a patient with subacute sclerosing panencephalitis (SSPE). The EEG is highly abnormal and reveals periodic bursts of high-amplitude, slow-wave complexes. Onset of the complexes is indicated by the *solid arrows*, whereas offset is indicated by the *open arrows*. The background rhythm is normal, except in the frontal lobes, where slow waves predominate. This is an example of "burst-suppression" on EEG and is highly characteristic of SSPE.

PATHOLOGY

GENERAL MEASLES

The principal pathologic features of measles infection are giant cells and cytoplasmic and nuclear inclusions (12,16). Giant cells are formed by the fusion of infected cells with noninfected cells (11). Inclusions are accumulations of insoluble materials. In the case of viral infections, the inclusions are typically viral proteins that have accumulated and coalesced within cells. Cellular inclusions and giant cell formation both reflect active viral replication (15).

Two types of giant cells occur in measles infection. The first is epithelial giant cells, which are found primarily in the respiratory epithelium. These vary in size, but generally consist of 3 to 36 nuclei per cell and contain nuclear and cytoplasmic inclusions (17). In addition to their presence in respiratory epithelium, these cells are also found in Koplik spots, within the exanthem, and throughout the gastrointestinal and respiratory tracts. Within these areas, where the virus actively replicates and where giant cells form, cellular necrosis and sloughing of epithelial cells also occur (1).

The second type of giant cells, referred to as *Warthin-Finkeldey cells*, are localized to the reticuloendothelial system, including the tonsils, adenoids, lymph nodes, thymus, Peyer patches, and appendix. Pathognomonic for measles infection, Warthin-Finkeldey cells vary in size, but can contain as many as 100 nuclei per cell, along with cytoplasmic and nuclear inclusions (11).

EXANTHEM AND ENANTHEM

The measles enanthem, Koplik spots (a pathognomic oral mucosal lesion), and the exanthem are caused by a T-cell–mediated hypersensitivity reaction to viral antigens within the mucous membranes and skin. The measles virus probably replicates simultaneously in both skin and mucosa. Koplik spots, however, can be detected several days earlier than the exanthem because the mucosal epithelium is thinner and more translucent than the skin. Electron microscopic examination of Koplik spots and skin lesions reveals syncytial giant cells with intranuclear and cytoplasmic inclusions that contain aggregates of microtubules, characteristic of paramyxovirus infection.

Evidence that the exanthem is immune mediated lies in the fact that patients with deficiencies in T-cell–mediated immunity do not develop a rash (1).

GESTATIONAL MEASLES

When measles infection occurs during pregnancy, the virus targets the placental syncytial trophoblastic cells and the decidua, while leaving the fetus uninfected. This pattern of infection can induce placental damage and subsequent fetal hypoxia, ultimately leading to fetal death or spontaneous abortion (18).

MEASLES ENCEPHALITIS

Encephalitis is an inflammation of the brain (19). Measles can induce encephalitis in at least three different paradigms, each with a different pathogenesis and pathologic findings. First, measles can directly infect the brain in the course of an acute systemic measles infection. This is referred to as *primary measles encephalitis* (20). In this disease, the virus invades and replicates within brain cells. This brain infection typically occurs during the exanthem phase of the systemic illness. The viral brain infection directly injures neurons, triggers a lymphocytic infiltration within the brain parenchyma and meninges, and often induces cerebral edema. In primary measles encephalitis, infectious measles virus can be isolated from brain and CSF (17).

A second form of measles-associated brain inflammation is immune mediated, which does not involve direct viral infection of the brain. This is referred to as *measles-induced acute disseminated encephalomyelitis* (ADEM) or postinfectious encephalomyelitis (PIE) (12,17). This is primarily a demyelinating disorder. Mild perivascular infiltrates of mononuclear leukocytes, petechial hemorrhages, microglial proliferation, and perivascular demyelination are often seen (14). Myelin basic protein concentrations are elevated in the CSF (16,21). Unlike primary measles encephalitis, measles-induced ADEM does not typically begin during the exanthem phase of systemic measles, but instead begins during the resolution phase or even weeks or months after the exanthem has cleared. Infectious measles virus cannot be isolated from the brain or CSF in measles-associated ADEM because the disease is postinfectious (20,22). Meningeal inflammation and neuronal damage are usually not prominent in measles-associated ADEM (1).

The third form of brain inflammation associated with measles is *subacute sclerosing panencephalitis* (SSPE). This disease is caused by a persistent measles infection of the brain (13). The measles virus is not a wild type, however, but a genetic variant (23). SSPE occurs almost exclusively in people who were infected with measles during the first 2 years of life, suggesting that pathogenesis involves an immature immune system (1). Disease symptoms begin years after the primary measles infection. Pathologic changes include brain atrophy and the presence of viral inclusion bodies within neurons and glial cells (11,19).

CLINICAL MANIFESTATIONS

CLASSIC MEASLES INFECTION

The classic measles infection includes four phases: incubation, prodrome, exanthem, and recovery. The incubation period is usually asymptomatic and lasts 10 to 12 days. The prodrome first presents with fever and malaise, followed 24 hours later with coryza, cough, and conjunctivitis. Symptoms worsen during the next 2 to 3 days, and the conjunctival infection becomes more notable, often leading to photophobia. Toward the end of the prodrome phase and approximately 1 to 2 days before the exanthem phase, Koplik spots appear, which are slightly raised white lesions on a bed of erythema that occur within the oral mucosa. Initially, less than a dozen Koplik spots are localized to the mucosa near the posterior molars. Koplik spots multiply over the next 24 hours to cover the entire mucous membrane of the cheek. In some cases, they extend to the lips and involve the eyelids. At this point, their appearance is often described as "grains of salt on a wet background" (1,12).

Next is the exanthem phase, which typically begins as the Koplik spots are resolving. Initial lesions are small red macules 1 to 2 mm in diameter, which usually first appear on the face and neck, especially on the forehead and behind the ears. They enlarge over the next 2 to 3 days and form maculopapules of 1 cm or greater, and often become confluent. By the second day, the rash travels to the trunk and upper extremities, and by the third day the lower extremities are affected. The exanthem begins to fade by the third or fourth day, leaving a brownish stain that can persist for 10 days. In the recovery phase, the patient gradually improves, but symptoms, especially cough, fever, and malaise can linger for days to weeks (16,17).

Common complications of measles include pneumonia, otitis media, diarrhea, thrombocytopenia, laryngotracheobronchitis (croup), keratoconjunctivitis, and pericarditis or myocarditis. Among these, otitis media is the most common complication, whereas bronchopneumonia is the most common cause of death from measles. Secondary pneumonia often results from a bacterial superinfection (12,14).

PRIMARY MEASLES ENCEPHALITIS

Approximately 1 to 3 of 1,000 patients with measles will develop encephalitis, which usually has its onset within 7 days of the prodrome. Signs and symptoms include fever, headache, mental status changes, motor deficits, and seizures (24). The CSF is usually abnormal with a lymphocytic pleocytosis and a mildly elevated protein content (20). Brain edema and increased intracranial pressure can induce substantial secondary brain injury (19). The prognosis for patients with primary measles encephalitis is guarded. Of these patients, 10% to 15% will die, and an additional 25% will be left with permanent neurologic sequelae, including seizures and mental retardation (12,17).

ACUTE DISSEMINATED ENCEPHALOMYELITIS

Measles-associated ADEM, or postinfectious encephalomyelitis, is most common in children and adolescents, but can occur in adults and infants (15,25). ADEM typically presents late in the course of systemic measles, or can be delayed in onset for weeks or months after the measles infection has resolved. Signs and symptoms generally include motor and sensory deficits, ataxia, and mental status changes (24). In patients with myelitis, back pain and bladder and bowel dysfunction are prominent. The prognosis in ADEM is better than in primary measles encephalitis. Some patients with measles-induced ADEM are left with substantial and permanent neurologic sequelae, however.

SUBACUTE SCLEROSING PANENCEPHALITIS

SSPE is a progressive neurologic disease caused by a persistent measles virus infection within the brain. Because of widespread use of the measles vaccine in the United States, SSPE has virtually disappeared from this country (26,27). Most cases in the United States occur in children who were born and raised in other countries, where measles infections and SSPE remain common (28).

SSPE typically develops 7 to 10 years after the initial measles infection. Because one of the strongest risk factors for SSPE is measles infection before age 2 years, most of these cases are seen in patients >20 years. The disease is characterized by intellectual and behavioral deterioration and seizures. Initial symptoms are often psychiatric in nature, and include decreased attention span, personality changes, and academic difficulty. Weeks to years later, the patient develops motor symptoms, including myoclonus, and long tract motor or sensory disease. The patient then develops a relentless intellectual disintegration and seizures. Most patients with SSPE progress to severe convulsions, dementia, coma, and death (11,13).

The pathogenesis of SSPE is unknown. Apparently, the measles viral genome becomes mutated in such a way that the virus is not infectious, yet large quantities of viral protein are produced (23). Pathologic analysis shows demyelination and infection of neurons as well as measles virus-specific inclusions within the cytoplasm and nuclei of neurons and glia (15).

Laboratory examination can confirm the diagnosis of SSPE. The CSF and serum of patients contain extremely high levels of antimeasles antibodies (CSF >1:160, serum >1:1280), a pathognomonic feature of SSPE (17,28). Additionally, measles virus-specific oligoclonal bands are produced from central nervous system (CNS) resident B cells (15). The EEG may show a "burst suppression" pattern, where bursts of abnormal sharp and slow waves arise from a normal background, followed by a relatively flat pattern. SSPE is one of the rare disorders in which a burst-suppression pattern occurs in a conscious patient. As the disease progresses, background activity deteriorates to diffuse slow waves. Brain imaging shows global atrophy and focal leukodystrophy (28).

SPECIAL SITUATIONS

Measles Infection During Pregnancy

Measles during pregnancy can cause substantial problems for both the mother and the fetus. Epidemiologic studies indicate that pregnant women who become infected with measles often have a severe disease course, usually caused by pneumonia. The mortality rate for pregnant women with measles is 3% to 15%. The fetus is also at risk. Measles infection during pregnancy puts the fetus in jeopardy for spontaneous abortion and low birthweight. Little evidence indicates that measles infection leads to congenital malformations (1,29).

Measles Infection in the Immunocompromised Host

Suppression of T-cell–mediated immunity, resulting from bone marrow transplantation, chemotherapy, immunosuppressive doses of steroids, or human immunodeficiency virus (HIV) is associated with increased severity of measles. Immunocompromised patients with measles have much higher rates of pneumonitis, encephalitis, and death. The clinical presentation in immunocompromised hosts can be atypical, including a range of rash appearances or failure to develop a rash (30). In the absence of a rash, lung biopsy may be necessary to make a diagnosis. Complications from measles infections are most severe when the immunodeficiency is caused by T-cell deficiency. Patients with B-cell immune deficiencies or those with defects in macrophage function do not have increased complications caused by measles infection (12,17).

Measles inclusion body encephalitis (MIBE) is a progressive CNS infection that occurs 5 weeks to 6 months after acute measles infection or vaccination in immunocompromised patients (31–33). Symptoms begin with mental status changes and seizures in the absence of fever. Death occurs in >80% of cases, generally within weeks of onset (12). Although the pathogenic mechanism is unknown, it is associated with virus spread to the brain because of the immunocompromised patient's inability to restrict the virus (15). Measles virus has been detected in MIBE cases via polymerase chain reaction (PCR) (34). Electron microscopy of biopsy demonstrates cellular inclusions characteristic of paramyxovirus within neurons, oligodendrocytes, and astrocytes, thus confirming the viral presence. Unlike SSPE, MIBE is not associated with a hyperimmune antibody response to measles proteins and no oligoclonal bands are present (14).

DIAGNOSTIC APPROACH

The classic presentation has historically been used to make the clinical diagnosis of measles and is sufficient during outbreaks (35). Not all signs and symptoms are present, however, in every infected individual. The Centers for Disease Control and Prevention (CDC) recommends the following three criteria to diagnose measles based on symptoms: (*a*) generalized maculopapular rash lasting three or more days, (*b*) fever of at least 38.3°C, and (*c*) the presence of cough, coryza, or conjunctivitis (36).

The differential diagnosis is different during each stage of infection. The prodrome resembles the common cold, with fever additionally present in measles infection, and can be confused with influenza, adenovirus, dengue virus, or respiratory syncytial virus infection (17). The differential diagnosis during the exanthem includes mycoplasma pneumoniae, human herpes virus-6 (HHV-6) infection, Rocky Mountain spotted fever, rubella, scarlet fever, infectious mononucleosis, Kawasaki disease, toxic shock syndrome, dengue, drug eruption, and other causes of rash and fever (16,37). The intensity of the measles exanthem and the brown discoloration of the rash usually distinguish measles from erythema infectiosum, rubella, roseola infantum, and enterovirus infection (17).

The clinical diagnosis is most often confirmed by serology. The WHO global measles laboratory network uses IgM testing for diagnosis (38). In countries such as the United States where prevalence of measles is very low, this method often yields false–positive results. Therefore, in low-prevalence countries, a paired acute and convalescent sera for antimeasles IgG and IgM is recommended and should show a substantial increase in antimeasles IgG antibody concentration (35). IgM antibodies can be detected 72 hours after onset of the rash and up to 1 month after its resolution. IgG antibodies generally do not appear until 7 days after onset of the rash, and peak at 14 days (16).

In some cases, the presentation of measles differs from the classic clinical picture. In these cases, laboratory testing should be used to confirm the diagnosis. This is especially applicable in infants, who may still have transplacentally acquired immunoglobulins, or in adults who have previously received an inactivated measles vaccine. In this case, diagnosis during the prodrome or early exanthem (the time period where serologic testing cannot yet be done) can be attained through examination of exfoliated cells from pharynx, nasal and buccal mucosa, conjunctiva, or urinary tract by direct staining for epithelial giant cells or identification of measles antigens by immunofluorescence (1).

Another diagnostic method is cell culture of the virus. Measles virus can be isolated from urine, blood, throat, or nasopharyngeal secretions and cultured. This is not the method of choice, however, because it is difficult to isolate the virus outside of a specific time period (1 to 5 days after rash appearance) (35).

Viral isolates are sometimes genotyped, but not usually for diagnostic purposes. Viral genotyping of measles is principally used to determine if the virus originated endemically or was imported. Genome sequencing can also differentiate between wild-type and vaccine virus infection.

TREATMENT

Treatment for measles virus infection is supportive, because no standard antiviral therapy is available. Ribavirin is effective against measles virus *in vitro*, which has been given via the intravenous and aerosol routes to treat complicated measles cases in children and adults (34,39). No conclusive results regarding its efficacy are available, however, and ribavirin has not been approved by the US Food and Drug Administration (FDA) for treatment of measles (37).

Supportive measures include fluid replacement and treatment of cough and coryza. During the febrile period, activity is discouraged. Fluids should be administered to maintain hydration. Acetaminophen can help to control fever, and air humidification can improve symptoms of croup or other dry cough (17).

When bacterial superinfection occurs, antimicrobial therapy should be directed against the most likely agents, which are *Streptococcus pneumoniae, Haemophilus influenzae, Staphylococcus aureus,* and *Streptococcus pyogenes.* Therapy should be further selected based on Gram stain and culture of appropriate specimens. In young infants where sputum or smears are not obtainable, broad-spectrum antibiotics against the most likely pathogens should be used (1).

Vitamin A supplementation should be considered in immunocompromised children, children with vitamin A deficiency, and young children between 6 months and 2 years of age. Clinical studies in the United States indicate that vitamin A levels are low in many measles cases. Additionally, increased morbidity and mortality have been linked to vitamin A deficiency (40,41). The WHO recommends that vitamin A be given to measles-infected children in areas where mortality from measles >1% or where vitamin A deficiency is prevalent (42). Recommended is oral dosing of vitamin A is 100,000 IU for children 6 months to 1 year of age, and 200,000 IU for children 1 year of age and older (37).

Immunoglobulin treatment can be given as a prophylactic measure in susceptible persons (especially, pregnant women and infants) within 6 days of exposure. The recommended dose is 0.25 mL/kg body weight (maximal dose 15 mL) (1,17).

MEASLES ENCEPHALITIS

Treatment for primary measles encephalitis is largely supportive. This includes careful monitoring of the patient's fluid and electrolyte balance. Intravenous mannitol or other osmotically active agents are indicated in patients with severe cerebral edema. Seizures in encephalitis should be treated aggressively with anticonvulsants. Ribavirin is effective against measles virus *in vitro*. No controlled trials of ribavirin in primary measles encephalitis have been conducted, however, and ribavirin is not approved by the FDA for treatment of measles (37).

Treatment for measles-associated ADEM is based on the notion that this is a postinfectious disease and is immune mediated. Thus, the goal of treatment is not to eliminate virus, but to temper the immune response. Recommended treatments include intravenous corticosteroids, followed by oral corticosteroids, and administration of intravenous immunoglobulin (IVIG) (43).

SUBACUTE SCLEROSING PANENCEPHALITIS

No established effective therapy for SSPE is known. Over the course of the past decade, however, multiple case reports and uncontrolled studies have suggested that a combination of antiviral medications (ribavirin and inosine pranobex) and immunomodulators (interferon) may stabilize or reverse the disease in some patients (44–46). The FDA has added inosine pranobex to its list of orphan products designations and approvals for the treatment of SSPE. The myoclonic seizures that frequently accompany SSPE should be treated aggressively with anticonvulsants. Valproic acid and topiramate are commonly successful at containing myoclonic seizures.

CLINICAL RECOMMENDATIONS OF THE VIGNETTE

The, the Thai boy with SSPE, was initially treated with valproic acid in an attempt to control the myoclonic jerks. Valproic acid worsened, rather than improved, the movement disorder however. He was then treated with phenytoin, which did decrease the frequency of the drop attacks.

Over the course of the next several months, the boy's neurologic status rapidly deteriorated, and he became stuporous. Repeat MRI scan revealed marked diffuse cortical atrophy (Fig. 150-1) that had not been present on the initial study 3 months earlier. In addition, the white matter abnormalities that had been evident only unilaterally on the initial scan were bilateral on the follow-up scan. The patient died 1 week after an acute deterioration and 9 months after onset of initial symptoms.

It is likely that this patient was infected with measles during the first several years of life, when he lived in an orphanage in Thailand. The risk of SSPE is much greater when a child's measles infection occurs during the first 2 years of life than when it occurs later. Throughout his infancy and toddler years, this child lived in Thailand, where measles remains endemic and where immunizations are often nonprotective. Thus, this case highlights that, whereas measles has been virtually eliminated from the United States, the virus remains endemic throughout much of the developing world, where it continues to exact a heavy toll on human health and life.

SUMMARY

Measles is a highly communicable viral infection. Signs and symptoms in classic cases include fever, malaise, coryza, cough, conjunctivitis, a characteristic enanthem (Koplik's spots), and exanthem (maculopapules that spread to confluency). Complications from measles are common and often life-threatening. Pneumonia and encephalitis induced by measles infections are often severe and fatal. Subacute sclerosing panencephalitis is a dreaded delayed-onset complication of measles infection that leads to dementia, seizures, movement abnormalities, and death in most of its victims. The measles vaccine has substantially reduced the incidence of measles and SSPE in the United States and other developed countries. Measles and its complications, however, continue to pose major public health problems throughout much of the developing world.

REFERENCES

1. Gershon AA. Chickenpox, measles and mumps. In: Remington JS, Klein JO, eds. *Infectious Diseases of the Fetus & Newborn Infant.* Philadelphia: WB Saunders; 1995:565–618.
2. Bryce J, Boschi-Pinto C, Shibuya K, et al. WHO estimates of the causes of death in children. *Lancet.* 2005;365:1147–1152.
3. Murray CJ, Lopez AD. Mortality by cause for eight regions of the world: Global burden of disease study. *Lancet.* 1997;349(9061):1269–1276.
4. Enders G. Paramyxoviruses. In: Baron S, ed. *Medical Microbiology.* Galveston, TX: University of Texas Medical Branch; 1996.
5. Kempe H, Fulginiti VA. The pathogenesis of measles virus infection. *Arch Gesamte Virusforsch.* 1965;16:103–128.
6. Hutchins S, Markowitz L, Atkinson W, et al. Measles outbreaks in the United States, 1987 through 1990. *Pediatr Infect Dis J.* 1996;15:31–38.
7. Yip FY, Papania MJ, Redd SB. Measles outbreak epidemiology in the United States, 1993–2001. *J Infect Dis.* 2004;189[Suppl 1]:S54–S60.
8. Parker AA, Staggs W, Dayan GH, et al. Implications of a 2005 measles outbreak in Indiana for sustained elimination of measles in the United States. *N Engl J Med.* 2006;355:447–455.
9. MMWR Centers for Disease Control and Prevention (CDC). Measles—United States, 1999. *MMWR Morb Mortal Wkly Rep.* 2000;49(25):557–560.
10. Katz SL, Hinman AR. Summary and conclusions: Measles elimination meeting 16–17 March 2000. *J Infect Dis.* 2004;189[Suppl]:s43–s47.
11. Shiff, GM. Rubeola (measles) and subacute sclerosing panencephalitis virus. In: Gorbach JL, Bartlett JG, Blacklow NR, eds. *Infectious Diseases.* Philadelphia: WB Saunders; 2004: 2018–2022.
12. Perry RT, Halsey NA. The clinical significance of measles: A review. *J Infect Dis.* 2004;189[Supp 1]s4–s16.
13. Asher AM. Slow viral infections of the central nervous system. In: Gorbach SL, Bartlett JG, Blacklow NR, eds. *Infectious Diseases.* Philadelphia: WB Saunders; 2004:1320–1332.
14. Ota MO, Moss WJ, Griffin DE. Emerging diseases: Measles. *J Neurovirol.* 2005;11:447–454.
15. Rima BK, Duprex WP. Morbilliviruses and human disease. *J Pathol.* 2006;208:199–214.
16. Griffin D. Measles virus. In: Knipe DM, Howel PM, eds. *Fields Virology*, 4th ed. Philadelphia: Lippincott Williams & Wilkins; 2001:1401–1441.
17. Cherry JD. Measles virus. In: Feigin RD, Bherry RD, eds. *Textbook of Pediatric Infectious Diseases.* Philadelphia: WB Saunders; 2004:2283–2304.
18. Moroi K, Saito S, Kurata T, et al. Fetal death associated with measles virus infection of the placenta. *Am J Obstet Gynecol.* 1991;164:1107.
19. Bonthius DJ, Karacay B. Meningitis and encephalitis in children. An update. *Neurology Clinics of North America.* 2002;20:1013–1038.
20. Hosoya M. Measles encephalitis: Direct viral invasion or autoimmune-mediated inflammation? *Intern Med.* 2006;45:841–842.
21. Jin K, Sato S, Saito R, et al. MRI findings from a case of fulminating adult-onset measles encephalitis. *Intern Med.* 2006;45:783–787.
22. Gendelman HE, Wolinsky JS, Johnson RT, et. al. Measles encephalomyelitis: Lack of evidence of viral invasion of the central nervous system and quantitative study of the nature of demyelination. *Ann Neurol.* 1984;15:353–360.
23. Rima BK, Duprex WP. Molecular mechanisms of measles virus persistence. *Virus Res.* 2005;111:132–146.
24. Murthy SN, Faden HS, Cohen ME, et al. Acute disseminated encephalomyelitis in children. *Pediatrics.* 2002;110(2 Pt1):e1–e7.
25. Kaneko M, Yamashita Y, Nagamitsu S, et al. Severe infantile measles encephalitis occurred three months after neonatal measles. *Neuropediatrics.* 2002;33:274–277.
26. MMWR. Subacute sclerosing panencephalitis surveillance—Unites States. *MMWR Morb Mortal Wkly Rep.* 1982;31:585.
27. Bellini WJ, Rota JS, Lowe LE, et al. Subacute sclerosing panencephalitis: More cases of this fatal disease are prevented by measles immunization than was previously recognized. *J Infect Dis.* 2005;192:1686–1693.
28. Bonthius DJ, Stanek N, Grose C. Subacute sclerosing panencephalitis, a measles complication, in an internationally adopted child. *Emerg Infect Dis.* 2000;6:377–381.
29. Ornoy A, Tenenbaum A. Pregnancy outcome following infections by coxsackie, echo, measles, mumps, hepatitis, polio and encephalitis viruses. *Reprod Toxicol.* 2006;21:446–457.
30. Kaplan LJ, Daum RS, Smaron M, et al. Severe measles in immunocompromised patients. *JAMA.* 1992;267:1237.
31. Colamaria V, Marradi P, Merlin D, et al. Acute measles encephalitis of the delayed type in an immunosuppressed child. *Brain Dev.* 1989;11:322–326.
32. Poon TP, Tchertkoff V, Win H. Subacute measles encephalitis with AIDS diagnosed by fine needle aspiration biopsy. A case report. *Acta Cytol.* 1998;42:729–733.
33. Bitnum A, Shannon P, Durward A, et al. Measles inclusion-body encephalitis caused by the vaccine strain of measles virus. *Clin Infect Dis.* 1999;29:855–861.
34. Mustafa MM, Weitman SD, Winick NJ, et al. Subacute measles encephalitis in the young immunocompromised host: Report of two cases diagnosed by polymerase chain reaction and treated with ribavirin and review of the literature. *Clin Infect Dis.* 1993;16:654–660.
35. Gellini WJ, Helfand RF. The challenges and strategies for laboratory diagnosis of measles in an international setting. *J Infect Dis.* 2003;187[Suppl 1]:s283.
36. Centers for Disease Control. Classification of measles cases and categorization of measles elimination program. *MMWR Morb Mortal Wkly Rep.* 1983;31:707–711.
37. American Academy of Pediatrics. Measles. In: Pickering LK, Baker CJ, Long SS, et al. eds. *Red Book: 2006 Report of the Committee on Infectious Diseases*, 27th ed. Elk Grove Village, IL: American Academy of Pediatrics; 2006:441–452.
38. Featherstone D, Brown D, Sanders R. Development of the global measles laboratory network. *J Infect Dis.* 2003;187[Suppl 1]:s264.
39. Forni AL, Schluger NW, Roberts RB. Severe measles pneumonitis in adults: Evaluation of clinical characteristics and therapy with intravenous ribavirin. *Clin Infect Dis.* 1994;19:454–462.
40. Frieden TR, Sowell AL, Henning KJ, et al. Vitamin A levels and severity of measles. New York City. *Am J Dis Child.* 1992;146:182–186.
41. Barclay AJ, Foster A, Sommer A. Vitamin A supplements and mortality related to measles: A randomised clinical trial. *BMJ.* 1987;294:194–196.
42. WHO and UNICEF. Expanded Programme on Immunization. Joint WHO/UNICEF statement on vitamin A for measles. *Wkly Epidemiol Rec.* 1987;62:133–134.
43. Banwell BL. Acquired demyelination of the central nervous system. In: Maria B, ed. *Current Management in Child Neurology*, 3rd ed. London: BC Decker; 2005:486–493.
44. Anlar B, Aydin OF, Guven A, et al. Retrospective evaluation of interferon-beta treatment in subacute sclerosing panencephalitis. *Clin Ther.* 2004;26:1890–1894.
45. Solomon T, Hart CA, Vinjamuri S, et al. Treatment of subacute sclerosing panencephalitis with interferon-alpha, ribavirin, and inosiplex. *J Child Neurol.* 2002;17:703–705.
46. Gascon GG, and International Consortium on Subacute Sclerosing Panencephalitis. Randomized treatment study of inosiplex versus combined inosiplex and intraventricular interferon-alpha in subacute sclerosing panencephalitis (SSPE): International multicenter study. *J Child Neurol.* 2003;18:819–827.

CHAPTER **151**

Mumps

Wendy L. Hobson-Rohrer • James F. Bale, Jr.

OBJECTIVES

- To discuss the epidemiology of mumps virus infection
- To describe the clinical manifestations of mumps virus infection
- To explain the application of appropriate diagnostic methods to detect mumps virus
- To explore the management of mumps virus infections of the nervous system

CASE VIGNETTE

A 15-year-old boy experienced the gradual onset of malaise, anorexia, and low-grade fever. Ear pain and swelling of the parotid gland ensued. Seven days after the illness began, he had the abrupt onset of headache, vomiting, back pain, and stiff neck. On neurologic examination, he had positive Kernig and Brudzinski signs. Cerebrospinal fluid (CSF) examination revealed a white blood cell (WBC) count of 58/μL (all lymphocytes), glucose of 45 mg/dL, and protein of 63 mg/dL. Brain magnetic resonance imaging (MRI) study findings were normal. During the subsequent 5 days, vomiting and headache subsided and, in 2 weeks, the boy returned to school. He recovered completely.

DEFINITION

Mumps virus, a member of the RNA paramyxovirus family (*Paramyxoviridae*), causes systemic infections and, occasionally, neurologic disease in children or adults.

EPIDEMIOLOGY, ETIOLOGY, AND PATHOGENESIS

Mumps virus, previously a major cause of meningitis and mild encephalitis worldwide, accounted for as many as 30% of the cases of aseptic meningitis and encephalitis in the United States before licensure of the mumps vaccine in the 1960s (1). In the prevaccine era, the annual incidence of mumps infection was as high as 2,000 cases per 100,000 population in the United States; mumps remains a serious concern in many regions of the world (2). Periodic resurgences in the United States and other developed countries with vaccination programs indicate that a substantial proportion of the population remains vulnerable to mumps virus infection (3–5).

Mumps virus infections peak in winter and early spring, although cases can occur year round. The virus spreads through person-to-person contact. During the prevaccine era epidemics, most persons with mumps were young, school-aged children, but recent outbreaks have affected persons in their teens or beyond (6). Infected persons shed the virus in saliva and upper respiratory secretions and transmit the virus to others through respiratory droplets or fomites. Aseptic meningitis and encephalitis develop in as many as 10% and 0.3% of persons with mumps parotitis, respectively (2,6,7). Infected persons experience viremia that disseminates the virus to many tissues, including the salivary glands, testes, liver, pancreas, and, occasionally, the brain. At least one third of mumps virus infections occur without symptoms.

CLINICAL MANIFESTATIONS

After an incubation period of approximately 2 weeks, children or adults with mumps experience low-grade fever, anorexia, malaise, and headache (2,6). Thereafter, parotitis, the cardinal manifestation of mumps, appears, causing parotid gland enlargement, earache, and facial tenderness; fever can be as high as 40ºC. Other systemic features of mumps include orchitis, epididymitis, prostatitis, oophoritis, hepatitis, pancreatitis, or thyroiditis. Mumps virus-induced aseptic meningitis or mild encephalitis usually appears 3 to 14 days after onset of parotitis, often after fever and parotitis resolve (2,6,7). Central nervous system (CNS) features can be concurrent with, or occur before, parotitis, and many patients with mumps aseptic meningitis have no history of parotid gland swelling. Signs of aseptic meningitis, consisting of headache, photophobia, meningismus, and somnolence, tend to begin abruptly (7). Signs of mumps encephalitis include seizures, focal deficits (e.g., aphasia), irritability, or motor deficits, including polymyelitis-like paralysis (8). Patients with encephalitis are more often male.

DIAGNOSTIC APPROACH

Infection can be confirmed by detecting mumps virus in saliva, throat washings, urine, or CSF, or by detecting mumps virus-specific IgM in serum (6). Mumps virus RNA can be detected by reverse transcription (RT) polymerase chain reaction (PCR), indicating a role for PCR in atypical cases or cases lacking parotitis. The CSF features of mumps meningitis or encephalitis are nonspecific, consisting of a lymphocytic pleocytosis (<100 to >1,000 cells/uL), normal or mildly elevated protein content, or normal or mildly depressed glucose content (2,7).

TREATMENT AND PROGNOSIS

Treatment consists of support care. Anticonvulsants are necessary should seizures ensue. Patients with CNS mumps usually recover completely in 5 to 10 days; sequelae are uncommon. Patients, however, can have permanent sensorineural hearing loss, optic atrophy, facial paresis, or behavioral abnormalities. Rates of sensorineural hearing loss after mumps have ranged from 4% to as high as 36% (2). Rarely, hydrocephalus develops as late sequelae of ependymitis and aqueductal obstruction (9).

CLINICAL RECOMMENDATIONS OF THE VIGNETTE

In the United States and other nations with compulsory immunization for mumps, mumps is a rare cause of aseptic meningitis or encephalitis. As the mumps resurgence of 2006 in the United States illustrated, many persons remain susceptible to mumps virus infection and its complications (4). In this 15-year-old boy, other common causes of aseptic meningitis, such as the nonpolio enteroviruses, deserve consideration. As with mumps, enteroviral meningitis requires supportive care only. If this adolescent had experienced seizures, however, he would have required CSF PCR for herpes simplex virus (HSV) type 1 and empiric acyclovir therapy and evaluation by MRI. If the HSV PCR result was negative and studies confirmed mumps virus infection, acyclovir could be discontinued. No data describe a role for acylovir or other antiviral medications in mumps virus infections. Corticosteroids can be considered in rare cases of encephalomyelitis with spinal cord involvement.

The association of parotitis and neurologic symptoms suggests mumps virus, a condition that should be considered strongly in nonimmunized persons or during periodic outbreaks. Management consists primarily of supportive care, and most affected persons recover completely.

SUMMARY

Although mumps virus infections are uncommon in regions with compulsory immunization programs, recent US outbreaks confirm that large segments of the population remain susceptible to infection. Most infected persons recover without sequelae.

REFERENCES

1. CDC. Mumps surveillance, January 1977–1982. Public Health Service, 1984.
2. Galazka AM, Robertson SE, Kraigher A. Mumps and mumps vaccine: A global review. *Bull WHO.* 1999;77:3–14.
3. Cochi SL, Perblud SR, Orenstein WA. Perspectives on the relative resurgence of mumps in the United States. *Am J Dis Child.* 1988;142:499–507.
4. Waxman MA, Abrahamian FM, Talan DM, et al. Update on emerging infections from the Centers for Disease Control and Prevention. Multistate outbreak of mumps—United States, January 1–May 2, 2006. *Ann Emerg Med.* 2006;48:332–335.
5. Mackenzie DG, Craig G, Hallam NF, et al. Mumps in a boarding school: Description of an outbreak and control measures. *Br J Gen Pract.* 2006;56:526–529.
6. American Academy of Pediatrics. Mumps. In: Pickering LK, Baker CJ, Long SS, et al., eds. *Red Book: 2006 Report of the Committee on Infectious Diseases,* 27th ed. Elk Grove Village, IL: American Academy of Pediatrics; 2006:464–468.
7. McLean DM, Larke RPB, Cobb C, et al. Mumps and enteroviral meningitis in Toronto, 1966. *Can Med Assoc J.* 1967;96:1355–1361.
8. Thomas FB, Perkins RL, Saslaw S. Paralytic mumps virus infection in two sisters. *Ann Intern Med.* 1968;121:45–49.
9. Bray PF. Mumps: A cause of hydrocephalus? *Pediatrics.* 1972;49:446–449.

CHAPTER 152

Rubella

Amanda Snodgrass • Charlotte T. Jones

OBJECTIVES

- To describe the clinical symptoms of rubella, both congenital rubella syndrome (CRS) and postnatally acquired rubella
- To explain the neurologic complications associated with rubella, including encephalitis and progressive panencephalitis
- To discuss the diagnostic and treatment strategies of rubella
- To highlight the importance of rubella vaccination

CASE VIGNETTE

The patient was born at 39 weeks to a 29-year-old G1 mother who received no prenatal care. He is microcephalic and small for gestational age. On physical examination, he is found to have purpuric skin lesions, bilateral cloudy corneas, and hepatosplenomegaly. He also has a cardiac murmur. Echocardiogram reveals a patent ductus arteriosus.

DEFINITION

Rubella generally is a mild, exanthematous, infectious illness that was first grouped with other clinically similar diseases such as measles and scarlet fever. It was described, however, as a distinct entity in the early 19th century by two German physicians and, thus, is sometimes referred to as *German measles.* Once acquired, the virus has minimal morbidity and mortality. Rubella became especially significant in 1941, however, when Australian ophthalmologist Normal McAlister Gregg reported congenital cataracts in babies born to mothers who had rubella during early pregnancy. This was the first recognition of congenital rubella syndrome (CRS).

EPIDEMIOLOGY

Acquired rubella is transmitted through direct or droplet contact from nasopharyngeal secretions. A peak incidence occurs in late winter and early spring, with the largest number of cases in the United States being in March, April, and May. Maximal viral shedding and, therefore, maximal transmissibility, extends from a few days before to 7 days after the onset of the rash. Rubella virus, however, has been found in nasopharyngeal secretions from 7 days before to 14 days after onset of the rash. Some infants with congenital rubella can shed the virus in nasopharyngeal secretions and urine for a year or more, making it possible for them to transmit the virus for an extended period. The incubation period for acquired rubella is approximately 16 to 18 days (1). Persons infected with rubella generally have lifelong immunity against clinical illness, but asymptomatic and symptomatic reinfection can occur. This reinfection has rarely resulted in congenital rubella (2).

Damage to the fetus from maternal rubella infection is directly correlated with the time in gestation in which the mother is infected. Infection in the first 12 weeks of pregnancy is the time most detrimental to the fetus, with as many as 90% infected and most of these symptomatic (3). Maternal infection during or after the fourth month of gestation has a much lower rate of fetal infection, as low as 5%, however, and, of those infected, the damage is much less severe (2).

Before widespread implementation of vaccine, rubella had an epidemic cycle with 6- to 9-year intervals. The last epidemic in the United States was 1964–1965, with as many as 20,000 cases of congenital rubella. Congenital rubella was not a reportable disease until 1966, so these numbers are not complete (1). The incidence of rubella has decreased by 99% in the United States since the prevaccine era. Outbreaks still occur, however, particularly on college campuses and in prisons, hospitals, office settings, and among the Amish. In fact, approximately 10% of the adolescent and young adult population in the United States remains susceptible to rubella. Some immigrant populations may have an even higher ratio of those susceptible, particularly adolescent and adult males from Latin America (2).

ETIOLOGY AND PATHOGENESIS

Rubella is in the *Rubivirus* genus of the *Togaviridae* family. It is an enveloped, positive-stranded RNA virus with only one antigenic type, and humans are the only known host (4). Rubella is transmitted from person-to-person through respiratory droplets, with the primary site of infection being the respiratory epithelium (1). The virus replicates in the nasopharynx and regional lymph nodes. A viremia occurs 5 to 7 days after exposure, with subsequent spread throughout the body, with resultant macular rash. Transmission from mother to fetus occurs during viremia when the infection crosses the placenta (4). When maternal infection occurs in the first trimester, placental infection regularly occurs and often persists throughout the remainder of pregnancy (1). Fetal damage occurs via destruction of cells and mitotic arrest (4). In addition to nasopharyngeal secretions, rubella virus has been recovered from serum, lymph nodes, urine, cerebrospinal fluid (CSF), conjunctival sac, breast milk, synovial fluid and lungs, and from skin at sites with and without rash (1).

PATHOLOGY

Few data are available regarding histologic findings in uncomplicated, postnatally acquired rubella. Extensive data, however is available on the gross and microscopic findings in congenital rubella. The damage from CRS is widespread and can include nearly all organ systems. These defects result from specific cell damage, as well as cellular deficiency. Also of great importance is the subsequent generalized vascular damage. In addition, there is a noncytolytic cellular infection, which results in mitotic arrest and a reduction of total number of cells in many organs (1). Neuropathologic findings include parenchymal lesions, delayed myelination, and intracranial calcifications (11). The parenchymal lesions are a result of extensive vascular damage with mineralization and intima proliferation, leading to small foci of necrosis. Except for visualizing calcifications, MRI is more sensitive than computed tomography (CT) in detecting these lesions (6).

CLINICAL MANIFESTATIONS

POSTNATALLY ACQUIRED RUBELLA

Postnatally acquired rubella is a relatively mild disease, and 30% to 50% of cases are subclinical or even asymptomatic (4). Common symptoms, when present, include a generalized erythematous maculopapular rash, lymphadenopathy, a low-grade fever, malaise; other symptoms resemble an upper respiratory infection. The lymphadenopathy is often in the suboccipital, postauricular, and cervical regions, and it can appear 1 week before the rash and last for several weeks after the rash is gone (2,4). The rash usually begins on the face and then spreads centrifugally from head to hands and feet, lasting approximately 3 days (4). The rash is sometimes pruritic, more often in adults than children. It can be confused with acne on the adolescent's face (1). As compared with the rash of measles, the rash of rubella is fainter and does not coalesce. In children, the rash is typically the only symptom. Adolescents and adults, particularly females, can experience the additional abovementioned symptoms in a prodrome for 1 to 5 days preceding the onset of the rash. Other less-common symptoms reported in rubella include conjunctivitis, testalgia, and orchitis. Forschheimer spots, small reddish spots on the soft palate, may appear on the soft palate (4).

Complications of acquired rubella include joint involvement, thrombocytopenia, and neurologic manifestations (2,4). Arthritis or arthralgia are rare in children and adult males with rubella, but are common in infected adult women, up to 70%, that they are considered by many to be a feature of the disease rather than a complication. The joints of the fingers, wrists, and knees are those commonly affected. The onset of these symptoms usually coincides with the onset of the rash and can last up to 1 month. Chronic arthritis secondary to rubella infection is rare (4).

Hemorrhagic manifestations, namely thrombocytopenic purpura, occur in approximately 1 of 3,000 cases of rubella. Gastrointestinal, cerebral, or intrarenal hemorrhage can occur (1,4). The average time of onset of purpura is 4 days after the onset of the rash, but it can occur anytime from the appearance of the rash to up to 2 weeks later. This manifestation is usually self-limited, and can last anywhere from a few days to several weeks or months. Most patients recover from this complication (1).

Neurologic complications of rubella are rare and include encephalitis, peripheral neuritis, and progressive panencephalitis. Polyradiculoneuritis and Guillain-Barré syndrome have also been reported, but very rarely (7,8). The most common of these neurologic complications is postinfectious encephalomyelitis, which occurs in approximately 1 of 5,000 to 6,000 cases of rubella, more frequently in adult females (1,4,7,9). It clinically resembles the encephalitis secondary to measles virus, although that of rubella is thought to be less severe (1). Rubella is certainly associated with morbidity and mortality. Because of the case-oriented nature of studies, it is difficult, however, to cite the true proportion of patients who experience morbidity or mortality. Case series of very small numbers of patients have reported between 0 and 50% mortality (8).

The onset of encephalitis usually occurs from 4 to 6 days after the onset of the rash, but can arise up to 2 weeks after the rash appears (1,9,10). Symptoms vary and can arise gradually or abruptly. They can include headache, vomiting, lethargy, dizziness, stiff neck, ataxia, and generalized or focal seizures. Patients can present with varying levels of consciousness, behavioral alterations, delirium, or coma (9–11). CSF evaluation reveals a mild pleocytosis, predominately lymphocytes, with normal to slightly elevated protein and normal glucose and chloride. CSF pressure is generally within the normal limits (9,11). Electroencephalogram (EEG) reveals slow wave activity, which can be diffuse or localized and persist long after recovery (10–12). Prognosis overall is good, with as many as 75% recovering normal function and intellectual ability, usually within 2 to 3 weeks (11). Coma and convulsions are poor prognostic indicators. In the fatal cases, death usually occurs within 3 days of the onset of encephalitis (9,12).

With few fatal cases of rubella encephalitis and, therefore, few postmortem reports, pathologic findings are not well reported or understood. The few autopsies performed have revealed cerebral edema, diffuse nonspecific neural degeneration, and perivascular infiltrates of lymphocytes and plasma cells. Of note, demyelination has not been found, which is in contrast to the otherwise similar encephalopathy associated with measles. This may be because of the rapid progression to death before demyelination becomes evident (9–11). Progressive rubella panencephalitis can also occur and is described in detail in the following section with the neurologic manifestations of congenital rubella.

CONGENITAL RUBELLA SYNDROME (CRS)

When a woman contracts the virus early in pregnancy, it can lead to miscarriage, fetal death, or a number of congenital anomalies referred to as *congenital rubella syndrome.* Some babies do escape with little to no anomalies, however, and the degree of damage to the fetus is strongly related to the time in gestation at which the mother contracts the illness. Infection before the 12th week of gestation yields nearly a 90% risk of CRS, whereas infection after the 24th week is usually benign (3).

Congenital infection with rubella can involve virtually any organ system. Some of these are obvious anomalies from the time of birth, whereas others may not be present until the second or third decade of life. The most common manifestation of CRS apparent at birth is generalized growth retardation, with over half being small for gestational age. Sometimes, this growth delay continues throughout life, leading to severe failure to thrive. Other anomalies and processes that may be apparent at birth include microcephaly, thrombocytopenia, encephalitis, and hepatitis (1).

The most frequent anomalies in CRS are auditory, ophthalmologic, cardiac, and neurologic. Deafness is the most common manifestation, with almost all patients having some degree of hearing impairment (1). In fact, it is often the only expression of the disease, especially if infection occurred after the fourth month of gestation (4). Patients display sensorineural hearing loss, which is often progressive, secondary to damage to the organ of Corti (5). Hearing loss is usually bilateral, but it can be unilateral. This finding is missed at times, especially if the child otherwise appears asymptomatic. This can lead to a child being mislabeled as mentally retarded (1).

Ophthalmologic findings in CRS include cataracts, microphthalmia, retinopathy, and congenital glaucoma (1,4). Approximately one third of patients with CRS will have cataracts, and most are apparent at birth. Some are not obvious until later in infancy. Cataracts can be unilateral or bilateral, and either diffuse or central with a surrounding clear zone.

Microphthalmia is typically unilateral and is much less common. When it does occur, it is usually associated with cataracts. Retinopathy also affects about one third of patients with CRS, and consists of pigmentary defects. It rarely affects visual acuity, however. Congenital glaucoma occurs only in approximately 5% of patients with CRS, but it is imperative that this defect be recognized early to preserve sight (1).

The most common cardiac defects associated with CRS, in descending order of frequency, include patent ductus arteriosus, pulmonary artery stenosis, and pulmonary valvular stenosis. Ventricular septal defect and coarctation of the aorta can also occur (4). In severe CRS, myocarditis may be present, and may actually be the cause of death (1).

Neurologic findings associated with CRS include meningoencephalitis, microcephaly, behavioral disorders, and mental retardation. Some older children and adolescents with CRS have developed a rubella-associated progressive panencephalitis (5). Some speculations exist of an association with schizophrenialike symptoms in adults with CRS (11,13). Some symptoms, such as lethargy, irritability, and motor retardation, are apparent at birth, whereas others do not manifest until development progresses. These latter symptoms include mental retardation, motor disabilities, abnormal posture and movements, and seizures (11).

The most prominent pathologic lesion in CRS brains is tissue damage with microcalcifications or ischemic necrosis, which is secondary to obstructive vasculopathy (14). Neuroimaging studies are often abnormal, with intracranial calcifications, delayed myelination, and ventriculitis. CSF of the newborn with CRS reveals mild pleocytosis and elevated protein (5).

Of infants with CRS, 10% to 29% may have active meningoencephalitis at birth, with positive examination findings of full anterior fontanelle, irritability, hypotonia, seizures, lethargy, and head retraction and arching of the back. The severity and persistence of this meningoencephalitis correlates with subsequent mental and motor retardation. The incidence of true microcephaly is rare, but those children have a poor prognosis for normal mental development (1).

Microcephaly follows suit with the nature of rubella, which is a tendency of affected organs to be small because of a decrease in the total number of cells (11). Positive findings on imaging studies, including enlargement of lateral ventricles, reduced gray matter, intracranial calcification, and linear hyperechogenicity in the basal ganglia region, may predict microcephaly (7). Approximately 10% to 20% of children with CRS have behavioral disorders. This does not seem to be related to meningoencephalitis, but can be common in deaf children. Some degree of mental retardation in found in 10% to 20% of children with CRS (1).

Additional complications of CRS include radiolucent bone disease, which primarily affects the metaphyses of long bones, and is present in as many as 10% to 20% of babies with CRS (1). Thrombocytopenia is found in 5% to 10%, whereas another 5% to 10% experience extramedullary hematopoiesis. The latter expresses itself as a purpuric rash described as a "blueberry muffin" appearance. This is mainly associated with severe disease and has a poor prognosis. Approximately 10% to 20% will have hepatosplenomegaly. Some will appear jaundiced, with a predominately direct hyperbilirubinemia. They may also be in respiratory distress from the ongoing viral process in the lungs, and perhaps secondary to myocarditis (1).

Some effects of CRS have a delayed onset, as late as the second or third decade of life. These can include hearing loss, ocular damage, vascular effects, progressive rubella panencephalitis, and endocrinopathies (e.g., diabetes mellitus and thyroid dysfunction) (1,15). Insulin-dependent diabetes mellitus is the most common delayed manifestation of CRS, with approximately 20% of patients affected by the third decade (7,15).

PROGRESSIVE RUBELLA PANENCEPHALITIS

Progressive rubella panencephalitis (PRP), which can result from either congenitally or postnatally acquired rubella infection, was first described in 1975 (16,17). It is pathologically and clinically similar to the subacute sclerosing panencephalitis (SSPE) associated with measles virus. PRP was first documented in adolescent patients with CRS, but has since been reported in postnatally acquired rubella (11). This sequela of rubella is caused by persistence of the virus in the brain and is uniformly fatal. It usually presents in the second decade of life and progresses over 8 to10 years. It is clinically and pathologically distinct from the acute encephalitis that can occur with onset of rubella (15).

Initial symptoms of PRP include intellectual decline, behavioral changes, and ataxia. As the disease progresses over the next several years, symptoms evolve to include seizures, spasticity, dysarthria, nystagmus, and truncal and limb ataxia. These patients demonstrate a slow neurologic degeneration (5,15). Of note, the early cerebellar symptoms and the absence of myoclonus in PRP help to distinguish it from SSPE (19).

CSF evaluation in PRP reveals elevated protein, which is predominantly caused by oligoclonal production of rubella-specific IgG antibodies. A high CSF-to-serum ratio of this antibody is seen, suggesting intrathecal production (10,15,18). Rubella-specific immune complexes have been detected in serum, and rubella virus has been isolated from brain tissue and circulating lymphocytes by cocultivation (15,18). More recently, reverse transcriptase polymerase chain reaction (RT-PCR) has become available for diagnosis and epidemiologic studies of rubella. In fact, rubella RNA has been detected in amniotic fluid by RT-PCR, with a sensitivity as high as 87% to 100%. It has also been detected in lens aspirates and oral fluid of infected persons (7). Neuropathologic changes in PRP include dilation of the lateral ventricles and extensive destruction of white matter. Grossly, the white matter becomes mottled to grayish in color and gelatinous in consistency, whereas microscopically, loss of myelin and severe gliosis are noted. Neuronal loss can be widespread, with near complete destruction of Purkinje cells. Immunoglobulin deposits are found in blood vessels and subacute to chronic inflammatory change seen in the leptomeninges, perivascular cuffs, and throughout the parenchyma (11,18). Pathogenesis of PRP, as with other neurologic consequences of rubella, remains poorly understood, but this evidence suggests an immunologic etiology.

DIAGNOSTIC APPROACH

DIFFERENTIAL DIAGNOSIS

Because no pathognomonic finding in acquired rubella exist, it is important to gather a complete history. With the high clinical expression rate of exanthem, it is unusual not to have a contact case or other known cases in the community. Also, the incubation period of rubella is long, approximately 18 days, as opposed to 3 to 7 days in common enteroviruses and respiratory viruses. A fever >38.5°C (101.5°F) is unusual in rubella, but common in enteroviral exanthems, measles, and *Mycoplasma pneumoniae infections.* The age of the patient is significant because rubella is now most common in the adolescent and young adult population. Season is also important to consider, because rubella is common in winter and early spring. On the other hand, enteroviral exanthems, which are the greatest impersonators of rubella in young children, are found in the summer and fall (1).

The suboccipital and posterior auricular lymphadenopathy in rubella has been considered by some to be pathognomonic. Such lymphadenopathy, however, is actually common with enteroviral illnesses in young children. Because enteroviral illnesses are less overwhelming in adolescents and adults, this lymphadenopathy bears more significance. Still, the differential diagnosis for such lymphadenopathy must include acquired toxoplasmosis, infectious mononucleosis, and *M. pneumoniae* infection (1).

Congenital rubella should be included in the differential diagnosis of any baby born with intrauterine growth retardation without known reason or with stigmata suggestive of CRS. Immediate virologic and serologic studies should be performed for rubella and other infectious agents. Babies born following maternal infection should be tested and followed up periodically, even if the child is seemingly normal, because deafness and subtle neurologic defects are sometimes missed (1).

DEFINITIVE DIAGNOSIS

Because many illnesses that exhibit a rash can mimic rubella, and as many as half of all cases of rubella may be subclinical, the only reliable proof of acute rubella infection is serologic or virologic evidence. This can include the presence of rubella-specific IgM antibody, a significant rise in IgG antibody from paired acute and convalescent sera, or a positive viral culture for rubella (4).

Serology is the most common route of confirmation of rubella infection. When a case is suspected, serum should be collected as soon as possible and checked for the presence of rubella IgM. A sample should also be held and measured concurrently with convalescent titers drawn 14 to 21 days later (4). Seroconversion or a rise of rubella IgG of fourfold or greater indicates recent infection (2). A neonate can have rubella IgG simply from transplacental passage of maternal IgG. Postnatal persistence of rubella-specific IgG beyond 6 to 12 months, however, confirms the diagnosis of congenital rubella (5). Serum rubella IgM tests can yield false–positive findings in the presence of parvovirus, with a positive heterophile test for infectious mononucleosis, or with a positive rheumatoid factor (4).

Enzyme-linked immunosorbent assays (ELISA) is currently the most commonly used technique for detecting rubella antibodies. It is highly sensitive and specific, and it is widely available and relatively easy to perform. It can also be modified to measure IgM antibodies. ELISA has replaced the hemagglutination inhibition (HI) test, which was formerly the standard test. Although HI is also sensitive and specific, quickness and simplicity make ELISA the test of choice (4).

Rubella virus can be isolated from nasopharyngeal, blood, urine, CSF, and throat swab specimens in both acquired and congenital rubella. Virus can be detected in acquired rubella from 1 week before until 2 weeks after the onset of the rash, and can be detected for a year or more in congenitally infected infants. Although isolation of the virus is diagnostic, these cultures are labor intensive and, therefore, not performed in many laboratories. Viral isolation, however, is a valuable tool in epidemiologic studies and should be attempted (13).

Other tests that may suggest congenital rubella infection include direct hyperbilirubinemia, elevated serum transaminases, and thrombocytopenia (3). Also in CRS, imaging studies may reveal cerebral atrophy, intracranial calcifications, periventricular leukomalacia, or subependymal cystic lesions (3,19).

TREATMENT

POSTNATALLY ACQUIRED RUBELLA

In uncomplicated postnatally acquired cases of rubella, no specific treatment is necessary. However, patients may benefit from starch baths for pruritus and aspirin for arthritis. Even with complications such as encephalitis and thrombocytopenia, care is still supportive. Management of encephalitis should include maintenance of fluids and electrolytes, and although thrombocytopenia is usually self-limited, severe bleeding may occur. In this case, intravenous immunoglobulin should be considered (1).

CONGENITAL RUBELLA SYNDROME

As with postnatally acquired rubella, the treatment for congenital rubella is predominately supportive. The clinical manifestations of CRS are varied, and some babies may even initially appear asymptomatic. Other neonates, however, may have several severe complications from birth, including pneumonia, thrombocytopenia, eye findings, heart defects, hyperbilirubinemia, and hepatosplenomegaly. Respiratory distress is caused by damage from the persistent viral infection and should be managed as is other neonatal respiratory disease with assisted ventilation, as needed. Thrombocytopenia can yield severe purpura and petechiae, but true hemorrhagic emergencies are uncommon. In such a case, corticosteroid therapy is not indicated, but intravenous immunoglobulin may be considered. Eye findings in neonates with CRS may include corneal clouding, suggesting infantile glaucoma. This finding necessitates immediate referral to an ophthalmologist. Cataracts and retinopathy may also be present, but these can be treated later. Management of cardiac findings and hyperbilirubinemia should be no different than in neonates without rubella. Hepatosplenomegaly is marked at times, but is of no therapeutic concern (1).

Neonates with CRS who survive the newborn period have high rates of sequelae affecting the cardiovascular, neurologic, and endocrine systems, as well as vision and hearing. Some of these, including diabetes mellitus, are not even apparent until the second or third decade of life. Other delayed sequelae that should be monitored include thyroid dysfunction and growth hormone deficiency (3,19). Progressive sensorineural hearing loss can develop, so those with known or even suspected CRS should have serial audiometry (19). Hearing disability is the most frequent and many times the only clinical manifestation of congenital rubella, so deafness in a child who had suspected CRS but was clinically asymptomatic at birth can be missed. Once identified, a child with hearing disability should be enrolled in an education program before or during the second year of life, and also be fitted for appropriate auditory amplification devices. No child with CRS should be labeled mentally retarded until a complete audiologic evaluation has been performed (1).

As stated above, the eye finding warranting the most immediate concern is glaucoma. The child should also be watched, however, for cataracts, retinopathy, and strabismus. These are treated as they would be in a child without rubella, which includes cataract surgery after the first year of life. Congenital heart defects secondary to CRS should be managed by a cardiologist the same as in a patient without rubella. In patients with low levels of IgG, immune globulin may be considered (1). Some delayed neurologic consequences of CRS that should be monitored include microcephaly, language delay, autistic features, and developmental or mental retardation (19).

EXPOSURES

Complete care of the patient with rubella should include counseling on the dangers of exposure to a pregnant woman and the potential serious consequences to her unborn fetus. A child with postnatally acquired rubella should be excluded from school or child care for 7 days after the onset of the rash. In the hospital setting, the patient with known acquired rubella should be under droplet precautions for the same time period. For a child with proved or suspected congenital rubella, contact isolation should be observed until the child is at least 1 year of age, or until nasopharyngeal and urine culture results after 3 months of age are repeatedly negative (2).

If a pregnant woman is exposed to rubella, a blood sample should be collected immediately and tested for rubella antibody. A sample should also be kept for further testing, if needed. The presence of rubella antibody in the first sample indicates that the mother is most likely immune (2). If the antibody is absent, the woman should be monitored for symptoms of rash, fever, or lymphadenopathy. Should she become symptomatic, a nasopharyngeal specimen should be cultured for rubella virus (1). Otherwise, a second blood sample should be collected 2 to 3 weeks later and tested in tandem with the first sample. If this test finding is still negative, a third sample should be collected 6 weeks after the initial one, and the first and third samples should be tested concurrently. If the antibody is not found in either sample, infection has not occurred. Antibody detected in the second or third sample, however, represents seroconversion and indicates recent infection (2). False-positive results do occur, however, so the test should be repeated for confirmation, possibly in a different laboratory. Some would suggest therapeutic abortion for rubella infection early in pregnancy (1). When this is not possible, the use of immunoglobulin is controversial. Data are limited, but some have reported positive results, whereas others have documented infants with congenital rubella whose mothers received immunoglobulin shortly after exposure (1,2).

VACCINE

The RA 27/3 strain is a live rubella virus vaccine grown in human diploid cell cultures and is the only rubella vaccine licensed for use in the United States. It is available alone, with mumps vaccine, or with measles and mumps. It is safer and more immunogenic than previous strains, with 95% or more of vacinees having serologic evidence of immunity. Immunity is generally lifelong, but cases of reinfection have been reported (2,4).

The Advisory Committee on Immunization Practices (ACIP) recommends the rubella vaccine be given in combination with vaccines for measles and mumps (MMR) between the ages of 12 and 15 months. A second dose is recommended before school entry at 4 to 6 years of age. This dose is primarily for the measles component, but the ACIP recommends that the MMR be given when any of the components are indicated (4). Emphasis should be placed on immunizing all susceptible adolescents and adults, particularly women of childbearing age who are not pregnant. Anyone born in or after 1957 who has not been vaccinated and does not have serologic evidence of immunity should be immunized. Efforts should also be made to immunize males and females in at-risk populations, such as recent immigrants, college students, military recruits, and health care professionals (2). Vaccine should also be administered to postpartum women who are rubella susceptible before leaving the hospital after giving birth (1).

Rubella is a very safe vaccine. In fact, most of the adverse affects following MMR administration, including rash and fever, are attributable to the measles component. Adults, especially women, may complain of transient arthritis, arthralgia, and paresthesias following rubella vaccination. As many as 25% of postpubertal females may complain of arthralgia and approximately 10% develop acute arthritis, but transient peripheral neuritic complaints, such as paresthesias and pain in the arms and legs, are much less common (2,4).

Pregnancy is a contraindication to rubella vaccine, and a woman should be advised to not become pregnant for 3 months after immunization. If the vaccine is given by mistake or if she becomes pregnant shortly after vaccine administration, she should be counseled on the theoretic risks to her fetus. No evidence, however, indicates that rubella vaccine causes fetal defects, and therapeutic abortion is not indicated. Those with altered immune states should not receive the immunization, although patients with human immunodeficiency virus (HIV) who are not severely immunocompromised may be considered for the vaccine. Patients who have been on high doses of corticosteroids for >14 days should be off of the steroids for 1 month before receiving the vaccine. Other contraindications include febrile illness and recent administration of blood products, including immune serum globulin. Women who have received human anti-Rho(D) immune globulin in the postpartum period can be immunized, however, but they should be tested 8 or more weeks later to determine antibody response. Breastfeeding is not a contraindication to rubella vaccination (2,4).

CLINICAL RECOMMENDATIONS OF THE VIGNETTE

The patient has congenital rubella syndrome. Because it can affect nearly all organ systems, he should have a full evaluation. Of immediate concern, he should be monitored for respiratory distress and signs of encephalitis. He should be thoroughly evaluated by an ophthalmologist. He should also receive his first of a series of audiometry examinations. Thrombocytopenia should be closely monitored, but true hemorrhagic emergencies are uncommon. His hepatosplenomegaly is likely of no clinical concern. His cardiac diagnosis should be handled as it would in a patient without CRS, as would hyperbilirubinemia should it develop. The child should be monitored throughout his life for the late-developing sequelae of CRS, including progressive sensorineural hearing loss, diabetes mellitus, behavioral problems, and progressive rubella panencephalitis.

SUMMARY

Rubella virus, when acquired postnatally, is a mild disease with minimal morbidity and mortality. Up to half of cases may even be asymptomatic. The most common expression is a generalized erythematous maculopapular rash. Also experienced may be lymphadenopathy, a low-grade fever, and symptoms resembling an upper respiratory infection. Some, particularly adolescent and adult females, may experience joint involvement. Treatment is symptomatic. Neurological complications can include encephalitis, peripheral neuritis, and progressive panencephalitis.

Conversely, consequences of a maternal infection early in gestation can be devastating to the fetus. Congenital rubella syndrome can affect virtually all organ systems. The most common anomalies are auditory, ophthalmologic, cardiac, and neurologic. Deafness is the most common, and sometimes only, manifestation. This hearing impairment can be progressive and should be monitored throughout life. Ophthalmologic consequences include cataracts, retinopathy, and congenital glaucoma, with the latter needing the most immediate intervention. Cardiac defects can include patent ductus arteriosus, pulmonary artery stenosis, and pulmonary valvular stenosis. Neurologic findings consist of meningoencephalitis, microcephaly, behavioral disorders, and mental retardation. Meningoencephalitis and microcephaly may be present at birth, whereas the latter two may not be apparent until later in life. Some late-developing sequelae of CRS include progressive sensorineural hearing loss, diabetes mellitus, behavioral problems, and progressive rubella panencephalitis.

Progressive rubella panencephalitis can develop in patients who were infected either postnatally or congenitally. It is caused by the persistence of the virus in the brain, and it usually presents in the second decade of life and progresses over 8 to 10 years. It is a uniformly fatal disease process.

Rubella was formerly a widespread disease with epidemics occurring in 6- to 9-year cycles. After the rubella vaccine was developed in the late 1960s, however, rubella activity has decreased by 99%. The vaccine is recommended in two doses, one at 12 to 15 months and the second at 4 to 6 years before school entry. All susceptible adolescents and adults, particularly women of childbearing age, should also be vaccinated. This vaccine process has proved effective and should be continued to combat rubella, particularly the deleterious effects of CRS and PRP.

REFERENCES

1. Feigin R, Cherry J. *Textbook of Pediatric Infectious Diseases.* 4th ed. Philadelphia: WB Saunders; 1998.
2. Pickering L, ed. *Red Book: 2003 Report on the Committee on Infectious Diseases*, 26th ed. Elk Grove Village, IL: American Academy of Pediatrics; 2003.
3. Bale J. Viral Infections of the nervous system. In: Swaiman K, Ashwal S, eds. *Pediatric Neurology: Principles & Practice.* 3rd ed. Philadelphia: Mosby; 1999:1001–1024.
4. Atkinson W, Wolfe C, Humiston S, et al., eds. *Epidemiology and Prevention of Vaccine-Preventable Diseases*, 6th ed. Atlanta, GA: CDC, 2000.
5. Griffith B, Booss J. Neurologic infections of the fetus and newborn. *Neurol Clin.* 1994;12(3):541–564.
6. Sugita K, Ando M, Makino M, et al. Magnetic resonance imaging of the brain in congenital rubella virus and cytomegalovirus infections. *Neuroradiology.* 1991;33(3):239–242.
7. Banatvala J, Brown D. Rubella. *Lancet.* 2004;363:1127–1137.
8. Chang D, Park J, Chung K. Encephalitis and polyradiculoneuritis following rubella virus infection—A case report. *J Korean Med Sci.* 1997;12(2):168–170.
9. Cifarelli P, Freireich A. Rubella encephalitis. *New York State Journal of Medicine.* 1966;66(9): 1117–1122.
10. Bosley A, Hart R. Rubella encephalopathy. *J Infect.* 1985;11(3):239–240.
11. Frey T. Neurological aspects of rubella virus infection. *Intervirology.* 1997;40:167–175.
12. Lau K, Lai S, Lai J, et al. Acute encephalitis complicating rubella. *Hong Kong Med J.* 1998 Sep;4(3):325–328.
13. Brown A, Susser E. In utero infection and adult schizophrenia. *Ment Retard Dev Disabil Res Rev.* 2002;8:51–57.
14. Parisot S, Droulle P, Feldmann M, et al. Unusual encephaloclastic lesions with paraventricular calcification in congenital rubella. *Pediatr Radiol.* 1991;21:229–230.
15. Sever J, South M, Shaver K. Delayed manifestations of congenital rubella. *Rev Infect Dis.* 1985;7[Suppl 1]:S164–S169.
16. Townsend J, Baringer J, Wolinsky J, et al. Progressive rubella panencephalitis: Late onset after congenital rubella. *N Engl J Med.* 1975;272(19):990–993.
17. Weil M, Itabashi H, Cremer N, et al. Chronic progressive panencephalitis due to rubella virus simulating subacute sclerosing panencephalitis. *N Engl J Med.* 19758;292(19): 994–998.
18. Wolinsky J. Subacute sclerosing panencephalitis, progressive rubella panencephalitis, and multifocal leukoencephalopathy. *Research Publications—Association for Research in Nervous and Mental Disease.* 1990;68:259–268.
19. Bale J. Congenital infections. *Neurologic Clinics of North America.* 2002;20(4):1039–1060.

CHAPTER 153

Varicella-Zoster Infections

Daniel J. Bonthius • Charles Grose

OBJECTIVES

- To describe the similarities and differences between varicella and zoster
- To discuss the common neurologic complications of varicella
- To describe the potential clinical problems of varicella-zoster virus infection during pregnancy
- To discuss the diagnostic approach and treatment options for varicella-zoster infections

CASE VIGNETTE

The patient, a 4-year-old boy, was in his usual state of good health until he developed a moderate fever and irritability. The following day, a skin rash appeared, consisting of 2- to 3-mm vesicular papules on an erythematous base. The skin lesions were pruritic and appeared as successive crops on the face, trunk, and extremities. Over the next 4 days, the patient's skin had lesions at different stages of development. Some consisted of newly formed lesions with a vesicle, whereas others were crusting. By the fifth day after the skin eruption, no new lesions were present, and all of the observable lesions were crusted.

Apart from the resolving skin lesions, the patient appeared and felt well for the next 2 days. On the third day, however, the patient awoke from a nap and could not walk. On examination, his sensorium was normal, as was his strength in all four extremities. He was acutely ataxic in his trunk and all four limbs, however. He was moderately dysarthric. He had mild horizontal nystagmus, but the cranial nerves were otherwise intact. Muscle stretch reflexes were normal.

The patient had a magnetic resonance imaging (MRI) scan of the brain, in which finding was normal. Lumbar puncture revealed normal cerebrospinal fluid (CSF) components and a normal opening pressure. A urine drug screen was negative. Within 3 days of the onset of ataxia, the patient's condition substantially improved. Mild ataxia remained for several additional weeks, then resolved completely. The patient had no permanent dermatologic or neurologic sequelae.

DEFINITION

Varicella-zoster virus (VZV) is a member of the *Herpesviridae* family of viruses, which is composed of >120 viruses. For most members of this family, infection is restricted to a single host species and is spread in the population by direct contact or aerosols. The hallmark of herpesvirus infections is the establishment of a lifelong latent infection that can reactivate one or more times to cause disease. In addition to VZV, other members of the herpesvirus family that cause human disease include herpes simplex virus (HSV) types 1 and 2, Epstein-Barr virus (EBV), human cytomegalovirus (CMV), and human herpesvirus (HHV) 6, 7, and 8 (1).

Varicella, also known as *chicken pox,* is the clinical condition induced by a primary infection with VZV. It is a systemic disorder. *Zoster,* also known as *shingles, herpeszoster,* and *acute posterior ganglionitis,* is caused by reactivation of VZV from specific cerebral ganglia or ganglia of the posterior nerve roots. It is a localized disorder.

EPIDEMIOLOGY

VZV is a highly contagious virus and humans are its only host. Transmission occurs most often when aerosolized droplets from nasopharyngeal secretions of an infected person contact the mucosa of a susceptible individual. Horizontal transmission can also occur by direct contact with vesicular fluid from a patient with varicella or zoster. The virus can also be transmitted vertically by transplacental passage of the virus from mother to fetus during maternal viremia.

The incubation period for VZV is usually approximately 2 weeks, but ranges from 10 to 21 days after contact with the virus. People infected with VZV are most contagious from 1 or 2 days before the onset of rash to shortly after its onset. People remain contagious until all of the skin lesions have crusted.

VZV is among the most contagious of all human pathogens. In the prevaccine era, the Centers for Disease Control and Prevention (CDC) estimated that 4 million cases of chicken pox occurred each year in the United States. Since introduction of the vaccine, the incidence of varicella disease has fallen by 85% (2). Among susceptible people, VZV infection remains hard to avoid. When the virus infects one member of a household, >90% of susceptible individuals within that household will be infected (3).

In temperate regions of the world in the prevaccine era, varicella was almost exclusively a childhood disease. Its incidence had a clear seasonal distribution and peaked during the late winter and early spring months. Within tropical climates, people have tended to acquire the virus at later ages, with a greater proportion of cases occurring in adults. Since the implementation of universal immunization of American children in 1995, a greater proportion of cases are occurring among adolescents and adults. However, the overall incidence for all age groups has been reduced substantially (4).

Once infected with VZV, patients typically develop life-long immunity. The immunity involves both cellular and humoral components, although cellular immunity is most important for limiting the extent of the primary infection and for preventing reactivation of VZV with consequent zoster.

Risk of severe disease from infection with VZV—both varicella and zoster—is greatest in the immunocompromised. Children with T-lymphocyte deficiency or dysfunction are at particularly high risk for disseminated varicella or zoster. Thus, acquired immunodeficiency syndrome (AIDS) and congenital T-lymphocyte defects are disorders that carry a high risk of severe complications from VZV infection.

ETIOLOGY AND PATHOGENESIS

People become infected with VZV when the virus contacts the mucosa of the upper respiratory tract or conjunctiva. From this initial site of entry, the virus disseminates via the blood stream and reaches the skin in mononuclear cells. Infection of the skin leads to the generalized rash of varicella. Although the skin is typically the most evidently infected organ, multiple organs, including the central nervous system (CNS), can be infected. The virus infects and becomes latent within sensory ganglia, including dorsal root ganglia and cranial nerve ganglia (5).

VZV presents many proteins to the immune system. Antibodies directed against viral glycoproteins can neutralize the ability of virus to infect cells. In addition, the cellular immune response plays a critical role in containing the infection by limiting the extent of primary infection and by preventing reactivation of virus and the onset of zoster (6).

Within the sensory ganglia, VZV can remain latent for multiple years before reactivating. During this latent phase, the virus evades the host immune system by limiting expression of viral proteins and by downregulating expression of major histocompatibility complex (MHC) class I antigens on the surface of infected cells (6). When cells are infected with viruses, the function of MHC class I molecules is to present viral proteins to cytotoxic T cells that can kill the infected cells. By reducing the expression of MHC class I proteins on cell surfaces, the virus limits presentation of viral antigens to the cytotoxic T cells and, thus, can escape destruction by the immune system (7).

PATHOLOGY

VARICELLA (CHICKENPOX)

Chicken pox is caused by a primary infection with VZV. This disorder is associated with a widespread vesicular exanthem that occurs without respect to dermatomal distribution.

Varicella can induce aseptic meningitis, in which case the neuropathologic findings consist of scattered inflammatory cells within the meninges. In these cases, virus is virtually never isolated from CSF or brain.

Children treated with salicylates during a varicella infection are at risk for Reye syndrome. Pathologic specimens in Reye syndrome reveal fatty livers and brain edema.

Some children, especially immunocompromised children and neonates, can develop encephalitis during a primary varicella infection. Neuropathologic specimens reveal widespread infection of multiple cell types, including neurons, oligodendrocytes, meningeal cells, ependymal cells, and cells of the blood vessel wall (8).

Latency

After the rash of chickenpox resolves, the virus enters a latent phase within the ganglia of the peripheral nervous system, where it persists for the duration of the host's life. During latency, the virus is not infectious and does not transcribe most of its genes. In this way, the virus avoids detection by the host immune system. Unlike retroviruses, VZV does not incorporate its nucleic acid into host DNA. Instead, the virus remains extrachromosomal, but in a noninfectious form (9).

While in this latent phase, the virus is present almost exclusively within neurons. Despite the viral presence, the infected neurons undergo little morphologic change, and the immune system is not activated.

ZOSTER (SHINGLES)

After a period of latency within ganglia neurons, VZV can reactivate and spread along axons to the skin, where it causes a vesicular rash with a dermatomal distribution. The pathologic hallmark of zoster is hemorrhage, necrosis, and inflammation of the affected ganglia (10). In contrast to latent VZV, during which the virus resides exclusively in neurons, zoster is marked by viral infection of neurons, satellite cells, and fibroblasts of the ganglia (11).

CLINICAL MANIFESTATIONS

VARICELLA

Varicella, the disease resulting from a primary infection with VZV, typically begins with fever, pharyngitis, and malaise. Usually, within 24 hours, this prodrome is followed by a vesicular and pruritic rash. Lesions usually occur first on the scalp and face, then spread to the trunk, followed by the extremities. Over the course of the next several days, new vesicular lesions appear as the older ones develop a crust. The course of this disease in an otherwise healthy child is typically 5 to 7 days. Most children have no serious complications during the infection, recover fully, and never have a symptomatic infection with the virus again.

The most common complication of varicella is bacterial superinfection of skin lesions. The bacterial organisms most commonly implicated are *Staphylococcus aureus* and *Streptococcus pyogenes* (12). These bacterial superinfections can worsen the scarring associated with the varicella skin lesions. The secondary bacterial infections can further complicate varicella by transforming into serious infections of their own, including cellulites, necrotizing fasciitis, toxic shock syndrome, sepsis, and osteomyelitis (13).

Adults are typically more severely ill with varicella than are children. In particular, varicella pneumonia is rare in childhood, but is relatively common in adolescents and adults. Of adults with varicella, approximately 16.3% have radiographic evidence of pneumonitis (14). Respiratory symptoms of varicella pneumonia usually have their onset within a few days of rash development and include cough, dyspnea, and occasionally hemoptysis. The chest X-ray study typically reveals a diffuse interstitial nodular infiltrate. Before antiviral therapies were available, varicella pneumonia carried a mortality rate of 30%. The availability of antiviral therapy and advancements in critical care have reduced the mortality rate to <10% (15).

Neurologic complications are not rare in association with varicella. In childhood, the most common neurologic complication is acute cerebellar ataxia, whereas in adulthood and infancy, the most common neurologic complication is encephalitis.

ACUTE CEREBELLAR ATAXIA

Acute cerebellar ataxia has an incidence of approximately 1 of 4,000 varicella cases (16). It most commonly affects children ages 2 to 7 years, but can affect adolescents and adults. Ataxia can develop from several days before, to several weeks after, the onset of the rash. Most commonly, the ataxia occurs late in the course of the rash or just after the rash has cleared. The onset of ataxia is often explosive and maximal at onset. Commonly, a previously healthy child awakens from a nap with marked ataxia and is unable to walk. The degree of ataxia can worsen somewhat during the first hours after onset, but a waxing and waning or a slowly progressive course would not be typical.

The ataxia may be accompanied by lethargy, vomiting, headache, and nystagmus. Commonly, however, the ataxia occurs in isolation. In particular, cerebral cortical function is normal, even if the cerebellar ataxia is profound.

The CSF is usually normal, but may show a moderate lymphocytic pleocytosis, usually with <100 cell/μL, and a mildly elevated protein concentration. MRI scan of the brain also usually appears normal, but may show evidence of demyelination within the cerebellum or its peduncles.

The ataxia typically begins to remit after several days. Most patients fully recover without any sequelae within several weeks. For some patients, however, multiple months are required for full recovery, and occasional cases have persistent cerebellar dysfunction (17).

The pathogenesis of VZV-induced acute cerebellar ataxia is unclear. One possible mechanism is direct viral infection of the cerebellum. That VZV-specific antigens and antibodies can be identified within the CSF of patients with varicella-associated cerebellar ataxia suggests that VZV can replicate within the CNS and favors the notion that cerebellar infection underlies the ataxia (18). Alternatively, the mechanism can be a parainfectious immune-mediated demyelinating process. That many cases of cerebellar ataxia have their onset after the rash and fever have subsided suggests that the virus is no longer present and favors the notion that the ataxia is postinfectious and immune-mediated.

ENCEPHALITIS

Among the most serious complications of varicella is encephalitis, which has an incidence of approximately 2 episodes per 10,000 varicella cases and affects adults and infants more often than children (13). As with acute cerebellar ataxia, varicella-associated encephalitis typically begins late in the course of the rash or just after its clearance. Signs and symptoms commonly include headache, fever, vomiting, altered mental status, seizures, and focal motor or sensory deficits (19).

The CSF is usually abnormal with an elevated opening pressure, lymphocytic pleocytosis, and elevated protein concentration. Electroencephalography (EEG) typically reveals diffuse slow-wave activity, consistent with diffuse cerebral dysfunction. Neuroimaging studies often show edema and focal areas of abnormal signal consistent with demyelination.

Mortality rates approach 10%, and 15% of survivors have long-term neurologic sequelae, the most common of which is epilepsy. Most patients with varicella-associated encephalitis, however, have a complete recovery (8).

REYE SYNDROME

Reye syndrome is a life-threatening disorder of mitochondrial function that accompanies or immediately follows a viral infection. Varicella has been especially implicated in this disorder. The pathogenesis of Reye syndrome is unknown, but has been clearly linked to the use of salicylates during viral infections. When varicella is the precipitating infection, the signs of Reye syndrome typically begin 3 to 6 days after the onset of rash. Initial symptoms usually include vomiting and headache. The disease can rapidly progress to include signs of agitation, delirium, decorticate posturing, and hyperventilation. Intracranial hypertension and liver dysfunction eventually become prominent signs (20).

Laboratory studies can provide valuable clues to the diagnosis of Reye syndrome. Blood abnormalities typically include hyperammonemia, hypoglycemia, and elevated concentrations of liver enzymes. Bilirubin levels, however, do not usually rise, and jaundice does not occur. The CSF is under abnormally high pressure, but its cellular and chemical components are normal. EEG is diffusely slow, consistent with a diffuse encephalopathy. Liver biopsy is diagnostic and shows panlobular accumulation of lipid and depletion of succinic acid dehydrogenase and glycogen.

Prognosis in Reye syndrome is guarded. The encephalopathy can progress to coma, and the intracranial hypertension can induce cerebral herniation and death. Thus, to reverse intracranial hypertension, aggressive steps must often be taken, including controlled mechanical hyperventilation, and administration of osmotic agents.

As late as several decades ago, Reye syndrome was a frequent and dreaded complication of viral illnesses and a major cause of death in children with varicella. Since the identification of salicylates as a precipitating factor in the cause of Reye syndrome, the incidence of this disorder has declined substantially (21).

POST-VARICELLA ARTERIOPATHY

For approximately 1 year following varicella infection, otherwise healthy children appear to be at increased risk for an arterial ischemic stroke. The precise mechanism underlying this association between previous varicella and ischemic stroke is unknown. Examination of diseased cerebral arteries at autopsy in children who had strokes following varicella, however, has revealed evidence of the virus within the vessel walls. Thus, it is believed that the virus induces an arteriopathy of cerebral vessels. The virus likely reaches the vessels by traveling along the trigeminal nerve from its dormant location in the trigeminal ganglion (22).

In post-varicella strokes, arteriograms typically reveal unilateral stenosis of the distal internal carotid artery and proximal segment of the anterior cerebral artery and middle cerebral artery. Brain imaging almost always reveals infarcts within the vascular territory of their lenticulostriate branches. Thus, the structures typically affected are the internal capsule and the basal ganglia.

Based on the rationale that virus is present in the vessel walls and is likely inducing inflammation and arteriopathy, both acyclovir and corticosteroids are usually used to treat post-varicella stroke. Recent evidence suggests, however, that the arteriopathy is monophasic and does not progress after the stroke. Thus, whether anti-inflammatory and antiviral medications are of any benefit is unclear (23).

HERPES ZOSTER (SHINGLES)

Following a case of chicken pox, VZV becomes latent in the peripheral nervous system ganglia of virtually all infected people. Within these ganglia, the virus persists for the lifetime of the host. As the host ages, the likelihood of viral reactivation increases. On reactivation, the virus spreads in a retrograde transaxonal fashion to the skin, where it causes a rash with a dermatomal distribution (8). The rash can occur in any dermatome, but those of the thorax and face are most commonly affected. Besides inducing skin rash within the affected dermatomes, herpes zoster also causes severe radicular pain. In some cases, the pain persists for weeks or months after the rash has resolved, a condition referred to as *postherpetic neuralgia.* Zoster is virtually always monophasic. The disease recurs in <5% of patients.

SPECIAL SITUATIONS

VARICELLA INFECTION DURING PREGNANCY

Varicella infection during pregnancy poses substantial risks to both the mother and the fetus. Vaccinating VZV-susceptible women before pregnancy can protect both the mother and fetus against VZV-induced morbidity and mortality.

Women who contract varicella while pregnant are at risk for severe infections. In particular, VZV-induced pneumonia is relatively common and harsh during pregnancy. Smoking and the presence of >100 skin lesions in pregnant women are risk factors for the development of VZV-induced pneumonia. The principal signs of varicella pneumonia in pregnancy are fever, dyspnea, cough, and tachypnea. The clinical course can rapidly progress to hypoxia and respiratory failure. In untreated pregnant women, the mortality rate of VZV-induced pneumonia is >40% (24). The mainstays of treatment are acyclovir and supportive care, often including intubation and mechanical ventilation.

Along with the mother, the fetus is also endangered by maternal varicella infection (25). Varicella can cross the placenta and infect the embryo or fetus. If this infection occurs during the first or second trimesters of pregnancy, congenital varicella syndrome can result. Clinical manifestations of the syndrome include limb hypoplasia, chorioretinitis, cataracts, microphthalmia, cutaneous scars (cicatrix), and CNS malformation and dysfunction. These CNS abnormalities can include microcephaly, hydrocephalus, Horner syndrome, cranial neuropathies, mental retardation, cerebral palsy, and epilepsy. Neuroimaging studies often reveal intracranial calcifications, cortical dysplasia, or hydranencephaly (26). Congenital varicella syndrome is rare, however. Only 2% of maternal varicella infections occurring during the first 20 weeks of gestation lead to fetal varicella syndrome (27).

Varicella poses a special risk to the developing child, not only when the infection occurs *prenatally*, but also when it occurs *perinatally*. The infant infected with varicella around the time of birth is at high risk of substantial morbidity and mortality (13). Neonates can acquire the virus from their mothers via either vertical or horizontal transmission. The temporal window of vulnerability for maternal varicella extends from approximately 4 days before delivery to 2 weeks after delivery. The greatest risk occurs when the infant is delivered after the onset of maternal viremia, but before development of maternal antibodies. These infants will typically appear healthy at birth, but can develop severe varicella 5 to 10 days after delivery. Infection in this scenario often includes multiple visceral organ involvement, including lung, liver, and brain disease, and has a mortality rate of 30% (28). Infants delivered during the high-risk window should be treated with intravenous acyclovir.

VARICELLA-ZOSTER INFECTIONS IN THE IMMUNOCOMPROMISED HOST

Varicella infections are generally more severe in patients whose immune systems are compromised (Cohen et al., [6]). Patients with an underlying malignancy, steroid use, immunosuppressive therapy, human immunovirus (HIV) infection, or solid organ transplantation are particularly susceptible to disseminated varicella because of impaired cellular immunity. In these immunocompromised patients, disseminated varicella can manifest itself as extensive skin lesions, pneumonia, hepatitis, and encephalitis. Disseminated varicella in immune compromised patients can have a mortality rate as high as 50% (29).

As with varicella, zoster is more severe in the immunocompromised host. Zoster has a much higher incidence among immunosuppressed patients than among immunocompetent ones. Furthermore, when zoster occurs in the immunosuppressed patient, its clinical impact is often worsened. Immunocompromised patients often experience zoster simultaneously in more than one dermatome, a phenomenon that virtually never occurs in immunocompetent patients. In addition, immunocompromised patients can experience multiple recurrences of zoster. Furthermore, zoster is not always restricted to the skin and peripheral nerves in immunocompromised patients, and, instead, can become disseminated. Pneumonia, encephalitis, and hepatitis can accompany dissemination in the course of viral reactivation.

A manifestation of herpes zoster that is unique to immunocompromised hosts is *abdominal zoster* (30). Hours to days before the onset of the cutaneous rash, these patients develop severe abdominal pain. The diagnosis does not typically become apparent until the skin rash of zoster appears, usually in a thoracic dermatome. In this condition, abdominal visceral involvement is common, and the mortality rate is high (13).

DIAGNOSTIC APPROACH

For most cases of varicella, the clinical history and the characteristic exanthem are sufficient to provide the diagnosis. That many individuals with a presumed second episode of varicella are seronegative before this second episode suggests, however, that the initial diagnosis of varicella was incorrect and that clinical features alone can be misleading (31).

For several days after the onset of rash, VZV can be obtained from vesicular fluid. Only rarely, however, can the virus be recovered from other sites of infection, such as the respiratory tract.

Furthermore, because the virus is highly labile, only approximately half of all culture from active skin lesions is positive.

Varicella-zoster viral antigens from skin scrapings can be detected by fluorescence microscopy. This method is more sensitive than culturing techniques. Furthermore, in contrast to the Tzanck smear, detection of varicella-zoster antigen can differentiate varicella-zoster from HSV, which can cause similar skin lesions (6).

PCR can be used to detect VZV DNA in vesicular swabs, scabs from crusted lesions, biopsy tissues, or in CSF in patients with CNS involvement. The PCR method is very sensitive and specific. Furthermore, PCR followed by restriction of endonuclease digestion can distinguish vaccine strain from wild-type.

Serologic testing for anti-VZV IgG antibodies can retrospectively confirm a diagnosis of varicella and can evaluate for adequate seroconversion following vaccination. Detection of anti-VZV IgM antibodies is not a reliable method of confirmation, but a positive result is consistent with an ongoing or recent varicella infection (4).

TREATMENT

Varicella vaccine is recommended for all children between 12 and 18 months of age. The vaccination has very few side effects, the most common being mild irritation at the injection site. Because the vaccine has been given since 1995, community-acquired chickenpox is becoming a less-common illness in the United States and Europe (32). For adults who have never had chickenpox or prior vaccination, two doses of vaccine 1 month apart are recommended.

Varicella zoster immune globulin (VZIG) is no longer produced in the United States. Instead of VZIG, prophylaxis of immunocompromised children who are varicella susceptible is accomplished via administration of oral acyclovir (40 mg/kg/day for a maximum 800 mg three times per day), beginning immediately after exposure to chickenpox and continuing for 10 days. Treatment of acute chickenpox in immune compromised children requires intravenous administration of acyclovir (30 mg/kg/day, divided every 8 hours). Treatment is usually continued for 5 to 7 days, until no new vesicles form. The most prominent side effect of intravenous acyclovir is renal toxicity. Therefore, serum creatinine levels should be checked approximately every 3 days.

Nonimmune healthy adults occasionally contract chickenpox. Because chickenpox in adults has a relatively high risk of serious complications, including pneumonia, treatment is recommended as soon as the vesicular rash appears. Pregnant women with chickenpox are at a particularly high risk of developing pneumonia. Adults can be treated with oral tablets, either famciclovir (500 mg three times daily) or valacyclovir (1,000 mg three times daily for 5 to 7 days). These are the same medications as indicated for treatment of acute zoster in older adults. Because it is difficult to predict which patients with acute zoster will develop more severe disease with subsequent postherpetic neuralgia, treatment of all patients with acute zoster may be considered.

CLINICAL RECOMMENDATIONS OF THE VIGNETTE

The patient initially had a classic onset and clinical course of varicella. His age at onset (early childhood), prodromal symptoms (fever and irritability), exanthem (crops of vesicular lesions on an erythematous base), progression (emergence of new lesions with crusting of others), and disease duration (5 days) were all highly typical of chicken pox.

Three days after the skin lesions had resolved, the patient developed the most common neurologic complication of varicella in childhood—acute cerebellar ataxia. The clinical signs and disease course in this patient were again classic. Neurologic abnormalities were restricted to ataxia, which was substantial at onset and resolved within several days.

In light of the close temporal proximity of the ataxia onset to the varicella infection, it was reasonable to conclude that the ataxia was etiologically related to the varicella. Thus, it is debatable whether the MRI scan and lumbar puncture were necessary for this patient. Both tests yielded normal results, which is typical of varicella-induced acute cerebellar ataxia. The urine drug screen was indicated for this patient, because acute ataxia in a young child can be caused by drug ingestion, a condition that can be life-threatening and often has a specific treatment.

The child was not treated with any specific therapy, nor was any indicated. Administration of acyclovir within 24 hours of rash onset might have modestly decreased symptoms (33), but its use is not recommended in otherwise healthy children with varicella (4). The child's parents should be warned not to administer salicylates or salicylate-containing products to the child, because of the risk of Reye syndrome. Instead, acetaminophen may be used to control fever.

SUMMARY

Varicella-zoster virus is a highly contagious pathogen that infects millions of people annually worldwide. Primary infection with the virus induces varicella (chickenpox), the most prominent clinical sign of which is a generalized exanthem consisting of vesicles on an erythematous base. After varicella resolves, the virus becomes latent in neurons of cranial and spinal ganglia. In some individuals, especially immunocompromised patients and the elderly, the virus can reactivate to produce a dermatomal rash and radicular pain, a condition referred to as *herpes zoster* or *shingles*. The incidence of varicella has declined substantially in the United States since introduction of the varicella vaccine.

Although varicella is usually a self-limited infection from which the patient fully recovers, it can be associated with serious complications. These include pneumonitis, encephalitis, Reye syndrome, disseminated VZV infection, vasculopathy with stroke, and bacterial superinfection of skin lesions. Immunocompromised patients, especially those with defects of cell-mediated immunity, are at particularly high risk for potentially life-threatening complications from VZV infection. Children with varicella can develop acute cerebellar ataxia, a condition that produces profound ataxia, but is usually self-limited and reversible.

Special concerns regarding VZV infection arise during pregnancy. Pregnant women are susceptible to pneumonia during VZV infection, whereas the fetus is vulnerable to congenital varicella syndrome and the newborn is at risk for disseminated varicella.

Antiviral medications, including acyclovir, famciclovir, and valacyclovir can impair VZV replication and improve outcome of the infection in some situations. Salicylates should not be used in cases of varicella because of the risk of Reye syndrome.

REFERENCES

1. Flint SJ, Enquist LW, Racaniello VR, et al. Herpesviruses. In: *Principles of Virology: Molecular Biology, Pathogenesis and Control of Animal Viruses*, 2nd ed. Washington, DC: ASM Press; 2004:810–813.
2. MMWR. Decline in annual incidence of varicella: Selected states, 1990–2001. *MMWR Morb Mortal Wkly Rep.* 2003;52:884.
3. Wharton M. The epidemiology of varicella-zoster infections. *Infect Dis Clin North Am.* 1996;10:571–581.
4. American Academy of Pediatrics. Varicella-zoster Infections. In: Pickering L, ed. *2006 Red Book: Report of the Committee on Infectious Diseases*, 27th ed. Elk grove Village, IL: American Academy of Pediatrics; 2006:711–725.
5. Straus SE, Ostrove JM, Inchauspe G, et al. NIH conference. Varicella-zoster virus infections. Biology, natural history, treatment, and prevention. *Ann Intern Med.* 1988;108:221–237.
6. Cohen JI, Brunell PA, Straus SE, et al. Recent advances in varicella-zoster virus infection. *Ann Intern Med.* 1999;130:922–932.
7. Cohen JI. Infection of cells with varicella-zoster virus down-regulates surface expression of class I major histocompatibility complex antigens. *J Infect Dis.* 1998;177:1390–1393.
8. Kleinschmidt-DeMasters BK, Gilden D. Varicella-zoster virus infections of the nervous system: Clinical and pathologic correlates. *Arch Pathol Lab Med.* 2001;125:770–780.
9. Cohrs R, Mahalingam R, Dueland AN, et al. Restricted transcription of varicella-zoster virus in latently infected human trigeminal and thoracic ganglia. *J Infect Dis.* 1992; 166[Suppl 1]:S24–S29.
10. Nagashima K, Nakazawa M, Endo H. Pathology of the human spinal ganglia in varicella-zoster virus infection. *Acta Neuropathol.* 1975;33:105–117.
11. Ghatak NR, Zimmerman HM. Spinal ganglion in herpes zoster. *Arch Pathol.* 1973;95:411–415.
12. Aebi C, Ahmed A, Ramilo O. Bacterial complications of primary varicella in children. *Clin Infect Dis.* 1996;23:698–705.
13. Gnann JW. Varicella-Zoster virus: Atypical presentations and unusual complications. *J Infect Dis.* 2002;186[Suppl 1]:S91–S98.
14. Weber DM, Pellecchia JA. Varicella pneumonia: Study of prevalence in adult men. *JAMA.* 1965;192:572–578.
15. Haake DA, Zakowski PC, Haake DL, et al. Early treatment with acyclovir for varicella pneumonia in otherwise healthy adults: Retrospective controlled study and review. *Review of Infectious Diseases.* 1990;12:788–798.
16. Guess HA. Population-based studies of varicella complications. *Pediatrics.* 1986;78:723–727.
17. Fenichel GM. Acute cerebellar ataxia. In: *Clinical Pediatric Neurology: A Signs and Symptoms Approach*, 4th ed. Philadelphia: WB Saunders; 2001:228–229.
18. Echevarria JM, Tellez A, Martinex-Martin D. Subclass distribution of the serum and intrathecal IgG antibody responses in varicella-zoster virus infections. *J Infect Dis.* 1990;162: 621–626.
19. Bonthius DJ, Karacay B. Meningitis and encephalitis in children: An update. *Neurology Clinics of North America.* 2002;20:1013–1038.
20. Hurwitz ES, Barrett MJ, Bregman D, et al. Public health service study on Reye's syndrome and medications: Report on the main study. *JAMA.* 1987;257:1905–1911.
21. Belay ED, Bresee JS, Holman RC, et al. Reye's syndrome in the United States from 1981 through 1997. *N Engl J Med.* 1999;340:1377–1382.
22. Gilden DH, Cohrs RJ, Mahalingam R. VZV vasculopathy and postherpetic neuralgia: Progress and perspective on antiviral therapy. *Neurology.* 2005;64:21–25.
23. Lanthier S, Armstrong D, Domi T, et al. Post-varicella arteriopathy of childhood: Natural history of vascular stenosis. *Neurology.* 2005;64:660–663.
24. Harger JH, Ernest JM, Thurnau GR, et al. Risk factors and outcome of varicella-zoster virus pneumonia in pregnant women. *J Infect Dis.* 2002;185:422–427.
25. Derrick CW, Lord L. In utero varicella-zoster infections. *South Med J.* 1998;91:1064–1066.
26. Bale J. Congenital infections. *Neurology Clinics of North America.* 2002;20:1039–1060.
27. Pastuszak AL, Levy M, Schiek B, et al. Outcome after maternal varicella infection in the first 20 weeks of pregnancy. *N Engl J Med.* 1994;330:901–905.
28. Preblud SR, Bregman DJ, Vernon LL. Deaths from varicella in infants. *Pediatr Infect Dis.* 1985;4:503–507.
29. Preblud SR. Varicella: Complications and costs. *Pediatrics.* 1986;78:728–735.
30. Rogers SY, Irving W, Harris A, et al. Visceral varicella zoster infection after bone marrow transplantation without skin involvement and the use of PCR for diagnosis. *Bone Marrow Transplant.* 1995;15:805–807.
31. Wallace MR, Chamberlin CJ, Zerboni L, et al. Reliability of a history of previous varicella infection in adults. *JAMA.* 1997;278:1520–1522.
32. Grose C. Varicella vaccination of children in the United States: Assessment after the first decade 1995–2005. *J Clin Virol.* 2005;33:89–95.
33. Harris D, Redhead J. Should acyclovir be prescribed for immunocompetent children presenting with chickenpox? *Arch Dis Child.* 2005;90:648–650.

CHAPTER **154**

Erythema Infectiosum (Fifth Disease)

Daniel J. Bonthius • Bahri Karaçay

OBJECTIVES

- To identify the ways in which parvovirus B19 can be transmitted to humans
- To discuss the pathogenesis of erythema infectiosum
- To identify the diagnostic tests for parvovirus B19 infection in immunocompetent and immunocompromised patients
- To discuss treatment options for patients infected with parvovirus B19

CASE VIGNETTE

A 15-month-old boy was in his usual state of excellent health until he developed mild irritability on the afternoon of admission. He was laid down for a nap. Thirty minutes later, his mother heard some unfamiliar noises in his bedroom and found him having a generalized tonic–clonic seizure. The seizure was self-limited and had stopped spontaneously within 5 minutes of its onset. The child was transported by ambulance to the local emergency room, where he was initially lethargic and febrile with a temperature of 39.1°C. The lethargy abated after 15 minutes, but he remained irritable. He received acetaminophen, which eliminated the fever and the irritability. He had a head computed tomographic (CT) scan, lumbar puncture, and several blood tests, including a complete blood count (CBC), serum electrolyte analysis, serum glucose concentration, and erythrocyte sedimentation rate, all of which were unremarkable. Diagnosed with a probable viral syndrome, he was discharged from the emergency department.

For the next 6 days, the patient continued to have intermittent fevers, which were treated successfully with acetaminophen. He had no further seizures. One week after the onset of symptoms, he developed an intensely red facial rash with a "slapped cheek" appearance. On that same day, he became afebrile. The following day, he developed a symmetric lacelike macular rash over his trunk and proximal extremities. This rash persisted 4 days, then disappeared. He had no further signs or symptoms, and he recovered fully.

DEFINITION

Erythema infectiosum is the most common clinical presentation of infection with parvovirus B19. The disorder is also commonly referred to as "fifth disease," which derives its name from a list of common childhood exanthems that were named in the order of the dates in which they were first reported. The list of six diseases includes measles, scarlet fever, rubella, Duke (fourth) disease, fifth disease, and roseola (sixth) disease.

The parvoviruses are a family of viruses, referred to as the *Parvoviridae* family. The members of this viral family are broadly defined by their small sizes. (Their name is derived from *parvum*, which is Latin for "small.") Each of the parvoviruses form small capsids, which are typically approximately 25 nm in diameter, and each contains a genome consisting of single-stranded DNA. Parvovirus B19 acquired its specific name when a virologist noted an unusual reaction induced by the virus's presence in position 19 of plate B on which she was working.

EPIDEMIOLOGY

Parvovirus B19 has a global distribution, as does the most common disease that it causes—erythema infectiosum. The virus is a common cause of infection in humans, who are the only known hosts. Parvovirus B19 has infected virtually all of the world's human populations, the only exceptions being a few isolated tribes in the Amazon basin of Brazil and in remote islands off the African coast (1,2).

Parvovirus B19 infections are ubiquitous. Infection with the virus is common in childhood. Half of 15-year-old adolescents have specific anti-parvovirus B19 antibodies. Infection continues in the adult population, so that >90% of elderly people are seropositive (3).

Parvovirus B19 can be transmitted by percutaneous exposure to blood or blood products or by vertical transmission from mother to fetus. By far the most common mode of spread is by respiratory droplet. Infection rates among susceptible household contacts are high, and outbreaks of erythema infectiosum can occur in elementary and junior high schools.

In temperate climates, infections with parvovirus B19 most commonly occur in the late winter and early spring. People with erythema infectiosum are most infectious before the onset of rash or joint symptoms. The incubation period for parvovirus B19—from acquisition of the virus to the onset of symptoms—is typically between 4 and 14 days, but can be as long as 3 weeks (4).

ETIOLOGY AND PATHOGENESIS

Erythema infectiosum is caused by infection with human parvovirus B19, a single-stranded DNA virus (5). The only known natural host cell of parvovirus B19 is the human erythrocyte precursor. This unique tropism of parvovirus B19 is caused by the expression of globoside (also called *erythrocyte P antigen*), a glycolipid that acts as a cellular receptor for the virus, on the surface of human erythroid progenitor cells. Rare individuals (1 of 200,000) who lack globoside are not susceptible to infection with parvovirus B19 (6).

When parvovirus B19 infects erythroid progenitor cells, erythropoiesis is temporarily suppressed. Reticulocyte counts temporarily drop to zero within approximately 1 week of infection. Because (*a*) erythrocytes have a long half-life and (*b*) the infection is typically short lived, however, hemoglobin levels usually remain stable (7).

The viral genome encodes only three proteins. The nonstructural protein, NS1, promotes viral replication and is cytotoxic to host cells (8). The two structural proteins, viral protein 1 (VP1) and viral protein 2 (VP2) constitute the viral capsid. These viral capsid proteins, especially VP1, contain many epitopes that can be recognized by neutralizing antibodies. As a result, the viral capsid is highly immunogenic. Antibody production is the dominant form of immune response in parvovirus B19 infection. Antibody production coincides with viral clearance from the blood, and IgG antibodies provide lasting protection against reinfection (9).

PATHOLOGY

The early systemic *flulike* symptoms of parvovirus B19 infections correspond to parvoviremia. The rash and arthropathy that follow are caused by the deposition of immune complexes in the skin and joints.

CLINICAL MANIFESTATIONS AND SPECIAL SITUATIONS

ERYTHEMA INFECTIOSUM (FIFTH DISEASE)

Most parvovirus B19 infections are asymptomatic. Among symptomatic cases of parvovirus B19 infections, erythema infectiosum is the most common.

Erythema infectiosum typically begins with mild, nonspecific systemic symptoms, including fever, headache, myalgias, and malaise. The fevers can be relatively intense and sometimes trigger febrile seizures in young children. Approximately 7 to 10 days following the onset of the systemic symptoms, a distinctive facial rash arises that produces a "slapped cheek" appearance. The onset of this rash often coincides with termination of the systemic symptoms. Several days after the facial rash appears, a lacy and pruritic full-body rash may arise and last for several weeks. The illness is self-limiting. Most healthy people recover fully and have lasting immunity to reinfection (4).

Although the distinctive facial rash is a common component of parvovirus B19 infections in young children, the rash may be absent or less characteristic in older children and adults. In contrast, polyarthritis and polyarthropathy are uncommon in children, but are commonly observed in adults with parvovirus B19. In some adults, parvovirus B19 infection will induce a polyarthropathy syndrome, in which the patient has arthralgia and arthritis in the absence of other manifestations of erythema infectiosum.

HYDROPS FETALIS

In a pregnant woman, parvovirus B19 can cross the placenta and infect the fetal liver, which is the site of erythrocyte production during much of fetal life. Within the fetal liver, parvovirus B19 can substantially impair erythrocyte production, leading to severe fetal anemia and congestive heart failure. The combination of heart failure and anemia leads to fetal swelling, a condition referred to as *hydrops fetalis* (10). These circumstances can lead to fetal loss or to multiorgan system dysfunction and severe permanent injury.

Seroprevalence data suggest that half of all pregnant women are susceptible to parvovirus B19 infection. The risk of infection is greatest in epidemic years and is correlated with the extent to which the pregnant woman has contact with children. The estimated risk of transplacental infection among women who are infected during pregnancy is 30% (9).

Most parvovirus B19 infections during pregnancy do not lead to fetal loss or to hydrops fetalis. Among infected pregnant women, the risk of fetal loss is 5% to 9%. Infection during the second trimester poses the greatest risk to the fetus (11). Although several cases of developmental anomalies of the eyes and central nervous system (CNS) in infants exposed to parvovirus B19 during fetal life have been reported, the relationship may be coincidental. Parvovirus B19 has not been proved a teratogen.

APLASTIC CRISIS

Because parvovirus B19 suppresses erythropoiesis, patients with hematologic disorders can be at particularly high risk of complications from the infection. This is particularly true of those hematologic disorders that cause an increased rate of erythrocyte destruction, such as sickle cell disease and hereditary spherocytosis. In these patient populations, parvovirus B19 infection can abruptly interrupt red cell production, thus provoking severe anemia. This *aplastic crisis* can provoke congestive heart failure, strokes, and acute splenic sequestration. Although usually self-limited, the anemia can be severe and fatal (12).

Patients with aplastic crisis typically have the prodromal illness of fever, myalgias, and malaise that is typical of erythema infectiosum. The rash is usually absent, however. Because patients infected with parvovirus B19 develop long-lasting protective immunity, the aplastic crisis is usually a nonrecurring event in the patient's life (13).

PERSISTENT PARVOVIRUS B19 INFECTION

Inability to produce protective antibodies allows parvovirus B19 to persist. Thus, patients with immunodeficiency states, including those from congenital, iatrogenic, or infectious causes, can become persistently infected with parvovirus B19. This phenomenon has been observed in a variety of patients in which antibody production is impaired, including inherited immunodeficiency states, patients who have received organ transplantations, patients receiving cytotoxic chemotherapy, and patients with acquired immunodeficiency syndrome (AIDS).

In the absence of an antibody response, erythema infectiosum does not develop, because the rash that defines this disease entity depends on production of antigen–antibody complexes. Instead, pure red cell aplasia is often the principal manifestation of persistent parvovirus B19 infection. The anemia in this condition is often severe, requiring blood transfusions (14).

NEUROLOGIC DISORDERS ASSOCIATED WITH PARVOVIRUS B19 INFECTION

Little question exists that parvovirus B19 infection can induce febrile seizures. Evidence in support of this concept lies in that seizures have occurred in many patients during the febrile phase of illnesses in which the classic exanthem and serologic conversion characteristic of erythema infectiosum later appear. Furthermore, fever is a well-documented sign of parvovirus B19 infection, and fever is the root cause of febrile seizures. Thus, the clinical course, laboratory evidence, and the scientific rationale all support an etiologic linkage between parvovirus B19 infection and febrile seizures.

In addition to febrile seizures, multiple other neurologic disorders have also been associated with parvovirus B19 infection. Documented cases of these other neurologic disorders occurring in association with parvovirus B19 are relatively few, however, and the causative role of the virus in these neurologic diseases remains unproved. The neurologic disorders in which parvovirus B19 can play a causal role include encephalitis, meningitis, convulsions, cerebellar ataxia, transverse myelitis, neuropathy, brachial plexitis, Guillain-Barré syndrome, and carpal tunnel syndrome (15,16).

DIAGNOSTIC APPROACH

Because parvovirus B19 is difficult to propagate in standard cell culture, laboratory diagnosis of the infection relies on serologic and DNA tests. In the immunocompetent patient, detection of IgM antibody directed specifically against parvovirus B19 is the strongest diagnostic test (4). IgM antibodies against parvovirus B19 can be detected in almost all cases of erythema infectiosum at the time of presentation and within a few days after the onset of transient aplastic crisis. A positive IgM antibody test suggests that the infection occurred within the previous 4 months. Serum IgG antibody is also reliably produced and detectable within 7 days of a parvovirus B19 infection in immunocompetent hosts. IgG antibodies persist for life, however. Thus, the presence of anti-parvovirus B19 IgG antibodies may reflect a previous infection and does not necessarily indicate a recent or ongoing acute infection.

For patients with persistent parvovirus B19 infection, serologic studies cannot be relied on for diagnosis because antibody production is absent or minimal. Thus, the optimal method for detecting chronic parvovirus B19 infection in the immunocompromised patient is by nucleic acid hybridization or polymerase chain reaction (PCR) assay (12). A problem with interpretation of the PCR assay is that low levels of parvovirus B19 DNA can be detected in serum for up to months or years following the acute phase of the infection. PCR detection of parvovirus B19 DNA, therefore, does not necessarily indicate a recent acute infection. The opposite problem plagues the nucleic acid hybridization technique. Nucleic acid hybridization is less sensitive than PCR and will generally be positive for only 2 to 4 days following onset of the infection. Thus, the nucleic acid hybridization technique may yield false–negative results.

For diagnosis of parvovirus B19 infection during pregnancy, both antibody tests and DNA assays may be useful (17). Viral DNA can be detected in amniotic fluid and umbilical cord blood. Likewise, IgM antibodies can be detected in umbilical cord blood and in maternal serum.

TREATMENT

Most children and adults with parvovirus B19 infections do not require any specific therapy. Only supportive care for treatment of the fevers, myalgias, malaise, and headaches is indicated.

Patients with acute aplastic crisis caused by parvovirus B19 infection often have anemia that is symptomatic at best and life-threatening at worst. These patients may benefit greatly from a blood transfusion.

Commercial immune globulins are a rich source of anti-parvovirus antibodies. Thus, patients with persistent parvovirus B19 infection caused by immunodeficiency may respond favorably to intravenous immune globulin (IVIG) therapy (18). Administration of a 5-day course of IVIG at a dose of 0.4 g/kg body weight to an immunodeficient patient with chronic parvovirus B19 infection and anemia often triggers a prompt decline in serum viral DNA levels and an increase in reticulocyte counts and hemoglobin levels. Because the rash of fifth disease is caused by formation of antigen–antibody complexes, immunoglobulin therapy to immunocompromised patients with chronic parvovirus B19 infection can trigger a rash. In cases in which immunodeficiency is iatrogenic, persistent parvovirus B19 infection might be rapidly and effectively terminated by temporarily discontinuing the immunosuppressive therapy.

Some cases of hydrops fetalis will resolve spontaneously. Intrauterine blood transfusions have been used effectively to restore fetal hemoglobin levels and to avoid the secondary fetal heart failure and systemic swelling. Alternatively, administration of immune globulin into the fetal peritoneal cavity may be an effective method of treating fetal hydrops while avoiding the risks of intrauterine blood transfusion (19).

CLINICAL RECOMMENDATIONS OF THE VIGNETTE

The patient had a classic clinical course for erythema infectiosum (fifth disease). The only slightly unusual feature of this case was that the patient presented with a febrile seizure. Although febrile seizures can certainly occur in the context of erythema infectiosum, most children with the disorder do not have seizures—febrile or otherwise.

The patient had a head CT scan, lumbar puncture, and multiple blood tests. Whether any of these laboratory tests were necessary is debatable. The child had a simple febrile seizure, from which he quickly and fully recovered. Following treatment of the fever, he had a normal level of consciousness and was no longer irritable. Many pediatricians and pediatric neurologists would not feel that laboratory testing was necessary in this setting.

Other than symptomatic treatment of the fever, the child did not receive any therapy, such as immunoglobulin, for parvovirus B19 infection, nor did he require it. As is true of most immunocompetent children infected with parvovirus B19, the patient mounted an immune response against the virus and cleared it. The "slapped cheek" exanthem announced that antibodies against parvovirus B19 had been formed. Unless the child develops an immune disorder, he will never again be infected with parvovirus B19.

SUMMARY

Parvovirus B19 is a ubiquitous pathogen that infects many individuals worldwide. In most cases of childhood infection, the virus causes erythema infectiosum, a benign and self-limited viral syndrome identifiable by its characteristic exanthem, the "slapped cheeks" rash. In patients who are not healthy normal children, the virus can induce more sinister diseases, including aplastic crisis in patients with hematologic disorders, persistent infection with anemia in immunocompromised patients, and hydrops fetalis in unborn children. Parvovirus B19 infection is a common cause of febrile seizures in children and has also been associated with a variety of other neurologic diseases, including meningitis, encephalitis, and transverse myelitis. The diagnostic approach to parvovirus B19, which depends on the clinical setting, includes serology and DNA assays. Much remains to be learned about parvovirus B19 infections, including the pathogenesis by which it induces diseases and identification of specific antiviral therapies.

REFERENCES

1. Schwartz TF, Gurtler LG, Zoulek G, et al. Seroprevalence of human parvovirus B19 infection in Sao Tome and Principe, Malawi and Mescarene Islands. *Zentralbl Bakteriol.* 1989;271:231–236.
2. De Freitas RB, Wong D, Boswell F, et al. Prevalence of human parvovirus B19 and rubella virus infections in urban and remote rural areas in northern Brazil. *J Med Virol.* 1990;32:203–208.
3. MMWR. Risks associated with human parvovirus B19 infection. *MMWR Morb Mort Wkly Rep.* 1989;38:81–88, 93–97.
4. American Academy of Pediatrics. Parvovirus B19 (*Erythema infectiosum*, fifth disease). In: Pickering L, ed. *2006 Red Book: Report of the Committee on Infectious Diseases*, 27th ed. Elk grove Village, IL: American Academy of Pediatrics; 2006:484–487.
5. Flint SJ, Enquist LW, Racaniello VR, et al. Parvoviruses. In: *Principles of Virology. Molecular Biology, Pathogenesis, and Control of Animal Viruses*, 2nd ed. Washington, DC: ASM Press; 2004:817–821.
6. Brown KE, Hibbs JR, Gallinella G, et al. Resistance to human parvovirus B19 infection due to lack of virus receptor (erythrocyte P antigen). *N Engl J Med.* 1994;330:1192–1196.
7. Weir E. Parvovirus B19 infection: Fifth disease and more. *CMAJ.* 2005;172:743.
8. Moffatt S, Yaegashi N, Tada K, et al. Human parvovirus B19 nonstructural (NS1) protein induces apoptosis in erythroid lineage cells. *J Virol.* 1998;72:3018–3028.
9. Corcoran A, Doyle S. Advances in biology, diagnosis and host-pathogen interactions of parvovirus B19. *J Med Microbiol.* 2004;53:459–475.
10. Morey AL, Keeling JW, Porter HJ, et al. Clinical and histopathological features of parvovirus B19 infection in the human fetus. *British Journal of Obstetrics and Gynaecology.* 1992;99:566–574.
11. Valeur-Jensen AK, Pedersen CB, Westergaard T, et al. Risk factors for parvovirus B19 infection in pregnancy. *JAMA.* 1999;281:1099–1105.
12. Young NS, Brown KE. Parvovirus B19. *N Engl J Med.* 2004;350:586–597.
13. Serjeant BE, Hambleton RR, Kerr S, et al. Hematological response to parvovirus B19 infection in homozygous sickle cell disease. *Lancet.* 2001;358:1779–1780.
14. Heegaard ED, Schmiegelow K. Serologic study on parvovirus B19 infection in childhood acute lymphoblastic leukemia during chemotherapy: Clinical and hematologic implications. *J Pediatr Hematol Oncol.* 2002;24:368–373.
15. Barah F, Vallely PJ, Cleator GM, et al. Neurological manifestations of human parvovirus B19 infection. *Rev Med Virol.* 2003;13:185–199.
16. Hsu D, Sandborg C, Hahn JS. Frontal lobe seizures and uveitis associated with acute human parvovirus B19 infection. *J Child Neurol.* 2004;19:304–306.
17. Koch WC, Harger JH, Barnstein B, et al. Serologic and virologic evidence for frequent intrauterine transmission of human parvovirus B19 with a primary maternal infection during pregnancy. *Pediatr Infect Dis J.* 1998;17:489–494.
18. Kurtzman G, Frickhofen N, Kimball J, et al. Pure red-cell aplasia of 10 years' duration due to persistent parvovirus B19 infection and its cure with immunoglobulin therapy. *N Engl J Med.* 1989;321:519–523.
19. Matsuda H, Sakaguchi K, Shibasaki T, et al. Intrauterine therapy for parvovirus B19 infected symptomatic fetus using B19 IgG-rich high titer gammaglobulin. *J Perinat Med.* 2005;33:561–563.

CHAPTER 155

Neurologic Complications of Henoch-Schonlein Purpura

William E. Bell • Jacob A. Lohr

OBJECTIVES

- To explain the immune-mediated pathophysiology of Henoch-Schonlein purpura
- To describe the clinical signs, variations in presentation, and laboratory abnormalities of the disease
- To explain the neurologic complications of the disease and their pathogenesis
- To discuss the treatment of the neurologic complications of Henoch-Schonlein purpura

CASE VIGNETTE

A 5-year-old boy has had cramping abdominal pain for 4 days. On the day of admission, he develops palpable purpura on both legs and buttocks. He has gross hematuria and his blood pressure is 142/94 mm Hg. Soon after admission, the child has a generalized convulsion, stopped after 6 minutes with intravenous lorazepam. On beginning to respond, he has "searching" eye movements and complains of inability to see. His vision recovers within 20 minutes.

DEFINITION

Henoch-Schonlein purpura is the most common noninfectious systemic vasculitis of childhood. The illness is a small-vessel, immune complex leukocytoclastic vasculitis with a predilection to affect arterioles and capillaries of the skin, the intestinal tract, the joints, and the kidneys. The pathologic hallmark of the disease is the deposition of IgA and, to a lesser degree, complement in cutaneous and visceral blood vessels, which can be demonstrated by direct immunofluorescent staining. The deposition of IgA in the kidneys is similar to that seen in IgA nephropathy.

The immune complex vascular deposits provoke a leukocytoclastic vasculitis consisting of perivascular collections of neutrophils, fibrinoid degeneration of the vessel wall, and local extravasation of red blood cells into tissues. The vascular inflammatory reaction is associated with slightly raised skin lesions referred to as *palpable purpurea,* which occur without a coagulopathy or reduced platelet count. The antigenic stimulus leading to this autoimmune process remains unknown, although a preceding viral illness is often suspected. In honor of the early descriptions by Berlin physicians, Johannes Schonlein in 1837 and Eduard Henoch in 1868, the disease is now called *Henoch-Schonlein purpura.* In earlier times, the disorder was often referred to as *anaphylactoid purpura.*

EPIDEMIOLOGY

Henoch-Schonlein purpura is most common in children between 3 and 7 years of age and is infrequent in adults. The annual incidence is approximately 10 cases per 100,000 children aged 14 years and younger (1). The illness is usually self-limiting, lasting 3 to 5 weeks in most. The intensity of the renal involvement is the most important factor determining the duration and the severity at the illness.

CLINICAL MANIFESTATIONS

The clinical manifestations of Henoch-Schonlein purpura vary from patient to patient, but involve a cutaneous petechial or purpuric rash, cramping abdominal pain, arthritis, and glomerulonephritis. At presentation, only about 20% of affected children exhibit all four of the cardinal features. When the three most common manifestations, including rash, abdominal pain, and arthritis, all develop during the illness, the time period between the initial symptoms and the presence of all three features is usually <3 weeks. Nephritis of some degree eventually is found in most, but usually somewhat later. In unusual cases, hematuria can be the presenting feature of the illness. The cutaneous rash is classically purpuric; in children, however, it initially can be urticarial and associated with local edema before becoming purpuric. The rash is generally most intense over the legs and buttocks and is found in almost all children, but is not always the initial sign. Abdominal pain, sometimes the presenting symptom, is the second most common feature of the illness, followed in frequency by arthritis and renal involvement. The relative, but not invariable, absence of pulmonary pathology in Henoch-Schonlein purpura is an important aspect differentiating this condition from certain other immune complex diseases.

Henoch-Schonlein purpura is uncommonly seen in infants <12 months of age; when it does occur, however, it is usually characterized by a facial purpuric eruption with facial edema, unlike the customary location of the rash in older children. Although the number of cases reported in early infancy is limited, it is believed that the frequency of symptomatic gastrointestinal and renal involvement in this age group is less than is found in the more typical older age group (2).

Cramping abdominal pain accompanied by gross blood in the stool or blood identified by guaiac testing is a diagnostic hallmark of Henoch-Schonlein purpura. Submucosal hemorrhages accompanied by bowel wall edema give rise to the abdominal symptoms and can serve as a lead-point for the development of intussusception in 3% or less of children with this condition. Intussusception occurring with Henoch-Schonlein purpura is ileoileal in about 50% of cases, whereas intussusception found in otherwise healthy children is ileocolic in location in up to 90% of cases. The ileoileal site is less likely to be reduced by nonsurgical means.

Arthritis, not usually a presenting sign, evolves during the course of the illness in most cases. One or two joints are typically affected with pain and swelling resulting in a limp or refusal to walk. A predilection exists for the knee and ankle to be affected, whereas large joints in the upper limbs are often less involved.

Nephritis is the least consistently present feature and the one most variable in regard to its degree of clinical significance in Henoch-Schonlein purpura. The prognosis of the disease is largely determined by the severity of renal involvement and, perhaps, by the effectiveness of therapy. Renal injury is not usually the initial or presenting finding and may first become apparent as late as 3 months after onset. In most cases, clinical evidence of nephritis is mild, with only microscopic hematuria, with or without low-grade proteinuria. Less often, the renal insult is more intense with macroscopic hematuria, nephrotic-range proteinuria, red blood cell casts in urine, oliguria, azotemia, and systemic hypertension. Severe nephritis increases the possibility of chronic renal sequelae, including end-stage renal failure in some. Renal function compromise and hypertension are the primary indications for aggressive treatment of Henoch-Schonlein purpura. Another possible genitourinary manifestation of the illness is scrotal erythema, swelling, and tenderness.

DIAGNOSTIC APPROACH

Few laboratory findings are considered diagnostic of Henoch-Schonlein purpurea, with the exception of tissue biopsy (skin or kidney) showing IgA deposits in vessel walls, combined with a compatible clinical syndrome. Laboratory findings that can be informative include a mild leukocytosis, which is found in many, but not all. Erythrocyte sedimentation rate (ESR) and C-reactive protein (CRP) are markedly elevated in most cases, but exceptions do occur, and a normal ESR does not exclude the diagnosis. Thrombocytosis is prevalent in the second or third week of illness. Serum complement levels usually remain normal, although a mild reduction in C3 can occur. Serum IgA levels are increased in more than half of the cases during active inflammation (1). Tissue biopsy showing IgA deposits in vessel walls can be useful in select instances, but is not required in most who present with typical clinical and laboratory findings.

The diagnosis of Henoch-Schonlein purpura is readily apparent when it presents with palpable purpura in the typical distribution, abdominal pain, and blood in the stools, and a normal or raised platelet count. The diagnosis becomes more problematic when abdominal complaints precede the rash or in unusual instances when nephritis is the initial manifestation leading to the assumption that other forms of acute nephritis are the more likely cause. The abdominal presentation can initially raise concern of acute appendicitis or inflammatory bowel disease. Acute onset of arthritis can sometimes support the possibility of juvenile rheumatoid arthritis, and the purpuric skin eruption initially may be assumed to be a manifestation of child abuse, especially in infants in whom the rash is often facial and associated with edema (3). Meningococcemia is included in the differential diagnosis, but is usually a more highly febrile illness and is accompanied by signs compatible with septicemia.

The prognosis among children with Henoch-Schonlein purpura is regarded to be favorable with >70% having recovered within 6 weeks after onset. This includes those with mild renal involvement, although patients with severe renal compromise often experience a more prolonged and more complicated clinical course. Recurrences, which can include any of the features of the disorder, occur in about a third of patients. These recurrences are ordinarily less severe than the initial presentations.

Treatment is primarily symptomatic for most children with Henoch-Schonlein purpura, including those with mild degrees of nephritis. Evidence suggests a benefit of corticosteroids for relief of arthritis symptoms and gastrointestinal pain, but not for prevention of recurrences. More severe renal compromise and hypertension require more aggressive therapeutic measures. Recent studies indicate that the prognosis when nephritis is intense can be improved with prolonged corticosteroid therapy, sometimes combined with azathioprine or cyclophosphamide (4,5).

NEUROLOGIC COMPLICATIONS

Neurologic complications, except for headache and irritability, are infrequent and are estimated to occur in 3% to 5% of cases. Either the central nervous system (CNS) or the peripheral nervous system (PNS) can be affected, the latter especially being rarely encountered. Among the few children who develop intussusception, it has been observed that lethargy disproportionate to fluid and electrolyte abnormalities is frequent. The cause of this finding is unclear. Headache and intense irritability are common, the latter to be expected in the young child with abdominal pain or joint pain.

Cranial or PNS involvement is decidedly rare and the pathogenesis of neuropathy with Henoch-Schonlein purpura is poorly understood. Cranial and peripheral mononeuropathies with damage to the facial nerve, the sciatic nerve, the common peroneal nerve, or the femoral nerve have been described and a variety of causative mechanisms have been proposed (6,7). An acute mononeuropathy in a child with Henoch-Schonlein purpura could result from ischemic or hemorrhagic injury to the nerve structure secondary to the vascular inflammatory process. In addition, a compression neuropathy from a localized area of swelling or an adjacent hematoma might explain an isolated neuropathy. Prolonged sitting with leg-crossing in a child no longer ambulating because of arthritic pain could possibly explain a common peroneal palsy with foot drop, although, this condition is much more often seen in adults with no underlying disease. Brachial plexus neuropathy as well as Guillain-Barré syndrome have been described with Henoch-Schonlein purpura and are less easily explained on the basis of an inflammatory vasculitis (8). These more generalized neuropathies in otherwise normal children are generally assumed to be postinfectious, immune-mediated disorders. If the preceding antigenic stimulus giving rise to Henoch-Schonlein purpura is a viral illness as proposed by many, it is possible that brachial plexis neuropathy or Guillain-Barré syndrome complicating Henoch-Schonlein purpura is an immune-mediated process provoked by the preceding infection and not determined by the inflammatory vasculitis associated with this condition.

Central nervous system involvement has been characterized by Belman et al. (6) It includes mental status changes, seizures of various types, and multiple types of focal neurologic defects, such as hemiparesis, chorea, ataxia, aphasia, and cortical blindness. Most brain insults with Henoch-Schonlein purpura are believed to be complications of nephritis and its attendant hypertension, volume depletion, azotemia, and electrolyte abnormalities. The vasculitic process with blood extravasation into tissues has been postulated to affect the brain microvasculature on rare occasions. That cerebral vascular inflammation can occur in this disease is supported by reported cases in which mental status changes, seizures, or focal neurologic deficits occurred early in the clinical course, before onset of renal disease or hypertension.

Seizures can be generalized and convulsive, simple partial or complex partial, or even in the form of status epilepticus. A given seizure episode can subside without subsequent neurologic deficits or be followed by a persistent hemiparesis or hemianopsia, indicating that the convulsive episode was the initial presentation of an ischemic or hemorrhagic stroke. The sudden onset of a generalized, convulsive seizure, which is immediately followed by transient bilateral blindness, is strongly suggestive that hypertension was the precipitating factor. This sequence is sometimes associated with a temporary posterior leukoencephalopathy on magnetic resonance imaging (MRI).

Mental status changes can also precede renal compromise or hypertension and are followed by resolution on subsequent improvement of the basic illness. Behavior changes, irritability, lethargy, emotional lability, and mental confusion have been described.

Subarachnoid hemorrhage, subdural hemorrhage, and ischemic strokes complicating Henoch-Schonlein purpura can be followed by eventual resolution and recovery or, less often, will result in permanent neurologic sequelae. Sokol et al. (9) reported the case of an adolescent with Henoch-Schonlein purpura with an ischemic stroke who was found to have antiphospholipid antibody in serum and cerebrospinal fluid (CSF). Whether this represents two unrelated factors acting in concert or the abnormal antibody is an indicator of the predisposition to stroke among those with Henoch-Schonlein purpura remains uncertain.

TREATMENT

No definite guidelines exist regarding treatment of children with Henoch-Schonlein purpura who develop neurologic complications during the active course of the illness. Recommended treatment is by conservative means only for those with the illness who do not have significant renal impairment or hypertension. Among those who develop seizures, strokes, other focal brain disorders, mental state changes, or a mononeuropathy in whom cerebral or neural inflammatory vasculitis is presumed to be causative, a brief course of corticosteroid therapy should be considered, recognizing that such therapy can induce or enhance a rise in blood pressure.

CLINICAL RECOMMENDATIONS OF THE VIGNETTE

The patient has the most threatening component of Henoch-Schonlein purpura—severe nephritis and hypertension. His seizure is attributed to an acute rise in blood pressure. His convulsive attack ceased with intravenous lorazepam and his management in the intensive care unit was designed to lower his blood pressure, control his fluid intake, and maintain electrolyte balance. He responded to these measures and corticosteroid therapy and no further seizures occurred.

SUMMARY

Henoch-Schonlein purpura is a small-vessel, immune complex leukocytoclastic vasculitis that affects young children, in most cases. The disorder can be quickly recognized when it presents with signs of joint inflammation, abdominal pain, and the characteristic purpuric rash in the absence of thrombocytopenia. It is more of a diagnostic challenge when the initial symptom is severe cramping abdominal pain. Neurologic complications of Henoch-Schonlein purpura are infrequent, but can occur secondary to acute hypertension or the metabolic derangements stemming from acute renal failure. Even less common are central or peripheral nervous system lesions provoked by immune complex vasculitis affecting nervous system structures.

REFERENCES

1. Calvino M, Llorca J, Garcia-Porrua C, et al. Henoch-Schonlein purpura in children from northwestern Spain. A 20-year epidemiologic and clinical study. *Medicine.* 2001;80:279–290.
2. Al-Sheyyab M, El-Shanti H, Ajlouni S, et al. The clinical spectrum of Henoch-Schonlein purpura in infants and young children. *Eur J Pediatr.* 1995;154(12):969–972.
3. Brown J, Melinkovich P. Henoch-Schonlein purpura misdiagnosed as suspected child abuse. A case report and literature review. *JAMA.* 1986;256:617–618.
4. Foster BJ, Bernard C, Drummond K, et al. Effective therapy for severe Henoch-Schonlein purpura nephritis with prednisone and azathioprine. A clinical and histopathologic study. *J Pediatr.* 2000;136:370–375.
5. Kawasaki Y, Suzuki J, Nozawa R, et al. Efficacy of methylprednisolone and urokinase pulse therapy for severe Henoch-Schonlein nephritis. *Pediatrics.* 2003;111:785–789.
6. Belman A, Leicher C, Moshe S, et al. Neurologic manifestations of Henoch-Schonlein purpura. Report of three cases and review of the literature. *Pediatrics.* 1985;75:687–692.
7. Ritter F, Seay A, Lahey M. Peripheral mononeuropathy complicating anaphylactoid purpura. *J Pediatr.* 1983;103:77–78.
8. Sanghri L, Sharma R. Guillain-Barré syndrome and presumed allergic purpura. *Archives of Neurology and Psychiatry.* 1956;76:497.
9. Sokol D, McIntyre J, Short R, et al. Henoch-Schonlein purpura and stroke. Antiphosphatidyl-ethanolamine antibody in CSF and serum. *Neurology.* 2000;55:1379–1381.

CHAPTER **156**

Neurologic Complications of the Hemolytic Uremic Syndrome

William E. Bell • Jacob A. Lohr

OBJECTIVES

- To describe the common mode of presentation and the clinical and laboratory abnormalities of the hemolytic uremic syndrome
- To discuss the pathogenesis of the thrombotic microangiopathies and how to manage them
- To explain the common and the unusual causes of the hemolytic uremic syndrome
- To describe the types of neurologic complications that can occur in children with the hemolytic uremic syndrome and their pathogenesis

CASE VIGNETTE

A 4-year-old girl had been well until onset of cramping abdominal pain, followed by watery diarrhea. On day 6 of the illness, the diarrhea becomes grossly bloody. She is admitted to the hospital, found to be lethargic, but combatable when stimulated; laboratory studies reveal evidence of a microangiopathic hemolytic anemia and thrombocytopenia. The child is then found to be oliguric, have azotemia, and blood pressure of 150/94 mm Hg. Within hours after admission, she develops intractable status epilepticus that is poorly responsive to anticonvulsant drugs. Additional laboratory results then become available.

DEFINITION AND EPIDEMIOLOGY

The hemolytic uremic syndrome was first described by Gasser et al. (1) in Germany in 1955 and became popularized in the western hemisphere by the publication of Gianantonio et al. (2) from Buenos Aires, Argentina in 1964. It is a disease that affects all age groups, with most childhood cases occurring in those <10 years of age with a mean of 3 years and with a mortality rate of approximately 3%. A variety of causes of the condition exist, but >90% of cases are the result of colonic infection with enterohemorrhagic *Escherichia coli* O157 H7, an organism that elaborates shiga exotoxins 1 and 2, also known as *verotoxin* because of its ability to damage vero cells or African green monkey cells in tissue culture.

ETIOLOGY AND PATHOGENESIS

Cattle are the primary reservoir of the organism, which can also be found in other large farm animals. Chronic human intestinal carriers of this bacillus are not known to occur, but acute human contamination with *E. coli* O157 H7 resulting in serious disease can derive from several sources. Consumption of inadequately cooked ground beef has been the most highly publicized method of acquiring the organism and, more recently, by direct contact with infected animals at petting zoos or dairy farms (3). The organism can also be acquired from unpasteurized milk or from contaminated water sources. Symptomatic patients can also transmit *E. coli* O157 H7 to others, especially in the early diarrheal stages when only a relatively small number of organisms in the intestinal tract can cause illness, thus rendering them highly contagious, at least for the initial days of illness. The remaining 5% to 10% of cases of hemolytic uremic syndrome are caused by other toxin-producing serotypes of *E. coli*, *Shigella dysenteriae*, *Streptococcus pneumoniae*, and the rare genetically determined, noninfectious form of the disease.

E. coli O157 H7-induced diarrhea becomes hemorrhagic in up to 90% of cases, but only about 10% of those infected will proceed to have the hemolytic uremic syndrome, some mildly and transiently affected but at least 50% will require dialysis because of acute renal failure. The illness begins with cramping abdominal pain and transient fever followed by watery diarrhea. Within 1 to 6 days, diarrhea becomes hemorrhagic and fever has usually subsided by this time. Among the 10% destined to develop the hemolytic uremic syndrome, evidence of nephropathy and hemolytic anemia will begin to appear 5 to 8 days after onset of bloody diarrhea. By this stage of the illness, the causative organisms will no longer be found in stools in 60% to 70% of cases. Etiologic diagnosis, if needed thereafter, will be on the basis of the serologic testing of blood for rising titers of specific IgM and IgG antibodies.

PATHOLOGY

The pathologic sequence of this condition begins with adherence of the *E. coli* O157 H7 to epithelial cells in the colon, followed by bacterial invasion and damage to underlying intestinal tissues. Bacterial elaboration of verotoxin, probably in concert with gram-negative endotoxin, causes damage of the colonic epithelium and vascular endothelium. The process allows entrance of exotoxin into the systemic circulation where it becomes attached to endothelial cells of the glomerular vasculature and that of other visceral tissues. The renal endothelial adherence of exotoxin enhances secretion of Von Willebrand factor multimers from endothelial cells, culminating in the adherence of platelets to the vessel walls and, with a complex interaction with neutrophils, leads to endothelial cell damage and platelet thromboses, a process referred to as *thrombotic microangiopathy* (4). The usurpation of platelets rapidly leads to thrombocytopenia; turbulent blood flow through the damaged microcirculation results in mechanical red blood cell fragmentation seen as schistocytes and helmet cells on peripheral blood smear, which is called *microangiopathic hemolytic anemia.* Thrombocytopenia and a rapidly falling hemotocrit are usually found along with a strikingly increased serum lactate dehydrogenase level, which is probably derived from ischemic tissue damage (4). As renal failure ensues, other common laboratory findings that can contribute to neurologic dysfunction can include progressive azotemia, hyponatremia, hypocalcemia, hyperkalemia, and metabolic acidosis.

CLINICAL MANIFESTATIONS

Certain risk factors are believed to increase the probability of the hemolytic uremic syndrome occurring in children with enterohemorrhagic *E. coli*-induced diarrhea. Antibiotic therapy during the early diarrheal stage is believed by many, but doubted by some, to increase intestinal production of exotoxin from dying bacteria and, thereby, increasing the probability of the development of renal damage. Molbak et al. (5) have proposed that subtherapeutic doses of antimicrobial agents can bring about an increase in bacteria-derived exotoxin within the infected colon. Although debate continues, current recommendations are to avoid antibiotic therapy as well as use of antimotility agents in the acute stage with diarrhea. The initial peripheral blood neutrophil count has been correlated with risk of development of hemolytic uremic syndrome, a finding that also correlates with proposed mechanisms of pathogenesis of neutrophils in the acute enteropathy and within the kidney. One study found that among patients in the diarrheal stage with an initial white blood cell count (WBC) <8,700 cells/mm^3, none developed hemolytic uremic syndrome, whereas among those with initial WBC counts over 14,300/mm^3, 35% developed hemolytic uremic syndrome (6).

Extrarenal microangiopathic pathology is common in this disorder and may or may not result in significant clinical findings (7). Neurologic injury, most often caused by the metabolic abnormalities or hypertension, is the most important extrarenal manifestation, occurring in 30% to 50% of cases. With modern day intensive care unit (ICU) care and improved methods of dialysis, central nervous system (CNS) disease has become one of the most common causes of death from this disease. Pancreatic microangiopathy is found in about 20% of cases of hemolytic uremic syndrome at autopsy and, among survivors, can result in diabetes mellitus, although this is unusual. Hepatomegaly is common and is usually accompanied by elevation of liver transaminases stemming from ischemic hepatic insults. Cholestatic jaundice is unusual and any hepatic manifestation has a favorable outcome. Myocardial dysfunction in the acute stage of the illness occurs infrequently, although pathology of the coronary microvasculature has been described in autopsy studies. The same applies to the lungs where pulmonary hemorrhage and edema are rare findings.

DIAGNOSTIC APPROACH

Diagnosis of hemolytic uremic syndrome is usually not difficult, although initial findings with bloody diarrhea preceding renal failure can be compatible with other bacterial pathogens, intussusception, or inflammatory bowel disease. The most commonly discussed condition in differential diagnosis is thrombotic thrombocytopenic purpura, another thrombotic microangiopathy. Most often encountered in adults, it is not usually preceded by bloody diarrhea, and has more consistent CNS signs and fever. Unlike hemolytic uremic syndrome, most individuals with thrombotic thrombocytopenic purpura will be found during the active stage to have a deficiency of a Von Willebrand-cleaving protease, which is the causative mechanism leading to the microangiopathic syndrome.

Atypical, nondiarrheal forms of hemolytic uremic syndrome are rare; they are heterogeneous relative to cause, usually more severe, sometimes associated with relapses, and have a higher mortality rate compared with those with the diarrheal disease caused by *E. coli* O157 H7. Enteropathogenic *E. coli* urinary tract infection has been found to be a rare cause of the hemolytic uremic syndrome (8), and numerous cases of invasive infection with *S. pneumoniae* have now been found to precede the onset of the nondiarrheal form of the condition. *S. pneumoniae*-associated hemolytic uremic syndrome usually affects younger children than the diarrheal-associated disorder and the illness is more intense, with 75% requiring dialysis. Most reported cases have presented with pneumonia, usually with empyema, and rarely with meningitis. The toxic factor inducing hemolytic uremic syndrome with pneumococcal infection is uncertain, but it is believed to be an effect of neuraminidase released by the organism (9).

Familial or genetically determined atypical hemolytic uremic syndrome is a nondiarrheal, autosomal recessive condition that occurs in early infancy and is characterized by recurrent attacks and with a low serum complement level, thus, is referred to as *hypocomplementemic hemolytic uremic syndrome* (10). Some have been found to be related to a deficiency of complement factor H, a molecule that normally inhibits complement consumption in response to a variety of stimuli. The clinical findings are similar to those of typical diarrheal hemolytic uremic syndrome, but with 1 relapsing microangiopathic hemolytic anemia and nephropathy that rapidly proceeds to end-stage renal failure.

TREATMENT

Treatment of the hemolytic uremic syndrome includes the avoidance of antibiotics and antimotility preparations. Most affected children require ICU care, with close attention to fluid and electrolyte management and control of hypertension, which is estimated to occur in 25% to 30% of cases and which is determined by renal involvement severity. Dialysis is required in at least 50% of patients. Red blood cell transfusion is determined by the degree of anemia. Plasma exchange has not been consistently beneficial in this condition. When the colonic damage is extensive, colectomy may be necessary, but this is a rare event.

NEUROLOGIC COMPLICATIONS

The frequency with which neurologic complications occur with hemolytic uremic syndrome has varied in recently published series, although the consensus is that 30% to 40% of patients with the disorder will experience significant neurologic dysfunction during the course of the illness. In a report describing 60 children by Bale et al. (11), 48% had major CNS signs, including seizures, coma, or both during the illness. In an early study by Gianantonio et al. (2), among 58 children with hemolytic uremic syndrome, 48 had neurologic complications. The high incidence of CNS dysfunction was perhaps explained by the far less advanced care of acute renal failure and its metabolic abnormalities that characterized medical care in all centers at that time.

A wide spectrum of neurologic abnormalities has been described in persons with the hemolytic uremic syndrome implicating either diffuse or focal insults to the brain. Seizures can be single or recurrent or as intractable status epilepticus. Seizures in most reported cases have been convulsive and generalized and, less often, partial in type. Alterations in responsiveness are the next most common CNS manifestation and range from lethargy to stupor to frank and prolonged, but possibly reversible, coma (12). Onset of hemiparesis or hemiplegia can be accompanied by homonymous field defects or aphasia, depending on the location of the causative lesion. Bilateral hypertonicity with hyperreflexia has also been described in patients with retained consciousness.

Diffuse cerebral edema manifested by headache, vomiting, decline in responsiveness, false localizing abducens palsy, or signs of transtentorial herniation can be seen with more severe CNS involvement. Less severe evidence of CNS dysfunction can be associated with vertigo, diplopia, mental confusion, hallucinations, ataxia, or behavioral abnormalities.

Most children with hemolytic uremic syndrome do not have CSF examinations, including those with neurologic complications. Sheth et al. (13) reported the CSF findings in 11 of their series of 15 children with abnormal neurologic signs. None had CSF pleocytosis and four had increased CSF protein content. Among this group of 15 children, electroencephalogram (EEG) finding was abnormal in all 9 patients in whom the test was performed, most showing diffuse slowing, suggestive of a metabolic encephalopathy.

Neuroimages involving cranial computed tomography (CT) and magnetic resonance imaging (MRI) are important in those with neurologic complications to understand the underlying pathology. MRI, especially, is useful to demonstrate single or multiple infarcts, which can be either deep-seated in the basal ganglia or thalamus or more superficial in location. Infarcts can be either ischemic or hemorrhagic and can stem from involvement of the microcirculation or, less often, affecting large or major cerebral arteries. When cerebral infarcts are discovered, magnetic resonance angiography (MRA) can be an additional useful diagnostic technique (10). In addition, neuroimages can play an important role in excluding other unsuspected findings, such as intracranial venous thrombosis, subdural hematoma, or even brain abscess, all having been described in children with the hemolytic uremic syndrome. Diffusion MRI might also be considered to determine whether cerebral edema is vasogenic or cellular in type, whereas perfusion MRI might provide some indication of the integrity at the capillary blood flow.

Risk factors that predispose to the development of CNS complications in hemolytic uremic syndrome are somewhat unclear. One study found that the early use of intestinal antimotility drugs was one such factor (14). Excessive volume of hypotonic fluid administration has been proposed to be a risk factor, but the major determining factor that is believed to explain most neurologic complications of the hemolytic uremic syndrome is the severity of the numerous metabolic abnormalities that accompany acute renal failure. Bale et al. (11), Sheth et al. (13), and others have found that the more severe the metabolic disturbance, the greater is the probability of CNS involvement. Anemia, azotemia, metabolic acidosis, hyperkalemia, hyponatremia, hypocalcemia, and systemic hypertension in various combinations are commonly encountered in children with acute, rapidly progressive renal failure and can directly or indirectly predispose to the neurologic events that occur with this condition.

The development of bacteremia secondary to intestinal mucosal compromise is another, although not often considered, possible risk factor for the occurrence of neurologic complications. Transient bacteremia is probably common in children with necrotizing intestinal disease and renal failure requiring dialysis. Anaerobic bacterial meningitis has been described, as has been *Clostridium septicum* cerebritis and brain abscess (15–17). *E. coli* O157 H7 bacteremia is probably infrequent in children with hemolytic uremic syndrome but has been found in isolated cases.

Although metabolic abnormalities and hypertension are believed to account for most neurologic complications with the hemolytic uremic syndrome, the pathogenesis of vascular insults, including ischemic and hemorrhagic strokes, is less well defined. The neuropathology thus far described among those with neurologic complications has been mainly cerebral edema and hypoxic-ischemic in type (18,19). Thrombotic microangiopathy affecting the cerebral vasculature has been infrequently found and some have questioned its occurrence. Upadhyaya et al. (20), in an early study in 1980, described a series of patients with hemolytic uremic syndrome that included some up to 22 years of age. Pathology at autopsy in some revealed cerebral microangiopathy. It is not known whether the illness was preceded by bloody diarrhea in these patients and the authors state that they were uncertain whether hemolytic uremic syndrome or thrombotic thrombocytopenic purpura was the underlying condition.

Single or multiple small infarcts in white matter of the brain have definitely been described with the hemolytic uremic syndrome. Infarcts in the distribution of major cerebral vessels have been reported much less frequently and have been both bland ischemic or hemorrhagic infarcts (21,22). Thrombocytopenia or, less likely, vitamin K deficiency could contribute to the conversion of an ischemic infarct into a hemorrhagic lesion. Thus far, the cause of large cerebral vessel thrombosis with this disease remains unexplained.

Most ophthalmologic manifestations associated with the hemolytic uremia syndrome appear to be secondary to cerebral hemisphere vascular lesions or the result of intracranial hypertension. Lesions of the optic nerves or retina do occur, in addition to vitreous hemorrhage. Vascular ischemic insults can lead to optic atrophy with visual loss, retinal infarcts, or retinal hemorrhagic lesions (23). Ocular abnormalities complicating this illness are usually seen in those with clinical CNS complications, and as with the latter, can be transient or permanent.

CLINICAL RECOMMENDATIONS OF THE VIGNETTE

The 4-year-old patient had the hemolytic uremic syndrome, with rapidly progressive renal failure and systemic hypertension. Her status epilepticus was explained by laboratory results that showed marked hyponatremia, hypocalcemia, a rising blood urea nitrogen (BUN), and hematocrit of 16. CT scan revealed no focal lesions, and seizures were rapidly controlled by correction of her metabolic abnormalities. She required dialysis for several days and eventually had complete recovery.

SUMMARY

Hemolytic uremic syndrome is a disorder usually seen in young children. Most cases in the United States are cause by *E. coli* O157 H7, although other shiga toxin-producing bacilli as well as *S. pneumoniae* can cause the illness. Hemolytic uremic syndrome is characterized by acute diarrhea, which soon becomes hemorrhagic, and is followed by microangiopathic hemolytic anemia, thrombocytopenia, and nephropathy. Neurologic complications are common among children with this condition, mostly with CNS involvement provoked by the multiple abnormalities and systemic hypertension that often accompany the illness. Thrombotic microangiopathy affecting the brain or spinal cord is believed to be infrequent, if occurring at all, and is more characteristic of thrombotic thrombocytopenic purpura.

REFERENCES

1. Gasser C, Gautier E, Steck A. Hemolytic-uremic syndrome: Bilateral necrosis of the renal cortex in acute acquired hemolytic anemia. *Schweiz Med Wchnschr.* 1955;85: 905–909.
2. Gianantonio C, Vitacco M, Mendilaharzv F, et al. The hemolytic-uremic syndrome. *J Pediatr.* 1964;64:478–491.
3. Crump JA, Sulka AC, Langer AJ, et al. An outbreak of *Escherichia coli* O157 H7 infections among visitors to a dairy farm. *N Engl J Med.* 2002;347:555–560.
4. Moake JL. Thrombotic microangiopathies. *N Engl J Med.* 2002;347:589–600.
5. Molbak K, Mead PS, Griffin PM. Antimicrobial therapy in patients with *Escherichia coli,* O157 H 7 infection. *JAMA.* 2002;288:1014–1016.
6. Wong CS, Jelacic S, Habeeb RL, et al. The risk of the hemolytic uremic syndrome after antibiotic treatment of *Escherichia coli* O157 H 7. *N Engl J Med.* 2000;342:1930–1936.
7. Siegler RL. Spectrum of extrarenal involvement in postdiarrheal hemolytic-uremic syndrome. *J Pediatr.* 1994;125:511–518.
8. Starr M, Bennett-Wood V, Bigham AK, et al. Hemolytic-uremic syndrome following urinary tract infection with enterohemorrhagic *Escherichia coli*: Case report and review. *Clin Infect Dis.* 1998;27:310–315.
9. Brandt J, Wong C, Mihm S, et al. Invasive pneumococcal disease and hemolytic uremic syndrome. *Pediatrics.* 2002;110:371–376.
10. Landau D, Shaler H, Levy-Finer G, et al. Familial hemolytic uremic syndrome associated with complement factor H deficiency. *J Pediatr.* 2001;138:412–417.
11. Bale JF, Jr., Bradsher C, Siegler RL. CNS manifestations of the hemolytic-uremic syndrome. Relationship to metabolic alterations and prognosis. *Am J Dis Child.* 1980;134:869–872.
12. Steele BT, Murphy N, Chuang SH, et al. Recovery from prolonged coma in hemolytic uremic syndrome. *J Pediatr.* 1983;102:402–404.
13. Sheth KJ, Swick HM, Haworth N. Neurologic involvement in hemolytic-uremic syndrome. *Ann Neurol.* 1986;19:90–93.
14. Cimolai N, Morrison BJ, Carter JE. Risk factors for the central nervous system manifestations of gastroenteritis-associated hemolytic-uremic syndrome. *Pediatrics.* 1992;90:616–621.
15. Broughton RA, Lee EY. Clostridium sepsis and meningitis as a complication of the hemolytic-uremic syndrome. *Clin Pediatr.* 1993;32:750–752.
16. Chiang V, Adelson PD, Povssaint TY, et al. Brain abscesses caused by *Clostridium septicum* as a complication of hemolytic-uremic syndrome. *Pediatr Infect Dis J.* 1995;14:72–74.
17. Randall JM, Hall R, Coulthard MG. Diffuse pnenumocephalus due to clostridium septicum cerebritis in hemolytic uraemic syndrome. CT demonstration. *Neuroradiology.* 1993;35: 218–220.
18. Hahn JS, Havens PL, Higgens JJ, et al. Neurological complications of hemolytic-uremic syndrome. *J Child Neurol.* 1989;4:108–113.
19. Rooney JR, Anderson RM, Hopkins IJ. Clinical and pathological aspects of the central nervous system involvement in the hemolytic uremic syndrome. *Australian Paediatric Journal.* 1971;7:28–33.
20. Upadhyaya K, Barwick K, Fishaut M, et al. The importance of nonrenal involvement in hemolytic-uremic syndrome. *Pediatrics.* 1980;65(1):115–120.
21. Crisp DE, Siegler RL, Bale JF, et al. Hemorrhagic cerebral infarction in the hemolytic-uremic syndrome. *J Pediatr.* 1981;99:273–276.
22. Trevathan E, Dooling EC. Large thrombotic strokes in hemolytic-uremic syndrome. *J Pediatr.* 1987;111:863–866.
23. Siegler RL, Brewer ED, Swartz M. Ocular involvement in hemolytic-uremic syndrome. *J Pediatr.* 1988;112:594–598.

CHAPTER **157**

Nonaccidental Head Trauma in Infants: The "Shaken Baby Syndrome"

Paula Gerber • Kathryn A. Coffman • John B. Bodensteiner

OBJECTIVES

- To describe the clinical presentation of shaken baby syndrome
- To explain the risk factors for abusive head injury in infants
- To describe the epidemiology, biomechanics, pathology, and imaging findings characteristic of shaken baby syndrome
- To discuss treatment strategies for shaken baby syndrome

CASE VIGNETTE

A 9-month-old girl is brought in to the emergency room after a reported ground-level fall onto soft carpet. She was previously healthy, twin B of an uncomplicated pregnancy, with age-appropriate development. She lives with her parents and twin brother, and attends a small home daycare during the week. In the emergency room, she is found to be stuporous, afebrile, and without external signs of trauma. Pupils are equal and reactive, and funduscopic examination reveals bilateral retinal hemorrhages. Tone is depressed and she withdraws to pain in all four extremities. A noncontrast computed tomographic (CT) scan reveals a large right subdural hematoma with right-to-left midline shift.

DEFINITION

Caffey (1) described the "shaken baby syndrome" (SBS) in 1972. The syndrome consists of retinal hemorrhages, subdural, subarachnoid, or both hemorrhage in an infant with little sign of external trauma. Other names given to this syndrome are the *whiplash shake syndrome* and the shaken impact syndrome (see below).

EPIDEMIOLOGY

The incidence of nonaccidental traumatic brain injury (TBI) in children <2 years of age is estimated to be 17 of 100,000 person-years versus 15.3 of 100,000 person-years for accidental TBI (2). A relatively higher incidence is found of nonaccidental TBI in male children, and in children aged 12 months and under compared with older children (2). Children of ethnic minority descent have been reported to have a higher incidence of both accidental and nonaccidental TBI, which may reflect socioeconomic factors. Other risk factors include young or unmarried mothers, a maternal education level of high school or lower, unstable family situations, low socioeconomic status, multiple birth pregnancies, and disability or prematurity of the child. Having extended family in the home and having a parent in the military have also been found to increase the risk of inflicted TBI (2–4). The most frequent perpetrators are fathers, followed closely by mother's boyfriends, then female babysitters, and lastly mothers (2–5).

CLINICAL MANIFESTATIONS

The classic presentation of nonaccidental head trauma in infants is the so-called *shaken baby syndrome*, consisting of retinal hemorrhages, subdural, subarachnoid, or both hemorrhage in an infant with little sign of external trauma. The mechanism of injury in the syndrome has been a matter of debate. The syndrome was originally described by Caffey in 1972 (1). Apparently, a nursemaid admitted to having shaken several such children while holding them by the arms or trunk, leading to the theory that the injury pattern resulted from shear forces tearing the bridging veins in the subdural space. Some authors have challenged this model, reporting that shaking alone is not sufficient to cause the pattern of injury seen in these patients, and that some impact is required (see below) (6). Others have described a *whiplash-shake syndrome* with significant cervical spine injury, with subdural and epidural hematomas and contusions of the cord at the cervicomedullary junction (7). According to this model, damage to the cervicomedullary junction, particularly the respiratory centers, is an important mechanism contributing to morbidity and mortality (7,9). Lastly, a similar *tin ear syndrome* has been reported, with unilateral ear bruising, ipsilateral cerebral edema, and retinal hemorrhage after blunt trauma to the ear (10). Regardless of the actual mechanism of injury, these patterns should raise suspicion for nonaccidental trauma.

Other *red flags* that may indicate inflicted head trauma in infants include a history that changes over time or between caregivers; also, a developmentally incompatible history (e.g., a 6-month-old child who tried to climb out of his crib and fell) is suspicious (3). In the situation where no trauma or only minor trauma is reported to the treating physicians, a positive predictive value of 0.92 exists for abuse (11). Some authors have reported that children with diffuse brain injury, such as that seen after shaking injury, will not present with a lucid interval; they will lose consciousness immediately (12). A lucid interval, however, has been described in young children with fatal diffuse brain injury caused by accidental falls, so this is not a reliable distinguishing feature (12,13).

External signs of abuse or neglect should be sought. In SBS, however, external signs of trauma often are lacking. Altered level of consciousness, irritability, bulging fontanel, focal neurologic signs, and seizures indicate a high likelihood of intracranial injury (14). A skeletal series is recommended to look for fractures indicating previous abuse. The most frequent fractures seen are through the metaphysis of the tibia, distal femora, and proximal humeri, where the immature bone is more susceptible to injury. Posterior rib fractures are highly specific for abuse as well (12).

Retinal hemorrhage (RH) usually indicates an inflicted injury, unless the presenting history is a severe trauma, such as a motor vehicle accident (12,15). RH are reported in only 10% of accidental TBI in children <24 months of age, versus 60% in inflicted TBI (16). A 2002 series of 16 infants with subdural hemorrhage after traffic accidents found only 3 who also had RH (17). Thus, it is believed that the average fall or injury occurring in the home would not be sufficient to cause this pattern of hemorrhage (18). It should also be noted that RH can sometimes be seen in association with papilledema, subarachnoid hemorrhage, coagulopathy, galactosemia, hypertension, after cardiopulmonary resuscitation, and up to 1 month after vaginal delivery (19). A rare metabolic disorder, *glutaric aciduria type 1*, can present with RH, acute subdural hematoma, and chronic subdural effusions. Nevertheless, statistically, RH in infants are still more likely to be seen after inflicted TBI (15,16,20).

RH in children with abusive head injury are more likely to be bilateral and multiple, to extend to the periphery of the retina, and to be associated with pre-RH and premacular RH (12,16). RH in these children can also be associated with retinal detachments, tears, folds, and vitreous hemorrhage. In contrast, RH associated with accidental trauma, tend to be unilateral, few in number, and found at the posterior pole (16,17,21). RH associated with increased intracranial pressure (IC P) also tend to be at the posterior pole, and associated with papilledema (12,17). Bilateral RH have been reported in children observed by a second party, fatal accidental short falls from playground equipment. The number of cases reported in this particular study was small (3/18), and >75,000 injury reports over a period of 11.5 years were searched to identify the 18 deaths. Formal ophthalmologic examinations were not documented. Age ranged from 12 months to 13 years, with a median age of 4.5 years (22). Most cases of SBS occur in children <12 months of age (2). Thus, this data should be interpreted with caution with regard to the typical infant with SBS. It is probably most prudent to view RH, regardless of the pattern, as suggestive of rotational acceleration injury, while remaining aware of possible exceptions. It is important to take into account the biomechanics of the reported trauma, and decide if the injury pattern fits.

BIOMECHANICS AND PATHOPHYSIOLOGY

Head trauma occurs when a mechanical load is delivered to the head. In most cases, this is a dynamic load, which can be of two types: *impact* or *impulsive*. An *impact* load, obviously, is delivered at a point of impact and can lead to immediate contact effects, such as skull fracture, contusion, or epidural hematoma. Small, focal subdural hemorrhage may also be seen underlying a point of impact (23,24). Possible remote impact injuries include contrecoup injuries and basilar skull fractures (23,25). *Impulse* is defined as a change in momentum caused by a force applied over an interval of time (i.e., acceleration or deceleration). This leads to tissue *strain*, which can be of three types: tension, compression, or shear (see Fig. 157-1) (25). Shearing forces on the bridging veins and the retina, caused by acceleration or deceleration in jury, are thought to be the cause of diffuse subdural hemorrhage and RH in SBS (1,12,23,24,25,35).

The brain has the unique property of *viscoelasticity*, which means that its tolerance to strain changes with the rate of delivery of the strain. This means that, not only the magnitude of acceleration or deceleration, but also the rate at which it occurs will determine the nature of the injury. For instance, falling and striking a hard surface leads to a rapid deceleration and impact load that can cause a superficial injury (e.g., a skull fracture) and possibly an underlying focal hemorrhage. Higher magnitude or duration of deceleration can cause more diffuse shearing injury. Brief, anterior-posterior acceleration and deceleration of high magnitude is thought to cause diffuse subdural hemorrhage (i.e., not directly underlying an impact site), whereas prolonged acceleration and deceleration of relatively lower magnitude in the coronal plane is more likely to lead to diffuse axonal injury (23,26). An example of this is striking the soft cushion of a headrest in a high-speed motor vehicle accident, which reduces impact effects but prolongs the duration of deceleration (25).

Violent shaking is presumed to cause severe acceleration or deceleration injury as the head whips back and forth. Infants, in particular, are at risk because of their relatively large heads,

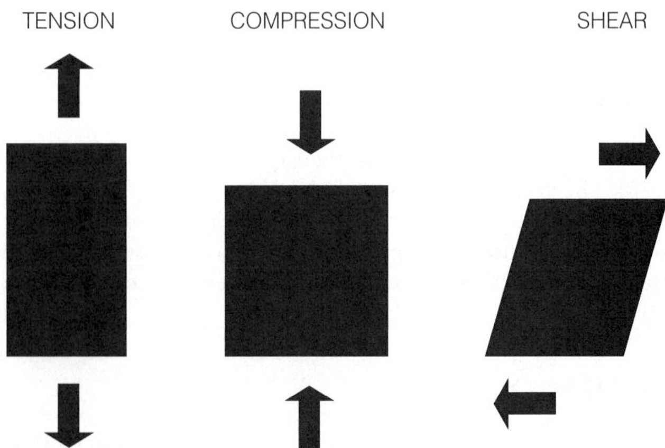

FIGURE 157-1. Patterns of tissue strain induced by acceleration/deceleration injury.

weak neck muscles, and relatively large subarachnoid spaces (6). Their brains are relatively "soft" because of immature myelination and small axonal size. They are more susceptible to impact effects as well. Their thin, soft skulls more readily transmit impulse forces to deeper structures (12).

Some have questioned the theory that shaking alone is sufficient to cause the injuries seen in SBS. One biomechanical model using dolls showed that the average adult shaking an infant would not achieve the degree of angular acceleration necessary to cause the pattern of injury seen in SBS; whereas shaking followed by impact would. These authors have proposed renaming the syndrome *shaken impact syndrome* (6). The exact mechanism of injury in SBS remains a subject of some controversy (27,28).

Following acute TBI, there is frequently a loss of cerebral blood flow autoregulation and a disruption in ion homeostasis. Both of these factors contribute to brain swelling seen after TBI, which usually develops over the first 24 to 72 hours following the injury. In particular, ipsilateral edema of an entire hemisphere is often seen in association with an acute subdural hematoma. This phenomenon is not entirely understood, but it is believed to be related to loss of autoregulation with increased blood flow, and subsequent disruption of the blood–brain barrier. Defective ion transport and excitatory amino acids, leading to cellular toxicity, have also been implicated. A region of brain with defective autoregulation will be at greater risk for ischemic or hyperemic injury secondary to changes in cerebral perfusion pressure. Infants appear to be more susceptible to these processes, perhaps because of immature autoregulation and a greater risk for postinjury apnea and hypotension (19,25,29).

NEUROIMAGING FINDINGS

Imaging modalities in suspected child abuse cases should include skull radiographs and CT imaging, to evaluate for skull fractures and intracranial hemorrhage, respectively (30). Magnetic resonance imaging (MRI) is increasingly being recognized as an important modality, because of its sensitivity to hypoxic-ischemic injury and white matter injury (30–32).

Subdural hemorrhage is a characteristic finding of SBS. These are most commonly seen along the interhemispheric fissure and over the convexities (33,34) (Fig. 157-2). Subarachnoid hemorrhage can be seen as well, typically along the falx cerebri or focally within sulci along the hemispheres (30).

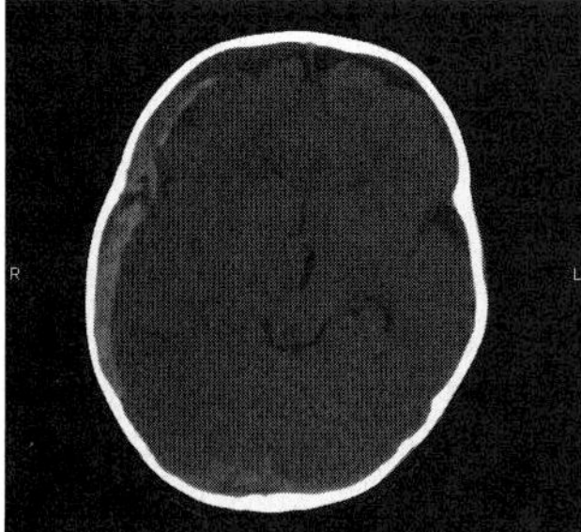

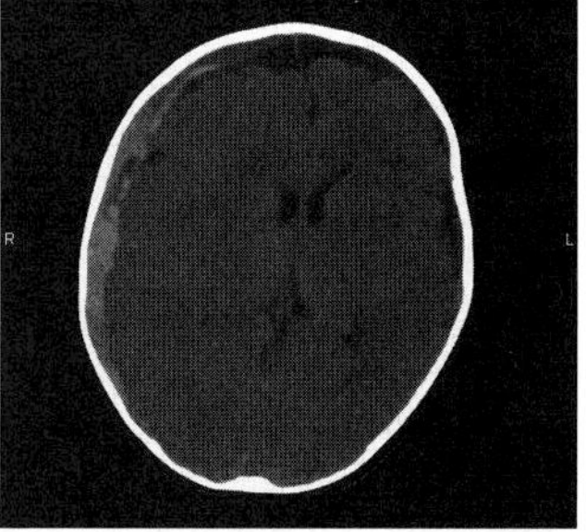

FIGURE 157-2. Noncontrast computed tomographic (CT) scan of the head of a 9-month-old girl shows a large right subdural hematoma with right-to-left midline shift. The varied density of the hematoma can be seen with hyperacute hemorrhage, an evolving subdural hemorrhage, or repetitive trauma with hemorrhage of different ages.

Epidural hemorrhage and intraparenchymal hemorrhage are seen less commonly (33,34).

Shear injury or diffuse axonal injury is classically associated with severe, high-velocity motor vehicle accidents, but can be seen in non-accidental TBI as well (30,33,34). It is an important marker for demonstrating severe accelerational injury. MRI is the modality of choice for detecting this, and gradient echo sequences should be included to detect small white matter hemorrhages. Diffusion-weighted imaging can detect nonhemorrhagic injury (31,32). Shearing injuries commonly involve the subcortical white matter, the corpus callosum, the brainstem, and the internal capsule (30).

Hypoxic-ischemic injury is an important consequence of SBS as well. This is best demonstrated with MRI diffusion-weighted imaging, which shows diffusion restriction in the area of injury. Injuries can be multifocal and widespread, and do not necessarily respect vascular territories. Cerebral edema, related to ischemia or caused by the mechanisms described above, is commonly seen. On CT scan, diffuse loss of gray-white differentiation and hypodensity in the hemisphere underlying a subdural hematoma, sometimes extending into the contralateral frontal lobe, is seen. MRI demonstrates diffusion restriction and T2 hyperintensity in the area of edema (Fig. 157-3) (4,30,33–35).

Children with inflicted injuries are also more likely to show enlarged subarachnoid or subdural spaces (often these are difficult to distinguish radiographically). Enlarged subarachnoid spaces can represent either brain atrophy or communicating hydrocephalus, reflecting previous head injuries (33,35). This phenomenon has also been reported underlying acute subdural hemorrhage. Subdural fluid collections (*hygromas*) can also develop after trauma from a tear in the arachnoid and accumulation of cerebrospinal fluid (35).

Benign extracerebral fluid collections (also known as *benign macrocephaly* or *external hydrocephalus*) are a source of controversy. These are defined as asymptomatic, enlarged subarachnoid spaces, without ventricular dilatation, in young children with rapidly growing heads (36,37). This is likely related to immaturity of the arachnoid villi with transient communicating hydrocephalus (35). Some studies have shown a predisposition in these children toward subdural hemorrhage after minor traumas, and have argued that this finding may be evidence against inflicted trauma (36,38). Others, however, have reported no increased frequency of subdural hematomas over time in these children (35,39). In general, all subdural hemorrhage should be viewed with a high index of suspicion. Consultation with an experienced neuroradiologist can help in distinguishing these confusing findings (37,40).

PATHOLOGY

In autopsy series, the most common findings in infants with nonaccidental head trauma are subdural hemorrhage, retinal hemorrhage, and skull fracture. Very young infants (2 to 3 months of age) tend to show patterns of apnea and hypoxia, craniocervical junction injury, skull fractures, and comparatively smaller subdural hemorrhages. Older children tend to show larger subdural hematomas and more severe extracranial injuries. Classic markers for diffuse axonal injury are relatively rare, but some authors suggest that this is because of differences in axonal injury patterns in an immature brain (8,9,12,41). Cause of death is most commonly raised ICP secondary to

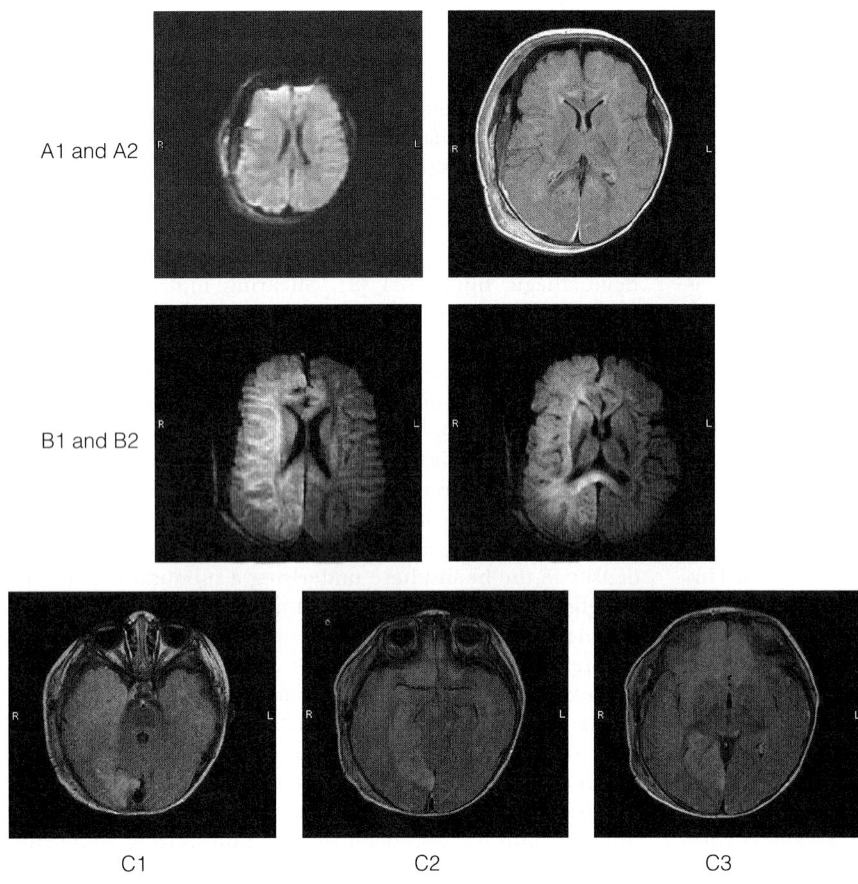

FIGURE 157-3. Magnetic resonance imaging (MRI) of the brain of a 9-month-old girl within the first 24 hours after admission with a right subdural hematoma shows no diffusion restriction and no T2 signal abnormality (fluid-attenuated inversion recovery [FLAIR] sequence shown) in the underlying parenchyma (**A1** and **A2**). Repeat MRI on hospital day 6 shows extensive diffusion restriction (**B1** and **B2**) and T2 hyperintensity on FLAIR images (**C1-C3**) involving the entire right hemisphere and part of the left inferior frontal lobe. The abnormality crosses multiple vascular territories. Magnetic resonance angiography (MRA) of the head and neck were normal.

severe brain edema; severe hypoxic brain damage is also common. It has been postulated that damage at the craniocervical junction leads to apnea and subsequent hypoxic injury (7–9).

OUTCOMES

Outcomes for these children are poor, with an estimated mortality rate from 15% to 38% (2). Survivors frequently have cognitive impairment and focal neurologic deficits (19). A lower Glasgow Coma Scale at presentation, a prolonged duration of impaired consciousness, and a higher number of lesions on imaging studies all correlate with worse outcomes (42). In addition, abused children who are returned home have a high rate of repeat abuse; estimates range from 31% to 43% (43,44).

TREATMENT

Initial treatment of these infants should include neuroimaging and, if necessary, urgent neurosurgical evaluation. Patients should be treated in the intensive care unit with fluid resuscitation, anticonvulsants, and intubation and ventilation, if necessary (4).

Physicians have a duty to report any suspected case of abuse to the proper authorities. An investigation may be uncomfortable for the family and the treating physician, but an investigation that turns out negative is preferable to missing a case of abuse and putting a child at risk (45). The high rates of repeat abuse mandate strict vigilance on the part of physicians to protect children from further harm or death (43,44).

Once stabilized, multidisciplinary care involving pediatric intensive care, neurology, neurosurgery, ophthalmology, forensic pediatrics, and social work is recommended. If the child survives, he or she will require appropriate therapies and rehabilitation efforts for any neurologic deficits.

CLINICAL RECOMMENDATIONS OF THE VIGNETTE

The patient was intubated in the emergency room and evaluated by neurosurgery, and an immediate craniotomy and drainage of the subdural hematoma were performed. She was admitted to the pediatric intensive care unit. A skeletal series was negative for signs of fracture. A bone scan showed a questionable tibial fracture. Ophthalmology was consulted for evaluation of RH. Forensic pediatrics was consulted because of a suspicion for a nonaccidental injury, and the case was reported to Child Protective Services, who opened an investigation. On hospital day 4, the patient was seen to have partial seizure activity involving the left arm, and she was treated with fosphenytoin. Despite adequate levels of phenytoin, she had continued seizure activity requiring loading with phenobarbital, which controlled the seizures. As she became more alert, a left hemianopia and left hemiparesis became evident. An MRI scan on admission had not shown any signs of parenchymal injury, but a repeat MRI scan on hospital day 6 showed diffuse diffusion restriction involving the entire right hemisphere and the left inferior frontal lobe, consistent with severe neuronal injury (Fig. 157-3).

She gradually had improvement in her level of consciousness, and was able to be extubated. Physical and occupational therapy worked with the patient and the family for treatment of her left hemiparesis. At the time of discharge, the family was still under investigation by Child Protective Services, and the patient was not discharged under the care of her parents.

SUMMARY

Nonaccidental head trauma in infants is common, and is the leading cause of infant death from injury. Clinical features that suggest inflicted trauma include the SBS, consisting of RH, subdural, subarachnoid, or both hemorrhage in an infant with little sign of external trauma. Although some controversy surrounds this topic, in general, the average short fall in the home is not expected to produce either subdural or retinal hemorrhage. Also, a lack of a reported history of trauma or an inconsistent history should raise suspicion. In addition to intracranial injury, these infants have cervical spine injuries and may have fractures of the extremities or ribs.

Acceleration or deceleration, especially of the rotational type, is believed to be the mechanism of injury in SBS (although controversy remains). This leads to shearing forces that can damage blood vessels and the brain parenchyma. After trauma and hemorrhage, there is loss of cerebral vessel autoregulation and breakdown of the blood–brain barrier, leading to brain edema.

Neuroimaging and autopsy findings show subdural hemorrhage and retinal hemorrhage, as well as damage to the lower brainstem and the cervical spine. Cellular damage, reflected by loss of gray-white differentiation on CT and diffusion restriction on MRI, can involve large volumes of tissue, without respecting vascular territories. Signs of hypoxia are seen on autopsy, suggesting that apnea may play a role in the injury process.

Outcomes for these children are poor, with high morbidity and mortality. Treatment should focus on initial stabilization and neurosurgical intervention, if necessary, followed by aggressive rehabilitation efforts to address neurologic deficits. All cases of suspected child abuse should be reported to the proper authorities.

REFERENCES

1. Caffey J. On the theory and practice of shaking infants: Its potential residual effects of permanent brain damage and mental retardation. *Am J Dis Child.* 1972;124:161–169.
2. Keenan HT, Runyan DK, Marshall SW, et al. A population-based study of inflicted traumatic brain injury in young children. *JAMA.* 2003;290(5):621–626.
3. Overpeck MD, Brenner RA, Trumble AC, et al. Risk factors for infant homicide in the United States. *N Engl J Med.* 1998;339(17):1211–6121.
4. Duhaime AC, Christian CW, Rorke LB, et al. Nonaccidental head injury in infants—the "shaken baby syndrome." *N Engl J Med.* 1998;338(25):1822–1829.
5. Starling SP, Holden JR, Jenny C. Abusive head trauma: The relationship of perpetrators to their victims. *Pediatrics.* 1995;95(2):259–262.
6. Duhaime AC, Gennarelli TA, Thibault LE, et al. The shaken baby syndrome: A clinical, pathological, and biomechanical study. *J Neurosurg.* 1987;66:409–415.
7. Hadley MN, Sonntag VKH, Rekate HL, et al. The infant whiplash-shake injury syndrome: A clinical and pathological study. *Neurosurgery.* 1989;24:536–540.
8. Geddes JF, Hackshaw AK, Vowles GH, et al. Neuropathology of inflicted head injury in children. Part I: Patterns of brain damage. *Brain.* 2001;124:1290–1298.
9. Geddes JF, Hackshaw AK, Vowles GH, et al. Neuropathology of inflicted head injury in children. Part II: Microscopic brain injury in infants. *Brain.* 2001;124:1299–1306.
10. Hanigan WC, Peterson RA, Njus G. Tin ear syndrome: Rotational acceleration in pediatric head injuries. *Pediatrics.* 1987;80(5):618–622.
11. Hettler J, Greenes DS. Can the initial history predict whether a child with a head injury has been abused? *Pediatrics.* 2003;111(3):602–607.
12. Case ME, Graham MA, Handy TC, et al. Position paper on fatal abusive head injuries in infants and young children. *Am J Forensic Med Pathol.* 2001;22(2):112–122.
13. Denton SD, Mileusnic D. Delayed sudden death in an infant following an accidental fall. *Am J Forensic Med Pathol.* 2003;24:371–376.
14. Schutzman SA, Barnes P, Duhaime AC, et al. Evaluation and management of children younger than two years old with apparently minor head trauma: Proposed guidelines. *Pediatrics.* 2001;107(5):983–993.
15. Gilliland MG, Luckenbach MW, Chenier TC. Systemic and ocular findings in 169 prospectively studied child deaths: Retinal hemorrhages usually mean child abuse. *Forensic Sci Int.* 1994;68(2):117–132.
16. Bechtel K, Stoessel K, Leventhal JM, et al. Characteristics that distinguish accidental from abusive injury in hospitalized young children with head trauma. *Pediatrics.* 2004;114(1):165–168.
17. Vinchon M, Noizet O, Defoort-Dhellemmes S, et al. Infantile subdural hematomas due to traffic accidents. *Pediatr Neurosurg.* 2002;37:245–243.
18. Duhaime AC, Alario AJ, Lewander WJ, et al. Head injury in very young children: Mechanisms, injury types and ophthalmologic findings in 100 hospitalized patients younger than 2 years of age. *Pediatrics.* 1992;90(2):179–185.
19. Graham DI, Gennarelli TA, McIntosh TK. Trauma. In: Graham DI, Lantos PL, eds. *Greenfield's Neuropathology,* 7th ed. Vol 1. London, England: Arnold; 2002:823–898.
20. Johnson DL, Braun D, Friendly D. Accidental head trauma and retinal hemorrhage. *Neurosurgery.* 1993;33:231–235.
21. Christian CW, Taylor AA, Hertle RW, et al. Retinal hemorrhages caused by accidental household trauma. *J Pediatr.* 1999;135(1):125–127.
22. Plunkett J. Fatal pediatric head injuries caused by short distance falls. *Am J Forensic Med Pathol.* 2001;22(1):1–12.
23. Hymel KP, Bandak FA, Partington MD, et al. Abusive head trauma? A biomechanics-based approach. *Child Maltreat.* 1998;3(2):116–128.
24. Hymel KP, Jenny C, Block RW. Intracranial hemorrhage and rebleeding in suspected victims of abusive head trauma: Addressing the forensic controversies. *Child Maltreat.* 2002;7(4):329–348.
25. Gennarelli TA, Meaney DF. Mechanisms of primary head injury. In: Wilkins RH, Rengachary SS, eds. *Neurosurgery,* 2nd ed. Vol. II. New York: McGraw-Hill 1996:2607–2637.
26. Wilkins B. Head injury-abuse of accident? *Arch Dis Child.* 1997;76:393–397.
27. Donohoe M. Evidence-based medicine and the shaken baby syndrome. Part 1: Literature review, 1966–1998. *Am J Forensic Med Pathol.* 2003;24:239–242.
28. Leestma J. Case analysis of brain-injured admittedly shaken infants, 54 cases, 1969–2001. *Am J Forensic Med Pathol.* 2005;26:199–212.
29. Popp AJ, Feustel PJ, Kimelberg HK. Pathophysiology of traumatic brain injury. In: Wilkins RH, Rengachary SS, eds., *Neurosurgery,* 2nd ed. Vol. II. New York: McGraw-Hill 1996:2633–2637.
30. Poussaint TY, Moeller KK. Imaging of pediatric head trauma. *Neuroimaging Clinics of North America.* 2002;12:271–294, ix.
31. Chan YL, Chu WC, Wong GW, et al. Diffusion-weighted MRI in shaken baby syndrome. *Pediatr Radiol.* 2003;33:574–577.
32. Parizel PM, Ceulemans B, Laridon A, et al. Cortical hypoxic-ischomic brain damage in shaken-baby (shaken impact) syndrome: Value of diffusion-weighted MRI. *Pediatr Radiol.* 2003;33:868–871.
33. Ewing-Cobbs L, Prasad M, Kramer L, et al. Acute neuroradiologic findings in young children with inflicted or noninflicted traumatic brain injury. *Childs Nerv Syst.* 2000;16(1):25–33.
34. Ewing-Cobbs L, Kramer L, Prasad M, et al. Neuroimaging, physical and developmental findings after inflicted and noninflicted traumatic brain injury in young children. *Pediatrics.* 1998;102(2):300–306.
35. Hymel KP, Rumack CM, Hay TC, et al. Comparison of intracranial computed tomography (CT) findings in pediatric abusive and accidental head trauma. *Pediatr Radiol.* 1997;27:743–747.
36. Ravid S, Maytal J. External hydrocephalus: A probable cause for subdural hematoma in infancy. *Pediatr Neurol.* 2003;28(2):139–141.
37. Maytal J, Alvarez LA, Elkin C, et al. External hydrocephalus: Radiologic spectrum and differentiation from cerebral atrophy. *AJR Am J Roentgenol.* 1987;148:1223–1230.
38. Papasian NC, Frim DM. A theoretical model of benign external hydrocephalus that predicts a predisposition towards extra-axial hemorrhage after minor head trauma. *Pediatr Neurosurg.* 2000;33:188–193.
39. Hamza M, Bodensteiner JB, Noorani PA, et al. Benign extracerebral fluid collections: A cause of macrocrania in infancy. *Pediatr Neurol.* 1987;3(4):218–221.
40. Kuzma BB, Goodman JM. Differentiating external hydrocephalus from chronic subdural hematoma. *Surg Neurol.* 1998;50:86–88.
41. Kinney HC, Armstrong DD. Perinatal neuropathology. In: Graham DI, Lantos PL, eds. *Greenfield's Neuropathology,* 7th ed. Vol. 1. London, England: Arnold; 2002:519–606.
42. Prasad MR, Ewing-Cobbs L, Swank PR, et al. Predictors of outcome following traumatic brain injury in young children. *Pediatr Neurosurg.* 2002;36:64–74.
43. Ellaway BA, Payne EH, Rolfe K, et al. Are abused babies protected from further abuse? *Arch Dis Child.* 2004;89:845–846.
44. MacMillan HL, Thomas BH, Jamieson E, et al. Effectiveness of home visitation by public-health nurses in prevention of the recurrence of child physical abuse and neglect: A randomized controlled trial. *Lancet.* 2005;365(9473):1786–1793.
45. Luerssen TG, Bruce DA, Humphreys RP. Position statement on identifying the infant with nonaccidental central nervous system injury (the whiplash-shake syndrome). *Pediatr Neurosurg.* 1993;19(4):170.

CHAPTER **158**

Neurologic Complications of Cystic Fibrosis

William E. Bell • Jacob A. Lohr

OBJECTIVES

- To explain the basic pathophysiology of cystic fibrosis
- To describe the variable genetic mechanisms that cause cystic fibrosis
- To provide an aware of the major organ systems affected in cystic fibrosis and the clinical presentations that result
- To discuss the neurologic abnormalities that can result from complications of cystic fibrosis

CASE VIGNETTE

A 3-year-old boy attended a picnic with his parents on a warm, humid summer day. The child has not grown well in the past year, attributed by his pediatrician to his "asthmalike" recurrences. After playing with other children on the day of the picnic, the child wished to rest and tells his mother he does not feel well. He then becomes confused and soon thereafter has a brief, generalized convulsion and is taken to the nearby emergency department. On entrance to the emergency department, he is responsive, his skin is flushed, and his shirt is moist with sweat. An intravenous line with glucose and isotonic saline is begun, blood is drawn for laboratory tests, and a head computed tomographic (CT) scan is performed.

DEFINITION

Cystic fibrosis is an autosomal-recessive disease caused by a gene mutation located on chromosome 7. Although the illness had been described long before, credit is given to Dorothy Andersen at Columbia University in New York for the first accurate clinical and pathologic description of cystic fibrosis in 1938 (1). Before Andersen's report, cystic fibrosis was widely believed to be caused by vitamin A deficiency because signs of vitamin A deficiency eventually emerged in most children with the disease. After 1944, the term *mucoviscidosis* became popular because of the thick, tenacious secretions found in the respiratory airways and pancreas in these children at autopsy. The first hint of the genetically determined protein defect in cystic fibrosis, not identified until 46 years later, appeared in 1953 when di Sant Agnese et al. (2) discovered that sweat of patients with the condition contained increased levels of chloride ions, an event that provided the diagnostic test for the illness.

The mutant gene for cystic fibrosis was characterized by Riordan et al. (3), in 1989, allowing the development of genetic DNA analysis as a diagnostic measure. The cystic fibrosis gene encodes a protein referred to as the *cystic fibrosis transmembrane conductance regulator* (CFTR protein and gene), which is the primary chloride channel of epithelial cells. Those who inherit double copies of the mutant CFTR gene will experience classic cystic fibrosis. Persons with one mutant gene will retain partial CFTR gene/protein function and have less severe or sometimes minimal pancreatic involvement, this situation is encountered in 10% to 15% of cases of cystic fibrosis. Either type of inheritance will be associated with increased sweat chloride levels, but usually less elevated in those with a single mutant gene copy. The clinical effect of the gene/protein defect is the result of abnormal electrolyte transfer across epithelial surfaces producing desiccated thick viscid secretions in sinuses, exocrine ducts of the pancreas, and airways in the lungs leading to airway obstruction. Sweat glands are likewise affected with diminished reabsorption of sodium and chloride across sweat ductal epithelium accounting for the high chloride content of sweat.

A rare point mutation in the CFTR gene was described by Highsmith et al. (4) in 1994 in which affected patients were found to have chronic obstructive pulmonary disease with characteristic colonization of pulmonary airways with *Staphylococcus aureus* and *Pseudomonas aeruginosa*, but with nondiagnostic, <60 mEq/L, sweat chloride values.

Because of the known wide variation of severity and rate of progression of the clinical illness with cystic fibrosis, even among those with the same gene mutation, current research is being directed to the interaction of so-called susceptibility genes, which generate the presence of a given disease, and modifier genes, which are fundamentally different from susceptibility genes but modify the disease phenotype relative to severity of clinical manifestations of an illness (5). Thus, the variations in clinical features that are recognized with cystic fibrosis can be determined by both the basic genetic mechanism of inheritance and, apparently, by the impact of unrelated genes on the expression of various organ involvements.

EPIDEMIOLOGY

The incidence of cystic fibrosis in the United States is 1 Of 3,400 live births. The disorder is less common, but not rare, among blacks, Native Americans, and Hispanics. The mean age at diagnosis of the illness in the United States has been stated to be between ages 3 and 4 years at which time almost 50% will have clinical evidence of advanced malnutrition. Recent studies suggest a much earlier age at which diagnosis is now established (2), in part, because neonatal screening is becoming more widely used. The current mean age of survival in this country has risen in the recent decades to approximately 33 years.

ETIOLOGY, PATHOGENESIS, AND PATHOLOGY

Respiratory tract disease is usually the initial cause of early symptoms and signs in infancy or early childhood and ultimately is the main cause of morbidity and mortality with cystic fibrosis. Thick, viscid mucus resulting from the basic electrolyte transport abnormality of epithelial cell surfaces leads to respiratory airway obstruction and subsequent airway colonization with *S. aureus*, *P. aeruginosa*, and other organisms. Bacterial infection adds an ongoing endobronchial inflammatory component to the pathology. Cough, episodic wheezing, and exercise intolerance are the usual early symptoms, followed by crackles found on examination and persistent hyperexpansion on chest X-ray study. Symptoms and signs are gradually progressive with aging and are punctuated by episodic exacerbation of airway inflammation with acute worsening of symptoms and with respiratory compromise. Upper airway inflammation manifested by chronic persistent sinusitis, characterized more by radiologic than clinical findings, will develop in most children with cystic fibrosis over time. Pneumothorax is a possible but unusual complication seen later in childhood or in older patients. Older children and adults with far advanced respiratory failure and pulmonary hypertension can develop cor pulmonale and eventual cardiac failure.

The presence or severity of pancreatic exocrine insufficiency in children with cystic fibrosis is much more variable than the respiratory tract disease. Steatorrhea with fat and protein malabsorption will occur in about 50% of cases soon after birth or in the first few months of life and will have developed in up to 90% by the end of the first decade. Malabsorption is a major cause of growth failure among affected children and, if untreated, can lead to depletion of fat-soluble vitamins, including vitamins A, D, E, and K. Cystic fibrosis-related insulin-dependent diabetes mellitus is infrequent in adolescents, but becomes more common among adult survivors of the illness. Approximately 10% to 15% of neonates with cystic fibrosis present with meconium ileus, which affects the distil ileum where thick inspissated meconium lead to obstruction which can be complicated by volvulus, intestinal perforation, and peritonitis. Cholestasis with an elevated serum conjugated bilirubin and jaundice is seen in about 5% of neonates with cystic fibrosis and eventually subsides spontaneously. A higher percentage of neonates and young infants will have elevated serum alanine aminotransferase (ALT) or alkaline phosphatase levels, not associated with, or followed by, significant liver disease.

CLINICAL MANIFESTATIONS, DIAGNOSTIC APPROACH, AND TREATMENT

Diagnosis of cystic fibrosis is sometimes suspected when there is a family history of the disease, but more often is considered in a child with persistent or recurrent respiratory symptoms. Growth failure, with or without clinically apparent diarrhea, is also a frequent reason to consider the possibility of this diagnosis. Less common presenting findings suggestive of the diagnosis include neonatal cholestasis, chronic sinusitis, rectal prolapse in early childhood, and parent discovery of a "salty taste" on kissing the child. The customary laboratory method to establish the diagnosis of cystic fibrosis is the sweat electrolyte test. Genetic DNA analysis can now be done, but is not necessary in many cases (6).

Prenatal diagnosis of cystic fibrosis is available for families with an affected child. The procedure is done by DNA analysis of a chorionic villus sample obtained at about 10 weeks gestation or by amniocentesis at approximately 16 weeks.

Neonatal cystic fibrosis screening can be accomplished using the immunoreactive trypsinogen analysis on a dried blood specimen and has recently been recommended for routine use by the American College of Medical Genetics (7). The test is claimed to have a 90% detection rate and can be confirmed by a variety of back-up methods, including DNA analysis. Proponents of the neonatal screening test point out that almost 50% of children will have advanced malnutrition at the time of diagnosis of the disease, which predisposes to later cognitive limitations (8). Diagnosis of cystic fibrosis by neonatal screening would allow early administration of pancreatic enzyme replacement, early addition of fat-soluble vitamins, and appropriate pulmonary therapy to minimize bacterial colonization.

The epithelial chloride transport defect with cystic fibrosis is expressed in sweat glands resulting in a high salt content of sweat, the basis of the sweat chloride test for diagnosis. Normally, salt is largely reabsorbed as sweat from glands in the skin is transported along their ducts to the skin surface, resulting in a hypotonic content of chloride, usually <20 mEq/L. With cystic fibrosis, chloride is poorly reabsorbed across the ductal epithelium, resulting in sweat chloride levels of 60 to 120 mEq/L, the range considered to be diagnostic of cystic fibrosis in persons with a compatible history. The procedure is done by pilocarpine iontophoresis and at least 100 mg of sweat is desired for a reliable study. The sweat chloride test is not considered to be consistently reliable in the neonate in the first 2 weeks of life because of the possibility of insufficient sweat obtained at this age (9). The sweat chloride test is extremely useful in clinical practice, although both false–positive and false–negative test results can occur. Some of the better known causes of a false–positive sweat chloride test findings include laboratory error, adrenal insufficiency, anhydrotic ectodermal dysplasia, malnutrition, hypothyroidism, and a rare degenerative brain disease called *fucosidosis, type 1.* By far the most common cause of a false–negative test result is inadequate sweat collection. False–negative test results also can occur by laboratory error, with soft tissue edema, and in association with the rare CFTR gene mutation with a nondiagnostic sweat test described by Highsmith et al. (4).

NEUROLOGIC COMPLICATIONS

The basic chloride channel protein defect that characterizes cystic fibrosis apparently is not associated with clinical neurologic abnormalities, although a variety of brain and ophthalmologic abnormalities can develop secondary to the nutritional consequences of the disease. Clinical signs of fat-soluble vitamin deficiencies in patients with exocrine pancreatic insufficiency or intrinsic hepatic disease have been recognized for decades. More recently, the cognitive considerations and restriction of head growth in children with delayed diagnosis of cystic fibrosis have been emphasized and are believed to be on the basis of reduced serum vitamin E levels that develop earlier than other fat-soluble vitamin deficiencies in infants with fat malabsorption (10). Numerous earlier studies of infants with prolonged, severe pancaloric malnutrition without overt malabsorption have shown a stunting effect on brain function and brain growth (11,12). This might suggest that the impact on cognitive function that can occur with delayed diagnosis of cystic fibrosis may be multifactorial, but with vitamin E deficiency playing a major role. The recent emphasis on the potential brain effects in infancy that can complicate uncontrolled exocrine pancreatic insufficiency has been directed to the urgent need for neonatal cystic fibrosis screening and was actually preceded by studies years before that revealed axonal and neuronal damage at the nucleus gracilis in the medulla and in the spinal cord, presumed even then to be related to vitamin E deficiency (13,14).

Trace metals, including copper and zinc, can become deficient with malabsorption. Copper hepatic stores in the neonate are normally markedly elevated compared with the older child or adult and are usually sufficient to prevent symptomatic deficiency, at least for the first 6 months after birth (15). Clinical features of copper deficiency are a hypochromic microcytic anemia refractory to iron therapy, neutropenia, and osteopenia. Zinc deficiency is a more practical concern in infants with malabsorption, especially with the premature infant, because a high percentage of zinc stores in the liver is established in the last trimester of pregnancy. Zinc is important in many cerebral enzyme systems and its deficiency can have an adverse effect on brain function and behavior, more widely recognized in older children than in infancy. Rash such as that of acrodermatitis enteropathica, which is most prominent in the perioral region and the diaper area, has been described with cystic fibrosis (16). Klebs et al. (17) found among infants with cystic fibrosis who were not receiving pancreatic enzyme replacement, that 29% had deficient zinc levels. Among infants with cystic fibrosis who become zinc deficient, any adverse effect on brain function would probably be subtle and overshadowed by other nutritional deficiencies that occur with this disease.

Deficiency of fat-soluble vitamins in children with cystic fibrosis with pancreatic insufficiency was a common, perhaps almost universal, cause of clinical signs in the early years of the 20th century. This is now largely preventable; in the absence of universal screening and delay in diagnosis, however, vitamin deficiencies are still an important concern, especially relative to vitamin E.

In addition to malabsorption of fat-soluble vitamins, vitamin B_{12} deficiency can be a complication of distil ileal resection (18), which is sometimes required in neonates with meconium ileus. Vitamin B_{12} deficiency in infants and young children is easily overlooked because of the atypical features of the condition, which include growth failure, vomiting, lethargy, hypotonia, developmental regression, and movement abnormalities, including tremors, chorea, and myoclonus (19).

Vitamin A deficiency in cystic fibrosis has been a cause of increased intracranial pressure (ICP), with bulging fontanel, suture separation, and rapid head enlargement (20,21). Disturbed cerebrospinal fluid (CSF) absorption via the arachnoid villi has been postulated, but not proved to explain the intracranial hypertension in these cases. Increased ICP can precede the more common ocular signs of vitamin A deficiency or the eye signs can be found when the fontanel becomes tense. An additional cause of acute increase in ICP (pseudotumor cerebri) has been described with rapid "catch-up" somatic growth after nutritional restoration in emaciated children (22).

Vitamin A is important in the maintenance of epithelial surfaces and its deficiency leads to dryness of the conjunctiva and cornea referred to as *xerophthalmia.* Ulceration and softening of the cornea is called *keratomalacia,* which has a detrimental effect on vision. Bitot's spots are a consequence of conjunctival dryness and appear as foamy circular or triangular patches adjacent to the limbus of the cornea. Retinal function also depends on vitamin A and its deficiency can result in a disturbance in dark adaptation causing poor vision in dim light referred to as *night blindness.* Unlike night blindness with retinitis pigmentosa in which funduscopic examination reveals a retinal abnormality, the fundus examination with vitamin A deficiency night blindness is normal. The photoreceptor pigment in rods in the retina called *rhodopsin* is sensitive to low-intensity light and requires vitamin A for its normal function.

Significant clinical bleeding caused by vitamin K deficiency is now uncommon among children with cystic fibrosis who receive routine vitamin K supplements. Serious hemorrhage has previously been described with this disease and can affect the brain as well as the intestinal tract and other sites (23,24). Conway et al. (25), in the United Kingdom, have recently shown that vitamin K deficiency is common among children with cystic fibrosis with pancreatic insufficiency who do not get supplemental vitamin K. In this study group of children with cystic fibrosis, 30% had both decreased serum vitamin K levels and increased proteins induced in vitamin K absence (PIVKA-II) levels, whereas 58% had reduced vitamin K levels. PIVKA-II, the under carboxylated, functionally inactive form of vitamin K-dependent coagulation factors are produced and released from the liver when vitamin K is deficient. Because bleeding in older children often occurs within the brain in those with vitamin K deficiency, the results of this study indicate the importance of maintaining adequate vitamin K serum levels in children with pancreatic insufficiency.

Infants and children with cystic fibrosis who are physically active in a hot climate or have sustained fever secondary to an infectious illness are at risk of acute salt depletion by the normal heat loss mechanism of sweating, sometimes compounded by the offering of hypotonic or salt-free fluids to the child by parents or other care-givers (26). The serum sodium can drop to <120 mEq/L and serum chloride can become markedly reduced to between 50 and 90 mEq/L. Symptoms are variable, but can include irritability, vomiting, confusion, seizures, lethargy, coma, and shock. On rare occasions, this sequence can comprise the event leading to the initial diagnosis of cystic fibrosis. Severe salt loss can also occur in the neonate requiring distal small bowel resection and ileostomy placement for meconium ileus. Intestinal losses of sodium from an ileostomy can be up to sixfold greater than occurs in healthy children and sodium depletion should be prevented by the administration of supplementary salt and sometimes sodium bicarbonate in amounts determined by laboratory studies (27).

Other considerations of a neurologic nature in children with cystic fibrosis include transient symptoms that can occur with intense paroxysmal coughing. After violent coughing, some children with advanced lung disease will experience lightheadedness, syncope, or brief visual aberrations, even with temporary visual dimness or loss of vision (28). Back pain has been claimed to be common among older children or adolescents with cystic fibrosis and is related to the severity of the lung disease (28). Extrapulmonary infections are apparently no more common among children with cystic fibrosis than in otherwise healthy children despite the chronic airway bacterial colonization that becomes characteristic of the disease. This also seems to be true of central nervous system (CNS) infections. For example, brain abscess has only rarely been reported among patients with cystic fibrosis and most of these have been in older adolescents or adults (29,30).

CLINICAL RECOMMENDATIONS OF THE VIGNETTE

The patient had a normal CT scan and promptly improved with his saline infusion. Laboratory results included a serum sodium of 118 and chloride of 70 mEq/L. It was initially assumed that he had Addison disease; however, his serum potassium was normal as was his blood glucose level. A sweat chloride test performed the following day revealed a chloride content of 104 mEq/L and the diagnosis of cystic fibrosis was confirmed.

SUMMARY

Studies in the past two decades have yielded major advances in the understanding of the genetic mechanisms, the basic pathophysiology, the diagnostic usefulness and limitations of the sweat chloride test, and the applicability of neonatal screening for cystic fibrosis. It is an autosomal-recessive disease in which a gene mutation creates an abnormality of electrolyte transport across epithelial surfaces. The primary effect of this defect is within the pulmonary airways, resulting in viscous secretions that cause slowly progressive pulmonary obstructive disease and within exocrine pancreatic ducts leading to variable degrees of fat malabsorption. With current earlier diagnosis and established treatment programs for this disease, significant neurologic complications have become uncommon. Depletion of fat-soluble vitamins, including A, D, E, and K, as well as depletion of zinc and copper can now be managed to prevent neurologic complications. Eventual widespread application of neonatal screening can be expected to further improve the health and survival of persons with this disease.

REFERENCES

1. Andersen DH. Cystic fibrosis of the pancreas and its relation to celiac disease. A clinical and pathologic study. *Am J Dis Child.* 1938;56:344–399.
2. di Sant Agnese P, Darling RC, Perera GA, et al. Abnormal electrolyte composition of sweat in cystic fibrosis of pancreas: Clinical significance and relationship to disease. *Pediatrics.* 1953;12:549–563.
3. Riordan J, Rommens JM, Kerem B, et al. Identification of the cystic fibrosis gene: Cloning and characterization complementary DNA. *Science.* 1989;245(4922):1066–1073.
4. Highsmith WE, Burch LH, Zhou Z, et al. A novel mutation in the cystic fibrosis gene in patients with pulmonary disease but normal sweat chloride concentrations. *N Engl J Med.* 1994;331:974–980.
5. Drumm ML, Konstan MW, Schluchter MD, et al. Genetic modifiers of lung disease in cystic fibrosis. *N Engl J Med.* 2005;353:1443–1453.
6. Accurso FJ, Sontag MK, Wagener JS. Complications associated with symptomatic diagnosis in infants with cystic fibrosis. *J Pediatr.* 2005;147:S37–S41.
7. Natowicz M. Newborn screening-setting evidence-based policy for protection. *N Engl J Med.* 2005;353:867–870.
8. Farrell PM, Kosorak MR, Rock MJ, et al. Early diagnosis of cystic fibrosis through neonatal screening prevents severe malnutrition and improves long-term growth. *Pediatrics.* 2001; 107:1–13.
9. Parad RB, Comeau AM, Dorkin HL, et al. Sweat testing infants detected by cystic fibrosis newborn screening. *J Pediatr.* 2005;147:S69–S72.
10. Koscik RL, Lai HJ, Laxova A, et al. Preventing early, prolonged vitamin E deficiency: An opportunity for better cognitive outcomes via early diagnosis through neonatal screening. *J Pediatr.* 2005;147:S51–S56.
11. Chase HP, Martin HP. Undernutrition and child development. *N Engl J Med.* 1970:282: 934–939.
12. Cravioto J, Delicardie ER. Mental performance in school age children. Findings after recovery from early severe malnutrition. *Am J Dis Child.* 1970;120:404–410.
13. Cavalier SJ, Gambetti P. Dystrophic axons and spinal cord demyelination in cystic fibrosis. *Neurology.* 1981;31:714–718.
14. Sung JH, Park SH, Mastri AR, et al. Axonal dystrophy in the gracile nucleus in congenital biliary atresia and cystic fibrosis (mucoviscidosis): Beneficial effect of vitamin E therapy. *J Neuropath Exp Neurol.* 1980;39:584–597.
15. Cordano A, Graham GG. Copper deficiency complicating severe chronic intestinal malabsorption. *Pediatrics.* 1966;38:596–604.
16. Hansen RC, Lemen R, Revsin B. Cystic fibrosis manifesting with acrodermatitis enteropathica-like eruption. Association with essential fatty acid and zinc deficiencies. *Arch Dermatol.* 1983;119:51.
17. Klebs NF, Sontag M, Accurso FJ, et al. Low plasma zinc concentration in young infants with cystic fibrosis. *J Pediatr.* 1998;133:761–764.
18. Rasmussen SA, Fernhoff PM, Scanlon KS. Vitamin B_{12} deficiency in children and adolescents. *J Pediatr.* 2001;138:10–17.
19. Emory ES, Homan AC, Colletti RB. Vitamin B12 deficiency: A cause of abnormal movements in infancy. *Pediatrics.* 1997;99:255–256.
20. Abernathy RS. Bulging fontanel as presenting sign in cystic fibrosis. Vitamin A metabolism and effect on cerebrospinal fluid pressure. *Am J Dis Child.* 1976;130:1360–1362.
21. Keating JP, Feigin RD. Increased intracranial pressure associated with probable vitamin A deficiency in cystic fibrosis. *Pediatrics.* 1970;46:41–46.
22. Bray PF, Herbst JJ. Pseudotumor cerebri as a sign of "catch-up" growth in cystic fibrosis. *Am J Dis Child.* 1973;126:78–79.
23. Torstenson OL, Humphrey GB, Edson JR, et al. Cystic fibrosis presenting with severe hemorrhage due to vitamin K malabsorption. A report of 3 cases. *Pediatrics.* 1970;45:857–861.
24. Walters TR, Koch HF. Hemorrhagic diathesis and cystic fibrosis in infancy. *Am J Dis Child.* 1972;124:641–642.
25. Conway SP, Wolfe SP, Brownlee KG, et al. Vitamin K status among children with cystic fibrosis and its relationship to bone density and bone turnover. *Pediatrics.* 2005;115:1325–1331.
26. Finberg L, Bernstein J. Acute hyponatremic dehydration. *J Pediatr.* 1971;79:499–503.
27. Schwarz KB, Ternberg JL, Bell MJ, et al. Sodium needs of infants and children with ileostomy. *J Pediatr.* 1983;102:509–513.
28. Rose J, Gamble J, Schultz A, et al. Back pain and spinal deformity in cystic fibrosis. *Am J Dis Child.* 1987;141:1313–1316.
29. Duffner PK, Cohen ME. Cystic fibrosis with brain abscess. *Arch Neurol.* 1979;36:27–28.
30. Fischer EG, Schwachman H, Wepsic JC. Brain abscess and cystic fibrosis. *J Pediatr.* 1979;95: 385–388.

CHAPTER **159**

Neurologic Consequences of Vaccines in Children

Leslie Allen • Charlotte T. Jones

OBJECTIVES

- To define neurologic complications of routine childhood vaccines
- To discuss contraindications to vaccine administration
- To report adverse events
- To discuss physician responsibility in vaccine administration

CASE VIGNETTE

A 12-year-old girl presents to the neurology clinic. Her mother writes, "She began to stop talking, playing with things, picking up stuff, she forgot potty training, she forgot everything after she took the measles, mumps, and rubella [MMR] shot." Her mother had noted loss of developmental skills since 17 months of age; she had attributed this to the MMR vaccine.

EPIDEMIOLOGY

Morbitity and Mortality Weekly Report released a summary of the Vaccine Adverse Event Reporting System (VAERS) data from 1991 to 2001. During this 10-year period, 110,421 nonserious reactions and 18,296 serious reactions were reported following vaccine administration. A serious reaction was defined as an event that required hospitalization, led to permanent disability, life-threatening illness, or death. Most adverse events (82%) were reported by the manufacturer, state health coordinator, or health care provider. The most commonly reported adverse events were fever, injection-site hypersensitivity, and rash. These three reactions make up approximately 50% of all reported adverse events of immunizations (1).

VACCINES

DIPHTHERIA, TETANUS, AND PERTUSSIS VACCINE (DTP/DTaP)

DTaP vaccine is given in five doses at ages 2 months, 4 months, 6 months, 15 months, and 4 years. The vaccine, a combination of tetanus and diphtheria toxoid and acellular (DTaP) or cellular pertussis (DTP), is given intramuscularly (2).

Neurologic Consequences of Components

- Diphtheria component has no known neurologic consequences (3).
- Tetanus vaccine is associated with Guillain-Barré syndrome (GBS) and brachial neuritis (3).
- Pertussis vaccine is associated with febrile seizures, periods of inconsolable crying or screaming, hypotonic–hyporesponsive episodes, and encephalopathy (4).

FEBRILE SEIZURES. Results from a study published by the *New England Journal of Medicine* (August 30, 2001) found a significantly elevated risk of febrile seizures on the day the DTP vaccine was injected. Of 100,000 children receiving the vaccine, approximately 6 to 9 would have a febrile seizure. The study concluded that these children were at no greater risk for epilepsy or neurodevelopmental disorders than those children who have febrile seizures in the absence of vaccines (5). From 1991 to 2001 when the pertussis component was changed from whole cell to acellular, reports of serious and nonserious reactions decreased by 50% in children <7 years of age (1).

HYPOTONIC–HYPORESPONSIVE EPISODES. Hypotonic–hyporesponsive episodes (HHE) are defined as a shocklike state (2). Hypotonic–hyporesponsive episodes are estimated to occur from 3.5 to 291 cases per 100,000 DTP vaccines administered (4). A study done to assess permanent disability from HHE concluded, no serious neurologic evidence or intellectual impairment was found (2).

INCONSOLABLE CRYING. This phenomenon is defined as inconsolable crying for 3 or more hours (2). It has been estimated to occur from 0.1% to 6% of DTP administrations (4).

ACUTE ENCEPHALOPATHY. Acute encephalopathy is estimated to occur from 0 to 10.5 per million immunizations (4).

Equivocal Evidence

- Chronic neurologic damage, aseptic meningitis, erythema multiforme, hemolytic anemia, juvenile diabetes mellitus, attention deficit disorder (ADD), learning disabilities, peripheral mononeuropathy, thrombocytopenia, radiculoneuritis, and thrombocytopenia purpura (4).

No Correlation

- Infantile spasms, hypsarrhythmia, Reye syndrome, and sudden infant death syndrome (SIDS) (4).

Contraindications to DTP/DTaP Vaccine

- Previous anaphylactic reaction, encephalopathy within 7 days of previous dose, moderate to severe otitis media (OM), vomiting, diarrhea, or moderate to severe illness (with or without fever) (6).

Precautions for DTP/DTaP Vaccine

- Fever (<105°F) within 48 hours of previous dose, collapse, or shocklike state (HHE) within 48 hours, persistent inconsolable crying for 3 or more hours within 48 hours of immunization, family history of adverse event, and GBS within 6 weeks of dose (6).
- If a child had a seizure within 3 days of the vaccine, has a seizure disorder, or had a fever of >105°F, then consider acetaminophen 4 hours before vaccine injection and every 4 hours for 24 hours after injection of the vaccine (6).
- A progressive neurologic disorder or children with a history of seizures may delay DTaP immunization. An increased risk exists of seizure activity after DTaP in children with a history of seizures (2).

MEASLES, MUMPS, AND RUBELLA (MMR) VACCINE

MMR vaccine is given in two doses at 15 months and 4 years. This is a live-attenuated vaccine. MMR is given subcutaneously (2).

Neurologic Consequences of Components

- Measles vaccine is associated with febrile seizures and measles encephalopathy or encephalitis (3). Transient thrombocytopenia has also occurred with its administration (2). Acute disseminated encephalomyelitis may follow measles vaccine injection; however, the risk is 10 times higher with natural infection (7).
- Mumps vaccine is not associated with neurologic consequences in the United States; however, the vaccine in other countries has been associated with aseptic meningitis and sensorineural deafness (3).
- Rubella (RA 27/3) has been associated with acute arthritis in adult women (4).

FEBRILE SEIZURES. The estimated risk of febrile seizures after the MMR vaccine is approximately 25 to 34 per 100,000 doses administered. The risk of febrile seizures increases on days number 8 through 14 after vaccine administration. A child who experiences a febrile seizure after the MMR vaccine has the same risk of developing epilepsy or neurodevelopmental delays as a child who experiences a non-vaccine related febrile seizure (5).

ACUTE ARTHRITIS. Approximately 13% to 15% of women receiving the RA 27/3 vaccine develop acute arthritis. The incidence rate in children and adolescents is reportedly lower (4).

Equivocal Evidence

- Rubella (RA 27/3) may be associated with radiculoneuritis thrombocytopenic purpura, or other neuropathies (4).

No Correlation

- Autism. In 2001 the Immunization Safety Review Committee concluded that no correlation is seen between the MMR vaccine and developing autism. In 2004, the Committee once again revisited this issue and confirmed their initial statement that the MMR vaccine is not associated with the development of autism (8).

Contraindications to MMR Vaccine

- Anaphylactic reaction to previous MMR vaccine or neomycin, moderate to severe diarrhea, vomiting, OM, or illness (with or without fever), immune globulin products simultaneously, hematologic or solid tumors, congenital immunodeficiency, long-term immunosupression (>14 days), and pregnancy (6).

Precautions for MMR Vaccine

- Thrombocytopenia, history of thrombocytopenia purpura, previous reaction to gelatin.
- Note: MMR vaccines should be given to all patients with human immunodeficiency virus (HIV) who are not severely immunocompromised (6).

POLIO (IPV/OPV)

Inactivated poliovirus vaccine (IPV) is given in four doses at 2 months, 4 months, 6 months, and 4 years. IPV is given either intramuscularly or subcutaneously (2).

Neurologic Consequences

- Oral polio vaccine (OPV) has been shown to cause vaccine-associated paralytic polio, especially after the first dose (1).
- IPV has no known neurologic complications (3).

VACCINE ASSOCIATED PARALYTIC POLIO (VAPP). VAPP occurs in approximately 1 per 2.4 million doses of OPV, with prevalence after the first dose. IPV is not associated with VAPP. In July 1999, the Advisory Committee on Immunization Practices (ACIP) recommended that IPV replace OPV in the immunization schedule to prevent VAPP (1).

No Correlation

- IPV is not associated with Guillain-Barré syndrome (3).

Contraindications to OPV

- Moderate to severe diarrhea, OM, vomiting, or illness (with or without fever), HIV infection in a household contact or the recipient, household contact with immunodeficiency, recipient with solid or hematologic tumor, or recipient with immunodeficiency (6).

Contraindications to IPV

- Anaphylactic reaction to neomycin or streptomycin; moderate to severe diarrhea, OM, vomiting, or illness (with or without fever) (6).

Precautions for OPV

- Recommendations are that OPV only be used in the following circumstances: mass vaccine campaigns to control outbreaks, unvaccinated children who will be traveling in <4 weeks to endemic polio regions, and unvaccinated children whose consent cannot be obtain for IPV. OPV should only be used for dose no. 3 or no. 4 and only after informed consent regarding VAPP (9).

HAEMOPHILUS INFLUENZAE TYPE B VACCINE (HIB)

Hib is given in four doses at 2 months, 4 months, 6 months, and 1 year. This vaccine is a polysaccharide protein conjugate. Hib is given intramuscularly (2).

Neurologic Consequences

- Hib has not been linked with neurologic consequences.

Equivocal Evidence

- Guillian Barré syndrome has been reported after vaccination; Institute of Medicine (IOM), however, has neither accepted nor rejected a causal relationship (1).

Contraindications to Hib

- Moderate to severe diarrhea, OM, vomiting, or illness (with or without fever) (6).

HEPATITIS B VACCINE (HEPB)

Hepatitis B vaccine is given in three doses at birth, 2 months, and 6 months. This vaccine is a recombinant viral antigen. HepB vaccine is given intramuscularly (2).

Neurologic Consequences

- Plasma derived HepB vaccine (1982–1988) was associated with Guillain-Barré syndrome, Bell's palsy, and brachial plexitis (3).

Equivocal Evidence

- Recombinant hepatitis B vaccine (1987 to present) may be associated with the first episode of central nervous system (CNS) demyelinating disorder, acute disseminated encephalomyelitis (ADEM), optic neuritis, transverse myelitis, GBS, and brachial neuritis (10). One case of cerebellar ataxia has been reported (3).

No Correlation

- Onset of multiple sclerosis or multiple sclerosis relapse (10).

Contraindications to HepB Vaccine

- Anaphylactic reaction to baker's yeast or previous dose of HepB vaccine, moderate to severe diarrhea, OM, vomiting or illness (with or without fever) (6).

Considerations

- If an infant's mother is HepB positive, then give the first HepB vaccine and Hepatitis B Immune Globulin (HBIG). If the infant is <2 kg, however, then this dose does not serve as dose no. 1 in the three-part series (6).

VARICELLA VACCINE

Varicella vaccine is given in one dose at 1 year of age. This is a live vaccine. Varicella vaccine is given subcutaneously (2).

Neurologic Consequences

- Varicella vaccine can be associated with a mild case of chickenpox followed by acute cerebellar ataxia. Complete spontaneous resolution can be expected (3). The frequency of this complication is unknown at this time.

Contraindications to Varicella Vaccine

- Pregnant recipient, anaphylactic reaction to neomycin, moderate to severe diarrhea, OM, vomiting, or illness (with or without fever), symptomatic HIV recipient, household member with immunodeficiency, recipient with hematologic, solid tumor, congenital immunodeficiency, or long-term immunosuppression (6).
- Do not administer vaccine for at least 5 months after blood transfusion, plasma transfusion, intravenous gamma globulin (IVIG), or varicella zoster immune globulin (VZIG) (6).

PNEUMOCOCCAL VACCINE

Pneumococcal vaccine is given in four doses at 2 months, 4 months, 6 months, and 1 year. It is a polysaccharide protein conjugate. Pneumococcal vaccines are given either intramuscularly or subcutaneously (2).

Neurologic Consequences

- Pneumococcal vaccine has no known associated neurologic consequences.

Contraindications to Pneumococcal Vaccine

- Moderate to severe diarrhea, OM, vomiting, or illness (with or without fever) (6).

HEPATITIS A VACCINE

Hepatitis A vaccine is not a routine vaccination in many states. In October 2005, however, the ACIP voted to recommend vaccination for children 12 to 35 months of age. This recommendation is being considered by CDC and the Department of Health and Human Services (11). Hepatitis A vaccine is administered in two doses separated by 6 months. This is an inactivated vaccine. Hepatitis A vaccine is given intramuscularly (2).

Neurologic Consequences

- Hepatitis A vaccine has no known associated neurologic consequences.

Contraindications to Hepatitis A Vaccine

- Moderate to severe diarrhea, OM , vomiting, or illness (with or without fever), and previous allergic reaction to alum or 2-phenoxyethanol (6).

INFLUENZA VACCINE

Influenza vaccine is given annually. It is an inactivated virus. The influenza vaccine is given intramuscularly (2).

Neurologic Consequences

- Influenza vaccine given in 1976 was associated with GBS (12).

GUILLAIN-BARRÉ SYNDROME. The VAERS estimates that the relative risk of developing GBS after the influenza vaccine is 1.7. In 1993–1994 VAERS reported the highest number of reported GBS cases. Data from 1991–2001 show that the greatest number of cases reported were women >18 years of age (1).

Equivocal Evidence

- Influenza vaccine administered after 1976 may be associated with GBS, onset of multiple sclerosis, optic neuritis, or other demyelinating neurological disorders (12).

No Correlation

- Influenza vaccine is not associated with relapse of multiple sclerosis (12).
- Influenza vaccine does not cause demyelinating disorders in children aged 6 moths to 23 months (12).

MENINGOCOCCAL VACCINE (A,C,Y, AND W135)

Neurologic Consequences

- Concern at this time is that Menactra Meningococcal Vaccine causes GBS. As of September 30, 2005, five cases of GBS have been reported (13).

REPORTING ADVERSE EVENTS

Physicians are obligated to report all adverse events of vaccines to VAERS. The National Childhood Vaccine and Injury Act of 1986 set forth reportable events, timeframes for reporting, and timeframes for client compensation. If an event is not listed in this table it must still be reported. This table can be found in Appendix IV of the *2003 Red Book.* A VAERS report can be sent via the web at www.vaers.org or by mail (2).

PHYSICIANS' ROLE IN IMMUNIZATION

In a clinical report in *Pediatrics* May 2005, Dr. Diekema, addresses the problem of parental refusal for children's immunizations. In this article, Dr. Diekema offers advice on issues that face physicians when parents refuse immunizations.

Parents often refuse immunizations because they do not feel the benefits of immunizing their child outweigh the risks. In this situation, the physician should attempt to counsel the parents regarding their fears of immunizations. Multiple web sites listed in the 2003 *Red Book* are available to parents to learn more about vaccines.

Physicians can protect themselves by documenting conversations regarding vaccines. The parents should also be asked to sign a refusal waiver. It is advised that pediatricians not discharge patients based on vaccine refusal; however, should a physician decide to terminate the patient relationship, then the patient's family must be given sufficient notice (14).

CLINICAL RECOMMENDATIONS OF THE VIGNETTE

On examination, the patient was found at 12 years of age to have a head circumference of 51.9 cm. She had no language and exhibited characteristic wringing hand movements. DNA analysis was sent confirming a diagnosis of Rett syndrome. The family was counseled on the diagnosis of their daughter's condition and that the vaccine they had associated with their daughter's regression was not the cause. Although a temporal relationship was found between the vaccine and the child's regression, it was only coincidental. As this case demonstrates, other causes should be explored before attributing the cause of a child's neurologic problems to vaccines.

SUMMARY

Preventable childhood infections can cause devastating neurologic consequences. Much less frequently, vaccines intended to prevent these diseases can be associated with neurologic sequelae. Childhood vaccination should only be withheld for a true allergic reaction or a degenerative or progressive neurologic disorder that is undiagnosed at the time of immunization.

REFERENCES

1. Zhou W, Pool V, Iskander J. Surveillance for Safety after Immunization: Vaccine Adverse Events Reporting System (VAERS)—United States 1991–2001. *MMWR Surveill Summ.* 2003;52:1–24.
2. Pickering L. *Red Book: 2003 Report of the Committee on Infectious Diseases*, 26th ed. Elk Grove Village, IL: American Academy of Pediatrics; 2003:8,24,40–41,426,482.
3. Fenichel G. Assessment: Neurologic risk of immunization. *Neurology.* 1999;52:1546–1552.
4. Howson CP, Fineberg HV. Adverse events following pertussis and rubella vaccines. Summary of a report of the Institute of Medicine. *JAMA.* 1992;267(3):392–396.
5. Barlow WE, Davis RL. The risk of seizures after receipt of whole cell pertussis or measles, mumps, and rubella vaccine. *N Engl J Med.* 2001;345(9):656–661.
6. *Guide to Contraindications to Childhood Vaccines, 2000.* Atlanta: Centers for Disease Control 2000.
7. Scott TFM. Postinfectious and vaccinal encephalitis. *Med Clin North Am.* 1967;51:701–716.
8. *Immunization Safety Review: Vaccines and Autism (Free Executive Summary).* Washington, DC: Immunization Review Committee; 2004.
9. Notice to Readers: Recommendations of the Advisory Committee on Immunization Practices: Revised Recommendations for Routine Poliomyelitis Vaccination. *MMWR Morb Mortal Wkly Rev.* 1999;48(27):590.
10. Stratton K, Almario DA, McCormick MC. *Hepatitis B Vaccine and Demyelinating Neurologic Disorders.* Washington, DC: The National Academies Press; 2002.
11. Frenck Robert. Universal hepatitis A immunization recommendation made by ACIP. Frenck, *American Academy of Pediatrics News.* 2005;26:1–13.
12. Stratton K, Almario DA, Wizemann T, et al. *Immunization Safety Review: Influenza Vaccines and Neurological Complications.* Washington, DC: The National Academies Press; 2004.
13. Food and Drug Administration. FDA and CDC issue Alert on Menactra Meningococcal Vaccine and Guillain Barré Syndrome. *FDA News.* 2005, September 30.
14. Diekema DS. Responding to parental refusals of immunization of children. *Pediatrics.* 2005;115(5):1428–1431.

CHAPTER 160

Acute Radiation Syndrome

Guillermo Linares-Tapia • J. Javier Provencio

OBJECTIVES

- To identify the clinical manifestations of acute radiation toxicity in humans
- To describe the pathologic changes that occur after high-dose radiation poisoning
- To identify the diagnostic approach to a patient in whom radiation toxicity is suspected
- To identify treatments for patients with radiation toxicity
- To explore potential therapeutic interventions that may hold promise in the future to improve outcome after lethal dose radiation

CASE VIGNETTE

A former Soviet KGB spy, Alexander Litvinenko, who was a prominent critic of Russian president Vladimir Putin fell ill on November 1, 2006 in London, England after a meeting with two former Russian associates. He was admitted to the hospital claiming he had been poisoned and died 23 days later of an illness that was initially suspected to be radiation poisoning from thallium. After analysis of blood and other body fluids showed no traces of thallium, the physicians investigated other possible causes of his illness. One day after his death, they identified large quantities of polonium-210, a rare radioactive substance that is very hard to detect.

His death was heralded by loss of his hair, gastrointestinal distress, bone marrow suppression, and later encephalopathy and cardiac arrest. His hospital care was supportive, but it was felt very early in the course of his illness that his radiation poisoning syndrome would be fatal.

EPIDEMIOLOGY

The incidence and prevalence of the *radiation syndromes*, both acute and delayed, have been a reflection of the advances in technology over the course of modern human history. Radium dial painters, underground miners, and patients having dental procedures were exposed to radioactive sources without much evidence of acute central nervous system (CNS) toxicity. The era of therapeutic radiation, however, exposed patients to higher doses of radiation with the intent of curing or palliating symptoms from varied conditions, such as tinea capitis, ankylosing spondylitis, and thymic hyperplasia, among others (1).

Accidental exposures as a result of nuclear testing provided a new understanding of the phenomenology of radiation toxicity, including that of the nervous system. Pacific Islanders residing in the Marshal Islands in the early era of nuclear testing and the inhabitants of Chernobyl in 1986 were unintentionally exposed to radiation as a result of new technologies (2). Atomic bomb survivors in Hiroshima and Nagasaki numbered 283,500 according to the Japanese National Census of 1950, providing more than half a century of observations and long-term follow up on this cohort (2).

In recent years, the increased utilization of radiation therapies for the treatment of CNS tumors and other neoplasms located in the vicinity of the nervous system has caused an exponential growth in the number of patients who receive high doses of radiation (3). In fact, neurotoxicity is often the dose-limiting factor for the treatment of neural and nonneural tumors.

PATHOGENESIS AND HISTOPATHOLOGY

A few differences in the type of radiation exposure have important implications. Radiation can manifest either as waves (gamma rays or x-rays) and particles (alpha and beta particles). The penetration of these particles into tissues is variable. Alpha particles, for instance, cannot penetrate barriers as simple as a piece of paper, whereas gamma rays can penetrate concrete walls of a few feet thickness. The standard unit of radiation as it is absorbed into the body is the gray (Gy). This measure does not take into account the special qualities of different types of radiation. Because of this, a unit called the sievert (Sv) has been applied to take into account both the Gy and the biological effect of the dose of radiation. In addition, the field of radiation is an important determinant of toxicity. It is not unusual for radiation oncologists to administer lethal doses of radiation to a small field inside the body where a tumor resides without serious systemic consequences. The discussion in this chapter is limited to whole body radiation exposure because this is the most likely scenario in an environmental catastrophe, an industrial accident, or a human-constructed terrorist act (4).

The mechanisms by which radiation damages nervous tissue are not completely understood. The central and peripheral nervous tissue's response to radiation bears some similarities to the response of other tissues and organs, culminating in rapid and irreversible cell injury in cases of high-dose exposures and various degrees of inflammation and gliosis in moderate and

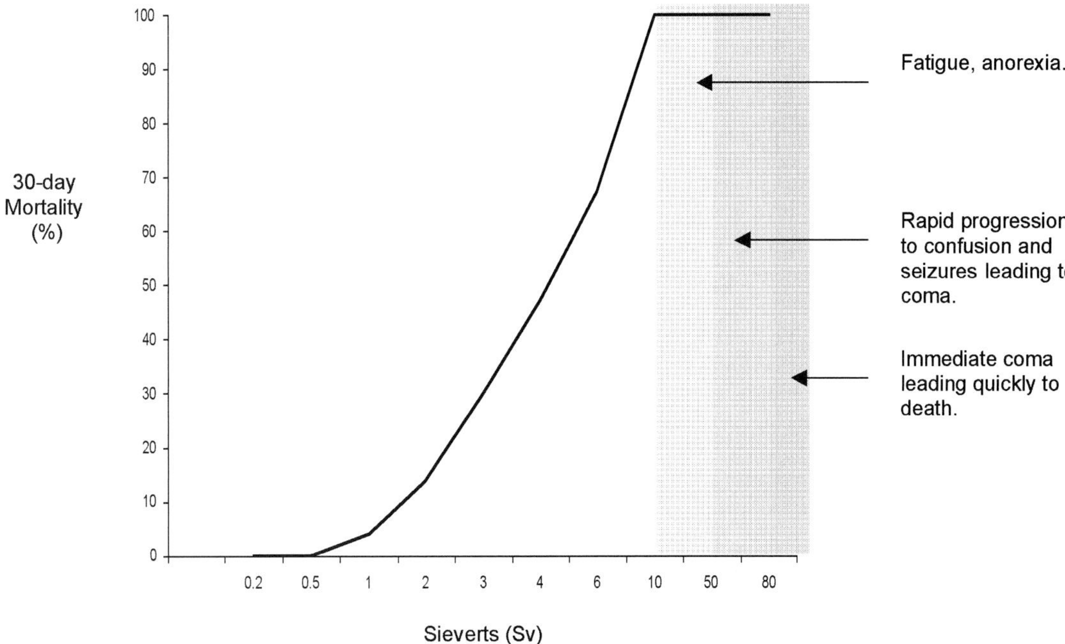

FIGURE 160-1. Dose of radiation in adults causing neurologic deterioration. This graph shows the superimposition of the mortality of radiation exposure with the neurologic sequelae of the exposure. The mortality of patients who experience early neurologic findings is nearly 100% by 30 days after exposure. Sievert (*Sv*) is the dose equivalent correction taking into account type of radiation and type of biological tissue exposed. For gamma radiation in humans, 1 Sv = 1 Gy.

low exposures (5). The risk of CNS injury increases in cases of fewer but greater doses of radiation. *Systemic acute radiation syndromes* occur at exposures of >1 Gy. Acute CNS dysfunction occurs with exposures of 50 Gy and higher, leading to death within the first 36 hours after exposure (6). Figure 160-1 summarizes the doses of radiation, mortality, and consequent neurologic toxicity. Notice that all of the doses of radiation that lead to acute neurologic deterioration are lethal.

High doses of radiation can lead to ultra-acute, reversible encephalopathy, which may be caused by direct release of certain neurochemicals from synapses. Acute toxicity seems likely to be vascular in origin, resulting from disruption of the blood–brain barrier and impairment of cerebral blood flow causing ischemia (7). The ensuing cerebral edema, as evidenced by shallow sulci, flattened convolutions, and herniations, has a progression directly related to the amount of radiation exposure. Histopathologic evidence of blood vessel thickening, hyaline changes, and intravascular thrombosis has been reported (3). Postmortem investigations have shown severe endothelial damage with perivascular edema and hemorrhage. With doses >1,000 Gy, direct neuronal injury is seen (5). Delayed toxicity may be more closely linked to selective oligodendroglia damage and subsequent demyelination (6). Nucleic acid damage and inhibition of the normal repair mechanisms lead to tumor formation and changes in neurongenesis (3,8).

CLINICAL MANIFESTATIONS

RADIATION SYNDROMES OF THE CENTRAL NERVOUS SYSTEM

Acute encephalopathy is manifested by nausea, vomiting, headache, vertigo, and mental status changes. Preexisting neurologic injuries may become apparent for the first time or worsen, leading to pronounced focal neurologic deficits. *Acute Necrotizing Leukoencephalopathy* presents as seizures, motor deficits, spasticity, and ataxia. Nonlethal doses result in transient cognitive impairment within a few weeks of exposure. Fatigue, short-term memory impairment, deficits in attention and concentration, as well as executive function are the hallmark of acute-subacute injury (9).

Delayed complications, such as radiation necrosis, severe leukoencephalopathy, dementia, and brain tumors occur months to years after the original exposure. Radiation vasculopathy, commonly causing accelerated atheromatous plaque formation, makes stroke a significant source of morbidity for those exposed to neurotoxic doses of radiation (10). Myelopathy caused by radiation damage and hemorrhagic lesions of the spinal chord have also been reported. Lhermitte sign is common among patients who have received radiation in the vicinity of the spinal chord, as are more severe manifestations of injury. Myelopathy symptoms, however, are more likely to be reversible (11).

The peripheral nervous system is generally regarded to be less susceptible to radiation toxicity. Neuropathies of the brachial plexus, lumbosacral plexus, and peripheral nerves are observed as part of the delayed effects of radiation exposure. In certain cases, symptoms appear after more than 6 months to a year after exposure. Demyelination caused by Schwann cell damage, fibrosis, and blood vessel changes, have been reported in doses of 60 Gy and higher (12,13).

SPECIAL SITUATIONS

The clinical manifestations of radiation injury to the brain depend both on the magnitude of the exposure and the host's inherent risk profile. The immature and variably myelinated brain of children is more vulnerable to radiation damage. The elderly represent another population at risk for acute injury at lower doses. Given the vascular pathophysiology of injury, it stands to reason that patients with a higher burden of small vessel disease of the brain are at increased risk (14).

Prenatal exposure to radiation at the time when embryonic nervous tissue is being formed results in severe injury, including architectural distortion of the granular and molecular layers of the cerebellum as well as altered neuronal migration (15). Mental retardation and small head size, along with an increased incidence of seizures and low IQ, have been reported in atomic bomb survivors exposed in the prenatal period (16).

No clear evidence indicates that gonadal irradiation during the atomic explosions of Hiroshima and Nagasaki has led to an increase in malignancies in individuals conceived after the explosion (17). The United Nations Scientific Committee on the Effects of Atomic Radiation (UNSCEAR) reported the total hereditary risk to be 0.3% to 0.5% per gray to the first generation after the explosion. Neurodegenerative conditions, such as dementing illnesses, Huntington's disease, and phakomatoses were part of the UNSCEAR model (2).

DIAGNOSTIC APPROACH

The diagnosis of acute radiation poisoning is largely a matter of fitting a set of stereotyped symptoms with a known exposure to radiation and following up with appropriate testing. Because hair loss and gastrointestinal symptoms are early and dramatic findings in patients after large-dose radiation exposure, these two symptoms should lead to a detailed history of possible exposure to a radioactive source.

Within the first few hours of radiation exposure, symptoms can be vague and flulike. Few patients come to medical attention this early unless there is a known radiation exposure or a very large dose. Within hours, diarrhea and hair loss are manifest. At this point, physicians should explore the medical history to determine if a possible radiation source can be identified. Certain populations are at increased risk of radiation exposure. People who work in radiation facilities, such as nuclear power plants or medical offices where radiation is used in patient care, are at very high risk. Patients getting treatments for cancer or hyperthyroidism who are treated with radiation are also susceptible. Miners who work in areas of high natural radiation and poor ventilation may also be at risk. It should be noted that chronic exposure to radiation followed by a transient increase in radiation acutely may show the same symptoms of acute high-dose radiation. In third world countries, thallium is used as a pesticide. Numerous cases of poisoning have been found in the literature.

In addition to determining exposure risks, establishing if home contacts or work mates are also affected may provide clues about the source of radiation. In facilities that commonly use radiation, safeguards are in place to limit cumulative radiation dose. The monitoring of this radiation by dosimetry may provide a method to test if ambient radiation levels have increased in the work setting.

After taking a careful history, patients who still are felt to be at risk for radiation can be tested in a number of ways. First, whole body examination with a Geiger counter may reveal increased radiation (4). Testing of blood and other body fluids for radioactivity using scintillation counters may help determine the source of the radiation. It must be noted that these tests are helpful only in situations where the radiation comes from a solid radiation source inside the body. Most of these come from medical treatments where radioactive material is implanted in the body to provide a source of continuous radiation. Some patients who inhale radon gas will also test positive on these tests. It is important to note that patients who experience a single large dose of radiation from an ionizing source outside the body may not have any evidence of radiation on their body at the time that their symptoms bring them to medical attention. In addition, patients who, as in the rare case of polonium-210 poisoning, have an alpha ray source as the cause of the damage may not be positive for external radiation on testing. Finally, if specific agents, such as thallium are suspected, colorimetric evaluation can be undertaken, but the rate of false–positive test results was considered very high.

TREATMENT

Treatment of acute radiation exposure is limited. A few remedies exist for specific agents that can cause radiation illness focused on competing against the biological substrate with which the radioactive chemical interacts. The most notable of these is potassium iodide, which can be given to patients who have internal exposure to iodine 125 or 131. Other treatments, such as Prussian blue, for exposure to cesium 137 and aluminum phosphate for strontium 90 exposure offer some decrease in radioactive exposure for small-dose radiation. Unfortunately, no well studied therapies for massive exposure to external radiation exist. In particular, no therapy is directed at the encephalopathy caused by radiation.

Neumune, androst-5-ene-3beta,17beta-diol or 5-androstene-diol, has been investigated in patients who receive sublethal doses of radiation to the bone marrow. Studies have shown a shorter time to recovery of bone marrow (18,19). In addition, butylated-hydroxytoluene (BHT), a food additive, has been tested in animal models of radiation injury for its antioxidant effects without much success (20).

The care of patients with radiation exposure is first to try to decontaminate the patient so that further exposure is limited. This can be done by removing the clothes and wiping the patient off with a wet cloth. After this, the supportive care is defined by the patient's symptoms. No specific treatment yet exists for the neurologic disease.

CLINICAL RECOMMENDATIONS OF THE VIGNETTE

As is apparent with the patient, high-dose radiation exposure is usually lethal; care was supportive until his death. After his death, the goal of the medical community has been to try to identify the source of the radiation and to determine if others have been exposed. In fact, one of the diners at the table with Mr. Litvinenko was also exposed to a lower dose of radiation and had to be hospitalized. From a neurologist's perspective, little can be done, but manage the delirium and the possible seizures with standard medicines. This can be emotionally difficult in large-dose radiation, knowing that the patient is surely going to die.

SUMMARY

Radiation exposure has been a source of significant mortality for a small group of people exposed to very high doses since Marie Curie first described radiation. Industrial exposures had affected the largest group of patients until the bombing of two cities in Japan during World War II. Since that time, we have seen small affected groups owing to a nuclear reactor accident. Individuals are most at risk in the setting of medical care. Clearly, the most frightening aspect of radiation exposure for the lay person is the risk that it can be used as a terrorist device.

Little treatment is available to counteract the effects of acute large-dose radiation exposure. Supportive measures are important in patients who have smaller dose exposure. Those patients who present with neurologic symptoms early, likely have received a very large dose of radiation and will likely die regardless of their neurologic treatment. Although antioxidants, such as BHT, have been used unsuccessfully so far, hope remains that in the future a treatment may become available.

REFERENCES

1. Pimperl LC. Radiation as a nervous system toxin. *Neurol Clin.* 2005;23(2):591–597.
2. The United Nations Scientific Committee on the Effects of Atomic Radiation 2000 report. New York: United Nations; 2000:2–17.
3. Schiff D. Central nervous system toxicity from cancer therapies. *Hematol Oncol Clin North Am.* 2006;20(6):1377–1398.
4. Mettler FA, Jr., Voelz GL. Major radiation exposure—What to expect and how to respond. *N Engl J Med.* 2002;346(20):1554–1561.
5. Fajardo LF, Berthrong M, Anderson RE. Nervous system. In: *Radiation Pathology.* New York: Oxford University Press; 2001:351–363.
6. Fajardo LF, Berthrong M, Anderson RE. Acute radiation syndrome. In: *Radiation Pathology.* New York: Oxford University Press; 2001:43–51.
7. Behin A, Delattre JY. Neurologic sequelae of radiotherapy on the nervous system. In: Schiff D, Wen PY, eds. *Cancer Neurology in Clinical Practice.* Totowa, NJ: Humana; 2002:173–191.
8. Monje ML, Palmer T. Radiation injury and neurogenesis. *Curr Opin Neurol.* 2003;16(2): 129–134.
9. Dropcho E. Central nervous system injury by therapeutic irradiation. *Neurol Clin.* 1991;9: 969–988.
10. Schiff D, Shin DM, Moots PL, et al. Neurologic complications of head and neck cancer. In: Schiff D, Wen PY, eds. *Cancer Neurology in Clinical Practice.* Totowa NJ: Humana; 2003: 425–434.
11. Schultheiss T, Kun L, Ang K. Radiation response of the central nervous system. *Int J Radiat Oncol Biol Phys.* 1995;31:1093–1112.
12. Olsen N, Pfeiffer P, Johannsen L. Radiation-induced brachial plexopathy: Neurological follow-up in 161 recurrence-free breast cancer patients. *Int J Radiat Oncol Biol Phys.* 1993;26:43–49.
13. van Vulpen M, Kal HB, Taphoorn MJ, et al. Changes in blood–brain barrier permeability induced by radiotherapy: Implications for timing of chemotherapy? *Oncol Rep.* 2002;9(4): 683–688.
14. Stryker J, Sommerville K, Perez R. Sacral plexus injury after radiotherapy for carcinoma of cervix. *Cancer.* 1990;66: 1488–1492.
15. Cowen D, Geller L. Long-term pathological effects of prenatal X: Irradiation on the central nervous system of the rat. *J Neuropathol Exp Neurol.* 1960;19: 488–527.
16. Otake M, Yoshimaru H, Schull W. Severe mental retardation among the prenatally exposed survivors of the atomic bombing of Hiroshima and Nagasaki: A comparison of the T65DR and DS86 dosimetry systems. Hiroshima: Radiation Effects Research Foundation; 1987:TR 16–87.
17. Yoshimoto Y. Cancer risk among children of atomic bomb survivors. *JAMA.* 1990;264: 596–600.
18. Whitnall MH, Inal CE, Jackson WE 3rd. In vivo radioprotection by 5-androstenediol: Stimulation of the innate immune system. *Radiat Res.* 2001;156(3):283–293.
19. Loria RM, Conrad DH, et al. Androstenetriol and androstenediol: Protection against lethal radiation and restoration of immunity after radiation injury. *Ann N Y Acad Sci.* 2000;917: 860–867.
20. Grillo CA, Dulout FN. The effect of butylated hydroxytoluene on the chromosomal damage induced by bleomycin in Chinese hamster ovary cells. *Mutat Res.* 1997;375:83–89.

CHAPTER 161

Nerve Agents

Christopher P. Holstege • Sarice L. Bassin

OBJECTIVES

- To review the pathophysiology associated with nerve agent toxicity
- To describe the signs and symptoms associated with nerve agent toxicity
- To explain the unique neurologic effects associated with nerve agents
- To explore the treatment options for nerve agent toxicity

CASE VIGNETTE

On March 20, 1995, five two-man teams of the Aum Shinrikyo cult carried out a nerve agent attack in Tokyo, Japan (1–3). At 0755, during peak commuting time, the assailants placed sarin-filled bags on the subway train floor and pierced them with sharpened umbrella tips. The first emergency call was received by the Tokyo fire department at 0809 and, in the ensuing hour, emergency medical authorities were inundated with calls for aid from multiple subway stations. A total of 131 ambulances and 1,364 emergency medical technicians were dispatched, with 688 people transported to hospitals by emergency rescue vehicles. More than 4,000 people found their own way to medical facilities using taxis, private cars, or on foot. The lack of emergency decontamination facilities and protective equipment resulted in a further secondary exposure of medical staff (135 ambulance staff and 110 staff in the main receiving hospital reported symptoms). Having initially been misinformed that a gas explosion had caused burns and carbon monoxide poisoning, medical centers nevertheless began treating for organophosphate exposure based on the typical symptomatology they encountered. An official announcement by the police that sarin had been identified came to the hospitals via television news, reportedly 3 hours after the release. Overall, 12 people died, 54 were severely injured, and approximately 980 were mildly to moderately affected. Most of the 5,000 seeking help were worried that they might have been exposed, many with psychogenic symptoms.

DEFINITION

The nerve agents are organophosphates and have chemical structures similar to the more familiar organophosphate pesticides, such as malathion (4). A number of nerve agents have been manufactured, including tabun, soman, sarin, cyclosarin, VX, and the Russia V-type agent designated *VR*. These agents are among the most potent toxins known to mankind. Tabun, sarin, soman, and cyclosarin are more volatile than the V-agents and evaporate from the skin more rapidly, therefore failing to penetrate skin unless occluded. Sarin is the most volatile of the nerve agents, possessing a volatility similar to water. The less volatile an agent is, the more persistent it is on terrain and material. The vapor densities of all these agents are heavier than air and, subsequently, they sink to the ground.

EPIDEMIOLOGY AND HISTORY

The discovery of nerve agents occurred in the 1930s when German scientists were attempting to improve on existing organophosphate pesticides (4). The German military manufactured the nerve agents tabun, sarin, and soman, but for unclear reasons their use in combat never occurred during World War II. The Iraqi military used nerve agents against the Iranian military in the mid-1980s, which was the first known use of these agents on a battlefield (5). In 1988, Iraq used sarin against the Kurds (6). In 1994, a terrorist sarin gas attack occurred in Matsumoto, Japan, resulting in the deaths of 7 people with >200 exposed civilians seeking medical attention (7). In 1995, another terrorist sarin gas attack occurred in Japan, resulting in 12 deaths with >5,000 civilians presenting to medical facilities believing they had been exposed (1–3). In 1996, the United States government acknowledged that troops operating during the Gulf War in 1991 were potentially exposed to sarin after an Iraqi chemical weapons dump was destroyed at Khamisiyah (8). On May 17, 2004, a roadside bomb containing sarin detonated near a US military convoy in Iraq, resulting in two military personnel requiring treatment for exposure.

PATHOPHYSIOLOGY

Acetylcholine (ACh) is a neurotransmitter found throughout the nervous system, including the central nervous system (CNS), the autonomic nervous system, and at the skeletal muscle motor end-plate (Fig. 161-1) (9). ACh acts in both the CNS and peripheral nervous system (PNS) by binding to, and activating, muscarinic and nicotinic cholinergic receptors. Muscarinic receptors are G-protein coupled receptors that act at visceral smooth muscle, cardiac muscle, and secretory glands. Nicotinic receptors are ligand-gated ion channels located in autonomic ganglia and neuromuscular junctions.

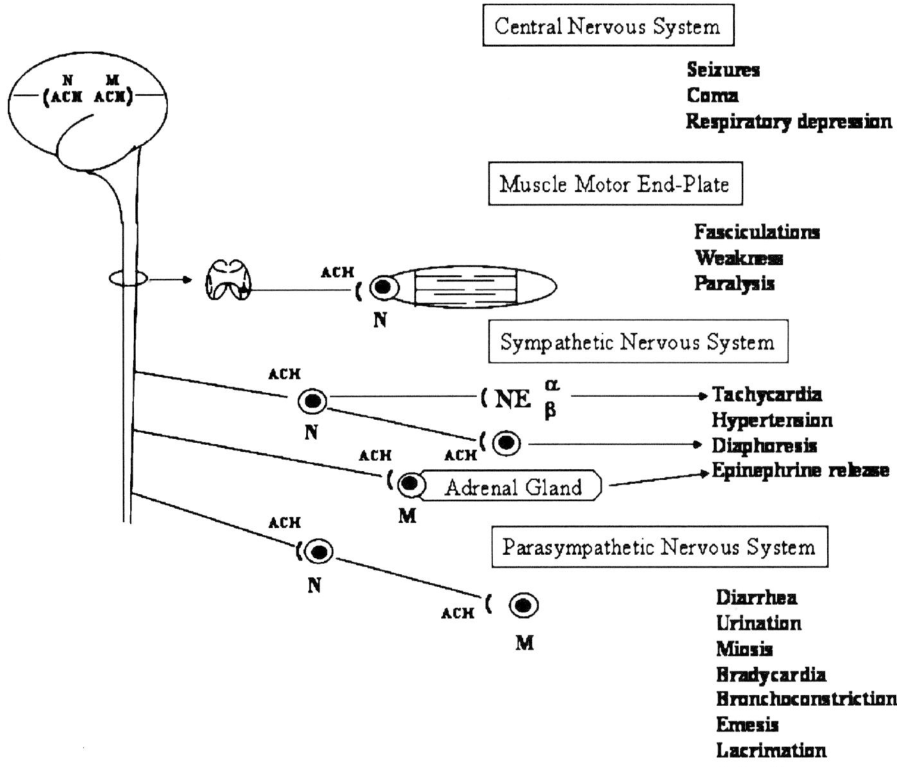

FIGURE 161-1. Clinical effects seen in nerve agent poisoning caused by access of acetylcholine in the central, autonomic, and peripheral nervous systems. M, muscarinic; N, nicotinic; NE, norepinephrine; ACH, acetylcholine.

The enzyme, acetylcholinesterase (AChE), terminates the activity of ACh within the synaptic cleft. ACh binds to AChE's active site where the enzyme hydrolyzes ACh to choline and acetic acid. These hydrolyzed products rapidly dissociate from AChE so that the enzyme is free to act on another molecule. Nerve agents act by binding the AChE active site (Fig. 161-2), rendering the enzyme incapable of inactivating ACh. As a result, ACh accumulates in the synapse and excessive stimulation occurs.

Over time, a portion of the bound nerve agent is cleaved, producing a stable, covalent bond between the nerve agent and AChE. This process is called *aging*. The time it takes for aging to occur depends on the nerve agent. Aging occurs within 2 minutes for soman, but takes hours for the other nerve agents. Before aging occurs, AChE reactivators, such as pralidoxime chloride, can remove the nerve agent and restore enzyme function. Once this aged covalent bond forms, however, AChE cannot be reactivated and activity is not restored until new enzyme is synthesized.

CLINICAL MANIFESTATIONS

The onset, severity, and clinical effects of nerve agent poisoning vary widely (Table 161-1) (9). Both the dose of nerve agent and the route of exposure are factors in determining the clinical effects. The two most prevalent routes of exposure are via dermal droplet contact and via gas inhalation or absorption. The progression of the signs and symptoms can range from a mild and gradual intoxication to cardiopulmonary collapse, seizures, and death within minutes.

RESPIRATORY

The respiratory system effects of nerve agents tend to be dramatic and are considered to be the major factor leading to the death of the victim. The development of respiratory failure results from the triad of increased airway resistance, neuromuscular failure, and depression of the central respiratory centers (10). Intoxication can present with profuse watery nasal discharge, nasal hyperemia, marked salivation, and bronchorrhea. Animal studies have reported weakness of the tongue and pharyngeal muscles, leading to airway obstruction (11). Laryngeal muscle paralysis can result in vocal cord dysfunction and subsequent stridor. A prolonged expiratory phase, cough, and wheezing can manifest as a consequence of lower respiratory tract bronchorrhea and bronchoconstriction. As systemic absorption occurs, respiratory muscle weakness ensues. Nerve agent-induced central apnea can contribute to the death of the patient if supportive therapy is not initiated.

CENTRAL NERVOUS SYSTEM

AChE receptors are found throughout the CNS, with highest concentrations within the reticular-activating system, basal ganglia, limbic system, cortical and cerebellar projections, the retina, and within the ventral and dorsal synapses of the spinal cord. Because of the ubiquity of these receptors, nerve agent poisoning can produce great variation in neurologic signs and symptoms. Headache, vertigo, paresthesias, anxiety, insomnia, depression, excessive dreaming, and emotional liability have all been reported following AChE inhibitor exposures (12). A rapidly progressive decrease in the level of consciousness resulting in coma is seen with the time from exposure to coma reported to be as fast as a few seconds (10).

Nerve agent poisoning is associated with seizure initiation, status epilepticus, seizure-related brain damage (SRBD), and subsequent death (7,13). The exact mechanism of seizure

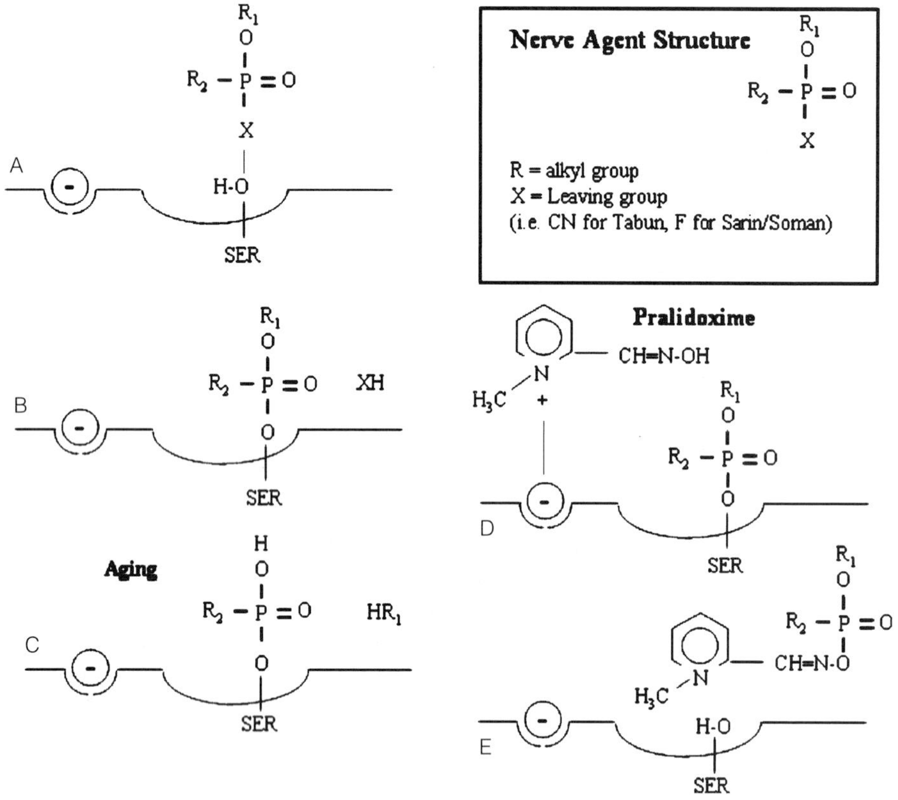

FIGURE 161-2. Schematic illustration of acetylcholinesterase (AChE) in which the site (−) normally attracts acetylcholine, according to the following: 1. The nerve agent binds to the serine hydroxyl group. 2. The leaving group (*X*) is cleaved to allow phosphorylation of AChE. 3. Aging occurs as a result of the leaving of one of the *R* groups and the formation of a stable covalent bond. 4. Pralidoxime binds to the anionic site before aging occurs. 5. Rejuvenation of AChE by removal of the nerve agent by pralidoxime. SER, serine residue.

activity has not been fully delineated, but excessive stimulation of cholinergic neurons, stimulation of glutamate (*N*-methyl-d-aspartate [NMDA]) excitatory neurotransmitter receptors, and antagonism of γ-aminobutyric acid (GABA)-mediated systems have been implicated mechanisms (9). Based on current evidence, the pathophysiologic progression of nerve agent-induced seizures can be divided into three phases: an early cholinergic phase that lasts from the time of exposure to approximately 5 minutes after seizure onset; a transitional phase of progressively mixed cholinergic or noncholinergic modulation that begins >5 minutes after seizure onset and lasts until approximately 40 minutes; and a predominantly noncholinergic phase beginning approximately 40 minutes (14,15). These phases result from the cholinergic-induced seizure activity itself recruiting other excitatory neurotransmitter systems (i.e., NMDA) that can eventually maintain the seizures independent of the initial cholinergic drive (14,16). The activation of NMDA receptors can lead to massive intracellular calcium fluxes into the cytoplasm, resulting in excitotoxin-mediated cell death and contributing to the profound SRBD that has been extensively noted in animal studies (16–18).

TABLE 161-1. Signs and Symptoms of Acute Nerve Agent Poisoning

MUSCARINIC MANIFESTATIONS

Ophthalmic: Conjunctival injection, lacrimation, miosis, blurred vision, diminished visual acuity, ocular pain
Respiratory: Rhinorrhea, stridor, wheezing, cough, excessive sputum, chest tightness, dyspnea, apnea
Cardiovascular: Bradydysrhythmias, hypotension
Dermal: Flushing, diaphoresis, cyanosis
Gastrointestinal: Nausea, vomiting, salivation, diarrhea, abdominal cramping, tenesmus, fecal incontinence
Genitourinary: Frequency, urgency, incontinence

NICOTINIC MANIFESTATIONS

Cardiovascular: Tachydysrhythmias, hypertension
Striated muscle: fasciculations, twitching, cramping, weakness, paralysis

CENTRAL NERVOUS SYSTEM MANIFESTATIONS

Anxiety, restlessness, depression, confusion, ataxia, tremors, seizures, coma, areflexia

CARDIOVASCULAR

The cardiovascular effects from nerve agent poisoning are variable and can be caused by either direct cholinergic effects at the heart or nicotinic effects at the autonomic ganglia (7). Experiments in rats indicate that soman-induced hypertension depends entirely on central muscarinic stimulation (19). Cardiotoxicity resulting from AChE inhibitors has been divided into three phases. Initially, a period of intense sympathetic activity results in sinus tachydysrhythmias, with or without hypertension. Victims may subsequently develop bradydysrhythmias, prolongation of the PR interval, atrioventricular blocks, and hypotension as parasympathetic tone predominates. The third phase occurs with QT prolongation and progression to polymorphous ventricular tachycardia (torsades de pointes). The cause of the QT prolongation has not been elucidated. The above phases can occur at any time while the patient is manifesting clinical signs of toxicity and do not necessarily follow sequentially.

MUSCULOSKELETAL

Skeletal muscle activity is initiated at nicotinic receptors at motor endplates. With early or minimal exposure to AChE inhibitors, symptoms can be vague and consist of muscular weakness and difficulty with ambulation. With increasing exposure, these agents resemble succinylcholine in that they cause muscular fasciculations and subsequent paralysis. This is especially problematic because this paralysis can mask seizure activity.

OPHTHALMOLOGIC

Nerve agent vapors rapidly penetrate the conjunctiva and stimulate muscarinic receptors. This causes constriction of both the ciliary and sphincter muscles, as well as stimulation of the lacrimal gland. As a result, victims of nerve agent poisoning experience lacrimation, blurred vision, and miosis. Miosis can develop immediately after vapor exposure or after direct ocular contact with liquid and is the most consistent clinical finding associated with nerve agent vapor exposure. In the Japan sarin attacks, miosis was reported in 89% to 99% of the victims (20). Following dermal absorption, however, miosis can be absent or delayed after other systemic signs and symptoms. Dark adaptation is lost because of pupillary inability to dilate. Miosis persists for a variable period, depending on the amount of exposure, with pupillary constriction reportedly lasting up to 45 days (21). Patients will frequently complain of eye pain, headache, nausea, and vomiting caused by ciliary spasm that is exacerbated by attempting to focus on close objects.

DERMAL

The sweat glands are innervated by sympathetic muscarinic receptors. After AChE inhibitor intoxication, profuse diaphoresis occurs. This effect can be diffuse after systemic absorption or localized only to the area of dermal droplet exposure.

GASTROINTESTINAL

Muscarinic receptors stimulate secretion from the salivary glands, pancreas, and small and large intestinal goblet cells. Muscarinic receptors also stimulate gastric parietal cell acid and chief cell pepsinogen release, gallbladder contraction, and decreased intestinal ion and water absorption. Cholinergic innervation causes an increase in gastric and intestinal motility and a relaxation of reflex anal sphincter tone. As a result, profuse watery salivation and gastrointestinal hyperactivity, with resultant nausea, vomiting, abdominal cramps, tenesmus, and uncontrolled defecation, are characteristic features of systemic AChE blockade. Even with exposure to vapor, as opposed to ingestion and dermal absorption, the Tokyo sarin gas victims reportedly experienced nausea (67%), vomiting (41%), and diarrhea (6%).

GENTITOURINARY

Cholinergic stimulation of the detrusor muscle causes contraction of the urinary bladder and relaxation of the trigone and sphincter muscles. The overall effect is involuntary urination.

DIAGNOSTIC APPROACH

A physician's bedside observations of end-organ toxicity are most helpful for making clinical decisions about nerve agent poisoning. The toxicology laboratory is useful, but has limitations. Of note, 25% of the moderately to severely poisoned patients in the Tokyo sarin attack had normal admission plasma cholinesterase activity (12).

The clinical laboratory can measure neither serum or urine concentrations of nerve agents or their metabolites nor the concentration of AChE in synapses. Instead, the nervous system's AChE activity is approximated by measuring plasma and erythrocyte cholinesterase activity. Plasma- or *pseudocholinesterase* is made in the liver and rapidly inactivated by nerve agents. Its activity is also depressed by liver disease, pregnancy, infection, and oral contraceptive use. The liver regenerates the enzyme rapidly. Erythrocyte (red blood cells [RBC]) or "true" cholinesterase is similar to the enzyme found at the neuronal synapse. Its regeneration, however, depends on replacing RBC in the circulation. It regenerates at approximately 1% per day and is slower than neuronal enzyme regeneration. Therefore, RBC and plasma cholinesterase activity may not always reflect neuronal enzyme activity.

In general, systemic signs and symptoms have been reported when RBC enzyme activity falls below 40%. Correlation between RBC enzyme activity and clinical effects is hindered by: (*a*) wide normal range, (*b*) route of exposure (vapor or dermal), (*c*) exposure dose, and (*d*) selective inhibition of RBC or plasma cholinesterase activity. The wide normal range for RBC enzyme activity makes interpretation of mild to moderate exposures difficult without a baseline measurement (22). Cholinesterase activity correlates poorly with severity of local effects after vapor exposures. On the other hand, when RBC enzyme activity is depressed 20% to 25% of normal, it tends to correlate with severe systemic toxic effects (12).

Various organophosphate compounds selectively inhibit either plasma or RBC cholinesterase. With mild to moderate exposure, nerve agents tend preferentially to inhibit RBC cholinesterase activity more than plasma (e.g., VX: 70% RBC inhibition, 20% plasma inhibition; sarin: 80% RBC, 30% plasma) (4). This selective inhibition is lost after large nerve agent exposures and the activity of both enzymes will be near zero. Treatment should never be withheld from a symptomatic patient, awaiting laboratory confirmation in suspected nerve agent poisoning. Conversely, pharmacologic treatment is not justified for patients with depressed cholinesterase activity and no clinical signs.

TREATMENT

DECONTAMINATION

Patient decontamination is a fundamental aspect of the management to both terminate toxin exposure and prevent secondary contamination of staff (23). Decontamination begins with clothing removal. Clothing can release nerve agents for up to 30 minutes after it has come in contact with poisonous vapor. Sarin liquid that contaminates clothing will continue to vaporize, thereby posing a risk to both the person wearing the contaminated garments and those in their immediate environment. Therefore, clothing should be quickly removed and carefully disposed of in double layer plastic bags (24).

Despite this first step, nerve agents can continue to penetrate the deeper layers of skin where they continue to be absorbed. Thorough washing of the body with soap and copious water and conjunctival irrigation should commence, with care taken not to cause injury to the skin that would further enhance absorption. Medical personnel assisting with decontamination should wear goggles, respirators, and protective clothing, including butyl rubber gloves, if available. Because nerve agents are lipophilic, latex gloves provide only partial protection. Bleach or 5% sodium hydrochlorite can be used to decontaminate scissors or other items used in clothing removal and patient decontamination.

INITIAL ASSESSMENT AND MANAGEMENT

Lifesaving treatment of severe nerve agent poisoning should initially focus on a patent airway, adequate ventilation, and aggressive atropine administration (10). Early endotracheal intubation is crucial in the critically ill patient. If rapid sequence intubation is performed, succinylcholine should be avoided because it is metabolized by AChE and subsequent neuromuscular blockade would be prolonged. Initial attempts at ventilation can be difficult because of the intense nerve agent-induced bronchoconstriction. Copious secretions in the upper and lower airways must be suctioned. Intravenous access should be obtained immediately. Aggressive atropine use will improve ventilation by drying secretions and decreasing airways resistance. Because it has been demonstrated that a dissociation exists between motor convulsant activity, or lack thereof, and electroencephalographic (EEG) activity, continuous EEG monitoring should be performed (7,14). Appropriate laboratory tests should be obtained, including plasma and RBC cholinesterase levels.

ANTIDOTE THERAPY

Atropine

Atropine is the initial drug of choice in the symptomatic nerve agent victim. Atropine acts as a muscarinic receptor antagonist and blocks neuroeffector sites on smooth muscle, cardiac muscle, secretory gland cells, peripheral ganglia, and in the CNS. Atropine, therefore, is useful in alleviating bronchoconstriction and bronchorrhea, tenesmus, abdominal cramps, nausea and vomiting, bradydysrythmias, and seizure activity. Atropine can be administered by either the intravenous, intramuscular, or endotracheal route. The dose varies with the severity of exposure, but typically even the worst reported cases require $<$20 mg in the first 24 hours (10). For the mildly and moderately symptomatic patient, 2.0 mg for adults and 0.02 mg/kg for children (minimum of 0.1 mg) is administered every 5 minutes, as needed, to alleviate signs and symptoms, such as bronchoconstriction or bronchorrhea. In the severely poisoned patient, dosages may need to be increased and given more frequently.

Tachycardia is an effect of nerve agent poisoning and is not a contraindication to atropine administration. Drying of the respiratory secretions and resolution of bronchoconstriction are the therapeutic endpoints used to determine the appropriate dose of atropine. If bag-assisted ventilation is difficult or secretions continue, then the atropine dose must be increased. Atropine has no effect on the nicotinic receptors and, therefore, has no effect on autonomic ganglia and neuromuscular junction. Therefore, muscle weakness, fasciculations, tremors, and paralysis are not an indication for further atropine dosing. It does have a partial effect on the CNS and is helpful in aborting seizures.

Miosis is a poor clinical sign to follow for guiding repeat doses of atropine. If the resolution of miosis is used as the endpoint of atropine dosing, an anticholinergic syndrome can develop. Ophthalmic instillation of atropine to alleviate miosis is not recommended because it actually worsens vision, resulting in photophobia and blurred vision caused by the subsequent mydriasis and the loss of accommodation (25). The only recommended indication for a topical ophthalmic mydriatics or cycloplegic agent is relief of intractable eye pain caused by ciliary spasm.

Pralidoxime Chloride

Pralidoxime chloride (2-PAMCL, Protopam Chloride) reactivates AChE by exerting a nucleophilic attack on the phosphorus, resulting in an oxime–phosphate bond that splits from the AChE leaving the regenerated enzyme (Fig. 161-2) (9). This reactivation is clinically most apparent at skeletal neuromuscular junctions, with less activity at muscarinic sites. Pralidoxime, therefore, must be administered concurrently with adequate atropine doses. In addition, the process of aging will prevent pralidoxime from regenerating the AChE active site and, as a result, is ineffective after aging has occurred. Therefore, the sooner the administration of pralidoxime, the greater the clinical effect.

The recommended initial dose of pralidoxime is 1.0 g for adults or 15 to 25 mg/kg for children by intravenous route. Slow administration over 15 to 30 minutes has been advocated to minimize side effects, including hypertension, headache, blurred vision, epigastric discomfort, nausea, and vomiting. In multiple animal models, the pralidoxime serum concentration to achieve therapeutic efficacy was reported to be 4 mg/L (26). The above dose will attain these levels, but pralidoxime is rapidly excreted and the concentration falls below 4 mg/L within 2 hours (27). Subsequently, repeat pralidoxime should be administered at hourly intervals if progressive worsening or serious signs of toxicity persist. It has been recently suggested that, after 2 to 3 intermittent intravenous boluses, a continuous intravenous infusion at a rate of 500 mg/hour should be used to achieve a steady state and control recurrence of symptoms in severe organophosphate poisoning. Continuous intravenous infusion for insecticide organophosphate poisoning has shown to be safe and effective (27). In the available case reports, however, severe toxic effects following nerve agent exposure rarely lasted more than a couple hours and prolonged pralidoxime therapy may not be necessary.

Adequate hydration should be maintained during therapy to facilitate renal excretion of pralidoxime. Theoretically, dosing should be lowered for patients with renal failure. If medical personnel are unable initially to obtain intravenous access, a solution for intramuscular use can be made by mixing the contents of a 1-g vial with 3 mL of sterile saline. Intramuscular administration to a patient with an adequate blood pressure will produce a therapeutic plasma concentration of 4 mg/L within 10 minutes.

Anticonvulsants

Effective and rapid management of nerve agent-induced seizures is critical. Pretreatment with a carbamate (e.g., pyridostigmine) to shield a fraction of AChE from irreversible inhibition, in conjunction with atropine and pralidoxime, has been shown to increase significantly the survival rate of experimental animals (14). This combined treatment regimen, however, does not ameliorate nerve agent-induced seizure activity without the addition of a benzodiazepine (13).

All centrally acting anticholinergic agents (i.e., atropine and scopolamine) can block onset or terminate seizures if given before or within 5 minutes of seizure onset in animal models, but are ineffective alone if treatment is delayed more than 40 minutes after seizure onset (17,28). Benzodiazepines are effective in treating nerve agent-induced seizures. Diazepam blocks seizure onset, yet seizures can occur after an initial period of anticonvulsant effect at doses <2.5 mg/kg in animal models. Diazepam alone can terminate ongoing seizures when given within 5 minutes after seizure onset, but doses up to 20 mg/kg are ineffective when treatment was delayed more than 40 minutes (14). Diazepam gel is easily administered rectally, which may be beneficial if intravenous access is delayed. Midazolam is more potent and rapidly acting as an anticonvulsant than diazepam, both via parenteral and intranasal routes (29,30). Because of its high water solubility, midazolam can be safely injected intramuscularly with very rapid absorption (31).

The combination of a benzodiazepine and an anticholinergic agent is effective in terminating seizures in mice, regardless of whether treatment was administered 5 or 40 minutes after seizure onset (32). Phenytoin, fosphenytoin, carbamazepine, valproic acid, felbamate, lamotrigine, magnesium sulfate, pentobarbital, and ketamine have no therapeutic anticonvulsant effectiveness for nerve agent-induced seizures (14,33).

In animal models, successful control of seizure activity, regardless of the pharmacologic agents used, was predictive of survival of the lethal effects of nerve agent exposure, a more rapid behavioral recovery, and greater protection from neuropathology (28). Numerous epidemiologic studies have shown that the duration of human seizures correlates with outcome, with longer seizures being more refractory to treatment and associated with cognitive decline (34,35). It, therefore, is clinically prudent to expeditiously and aggressively treat nerve agent-induced seizures.

CLINICAL RECOMMENDATIONS OF THE VIGNETTE

The hallmark findings of miosis, profuse diaphoresis, bronchorrhea, bronchospasm, intractable seizures, and muscle weakness should clue the clinician into the possibility of nerve agent poisoning. The clinical syndrome of nerve agent toxicity varies widely, ranging from the classic cholinergic syndrome to flaccid paralysis and status epilepticus. All nerve agents are capable of producing marked neuropathology. Seizure control is strongly associated with protection against acute lethality and brain pathology.

The mainstays of therapy of nerve agent-poisoned patients are atropine, pralidoxime, and benzodiazepines. Tachycardia is *not* a contraindication to treatment with atropine in nerve agent toxicity. Atropine should be administered to alleviate respiratory distress, symptomatic bradycardia, and used as an adjunct to benzodiazepines and pralidoxime to alleviate seizure activity.

SUMMARY

The threat of nerve agent exposure in both combat and terrorist acts has become a greater concern over the past decade. Physicians should to be familiar with the mechanisms of action, clinical course, and treatment of nerve agent intoxication. Initial management should focus on supportive care, with an emphasis toward aggressive airway maintenance. Atropine should be titrated, with the goals of drying secretions and resolving bronchoconstriction. Early treatment with pralidoxime chloride will maximize efficacy. Benzodiazepine, in addition to atropine, should be administered if seizures develop or are suspected. Early, aggressive medical therapy is the key to prevention of the morbidity and mortality associated with nerve agent poisoning.

REFERENCES

1. Okumura T, Suzuki K, Fukuda A, et al. The Tokyo subway sarin attack: Disaster management. Part 3: National and international responses. *Acad Emerg Med.* 1998;5(6):625–628.
2. Okumura T, Suzuki K, Fukuda A, et al. The Tokyo subway sarin attack: Disaster management. Part 2: Hospital response. *Acad Emerg Med.* 1998;5(6):618–624.
3. Okumura T, Suzuki K, Fukuda A, et al. The Tokyo subway sarin attack: Disaster management. Part 1: Community emergency response. *Acad Emerg Med.* 1998;5(6):613–617.
4. Holstege CP, Kirk M, Sidell FR. Chemical warfare. Nerve agent poisoning. *Crit Care Clin.* 1997;13(4):923–942.
5. Newmark J. The birth of nerve agent warfare: Lessons from Syed Abbas Foroutan. *Neurology.* 2004;62(9):1590–1596.
6. Black RM, Clarke RJ, Read RW, et al. Application of gas chromatography-mass spectrometry and gas chromatography-tandem mass spectrometry to the analysis of chemical warfare samples, found to contain residues of the nerve agent sarin, sulphur mustard and their degradation products. *J Chromatogr A.* 1994;662(2):301–321.
7. Okudera H. Clinical features on nerve gas terrorism in Matsumoto. *J Clin Neurosci.* 2002;9(1):17–21.
8. Gray GC, Smith TC, Knoke JD, et al. The postwar hospitalization experience of Gulf War Veterans possibly exposed to chemical munitions destruction at Khamisiyah, Iraq. *Am J Epidemiol.* 1999;150(5):532–540.
9. Holstege CP, Dobmeier SG. Nerve agent toxicity and treatment. *Current Treatment Options in Neurology.* 2005;7(2):91–98.
10. Sidell FR. Soman and sarin: Clinical manifestations and treatment of accidental poisoning by organophosphates. *Clin Toxicol.* 1974;7(1):1–17.
11. Grob D. The manifestations and treatment of poisoning due to nerve gas and other organic phosphate anticholinesterase compounds. *Arch Intern Med.* 1956;98(2):221–239.
12. Okumura T, Takasu N, Ishimatsu S, et al. Report on 640 victims of the Tokyo subway sarin attack. *Ann Emerg Med.* 1996;28(2):129–135.
13. Auta J, Costa E, Davis J, Guidotti A. Imidazenil: A potent and safe protective agent against diisopropyl fluorophosphate toxicity. *Neuropharmacology.* 2004;46(3):397–403.
14. Shih T, McDonough JH, Jr., Koplovitz I. Anticonvulsants for soman-induced seizure activity. *J Biomed Sci.* 1999;6(2):86–96.
15. McDonough JH, Jr., Shih TM. Neuropharmacological mechanisms of nerve agent-induced seizure and neuropathology. *Neurosci Biobehav Rev.* 1997;21(5):559–579.
16. de Groot DM, Bierman EP, Bruijnzeel PL, et al. Beneficial effects of TCP on soman intoxication in guinea pigs: Seizures, brain damage and learning behaviour. *J Appl Toxicol.* 2001;21[Suppl 1]:S57–S65.
17. Shih TM, McDonough JH. Efficacy of biperiden and atropine as anticonvulsant treatment for organophosphorus nerve agent intoxication. *Arch Toxicol.* 2000;74(3):165–172.
18. Bhagat YA, Obenaus A, Hamilton MG, et al. Neuroprotection from soman-induced seizures in the rodent: Evaluation with diffusion- and T2-weighted magnetic resonance imaging. *Neurotoxicology.* 2005;26(6):1001–1013.
19. Letienne R, Julien C, Barres C, et al. Soman-induced hypertension in conscious rats is mediated by prolonged central muscarinic stimulation. *Fundam Clin Pharmacol.* 1999;13(4):468–474.
20. Ohbu S, Yamashina A, Takasu N, et al. Sarin poisoning on Tokyo subway. *South Med J.* 1997;90(6):587–593.
21. Rengstorff RH. Accidental exposure to sarin: Vision effects. *Arch Toxicol.* 1985;56(3):201–203.
22. Coye MJ, Barnett PG, Midtling JE, et al. Clinical confirmation of organophosphate poisoning by serial cholinesterase analyses. *Arch Intern Med.* 1987;147(3):438–442.
23. Nozaki H, Hori S, Shinozawa Y, et al. Secondary exposure of medical staff to sarin vapor in the emergency room. *Intensive Care Med.* 1995;21(12):1032–1035.

24. Facts about sarin. Atlanta, GA: Centers for Disease Control and Prevention (CDC); 2006.
25. Nozaki H, Aikawa N. Sarin poisoning in Tokyo subway. *Lancet.* 1995;345(8962):1446–1447.
26. Zvirblis P, Kondritzer AA. Prophylaxis against sarin poisoning in the rat by oral administration of pralidoxime chloride. *J Pharmacol Exp Ther.* 1967;157(2):432–434.
27. Medicis JJ, Stork CM, Howland MA, et al. Pharmacokinetics following a loading plus a continuous infusion of pralidoxime compared with the traditional short infusion regimen in human volunteers. *J Toxicol Clin Toxicol.* 1996;34(3):289–295.
28. McDonough JH, Jr., Zoeffel LD, McMonagle J, et al. Anticonvulsant treatment of nerve agent seizures: Anticholinergics versus diazepam in soman-intoxicated guinea pigs. *Epilepsy Res.* 2000;38(1):1–14.
29. Gilat E, Goldman M, Lahat E, et al. Nasal midazolam as a novel anticonvulsive treatment against organophosphate-induced seizure activity in the guinea pig. *Arch Toxicol.* 2003; 77(3):167–172.
30. Shih TM, Duniho SM, McDonough JH. Control of nerve agent-induced seizures is critical for neuroprotection and survival. *Toxicol Appl Pharmacol.* 2003;188(2):69–80.
31. Rey E, Treluyer JM, Pons G. Pharmacokinetic optimization of benzodiazepine therapy for acute seizures. Focus on delivery routes. *Clin Pharmacokinet.* 1999;36(6):409–424.
32. Koplovitz I, Schulz S, Shutz M, et al. Combination anticonvulsant treatment of soman-induced seizures. *J Appl Toxicol.* 2001;21[Suppl 1]:S53–S55.
33. McDonough JH, Benjamin A, McMonagle JD, et al. Effects of fosphenytoin on nerve agent-induced status epilepticus. *Drug Chem Toxicol.* 2004;27(1):27–39.
34. Towne AR, Pellock JM, Ko D, et al. Determinants of mortality in status epilepticus. *Epilepsia.* 1994;35(1):27–34.
35. Lothman EW, Bertram EH, 3rd. Epileptogenic effects of status epilepticus. *Epilepsia.* 1993;34[Suppl 1]:S59–S70.

CHAPTER 162

Botulinum Toxin

Andreas H. Kramer • Vern C. Juel

OBJECTIVES

- To describe the characteristic clinical manifestations of botulism, especially those features that distinguish it from other causes of acute neuromuscular weakness, such as Guillain-Barré syndrome or myasthenia gravis
- To explain the public health implications associated with a case of botulism. Early communication with the state health department is essential
- To identify atypical features of the clinical presentation that could potentially be consistent with deliberate release of botulinum toxin
- To discuss the diagnostic tests required in a case of suspected botulism
- To emphasize that, in most cases, initiation of therapy should *not* be delayed while awaiting the results of definitive diagnostic testing
- To describe the factors that mandate timely endotracheal intubation

CASE VIGNETTE

A 37-year-old man presented to the emergency department with a 24-hour history of blurred vision, difficulty swallowing, and slurred speech. Vital signs were normal, with the exception of a respiratory rate of 22 breaths per minute. He was awake and oriented, although his speech was difficult to understand because of dysarthria. He was noted to be mildly diaphoretic and using accessory muscles of respiration. Neurologic examination was notable for minimally reactive pupils, bilateral ptosis, inability to gaze upward, weakness of the facial muscles, inability to lift his head off the bed, and 4-/5 motor power in his upper extremities. Muscle tone, sensation, and reflexes were normal. Complete blood count (CBC), basic metabolic panel, and electrocardiogram (ECG) findings were unremarkable. Chest radiography revealed low lung volumes and bibasilar atelectasis. Forced vital capacity was found to be only 700 mL. The previous day, he had been at a local political rally, where a variety of different home-made foods had been served.

DEFINITION

Botulism is characterized by the development of potentially life-threatening paralysis, induced by the effects of a neurotoxin released by the bacterium *Clostridium botulinum*. Humans can be exposed to this neurotoxin in a number of different ways, but the clinical manifestations are consistent. With a mean lethal dose (LD_{50}) of only 1 ng/kg of body weight, botulinum toxin is widely regarded as the most lethal substance in nature. In recent years, increasing concern has arisen about the potential use of botulinum toxin as a biological weapon. The Center for Disease Control and Prevention (CDC) has classified botulism as a high priority, "category A" bioterrorism agent that poses a risk to national security (1).

EPIDEMIOLOGY AND ETIOLOGY

C. botulinum is a gram-positive, anaerobic, spore-forming bacterium that is ubiquitous in nature, being particularly abundant in soil. The organisms *C. baratii* and *C. butyricum* are genetically distinct from *C. botulinum*, but have similar properties, in that they also produce neurotoxins and, occasionally, are responsible for causing botulism (2).

Through the formation of spores, *C. botulinum* can survive harsh environmental conditions. Heating to >120°C is necessary to kill the spores, although approximately 85°C is sufficient to denature the toxin. Modern canning techniques were developed in large part to specifically combat botulism. When ideal conditions are met (anaerobic environment, alkaline pH, temperature 25°C to 37°C, low sugar, and salt concentration), the spores germinate and the organism can produce toxin (3).

Eight different toxins (A, B, C_1, C_2, D, E, F, and G) have been identified. The clinical syndrome of botulism is caused exclusively by toxins A, B, E and, rarely, F. The severity of the condition can vary, depending on the particular toxin involved, with evidence that recovery time is somewhat longer for type A than for the others (3). Most cases in the western United States are caused by toxin A, whereas those in the eastern United States and Europe are largely caused by toxin B (4). Exposure to toxin E has frequently been described in association with the traditional Native Alaskan practice of fermenting a variety of foods (5).

Botulism is usually classified according to how exposure to the toxin occurs. The four naturally occurring forms include foodborne botulism, wound botulism, infant botulism, and, rarely, adult infectious botulism. The two other forms now recognized are (*a*) inhalational botulism, which could theoretically occur if the toxin were to become aerosolized; and (*b*) inadvertent, iatrogenic botulism, which can rarely complicate the use of botulinum toxin for therapeutic purposes. Foodborne botulism, the most well-known form, is responsible about 20 to 25 cases per year in the United States. Improperly canned foods, particularly those containing fish, fruits, and vegetables, are often implicated. Because botulinum toxin is heat labile, foodborne botulism generally always occurs with consumption of uncooked food. Although botulism is often sporadic, outbreaks arising in restaurants or at public events are sometimes responsible for a cluster of cases. Once ingested, the toxin is absorbed quickly from the gastrointestinal tract and disseminates throughout the body. Clinical sequelae typically occur within 1 to 2 days (5).

Wound botulism was originally described as being caused by infections of surgical wounds (6). Until recently, it was considered rare, accounting for <5% of cases in the United States. A significant increase in the incidence of wound botulism has been seen in the past 20 years, however, occurring almost exclusively among injection drug users. A particularly strong association has been described with the use of black tar heroin, especially when it is injected subcutaneously ("skin-poppers") or intramuscularly, rather than into a vein. This mode of administration is often used by those who have difficulty with intravenous access (e.g., sclerosis of veins from repeated injection) or wish to avoid track marks. Anaerobic conditions promote the formation of soft tissue abscesses and allow the growth of *C. botulinum.* Exactly how black tar heroin becomes contaminated with *C. botulinum* has not been resolved, but it is thought to occur when the drug is mixed and diluted with other materials to provide more bulk (7,8).

Infant botulism was first described in 1976 (9,10), and is actually the most common form of the disease, with 80 to 100 cases occurring annually in the United States. Spores are ingested and germinate to produce the toxin *in situ* in the small intestine. The immature bowel of infants is thought to be particularly vulnerable to colonization by *C. botulinum.* The source of ingestion is usually never identified, although honey consumption has been identified as a risk factor (11).

Adult infectious botulism is extremely rare, and has a pathogenesis similar to that of infant botulism. Most patients have a functional or anatomic abnormality of their gastrointestinal tract, as well as recent antibiotic use. These factors combine to permit *C. botulinum* to compete with the usual bowel flora (12).

Two potential forms of botulism, hypothetically, could be utilized for bioterrorism. First, deliberate contamination of food products would potentially cause botulism among a cluster of individuals. A lingering concern is whether it is possible for the toxin to contaminate municipal water supplies. This is thought to be unlikely, in large part because of the vulnerability of the toxin to standard water treatments (1,13). To date, botulism caused by contaminated water has never been reported. Second, if the toxin were to be successfully aerosolized, a much larger population could be at risk. Only three human cases of inhalational botulism have been reported, occurring accidentally in West German laboratory workers who performed autopsies on animals that had been subjected to type A botulinum aerosol (14). It is not clear how stable botulinum toxin is when aerosolized, but its potential to cause disease after inhalation has been demonstrated in primates (15). Estimate is that the release of toxin in this fashion could affect 10% of people within a 500 m radius (1). The onset of symptoms with inhalational botulism appears to be slightly more gradual than with foodborne botulism.

During World War II, intelligence reports suggested that Germany had succeeded in weaponizing botulinum toxin. This led to the production of more than 1 million doses of vaccine for Allied troops preparing to invade (1). Several governments, including the United States, have subsequently performed research with botulinum toxin. Following the first Gulf War in 1991, it was discovered that the Iraqi military had loaded several thousand liters of concentrated botulinum toxin into military weapons (16). The Japanese cult Aum Shinrikyo, infamous for their use of the nerve agent sarin, attempted to use aerosolized botulinum toxin on several occasions between 1990 and 1995 (15).

Deliberate release of botulinum toxin would need to be differentiated from naturally occurring outbreaks of foodborne botulism. Most such outbreaks are small, with only a few individuals affected (1,5). The largest documented outbreak in the United States involved 59 cases (17). Thus, an unusually large number of individuals with symptoms should raise concerns about a possible terrorist act. Given that toxins A, B, and E account for almost all cases of foodborne botulism in the United States (5), the identification of an uncommon type (i.e., C, D, F, or G) would also be suspicious. Although toxins C, D, and G have never been found to cause disease in humans, they have been used in animal experiments to induce botulism, both via ingestion and inhalation (18–20). The presence of a particular toxin type in an unusual geographic area (e.g., type B botulism in the western United States) should also be investigated closely.

PATHOGENESIS

The various botulinum toxins consist of a heavy (100 kd) and light (50 kd) polypeptide chain held together by a disulfide bond. After uptake from the gastrointestinal tract or lungs, the toxin becomes widely disseminated and binds to presynaptic nerve terminals at neuromuscular junctions and in autonomic ganglia. Binding to the nerve terminal occurs via the heavy chain, and is followed by endocytosis of the toxin and subsequent cleavage of the disulfide bond. The liberated light chain, in turn, functions as a protease, which breaks down proteins that are required for fusion of acetylcholine-containing vesicles to the terminal membrane. The resulting failure of acetylcholine release into the synapse results in blockade of neuromuscular junctions and autonomic ganglia (21).

CLINICAL MANIFESTATIONS

Depending on the degree of exposure to the toxin, manifestations can range from relatively mild weakness to life-threatening respiratory failure. Symptoms usually develop within the first 2 days, but can occasionally be delayed for up to a week. Foodborne botulism is often preceded by gastrointestinal complaints, with prominent nausea, vomiting, and abdominal discomfort. It has been suggested that these symptoms might be caused by other bacterial products, rather than botulinum toxin itself. Thus, in the event of deliberate contamination of food products, the gastrointestinal symptoms might be absent (22).

Invariably, the initial neurologic signs and symptoms involve bilateral cranial nerve palsies, with common manifestations being diplopia, ptosis, dysarthria, and dysphagia. The presence of bulbar findings is so characteristic (e.g., dysphagia is present in 96% of cases) (4) that their absence should prompt a search for an alternative diagnosis. Cranial nerve palsies are followed by the development of a descending, flaccid. paralysis, which progresses to involve not only the upper and lower extremities, but also the respiratory musculature. Dyspnea has been identified as the best predictor identifying patients at high risk of death (23). Because of the frequent facial muscle weakness and ptosis, patients can look expressionless, giving them a deceptively calm appearance, even in the presence of markedly impaired respiratory function (2).

Worsening inspiratory muscle strength leads to progressive atelectasis and hypoxemia. The prominent bulbar involvement combined with a weak cough can result in failure to effectively clear laryngeal and pharyngeal secretions. Closure of the weakened glottis during inspiration can further contribute to upper airway obstruction. Because of the potential for airway compromise, respiratory failure sometimes occurs sooner than might otherwise be predicted based on vital capacity and maximal inspiratory pressure measurements. Return of strength requires the formation of new neuromuscular junctions, such that recovery can be very slow (24,25). If respiratory failure develops, mechanical ventilation is usually required for several weeks (26).

Autonomic manifestations are more common with toxins B and E, most often including dilatation of pupils, dry mouth, postural hypotension, urinary retention, and constipation. In one study, decreased heart rate variation and reduced plasma norepinephrine levels were described (27). Impaired reflexes gradually develop, but sensory findings are absent. Because the toxin does not cross the blood–brain barrier, no central nervous system (CNS) manifestations should occur.

DIAGNOSIS

Although the manifestations are remarkably consistent, diagnosis is often delayed, probably because botulism is a rare condition with which most clinicians have had little clinical experience (28,29). A high index of suspicion and early diagnosis are essential for a number of reasons: First, the efficacy of the antitoxin is time-dependent, and prompt administration may limit the severity of the condition. Second, botulism can be fulminant, with the patient's condition deteriorating to the point of necessitating mechanical ventilation within hours. Third, other individuals may have been exposed and, therefore, require urgent medical attention. Fourth, whether it is naturally occurring, foodborne botulism or deliberate release of botulinum toxin, timely recognition may help prevent others from becoming exposed. Thus, when the possibility of botulism is considered, the state health department must be notified as soon as possible (links can be found at www.astho.org).

The differential diagnosis of botulism includes any disorder that causes an acute onset of generalized weakness. Because of the prominent bulbar manifestations, the most common conditions for which botulism is initially mistaken are myasthenia gravis and the Miller-Fisher variant of Guillain-Barré syndrome (GBS) (28). Unlike botulism, however, neither myasthenia gravis nor Lambert-Eaton myasthenic syndrome commonly present with onset over hours, and myasthenia gravis has no autonomic involvement. A significant improvement in the neurologic examination with edrophonium suggests myasthenia gravis, but false–positive results in the setting of botulism have repeatedly been reported (30,31). GBS is normally easily distinguished from botulism, in that there is sensory involvement, ascending rather than descending paralysis, and early areflexia. The Miller-Fisher variant, however, is responsible for a small proportion of cases and creates confusion because of the early bulbar findings. One useful feature of Miller-Fisher syndrome, which may be useful in distinguishing it from botulism, is ataxia. Tick paralysis can present in a similar fashion to botulism, although the weakness is more often ascending than descending. Careful examination often still reveals the tick to be attached, most commonly to the scalp or neck. Poliomyelitis usually presents with fever and asymmetric weakness.

Currently, no rapid confirmatory test exists to verify the diagnosis of botulism. Consequently, obtaining a careful history regarding possible sources of exposure, including the consumption of high-risk foods or a history of injection drug use, is important. Ancillary diagnostic tests are helpful, especially at ruling out other disorders in the differential diagnosis. Cerebral imaging should be performed if brainstem ischemia is considered a possibility. The absence of cells or protein on lumbar puncture argues against a diagnosis of GBS. If the clinical suspicion for botulism remains high after these investigations, consideration should be given to initiating treatment before obtaining a definitive diagnosis.

Electrophysiologic studies can be useful in localizing the source of weakness to the presynaptic aspect of the neuromuscular junction and in supporting the diagnosis of botulism. Sensory nerve conduction study findings are normal. Motor nerve conduction velocities are also normal, but the amplitude of compound muscle action potentials is reduced in clinically affected muscles. After exercise and posttetanic facilitation with high frequency (20 to 50 Hz), repetitive motor nerve stimulation occurs in both botulism and Lambert-Eaton syndrome, although the facilitation may be less prominent and more sustained in botulism (32,33). Needle electromyography (EMG) may reveal low-amplitude, short-duration motor unit potentials with an unstable firing pattern, although this is a nonspecific finding. Positive sharp waves and fibrillation potentials are present in about half of the cases (34). Single-fiber EMG is the most sensitive electrodiagnostic test for neuromuscular junctional disorders, although it cannot reliably distinguish between presynaptic junctional disorders.

Depending on the suspected route of exposure, cultures of stool, gastric fluids, wounds, and sputum should be sent in anaerobic culture media. Similarly, serum, stool, and any potentially contaminated food should be sent to an appropriate laboratory (as directed by the local or state health department) to assess for the presence of botulinum toxin. The classic test for the toxin is a mouse bioassay, in which the biologic fluid is inoculated into the peritoneum of either mice pretreated with antitoxin or control animals. This bioassay is also used to determine the specific type of toxin. It is essential that serum be drawn from the patient before administration of the antitoxin, otherwise the mouse bioassay finding may be falsely negative. False–positive results in mouse bioassays have been reported in the setting of GBS (35). The sensitivity and specificity of diagnostic testing for botulism decreases with delays in sending samples and is increased by concomitantly searching for both the toxin and the organism (2,36). Because the results of the mouse bioassay are generally not available for at least 24 to 48 hours, initiation of treatment should not be delayed while waiting for results. A more rapid enzyme-linked immunosorbent assay (ELISA) for botulinum toxin is currently being developed, but is not yet widely available (37). The American Society for Microbiology has published *Sentinel Laboratory Guidelines* with detailed descriptions of how specimens should be collected (38).

TREATMENT

The mortality related to botulism has decreased dramatically in the past 50 years with the development of intensive care units and the provision of mechanical ventilation. The current case fatality is approximately 5% to 10% (23). Supportive care for botulism is similar to that of other conditions causing neuromuscular respiratory failure. Serial testing of vital capacity can help determine the optimal timing for endotracheal intubation, the goal being to do so under controlled circumstances rather than emergently in the setting of respiratory arrest. Hypercapnia is a late feature of neuromuscular respiratory failure, and it is generally important to not wait for it to develop before intervening. Intubation must be considered with vital capacities decreasing below 15 mL/kg. Given that recovery from botulism takes several weeks, these patients are ideal candidates for early tracheostomy and percutaneous gastrostomy for improved comfort. In one case series, early tracheostomy appeared to reduce the overall duration of mechanical ventilation (26). The predictably long hospital course mandates meticulous intensive care unit treatment, with particular attention to the prevention of nosocomial complications (e.g., ventilator-associated pneumonia, deep venous thrombosis, and decubitus ulcers). No role exists for antibiotics in either foodborne or inhalational botulism. Gastric lavage or activated charcoal may help remove recently ingested contaminated food from the gastrointestinal tract.

Either a trivalent (for types A, B, and E) or bivalent (for types A and B) antitoxin can be obtained from the CDC via state health departments (1,39). The benefit of antitoxin has been demonstrated in retrospective and observational studies (26,40,41). Because the antitoxin neutralizes only unbound toxin, administration as early as possible is required to maximize its benefit. Largely because it is obtained from equine serum, the main risk of the antitoxin is an allergic reaction. The chance of serum sickness or even anaphylaxis has been found to be approximately 9% (42), although numerous patients in this study received repeated doses, a practice that is no longer advocated. Skin testing is recommended before administration of the antitoxin. If a significant wheal and flare reaction occurs, desensitization can be attempted, beginning with 0.01 to 0.1 mL and doubling the previous dose every 20 minutes, until 1.0 to 2.0 mL is given without significant effect (39). Because circulating antitoxins have a half-life of 5 to 8 days, only a single dose is necessary, with a 10 mL vial administered intravenously (1). Treatment with the antitoxin is thought to be safe in children and during pregnancy (43,44). A deliberate terrorist attack would not necessarily involve serotypes A, B, or E, such that the trivalent antitoxin may not be effective. For such a circumstance, the US Army also has an investigational heptavalent (A, B, C, D, E, F, and G) antitoxin available, which was used during an outbreak of foodborne botulism in Egypt in 1991 (39,45).

The equine antitoxin available for adults has generally not been used in infants. Botulism immune globulin intravenous (BIG-IV) is a bivalent human-derived product that has recently become available for the treatment of infant botulism, and is effective against toxins A and B. In a randomized, controlled trial, treatment with BIG-IV within 72 hours of admission markedly reduced the duration of hospitalization, need for mechanical ventilation, and nosocomial complications (46). At present, BIG-IV is only available through the California Department of Health Services. It has not been approved for use in adults, but may be an alternative, particularly in patients who have a pronounced allergic reaction to skin testing with the equine antitoxin. A recombinant version of botulism immune globulin is currently under development (47).

CLINICAL RECOMMENDATIONS OF THE VIGNETTE

Regardless of arterial blood gas results, this patient requires admission to an intensive care unit, and strong consideration of endotracheal intubation. If possible, electrophysiologic studies should be performed as soon as possible. Along with the clinical findings, electrodiagnostic testing should help to distinguish botulism from subacute peripheral neuropathic disorders, such as the Miller-Fisher variant of GBS, and from postsynaptic junctional disorders, such as myasthenia gravis. The state health department must be notified, especially because other individuals may have been, or still become, exposed if the diagnosis is confirmed to be botulism. If other cases are identified, the possibility of deliberate release of botulinum toxin should be investigated and excluded. Gastric contents, stool, and serum need to be sent for toxin bioassay. In addition, stool should be cultured under anaerobic conditions. Sufficient clinical suspicion exists to justify the empiric use of the antitoxin in this case.

SUMMARY

Botulism is the paralytic disorder resulting from intoxication with neurotoxins released by *C. botulinum.* Forms of human botulism include foodborne, wound, infant, adult infectious, inhalational, and iatrogenic disease. Deliberate toxin releases for bioterrorism should be suspected when (*a*) a large number of cases occur in a botulism outbreak, (*b*) botulism occurs in a geographic region where disease related to that serotype is atypical, or (*c*) human botulism occurs with toxin serotypes that do not normally cause human disease. Clinical features of botulism are owing to the effects of toxin at the neuromuscular junction and autonomic ganglia and include bulbar paralysis, ophthalmoplegia, respiratory failure, and orthostatic hypotension. A clinical diagnosis may be supported by electrodiagnostic testing, including repetitive nerve stimulation studies and single-fiber EMG. Although immunologic diagnostic methods are being developed, the mouse bioassay remains confirmatory and defines the toxin serotype. Given that neuromuscular respiratory failure is common in botulism, close monitoring and support of breathing are important. Several antisera are available for treatment, and these should be administered as early as possible to reduce the amount of unbound toxin and the extent of paralysis. All cases of suspected botulism should be reported to the hospital epidemiologist or infection control officer and to local or state health departments or the CDC.

REFERENCES

1. Arnon SS, Schechter R, Inglesby TV, et al. Botulinum toxin as a biological weapon. *JAMA.* 2001;285:1059–1070.
2. Sobel J. Botulism. *Clin Infect Dis.* 2005;41:1167–1173.
3. Woodruff BA, Grifin PM, McCroskey LM, et al. Clinical and laboratory comparison of botulism from toxin types A, B, and E in the United States, 1975–1988. *J Infect Dis.* 1992;166: 1281–1286.
4. Shapiro RL, Hatheway C, Swerdlow DL. Botulism in the United States: A Clinical and Epidemiologic Review. *Ann Intern Med.* 1998;129:221–228.
5. Sobel J, Tucker, N, Sulka A, et al. Foodborne botulism in the United States, 1990–2000. *Emerg Infect Dis.* 2004;10:1606–1611.
6. Merson MH, Dowel VR, Jr. Epidemiologic, clinical and laboratory aspects of wound botulism. *N Engl J Med.* 1973;289:1005–1010.
7. Passaro DJ, Werner SB, McGee J, et al. Wound botulism associated with black tar heroin among injecting drug users. *JAMA.* 1998;279:859–863.
8. Werner SB, Passaro D, McGee J, et al. Wound botulism in California, 1951–1998: Recent epidemic in heroin injectors. *Clin Infect Dis.* 2000;31:1018–1024.
9. Pickett J, Berg B, Chaplin E, et al. Syndrome of botulism in infancy: Clinical and electrophysiologic study. *N Engl J Med.* 1976;295:770–772.
10. Midura TF, Arnon SS. Infant botulism. Identification of Clostridium botulinum and its toxins in faeces. *Lancet.* 1976;2(7992):934–936.
11. Spika JS, Shaffer N, Hargrett-Bean N, et al. Risk factors for infant botulism in the United States. *Am J Dis Child.* 1989;143:828–832.
12. McCroskey LM, Hatheway CL. Laboratory findings in four cases of adult botulism suggest colonization of the intestinal tract. *J Clin Microbiol.* 1998;26(5)1052–1054.
13. Siegel LS. Destruction of botulinum toxin in food and water. In: Hauschild AH, Dodds KL, eds. *Clostridium Botulinum: Ecology and Control in Foods.* New York, NY: Marcel Dekker; 1993: 323–341.
14. Holzer VE. Botulismus durch inhalation. *Med Klin.* 1962;57:1735–1738.
15. WuDunn S, Miller J, Broad WJ. How Japan germ terror alerted world. *New York Times.* May 26, 1998;A1,A10.
16. Zilinskas RA. Iraq's biological weapons: The past as future? *JAMA.* 1997;278:418–424.
17. Terranova W, Breman JG, Locey RP, et al. Botulism type B: Epidemiological aspects of an extensive outbreak. *Am J Epidemiol.* 1978;109:150–156.
18. Franz DR, Pitt LM, Clayton MA, et al. Efficacy of prophylactic and therapeutic administration of antitoxin for inhalation botulism. In: Das Gupta BR, ed. *Botulinum and Tetanus Neurotoxins: Neurotransmission and Biomedical Aspects.* New York: Plenum; 1993:473–476.
19. Gunnison JB, Meyer KF. Susceptibility of monkeys, goats and small animals to oral administration of botulinum toxin types B, C and D. *J Infect Dis.* 1930;46:335–340.
20. Middlebrook JL, Franz DR. Botulinum toxins. In: Sidell FR, Takafujl ET, Franz DR, eds. *Medical Aspects of Chemical and Biological Warfare.* Washington, DC: Office of the Surgeon General; 1997:643–654.
21. Simpson LL. Identification of the major steps in botulinum toxin action. *Annu Rev Pharmacol Toxicol.* 2004;44:167–193.
22. Bleck TP. Botulinum toxin as a biological weapon. In: Mandell, Bennett, Dolin, eds. *Principles and Practice of Infectious Diseases,* 6th ed. Philadelphia: Elsevier Churchill Livingstone; 2005.
23. Varma JK, Katsitadze G, Moiscrafishvili M, et al. Signs and symptoms predictive of death in patients with foodborne botulism—Republic of Georgia 1980–2002. *Clin Infect Dis.* 2004;39:357–362.
24. Duchen LW. Motor nerve growth induced by botulinum toxin as a regenerative phenomenon. *Proceedings of the Royal Society of Medicine.* 1972;65:196–197.
25. De Pavia A, Meunier FA, Molgo J, et al. Functional repair of motor endplates after botulinum neurotoxin type A poisoning: Biphasic switch of synaptic activity between nerve sprouts and their parent terminals. *Proc Natl Acad Sci U S A.* 1999;96:3200–3205.
26. Sandrock CE, Murin S. Clinical predictors of respiratory failure and long-term outcome in black tar heroin-associated wound botulism. *Chest.* 2001;120:562–566.
27. Chen JT, Chen CC, Lin KP, et al. Botulism: Heart rate variation, sympathetic skin responses, and plasma norepinephrine. *Can J Neurol Sci.* 1999;26(2):123–126.
28. St. Louis ME, Peck SH, Bowering D, et al. Botulism from chopped garlic: Delayed recognition of a major outbreak. *Ann Intern Med.* 1988;108:363–368.
29. Cosgrove SE, Perl TM, Song X, et al. Ability of physicians to diagnose and manage illness due to category A bioterrorism agents. *Arch Intern Med.* 2005;165:2002–2006.
30. Angulo FJ, Getz J, Taylor JP, et al. A large outbreak of botulism: The hazardous baked potato. *J Infect Dis.* 1998;178:172–177.
31. Edell TA, Sullivan CP, Osborn KM, et al. Wound botulism associated with a positive tensilon test. *West J Med.* 1983;139:218–219.
32. Cherington M. Botulism: Update and review. *Semin Neurol.* 2004;24:155–163.
33. Fakadej AV, Gutmann L. Prolonged post-tetanic facilitation in infant botulism. *Muscle Nerve.* 1982;5:727–729.
34. Cornblath DR, Sladky JT, Sumner AJ. Clinical electrophysiology of infantile botulism. *Muscle Nerve.* 1983;6:448–452.
35. Notermans SHW, Wokke JHJ, van den Berg LH. Botulism and Guillain-Barre syndrome. *Lancet.* 1992;340:303.
36. Woodruff BA, Griffin PM, McCroskey LM, et al. Clinical and laboratory comparison of botulism from toxin type A, B, and E in the United States, 1975–1988. *J Infect Dis.* 1992;166: 1281–1286.
37. Caya JG, Agni R, Miller JE. Clostridium botulinum and the clinical laboratorian: A detailed review of botulism, including biological warfare ramifications of botulinum toxin. *Arch Pathol Lab Med.* 2004;128:653–662.
38. www.asm.org/ASM/files/LEFTMARGINHEADERLIST/downloadfilename/0000000522/BotulismFinalVersion73003.pdf
39. U.S. Army Medical Research Institute of Infectious Diseases: Botulinum. In: *USAMRIID'S Medical Management of Biological Casualties Handbook,* 5th ed. Fort Detrick, MD: USA RIID; 2004:81–87.
40. Tacket CO, Shandera WX, Mann JM, et al. Equine antitoxin use and other factors that predict outcome in type A foodborne botulism. *Am J Med.* 1984;76:794–798.
41. Chang GY, Ganguly G. Early antitoxin treatment in wound botulism results in better outcome. *Eur J Neurol.* 2003;49:151–153.
42. Black RE, Gunn RA. Hypersensitivity reactions associated with botulinal antitoxin. *Am J Med.* 1980;69:567–570.
43. Keller MA, Miller VH, Berkowitz CD, et al. Wound botulism in pediatrics. *Am J Dis Child.* 1982;136:320–322.
44. Robin L, Herman D, Redett R. Botulism in a pregnant woman. *N Engl J Med.* 1996;335: 823–824.
45. Hibbs RG, Weber JT, Corwin A, et al. Experience with the use of an investigational $F(ab)_2$ heptavalent botulism immune globulin of equine origin during an outbreak of type E botulism in Egypt. *Clin Infect Dis.* 1996;23:337–340.
46. Arnon SS, Schechter R, Maslanka SE, et al. Human botulism immune globulin for the treatment of infant botulism. *N Engl J Med.* 2006;354:445–447.
47. Nowakowski A, Wang C, Powers DB, et al. Potent neutralization of botulinum neurotoxin by recombinant oligoclonal antibody. *Proc Natl Acad Sci U S A.* 2002;99:11346–11350.

CHAPTER **163**

Cyanide

Mark A. Kirk • Jeffery J. Fletcher

OBJECTIVE

- To identify the common sources of cyanide exposure
- To describe the signs and symptoms associated with cyanide toxicity
- To discuss the diagnostic studies useful to diagnose cyanide poisoning
- To describe the immediate therapeutic actions used to treat acute cyanide poisoning
- To explain the neurologic sequelae of cyanide poisoning

CASE VIGNETTE

A 60-year-old federal judge is witnessed to collapse while at his desk working in the local courthouse. He was recently involved in a high profile, organized crime case where the defendant threatened to "get even with you if I am found guilty." His office assistant witnessed him drink a glass of cola while eating his lunch at his desk. He immediately began to complain of nausea and headache. He then became agitated and collapsed unconscious. When emergency medical services (EMS) arrived, he was unresponsive to painful stimuli; his heart rate (HR) was 44 beats per minute, and systolic blood pressure (BP) was 64 mm Hg. The patient had two generalized tonic–clonic seizures while in the ambulance on transport to the emergency department. He is subsequently intubated, without pharmacologic agents, for apnea and failure to protect his airway. Neurologic examination shows the patient to be comatose, with dilated, sluggishly reactive pupils; partially intact brainstem reflexes; and flaccid tone, with absent muscle stretch reflexes. While looking for retinal hemorrhages on the funduscopic examination, exceptionally red blood vessels with spontaneous venous pulsations are noted. The suggestion of an apocalyptic intracranial event leads to computed tomographic (CT) scan of the brain, which is normal. Other diagnostic tests of note were a pH of 7.01, $P\text{CO}_2$ of 21 and $P\text{O}_2$ of 575 on an arterial blood gas. The electrolytes were normal, except for a serum bicarbonate of 6 mEq/L and an anion gap of 34. A lactic acid level was reported to be 10 mmol/L. The patient's office assistant thought he had a heart attack and began rescue breathing that she learned in a cardiopulmonary resuscitation (CPR) class. She now complains of cephalgia, nausea, and anxiousness.

DEFINITION

Cyanide (C-N) is a highly toxic and rapidly acting chemical. The most clinically significant forms are salts (e.g., potassium cyanide [KCN] and sodium cyanide [NaCN]) and gases (e.g., hydrogen cyanide). Cyanide is also a naturally occurring substance in plants. Its highly toxic effects are the result of inhibiting cellular respiration causing cellular asphyxiation. Cyanide has a well-known reputation as a highly toxic chemical and specific antidotes are available to treat suspected poisonings.

EPIDEMIOLOGY

Acute cyanide poisoning most often occurs from workplace accidents, smoke inhalation, suicide attempts, or malicious acts. The American Association of Poison Control Centers Toxic Exposure Surveillance System (TESS) reported 257 exposures and 8 deaths in 2004 (1). The diagnosis of cyanide poisoning is challenging, however, and it is thought that many cases of cyanide toxicity may be misdiagnosed as other causes of acute death, such as pulmonary embolus, myocardial infarction, or arrhythmia.

Cyanide has many industrial uses. The National Occupational Exposure Survey indicates that >250,000 workers are potentially exposed to cyanide compounds. The National Institute for Occupational Safety and Health (NIOSH) lists the following populations at high risk for cyanide exposure: workers involved in electroplating, metallurgy, pesticide application, steel manufacturing, gas works applications, metal cleaning, manufacturing of electronic computing equipment, research and development laboratories, newspaper and commercial printing, manufacturing of industrial inorganic chemicals, production of adhesives and sealants, the construction of furniture, direct application of herbicidal formulations, handling treatment or disposal of thiocyanate-containing wastes from industrial processes, hazardous waste sites, cyanide-containing road salts, industrial waste waters from coal processing, extraction of gold and silver, and hospital employees (2).

Cyanide is a significant product of combustion from burning polyurethane, synthetic polymers, nitrocellulose, wool, and silk in home and building fires. Therefore, victims of smoke inhalation and firefighters are at risk of cyanide poisoning.

Because of its use in judicial executions and spy movies, cyanide is well known to the general public as a highly toxic chemical. Cyanide is used in suicide attempts, especially by chemist and laboratory technicians where reagents containing cyanide salts are readily available. It is easily accessible (even via the internet) and frequently used for intentional poisonings, such as tainting over-the-counter medications and food, or in mass suicides (e.g., Jonestown). Hydrogen cyanide is included among the class of agents known be used as chemical warfare. According to the World Health Organization (WHO), hydrogen cyanide was reportedly used against the Kurds in the Iran-Iraq war in the 1980s. Zyklon B (hydrogen cyanide) was used in the Nazi gas chambers during the World War II. Cyanide has been developed as a battlefield chemical weapon. Because of the high volatility of cyanide gas (HCN), it is difficult to obtain high concentrations outdoors, making it a less than optimal agent for mass inhalational exposure on the battlefield. Its intentional release into small confined spaces or building ventilation systems, however, remains a concern.

Additional sources of cyanide poisoning include ingestions of foods containing cyanogenic glycosides, such as apricot pits, lima beans, certain cereal grains, and cassava. According to the World Health Organization (3), in 2004, some populations in Africa have had outbreaks of acute cyanide poisoning from improper processing of cassava and populations in developing countries that consume large amounts of cassava have acquired tropical ataxic neuropathy, a demyelinating disease from chronic cyanide poisoning. Nitroprusside is an iatrogenic cause of parenteral cyanide toxicity when used as an intravenous infusion to control blood pressure.

ETIOLOGY AND PATHOGENESIS

Cyanide toxicity most commonly occurs from inhalation of cyanide gas or ingestion of cyanide salts. It can also cause toxicity through dermal absorption and parenteral exposure (4,5). Small exposures can lead to symptoms and, with acute toxicity, symptoms typically evolve over minutes to hours. Oral ingestion of 200 mg and airborne exposure of 270 ppm (μg/mL) of cyanide are rapidly lethal (within minutes).

Cyanide acts as a cellular asphyxiant, in large part by inhibiting mitochondrial cytochrome oxidase, which leads to the inability to utilize oxygen (6,7). Hyperlactemia ensues from failure of aerobic metabolism. In addition to its inhibitory action on cytochrome oxidase, cyanide toxicity also involves inhibition of various other enzymes, causes oxidative stress, and augments excitotoxic mechanisms in the central nervous system (CNS). The inability to utilize oxygen can lead to elevated venous oxygen saturation >90%. Cyanide is also thought to inhibit succinic acid dehydrogenase, superoxide dismutase, and carbonic anhydrase. Neurologic injury is mediated through many of the same mechanisms mentioned above, including failure of aerobic metabolism and increased oxidative stress.

Additionally, cyanide appears to enhance N-methyl-d-aspartate (NMDA) receptor activity, increasing cytosolic calcium concentration, which leads to increased reactive oxygen species and formation of nitrous oxide. Mitochondrial dysfunction is exacerbated and pathways leading to cellular apoptosis are activated.

PATHOLOGY

Because cellular asphyxiation is thought to be the major pathophysiologic mechanism involved in the toxicity of cyanide, the heart and CNS are most affected, especially those regions most sensitivity to hypoxic-ischemic insults. Imaging studies indicate the basal ganglia, cerebellum, and sensorimotor cortex are affected most severely in cyanide poisoning (8,9). These are known to be highly oxygen-sensitive regions of the brain. Pathologicl studies have also confirmed extensive destruction in the basal ganglia (10). Interestingly, the hippocampus, which is potentially the most oxygen-sensitive structure in the CNS, seems to be spared with acute cyanide poisoning but may be involved in delayed or chronic complications (11). Rat studies have suggested that different neuronal populations undergo different destructive mechanisms, with necrosis predominating in the subcortical structures and apoptosis in the cortex (12). Although certain regions of the brain seem to be more susceptible to the effects of cyanide, the syndrome of severe acute cyanide toxicity may affect all regions of the brain and cause death by neurologic criteria. Cyanide toxicity occurs in virtually all organs systems. Subendocardial, subepicardial hemorrhage, and petechial hemorrhage in the intestine have been described (13). Bronchial inflammation and evidence of cardiogenic and acute lung injury are seen at autopsy.

CLINICAL MANIFESTATIONS

GENERAL

The amount of cyanide (dose), route of exposure, and preexisting conditions determine the onset and severity of the toxic effects. Those most susceptible to toxicity include children, the elderly, and patients with underlying coronary artery disease, pulmonary disease, seizure disorders, and other chronic diseases. The fetus of a pregnant women and children are thought to be at higher risk for more severe symptoms when exposed to cyanide. Patients with motor neuron disease may also be at higher risk, possibly because of a preexisting excitotoxic mechanism thought to play a role in their disease process.

Significant exposure causes abrupt onset of profound toxic effects (*knock-down*) that can include syncope, seizures, coma, gasping respirations, and cardiovascular collapse, potentially causing death within minutes. Milder symptoms from low concentrations cause multiple symptoms without knock-down (e.g., nausea, dyspnea, palpitations, chest tightness, headache, dizziness, syncope, anxiousness). Inhalation exposure causes a rapid onset of symptoms potentially leading to death in minutes. In lower doses that only cause mild symptoms, however, effects can peak within minutes and resolve once the individual is removed from exposure. Effects of ingestion can be rapid (within minutes), but because of slower absorption into the systemic circulation, onset can be delayed. Dermal absorption can be delayed (hours).

NEUROLOGIC

With acute inhalation of cyanide, neurologic symptoms typically develop rapidly over seconds to minutes, but can be delayed for several minutes to hours if ingested. Initially, symptoms of anxiety and a hyperadrenergic state may predominant. Cephalgia and hyperactive encephalopathy can subsequently progress to more impaired levels of consciousness with progression to coma. Bradycardia and hypotension consistent with neurogenic shock develop in advanced cases, although the etiologic factors involved in cardiovascular collapse are related to the dysfunction of multiple organ systems. With acute, severe intoxication, these symptoms can progress so rapidly that hypoactive encephalopathy with stupor, then coma, may be the initial manifestation. Apnea is not uncommon. Seizures of various ictal semiology and status epilepticus have also been reported during cyanide intoxication and they can aggravate systemic hemodynamic instability. On funduscopic examination, the arteries and veins may appear exceptionally red because of high oxygen concentrations. Because of the lethal outcomes in cyanide poisoning, most literature focuses on acute exposure. Delayed neurologic sequelae in survivors correlates with areas of damage seen on neuroimaging studies. Akinetic-rigid syndromes and dystonia tend to develop within weeks to months after the acute poisoning. Radiographic changes may not appear for several weeks after the onset of symptoms. These symptoms may regress with time, but it is not uncommon for them to be persistent.

Some populations can have chronic cyanide exposure from cyanide-containing food or prolonged occupational exposure, which is known to deplete dopamine. Tobacco smoking can also cause more chronic cyanide exposure. The levels of cyanide may be sufficient in these cases to cause more indolent symptoms, such as tobacco amblyopia, parkinsonism, ataxia, and optic neuropathy.

SYSTEMIC

Cardiovascular collapse is a major feature of acute cyanide toxicity. Neurogenic, cardiogenic, and primary vasomotor tone abnormalities all contribute. The terminal effect is bradycardia and hypotension, although tachycardia and hypertension can be early and transient manifestations. Other findings include abdominal pain, nausea and vomiting, dyspnea, acute lung injury, and pulmonary edema (cardiogenic and, likely, neurogenic). Cyanide toxicity should be suspected in all patients who are acyanotic, but otherwise appear hypoxic. Observations, such as skin color and odor are often noted in the literature, but these observations should be considered unreliable. The characteristic "bitter almonds" odor of cyanide is not helpful, because many people cannot smell cyanide and various other descriptive terms have been used for its odor (e.g., dirty socks or bleach-like).

DIAGNOSTIC APPROACH

Because of the high morbidity and mortality of cyanide poisoning, it is important not to wait for the results of laboratory, imaging, and other diagnostic studies to initiate empiric therapy. Cyanide is rapidly fatal and no laboratory analyses or diagnostic imaging studies are readily available to confirm cyanide poisoning sufficiently quickly to guide management decisions. Diagnostic testing is best used to confirm poisoning. The history is a valuable part of the diagnostic algorithm. High risk occupations, suicide attempts in chemists, suspicious circumstances, and the abrupt onset of profound toxic effects (knockdown) (e.g., syncope, seizures, coma, gasping respirations, and cardiovascular collapse) should lead to serious consideration of the diagnosis of cyanide poisoning. Elevated anion gap metabolic acidosis, hyperlactemia, small arterial-venous oxygen saturation difference, and elevated venous oxygen saturation are all commonly seen, however these are not specific to cyanide toxicity. Conditions such as sepsis or other toxic exposures can be associated with similar laboratory findings. ECG abnormalities may be seen, but they are nonspecific. Blood cyanide levels can confirm toxicity, but these results will not likely be available for days. Baud et al. (14) demonstrated in a small group of patients with strong clinical suspicion of cyanide toxicity, that a plasma lactic acid concentration level >8 mmol/L was strongly correlated with a blood cyanide concentration >1 mg/L. Therefore, suspicion of cyanide poisoning should be high when lactic acid levels are >8 mmol/L (or 10 mmol/L, if history of smoke inhalation). Plasma thiocyanate levels are of little value in assessing acute poisoning because they do not correlate with symptoms.

TREATMENT

Cyanide is extremely toxic and can be rapidly fatal within minutes of acute exposure to high concentrations. First responders and clinicians must act quickly to initiate therapy, because delays of more than 5 to 10 minutes can be associated with failure of therapy and high morbidity and mortality. A high index of suspicion is needed in many cases and therapy should not be delayed pending results of diagnostic work when acute, severe poisoning is suspected. Consultation with a toxicologist is essential, if available.

If the patient has skin or clothing contamination, a decontamination procedure (clothing removal and soap and water shower) should take place in the emergency department before transfer to the intensive care unit. Protective gloves, eyewear, and water-insoluble gowns should be used until the patient is adequately decontaminated. People with only a skin exposure to gas or vapor pose little risk of contaminating others; however, clothing can carry gas or vapor. After decontamination, standard precautions are adequate. Patients ingesting cyanide-containing substances can potentially off-gas hydrogen cyanide gas. Precautions should be taken to ensure the stomach is emptied of any liquid and that the patient's vomitus is handled carefully.

Acute cyanide poisoning needs to be recognized as a medical emergency with potential for rapid deterioration. Supportive care alone (100% oxygen and observation) without administration of the cyanide antidote kit may be sufficient for patients who are asymptomatic or only have minimal suggestive symptoms. The airway breathing circulation (ABC) survey should be performed first in any unstable patient. Endotracheal intubation for control of ventilation in the face of acidosis and to reduce oxygen debt may be indicated. Evidence suggests that administering 100% oxygen may be beneficial, despite cyanide's impairment of oxygen utilization and high arterial oxygen saturation. Adequate intravenous venous access should be established. In severe poisoning, consider central venous line placement for measurement of central venous pressure or potential right-sided heart catheterization and arterial line placement for continuous monitoring of the patient's cardiovascular parameters and to follow acid-base status.

For a symptomatic patient with witnessed ingestion or when a high suspicion exists of cyanide exposure, the cyanide antidote kit should be administered. The cyanide antidote kit contains both sodium thiosulfate and nitrites. Although both detoxify cyanide individually, they are synergistic in treating cyanide poisoning.

Amyl nitrite and sodium nitrite, available in the cyanide antidote kit in the United States, induces methemoglobin. This methemoglobin binds to cyanide to form cyanomethemoglobin. Amyl nitrite ampules are contained in the kit and can be used (inhaled or introduced into the ventilator system) when obtaining intravenous access is delayed. Sodium thiosulfate is a substrate for the body's detoxifying enzyme, rhodanese. It converts highly toxic cyanide to thiocyanate, which is renally eliminated.

Recommendations for administering the cyanide antidote kit

- If intravenous (IV) treatment is **not** available: Amyl nitrite pearls, crush and place in bag-valve mask
- If IV treatment **is** available:
  - o Sodium nitrite, 300 mg IV over 5 minutes (Complications: Hypotension, methemoglobinemia), **and**
  - o Sodium thiosulfate, 12.5 g IV (Complications: NONE)
  - o Doses of s sodium nitrite and sodium thiosulfate can be repeated in 30 minutes.

Intravenous infusion of sodium nitrite can cause hypotension and excessive methemoglobinemia (especially if patient is anemic). Methemoglobinemia decreases oxygen-carrying capacity, therefore, it can be harmful to patients with smoke inhalation who have elevated carboxyhemoglobin levels. Patients with smoke inhalation suspected of having coexisting cyanide toxicity (especially if lactic acid level >10 mmol/L), should receive only the thiosulfate infusion and not nitrites. The Centers for Disease Control and Prevention (CDC) recommends empirically administering sodium thiosulfate alone for mass casualty events suspected to be from cyanide poisoning. Hydroxcobalamin is a promising antidote used in other countries that will likely be approved in the United States in the near future.

The optimal arterial pH at which to institute bicarbonate in metabolic acidosis caused by elevated lactic acid remains controversial. Bicarbonate can exacerbate intracellular acidosis despite raising arterial pH and does not necessarily augment the effects of vasopressor and inotropes more than fluids.

Hyperbaric oxygen therapy has been used for cyanide poisoning, although no convincing data exist for its clinical benefits. Therefore, hyperbaric oxygen should never be used in place of normobaric oxygen and cyanide antidotes.

Acute cyanide poising can merit a neurologic consultation when a patient presents with seizures, unexplained encephalopathy or coma, or acute brain injury, or when death by neurologic criteria is suspected. An electroencephalogram (EEG) is required when patients have had events suspicious for seizures and do not awaken to their baseline neurologic status. For status epilepticus, benzodiazepines remain the mainstay of therapy. Addition of a maintenance antiepileptic medication for at least 7 days is reasonable. For refractory status epilepticus, continuous EEG monitoring is required. High-dose benzodiazepines to achieve seizure freedom are preferred to propofol infusion. Propofol infusion syndrome can cause similar features to cyanide toxicity, including mitochondrial dysfunction. Parkinsonism seen in survivors, especially as a delayed syndrome, is usually resistant to dopaminergic medications because of the destruction of the target nuclei. Importantly, patients who die from cyanide toxicity or have devastating neurologic injury should be considered candidates for organ donation after death by neurologic criteria or after cardiac death.

CLINICAL RECOMMENDATIONS OF THE VIGNETTE

Sudden onset coma and hemodynamic instability suggest a severe, acute intracranial (subarachnoid hemorrhage) or cardiovascular event with anoxic brain injury. Postictal states can also appear similar. A toxic exposure should be considered when the possibility exists of more than one victim involved or other features of the history are suggestive. This reinforces the importance of a detailed history and formulation of a broad differential diagnosis while evaluating for common disorders. The history and examination of the patient suggest possible toxic exposure, specifically the sudden onset of severe illness, an additional victim, red appearing blood vessels on funduscopic examination, and negative head CT finding. Cyanide exposure via ventilation systems in government building is a concerning potential terrorist act.

In addition to hemodynamic support, the patient should be treated with 100% oxygen and have the cyanide antidote kit administered without waiting for confirmatory diagnostic tests. The patient needs an EEG to evaluate for ongoing seizure activity. Additional recommendations about diagnosis, acute treatment, and intensive care are available by consulting a medical toxicologist via the regional poison center or medical toxicology clinical service. Because this appears to be severe poisoning, prognostication of coma with somatosensory evoked potentials could be considered early in the course, although they have not been studied specifically in toxic encephalopathies.

SUMMARY

Cyanide poisoning is rare, but neurologists need to maintain a high clinical suspicion when patients present with a history suggestive of possible exposure. It can be rapidly lethal following acute exposure and treatment should not be delayed in these cases pending cyanide levels of other laboratory test that are not immediately available. Exposure may occur from accidental workplace exposures, suicide attempts, or intentional malicious acts (e.g., homicide or terrorism). Physicians need to recognize cyanide toxicity as a potential cause of unexplained encephalopathy, seizures, and coma. They also need to be familiar with the treatment algorithms, including the cyanide antidote kit. Management of seizures and prognostication of coma may be required.

REFERENCES

1. Watson WA, Litovitz TL, Rodgers GC, et al. 2004 annual report of the American Association of Poison Control Centers Toxic Exposure Surveillance System. *Am J Emerg Med.* 2005;23(5):589–666.
2. Agency for Toxic Substances and Disease Registry (ATSDR). Toxicological profile for cyanide (Draft for public comment). Atlanta, GA: U.S. Department of Health and Human Services, Public Health Service. 2004.
3. World Health Organization. Hydrogen Cyanide and Cyanides Human Health Aspects Concise International Chemical Assessment Document, No. 61. Geneva, 2004.
4. Blanc P, Hogan M, Mallin K, et al. Cyanide intoxication among silver-reclaiming workers. *JAMA.* 1985;253:367–371.

5. Singh BM, Coles N, Lewis P, et al. The metabolic effects of fatal cyanide poisoning. *Postgrad Med J.* 1989;65:923–925.
6. Pettersen JC, Cohen SD. The effects of cyanide on brain mitochondrial cytochrome oxidase and respiratory activities. *J Appl Toxicol.* 1993;13:9–14.
7. Way JL. Cyanide intoxication and its mechanism of antagonism. *Annu Rev Pharmacol Toxicol.* 1984;24:451–481.
8. Rosenow F, Herholz K, Lanfermann H, et al. Neurological sequelae of cyanide intoxication—The patterns of clinical, magnetic resonance imaging, and positron emission tomography findings. *Ann Neurol.* 1995;38:825–828.
9. Shou Y, Gunasekar PG, Borowitz JL, et al. Cyanide-induced apoptosis involves oxidative-stress-activated NF-kappaB in cortical neurons. *Toxicol Appl Pharmacol.* 2000;164:196–205.
10. Kanthasamy AG, Borowitz JL, Pavlakovc G, et al. Dopaminergic neurotoxicity of cyanide: Neurochemical, histological, and behavioral characterization. *Toxicol Appl Pharmacol.* 1994;126(1):156–163.
11. Rachinger J, Fellner FA, Stieglbauer K, et al. MR changes after acute cyanide intoxication. *AJNR Am J Neuroradiol.* 2002;23:1398–1401.
12. Prabhakaran K, Li L, Borowitz JL, et al. Cyanide induces different modes of death in cortical and mesencephalon cells. *J Pharmacol Exp Ther.* 2002;303:510–519.
13. Fernando GC, Busuttil A. Cyanide ingestion: Case studies of four suicides. *Am J Forensic Med Pathol.* 1991;12:241–246.
14. Baud FJ, Borron SW, Megarbane B, et al.: Value of lactic acidosis in the assessment of the severity of acute cyanide poisoning. *Crit Care Med.* 2002;30:2044–2050.

CHAPTER **164**

Smallpox

Richard A. Zuckerman • Barnett R. Nathan

OBJECTIVES

- To describe the history, epidemiology, etiology, pathogenesis, and pathology of vaccinia and variola infections with regard to neurologic disease
- To define the unique clinical characteristics of vaccinia-associated neurologic disease and to compare them with natural infection with variola
- To describe the approach to diagnosis of neurologic disease caused by vaccinia and variola
- To discuss the treatment of neurologic manifestations of vaccinia and variola

CASE VIGNETTE

A 27-year-old military trainee presents with acute onset of fever, followed by confusion and altered mental status. He had received his immunization for smallpox 2 weeks previously. He was noted by his friends to be emotionally labile and forgetful, and eventually he was found wandering aimlessly. When he was brought to the emergency department, he was noted to have confusion and paranoia. Physical examination was normal, with a dry scab at the site of immunization; neurologic examination was without focal deficits, but he was not oriented to place and was unable to complete simple tasks, including serial 7s. Complete blood count (CBC), metabolic panel, toxin screen, thyroid-stimulating hormone (TSH), chest X-ray, and urinalysis were all normal; rapid human immunodeficiency virus (HIV) test and rapid plasma reagin (RPR) were negative. Computed tomographic (CT) scan of the head showed diffuse white matter changes, and lumbar puncture (LP) showed a white blood cell count (WBC) of 35 WBC (80% lymphocytes), glucose 65, protein 83; Gram stain was negative.

The patient was started on intravenous ceftriaxone and acyclovir. Within 12 hours, he developed left leg weakness and then had a generalized tonic–clonic seizure. Magnetic resonance imaging (MRI) of the head, with and without gadolinium, showed multiple bilateral white matter lesions suggestive of a demyelinating process. An electroencephalogram (EEG) suggested effects of benzodiazepines, and it showed no epileptiform discharges. Over the ensuing days, he became progressively more somnolent, but otherwise remained clinically stable. Ceftriaxone and acyclovir were discontinued when culture and herpes simplex virus (HSV) results were negative. Intravenous steroids were started because of the concern for immune-mediated demyelinating process.

DEFINITION

On May 8, 1980, the World Health Organization (WHO) declared that smallpox, which is caused by variola virus, had been officially eradicated. In recent years, however, new concern has arisen for the potential use of variola as an agent of biological warfare or terrorism. This has prompted a resurgence in reintroducing smallpox vaccination with the related orthopoxvirus, vaccinia, as a protective countermeasure. In the coming years, the generalist will more likely encounter postvaccination sequelae, so this chapter primarily focuses on the current most clinically useful information regarding the neurologic sequelae of smallpox vaccination. In tandem, the chapter will reference the potential manifestations that could be encountered in the rare, but worrisome, event that wild-type variola infection be encountered.

Vaccinia-associated neurologic complications have been classified into distinct entities based on histopathologic findings and the age groups affected. In children <2 years of age, a rapidly progressive, *postvaccinal encephalopathy* is the most common finding, whereas in adults, postvaccinial encephalomyelitis (PVE) or *microglial encephalomyelitis* predominates (1). This is commonly a demyelinating entity similar to acute disseminated encephalomyelitis (ADEM). It is important to note that most information about variola and vaccinia are from historical sources, so the quality of the information is a function of the technology and archival processes of the times.

EPIDEMIOLOGY

The development of a vaccination for protection against the worldwide epidemic of smallpox was borne from the ancient practice of variolation, the process of inoculating persons with material from the scab of a patient with smallpox to develop an attenuated form of the disease. In the late 18th century, Jenner discovered that inoculation with the cowpox (vaccinia) virus was associated with significantly less morbidity and mortality than variolation and also provided protection from smallpox disease. His discovery of vaccination is heralded as one of the great medical achievements in history. Nevertheless, the disease remained widespread until the 1960s, when the WHO embarked upon the "Intensified Smallpox Eradication Programme."

A broad vaccination campaign is not without potential adverse events, so much of the data regarding adverse reactions to the smallpox vaccination were acquired during vaccination campaigns between the 1940s and 1970s. Additional information has been recently acquired from the vaccination campaign in 2002–2005, in which >750,000 US civilian and military personnel were immunized (2).

Multiple strains of vaccinia have been used for vaccination, and it is clear that some strains are associated with higher rates of adverse events than others (3). In the United States, the New York City Board of Health (NYCBH) strain has been used for decades and appears to be associated with the lowest frequency of adverse neurologic events compared with some of the strains used in Europe (Bern, Copenhagen, Lister).

In the past century, neurologic complications of vaccinia were more frequently encountered than in variola infection. This is not because of a high risk of neurologic complication from the vaccine, but rather the extremely large number of people who receive the inoculation. In fact, the incidence of serious neurologic reactions to the NYCBH strain is less than 10 cases per million people vaccinated (4). What is most striking and receives the most attention, is that the case fatality rate among those with neurologic complications (principally, encephalomyelitis) approaches 25% (4). The primary significance of this is the consideration for mass vaccination and the potential for very rare, but serious, events to occur.

The risk of the postvaccinal encephalopathy that presents in children <2 years of age is likely greatest in the very young, those children <1 year of age, with an incidence of approximately 11 cases per million vaccines (4), a rate more frequent than PVE in older children or adults. Hence, the recommendation in the 1960s to delay vaccination for smallpox until after age 2 years.

Older children (5 to 9 years) and adults may be at greater risk for PVE than in the younger children (5). It is also likely that those receiving a primary vaccine, rather than a revaccination, are at greater risk for developing a neurologic complication (4). Few data are available on the risk of neurologic complications of vaccination in immunocompromised individuals, such as those with HIV, and the widespread use of immunosuppressing drugs was not an issue during prior smallpox vaccination programs.

As mentioned, neurologic complications from primary variola infection are rare (5). Between 1 of 500 and 2,000 patients may develop an encephalitis during the acute smallpox infection (4). Although the reported incidence of neurologic complications of variola may be equal to, or exceed, those of the smallpox vaccination, the absolute numbers are small because few wild-type smallpox infections have occurred when compared with the magnitude of people vaccinated during a mass immunization campaign. In <1% of smallpox cases, myelitis, meningitis, brainstem encephalitis, peripheral neuropathies, and ascending paralysis have historically been reported (6). These reports predate modern medicine; they are based on case series from the 18th through the early 20th centuries, so it is not clear if these neurologic syndromes are caused by infection from variola or a secondary complication of the disease.

ETIOLOGY, PATHOGENESIS, AND PATHOLOGY

Variola and vaccinia are members of the *orthopoxvirus* genera of *Poxviridae.* The smallpox vaccine contains live vaccinia virus, which is inoculated into the skin using the multipuncture technique. A local reaction occurs, with a range of local and more generalized reactions reported to be normal as the host develops systemic humoral and cellular immune responses (7). Headache is commonly reported in the absence of neurologic dysfunction (8). In normal vaccination, transient viremia can occur, typically by the sixth day, but is rapidly cleared in immunocompetent hosts. Vaccinia infection can be transmitted by contact transmission from the lesion of a vaccinee in the time before the scab falls off, but is a rare occurrence, particularly if appropriate contact precautions are taken.

In children, the syndrome of postvaccinal encephalopathy usually occurs earlier, 6 to 10 days after vaccination, and likely represents cerebral damage as a result of vascular changes. Associated histopathologic changes include generalized cerebral edema, mild lymphocytic meningeal infiltration, widespread ganglion degenerative changes, and, occasionally, perivascular hemorrhages (10).

In adults, PVE usually begins approximately 11 to 15 days (mean of 12 days) (9) after vaccination, consistent with an immune-mediated phenomenon. Clinical characteristics are described below. It is felt that PVE is an abnormal host response to viral or virus-induced antigens because virus has not been recovered from most fatal cases (9). The histopathology of PVE is consistent with this description: mild meningeal inflammation, perivascular demyelination, and cellular infiltration with lymphocytes and pleomorphic microglia (9–11).

Natural infection with variola was usually acquired via the respiratory tract, but inoculation of the skin or conjunctiva or infection through the placenta has also been described. After spread to regional lymph nodes, transient viremia occurs and clinical symptoms appear. As previously described, encephalitis can be common with variola, but because of the lack of serious neurologic complications little has been described about the pathophysiology.

CLINICAL MANIFESTATIONS

The clinical history of smallpox (variola) and cowpox (vaccinia) have been closely integrated since Jenner developed the smallpox vaccine from a cowpox lesion in 1796. A clinical description of variola, in particular with regard to the neurologic manifestations, would not be complete without also describing vaccinia-associated syndromes.

VACCINIA

PVE is the most common neurologic complication of the smallpox vaccine. The clinical syndrome was described in the early 1920s with a cluster of case reports in a number of diverse locations (12). The histopathologic correlate was first described in the literature by Turnbull in 1926 (11). An excellent description of the syndrome, circa 1929 is still clinically relevant (12):

> The symptoms in this complication usually appear suddenly and have their onset in 70 per cent of the cases from the tenth to the thirteenth day, inclusive, following vaccination. That is, they

appear when the vaccination, usually primary, is at its height. The symptoms as recorded for different cases vary somewhat, but four symptoms are quite constantly noted, namely: (i) fever (104°F., or higher in severe cases); (ii) vomiting; (iii) headache; (iv) stupor or coma. The stupor may develop within a few hours after the onset of the symptoms and is always present in fatal cases. Symptoms of meningeal irritation are usually present in conscious cases, absent in others. Convulsions are common in young children, as are also cramps or spasms. Trismus has been occasionally observed, and is worthy of note, as it may lead to confusion of the ailment with tetanus. Varying degrees of paresis or paralysis are noted in some cases. The eye muscles usually escape. The Babinski is usually positive, a point considered as of high diagnostic significance. Death, which follows in from 30 to 40 per cent of the cases, usually occurs from the third to the tenth day following the onset of symptoms. Recovery, when it takes place, is usually rapid and complete; however, some degree of crippling has been noted in a few cases.

Although there is little modern experience with PVE, the clinical presentation and the pathology at autopsy suggest that the syndrome has much in common with ADEM, which is typically a postinfectious or postvaccination syndrome characterized by a wide variety of CNS signs and symptoms. PVE has been described most commonly presenting with stupor and coma, seizure and status epilepticus, headache, dizziness, neck pain, and fever and vomiting (4,5). As stated, these symptoms typically develop 11 to 15 days (9) after the vaccination, but can occur up to a month after the initial exposure. Several days later, some patients can acquire more focal and severe deficits, including paraparesis, hemiparesis, eye movement abnormalities and other cranial nerve deficits, ataxia, movement disorders, mutism, and hallucinations. This acute phase typically lasts about 1 week. In those who have survived, recovery was often complete; however, permanent neurological sequelae could persist (Table 164-1). Predictors on presentation of poor neurologic outcomes included altered mental status, confusion, seizures, and coma. Those who developed myelitis were also at risk for permanent weakness (4). Much of the mortality associated with PVE may well be a consequence of secondary infectious complications of the syndrome, such as pneumonia, sepsis, and urinary tract infections. Whereas the mortality rate of PVE is in line with percentages quoted for ADEM (0% to 30%) (13), a strong likelihood is that many of the secondary complications described above could be ameliorated by modern acute and critical care medicine.

TABLE 164-1. Permanent Neurological Sequelae[a]

Cranial nerve palsy (VI)
"Brain damage," severe
Deafness, unilateral
Epilepsy
Hemiparesis
Movement disorders[b]
Neurotic disorder[c]
Optic neuritis[d]
Paraparesis
Psychosis

[a]For which 1 to 3 cases were reported.
[b]Chorea or ballismus.
[c]Approximate equivalent terms for psychasthenia.
[d]And other spinal cord problems.
(From Abrahams BC, Kaufman DM. Anticipating smallpox and monkeypox outbreaks: Complications of the smallpox vaccine. *Neurologist* 2004;10(15):265–274, with permission.)

Less severe CNS symptomatology can also be seen, including headache, fever, nuchal rigidity, and photophobia. These symptoms typically arise 5 to 7 days after vaccination and then resolve without sequelae (14).

Although none of the Centers for Disease Control and Prevention (CDC) contraindications for smallpox vaccine are related to a known risk of acquiring neurologic complications, they bear mentioning here. Smallpox vaccination in the setting before outbreak is contraindicated for persons who have the following conditions or have a close contact with the following conditions: (*a*) a history of atopic dermatitis (commonly referred to as eczema), irrespective of disease severity or activity; (*b*) active acute, chronic, or exfoliative skin conditions that disrupt the epidermis; (*c*) pregnant women or women who desire to become pregnant in the 28 days after vaccination; and (*d*) persons who are immunocompromised as a result of HIV or acquired immunodeficiency syndrome (AIDS), autoimmune conditions, cancer, radiation treatment, immunosuppressive medications, or other immunodeficiencies (15).

Very young children (<2 years of age) may develop postvaccinal encephalopathy rather than the encephalomyelitis. This syndrome can present with a variety of acute and fulminant CNS signs, such as seizures, hemiplegia, and aphasia (9). Cerebrospinal fluid (CSF) is typically normal, although it may be under especially high pressure. Symptoms usually occur 6 to 10 days after vaccination, typically presenting 5 days or so before one would expect to see PVE. Patients can have a complete recovery, usually in 24 to 48 hours (14), although some die or are left with cerebral impairment and hemiplegia (9).

VARIOLA

Neurologic complications of variola infection are uncommon. The nonneurologic clinical course bears mentioning because most clinicians have little experience with the primary disease. The incubation period of smallpox averages 12 days, with a range of 7 to 17 days. During the incubation period, the patient is typically asymptomatic. The prodromal stage follows and can be severe, but nonspecific, with flulike symptoms, including fever, malaise, headache, muscle pain, backache, and nausea and vomiting. The patient usually feels better once the prodromal stage is coming to an end with defervescence of the fever. At this point, the rash appears and the patient becomes infectious. The rash, or enanthem, is composed of small red spots on the tongue and in the mouth. These lesions grow and ulcerate, releasing large amounts of virus into the saliva. This coincides with the appearance of the cutaneous rash and when the patient is most contagious. The cutaneous rash, or exanthema, occurs on all parts of the body within 24 hours. The cutaneous rash is initially macular, then progresses to papular, then finally vesicular. The vesicles frequently have a central depression or umbilication (Figs. 164-1 and 164-2). Finally, the vesicles mature into pustules. These pustules are deeply embedded in the dermis and this makes them feel like beads under the skin. The entire body usually develops the rash simultaneously. The rash can be distinguished from chickenpox (varicella) by the appearance at any given time and the character of the distribution of the pox. In smallpox, the rash is all of the same stage at any given time and is centrifugal, or seen most heavily on the extremities (including the palms and soles) and the face,

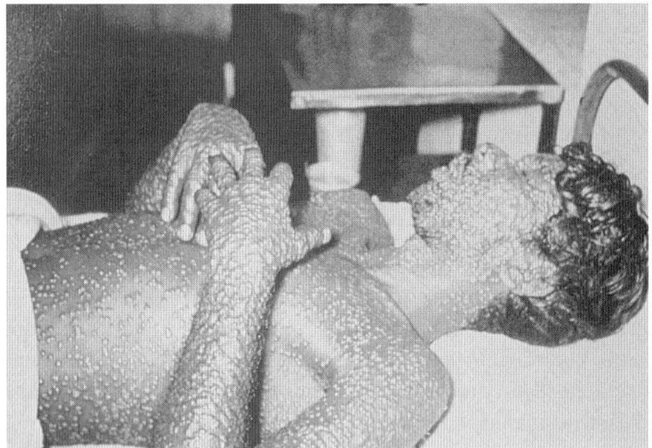

FIGURE 164-1. Man with smallpox. (From Centers for Disease Control and Prevention (CDC)/National Immunization Program (NIP)/Barbara Rice, with permission.)

whereas in chickenpox, the pox can be of various stages and located more in the core, or the trunk.

Mortality from smallpox has historically been approximately 30%, with increased mortality in children <1 year of age. In an analysis of historical case series, Martin (16) describes much of the mortality as multifactorial, including renal failure, shock secondary to volume depletion, and hypoxia secondary to viral pneumonia and airway compromise. Because of the loss of skin integrity from the vesicular and pustular stages, the patient with smallpox resembles a burn victim in as much as they become severely volume depleted and develop a prerenal syndrome and shock.

DIAGNOSTIC APPROACH

Diagnostic investigation when suspecting PVE should proceed as for a patient suspected of having a CNS infection, especially if the patient presents with fever, altered mental status, and meningeal signs. Most of the workup should be performed to rule out other causes that would explain the patient's presentation. In persons with a recent history of vaccination, clinical suspicion should be high. Sejvar et al. (1) have established a case definition for encephalitis or encephalomyelitis for use in the *Smallpox Adverse Events Monitoring and Response Activity*, which helps to define if the encephalitis or encephalomyelitis is confirmed, probable, and suspected (Table 164-2) (1). Outside of the histopathologic criteria for a confirmed case, the definition is based solely on clinical, laboratory, EEG, and imaging studies.

There is little modern experience with PVE, but it is likely that computerized axial tomography findings will be normal, because commonly it is in ADEM. If no focal lesions are seen on CT scanning, then proceed to lumbar puncture. Historical evidence suggests that the CSF may be moderately abnormal, with an increased opening pressure, an average of 100 WBC/mm^2, and a normal protein and glucose (5). EEG may show diffuse background slowing. If similar to ADEM, MRI likely will show high signal on T2 or fluid-attenuated inversion recovery (FLAIR) imaging in the white matter (demyelinating lesions); in ADEM, however, the corpus callosum is usually not involved. In ADEM, extensive edema around these lesions may be seen and few MRI lesions may enhance after gadolinium administration. In ADEM, white matter involvement predominates, although gray matter can also be affected, particularly basal ganglion, thalami, and brainstem (13).

In the modern era, polymerase chain reaction (PCR) of CSF can be used to look for virus components, but the sensitivity of this method is not clear, given the few clinical cases since PCR has been available. Additionally, because PVE is felt to be a primarily immunologic phenomenon, the presence of virus is felt to be unlikely. Nevertheless, if encountering a suspected case of PVE from vaccinia, CSF should be saved for potential testing by the CDC.

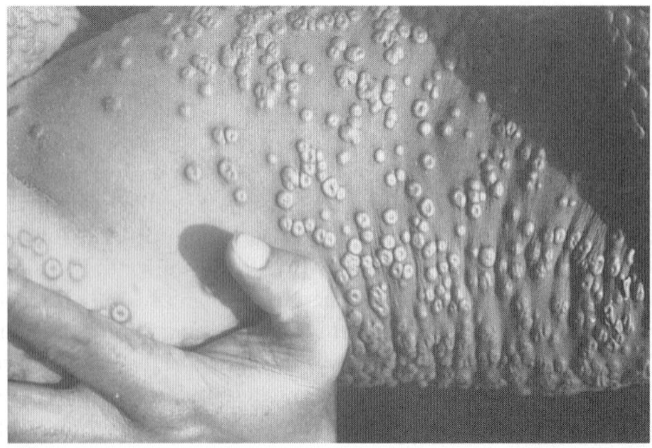

FIGURE 164-2. Smallpox lesions on skin of trunk. (From Centers for Disease Control and Prevention (CDC), James Hicks, with permission.)

TREATMENT

Treatment of PVE has not been established. Treatment should be directed at the acute complications (status epilepticus, increased intracranial pressure [ICP]) with anticonvulsants and maneuvers to lower elevated ICP. Quality intensive care to mitigate complications, therefore, is the best course of action.

Some evidence suggests that treatment with intravenous corticosteroids may be useful in patients with PVE, typically in doses of approximately 1,000 mg/day of methylprednisolone for 5 days to a week. This would then be followed by an oral taper with prednisone over 4 to 8 weeks (14). Plasma exchange has been used successfully in the treatment of ADEM (17,18); however, because of the likely significant role of T cells in PVE, it may not be efficacious (14).

Using vaccinia immune globulin (VIG, also known as *antivaccinia gamma globulin* [AGG]) at the time of smallpox vaccination has been successful in reducing the incidence of PVE (14,19). VIG is obtained from recently vaccinated individuals. It has not demonstrated efficacy in ameliorating the signs and symptoms of PVE once it has been established. Intravenous immunoglobulin (IVIg) may also provide similar prophylactic effects as VIG; however, the role of IVIg in smallpox vaccination has not yet been established. Although VIG is recommended as the first-line therapy for vaccinia-associated complications, the antiviral cidofovir is recommended as a second-line agent (7). Cidofovir is active *in vitro* against orthopoxviruses, but has not been approved for this use. The CDC has issued guidelines for the use of cidofovir in rare cases

TABLE 164-2. Case Definition: Encephalitis/Encephalomyelitis, for Use in the Smallpox Adverse Events Monitoring and Response Activity

CASE DEFINITION FOR ACUTE ENCEPHALITIS

A. **A confirmed case of encephalitis** is defined by demonstration of acute cerebral inflammation (± meninges) or demyelination by histopathology
B. **A probable case of encephalitis** is defined by the acute onset of:
   1. Encephalopathy (e.g., depressed or altered level of consciousness, lethargy, or personality change lasting ≥24 hours)

AND

   2. Additional clinical evidence suggestive of cerebral inflammation, including 2 or more of the following:
      a. Fever (temperature ≥38°C) or hypothermia (temperature ≤35°C)
      b. Meningismus (i.e., nuchal rigidity, photophobia/phonophobia)
      c. CSF pleocytosis (>5 white blood cells/mm^3)
      d. Presence of focal neurologic deficit
      e. Electroencephalography findings consistent with encephalitis
      f. Neuroimaging findings on magnetic resonance imaging (MRI) consistent with acute inflammation (± meninges) or demyelination of the nervous system
      g. Seizures, either new onset or exacerbation of previously controlled seizures

AND

   3. No alternative (investigated) etiologies are found for presenting sign and symptoms

C. **A suspected case of encephalitis** is defined as the presence of the acute onset of
   1. Encephalopathy, as outlined for a probable case

AND

   2. One of the criteria listed for probable encephalitis as clinical evidence suggestive of cerebral inflammation

AND

   3. No alternative (investigated) etiologies are found for presenting signs and symptoms

CASE DEFINITION FOR ACUTE MYELITIS

A. **A confirmed case of myelitis** is defined by demonstration of acute spinal cord inflammation (± meninges) or demyelination by histopathology
B. **A probable case of myelitis** is defined by the acute onset of:
   1. Myelopathy (development of sensory, motor, or autonomic dysfunction attributable to the spinal cord, including upper- and lower-motor neuron weakness, sensory level, bowel or bladder dysfunction)

AND

   2. Additional evidence suggestive of spinal cord inflammation, including 2 or more of the following:
      a. Fever (temperature ≥38°C) or hypothermia (temperature ≤35°C)
      b. CSF pleocytosis (>5 white blood cells/mm^3)
      c. Presence of focal neurologic deficit
      d. Electromyographic studies suggestive of central (spinal cord) dysfunction
      e. Neuroimaging findings on MRI demonstrating acute inflammation (± meninges) or demyelination of the spinal cord

AND

   3. No alternative (investigated) etiologies are found for presenting sign and symptoms

C. **A suspected case of myelitis** is defined as presence of the acute onset of:
   1. Myelopathy as outlined for a probable case

AND

   2. One of the criteria listed for probable myelitis, as evidence suggestive of spinal cord inflammation

AND

   3. No alternative (investigated) etiologies are found for presenting sign and symptoms

CASES FULFILLING THE CRITERIA FOR BOTH ENCEPHALITIS AND MYELITIS IN ANY CATEGORY WOULD BE CLASSIFIED AS ENCEPHALOMYELITIS.

CSF, cerebrospinal fluid.
(From Sejvar JJ, Labutta RJ, Chapman LE, et al. Neurologic adverse events associated with smallpox vaccination in the United States, 2002–2004. *JAMA.* 2005;294(21):2744–2750, with permission.)

of vaccinia-associated complications, but only under direction of the CDC and Department of Defense (7).

No approved therapies exist for variola infection, although novel agents are being developed. VIG may have some benefit, but is not available for widespread use because of limited supply. Cidofovir may also be an effective agent, but experience must be extrapolated from animal models of other poxvirus infections.

It is important also to mention prevention of variola in the event of identified disease within the population. Immunization with vaccinia has been shown to provide protection from disease in some persons and also likely decreases the severity of infection if given by the fourth day after exposure (20). The United States government has stockpiled vaccinations for this purpose.

CLINICAL RECOMMENDATIONS OF THE VIGNETTE

A diagnosis of PVE in the patient was considered secure given the 2-week time period from vaccination as well as the consistent clinical, laboratory, and imaging findings that fit the case definition for probable encephalomyelitis (1). In this acute setting, the patient should be started on phenytoin or other anticonvulsant for the seizures and the high-dose steroids continued. Consideration should be given for plasmapheresis and immunoglobulin therapy, but should not be initiated until the patient is clinically stable. Aggressive supportive care and prevention of nosocomial and iatrogenic complications are requisite. Finally, it is important to report all potential vaccine adverse events to the US Food and Drug Administration (FDA) or CDC Vaccine Adverse Event Response System (VAERS).

SUMMARY

Smallpox disease has been eradicated from the globe, but concerns remain for potential release of the virus into the population as an agent of biological warfare. Thus, a general knowledge of the clinical manifestations of variola is important. Additionally, because vaccination of a considerable number of persons is probable, knowledge of the potential adverse effects of this intervention is essential. The neurologic complications of vaccinia and variola are rare, but early diagnosis, treatment, and prophylaxis may improve clinical outcome because of improvements in supportive care. As the ethical debate over the widespread use of the vaccination continues, it behooves clinicians to remain current regarding these potentially devastating viruses.

REFERENCES

1. Sejvar JJ, Labutta RJ, Chapman LE, et al. Neurologic adverse events associated with smallpox vaccination in the United States, 2002–2004. *JAMA.* 2005;294(21):2744–2750.
2. Poland GA, Grabenstein JD, Neff JM. The US smallpox vaccination program: A review of a large modern era smallpox vaccination implementation program. *Vaccine.* 2005;23(17–18):2078–2081.
3. Kretzschmar M, Wallinga J, Teunis P, et al. Frequency of adverse events after vaccination with different vaccinia strains. *PLoS Med.* 2006;3(8):e272.
4. Abrahams BC, Kaufman DM. Anticipating smallpox and monkeypox outbreaks: Complications of the smallpox vaccine. *Neurologist.* 2004;10(5):265–274.
5. Booss J, Davis LE. Smallpox and smallpox vaccination: Neurological implications. *Neurology.* 2003;60(8):1241–1245.
6. Wilson SAK, Bruce AN. Encephalitis of fevers, exanthems, and known infections. In: Bruce AN, ed. *Neurology.* Baltimore: Williams & Wilkins; 1941:55–80.
7. Smallpox. In: Atkinson W, Hamborsky J, McIntyre L, et al., eds. *Centers for Disease Control and Prevention Epidemiology and Prevention of Vaccine-Preventable Diseases,* 9th ed. Washington, DC: Public Health Foundation; 2006:281–306.
8. Sejvar J, Boneva R, Lane JM, et al. Severe headaches following smallpox vaccination. *Headache.* 2005;45(1):87–88.
9. Fenner F, Henderson DA, Arita I, et al. *Smallpox and Its Eradication.* Geneva, Switzerland: World Health Organization; 1988.
10. de Vries E. Postvaccinial perivenous encephalitis. A pathological anatomical study on the place of postvaccinial perivenous encephalitis in the group encephalitides (the disease of Turnbull-Lucksch-Bastiaanse). *Folia Psychiatr Neurol Jpn.* 1960;[Suppl 5]:1–181.
11. Turnbull HM, McIntosh J. Encephalo-myelitis following vaccination. *Br J Exp Path.* 1926;7:181–222.
12. Defries RD, McKinnon NE. Vaccination and encephalitis. *Can Med Assoc J.* 1929; 21(5):516–520.
13. Garg RK. Acute disseminated encephalomyelitis. *Postgrad Med J.* 2003;79(927):11–17.
14. Miravalle A, Roos KL. Encephalitis complicating smallpox vaccination. *Arch Neurol.* 2003;60(7):925–928.
15. Cono J, Casey CG, Bell DM. Smallpox vaccination and adverse reactions. Guidance for clinicians. *MMWR Recomm Rep.* 2003;52(RR–4):1–28.
16. Martin DB. The cause of death in smallpox: An examination of the pathology record. *Mil Med.* 2002;167(7):546–551.
17. Lin CH, Jeng JS, Yip PK. Plasmapheresis in acute disseminated encephalomyelitis. *J Clin Apheresis.* 2004;19(3):154–159.
18. Miyazawa R, Hikima A, Takano Y, et al. Plasmapheresis in fulminant acute disseminated encephalomyelitis. *Brain Dev.* 2001;23(6):424–426.
19. Kleiman M, Brunquell P. Acute disseminated encephalomyelitis: response to intravenous immunoglobulin. *J Child Neurol.* 1995;10(6):481–483.
20. Henderson DA, Inglesby TV, Bartlett JG, et al. Smallpox as a biological weapon: Medical and public health management. Working Group on Civilian Biodefense. *JAMA.* 1999; 281(22):2127–2137.

PART XXII Psychiatry

CHAPTER 165

Depression and Neurology

Richard Wolin • Steven L. Dubovsky • Richard Cowan

Primary mood disorders (depressive and bipolar mood disorders) share with other disorders of the nervous system neuroanatomic, neurochemical, psychological, emotional, behavioral, and social dimensions. In addition, the neurobiology of certain neurologic illnesses cause depression (and some cause mania), whereas some neurologic medications cause depression or mania as side effects. Comorbid depression complicates the course of neurologic illnesses, and its treatment can improve the outcome of the medical disorders. It is extremely important, therefore, for physicians to be aware of new developments in the diagnosis and treatment of depression.

OBJECTIVES

- To discuss the diagnosis and treatment of unipolar depression that occurs in the context of neurologic disease
- To review advances in knowledge of the neurobiology, neuroanatomy, genetics, and psychopharmacology of depression in the neurologic setting
- To illustrate ways in which depression can affect the morbidity and mortality of neurologic disorders

CASE VIGNETTE

A 54-year-old woman with a 17-year history of multiple sclerosis (MS) complains of visual impairment, cognitive dysfunction, impairment of gait, problems with bladder control, and depressive symptoms that include sadness, irritability, decreased energy, loss of appetite, insomnia, and decreased enjoyment of her usual activities. The patient has recently been divorced. Her medical history includes hypothyroidism and head trauma with brief loss of consciousness in a motor vehicle accident 30 years previously. She has been treated for the past 3 years with interferon.

Neurologic examination demonstrates impaired short-term memory, bilateral decreased visual acuity, and slightly hyperactive muscle stretch reflexes bilaterally. On mental status examination, the patient has a reduced level of psychomotor activity. Her speech appears ruminative around negative thoughts, but there may also be an element of perseveration. Her affect is depressed. She is preoccupied with a recent divorce. She has obvious difficulty with attention and short-term memory. Neuropsychological assessment demonstrates impaired auditory and visual processing speed, abstraction and psychomotor problem-solving, as well as constructional apraxia, reduced visual perceptual processing speed, and decreased visual memory.

DEFINITION

Mood disorders are categorized broadly as unipolar (no history of mania or hypomania) or bipolar. The *Diagnostic and Statistical Manual of Mental Disorders*, fourth edition, text revision (DSM-IV-TR) (1) distinguishes between mood episodes and mood disorders. An *episode* is a period lasting at least 2 weeks during which there are sufficient symptoms for full criteria to be met for the episode. *A major depressive episode* is diagnosed if depressed mood or anhedonia (irritability may substitute for depressed mood in juvenile patients) has been present for at least 2 weeks. At least four additional symptoms from the following list also should be present for a major depressive episode to be diagnosed formally:

Vegetative:	Weight loss of 5% of body weight
	Increase or decrease in appetite
	Insomnia or hypersomnia
	Fatigue or apathy
Motor:	Psychomotor agitation or retardation
Cognitive:	Diminished ability to think or concentrate, indecisiveness
Psychological:	Worthlessness, guilt, recurrent thoughts of death or suicide

The lifetime risk of suicide in mood disorders is as high as 10% to 15% (2), which is significantly higher than the risk in other disorders. Neuropsychological deficits are more common in depressed patients who have made highly lethal suicide attempts than in those who have made low lethal attempts and nonpatients, suggesting that impaired executive function may exist in people at risk for severe suicide attempts (3). It, therefore, is particularly important to evaluate all depressed neurologic patients for suicide risk. Although it is difficult to predict suicide with certainty, the following factors indicate the need for rapid psychiatric consultation to clarify the risk (4).

Demographic factors
- Male sex
- Recent loss
- Never married
- Older age

Symptoms
  Severe depression
  Anxiety
  Hopelessness
Bipolar disorder
  Psychosis, especially with command hallucinations
Current substance use
History
  History of suicide attempts, especially if multiple or severe attempts
  Family history of suicide
Suicidal thinking
  Presence of a specific plan
  Means available to carry out the plan
  Absence of factors that would keep the patient from completing the plan
  Rehearsal of the plan

DSM-IV-TR adds a number of *specifiers* to a major depressive episode that may indicate dimensions of depression that predict certain outcomes or responses to treatment. Melancholic features are defined by either pervasive anhedonia (loss of pleasure in all, or nearly all, activities) or lack of reactivity to usually pleasurable stimuli (does not feel much better, even temporarily, when something good happens). In addition, three or more of the following are required for the diagnosis, although the evidence that melancholia with two of these symptoms is substantially different from melancholia associated with three symptoms is not strong:

1. Distinct quality of depressed mood (i.e., the depressed mood is experienced as distinctly different from the kind of feeling experienced after the death of a loved one)
2. Depression regularly worse in the morning
3. Early morning awakening (at least 2 hours before usual time of awakening)
4. Marked psychomotor retardation or agitation
5. Significant anorexia or weight loss
6. Excessive or inappropriate guilt

Melancholic depression is thought by some experts to reflect a more severe depressive episode that may be less likely to respond to selective serotonin reuptake inhibitors (SSRI) than to tricyclic antidepressants (TCA), venlafaxine or duloxetine. A review of 18 clinical trials comparing SSRI with TCA and 5 comparing SSRI with placebo found, however, that SSRI were as effective as TCA for severe depression (5). Similarly, a review of 315 randomized, controlled trials comparing newer antidepressants with older antidepressants, placebo or psychosocial interventions in depression found that SSRI and TCA had similar response rates and similar dropout rates, although specific side effects differed (6).

In contrast to the *typical* depressive symptoms of melancholia, atypical features are present when two kinds of symptoms have been present during the most recent 2 weeks of a major depressive episode:

A. Mood reactivity (i.e., mood brightens in response to actual or potential positive events)
B. Two (or more) of the following features:
   1. Significant weight gain or increase in appetite
   2. Hypersomnia
   3. Leaden paralysis (inability to get oneself to do things that one wants to do)
   4. Long-standing pattern of interpersonal rejection sensitivity (i.e., the capacity to be cheered up temporarily by positive events) that results in significant social or occupational impairment

Psychotic features are present when a major depressive episode is associated with hallucinations or delusions. Although such symptoms are traditionally thought to be rare, especially in outpatient practice, numerous studies have found a prevalence of psychosis, which may be severe or relatively subtle, in as many as 50% of depressed patients (7). The presence of psychosis, at least when it is more marked, is an indication for treatment with a combination of an antidepressant and an antipsychotic drug or with electroconvulsive therapy (ECT).

Whereas a single major depressive episode can be acute or chronic and can have a unipolar or bipolar outcome, major depressive disorder is characterized by recurrent major depressive episodes without any manic or hypomanic symptoms. Major depressive disorder, therefore, is equivalent to recurrent unipolar depression.

Major depressive disorder can be chronic as well as recurrent. Dysthymia (dysthymic disorder) is a form of chronic unipolar depression. DSM-IV-TR criteria for dysthymic disorder include at least 2 years' duration of depressed mood (or irritable mood in children) and two of the additional symptomatic criteria for major depressive disorder as opposed to four of these symptoms to diagnose a major depressive episode. Dysthymia is meant to convey a milder form of chronic depression, but because the number of symptoms experienced by chronically depressed patients fluctuates over time, the same patient may meet criteria for dysthmic disorder at one point and chronic major depression at another. In addition, dysthymic disorder is associated with as much functional impairment as chronic major depression, and a substantial difference in treatment response between these conditions does not seem to exist.

The clinical importance of distinguishing between these two kinds of chronic depression, therefore, remains to be clarified. About 70% of patients feel more depressed during the winter in the northern hemisphere. In DSM-IV-TR, a seasonal pattern of major depressive episodes (i.e., seasonal affective disorder) is said to be present when depressive episodes regularly occur at a particular time of year (usually, the fall or winter, but in a few cases in the spring and summer), not in association with a seasonal stressor, such as starting school in the fall). A full remission of depression should occur at other times of the year, with at least two major depressive episodes in the previous 2 years having a seasonal onset and seasonal episodes substantially outnumbering nonseasonal episodes. Seasonality of mood disorders appears to be driven by changes in available daylight, and seasonal affective disorder can be treated effectively with artificial bright light.

At one time, the term *secondary depression* was used to refer to depression caused by another illness, a medication, or some other substance. In DSM-IV-TR, the first condition is called *depression* because of a general medical condition, and the latter two are called *substance-induced depression.* Although not a formal diagnosis, secondary depression now refers to depression that occurs in the context of another psychiatric or medical disorder, whereas primary depression refers to depression that is not associated with other conditions.

EPIDEMIOLOGY

In the United States, the lifetime risk of a major depressive episode is said to be approximately 6% (8). The point prevalence of major depression ranges from 2.6% to 5.5% in men and from 6.0% to 11.8% in women (9). The prevalence of dysthymia is 3% to 4% (9). Most studies have found unipolar depression to be twice as common in women as in men (10). The meaning of the gender difference, which is not apparent until adolescence, remains to be clarified, but probably involves differences in role stress as much as hormonal effects. The prevalence of major depression in primary care practice is 4.8% to 9.2%, and the prevalence of all depressive disorders in primary care practice is 9% to 20%, which makes mood disorders the most common psychiatric problems in primary care (11), and its presence increases the use of general health services (12).

In worldwide surveys, depression is the fourth most important cause of disability and the fourth most costly medical illness (4). Depressed patients spend more time in bed because of poor health and have more bodily pain than patients with diabetes, hypertension, arthritis, or chronic lung disease and have as much functional disability as patients with heart disease. In a study of general medical patients in a health maintenance organization, patients with depressed mood or anhedonia of 2 weeks' duration, but with an insufficient number of additional symptoms to meet full criteria for major depressive disorder (MDD), still had 7.7 times as much impairment of social, family, and work functioning as did patients without any depressive symptoms (13). Primary care physicians spend more time treating depression than hypertension, arteriosclerotic heart disease, and diabetes mellitus.

ETIOLOGY AND PATHOGENESIS

NEUROBIOLOGY

Theories linking disordered chemistry to disordered mood go back to at least the fourth century BC, when Hippocrates hypothesized that mood depends on a balance among the four bodily humors—blood, phlegm, yellow bile, and black bile, found in the heart, brain, liver, and spleen, respectively (4). Hippocrates proposed that depression was caused by an excess of black bile in the spleen. Because the spleen occupied a position in the body analogous to the position of Saturn in the heavens, it was believed that those born under the sign of Saturn were susceptible to depression. These ideas are the basis of references to an attitude of depressive hostility as spleen and to morose people as saturnine.

Modern studies of the neurobiology of major depression have traditionally focused on biogenic amine and other neurotransmitters, receptors, and, more recently, intracellular signaling. The monoamine hypothesis, which was first proposed in 1965, holds that monoamines such as norepinephrine (NE) and serotonin (5-HT) are deficient in depression and that the therapeutic action of antidepressants depends on increasing synaptic availability of these monoamines (14). The monoamine depletion hypothesis was originally derived from observations that antidepressants block reuptake inhibition of NE, 5-HT, or dopamine (DA). This hypothesis is limited, however, by several factors (15). Monoamine precursors, such as tyrosine or tryptophan, by themselves do not reliably improve mood. Depletion of serotonin can aggravate depression that has been in remission, but it does not predictably cause depression, and when it does cause depression, the depression is not sustained. Some substances that are monoamine reuptake inhibitors (e.g., amphetamines and cocaine) do not have reliable antidepressant properties, and antidepressant medications exist (e.g., iprindole, mianserin, mirtazapine, ketanserin) that have no effect on monoamine reuptake. In the case of monoamine reuptake inhibitors that are antidepressants, reuptake inhibition is immediate, whereas the onset of antidepressant effect is delayed a month or more. Tianeptine, a tricyclic antidepressant that enhances serotonin reuptake and reduces synaptic serotonin is as effective an antidepressant as the serotonin reuptake inhibitors, which have the opposite effect.

Although initial reports of decreased 24-hour urinary excretion of the NE metabolite 3-methoxy-4-hydroxyphenylglycol (MHPG) seemed to support a hypothesized reduction of noradrenergic neurotransmission in major depression, subsequent reports suggest that activity of NE in the locus coeruleus and the sympathetic nervous system is increased at baseline, consistent with high levels of arousal. Siever and Davis (16) suggested that depression is associated not with consistently elevated or reduced norepinephrine activity, but with uneven responsiveness to stresses that activate noradrenergic stress response systems. As with the heat produced by a furnace that is controlled by a poorly regulated thermostat, baseline noradrenergic activity is excessive, but acute stresses that call for mobilization of the stress response result in inadequate mobilization of additional noradrenergic transmission. The behavioral and affective correlates of this situation would be high levels of baseline anxiety with a sense of "spinning one's wheels" with inability to mount an organized response to important challenges.

A number of studies have found lower concentrations of 5-hydroxyindoleacetic acid (5-HIAA, the major 5-HT metabolite) in the cerebrospinal fluid (CSF) of depressed patients than in CSF of controls (17) and reduced platelet serotonin uptake in unmedicated major depression (18), suggesting hypofunction of a cellular serotonin transporter that is further supported by reports of linkage of a polymorphism of the serotonin transporter gene to major depression. Reduced [3H]-imipramine binding has been found in the brains of depressed patients who died of suicide and of natural causes, but this finding has been inconsistent (17), and another postmortem study reported decreased serotonin uptake sites as measured by [3H]-citalopram in both major depression and bipolar disorder (19). A confounding factor in many of these studies is that deficient serotonergic neurotransmission may be linked, not to the diagnosis of depression, but to a feature associated with it, such as suicide. Of seven studies, five demonstrated modestly reduced brain stem 5-HT and 5-HIAA in persons who committed suicide, regardless of diagnosis, and in 10 of 15 studies of CSF 5-HIAA, levels were lower in depressed patients who made a suicide attempt than in those who did not attempt suicide (20). A study of 22 drug-free depressed inpatients with a history of a suicide attempt found that current depressive episodes in patients whose past attempts caused more medical damage and were better planned were associated with lower CSF 5-HIAA (but no changes in other neurotransmitter metabolites) than were depressive episodes in patients who had made less lethal and less well-planned suicide attempts, which suggests that reduced 5-HIAA may be a marker of seriousness of suicidal ideation (21). Reduced central 5-HT turnover may be more reliably linked to unpredictable aggression, regardless of whether it is turned outward or inward (22), than it is to any specific depressive diagnosis.

Some investigations have found that CSF concentrations of the DA metabolite homovanillic acid (HVA) are lower in patients with major depression than in controls and that lower CSF HVA levels are found in more severely depressed patients, but results have not been consistent (17). The DA reuptake inhibitors nomifensine (no longer available), amineptine (available in Europe), and bupropion are antidepressants. Dopaminergic agonists, such as bromocriptine, pramipexole, and piribedil, and the DA-releasing stimulants methylphenidate and dextroamphetamine have antidepressant properties that make them useful adjuncts in the treatment of depression. As is true of 5-HT, however, any apparent dopaminergic hypofunction may have a greater impact on dimensions of mood disorders than on specific diagnoses. Because mobilization of goal-directed behavior is mediated by DA, underactivity of dopaminergic systems may be related to anhedonia, decreased drive, and motivation in depression. Unresponsive dopaminergic systems could be one reason why experience is unrewarding to depressed patients. Because elevated levels of DA metabolites have been observed in psychotic depression, hyperactivity of dopaminergic motivational and action systems could be related to manic or psychotic symptoms in mood disorders.

Reports of dysfunction in multiple neurotransmitters, including acetylcholine, substance P, and excitatory amino acids (in addition to the monoamines already discussed) suggest that rather than being related to any particular neurotransmitter disturbance, mood disorders may be disorders of the overall cohesiveness of multiple transmitter systems involved in responding to danger. Such dysfunction may be mediated by altered intracellular signaling leading to alterations in expression of genes for proteins that promote neuronal stability, such as brain-derived neruotrophic factor 23. Antidepressant therapies do not affect one of these systems in isolation, but produce adaptational changes in multiple systems, including enhancement of neuroprotective factors (24). Greater coordination between affective, cognitive, and behavioral systems associated with these transmitters may be associated with normalization of mental state.

GENETICS

Relatives of people with mood disorders are consistently two to three times as likely to have mood disorders as are relatives of controls (25). If one parent has a bipolar mood disorder, the risk that a child will have a unipolar or bipolar mood disorder is approximately 28%; if both parents have mood disorders, the risk is two to three times as great (26). Patients with mood disorders also have an elevated familial incidence of substance abuse, and patients who are depressed and anxious have more relatives who are depressed, anxious, or both (23,27). Kendler et al. (28) reported that 1,033 pairs of female twins had increased concordance for both major depression and generalized anxiety disorder, agoraphobia, and social phobia, leading to the hypothesis that a common trait predisposing to anxiety and depression may be inherited and that experience determines whether anxiety or depression will predominate clinically (29).

Concordance studies reliably demonstrate that the overall risk of mood disorders is three times as great in monozygotic (MZ) as in dizygotic (DZ) twins of probands with mood disorders (30). For bipolar disorder, concordance rates average 0.67 to 1.0 for MZ and 0.20 for DZ twins. Concordance rates for unipolar depression are generally around 0.50 in MZ twins and 0.20 in DZ twins. The greater difference in concordance rates between MZ and DZ twins in bipolar disorder may reflect a greater genetic influence in bipolar disorder. Because concordance rates for mood disorders in twin studies are <100%, any genetic factors that are present must interact with environmental influences to create the risk for development of the actual disorder (30). Reviews of twin studies suggest that 21% to 45% of the variance in the risk of depressive disorders can be attributed to genetic factors and 55% to 75% of the variance can be attributed to environmental factors (29). A substantial amount (60%) of the effect of genetic factors appears to be direct, but 40% seems to reflect genetic factors that increase the likelihood that people will put themselves in situations that lead to depression (e.g., becoming romantically involved with someone who is likely to leave). And loss seems to be the life stress that is most likely to lead to depression (29).

Because familial forms of bipolar disorder seem more likely than unipolar depression to have a dominant pattern of transmission, most linkage studies have been performed in bipolar disorder. These studies suggest linkage to markers on the X-chromosome in about one third of cases, and to a variety of markers on chromosomes 4p, 12q24, 18q22, and 21q21. Markers on chromosomes 18p11, 13q21, and 22q11 have been linked to both schizophrenia and bipolar disorder, suggesting overlapping etiologic factors in both conditions, perhaps involving susceptibility to psychosis.

NEUROPATHOLOGY

Pathologic studies of brains of patients with mood disorders are complicated by factors such as sample size, methods of brain fixation, and reliability of diagnoses. A few findings, however, have appeared to be reliable (19). For example, loss of glial cells in the left prefrontal cortex has been demonstrated in both bipolar and unipolar mood disorders, whereas decreased size and density of gray matter neurons in the same region were found in major depressive disorder. Loss of glial cells and neurons in the hippocampus has been repeatedly noted in mood disorders. This finding is important because failure to inhibit corticotrophin-releasing factor (CRF) in response to rising adrenal steroid production in some depressed patients leads to chronic hyperactivity of the hypothalamic-pituitary-adrenal (HPA) axis, with elevated cortisol turnover and loss of the normal diurnal variation in cortisol production (31). Because cortisol is toxic to hippocampal neurons, excessive HPA activity can result in hippocampal damage, which further dysregulates the HPA axis.

NEUROIMAGING

A variety of findings have emerged from structural and brain imaging studies of depressed patients (32). One of the most consistent generalized brain abnormalities in structural imaging studies of unipolar depression has been enlarged lateral ventricles, which are reported most frequently in late-onset MDD. Similar ventricular enlargement is also found in schizophrenia and Alzheimer's disease. This and other structural abnormalities may define a substrate of depressed patients more susceptible to chronicity, treatment resistance, and dementia syndrome of depression, as well as to later onset of dementia. Subcortical white matter and periventricular hyperintensities have been found on magnetic resonance imaging (MRI) in older but not younger unipolar depressed patients. Although enlarged lateral ventricles are more common in major depression with psychotic features, white matter hyperintensities are not (32). A substrate of neurologic dysfunction associated with white matter hyperintensities could also account for an increased risk of delirium with ECT, extrapyramidal side effects with neuroleptic medications, chronicity, and overall poor treatment response in patients with this MRI finding (33). Regional abnormalities most consistently reported in unipolar depression have included decreased size of the caudate, putamen, and possibly the cerebellum. Reduced frontal lobe volume has been variably reported. Loss of glial and other cells in the hippocampus is reversible after early episodes, but becomes irreversible after depression has been present for extended periods of time.

Functional brain imaging with positron emission tomography (PET) has demonstrated reduced metabolic activity in the frontal lobes (i.e., hypofrontality), especially the dorsolateral prefrontal cortex, in unipolar depression, with normalization by antidepressants (34). Asymmetries in cerebral blood flow have also been found in depression, but such findings have been variable. Most, but not all, major depressive disorder (SPECT) studies using technetium Tc-99m hexamethyl propylenamine oxime (Tc-99m HMPAO) have demonstrated reduced global cerebral blood flow in depressed patients compared with controls, with localized perfusion deficits frontal, prefrontal, cingulate, temporal, and sometimes parietal and subcortical regions (35). I-123 p-iodoamphetamine-SPECT in 12 rapid-cycling bipolar patients in manic, depressed, and euthymic states showed greater uptake in the right than in the left anterior temporal lobe in both the depressed and manic phase, but not during euthymia, which suggests state-dependent metabolic asymmetry in both poles of abnormal mood (36).

DEPRESSION AND NEUROLOGIC DISEASE

A number of neurological illnesses are associated with an increased risk of mood disorders (4). Depression is a complication of 20% to 50% of neurologic patients and, when it is present, it predicts a worse prognosis and reduced treatment response (37). Certain disorders in particular are associated with high rates of secondary depression.

STROKE

Between 8% and 75% (average 405 to 50%) of patients with cerebrovascular accidents develop major depression; in one study, depressed patients who had a stroke had eight times the mortality rate of matched nondepressed patients who had a stroke (38). Anatomic location of the stroke appears to have a marked effect on the prevalence of associated depression: left prefrontal and basal ganglia strokes more frequently result in depressive disorders than do right hemisphere lesions. The closer the lesion is to the left frontal pole, the more severe the depression tends to be. Less severe depression can be associated with right and left posterior primarily parietal lesions. On the other hand, right hemisphere lesions are more frequently associated with development of mania. The same relationship holds true in older patients: cerebrovascular and degenerative disease on the left side of the brain causes late-onset depression and disease on the right side of the brain is often associated with late-onset mania (4).

Recognition of stroke-induced mood disorders can be complicated in patients with aprosodia, which is usually associated with right hemisphere disease that might or might not be apparent (39). Clues to depression in neurologic patients who do not report a depressed mood include vegetative signs, such as sleep disturbance or loss of interest not explained by the illness, failure to improve as expected, negativism, unexplained withdrawal, a history of depression, and a family history of depression. An empiric trial of treatment for depression may be justified for patients who are not recovering as they should when these factors are present.

Poststroke depression typically lasts 3 to 12 months, but can become chronic (38). This condition, however, has repeatedly been demonstrated to respond to antidepressants, which also improve functional outcome. Extensive experience has accrued with nortriptyline, but hypotensive and anticholinergic side effects of the tricyclic antidepressants make the newer antidepressants better choices. Serotonin reuptake inhibitors have been shown to be effective (40). Bupropion is well tolerated by patients with stroke, but not well studied in stroke. ECT is effective and safe for poststroke depression in the absence of increased intracranial pressure.

HUNTINGTON'S DISEASE

The Huntington Study Group found that 58% of patients with definite Huntington's disease felt depressed. The rate was equally high in those with soft signs and patients who were as yet asymptomatic (2). Depression can precede chorea in half the patients and depression is common in patients even those who do not know they are at risk. Basal ganglia dysfunction can contribute to the development of depression, probably in combination with inherent risk factors, because 40% of depressed patients with Huntington's disease have a history of depression (28). The suicide rate is as high as 9% in Huntington's disease (9% versus 0.1% in the general population (4). Some of this excess suicide risk is probably related to knowing the ultimate consequences of the illness, but depression undoubtedly contributes substantially to suicide in this and other neurologic diseases.

In early stages of Huntington's disease, typical symptoms of depression predominate. In middle or advanced stages of Huntington's disease psychomotor retardation, bradykinesia, and apparent alexithymia may be more evident. These patients experience intense emotional pain, but they are unable to describe it. Other symptoms include social withdrawal, anhedonia, weight loss, sleep disturbance, poverty of speech, mutism, and masked facies.

No controlled studies have been done on the treatment of depression in Huntington's disease. Experience suggests, however, that antidepressants can be effective. Dopaminergic medications, such as stimulants and bupropion, could have the potential to increase tics, whereas SSRI, which reduce DA release, could be more appropriate first choices. The atypical antipsychotic drugs, which have antidepressant properties, could be useful for both depression and tics, although no published experience for this indication exists. ECT has not been found to worsen Huntington's disease or any other neurologic disorder other than space-occupying lesion.

PARKINSON DISEASE

Parkinson disease (PD), the most common movement disorder in the elderly, is complicated by depression in as many as 50% of patients. The high comorbidity of depression and PD may reflect the role of the basal ganglia and locus coeruleus in mood regulation (41). Although major depressive episodes are common, dysthymia also occurs frequently. Depression appears more common in the late stages of disease, but also can predate the onset of motor symptoms. Untreated depression in PD is associated with more cognitive and motor dysfunction and greater impairment and caretaker distress (34).

Selegiline, a selective inhibitor of the B form of monoamine oxidase (MAO-B) used as a standard treatment for PD at doses of 5 to 10 mg/day, has antidepressant doses that range from 20 to 50 mg/day (42). At these doses selegiline becomes a nonselective, however, inhibiting MAO-A as well as MAO-B and can interact with tyramine-containing foods and serotonergic substances. No reports have been published of experience with antidepressant doses of selegiline in combination with L-dopa, so it is not clear whether potential hypertensive interactions could occur. A transdermal delivery system does not appear to have the expected interactions (42), although it has not been combined with antiparkinsonian drugs in controlled trials.

Other dopaminergic medications are also initial considerations for depression in patients with PD. Bupropion is one obvious choice. For patients with depression associated with acute worsening of the neurologic illness or those requiring augmentation of an antidepressant for a partial response, a dopaminergic stimulant, such as dextroamphetamine or methylphenidate, should be considered. Conversely, the antidopaminergic effect of SSRI can be troublesome for patients with PD (43,44). Reports of worsening of PD with SSRI have been balanced by reports of efficacy, but until controlled trials demonstrate predictable benefit these medications should probably be considered second-line treatments for depression in the presence of PD (4,45). If an SSRI is otherwise well tolerated and effective but it causes or aggravates parkinsonism, the side effect can be treated with a dopaminergic medication, such as bupropion, a stimulant, or pramipexole.

ECT is not only effective for depression in PD, but it has been noted to improve motor symptoms independently of its antidepressant effect (46,47). In a few case series, maintenance ECT has produced sustained improvement for nondepressed patients with PD. Such benefit may be related to a dopaminergic action of ECT or perhaps to transient breakdown of the blood–brain barrier leading to increased entry of antiparkinsonian drugs into the brain. Demented patients may be more susceptible to post-ECT delirium, which can be minimized by administering treatments less frequently.

MULTIPLE SCLEROSIS

MS frequently is associated with changes in mood. Depression is more common when frontal and temporal lesions are present (48). More diffuse lesions, especially in the right hemisphere, can produce manic symptoms, which occur in as many as 10% of patients. Regardless of the location of lesions, medications used to treat MS (e.g., interferon) regularly cause depression, probably as a result of the impact of altered cytokine production on mood. Antidepressants can treat the latter depression and can reduce production of proinflammatory cytokines (49).

Patients with MS can be exquisitely sensitive to side effects of all medications, including antidepressants. The tricyclic antidepressants, therefore, are later choices. Bupropion and venlafaxine may have positive cognitive effects that are particularly beneficial for patients with MS (50). For patients with depression associated with acute exacerbations of disease, stimulants may prove useful and these medications can counteract some of the lassitude associated with MS; however, tolerance to these effects can develop after several months of treatment. Dopamine agonists, such as pramipexole or ropinirole, can be effective for depression and fatigue in MS, as can the activating MAO inhibitors, such as selegiline.

EPILEPSY

Depression is the most frequent psychiatric disorder in patients with epilepsy, with prevalence rates of 21% to 33% in patients with persistent seizures and 4% to 6% among seizure-free patients (51,52). Depression is the most common interictal psychiatric disorder, occurring in one half of patients, and suicide attempts are not uncommon. Persistent depression appears to be a direct manifestation of altered limbic activity, especially in temporal lobe epilepsy, and patients with complex partial seizures and depression have more left-sided than right-sided lesions. This probably explains why uncontrolled seizures are more likely than controlled seizures to be accompanied by depression.

Although seizure control would seem to be the first step in treating epilepsy-associated depression, some patients feel worse when their seizures remit. When remission of seizures does not induce a remission of depression, antidepressants can be effective (4). The choice of an antidepressant is determined by anticipated effects on the seizure disorder and possible interactions with anticonvulsants. All antidepressants have the potential to cause or aggravate seizures at a sufficiently high dose, but for a few antidepressants, this dose overlaps the therapeutic dose. Clomipramine, amoxapine, maprotiline, and amoxapine lower the seizure threshold at doses that are used in clinical practice in a dose-dependent manner, and overdose with amoxapine can cause intractable seizures. At doses >450 mg/day, the risk of seizures with bupropion increases about tenfold (from 0.4% to 4% to 5%); below this dose, bupropion is no more likely to cause seizures than any other antidepressant. Nevertheless, most clinicians avoid all of these antidepressants in epileptic patients. Paroxetine may or may not lower the seizure threshold, and the other SSRI appear not to have a significant impact on the seizure threshold.

Drug interactions are also important considerations in the depression in the presence of epilepsy. Medications that inhibit the CYP450 2D6 isoenzyme, such as paroxetine and fluoxetine, can substantially elevate levels of anticonvulsants that are metabolized by this isoenzyme, such as phenytoin and, to some extent, carbamazepine. Antidepressants that inhibit P450 3A4, such as fluvoxamine and nefazodone, can raise levels of 3A4 substrates such as carbamazepine. By the same token, anticonvulsants that induce 2D6 and 3A4, such as carbamazepine and phenytoin, will reduce serum levels of most antidepressants, requiring higher doses in many cases. The MAO inhibitors do not have these kinds of interactions and do not have a great impact on seizures, although it is necessary to follow dietary restrictions with them.

TREATMENT OF DEPRESSION IN NEUROLOGIC DISORDERS

In milder acute forms of depression, psychosocial therapies, such as cognitive behavior therapy (CBT), are as effective as antidepressants. CBT is also an established treatment for insomnia that is as, or more, effective than the newer hypnotics. For more severe or persistent depression, a somatic therapy (usually an antidepressant) is necessary. The following general principles amplify issues in specific neurologic illnesses noted earlier in this chapter.

Antidepressants are generally thought to work by inhibiting monoamine reuptake pumps and enhancing neurotransmission with norepinephrine, serotonin, or dopamine. Neurotransmitter reuptake inhibition is immediate, however, whereas the onset of action of antidepressants can take a month or more. In addition, some antidepressants (e.g., mianserin, available in Europe) and ECT have no direct effect on neurotransmitters, whereas tianeptine, an effective tricyclic antidepressant available in Europe, is a serotonin reuptake enhancer. The time course of down-regulation of 5-hydroxytryptamine-2 (5-HT2) and β-receptors by antidepressants is more consistent with the onset of clinical effect of these medications, but reports of these actions are inconsistent and at times contradictory. More recent research is investigating the effects of antidepressants on induction of neuroprotective and other genes (e.g., brain-derived neurotrophic factor [BDNF]) as a possible mechanism of action. For example, chronic treatment with antidepressants increases expression of the gene for BDNF and its protein, facilitates neurogenesis in the hippocampus, increases expression of neuromodulin (growth-associated protein 43), reduces somatostatin expression, upregulates cyclic adenosine monophosphate (cAMP) signaling, and increases expression of genes for cAMP responsive element binding protein (CREB) and c-Fos (53,54).

Several classes of antidepressants are available (50). The heterocyclic antidepressants (TCA, such as amitripyline and imipramine and tetracyclic antidepressants, such as maprotiline) are no longer considered first-line treatments because they are more anticholinergic than newer medications, they more consistently cause weight gain and hypotension, and they are more likely to be lethal in overdose. These medications, however, appear to be more effective than the newer antidepressants for migraine prophylaxis and they are more useful than the serotonin reuptake inhibitors for chronic pain.

The SSRI vary considerably in their structure and their potency in inhibiting CYP450 enzymes. All but fluvoxamine have elimination half-lives longer than a day and can be given in one daily dose. The SSRI are all effective for depressive and anxiety disorders, but although they are easier to use and better tolerated than the heterocyclics, they are not more effective. The SSRI, however, are more effective than other antidepressants beside clomipramine for the treatment of obsessive compulsive disorder. This class of medications sometimes reduces migraine headaches, possibly through blockade of platelet serotonin uptake, but in some patients their serotonergic action exacerbates migraines. The SSRI can reduce unpredictable agitation and aggression in brain-damaged patients.

Third generation antidepressants comprise a diverse group of medications. Trazodone is a 5-HT2 receptor antagonist without significant effects on 5-HT reuptake. Its short elimination half-life and sedative action have made it popular as a hypnotic for patients who should not take benzodiazepines and related sleeping pills; the same properties have made it impractical for routine treatment of depression, because it must be given in divided dose at levels that most patients cannot tolerate. Trazodone has a risk of priapism of approximately 1 or 6,000 that is not dose related. Nefazodone, which combines 5-HT2 blockade, serotonin reuptake inhibition, and 5-HT1A partial agonism, is unique along with the TCA trimipramine in not reducing and possibly increasing slow wave sleep. This medication has been found helpful in fibromyalgia. The proprietary form (Serzone) was withdrawn from the market because of reports of occasional severe and, at times fatal, hepatotoxicity; all preparations were withdrawn in most countries, but the generic form is still available in the United States. Bupropion, a norepinephrine and to a lesser extent a DA reuptake inhibitor, does not cause cardiac side effects or weight gain. As mentioned, the risk of seizures is approximately 4% at doses >450 mg/day, but lower doses do not have a risk of seizures higher than that of other antidepressants. Bupropion is a first choice for depression in patients with PD and dementia. Mirtazepine antagonizes 5-HT2, 5-HT3, and $\alpha 2$ receptors, actions that make it useful for depression in patients with carcinoid. Other patients receiving cancer chemotherapy who have nausea and weight loss, respond very well to this medication, and a chewable form is useful for patients with difficulty swallowing. On the other hand, patients who cannot tolerate weight gain or sedation have difficulty taking mirtazepine. Venlafaxine is a serotonin reuptake inhibitor at low doses. At higher doses it acquires norepinephrine reuptake inhibitor properties and as the dose rises further it inhibits DA reuptake. Duloxetine is a serotonin and a norepinephrine reuptake inhibitor at all doses. Both of these medications have relatively short half-lives that can result in significant withdrawal and rebound symptoms when the medication is discontinued and at times between doses, even with the sustained release form of venlafaxine. Both medications are useful for chronic pain.

Monoamine oxidase inhibitors (MAOI) inhibit MAO, an intracellular enzyme that oxidizes monoamines, such as norepinephrine, serotonin, and DA. Currently available MAOI irreversibly inhibit two major forms of monoamine oxidase: MAO-A is located in the gut, lungs and brain, whereas MAO-B is located in the brain and in blood platelets. Although an antidepressant effect is more likely with 80% or more inhibition of platelet MAO, it is not clear whether MAO inhibition is a mechanism of therapeutic action or a marker of a more important action elsewhere. Inhibition of intestinal MAO-A, however, impairs inactivation of dietary tyramine, which is a naturally occurring pressor amine found in certain foods. As a result, severe hypertension can occur when patients taking MAOI ingest tyramine-containing foods. Because MAO-B metabolizes serotonin, inhibition of this enzyme can lead to serotonin toxicity when MAOI are combined with serotonergic substances or foods. Reversible inhibitors of MAO-A (RIMA), such as moclobemide (not available in the United States), are displaced from MAO-A by tyramine, allowing the enzyme to metabolize the amine and eliminating hypertensive reactions at moderate doses. Selective MAO-B inhibitors, such as selegiline, do not affect tyramine absorption at antiparkinsonian doses (5 to 10 mg), but at antidepressant doses (20 to 50 mg), this drug is no longer selective and dietary restrictions are necessary. A selegiline patch has recently been approved that appears not to cause hypertensive reactions or serotonin syndrome at modest but not higher doses, presumably because inhibition of intestinal MAO is substantially lower than with oral doses.

Three MAOI classes are available in the United States. Hydrazines (phenelzine, isocarboxazid), non-hydrazines (tranylcypromine), and propargylamines (selegiline). With the exception of selegiline use in PD, MAOI are usually prescribed by psychiatrists. These medications are particularly useful for refractory depression, depression with prominent anxiety, and bipolar depression.

In uncomplicated major depression, the response rate to a single antidepressant is approximately 60%. Data are emerging suggesting that patients who have a partial response to an antidepressant may be more likely to benefit from augmenting with a medication in another class, whereas those who have had no response whatsoever may do better with a change of antidepressant. The best studied augmenting agent is lithium. Other agents with less empiric support that are in common use for increasing the response to an antidepressant in unipolar depression include stimulants, carbamazepine, lamotrigine, buspirone, and adding another antidepressant (e.g., maprotiline added to venlafaxine or a low dose of a tricyclic antidepressant added to an SSRI).

ECT is the most effective and fastest acting treatment for depression (55). ECT is effective in 90% of patients who have not received adequate pharmacologic treatment for depression, whereas the response rate is reduced to 50% in those who have been adequately treated with medications, indicating that treatment resistance is a feature of the patient as much as the illness (56).

Two important considerations when ECT is used in neurologic settings: *First*, the most common and important side effect of ECT is dose-dependent memory impairment. This usually consists of brief retrograde and anterograde amnesia around the time of the treatment; with continued treatment, however, memory impairment may become more generalized (57). Occasionally, an isolated, but significant element of autobiographical memory is lost, whereas other memories remain intact (58). Cognitive side effects of ECT can be reduced with right unilateral electrode placement, less frequent administration (e.g., twice rather than three times per week), and lower stimulus intensities, although with unilateral stimulus placement it appears that doses more >150% above the seizure threshold are more likely to be effective (56). Extensive clinical experience, autopsy studies of patients who received thousands of ECT over their lifetimes, neuroimaging studies, and animal research has repeatedly demonstrated that modified ECT (with the use of brief general anesthesia and muscle relaxants) as it is currently used does not cause neurologic injury (59,60).

The *second issue* concerns the use of ECT in patients with neurologic disease. As has already been noted, ECT improves parkinsonism separate from its antidepressant effect, probably through a dopaminergic action (61). Because induced seizures raise the seizure threshold, ECT can help abate seizure disorders, although prolonged seizures sometimes occur in patients with epilepsy following a single ECT (62). Conversely, because an electrical seizure is necessary for the therapeutic action of ECT, anticonvulsants can interfere with the response to ECT. Although delirium is an acute side effect of ECT, this treatment can be very effective in treating delirium of any cause (47). ECT does not worsen the long-term course of dementia, but demented patients tend to have more severe acute cognitive side effects. Deterioration has been reported in as many as 50% of patients with space-occupying lesions who receive ECT, but the other 50% tolerate the procedure. Increased intracranial pressure probably elevates the risk further because ECT itself acutely increases intracranial pressure.

Vagus nerve stimulation (VNS) was recently approved for refractory depression. A controlled study of VNS in major depression that was refractory to at least four different antidepressants found improvement that became apparent after a year of treatment in about 30% of patients (63). The finding that a few patients who did not benefit from other treatments (including ECT in half the sample) got at least partial relief with VNS indicates that VNS can be a valuable option for a few patients, although the number of patients studied so far is too small to determine exactly who benefits.

CLINICAL RECOMMENDATIONS OF THE VIGNETTE

Because of substantial insomnia and anorexia, the patient was treated with mirtazepine and the dose was gradually increased to 30 mg at bedtime. Her sleep and appetite improved rapidly, and she gained 4 kg over the next 3 months. She still complained, however, of low energy, problems concentrating, and mood swings. Lamotrigine was added and, as the dose was slowly increased to 100 mg per day, the residual symptoms remitted. On this regimen, she was able to continue interferon without a return of depression. She then decided that psychotherapy was needed to address losses involved with the illness and changed relationships resulting from physical disability.

SUMMARY

Depression is a problem for as many as half of all neurologic patients. When it is present, it can have a profound impact on response to treatment for the neurologic disorder. In some cases, depression is a component of the primary illness, whereas in others it is a separate disorder or it represents a side effect of neurologic treatment. In all of these situations, depression has a gratifying response to treatment, which then can improve the neurologic outcome—and, certainly, also the quality of life.

The armamentarium of antidepressants has been greatly expanded in recent years, resulting in the availability of an appropriate treatment for most patients. Patients who do not respond as expected to a single antidepressant should have either augmentation of that medication or a change to a different antidepressant. ECT is usually administered to patients who cannot tolerate, or who have a poor response to, antidepressants. The oldest somatic therapy in psychiatry, ECT, is a consideration for most severely depressed neurologic patients regardless of the psychiatric illness. Patients with complicated or severe depression, family turmoil, or depression accompanied by another psychiatric disorder, such as substance abuse, should have psychiatric consultation to determine the best course of treatment.

REFERENCES

1. Bhandari M, Busse JW, Jackowski D, et al. Association between industry funding and statistically significant pro-industry findings in medical and surgical randomized trials. *Can Med Assoc J.* 2004;170:477–480.
2. Mueller TI, Leon AC. Recovery, chronicity, and levels of psychopathology in major depression. *Psychiatr Clin North Am.* 1996;19(1):85–102.
3. Keilp JG, Sackeim HA, Brodsky BS, et al. Neuropsychological dysfunction in depressed suicide attempters. *Am J Psychiatry.* 2001;158:735–741.
4. Dubovsky SL, Dubovsky AN. *Concise Guide to Mood Disorders.* Washington, DC: American Psychiatric Press; 2002.
5. Hirschfeld R. Efficacy of SSRIs and newer antidepressants in severe depression: Comparison with TCAs. *J Clin Psychiatry.* 1999;60:326–335.
6. Club AJ. Review: Newer and older antidepressants have similar efficacy and total discontinuation rates but different side effects. *ACP Journal Club.* 2000;133(1):10.
7. Dubovsky SL, Thomas MT. Psychotic depression: Advances in conceptualization and treatment. *Hospital and Community Psychiatry.* 1992;43:1189–1198.
8. Cassem EH. Depressive disorders in the medically ill: An overview. *Psychosomatics.* 1995;36(2):S2–S10.
9. Keller MB, Hanks DL, Klein D. Summary of the DSM-IV mood disorders field trial and issue overview. *Psychiatr Clin North Am.* 1996;19(1):1–27.
10. Kessler RC, McGonagle KA, Zhao S, et al. Lifetime and 12-month prevalence of DSM-III-R psychiatric disorders in the United States. Results from the National Comorbidity Study. *Arch Gen Psychiatry.* 1994;51(1):8–19.
11. McDaniel JS, Musselman DL, Proter MR. Depression in patients with cancer. *Arch Gen Psychiatry.* 1995;52:89–99.
12. Weissman MM, Leaf PJ, Bruce ML. The epidemiology of dysthymia in five communities: Rates, risks, comorbidity, and treatment. *Am J Psychiatry.* 1988;145:815–819.
13. Olfson M. Subthreshold psychiatric symptoms in a primary care group practice. *Arch Gen Psychiatry.* 1996;53:880–886.
14. Schildkraut JJ. The catecholamine hypothesis of affective disorders: A review of supporting evidence. *Am J Psychiatry.* 1965;122:509–514.
15. Salomon RM, Miller HL, Krystal JH, et al. Lack of behavioral effects of monamine depletion in healthy subjects. *Biol Psychiatry.* 1997;41:58–64.
16. Siever LJ, Davis KL. Overview: Toward a dysregulation hypothesis of depression. *Am J Psychiatry.* 1985;142:1017–1025.
17. Brown S-L, Steinberg RL, van Praag HM. The pathogenesis of depression: Reconsideration of neurotransmitter data. In: den Boer JA, Sitsen JMA, eds. *Handbook of Depression and Anxiety.* New York: Marcel Dekker; 1994:317–347.
18. Brown S-L, Bleich A, van Praag HM. The monoamine hypothesis of depression. The case for serotonin. In: Brown S-L, van Praag HM, eds. *The Role of Serotonin in Psychiatric Disorders.* New York: Brunner/Mazel; 1990:91–128.
19. Vawter MP, Freed WJ, Kleinman JE. Neuropathology of bipolar disorder. *Biol Psychiatry.* 2000;48:486–504.
20. Mann JJ, Arango V, Marzuk PM. Evidence for the 5-HT hypothesis of suicide. A review of post- mortem studies. *Br J Psychiatry.* 1989;155[Suppl 8]:7–14.
21. Mann JJ, Malone KM. Cerebrospinal fluid amines and higher-lethality suicide attempts in depressed inpatients. *Biol Psychiatry.* 1997;41:162–171.
22. McBride PA, Brown RP, DeMeo M. The relationship of platelet 5-HT2 receptor indices to major depressive disorder, personality traits, and suicidal behavior. *Biol Psychiatry.* 1994;35:295–308.
23. Dwivedi Y, Rizavi HS, Conley RR, et al. Altered gene expression of brain-derived neurotrophic factor and receptor tyrosine kinase B in postmortem brain of suicide subjects. *Arch Gen Psychiatry.* 2003;60:804–815.
24. Leonard BE. Effect of antidepressants on specific neurotransmitters: Are such effects relevant to the therapeutic action? In: den Boer JA, Sitsen JMA, eds. *Handbook of Depression and Anxiety.* New York: Marcel Dekker; 1994:379–404.
25. Gershon ES. Genetics. In: Goodwin FK, Jamison KR, eds. *Manic-Depressive Illness.* New York: Oxford University Press; 1990:373–401.
26. Jamison KR. Manic-depressive illness, genes, and creativity. In: Hall LL, ed. *Genetics and Mental Illness Evolving Issues for Research and Society.* New York: Plenum Press; 1996:111–132.
27. Gorman JM, Coplan JD. Comorbidity of depression and panic disorder. *J Clin Psychiatry.* 1996;57:[Suppl 10]:34–41.
28. Kendler KK, Neale MC, Kessler RC, et al. Major depression and generalized anxiety disorder. Same genes, (partly) different environments? *Arch Gen Psychiatry.* 1992;49:716–722.
29. Kendler KK, Kessler CC, Neale MC, et al. The prediction of major depression in women. Toward an integrated etiologic model. *Am J Psychiatry.* 1993;150:1139–1148.
30. Tsuang MT, Faraone SV. The inheritance of mood disorders. In: Hall LL, ed. *Genetics and Mental Illness Evolving Issues for Research and Society.* New York: Plenum Press; 1996: 79–109.
31. Gold PW, Licinio J, Wong ML, et al. Corticotropin releasing hormone in the pathophysiology of melancholic and atypical depression and the mechanisms of action of antidepressant drugs. *Ann N Y Acad Sci.* 1995;77:716–729.
32. Soares JC, Mann JJ. The anatomy of mood disorders: Review of structural neuroimaging studies. *Biol Psychiatry.* 1997;41:86–106.
33. Dupont RM, Jernigan TL, Heindel W, et al. Magnetic resonance imaging and mood disorders: Localization of white matter and other subcortical abnormalities. *Arch Gen Psychiatry.* 1995;52(9):747–755.
34. Buchsbaum MS, Wu J, Siegel BV, et al. Effect of sertraline on regional metabolic rate in patients with affective disorder. *Biol Psychiatry.* 1997;41:15–22.
35. Bonne O, Krausz Y, Gorfine M, et al. Cerebral hypoperfusion in medication resistant, depressed patients assessed by Tc99m HMPAO SPECT. *J Affect Disord.* 1996;41:163–171.
36. Gyulai L, Alavi A, Broich K, et al. I-123 iofetamine single-photon computed emission tomography in rapid cycling bipolar disorder: A clinical study. *Biol Psychiatry.* 1997;41: 152–161.
37. Kanner AM. Should neurologists be trained to recognize and treat comorbid depression of neurologic disorders? Yes. *Epilepsy & Behavior.* 2005;6:303–311.
38. Morris PLP, Robinson RG, Samuels J. Depression, introversion and mortality following stroke. *Aust N Z J Psychiatry.* 1993;27:443–449.
39. Ross ED. The aprosodias: Functional anatomic organization of the affective components of language in the right hemisphere. *Arch Neurol.* 1981;38(38):561–569.
40. Pollock BG, Mulsant BH, Sweet R, et al. An open pilot study of citalopram for behavioral disturbances of dementia. Plasma levels and real-time observations. *Am J Geriatr Psychiatry.* 1997;5(1):70–78.
41. Klassen T, Verhey FRJ, Rozendaal N. Treatment of depression in Parkinson's disease: A meta-analysis. *J Neuropsychiatry Clin Neurosci.* 1995;7:281–286.
42. Amsterdam JD. A double-blind, placebo-controlled trial of the safety and efficacy of selegiline transdermal system without dietary restrictions in patients with major depressive disorder. *J Clin Psychiatry.* 2003;64:208–214.
43. Dubovsky SL, Thomas M. Beyond specificity: Effects of serotonin and serotonergic treatments on psychobiological dysfunction. *J Psychosom Res.* 1995;39(4):429–444.
44. Tom T, Cummings JL. Depression in Parkinson's disease. Pharmacological characteristics and treatment [Review]. *Drugs Aging.* 1998;12(1):55–74.
45. Chouza C, Scaramelli A, Carmano JL. Parkinsonism, tardive dyskinesia, akathisia and depression induced by flunarizine. *Lancet.* 1986;1:1303–1304.
46. Moellentine C, Rummans TA, Ahlskog JE, et al. Effectiveness of ECT in patients with parkinsonism. *J Neuropsychiatry Clin Neurosci.* 1998;10:187–193.
47. Dubovsky SL. Using electroconvulsive therapy for patients with neurological disease. *Hospital and Community Psychiatry.* 1986;37:819–825.
48. Scott TF, Allen D, Price TRP. Characterization of major depression symptoms in multiple sclerosis patients. *J Neuropsychiatry Clin Neurosci.* 1996;8:318–323.
49. Capuron L, Hauser P, Hinze-Selch D, et al. Treatment of cytokine-induced depression. *Brain Behav Immun.* 2002;16:575–580.
50. Dubovsky SL. *Clinical Guide to Psychtropic Medications.* New York: WW Norton; 2005.
51. Rundell JR, Wise M G. Causes of organic mood disorder. *J Neuropsychiatry Clin Neurosci.* 1989;1(4):398–400.
52. Fann JR, Tucker GJ. Mood disorders with general medical condition. *Current Opinion in Psychiatry.* 1995;8:13–18.
53. Chen B, Wang JF, Sun X, et al. Regulation of GAP-43 expression by chronic desipramine treatment in rat cultured hippocampal cells. *Biol Psychiatry.* 2003;53:530–537.
54. Santarelli L, Saxe M, Gross C, et al. Requirement of hippocampal neurogenesis for the behavioral effects of antidepressants. *Science.* 2003;301:805–809.
55. Dubovsky SL. Electroconvulsive therapy. In: Kaplan HI, Sadock BJ, eds. *Comprehensive Textbook of Psychiatry,* 6th ed. Vol. VI. Baltimore: Williams & Wilkins; 1995:2129–2140.
56. Devanand DP, Sackeim HA, Prudic J. Electroconvulsive therapy in the treatment-resistant patient. *Psychiatr Clin North Am.* 1991;14:905–923.
57. Coleman EA, Sackeim HA, Prudic J, et al. Subjective memory complaints prior to and following electroconvulsive therapy. *Biol Psychiatry.* 1996;39(5):346–356.
58. McElhiney MC, Moody BJ, Steif BL, et al. Autobiographical memory and mood: Effects of electroconvulsive therapy. *Neuropsychology.* 1995;9(4):501–517.
59. Weiner RD. Does electroconvulsive therapy cause brain damage? *Behav Brain Sci.* 1984;7(1):1–53.
60. Devanand DP, Dwork AJ, Hutchinson ER, et al. Does ECT alter brain structure? *Am J Psychiatry.* 1994;151(7):957–970.
61. Aarsland D, Larsen JP, Waage O, et al. Maintenance electroconvulsive therapy for Parkinson's disease. *Convulsive Therapy.* 1997;13(4):274–277.
62. Regenold WT, Weintraub D, Taller A. Electroconvulsive therapy for epilepsy and major depression. *Am J Geriatr Psychiatry.* 1998;6(2):180–183.
63. Marangell LB, Rush AJ, George MS, et al. Vagus nerve stimulation (VNS) for major depressive episodes: One year outcomes. *Biol Psychiatry.* 2002;51:280–287.

CHAPTER **166**

The Anxiety Disorders: Clinical Presentation, Diagnosis, Treatment, and Beyond

Abigail L. Donovan • Joshua L. Roffman • Dan V. Iosifescu • Jeremiah M. Scharf • Theodore A. Stern

OBJECTIVES

- To discuss the common clinical presentations of anxiety disorders
- To describe the distinguishing characteristics of each anxiety disorder
- To explain how to distinguish medical illnesses with symptoms of anxiety from primary anxiety disorders
- To explain the first-line and second-line treatments for anxiety disorders

CASE VIGNETTE

A 26-year-old white woman presents to the emergency department (ED) with acute onset shortness of breath, palpitations, diaphoresis, dizziness, and a sense of impending doom. A previous episode 1 month earlier occurred when she was trapped in an elevator; none of her subsequent episodes were associated with small spaces. She has had two similar episodes in the past week. Her medical history is notable only for mitral valve prolapse and her psychiatric history is otherwise unremarkable. She takes no medications and has no allergies. She recently started a new job as a paralegal, which she says is demanding but going very well. Her family history is notable for coronary artery disease in both of her parents and non–insulin-dependent diabetes mellitus (NIDDM) in her father. Her mother suffers from anxiety.

On arrival to the ED, her blood pressure is 140/90 mm Hg, her pulse is 115 beats per minute, her respiratory rate is 18 breaths per minute, and her oxygen saturation is 98% on room air. An electrocardiogram (ECG) reveals sinus tachycardia with no ST- or T-wave changes. A chest X-ray study is unremarkable. All laboratory tests, including a complete metabolic panel, complete blood count, serum toxicology panel, and thyroid-stimulating hormone, are within normal limits. After 30 minutes, her symptoms gradually decrease, her vital signs normalize, and she feels fine. She feels embarrassed about coming to the ED, and causing "such a fuss over nothing." She asks to go home without further tests or follow-up.

DEFINITION

Anxiety is a normal human response to stress; from an evolutionary standpoint, it serves as an important warning of impending danger or threat. Normal anxiety is transitory and directly related to an environmental cue. Pathologic anxiety occurs, however, with no identifiable environmental stimulus or when the reaction to a stimulus is either excessive or inappropriate. Pathologic anxiety is disabling, rather than protective. Pathologic anxiety can be distinguished from a normal response by: the absence of an identifiable environmental trigger; by intense and persistent symptoms; and by impaired coping, so that the individual develops maladaptive behavioral strategies, including avoidance and withdrawal (1).

The clinical presentation of anxiety is significantly heterogeneous. Symptoms of anxiety can be categorized into four domains: physical, emotional, behavioral, and cognitive. *Physical symptoms* include tachycardia, tachypnea, dizziness, and diaphoresis (i.e., manifestations of autonomic arousal). *Emotional symptoms* range from mild irritability to terror, and can include a feeling of losing control, or "going crazy." *Behavioral symptoms* are characterized by avoidance, withdrawal, or compulsive acts, all of which are maladaptive attempts to reduce or to prevent distress. Finally, *cognitive symptoms* include persistent worries, apprehensions, or obsessions.

Anxiety disorders encompass a diverse group of conditions in which the feeling of anxiety is the common clinical feature.

Anxiety disorders can be further broken down into several distinct disorders. *Panic disorder* is characterized by recurrent panic attacks, in which the individual experiences a sudden onset of shortness of breath, chest pain, diaphoresis, or other symptoms of autonomic arousal. Panic disorder can also be accompanied by agoraphobia, literally a fear of open spaces. *Generalized anxiety disorder* (GAD) is characterized by persistent and excessive worrying. *Specific phobia,* formerly known as simple phobia, is fear of a specific object or situation. *Social phobia* is a fear of social interactions or events. *Obsessive-compulsive disorder* (OCD) is characterized by intrusive thoughts and by ruminations, as well as by intense behavioral urges. *Posttraumatic stress disorder* (PTSD) is defined by a persistent reexperiencing of a traumatic event.

EPIDEMIOLOGY

Anxiety disorders are among the most prevalent psychiatric disorders in the general population; the lifetime prevalence of anxiety disorders in the United States is 25% (2). The anxiety disorders share several epidemiologic characteristics in common. Panic disorder, GAD, specific phobia, and social phobia are all more frequently diagnosed in females in community samples, with a 2:1 female-to-male ratio (2). All of the anxiety disorders, with the exception of PTSD, have an average age of onset in adolescence to the mid-twenties; however, many individuals note that some anxiety symptoms date back to childhood. In addition, the disease course for all anxiety disorders is chronic, although the symptoms can wax and wane; stress can worsen the intensity of the symptoms. In general, anxiety disorders are responsive to a variety of treatments, although high rates of relapse are seen after discontinuation of treatment. Also, high rates of comorbidity exist, especially with depression and substance abuse disorders.

Several epidemiologic characteristics distinguish the anxiety disorders from each other (3). Specific phobia is one of the most common anxiety disorders; it has a lifetime prevalence of 10%. The age of onset varies according to the specific subtype of phobia. Phobias to the natural environment (including heights, animals, blood, and injections), all have an onset in childhood, whereas phobias to specific situations (e.g., airplanes, elevators, or enclosed spaces), have a bimodal distribution, with one peak in childhood and the second peak in the mid-twenties. Unlike other anxiety disorders which, although chronic, do respond well to treatment, phobias that persist well into adulthood have low remission rates (~20%). Social phobia is also very common and the prevalence ranges between 3% and 13%; this wide variance is likely caused by different thresholds used to determine impairment. PTSD has a lifetime prevalence of 1% to 14%. Unlike other anxiety disorders, the onset of PTSD can occur at any age. Symptoms usually occur within 3 months of the traumatic event; however, in some cases, symptoms are delayed for many months or years. GAD has a lifetime prevalence of 5%, whereas panic disorder has a lifetime prevalence of 3.5%. Panic disorder also has a staggering co-occurrence with agoraphobia; approximately one-third of patients with agoraphobia also have panic disorder. OCD is unique in that the prevalence is equal in males and females and is between 1% and 3% in the general population. The modal age at onset is slightly earlier for males than it is for females.

ETIOLOGY AND PATHOGENESIS

The exact pathogenesis of anxiety remains largely unknown and it is the focus of much active research. The current hypotheses regarding the pathophysiology of anxiety disorders are based on observations of the effectiveness of anxiolytic medications and subsequent analyses of the neurobiological effects of these agents.

Although the precise cause of anxiety disorders has yet to be clarified, it is apparent that a significant genetic contribution to this group of diseases exists. Current research estimates that heritability across anxiety disorders ranges between 30% and 40% (4). The strongest and most extensive evidence exists for the genetic contributions to panic disorder, where first-degree relatives have an approximately five-fold greater risk of developing the disorder than occurs in less closely related individuals (4).

NEUROPHYSIOLOGY

Several specific neurotransmitters and neuropeptides, as detailed below, act on a variety of brain circuits (including limbic structures and the locus coeruleus [LC]), in the mediation of anxiety responses.

Central Noradrenergic Systems

The physiologic symptoms of anxiety, including cardiac and neurologic hyperarousal, are all consistent with increased noradrenergic function. The LC is the key source of central nervous system (CNS) adrenergic innervation. Neurons in the LC are activated in anxiety states; stimulation of the LC can induce panic attacks. Alcohol and benzodiazepines decrease firing rates of noradrenergic neurons and pharmacologic blockade of the LC decreases panic attacks (2).

GABAergic Systems

γ-aminobutyric acid (GABA)-producing neurons within the limbic system, particularly in the septohippocampal pathway, participate in controlling worry and generalized anxiety. Furthermore, neuronal connections exist between the LC, the septohippocampal circuit, and limbic structures (e.g., the amygdala and hippocampus). When GABA receptors in the limbic system bind benzodiazepines, activation of this circuit decreases, with a subsequent reduction in amplified states of worry and vigilance (5).

Serotonin Systems and Neuropeptides

5-hydroxytryptamine$_{1A}$ (5-HT$_{1A}$) receptors are found in the superficial cortical layers, the hippocampus, and the amygdala; serotonin serves as a critical modifier of the systems outlined above. Neuropeptides, such as neuropeptide Y, C-reactive protein (CRP) and arginine vasopressin (AVP), may further modulate these systems (9). The efficacy of pharmacologic interventions with diverse mechanisms of action, including selective serotonin reuptake inhibitors (SSRIs), serotonin norepinephrine reuptake inhibitors (SNRIs), and benzodiazepines, is one piece of evidence to support the hypothesis that these neuronal circuits are interconnected and involved in the pathogenesis of anxiety.

COGNITIVE-BEHAVIORAL THEORY

Cognitive-behavioral explanations of anxiety focus on the interpretation of information, the emotions that are provoked, and the resulting behavior that defines anxiety. The central tenet is that certain types of thoughts and beliefs (cognitions) serve to activate anxiety and can lead to avoidance or to withdrawal (behaviors), causing the maintenance of both fear and dysfunctional thinking patterns (6). These cognitions are considered faulty when they over-predict the likelihood of negative events. Moreover, trying to decrease anxiety with avoidance or compulsive behavior is maladaptive because it actually reinforces the anxiety and leads to chronic hyperarousal. For example, the patient featured in the clinical vignette may believe that getting stuck in a elevator means that she is going to die (because if the elevator is malfunctioning, it must be about to fall). The belief triggered her anxiety and led her to avoid all elevators since that episode. As a result, she has not had a subsequent positive experience riding in an elevator and she remains deathly afraid of them.

PATHOLOGY

The neuroanatomic pathology associated with anxiety disorders is still unknown. Neuroimaging studies, however, have yielded important results that offer several clues to understanding the pathologic basis of anxiety disorders. These findings have generated compelling hypotheses for the neuroanatomic basis of both OCD and panic disorder.

Current research suggests that the pathophysiology of OCD involves dysfunction within frontosubcortical circuits. Numerous parallel and reciprocal circuits are largely composed of projections between the frontal cortex, striatum (e.g., the caudate, putamen, and nucleus accumbens), basal ganglia, and thalamus. Functional imaging studies have revealed that, in OCD, increased activity occurs in the orbitofrontal cortex (OFC), anterior cingulate (AC), caudate, and thalamus, as compared with healthy controls (7). Furthermore, subjects who experience a decrease in their symptoms after treatment display corresponding reductions in hyperactivity in these areas (7).

The OFC, which projects to the ventromedial caudate, is thought to mediate emotional responses to environmental stimuli; in OCD, OFC activity appears to be elevated. The elevated OFC activity produces a hyperactive orbitofrontal–subcortical circuit, leading to increased concern over environmental stimuli and giving rise to OCD symptoms (7). The efficacy of capsulotomy, a psychosurgery performed in severe cases of treatment-resistant OCD in which the connections between the frontal cortex and basal ganglia are interrupted, is further indirect evidence of the importance of these circuits in the pathogenesis of OCD (5).

Current hypotheses regarding the pathophysiology of panic disorder focus on dysfunction within the pathways that mediate fear responses. These hypotheses are based on the observation that the conditioned fear response has remarkably similar physiologic and behavioral manifestations compared with panic attacks. Functional neuroimaging and animal model studies have led to a proposed model of the fear pathway. It is hypothesized that sensory input of the feared stimulus travels to the anterior thalamus and then to the lateral nucleus of the amygdala. Signals are then sent to the central nucleus of the amygdala that, in turn, initiates the physiologic and behavioral response. This fear response is controlled through projections to the brainstem. Specifically, the central nucleus of the amygdala projects to the (*a*) parabrachial nucleus (leading to an increase in respiratory rate), (*b*) hypothalamus (causing sympathetic nervous system activation, the release of adrenocorticoids, and autonomic arousal), and (*c*) LC (leading to norepinephrine release and to further autonomic arousal) (8). The amygdala also sends projections to the periaqueductal gray region, which further mediates behavioral responses, including defensive behaviors and, possibly, avoidance. Current research suggests that patients with panic disorder may have hyperactive or hyperresponsive fear pathways, predisposing them to frequent panic attacks (8). The efficacy of SSRIs in panic disorder, and current knowledge of their mechanism of action provides further indirect evidence of the importance of these circuits. For example, 5-HT neurons inhibit activity in the LC and the periaqueductal gray area, causing decreased activation of the fear-response pathway (8).

The sensory information processing centers are also implicated in the pathogenesis of panic disorder. Animal models have revealed that the amygdala receives projections from the prefrontal cortex and other cortical regions that are involved in processing and evaluating sensory information. It is possible that, in panic disorder, dysfunction in these cortical processing pathways, leads to a misinterpretation of sensory information and to inappropriate activation of the fear response pathway in the amygdala (8).

CLINICAL MANIFESTATIONS

Anxiety disorders are associated with significant impairment in physical, vocational, social, and family function. Although these disorders may share some common clinical and pathologic manifestations, they can be differentiated from one another by several key characteristics, as defined in the *Diagnostic and Statistical Manual-Fourth Edition* (DSM-IV).

Panic disorder is characterized by recurrent and unexpected, or unprovoked, panic attacks. In addition, the individual has persistent concern about (*a*) having another panic attack, (*b*) the consequences of the panic attack, or (*c*) significant behavioral changes related to the panic attack. Panic attacks are characterized by discrete episodes, with an acute onset that generally peak within 10 minutes, and are associated with at least four symptoms of hyperarousal. The origin of these hyperarousal symptoms can be cardiac (e.g., palpitations, tachycardia, chest pain, or discomfort), pulmonary (e.g., shortness of breath or a choking sensation), gastrointestinal (e.g., nausea or abdominal distress), neurologic (e.g., dizziness, lightheadedness, paresthesias, or trembling), autonomic (e.g., sweating, chills, or hot flashes), or psychological (e.g., derealization, depersonalization, fear of losing control or going crazy, and a fear of dying). A significant number of individuals with panic disorder also have agoraphobia, which is a fear of places or situations from which escape may be difficult or embarrassing, or in which help may not be readily available in the event of a panic attack. Agoraphobia can lead to avoidance of such situations and eventually to an impairment of an individual's ability to leave his or her home. Panic disorder with agoraphobia can be extremely disabling and have an impact on an individual's work, social, and family life.

Generalized anxiety disorder is defined as excessive and persistent worry about a number of events or activities (including health, work, school, or family events), which the individual finds difficult to control. The worry is out of proportion to the magnitude of the issue or event. The anxiety is also accompanied by physiologic symptoms (including, sleep disturbance, restlessness, fatigue, irritability, or muscle tension). The symptoms must interfere with daily functioning at work, at home, or in social situations, and be present for >6 months (3).

A specific phobia is a marked and persistent fear (which the individual recognizes as excessive) of a clearly discernable object or situation. This persistent fear must also be accompanied by avoidance of the object or situation, which has a significant impact on the individual's daily function. When the individual is exposed to the object, he or she experiences symptoms of anxiety, which can include a situationally-bound panic attack (3). Specific phobias can be further divided into distinct subtypes based on the phobic object: animal type (e.g., snakes or spiders), natural environment type (e.g., heights or water), blood-injection-injury type, and situational type (e.g., airplanes or elevators). The most common specific phobias, in order of descending prevalence, are fear of animals, storms, heights, illnesses, injury, and death (3). The symptoms cannot be better accounted for by another disease (including, hypochondriasis, OCD, or paranoia).

Social phobia is a marked and persistent fear of social or performance situations in which the individual meets new people or is under potential scrutiny. Affected individuals fear that they will be embarrassed and humiliated or that others will recognize their anxiety. When the individual is in the feared social situation, he or she experiences anxiety, which can include a situationally-bound panic attack (3). This fear leads to an avoidance of social situations or to intense distress during social situations. The individual must also recognize that the fear is excessive. Moreover, the symptoms must have a significant impact on the patient's daily function. The symptoms also cannot be better accounted for by another disorder (including, agoraphobia, body dysmorphic disorder, or separation anxiety).

OCD is characterized by recurrent obsessions, compulsions, or both that interfere with the individual's daily function. Obsessions are persistent thoughts, impulses, or images that are intrusive and distressing to the individual. The obsessions are not merely exaggerated worries about existent problems. The affected individual tries to ignore, suppress, or neutralize the obsession with another thought or action. The individual recognizes that the obsession is inappropriate and also that the thoughts come from within his or her own mind, as opposed to a psychotic thought insertion. *Common obsessions* include fears of contamination, repeated doubts about locking doors or turning off appliances, and disturbing sexual imagery. *Compulsions* are repetitive behaviors or mental acts, which the individual feels impelled to perform in response to an obsessive thought or in accordance with an internally held, rigid rule system. The behaviors and acts are performed to decrease distress or to prevent a feared event. Common compulsions include handwashing, checking, counting, and repeating words. The affected individual recognizes that the obsessions or compulsions are illogical, but cannot stop them. These symptoms cause distress and take a significant amount of time to complete, or they must interfere with the individual's daily function.

PTSD occurs after an individual witnesses or has been exposed to a traumatic event (which involved death or serious injury) and the initial reaction includes intense fear or helplessness. PTSD is then characterized by a persistent reexperiencing of that traumatic event, through thoughts or images, dreams, feelings of the event reoccurring (flashbacks), and psychological or physiologic distress when exposed to stimuli associated with the trauma. The affected individual avoids reminders associated with the trauma (including, thoughts, activities, places, and people). The individual also experiences a numbing of responsiveness, as exemplified by diminished interest in previously significant activities, feelings of detachment from other people, blunted emotions, or a sense of a dismal future. In addition, the individual also has persistent symptoms of increased arousal (including, insomnia, irritability, angry outbursts, increased startle, and hypervigilance). These symptoms are all present for >1 month and they cause significant distress or impact on daily function.

DIAGNOSTIC APPROACH

More than 90% of patients with anxiety disorders present with somatic complaints (9); most patients will first seek treatment in primary care settings or in emergency rooms, as did the patient in the clinical vignette. In fact, anxiety is the presenting complaint for 11% of patients visiting their primary care physicians (10). Many medical illnesses can mimic the symptoms of anxiety; thus, anxiety disorders should be distinguished from the direct physiologic effects of an underlying medical condition. Several factors can be used to differentiate a medical illness that mimics anxiety (e.g., an organic anxiety syndrome) from a primary anxiety disorder (9) (Table 166-1).

A variety of medical conditions can cause organic anxiety symptoms, as detailed in Table 166-2. The diagnostic evaluation of the patient presenting with anxiety should focus on the medical, psychiatric, medication, and drug history, and then explore recent social stressors. It is important to take into account the anxiogenic effects of medical conditions and medications, as well as the effects of illicit substances and withdrawal from these agents. The patient's characteristics and presenting complaints can direct a targeted, yet thorough, physical and neurologic examination. An initial medical workup can

TABLE 166-1. Factors Used to Differentiate a Medical Illness with Anxiety Symptoms from a Primary Anxiety Disorder

	Primary Anxiety Disorder	*Organic Anxiety Symptoms*
Age of Onset	During the second to third decades of life	After the third decade of life
Family History	Relatives with anxiety disorders	No family history of anxiety
Childhood History	History of excessive worry, phobias, or separation anxiety	Normal childhood development
Social Stressors	Recent life events exacerbating the symptoms	Absence of significant life events
Behavioral Changes	Avoidance or withdrawal	No associated behavioral changes
Response to Medication	Good response to anxiolytic medication	Little or no response to anxiolytic medications

TABLE 166-2. Medical Conditions That Can Cause Symptoms of Anxiety

Endocrine	Hyperadrenalism, hyperthyroidism, hyperparathyroidism, carcinoid syndrome, hypoglycemia, Addison disease, Cushing syndrome
Drug Intoxication	Caffeine, cocaine, theophylline, sympathomimetics, anticholinergics, corticosteroids, thyroid hormones
Drug Withdrawal	Alcohol, narcotics, sedative-hypnotics, antihypertensives
Cardiovascular	Arrhythmias, congestive heart failure, anemia
Pulmonary	Chronic obstructive pulmonary disease, asthma, pulmonary embolism
Metabolic	Acidosis, hyperthermia, electrolyte abnormalities
Neurologic	Vestibular dysfunction, seizures (especially temporal lobe epilepsy), Parkinson disease, Huntington disease, Wilson disease, Sydenham chorea, dystonia disorders, frontotemporal dementia

include, but may not be limited to, a complete metabolic panel, thyroid function tests, a complete blood count, and an ECG.

In addition, primary anxiety disorders should be considered as part of the differential diagnosis for several medical and neurologic disorders. Specifically, anxiety disorders should be considered in patients with unexplained cardiac symptoms (e.g., repeated chest pain) or pulmonary symptoms (e.g., asthma attacks). Furthermore, patients who present to neurologists with memory or word-finding complaints may have an underlying anxiety disorder. Similarly, patients with panic disorder or PTSD might present for evaluation of temporal lobe epilepsy (and vice versa).

TREATMENT

Anxiety disorders are chronic and associated with significant morbidity and impaired quality of life. Anxiety disorders respond to both pharmacologic treatment and cognitive-behavioral therapy (CBT). Many patients benefit from a bimodal treatment that includes both medication and CBT. Most patients with anxiety disorders improve after treatment; however, high relapse rates are seen after discontinuation of treatment, suggesting that many individuals will benefit from maintenance therapy (11).

The mainstays of pharmacologic treatment for anxiety disorders are antidepressants and benzodiazepines.

SELECTIVE SEROTONIN REUPTAKE INHIBITORS

SSRIs are an appealing treatment option because of their favorable side effect profile, a broad spectrum of efficacy for anxiety as well as comorbid disorders (e.g., depression), a low potential for abuse, few drug interactions, and safety in overdose. The downside to use of SSRIs include a delayed onset of action (3 to 6 weeks), sexual dysfunction, a potential for increased anxiety on initiation of therapy, and restlessness. There have also been some cases, particularly in adolescents, of suicidal ideation correlated with the initiation of SSRI therapy. Given the potential for increased anxiety on initiation of treatment, the starting dose of SSRIs should be low and the dose can then be gradually increased, based on clinical response and side effects.

SSRIs are considered the first-line treatment for panic disorder, GAD, and OCD (12). SSRIs are also effective for social phobia and have been shown to reduce symptoms of PTSD.

Although most SSRIs may be efficacious in the treatment of anxiety disorders, paroxetine (Paxil) and escitalopram (Lexapro) have been US Food and Drug Administration (FDA)-approved for the treatment of GAD. Fluoxetine (Prozac), paroxetine (Paxil and Paxil CR), and sertraline (Zoloft) have been FDA-approved for the treatment of panic disorder. Fluoxetine (Prozac), fluvoxamine (Luvox), paroxetine (Paxil), and sertraline (Zoloft) have been FDA-approved for the treatment of OCD. Paroxetine (Paxil) and sertraline (Zoloft) have been FDA-approved for the treatment of PTSD. Paroxetine (Paxil and Paxil CR), and sertraline (Zoloft) have been FDA-approved for the treatment of social phobia.

The average effective doses for treatment of panic disorder, GAD, social phobia, and PTSD are in the typical antidepressant range (e.g., fluoxetine 20 to 40 mg/day, paroxetine 20 to 40 mg/day, paroxetine CR 25 to 50 mg/day, sertraline 50 to 150 mg/day, fluvoxamine 150 to 200 mg/day, citalopram 20 to 40 mg/day, and escitalopram 10 to 20 mg/day). SSRIs, however, are generally effective in OCD at higher doses compared with antidepressant doses: fluvoxamine (up to 300 mg/day), fluoxetine (up to 80 mg/day), sertraline (up to 200 mg/day), and paroxetine (up to 60 mg/day). Response to SSRI in OCD may also require a longer period of treatment (at least 8 to 10 weeks).

SEROTONIN-NOREPINEPHRINE REUPTAKE INHIBITORS AND ATYPICAL ANTIDEPRESSANTS

Venlafaxine is a dual serotonin and norepinephrine reuptake inhibitor and is efficacious for the treatment of panic disorder, GAD, and social phobia, at standard antidepressant doses (between 75 and 300 mg/day) (13). Venlafaxine (Effexor XR) has been FDA-approved for the treatment of GAD and social phobia. Duloxetine (Cymbalta) a newer SNRI, has been FDA-approved for the treatment of anxiety disorders and is effective for the treatment of GAD. Bupropion (Wellbutrin), an antidepressant with noradrenergic and dopaminergic activity, has previously been considered to be ineffective for the treatment of panic disorder based on a small study (14); however, a more recent study has demonstrated efficacy for panic disorder (15). It has also been found to be efficacious in reducing the symptoms of PTSD (12).

TRICYCLIC ANTIDEPRESSANTS

TCAs are pharmacologically active on a variety of neurotransmitters, including reuptake inhibition of norepinephrine, serotonin, and, to a lesser extent, dopamine, as well as being direct receptor blockers of norepinephrine (α_1 and α_2), serotonin, acetylcholine, and histamine (H_1). TCAs are the most extensively studied agents for the treatment of anxiety disorders. Their advantages include lower cost compared with SSRIs, and efficacy in SSRI nonresponders. The disadvantages include multiple side-effects (e.g., anticholinergic symptoms, orthostatic hypotension, cardiac conduction delay, weight gain, increased anxiety on initiation, restlessness, jitteriness), a delayed onset of action (3 to 6 weeks), and cardiotoxicity in overdose. Given these disadvantages, they are no longer considered as first-line treatment for anxiety disorders and should be used carefully, especially in older patients with concomitant medical conditions. Given the potential for increased anxiety on initiation, such as with an SSRI, treatment should be initiated with lower doses and gradually titrated up, guided by clinical response and side effects.

TCAs are effective for the treatment of panic disorder, GAD, OCD, and PTSD (12). Of note, TCAs have not been found to be effective for social phobia. Clomipramine is considered to have superior antipanic properties compared with other TCAs, perhaps related to its selectivity for serotonergic uptake (1). For the same reason, it is considered to be especially efficacious for the treatment of OCD. The average effective dose for panic disorder, GAD, and PTSD is in the typical antidepressant range (e.g., 100 to 300 mg/day for imipramine), whereas effective dosing for the treatment of OCD is considerably higher (e.g., clomipramine up to 250 mg/day). Blood levels of imipramine, nortriptyline, and desipramine can be checked after a steady-state is achieved (~5 days) and may be useful in cases of a poor response or side effects.

MONOAMINE OXIDASE INHIBITORS

MAOIs bind to the monoamine oxidase enzyme, resulting in noncompetitive, irreversible inhibition. MAOI, such as phenelzine and tranylcypromine, are powerful anxiolytic agents and they may be useful in treatment-resistant patients. MAOIs, however, have multiple side effects (including orthostatic hypotension, weight gain, and sexual dysfunction) and multiple drug interactions; they are toxic in overdose and they require dietary restriction to prevent hypertensive crisis. As such, their use is typically reserved for treatment-resistant individuals with severe anxiety. A more selective MAOI (transdermal selegiline, EMSAM) is currently FDA approved for the treatment of major depressive disorder and it may prove to have fewer drug–drug interactions and dietary restrictions than traditional MAOI (because of increased selectivity for MAO-B and the lower dose allowed by the transdermal delivery system). The efficacy of transdermal selegiline in anxiety disorders is not yet established, however.

MAOIs are effective for the treatment of panic disorder, GAD, and, in the case of phenelzine, social phobia (12). Phenelzine has also been shown to reduce symptoms of PTSD. Effective doses are similar to those for depression (for phenelzine between 60 and 90 mg/day and for tranylcypromine between 30 and 60 mg/day).

BENZODIAZEPINES

Benzodiazepines are frequently used alone or in conjunction with antidepressants for the treatment of anxiety disorders. They are especially useful because of their rapid onset of action, favorable side effect profile, and efficacy. The drawbacks of benzodiazepines include initial sedation and ataxia, increased sedation in the elderly, short-term memory impairment, withdrawal syndromes, and the potential for abuse. Benzodiazepines should be used with caution in the elderly, because they may be more sensitive to sedation, ataxia, risk of falls, and memory impairment. The elderly may also experience a paradoxic agitation from benzodiazepines.

Benzodiazepines are effective for panic disorder, GAD, and social phobia (12). In the case of OCD, benzodiazepines can be used successfully to treat comorbid anxiety, but are not effective for primary treatment of OCD. In PTSD, benzodiazepines can reduce anxiety and improve sleep, but they can also lead to disinhibition and irritability, and, possibly, delayed recovery. No evidence indicates that any one benzodiazepine is more effective than another for panic, GAD, social phobia, OCD, or PTSD. Agents with a short half-life (e.g., alprazolam), however, can lead to rebound anxiety between doses and to withdrawal symptoms. Longer-acting agents (e.g., clonazepam) may, therefore, be preferable. Typical doses of benzodiazepines in anxiety disorders are clonazepam 1 to 5 mg/day, diazepam 5 to 40 mg/day, and lorazepam 3 to 12 mg/day. The starting doses, however, should typically be much lower (e.g., clonazepam 0.25 mg/day, diazepam 2.5 mg/day, and lorazepam 1 mg/day).

Rapid taper of benzodiazepines can be associated with a withdrawal syndrome characterized by rebound anxiety, insomnia, weakness, hypertension, and tachycardia. In some severe cases, the withdrawal syndrome can cause confusion, seizures, and psychosis. Withdrawal syndromes can be seen after taking benzodiazepines for a few as 4 weeks. Benzodiazepines, therefore, should be tapered gradually, even over a period of months; furthermore, the greatest risk of withdrawal is at the end of the taper, so the taper should be slower near the end.

Before prescribing benzodiazepines, physicians need to consider the potential for abuse and dependence, and it is important to complete a thorough alcohol and substance abuse history. Although a history of substance abuse is not an absolute contraindication to benzodiazepine treatment, it should signal caution and the need for careful monitoring on the part of the clinician.

ADDITIONAL AGENTS

Atypical Antipsychotics

Atypical antipsychotic medications (with dopaminergic, serotonergic, and histaminergic activity) are not yet FDA-approved for the treatment of anxiety disorders. In clinical practice, however, many physicians find them useful for the treatment of anxiety, particularly in individuals with resistant disease or with histories of substance abuse.

Buspirone

Buspirone is a 5-HT_{1A} partial agonist that has been found effective in several studies for the treatment of GAD, treatment-resistant OCD, and hyperarousal in PTSD (9); however, the experience in clinical practice has not been as positive. Clinically, it is most commonly used as an adjunctive therapy (in doses of 15 to 60 mg/day, divided twice or three times daily).

Gabapentin

Gabapentin leads to increased release of nonsynaptic GABA and it has been shown to be moderately effective for panic disorder and social phobia in clinical trials, as well as for sleep disturbance in PTSD (16); clinical experience has found that it is most effective as an adjunctive treatment, rather than as monotherapy. Gabapentin should be started at 300 mg at bedtime or twice daily; typical doses for anxiety are 600 to 2,700 mg/day, usually divided twice or three times daily.

Valproate

Valproate has been an effective treatment for panic disorder and PTSD, whereas clinical studies have yielded mixed results for treatment of social phobia (16). Valproate requires careful monitoring of blood levels and its use can be associated with a variety of adverse effects (including, liver disease and toxicity in overdose). Valproate should be started at 250 mg twice daily; typical doses for anxiety are 500 to 2,000 mg/day, usually divided twice daily (and based on blood levels).

Beta-Blockers

Beta-blockers may be useful for adjuvant treatment for GAD, although they are not indicated for primary therapy. They are not clinically useful in the primary treatment of panic or PTSD, but they can block symptoms of autonomic arousal and can be used as adjunctive therapy (9). They may be particularly effective for performance anxiety (such as that triggered by public speaking or test-taking). Propranolol can be used for anxiety starting at 10 mg twice daily; typical doses are 10 to 60 mg daily.

COGNITIVE-BEHAVIORAL THERAPY

CBT is a time-limited therapy (typically 12 to 15 sessions) aimed at addressing the faulty cognitions and maladaptive behaviors that serve to perpetuate anxiety. In addition, a significant component of the therapy can include exposure to the feared stimulus and prevention of the behavioral response (exposure response prevention), leading to the gradual acclimation to, and eventual decrease of, anxiety symptoms. CBT is an effective treatment for all anxiety disorders (6) and is especially important for the treatment of specific phobia where pharmacotherapy has not proved effective.

Specific components of CBT can include educational interventions, cognitive restructuring, exposure-response-prevention, and anxiety management skills. Educational interventions include psychoeducation about the nature of the disorder (to demystify the somatic sensations associated with anxiety), education about the self-perpetuating patterns that maintain the disorder, and explanation of the role of avoidance in heightening the anxiety response. Cognitive restructuring is aimed at identifying maladaptive cognitive patterns and decreasing the catastrophic beliefs about the consequences of symptoms and more realistically estimating the probability of feared outcomes. Exposure-response-prevention entails the gradual exposure to situations or objects associated with anxiety aimed at extinguishing the conditioned response. Finally, anxiety management skills include muscle relaxation and slow breathing techniques that can be used to decrease the hyperarousal found in anxiety; these skills allow individuals to cope with the initial sensations of anxiety.

CLINICAL RECOMMENDATIONS OF THE VIGNETTE

The patient has panic disorder without agoraphobia. Her physical symptoms, the progressive course, the rapid resolution without medical intervention, and her family history are all consistent with panic disorder. Being trapped in an elevator triggered her initial panic attack, whereas her subsequent panic attacks were not provoked by a distressing stimulus. The recent stressor of a new job could play a role in her current presentation. The thorough physical examination and medical workup has ruled out potential medical causes of her symptoms (including cardiac, respiratory, and thyroid disease).

Although the patient is feeling better after her symptoms have subsided, they will likely return without further intervention. Thus, it is recommended that she be started on an SSRI, at a low dose, under the care of her primary care physician or a psychiatrist. She may also benefit from the time-limited use of a long-acting benzodiazepine during the initial period of treatment. She should be carefully monitored by a physician for any side effects, including an initial increase in anxiety and changes in mood or behavior. The dose of the SSRI can be increased, as her clinical response and side effects dictate.

SUMMARY

Anxiety disorders are prevalent and associated with a high degree of morbidity and functional impairment. They are a heterogeneous group of disorders that can frequently mimic medical conditions or be seen in conjunction with underlying medical disease. Anxiety disorders benefit from a range of pharmacologic and therapeutic interventions, including antidepressants, benzodiazepines, and CBT. These disorders are chronic and subject to relapse on cessation of treatment.

REFERENCES

1. Iosifescu DV, Pollack MH. Anxiety disorders. In: Stern TA, Herman JB, eds. *MGH Psychiatry Update and Board Preparation*, 2nd ed. New York: McGraw-Hill; 2004.
2. Fyer AJ, Gabbard GO, Pine DS, et al. Anxiety disorders. In: Kaplan HI, Sadock BJ, eds. *Comprehensive Textbook of Psychiatry*, 7th ed. Baltimore: Williams & Wilkins; 2000.
3. American Psychiatric Association. *Diagnostic and Statistical Manual of Mental Disorders*, 4th ed. DSM-IV-TR (Text Revision). Washington, DC: American Psychiatric Association; 2000.
4. Hettema JM, Neale MC, Kendler KS. A review and meta-analysis of the genetic epidemiology of anxiety disorders. *Am J Psychiatry.* 2001;158(10):1568–1578.
5. Charney DS, Bremner JD. The neurobiology of anxiety disorders. In: Charney DS, Nestler EJ, eds. *Neurobiology of Mental Illness*, 2nd ed. New York: Oxford University Press; 2004.
6. Otto MW, Reilly-Harrington NA, Harrington JA: Cognitive-behavioral strategies for specific disorders. In: Stern TA, Herman JB, Slavin PL, eds. *The MGH Guide to Primary Care Psychiatry*, 2nd ed. New York: McGraw-Hill; 2004.
7. Saxena S, Rauch SL. Functional neuroimaging and the neuroanatomy of obsessive-compulsive disorder. *Psychiatr Clin North Am.* 2000;23(3):563–584.
8. Gorman JM, Kent JM, Sullivan GM, et al. Neuroanatomical hypothesis of panic disorder, revised. *Am J Psychiatry.* 2000;157(4):493–505.
9. Iosifescu DV, Pollack MH. An approach to the anxious patient: symptoms of anxiety, fear, avoidance, or increased arousal. In: Stern TA, ed. *The Ten-Minute Guide to Psychiatric Diagnosis and Treatment.* New York: Professional Publishing Group, Ltd; 2005.
10. Lawrence L, McLemore T. 1981 Summary: National Ambulatory Medical Care Survey. *Adv Data.* 1983;16(88):1–9.
11. Pollack M, Otto M, Bernstein J, et al. Anxious patients. In: Stern TA, Fricchione GL, Cassem NH, et al., eds. *Massachusetts General Hospital Handbook of General Hospital Psychiatry*, 5th ed. Philadelphia: Mosby; 2004.
12. Hyman SE, Arana GW, Rosenbaum JF. *Handbook of Psychiatric Drug Therapy*, 4th ed. Boston: Little, Brown; 2000.
13. Taylor CB. Treatment of anxiety disorders. In: Schatzberg AF, Nemeroff CB, eds. *The American Psychiatric Press Textbook of Psychopharmacology*, 2nd ed. Washington, DC: American Psychiatric Press; 1998.
14. Sheehan DV, Davidson J, Manschreck T, et al. Lack of efficacy of new antidepressant (bupropion) in the treatment of panic disorder with phobias. *J Clin Psychopharmacol.* 1983;3(1):28–31.
15. Simon NM, Emmanuel N, Ballenger J, et al. Bupropion sustained release for panic disorder. *Psychopharmacol Bull.* 2003;37(4):66–72.
16. Ameringen MV, Mancini C, Pipe B, et al. Antiepileptic drugs in the treatment of anxiety disorders. *Drugs.* 2004;64(19):2199–2220.

CHAPTER 167

Delirium

Benjamin Liptzin • Steven V. Fischel • Sheldon Benjamin

OBJECTIVES

- To describe the signs and symptoms of delirium
- To discuss that delirium is most common in the elderly
- To clarify the most common causes of delirium, particularly medications and infections
- To explain how treating the underlying medical condition is key to treatment

CASE VIGNETTE

An 87-year-old woman has a 2-month history of "going downhill." Before that, she was driving with no problem and paying her bills accurately. She was unable to pack up her house for a long-planned move to a retirement community near her son. When she arrived, she was confused and did not know what city she was in. She was thought to be depressed and was started on escitalopram, but became incoherent and unable to play cards. She was admitted to a psychiatric inpatient unit because she was up at night trying to push out window screens so she could jump out. On examination, she was unable to remember any of three objects she was asked to recall. She was unable to write a complete sentence or copy a design and was totally perplexed by a clock drawing test. Given the absence of depressive symptoms, escitalopram was stopped. She was found to have a urinary tract infection and to be dehydrated, necessitating a transfer to medicine for treatment with intravenous fluids and antibiotics. Subsequently, she gradually began to return to her baseline. Eight months later she was living independently with her husband in the retirement community. Although she was able to converse and play cards, she was not able to return to managing the finances.

DEFINITION

According to the *Diagnostic and Statistical Manual of Mental Disorders*, Fourth Edition, Text Revision (DSM-IV-TR), delirium is

> "A disturbance of consciousness (i.e., reduced clarity of awareness of the environment) with reduced ability to focus, sustain or shift attention; a change in cognition (such as memory deficit, disorientation, language disturbance) or the development of a perceptual disturbance that is not better accounted for by a pre-existing, established, or evolving dementia; and the disturbance develops over a short period of time (usually hours to days) and tends to fluctuate during the course of the day" (1).

EPIDEMIOLOGY

Delirium is very common in general hospitals (2). In medical inpatients, the prevalence of delirium has been reported as 11% to 16%, and the incidence of new cases that develop while the patient is in the hospital ranged from 4% to 10%. Rates of postoperative delirium vary, but in one study were reported to be as high as 73%. Up to 80% of patients with terminal illness develop delirium near death. Among community-dwelling elderly, the prevalence of delirium has been reported as 1.1%. Episodes of delirium have been noted in 22% of community-dwelling patients with Alzheimer's disease.

Risk factors for delirium include preexisting cognitive impairment, older age, psychoactive drug use, severe illness or comorbidity, azotemia or dehydration, male gender, history of alcohol abuse, infection, fever, and metabolic abnormality (3). Most of these risk factors for delirium (e.g., older age) cannot be modified. Being aware of patients who are at risk can alert clinicians, however, to the need for careful monitoring to detect early symptoms of delirium and to treat reversible factors (4,5).

ETIOLOGY AND PATHOGENESIS

Delirium is the final common pathway for brain dysfunction owing to multiple causes. Almost any serious medical illness or drug intoxication can cause delirium in a vulnerable individual. The most common causes are medication-related side effects, infections, substance intoxication, substance withdrawal, postanesthesia or postoperative states, metabolic disorders including dehydration, electrolyte imbalances, hypoglycemia or hyperglycemia, kidney failure, hepatic failure, anemia, vitamin deficiencies, or endocrinopathies; cardiovascular disorders including congestive heart failure, myocardial infarction, cardiac arrhythmia, shock, or pulmonary emboli; central nervous system (CNS) disorders including head trauma, seizures, stroke, brain injury, meningitis, encephalitis, or space-occupying lesions such as a tumor, subdural hematoma, or abscess; fracture or other trauma; hypoxia or hypercapnia; obstructive sleep apnea; sleep deprivation; or sensory deprivation.

The side effects of medication can be exacerbated by changes in pharmacokinetics and pharmacodynamics in older patients. Changes in metabolism and excretion can result in a higher blood level than for a younger patient given the same oral dose. Older persons may also be more sensitive to the effects of a drug so that even at a "therapeutic" blood level, an older patient may develop delirium. An example of this is lithium toxicity in an older patient, even at therapeutic or very low blood levels. Medication toxicity is also more likely in older patients who may be on multiple drugs that interact or potentiate each other's effects.

The pathogenesis of delirium in not understood, but several hypotheses exist about the underlying mechanism. Brown (6) suggested that delirium is

> "A reversible dysregulation of neuronal membrane function 1. initiated by a functional lesion of the brain structures most sensitive to the insult in question–this is the principle of 'selective vulnerability'; 2. is intimately linked to the specific functions and properties of a few neurotransmitters; 3. is a progression of characteristic signs and symptoms as structures more resistant to deliriogenic impairment are progressively affected–the principle of 'progressive vulnerability.'

He suggested that a number of neurotransmitters may be involved in the development of delirium. Excess dopamine, which can be produced under conditions of hypoxia, can facilitate the excitotoxic effects of glutamate. He also noted that acetylcholine is an important neuromodulator of cortical and hippocampal neuronal function and can disrupt higher cognitive function if its release is altered or if its effects are pharmacologically blocked, for example by a medication with anticholinergic activity (6).

PATHOLOGY

No known structural pathology explains the symptoms of delirium. Functional hypotheses are described in the section above.

CLINICAL MANIFESTATIONS

The course of delirium varies widely in individual patients and depends on the cause of the delirium. Although delirium is generally thought of as having an acute onset, many patients experience a prodromal period with some symptoms of delirium before the onset of the full syndrome. Generally, the full syndrome appears within 2 days of the appearance of the patient's first new symptom. The resolution of delirium may take longer than the usual picture of a transient condition. Some patients may have residual symptoms for 6 months after an episode of delirium associated with hospitalization.

Several subtypes of delirium have been described and studied (7). The hypoactive type of delirium is characterized by decreased activity, unawareness, decreased alertness, somnolence, lethargy, staring into space, apathy, and sparse, slow, or decreased speech. The delirium in these patients is often undiagnosed, but they may be at increased risk of developing pressure skin ulcerations or aspiration pneumonia or at risk of not taking medication properly at home after hospital discharge. Neurologists refer to these patients as having an *acute confusional state* or *encephalopathy* in contrast to hyperactive patients whose condition they have diagnosed as delirium. Hyperactive symptoms include increased psychomotor activity, hypervigilance, hyperalertness, hallucinations, delusions, fast or loud speech, irritability, combativeness, impatience, swearing, singing, laughing, uncooperativeness, euphoria, anger, wandering, easy startling, distractibility, tangentiality, nightmares, or restlessness. Patients with these symptoms tend to be recognized and referred for psychiatric consultation because they may pull out catheters or intravenous lines, try to leave the hospital, or be at risk for falling. In contrast to these pure forms of delirium, most patients exhibit some features of hypoactive and of hyperactive delirium at different times and are considered to have a mixed type of delirium. Patients with hyperactive delirium tend to have a better outcome than those with hypoactive delirium.

Delirium is associated with significant morbidity and mortality. Hospitalizations tend to be longer and patients show worsening physical function. Patients with delirium are more likely to have poor functional recovery after a hip fracture. Delirious patients are more likely to develop urinary incontinence, falls, pressure sores, and other complications during hospitalization. For this and other reasons, patients with delirium have a higher risk of institutional placement. Overall, delirium is associated with a poorer long-term prognosis.

DIAGNOSTIC APPROACH

The key to diagnosing patients suspected of having delirium is to take a careful clinical history (8). The first step is the recognition that symptoms of delirium are present. These need to be differentiated from prior symptoms of cognitive impairment that were caused by dementia. The best way to clarify this is by talking with family or other caretakers to identify a change in mental status. Review of prior medical records is often helpful as well. The history should focus on any recent new medications or changes in medication dosage, or the use of alcohol or illicit drugs. Prescription and nonprescription medications can cause delirium in an older patient who may have increased sensitivity to a drug's effects. Changes in physical condition should be asked about, although delirium may be the initial presenting condition for an infection, congestive heart failure, and so on. Prior psychiatric history can identify patients whose symptoms may be caused by a recurrence of mania or depression. In the elderly, especially in those with dementia, the possibility of head trauma caused by an unwitnessed fall should be considered. Delirium in the post-myocardial infarction period may be the first indication of rapid arrhythmia. Individuals with dementia are especially susceptible to develop delirium in the setting of any of the above medical conditions. The development of delirium can trigger a diagnostic evaluation for dementia if treatment of the underlying cause of delirium does not return the patient to his or her customary mental status baseline.

Following the history the patient should be observed for behavioral symptoms of delirium, such as restlessness, suspiciousness, somnolence, hyperalertness, unstable mood, belligerence, distractibility, or hallucinations. Even if a patient seems completely normal when interviewed, it is important to review the medical record and ask nursing staff about any abnormal behavior or disorientation. It is not unusual for patients to seem pleasant and cooperative on rounds in the morning, but become agitated and disoriented at night. Mental status examination may reveal a panoply of cognitive deficits. In the setting of waxing and waning arousal and attention that characterizes delirium, deficits such as nonaphasic misnaming, constructional apraxia, right-left confusion, geographic disorientation, and memory impairment may be seen, without implying specific lesions in areas typically associated with these functions. Transient deficits in executive functions are common. Hallucinations, if present, are more likely to be visual rather than auditory. One indication of recovery from delirium may be the patient's ability to learn and recall new information (anterograde learning).

A thorough physical examination and laboratory evaluation need to be done to investigate for possible causes of the delirium. The physical examination should check vital signs and focus on the patient's neurologic, cardiac, and pulmonary systems. A standard laboratory assessment includes a complete blood count with differential and platelet count; serum chemistries including albumin, blood urea nitrogen (BUN), calcium, creatinine, electrolytes, and sedimentation rate; thyroid and liver function tests; a urinalysis and culture, if necessary; electrocardiogram; and chest X-ray. Serum drug levels may help identify potentially toxic levels of certain drugs, such as lithium, digitalis, tricyclic antidepressants, anticonvulsants, cyclosporine, or quinidine. If alcohol or drug intoxication is suspected, a urine toxicology screen should be done. Pulse oximetry can detect otherwise unsuspected hypoxemia. If a specific CNS disorder (e.g., head trauma, subdural hematoma, or brain tumor) is suspected, then a computed tomography (CT) or magnetic resonance imaging (MRI) scan should be done. An electroencephalogram (EEG) is indicated for patients suspected of having seizures, but otherwise the EEG in a delirious individual would be expected to reveal slowing, a nonspecific indicator of brain dysfunction.

One of the challenges in determining cause is that often multiple laboratory abnormalities turn up as part of the workup. Furthermore, the abnormalities may be just outside the normal range and, therefore, unlikely to be the cause of the patient's delirium. A judgment that some condition is etiologically related to the delirium may depend on the time course of symptoms. An abnormality that is likely to be etiologic should precede the onset of symptoms and should return to normal when the delirium clears. Any physicians caring for the patient with delirium should identify and correct any conditions that may be contributing to the delirium. On the other hand, it may be prudent to reduce the patient's medications to only essential ones, given the high likelihood than medications could be the cause of the delirium.

TREATMENT

The primary treatment for delirium is to identify and treat the underlying medical condition that is causing the delirium. Sometimes this may involve stopping some medication that a patient is on or substituting another drug within the therapeutic class, such as using a selective serotonin reuptake inhibitor (SSRI) rather than a tricyclic antidepressant.

Psychological and behavioral interventions may also be helpful in managing delirious patients. Carefully explaining to patients and family members what to expect in the postoperative period may reduce anxiety and improve the detection of symptoms of delirium so that proper treatment can be started. Having family members stay with the patient who becomes delirious can also provide reassurance and orientation. Nursing interventions can also be helpful in managing delirious patients. These include keeping the patient in a quiet room with lights on in the daytime and a night-light on after bedtime; avoiding excessive sensory stimulation but providing some gentle music or television; having orientation cues, such as a calendar or clock, clearly visible to the patient; correcting sensory impairments with eyeglasses or a hearing aid; keeping the patient near the nursing station for regular checks and staff interaction; encouraging family presence for reassurance and orientation; having available familiar objects from home, such as family pictures; explaining staff interventions in a clear, firm, but caring manner; carefully monitoring intake of fluids and food to ensure adequate intake; and using physical restraints only if the patient is unsupervised and at risk of falling or pulling out intravenous lines, urinary catheters, or other tubes. Any use should be consistent with hospital policy and include frequent nursing checks and adequate documentation.

The quietly confused patient can usually be treated safely using the above interventions. Patients who are highly agitated or psychotic will often require a pharmacologic intervention to help treat their behavioral disturbance, particularly on an inpatient medical or surgical unit.

An evidence-based practice guideline has been developed for pharmacologic management of alcohol withdrawal. This involves careful symptom monitoring using the *Clinical Interview for Withdrawal from Alcohol*, revised (CIWA-r) scale and then titrating the dose of benzodiazepine to treat the symptoms of withdrawal (9). Benzodiazepines have been recommended over most other sedative-hypnotics because of their documented efficacy, greater margin of safety, and low abuse potential.

If the delirium is not caused by alcohol withdrawal, but the patient is difficult to manage because of agitation, several treatment options are available. If the patient is clearly psychotic, the first choice is generally to use a neuroleptic drug despite the absence of controlled clinical trials. Haloperidol has been used extensively for many years, but more recently atypical neuroleptics (e.g., risperidone, olanzapine, or quetiapine) have also been used to reduce the incidence of extrapyramidal side effects. Haloperidol may have the advantage of being available for parenteral administration, but patients need to be monitored for prolongation of the QTc.

An alternative to neuroleptics for patients who are not psychotic and primarily require sedation, is the use of a short-acting benzodiazepine, such as lorazepam. Extensive clinical experience using lorazepam in delirium exists, but limited data from controlled clinical trials. Patients should be monitored for paradoxic reactions such as disinhibition, which can be confused with a worsening delirium. Adjunctive valproate has also been shown to control agitation when benzodiazepines or neuroleptics could not be used.

It has been hypothesized that cholinesterase inhibitors approved for use in Alzheimer's disease might be useful in delirium, given that serum anticholinergic activity may be elevated in patients with delirium. To date, there are anecdotal case reports but only one controlled clinical trial using a cholinesterase inhibitor to try to prevent and treat delirium which showed no benefit (10).

CLINICAL RECOMMENDATIONS OF THE VIGNETTE

The patient responded well to treatment of her dehydration and urinary tract infection (UTI) as well as to the minimizing of her other medications. She needs to be carefully monitored for a recurrence of delirium caused by another UTI or any new medical condition. She should also be periodically assessed for symptoms of dementia, which may become more evident over time. Although patients with delirium usually return to their baseline functioning, patients with dementia may not fully recover to that level. Her family needs to be educated about the nature of delirium and the need to observe for a recurrence of symptoms.

SUMMARY

Delirium is a common condition in hospitalized elderly patients. It is often unrecognized or the symptoms are attributed solely to a coexisting dementia. Prescribed medications or surgical interventions are often the iatrogenic cause of delirium. Careful assessment of patients is key to recognizing and monitoring the condition. Often no single cause is found. Patients need to be kept safe and well hydrated and fed until the underlying medical condition is successfully treated. Symptoms can persist for several months after the episode. Pharmacologic interventions may be needed for patients with agitation or psychotic symptoms.

REFERENCES

1. American Psychiatric Association. *Diagnostic and Statistical Manual of Mental Disorders*, Fourth Edition, Text Revision. Washington, DC: 1994.
2. Liptzin B. Delirium. In: Sadavoy J, Jarvik LF, Grossberg GT, et al., eds. *Textbook of Geriatric Psychiatry*, 3rd ed. New York: WW Norton; 2004.
3. Inouye S. Delirium in older persons. *N Engl J Med.* 2006;354:1157–1165.
4. Bergmann MA, Murphy KM, Kiely D, et al. A model for management of delirious postacute care patients. *J Am Geriatr Soc.* 2005;53:1817–1825.
5. Inouye S, Bogardus ST, Jr., Charpentier PA, et al. A multicomponent intervention to prevent delirium in hospitalized older patients. *N Engl J Med.* 1999;340:669–676.
6. Brown TM. Basic mechanisms in the pathogenesis of delirium. In: Stoudemire A, Fogel BS, Greenberg DB, eds. *Psychiatric Care of the Medical Patient*, 2nd ed. Washington, DC: American Psychiatric Press; 2000.
7. Liptzin B, Levkoff SE. An empirical study of delirium subtypes. *Br J Psychiatry.* 1992;161: 843–845.
8. American Psychiatric Association. Practice guideline for the treatment of patients with delirium. *Am J Psychiatry.* 1999;156[Suppl]:1–20.
9. Mayo-Smith MF. Pharmacological management of alcohol withdrawal: A meta-analysis and evidence-based practice guideline. *J Am Med Assoc.* 1997;278:144–151.
10. Liptzin B, Laki A, Garb JL, et al. Donepezil in the prevention and treatment of post-surgical delirium. *Am J Geriatr Psychiatry.* 2005;13:1100–1106.

CHAPTER 168

Somatoform Disorders

Thomas N. Wise • James R. Merikangas

OBJECTIVES

- To describe the essential features of the somatoform disorders
- To review distinguishing features of somatoform disorders
- To discuss the epidemiology of medically unexplained complaints
- To describe treatment approaches to the somatizing patient
- To describe prognostic factors regarding the somatoform disorders

CASE VIGNETTE

A 48-year-old divorced woman was sent for psychiatric consultation by her internist after she was convinced she had multiple sclerosis. She complained that she had numbness and tingling in her arms and, on occasion, her vision blurred. A medical secretary, she indicated she had read extensively about such symptoms and felt they best fit into the diagnosis of multiple sclerosis. The symptoms began after she had an argument with her husband from whom she recently divorced. Her neurologic examination findings were normal. The primary care physician suggested everything was normal and the symptoms may be secondary to anxiety. She responded angrily and requested a neurology consultation. Both the neurologic and ophthalmologic consultations found nothing suggestive of a demyelinating disorder.

The patient refused to accept a trial of antidepressant medication, but went to a major referral center in another city, which also found no evidence of a neurologic disorder. The patient was convinced that the physicians had missed something but agreed to see a psychiatrist.

Her history was significant in that she was raised in a physically abusive family. Unhappily married, she focused on her children and her career as a successful medical secretary. She had an unhappy marriage. After her children reached adulthood, she finally gathered the courage to separate from her husband. She stated she always imagined that being single again would allow her to have a more exciting life and find a better mate, but because of her social anxiety, she was unable to socialize and lived a drab, lonely existence. Within this context, she had agreed to see a psychiatrist for a single consultation.

The psychiatric consultation revealed that the patient was both anxious and depressed, but also resistant to the idea that her physical complaints could be related to a psychiatric disorder. She also reported symptoms indicating a longstanding social anxiety disorder that limited her ability to seek out social situations now that she was divorced. She refused to link such psychosocial issues to her physical symptoms. She noted “All of you physicians think my symptoms are not real.” She refused to follow up with further psychiatric treatment after her initial psychiatric consultation.

DEFINITION

The *Diagnostic and Statistical Manual of Mental Disorders*, Fourth Edition (DSM-IV) frames the essential feature of the somatoform disorders as the individual’s focus on physical complaints, whether subjective discomfort, pain, or an imagined physical defect that causes distress (1). The somatoform disorders include the following categories: somatization disorder; conversion disorder; pain disorder; hypochondriasis; body dysmorphic disorder, and two residual categories: undifferentiated somatoform disorder and somatoform disorder not otherwise specified.

The diagnostic elements for each of these categories are as follows:

Somatization disorder is a chronic, multisymptomatic disorder beginning in adolescence or young adulthood wherein the individual complains of multiple medical problems (2). Specifically, four pain symptoms, two gastrointestinal symptoms, one symptom of sexual difficulties, and one pseudoneurologic symptom are required. These multiple complaints lead to repetitive medical evaluations that often result in needless tests and surgical procedures. The symptoms are not consciously produced or “made up” by the patient, who genuinely believes that he or she is sick.

The undifferentiated somatoform disorder is a condition that lasts for at least 6 months and includes medically unexplained complaints of one or more physical conditions, such as fatigue, and gastrointestinal or urinary difficulties. It is essential that such complaints cause distress or impairment for the patient.

Conversion disorder denotes one or more voluntary motor or sensory dysfunctions suggestive of a neurologic or medical condition (3). The clinician must judge that psychological factors are associated with these symptoms, which are temporally linked to the disorder. As in the other somatoform disorders, the symptoms are not consciously feigned to avoid an external task.

The pain disorder denotes the clinical condition where pain is the predominant symptom and judged to have psychological factors that are important in the onset, severity, and maintenance of the symptom (4).

Hypochondriasis is a category wherein the individual is preoccupied with fears of having a serious illness or an individual's misinterpretation of normal bodily symptoms as a signal of a serious illness (5,6). This preoccupation often leads to multiple medical evaluations and reassurance is only transient. The duration of hypochondriasis must be for at least 6 months and not an obsessive-compulsive disorder or another somatoform disorder.

Body dysmorphic disorder differs from the other somatoform disorders in that it focuses on an imaginary defect in one's physical appearance (7). Even if there is some slight anomaly physically, the individual's concern is particularly excessive and leads to health care evaluations and requests for repeated cosmetic surgeries.

Somatoform disorder not otherwise specified is the residual category that includes conditions such as pseudocyesis, the false belief that one is pregnant, or hypochondriasis <6 months' duration.

The somatoform disorders often overlap with mood and anxiety disorders (8). Most patients with hypochondriasis report clinical significant anxiety or depression during their lifetime (9). Those with body dysmorphic disorders and pain disorders also have very high rates of comorbid mood disorders. It is complicated to separate to the physical symptoms within major mood disorders or generalized anxiety, such as fatigue, back pain, sensory changes (numbness and tingling), or headache, from similar complaints in somatoform disorders (10). Thus, individuals can have both an anxiety and a mood disorder with a concurrent somatoform category (11). To help such diagnostic conundrums, it is useful to focus on the affect of the patient. Does the patient have persistent anxiety or depressed mood that is producing difficulties in functioning or in a sense of well-being. Two questions will help identify most depressed patients. Ask, if during the past month, the patient has been (*a*) bothered by little interest or pleasure in doing things (anhedonia) and (*b*) feeling down, depressed, or hopeless (depressed mood). Affirmative responses to these questions are highly sensitive for a diagnosis of depression because most depressed patients endorse such problems, but is only moderately specific because only about 30% of those who affirm both in fact have a major depressive disorder (12). Follow-up questions that investigate whether any problems exist in sleep disturbance, low self-esteem, and decreased appetite greatly increase the sensitivity of such screening in a brief evaluation (13). Investigating whether a patient has a long history of being a "worrier" suggests the propensity for a concurrent anxiety disorder, although the clinician must further investigate the combination of emotional and physical symptoms that comprise the syndrome of generalized anxiety (14).

EPIDEMIOLOGY

Anywhere from 9% to 16% of community sampled individuals report worry that they might have a serious disease (15). Community surveys find that musculoskeletal discomfort, such as backache, joint pain, and headache, vary from 20% to 30% (16). Physical symptoms are generally reported at least 50% more often by women than by men (17). Such complaints rarely lead to medical evaluation because individuals tend to attribute them to causes that do not require medical attention.

Somatization disorder is seen even less frequently, with community rates of 1% (13). Gender differences are also found in the somatoform disorders in that hypochondriasis has equal gender ratios, but somatization disorder is found five times more frequently in women. The rates of body dysmorphic disorder may affect 1% of the general population, but are as high as 15% in individuals seeking cosmetic surgery (18). Conversion disorders are thought to be 1% to 4% in general hospital settings and perhaps higher in neurologic settings (19,20).

ETIOLOGY AND PATHOGENESIS

A common feature of the somatoform disorders is the propensity of the individual to worry and feel vulnerable. This has been termed as *neuroticism*, a personality trait that has genetic and environmental features (21). Early life experiences, such as being faced with parental illness, often organize the individual's anxiety into focused health anxiety. When such patients become depressed in the context of life adversity, their health worries can escalate into a diagnosable somatoform disorder (13,22). Parents of such patients may also take greater interest in them when they are ill or express physical complaints (23). The patient with a conversion disorder is often reported to be very suggestible. An acute life stress can provoke a psychological crisis wherein the physical symptom (paralysis or mutism) is expressed unconsciously rather than the emotional content. The maintaining factor of many of these disorders is the comorbid presence of a major mood disorder or anxiety disorder, such as generalized anxiety. Family studies in female patients with somatization disorder reveal elevated rates of antisocial personality and substance abuse in male family members (24). Evidence for organic pathophysiology in somatoform disorders is limited, but some data suggest that immune abnormalities can be found in the somatizing patient (13). Recent imaging data indicate that conversions symptoms may involve activation of subcortical limbic areas that could affect conscious recognition of emotional stimuli, which together foster psychogenic neurologic deficits (25,26).

CLINICAL MANIFESTATIONS

As noted, the central clinical manifestation of most somatoform disorders is the medically unexplained complaint (27). The persistence of such symptoms with undue concern and expansion to multiple symptoms should alert the clinician to consider somatoform disorders. With the pain complaints, the diagnosis is more complicated, because individuals will vary in their tolerance to musculoskeletal or other types of pain. Because pain is a subjective complaint, some authors have suggested that utilizing *nonorganic signs* or Waddell signs may help in establishing if the pain is "real," thus facilitating the process of attributing the painful physical symptom complaint to depression (28). Recent evidence, however, indicates that Waddell signs are not reliable and valid in making this distinction (29). It should be noted that partitioning pain into organic and nonorganic is a false dichotomy, because painful physical symptoms with a mood disorder likely have a biological or organic basis. All complaints of pain are "real," because pain is a subjective phenomenon, and the elimination of pain by treatment with antidepressants does not establish causation. For pain syndromes, opiates should be avoided, unless convincing evidence on examination or imaging indicates a neurologic disorder. Physical therapy and massage may be judiciously prescribed in conjunction with psychotherapy.

Increasing requests for evaluations and medication should heighten the concern of the clinician. The patient with a conversion reaction is often noted to have "la belle indifference," which is a lack of appropriate concern. Thus, an individual who complains of blindness or paralysis, but does not seem distressed or concerned in a setting of no observable medical cause should be considered a candidate for the diagnosis of conversion disorder. Many patients with conversion symptoms, however, do not exhibit this indifference (30). To diagnose body dysmorphic disorder, excess concern about a physical defect should also alert the clinician. This is also difficult and, at times subjective, because there is increasing cultural pressure for individuals to receive plastic surgery in the pursuit of "physical perfection." Nevertheless, repeated requests after a plastic surgical procedure or a cosmetic surgical procedure for minor changes or repeated requests for cosmetic surgery should alert the clinician that this might be a body dysmorphic disorder.

TREATMENT

The most important factor in the successful treatment of a patient with unexplained medical complaints, which may represent a somatoform disorder, malingering, or frank delusional disorder, is the doctor–patient relationship (31). Leaping to the conclusion that the condition is *psychosomatic*, and labeling it as such, is to guarantee a treatment failure. Patients will understand and respect a doctor who takes a comprehensive biopsychosocial approach from the start, and makes it clear that the search for health requires collaboration with the patient. The discussion of the patient's psychiatric history must be in the initial review of symptoms, or else it will appear as an attempt to attribute the problem to psychological weakness after the physician fails initially to find the biological cause. Medically unexplained complaints can be the result of the inability of patients to describe the symptoms, because of the diffuse nature of pain or discomfort, or the failure of the physician to ask the relevant questions in an organized and logical manner when taking the history. The review of systems must be complete, not just a "problem focused" approach, and must have adequate time allotted to the initial consultation. Do not depend on getting the proper diagnosis on the first visit, because laboratory tests are usually indicated, even if an internist who has provided "medical clearance" refers the patient (32). An erythrocyte sedimentation rate (ESR), complete blood count (CBC), VDRL or rapid plasma regain (RPR), antinuclear antibody (ANA), thyroid functions, and metabolic tests are a bare minimum.

A physical examination by a psychiatrist qualified to perform one inspires trust and fosters diagnostic explanation (33,34). The physician must feel qualified to perform such a procedure. Of course this is only practical if a nurse or assistant is present to make the situation appropriate for both doctor and patient. A physical examination must be complete as well, because multiorgan involvement in autoimmune and infectious disease is common, and frequently overlooked, if not specifically sought. Examples are systemic lupus erythematosis, thyroid disease, including Hashimoto thyroidits) syphilis, arteritis, fibromyalgia, thalamic pain syndromes, prophyria, sleep apnea, and peripheral neuropathy (including post-zoster and herpetic pain or multiple sclerosis, as in the vignette).

Clinicians must accept the individual's complaint as real in the sense that they are truly distressed about the nature and meaning of the physical problem, but this does not mandate the need for aggressive, inappropriate physical interventions. This should alert the clinician to offer both conservative reassurance and support, and to investigate comorbid psychiatric disorders (e.g., depression). For the somatization disorder wherein multiple complaints drive the patient to request multiple procedures and tests, very conservative management with regularly scheduled follow-up is essential (35).

CLINICAL RECOMMENDATIONS OF THE VIGNETTE

After seeking evaluations from many primary care physicians and specialists, the patient found an internist who listened to her complaints and empathized with her distress. He openly admitted he did not know the cause of her problems, but wanted to carefully follow them in a conservative medical manner because she had already undergone extensive medical evaluations. After two visits, he suggested that antidepressant medication might help her fatigue and a variety of painful physician complaints that she reported when he did a review of symptoms. She slowly improved with medication, support, and time. After a 4-year period, she was less symptomatic and actually began to increase her socialization. She never accepted that she had a fundamental psychiatric disorder, but did minimize her medical utilization and adhered to scheduled follow-up visits with her primary care physician.

This case example demonstrates the importance of accepting the patient's distress, admitting after appropriate evaluation that the cause of the symptoms are not clearly explained, and the necessity of maintaining regular follow-up visits without needless and invasive tests.

SUMMARY

Somatoform disorders are characterized by medically unexplained complaints that are very common in all forms of medical practice. They must be managed with an open mind to what are more ominous physical underpinnings, but have to be handled conservatively and on an ongoing basis. Aggressive attention to the comorbidity with depression and anxiety is needed, as well as an open and supportive approach without exposing the patient to unneeded tests, invasive studies, or needless surgery.

REFERENCES

1. *Diagnostic and Statistical Manual of Mental Disorders.* Fourth Edition. Text Revision. Washington, DC: American Psychiatric Association; 2000.
2. Yutzy SH, Cloninger CR, Guze SB, et al. DSM-IV field trial: Testing a new proposal for somatization disorder. *Am J Psychiatry.* 1995;152(1):97–101.
3. Owen C, Dein S. Conversion disorder: The modern hysteria. *Advances in Psychiatric Treatment.* 2006;12(2):152–157.
4. King SA. Review: DSM-IV and pain. *Clin J Pain.* 1995;11(3):171–176.

5. Barsky AJ, Klerman GL. Overview: Hypochondriasis, bodily complaints, and somatic styles. *Am J Psychiatry.* 1983;140(3):273–283.
6. Barsky AJ, Wyshak G, Klerman GL. Hypochondriasis. An evaluation of the DSM-III criteria in medical outpatients. *Arch Gen Psychiatry.* 1986;43(5):493–500.
7. Phillips KA. Body dysmorphic disorder: Diagnosis and treatment of imagined ugliness. *J Clin Psychiatry.* 1996;57[Suppl 8]:61–64; discussion 65.
8. Mayou R, Kirmayer LJ, Simon G, et al. Somatoform disorders: Time for a new approach in DSM-V. *Am J Psychiatry.* 2005;162(5):847–855.
9. Barsky AJ, Wyshak G, Klerman GL. Psychiatric comorbidity in DSM-III-R hypochondriasis. *Arch Gen Psychiatry.* 1992;49(2):101–108.
10. Ohayon MM, Schatzberg AF. Using chronic pain to predict depressive morbidity in the general population. *Arch Gen Psychiatry.* 2003;60(1):39–47.
11. Brawman-Mintzer O, Monnier J, et al. Patients with generalized anxiety disorder and a history of trauma: Somatic symptom endorsement. *Journal of Psychiatric Practice.* 2005;11(3): 212–215.
12. Lowe B, Kroenke K, Grafe K. Detecting and monitoring depression with a two-item questionnaire (PHQ-2). *J Psychosom Res.* 2005;58(2):163–171.
13. Kroenke K, Spitzer RL, Williams JB. The Patient Health Questionnaire-2: Validity of a two-item depression screener. *Med Care.* 2003;41(11):1284–1292.
14. Barsky AJ, Ahern DK, Bailey ED, et al. Hypochondriacal patients' appraisal of health and physical risks. *Am J Psychiatry.* 2001;158(5):783–787.
15. Noyes R, Jr., Carney CP, Hillis SL, et al. Prevalence and correlates of illness worry in the general population. *Psychosomatics.* 2005;46(6):529–539.
16. Rief W, Hessel A, Braehler E. Somatization symptoms and hypochondriacal features in the general population. *Psychosom Med.* 2001;63(4):595–602.
17. Kroenke K, Spitzer RL. Gender differences in the reporting of physical and somatoform symptoms. *Psychosom Med.* 1998;60(2):150–155.
18. Glaser DA, Kaminer MS. Body dysmorphic disorder and the liposuction patient. *Dermatol Surg.* 2005;31(5):559–560.
19. Stefansson JG, Messina JA, Meyerowitz S. Hysterical neurosis, conversion type: Clinical and epidemiological considerations. *Acta Psychiatr Scand.* 1976;53(2):119–138.
20. Marsden CD. Hysteria—A neurologist's view. *Psychol Med.* 1986;16(2):277–288.
21. Neeleman J, Bijl R, Ormel J. Neuroticism, a central link between somatic and psychiatric morbidity: Path analysis of prospective data. *Psychol Med.* 2004;34(3):521–531.
22. Craig TK, Boardman AP, Mills K, et al. The South London Somatisation Study. I: Longitudinal course and the influence of early life experiences. *Br J Psychiatry.* 1993;163: 579–588.
23. Craig TK, Bialas I, Hodson S, et al. Intergenerational transmission of somatization behaviour: 2. Observations of joint attention and bids for attention. *Psychol Med.* 2004;34(2): 199–209.
24. Guze SB. Genetics of Briquet's syndrome and somatization disorder. A review of family, adoption, and twin studies. *Ann Clin Psychiatry.* 1993;5(4):225–230.
25. Vuilleumier P. Hysterical conversion and brain function. *Prog Brain Res.* 2005;150:309–329.
26. Werring DJ, Weston L, Bullmore ET, et al. Functional magnetic resonance imaging of the cerebral response to visual stimulation in medically unexplained visual loss. *Psychol Med.* 2004;34(4):583–589.
27. Kroenke K. Patients presenting with somatic complaints: Epidemiology, psychiatric comorbidity and management. *International Journal of Methods of Psychiatric Research.* 2003;12(1): 34–43.
28. Waddell G, McCulloch JA, Kummel E, et al. Nonorganic physical signs in low-back pain. *Spine.* 1980;5(2):117–125.
29. Fishbain DA, Cole B, Cutler RB, et al. A structured evidence-based review on the meaning of nonorganic physical signs: Waddell signs. *Pain Medicine.* 2003;4(2):141–181.
30. Stone J, Smyth R, Carson A, et al. La belle indifference in conversion symptoms and hysteria: Systematic review. *Br J Psychiatry.* 2006;188:204–209.
31. Bensing JM, Verhaak PF. Somatisation: A joint responsibility of doctor and patient. *Lancet.* 2006;367(9509):452–454.
32. Stone J, Smyth R, Carson A, et al. Systematic review of misdiagnosis of conversion symptoms and "hysteria." *BMJ.* 2005;331(7523):989.
33. Sanders RD, Keshavan MS. Physical and neurologic examinations in neuropsychiatry. *Semin Clin Neuropsychiatry.* 2002;7(1):18–29.
34. Summers WK, Munoz RA, Read MR. The psychiatric physical examination. Part I: Methodology. *J Clin Psychiatry.* 1981;42(3):95–98.
35. Smith RC. A clinical approach to the somatizing patient. *J Fam Pract.* 1985;21(4):294–301.

CHAPTER 169

Suicide Risk Assessment

Howard S. Sudak

OBJECTIVES

- To describe the signs and symptoms indicating elevated risk of suicide
- To indicate the various measures clinicians should use to keep a patient safe
- To advise on ways to reduce suicide attempts and suicide completions
- To review theories regarding the causes of suicide

CASE VIGNETTE

A 56-year-old white married pediatrician is referred to a neurologist for evaluation of a mild bilateral tremor of his hands. His wife tells the neurologist that he has been sleeping poorly for the past few weeks; has a poor appetite with a 10 lb weight loss over this same period and has become preoccupied about their "precarious financial state." She does not understand this because their financial state is unchanged and they have more than an adequate income. He has had periods like this in the past, but they have just spontaneously cleared without medical attention after 1 or 2 months.

The neurologist's physical examination findings are normal, except for a slight bilateral hand tremor when his arms are fully extended forward. The patient tells him that he is worried that this is an early sign of a serious progressive neurologic disease and does not appear satisfied by the neurologist's reassurance that this appears to be either the result of his anxiety or a mild and not serious familial tremor. The patient requests a brain magnetic resonance imaging (MRI), a computed tomographic (CT) scan, and, should those prove negative, wonders if the neurologist can arrange a positron emission tomography (PET) scan and have his insurance cover the cost.

The neurologist is reluctant to follow his instructions and telephones the primary care physician who referred the patient to him. He informs the neurologist that the patient has a long history of alcohol and benzodiazepine abuse and has told his wife how hopeless he feels things are, especially their finances, and has said to her, "maybe I should end it all."

DEFINITION

Suicide risk assessment refers to the evaluation of a patient to determine which factors are present that indicate an increased risk for suicide so that a safe and appropriate disposition can be effected for him or her. Many different schemas exist for classifying such factors, including:

A. Dynamic versus static (i.e., changeable or otherwise): For instance, the following
   1. Demographic factors: age, race, gender, and so forth are static.
   2. Diagnostic factors: depressed, psychotic, agitated, are dynamic.
B. Acute versus long-term (1,2): For instance, the following
   1. Acute risk: recent serious suicidal attempt, current suicide plan, means to implement the plan, prior attempts, comorbid substance abuse, recent significant losses.
   2. Longer-term risk: suicide ideation, intent, and actual past attempts increase both short- and long-term risk, as does a family history of depression or suicide.
   3. Risk factors (longer term) versus warning signs (more immediate).
C. Classification according to categories (3): For instance, primary diagnosis; demographic and miscellaneous factors; personality factors; comorbidity; social factors, and other (Table 169-1)
   1. Subjective factors: In addition to gathering data for the objective factors already cited, the clinician's subjective sense of how much distress, anxiety, and desperation the patient is feeling provides important clues. The more the distress, the greater the risk (except this does not mean that a patient with a retarded depression is at low risk—quite the contrary).

Regardless of which classification is used, the responsibility of the nonpsychiatrist physician is to make an assessment of how much of a risk for a suicide attempt or completion the patient presents to be able to effect a safe and appropriate disposition for the patient. No way exists to determine with absolute certainty whether an individual patient will kill him- or herself or not. What is possible, and expected, of the physician is a careful exploration of the patient's risk factors for suicide so that his or her relative suicide risk can be ascertained and the patient properly treated. Although the standard of care for a nonpsychiatrist is based on what is expected of a reasonable physician in the same specialty, it is well to remember that the primary care doctor who treats his or her patient's anxiety or depression with medication is likely to be held to the same standards as would a psychiatrist.

TABLE 169-1. Risk Factors by Category

Primary Diagnosis	*Demographics and Miscellaneous*	*Personality*	*Comorbidity*	*Social Factors*	*Other Factors*
Bipolar	Male	Borderline	Substance abuse/ dependence	Divorced	Means available
Schizophrenia	Older age White race	Narcissistic	Alcohol abuse/ dependence	Widower	History of abuse
Major depressive episode	Prior depression or Suicide attempts	Antisocial	Anxiety	Lives alone	Few reasons to live
Dysthymia	Family history Depression or attempts	Conduct disorder	Axis III diagnosis	Isolated	Adverse events
Adjustment disorder with depression	Homosexual	Impulsive	Panic	Financial worries	Change of grades
Delirium or dementia	Suicidal ideation			Other losses	Change of friends
Any psychosis	Hopeless/helpless			No religion	Giving away possessions
Hallucinations/delusions: especially of poverty	Agitation/desperation				Guns in home

(Adapted from Sudak H. Suicide. In: Sadock BJ, Sadock VA, eds. *Kaplan and Sadock's Comprehensive Textbook of Psychiatry*, 8th ed. Philadelphia: Lippincott Williams & Wilkins; 2005:2448, with permission.)

EPIDEMIOLOGY

Epidemiologic factors in suicide are fairly well-known. Completed suicide rates are higher in males than females (3:1); whites more than nonwhites (2.5:1); older more than younger in white males (almost in direct proportion); slightly higher in Protestants and Jews than in Catholics (Hindus comparable to western religions and Muslims remarkably lower). Axis I disorders are more typical of completers than attempters. Suicide attempts, however, are more frequent in females than males (3:1); in younger (age 15 to 30 years) than older females; and more typically occur in patients with Axis II disorders. Interestingly, black male completion rates rise in proportion to age up until age 35 to 45 and then decline (in contrast to white rates); they also have gotten closer to average white male rates in recent years (from 4 or 5 to 1 to 2.5 to 3 to 1). Also, adolescent completion rates increased threefold for white males, age 15 to 19 years of age, black males, and black females. Also, 15–19 year old completion rates rose threefold for white males, black males and black females and twofold for white females, between 1950 and 1990. Rates then leveled off and significantly decreased from 1990 to the present (4).

The overall white male suicide completion rate has remained around 20 per 100,000 since 1900, with two major exceptions: they dropped significantly during World Wars I and II and increased significantly during the great depression of the 1930s. Subgroups, however, have undergone major changes: the adolescent increase described above was matched by a comparable, although less dramatic (because the age range is much broader), decrease in elderly rates from the 1950s to the 1990s. Thus, the overall rates were little changed. The 1950 rates were the highest in this century but, by 2000, the rates had fallen to the 1990 levels and have continued to decrease. The 2003 white adolescent male rates were approximately 25% lower than the 1990 rates—a very significant decrease.

ETIOLOGY AND PATHOGENESIS

Although theories abound, the cause(s) of suicide is not known. Some critical correlations to keep in mind, however, are that 90% to 95% of suicide completers have an Axis I or Axis II diagnosis and approximately 65% to 75% of completers suffer from a significant depressive disorder. Comorbidity of depression with alcohol or substance abuse increases the risk; also comorbid borderline personality disorder and antisocial disorder raise the risk. Axis III, comorbid medical conditions, also increase the risk of completed suicide. Among the depressive disorders, bipolar (manic-depressive) disorder has the highest lifetime prevalence of death by suicide, 15% to 20%, and such deaths are more likely to occur during the depressed phase. By themselves, schizophrenia, major depression, and borderline personality disorder all have increased lifetime prevalence of suicide (5). Genetic factors play a major role in the genesis of most of these disorders so that suicide, as a product of these illnesses, can be viewed as *genetic* also. Much interest exists in whether or not an independent genetic predisposition to suicide exists aside from that mediated by these disorders. Egeland and Sussex's Amish studies (6) and the Roy et al. twin studies (7) lend considerable support to such a hypothesis as does an intriguing recent study of genetic spermine or spermidine abnormalities in completers (8).

Psychological theories to account for suicide can be traced to antiquity. More recently, Freud, in "Mourning and Melancholia," wrote of introjecting the lost object (following a death) so that killing oneself also meant killing the other. Menninger (9) elaborated on this as he wrote of "the wish to kill, to be killed, and to die." Schneidman (10) wrote of "psychache" (i.e., psychic pain), and it is clear that hopelessness, despair, desperation, helplessness, guilt, worthlessness, anhedonia, and sadness are critically related to an individual's renouncing self-preservation in favor of death.

Why men kill themselves more often than women is not known, but the much higher rate of alcoholism in men may play a key role (11,12). Also women are more likely to use pills than men (thus, a larger safety margin), and men more likely to use faster, more violent, and more quickly fatal method (guns, stabbing, jumping). For both sexes, however, guns lead the list of methods, so that inquiring about the presence of guns in the home is an essential part of the history-taking of all depressed or possibly suicidal patients. A thorough inquiry into suicidal ideation, plans, and actual attempts should be part of the evaluation of all depressed patients. The huge increase in adolescent suicide over the past 60 years may relate to increased substance abuse, gun availability, family instability, religious breakdown, or more likely, to changes in the proportion of adolescents compared with the rest of the population (13). Why black rates are low is also poorly understood as is the paradoxic black male suicide pattern of a peak in middle years followed by a decrease. Elderly decreases in suicide rates are generally viewed as related to better medicines and medical care for the elderly and an improved quality of life because of factors such as social security.

PATHOLOGY

Separately, Mann et al. (14) and Nemeroff et al. (15) have posited stress-diathesis or stress models for depression and suicide. Mann et al. focus on serotonin and norepinephrine neurotransmitters, whereas Nemeroff et al. focus on the cortico-hypothalamic-pituitary axis. What these researchers have in common is that they believe that depressed or suicidal individuals may be born with a genetic predisposition to depression or impulsivity (the diathesis), but this diathesis may operate like a silent genotype until later in life (e.g., adolescence); if certain stressors occur, the phenotype becomes manifest and depression or impulsive behavior (e.g., suicide) is seen. Early childhood trauma or losses, if sufficiently severe, can also serve as the diathesis for a later reaction when stressed to produce depression or suicide. These hypotheses fit well with both biological and psychological perspectives of mental illness and suicide.

CLINICAL MANIFESTATIONS AND SPECIAL SITUATIONS

CHILDREN AND ADOLESCENTS

Suicide attempts are rare before puberty—either because of the technical aspects being too difficult for children or their cognitive or emotional immaturities making them unlikely to feel the sort of despair we associate with adult suicide (or because of their dependence on their parents being so profound that they look to them for relief of any and all pain). For teenagers, suicide is the second or third leading cause of death—not because their actual rates per 100,000 at risk are so high, but because they are generally so physically healthy, without heart disease, strokes, or cancer, so that even a relatively moderate rate of suicidal deaths ranks higher as a leading cause of death. Depression in teen-agers may or may not present in the adult manner (i.e., with sadness, anhedonia, change in sleep or eating habits, tearfulness, guilt, hopelessness, helplessness), but as a behavioral change (the "good boy" becomes "bad"; the good student's grades fall; prized belongings are given away; the abstemious student begins abusing substances; friends are changed or dropped). Shaffer et al. (16) write of the quiet and perfectionistic adolescent who never gets into trouble, but who cannot maintain his perfection as he gets older and the competition increases, and he decompensates into a suicidal crisis; they also warn of the conduct-disordered child who may be at special risk for impulsive suicidal behavior. Adolescents also appear to be especially sensitive to imitative ("copy-cat") suicides in which vulnerable adolescents become overtly suicidal following the death of a fellow student or after reading a romanticized, detailed, or lurid newspaper account of a prominent suicide.

ELDERLY

Elderly white male suicide rates are the highest of all; furthermore, the elderly have the fewest number of attempts per completion of any group. Therefore, when an older person makes an attempt, it is more likely to lead to death than in a younger individual. Although the elderly constituted 13% of the population in 2000, they accounted for 19% of the total suicides (17). As with adolescents, the elderly depressed may not present with classic symptomatology; they may merely show some sleep or appetite changes or be somatically preoccupied. The elderly are often inadvertently discriminated against by physicians who regard depression in the elderly as inevitable or irreversible—an incorrect assumption.

DIAGNOSTIC APPROACH

Unless an independent genetic predisposition to suicide is found to exist, suicidal behavior should be viewed as a symptom of an underlying disease or disorder rather than as a disease itself. Just as we sometimes are forced to treat a fever (e.g., if it becomes sufficiently high to threaten to cause brain damage) even if we do not know its cause, we sometimes "treat" the symptom of suicidality without knowing its underlying disease (e.g., by hospitalizing someone for protection). In general, we treat the underlying condition (the Axis I or II pathology) and, if successful, the suicidal wishes subside.

Because most completed suicides occur in patients who are depressed, the most fruitful diagnostic approach is to assess suicidality and suicide risk factors thoroughly in at least *every* depressed patient. Because half or more of those who kill themselves have seen their primary care physician in the month before their suicides, primary care physicians have a unique opportunity to detect suicidality in their patients before a suicide occurs. The suicide inquiry entails asking about ideation and any prior attempts in detail. Knowing the circumstances of the attempt: How potentially lethal was it? Was the intent really to die or something else? How likely was discovery before death would have occurred? Such queries are an important component. Many of the risk factors listed in Table 169-1 will have been ascertained in the process of taking a general medical history.

If the primary care physician works in a group setting where clinical psychologists or psychiatrists are available, he or she may elect to refer the patient to them for further evaluation and treatment. Although projective tests (e.g., Rorschach, Thematic Apperception Test [TAT]) are not particularly helpful in ascertaining suicide risk, depression or suicide rating scales may be quite useful (e.g., Hamilton Depression Scale, Beck's Suicide Intent Scale). The Hopelessness Scale (A. T. Beck) is the best current predictive paper and pencil test available. Obtaining an outside history may prove invaluable when the clinician is unsure how truthful the patient is being about his or her degree of suicidality. If the patient refuses permission, the clinician needs to decide at how much risk for acting on their suicidal impulses is the patient. If he or she is viewed as at significant risk, the clinician may (and should) waive confidentiality and contact the family to get further information and enlist their aid. Furthermore, even if no self-harm appears imminent, confidentiality does not preclude the clinician from *acquiring* information from family members or friends should they contact him or her.

TREATMENT

As discussed, treatment generally entails treating the underlying disorder. For acutely suicidal patients and for patients who have already made a serious attempt and are being treated in an emergency room, inpatient hospitalization on a psychiatric unit may be required. If the patient is unwilling to be admitted voluntarily, commitment may be required. Although patients sometimes kill themselves while so hospitalized, it is harder to do so than if not hospitalized. Inpatient care allows the patient time to begin treatment, while concomitantly providing a suitable level of observation to protect him or her. "Why now in and why now out?" are relevant questions for all suicidal patients: what prompted the suicide attempt in the first place and, before discharging a hospitalized suicidal patient, what has changed in his or her life to now make discharge safe?

Because most suicidal patients suffer from underlying depressive disorders, treatment suggestions will focus on these disorders. Although optimal treatment entails both psychotherapy and pharmacotherapy, they are discussed separately for clarity.

PSYCHOTHERAPY

Many types of psychotherapy have been successfully used to treat depressive disorders, including interpersonal, brief, psychodynamic (psychoanalytically oriented), cognitive-behavioral, and dialectic behavior psychotherapies. Dialectic behavior therapy, developed by Linehan et al. (18), is particularly effective for the treatment of borderline personality disorder (and is one of the few psychotherapies to have demonstrated an evidence-based reduction in suicidal behavior). Cognitive-behavior therapy, pioneered by Beck et al. (19), an evidence-based treatment for depression, has become a very popular approach since it appears to heal faster than most other psychotherapies and has been shown to be comparable to medication without psychotherapy in effectiveness.

PHARMACOTHERAPY AND OTHER SOMATIC THERAPIES

Despite not having shown to be superior to older antidepressants (e.g., monoamine-oxidase inhibitors, tricyclic antidepressants) in effectiveness, currently serotonin reuptake inhibitors (SSRI) or serotonin norepinephrine reuptake inhibitors (SNRI) are more likely to be used to treat depressive disorders because they are safer and better tolerated by patients. If an adequate dose for an adequate duration of one such antidepressant fails to relieve symptoms, patients are often switched to another agent, usually of a different type (i.e., if an SSRI was what was originally prescribed, change to an SNRI, and vice-versa). For patients who are bipolar, a mood stabilizer (e.g., lithium, valproic acid, lamotrigine, carbamazepine) is essential, but these agents may also be very helpful for patients who are bipolar, in depressed phase, and for patients who are not bipolar, but depressed, appearing to either enhance the antidepressant's effectiveness or to have antidepressant effects of their own. It should be noted that, regarding evidence-based therapy, the long-term use of lithium in bipolar patients (20) and clozapine in schizophrenic patients (21) are the only pharmacotherapies so far shown to decrease suicidal behavior. Electroconvulsive therapy (ECT) is generally reserved for severely depressed patients who are refractory to pharmacotherapy or elderly individuals who are unable to tolerate the undesirable side effects of many of the antidepressants. The role of transcranial magnetic stimulation (TMS) or implanted electrode stimulation therapies remains to be determined because they are so new that their definitive usefulness remains to be established.

CLINICAL RECOMMENDATIONS OF THE VIGNETTE

Clearly, whatever disease is reflected by the patient's tremor, it is not the primary problem. The patient reveals that he has vegetative signs typical of depression (insomnia and decreased appetite); he also reveals his marked anxiety or depressed feelings by his inability to be reassured by the neurologist and by his ruminations about his finances. He has a previous history of such symptomatology, also. The referring physician, when contacted, adds the history of substance abuse, hopelessness, and suicidal ideation. The clinician realizes that this unrealistic (according to the spouse) fixation about money probably represents a delusion of poverty, not uncommonly seen in psychotically depressed patients.

Clearly, this patient requires urgent intervention. The neurologist should inquire about a family history of depression and suicide; should ask if he has ever attempted suicide in the past (and, if so, what were the details of these). All suicidal patients should be asked if there are guns in the home and, if so, they should be removed. It is useful to ask the patient and his family if they are concerned that he might actually harm himself because an affirmative answer increases the risk. The risk is also clearly increased by the comorbid substance abuse history. Asking if there have been any manic or hypomanic periods would supply additional useful information.

What disposition should the neurologist try to effect? The first priority is the patient's safety. Assuming that no imminent suicidal threat exists (which might necessitate hospitalization) and that the patient's wife is comfortable taking him home, the patient needs a prompt referral to a psychiatrist. The neurologist might discuss the choice of psychiatrist with his internist and present this to the patient and his wife or, if deemed less urgent, might just send the patient back to the internist for further disposition. In any event, the patient needs to be seen a psychiatrist within 1 or 2 weeks and the wife needs to be cautioned to call the neurologist or internist back in the interim if she becomes more concerned and she should be instructed to go to their nearest emergency room should things seem more acute and she cannot reach these providers quickly.

SUMMARY

The assessment of suicidal risk entails an evaluation of the factors known to increase the risk for suicide, as given in Table 169-1. These factors are not simply additive nor are they equal in importance. Because more than 90% of completed suicides are in individuals with *Diagnostic and Statistical Manual of Mental Disorders*, Fourth Edition, Text Revision (DSM-IV-TR) Axis I disorders, this is probably the most important warning (along with current suicidal ideation, plan, or attempt, followed by a past attempt). Among these Axis I disorders, the depressions and schizophrenia carry the highest risks. For Axis II disorders, borderline, narcissistic, and antisocial personalities are highest. Comorbidity of alcohol or substance abuse or dependence with any of these Axis I or II disorders greatly increases the risk. Demographically, older, white, males carry the highest long-term risk. Recent losses (e.g., age-related, health, job, divorce or separation, empty-nesting, deaths) and social isolation all increase risk. Depressed adolescents may not present themselves clinically as adults do; they may show behavioral manifestations of their depression (e.g., emerging conduct disturbances, changing friends or grades) rather than sadness, tearfulness, and so on. Elderly depressed individuals may also present atypically, that is, with increased somatic concerns or with vegetative signs (sleep and appetite changes) in the absence of overt depressive symptoms. The more distress the patient communicates to the physician (hopelessness, helplessness, agitation, desperation, anxiety), the more the risk (especially if these feelings are palpable to the clinician).

Having evaluated these factors, the clinician needs to determine his or her next steps regarding maintaining safety for the patient and, if indicated, referring the patient to a mental health professional. Legally, the standard of care does not mandate that a physician be able to accurately predict suicide, only that the reasonably prudent physician has carefully appraised the risk factors for suicide, determined what constitutes a safe disposition for his or her patient, documents his or her evaluation in writing, and follows-up to ensure these recommendations have been carried out.

REFERENCES

1. Fawcett J. Predictors of early suicide: Identification and appropriate intervention. *J Clin Psychiatry.* 1998;49[Suppl]:7.
2. Simon RI, Hales RE. *Textbook of Suicide Assessment and Management.* Washington, DC: American Psychiatric Association; 2006.
3. Sudak HS. Suicide. In: Sadock BJ, Sadock VA. *Comprehensive Textbook of Psychiatry*, 8th ed. Philadelphia: Lippincott; 2005.
4. Http://www.cdc.gov. Suicide mortality tables. Cited 2006, May.
5. Inskip HM, Harris EC, Barraclough B. Lifetime risk of suicide for affective disorders, alcoholism, and schizophrenia. *Br J Psychiatry.* 1998;171:35.
6. Egeland J, Sussex JN. Suicide and family loading for affective disorders. *JAMA.* 1985; 254:9915.
7. Roy A, Rylander C, Sarchiapone M. Genetics of suicide, family studies and molecular genetics. *Ann NY Acad Sci.* 1997;836:135.
8. Sequeria A, Gwadry FG, French-Mullen JM, et al. Implication of SSAT by gene expression and genetic variation in suicide and major depression. *Arch Gen Psychiatry.* 2006;63: 35–48.
9. Menninger KA. Psychoanalytic aspects of suicide. *Int J Psychoanal.* 1933;4:336.
10. Schneidman ES. Suicide as psychache. *J Nerv Ment Dis.* 1993;181:147.
11. Rich CL, Ricketts, JE, Fowler RC, et al. Some differences between men and women who commit suicide. *Am J Psychiatry.* 1988;145:718.
12. Haw C, Hawton K, Casey D, et al. Alcohol dependence, excessive drinking and deliberate self-hate: Trends and patterns in Oxford, 1989–2002. *Soc Psychiatry Psychiatr Epidemiol.* 2005;40:964.
13. Holinger PC, Offer D. Toward the prediction of violent deaths in the young. In: Sudak HS, Rushforth NB, Ford AB, eds. *Suicide in the Young.* Boston: John Wright; 1984.
14. Mann JM, Waternaux C, Haas GL, et al. Toward a clinical model of suicidal behavior in psychiatric patients. *Am J Psychiatry.* 1999;156:181.
15. Nemeroff CB, Owens MJ, Bissett G. Reduced corticotropin releasing factor binding sites in the frontal cortex of suicide victims. *Arch Gen Psychiatry.* 1988;45:577.
16. Shaffer D, Gould MS, Fisher P. Psychiatric diagnoses in child and adolescent suicide. *Arch Gen Psychiatry.* 1996;53:339.
17. Duberstein P, Conwell Y. Preventing suicide in older adults. *Directions in Psychiatry.* 2000;20: 351.
18. Linehan MM, Tutek DA, Heard HL. Interpersonal outcomes of CBT for chronically suicidal borderline patients. *Am J Psychiatry.* 1994;151:1771.
19. Beck AT, Brown GK, Steer RA, et al. Suicide ideation at its worst point: A predictor of suicide in psychiatric outpatients. *Suicide Life Threat Behav.* 1999;29:1.
20. Geddes JR, Burgess S, Hawton K, et al. Long-term lithium therapy for bipolar disorder: Systematic review and meta-analysis of randomized controlled trials. *Am J Psychiatry.* 2004;161:217.
21. Meltzer HY, Okayli G. Reduction of suicidality during clozapine treatment of neuroleptically resistant schizophrenic patients: Impact on risk-benefit assessment. *Am J Psychiatry.* 1995;152:183.

CHAPTER 170

Commonly Used Psychotropic Medications

Alexander W. Thompson • Dan Major • Glenn Treisman

OBJECTIVES

- To describe common psychotropic medications
- To explain the basic differences between drugs in the same class
- To discuss the common and serious side effects of commonly used psychotropic medications
- To discuss clinical situations, including use of psychotropic medications in children, pregnancy, and geriatric patients

CASE VIGNETTE

A 72-year-old woman with mild dementia was hospitalized for an exacerbation of chronic obstructive pulmonary disease. She was started on steroids, a fluoroquinolone antibiotic, and nebulized bronchodilators. While in the emergency department, she was disoriented and was given diazepam (2 mg) for agitation. On the first night of hospitalization, she again became acutely agitated, pulling off her nebulizer mask, removing her peripheral line, and threatening nurses. On examination, she was disoriented, intermittently somnolent, paranoid, and described seeing people in her room who were not present.

DEFINITION

Drugs that are active in the central nervous system (CNS) and produce changes in mental function have been referred to as *psychotropic drugs*, implying altered (tropic-turning) rather than diminished function, and include those used to treat psychiatric illnesses as well as those used to alter mental function for other purposes. It has been difficult to create categories for these drugs, because they can be classified by structure, clinical utility, receptor activity, presumed mechanism of action, or by the subjective sensation they create. As an example, drugs in the general class of sedative-hypnotics are mostly drugs that enhance the actions of γ-aminobutyric acid (GABA), and have antianxiety and anticonvulsant properties, decrease activity and arousal, and induce a pleasant relaxed state that can turn depressive. They can be classified as *anxiolytics*, as *anticonvulsants*, as *benzodiazepines*, as *barbiturates*, as *GABA agonists*, and as *downers*. We will use categories based on the major clinical utility to psychiatry, understanding that each drug has many uses in different disciplines. It is also important to recognize that many medicines are used psychiatrically that would not traditionally be defined as psychotropics. Examples include clonidine use for opiate withdrawal and propranolol use for performance anxiety.

We have divided the drugs we discuss into the following categories: *antidepressants, mood stabilizers, antipsychotics, anxiolytics/hypnotics*, and *stimulants*.

EPIDEMIOLOGY

The use of drugs to alter mood and mental function predates history. Herbs, alcohol, and medicinal chemicals have been described through the history of medicine. Sedative-hypnotic drugs, starting with alcohol, bromides, and barbiturates and, most recently, benzodiazepines have been among the most popular drugs used by physicians. Opium- and cocaine-derived products have enjoyed similar popularity. The principal use of these compounds has been symptom-directed treatments and, because of liabilities over time, many have been avoided by the more scrupulous practitioners. With the development of specific therapeutic agents that were diagnosis directed and improved functioning and lessened disease prognosis over the past 40 years, psychotropic use has grown dramatically. From 1987 to 1997, a nearly fivefold increase occurred in the use of psychotropics to treat depression (1). One large health maintenance organization (HMO) found the rate of antidepressant prescriptions to adolescents doubled from 1994 to 2003 (2). The European Study of the Epidemiology of Mental Disorders found that 32.6% of patients with a (DSM-IV-TR) mental disorder for at least 1 year used psychotropics. Of the patients diagnosed with depression for over a year, only 21.2% received an antidepressant (3). A 15-center international epidemiologic survey found that most psychiatric conditions are not diagnosed and managed in the office of a psychiatrist (4).

ANTIDEPRESSANTS

The development of antidepressants began with two parallel discoveries. Imipramine was synthesized by Hafliger and Schindler in the late 1940s as part of an effort to develop new antihistamines. It is very similar in structure to the antipsychotic phenothiazines, and was tried as a sedative for patients who were psychotic, but Kuhn reported it had antidepressant properties in 1958 (5). Drugs synthesized as analogs of imipramine block the reuptake of serotonin and norepinephrine, and this ultimately led to the development of other serotonin reuptake inhibitors and other monoamine reuptake blockers. At very nearly the same time, the antituberculosis drug iproniazid was developed and noted to have antidepressant properties. It was discovered that the drug inhibited monoamine oxidase (MAO) and led to the development of monoamine oxidase inhibitors (MAOI) used as antidepressants and in Parkinson's disease.

TRICYCLIC ANTIDEPRESSANTS

Tricyclic antidepressants (TCA) are less popular than the newer and safer selective serotonin reuptake inhibitor (SSRI) antidepressants, but they have particular neurologic properties that make them useful, and it is possible they should receive wider use in psychiatry. They have efficacy in a variety of chronic pain disorders, are useful in migraine, and have prorectic and hypnotic activity. Imipramine and its metabolite desipramine, as well as amitriptyline and its metabolite nortriptyline, are effective TCA used for the treatment of depression. Numerous other TCA have been developed, with a variety of differing side effect profiles. Tricyclics are thought to work by inhibiting the reuptake of norepinephrine and serotonin. Tricyclics have anticholinergic (dry mouth, blurry vision, constipation, urinary retention), anithistaminergic (sedation and weight gain), antiadrenergic (orthostasis and dizziness), and cardiotoxic (quinidine-like effects and prolonged QT interval) side effects. Those side effects are more apparent in the parent compounds, amitriptyline and imipramine. A series of related antidepressants, such as clomipramine and doxepin, vary in the degree of specific side effects, and have utility in specific patients. Compared with other TCA, clomipramine is a more potent serotonergic reuptake inhibitor and primarily is used as a treatment for obsessive-compulsive disorder (OCD) when SSRI have failed. Doxepin is a potent antihistamine. It is very sedating and used topically for the treatment of pruritis. The frequency of side effects and lethality in overdose caused by arrhythmia limit the popularity of TCA. Nortriptyline has well established blood levels between 50 and 150 ng/mL for effectiveness. For amitriptyline, imipramine, and desipramine, there appears to be a linear relationship between response and blood level, and although the utility of the blood levels is debated for therapeutic purposes, because of metabolic variability, blood levels should be monitored for safety. Patients with significant risk should probably be monitored with electrocardiogram (ECG) before and during treatment.

SELECTIVE SEROTONIN REUPTAKE INHIBITORS

The SSRI, the most commonly prescribed antidepressants, include citalopram, escitalopram, fluoxetine, fluvoxamine, paroxetine, and sertraline. SSRI are indicated for major depression (fluoxetine, sertraline, paroxetine, citalopram, escitalopram), bulimia (fluoxetine), panic disorder (fluoxetine, sertraline, paroxetine), OCD (fluoxetine, fluvoxamine, sertraline, paroxetine), generalized anxiety disorder (paroxetine, escitalopram), posttraumatic stress disorder (sertraline, paroxetine), social phobia (sertraline, paroxetine), and premenstrual dysphoric disorder (fluoxetine, sertraline, paroxetine). As a class, they are well tolerated, well studied, and relatively safe in overdose. Table 170-1 highlights common side

TABLE 170-1. Adverse Reactions and Management Strategies for Selective Serotonin Reuptake Inhibitors

Common Adverse Reactions	*Management Techniques*
Nausea, constipation, diarrhea	Reassurance and conservative management
Sexual dysfunction (decreased libido, delayed ejaculation, anorgasmia)	Add bupropion or switch to another effective antidepressant. The use of sildenafil and cyproheptadine may be effective
Sleep disturbance	Add a sleeping agent or switch drugs
Weight gain	Consider switching agents. Some clinicians have had success adding topiramate
Agitation, nervousness, akathisia	Consider switching to another agent
	Less Common Adverse Reactions
Withdrawal syndrome	Paroxetine appears to be most likely to cause a withdrawal syndrome and slow tapering is necessary to avoid headache, gastrointestinal distress, and anxiety.
Hyponatremia	Appears more often in the elderly. Close monitoring before medication and with the onset of any mental state change is important.
Prolonged bleeding time	Because of decreased serotonin uptake by platelets. May be beneficial for patients with post myocardial infarction depressions.

(From Dording CM, Mischoulon D. The pharmacologic management of SSRI-induced side effects: A survey of psychiatrists. *Ann Clin Psychiatry.* 2002;14(3):143–147, with permission.)

effects and provides useful management strategies (6). If side effects are intolerable, switching to another SSRI can be successful.

BUPROPION

Bupropion (Wellbutrin) is effective for the treatment of major depression and smoking cessation. It is structurally similar to amphetamine and affects dopamine and norepinephrine. Bupropion can be stimulating, causing nervousness, agitation, and at times psychosis. Bupropion can cause some anxiety as a side effect, and it has generally not been thought to be as useful in the treatment of anxiety disorders. The risk of seizures is 0.4% and use should be cautioned in patients with a history of seizure. Bupropion has a low incidence of sexual side effects and often is added to an SSRI when there is SSRI-related sexual dysfunction. It does not alter cardiac conduction, cause orthostasis, or create anticholinergic side effects.

MIRTAZAPINE

Mirtazapine (Remeron) is an effective antidepressant indicated for the treatment of major depression. It has been reported to antagonize α_2 and serotonin receptors. It does not significantly antagonize acetylcholine or α_1 receptors and has few adverse interactions with other medications. It causes marked weight gain and sedation and, although this can limit the use of this drug, it may be a reason to choose this drug in a patient where weight loss and insomnia are a problem. This drug also has some activity in chronic pain.

TRAZODONE

Trazodone (Desyrel) is an antidepressant indicated for the treatment of major depression. Because of significant sedation and orthostasis, trazodone is seldom used at doses sufficiently high to be an effective antidepressant. Most clinicians will encounter or use this drug as a treatment for insomnia that is not habit forming. Doses for depression are probably in the 400 mg to 600 mg per day range, whereas the drug may aid sleep at doses of 50 to 200 mg a night. Priapism can occur in both men and woman and patients need to be warned of this potentially serious side effect.

SEROTONIN NOREPINEPHRINE REUPTAKE INHIBITORS

VENLAFAXINE

Venlafaxine (Effexor) is indicated for the treatment of major depression, generalized anxiety disorder, panic disorder, and social phobia. As with the tricyclics, it is a mixed serotonin and norepinephrine reuptake inhibitor. It has no appreciable anticholinergic, cardiac depressant, or sedative effects, however. The side effect profile is similar to SSRI, although more potential exists to cause sweating. There is the potential for elevated blood pressure, which should be monitored periodically. Also, as with paroxetine, withdrawal phenomena are common and a slow tapering should be used when discontinuing.

DULOXETINE

Duloxetine (Cymbalta) has been approved for the treatment of major depression and diabetic peripheral neuropathy. Although structurally different, its mechanism of action is like venlafaxine. Duloxetine is an effective antidepressant and has demonstrated efficacy in the treatment of chronic pain disorders. Some patients respond to treatment with this drug or venlafaxine when they have failed to respond to SSRI. Whether this is a specific property of the so-called SNRI drugs or simply trial and error is not clear. But, clinical experience shows that some patients respond to one agent and not another.

MONOAMINE OXIDASE INHIBITORS

The MAOI are indicated for the treatment of major depression. Monoamine oxidase metabolizes biogenic amines and is found as two subtypes, MAO-A and MAO-B. MAO-A primarily metabolizes serotonin, norepinephrine, and epinephrine and is found in the brain, liver, and gut. MAO-A, in the gut, metabolizes dietary tyramine. MAO-B metabolizes dopamine and is only found in the brain. The nonselective MAOI (tranylcypromine, phenelzine, isocarboxazid) irreversibly inhibit both MAO-A and MAO-B, leaving patients open to dangerous drug interactions (discussed below) (7). The selective MAO-B inhibitor, selegiline, is used in Parkinson disease and appears to avoid the drug interactions of the nonspecific MAOI. It has been less effective for depression until the recent development of a transdermal delivery system, which appears to improve the effectiveness of the drug, and it has recently been found effective and is indicated for the treatment of major depression (8) (Table 170-2).

USE OF ANTIDEPRESSANTS IN THE ELDERLY

Major depression and anxiety disorders are common in older patients. Geriatric patients are at risk for side effects from antidepressants (as well as all psychotropics) because of delayed renal and hepatic metabolism, comorbid medical conditions, concurrent medications, and, at times, underlying cognitive deficits. For that reason, lower doses should be used initially. Adequate dosing remains essential, and many elderly patients are treated with subtherapeutic doses of antidepressants, leaving them with side effects, but without benefit.

USE OF ANTIDEPRESSANTS IN CHILDREN

Evidence indicates that the use of antidepressants in children increases the likelihood of self-injurious feelings, which have been termed "suicide related events." Also, randomized double-blind, placebo-controlled trials demonstrate the effectiveness of antidepressants in major depression and OCD in children (9). Suicide is the fourth leading cause of death for children aged 1 to 19 years. Most adolescent suicides are related to psychiatric illness and most of those who complete suicide are not taking antidepressants. Depressed adolescents and children who receive treatment are less likely to commit suicide than those left untreated (10). Our recommendation for all patients is that antidepressants should be prescribed only after an accurate diagnosis is made and close follow-up is available, but that children and adolescents should not be denied antidepressant treatment.

TABLE 170-2. Summary Table for Commonly Used Antidepressants

Name	*Dose*	*Important Clinical Information*
Amitriptyline (Elavil)	50 to 300 mg qhs (Start: 25 mg qhs)	• Used in low dose for insomnia • Effective for pain syndromes
Bupropion (Wellbutrin)	Start: 100 mg bid titrating to 300 to 450 mg bid or tid	• Seizure risk • Stimulating; not good for anxiety
Citalopram (Celexa)	20 to 60 mg qam (Start: 20 mg qam)	• Less gastrointestinal distress than other SSRI • No clinical CYP interactions
Duloxetine (Cymbalta)	20 to 30 mg bid (Start: 20 mg bid)	• Side effect profile like SSRIs and venlafaxine
Escitalopram (Lexapro)	10 to 20 mg qam (Start: 10 mg qam)	• Less gastrointestinal distress than other SSRI • No clinical CYP interactions
Fluoxetine (Prozac)	20 to 80 mg qam (Start: 10 to 20 mg qam)	• More stimulating than other SSRI • Long half-life prevents withdrawal • Once weekly dosing option
Mirtazapine (Remeron)	30 to 45 mg qhs (Start: 15 mg qhs)	• Very sedating and appetite promoting • Neutropenia risk (1 in 1000)
Nortriptyline (Pamelor)	50 to 150 mg qhs (Start: 25 mg qhs)	• Combined with lithium, it is a well studied after ECT treatment • Effective for poststroke depression
Paroxetine (Paxil)	20 to 50 mg qhs (Start: 10 to 20 mg qhs)	• Anticholinergic and sedating side effects may occur • Withdrawal syndrome likely
Sertraline (Zoloft)	50 to 200 mg qam (Start: 25 to 50 mg qam)	• No clinical CYP interactions • Wide dosing range helpful
Trazodone (Desyrel)	50 to 150 mg qhs for sleep (Start: 25 mg qhs)	• Commonly used as sleep aid • Priapism risk
Venlafaxine (Effexor)	Start: 37.5 to 75 mg bid with titration to 300 to 375 mg daily	• Side effects generally like SSRI • Effective for anxiety disorders • Hypertension and withdrawal syndrome risk

qhs, at bedtime; bid, twice daily; tid, three times daily; qam, every morning; SSRI, selective serotonin reuptake inhibitors; ECT, electroconvulsive therapy; CYP, cytochrome P 450.

USE OF ANTIDEPRESSANTS IN PREGNANCY, POSTPARTUM, AND WHILE BREASTFEEDING

The use of any psychotropic during pregnancy and the postpartum period requires an evaluation of the risks of not treating the mother's psychiatric illness compared with the potential harm the medication may impose on the child. All antidepressant drugs enter breast milk. Sertraline has been recommended as the first-line treatment for breastfeeding mothers (11). An excellent discussion of this complicated topic can be found elsewhere (12).

MOOD STABILIZERS

Drugs used to treat bipolar disorder include antidepressants, neuroleptics, and a group of drugs that have predominantly antimanic activity and variable antidepressant activity. These drugs are often classed as *mood stabilizers*, but vary in how much they treat and prevent depression and mania. Although discussed below in a separate category, increasing evidence indicates that neuroleptic medications are mood stabilizers as well.

LITHIUM

Lithium has been termed the gold standard mood stabilizer and the one to which other treatments are compared. It is well studied as a prophylactic agent for both depressive episodes and manic episodes in patients with bipolar disorder. Also evidence suggests that lithium decreases suicide in patients with bipolar disorder (13). Many patients have breakthrough symptoms while on lithium or are unable to tolerate the frequent side effects (14). Commonly encountered side effects occur in almost all organ systems. Patients often experience tremor, gastrointestinal (GI) distress, delayed thyroid hormone release, renal concentrating problems, leukocytosis, ECG changes, acne, and weight gain. Initiating lithium requires checking blood counts, electrolytes, renal function, and thyroid function. These tests, along with lithium levels, should be followed every 6 months in a stable patient. Lithium toxicity causes neurologic damage, including (but not limited to) problems of balance, cognition, memory, tremor, ataxia, seizures, and focal neurologic deficits. Deficits are permanent with prolonged toxicity, and the narrow therapeutic index with this drug, combined with overdose, is a significant source of collaboration between psychiatrists and neurologists.

VALPROIC ACID

Valproic acid is a drug that has activity in both preventing and treating manic episodes in bipolar disorder. Many patients tolerate valproic acid, particularly the coated forms, better then lithium. Disagreement (based on opinions about the quality of evidence) is found to whether valproic acid is as effective an agent as lithium (13,14). Valproic acid has common side effects, including GI distress, weight gain, tremor sedation, and ataxia. Serious liver damage, thrombocytopenia, and platelet dysfunction must be watched for during treatment and complete blood counts, electrolytes, and liver function tests should be obtained before treatment.

LAMOTRIGINE

Lamotrigine is an anticonvulsant effective in preventing and treating episodes of mania and depression in bipolar disorder (types I and II). Compared with lithium, it may be more effective at preventing depressive episodes in bipolar patients and is less likely to be discontinued because of side effects (14). It is often considered particularly useful for patients with bipolar disorder type II (13). Although relatively free of side effects, the risk of the rare Stevens-Johnson syndrome is a very real issue in the use of this drug, and is ameliorated by slowing the speed of dose escalation.

CARBAMAZEPINE

Carbamazepine has been shown to be an effective agent in bipolar disorder, although recent studies suggest it may be less effective than lithium (15). Common side effects include stomach discomfort, dizziness, sedation, and blurred vision. Serious side effects include aplastic anemia, agranulocytosis, Stevens-Johnson syndrome, and hyponatremia. Because of its side effects, carbamazepine is less popular than other drugs for bipolar disorder.

OXCARBAZEPINE

Oxcarbazepine has limited data indicating it is as effective as lithium in the treatment of bipolar disorder. It is seldom used as the first agent tried, and tends to be used as a therapy in patients with complicated courses and treatment. Gabapentin, topiramate, levetiracetam, zonisamide, and tiagabine have not been demonstrated as effective treatments for bipolar disorder (15).

USE OF MOOD STABILIZERS IN PREGNANCY, POSTPARTUM, AND WHILE BREASTFEEDING

Lithium, valproic acid, and carbamazepine are associated with an increased risk of congenital malformations when used during pregnancy. Lamotrigine can be associated with a lower risk of malformations (16). All the mood stabilizers enter breast milk, although the degree absorbed by the infant and resulting effects varies with each drug (17). The importance of a planned pregnancy should be discussed with all women of childbearing age with bipolar disorder. The difficult decision regarding the use of mood stabilizers during pregnancy and whether or not to breastfeed requires the input of the patient, her obstetrician, and pediatrician (Table 170-3).

ANTIPSYCHOTICS (NEUROLEPTICS)

Drugs with specific antipsychotic action were also developed in the search for new antihistamines in the 1940s and 1950s. The drugs were initially mostly structurally in the phenothiazine class, and these drugs are often referred to as *phenothiazines* despite that the term refers to the structure of only a subset of the drugs. Additionally, the drugs were referred to as *major tranquilizers* or *neuroleptics*. The older agents, sometimes referred to as *typical antipsychotics* include haloperidol, chlorpromazine, perphenazine, and fluphenazine. What is "typical" about these drugs is the primary pharmacologic action of antagonizing dopamine 2 receptors. The antagonism of dopamine causes acute dystonia, parkinsonism, akathisia, neuroleptic malignant syndrome, tardive dystonia or dyskinesia, and hyperprolactinemia. Other pharmacologic effects include anticholinergic, antiadrenergic, and antihistaminergic actions. The higher potency (potency at the D2 receptor) typical antipsychotics (e.g., haloperidol) have little anticholinergic or antiadrenergic effects, but are more susceptible to antidopaminergic side effects. Less potent typical antipsychotics (chlorpromazine) have treatment-limiting sedation, dry mouth, constipation, blurry vision, and dizziness. Less-potent typical neuroleptic medications are used infrequently when managing long-term diseases such as schizophrenia. All of the typical neuroleptics are effective at treating the "positive" symptoms of

TABLE 170-3. Summary Table for Commonly Used Mood Stabilizers

Name	*Dose*	*Important Clinical Information*
Lithium	Start: 150 to 300 mg bid with doses up to 1,200 to 1,500 mg daily based on renal function	• Black box warning related to potential for toxicity and the need to check levels • Excreted unchanged by kidney • Therapeutic drug levels of 0.8 mEq/L to 1.2 mEq/L are well established
Valproic Acid	Start: 250 mg bid with end dose of 1,000 to 2,000 mg divided bid (maximal dose: 60 mg/kg/day divided bid)	• Black box warning regarding risk of hepatotoxicity, pancreatitis, and teratogenicity • Therapeutic drug levels are well established (80 to 120 μg/mL)
Lamotrigine (Lamictal)	Start: 25 mg daily for 2 weeks then 50 mg daily for 2 weeks with a final dose of 200 to 400 mg once or divided.	• Black box warning due to rash • No therapeutic drug levels • If used with valproic acid, the dose must be halved

bid, twice daily.

schizophrenia, including hallucinations, delusions, and grossly disorganized speech and behavior.

Atypical antipsychotics (aripiprazole, clozapine, olanzapine, quetiapine, risperidone, and ziprasidone) have varying mechanisms of action and affect other neurotransmitter systems in addition to dopamine. The relative decrease in acute and chronic side effects with the promise of improved efficacy has led to a reliance on these drugs as first-line treatments in psychotic disorders, mania, and agitation. Although they have less risk for extrapyramidal side effects, the atypical medications can create metabolic complications, including weight gain, hyperglycemia, and dyslipidemia.

COMPLIANCE AND EFFICACY

Atypical neuroleptics have not proved to be exceedingly better than the typical neuroleptics. The Clinical Antipsychotic Trial of Intervention Effectiveness (CATIE) randomly assigned schizophrenic patients, 18 to 65 years of age to 18-month treatment with olanzapine, quetiapine, ziprasidone, risperidone, or perphenazine. Only about 20% to 30% of the patients in any group completed the study. Olanzapine showed superiority, with a longer time of successful treatment, fewer hospitalizations, and a lower rate of discontinuation. No significant difference was noted between perphenazine and the other atypical neuroleptics. The difference between perphenazine and olanzapine was "moderate" (18).

USE IN DELIRIUM AND THE ELDERLY

Atypical neuroleptic **medication**s received a black box warning because of an increased risk of death in elderly patients with dementia. A follow-up study compared the risk of death in patients >65 years of age filling prescriptions for typical neuroleptics compared with those filling prescriptions for atypical neuroleptics. The results found that those taking typical neuroleptics had a significantly higher risk of death compared with those taking atypical neuroleptics (19) (Table 170-4).

ANXIOLYTICS, SEDATIVES, AND HYPNOTICS

BENZODIAZEPINES

Benzodiazepines are used for the temporary relief of anxiety, insomnia, seizures, and muscle spasms. The binding of benzodiazepines to the benzodiazepine receptor on the GABA-A complex in the CNS potentiates CNS inhibition. This mechanism of action is similar to barbiturates and ethanol and highlights the abusability of this class of drugs. Benzodiazepines are beneficial complements to antidepressants when treating panic disorder, social anxiety disorder, and generalized anxiety disorder. Patients with liver disease or underlying cognitive difficulties may experience excess sedation and delirium on benzodiazepines. The benzodiazepines most worrisome for these

TABLE 170-4. Summary Table of Commonly Used Antipsychotics

Name	*Dose*	*Important Clinical Information*
Risperidone (Risperdal)	Start: 0.5 to 1 mg qhs or bid titrating to 4 to 6 mg daily or bid	• Decanoate preparation available • Orally dissolvable tablet excellent for acute agitation • Hyperprolactinemia common
Olanzapine (Zyprexa)	Start: 5 to 10 mg daily titrating to 15 to 30 mg daily once or divided bid	• Has been found as effective as other mood stabilizers for treatment of bipolar disorder • Sedation, weight gain, and metabolic complications are common
Quetiapine (Seroquel)	Start: 20 mg bid titrating to 400 to 600 mg daily divided bid (maximal dose: 800 mg)	• Very sedating with a low incidence of extrapyramidal side effects • May be beneficial for the treatment of depression
Ziprasidone (Geodon)	Start: 20 mg bid titrating to 40 to 80 mg bid	• Carries a black box warning for QT prolongation
Aripiprazole (Abilify)	Start:10 to 15 mg daily titrating to 15 to 30 mg daily	• May have less metabolic complications than other atypicals • Also has an indication for bipolar disorder
Clozapine (Clozaril)	Start: 12.5 mg daily or bid titrating slowly to 300 to 450 mg daily in divided doses (maximal dose: 900 mg)	• Generally considered the most effective antipsychotic in treatment refractory patients • Use is limited by orthostasis, tachycardia, weight gain, and drooling • Risk of agranulocytosis requires blood counts weekly for the first 6 months and twice weekly for the next 6 months
Haloperidol (Haldol)	Start: 0.5 to 5 mg daily or bid titrating to 5 to 20 mg daily once or divided bid (maximal dose: 100 mg)	• Classic typical, high potency neuroleptic • Comes in an elixir and can be given orally, intravenously, or intramuscularly • In medically ill delirious patients with agitation, we recommend small doses (0.5 mg) intravenously • Also comes in a decanoate form

qhs, at bedtime; bid, twice daily.

effects include those with very long half-lives such as diazepam, chlordiazepoxide, chlorazepate, and flurazepam. Lorazepam, oxazepam, and temazepam are only metabolized by glucoronidation and have no active metabolites. In addition, withdrawal after long-term use must be gradual to avoid anxiety, insomnia, and agitation. Abrupt cessation of long-term, high-dose use can cause withdrawal phenomena such as seizures and delirium tremens.

NONBENZODIAZEPINE SEDATIVES

Zolpidem (Ambien) is a nonbenzodiazepine agent the US Food and Drug Administration (FDA) approved for the short-term treatment of insomnia. It acts by preferentially binding to the benzodiazepine receptor subunit responsible for sedation (α_1). Because of its specificity, zolpidem is not useful as an anticonvulsant or anxiolytic. Zolpidem has a relatively short half-life of 2 to 3 hours that limits daytime sedation. Reports exist of overuse in patients vulnerable to substance abuse and withdrawal phenomena similar to benzodiazepines and alcohol have been observed.

Zaleplon (Sonata) is another nonbenzodiazepine sleeping agent indicated for insomnia. As with zolpidem, it interacts with the benzodiazepine-1 receptor in the CNS. It has an elimination half-life of 1 hour, however, which lessens the risk of daytime sedation.

Eszopiclone (Lunesta) is the first sleeping agent approved for the long-term treatment of insomnia. Its mechanism of action is not well characterized, but probably involves the GABA–benzodiazepine receptor complex. There has not been evidence of tolerance, dependence, or withdrawal syndromes when the medicine is used for up to 6 months.

Ramelteon (Rozerem) is a melatonin receptor agonist indicated for the treatment of chronic insomnia. It has no effect on GABA or other neurotransmitters and does not appear to interact with other psychotropics. Although experience with this drug is limited, it harbors the potential to be a very useful nonabusable sleeping agent (20) (Table 170-5).

STIMULANT MEDICATIONS

The primary indications for amphetamine and "amphetamine like" stimulants (methylphenidate and dexmethylphenidate)

TABLE 170-5. Summary Table of Commonly Used Anxiolytics and Hypnotics

Name	*Dose*	*Important Clinical Information*
Alprazolam (Xanax)	Start: 0.25 mg to 0.5 mg tid (doses up to 10 mg daily could be used, but this is not recommended)	• Indicated for panic disorder and anxiety • Onset: intermediate; Elimination: 6 to 20 h • Equivalent dose: 0.5 mg
Clonazepam (Klonopin)	Start: 0.25 to 0.5 mg bid with doses up to 1 to 4 mg in panic disorder and up to 20 mg divided bid for seizures	• Indicated for panic disorder and seizure disorder • Has been effective in mania • Onset: intermediate; Elimination: 18 to 50 h • Equivalent dose: 0.25 mg
Diazepam (Valium)	Start: 2 to 10 mg bid to qid with doses varying widely based on the reason for use	• Many indications, including anxiety, seizures, alcohol withdrawal, and muscle spasm • Onset: fast; elimination: 30 to 100 h • Equivalent dose: 5 mg
Oxazepam (Serax)	Start: 10 mg bid or tid for anxiety. For insomnia, start with 15 mg at bedtime. As with other benzodiazepines, doses may vary widely	• Indicated for alcohol withdrawal and anxiety • Onset: slow • Elimination: 8 to 12 h • Equivalent dose: 15 mg • Typical Alcohol Withdrawal Taper: 30 mg every 6 h for 1 day, 30 mg every 8 h for 1 day, 15 mg every 6 h for 1 day, 15 mg every 8 h for 1 day, 15 mg every 12 h for 1 day, then discontinue based on close observation
Lorazepam (Ativan)	Anxiety: 2 to 3 mg bid or tid Insomnia: 2 to 3 mg qhs	• Indicated for insomnia, anxiety, preanesthesia, and status epilepticus • Safer in liver disease • Onset: intermediate; Elimination: 10 to 20 h • Equivalent dose: 1 mg
Eszopiclone (Lunesta)	Start: 1 to 2 mg at bedtime titrated to 3 mg if needed	• Approved for long-term use • No evidence of tolerance, withdrawal, or dependence over 6-month treatment
Zolpidem (Ambien)	Start: 5 mg at bedtime titrated to 10 mg if needed	• Short half life of 2 to 3 h
Zaleplon (Sonata)	Start: 10 mg at bedtime titrated to 20 mg if needed	• Essentially, like zolpidem • Has a very short half-life of 1 h
Ramelteon (Rozerem)	Start: 8 mg at bedtime	• Melatonin receptor agonist • Appears safe for long-term use in insomnia

tid, three times daily; bid, twice daily, qid, four times daily; qhs, at bedtime.

TABLE 170-6. Summary Table for Commonly Used Stimulants

Name	*Dose*	*Important Clinical Information*
Methylphenidate (Ritalin)	10 to 60 mg daily divided bid or tid	• Schedule II controlled substance • Long-acting preparation available marketed as Concerta
Amphetamine/ Dextroamphetamine (Adderall)	5 to 60 mg daily bid or tid	• Schedule II controlled substance • Long-acting preparation available marketed as Adderall XR
Modafinil (Provigil)	200 mg once daily	• Uncertain mechanism of action • Is not an amphetamine • Schedule IV controlled substance
Atomoxetine (Strattera)	40 mg daily titrating to a target dose of 80 mg daily	• A selective norepinephrine reuptake inhibitor • Is not a controlled substance • Black box warning regarding suicidality in children

bid, twice daily; tid, three times daily.

are the treatment of attention deficit/hyperactivity disorder (ADHD) and narcolepsy. These drugs stimulate the release of monoamines at the presynaptic neurons in the CNS. The amphetamines are classified as schedule II substances by the US Drug Enforcement Agency (DEA) (e.g., OxyContin, Dilaudid, and Demerol) and carry black box warnings regarding abuse potential. Stimulants may be useful for the treatment of depression, especially in the elderly and medically ill. Because of their potential to increase heart rate and blood pressure, care must be taken, however, when using stimulants in patients at risk for cardiovascular or cerebrovascular events. Common side effects include decreased appetite, weight loss, headaches, and insomnia. There can be growth suppression and the emergence of tics in children taking stimulants. Controversy exists over the appropriateness of stimulant use. Nearly 2.5 million children take stimulants. In addition, 10% of users of stimulant medications are >50 years of age. Opponents are concerned that ADHD is over diagnosed and patients are at risk from cardiovascular events (21). Proponents argue that, untreated, ADHD leads to high rates of academic failure, substance abuse, psychiatric disorders, and car accidents (22).

Modafinil is an "amphetamine related" stimulant approved for the treatment of narcolepsy and the daytime sleepiness associated with obstructive sleep apnea. Modafinil has shown some benefit in ADHD. One open label trial found modafinil effective for residual symptoms of depression (22). Modafinil is effective at treating daytime sleepiness associated with sleep apnea, but has been found ineffective for the treatment of fatigue in multiple sclerosis and excessive daytime sleepiness in Parkinson disease (24–26).

Pemoline (Cylert) is another "amphetamine related" stimulant with an unclear mechanism of action. It is indicated for ADHD, but its use is limited because of the risk of hepatic failure.

Atomoxetine is a new drug used as an alternative to amphetamine stimulants. Atomoxetine was developed as an antidepressant and is classified as a SNRI. It is only FDA indicated for the treatment of ADHD, however. Common side effects include dizziness, headache, insomnia, and GI distress (Table 170-6).

PSYCHOTROPIC DRUG INTERACTIONS

It is a Sisyphean ordeal to memorize the inhibitors, inducers, and substrates for each cytochrome P450 (CYP) enzyme. In addition, most of the interactions listed in the tables are theoretic and based on *in vitro* pharmacologic studies or case reports. A recent systematic review found that most of the data proposing drug interactions for antidepressants are of poor quality (single case reports) (27). To be clinically adept, it is helpful to understand frequent inhibitors and inducers, to know the most dangerous potential reactions, and to follow patients closely when medicines are combined. Below, we will discuss general trends and dangerous potential interactions in each category (Table 170-7).

ANTIDEPRESSANTS

Combining nonspecific MAOI with adrenergic drugs (e.g., decongestants, dextromethorphan, stimulants, meperidine) or tyramine-containing foods (e.g., aged meats and cheeses, fava beans, sauerkraut, tap beer) can cause a hypertensive crisis. A

TABLE 170-7. Common Inhibitors and Inducers and Drug Metabolism

Inhibitors (STTOPPPED)	**S**SRI (especially fluoxetine, fluvoxamine, and paroxetine), **T**CA, **T**agamet (cimetidine), **O**ld English (acute alcohol), **P**henothiazines, **P**sychostimulants (methylphenidate), **P**rotease Inhibitors (ritonavir), **E**rythromycin (macrolides), **D**epakote
Inducers	Carbamazepine (not oxcarbazepine), Phenobarbital, Primidone, cigarettes, Phenytoin and Fosphenytoin

SSRI, selective serotonin reuptake inhibitors; TCA, tricyclic antidepressants.

hypertensive crisis will present with extremely elevated blood pressure and end-organ damage, such as encephalopathy, intracerebral hemorrhage, myocardial infarction (MI), and death. Combining nonspecific MAOI with serotonergic drugs (SSRI, SNRI, cyclic antidepressants) may precipitate a serotonin syndrome manifest by tremor, delirium, myoclonus, fever, diarrhea, and possibly autonomic instability. MAOI must be stopped for at least 2 weeks before a serotonergic or adrenergic drug is started and other drugs must be stopped for at least 2 weeks (5 weeks for fluoxetine) before starting a nonspecific MAOI. The SSRI and TCA are both substrates and inhibitors of CYP enzymes. Thus, their combination could cause a serotonin syndrome or lethal tricyclic toxicity (arrhythmias).

MOOD STABILIZERS

Carbamazepine is metabolized by CYP 3A4 and induces its own metabolism along with other CYP enzymes. It has the potential to decrease levels of many psychotropic drugs and its level can be altered by enzyme inhibitors and inducers. Combining carbamazepine with clozapine or mirtazapine may increase the risk of bone marrow suppression. Valproic acid may increase levels of lamotrigine, causing a life-threatening rash. Lithium is neurotoxic and its combination with phenothiazines can worsen or bring about extrapyramidal side effects and delirium. Nonsteroidal anti-inflammatory drugs, thiazide diuretics, and angiotensin-converting enzyme (ACE) inhibitors can increase lithium levels.

ANTIPSYCHOTICS

Neuroleptic malignant syndrome can present with altered mental status, rigidity, fever, rhabdomyolosis, and autonomic instability. Although not associated with a particular drug interaction (but instead the use of dopamine antagonists in general), it can mimic other serious drug interactions (e.g., combining MAOI with TCA or SSRI) and should be on the differential diagnosis. Antipsychotic levels can be decreased by enzyme inducers. Cigarette smoking induces CYP1A2 and is common in patients with schizophrenia. CYP1A2 induction can decrease levels of antipsychotics such as clozapine and olanzapine. Combining clozapine with a benzodiazepine can cause life-threatening CNS depression.

HYPNOTICS, SEDATIVES, AND ANXIOLYTICS

Valproic acid inhibits glucoronidation and can increase levels of lorazepam, oxazepam, and temazepam. In addition, potent CYP inhibitors can increase levels of other benzodiazepines. The most dangerous interactions involve combinations with other CNS depressants.

STIMULANTS

The major concern with stimulants is avoiding concurrent use with an MAOI or with other stimulants. Methylphenidate and atomoxetine both have the potential to increase the levels of other psychotropics through CYP inhibition.

LIMITATIONS

We have only touched on the most common agents and only in the most superficial way. We have neglected many of the agents we use and many of the conditions we treat, including OCD, panic disorder, insomnia, pain, addiction, paraphilia, and many others as well as the many conditions for which behavioral treatments or psychotherapies are used. For further reading and more comprehensive information, we recommend the well-organized and useful Rosenbaum et al. *Handbook of Psychiatric Drug Therapy* (28), and for rapid online lookup, the Thomson Micromedex online drug reference (29).

CLINICAL RECOMMENDATIONS OF THE VIGNETTE

The patient calmed after receiving 0.5 mg haloperidol intravenously on two occasions. A standing nightly dose of 0.5 mg haloperidol was initiated and titrated over 3 days to 0.5 mg in the morning to 1 mg at bedtime. Her mental state improved over the next 3 days as her medical condition improved. A standing atypical agent could have been chosen because of favorable effects in the elderly and less chance of EPS (30). Before discharge, her mental state had returned to baseline and the haloperidol was discontinued.

SUMMARY

It is difficult for clinicians to keep pace with the growing number of psychotropic drugs and their myriad indications. As advances continue in the understanding and treatment of psychiatric conditions, the number and uses of psychotropic drugs will continue to grow. Developing a working knowledge of the major categories of psychotropic medications helps clinicians address the common issues encountered with many of them. Such an understanding increases the likelihood of avoiding complications and improving a patient's overall health.

REFERENCES

1. Olfson M, Marcus SC, Druss B, et al. National trends in the outpatient treatment of depression. *JAMA*. 2002;287(2):203–209.
2. Hunkeler EM, Fireman B, Lee J, et al. Trends in use of antidepressants, lithium, and anticonvulsants in Kaiser-Permanente insured youths, 1994–2003. *J Child Adolesc Psychopharmacol.* 2005;15(1):26–37.
3. Alonso J, Angermeyer MC, Bernert S, et al. Psychotropic drug utilization in Europe: Results from the European study of the epidemiology of mental disorders (ESEMeD) project. *Acta Psychiatr Scand Suppl.* 2004;(420):55–64.
4. Linden M, Lecrubier Y, Bellantuono C, et al. The prescribing of psychotropic drugs by primary care physicians: An international collaborative study. *J Clin Psychopharmacol.* 1999;19(2):132–140.
5. Baldessarini RJ. Drugs and the Treatment of Psychiatric Disorders. In Gilman AG, Rall TW, Nies AS, et al. eds. Goodman and Gilman's The Pharmacological Basis of Therapeutics. 8th edition. New York: Pergamon Press, 1990:383–435.
6. Dording CM, Mischoulon D. The pharmacologic management of SSRI-induced side effects: A survey of psychiatrists. *Ann Clin Psychiatry.* 2002;14(3):143–147.
7. Howland RH. MAOI antidepressant drugs. *J Psychosoc Nurs Ment Health Serv.* 2006;44(6): 9–12.
8. Feiger AD, Rickels K, Rynn MA, et al. Selegiline transdermal system for the treatment of major depressive disorder: An 8-week, double-blind, placebo-controlled, flexible-dose titration trial. *J Clin Psychiatry.* 2006 Sep;67(9):1354–1361.
9. McClellan JM, Werry JS. Evidence-based treatments in child and adolescent psychiatry: An inventory. *J Am Acad Child Adolesc Psychiatry.* 2003;42(12):1388–1400.
10. Valuck RJ, Libby AM, Sills MR, et al. Antidepressant treatment and risk of suicide attempt by adolescents with major depressive disorder. *CNS Drugs.* 2004;18(15):1119–1132.
11. Wisner KL, Parry BL, Piontek CM. Postpartum depression. *N Engl J Med.* 2002;347: 194–199.

12. Wisner KL, Zarin DA, Holmboe ES, et al. Risk-benefit decision making for treatment of depression during pregnancy. *Am J Psychiatry.* 2000;157(12):1933–1940.
13. Taylor MJ, Goodwin GM. Long-term prophylaxis in bipolar disorder. *CNS Drugs.* 2006;20(4):303–310.
14. Muzina DJ, Calabrese JR. Maintenance therapies in bipolar disorder: Focus on randomized controlled trials. *Aust N Z J Psychiatry.* 2005;39(8):652–661.
15. Marken PA, Pies RW. Emerging treatments for bipolar disorder: Safety and adverse effect profiles. *Ann Pharmacother.* 2006;40(2):276–285. Epub 2006 January 10.
16. Yonkers KA, Wisner KL, Stowe Z, et al. Management of bipolar disorder during pregnancy and the postpartum period. *Am J Psychiatry.* 2004;161:608–620.
17. Hale T. *Medications and Mother's Milk: A Manual of Lactational Pharmacology,* 11th ed. Amarillo: Pharmasoft Publishing; 2004.
18. Lieberman J, Stroup T, McEvoy J, et al. Effectiveness of antipsychotic drugs in patients with chronic schizophrenia. *N Engl J Med.* 2005;353:1209–1223.
19. Wang PS, Schneeweiss S, Avorn J, et al. Risk of death in elderly users of conventional vs. atypical antipsychotic medications. *N Engl J Med.* 2005;353(22):2335–2341.
20. Johnson MW, Suess PE, Griffiths RR. Ramelteon: A novel hypnotic lacking abuse liability and sedative adverse effects. *Arch Gen Psychiatry.* 2006;63(10):1149–1157.
21. Nissen SE. ADHD drugs and cardiovascular risk. *N Engl J Med.* 2006;354(14):1445–1448.
22. Anders T, Sharfstein S. ADHD drugs and cardiovascular risk. *N Engl J Med.* 2006;354(21): 2296–2298; author reply 2297–2298.
23. Thase ME, Fava M, DeBattista C, et al. Modafinil augmentation of SSRI therapy in patients with major depressive disorder and excessive sleepiness and fatigue: A 12-week, open-label, extension study. *CNS Spectrums.* 2006;11(2):93–102.
24. Keating GM, Raffin MJ. Modafinil: A review of its use in excessive sleepiness associated with obstructive sleep apnoea/hypopnoea syndrome and shift work sleep disorder. *CNS Drugs.* 2005;19(9):785–803.
25. Stankoff B, Waubant E, Confavreux C, et al; French Modafinil Study Group. Modafinil for fatigue in MS: A randomized placebo-controlled double-blind study. *Neurology.* 2005;64(7):1139-1143.
26. Ondo WG, Fayle R, Atassi F, et al. Modafinil for daytime somnolence in Parkinson's disease: A double blind, placebo controlled parallel trial. *J Neurol Neurosurg Psychiatry.* 2005;76(12): 1636–1639.
27. Nieuwstraten C, Labiris NR, Holbrook A. Systematic overview of drug interactions with antidepressant medications. *Can J Psychiatry.* 2006;51(5):300–316.
28. Rosenbaum JF, Arana GW, Hyman SE, et al. *Handbook of Psychiatric Drug Therapy,* 5th ed. Philadelphia: Lippincott Williams & Wilkins; 2005.
29. Micromedex® Healthcare Series, (electronic version). Thomson Micromedex, Greenwood Village, Colorado, USA. Available at: http://www.thomsonhc.com (accessed: November 1, 2006).
30. Tariot PN, Schneider L, Katz IR, et al. Quetiapine treatment of psychosis associated with dementia: A double-blind, randomized, placebo-controlled clinical trial. *Am J Geriatr Psychiatry.* 2006; 14(9):767–776.

CHAPTER 171

Commonly Used Drugs in the Neurology Realm

Roger E. Kelley

OBJECTIVES

- To identify commonly used drugs associated with potential neurologic side effects
- To provide an awareness of manifestations of such side effects
- To outline monitoring methodology to prevent such potential side effects
- To discuss outcome of some of the potential more serious adverse effects on the nervous system

CASE VIGNETTE

A 27-year-old right-handed man is brought to the emergency room with two generalized seizures observed by his girlfriend earlier in the day. He has recently been placed on bupropion (Wellbutrin, Zyban) for a combination of depression and to promote smoking cessation, initiated several weeks ago by his primary care physician. His primary care physician had asked him about ever having a "seizure disorder." According to the patient's girlfriend, the patient had denied this, but had mentioned to her later that he had been on phenytoin (Dilantin) in the past for epileptic seizures related to previous excessive alcohol consumption. He no longer viewed himself as having an epileptic tendency and had stopped the Dilantin, on his own, several years ago. General physical and neurologic examination findings were noted to be normal. Computed tomographic (CT) brain scan with and without contrast, was normal. Electroencephalogram (EEG), performed 1 week later, showed some nonspecific slowing and occasional sharp wave activity in the left temporal region. He was advised to stop the buproprion and to seek a neurologic consultation. He was also advised about seizure precautions, with no driving until cleared by the neurologist.

OVERVIEW

An increasing array of medications available in all fields of medicine can have a potential adverse effect on the nervous system. Typically, the most common central nervous system (CNS) side effects are lightheadedness, excessive sedation, confusion, or headache. These tend to be most prevalent with CNS active medications such as sedative/hypnotics, psychotropic medications, anticonvulsants, or agents that promote vasodilatation or vasoconstriction. In general, it is best for CNS active agents initially to be administered in the evening, if at all possible, and not preceding a busy work day or scheduled social activity. Some patients are particularly sensitive to medications and they will inform you of this when asked. It is always important to recognize that patients sensitive to medications have no particular reason to fabricate such information and this information needs to be factored into the choice of therapy. It is important for clinicians to recognize the reason why *alternative* medicines, such as herbal preparations and megavitamins are very popular with the general lay population and that books warning about the potential ill effects of a number of US Food and Drug Administration (FDA)-approved medications are also very popular.

This becomes the art of medicine when a medication is tailored to the patient's specific needs. For example, a woman of childbearing potential needs to be treated very cautiously in terms of potential teratogenetic agents. Elderly patients, in general, are often already on an array of formulations and they tend to be less tolerant of additional medications. Noncompliant patients with epilepsy tend to have increasing *add on* medications until it is determined that they are not taking the medications already prescribed. The same often goes for noncompliant hypertensive patients who end up becoming hypotensive with lightheadedness, and possibly syncopal, when they finally decide to take the multiple medications prescribed. This is why the medication history is so important and patients on multiple medications do themselves, and their caregivers, a great service by having an accurate list of their medications available at all times. Another important concept is that of drug–drug interaction. The *Physicians' Drug Reference* (PDR) provides a ready source of such information and it needs to be consulted for any new prescribed medication with which the prescriber is not overly familiar. Such an interaction can have both direct and indirect effect. For example, a number of the older enzyme-inducing anticonvulsants significantly interfere with the efficacy of oral contraceptives. Failure to recognize this, and take appropriate measures, might lead to an unwanted pregnancy and also to a potential for birth defects.

SPECIFIC MEDICATIONS

ANTICONVULSANTS

Almost all of the anticonvulsant medications can be associated with somnolence, confusion as well as ataxia and dysarthria (1). This is especially common when the levels are in the supratherapeutic range and the degree of symptoms tends to correlate with the blood level.

Phenytoin (Dilantin, Phenytek) can lead to ataxia, confusion, and somnolence when in a toxic range. It can also be associated with cerebellar degeneration, over the longer term, as well as peripheral neuropathy.

Carbamazepine (Tegretol, Carbatrol) can lead to encephalopthy secondary to either toxic drug range or cause significant hyponatremia from syndrome of inappropriate secretion of antidiuretic hormone (SIADH). Ataxia with toxic levels can be seen as well as diplopia.

Oxcarbazepine (Trileptal) can cause encephalopathy from either a toxic level or from hyponatremia, including SIADH.

Valproic acid (Depakote) can cause encephalopathy, either as a direct effect of the drug or secondarily as a result of hepatic toxicity, which can include an elevated serum ammonia level. In addition, progressive somnolence and ataxia can be seen at toxic levels of this drug. It is also not uncommonly associated with tremor.

Phenobarbital can promote sedation, coma, and even death because it is a barbiturate with the potential for respiratory arrest at toxic drug levels.

Primidone (Mysoline) is partially metabolized to phenobartital. Thus, elevated levels can promote somnolence, coma, or even death from respiratory depression.

Gabapentin (Neurontin) can promote sedation and ataxia, especially at high doses.

Pregabalin (Lyrica) is similar chemically to gabapentin and can also promote ataxia and sedation.

Topiramate (Topamax) can cause visual blurring, primarily through either promotion of glaucoma or myopia. The major potential CNS side effect, however, is cognitive disturbance, including mental clouding and word finding difficulty. This can be seen at relatively small doses (e.g., 25 or 50 mg/day). In addition, sensory disturbance with numbness and tingling can be of such severity that the patient stops the medication.

Tiagabine (Gabitril) is most commonly associated with mental clouding and somnolence to the degree that it may significantly limit its use.

Lamotrigine (Lamictal) is generally well tolerated from a cognitive standpoint. It tends to be well tolerated because of the mandatory slow titration schedule to prevent what can be severe skin reactions.

Levetiracetam (Keppra) is attractive because of the initial dose having the potential to be therapeutic. It can have significant neurobehavioral side effects, however, which appear to be more prevalent in children.

ANTI-PARKINSON MEDICATIONS

Carbidopa or levodopa (Sinemet) is generally recognized as the most effective agent for Parkinson disease, but it can promote confusion. It can also promote lightheadedness and *black out* spells because of its potential to promote orthostatic hypotension.

Amantadine (Symmetrel) is generally well tolerated, with little in terms of cognitive side effects. As with dopaminergic agents, however, it can promote orthostatic hypotension with lightheadedness.

Anticholinergics include trihexyphenidyl (Artane) and benztropine (Cogentin). They are well recognized for their potential to promote confusion and should be avoided in older patients, especially those with cognitive deficit.

Dopamine receptor agonists include bromocriptine (Parlodel), pergolide (Permax), ropirinole (Requip), and pramipexole (Mirapex). These agents have become popular because of their efficacy and their potential to delay the need for levodopa that may, over time, have a deleterious effect. The potential exists, however, to promote confusion to the point of psychosis, with hallucinations, somnolence to the point of uncontrolled sleep, and recent concerns have emerged about the potential for compulsive behavior, including gambling and sexual aggression.

To date, there has been an isolated case report of rhabdomyolysis with pramipexole and also recent reports of valvular heart disease and fibrotic reactions associated with ergot-derived dopamine agonists (2).

ANTIDEPRESSANT MEDICATIONS

Bupropion (Wellbutrin, Zyban) is a popular antidepressant agent because of efficacy and a reduced risk of inhibited sexual desire. It is well recognized, however, that it can lower the seizure threshold. This is reported to be dose dependent. The bottom line is that this agent should be avoided if any significant enhanced risk exists of an epileptic predisposition. It is important, however, to recognize that buproprion can increase the susceptibility in a patient with an underlying seizure disorder. Thus, evaluation for an ongoing epileptic potential needs to be assessed before concluding that buproprion is the sole culprit.

Amitriptyline (Elavil), a tricyclic antidepressant, is a popular agent for migraine headache, neuropathic pain, and depression. Amitriptyline can promote sedation, as can the other tricyclic agents, along with orthostatic hypotension with secondary lightheadedness. Also, the potential exists for cardiac conduction disturbance, which can also promote lightheadedness, and this is a considerable concern with agents of this class in patients with cardiac disease. Also, the potential exists for tricyclics to lower the seizure potential and they should be used with particular caution in susceptible patients (3).

Selective serotonin reuptake inhibitors (SSRI) are very popular agents for depression and anxiety disorder. In certain patients, they can promote sedation, whereas they can promote insomnia in others. Movement disorders (e.g., tremor and dystonia) have also been reported. In addition, the potential is seen for interaction with triptan agents, with concern about an enhanced risk of serotonin syndrome (4).

Lithium, which remains perhaps the most effective mood stabilizing agent for bipolar disease, is not uncommonly associated with tremor.

PSYCHOTROPIC MEDICATIONS

It is well recognized that antipsychotic medications (neuroleptics) can produce parkinsonism, dystonic reactions, akathisia, and tardive dyskinesia (5). The older agents are particularly susceptible to cause such adverse effects. These include haloperidol (Haldo), chlorpromazine (Thorazine), trifluoperazine (Stelazine), fluphenazine (Prolixin), and thioridazine (Mellaril).

The newer *atypical* antipsychotic agents are reported less likely to be associated with extrapyramidal side effects. These include quetiapine (Seroquel), risperidone (Risperidol), olanzapine (Zyprexa), ziprasidone (Geodon), and clozapine (Clozaril). These agents, however, have been associated with other potential problems, such as weight gain.

Neuroleptic malignant syndrome is a potentially life-threatening adverse reaction to neuroleptic medication. This relatively rare phenomenon consists of hyperpyrexia, skeletal muscle hypertonia, altered mental status, and autonomic dysfunction, which would be associated with elevated creatine kinase (CK), leukocytosis, and abnormal liver function tests. The risk of fatality is 20% to 30%. Neuroleptics also have the potential to lower the seizure threshold.

Benzodiazepines, such as diazepam (Valium), clonazepam (Klonopin), and lorazepam (Klonopin) have the potential to promote sedation, cognitive disturbance, and a withdrawal picture when taken on a chronic basis.

GASTROINTESTINAL AGENTS

It is well recognized that metoclopramide (Reglan), designed to promote gastrointestinal motility, can promote extrapyramidal side effects, such as parkinsonism.

The proton pump inhibitors have the potential to promote headache. These include esomeprazole (Nexium), omeprazole (Prilosec), pantoprazole (Protonix), and rabeprazole (Aciphex).

Of historical interest, clioquinol is an agent that has been used to treat chronic gastroenteritis and to prevent traveler's diarrhea. Although removed from the market after a number of cases of neurologic complication were reported in Japan, it was believed to be associated with combination of myelopathy and optic neuropathy somewhat akin to neuromyelitis optica. This apparent toxic CNS process had a subacute course, however, and recovery was reported to be incomplete following discontinuation of the drug.

ANTIMIGRAINE MEDICATIONS

Many of the prophylactic agents are now in the anticonvulsant class, including valproic acid and topiramate, which have been discussed previously. Other classes of prophylactic therapy include tricyclics, which have also been previously discussed. Beta-blockers, such as propranolol, timolol, and nadolol, as well as calcium channel blockers, such as verapamil, tend to have little in terms of CNS side-effects, although beta-blockers, such as propranolol, can be associated with depression.

Triptans are 5-hydroxytryptamine-1 (5-HT1) agonists whose abortive effect includes vasoconstriction. The first of these agents was sumatriptan (Imitrex). The later released agents include rizatriptan (Maxalt), zolmitriptan (Zomig), naratriptan (Amerge), eletriptan (Relapx), almotriptan (Axert), and frovatriptan (Frova). Because of the potential for vasoconstriction, the potential for cerebral ischemia exists. Thus, they are contraindicated with hemiplegic migraine as well as in patients at risk for, or with documented, ischemic cerebrovascular disease.

Ergotamines, such as dihydroergotamine, are also vasoconstrictors and the same concerns for cerebral ischemia as invoked for the triptans are in place. Furthermore, recurrent use of ergots can lead to *ergotism* characterized by muscle spasms, myoclonus, fasciculations, and even seizures with severe toxicity. The neurological sequelae of marked blood pressure elevation can also be seen with acute overdose of ergotamine.

Medication overuse headache, also known as *drug withdrawal* or *rebound* headache reflects the patient becoming acclimated to an abortive headache agent when it is taken too regularly. The most common culprits are formulations containing caffeine with other entities, such as the combination of aspirin, acetaminophen, and caffeine, which is readily obtained over the counter. The combination of caffeine, butalbital, and either acetaminophen or aspirin is probably the most notorious formulation for promoting rebound-type headache. This formulation is often avoided by neurologists because of this concern. The rebound pattern related to medication overuse can often be avoided, however, by keeping track of what is in the formulation and using no particular agent, or compound, more than twice a week. This mandates keeping track of ingredients because a number of formulations combine either aspirin or acetaminophen with caffeine and just alternating names does not prevent the potential for withdrawal headache for the same ingredient in different formulations.

ANTINEOPLASTIC AGENTS

Agents that have been associated with a subacute senosorimotor neuropathy include cisplatin, chlorambucil, vinca alkaloids, methotrexate, daunorubicin, as well as paclitaxel (Taxol) and docetaxel.

Vincristine is associated primarily with a sensory neuropathy, but the cranial nerves and autonomic nervous system can also be involved. Procarbazine, used for Hodgkin disease, other lymphomas, and other malignancies, as well as oligodendrogliomas, is associated with neuropathy in 10% to 15 % of treated patients. It can also be associated with ataxia.

Cisplatin is commonly associated with axonal neuropathy or dorsal root ganglia neuronal loss, which can be associated with Lhermitte's phenomenon. Manifestations can include numbness and tingling in the distal extremities, which can be painful. Also seen is tinnitus or high frequency hearing loss in up to one third of patients, which is associated with cochlear hair cell loss. These symptoms tend to be dose related and tend to improve once the drug is discontinued.

Both 5-fluorouracil (5-FU) and cytarabine (Ara-C) can be associated with cerebellar toxicity characterized by truncal ataxia, dysmetria, nystagmus, and dysarthria.

A number of the newer agents have been associated with some degree of cognitive compromise, especially manifested by forgetfulness.

Methotrexate, given intrathecally, can cause an acute paraplegia. In combination with radiation therapy, a necrotizing leukoencoephalopathy can been seen, characterized by dementia, pseudobulbar palsy, and incapacitating ataxia.

ANTI-HUMAN IMMUNODEFICIENCY VIRUS AGENTS

Zidovudine is recognized as a potential cause of mitochondrial related myopathy This needs to be distinguished from the type II muscle fiber atrophic myopathy seen as a complication of acquired immunodeficiency syndrome (AIDS) or AIDS-related complex (ARC).

A painful sensorimotor neuropathy can be seen as a complication of both didanosine and zalcitabine.

CARDIAC-RELATED MEDICATIONS

Nitrates, which are vasodilators, are well recognized to promote a vascular type headache.

Amiodarone (Pacerone), a cardiac antiarrhythmic agent, has several potential neurologic side effects, including optic neuropathy or neuritis, ataxia, and abnormal involuntary movements.

Cholesterol lowering agents, which have the potential to prevent both heart attack and stroke, are now commonly used and the agents of choice tend to be the statins. According to one study (6), the odds ratio for risk of idiopathic polyneuropathy associated with treatment with statins, for 2 years or longer, was 26.4. In addition, myalgia is reported in 2% to 5% of patients on statin therapy with myopathy in 0.1% to 0.2% (7). The greatest concern is for rhabdomyolysis and the 10-fold higher risk of myotoxicity with cerivastatin use, especially when combined with gemfibrozil (Lopid), which led to cerivastatin being removed from the market (8).

IMMUNOMODULATING THERAPY FOR MULTIPLE SCLEROSIS

Some isolated reports indicate an enhanced seizure predisposition in patients with multiple sclerosis receiving interferon-β_{1a} (9).

Both IFN-β_{1a} (Avonex®, Rebif) and IFN- β_{1a} (Betaseron) can be associated with an enhanced frequency of depression and for which it has be monitored. IFN- β_{1a} and β_{1b} have the potential for liver toxicity and this requires periodic monitoring, generally every 6 months. In addition, the potential for leucopenia exists, which also requires monitoring, and the reduction in immunosurveillance raises concern about their use in patients at significant risk for malignancy or who develop malignancy.

Glatiramer (Copaxone) has been reported to be associated with a meningitic reaction on an isolated basis.

Recently reintroduced natalizumab (Tysabri) is reported to have an association with progressive multifocal encephalopathy (PML) (10), with a risk of approximately 1 of 1,000 treated patients.

IMMUNOSUPPRESSANTS IN TRANSPLANT SURGERY

Both cyclosporine and tacrolimus (FK-506) can be associated with headache, confusion, seizures, and visual loss. This is often seen in association with pronounced white matter changes, in the posterior aspect of the brain, on magnetic resonance imaging (MRI) scan.

OTHER AGENTS WITH SPECIFIC TOXICITY

Penicillamine, used to treat Wilson disease, has the potential to promote myasthenia gravis.

Tramadol (Ultram), a commonly used pain medication, has the potential to lower the seizure threshold and can promote seizures in susceptible individuals.

Steroids are commonly used for inflammatory neurologic conditions. Their potential side effects are well recognized. Pertinent, from a neurologic standpoint, is their potential to promote agitation and psychosis, which might be reflective an underlying psychiatric disorder in at least some individuals, as well as the potential for steroid myopathy with prolonged use.

Acyclovir tends to be a very safe drug and it is often started empirically if any suggestion exists of herpes simplex encephalitis. The possibility of encephalopathy in association with acute renal failure is a potential adverse effect of this drug (11).

Intravenous immuneglobulin (IVIg) is now popular for autoimmune related neurologic illness. Although generally safe, and well tolerated, the potential is seen for headache in association with fever and myalagia, which tends to be reflective of the infusion rate. Aseptic meningitis has been reported and concern also exists about thromboembolic events in susceptible individuals (12).

Antithrombotics, such as antiplatelet agents and anticoagulants, are commonly used for ischemic stroke prevention and for intervention. By definition, they are associated with a heightened risk of bleeding, which can include intracranial hemorrhage. Recent studies looking at the combination of aspirin and clopidogrel (Plavix) for protection against cerebrovascular events found no clear benefit and a worrisome risk of bleeding.

Thrombolytic therapy with intravenous recombinant tissue plasminogen activator (rt-PA) is available for acute ischemic stroke intervention if the patient fulfills strict eligibility criteria, including initiation within 3 hours of onset of symptoms. The major concern, from a side effect standpoint, is the approximate 6.4% risk of significant intracranial hemorrhage.

CLINICAL RECOMMENDATIONS OF THE VIGNETTE

The patient presented represents the potential complications of medications. Experienced clinicians recognize that it is important to be very cautious with medications and properly instruct patients about potential serious side effects. Certain patients are particularly sensitive to medications. This can be difficult to predict *de novo*, but the cautious clinician can often detect this from the history. In other words, if a patient informs says that he or she could not "wake up" after a small dose of previously prescribed diazepam or amitriptyline, then it will not be unexpected they will have difficulty with other potentially sedating agents. The patient with seizure susceptibility should not be prescribed buproprion, and probably avoid tramadol and agents that have the potential to lower the seizure threshold, such as tricyclics, and needs to be assessed carefully for potential risks versus benefits. Patients on multiple medications need to be assessed for potential drug–drug interactions. Older patients typically are already on multiple medications and they need to have careful titration of new medications, when indicated. Obviously, it is a good rule of thumb to avoid the initiation of more than one medication at a time to be able to more accurately identify a drug reaction when one occurs.

SUMMARY

A look at the multitude of books on alternative medications, as well as the books of "bad medicines," helps to understand the scope of what many physicians, and the lay press, interpret as overprescibing and putting the patient at risk from an iatrogenic cause. Interest has heightened in this potential for drug reaction with the recent removal of two very popular cyclooxygenase (COX)-2 inhibitors from the market because of cardiovascular concerns. Many neurologists remember the panic generated when felbamate (Felbatol) hit the "6 o'clock news" with concerns about aplastic anemia. A more recent headline was the potential for natalizumab, a particularly potent medication for multiple sclerosis, to be associated with PML. It is a good idea for patients to have a laminated copy of their present medications that they can provide to every health care provider when they make their visit. It is also advantageous to build up the dose as tolerated with documentation, in your notes, that potential serious side effects of a newly prescribed medication were discussed and the patient was advised to immediately draw this to your attention, or seek immediate evaluation in an emergency room setting, if a serious reaction does occur. The agent natalizumab illustrates that, despite the advantages of newer medications, not all potential serious problems are detected during the clinical trial process in preparation for release by the FDA.

REFERENCES

1. Szoeke CE, Newton M, Wood, JM, et al. Update on pharmacogenetics in epilepsy: A brief review. *Lancet Neurol.* 2006;5:189–196.
2. Horvath J, Fross RD, Kleiner-Fisman G, et al. Severe multivalvular heart disease: A new complication of the ergot derivative dopamine agonists. *Mov Disord.* 2004;19:656–662.
3. Degner D, Grohmann R, Kropp S, et al. Severe adverse reactions of antidepressants: Results of the German multicenter drug surveillance program AMSP. *Pharmacopsychiatry.* 2004;37[Suppl 1]:S39–S45.
4. Boyer EW, Shannon M. The serotonin syndrome. *N Engl J Med.* 2005;352:1112–1120.
5. Bender S, Grohmann R, Engell RR, et al. Severe adverse drug reactions in psychiatric inpatients treated with neuroleptics. *Pharmacopsychiatry.* 2004;37[Suppl 1]:S46–S53.
6. Gaist D, Jeppesen U, Anderson M, et al. Statins and risk of polyneuropathy. A case-control study. *Neurology.* 2002;58:1333–1337.
7. Hamilton-Craig I. Statin-associated myopathy. *Med J Aust.* 2001;175:486–489.
8. Evans M, Rees A. The myotoxicity of statins. *Curr Opin Lipidol.* 2002;13:415–420.
9. Disease modifying therapies in multiple sclerosis: Report of the Therapeutics and Technology Assessment Subcommittee of the American Academy of Neurology and the MS Council for Clinical Practice Guidelines. *Neurology.* 2002;58:169–178.
10. Berger JR, Koralnid IJ. Progressive multifocal leukoencephalopathy and natalizumab—Unforeseen consequences. *N Engl J Med.* 2005;353:414–416.
11. Dalakas MC. The use of intravenous immunoglobulin in the treatment of autoimmune neuromuscular diseases: Evidence-based indications and safety profile. *Pharmacol Ther.* 2004;102:177–193.
12. Delluc A, Mocquard Y, Latour P, et al. Encephalopathy and acute renal failure during acyclovir treatment. *Rev Neurol.* 2004;160:704–706.

INDEX

Page numbers followed by *f* indicate figures; those followed by *t* indicate tables.

B

C

D

E

H

I

J

K

L

Q

R

S

U

V